Davis's

DRUG GUIDE FOR REHABILITATION PROFESSIONALS

CHARLES D. CICCONE, PT, PhD, FAPTA
Professor
Department of Physical Therapy
School of Health Sciences and Human Performance
Ithaca College
Ithaca, New York

F. A. DAVIS COMPANY • Philadelphia

F. A. Davis Company
1915 Arch Street
Philadelphia, PA 19103
www.fadavis.com

Printed in the United States of America

Last digit indicates print number: 10 9 8 7 6 5 4 3

Acquisitions Editor: Melissa Duffield
Manager of Content Development: George W. Lang
Developmental Editor: Jennifer P. Ajello
Art and Design Manager: Carolyn O'Brien

As new scientific information becomes available through basic and clinical research, recommended treatments and drug therapies undergo changes. The author(s) and publisher have done everything possible to make this book accurate, up to date, and in accord with accepted standards at the time of publication. The author(s), editors, and publisher are not responsible for errors or omissions or for consequences from application of the book, and make no warranty, expressed or implied, in regard to the contents of the book. Any practice described in this book should be applied by the reader in accordance with professional standards of care used in regard to the unique circumstances that may apply in each situation. The reader is advised always to check product information (package inserts) for changes and new information regarding dose and contraindications before administering any drug. Caution is especially urged when using new or infrequently ordered drugs.

Library of Congress Cataloging-in-Publication Data

Ciccone, Charles D., 1953–
Davis's drug guide for rehabilitation professionals / Charles D. Ciccone.
p. ; cm.
Drug guide for rehabilitation professionals
Includes bibliographical references and index.
ISBN 978-0-8036-2589-1
I. Title. II. Title: Drug guide for rehabilitation professionals.
[DNLM: 1. Pharmaceutical Preparations--Handbooks. 2. Physical Therapy Specialty--Handbooks. 3. Rehabilitation--Handbooks. QV 39]

615.1--dc23 2013001373

DEDICATION

For my wife Penny and my children Kate and Alex.

ACKNOWLEDGEMENTS

I am extremely grateful for the efforts of others who made this book possible. In particular, I need to thank Judith Hopfer Deglin and April Hazard Vallerand, who are the authors of *Davis's Drug Guide for Nurses.* Their outstanding resource served as the basis for much of the material in *Davis's Drug Guide for Rehabilitation Professionals*, and it would have been impossible to create a guide for physical therapists without drawing heavily on the wealth of information compiled by Drs. Deglin and Vallerand. I am also grateful for the feedback and excellent suggestions provided by Steven Tippet, Stephen Carp, Ellen Wruble, LeeAnne Carrothers, Andrew Priest, Thomas Freeland, Sam Pierce, David Morrisette, Dina Brooks, Michael Moran, and Leonard Elbaum, who reviewed the early versions of the material in this book. Finally, I am indebted to the F.A. Davis staff, especially Melissa Duffield, Margaret Biblis, George Lang, Elizabeth Stepchin, Jennifer Ajello, Stephanie Kelly, and Rob Allen. They were instrumental in bringing this project to completion, and I appreciate their commitment to providing useful resources that can enhance physical therapist practice.

CONTRIBUTORS

Judith Hopper Deglin, PharmD
Consultant Pharmacist
Hospice of Southeastern Connecticut
Uncasville, Connecticut

April Hazard Vallerand, PhD, RN, FAAN
College of Nursing
Wayne State University
Detroit, Michigan

Cynthia A. Sanoski, BS, PharmD, FCCP, BCPS
Chair, Department of Pharmacy Practice
Jefferson School of Pharmacy
Thomas Jefferson University
Philadelphia, Pennsylvania

REVIEWERS

Joel W. Beam, EdD, LAT, ATC
Associate Professor
Brooks College of Health
University of North Florida
Jacksonville, Florida

Dina Brooks, PhD, MSc, BSc (PT)
Professor
Department of Physical Therapy
University of Toronto
Toronto, Ontario, Canada

Ann Burkhardt, OTD, OTR/L, FAOTA
Associate Professor and Director
Division of Occupational Therapy
Long Island University
New York, New York

Stephen J. Carp, PT, PhD, GCS
Assistant Professor
Director of DPT Admissions and Outcomes Assessment
Department of Physical Therapy
Temple University
Philadelphia, Pennsylvania

LeeAnne Carrothers, PT, PhD
Physical Therapist
Physical Therapy
Alaska Regional Hospital
Anchorage, Alaska

Margarita V DiVall, PharmD, BCPS
Associate Clinical Professor and Director of Assessment
Department of Pharmacy Practice and School of Pharmacy
Northeastern University
Boston, Massachusetts

Steven Fehrer, PT, PhD
Assistant Professor
School of Physical Therapy and Rehabilitation Science
University of Montana
Missoula, Montana

Bruce Greenfield, PT, PhD, OCS
Associate Professor
Department of Rehabilitation Medicine
Emory University
Atlanta, Georgia

Michael Moran, PT, DPT, ScD
Professor
Department of Physical Therapy
Misericordia University
Dallas, Pennsylvania

David Morrisette, PT, PhD, OCS, ATC
Director and Professor
College of Health Professions
Division of Physical Therapy
Medical University of South Carolina
Charleston, South Carolina

Sam Pierce, PT, PhD, NCS
Associate Professor
Institute for Physical Therapy Education
Widener University
Chester, Pennsylvania

Andrew Priest, MPT, EdD
Chair and Professor
Department of Physical Therapy
Clarke College
Dubuque, Iowa

Steven Raymond Tippett, PhD, PT, SCS, ATC
Department Chair and Professor
Department of Physical Therapy and Health Science
Bradley University
Peoria, Illinois

Meghan Warren, PT, MPH, PhD
Assistant Professor
College of Health and Human Services
Physical Therapy and Athletic Training Programs
Northern Arizona University
Flagstaff, Arizona

Ellen Wruble Hakim, PT, DScPT, MS, CWS, FACCWS
Assistant Professor
Department of Physical Therapy
and Rehabilitation Science
University of Maryland School of Medicine
Baltimore, Maryland

Director, DPT Program
Associate Professor
Department of Physical Therapy
University of Delaware
Newark, Delaware

CONTENTS

ADDITIONAL ONLINE RESOURCES DavisPlus DavisPlus.fadavis.com

The following resources can be found online at http://davisplus.fadavis.com, key word: Ciccone.

Alphabetical List of Herbal/Natural Products Found Online

APPENDICES

HOW TO USE *Davis's Drug Guide for Rehabilitation Professionals*

Davis's Drug Guide for Rehabilitation Professionals is intended to provide rehabilitation specialists with an up-to-date and easy-to-use resource about specific medications. Although physical therapists do not typically prescribe drugs and administer drugs only a limited basis, clinicians need to be aware of drug indications, therapeutic effects, and potential adverse affects that can affect patient responses to physical rehabilitation. This guide consists of an alphabetical listing of more than 850 drug summaries, or "monographs," that contain pertinent information about each drug. Monographs are focused on specific issues that are most relevant to physical therapy practice. In particular, a section of each monograph organizes the Physical Therapy Implications according to three primary areas: Evaluation and Examination, Interventions, and Patient/Client-Related Instructions. This guide also includes supplemental material in 15 appendices that expand on the physical therapy implications and link this information to specific aspects of clinical practice. These 15 appendices can be found online along with a bonus content of 175 additional monographs, including herbal/natural products, at http://davisplus.fadavis.com, key word Ciccone. The following sections describe the organization of *Davis's Drug Guide for Rehabilitation Professionals* and explain how to quickly find the information you need.

Classifications Profile

Medications in the same therapeutic class often share similar therapeutic indications, mechanisms of action, and expected outcomes. The Classifications Profile, found online at http://davisplus.fadavis.com key word Ciccone, provides summaries of the major therapeutic classifications used in *Davis's Drug Guide for Rehabilitation Professionals*. It provides some basic information about the actions of drugs within the class and a list of drugs within each class. This section also indicates chapters from a companion resource (Ciccone CD: *Pharmacology in Rehabilitation*, 4th edition, FA Davis Company, Philadelphia, 2007) that may be helpful in providing physical therapists with additional information about each drug class.

Drug Monographs

Drug monographs are organized in the following manner:

High Alert Status: Some medications, such as chemotherapeutic agents, anticoagulants, and insulins, have a greater potential for harm than others. These medications have been identified by the Institute for Safe Medication Practices as **high alert drugs**. *Davis's Drug Guide for Rehabilitation Professionals* includes a high alert tab in the upper right corner of the monograph header of appropriate medications to alert the clinician to the medication's risk. The term "high alert" is also used in other parts of the monograph to identify specific areas of drug administration or response that may be problematic. Physical therapists should be especially careful about identifying possible adverse reactions in patients taking these high alert drugs.

Generic/Trade Name: The generic name appears first, with a pronunciation key, followed by an alphabetical list of trade names. Common names, abbreviations, and selected foreign names are also included. Because drug monographs in this guide appear alphabetically by generic names, physical therapists may need to consult the index at the back of this guide when presented with the trade name, which will then direct them to the appropriate generic name.

Classification: The therapeutic classification, which categorizes drugs by the disease state they are used to treat, appears first, followed by the pharmacologic classification, which is based on the drug's mechanism of action. Clinicians can consult the *classifications profile* (see above) to see what other drugs share the classification and indications for a given medication.

Controlled Substance Schedule: All drugs regulated by federal law are placed into one of five schedules, based on the drug's medicinal value, harmfulness, and potential for abuse or addiction; see Appendix O for a description of the schedules of controlled substances. Schedule I drugs, the most dangerous ones and those having no medicinal value, are not included in *Davis's Drug Guide* *for Rehabilitation Professionals*. Identifying the level of a controlled substance will give physical therapists an immediate indication of the abuse potential and possible risks associated with that drug.

Indications: Medications are approved by the Food and Drug Administration (FDA) for specific disease states. This section identifies the diseases or conditions for which the drug is commonly used and includes significant unlabeled (i.e., off-label prescription) uses as well. Physical therapists can use this information to see if a patient is taking the drug for an FDA-approved purpose or if the drug is being prescribed "off label" or in an experimental situation.

Action: This section contains a concise description of how the drug produces the desired therapeutic effect.

Adverse Reactions and Side Effects: Although it is not possible to include all reported reactions, major side effects that clinicians should be alert for are included. Life-threatening adverse reactions or side effects are in red text and CAPITALIZED, and the most frequent side effects are underlined. Those that are underlined generally have an incidence of 10% or greater. Those not underlined occur in fewer than 10% but more than 1% of patients. Although life-threatening reactions may be rare (fewer than 1%), they are included because of their significance. The following abbreviations are used for body systems:

CNS: central nervous system
EENT: eye, ear, nose, and throat
Resp: respiratory
CV: cardiovascular
GI: gastrointestinal
GU: genitourinary
Derm: dermatologic
Endo: endocrinologic
F and E: fluid and electrolyte
Hemat: hematologic
Metab: metabolic
MS: musculoskeletal
Neuro: neurologic
Misc: miscellaneous

Physical Therapy Implications: This section lists the primary ways that each drug can impact physical rehabilitation. Implications are organized into the following subsections:

Examination and Evaluation: This subsection identifies key aspects of drug therapy that can be accounted for when implementing the examination and evaluation processes. According to the *Guide to Physical Therapist Practice, Revised* (American Physical Therapy Association, Alexandria, Virginia, 2003), "examination" consists of obtaining the patient's history, performing a systems review, and using tests and measurements to gather data. Evaluation is likewise defined as the formation of clinical judgments based on the examination. Both examination and evaluation also help identify potential problems that may require consultation with another health care provider. Hence, many aspects of drug therapy can be identified and dealt with during the examination and evaluation processes. In particular, adverse reactions and drug side effects often become apparent when examining and evaluating the patient. Likewise, certain tests and measurements may help identify specific adverse drug reactions or help monitor the responses to these medications. This subsection therefore lists the key drug issues that therapists should be alert for during examination and evaluation. Issues are prioritized so that the more serious and life-threatening drug problems appear first, with important but less critical issues identified later in the list.

Interventions: This subsection identifies the primary physical therapy methods and techniques that are related to each drug. Whenever possible, specific physical therapy procedures are identified that can supplement the drug's effects and help improve outcomes. Conversely, physical therapists can sometimes implement interventions that help decrease or allay drug-related problems. Finally, this subsection addresses any rehabilitation interventions that may interact adversely with specific drugs, and explains why these interventions should be avoided.

Patient/Client-Related Instruction: This subsection includes key information that clinicians can impart to their patients and families to promote better outcomes. In particular, physical therapists can encourage patients to adhere to the recommended dose schedule and administration techniques for specific medications. Clinicians can also advise patients and their families to watch for signs of drug-related problems, and to contact the physician or nurse when these problems arise.

Pharmacokinetics: *Pharmacokinetics* refers to the way the body processes a medication by absorption, distribution, metabolism, and excretion. This section also includes information on the drug's half-life. For more information about pharmacokinetic variables, refer to Ciccone: *Pharmacology in Rehabilitation,* 4th edition (Philadelphia, F.A. Davis Company, 2007).

Absorption: *Absorption* describes the process that follows drug administration and its subsequent delivery to systemic circulation. If only a small fraction is absorbed following oral administration (diminished bioavailability), then the oral dose must be much greater than a dose administered directly into the blood stream (i.e., intravenous dose). Absorption into the systemic circulation also follows other routes of administration such as topical, transdermal, intramuscular, subcutaneous, rectal, and ophthalmic routes. Drugs administered intravenously are usually 100% bioavailable.

Distribution: This subsection comments on the drug's distribution in body tissues and fluids. Distribution becomes important in choosing one drug over another, as in selecting an antibiotic that will penetrate the central nervous system to treat meningitis or in avoiding drugs that cross the placenta or concentrate in breast milk. Information on protein binding is included for drugs that are >95% bound to plasma proteins, which has implications for drug-drug interactions.

Metabolism and Excretion: Drugs are primarily eliminated from the body either by hepatic conversion to less active or inactive compounds (metabolism or biotransformation) and subsequent excretion by the kidneys or by renal elimination of unchanged drug. Therefore, drug metabolism and excretion information is important in determining dosage regimens and intervals for patients with impaired renal or hepatic function. The creatinine clearance (CCr) helps quantify renal function and guides dosage adjustments.

Half-Life: The half-life of a drug is the amount of time it takes for the drug level to decrease by 50% and roughly correlates with the duration of action. Half-lives are given for drugs assuming the patient has normal renal or hepatic function. Conditions that alter the half-life are noted.

Time/Action Profile: The time/action profile table provides the onset of drug action, its peak effect, and its duration of activity. This can aid in planning physical therapy interventions to capitalize on beneficial drug effects; that is, provide treatments when patients are experiencing peak analgesic effects, decreased spasticity, improved cognition, and so forth. Conversely, clinicians may want to avoid seeing patients when certain effects, such as sedation, are peaking, or when the duration of activity has expired and beneficial effects have diminished.

Contraindications and Precautions: Situations in which drug use should be avoided or alternatives strongly considered are listed as contraindications. Hence, this section may help physical therapists recognize situations where drugs are used inappropriately. In general, most drugs are contraindicated in pregnancy or lactation, unless the potential benefits outweigh the possible risks to the mother or baby (e.g., anticonvulsants, antihypertensives, and antiretrovirals). Contraindications may be absolute (i.e., the drug in question should be avoided completely) or relative, in which certain clinical situations may allow cautious use of the drug. The precautions portion includes disease states or clinical situations in which drug use involves particular risks or in which dosage modification may be necessary. Extreme cautions are noted separately to draw attention to conditions under which use of the drug results in serious, potentially life-threatening consequences.

Interactions: Drug interactions are a significant risk for patients. As the number of medications a patient receives increases, so does the likelihood of drug-drug interactions. This section provides the most important drug-drug interactions and their physiologic effects. Significant drug-food and drug–natural product interactions are also noted, as are recommendations for avoiding or minimizing these interactions. Physical therapists can consult this section if they suspect that one of the drugs in a patient's regimen might be interacting with another drug, nutritional supplement, or food source.

Route and Dosage: Routes of administration are grouped together and include recommended doses for adults, children, and other more specific age groups such as geriatric patients. The recommended doses can give physical therapists a sense of how much a given patient is taking relative to the maximum dose (i.e., is the patient at the low, middle, or upper end of the dosage range). Dosage units are expressed in the terms in which they are usually prescribed. For example, penicillin G dosage is given in units rather than in milligrams. Dosing intervals are also provided in the manner in which they are frequently ordered. If a specific clinical situation (indication) requires a different dose or interval, this is listed separately for clarity. Specific dosing regimens for hepatic or renal impairment are also included.

Availability: This section lists the strengths and concentrations of available dose forms. Such information is useful for physicians and nurses when planning more convenient regimens (fewer tablets/capsules, less injection volume), determining whether certain dosing forms are available (suppositories, oral concentrates, sustained- or extended-release forms), or seeking ways to improve compliance and adherence (using flavored oral liquids and chewable tablets for children). Physical therapists may also consult this section to see if an alternative form or delivery route is available when a patient is having trouble taking the drug as originally prescribed. For example, a transdermal form may be available for a patient who is having trouble swallowing an orally administered drug.

abacavir (ah-back-ah-veer)

Ziagen

Classification

Therapeutic: antiretrovirals

Pharmacologic: nucleoside reverse transcriptase inhibitors

Indications

Management of HIV infection (AIDS) in combination with other antiretrovirals (not with lamivudine and/or tenofovir).

Action

Converted inside cells to carbovir triphosphate, its active metabolite. Carbovir triphosphate inhibits the activity of HIV-1 reverse transcriptase, which in turn terminates viral DNA growth. **Therapeutic Effects:** Slows the progression of HIV infection and decreases the occurrence of its sequelae. Increases CD4 cell counts and decreases viral load.

Adverse Reactions/Side Effects

CNS: headache, insomnia. **CV:** MYOCARDIAL INFARCTION. **GI:** HEPATOTOXICITY, <u>diarrhea</u>, <u>nausea</u>, <u>vomiting</u>, anorexia. **Derm:** rashes. **F and E:** LACTIC ACIDOSIS. **Misc:** HYPERSENSITIVITY REACTIONS.

PHYSICAL THERAPY IMPLICATIONS

Examination and Evaluation

- Be alert for signs of myocardial infarction. Seek immediate medical assistance if patient develops sudden chest pain, pain radiating into the arm or jaw, shortness of breath, dizziness, sweating, anxiety, and nausea.
- Monitor signs of hypersensitivity reactions, including pulmonary symptoms (tightness in the throat and chest, wheezing, dyspnea) or skin reactions (rash, pruritus, urticaria). Notify physician or nursing staff immediately if these reactions occur.
- Be alert for signs of hepatotoxicity, including anorexia, abdominal pain, severe nausea and vomiting, yellow skin or eyes, fever, sore throat, malaise, weakness, facial edema, lethargy, and unusual bleeding or bruising. Report these signs to the physician immediately.
- Monitor signs of lactic acidosis, including confusion, lethargy, stupor, shallow rapid breathing, tachycardia, hypotension, nausea, and vomiting. Notify physician immediately if these signs occur.

Interventions

- Implement resistive exercises and other therapeutic exercises as tolerated to maintain muscle strength and function, and prevent muscle wasting associated with HIV infection and AIDS.
- Because of the risk of MI and lactic acidosis, use extreme caution during aerobic exercise and other forms of therapeutic exercise. Assess exercise tolerance frequently (blood pressure, heart rate, fatigue levels), and terminate exercise immediately if any untoward responses occur (See Appendix L).

Patient/Client-Related Instruction

- Instruct patient and family or caregiver to recognize and seek immediate medical assistance if symptoms of MI develop (see symptoms listed above under Examination and Evaluation.
- Emphasize the importance of taking abacavir as directed even if the patient is asymptomatic, and that this drug must always be used in combination with other antiretroviral drugs. Do not take more than prescribed amount and do not stop taking without consulting health care professional.
- Inform patient that abacavir does not cure HIV or AIDS, or prevent associated or opportunistic infections. Abacavir does not reduce the risk of transmission of HIV to others through sexual contact or blood contamination. Caution patient to use a condom, and avoid sharing needles or donating blood to prevent spreading the AIDS virus to others.
- Instruct patient to report other troublesome side effects such as prolonged or severe headache, sleep loss, skin rash, or GI problems (diarrhea, nausea, vomiting, loss of appetite).

Pharmacokinetics

Absorption: Rapidly and extensively (83%) absorbed.
Distribution: Distributes into extravascular space and readily distributes into erythrocytes.
Metabolism and Excretion: Mostly metabolized by the liver; 1.2% excreted unchanged in urine.
Half-life: 1.5 hr.

TIME/ACTION PROFILE (blood levels)

ROUTE	ONSET	PEAK	DURATION
PO	unknown	unknown	unknown

Contraindications/Precautions

Contraindicated in: Hypersensitivity (rechallenge may be fatal); Lactation: Breastfeeding not recommended for HIV-infected patients.

Use Cautiously in: Coronary heart disease; OB: Safety not established; Pedi: Safety not established in children <3 mo.
Exercise Extreme Caution in: Patients positive for HLA-B*5701 allele (unless exceptional circumstances exist where benefits clearly outweigh the risks).

Interactions

Drug-Drug: Alcohol increases blood levels. May increase **methadone** metabolism in some patients; slight increase in **methadone** dosing may be needed.

Route/Dosage

PO (Adults): 300 mg twice daily.
PO (Children 3 mo–16 yr): 8 mg/kg twice daily (not to exceed 300 mg twice daily).

Availability

Tablets: 300 mg. **Oral solution (strawberry/banana flavor):** 20 mg/mL in 240-mL bottles.
In combination with: lamivudine and zidovudine (Trizivir). See Appendix B.

abarelix (a-ba-re-lix)

Plenaxis

Classification
Therapeutic: antineoplastics
Pharmacologic: gonadotropin-releasing hormone (GnRH) antagonists

Indications

Advanced prostate cancer when luteinizing hormone–releasing hormone (LHRH) agonists are inappropriate or surgical castration is refused and there is risk of neurologic compromise from metastatic disease, ureteral/bladder obstruction due to local/metastatic disease, or severe metastatic bone pain unresponsive to adequate opioid analgesia.

Action

Directly and competitively blocks pituitary GnRH receptors, thereby suppressing production of luteinizing hormone (LH) and follicle-stimulating hormone (FSH). This results in decreased production of testosterone by the testes, which is not accompanied by an initial increase in testosterone.
Therapeutic Effects: Suppressed spread of metastatic prostate cancer, with decreased neurologic complications, bladder outlet obstruction, and need for opioid analgesics.

Adverse Reactions/Side Effects

CNS: dizziness, fatigue, headache, sleep disturbances. **CV:** peripheral edema, prolonged QTc interval. **GI:** constipation, diarrhea, nausea, increased transaminases. **GU:** dysuria, urinary frequency. **Derm:** hot flushes. **Endo:** breast enlargement/nipple tenderness. **MS:** back pain. **Misc:** allergic reactions, decreased bone mineral density.

PHYSICAL THERAPY IMPLICATIONS

Examination and Evaluation

- Assess heart rate, ECG, and heart sounds, especially during exercise (See Appendices G, H). Report any rhythm disturbances or symptoms of increased arrhythmias, including palpitations, chest discomfort, shortness of breath, fainting, and fatigue/weakness.
- Assess peripheral edema using girth measurements, volume displacement, and measurement of pitting edema (See Appendix N). Report increased swelling in feet and ankles or a sudden increase in body weight due to fluid retention.
- Monitor signs of allergic reactions, including pulmonary symptoms (tightness in the throat or chest, wheezing, dyspnea, cough) or skin reactions (rash, pruritus, urticaria). Notify physician or nursing staff immediately if these reactions occur.
- Assess dizziness and drowsiness that might affect gait, balance, and other functional activities (See Appendix C). Report balance problems and functional limitations to the physician and nursing staff, and caution the patient and family/caregivers to guard against falls and trauma.
- Assess any back pain to rule out musculoskeletal pathology; that is, try to determine if pain is drug induced rather than caused by anatomic or biomechanical problems.

Interventions

- For patients who are medically able to begin exercise, implement appropriate resistive exercises and aerobic training to maintain muscle strength and aerobic capacity during cancer chemotherapy, or to help restore function after chemotherapy.
- Institute weight-bearing and resistance exercises as tolerated to maintain or increase bone mineral density.
- Because of possible changes in cardiac excitation (prolonged QTc interval), use caution during aerobic exercise and endurance conditioning. Assess exercise tolerance frequently (blood pressure,

heart rate, fatigue levels), and terminate exercise immediately if any untoward responses occur (See Appendix L).

Patient/Client-Related Instruction

- Advise patient about the likelihood of GI reactions (nausea, diarrhea, constipation). Instruct patient to report severe or prolonged GI problems.
- Instruct patient to report severe or prolonged problems with urination, including increased urinary frequency or painful and difficult urination.
- Advise patient about the likelihood of vasomotor symptoms (hot flashes); report severe or problematic vasomotor effects.
- Instruct patient or family/caregivers to report other troublesome side effects including severe or prolonged headache, fatigue, sleep disturbances, or breast enlargement and tenderness.

Pharmacokinetics

Absorption: Well absorbed following IM administration.
Distribution: Extensively distributed.
Protein Binding: 96–99%.
Metabolism and Excretion: Metabolized by hydrolysis of peptide bonds; 13% excreted unchanged in urine.
Half-life: 13.2 days.

TIME/ACTION PROFILE
(decrease in testosterone levels)

ROUTE	ONSET	PEAK	DURATION
IM	2 days	3 days (blood level)	1 mo*

*Testosterone levels at month reflect medical castration.

Contraindications/Precautions

Contraindicated in: Hypersensitivity; Adult females or children.
Use Cautiously in: Patients with preexisting QTc prolongation or concurrent use of Class IA antiarrhythmics (amiodarone, sotalol); Weight >225 lb (decreased effectiveness over time).

Interactions

Drug-Drug: None noted.

Route/Dosage

IM (Adults): 100 mg on days 1, 15, and 29 and then every 4 wk thereafter.

Availability

Sterile powder for suspension (requires reconstitution): 113 mg/vial (yields 100 mg/2-mL dose).

abatacept (a-bat-a-sept)

Orencia

Classification
Therapeutic: antirheumatics
Pharmacologic: fusion proteins

Indications

Reduction of signs/symptoms and disease progression in moderate to severely active rheumatoid arthritis which has progressed despite use of previous disease-modifying antirheumatic drug (DMARD).

Action

Inhibits T-cell activation (and the inflammatory process) by binding to specific receptors. **Therapeutic Effects:** Decreased progression of rheumatoid arthritis.

Adverse Reactions/Side Effects

CNS: headache, dizziness. **Misc:** HYPERSENSITIVITY REACTIONS, INCLUDING ANAPHYLAXIS, INFECTIONS, infusion-related events.

PHYSICAL THERAPY IMPLICATIONS

Examination and Evaluation

- Monitor signs of hypersensitivity reactions and anaphylaxis, including pulmonary symptoms (tightness in the throat and chest, wheezing, cough, dyspnea) or skin reactions (rash, pruritus, urticaria). Be especially alert for allergic-like responses that occur during and after administration (infusion-related events). Notify physician or nursing staff immediately if any hypersensitivity reactions occur.
- Periodically assess impairments (pain, range of motion), functional ability, and disability to help document whether antirheumatic drug therapy is successful.
- Assess dizziness that might affect gait, balance, and other functional activities (See Appendix C). Report balance problems and functional limitations to the physician and nursing staff, and caution the patient and family/caregivers to guard against falls and trauma.

Interventions

- Implement appropriate manual therapy techniques, physical agents, therapeutic exercises, and orthotic/assistive devices to reduce pain, improve function, and augment the effects of antirheumatic drug therapy.

- Help patients with arthritis explore other nonpharmacologic methods to reduce chronic arthritis pain, such as relaxation techniques, exercise, counseling, and so forth.

Patient/Client-Related Instruction

- Advise patient to guard against infection (frequent hand washing, etc.), and to avoid crowds and contact with persons with contagious diseases.
- Instruct patient to report other troublesome side effects, including severe or prolonged headache.

Pharmacokinetics

Absorption: IV administration results in complete bioavailability.
Distribution: Unknown.
Metabolism and Excretion: Unknown.
Half-life: 13 days.

TIME/ACTION PROFILE
(improvement in symptoms)

ROUTE	ONSET	PEAK	DURATION
IV	within 15 days–3 mo	6–12 mo	3 yr (maintenance of response)

Contraindications/Precautions

Contraindicated in: Hypersensitivity; Concurrent use of tumor necrosis factor (TNF) antagonists or anakinra; Lactation: Discontinue drug or provide formula.
Use Cautiously in: Patients with chronic obstructive pulmonary disease (↑ risk of exacerbations and other adverse events); Geri: ↑ risk of adverse reactions; Pedi: Safe use in children not established; OB: Use in pregnancy only if clearly needed.

Interactions

Drug-Drug: Concurrent use with **tumor necrosis factor (TNF) antagonists** may ↑ risk and severity of infections. May ↑ incidence and risk of adverse reactions from **live virus vaccines**.

Route/Dosage

IV (Adults): *<60 kg*—500 mg every 2 wk for 3 doses, then every 4 wk; *60–100 kg*—750 mg every 2 wk for 3 doses, then every 4 wk; *>100 kg*—1000 mg every 2 wk for 3 doses, then every 4 wk.

Availability

Lyophilized powder for intravenous administration: 250 mg/15-mL vial.

HIGH ALERT

abciximab (ab-six-i-mab)

ReoPro

Classification
Therapeutic: antiplatelet agents
Pharmacologic: glycoprotein IIb/IIIa inhibitors

Indications

Used with heparin and aspirin to decrease cardiac ischemic complications before or after percutaneous coronary intervention (PCI), including percutaneous transluminal coronary angioplasty (PTCA). **Unlabeled Use:** In combination with heparin and/or low-dose alteplase or reteplase to enhance coronary perfusion in patients with acute coronary syndromes (ACS).

Action

Binds to glycoprotein (GP) receptors on platelet surfaces (GP IIb/IIIa), resulting in decreased platelet aggregation. **Therapeutic Effects:** Decreased incidence of restenosis of coronary arteries and improved myocardial perfusion.

Adverse Reactions/Side Effects

CNS: abnormal thinking, dizziness, headache.
CV: hypotension, atrial fibrillation/flutter, bradycardia, complete AV block, supraventricular tachycardia, vascular disorder, chest pain, peripheral edema.
Hemat: BLEEDING, thrombocytopenia. **Misc:** ALLERGIC REACTIONS, INCLUDING ANAPHYLAXIS.

PHYSICAL THERAPY IMPLICATIONS

Examination and Evaluation

- Assess for signs of bleeding and thrombocytopenia, including bleeding gums, nosebleed, unusual bruising, black/tarry stools, hematuria, and a decrease in hematocrit or blood pressure. Notify physician or nursing staff immediately if these signs occur.
- Be alert for signs of allergic reactions and anaphylaxis, including pulmonary symptoms (tightness in the throat and chest, wheezing, cough, dyspnea) or skin reactions (rash, pruritus, urticaria). Notify physician or nursing staff immediately if these reactions occur.
- Assess heart rate, ECG, and heart sounds, especially during exercise (see Appendixes G, H). Report any rhythm disturbances or symptoms of increased arrhythmias, including palpitations, chest pain, shortness of breath, fainting, and fatigue/weakness.
- Assess blood pressure periodically, and compare to normal values (see Appendix F). Report low blood pressure (hypotension), especially if patient experiences dizziness, fatigue, or other symptoms.
- Assess peripheral edema using girth measurements, volume displacement, and measurement of pitting edema (see Appendix N). Report increased swelling in feet and ankles or a sudden increase in body weight due to fluid retention.
- Assess dizziness that might affect gait, balance, and other functional activities (see Appendix C). Report balance problems and functional limitations to the physician and nursing staff, and caution the patient and family/caregivers to guard against falls and trauma.

Interventions

- Use caution with any physical interventions that could increase bleeding, including wound débridement, chest percussion, joint mobilization, and application of local heat.
- Because of the risk of cardiac arrhythmias (bradycardia, atrial fibrillation, others), use caution during aerobic exercise and endurance conditioning. Assess exercise tolerance frequently (blood pressure, heart rate, fatigue levels), and terminate exercise immediately if any untoward responses occur (see Appendix L).

Patient/Client-Related Instruction

- Instruct patient to immediately report signs of GI bleeding, including abdominal pain, vomiting blood, blood in stools, or black, tarry stools.
- Remind patients to take medication as directed to reduce the risk of coronary infarction, even if they are asymptomatic.
- Counsel patients about additional interventions to help reduce the risk of heart disease, such as regular exercise, weight loss, sodium restriction, stress reduction, moderation of alcohol consumption, and smoking cessation.
- Instruct patient or family/caregivers to report other problematic side effects such as severe or prolonged headache or abnormal thinking.

Pharmacokinetics

Absorption: IV administration results in complete bioavailability.
Distribution: Unknown.
Metabolism and Excretion: Remains bound to platelet receptor sites for up to 10 days.
Half-life: 30 min.

TIME/ACTION PROFILE (effect on platelet function)

ROUTE	ONSET	PEAK	DURATION
IV	within min	2 hr	24–48 hr

Contraindications/Precautions

Contraindicated in: Hypersensitivity to abciximab or murine (mouse) protein; Active internal bleeding; Recent significant GI or GU bleeding (within 6 wk); History of CVA (within 2 yr) or CVA with neurologic sequelae; History of bleeding disorder; Recent (within 7 days) oral anticoagulant therapy (PT ≥1.2 times control); Platelet count <100,000 cells/mm^3; Recent trauma or major surgery (within 6 wk); Intracranial neoplasm; Aneurysm or AV malformation; Severe uncontrolled hypertension; History of vasculitis; Concurrent use of another parenteral GP IIb/IIIa inhibitor; Recent or concurrent dextran therapy.

Use Cautiously in: Patients weighing <75 kg or >65 yr (increased risk of bleeding); History of previous GI pathology; Concurrent thrombolytic or heparin therapy; PCI within 12 hr of onset of MI symptoms or PCI procedure lasting >70 min; OB/Lactation/Pedi: Safety not established.

Interactions

Drug-Drug: Risk of bleeding may be increased by concurrent **thrombolytics, warfarin, NSAIDs, cefoperazone, cefotetan, dipyridamole, dextran, clopidogrel, heparin, heparin-like drugs, valproates,** or **ticlopidine**, although concurrent use with **heparin** and **aspirin** is recommended.
Drug-Natural: Increased bleeding risk with **anise, arnica, chamomile, clove, feverfew, garlic, ginger, ginkgo,** ***Panax ginseng***, and others.

Route/Dosage

IV (Adults): 250 mcg (0.25 mg)/kg bolus 10–60 min prior to PCI, followed by 0.125 mcg/kg/min (up to 10 mcg/min) continuous infusion for 12 hr; *patients with unstable angina not responding to conventional therapy and who are planned to undergo PCI within 24 hr*—250 mcg (0.25 mg)/kg bolus followed by 10 mcg/min continuous infusion for 18–24 hr, ending 1 hr after PCI.

Availability

Injection: 2 mg/mL in 5-mL vials.

abobotulinum toxin A

(ab-oh-**bot**-yoo-**lye**-num **tox**-in aye)
Dysport

Classification
Therapeutic: antispasticity agents cosmetic agents
Pharmacologic: neurotoxins

Indications

Treatment of cervical dystonia in adults in order to decrease severity of abnormal head position and neck pain Temporary improvement of moderate to severe glabellar (frown) lines in adult patients <65 yr.

Action

Inhibits release of acetylcholine from peripheral cholinergic nerve endings, resulting chemical denervation of treated muscle. **Therapeutic Effects:** Localized reduction of muscle activity, with decreased spasticity in cervical dystonia. Decreased appearance of glabellar lines.

Adverse Reactions/Side Effects

Cervical dystonia

CNS: fatigue, headache. **EENT:** dysphonia, eye disorder. **GI:** dry mouth, dysphagia. **Local:** injection site pain. **MS:** muscular weakness, neck pain. **Misc:** SPREAD OF TOXIN EFFECT.

Glabellar lines

CNS: headache. **EENT:** nasopharyngitis, eyelid edema, eyelid ptosis, sinusitus. **Resp:** nasopharyngitis, dyspnea. **GI:** nausea, dysphagia. **Local:** injection site pain/reaction. **Misc:** SPREAD OF TOXIN EFFECT.

PHYSICAL THERAPY IMPLICATIONS (when treating cervical dystonia or spasticity)

Examination and Evaluation

- Assess dystonia, spasticity, ROM, and functional ability as the drug begins to take effect. Document whether changes in spasticity and tone are consistent with rehabilitation goals.
- Watch for signs that the effects of abotulinum toxin A spread beyond the site of local injection. Signs include generalized muscle weakness, difficulty breathing, vision disturbances, drooping eyelids (ptosis), urinary incontinence, difficulty swallowing, and problems speaking. These signs can occur hours to weeks after injection. Report these signs to the physician immediately.
- Monitor IM injection site for redness, swelling, and irritation. Report prolonged or excessive skin reactions to the physician.

Interventions

- Implement aggressive therapeutic exercises (neuromuscular re-education, postural stabilization, gait training, other task-specific training) to facilitate voluntary motor function and help patient adjust to reduced spasticity and tone.
- Provide appropriate assistive devices (walker, cane, crutches) while patient adjusts to reduced levels of spasticity. Specifically, make sure patient can ambulate and transfer safely while adjusting to reduced tone in the lower extremities.
- When indicated, incorporate serial casting and similar techniques to capitalize on drug effects and achieve maximal soft tissue lengthening and help reduce contractures.

Patient/Client-related Instruction

- Explain to patient and family/caregivers that treatment effects may only last 2–4 months. Periodic re-injection may be needed to sustain muscle relaxant effects.
- Instruct patient or family/caregivers to report any untoward responses such as severe or prolonged headache, drooping eyelids, vision problems, difficulty speaking, or GI problems (nausea, dry mouth, difficulty swallowing).

Pharmacokinetics

Absorption: Minimal but may be significant in selected populations.
Distribution: Unknown
Metabolism and Excretion: Unknown
Half-life: Unknown

TIME/ACTION PROFILE (improvement in spasticity/appearance of lines)

ROUTE	ONSET	PEAK	DURATION
IM	within 4 wk	unknown	up to 4 mo

Contraindications/Precautions

Contraindicated in: Hypersensitivity to botulinum toxin products or additives. Allergy to cow's-milk protein. Infection at injection site.
Use Cautiously in: Previous surgical facial alterations, marked facial asymmetry, known weakness/atrophy of muscle in question, inflammation or skin abnormality at injection site, ptosis; Peripheral motor neuropathic disorders (may exacerbate clinical effects and ↑ the risk of severe dysphagia and respiratory compromise); Hyperhydrosis (safety not established); Geri: Use cautiously; consider concurrent diseases and drug therapy; OB: Use only if potential benefit justifies potential risk to the fetus; Pedi: Safety and effectiveness not been established.

Interactions

Drug-Drug: Concurrent use of **aminoglycosides** or other **agents interfering with neuromuscular transmission** including **curare-like agents** or **muscle relaxants** may ↑ effect. Concurrent use of **anticholinergics** ↑ systemic anticholinergic effects.

Route/Dosage

Cervical dystonia

IM (Adults): 500 Units as a divided dose among affected muscles; may be repeated every 12–16 wk, based on return of symptoms (range 250 and 1000 Units). Increments may be made in 250 Unit steps according to response.

Glabellar lines

IM (Adults <65 yr): 50 Units, divided in five equal aliquots of 10 Units; may be repeated every 3 mo.

Availability

Freeze dried powder for reconstitution: 500 Unit/vial, 300 Unit/vial.

acarbose (aye-kar-bose)

Precose

Classification

Therapeutic: antidiabetics

Pharmacologic: alpha-glucosidase inhibitors

Indications

Management of type 2 diabetes in conjunction with dietary therapy; may be used with insulin or other hypoglycemic agents.

Action

Lowers blood glucose by inhibiting the enzyme alpha-glucosidase in the GI tract. Delays and reduces glucose absorption. **Therapeutic Effects:** Lowering of blood glucose in diabetic patients, especially postprandial hyperglycemia.

Adverse Reactions/Side Effects

GI: abdominal pain, diarrhea, flatulence, ↑ transaminases.

PHYSICAL THERAPY IMPLICATIONS

Examination and Evaluation

- Be alert for signs of hypoglycemia, especially during and after exercise. Common neuromuscular signs include anxiety; restlessness; tingling in hands, feet, lips, or tongue; chills; cold sweats; confusion; difficulty in concentration; drowsiness; excessive hunger; headache; irritability; nervousness; tremor; weakness; unsteady gait. Report persistent or repeated episodes of hypoglycemia.
- Assess blood pressure periodically (see Appendix F). A sudden or sustained increase in blood pressure (hypertension) may indicate problems in diabetes management, and should be reported to the physician.

Interventions

- Implement aerobic exercise and endurance training programs to maintain optimal body weight, improve insulin sensitivity, and reduce the risk of macrovascular disease (heart attack, stroke) and microvascular problems (reduced blood flow to tissues and organs that causes poor wound healing, neuropathy, retinopathy, and nephropathy).

Patient/Client-Related Instruction

- Encourage patient to monitor blood glucose before and after exercise, and to adjust food intake to maintain normal glycemic levels.
- Emphasize the importance of adhering to nutritional guidelines, and the need for periodic assessment of glycemic control (serum glucose and glycosylated hemoglobin levels) throughout the management of diabetes mellitus.
- Advise patient about symptoms of hyperglycemia (confusion, drowsiness; flushed, dry skin; fruit-like breath odor; rapid, deep breathing, polyuria; loss of appetite; unusual thirst). Drug dosages may need to be adjusted to prevent repeated episodes of hyperglycemia.
- Instruct patient to report troublesome GI problems, including severe or prolonged diarrhea, flatulence, and abdominal pain.

Pharmacokinetics

Absorption: <2% systemically absorbed; action is primarily local (in the GI tract).
Distribution: Unknown.
Metabolism and Excretion: Minimal amounts absorbed are excreted by the kidneys.
Half-life: 2 hr.

TIME/ACTION PROFILE (effect on blood glucose)

ROUTE	ONSET	PEAK	DURATION
PO	unknown	1 hr	unknown

Contraindications/Precautions

Contraindicated in: Hypersensitivity; Diabetic ketoacidosis; Cirrhosis; Serum creatinine >2 mg/dL; OB/Lactation/Pedi: Safety not established.
Use Cautiously in: Presence of fever, infection, trauma, stress (may cause hyperglycemia, requiring alternative therapy).

Interactions

Drug-Drug: Thiazide diuretics and **loop diuretics, corticosteroids, phenothiazines, thyroid preparations, estrogens (conjugated), progestins, hormonal contraceptives, phenytoin, niacin, sympathomimetics, calcium channel blockers,** and **isoniazid** may ↑ glucose levels in diabetic patients and lead to ↓ control of blood glucose. Effects are ↓ by **intestinal adsorbents**, including **activated charcoal** and **digestive enzyme preparations (amylase, pancreatin)**; avoid concurrent use. ↑ effects of **sulfonylurea hypoglycemic agents**. May ↓ absorption of **digoxin**; may require dosage adjustment.
Drug-Natural: Glucosamine may worsen blood glucose control. **Chromium** and **coenzyme Q10** may ↑ hypoglycemic effects.

Route/Dosage

PO (Adults): 25 mg 3 times daily; may be increased q 4–8 wk as needed/tolerated (range 50–100 mg

3 times daily; not to exceed 50 mg 3 times daily in patients ≤60 kg or 100 mg 3 times daily in patients >60 kg).

Availability (generic available)

Tablets: 25 mg, 50 mg, 100 mg.

acebutolol (a-se-byoo-toe-lol)

Monitan, Sectral

Classification

Therapeutic: antiarrhythmics (class II), antihypertensives

Pharmacologic: beta blockers

Indications

Treatment of hypertension (single agent or with other antihypertensives). Treatment of ventricular tachyarrhythmias. **Unlabeled Use:** Prophylaxis of MI, treatment of angina pectoris, management of anxiety, tremors, thyrotoxicosis, mitral valve prolapse, idiopathic hypertrophic subaortic stenosis.

Action

Blocks stimulation of $beta_1$ (myocardial)–adrenergic receptors. Does not usually affect $beta_2$ (pulmonary, vascular, or uterine) receptor sites. Mild intrinsic sympathomimetic activity (ISA). **Therapeutic Effects:** Decreased heart rate. Decreased AV conduction. Decreased blood pressure.

Adverse Reactions/Side Effects

CNS: fatigue, weakness, anxiety, depression, dizziness, drowsiness, insomnia, memory loss, nervousness, nightmares. **EENT:** blurred vision, stuffy nose. **Resp:** bronchospasm, wheezing. **CV:** BRADYCARDIA, CHF, PULMONARY EDEMA, hypotension, peripheral vasoconstriction. **GI:** constipation, diarrhea, nausea, vomiting. **GU:** erectile dysfunction, diminished libido, urinary frequency. **Derm:** rashes. **Endo:** hyperglycemia, hypoglycemia. **MS:** arthralgia, joint pain. **Misc:** drug-induced lupus syndrome.

PHYSICAL THERAPY IMPLICATIONS

Examination and Evaluation

- Assess heart rate, ECG, and heart sounds, especially during exercise (see Appendixes G, H). Although intended to treat certain arrhythmias, this drug can unmask or precipitate new arrhythmias (proarrhythmic effect). Report any rhythm disturbances or symptoms of increased arrhythmias, including palpitations, chest pain, shortness of breath, fainting, and fatigue/weakness.
- Assess routinely for signs of CHF and pulmonary edema such as dyspnea, rales/crackles, weight gain, peripheral edema, and jugular venous distention. Report these signs to the physician immediately.
- Assess blood pressure periodically, and compare to normal values (see Appendix F) to help document antihypertensive effects.
- Assess exercise tolerance and episodes of angina pectoris. Document improvements in these variables, but also report any decline in exercise tolerance or increased frequency/severity of anginal attacks.
- Assess symptoms of bronchospasm (wheezing, coughing, tightness in chest). Perform pulmonary function tests to quantify suspected changes in ventilation and respiration (See Appendices I, J, K). Repeated or prolonged bronchoconstriction may require a change in dose or medication.
- Monitor signs of peripheral vasoconstriction, such as extreme coldness in the hands and feet, cyanosis, and muscle cramping. Notify physician of severe or prolonged signs of vasoconstriction.
- Monitor signs of hypoglycemia (weakness, malaise, irritability, fatigue) or hyperglycemia (drowsiness, fruity breath, increased urination, unusual thirst). Medication may mask some signs of hypoglycemia, but dizziness and sweating may still occur. Patients with diabetes mellitus should check blood glucose levels frequently.
- Assess dizziness and drowsiness that might affect gait, balance, and other functional activities (see Appendix C). Report balance problems and functional limitations to the physician, and caution the patient and family/caregivers to guard against falls and trauma.
- Assess any joint or muscle pain to rule out musculoskeletal pathology; that is, try to determine if pain is drug induced rather than caused by anatomic or biomechanical problems.
- Monitor mood and personality changes, including depression, anxiety, nervousness, memory loss, or other changes in behavior. Notify physician if these changes become problematic.
- Monitor excessive fatigue or weakness. Beta blockers often cause some degree of fatigue and weakness, but any sudden or severe change in muscle strength or energy levels should be reported.
- Monitor signs of drug-induced lupus syndrome, including increased BP, fever, joint pain, skin rashes, and redness/irritation of the eye (uveitis). Notify physician promptly if these signs appear.

Interventions

- Because of an increased risk of cardiac arrhythmias and CHF, use caution during aerobic exercise and endurance conditioning. Likewise, monitor patients closely during treatment of angina and other cardiac problems. Terminate exercise if patient exhibits untoward symptoms (chest pain, shortness of breath, unusual fatigue), or displays other criteria for exercise termination (see Appendix L).
- Establish aerobic exercise workloads that account for the effects of beta blockers on heart rate. Some heart rate guidelines may not be appropriate

because beta blockers typically decrease maximal HR by 20–30 bpm. Use other guidelines such as rating of perceived exertion (RPE, modified Borg scale) to determine exercise workloads.

- To minimize orthostatic hypotension, patient should move slowly when assuming a more upright position.

Patient/Client-Related Instruction

- Remind patients to take medication as directed to control hypertension and other cardiac conditions, even if they are asymptomatic.
- Counsel patients about additional interventions to help control blood pressure and cardiac dysfunction including regular exercise, weight loss, sodium restriction, stress reduction, moderation of alcohol consumption, and smoking cessation.
- Instruct patient or family/caregivers to report other troublesome side effects such as severe or prolonged insomnia, nightmares, blurred vision, stuffy nose, skin rash, increased urinary frequency, sexual problems (decreased libido, erectile dysfunction), or GI problems (nausea, vomiting, constipation, diarrhea).

Pharmacokinetics

Absorption: Well absorbed following oral administration but rapidly undergoes metabolism.
Distribution: Minimal penetration of the CNS. Crosses the placenta and enters breast milk in small amounts.
Metabolism and Excretion: Mostly metabolized to diacetolol, which is also a beta blocker.
Half-life: 3–4 hr (8–13 hr for diacetolol).

TIME/ACTION PROFILE

ROUTE	ONSET	PEAK	DURATION
PO (effect on BP)	1–1.5 hr	2–8 hr	12–24 hr
PO (antiarrhythmic)	1 hr	4–6 hr	up to 10 hr

Contraindications/Precautions

Contraindicated in: Uncompensated CHF; Pulmonary edema; Cardiogenic shock; Bradycardia or heart block; Obstructive airway disease including asthma.
Use Cautiously in: Renal or hepatic impairment (dosage reduction recommended if CCr <50 mL/min/1.73 m^2); Geri: Increased sensitivity; Thyrotoxicosis (may mask symptoms); Diabetes mellitus (may mask symptoms of hypoglycemia); History of severe allergic reactions (intensity of reactions may be increased); OB/Lactation/Pedi: Safety not established; neonatal bradycardia, hypotension, hypoglycemia, and respiratory depression may occur rarely.

Interactions

Drug-Drug: General anesthetics, IV phenytoin, and **verapamil** may cause additive myocardial depression. Concurrent use with **digoxin** may increase bradycardia. **Antihypertensives,** acute ingestion of **alcohol**, or **nitrates** may cause additive hypotension. Use with **epinephrine** may result in unopposed alpha-adrenergic stimulation. Concurrent use with **thyroid preparations** may decrease effectiveness. Concurrent use with **insulin** may result in prolonged hypoglycemia. May decrease effectiveness of **theophylline**.

Route/Dosage

PO (Adults): 400–800 mg/day—single dose or twice daily (up to 1200 mg/day or 800 mg/day in geriatric patients).

Renal Impairment

PO (Adults): If CCr <50 mL/min/1.73 m^2, use 50% of normal dose. If CCr <25 mL/min/1.73 m^2, use 25% of normal dose.

Availability (generic available)

Capsules: 200 mg, 400 mg. **Tablets:** 100 mg, 200 mg, 400 mg.

acetaminophen

(a-seet-a-**min**-oh-fen)

✱ Abenol, Acephen, Aceta, Aminofen, Apacet, APAP, Apo-Acetaminophen, Aspirin Free Anacin, Aspirin Free Pain Relief, Children's Pain Reliever, Dapacin, Feverall, Extra Strength Dynafed E.X., Extra Strength Dynafed (Billups, P.J.), Genapap, Genebs, Halenol, Infant's Pain Reliever, Liquiprin, Mapap, Maranox, Meda, Neopap, Novo-Gesic, Oraphen-PD, ✱ Panadol, Paracetamol, Redutemp, Ridenol, Silapap, Tapanol, ✱ Tempra, Tylenol, Uni-Ace

Classification
Therapeutic: antipyretics, nonopioid analgesics

Indications

Mild pain. Fever.

Action

Inhibits the synthesis of prostaglandins that may serve as mediators of pain and fever, primarily in the CNS. Has no significant anti-inflammatory properties or GI toxicity. **Therapeutic Effects:** Analgesia. Antipyresis.

Adverse Reactions/Side Effects

GI: HEPATIC FAILURE, HEPATOTOXICITY (OVERDOSE). **GU:** renal failure (high doses/chronic use). **Hemat:** neutropenia, pancytopenia, leukopenia. **Derm:** rash, urticaria.

PHYSICAL THERAPY IMPLICATIONS

Examination and Evaluation

- Be alert for signs of hepatotoxicity and liver failure, including anorexia, abdominal pain, severe nausea and vomiting, yellow skin or eyes, fever, sore throat, malaise, weakness, facial edema, lethargy, and unusual bleeding or bruising. Notify physician immediately of these signs.
- Assess pain and other variables (range of motion, muscle strength) to document whether this drug is successful in helping manage the patient's pain and decreasing impairments.
- Monitor signs of leukopenia and neutropenia (fever, sore throat, signs of infection) or unusual weakness, fatigue, and excessive bleeding that might be due to anemia or other blood dyscrasias. Report these signs to the physician.
- Monitor signs of renal failure, including decreased urine output, increased blood pressure, muscle cramps/twitching, edema/weight gain from fluid retention, yellowish brown skin, and confusion that progresses to seizures and coma. Report these signs to the physician immediately.

Interventions

- Implement appropriate manual therapy techniques, physical agents, and therapeutic exercises to reduce pain and decrease the need for acetaminophen and other analgesics.
- Help patient explore other nonpharmacologic methods to reduce chronic pain, such as relaxation techniques, exercise, counseling, and so forth.

Patient/Client-Related Instruction

- Advise patient that analgesics are usually more effective if given before pain becomes severe; emphasize that adequate pain control will allow better participation in physical therapy.
- Instruct patient and family/caregivers about the signs of liver toxicity and renal failure (see above in Examination and Evaluation). Encourage early recognition and notification of the physician about these signs.
- Advise patient to reduce alcohol intake because alcohol increases the risk of liver toxicity.
- Caution patient about the use of over-the-counter products that contain aspirin, other NSAIDs, or acetaminophen while taking high doses of acetaminophen. Use of multiple analgesics increases the risk of toxicity and overdose.
- Instruct patient and family/caregivers to report severe or prolonged skin reactions such as rash, itching, and hives.

Pharmacokinetics

Absorption: Well absorbed following oral administration. Rectal absorption is variable.

Distribution: Widely distributed. Crosses the placenta; enters breast milk in low concentrations.

Metabolism and Excretion: 85–95% metabolized by the liver. Metabolites may be toxic in overdose situation. Metabolites excreted by the kidneys.

Half-life: Neonates: 2–5 hr. Adults: 1–3 hr.

TIME/ACTION PROFILE (analgesia and antipyresis)

ROUTE	ONSET	PEAK	DURATION
PO	0.5–1 hr	1–3 hr	3–8 hr*
rectal	0.5–1 hr	1–3 hr	3–4 hr

*Depends on dose.

Contraindications/Precautions

Contraindicated in: Previous hypersensitivity; Products containing alcohol, aspartame, saccharin, sugar, or tartrazine (FDC yellow dye #5) should be avoided in patients who have hypersensitivity or intolerance to these compounds.

Use Cautiously in: Hepatic disease/renal disease (lower chronic doses recommended); Chronic alcohol use/abuse; Malnutrition.

Interactions

Drug-Drug: Chronic high-dose acetaminophen (>2 g/day) may ↑ risk of bleeding with **warfarin** (PT should be monitored regularly and INR should not exceed 4). Hepatotoxicity is additive with other **hepatotoxic substances**, including **alcohol**. Concurrent use of **sulfinpyrazone**, **isoniazid**, **rifampin**, **rifabutin**, **phenytoin**, **barbiturates**, and **carbamazepine** may ↑ the risk of acetaminophen-induced liver damage (limit self-medication); these agents will also ↓ therapeutic effects of acetaminophen. Concurrent **NSAIDs** ↑ the risk of adverse renal effects (avoid chronic concurrent use). **Propranolol** ↓ metabolism and may ↑ effects. May ↓ effects of **lamotrigine** and **zidovudine**.

Route/Dosage

Children ≤12 yr should not receive >5 doses/24 hr without notifying physician or other health care professional.

PO (Adults and Children >12 yr): 325–650 mg q 4–6 hr or 1 g 3–4 times daily or 1300 mg q 8 hr (not to exceed 4 g or 2.5 g/24 hr in patients with hepatic/renal impairment).

PO (Children 1–12 yr): 10–15 mg/kg/dose q 4–6 hr as needed (not to exceed 5 doses/24 hr).

PO (Infants): 10–15 mg/kg/dose q 4–6 hr as needed (not to exceed 5 doses/24 hr).

PO (Neonates): 10–15 mg/kg/dose q 6–8 hr as needed.

Rectal (Adults and Children >12 yr): 325–650 mg q 4–6 hr as needed or 1 g 3–4 times/day (not to exceed 4 g/24 hr).

Rectal (Children 1–12 yr): 10–20 mg/kg/dose q 4–6 hr as needed.
Rect (Infants): 10–20 mg/kg/dose q 4–6 hr as needed.
Rectal (Neonates): 10–15 mg/kg/dose q 6–8 hr as needed.

Availability (generic available)

Chewable tablets (fruit, bubblegum, or grape flavor): 80 mg OTC, 160 mg OTC. **Tablets:** 160 mg OTC, 325 mg OTC, 500 mg OTC, 650 mg OTC. **Caplets:** 325 mg OTC, 500 mg OTC. **Solution (berry, fruit, and grape flavor):** 100 mg/mL OTC. **Liquid (mint):** 160 mg/5 mL OTC, 500 mg/15 mL OTC. **Elixir (grape and cherry flavor):** 160 mg/5 mL OTC. **Drops:** 100 mg/mL OTC. **Suspension:** 100 mg/mL OTC, 160 mg/5 mL OTC. **Syrup:** 160 mg/5 mL OTC. **Suppositories:** 80 mg OTC, 120 mg OTC, , 325 mg OTC, 650 mg OTC. ***In combination with:*** many other medications. See Appendix B.

acetazolamide

(a-set-a-**zole**-a-mide)

✱ Acetazolam, AK-Zol, Apo-Acetazolamide, Dazamide, Diamox, Diamox Sequels, Storzolamide

Classification

Therapeutic: anticonvulsants, antiglaucoma agents, diuretics, ocular hypotensive agents

Pharmacologic: carbonic anhydrase inhibitors

Indications

Lowering of intraocular pressure in the treatment of glaucoma. Management of acute altitude sickness. **Unlabeled Use:** Diuretic. Adjunct to the treatment of refractory seizures. Reduce cerebrospinal fluid production in hydrocephalus. Prevention of renal calculi composed of uric acid or cystine.

Action

Inhibition of carbonic anhydrase in the eye results in decreased secretion of aqueous humor. Inhibition of renal carbonic anhydrase, resulting in self-limiting urinary excretion of sodium, potassium, bicarbonate, and water. CNS inhibition of carbonic anhydrase and resultant diuresis may decrease abnormal neuronal firing. Alkaline diuresis prevents precipitation of uric acid or cystine in the urinary tract. **Therapeutic Effects:** Lowering of intraocular pressure. Control of some types of seizures. Prevention and treatment of acute altitude sickness. Prevention of uric acid or cystine renal calculi.

Adverse Reactions/Side Effects

CNS: depression, tiredness, weakness, drowsiness. **EENT:** transient nearsightedness. **GI:** anorexia, metallic taste, nausea, vomiting, melena. **GU:** crystalluria, renal calculi. **Derm:** STEVENS-JOHNSON SYNDROME, rashes. **Endo:** hyperglycemia. **F and E:** hyperchloremic acidosis, hypokalemia, growth retardation (in children receiving chronic therapy). **Hemat:** APLASTIC ANEMIA, HEMOLYTIC ANEMIA, LEUKOPENIA. **Metab:** weight loss, hyperuricemia. **Neuro:** paresthesias. **Misc:** ALLERGIC REACTIONS, INCLUDING ANAPHYLAXIS.

PHYSICAL THERAPY IMPLICATIONS

Examination and Evaluation

- Monitor signs of hypersensitivity reactions and anaphylaxis, including pulmonary symptoms (tightness in the throat and chest, wheezing, cough, dyspnea) or skin reactions (rash, pruritus, urticaria). Be especially alert for dermatitis, exfoliation, and other severe skin reactions that might indicate Stevens-Johnson syndrome. Notify physician immediately about any hypersensitivity reactions.
- Be alert for signs of aplastic or hemolytic anemia (unusual fatigue, weakness, dizziness, pallor, jaundice, abdominal pain), leukopenia (fever, sore throat, mucosal lesions, signs of infection), or fatigue and poor health that might be due to other anemias and blood dyscrasias. Report these signs immediately to the physician.
- Monitor any changes in vision to help document drug effectiveness in decreasing glaucoma.
- If used as an anticonvulsant, document the number, duration, and severity of seizures to help determine if this drug is effective in reducing seizure activity.
- Assess signs of parasthesia (numbness, tingling) or muscle twitching. Perform objective tests including electroneuromyography and sensory testing to document any drug-related neuropathic changes.
- Monitor and report signs of renal calculi and kidney stones, including severe pain in the side and back, pain on urination, bloody urine, and a persistent urge to urinate.
- Monitor signs of hyperglycemia, including confusion, drowsiness, flushed, dry skin, fruit-like breath odor, rapid/deep breathing, polyuria, loss of appetite; and unusual thirst. Insulin dosages may need to be adjusted to prevent repeated episodes of hyperglycemia.
- Monitor signs of acid-base and electrolyte imbalances (acidosis, hypokalemia), including

headache, lethargy, stupor, seizures, vision disturbances, increased respiration, cardiac arrhythmias, weakness, GI symptoms, and muscular problems (weakness, cramping, hyperexcitability, tetany). Notify physician immediately if these signs occur.
- Monitor daytime drowsiness, depression, tiredness, or weakness. Repeated or excessive symptoms may require change in dose or medication.
- Periodically assess height (in children) and body weight. Report a rapid or unexplained weight loss, or stunted growth in children.

Interventions

- Guard against falls and trauma (hip fractures, head injury, and so forth), especially if glaucoma or other vision problems affect gait and mobility.
- Implement fall prevention strategies, especially if vision is impaired (See Appendix E).

Patient/Client-Related Instruction

- Advise patient to avoid alcohol and other CNS depressants because of the increased risk of sedation and adverse effects.
- Advise patients on prolonged antiseizure therapy not to discontinue medication without consulting health care professional. Abrupt withdrawal may cause increased seizures.
- Instruct patient and family/caregivers to report other troublesome side effects such as severe or prolonged skin rash or GI problems (nausea, vomiting, loss of appetite, abnormal taste).

Pharmacokinetics

Absorption: Dose dependent; erratic with doses >10 mg/kg/day.
Distribution: Crosses the placenta and blood-brain barrier; enters breast milk.
Protein Binding: 95%.
Metabolism and Excretion: Excreted mostly unchanged in urine.
Half-life: 2.4–5.8 hr.

TIME/ACTION PROFILE (lowering of intraocular pressure)

ROUTE	ONSET	PEAK	DURATION
PO	1–1.5 hr	2–4 hr	8–12 hr
PO-ER	2 hr	8–18 hr	18–24 hr
IV	2 min	15 min	4–5 hr

Contraindications/Precautions

Contraindicated in: Hypersensitivity or cross-sensitivity with sulfonamides may occur; Hepatic disease or insufficiency; Concurrent use with ophthalmic carbonic anhydrase inhibitors (brinzolamide, dorzolamide) is not recommended; OB: Avoid during first trimester of pregnancy.

Use Cautiously in: Chronic respiratory disease; Electrolyte abnormalities; Gout; Renal disease (dosage reduction necessary for ClCr <50 mL/min); Diabetes mellitus; OB: Use with caution during second or third trimester of pregnancy; Lactation: Safety not established.

Interactions

Drug-Drug: Excretion of **barbiturates**, **aspirin**, and **lithium** is ↑ and may lead to ↓ effectiveness. Excretion of **amphetamine**, **quinidine**, **procainamide**, and possibly **tricyclic antidepressants** is ↓ and may lead to toxicity. May ↑ **cyclosporine** levels.

Route/Dosage

PO (Adults): *Glaucoma (open angle)*—250–1000 mg/day in 1–4 divided doses (up to 250 mg q 4 hr) or 500-mg extended-release capsules twice daily. *Epilepsy*—4–16 mg/kg/day in 1–4 divided doses (maximum 30 mg/kg/day or 1 g/day). *Altitude sickness*—250 mg 2–4 times daily started 24–48 hr before ascent, continued for 48 hr or longer to control symptoms. *Antiurolithic*—250 mg at bedtime. *Edema*—250–375 mg/day. *Urine alkalinization*—5 mg/kg/dose repeated 2–3 times over 24 hr.
PO (Adults): *Glaucoma (open angle)*—250–1000 mg/day in 1–4 divided doses (up to 250 mg q 4 hr) or 500-mg extended-release capsules twice daily. *Epilepsy*—4–16 mg/kg/day in 1–4 divided doses (maximum 30 mg/kg/day or 1 g/day). *Altitude sickness*—250 mg 2–4 times daily started 24–48 hr before ascent, continued for 48 hr or longer to control symptoms. *Antiurolithic*—250 mg at bedtime. *Edema*—250–375 mg/day. *Urine alkalinization*—5 mg/kg/dose repeated 2–3 times over 24 hr.
PO (Children): *Glaucoma*—8–30 mg/kg (300–900 mg/m²/day) in 3 divided doses (usual range 10–15 mg/kg/day). *Edema*—5 mg/kg/dose once daily. *Epilepsy*—4–16 mg/kg/day in 1–4 divided doses (maximum 30 mg/kg/day or 1 g/day).
PO (Neonates): *Hydrocephalus*—5 mg/kg/dose q 6 hr increased by 25 mg/kg/day up to a maximum of 100 mg/kg/day.
IV (Adults): *Glaucoma (closed angle)*—250–500 mg, may repeat in 2–4 hr to a maximum of 1 g/day. *Edema*—250–375 mg/day.
IV (Children): *Glaucoma*—5–10 mg/kg q 6 hr, not to exceed 1 g/day. *Edema*—5 mg/kg/dose once daily.
IV (Neonates): *Hydrocephalus*—5 mg/kg/dose q 6 hr increased by 25 mg/kg/day up to a maximum of 100 mg/kg/day.

Availability

Tablets: 125 mg, 250 mg. **Extended-release capsules:** 500 mg. **Injection:** 500 mg/vial.

acetohydroxamic acid
(a-seat-oh-hye-drox-**am**-ik **as**-id)
AHA, Lithostat

Classification
Therapeutic: anti-infectives (adjunct)
Pharmacologic: urease inhibitors

Indications
Adjunct therapy in chronic urea-splitting urinary tract infection.

Action
Reversibly inhibits the bacterial enzyme urease, which results in decreased hydrolysis of urea and subsequent production of ammonia in urine infected with urea-splitting bacteria. **Therapeutic Effects:** Decreased urinary ammonia levels and decreased urine pH, which increases the efficacy of anti-infective therapy and cure rates. Does not directly alter pH or have any direct antibacterial activity.

Adverse Reactions/Side Effects
CNS: headache, anxiety, depression, malaise, nervousness, tremulousness. **CV:** palpitations, superficial phlebitis of the lower extremities. **Derm:** alopecia, rash (in association with alcohol). **GI:** anorexia, nausea, vomiting. **Hemat:** anemia, hemolytic anemia.

PHYSICAL THERAPY IMPLICATIONS

Examination and Evaluation
- Be alert for signs of hemolytic anemia (unusual fatigue, weakness, dizziness, pallor, jaundice, abdominal pain) or fatigue and poor health that might be due to other anemias and blood dyscrasias. Report these signs immediately to the physician.
- Monitor and report signs of phlebitis in the lower extremities, including local pain, swelling, and inflammation.
- Monitor anxiety, depression, nervousness, or malaise. Repeated or excessive symptoms may require change in dose or medication.

Interventions
- Always wash hands thoroughly and disinfect equipment (whirlpools, electrotherapeutic devices, treatment tables, and so forth) to help prevent the spread of infection. Use universal precautions or isolation procedures as indicated for specific patients.

Patient/Client-Related Instruction
- Advise patient to avoid alcohol because of the increased risk of skin rash.
- Instruct patient and family/caregivers to report other troublesome side effects such as severe or prolonged headache, skin rash, hair loss, palpitations, or GI problems (nausea, vomiting, loss of appetite).

Pharmacokinetics
Absorption: Well absorbed following oral administration.
Distribution: Distributed throughout body water.
Metabolism and Excretion: 36–65% excreted unchanged in urine.
Half-life: 5–10 hr (increased in renal impairment).

TIME/ACTION PROFILE (effect on urine)

ROUTE	ONSET	PEAK	DURATION
PO	4–8 hr	0.25–1 hr*	6–8 hr

*Blood levels

Contraindications/Precautions
Contraindicated in: Urinary tract infection with non–urea-splitting organisms; Urinary tract infections that can be controlled by culture-specific oral antibiotics; Serum creatinine >2.5 mg/dL or CCr <20 mL/min; OB: Causes birth defects; women of childbearing potential must use adequate contraception; Lactation: Safety not established.
Use Cautiously in: Renal impairment (increased risk of adverse reactions; dosage reduction recommended); Hepatic impairment; Preexisting thrombophlebitis or phlebothrombosis (increased risk of adverse reactions).

Interactions
Drug-Drug: Decreases absorption of **iron**. **Iron** decreases the absorption of acetohydroxamic acid. Concurrent ingestion of **alcohol** increases the incidence of rash.

Route/Dosage
PO (Adults): 250 mg 3–4 times daily (total dose 10–15 mg/kg/day) (maximum daily dose = 1500 mg).
PO (Children): 10 mg/kg/day in divided doses; further titration may be necessary.

Renal Impairment
PO (Adults): *Serum creatinine 1.8–2.5 mg/dL*—do not exceed 1000 mg/day (given at 12- hr intervals; further adjustments may be necessary).

Availability
Tablets: 250 mg.

acetylcysteine (a-se-til-sis-teen)

Acetadote, ✱Mucomyst, Mucosil

Classification

Therapeutic: antidotes (for acetaminophen toxicity), mucolytics

Indications

PO: Antidote for the management of potentially hepatotoxic overdosage of acetaminophen (should be administered within 24 hr of ingestion). **IV:** Antidote for the management of potentially hepatotoxic overdosage of acetaminophen (should be administered within 8–10 hr of ingestion). **Inhaln:** Mucolytic in the management of conditions associated with thick viscid mucous secretions. **Unlabeled Use:** Prevention of radiocontrast-induced renal dysfunction (oral).

Action

PO: Decreases the buildup of a hepatotoxic metabolite in acetaminophen overdosage. **IV:** Decreases the buildup of a hepatotoxic metabolite in acetaminophen overdosage. **Inhaln:** Degrades mucus, allowing easier mobilization and expectoration. **Therapeutic Effects: PO:** Prevention or lessening of liver damage following acetaminophen overdose. **Inhaln:** Lowers the viscosity of mucus.

Adverse Reactions/Side Effects

CNS: drowsiness. **CV:** vasodilation. **EENT:** rhinorrhea. **Resp:** bronchospasm, bronchial/tracheal irritation, chest tightness, increased secretions. **GI:** nausea, vomiting, stomatitis. **Derm:** pruritus, rash, urticaria, clamminess. **Misc:** allergic reactions (primarily with IV), including anaphylaxis, ANGIOEDEMA, chills, fever.

PHYSICAL THERAPY IMPLICATIONS

Examination and Evaluation

- Monitor signs of angioedema, including rashes, raised patches of red or white skin (welts), burning/itching skin, swelling in the face, and difficulty breathing. Notify physician of these signs immediately.
- Monitor other signs of allergic reactions and anaphylaxis, especially after IV administration. Signs include pulmonary symptoms (tightness in the throat and chest, wheezing, cough, dyspnea) and skin reactions (rash, pruritus, urticaria). Notify physician or nursing staff immediately if these reactions occur.
- Monitor signs of bronchospasm and respiratory irritation, including wheezing, cough, dyspnea, increased secretions, and tightness in the chest and throat. Report excessive or prolonged respiratory problems to the physician.
- When used as a mucolytic, assess the quantity and consistency of sputum to help document whether this drug is successful in reducing the viscosity of respiratory secretions.

Interventions

- When implementing airway clearance techniques, attempt to intervene when the drug has produced maximum mucolytic effects. Peak responses typically occur 5–10 min after inhalation.

Patient/Client-Related Instruction

- If treating acetaminophen overdose, make sure patient understands the purpose of drug therapy, and that the patient should consult the physician before resuming use of products containing acetaminophen.
- When used as a mucolytic, counsel patient on proper inhalation techniques, and advise patient not to exceed the recommended dose or frequency of inhalations. Contact physician immediately if bronchospasm or other respiratory symptoms are increased by drug inhalation.
- Instruct patient and family/caregivers to report other troublesome side effects such as severe or prolonged drowsiness, chills, fever, nasal inflammation, or GI problems (nausea, vomiting, irritation in/around the mouth).

Pharmacokinetics

Absorption: Absorbed from the GI tract following oral administration. Action is local following inhalation; remainder may be absorbed from pulmonary epithelium.
Distribution: Crosses the placenta; 0.47 L/kg.
Protein Binding: 83% bound to plasma proteins.
Metabolism and Excretion: Partially metabolized by the liver, 22% excreted renally.
Half-life: *Adult*—5.6 hr (↑ in hepatic impairment); *newborns*—11 hr.

TIME/ACTION PROFILE

ROUTE	ONSET	PEAK	DURATION
PO (antidote)	unknown	30–60 min	4 hr
Inhalation (mucolytic)	1 min	5–10 min	short

Contraindications/Precautions

Contraindicated in: Hypersensitivity.
Use Cautiously in: Severe respiratory insufficiency, asthma or history of bronchospasm; History of GI bleeding (oral only); OB/Lactation: Safety not established.

Interactions

Drug-Drug: Activated charcoal may adsorb orally administered acetylcysteine and decrease its effectiveness as an antidote.

Route/Dosage

Acetaminophen Overdose

PO (Adults and Children): 140 mg/kg initially, followed by 70 mg/kg q 4 hr for 17 additional doses.
IV (Adults and Children): *Loading dose*—150 mg/kg over 15 min initially followed by *first maintenance*

dose—50 mg/kg over 4 hr, then *second maintenance dose*—100 mg/kg over 16 hr.

Mucolytic

Inhaln (Adults and Children): *Nebulization via face mask*—3–5 mL of 20% solution or 6–10 mL of the 10% solution 3–4 times daily (range:1–10 mL of 20% solution or 2–20 mL of 10% solution q 2–6 hr); *nebulization via tent or croupette*—volume of 10–20% solution required to maintain heavy mist; *direct instillation*—1–2 mL of 10–20% solution q 1–4 hr; *intratracheal instillation via tracheostomy*—1–2 mL of 10–20% solution q 1–4 hr (up to 2–5 mL of 20% solution via tracheal catheter into particular segments of the bronchopulmonary tree).

Unlabeled Use (prevention of radiocontrast-induced renal dysfunction)

PO (Adults): 600 mg twice daily for 2 days, beginning the day before the procedure.

Availability (generic available)

Solution for inhalation: 10% in 4-, 10-, and 30-mL vials; 20% in 4-, 10-, 30-, and 100-mL vials. **Solution for injection:** 20% in 30-mL vials.

acitretin (a-si-**tre**-tin)

Soriatane

Classification
Therapeutic: antipsoriatics
Pharmacologic: retinoids

Indications

Severe psoriasis unresponsive to other therapies.

Action

Mechanism of action is not known. **Therapeutic Effects:** Improvement in psoriatic lesions.

Adverse Reactions/Side Effects

CNS: depression, fatigue, headache, pseudotumor cerebri (benign intracranial hypertension), rigors, sleep disorders. **EENT:** decreased night vision/night blindness, dry eyes, dry mouth, irritation, blurred vision, intolerance to contact lenses, loss of lashes and brows, photophobia, taste disturbances, tinnitus. **CV:** edema. **GI:** HEPATOTOXICITY, abdominal pain, anorexia, diarrhea, gingivitis, nausea, PANCREATITIS, stomatitis, vomiting. **Derm:** alopecia, dermatitis, dry skin, nail disorder, peeling, pruritus, rash, sunburn, sweating. **GU:** hematuria. **Hemat:** anemia. **Metab:** hyperglycemia, hypoglycemia, hyperkalemia, hyperlipidemia (↑ triglycerides, ↑ total cholesterol, ↓ HDL), hyper/hypomagnesemia, hypernatremia, hyperphosphatemia, hyperuricemia. **MS:** arthralgia, hyperostosis, myalgia. **Misc:** cheilitis, hot flashes, paresthesia. **Resp:** epistaxis.

PHYSICAL THERAPY IMPLICATIONS

Evaluation and Examination

- Be alert for signs of hepatotoxicity (anorexia, abdominal pain, severe nausea and vomiting, yellow skin or eyes, fever, sore throat, malaise, weakness, facial edema, lethargy, unusual bleeding or bruising), or signs of pancreatitis (upper abdominal pain after eating, indigestion, weight loss, oily stools). Report these signs to the physician immediately.
- Assess skin for any changes in psoriasis to help document the effects of drug therapy.
- Monitor signs of anemia, including unusual fatigue, pallor, shortness of breath with exertion, and bruising. Notify physician immediately if these signs occur.
- Monitor signs of hypoglycemia (weakness, malaise, irritability, fatigue) or hyperglycemia (drowsiness, fruity breath, increased urination, unusual thirst). Patients with diabetes mellitus should check blood glucose levels frequently.
- Monitor signs of electrolyte imbalances, including high plasma potassium levels (bradycardia, fatigue, weakness, numbness, tingling), high phosphate levels (ectopic calcification), or any lethargy, irritability, insomnia, palpitations, muscle tremors, and confusion that might be due to other electrolyte imbalances. Notify physician of these signs.
- Assess any muscle or joint pain to rule out musculoskeletal pathology; that is, try to determine if pain is drug induced rather than caused by anatomic or biomechanical problems.
- Be alert for signs of paresthesias (numbness, tingling, decreased muscle strength). Establish baseline electroneuromyographic values at the beginning of drug treatment whenever possible, and reexamine these values periodically to document drug-induced changes in peripheral nerve function.
- Monitor depression, sleep disorders, or shivering-like reactions (rigors). Repeated or excessive symptoms may require change in dose or medication.
- Assess peripheral edema using girth measurements, volume displacement, and measurement of pitting edema (See Appendix N). Report increased swelling in feet and ankles or a sudden increase in body weight due to fluid retention.

Interventions

- Implement ultraviolet light therapy when indicated to help treat psoriasis and augment the effects of drug therapy.

Patient/Client-Related Instruction

- Instruct patient and family/caregivers to report other troublesome side effects such as severe or prolonged headache, vision disturbances, ringing/buzzing in the ears (tinnitus), nosebleeds, bloody urine, hot flashes, skin reactions (rash, hair loss, itching, dermatitis, peeling, increased sweating), or GI problems (nausea, diarrhea, loss of appetite, abdominal pain).

Pharmacokinetics

Absorption: Well absorbed (72%) following oral administration.
Distribution: Crosses the placenta; remainder of distribution unknown.
Protein Binding: Highly protein bound (99.9%).
Metabolism and Excretion: Mostly metabolized by the liver; metabolites excreted in feces (34–54%) and urine (16–53%).
Half-life: 49–63 hr.

TIME/ACTION PROFILE (antipsoriatic effect)

ROUTE	ONSET	PEAK	DURATION
PO	unknown	up to 3 mo	unknown

Contraindications/Precautions

Contraindicated in: Hypersensitivity to retinoids or parabens; Concurrent use of alcohol, in any form; Patients taking methotrexate or a tetracycline; Chronically elevated blood lipids; Severe hepatic or renal impairment; OB/Lactation/Pedi: Safety not established.
Use Cautiously in: Concurrent phototherapy (intensity of treatment may need to be altered).
Exercise Extreme Caution in: Women of childbearing age.

Interactions

Drug-Drug: May ↓ effectiveness of **hormonal contraceptives** (especially microdosed progestin preparations). May ↑ hypoglycemic effects of **sulfonylureas**. **Alcohol** ↑ conversion to a very long-acting compound (avoid use of alcohol during acitretin therapy and for 2 mo after discontinuation). Concurrent use with high doses of **vitamin A** ↑ risk of hypervitaminosis A. **Methotrexate** ↑ risk of hepatotoxicity (avoid concurrent use). **Tetracyclines** may ↑ intracranial pressure (avoid concurrent use).
Drug-Food: Food ↑ absorption.

Route/Dosage

PO (Adults): 25 or 50 mg once daily with a meal.

Availability

Capsules: 10 mg, 25 mg.

acyclovir (ay-**sye**-kloe-veer)

Avirax, Zovirax

Classification
Therapeutic: antivirals
Pharmacologic: purine analogues

Indications

PO: Recurrent genital herpes infections. Localized cutaneous herpes zoster infections (shingles) and chickenpox (varicella). **IV:** Severe initial episodes of genital herpes in nonimmunosuppressed patients. Mucosal or cutaneous herpes simplex infections or herpes zoster infections (shingles) in immunosuppressed patients. Herpes simplex encephalitis. **Topical:** *Cream*—Recurrent herpes labialis (cold sores). *Ointment*—Treatment of limited non–life-threatening herpes simplex infections in immunocompromised patients (systemic treatment is preferred).

Action

Interferes with viral DNA synthesis. **Therapeutic Effects:** Inhibition of viral replication, decreased viral shedding, and reduced time for healing of lesions.

Adverse Reactions/Side Effects

CNS: SEIZURES, dizziness, headache, hallucinations, trembling. **GI:** diarrhea, nausea, vomiting, elevated liver enzymes, hyperbilirubinemia, abdominal pain, anorexia. **GU:** RENAL FAILURE, crystalluria, hematuria, renal pain. **Derm:** acne, hives, skin rashes, unusual sweating, STEVENS-JOHNSON SYNDROME. **Endo:** changes in menstrual cycle. **Hemat:** THROMBOTIC THROMBOCYTOPENIC PURPURA/HEMOLYTIC UREMIC SYNDROME (HIGH DOSES IN IMMUNOSUPPRESSED PATIENTS). **Local:** pain, phlebitis, local irritation. **MS:** joint pain. **Misc:** polydipsia.

PHYSICAL THERAPY IMPLICATIONS

Examination and Evaluation

- Be alert for new seizures or increased seizure activity, especially at the onset of drug treatment. Document the number, duration, and severity of seizures, and report these findings to the physician immediately.
- Monitor signs of renal failure, including decreased urine output, increased blood pressure, muscle cramps/twitching, edema/weight gain from fluid retention, yellowish brown skin, and confusion that progresses to seizures and coma. Report these signs to the physician immediately.
- Monitor signs of thrombotic thrombocytopenic purpura (purplish spots on the skin, decreased consciousness, fatigue, weakness, shortness of breath on exertion, tachycardia) and hemolytic uremic syndrome (bloody diarrhea and vomiting, decreased urine output). Report these signs to the physician immediately.
- Monitor rashes or other skin reactions (hives, acne, abnormal sweating, exfoliation). Notify physician

immediately as certain skin reactions may indicate serious hypersensitivity reactions such as Stevens-Johnson syndrome or erythema multiforme.

- Assess any joint pain to rule out musculoskeletal pathology; that is, try to determine if pain is drug induced rather than caused by anatomic or biomechanical problems.
- Assess dizziness or trembling that might affect gait, balance, or other functional activities (See Appendix C). Report balance problems and functional limitations to the physician, and caution the patient and family/caregivers to guard against falls and trauma.
- Assess skin and mucosal lesions to help determine if drug therapy is successful in controlling infection.
- Monitor IV injection site for pain, swelling, and irritation. Report prolonged or excessive injection site reactions to the physician.

Interventions

- Avoid contact with cutaneous or mucosal lesions when treating patient.
- Always wash hands thoroughly and disinfect equipment (whirlpools, electrotherapeutic devices, treatment tables, and so forth) to help prevent the spread of infection. Employ universal precautions as indicated for specific patients.

Patient/Client-Related Instruction

- Advise patient to take or apply medication as directed. Acyclovir should not be used more frequently or longer than prescribed.
- Remind patient that acyclovir does not cure herpes infections. The virus lies dormant in the ganglia, and acyclovir will not prevent the spread of infection to others.
- Instruct patient and family/caregivers to report other troublesome side effects, including severe or prolonged headache, hallucinations, menstrual problems, or GI problems (diarrhea, nausea, vomiting, loss of appetite, abdominal pain).

Pharmacokinetics

Absorption: Despite poor absorption (15–30%), therapeutic blood levels are achieved.
Distribution: Widely distributed. CSF concentrations are 50% of plasma. Crosses placenta; enters breast milk.
Protein Binding: <30%.
Metabolism and Excretion: >90% eliminated unchanged by kidneys; remainder metabolized by liver.
Half-life: *Neonates*—4 hr; *Children 1–12 yr*—2–3 hr; *Adults*—2–3.5 hr (↑ in renal failure).

TIME/ACTION PROFILE (antiviral blood levels)

ROUTE	ONSET	PEAK	DURATION
PO	unknown	1.5–2.5 hr	4 hr
IV	prompt	end of infusion	8 hr

Contraindications/Precautions

Contraindicated in: Hypersensitivity to acyclovir or valacyclovir.
Use Cautiously in: Preexisting serious neurologic, hepatic, pulmonary, or fluid and electrolyte abnormalities; Renal impairment (dose alteration recommended if CCr <50 mL/min); Geri: Due to age-related ↓ in renal function; Obese patients (dose should be based on ideal body weight); Patients with hypoxia; OB/Lactation: Safety not established.

Interactions

Drug-Drug: Probenecid ↑ blood levels of acyclovir. ↑ blood levels and risk of toxicity from **theophylline**; dose adjustment may be necessary. ↓ blood levels and may ↓ effectiveness of **valproic acid** or **hydantoins**. Concurrent use of other **nephrotoxic drugs** ↑ risk of adverse renal effects. **Zidovudine** and IT **methotrexate** may ↑ risk of CNS side effects.

Route/Dosage

Initial Genital Herpes

PO (Adults and Children): 200 mg q 4 hr while awake (5 times/day) for 7–10 days or 400 mg q 8 hr for 7–10 days; maximum dose in children: 80 mg/kg/day in 3–5 divided doses.
IV (Adults and Children): 5 mg/kg q 8 hr or 750 mg/m^2/day divided q 8 hr for 5–7 days.

Chronic Suppressive Therapy for Recurrent Genital Herpes

PO (Adults and Children): 400 mg twice daily or 200 mg 3–5 times/day for up to 12 mo. Maximum dose in children: 80 mg/kg/day in 2–5 divided doses.

Intermittent Therapy for Recurrent Genital Herpes

PO (Adults and Children): 200 mg q 4 hr while awake (5 times/day) or 400 mg q 8 hr or 800 mg q 12 hr for 5 days, start at first sign of symptoms. Maximum dose in children: 80 mg/kg/day in 2–5 divided doses.

Acute Treatment of Herpes Zoster in Immunosuppressed Patients

PO (Adults): 800 mg q 4 hr while awake (5 times/day) for 7–10 days. Prophylaxis—400 mg 5 times/day.
PO (Children): 250–600 mg/m^2/dose 4–5 times/day.

Herpes Zoster in Immunocompetent Patients

PO (Adults and Children): 4000 mg/day in 5 divided doses for 5–7 days, maximum dose in children: 80 mg/kg/day in 5 divided doses.

Chickenpox

PO (Adults and Children): 20 mg/kg (not to exceed 800 mg/dose) qid for 5 days. Start within 24 hr of rash onset.

Mucosal and Cutaneous Herpes Simplex Infections in Immunosuppressed Patients

IV (Adults and Children >12 yr): 5 mg/kg q 8 hr for 7 days.

IV (Children <12 yr): 10 mg/kg q 8 hr for 7 days.

Topical (Adults): 0.5 in. ribbon of 5% ointment for every 4-square-in. area q 3 hr (6 times/day) for 7 days.

Herpes Simplex Encephalitis

IV (Adults): 10 mg/kg q 8 hr for 14–21 days.

IV (Children 3 mo–12 yr): 10 mg/kg q 8 hr for 14–21 days.

IV (Children birth–3 mo): 20 mg/kg q 8 hr for 14–21 days.

IV (Neonates, premature): 10 mg/kg q 12 hr for 14–21 days.

Varicella Zoster Infections in Immunosuppressed Patients

IV (Adults): 10 mg/kg q 8 hr for 7–10 days.

IV (Children <12 yr): 10 mg/kg q 8 hr for 7–10 days.

Renal Impairment

PO, IV (Adults and Children): *CCr >50 mL/min/1.73 m²*—no dosage adjustment needed; *CCr 25–50 mL/min/1.73 m²*— administer normal dose q 12 hr; *CCr 10–25 mL/min/1.73 m²*— administer normal dose q 24 hr; *CCr 0–10 mL/min/1.73 m²*—50% of dose q 24 hr.

IV (Neonates): *SCr 0.8–1.1 mg/dL:* Administer 20 mg/kg/dose q 12 hr; *SCr 1.2–1.5 mg/dL:* administer 20 mg/kg/dose q 24 hr; *SCr >1.5 mg/dL:* administer 10 mg/kg/dose q 24 hr.

Herpes labialis

Topical (Adults and Children >12 yr): Apply 5 times/day for 4 days; start at first symptoms.

Availability (generic available)

Capsules: 200 mg. **Tablets:** 400 mg, 800 mg. **Suspension (banana flavor):** 200 mg/5 mL. **Powder for injection:** 500 mg/vial, 1000 mg/vial. **Solution for injection:** 25 mg/mL in 20-m and 40-mL vials, 50 mg/mL in 10-mL and 20-mL vials. **Cream:** 5% in 2-g and 5-g tubes. **Ointment:** 5% in 15-g tubes.

adalimumab (a-da-li-mu-mab)

Humira

Classification

Therapeutic: antirheumatics

Pharmacologic: DMARDs, monoclonal antibodies

Indications

Treatment of moderately to severely active rheumatoid arthritis in patients who have responded inadequately to other DMARDs; may be used with methotrexate or other DMARDs. Psoriatic arthritis. Active ankylosing spondylitis. Crohn's disease.

Action

Neutralizes and prevents the action of tumor necrosis factor (TNF), resulting in anti-inflammatory and antiproliferative activity. **Therapeutic Effects:** Decreased pain and swelling with decreased rate of joint destruction in patients with rheumatoid arthritis, psoriatic arthritis, and ankylosing spondylitis. Reduced signs and symptoms of Crohn's disease.

Adverse Reactions/Side Effects

CNS: headache. **CV:** hypertension. **GI:** abdominal pain, nausea. **GU:** hematuria. **Derm:** rash. **Hemat:** neutropenia, thrombocytopenia. **Local:** injection site reactions. **Metab:** hypercholesterolemia, hyperlipidemia. **MS:** back pain. **Misc:** ALLERGIC REACTIONS, INCLUDING ANAPHYLAXIS, INFECTIONS (INCLUDING REACTIVATION TUBERCULOSIS).

PHYSICAL THERAPY IMPLICATIONS

Examination and Evaluation

- Monitor signs of allergic reactions and anaphylaxis, including pulmonary symptoms (tightness in the throat and chest, wheezing, cough, dyspnea) or skin reactions (rash, pruritus, urticaria). Notify physician immediately if these reactions occur.
- Report any signs of infection, especially dormant tuberculosis that is reactivated by drug therapy (reactivation tuberculosis). Signs include fatigue, chills, fever, night sweats, loss of appetite, and pulmonary pathology (persistent cough, coughing up blood, chest pain when breathing and coughing).
- Monitor and report signs of neutropenia (fever, sore throat, signs of infection) or thrombocytopenia (bruising, nose bleeds, and bleeding gums). Periodic blood tests may be needed to monitor WBC and RBC counts.
- Assess any new or increased back pain, joint pain, or other musculoskeletal problems to rule out musculoskeletal pathology; that is, try to determine if pain is drug induced rather than caused by arthritis or anatomic and biomechanical problems.
- Assess blood pressure periodically, and compare to normal values (see Appendix F). Report a sustained increase in BP (hypertension).
- If treating arthritic conditions, periodically assess impairments (pain, range of motion), functional ability, and disability to help document whether antirheumatic drug therapy is successful.
- If treating inflammatory bowel diseases, monitor any changes in symptoms (decreased abdominal pain, decreased diarrhea, improved appetite) to help determine if drug therapy is successful.

- If treating psoriasis, monitor skin responses to help determine if drug therapy is successful in resolving this condition.
- Assess the subcutaneous injection site for pain, swelling, and irritation. Report prolonged or excessive injection site reactions to the physician.

Interventions

- If treating arthritic conditions, implement appropriate manual therapy techniques, physical agents, therapeutic exercises, and orthotic/assistive devices to reduce pain, improve function, and augment the effects of antirheumatic drug therapy.
- Help patients with arthritis explore other nonpharmacologic methods to reduce chronic arthritis pain, such as relaxation techniques, exercise, counseling, and so forth.

Patient/Client-Related Instruction

- Advise patient to guard against infection (frequent hand washing, etc.), and to avoid crowds and contact with persons with contagious diseases.
- Advise patient that this drug may cause problems in fat metabolism (hyperlipidemia, hypercholesterolemia). Remind patient that periodic blood tests may be needed to monitor plasma lipids.
- Instruct patient to report other troublesome side effects including severe or prolonged headache, skin rashes, bloody urine, or GI problems (abdominal pain, nausea).

Pharmacokinetics

Absorption: 64% absorbed after SC administration.
Distribution: Synovial fluid concentrations are 31–96% of serum.
Metabolism and Excretion: Unknown.
Half-life: 14 days (range 10–20 days).

TIME/ACTION PROFILE (improvement)

ROUTE	ONSET	PEAK	DURATION
SC	8–26 wk	131 hr*	2 wk†

*Blood level
†Following discontinuation

Contraindications/Precautions

Contraindicated in: Hypersensitivity; Concurrent use of anakinra; Active infection (including chronic or localized); Lactation: Potential for serious side effects in the infant; discontinue drug or provide formula.
Use Cautiously in: History of recurrent infection or underlying illness/treatment predisposing to infection; Patients residing, or who have resided, where tuberculosis or histoplasmosis is endemic; Preexisting or recent-onset CNS demyelinating disorders; History of lymphoma; Geri: ↑ risk of infection/malignancy; OB: Use only if clearly needed; Pedi: Safety not established.

Interactions

Drug-Drug: Concurrent use with **anakinra** or other **TNF-blocking agents** ↑ risk of serious infections and is contraindicated. **Live vaccinations** should not be given concurrently.

Route/Dosage

Rheumatoid Arthritis, Ankylosing Spondylitis, and Psoriatic Arthritis

SC (Adults): 40 mg every other week; patients not receiving concurrent methotrexate may receive additional benefit by increasing dose to 40 mg once weekly.

Crohn's Disease

SC (Adults): 160 mg initially on day 1 (given as 4 40-mg injections in 1 day or as 2 40-mg injections given in 2 consecutive days), followed by 80-mg 2 wks later on day 15. Two weeks later (day 29) begin maintenance dose of 40 mg every other week. Aminosalicylates, corticosteroids, and/or immunomodulatory agents may be continued during therapy.

Availability

Solution for SC injection (prefilled syringes): 40 mg/0.8 mL. **Prefilled pen:** 40 mg/0.8 mL.

adefovir (a-def-oh-veer)

Hepsera

Classification
Therapeutic: antivirals
Pharmacologic: nucleotides

Indications

Treatment of chronic hepatitis B in patients with evidence of active viral replication and either evidence of persistently elevated liver function tests or active disease (should be used with lamivudine to ↓ risk of resistance).

Action

Converted to adefovir diphosphate which inhibits viral DNA polymerase (reverse transcriptase). Incorporation into viral DNA causes termination of the DNA chain.
Therapeutic Effects: Decreased progression/sequelae of chronic hepatitis B infection.

Adverse Reactions/Side Effects

CNS: headache. **Resp:** cough, pharyngitis, sinusitis.
GI: dyspepsia, HEPATOMEGALY WITH STEATOSIS, abdominal

pain, diarrhea, flatulence, increased liver enzymes, nausea, vomiting. **GU:** hematuria, nephrotoxicity. **Derm:** pruritus, rash. **F and E:** LACTIC ACIDOSIS. **MS:** weakness. **Misc:** fever, HIV resistance.

PHYSICAL THERAPY IMPLICATIONS

Examination and Evaluation

- Be alert for signs of enlarged, fatty liver (hepatomegaly with steatosis) that can progress to liver dysfunction and liver failure. Signs of liver disease include anorexia, abdominal pain, abdominal swelling (ascites), severe nausea and vomiting, yellow skin or eyes, fever, sore throat, malaise, weakness, facial edema, lethargy, and unusual bleeding or bruising. Notify physician of these signs immediately.
- Monitor signs of lactic acidosis, including confusion, lethargy, stupor, shallow rapid breathing, tachycardia, hypotension, nausea, and vomiting. Notify physician immediately if these signs occur.
- Monitor signs of nephrotoxicity, including blood or pus in urine, decreased urine output, weight gain from fluid retention, and fatigue. Report these signs to the physician.

Interventions

- Always wash hands thoroughly and disinfect equipment (whirlpools, electrotherapeutic devices, treatment tables, and so forth) to help prevent the spread of infection. Employ universal precautions as indicated for specific patients.
- Because of the risk of lactic acidosis, use caution during aerobic exercise and other forms of therapeutic exercise. Assess exercise tolerance frequently (blood pressure, heart rate, fatigue levels), and terminate exercise immediately if any untoward responses occur (See Appendix L).

Patient/Client-Related Instruction

- Instruct patient and family/caregivers to report other troublesome side effects, including severe or prolonged headache, cough, nasopharyngeal inflammation, fever, skin problems (rash, itching), or GI problems (diarrhea, nausea, vomiting, indigestion, loss of appetite, abdominal pain, flatulence).

Pharmacokinetics

Absorption: Rapidly converted from prodrug form (adefovir dipivoxil) to adefovir following oral administration; 59% bioavailable.
Distribution: 0.35–0.39 L/kg.
Metabolism and Excretion: Elimination is primarily renal as unchanged drug.
Half-life: 7.5 hr.

TIME/ACTION PROFILE (blood levels)

ROUTE	ONSET	PEAK	DURATION
PO	unknown	1–4 hr	unknown

Contraindications/Precautions

Contraindicated in: Hypersensitivity; Lactation: Provide formula or discontinue drug.
Use Cautiously in: Unrecognized HIV infection (may foster resistance); Patients with renal impairment or at risk of renal impairment (↑ risk of nephrotoxicity; dose adjustment recommended if CCr <50 mL/min); Liver disease or risk factors for liver disease (↑ risk of hepatotoxicity); Women, obese patients, patients with previous nucleoside exposure (↑ risk of lactic acidosis and hepatotoxicity); Geri: Greater risk of side effects due to greater risk of renal or cardiac disorders; OB: Pregnant patients should be enrolled in the pregnancy registry for fetal outcome (1-800-258-4263); Pedi: Children <12 yr (safety not established).

Interactions

Drug-Drug: Drugs that are renally excreted or alter renal function should be used cautiously as they may affect blood levels. **Ibuprofen** may increase blood levels.

Route/Dosage

PO (Adults and Children ≥12 yr): 10 mg once daily.

Renal Impairment

PO (Adults): *CCr 30–49 mL/min*—10 mg every 48 hr; *CCr 10–29 ml/min*—10 mg every 72 hr; *Hemodialysis patients*—10 mg every 7 days following dialysis.

Availability

Tablets: 10 mg.

adenosine (a-den-oh-seen)

Adenocard, Adenoscan

Classification
Therapeutic: antiarrhythmics

Indications

Conversion of paroxysmal supraventricular tachycardia (PSVT) to normal sinus rhythm when vagal maneuvers are unsuccessful. As a diagnostic agent (with noninvasive techniques) to assess myocardial perfusion defects occurring as a consequence of coronary artery disease.

Action

Restores normal sinus rhythm by interrupting reentrant pathways in the AV node. Slows conduction time through the AV node. Also produces coronary artery vasodilation. **Therapeutic Effects:** Restoration of normal sinus rhythm.

Adverse Reactions/Side Effects

CNS: apprehension, dizziness, headache, head pressure, light-headedness. **EENT:** blurred vision, throat tightness. **Resp:** shortness of breath, chest pressure, hyperventilation. **CV:** facial flushing, transient arrhythmias, chest pain, hypotension, palpitations. **GI:** metallic taste, nausea. **Derm:** burning sensation, sweating. **MS:** neck and back pain. **Neuro:** numbness, tingling. **Misc:** heaviness in arms, pressure sensation in groin.

PHYSICAL THERAPY IMPLICATIONS

Examination and Evaluation

- Assess heart rate, ECG, and heart sounds, especially during exercise (See Appendices G, H). Although intended to treat certain arrhythmias, this drug can precipitate new, transient arrhythmias (proarrhythmic effect). Report any rhythm disturbances or symptoms of increased arrhythmias, including palpitations, chest pain, shortness of breath, hyperventilation, fainting, and fatigue/weakness.
- Assess blood pressure periodically, and compare to normal values (See Appendix F). Report low blood pressure (hypotension), especially if patient experiences dizziness, light-headedness, or other symptoms.
- Assess any neck or back pain to rule out musculoskeletal pathology; that is, try to determine if pain is drug induced rather than caused by anatomic or biomechanical problems.
- Assess signs of parasthesia (numbness, tingling). Perform objective tests, including electroneuromyography and sensory testing to document any drug-related neuropathic changes.
- Assess dizziness that might affect gait, balance, and other functional activities (See Appendix C). Report balance problems and functional limitations to the physician and nursing staff, and caution the patient and family/caregivers to guard against falls and trauma.

Interventions

- Because of an increased risk of cardiac arrhythmias, use caution during aerobic exercise and endurance conditioning. Terminate exercise if patient exhibits untoward symptoms (chest pain, shortness of breath, etc.) or displays other criteria for exercise termination (See Appendix L).

Patient/Client-Related Instruction

- Remind patients to take medication as directed to control arrhythmias even if they are asymptomatic.
- Counsel patients about additional interventions to help control cardiac dysfunction, including regular exercise, weight loss, sodium restriction, stress reduction, moderation of alcohol consumption, and smoking cessation.
- Instruct patient or family/caregivers to report other troublesome side effects such as severe or prolonged headache, apprehension, blurred vision, facial flushing, throat tightness, skin reactions (increased sweating, burning sensation), or GI problems (nausea, metallic taste).

Pharmacokinetics

Absorption: Following IV administration, absorption is complete.
Distribution: Taken up by erythrocytes and vascular endothelium.
Metabolism and Excretion: Rapidly converted to inosine and adenosine monophosphate.
Half-life: <10 sec.

TIME/ACTION PROFILE (antiarrhythmic effect)

ROUTE	ONSET	PEAK	DURATION
IV	immediate	unknown	1–2 min

Contraindications/Precautions

Contraindicated in: Hypersensitivity; 2nd- or 3rd-degree AV block or sick sinus syndrome, unless a functional artificial pacemaker is present.
Use Cautiously in: Patients with a history of asthma (may induce bronchospasm); Unstable angina; OB/Lactation: Safety not established.

Interactions

Drug-Drug: Carbamazepine may ↑ risk of progressive heart block. **Dipyridamole** ↑ effects of adenosine (dosage reduction of adenosine recommended). Effects of adenosine ↑ by **theophylline** or **caffeine** (larger doses of adenosine may be required). Concurrent use with **digoxin** may ↑ risk of ventricular fibrillation.

Route/Dosage

IV (Adults and Children >50 kg): *Antiarrhythmic*—6 mg by rapid IV bolus; if no results, repeat 1–2 min later as 12-mg rapid bolus. This dose may be repeated (single dose not to exceed 12 mg). *Diagnostic use*—140 mcg/kg/min for 6 min (0.84 mg/kg total).
IV (Children <50 kg): *Antiarrhythmic*—0.05–0.1 mg/kg as a rapid bolus, may repeat in 1–2 min; if response is inadequate, may increase by 0.05–0.1 mg/kg until sinus rhythm is established or maximum dose of 0.3 mg/kg is used.

Availability (generic available)

Injection: 6 mg/2-mL vial (Adenocard), 3 mg/1 mL in 30-mL vial (Adenoscan).

albuterol (al-byoo-ter-ole)

Airet, Apo-Salvent, Gen-Salbutamol, Novo-Salmol, Proventil, Proventil HFA, Ventodisk, Ventolin, Ventolin HFA, Ventolin nebules, Ventolin rotacaps

Other Names:
salbutamol

Classification
Therapeutic: bronchodilators
Pharmacologic: adrenergics

Indications

Used as a bronchodilator to control and prevent reversible airway obstruction caused by asthma or COPD. **Inhaln:** Used as a quick-relief agent for acute bronchospasm and for prevention of exercise-induced bronchospasm. **PO:** Used as a long-term control agent in patients with chronic/persistent bronchospasm.

Action

Binds to $beta_2$-adrenergic receptors in airway smooth muscle, leading to activation of adenyl cyclase and increased levels of cyclic-3,′,5,′ adenosine monophosphate (cAMP). Increases in cAMP activate kinases, which inhibit the phosphorylation of myosin and decrease intracellular calcium. Decreased intracellular calcium relaxes smooth muscle airways. Relaxation of airway smooth muscle with subsequent bronchodilation. Relatively selective for $beta_2$ (pulmonary) receptors. **Therapeutic Effects:** Bronchodilation.

Adverse Reactions/Side Effects

CNS: nervousness, restlessness, tremor, headache, insomnia (Pedi: occurs more frequently in young children than adults), hyperactivity in children. **CV:** chest pain, palpitations, angina, arrhythmias, hypertension. **GI:** nausea, vomiting. **Endo:** hyperglycemia. **F and E:** hypokalemia.

PHYSICAL THERAPY IMPLICATIONS

Examination and Evaluation

- Assess pulmonary function at rest and during exercise (see Appendixes I, J, K) to document effectiveness of medication in controlling bronchospasm.
- Monitor signs of paradoxical bronchospasm (wheezing, cough, dyspnea, tightness in chest and throat), especially at higher or excessive doses. If condition occurs, advise patient to withhold medication and notify physician immediately.
- Assess blood pressure periodically and compare to normal values (see Appendix F). Report a sustained increase in blood pressure (hypertension) to the physician.
- Assess heart rate, ECG, and heart sounds, especially during exercise (see Appendixes G, H). Report any rhythm disturbances or symptoms of increased arrhythmias, including palpitations, chest discomfort, shortness of breath, fainting, and fatigue/weakness.
- Monitor and report signs of CNS toxicity, including nervousness, restlessness, tremor, or hyperactivity. Sustained or severe CNS signs may indicate overdose or excessive use of this drug.
- Monitor signs of hyperglycemia, including drowsiness, fruity breath, increased urination, and unusual thirst. Patients with diabetes mellitus should check blood glucose levels frequently.
- Monitor and report any muscle weakness, aches, or cramps that might indicate low potassium levels (hypokalemia).

Interventions

- When implementing airway clearance techniques or respiratory muscle training, attempt to intervene when the airway is maximally bronchodilated. Peak responses typically occur 60–90 min after inhalation or 2–3 hr after oral administration.
- Use caution during aerobic exercise and endurance conditioning because of the risk of cardiovascular stimulation. Cardiac effects should be minimal at lower oral doses or occasional inhaled use. Cardiovascular effects such as arrhythmias, angina pectoris, or increased blood pressure may occur at higher doses or during excessive use, and are caused by inadvertent stimulation of beta receptors on the heart.

Patient/Client-Related Instruction

- Advise patient to not exceed the recommended dose or frequency of inhalations. Contact physician immediately if bronchospasm is not relieved by medication or is accompanied by diaphoresis, dizziness, or other symptoms.
- Counsel patient on proper use of inhaler or nebulizer; observe use of these devices whenever possible to ensure proper technique.
- Instruct patient and family/caregivers to report troublesome side effects such as severe or prolonged headache, sleep loss, or GI problems (nausea, vomiting).

Pharmacokinetics

Absorption: Well absorbed after oral administration but rapidly undergoes extensive metabolism.
Distribution: Small amounts appear in breast milk.
Metabolism and Excretion: Extensively metabolized by the liver and other tissues.
Half-life: Oral 2.7–5 hr; Inhalation: 3.8 hr.

TIME/ACTION PROFILE (bronchodilation)

ROUTE	ONSET	PEAK	DURATION
PO	15–30 min	2–3 hr	4–6 hr or more
PO–ER	30 min	2–3 hr	12 hr
inhalation	5–15 min	60–90 min	3–6 hr

Contraindications/Precautions

Contraindicated in: Hypersensitivity to adrenergic amines; Hypersensitivity to fluorocarbons (some inhalers).

Use Cautiously in: Cardiac disease; Hypertension; Hyperthyroidism; Diabetes; Glaucoma; Seizure disorders; Excess inhaler use may lead to tolerance and paradoxical bronchospasm; OB/Lactation/Pedi: Safety not established for pregnant women near term, breastfeeding women, and children <2 yr; Geri: Increased risk adverse reactions; may require dosage reduction.

Interactions

Drug-Drug: Concurrent use with other **adrenergic agents** will have ↑ adrenergic side effects. Use with **MAO inhibitors** may lead to hypertensive crisis. **Beta blockers** may negate therapeutic effect. May decrease serum **digoxin** levels. Cardiovascular effects are potentiated in patients receiving **tricyclic antidepressants**. Risk of hypokalemia ↑ concurrent use of **potassium-losing diuretics**. Hypokalemia ↑ the risk of **digoxin** toxicity.

Drug-Natural: Use with caffeine-containing herbs (**cola nut, guarana, tea, coffee**) ↑ stimulant effect.

Route/Dosage

PO (Adults and Children ≥12 yr): 2–4 mg 3–4 times daily (not to exceed 32 mg/day) or 4–8 mg of extended-release tablets twice daily.

PO (Geriatric Patients): Initial dose should not exceed 2 mg 3–4 times daily, may be increased carefully (up to 32 mg/day).

PO (Children 6–12 yr): 2 mg 3–4 times daily or 0.3–0.6 mg/kg/day as extended-release tablets divided twice daily; may be carefully increased as needed (not to exceed 8 mg/day).

PO (Children 2–6 yr): 0.1 mg/kg 3 times daily (not to exceed 2 mg 3 times daily initially); may be carefully increased to 0.2 mg/kg 3 times daily (not to exceed 4 mg 3 times daily).

Inhalation (Adults and Children ≥4 yr): *Via metered-dose inhaler*—2 inhalations q 4–6 hr or 2 inhalations 15 min before exercise (90 mcg/spray); some patients may respond to 1 inhalation. *NIH Guidelines for acute asthma exacerbation: Children*—4–8 puffs q 20 min for 3 doses then q 1–4 hr; *Adults*—4–8 puffs q 20 min for up to 4 hr then q 1–4 hr prn.

Inhalation (Adults and Children >12 yr): *NIH Guidelines for acute asthma exacerbation via nebulization or IPPB*—2.5–5 mg q 20 min for 3 doses then 2.5–10 mg q 1–4 hr prn; *Continuous nebulization*—10–15 mg/hr.

Inhalation (Children 2–12 yr): *NIH Guidelines for acute asthma exacerbation via nebulization or IPPB*—0.15 mg/kg/dose (minimum dose 2.5 mg) q 20 min for 3 doses then 0.15–0.3 mg/kg (not to exceed 10 mg) q 1–4 hr prn *or* 1.25 mg 3–4 times daily for children 10–15 kg *or* 2.5 mg 3–4 times daily for children >15 kg; *Continuous nebulization*—0.5–3 mg/kg/hr.

Inhalation (Adults and Children ≥4 yr): *Via Rotahaler inhalation device*—200 mcg (as Ventolin Rotacaps) q 4–6 hr (up to 400 mcg q 4–6 hr). May also be given 15 min before exercise.

Availability (generic available)

Tablets: 2 mg, 4 mg. **Extended-release tablets:** 4 mg, 8 mg. **Oral syrup (strawberry flavored):** 2 mg/5 mL. **Metered-dose aerosol:** 90 mcg/inhalation in 6.7-g, 8.5-g, 17-g, and 18-g canisters (200 metered inhalations), 100 mcg/spray. **Inhalation solution:** 0.63 mg/3 mL, 1.25 mg/3 mL, 0.83 mg/mL in vials and 3 mL unit dose, 1 mg/mL, 2 mg/mL, 5 mg/mL. **Powder for inhalation (Ventodisk):** 200 mcg, 400 mcg. ***In combination with:*** ipratropium (Combivent, DuoNeb). See Appendix B.

alclometasone (topical)

(al-kloe-**met**-a-sone)

Aclovate

Classification

Therapeutic: anti-inflammatories (steroidal)

Pharmacologic: corticosteroids

Indications

Management of inflammation and pruritus associated with various allergic/immunologic skin problems.

Action

Suppresses normal immune response and inflammation. **Therapeutic Effects:** Suppression of dermatologic inflammation and immune processes.

Adverse Reactions/Side Effects **Derm:** allergic contact dermatitis, atrophy, burning, dryness, edema, folliculitis, hypersensitivity reactions, hypertrichosis, hypopigmentation, irritation, maceration, miliaria, perioral dermatitis, secondary infection, striae. **Misc:** adrenal suppression (use of occlusive dressings, long-term therapy).

PHYSICAL THERAPY IMPLICATIONS

Examination and Evaluation

- Assess the area being treated to help document whether drug therapy is successful in resolving skin conditions.
- Monitor any new or increased reactions at the site of application, including inflammation, irritation, infection, burning, swelling, exfoliation, and rash. Report severe or prolonged skin reactions to the physician.
- Report signs of adrenal suppression, including hypotension, weight loss, weakness, nausea, vomiting, anorexia, lethargy, confusion, and restlessness.

Interventions

- Protect skin from breakdown, especially over bony prominences.

Patient/Client-Related Instruction

- Advise patients on long-term treatment to consult physician before stopping this medication. Stopping the medication suddenly may result in adrenocortical shock (severe hypotension, hypoglycemia, weakness, vomiting). If these signs appear, notify physician immediately; may be life threatening.
- Check that the patient and family or caregivers understand topical application procedures, and adhere to the recommended dosing schedule.

Pharmacokinetics

Absorption: Minimal. Prolonged use on large surface areas or large amounts applied or use of occlusive dressings may increase systemic absorption.
Distribution: Remains primarily at site of action.
Metabolism and Excretion: Usually metabolized in skin.
Half-life: Unknown.

TIME/ACTION PROFILE (response depends on condition being treated)

ROUTE	ONSET	PEAK	DURATION
topical	min–hrs	hrs–days	hrs–days

Contraindications/Precautions

Contraindicated in: Hypersensitivity or known intolerance to corticosteroids or components of vehicle (ointment base or preservatives); Untreated bacterial or viral infections.
Use Cautiously in: Hepatic dysfunction; Diabetes mellitus, cataracts, glaucoma, or tuberculosis (if significant systemic absorption occurs, condition may worsen); Patients with preexisting skin atrophy; OB/Lactation: Chronic use at high-dosages may result in adrenal suppression in mother and growth suppression in children; Pedi: Children may be more susceptible to adrenal and growth suppression).

Interactions

Drug-Drug: None significant.

Route/Dosage

Topical (Adults): Apply to affected area(s) 2–3 times daily (depends on condition being treated).

Availability

Cream: 0.05% Rx. **Ointment:** 0.05% Rx.

HIGH ALERT

aldesleukin (al-dess-loo-kin)

Proleukin

OTHER NAMES:
interleukin-2, IL-2

Classification
Therapeutic: antineoplastics
Pharmacologic: interleukins

Indications

Management of metastatic renal cell carcinoma.

Action

Increases cellular immunity (noted as lymphocytosis and eosinophilia), increases the production of cytokines (including tumor necrosis factor, interleukin-1, and gamma interferon), and inhibits tumor growth. **Therapeutic Effects:** Regression of renal cell carcinoma.

Adverse Reactions/Side Effects

Resp: APNEA, RESPIRATORY FAILURE, dyspnea, pulmonary congestion, pulmonaryedema, hemoptysis, pleural effusion, pneumothorax, tachypnea, wheezing. **CV:** CARDIAC ARREST, CHF, MI, STROKE, arrhythmias, hypotension, tachycardia, myocardial ischemia, pericardial effusion, thrombosis. **GI:** BOWEL PERFORATION, diarrhea, jaundice, nausea, stomatitis, vomiting, ascites, hepatomegaly. **GU:** oliguria/anuria, proteinuria, dysuria, hematuria, renal failure. **Derm:** EXFOLIATATIVE DERMATITIS, pruritus. **F and E:** acidosis, hypocalcemia, hypokalemia, hypomagnesemia, hypophosphatemia, alkalosis, hyperkalemia, hyperuricemia, hyponatremia. **Hemat:** anemia, coagulation disorders, leukopenia, thrombocytopenia, eosinophilia, leukocytosis. **Misc:** CAPILLARY LEAK SYNDROME, chills, fever, weight gain, weight loss.

PHYSICAL THERAPY IMPLICATIONS

Examination and Evaluation

- Continually monitor for signs of MI and cardiac arrest (sudden chest pain, pain radiating into the arm or jaw, shortness of breath, dizziness, sweating, anxiety, nausea) or stroke (sudden severe headache, confusion, nausea, vomiting, paralysis, numbness, speech problems, visual disturbances). Seek immediate medical assistance if patient develops these signs.

- Assess respiration, and notify physician immediately if patient exhibits any interruption in respiratory rate (apnea), signs of respiratory failure (rapid labored breathing, cyanosis, confusion, irritability, sleepiness, headache, oxygen desaturation), or other signs of acute or severe pulmonary pathology (coughing up blood, sudden severe chest pain, abnormal breath sounds). Monitor pulse oximetry and perform pulmonary function tests (See Appendices I, J, K) to quantify suspected changes in ventilation and respiratory function.
- Monitor signs of CHF such as dyspnea, rales/crackles, peripheral edema, jugular venous distention, and exercise intolerance; report these signs to the physician immediately.
- Assess blood pressure and report signs of capillary leak syndrome, including hypotension, generalized edema, light-headedness, fainting, and nasal congestion.
- Watch for signs of exfoliative dermatitis such as itching, scaling, redness, warmth, and rapid skin loss. Report these signs to the physician immediately.
- Monitor signs of leukopenia (fever, sore throat, signs of infection), thrombocytopenia (bruising, nose bleeds, bleeding gums), or unusual weakness and fatigue that might be due to anemia or other blood dyscrasias. Report these signs to the physician.
- Assess heart rate, ECG, and heart sounds, especially during exercise (See Appendices G, H). Report any rhythm disturbances or signs of increased arrhythmias, including palpitations, chest discomfort, shortness of breath, fainting, and fatigue/weakness.
- Monitor signs of venous thrombosis and thromboembolism (shortness of breath, chest pain, cough, bloody sputum). Notify physician immediately, and request objective tests (Doppler ultrasound, lung scan, others) if thrombosis is suspected.
- Monitor any urinary problems or signs of renal failure, including decreased urine output, increased blood pressure, muscle cramps/twitching, edema/weight gain from fluid retention, yellowish brown skin, and confusion that progresses to seizures and coma. Report these signs to the physician immediately.
- Monitor neuromuscular signs of acid-base and electrolyte imbalances (acidosis, alkalosis, hypocalcemia, hypokalemia, etc.), including headache, lethargy, weakness, cramping, and muscle hyperexcitability and tetany. Notify physician immediately if these signs occur.
- Monitor body weight and report any sudden or substantial weight gain or loss.

Interventions

- For patients who are medically able to begin exercise, implement appropriate resistive exercises and aerobic training to maintain muscle strength and aerobic capacity during cancer chemotherapy, or to help restore function after chemotherapy.
- Because of the risk severe cardiovascular events (MI, stroke, CHF), use extreme caution during aerobic exercise and other forms of therapeutic exercise. Assess exercise tolerance frequently (blood pressure, heart rate, fatigue levels), and terminate exercise immediately if any untoward responses occur (See Appendix L).
- Design and implement breathing exercises as tolerated to maximize ventilation and prevent respiratory failure.

Patient/Client-related Instruction

- Advise patient and family or caregiver about the signs of MI, respiratory failure, and other severe reactions such as bowel perforation, capillary leak syndrome, and exfoliative dermatitis (see above under Examination and Evaluation). Instruct patient and family/caregivers to seek immediate medical assistance if these signs develop.
- Advise patient about the likelihood of other GI reactions (nausea, vomiting, diarrhea, irritation of the oral mucosa). Instruct patient to report severe or prolonged GI problems, or signs of liver toxicity (yellow skin or eyes, abdominal pain, severe nausea and vomiting, fever, sore throat, malaise, weakness, facial edema).

Pharmacokinetics

Absorption: IV administration results in complete bioavailability.
Distribution: Rapidly distributes to intravascular, extracellular space; 70% is taken up by the liver, kidneys, and lungs.
Metabolism and Excretion: Metabolized to amino acids by renal tubular cells.
Half-life: 85 min.

TIME/ACTION PROFILE (tumor regression after completion of first course)

ROUTE	ONSET	PEAK	DURATION
IV	4 wk	unknown	12 mo

Contraindications/Precautions

Contraindicated in: Hypersensitivity to aldesleukin or mannitol; Cross-sensitivity to *Escherichia coli*—derived proteins may occur; Patients with any history of cardiac or pulmonary disease as assessed by abnormal thallium stress testing or abnormal pulmonary function testing; Patients who have experienced any of the following toxicities during previous courses of aldesleukin—sustained ventricular tachycardia (≥5 beats), angina pectoris or MI as indicated by ECG changes, respiratory problems requiring more than 72 hr of intubation, pericardial tamponade, renal toxicity requiring more than 72 hr of dialysis, CNS dysfunction consisting of more than 48 hr of coma or psychosis, intractable seizures, bowel perforation or ischemia, GI bleeding requiring surgical intervention; Patients who have had allograft organ transplantation (increased risk of rejection).

Use Cautiously in: Patients with a history of cardiovascular, respiratory, hepatic, or renal disease; Patients with a history of seizures or suspected CNS metastases (symptoms may be exaggerated and seizures may occur); Patients with child-bearing potential; OB/Lactation/Pedi: Safety not established.

Interactions

Drug-Drug: Corticosteroids decrease antineoplastic effectiveness. Avoid concurrent use with aldesleukin. Additive hypotension may occur with **antihypertensives**. Concurrent **cardiotoxic, hepatotoxic, myelotoxic**, or **nephrotoxic drug therapy** increases the risk of toxicity in these organs.

Route/Dosage

IV (Adults): 600,000 IU/kg (0.037 mg/kg) every 8 hr for 14 doses. Cycle is repeated once after a 9-day rest period to a total of 28 doses. After a rest period of 7 wk, patients who have had a beneficial response may be evaluated for additional courses.

Availability

Vials: containing 22 million IU.

alefacept (a-le-fa-sept)

Amevive

Classification

Therapeutic: antipsoriatics, immunosuppressants

Pharmacologic: fusion proteins (rDNA)

Indications

Treatment of moderate to severe chronic plaque psoriasis in patients who are candidates for systemic therapy or phototherapy.

Action

Inhibits the activation of T lymphocytes by binding to specific surface antigens. **Therapeutic Effects:** Reduction in size and severity of psoriatic lesions.

Adverse Reactions/Side Effects

CNS: dizziness, chills. **Derm:** pruritus. **GI:** fatty liver, hepatitis, increase in liver enzymes, LIVER FAILURE, nausea. **Hemat:** LYMPHOPENIA. **Local:** injection site reactions. **MS:** myalgia. **Resp:** pharyngitis, cough. **Misc:** HYPERSENSITIVITY REACTIONS (ANGIOEDEMA, urticaria), IMMUNOSUPPRESSION, INFECTION, MALIGNANCIES.

PHYSICAL THERAPY IMPLICATIONS

Examination and Evaluation

- Monitor signs of hypersensitivity reactions and angioedema, including pulmonary symptoms (tightness in the throat and chest, wheezing, cough, dyspnea) or skin reactions (rash, pruritus, urticaria, swelling in the face). Notify physician immediately if any hypersensitivity reactions occur.
- Monitor signs of malignancy, including a change in bowel or bladder habits, nonhealing sores, unusual bleeding or discharge, a lump in the breast or other parts of the body, chronic indigestion or difficulty in swallowing, obvious changes in a wart or mole, and persistent coughing or hoarseness. Report these signs to the physician immediately.
- Be alert for signs of hepatitis and liver failure, including anorexia, abdominal pain, severe nausea and vomiting, yellow skin or eyes, fever, sore throat, malaise, weakness, facial edema, lethargy, and unusual bleeding or bruising. Notify physician immediately if these signs occur.
- Monitor signs of decreased lymphocytes (lymphopenia) or immunosuppression, including infections, fever, sore throat, and white patches in the throat or mouth. Report these signs to the physician immediately.
- Assess skin for any changes in psoriasis to help document the effects of drug therapy.
- Assess dizziness that might affect gait, balance, and other functional activities (See Appendix C). Report balance problems and functional limitations to the physician, and caution the patient and family/caregivers to guard against falls and trauma.
- Assess any muscle pain to rule out musculoskeletal pathology; that is, try to determine if pain is drug induced rather than caused by anatomic or biomechanical problems.
- Monitor injection site for pain, swelling, and irritation. Report prolonged or excessive injection-site reactions to the physician.

Interventions

- Implement ultraviolet light therapy when indicated to help treat psoriasis and augment the effects of drug therapy.

Patient/Client-Related Instruction

- Advise patient to guard against infection (frequent hand washing, etc.), and to avoid crowds and contact with persons with contagious diseases.

- Instruct patient to report other troublesome side effects including severe or prolonged nausea, cough, chills, or skin reactions (rash, hives, itching).

Pharmacokinetics

Absorption: 63% absorbed following IM administration.
Distribution: 0.094 L/kg.
Metabolism and Excretion: Unknown.
Half-life: 270 hr.

TIME/ACTION PROFILE (improvement in psoriatic lesions)

ROUTE	ONSET	PEAK	DURATION
IM, IV	2 mo	unknown	2 mo*

*Following discontinuation

Contraindications/Precautions

Contraindicated in: Hypersensitivity; Concurrent immunosuppressant or phototherapy; Active infection; History of malignancy; Patients with CD4+ T-lymphocyte count below normal; Lactation or children.
Use Cautiously in: Patients with chronic or recurrent infections; Patients at high risk for malignancy; OB: Safety not established); Geri: May have increased risk of serious infections or malignancy.

Interactions

Drug-Drug: Unknown.

Route/Dosage

IM (Adults): 15 mg once weekly for 12 wk; after at least a 12-wk rest; a second course may be given as long as the CD4+ T-lymphocyte counts are normal; **IV (Adults)** 7.5 mg once weekly for 12 wk; after at least a 12-wk rest, a second course may be given as long as the CD4+ T-lymphocyte counts are normal.

Availability

Lyophilized powder for IM administration: 15 mg/vial.

HIGH ALERT

alemtuzumab

(a-lem-**too**-zoo-mab)
Campath

Classification
Therapeutic: antineoplastics
Pharmacologic: monoclonal antibodies

Indications

Treatment of B-cell chronic lymphocytic leukemia in patients who have been treated with alkylating agents and in whom fludarabine therapy has failed.

Action

Binds to the CD52 antigen found on the surface of B and T lymphocytes and other white blood cells; resulting in lysis. **Therapeutic Effects:** Lysis of leukemic cells with eventual improvement in hematologic parameters.

Adverse Reactions/Side Effects

CNS: depression, dizziness, drowsiness, fatigue, headache, weakness. **Resp:** bronchospasm, cough, dyspnea. **CV:** hypertension, hypotension, tachycardia. **GI:** abdominal pain, anorexia, constipation, stomatitis. **Derm:** rash, sweating. **F and E:** edema. **Hemat:** NEUTROPENIA, PANCYTOPENIA/MARROW HYPOPLASIA, anemia, lymphopenia, thrombocytopenia. **MS:** back pain, skeletal pain. **Misc:** infusion-related events, infection, sepsis.

PHYSICAL THERAPY IMPLICATIONS

Examination and Evaluation

- Monitor signs of bone marrow suppression, including neutropenia (fever, sore throat, signs of infection), thrombocytopenia (bruising, nose bleeds, bleeding gums), or unusual weakness and fatigue that might be due to anemia or other blood dyscrasias. Report these signs to the physician or nursing staff immediately.
- Report allergy-like responses (wheezing, tightness in the throat or chest, urticaria, other skin reactions) that occur during and after administration (infusion-related events).
- Assess blood pressure (BP) and compare to normal values (See Appendix F). Report changes in BP, either a problematic decrease in BP (hypotension), or a sustained increase in BP (hypertension).
- Assess heart rate (HR), ECG, and heart sounds, especially during exercise (See Appendices G, H). Report a rapid HR rate (tachycardia) or signs of other arrhythmias, including palpitations, chest discomfort, shortness of breath, fainting, and fatigue/weakness.
- Monitor signs of bronchospasm (wheezing, coughing, tightness in chest) or other prolonged or severe respiratory problems (difficult or labored breathing). Perform pulmonary function tests and monitor breath sounds to quantify suspected changes in ventilation and respiration (See Appendices I, J, K).
- Assess peripheral edema using girth measurements, volume displacement, and measurement of pitting edema (See Appendix N). Report increased swelling in feet and ankles or a sudden increase in body weight due to fluid retention.
- Assess any joint, back, or other skeletal pain to rule out musculoskeletal pathology; that is, try to determine if pain is drug induced rather than caused by anatomic or biomechanical problems.

- Assess dizziness, drowsiness, or weakness that might affect gait, balance, and other functional activities (See Appendix C). Report balance problems and functional limitations to the physician and nursing staff, and caution the patient and family/caregivers to guard against falls and trauma.
- Monitor and report depression or other changes in mood and behavior.

Interventions

- For patients who are medically able to begin exercise, implement appropriate resistive exercises and aerobic training to maintain muscle strength and aerobic capacity during cancer chemotherapy, or to help restore function after chemotherapy.
- Because of potential adverse changes in BP and HR, use caution during aerobic exercise and endurance conditioning. Terminate exercise if patient exhibits untoward symptoms (chest pain, shortness of breath, etc.), or displays other criteria for exercise termination (See Appendix L).

Patient/Client-Related Instruction

- Advise patient to guard against infection (frequent hand washing, etc.), and avoid crowds and contact with persons with contagious diseases.
- Advise patient that rash and other skin reactions (sweating, pruritus) are likely. Report severe or unexpected skin reactions to the physician.
- Advise patient about the likelihood of GI reactions (abdominal pain, constipation, loss of appetite, inflammation of mucous membranes). Instruct patient to report severe or prolonged GI problems.
- Instruct patient or family/caregivers to report other severe or prolonged side effects such headache, fever, or other signs of infection.

Pharmacokinetics

Absorption: IV administration results in complete bioavailability.
Distribution: Binds to CD52 receptors.
Metabolism and Excretion: Unknown.
Half-life: 12 days.

TIME/ACTION PROFILE (hematologic parameters)

ROUTE	ONSET	PEAK	DURATION
IV	unknown	2–4 mos*	7–11 mos†

*Median time to response.
†Duration of response.

Contraindications/Precautions

Contraindicated in: Hypersensitivity; Systemic infections; Underlying immunodeficiency, including HIV infection; Lactation: Discontinue breastfeeding during and for 3 mo following last dose of alemtuzumab.
Use Cautiously in: Patients with ischemic heart disease or in patients on antihypertensive medications; Women and men with reproduction potential should use contraception during treatment and for 6 mo after therapy; OB: Should be administered only if clearly needed.

Interactions

Drug-Drug: Additive bone marrow depression with other **antineoplastics** or **radiation therapy**. May ↓ antibody response to and increase the risk of adverse reactions to **live-virus vaccines**.

Route/Dosage

IV (Adults): 3 mg/day initially, as tolerated increase dose to 10 mg/day and then 30 mg/day given 3 times weekly for up to 12 weeks; single doses should not exceed 30 mg or more than 90 mg/wk.

Availability

Solution for injection (requires further dilution): 30 mg/3 mL in single-use ampules.

alendronate (a-len-drone-ate)

Fosamax

Classification
Therapeutic: bone resorption inhibitors
Pharmacologic: biphosphonates

Indications

Treatment and prevention of postmenopausal osteoporosis. Treatment of osteoporosis in men. Treatment of Paget's disease of the bone. Treatment of corticosteroid-induced osteoporosis in patients (men and women) who are receiving ≥7.5 mg of prednisone/day (or equivalent) with evidence of decreased bone mineral density.

Action

Inhibits resorption of bone by inhibiting osteoclast activity. **Therapeutic Effects:** Reversal of the progression of osteoporosis with decreased fractures. Decreased progression of Paget's disease.

Adverse Reactions/Side Effects

CNS: headache. **EENT:** blurred vision, conjunctivitis, eye pain/inflammation. **CV:** atrial fibrillation. **GI:** abdominal distention, abdominal pain, acid regurgitation, constipation, diarrhea, dyspepsia, dysphagia, esophageal ulcer, flatulence, gastritis, nausea, taste perversion, vomiting. **Derm:** erythema, photosensitivity, rash. **MS:** musculoskeletal pain, osteonecrosis (primarily of jaw).

PHYSICAL THERAPY IMPLICATIONS

Examination and Evaluation

- Assess heart rate, ECG, and heart sounds (See Appendices G, H). Report rhythm disturbances such as atrial fibrillation, or symptoms of increased arrhythmias, including palpitations, chest discomfort, shortness of breath, fainting, and fatigue/weakness.

- Assess any muscle or joint pain. Report persistent or increased musculoskeletal pain to determine presence of bone or joint pathology including fracture. Be especially aware of possible mouth and jaw pain due to osteonecrosis of the jaw.

Interventions

- Institute weight-bearing and resistance exercises as tolerated to maintain or increase bone mineral density. Start with low impact or aquatic programs in patients with extensive demineralization, and increase exercise intensity slowly to prevent fractures.
- Protect against falls and fractures (See Appendix E). Modify home environment (remove throw rugs, improve lighting, etc.) and provide assistive devices (cane, walker) or other protective devices as needed to improve balance and prevent falls.
- Because of the risk of cardiac arrhythmias (atrial fibrillation, others), use caution during aerobic exercise and endurance conditioning Terminate exercise if patient exhibits untoward symptoms (chest pain, shortness of breath, unusual fatigue), or displays other criteria for exercise termination (See Appendix L).
- Causes photosensitivity; use care if administering UV treatments.

Patient/Client-Related Instruction

- Encourage patient to modify behaviors that increase the risk of osteoporosis (stop smoking, reduce alcohol consumption).
- Advise patient about the benefits of proper diet in sustaining bone mineralization. If necessary, refer patient for nutritional counseling about supplemental calcium and vitamin D.
- Instruct patient on the importance of taking this drug exactly as directed, and to remain upright for 30 min following dose to facilitate passage to stomach and minimize risk of esophageal irritation.
- Instruct patient to notify physician about any vision disturbances or eye pain and inflammation.
- Advise patient about photosensitivity, and to use sunscreens, protective clothing, and avoid prolonged sun exposure. Instruct patient to report any rashes or other skin reactions.
- Instruct patient to report other severe or prolonged side effects such as headache, difficulty swallowing, retrosternal pain, new/worsening heartburn, or other GI problems (nausea, vomiting, diarrhea, constipation).

Pharmacokinetics

Absorption: Poorly absorbed (0.6–0.8%) after oral administration.
Distribution: Transiently distributes to soft tissue, then distributes to bone.
Metabolism and Excretion: Excreted in urine.
Half-life: 10 yr (reflects release of drug from skeleton).

TIME/ACTION PROFILE (inhibition of bone resorption)

ROUTE	ONSET	PEAK	DURATION
PO	1 mo	3–6 mo	3 wk–7 mo*

*After discontinuation of alendronate.

Contraindications/Precautions

Contraindicated in: Renal insufficiency (CCr <35 mL/min); OB/Lactation: Safety not established.
Use Cautiously in: Patients with active GI pathology (dysphagia, esophageal disease, gastritis, duodenitis, ulcers); Preexisting hypocalcemia or vitamin D deficiency; Concurrent dental surgery (may ↑ risk of jaw osteonecrosis).

Interactions

Drug-Drug: Calcium supplements, **antacids**, and **other oral medications** ↓ the absorption of alendronate. Doses >10 mg/day ↑ risk of adverse GI events when used with **NSAIDs**. IV **ranitidine** ↑ blood levels.
Drug-Food: Food significantly ↓ absorption. **Caffeine (coffee, tea, cola)**, **mineral water**, and **orange juice** also ↓ absorption.

Route/Dosage

PO (Adults): *Treatment of osteoporosis*—10 mg once daily or 70 mg once weekly. *Prevention of osteoporosis*—5 mg once daily or 35 mg once weekly. *Paget's disease*—40 mg once daily for 6 mo. Retreatment may be considered for patients who relapse. *Treatment of corticosteroid-induced osteoporosis in men and premenopausal women*—5 mg once daily. *Treatment of corticosteroid-induced osteoporosis in postmenopausal women not receiving estrogen*—10 mg once daily.

Availability (generic available)

Tablets: 5 mg, 10 mg, 35 mg, 40 mg, 70 mg. **Oral solution (raspberry flavor):** 70 mg/75 mL. ***In combination with***: cholecalciferol (Fosamax plus D) (See Appendix B).

HIGH ALERT

alfentanil (al-fen-ta-nil)

Alfenta, 🍁Rapifen

Classification
Therapeutic: analgesic adjuncts, opioid analgesics
Pharmacologic: opioid agonists

Schedule II

Indications
Analgesic adjunct used to maintain anesthesia with barbiturate/nitrous oxide/oxygen. Analgesic (continuous IV infusion) with nitrous oxide/oxygen while maintaining general anesthesia. Primary induction anesthetic when endotracheal intubation and mechanical ventilation are required.

Action
Binds to opiate receptors in the CNS, altering the response to and perception of pain while causing generalized CNS depression. **Therapeutic Effects:** Relief of moderate to severe pain. Anesthesia.

Adverse Reactions/Side Effects
CNS: dizziness, sleepiness. **EENT:** blurred vision. **Resp:** apnea, respiratory depression. **CV:** bradycardia, hypotension, tachycardia, arrhythmias, hypertension. **GI:** nausea, vomiting. **MS:** thoracic muscle rigidity, skeletal muscle rigidity.

PHYSICAL THERAPY IMPLICATIONS

Examination and Evaluation
- Assess respiration, and notify physician immediately if patient exhibits any interruption in respiratory rate (apnea) or signs of respiratory depression, including decreased respiratory rate, confusion, bluish color of the skin and mucous membranes (cyanosis), and difficult, labored breathing (dyspnea). Monitor pulse oximetry and perform pulmonary function tests (See Appendix I) to quantify suspected changes in ventilation and respiratory function. Apnea or excessive respiratory depression requires emergency care.
- Be alert for excessive sedation, and notify physician or nurse immediately if patient is unconscious or extremely difficult to arouse.
- Use appropriate pain scales (visual analog scales, others) to document whether this drug is successful in helping manage the patient's pain.
- Assess blood pressure (BP) and compare to normal values (See Appendix F). Report changes in BP, either a problematic decrease in BP (hypotension), or a sustained increase in BP (hypertension).
- Assess heart rate, ECG, and heart sounds, especially during exercise (See Appendices G, H). Report any rhythm disturbances or symptoms of arrhythmias, including palpitations, chest discomfort, shortness of breath, fainting, and fatigue/weakness.
- Assess dizziness that might affect gait, balance, and other functional activities (See Appendix C). Report balance problems and functional limitations to the physician and nursing staff, and caution the patient and family/caregivers to guard against falls and trauma.
- Be alert for residual muscle rigidity and decreased thoracic and limb movements after rapid IV administration. Report a sustained increase in muscle tone.

Interventions
- Implement appropriate manual therapy techniques, physical agents, and therapeutic exercises to reduce pain and help wean patient off opioid analgesics as soon as possible.
- Because of the risk of respiratory depression, arrhythmias, and abnormal BP responses, use caution during aerobic exercise and other forms of therapeutic exercise. Assess exercise tolerance frequently (BP, heart rate, respiratory rate, fatigue levels), and terminate exercise immediately if any untoward responses occur (See Appendix L).
- Help patient explore other nonpharmacologic methods to reduce chronic pain (relaxation techniques, exercise, counseling, and so forth).
- Guard against falls and trauma (hip fractures, head injury). Implement fall prevention strategies (See Appendix E), especially if patient exhibits sedation, dizziness, or blurred vision.
- To minimize orthostatic hypotension, patient should move slowly when assuming a more upright position.

Patient/Client-Related Instruction
- Advise patient that opioid analgesics are usually more effective if given before pain becomes severe; emphasize that adequate pain control will allow better participation in physical therapy.
- Educate patient about the dangers of opioid overdose; encourage patient to adhere to proper dosing schedule.
- Emphasize that the risk of physical addiction (tolerance and dependence) is usually minimal during short-term treatment of pain. Advise patient that addiction is more likely during excessive or inappropriate use of opioid analgesics.
- Advise patient to avoid alcohol and other CNS depressants because of the increased risk of sedation and decreased CNS function.
- Instruct patient to report other troublesome side effects such as severe or prolonged blurred vision or GI problems (nausea, vomiting).

Pharmacokinetics
Absorption: Following IV administration, absorption is essentially complete.
Distribution: Does not penetrate adipose tissue. Crosses placenta, enters breast milk.
Metabolism and Excretion: >95% metabolized by the liver.
Half-life: 60–130 min (↓ in children).

TIME/ACTION PROFILE (analgesia and respiratory depression)

ROUTE	ONSET	PEAK	DURATION
IV	immediate	1–1.5 min	5–10 min*

*↓ in children.

Contraindications/Precautions

Contraindicated in: Hypersensitivity; Known intolerance.

Use Cautiously in: Debilitated, geriatric, or severely ill patients; Diabetes; Severe pulmonary or hepatic disease; CNS tumors; Increased intracranial pressure; Head trauma; Adrenal insufficiency; Undiagnosed abdominal pain; Hypothyroidism; Alcoholism; Cardiac disease (arrhythmias); OB/Lactation/Pedi: Safety not established; Geri: Older patients may be more susceptible to side effects.

Interactions

Drug-Drug: alcohol, antihistamines, antidepressants, and other **sedative/hypnotics**—concurrent use ↑ CNS depression. **MAO inhibitors** should be avoided for 14 days before use. **Cimetidine** or **erythromycin** may ↑ duration of recovery. Concurrent use with **benzodiazepines, antihypertensives, alcohol**, or **diuretics** may ↑ risk of hypotension. **Nalbuphine, buprenorphine, butorphanol**, or **pentazocine** may ↓ analgesia. Concurrent use of **protease inhibitor antiretrovirals** may ↑ risk of CNS depression. **Naltrexone** and **naloxone** will block all effects of alfentanil.

Drug-Natural: Concomitant use of kava, valerian can ↑ CNS depression.

Route/Dosage

Incremental Injection (Duration of Anesthesia <30 min)—Induction Period

IV (Adults): 8–20 mcg/kg.

Incremental Injection (Duration of Anesthesia <30 min)—Maintenance Period

IV (Adults): 3–5 mcg/kg every 5–20 min or 0.5–1 mcg/kg/min (total dose 8–40 mcg/kg).

Incremental Injection (Duration of Anesthesia 30–60 min)—Induction Period

IV (Adults): 20–50 mcg/kg.

Incremental Injection (Duration of Anesthesia 30–60 min)—Maintenance Period

IV (Adults): 5–15 mcg/kg every 5–20 min (up to total dose of 75 mg/kg).

Continuous Infusion (Duration of Anesthesia >45 min)—Induction

IV (Adults): 50–75 mcg/kg.

Continuous Infusion (Duration of Anesthesia >45 min)—Maintenance

IV (Adults): 0.5–3 mcg/kg/min (average rate 1–1.5 mcg/kg/min). Infusion rate should be decreased by 30–50% after first hour of maintenance. If lightening occurs, infusion rate may be increased up to 4 mcg/kg/min or boluses of 7 mcg/kg may be administered.

Pediatric dose (unlabeled)

IV (Children): *Induction*—12.5–50 mcg/kg initially, followed by supplemental doses of 10–15 mcg or infusion at 0.5–1.5 mcg/kg/min.

Anesthetic Induction (Duration of Anesthesia >45 min)

IV (Adults): 130–245 mcg/kg followed by 0.5–1.5 mcg/kg/min or general anesthesia.

Monitored Anesthesia Care (MAC)—Induction

IV (Adults): 3–8 mcg/kg.

Monitored Anesthesia Care (MAC)—Maintenance

IV (Adults): 3–5 mcg/kg every 5–20 min *or* 0.25–1 mcg/kg/min (total dose 3–40 mg/kg).

Availability

Injection: 500 mcg/mL in 2-, 5-, 10-, and 20-mL ampules Rx.

HIGH ALERT

alfuzosin (al-fyoo-zo-sin)

Uroxatral

Classification

Therapeutic: urinary tract antispasmodics

Pharmacologic: peripherally acting antiadrenergics

Indications

Management of symptomatic benign prostatic hyperplasia (BPH).

Action

Selectively blocks $alpha_1$-adrenergic receptors in the lower urinary tract to relax smooth muscle in the bladder neck and prostate. **Therapeutic Effects:** Increased urine flow and decreased symptoms of BPH.

Adverse Reactions/Side Effects

CNS: dizziness, fatigue, headache. **Resp:** bronchitis, sinusitis, pharyngitis. **CV:** orthostatic hypotension. **GI:** abdominal pain, constipation, dyspepsia, nausea. **GU:** erectile dysfunction.

PHYSICAL THERAPY IMPLICATIONS

Examination and Evaluation

- Assess blood pressure when patient assumes a more upright position (lying to standing, sitting to standing, lying to sitting). Document orthostatic hypotension and contact physician when systolic blood pressure (BP) falls >20 mm Hg, or diastolic BP falls >10 mm Hg.

- Assess dizziness that might affect gait, balance, and other functional activities (See Appendix C). Report balance problems and functional limitations to the physician, and caution the patient and family/caregivers to guard against falls and trauma.
- Monitor signs of prostate hypertrophy such as difficulty starting a urine stream, painful urination, weak urine flow, feeling that the bladder is not completely empty, frequent nighttime urination, and an urge to urinate again soon after urinating. Document any change in symptoms to help assess the effects of drug therapy.

Interventions

- To minimize orthostatic hypotension, patient should move slowly when assuming a more upright position.

Patient/Client-Related Instruction

- Advise patient that sexual function may be affected, and to consult physician if erectile dysfunction becomes problematic.
- Instruct patient or family/caregivers to report other troublesome side effects such as severe or prolonged headache, fatigue, respiratory irritation, or GI problems (nausea, constipation, abdominal pain, indigestion).

Pharmacokinetics

Absorption: 49% absorbed following oral administration; food enhances absorption.
Distribution: Unknown.
Metabolism and Excretion: Mostly metabolized by the liver (CYP3A4 enzyme system); 69% eliminated in feces, 24% in urine.
Half-life: 10 hr.

TIME/ACTION PROFILE

ROUTE	ONSET	PEAK	DURATION
PO-ER	within hr	8 hr	24 hr

Contraindications/Precautions

Contraindicated in: Hypersensitivity; Moderate to severe hepatic impairment; Potent inhibitors of the CYP3A4 enzyme system; Concurrent use of other alpha-adrenergic blocking agents; Severe renal impairment; OB/Pedi: No indications for women and children.
Use Cautiously in: Congenital or acquired QTc prolongation or concurrent use of other drugs known to prolong QTc; Mild hepatic impairment; Geri: Consider age-related changes in body mass, cardiac, renal and hepatic function when prescribing.

Interactions

Drug-Drug: Ketoconazole, itraconazole, and **ritonavir** ↓ metabolism and significantly ↑ levels and effects (concurrent use in contraindicated). Levels are also ↑ by **cimetidine, atenolol,** and **diltiazem.** Alfuzosin ↑ levels and may ↑ effects of **atenolol** and **diltiazem** (monitor BP pressure and heart rate). ↑ risk of hypotension with **antihypertensives, nitrates,** and acute ingestion of **alcohol.**

Route/Dosage

PO (Adults): 10 mg once daily.

Availability

Extended-release tablets: 10 mg.

aliskiren (a-lis-ki-ren)
Tekturna

Classification
Therapeutic: antihypertensives
Pharmacologic: direct renin inhibitor

Indications

Treatment of hypertension (alone or with other agents).

Action

Inhibition of renin results in decreased formation of angiotensin II, a powerful vasoconstrictor.
Therapeutic Effects: Decreased blood pressure.

Adverse Reactions/Side Effects

Resp: cough. **GI:** abdominal pain, diarrhea ↑ (in females and elderly), dyspepsia, reflux. **Misc:** ANGIOEDEMA.

PHYSICAL THERAPY IMPLICATIONS

Examination and Evaluation

- Monitor signs of angioedema including rashes, raised patches of red or white skin (welts), burning/itching skin, swelling in the face, and difficulty breathing. Notify physician of these signs immediately.
- Assess blood pressure periodically, and compare to normal values (see Appendix F) to help document antihypertensive effects.

Interventions

- Avoid physical therapy interventions that cause systemic vasodilation (large whirlpool, Hubbard tank). Additive effects of this drug and the intervention may cause a dangerous fall in blood pressure.

Patient/Client-Related Instruction

- Remind patients to take medication as directed to control hypertension even if they are asymptomatic.
- Counsel patients about additional interventions to help control blood pressure, including regular exercise, weight loss, sodium restriction, stress reduction, moderation of alcohol consumption, and smoking cessation.

- Instruct patient to notify physician of a prolonged dry cough; drug therapy may need to be altered to resolve this side effect.
- Instruct patient or family/caregivers to report severe or prolonged GI problems such as diarrhea, indigestion, heartburn, and abdominal pain.

Pharmacokinetics

Absorption: Poorly absorbed (bioavailability 2.5%).
Distribution: Unknown.
Metabolism and Excretion: 2% excreted unchanged in urine, remainder is probably metabolized (CYP3A4 enzyme system).
Half-life: 24 hr.

TIME/ACTION PROFILE (antihypertensive effect)

ROUTE	ONSET	PEAK	DURATION
PO	unknown	2 wk	24 hr

Contraindications/Precautions

Contraindicated in: Hypersensitivity; OB: May cause fetal injury or death; Concurrent use with cyclosporine.
Use Cautiously in: Salt or volume depletion (correct before use); Severe renal impairment; Pedi: Safety not established.

Interactions

Drug-Drug: Blood levels are ↓ by **irbesartan**. Blood levels are ↑ by **atorvastatin**, **ketoconazole**, and **cyclosporine** (concurrent use with cyclosporine not recommended). ↓ blood levels and may ↓ effects of **furosemide**. Antihypertensive effects may be ↑ by other **antihypertensives**, **diuretics**, and **nitrates**. ↑ risk of hyperkalemia with concurrent use of ACE **inhibitors, angiotensin II receptor antagonists, potassium supplements, potassium-sparing diuretics,** or **potassium-containing salt substitutes.**
Drug-Food: High-fat meals significantly ↓ absorption.

Route/Dosage

PO (Adults): 150 mg/day initially; may be increased to 300 mg/day.

Availability

Tablets: 150 mg, 300 mg. ***In combination with:*** hydrochlorothiazide (Tekturna HCT) (See Appendix B).

alitretinoin (a-li-tret-i-noyn)

Panretin

Classification

Therapeutic: antineoplastics
Pharmacologic: retinoids

Indications

Topical treatment of cutaneous lesions from AIDS-related Kaposi's sarcoma (KS).

Action

Binds to and activates retinoid receptors, resulting in inhibition of KS cells. **Therapeutic Effects:** Decreased cutaneous lesions of KS.

Adverse Reactions/Side Effects **Local:** <u>pain</u>, <u>pruritus</u>, <u>rash</u>, edema, exfoliative, dermatitis, paresthesia.

PHYSICAL THERAPY IMPLICATIONS

Examination and Evaluation

- Assess the area being treated to help document whether drug therapy is successful in reducing skin lesions.
- Monitor any new or increased reactions at the site of application, including inflammation, irritation, burning, swelling, numbness, tingling, exfoliation, and rash. Report severe or prolonged skin reactions to the physician.

Interventions

- Protect skin from breakdown, especially over bony prominences.

Patient/client-Related Instruction

- Check that the patient and family or caregivers understand topical application procedures, and adhere to the recommended dosing schedule.

Pharmacokinetics

Absorption: Small amounts are absorbed.
Distribution: Unknown.
Metabolism and Excretion: Some metabolism occurs.
Half-life: Unknown.

TIME/ACTION PROFILE (response of KS lesions)

ROUTE	ONSET	PEAK	DURATION
topical	2 wk	4–14 wk	unknown

Contraindications/Precautions

Contraindicated in: Hypersensitivity to retinoids; OB: Potential for birth defects; Lactation: Use breast milk alternative.
Use Cautiously in: Patients with childbearing potential; Pedi: Safety not established.

Interactions

Drug-Drug: Do not use concurrently with insect-repellent products containing **N,N-diethyl-m-toluamide (DEET)**. Alitretinoin increases **DEET** absorption.

Route/Dosage

Topical (Adults): Apply generous coating twice daily to KS lesions initially; application may be increased to 3–4 times daily.

Availability

Topical gel: 0.1% in 60-g tubes.

allopurinol (al-oh-pure-i-nole)

Aloprim, Apo-Allopurinol, Lopurin, Purinol, Zyloprim

Classification

Therapeutic: antigout agents, antihyperuricemics

Pharmacologic: xanthine oxidase inhibitors

Indications

PO: Prevention of attack of gouty arthritis and nephropathy. **PO, IV:** Treatment of secondary hyperuricemia, which may occur during treatment of tumors or leukemias.

Action

Inhibits the production of uric acid by inhibiting the action of xanthine oxidase. **Therapeutic Effects:** Lowering of serum uric acid levels.

Adverse Reactions/Side Effects

CV: hypotension, flushing, hypertension, bradycardia, and heart failure (reported with IV administration). **CNS:** drowsiness. **GI:** diarrhea, hepatitis, nausea, vomiting. **GU:** renal failure, hematuria. **Derm:** rash (discontinue drug at first sign of rash), urticaria. **Hemat:** bone marrow depression. **Misc:** hypersensitivity reactions.

PHYSICAL THERAPY IMPLICATIONS

Examination and Evaluation

- Monitor signs of hypersensitivity reactions, including pulmonary symptoms (tightness in the throat and chest, wheezing, cough, dyspnea) or skin reactions (rash, pruritus, urticaria). Be especially alert for skin rash, and notify physician or nursing staff immediately of any signs of hypersensitivity.
- Monitor signs of renal failure, including decreased urine output, bloody urine, increased blood pressure (BP), muscle cramps/twitching, edema/weight gain from fluid retention, yellowish brown skin, and confusion that progresses to seizures and coma. Report these signs to the physician immediately.
- Assess BP and compare to normal values (See Appendix F). Report changes in BP, either a problematic decrease in BP (hypotension) or a sustained increase in BP (hypertension).
- Assess signs of congestive heart failure (dyspnea, rales/crackles, peripheral edema, jugular venous distention, exercise intolerance). Report these signs to the physician immediately.
- Assess heart rate, ECG, and heart sounds, especially during exercise (See Appendices G, H). Report an abnormally slow heart rate (bradycardia) or symptoms of other arrhythmias such as including palpitations, chest discomfort, shortness of breath, fainting, and fatigue/weakness.
- Monitor signs of bone marrow depression including fatigue, dizziness, fever, chills, sore throat, shortness of breath, chest pain, pallor, and unusual bruising or bleeding. Report these signs to the physician.
- If treating gouty arthritis, periodically assess impairments (pain, range of motion), functional ability, and disability to help document whether drug therapy is successful.

Interventions

- If treating arthritic conditions, implement appropriate manual therapy techniques, physical agents, therapeutic exercises, and orthotic/assistive devices to reduce pain, improve function, and augment the effects of drug therapy.
- Because of the risk of arrhythmias, heart failure, and abnormal BP responses, use caution during aerobic exercise and other forms of therapeutic exercise. Assess exercise tolerance frequently (BP, heart rate, fatigue levels), and terminate exercise immediately if any untoward responses occur (See Appendix L).

Patient/Client-Related Instruction

- Advise patient to guard against infection (frequent hand washing, etc.), and to avoid crowds and contact with persons with contagious diseases.
- Advise patient about the likelihood of GI reactions such as nausea, vomiting, and diarrhea. Instruct patient to report severe or prolonged GI problems, or signs of hepatitis such as yellow skin or eyes, abdominal pain, severe nausea and vomiting, fever, sore throat, malaise, weakness, and facial edema.
- Instruct patient and family/caregivers to report other troublesome side effects such as severe or prolonged drowsiness or skin reactions (flushing, itching).

Pharmacokinetics

Absorption: Well absorbed (80%) following oral administration.
Distribution: Widely distributed in tissue and breast milk.
Protein Binding: <1%.
Metabolism and Excretion: Metabolized to oxypurinol, an active compound with a long half-life. 12% excreted unchanged, 76% excreted as oxypurinol.
Half-life: 1–3 hr (oxypurinol 18–30 hr).

TIME/ACTION PROFILE (hypouricemic effect)

ROUTE	ONSET	PEAK	DURATION
PO, IV	1–2 days	1–2 wk	1–3 wk*

*Duration after discontinuation of allopurinol.

Contraindications/Precautions

Contraindicated in: Hypersensitivity.
Use Cautiously in: Acute attacks of gout; Renal insufficiency (dose reduction required if CCr <20 mL/min); Dehydration (adequate hydration necessary); OB/Lactation: Rarely used; Geri: Begin at lower end of dosage range.

Interactions

Drug-Drug: Use with **mercaptopurine** and **azathioprine** ↑ bone marrow depressant properties—doses of these drugs should be ↓. Use with **ampicillin** or **amoxicillin** ↑ risk of rash. Use with **oral hypoglycemic agents** and **warfarin** ↑ effects of these drugs. Use with **thiazide diuretics** or **ACE inhibitors** ↑ risk of hypersensitivity reactions. Large doses of allopurinol may ↑ risk of **theophylline** toxicity. May ↑ **cyclosporine** levels.

Route/Dosage

Management of Gout

PO (Adults and Children >10 yr): *Initially*—100 mg/day; increase at weekly intervals based on serum uric acid (not to exceed 800 mg/day). Doses >300 mg/day should be given in divided doses; *Maintenance dose*—100–200 mg 2–3 times daily. Doses of ≤300 mg may be given as a single daily dose.

Management of Secondary Hyperuricemia

PO (Adults and Children >10 yr): 600–800 mg/day in 2–3 divided doses starting 1–2 days before chemotherapy or radiation.
PO (Children 6–10 yr): 10 mg/kg/day in 2–3 divided doses (maximum 800 mg/day) or 300 mg daily in 2–3 divided doses.
PO (Children <6 yr): 10 mg/kg/day in 2–3 divided doses (maximum 800 mg/day) or 150 mg daily in 3 divided doses.
IV (Adults and Children >10 yr): 200–400 mg/m^2/day (up to 600 mg/day) as a single daily dose or in divided doses q 8–24 hr.
IV (Children <10 yr): 200 mg/m^2/day initially as a single daily dose or in divided doses q 8–24 hr (maximum dose 600 mg/day).

Renal Impairment

(Adults and Children): *CCr >50 mL/min*—No dosage change; *CCr 10–50 mL/min*—Reduce dosage to 50% of recommended; *CCr <10 mL/min*—Reduce dosage to 30% of recommended.

Availability (generic available)

Tablets: 100 mg, 300 mg. **Injection:** 500 mg/vial.

almotriptan (al-moe-trip-tan)

Axert

Classification
Therapeutic: vascular headache suppressants
Pharmacologic: 5-HT_1 agonists

Indications

Acute treatment of migraine headache.

Action

Acts as an agonist at specific 5-HT_1 receptor sites in intracranial blood vessels and sensory trigeminal nerves.
Therapeutic Effects: Cranial vessel vasoconstriction with associated decrease in release of neuropeptides and resultant decrease in migraine headache.

Adverse Reactions/Side Effects

CNS: drowsiness, headache. **CV:** CORONARY ARTERY VASOSPASM, MI, myocardial ischemia, VENTRICULAR FIBRILLATION, VENTRICULAR TACHYCARDIA. **GI:** dry mouth, nausea. **Neuro:** paresthesia.

PHYSICAL THERAPY IMPLICATIONS

Examination and Evaluation

- Continually monitor for signs of coronary artery vasospasm and MI, including sudden chest pain, pain radiating into the arm or jaw, shortness of breath, dizziness, sweating, anxiety, and nausea. Seek immediate medical assistance if patient develops these signs.
- Assess heart rate, ECG, and heart sounds, especially during exercise (See Appendices G, H). Report any rhythm disturbances or symptoms of increased arrhythmias, including palpitations, chest discomfort, shortness of breath, dizziness, and fatigue/weakness. Seek immediate medical assistance if patient exhibits signs associated with ventricular fibrillation such as fainting and loss of consciousness.
- Assess the frequency and severity of headaches, and document whether drug therapy is successful in decreasing migraine attacks.
- Assess signs of paresthesia such as numbness and tingling. Perform objective tests, including electroneuromyography and sensory testing to document any drug-related neuropathic changes.

Interventions

- Because of the risk of MI and serious arrhythmias, use extreme caution during aerobic exercise and other forms of therapeutic exercise. Assess exercise tolerance frequently (blood pressure, heart rate, fatigue levels), and terminate exercise immediately if any untoward responses occur (See Appendix L).

♣ = Canadian drug name; *CAPITALS indicate life-threatening; underlines indicate most frequent.

Patient/Client-Related Instruction

- Advise patient and family or caregiver about the signs of MI and arrhythmias (see above under Examination and Evaluation), and to seek immediate medical assistance if these signs develop.
- Advise the patient to bring this drug to each therapy session; almotriptan drug is most effective when taken at the first signs of a migraine attack. Patients should also adhere to the correct dosing procedures; that is, a second dose can be taken 2 hr after the first dose, but patients should not exceed 2 doses in each 24-hr period.
- Instruct patient to report other troublesome side effects such as severe or prolonged headache, drowsiness, or GI problems (nausea, dry mouth).

Pharmacokinetics

Absorption: Well absorbed following oral administration (70%).
Distribution: Unknown.
Metabolism and Excretion: 40% excreted unchanged in urine; 27% metabolized by monoamine oxidase-A (MAO-A); 12% metabolized by cytochrome P450 hepatic enzymes (3A4 and 2D6); 13% excreted in feces as unchanged and metabolized drug.
Half-life: 3–4 hr.

TIME/ACTION PROFILE (blood levels)

ROUTE	ONSET	PEAK	DURATION
PO	unknown	1–3 hr	unknown

Contraindications/Precautions

Contraindicated in: Hypersensitivity; Ischemic cardiovascular, cerebrovascular, or peripheral vascular syndromes; History of significant cardiovascular disease; Uncontrolled hypertension; Should not be used within 24 hr of other 5-HT$_1$ agonists or ergot-type compounds (dihydroergotamine); Basilar or hemiplegic migraine; Concurrent MAO-A inhibitor therapy or within 2 wk of discontinuing MAO-A inhibitor therapy.
Use Cautiously in: Cardiovascular risk factors (hypertension, hypercholesterolemia, cigarette smoking, obesity, diabetes, strong family history, menopausal women or men >40 yr); use only if cardiovascular status has been evaluated and determined to be safe and first dose is administered under supervision; Impaired hepatic or renal function; OB/Lactation/Pedi: Safety not established.

Interactions

Drug-Drug: Concurrent use with **MAO-A inhibitors** increases blood levels and the risk of adverse reactions (concurrent use or use within 2 wk or MAO inhibitor is contraindicated). Concurrent use with other **5-HT$_1$ agonists or ergot-type compounds (dihydroergotamine)** may result in additive vasoactive properties (avoid use within 24 hr of each other). Concurrent use with **SSRI antidepressants** may result in weakness, hyperreflexia, and incoordination. Blood levels and effects may be increased by **ketoconazole, itraconazole, ritonavir,** and **erythromycin** (inhibitors of CYP3A4 enzymes).

Route/Dosage

PO (Adults): 6.25–12.5 mg initially, may repeat in 2 hr; not to exceed 2 doses per 24-hr period.

Hepatic/Renal Impairment

PO (Adults): 6.25 mg initially, may repeat in 2 hr; not to exceed 2 doses per 24-hr period.

Availability

Tablets: 6.25 mg, 12.5 mg.

alosetron (a-low-se-tron)

Lotronex

Classification
Therapeutic: anti-irritable bowel syndrome agents
Pharmacologic: 5-HT$_3$ antagonists

Indications

Treatment of severe diarrhea-predominant irritable bowel syndrome (IBS) in women who have chronic symptoms (≥6 mo), no other GI pathology, and have had no response to conventional therapy.

Action

5-HT$_3$ receptors are nonselective cation channels responsible for regulation of visceral pain, colonic transit, and GI secretions. Alosetron inhibits the activation of these channels. **Therapeutic Effects:** Increased colonic transit time without affecting orocecal transit time resulting in decreased pain/discomfort and diarrhea associated with IBS.

Adverse Reactions/Side Effects

GI: ACUTE ISCHEMIC COLITIS, TOXIC MEGACOLON, constipation, abdominal discomfort, abdominal distention, flatulence, nausea, GI viral infections, hemorrhoids, regurgitation or reflux.

PHYSICAL THERAPY IMPLICATIONS

Examination and Evaluation

- Be alert for signs of severe GI reactions such as acute ischemic colitis or toxic megacolon. Signs include sudden abdominal pain, abdominal distention, bloody diarrhea, fever, vomiting, tachycardia, and shock. See immediate medical assistance if these signs occur.
- Monitor GI symptoms (diarrhea, abdominal pain, cramps) to help document whether drug therapy is successful in reducing these symptoms.

Patient/Client-Related Instruction

- Advise patient to avoid alcohol and foods that may increase GI irritation and diarrhea.
- Instruct patient to report other bothersome GI side effects such as constipation, nausea, flatulence,

hemorrhoids, heartburn, indigestion, and abdominal pain and distension.

Pharmacokinetics

Absorption: 50–60% absorbed following oral administration.
Distribution: 65–95 L.
Protein Binding: 82% bound to plasma proteins.
Metabolism and Excretion: Extensively metabolized by the liver; 13% excreted unchanged in urine.
Half-life: 1.5 hr.

TIME/ACTION PROFILE (pain/discomfort, diarrhea)

ROUTE	ONSET	PEAK	DURATION
PO	within 1–2 wks	up to 6 wk	1 wk*

*Following discontinuation.

Contraindications/Precautions

Contraindicated in: Hypersensitivity; Constipation; History of chronic/severe constipation or complications due to constipation; History of GI obstruction, stricture, toxic megacolon, perforation, and/or adhesions; History of ischemic colitis, decreased intestinal circulation, thrombophlebitis, or coagulation defects; History of Crohn's disease/ulcerative colitis/diverticulitis; Severe hepatic impairment; Patients taking fluvoxamine.
Use Cautiously in: Men—safety not established; Mild-to-moderate hepatic impairment; Patients who are elderly, debilitated, or taking medications that decrease GI motility; OB/Lactation/Pedi: Safety not established.

Interactions

Drug-Drug: Blood levels of alosetron can be increased by **fluvoxamine** (concomitant use is contraindicated). Blood levels of alosetron can be increased by **amiodarone**, **cimetidine**, **ciprofloxacin**, **clarithromycin**, **itraconazole**, **ketoconazole**, **ofloxacin**, **protease inhibitors**, **telithromycin**, and **voriconazole** (use concomitantly with caution).

Route/Dosage

PO (Adults): *Women*—0.5 mg twice daily.

Availability

Tablets: 0.5 mg, 1 mg.

alprazolam (al-pray-zoe-lam)

Apo-Alpraz, Novo-Alprazol, Niravam, Nu-Alpraz, Xanax, Xanax XR

Classification
Therapeutic: antianxiety agents
Pharmacologic: benzodiazepines

Schedule IV

Indications

Treatment of Generalized anxiety disorder (GAD); Panic disorder; Management of anxiety associated with depression. **Unlabeled Use:** Management of symptoms of premenstrual syndrome (PMS). Insomnia, irritable bowel syndrome (IBS), and other somatic symptoms associated with anxiety. Used as an adjunct with acute mania, acute psychosis.

Action

Acts at many levels in the CNS to produce anxiolytic effect. May produce CNS depression. Effects may be mediated by GABA, an inhibitory neurotransmitter.
Therapeutic Effects: Relief of anxiety.

Adverse Reactions/Side Effects

CNS: dizziness, drowsiness, lethargy, confusion, hangover, headache, mental depression, paradoxical excitation. **EENT:** blurred vision. **GI:** constipation, diarrhea, nausea, vomiting, weight gain. **Derm:** rashes. **Misc:** physical dependence, psychologic dependence, tolerance.

PHYSICAL THERAPY IMPLICATIONS

Examination and Evaluation

- Monitor daytime drowsiness and "hangover" symptoms (headache, nausea, irritability, lethargy, dysphoria). Repeated or excessive symptoms may require change in dose or medication.
- Assess dizziness that might affect gait, balance, and other functional activities (See Appendix C). Report balance problems and functional limitations to the physician, and caution the patient and family/caregivers to guard against falls and trauma.
- Report any behavioral or personality changes such as confusion, decreased mental acuity, or excessive excitation.

Interventions

- Guard against falls and trauma (hip fractures, head injury, and so forth). Implement fall-prevention strategies, especially in older adults or if drowsiness and dizziness carry over into the daytime (See Appendix E).
- Help patient explore nonpharmacologic methods to reduce anxiety and depression, such as relaxation techniques, exercise, counseling, support groups, and so forth.

Patient/Client-Related Instruction

- Instruct patients on prolonged treatment to not discontinue medication without consulting their physician. Abrupt withdrawal can cause insomnia, unusual irritability or nervousness, and seizures.

- Advise patient or family/caregivers about the potential risk of tolerance and physical/psychologic dependence. Emphasize that addiction is more likely during prolonged, excessive, or inappropriate use of this drug.
- Advise patient to avoid alcohol and other CNS depressants because of the increased risk of sedation and adverse effects.
- Instruct patient to report other bothersome side effects such as severe or prolonged headache, blurred vision, rash, weight gain, or GI problems (nausea, vomiting, diarrhea, constipation).

Pharmacokinetics

Absorption: Well absorbed (90%) from the GI tract; absorption is slower with extended-release tablets.
Distribution: Widely distributed, crosses blood-brain barrier. Probably crosses the placenta and enters breast milk. Accumulation is minimal.
Metabolism and Excretion: Metabolized by the liver (CYP3A4 enzyme system) to an active compound that is subsequently rapidly metabolized.
Half-life: 12–15 hr.

TIME/ACTION PROFILE (sedation)

ROUTE	ONSET	PEAK	DURATION
PO	1–2 hr	1–2 hr	up to 24 hr

Contraindications/Precautions

Contraindicated in: Hypersensitivity; Cross-sensitivity with other benzodiazepines may exist; Preexisting CNS depression; Severe uncontrolled pain; Angle-closure glaucoma, obstructive sleep apnea, pulmonary disease; Pregnancy and lactation; Concurrent itraconazole or ketoconazole; OB/Lactation: Use in pregnancy or lactation may cause CNS depression, flaccidity, feeding difficulties, and seizures in infant.
Use Cautiously in: Renal Impairment, Hepatic dysfunction (↓ dose required); Concurrent use with nefazodone, fluvoxamine, cimetidine, fluoxetine, hormonal contraceptives, propoxyphene, diltiazem, isoniazid, erythromycin, clarithromycin, grapefruit juice (↓ dose may be necessary); History of suicide attempt or alcohol/drug dependence, debilitated patients (↓ dose required); Pedi: Safety and efficacy not established. Decreased dosage and frequent monitoring required; Geri: Elderly patients have increased sensitivity to benzodiazepines. Appears on Beers" list and is associated with increased risk of falls (↓ dose required) and excessive CNS effects.

Interactions

Drug-Drug: Alcohol, **antidepressants**, other **benzodiazepines**, **antihistamines**, and **opioid analgesics**—concurrent use results in ↑ CNS depression. **Hormonal contraceptives**, **disulfiram**, **fluoxetine**, **isoniazid**, **metoprolol**, **propoxyphene**, **propranolol**, **valproic acid**, **CYP3A4 inhibitors (erythromycin**, **ketoconazole**, **itraconazole**, **fluvoxamine**, **cimetidine**, **nefazodone)** ↓ metabolism of alprazolam, ↑ blood levels and ↑ its actions (dose adjustments may be necessary). May ↓ efficacy of **levodopa**. **CYP3A4 inducers (rifampin**, **carbamazepine**, or **barbiturates)** ↑ metabolism and ↓ effects of alprazolam. Sedative effects may be ↓ by **theophylline**. **Cigarette smoking** ↓ blood levels and effects.
Drug-Natural: Kava-kava, **valerian**, or **chamomile** can ↑ CNS depression.
Drug-Food: Concurrent ingestion of **grapefruit juice** ↑ blood levels.

Route/Dosage

Anxiety

PO (Adults): 0.25–0.5 mg 2–3 times daily (not >4 mg/day; begin with 0.25 mg 2–3 times daily in geriatric/debilitated patients).

Panic Attacks

PO (Adults): 0.5 mg 3 times daily; may be increased by 1 mg or less every 3–4 days as needed (not >10 mg/day). *Extended-release tablets (Xanax XR)*—0.5–1 mg once daily in the morning, may be increased every 3–4 days by not more than 1 mg/day; up to 10 mg/day (usual range 3–6 mg/day).

Availability (generic available)

Tablets: 0.25 mg, 0.5 mg, 1 mg, 2 mg. **Extended-release tablets:** 0.5 mg, 1 mg, 2 mg, 3 mg. **Orally disintegrating tablets (orange):** 0.25 mg, 0.5 mg, 1 mg, 2 mg.

HIGH ALERT

alteplase (al-te-place)

Activase, Activase rt-PA, Lysatec rt-PA, Cathflo Activase

Other Names:
Tissue plasminogen activator (T-PA)

Classification
Therapeutic: thrombolytics
Pharmacologic: plasminogen activators

Indications

Acute myocardial infarction (MI). Acute ischemic stroke. Pulmonary embolism (PE). Occluded central venous access devices. **Unlabeled Use:** Deep venous thrombosis (DVT). Acute peripheral arterial thrombosis.

Action

Directly converts plasminogen to plasmin, which then degrades clot-bound fibrin. **Therapeutic Effects:** Lysis of thrombi in coronary arteries, with improvement of ventricular function, and reduced risk of heart failure or death. Lysis of pulmonary emboli. Lysis of thrombi causing ischemic stroke, reducing risk of neurologic sequelae. Restoration of cannula or catheter function.

Adverse Reactions/Side Effects

CNS: INTRACRANIAL HEMORRHAGE. **EENT:** epistaxis, gingival bleeding. **Resp:** bronchospasm, hemoptysis. **CV:** reperfusion arrhythmias, hypotension, RECURRENT ISCHEMIA/THROMBOEMBOLISM. **GI:** GI BLEEDING, nausea, RETROPERITONEAL BLEEDING, vomiting. **GU:** GU TRACT BLEEDING. **Derm:** ecchymoses, flushing, urticaria. **Hemat:** BLEEDING. **Local:** hemorrhage at injection site, phlebitis at injection site. **MS:** musculoskeletal pain. **Misc:** ALLERGIC REACTIONS, INCLUDING ANAPHYLAXIS, fever.

PHYSICAL THERAPY IMPLICATIONS

Examination and Evaluation

- Assess for signs of bleeding and hemorrhage (bleeding gums; nosebleed; unusual bruising; coughing up blood; black, tarry stools; hematuria; fall in hematocrit or blood pressure). Be especially alert for signs of intracranial bleeds, including sudden severe headache, confusion, nausea, vomiting, paralysis, numbness, speech problems, visual disturbances. Notify physician or nursing staff immediately if these signs occur.
- Be alert for signs of recurrent cardiac ischemia (chest pain, pain radiating into the arm or jaw, shortness of breath, dizziness, sweating, anxiety) or recurrent cerebral ischemia (sudden dizziness, vertigo, slurred speech, incoordination, numbness). Notify physician or nursing staff immediately if these signs occur.
- Monitor signs of recurrent thromboembolism and PE (shortness of breath, chest pain, cough, bloody sputum). Notify physician immediately, and request objective tests (Doppler ultrasound, lung scan, others) if PE is suspected.
- Monitor signs of allergic reactions or anaphylaxis, including pulmonary symptoms (tightness in the throat and chest, wheezing, cough, dyspnea) or skin reactions (rash, pruritus, urticaria). Notify physician or nursing staff immediately if these reactions occur.
- Assess heart rate, ECG, and heart sounds when cardiac perfusion is restored (see Appendices G, H). Report any rhythm disturbances or symptoms of increased arrhythmias, including palpitations, chest discomfort, shortness of breath, fainting, and fatigue/weakness.
- Assess blood pressure, especially for the first few days after infusion. Report low blood pressure (hypotension), especially if patient experiences dizziness or syncope.
- Assess any muscle of joint pain to rule out musculoskeletal pathology or hemorrhage; that is, try to determine if pain is drug induced rather than caused by anatomic or biomechanical problems. Be especially concerned about back pain that could indicate retroperitoneal bleeding.
- Assess injection site during and after IV administration, and report signs of bleeding or phlebitis (local pain, swelling, inflammation).

Interventions

- Use caution with any physical interventions that could increase bleeding, including wound débridement, chest percussion, joint mobilization, and application of local heat.
- Use extreme caution during aerobic exercise in patients with recent MI or ischemic stroke. Assess exercise tolerance frequently (blood pressure, heart rate, fatigue levels, neurologic signs), and terminate exercise immediately if any untoward responses occur (see Appendix L).
- For patients with DVT, recommend or implement other physical methods to decrease DVT and prevent recurrent thromboembolism, including graduated compression stockings and intermittent pneumatic compression pumps.

Patient/Client-Related Instruction

- Advise patient and family or caregiver about the signs of intracranial hemorrhage and other bleeds (see above under Examination and Evaluation), and to seek immediate medical assistance if these signs develop.
- Instruct patient or family/caregivers to report other side effects such as severe or prolonged fever, rashes, itching, or GI problems (nausea, vomiting).

Pharmacokinetics

Absorption: Complete after IV administration. Intracoronary administration or administration into occluded catheters or cannulae has a more localized effect.
Distribution: Unknown.
Metabolism and Excretion: Rapidly metabolized by the liver.
Half-life: 35 min

TIME/ACTION PROFILE (fibrinolysis)

ROUTE	ONSET	PEAK	DURATION
IV	30 min	60 min	unknown

Contraindications/Precautions

Contraindicated in: Active internal bleeding; History of cerebrovascular accident; Recent (within 2 mo)

intracranial or intraspinal injury or trauma; Intracranial neoplasm, arteriovenous malformation, or aneurysm; Severe uncontrolled hypertension; Known bleeding tendencies; Hypersensitivity.
Use Cautiously in: Recent (within 10 days) major surgery, trauma, GI or GU bleeding; Left heart thrombus; Severe hepatic or renal disease; Hemorrhagic ophthalmic conditions; Septic phlebitis; Previous puncture of a noncompressible vessel; Subacute bacterial endocarditis or acute pericarditis; Geriatric patients (>75 yr; increased risk of intracranial bleeding); OB/Lactation/Pedi: Safety not established.
Exercise Extreme Caution in: Patients receiving concurrent anticoagulant therapy (increased risk of intracranial bleeding).

Interactions

Drug-Drug: Aspirin, other **NSAIDs**, **warfarin**, **heparin** and **heparin-like agents**, **abciximab**, **eptifibatide**, **tirofiban**, **clopidogrel**, **ticlopidine**, or **dipyridamole**—concurrent use ↑ risk of bleeding, although these agents are frequently used together or in sequence. Effects may be ↓ by **antifibrinolytic agents**, including **aminocaproic acid** or **tranexamic acid**.
Drug-Natural: ↑ anticoagulant effect and bleeding risk with **anise**, **arnica**, **chamomile**, **clove**, **dong quai**, **fenugreek**, **feverfew**, **garlic**, **ginger**, **ginkgo**, ***Panax ginseng***, **licorice**, and others.

Route/Dosage

Myocardial Infarction (Accelerated or Front-Loaded Regimen)

IV (Adults): 15-mg bolus, then 0.75 mg/kg (up to 50 mg) over 30 min, then 0.5 mg/kg (up to 35 mg) over next 60 min; usually accompanied by heparin therapy.

Myocardial Infarction (Standard Regimen)

IV (Adults >65 kg): 60 mg over 1st hr (6–10 mg given as a bolus over first 1–2 min), 20 mg over the 2nd hr, and 20 mg over the 3rd hr for a total dose of 100 mg.
IV (Adults <65 kg): 0.75 mg/kg over 1st hr (0.075–0.125 mg/kg given as a bolus over first 1–2 min), 0.25 mg/kg over the 2nd hr, and 0.25 mg/kg over the 3rd hr for a total dose of 1.25 mg/kg (not to exceed 100 mg total).

Acute Ischemic Stroke

IV (Adults): 0.9 mg/kg (not to exceed 90 mg), given as an infusion over 1 hr, with 10% of the dose given as a bolus over the 1st min.

Pulmonary Embolism

IV (Adults): 100 mg over 2 hr; follow with heparin.

Occluded Venous Access Devices

IV (Adults and Children >30 kg): 2 mg/2 mL instilled into occluded catheter; if unsuccessful, may repeat once after 2 hr.
IV (Adults and Children <30 kg): 110% of the lumen volume (not to exceed 2 mg in 2 mL) instilled into occluded catheter; if unsuccessful, may repeat once after 2 hr.

Availability

Powder for injection: 2-mg vial, 20 mg/vial, 50 mg/vial.

HIGH ALERT

altretamine (al-tret-a-meen)

Hexalen, Hexastat

Other Names:
hexamethylmelamine

Classification
Therapeutic: antineoplastics

Indications

Management of ovarian cancer unresponsive to treatment with other agents.

Action

Mechanism unknown, but may disrupt DNA and RNA synthesis. **Therapeutic Effects:** Death of rapidly replicating cells, particularly malignant ones.

Adverse Reactions/Side Effects

CNS: SEIZURES, fatigue. **GI:** nausea, vomiting, anorexia, hepatic toxicity. **GU:** renal toxicity. **Derm:** alopecia, pruritus, skin rash. **Endo:** gonadal suppression. **Hemat:** anemia, leukopenia, thrombocytopenia. **Neuro:** peripheral neuropathy.

PHYSICAL THERAPY IMPLICATIONS

Examination and Evaluation

- Be alert for new seizures or increased seizure activity. Document the number, duration, and severity of seizures, and report these findings to the physician immediately.
- Assess signs of peripheral neuropathy such as numbness, tingling, and decreased muscle strength. Establish baseline electroneuromyographic values using EMG and nerve conduction at the beginning of drug treatment whenever possible, and reexamine these values periodically to document drug-induced changes in peripheral nerve function.
- Watch for signs of leukopenia (fever, sore throat, signs of infection), thrombocytopenia (bruising, nose bleeds, bleeding gums), or unusual weakness and fatigue that might be due to anemia. Report these signs to the physician or nursing staff.
- Monitor signs of renal toxicity, including blood or pus in urine, decreased urine output, weight gain from fluid retention, and fatigue. Report these signs to the physician or nursing staff.

Interventions

- For patients who are medically able to begin exercise, implement appropriate resistive exercises, and aerobic training to maintain muscle strength and aerobic capacity during cancer chemotherapy, or to help restore function after chemotherapy.

Patient/Client-Related Instruction

- Advise patient to guard against infection (frequent hand washing, etc.), and avoid crowds and contact with persons with contagious diseases.
- Advise patient about the likelihood of GI reactions (nausea, vomiting, loss of appetite). Instruct patient or family and caregivers to report severe or unexpected GI reactions, and also to report signs of hepatotoxicity, including abdominal pain, severe nausea and vomiting, yellow skin or eyes, fever, sore throat, malaise, weakness, facial edema, lethargy, and unusual bleeding or bruising.
- Advise patient that rash and other skin reactions (itching, hair loss) are likely. Report severe or unexpected skin reactions to the physician.

Pharmacokinetics

Absorption: Well absorbed following oral administration. Requires metabolism for conversion to antineoplastic compounds.
Distribution: Reaches high concentrations in liver, kidney, and small intestine. Poor penetration into brain.
Metabolism and Excretion: Mostly metabolized by the liver to compounds with antineoplastic activity.
Half-life: 4.7–10.2 hr.

TIME/ACTION PROFILE (effects on blood counts)

ROUTE	ONSET	PEAK	DURATION
PO	unknown	3–4 wk	6 wk

Contraindications/Precautions

Contraindicated in: Hypersensitivity; OB/Lactation: Contraindicated due to risk to fetus/infant.
Use Cautiously in: Preexisting neurologic diseases; Patients with childbearing potential; Infections; Decreased bone marrow reserve; Other chronic debilitating illnesses; Pedi: Safety not established.

Interactions

Drug-Drug: Concurrent use with **MAO inhibitors** may produce orthostatic hypotension. May decrease antibody response and increase risk of adverse reactions from **live-virus vaccines**. Additive bone marrow depression may occur with other **antineoplastics** or **radiation therapy. Cimetidine** increases blood levels and risk of toxicity.

Route/Dosage

PO (Adults): 65 mg/m² 4 times daily (after meals and at bedtime) for 14 or 21 days of each 28-day cycle. Dosage reduction to 50 mg/m² 4 times daily (after meals and at bedtime) recommended after 14 or more days' rest for any of the following: GI intolerance, severe bone marrow depression, or progressive neurologic toxicity.

Availability

Capsules: 50 mg, 100 mg.

amantadine (a-man-ta-deen)

Symmetrel

Classification

Therapeutic: antiparkinson agents, antivirals

Indications

Symptomatic initial and adjunct treatment of Parkinson's disease. Prophylaxis and treatment of influenza A viral infections.

Action

Potentiates the action of dopamine in the CNS. Prevents penetration of influenza A virus into host cell.
Therapeutic Effects: Relief of Parkinson's symptoms. Prevention and decreased symptoms of influenza A viral infection.

Adverse Reactions/Side Effects

CNS: ataxia, dizziness, insomnia, anxiety, confusion, depression, drowsiness, psychosis, seizures. **GI:** nausea, vomiting, anorexia, constipation. **EENT:** blurred vision, dry mouth. **Resp:** dyspnea. **CV:** hypotension, CHF, edema. **GU:** urinary retention. **Derm:** mottling, livedo reticularis, rashes. **Hemat:** leukopenia, neutropenia.

PHYSICAL THERAPY IMPLICATIONS

Examination and Evaluation

- Be alert for new seizures or increased seizure activity, especially at the onset of drug treatment. Document the number, duration, and severity of seizures, and report these findings to the physician immediately.
- If treating Parkinson's disease, assess patient's motor function to help document anti-Parkinson effects, especially when starting drug therapy, or during dosing changes or addition of other anti-Parkinson drugs. Motor function should be assessed at different times of the day, such as when drugs are reaching peak therapeutic levels (i.e., 30–60 min after oral dose), as well as when drug effects are minimal (just before the next dose).

- Assess blood pressure (BP) periodically and compare to normal values (See Appendix F). Report low blood pressure (hypotension), especially if patient experiences dizziness, fatigue, or other symptoms.
- Assess signs of congestive heart failure, including dyspnea, rales/crackles, peripheral edema, jugular venous distention, and exercise intolerance. Report these signs to the physician.
- Assess peripheral edema using girth measurements, volume displacement, and measurement of pitting edema (See Appendix N). Report increased swelling in feet and ankles or a sudden increase in body weight due to fluid retention.
- Monitor signs of leukopenia or neutropenia including fever, sore throat, and signs of infection. Report these signs to the physician.
- Be alert for anxiety, confusion, depression, psychosis, or other alterations in mental status. Notify physician promptly if these symptoms develop.
- Be alert for ataxia or dizziness that might affect gait, balance, or other functional activities. Report balance problems and functional limitations to the physician, and caution the patient and family/caregivers to guard against falls and trauma.

Interventions

- Because of the risk of CHF and abnormal BP responses, use caution during aerobic exercise and other forms of therapeutic exercise. Assess exercise tolerance frequently (BP, heart rate, fatigue levels), and terminate exercise immediately if any untoward responses occur (See Appendix L).
- For patients with Parkinson's disease:
  - Guard against an increased risk of falls and trauma (hip fractures, head injury, and so forth) due to a combination of Parkinson's symptoms (postural instability, rigidity) and drug side effects (dizziness, ataxia). Implement fall prevention strategies whenever possible (See Appendix E).
  - Implement therapeutic exercises (coordination exercises, gait training, cardiovascular conditioning) to compliment the effects of drug therapy and help achieve optimal function.
- If treating influenza, always wash hands thoroughly and disinfect equipment (whirlpools, electrotherapeutic devices, treatment tables, and so forth) to help prevent the spread of infection. Employ universal precautions as indicated for specific patients.

Patient/Client-Related Instruction

- Instruct patient and family/caregivers to report other troublesome side effects, including severe or prolonged sleep loss, urinary retention, blurred vision, skin problems (rash, discoloration), or GI problems (nausea, vomiting, constipation, dry mouth, loss of appetite).

Pharmacokinetics

Absorption: Well absorbed from the GI tract.
Distribution: Distributed to various body tissues and fluids. Crosses blood-brain barrier and enters breast milk.
Metabolism and Excretion: Excreted unchanged in the urine.
Half-life: 10–28 hr.

TIME/ACTION PROFILE (antiparkinson effect)

ROUTE	ONSET	PEAK	DURATION
PO	within 48 hr	up to 2 wk	unknown

Contraindications/Precautions

Contraindicated in: Hypersensitivity.
Use Cautiously in: Seizure disorders; Liver disease; Psychiatric problems; Congestive heart failure; Renal impairment (dosage reduction/increased dosing interval required if CCr ≤50 mL/min); May increase susceptibility to rubella infections; OB/Lactation: Safety not established; Geri: Increased sensitivity to adverse effects.

Interactions

Drug-Drug: Concurrent use of **antihistamines, phenothiazines, quinidine, disopyramide,** and **tricyclic antidepressants** may increase anticholinergic effects (dry mouth, blurred vision, constipation). Increased risk of adverse CNS reactions with **alcohol.** Increased risk of CNS stimulation with other **CNS stimulants.**

Route/Dosage

Parkinson's Disease

PO (Adults): 100 mg 1–2 times daily (up to 400 mg/day).

Influenza A Viral Infection

PO (Adults and Children >12 yr): *Treatment*—200 mg/day as a single dose or 100 mg bid (not >100 mg/day in geriatric patients); *Prophylaxis*—100 mg/day in 1–2 divided doses.
PO (Children 10–12 yr): 100 mg q 12 hr *or* 5 mg/kg/day in 1–2 divided doses; not to exceed 200 mg/day.
PO (Children 1–9 yr): 5 mg/kg/day in 1–2 divided doses; not to exceed 150 mg/day.

Renal Impairment

PO (Adults): *CCr 30–50 mL/min*—200 mg on the first day, then 100 mg once daily; *CCr 15–29 mL/min*—200 mg on the first day, then 100 mg every other day; *<15 mL/min or hemodialysis patients*—200 mg once every 7 days.

Availability (generic available)

Liquid-filled capsules: 100 mg. **Tablets:** 100 mg. **Syrup (raspberry flavor):** 50 mg/5 mL.

ambrisentan (am-bri-sen-tan)

Letairis

Classification

Therapeutic: antihypertensives

Pharmacologic: endothelin receptor antagonists

Indications

Pulmonary arterial hypertension.

Action

Antagonizes endogenous endothelin, resulting in vasodilation. **Therapeutic Effects:** Improved exercise capacity and delayed clinical worsening.

Adverse Reactions/Side Effects

CNS: headache. **GI:** HEPATOTOXICITY. **F and E:** fluid retention. **Hemat:** ↓ hemoglobin. **Misc:** ↓ sperm count.

PHYSICAL THERAPY IMPLICATIONS

Examination and Evaluation

- Be alert for signs of hepatotoxicity including anorexia, abdominal pain, severe nausea and vomiting, yellow skin or eyes, fever, sore throat, malaise, weakness, facial edema, lethargy, and unusual bleeding or bruising. Report these signs to the physician immediately.
- Assess exercise tolerance, and document possible benefits of drug therapy in reducing pulmonary hypertension and improving exercise capacity.

Interventions

- Design and implement aerobic exercise and endurance training programs as tolerated to improve exercise tolerance, reduce pulmonary impairments, and augment the effects of drug therapy.

Patient/Client-related Instruction

- Instruct patient or family/caregivers to report other troublesome side effects such as severe or prolonged headache or fluid retention.

Pharmacokinetics

Absorption: Absorbed following oral administration, Bioavailability unknown.
Distribution: Unknown.
Protein Binding: 99%.
Metabolism and Excretion: Highly metabolized.
Half-life: 15 hr (effective half-life 9 hr).

TIME/ACTION PROFILE (blood levels)

ROUTE	ONSET	PEAK	DURATION
PO	unknown	2 hr	24 hr

Contraindications/Precautions

Contraindicated in: OB: Pregnancy or lactation; Moderate/severe hepatic impairment.
Use Cautiously in: Mild hepatic impairment; Concurrent use of cyclosporine or strong inhibitors of CYP2C19 and CYP3A; Pedi: safety and efficacy in children has not been established.

Interactions

Drug-Drug: Blood levels may be ↑ by **cyclosporine**, strong **CYP3A inhibitors** including **ketoconazole** and strong **2C19 inhibitors** including **omeprazole**.

Route/Dosage

PO (Adults): 5 mg once daily, may be increased to 10 mg once daily.

Availability

Tablets: 5 mg, 10 mg.

amcinonide (am-sin-oh-nide)

Cyclocort

Classification

Therapeutic: anti-inflammatories (steroidal)

Pharmacologic: corticosteroids

Indications

Management of inflammation and pruritus associated with various allergic/immunologic skin problems.

Action

Suppresses normal immune response and inflammation. **Therapeutic Effects:** Suppression of dermatologic inflammation and immune processes.

Adverse Reactions/Side Effects

Derm: allergic contact dermatitis, atrophy, burning, dryness, edema, folliculitis, hypersensitivity reactions, hypertrichosis, hypopigmentation, irritation, maceration, miliaria, perioral dermatitis, secondary infection, striae. **Misc:** adrenal suppression (use of occlusive dressings, long-term therapy).

PHYSICAL THERAPY IMPLICATIONS

Examination and Evaluation

- Assess the area being treated to help document whether drug therapy is successful in resolving skin conditions.

- Monitor any new or increased reactions at the site of application, including inflammation, irritation, infection, burning, swelling, exfoliation, and rash. Report severe or prolonged skin reactions to the physician.
- Report signs of adrenal suppression, including hypotension, weight loss, weakness, nausea, vomiting, anorexia, lethargy, confusion, and restlessness.

Interventions

- Protect skin from breakdown, especially over bony prominences.

Patient/Client-Related Instruction

- Advise patients on long-term treatment to consult physician before stopping this medication. Stopping the medication suddenly may result in adrenocortical shock (severe hypotension, hypoglycemia, weakness, vomiting). If these signs appear, physician immediately; may be life threatening.
- Check that the patient and family or caregivers understand topical application procedures, and adhere to the recommended dosing schedule.

Pharmacokinetics

Absorption: Minimal. Prolonged use on large surface areas or large amounts applied or use of occlusive dressings may increase systemic absorption.
Distribution: Remains primarily at site of action.
Metabolism and Excretion: Usually metabolized in skin.
Half-life: Unknown.

TIME/ACTION PROFILE (response depends on condition being treated)

ROUTE	ONSET	PEAK	DURATION
topical	min–hrs	hrs–days	hrs–days

Contraindications/Precautions

Contraindicated in: Hypersensitivity or known intolerance to corticosteroids or components of vehicle (ointment or cream base, preservative); Untreated bacterial or viral infections.
Use Cautiously in: Hepatic dysfunction; Diabetes mellitus, cataracts, glaucoma, or tuberculosis (use of large amounts of high-potency agents may worsen condition); Patients with preexisting skin atrophy; OB/Lactation/Pedi: Chronic high-dose usage may result in adrenal suppression in mother, growth suppression in children; children may be more susceptible to adrenal and growth suppression.

Interactions

Drug-Drug: None significant.

Route/Dosage

Topical (Adults): Apply to affected area(s) 2–3 times daily (depends on preparation and condition being treated).
Topical (Children): Apply to affected area(s) 2–3 times daily (depends on preparation and condition being treated).

Availability (generic available)

Cream: 0.1%. **Lotion:** 0.1%. **Ointment:** 0.1%.

amikacin (am-i-kay-sin)

Amikin

Classification
Therapeutic: anti-infectives
Pharmacologic: aminoglycosides

Indications

IM, IV: Treatment of serious infections for which treatment with less toxic anti-infectives is contraindicated or known to be ineffective. **Unlabeled Use:** Part of combination treatment of *Mycobacterium avium* complex infections. **Intrathecal:** With parenteral amikacin in the management of CNS infections. **Inhaln:** By aerosol nebulization for the prevention of serious pneumonia in high-risk populations.

Action

Inhibits protein synthesis in bacteria at the level of the 30S ribosome. Resists the action of enzymes known to inactivate other aminoglycosides. **Therapeutic Effects:** Bactericidal action against susceptible bacteria. **Spectrum:** Notable for activity against *Pseudomonas aeruginosa*, *Klebsiella pneumoniae*, *Escherichia coli*, *Proteus*, *Providencia*, *Enterobacter*, *Citrobacter freundii*, *Serratia*, *Acinetobacter*, *Mycobacterium*. Amikacin is also active against staphylococci (including methicillin-resistant strains). Acts synergistically with beta-lactam anti-infectives against gram-negative organisms. In the treatment of enterococcal infections, synergy with a penicillin is required.

Adverse Reactions/Side Effects

CNS: vertigo. **EENT:** ototoxicity (vestibular and cochlear). **GU:** nephrotoxicity. **Neuro:** enhanced neuromuscular blockade. **Resp:** apnea. **Misc:** hypersensitivity reactions.

PHYSICAL THERAPY IMPLICATIONS

Examination and Evaluation

- Assess respiration and notify physician immediately if patient exhibits any interruption in respiratory rate (apnea) or other signs of respiratory failure (rapid labored breathing, cyanosis, confusion, irritability, sleepiness, headache, oxygen desaturation).
- Monitor signs of hypersensitivity reactions, including pulmonary symptoms (tightness in the throat and chest, wheezing, cough dyspnea) or

skin reactions (rash, pruritus, urticaria). Notify physician or nursing staff immediately if these reactions occur.

- Assess any residual muscle weakness that might occur following surgery, especially when neuromuscular junction (NMJ) blockers were used during general anesthesia (this drug enhances the effects of NMJ blockers). Report prolonged muscle weakness to the physician.
- Monitor signs of ototoxicity (hearing loss, tinnitus, dizziness). Report these signs to the physician, and caution the patient and family/caregivers to guard against falls and trauma.

Interventions

- Always wash hands thoroughly and disinfect equipment (whirlpools, electrotherapeutic devices, treatment tables, and so forth) to help prevent the spread of infection. Use universal precautions or isolation procedures as indicated for specific patients.

Patient/Client-Related Instruction

- Advise patient to report signs of nephrotoxicity, including blood or pus in urine, decreased urine output, fatigue, and weight gain from fluid retention.

Pharmacokinetics

Absorption: Poorly absorbed from the GI tract. Well absorbed after IM administration; IV administration results in complete bioavailability.
Distribution: Widely distributed throughout extracellular fluid. Crosses the placenta; small amounts enter breast milk. Poor penetration into CSF (increased when meninges inflamed).
Metabolism and Excretion: Excretion is mainly (>90%) renal; minimal amounts are metabolized by the liver.
Half-life: Infants >7 days: 4–5 hr; Children: 1.6–2.5 hr; Adolescents: 0.5–2.5 hr; Adults: 2–3 hr (increased in renal impairment, decreased in patients with burns).

TIME/ACTION PROFILE (peak blood levels)

ROUTE	ONSET	PEAK	DURATION
IM	rapid	0.75–2 hr	12–24 hr
IV	rapid	within 30 min of 30 min infusion	12–24 hr

Contraindications/Precautions

Contraindicated in: Hypersensitivity to amikacin, other aminoglycosides, or bisulfites.
Use Cautiously in: Renal or auditory impairment of any kind (dosage adjustments necessary—blood level monitoring useful in preventing ototoxicity and nephrotoxicity); Neuromuscular diseases such as myasthenia gravis or Parkinson's disease; Patients with burns (may require larger, more frequent doses); OB: May cause fetal nephrotoxicity or deafness; Lactation: Safety not established; Pedi: Neonates have prolonged half-life due to renal immaturity; Geri: Cautious use due to age-related renal impairment; may be difficult to assess vestibular and auditory function in geriatric or debilitated patients.

Interactions

Drug-Drug: Inactivated by **extended-spectrum penicillins** when coadministered to patients with renal insufficiency. May potentiate effects of **inhalation anesthetics** or **neuromuscular blockers**. Increased incidence of ototoxicity with **loop diuretics**. Increased incidence of nephrotoxicity with other **nephrotoxic drugs**, such as **amphotericin**, **vancomycin**, **acyclovir**, **cisplatin**, or **cephalosporins**.

Route/Dosage

IM, IV (Adults and Children): 15 mg/kg/day divided q 8–12 hr (not to exceed 1.5 g/day). Mycobacterium avium *complex infection:* 7.5–15 mg/kg/day divided q 12–24 hr.
IM, IV (Neonates): *Loading dose*—10 mg/kg. *Maintenance dose*—7.5 mg/kg q 12 hr.

Renal Impairment

IM, IV (Adults): *Loading dose*—7.5 mg/kg; further dosing based on serum levels.

Availability (generic available)

Injection: 50 mg/mL Rx; 62.5 mg/mL Rx; 250 mg/mL Rx.

amiloride (a-mill-oh-ride)

Midamor

Classification

Therapeutic: diuretics, potassium-sparing diuretics

Indications

Counteracts potassium loss caused by other diuretics. Used with other agents to treat edema or hypertension.

Action

Inhibition of sodium resorption in the kidney, saving potassium and hydrogen ions. **Therapeutic Effects:** Weak diuretic and antihypertensive response when compared with other diuretics. Conservation of potassium.

Adverse Reactions/Side Effects

CNS: dizziness, headache. **CV:** arrhythmias. **GI:** constipation, nausea, vomiting. **F and E:** hyperkalemia, hyponatremia. **MS:** muscle cramps. **Misc:** allergic reactions.

PHYSICAL THERAPY IMPLICATIONS

Examination and Evaluation

- Monitor signs of fluid or electrolyte imbalances (hyperkalemia, hyponatremia), including dizziness, drowsiness, headache, blurred vision, confusion, hypotension, or muscle cramps and weakness. Report excessive or prolonged symptoms to the physician.
- Assess dizziness that might affect gait, balance, and other functional activities (See Appendix C). Report balance problems and functional limitations to the physician, and caution the patient and family/ caregivers to guard against falls and trauma.
- Assess heart rate, ECG, and heart sounds, especially during exercise (See Appendixes G, H). Report any rhythm disturbances or symptoms of increased arrhythmias, including palpitations, chest discomfort, shortness of breath, fainting, and fatigue/ weakness.
- Assess blood pressure periodically and compare to normal values (See Appendix F) to help document antihypertensive effects.
- When used to treat edema, help determine drug effects by assessing peripheral edema using girth measurements, volume displacement, and measurement of pitting edema (See Appendix N). Also monitor signs of pulmonary edema such as dyspnea and rales/crackles (See Appendix K). Document whether peripheral and pulmonary symptoms are controlled adequately by diuretic therapy.
- Monitor signs of allergic reactions, including pulmonary symptoms (tightness in the throat and chest, wheezing, cough, dyspnea) or skin reactions (rash, pruritus, urticaria). Notify physician immediately if these reactions occur.

Interventions

- Implement fall prevention strategies, especially in older adults or if patient exhibits sedation, dizziness, blurred vision, or other impairments that affect gait and balance (See Appendix E).
- Use caution during aerobic exercise, especially in hot environments. Increased sweating will cause fluid and electrolyte loss, and may exaggerate arrhythmias and diuretic side effects (dizziness, muscle cramps, and so forth).
- To minimize orthostatic hypotension, patient should move slowly when assuming a more upright position.

Patient/Client-Related Instruction

- Remind patients to take medication as directed to control hypertension and other cardiac conditions even if they are asymptomatic.
- Counsel patients about additional interventions to help control blood pressure and cardiac dysfunction, including regular exercise, weight loss, sodium restriction, stress reduction, moderation of alcohol consumption, and smoking cessation.
- Instruct patient or family and caregivers to report troublesome GI problems such as severe or prolonged nausea, vomiting, or constipation.

Pharmacokinetics

Absorption: 30–90% absorbed.
Distribution: Widely distributed.
Metabolism and Excretion: 50% eliminated unchanged in urine; 40% excreted in the feces.
Half-life: 6–9 hr.

TIME/ACTION PROFILE (diuretic effect)

ROUTE	ONSET	PEAK	DURATION
PO	2 hr*	6–10 hr*	24 hr*

*Single dose

Contraindications/Precautions

Contraindicated in: Hypersensitivity; Hyperkalemia; Concurrent use of potassium supplements or other potassium-sparing agents.
Use Cautiously in: Hepatic dysfunction; Patients with diabetes mellitus (increased risk of hyperkalemia); Renal insufficiency; OB/Lactation/Pedi: Safety not established.

Interactions

Drug-Drug: ↑ risk of hypotension with acute ingestion of **alcohol**, other **antihypertensive agents**, or **nitrates**. Use with **ACE inhibitors, angiotensin II receptor antagonists, indomethacin, potassium supplements**, or **cyclosporine** ↑ risk of hyperkalemia. ↓ **lithium** excretion. Effectiveness may be ↓ by **NSAIDs**.

Route/Dosage

PO (Adults): 5–10 mg/day (up to 20 mg).

Availability

Tablets: 5 mg. ***In combination with:*** hydrochlorothiazide (Moduretic, [Moduret]). See Appendix B.

aminocaproic acid

(a-mee-noe-ka-**pro**-ik)
Amicar, epsilon aminocaproic acid

Classification
Therapeutic: hemostatic agents
Pharmacologic: fibrinolysis inhibitors

Indications

Management of acute, life-threatening hemorrhage due to systemic hyperfibrinolysis or urinary fibrinolysis.

Unlabelled Use: Prevention of recurrent subarachnoid hemorrhage. Prevention of bleeding following oral surgery in hemophiliacs. Management of severe hemorrhage caused by thrombolytic agents.

Action

Inhibits activation of plasminogen. **Therapeutic Effects:** Inhibition of fibrinolysis. Stabilization of clot formation.

Adverse Reactions/Side Effects

CNS: dizziness, malaise. **EENT:** nasal stuffiness, tinnitus. **CV:** arrhythmias, hypotension (IV only). **GI:** anorexia, bloating, cramping, diarrhea, nausea. **GU:** diuresis, renal failure. **MS:** myopathy.

PHYSICAL THERAPY IMPLICATIONS

Examination and Evaluation

- Be alert for nosebleeds, bleeding gums, or other unusual bleeding or bruising that might indicate inadequate drug effects. Report signs of bleeding to the physician immediately.
- Assess any signs of myopathy such as muscle pain, tenderness, or weakness. Report any unexplained musculoskeletal symptoms to the physician.
- Assess heart rate, ECG, and heart sounds, especially during exercise (See Appendices G, H). Report any rhythm disturbances or symptoms of increased arrhythmias, including palpitations, chest discomfort, shortness of breath, fainting, and fatigue/weakness.
- Assess blood pressure, especially after IV administration. Compare to normal values (See Appendix F), and report low blood pressure (hypotension).
- Monitor signs of renal failure, including decreased urine output, increased blood pressure, muscle cramps/twitching, edema/weight gain from fluid retention, yellowish-brown skin, and confusion that progresses to seizures and coma. Report these signs to the physician immediately.
- Assess dizziness that might affect gait, balance, and other functional activities (See Appendix C). Report balance problems and functional limitations to the physician and nursing staff, and caution the patient and family/caregivers to guard against falls and trauma.

Interventions

- Because of the risk of arrhythmias, use caution during aerobic exercise and other forms of therapeutic exercise. Assess exercise tolerance frequently (blood pressure, heart rate, fatigue levels), and terminate exercise immediately if any untoward responses occur (See Appendix L).
- In patients with drug-induced myopathy, implement gradual strengthening and other therapeutic exercises to facilitate recovery from muscle pain and weakness. Use caution during early stages to avoid fatigue of affected muscles, and implement assistive devices (walker, cane, crutches) as needed to prevent falls and assist mobility. Increase exercise intensity as tolerated; recovery from myopathy typically takes 4–6 weeks, but can be longer in older patients or people with comorbidities.

Patient/Client-related Instruction

- Instruct patient and family/caregivers to report other troublesome side effects such as severe or prolonged malaise, nasal congestion, ringing/buzzing in the ears (tinnitus), excessive urination, or GI problems (nausea, vomiting, loss of appetite, bloating, cramping).

Pharmacokinetics

Absorption: Rapidly absorbed following oral administration.
Distribution: Widely distributed.
Metabolism and Excretion: Mostly eliminated unchanged by the kidneys.
Half-life: Unknown.

TIME/ACTION PROFILE (peak blood levels)

ROUTE	ONSET	PEAK	DURATION
PO	unknown	2 hr	N/A
IV	unknown	2 hr	N/A

Contraindications/Precautions

Contraindicated in: Active intravascular clotting.
Use Cautiously in: Upper urinary tract bleeding; Cardiac, renal, or liver disease (dosage reduction may be required); Disseminated intravascular coagulation (should be used concurrently with heparin); OB/Lactation: Safety not established; Pedi: Do not use products containing benzyl alcohol with neonates.

Interactions

Drug-Drug: Concurrent use with **estrogens, conjugated** may result in a hypercoagulable state. Concurrent use with **clotting factors** may ↑ risk of thromboses.

Route/Dosage

Acute Bleeding Syndromes due to Elevated Fibrinolytic Activity

PO (Adults): 5 g 1st hr, followed by 1–1.25 g q hr for 8 hr or until hemorrhage is controlled; or 6 g over 24 hr after prostate surgery (not > 30 g/day).
IV (Adults): 4–5 g over 1st hr, followed by 1 g/hr for 8 hr or until hemorrhage is controlled; or 6 g over 24 hr after prostate surgery (not >30 g/day).

PO, IV (Children): 100 mg/kg or 3 g/m^2 over 1st hr, followed by continuous infusion of 33.3 mg/kg/hr; or 1 g/m^2/hr (total dosage not >18 g/m^2/24 hr).

Subarachnoid Hemorrhage

PO (Adults): *To follow IV*—3 g q 2 hr (36 g/day). If no surgery is performed, continue for 21 days after bleeding stops, then decrease to 2 g q 2 hr (24 g/day) for 3 days, then 1 g q 2 hr (12 g/day) for 3 days.
IV (Adults): 36 g/day for 10 days followed by PO.

Prevention of Bleeding Following Oral Surgery in Hemophiliacs

PO (Adults): 75 mg/kg (up to 6 g) immediately after procedure, then q 6 hr for 7–10 days; syrup may also be used as an oral rinse of 1.25 g (5 ml) 4 times a day for 7–10 days.
IV, PO (Children): *Also for epistaxis*—50–100 mg/kg/dose administered IV every 6 hr for 2–3 days starting 4 hr before the procedure. After completion of IV therapy, aminocaproic acid should be given as 50–100 mg/kg/dose orally every 6 hr for 5–7 days.

Availability

Tablets: 500 mg. **Syrup (raspberry flavor):** 1.25 g/5 mL. **Injection:** 250 mg/mL.

aminophylline (am-in-off-i-lin)

Phyllocontin, Truphylline

Classification
Therapeutic: bronchodilators
Pharmacologic: xanthines

Indications

Long-term control of reversible airway obstruction caused by asthma or COPD. Increases diaphragmatic contractility. **Unlabeled Use:** Respiratory and myocardial stimulant in premature infant apnea (apnea of prematurity).

Action

Inhibit phosphodiesterase, producing increased tissue concentrations of cyclic adenosine monophosphate (cAMP). Increased levels of cAMP result in Bronchodilation, CNS stimulation, Positive inotropic and chronotropic effects, Diuresis, Gastric acid secretion. Aminophylline is a salt of theophylline and releases free theophylline after administration. **Therapeutic Effects:** Bronchodilation.

Adverse Reactions/Side Effects

CNS: SEIZURES, anxiety, headache, insomnia, irritability. **CV:** ARRHYTHMIAS, tachycardia, angina, palpitations. **Derm:** rash. **GI:** nausea, vomiting, anorexia. **Neuro:** tremor.

PHYSICAL THERAPY IMPLICATIONS

Examination and Evaluation

- Be alert for new seizures or increased seizure activity, especially at the onset of drug treatment. Document the number, duration, and severity of seizures, and report these findings to the physician immediately.
- Assess heart rate, ECG, and heart sounds, especially during exercise (See Appendices G, H). Report a rapid heart rate (tachycardia) or signs of other arrhythmias, including palpitations, chest pain, shortness of breath, fainting, and fatigue/weakness.
- Assess pulmonary function periodically by measuring lung volumes, breath sounds, respiratory rate, and other symptoms (wheezing, dyspnea, shortness of breath) (See Appendices I, J, K). Report changes in pulmonary function to help document the effects of drug therapy in treating or preventing bronchoconstriction.
- Monitor and report signs of CNS toxicity, including tremor, anxiety, irritability, or other changes in mood or behavior. Sustained or severe CNS signs may indicate overdose or excessive use of this drug.

Interventions

- Because of the risk of cardiovascular stimulation, use caution during aerobic exercise and endurance conditioning. Assess exercise tolerance frequently (blood pressure, heart rate, fatigue levels), and terminate exercise immediately if any untoward responses occur (See Appendix L).

Patient/Client-Related Instruction

- Because of the risk of cardiovascular and CNS stimulation, caution patient to avoid taking more than the recommended dose. Instruct patient to contact physician immediately if bronchospasm is not relieved by medication or worsens after treatment.
- Advise patient to minimize intake of caffeine or other xanthine-containing foods or beverages (colas, coffee, tea, chocolate), and to reduce intake of charcoal-broiled foods.
- Instruct patient and family/caregivers to report other troublesome side effects such as severe or prolonged headache, sleep loss, skin rash, or GI problems (nausea, vomiting, loss of appetite).

Pharmacokinetics

Absorption: Aminophylline releases theophylline after administration; well absorbed from oral dosage forms; absorption from extended-release dosage forms is slow but complete.

Distribution: Widely distributed as theophylline; crosses the placenta; breast milk concentrations are 70% of plasma levels; not distributed into adipose tissue.
Metabolism and Excretion: Aminophylline is converted to theophylline; theophylline is metabolized by the liver (90%) to caffeine, which may accumulate in neonates; metabolites are renally excreted; 10% excreted unchanged by the kidneys.
Half-life: *Theophylline*—Premature infants: 20–30 hr; Term infants: 11–25 hr; Children 1–4 yr: 3.4 hr; Children 6–17 yr: 3.7 hr; Adults: 9–10 hr (increased in patients >60 yr, patients with congestive heart failure or liver disease; decreased in cigarette smokers).

TIME/ACTION PROFILE (bronchodilation)

ROUTE	ONSET*	PEAK	DURATION
PO	15–60 min	1–2 hr	6–8 hr
PO-ER	unknown	4–7 hr	8–12 hr
IV	rapid	end of infusion	6–8 hr

*Provided that a loading dose has been given and steady-state blood levels exist.

Contraindications/Precautions
Contraindicated in: Hypersensitivity to aminophylline or theophylline.
Use Cautiously in: Cardiac arrhythmias; heart failure, liver disease, or hypothyroidism (dosage reduction required); Peptic ulcer disease; Seizure disorder; OB/Lactation: Safety not established; Pedi: Dosage reduction required in children <1 yr; Geri: Initial dosage reduction may be necessary in geriatric (>60 yr) or debilitated patients.

Interactions
Drug-Drug: Additive CV and CNS side effects with **adrenergics (sympathomimetic)**. May ↓ the therapeutic effect of **lithium** and **phenytoin**. Smoking, **barbiturates, carbamazepine, phenytoin, nevirapine,** and **rifampin** may ↑ metabolism and may ↓ effectiveness. **Erythromycin, beta blockers, clarithromycin, calcium channel blockers, cimetidine, hormonal contraceptives, disulfiram, doxycycline, estrogens, fluvoxamine, isoniazid, ketoconazole, mexiletine, nefazodone, protease inhibitors, quinidine,** some **fluoroquinolones,** and large doses of **allopurinol** ↓ metabolism and may lead to toxicity.
Drug-Natural: Caffeine-containing herbs (**cola nut, guarana, maté, tea, coffee**) may ↑ serum levels and risk of CNS and CV side effects. ↓ serum levels and effectiveness with **St. John's wort**.
Drug-Food: Excessive regular intake of **charcoal-broiled foods** may ↓ effectiveness.

Route/Dosage
Dose should be determined by theophylline serum level monitoring. Loading dose should be decreased or eliminated if theophylline preparation has been used in preceding 24 hr. Aminophylline is 80% theophylline (100 mg aminophylline = 80 mg theophylline). Extended-release (controlled-release, sustained-release) products may be given q 8–24 hr.
PO (Adults and Children): See theophylline monograph for oral doses.
IV (Adults): *Loading dose*—6 mg/kg (4.7 mg/kg of theophylline) given over 20–30 min, followed by 0.7 mg/kg/hr (0.56 mg/kg/hr of theophylline) via continuous infusion (nonsmoking adults); an infusion rate of 0.9 mg/kg/hr (0.72 mg/kg/hr of theophylline) should be used for adults who smoke.
IV (Geriatric Patients and Adult Patients with Cor Pulmonale): *Loading dose*—6 mg/kg (4.7 mg/kg of theophylline) given over 20–30 min, followed by 0.6 mg/kg/hr (0.47 mg/kg/hr of theophylline) via continuous infusion.
IV (Adults with Congestive Heart Failure or Liver Failure): *Loading dose*—6 mg/kg (4.7 mg/kg/hr of theophylline) given over 20–30 min, followed by 0.5 mg/kg/hr (0.39 mg/kg/hr of theophylline) via continuous infusion.
IV (Children 12–16 yr): *Loading dose:* 6 mg/kg (4.7 mg/kg of theophylline) given over 20–30 min, followed by 0.7 mg/kg/hr (0.56 mg/kg/hr of theophylline) via continuous infusion.
IV (Children 9–12 yr): *Loading dose:* 6 mg/kg (4.7 mg/kg of theophylline) given over 20–30 min, followed by 0.9 mg/kg/hr (0.72 mg/kg/hr of theophylline) via continuous infusion.
IV (Children 1–9 yr): *Loading dose:* 6 mg/kg (4.7 mg/kg of theophylline) given over 20–30 min, followed by 1–1.2 mg/kg/hr (0.8–0.96 mg/kg/hr of theophylline) via continuous infusion.
IV (Children 6 mo–1 yr): *Loading dose:* 6 mg/kg (4.7 mg/kg of theophylline) given over 20–30 min, followed by 0.6–0.7 mg/kg/hr (0.48–0.56 mg/kg/hr of theophylline) via continuous infusion.
IV (Children 6 wk–6 mo): *Loading dose:* 6 mg/kg (4.7 mg/kg of theophylline) given over 20–30 min, followed by 0.5 mg/kg/hr (0.4 mg/kg/hr of theophylline) via continuous infusion.

Availability
Tablets: 100 mg Rx, 200 mg Rx. **Extended-release tablets:** 225 mg Rx, 350 mg Rx. **Oral solution:** 105 mg/5 mL Rx. **Suppositories:** 250 mg Rx, 500 mg Rx. **Injection:** 25 mg/mL Rx.

HIGH ALERT

amiodarone (am-ee-**oh**-da-rone)
Cordarone, Pacerone

Classification
Therapeutic: antiarrhythmics (class III)

Indications

Life-threatening ventricular arrhythmias unresponsive to less toxic agents. **Unlabeled Use: PO:** Management of supraventricular tachyarrhythmias. **IV:** As part of the Advanced Cardiac Life Support (ACLS) and Pediatric Advanced Life Support (PALS) guidelines for the management of ventricular fibrillation/pulseless ventricular tachycardia after cardiopulmonary resuscitation and defibrillation have failed; also for other life-threatening tachyarrhythmias.

Action

Prolongs action potential and refractory period. Inhibits adrenergic stimulation. Slows the sinus rate, increases PR and QT intervals, and decreases peripheral vascular resistance (vasodilation). **Therapeutic Effects:** Suppression of arrhythmias.

Adverse Reactions/Side Effects

CNS: confusional states, disorientation, hallucinations, dizziness, fatigue, malaise, headache, insomnia. **EENT:** corneal microdeposits, abnormal sense of smell, dry eyes, optic neuritis, optic neuropathy, photophobia. **Resp:** ADULT RESPIRATORY DISTRESS SYNDROME (ARDS), PULMONARY FIBROSIS, PULMONARY TOXICITY. **CV:** CHF, WORSENING OF ARRHYTHMIAS, bradycardia, hypotension. **GI:** LIVER FUNCTION ABNORMALITIES, anorexia, constipation, nausea, vomiting, abdominal pain, abnormal sense of taste. **GU:** decreased libido, epididymitis. **Derm:** TOXIC EPIDERMAL NECROLYSIS (RARE), photosensitivity, blue discoloration. **Endo:** hypothyroidism, hyperthyroidism. **Neuro:** ataxia, involuntary movement, paresthesia, peripheral neuropathy, poor coordination, tremor.

PHYSICAL THERAPY IMPLICATIONS

Examination and Evaluation

- Assess heart rate, ECG, and heart sounds, especially during exercise (see Appendices G, H). Although intended to treat certain arrhythmias, this drug can unmask or precipitate new arrhythmias (proarrhythmic effect). Report any rhythm disturbances or symptoms of increased arrhythmias, including palpitations, chest pain, shortness of breath, fainting, and fatigue/weakness.
- Watch for signs of congestive heart failure, including dyspnea, rales/crackles, peripheral edema, jugular venous distention, and exercise intolerance. Report these signs to the physician or nursing staff immediately.
- Watch for signs of pulmonary toxicity, pulmonary fibrosis, and ARDS. Signs include rales/crackles, decreased breath sounds, pleuritic friction rub, fatigue, dyspnea, tachypnea, cough, wheezing, pleuritic pain, fever, hemoptysis, and hypoxia. Monitor pulse oximetry and perform pulmonary function tests (See Appendices I, J, K) to quantify suspected changes in ventilation and respiratory function. Notify physician or nursing staff immediately of any pulmonary dysfunction.
- Be alert for signs of liver function abnormalities, as indicated by anorexia, abdominal pain, severe nausea and vomiting, yellow skin or eyes, fever, sore throat, malaise, weakness, facial edema, lethargy, and unusual bleeding or bruising. Report these signs to the physician or nursing staff immediately.
- Monitor rashes or other skin reactions (hives, acne, abnormal sweating, exfoliation). Notify physician or nursing staff immediately because certain skin reactions may indicate rare but serious hypersensitivity reactions (toxic epidermal necrosis).
- Assess blood pressure periodically, and compare to normal values (see Appendix F). Report low blood pressure (hypotension), especially if patient experiences dizziness or syncope.
- Monitor and report any increase or decrease in metabolism that might indicate thyroid disorders. Signs of hyperthyroidism include tachycardia, nervousness, heat intolerance, weight loss, and muscle wasting. Hypothyroidism is typically indicated by bradycardia, lethargy, cold intolerance, weight gain, and muscle weakness.
- Assess signs of peripheral neuropathy and paresthesia such as numbness, tingling, and decreased muscle strength. Perform objective tests including electroneuromyography and sensory testing to document any drug-related neuropathic changes.
- Monitor changes in mood and behavior, such as confusion, disorientation, and hallucinations. Notify physician if these changes become problematic.
- Assess dizziness, ataxia, or poor coordination that might affect gait, balance, and other functional activities (See Appendix C). Report balance problems and functional limitations to the physician and nursing staff, and caution the patient and family/caregivers to guard against falls and trauma.

Interventions

- Because of the risk of CHF, arrhythmias, and pulmonary toxicity, use extreme caution during aerobic exercise and other forms of therapeutic exercise. Assess exercise tolerance frequently (blood pressure, heart rate, fatigue levels), and terminate exercise immediately if any untoward responses occur (see Appendix L).

- Causes photosensitivity; use care if administering UV treatments. Advise patient to avoid direct sunlight and use sunscreens and protective clothing.

Patient/Client-Related Instruction

- Advise patient and family/caregivers about the signs of CHF, cardiac arrhythmias, and ARDS (See above under Examination and Evaluation), and to seek immediate medical assistance if these signs develop
- Instruct patient and family/caregivers to report other side effects such as severe or prolonged headache, sleep loss, vision problems, altered sense of smell, tremor, involuntary movements, fatigue, decreased libido, scrotal pain, skin discoloration, or GI problems (nausea, vomiting, constipation, abdominal pain, altered taste, loss of appetite).

Pharmacokinetics

Absorption: IV administration results in complete bioavailability. Slowly and variably absorbed from the GI tract (35–65%).
Distribution: Distributed to and accumulates slowly in body tissues. Reaches high levels in fat, muscle, liver, lungs, and spleen. Crosses the placenta and enters breast milk.
Protein Binding: 96% bound to plasma proteins.
Metabolism and Excretion: Metabolized by the liver, excreted into bile. Minimal renal excretion. One metabolite has antiarrhythmic activity.
Half-life: 13–107 days.

TIME/ACTION PROFILE (suppression of ventricular arrhythmias)

ROUTE	ONSET	PEAK	DURATION
PO	2–3 days (up to 2–3 mos)	3–7 hr	wks–mos
IV	2 hr	3–7 hr	unknown

Contraindications/Precautions

Contraindicated in: Patients with cardiogenic shock; Severe sinus node dysfunction; 2nd- and 3rd-degree AV block; Bradycardia (has caused syncope unless a pacemaker was in place); Hypersensitivity to amiodarone or iodine; OB: Can cause fetal hypo- or hyperthyroidism; Lactation: Enters breast milk and can cause harm to the neonate; use an alternative to breast milk; Pedi: Safety not established; products containing benzyl alcohol should not be used in neonates.
Use Cautiously in: History of CHF; Thyroid disorders; Corneal refractive laser surgery; Severe pulmonary or liver disease; Geri: Appears on Beers list. Potential to affect QT interval and cause torsades de pointes. Initiate therapy at the low end of the dosing range due to decreased hepatic, renal, or cardiac function; comorbid disease; or other drug therapy.

Interactions

Drug-Drug: Increased risk of QT prolongations with **fluoroquinolones**, **macrolides**, and **azole antifungals** (undertake concurrent use with caution). ↑ blood levels and may lead to toxicity from **digoxin** (↓ dose of digoxin by 50%). ↑ blood levels and may lead to toxicity from other **class I antiarrhythmics (quinidine, procainamide, mexiletine, lidocaine,** or **flecainide**—↓ doses of other drugs by 30–50%). ↑ blood levels of **cyclosporine**, **dextromethorphan**, **methotrexate**, **phenytoin**, and **theophylline**. **Phenytoin** ↓ amiodarone blood levels. ↑ activity of **warfarin** (↓ dose of warfarin by 33–50%). ↑ risk of bradyarrhythmias, sinus arrest, or AV heart block with **beta blockers** or **calcium channel blockers**. **Cholestyramine** may ↓ amiodarone blood levels. **Cimetidine** and **ritonavir** ↑ amiodarone blood levels. Risk of myocardial depression is ↑ by **volatile anesthetics**.
Drug-Natural: St. John's wort induces enzymes that metabolize amiodarone; may ↓ levels and effectiveness. Avoid concurrent use.
Drug-Food: Grapefruit juice inhibits enzymes in the GI tract that metabolize amiodarone resulting in ↑ levels and risk of toxicity; avoid concurrent use.

Route/Dosage

Ventricular Arrhythmias

PO (Adults): 800–1600 mg/day in 1–2 doses for 1–3 wk, then 600–800 mg/day in 1–2 doses for 1 mo, then 400 mg/day maintenance dose.
PO (Children): 10 mg/kg/day (800 mg/1.72 m^2/day) for 10 days or until response or adverse reaction occurs, then 5 mg/kg/day (400 mg/1.72 m^2/day) for several weeks, then decreased to 2.5 mg/kg/day (200 mg/1.72 m^2/day) or lowest effective maintenance dose.
IV (Adults): 150 mg over 10 min, followed by 360 mg over the next 6 hr and then 540 mg over the next 18 hr. Continue infusion at 0.5 mg/min until oral therapy is initiated. If arrhythmia recurs, a small loading infusion of 150 mg over 10 min should be given; in addition, the rate of the maintenance infusion may be increased. *Conversion to initial oral therapy*—If duration of IV infusion was <1 wk, oral dose should be 800–1600 mg/day; if IV infusion was 1–3 wk, oral dose should be 600–800 mg/day; if IV infusion was >3 wk, oral dose should be 400 mg/day. *ACLS guidelines for*

pulseless VFib/VTach—300 mg IV push, may repeat once after 3–5 min with 150 mg IV push (maximum cumulative dose 2.2 g/24 hr; unlabeled).
IV Intraosseous: (Children and infants): *PALS guidelines for pulseless VFib/Vtach* 5 mg/kg as a bolus; *perfusion tachycardia*—5 mg/kg loading dose over 20–60 min (maximum of 15 mg/kg/day; unlabeled).

Supraventricular Tachycardia

PO (Adults): 600–800 mg/day for 1 wk or until desired response occurs or side effects develop, then decrease to 400 mg/day for 3 wk, then maintenance dose of 200–400 mg/day.
PO (Children): 10 mg/kg/day (800 mg/1.72 m^2/day) for 10 days or until response or side effects occur, then 5 mg/kg/day (400 mg/1.72 m^2/day) for several weeks, then decreased to 2.5 mg/kg/day (200 mg/1.72 m^2/day) or lowest effective maintenance dose.

Availability (generic available)

Tablets: 200 mg, 400 mg. **Injection:** 50 mg/mL in 3-, 9-, and 18-mL vials.

amitriptyline

(a-mee-**trip**-ti-leen)
Apo-Amitriptyline, Elavil, Levate

Classification
Therapeutic: antidepressants
Pharmacologic: tricyclic antidepressants

Indications

Depression. **Unlabeled Use:** Anxiety, insomnia, treatment-resistant depression. Chronic pain syndromes (i.e., fibromyalgia, neuropathic pain/chronic pain, headache, low back pain).

Action

Potentiates the effect of serotonin and norepinephrine in the CNS. Has significant anticholinergic properties. **Therapeutic Effects:** Antidepressant action.

Adverse Reactions/Side Effects

CNS: lethargy, sedation. **EENT:** blurred vision, dry eyes, dry mouth. **CV:** ARRHYTHMIAS, hypotension, ECG changes. **GI:** constipation, hepatitis, paralytic ileus, increased appetite, weight gain. **GU:** urinary retention, ↓ libido. **Derm:** photosensitivity. **Endo:** changes in blood glucose, gynecomastia. **Hemat:** blood dyscrasias.

PHYSICAL THERAPY IMPLICATIONS

Examination and Evaluation

- Assess heart rate, ECG, and heart sounds, especially during exercise (see Appendices G, H). Report any rhythm disturbances or symptoms of increased arrhythmias, including palpitations, chest discomfort, shortness of breath, fainting, and fatigue/weakness.
- Be alert for increased depression and suicidal thoughts and ideology, especially when initiating drug treatment or in children and teenagers. Notify physician or mental health professional immediately if patient exhibits worsening depression or other changes in mood and behavior.
- If used to treat chronic pain, assess pain levels periodically to help determine drug efficacy.
- Measure blood pressure periodically, and compare to normal values (see Appendix F). Report low blood pressure (hypotension), especially if patient experiences dizziness or syncope.
- Watch for signs of leukopenia (fever, sore throat, signs of infection), thrombocytopenia (bruising, nose bleeds, bleeding gums), or unusual weakness and fatigue that might be due to anemia or other blood dyscrasias. Report these signs to the physician.
- Monitor signs of hypoglycemia (weakness, malaise, irritability, fatigue) or hyperglycemia (drowsiness, fruity breath, increased urination, unusual thirst). Patients with diabetes mellitus should check blood glucose levels frequently.
- Periodically assess body weight and other anthropometric measures (body mass index, body composition). Report a rapid or unexplained weight gain or increased body fat.

Interventions

- Guard against falls and trauma (hip fractures, head injury, and so forth), and implement fall prevention strategies (See Appendix E).
- Because of the risk of cardiac arrhythmias, use caution during aerobic exercise and endurance conditioning. Advise patient to also report any signs of increased arrhythmias, including palpitations, chest discomfort, shortness of breath, fainting, and fatigue/weakness.
- To minimize orthostatic hypotension, patient should move slowly when assuming a more upright position.
- Help patient explore nonpharmacologic methods to reduce depression (exercise, counseling, support groups, and so forth).
- If treating neuropathic pain or other pain syndromes, implement appropriate interventions (physical agents, manual techniques, therapeutic exercise) to manage pain and reduce the need for drug therapy. Help patient also explore other nonpharmacologic methods to reduce chronic pain (relaxation techniques, imagery, counseling, and so forth).
- Causes photosensitivity; use care if administering UV treatments. Advise patient to avoid direct sunlight and use sunscreens and protective clothing.

Patient/Client-Related Instruction

- Advise patient that antidepressant effects may not occur immediately; it may take 2 weeks or more before an improvement in mood is observed.
- Advise patient to avoid alcohol and other CNS depressants because of the increased risk of sedation and adverse effects.
- Advise patient about the risk of daytime drowsiness and decreased attention and mental focus. Use care if driving or in other activities that require strong concentration.
- Advise patient that this medication should be tapered at the completion of long-term therapy. Abrupt discontinuation may cause nausea, vomiting, diarrhea, headache, trouble sleeping with vivid dreams, and irritability.
- Instruct patient to report severe or prolonged constipation, or signs of liver dysfunction and hepatitis (yellow skin or eyes, abdominal pain, severe nausea and vomiting, fever, sore throat, malaise, weakness, facial edema).
- Instruct patient to report other severe or prolonged side effects such as dry eyes/mouth, blurred vision, difficult urination, lethargy, decreased libido, or increased breast growth in men (gynecomastia).

Pharmacokinetics

Absorption: Well absorbed from the GI tract.
Distribution: Widely distributed.
Protein Binding: 95% bound to plasma proteins.
Metabolism and Excretion: Extensively metabolized by the liver. Some metabolites have antidepressant activity. Undergoes enterohepatic recirculation and secretion into gastric juices. Probably crosses the placenta and enters breast milk.
Half-life: 10–50 hr.

TIME/ACTION PROFILE (antidepressant effect)

ROUTE	ONSET	PEAK	DURATION
PO	2–3 wk (up to 30 days)	2–6 wk	days–wks

Contraindications/Precautions

Contraindicated in: Angle-closure glaucoma; Known history of QTc prolongation, recent MI, heart failure.
Use Cautiously in: May ↑ risk of suicide attempt/ideation, especially during dose early treatment or dose adjustment; risk may be greater in children or adolescents; Patients with preexisting cardiovascular disease; Prostatic hyperplasia (increased risk of urinary retention); History of seizures (threshold may be ↓); OB: Use only if clearly needed and maternal benefits outweigh risk to fetus; Lactation: May cause sedation in infant; Pedi: Safety not established in children <12 yr; Geri: Appears on Beers list. Geriatric patients are at increased risk of adverse reactions, including falls secondary to sedative and anticholinergic effects.

Interactions

Drug-Drug: Amitriptyline is metabolized in the liver by the cytochrome P450 2D6 enzyme, and its action may be affected by drugs that compete for metabolism by this enzyme, including other **antidepressants, phenothiazines, carbamazepine, class 1C antiarrhythmics,** including **propafenone**, and **flecainide**; when these drugs are used concurrently with amitriptyline, dosage ↓ of one or the other or both may be necessary. Concurrent use of other drugs that inhibit the activity of the enzyme, including **cimetidine, quinidine, amiodarone**, and **ritonavir**, may result in ↑ effects of amitriptyline. May cause hypotension, tachycardia, and potentially fatal reactions when used with **MAO inhibitors** (avoid concurrent use—discontinue 2 wk before starting amitriptyline). Concurrent use with **SSRI antidepressants** may result in ↑ toxicity and should be avoided (**fluoxetine** should be stopped 5 wk before starting amitriptyline). Concurrent use with **clonidine** may result in hypertensive crisis and should be avoided. Concurrent use with **levodopa** may result in delayed or ↓ absorption of levodopa or hypertension. Blood levels and effects may be ↓ by **rifamycins (rifampin, rifapentine**, and **rifabutin**). Concurrent use with **moxifloxacin** ↑ risk of adverse cardiovascular reactions. ↑ CNS depression with other **CNS depressants,** including **alcohol, antihistamines, clonidine, opioids**, and **sedative/hypnotics. Barbiturates** may alter blood levels and effects. **Adrenergic** and **anticholinergic** side effects may be ↑ with other agents having **anticholinergic** properties. **Phenothiazines** or **oral contraceptives** ↑ levels and may cause toxicity. **Nicotine** may ↑ metabolism and alter effects.
Drug-Natural: St. John's wort may decrease serum concentrations and efficacy. Concomitant use of **kava-kava, valerian**, or **chamomile** can increase CNS depression. Increased anticholinergic effects with **jimson weed** and **scopolia**.

Route/Dosage

PO (Adults): 75 mg/day in divided doses; may be increased up to 150 mg/day *or* 50–100 mg at bedtime, may increase by 25–50 mg up to 150 mg (in hospitalized patients, may initiate with 100 mg/day, increasing total daily dose up to 300 mg).
PO (Geriatric Patients and Adolescents): 10 mg tid and 20 mg at bedtime *or* 25 mg at bedtime initially, slowly increased to 100 mg/day as a single bedtime dose or divided doses.

Availability (generic available)

Tablets: 10 mg, 25 mg, 50 mg, 75 mg, 100 mg, 150 mg. **Syrup:** 10 mg/5 mL.

amlodipine (am-loe-di-peen)

Norvasc

Classification

Therapeutic: antihypertensives

Pharmacologic: calcium channel blockers

Indications

Alone or with other agents in the management of hypertension, angina pectoris, and vasospastic (Prinzmetal's) angina.

Action

Inhibits the transport of calcium into myocardial and vascular smooth muscle cells, resulting in inhibition of excitation-contraction coupling and subsequent contraction. **Therapeutic Effects:** Systemic vasodilation resulting in decreased blood pressure. Coronary vasodilation resulting in decreased frequency and severity of attacks of angina.

Adverse Reactions/Side Effects

CNS: headache, dizziness, fatigue. **CV:** peripheral edema, angina, bradycardia, hypotension, palpitations. **GI:** gingival hyperplasia, nausea. **Derm:** flushing.

PHYSICAL THERAPY IMPLICATIONS

Examination and Evaluation

- Assess heart rate, ECG, and heart sounds, especially during exercise (See Appendices G, H). Report any rhythm disturbances or symptoms of increased arrhythmias, including palpitations, chest pain, shortness of breath, fainting, and fatigue/weakness.
- Assess blood pressure periodically, and compare to normal values (see Appendix F) to help document antihypertensive effects.
- Assess episodes of angina pectoris at rest and during exercise. Document whether drug therapy is helpful in reducing the frequency and severity of anginal attacks.
- Assess peripheral edema using girth measurements, volume displacement, and measurement of pitting edema (see Appendix N). Report increased swelling in feet and ankles due to peripheral vasodilation.
- Assess dizziness and fatigue that might affect gait, balance, and other functional activities (See Appendix C). Report balance problems and functional limitations to the physician, and caution the patient and family/caregivers to guard against falls and trauma.

Interventions

- Design and implement aerobic exercise and endurance training programs to normalize blood pressure, improve coronary perfusion, reduce angina, and improve myocardial pumping ability.
- Because of the risk of cardiac arrhythmias and angina pectoris, use caution during aerobic exercise and other forms of therapeutic exercise. Assess exercise tolerance frequently (blood pressure, heart rate, fatigue levels), and terminate exercise immediately if any untoward responses occur (See Appendix L).
- To minimize orthostatic hypotension, patient should move slowly when assuming a more upright position.

Patient/Client-Related Instruction

- Remind patients to take medication as directed to control hypertension and other cardiac conditions, even if they are asymptomatic.
- Counsel patients about additional interventions to help control blood pressure and cardiac dysfunction, including regular exercise, weight loss, sodium restriction, stress reduction, moderation of alcohol consumption, and smoking cessation.
- Instruct patient or family/caregivers to report other troublesome side effects such as severe or prolonged headache, fatigue, nausea, or warmth/flushing of the skin.

Pharmacokinetics

Absorption: Well absorbed after oral administration (64–90%).
Distribution: Probably crosses the placenta.
Protein Binding: 95–98%.
Metabolism and Excretion: Mostly metabolized by the liver.
Half-life: 30–50 hr (↑ in geriatric patients and patients with hepatic impairment).

TIME/ACTION PROFILE (cardiovascular effects)

ROUTE	ONSET	PEAK	DURATION
PO	unknown	6–9	24 hr

Contraindications/Precautions

Contraindicated in: Hypersensitivity; Blood pressure <90 mm Hg.
Use Cautiously in: Severe hepatic impairment (dosage reduction recommended); Aortic stenosis; History of CHF; OB/Lactation/Pedi: Safety not established; Geri: Dose reduction recommended; increased risk of hypotension.

Interactions

Drug-Drug: Additive hypotension may occur when used concurrently with **fentanyl**, other **antihypertensives**, **nitrates**, acute ingestion of **alcohol**, or **quinidine**. Antihypertensive effects may be ↓ by concurrent use of **nonsteroidal anti-inflammatory agents**. May ↑ risk of neurotoxicity with **lithium**.
Drug-Food: Grapefruit juice ↑ serum levels and effect.

Route/Dosage

PO (Adults): 5–10 mg once daily; *antihypertensive in fragile or small patients or patients already receiving other antihypertensives*—initiate at 2.5 mg/day, increase as required/tolerated (up to 10 mg/day) as an antihypertensive therapy with 2.5 mg/day in patients with hepatic insufficiency.
PO (Geriatric Patients): *Antihypertensive*—Initiate therapy at 2.5 mg/day, increase as required/tolerated (up to 10 mg/day); *antianginal*—initiate therapy at 5 mg/day, increase as required/tolerated (up to 10 mg/day).

Hepatic Impairment

PO (Adults): *Antihypertensive*—Initiate therapy at 2.5 mg/day, increase as required/tolerated (up to 10 mg/day); *antianginal*—initiate therapy at 5 mg/day, increase as required/tolerated (up to 10 mg/day).

Availability (generic available)

Tablets: 2.5 mg, 5 mg, 10 mg. ***In combination with:*** atorvastatin (Caduet), benazepril (Lotrel), olmesartan (Azor), and valsartan (Exforge). See Appendix B.

amobarbital (am-oh-bar-bi-tal)

Amytal

Classification

Therapeutic: sedative/hypnotics
Pharmacologic: barbiturates

Schedule II

Indications

Preoperative sedative and in other situations in which sedation may be required. Hypnotic for short-term treatment of insomnia. **Unlabeled Use:** Psychiatric interviews. Wada testing (intracarotid administration to determine hemispheric locus of language dominance prior to epilepsy surgery).

Action

Produces all levels of CNS depression: Depresses sensory cortex, Decreases motor activity, Alters cerebral function. Inhibits transmission in the CNS and raises seizure threshold. **Therapeutic Effects:** Hypnosis, Sedation.

Adverse Reactions/Side Effects

CNS: drowsiness, abnormal thinking, agitation, ataxia, CNS depression, confusion, dizziness, headache, nightmares, vertigo. **Resp:** BRONCHOSPASM (IV ONLY), LARYNGOSPASM (IV ONLY), apnea, respiratory depression. **CV:** bradycardia, hypotension, syncope. **GI:** constipation, nausea, vomiting. **Derm:** ANGIOEDEMA, exfoliative dermatitis, purpura, rash. **Local:** pain or sterile abscess at IM site, phlebitis at IV site. **MS:** hyperkinesia. **Misc:** HYPERSENSITIVITY REACTIONS, INCLUDING STEVENS-JOHNSON SYNDROME, fever.

PHYSICAL THERAPY IMPLICATIONS

Examination and Evaluation

- Monitor signs of hypersensitivity reactions and angioedema, including pulmonary symptoms (tightness in the throat and chest, wheezing, cough, dyspnea) or skin reactions (rash, pruritus, urticaria, burning/itching skin). Be especially alert for exfoliation and other severe skin reactions that might indicate Stevens-Johnson syndrome. Notify physician or nursing staff immediately if these reactions occur.
- Assess symptoms of bronchospasm and laryngospasm (wheezing, coughing, tightness in chest), especially after IV administration. Perform pulmonary function tests (See Appendices I, J, K) to quantify suspected changes in ventilation and respiratory function, or if patient exhibits signs of respiratory depression (dyspnea, hypoxia).
- Assess blood pressure periodically, and compare to normal values (See Appendix F). Report low blood pressure (hypotension), especially if patient experiences dizziness or syncope.
- Assess heart rate, ECG, and heart sounds, especially during exercise (See Appendices G, H). Report an abnormally slow heart rate (bradycardia) or symptoms of other arrhythmias, including palpitations, chest discomfort, shortness of breath, fainting, and fatigue/weakness.
- Monitor respiration, and notify physician or nursing staff immediately if patient exhibits any interruption in respiratory rate (apnea) or signs of respiratory depression (rapid labored breathing, cyanosis, confusion, irritability, sleepiness, headache, oxygen desaturation).
- Assess dizziness, syncope, and vertigo that might affect gait, balance, and other functional activities (See Appendix C). Report balance problems and functional limitations to the physician and nursing staff, and caution the patient and family/caregivers to guard against falls and trauma.
- Monitor excessive sedation or changes in mood and behavior such as agitation, hyperactivity, confusion, or abnormal thoughts. Notify physician if these changes become problematic.
- Assess injection site following IV or IM administration, and report excessive or prolonged local pain, swelling, and inflammation.

= Canadian drug name; *CAPITALS indicate life-threatening; underlines indicate most frequent.

Interventions

- Guard against falls and trauma (hip fractures, head injury, and so forth), especially if drowsiness and confusion carry over into the daytime. Implement fall prevention strategies, especially if balance is impaired (See Appendix E).
- Because of the risk of arrhythmias, use caution during aerobic exercise and other forms of therapeutic exercise. Assess exercise tolerance frequently (blood pressure, heart rate, fatigue levels), and terminate exercise immediately if any untoward responses occur (See Appendix L).
- Help patient explore nonpharmacologic methods to induce sleep, such as relaxation techniques, reduced caffeine intake, and so forth.

Patient/Client-Related Instruction

- Advise patient to avoid alcohol and other CNS depressants because of the increased risk of sedation and other adverse effects.
- Remind patient that this drug is typically recommended for only occasional use as a preoperative sedative or for short-term use (2 wk or less) to treat insomnia. Long-term use can cause tolerance and dependence.
- Instruct patient or family/caregivers to report other severe or prolonged side effects such headache, nightmares, fever, or GI problems (nausea, vomiting, constipation).

Pharmacokinetics

Absorption: Well absorbed after IM administration.
Distribution: Rapidly and widely distributed; concentrates in brain, liver, and kidneys. Readily crosses placenta; small amounts enter breast milk. Moderately bound to plasma proteins.
Metabolism and Excretion: Mostly metabolized by the liver.
Half-life: 16–40 hr.

TIME/ACTION PROFILE (sedation)

ROUTE	ONSET	PEAK	DURATION
Oral	0.75–1 hr	unknown	6–8 hr
IM	30–45 min	rapid	6–8 hr
IV	several min	rapid	6–8 hr

Contraindications/Precautions

Contraindicated in: Hypersensitivity; Dyspnea or airway obstruction; Comatose patients; Preexisting CNS depression; Severe hepatic dysfunction; Porphyria; OB/Lactation: Not recommended.
Use Cautiously in: History of suicide attempts or substance abuse; Debilitated patients (use smaller doses); Patients using alcohol or drugs that cause CNS depression; Patients with hepatic or renal impairment (dosage should be reduced); Acute or chronic pain (paradoxical excitement may occur); Hypoadrenalism (decreases effects of corticosteroids); Pedi: Safety not established in children <6 yr; Geri: Appears on Beers list. Geriatric patients are at increased risk for excitement, confusion, CNS depression; use smaller doses).

Interactions

Drug-Drug: Additive CNS depression with other **CNS depressants**, including **alcohol**, **antidepressants**, **antihistamines**, **opioid analgesics**, and other **sedative/hypnotics**. Sedation may be prolonged with **MAO inhibitors** and **valproic acid**. Induces hepatic enzymes that metabolize other drugs, decreasing their effectiveness, including **hormonal contraceptives**, **furosemide**, **disopyramide**, **propafenone**, **methadone**, **cimetidine**, **cyclosporine**, **tacrolimus**, **rifampin**, **estrogen**, **chloramphenicol**, **acebutolol**, **propranolol**, **metoprolol**, **timolol**, **doxycycline**, **corticosteroids**, **tricyclic antidepressants**, **warfarin**, **theophylline**, and **quinidine**.
Drug-Natural: Concomitant use of **kava**, **valerian**, **skullcap**, **chamomile**, or **hops** can increase CNS depression. **St. John's wort** may decrease barbiturate effect.

Route/Dosage

IM, IV (Adults): *Sedative*—30–50 mg 2–3 times daily; *hypnotic*—65–200 mg at bedtime.
IV (Adults): *Psychiatric interviews (unlabeled use)* 50–100 mg/min for total dose of 200–1000 mg or until patient experiences drowsiness, impaired attention, slurred speech, or nystagmus.
IA (Adults): *Wada test (unlabeled use)* 100 mg over 4–5 sec via percutaneous transfemoral catheter.
IM, IV (Children 6–12 yr): *Sedative*—65–500 mg (3–5 mg/kg), depending on response.
IM (Children ≥6 yr): *Hypnotic*—2–3 mg/kg/dose.

Availability (generic available)

Injection: 500-mg vials.

amoxapine (a-mox-a-peen)

Asendin

Classification

Therapeutic: antidepressants

Indications

Treatment of various types of depression. **Unlabeled Use:** Anxiety, insomnia, neuropathic and chronic pain syndromes.

Action

Potentiates the effects of serotonin and norepinephrine in the CNS. Has significant anticholinergic properties. Also has antianxiety effect related to sedative properties. **Therapeutic Effects:** Antidepressant and antianxiety action.

A

Adverse Reactions/Side Effects

CNS: NEUROLEPTIC MALIGNANT SYNDROME, fatigue, sedation, extrapyramidal reactions, tardive dyskinesia. **EENT:** blurred vision, dry eyes, dry mouth. **CV:** ARRHYTHMIAS, hypotension, ECG changes. **GI:** constipation, increased appetite, weight gain, paralytic ileus. **GU:** testicular swelling, urinary retention. **Derm:** photosensitivity, rash. **Endo:** gynecomastia, sexual dysfunction. **Hemat:** blood dyscrasias. **Misc:** fever.

PHYSICAL THERAPY IMPLICATIONS

Examination and Evaluation

- Assess heart rate, ECG, and heart sounds, especially during exercise (See Appendices G, H). Report any rhythm disturbances or symptoms of increased arrhythmias, including palpitations, chest discomfort, shortness of breath, fainting, and fatigue/weakness.
- Watch for signs of neuroleptic malignant syndrome, including hyperthermia, diaphoresis, generalized muscle rigidity, altered mental status, tachycardia, changes in blood pressure (BP), and incontinence. Symptoms typically occur within 4–14 days after initiation of drug therapy, but can occur at any time during drug use. Report these signs to the physician immediately.
- Be alert for increased depression, especially in the initial period of drug therapy, and in children and teenagers. Notify physician immediately if patient exhibits signs of worsening depression or expresses thoughts of suicide.
- Assess motor function, and be alert for extrapyramidal symptoms. Report these symptoms immediately, especially tardive dyskinesia, because this problem may be irreversible. Common extrapyramidal symptoms include:
  - Tardive dyskinesia (uncontrolled rhythmic movement of mouth, face, and extremities, lip smacking or puckering, puffing of cheeks, uncontrolled chewing, rapid or worm-like movements of tongue).
  - Pseudoparkinsonism (shuffling gait, rigidity, tremor, pill-rolling motion, loss of balance control, difficulty speaking or swallowing, mask-like face)
  - Akathisia (restlessness or desire to keep moving)
  - Other dystonias and dyskinesias (dystonic muscle spasms, twisting motions, twitching, inability to move eyes, weakness of arms or legs)
- If used to treat chronic pain, assess pain levels periodically to help determine drug efficacy.
- Measure blood pressure periodically, and compare to normal values (See Appendix F). Report low BP (hypotension), especially if patient experiences dizziness or syncope.
- Watch for signs of leukopenia (fever, sore throat, signs of infection), thrombocytopenia (bruising, nose bleeds, and bleeding gums), or unusual weakness and fatigue that might be due to anemia or other blood dyscrasias. Report these signs to the physician.
- Report excessive sedation and fatigue, especially in older adults. Determine if these side effects might impair gait, balance, and other functional activities.
- Periodically assess body weight and other anthropometric measures (body mass index, body composition). Report a rapid or unexplained weight gain or increased body fat.

Interventions

- Guard against falls and trauma (hip fractures, head injury, and so forth), and implement fall prevention strategies (See Appendix E).
- Because of the risk of cardiac arrhythmias, use caution during aerobic exercise and endurance conditioning. Advise patient to also report any signs of increased arrhythmias, including palpitations, chest discomfort, shortness of breath, fainting, and fatigue/weakness.
- To minimize orthostatic hypotension, patient should move slowly when assuming a more upright position.
- Help patient explore nonpharmacologic methods to reduce depression (exercise, counseling, support groups, and so forth).
- If treating neuropathic pain or other pain syndromes, implement appropriate interventions (physical agents, manual techniques, therapeutic exercise) to manage pain and reduce the need for drug therapy. Help patient also explore other nonpharmacologic methods to reduce chronic pain (relaxation techniques, imagery, counseling, and so forth).
- Causes photosensitivity; use care if administering UV treatments. Advise patient to avoid direct sunlight and use sunscreens and protective clothing.

Patient/Client-Related Instruction

- Advise patient that antidepressant effects may not occur immediately; it may take 2 wk or more before an improvement in mood is observed.
- Advise patient to avoid alcohol and other CNS depressants because of the increased risk of sedation and adverse effects.
- Advise patient that this medication should be tapered at the completion of long-term therapy. Abrupt discontinuation may cause nausea, vomiting, diarrhea, headache, trouble sleeping with vivid dreams, and irritability.
- Instruct patient to report other troublesome side effects such as severe or prolonged dry eyes/mouth, blurred vision, rash, difficult urination, fever, constipation, sexual dysfunction, testicular swelling, or increased breast growth in men (gynecomastia).

Pharmacokinetics

Absorption: Well absorbed following oral administration.
Distribution: Widely distributed; enters breast milk.
Protein Binding: 92% bound to plasma proteins.
Metabolism and Excretion: Extensively metabolized by the liver.
Half-life: 8 hr.

TIME/ACTION PROFILE (antidepressant effect)

ROUTE	ONSET	PEAK	DURATION
PO	within 1–2 wk	2–6 wk	days–wks

Contraindications/Precautions

Contraindicated in: Angle-closure glaucoma; Recent MI; Prolongation of QTc interval; Cardiac arrhythmia; Heart failure.
Use Cautiously in: Preexisting cardiovascular disease; Prostatic hyperplasia (increased susceptibility to urinary retention); History of seizures (threshold may be lowered); May ↑ risk of suicide attempt/ideation, especially during dose early treatment or dose adjustment; OB: Use only if clearly needed and maternal benefits outweigh risk to fetus; Lactation: May result in sedation in infant; discontinue drug or bottle feed; Pedi: Suicide risk, especially at initiation of therapy, may be greater in children and adolescents; Geri: May be more susceptible to adverse effects; dosage reduction required.

Interactions

Drug-Drug: Amoxapine is metabolized in the liver by the cytochrome P450 2D6 enzyme, and its action may be affected by drugs that compete for metabolism by this enzyme, including other **antidepressants, phenothiazines, carbamazepine,** and **class 1C antiarrhythmics,** including **propafenone,** and **flecainide**; when these drugs are used concurrently with amoxapine, dosage reduction of one or the other or both may be necessary. Concurrent use of other drugs that inhibit the activity of the enzyme, including **cimetidine, quinidine, amiodarone,** and **ritonavir** may result in ↑ effects of amoxapine. May cause hypotension, tachycardia, and potentially fatal reactions when used with **MAO inhibitors** (avoid concurrent use—discontinue 2 wk before starting amoxapine). Concurrent use with **SSRI antidepressants** may result in ↑ toxicity and should be avoided (**fluoxetine** should be stopped 5 wk before starting amoxapine). Concurrent use with **clonidine** may result in hypertensive crisis and should be avoided. Concurrent use with **levodopa** may result in delayed/decreased absorption of levodopa or hypertension. Blood levels and effects may be ↓ by **rifamycins (rifapentine, rifampin, rifabutin)**. **Cimetidine, fluoxetine, phenothiazines,** or **oral contraceptives** ↑ levels and may cause toxicity. Increased risk of extrapyramidal reactions with other drugs causing extrapyramidal reactions (**phenothiazines**).

Route/Dosage

PO (Adults): 50 mg 2–3 times daily, increase to 100 mg 2–3 times daily by end of 1 week (not to exceed 300 mg daily in outpatients, 600 mg daily in divided doses in hospitalized patients). Once optimal dose is achieved, may be given as a single bedtime dose; no single dose to exceed 300 mg.
PO (Geriatric Patients): 25 mg 2–3 times daily, may be increased to 50 mg 2–3 times daily (not >300 mg/day).

Availability (generic available)

Tablets: 25 mg, 50 mg, 100 mg, 150 mg.

amoxicillin (a-mox-i-sil-in)

Amoxil, Apo-Amoxi, DisperMox, Moxatag, Novamoxin, Nu-Amoxi, Trimox, Wymox

Classification
Therapeutic: anti-infectives, antiulcer agents
Pharmacologic: aminopenicillins

Indications

Treatment of Skin and skin structure infections, Otitis media, Sinusitis, Respiratory infections, Genitourinary infections. Endocarditis prophylaxis. Postexposure inhalational anthrax prophylaxis. Management of ulcer disease due to *Helicobacter pylori*. **Unlabeled Use:** Lyme disease in children <8 yr.

Action

Binds to bacterial cell wall, causing cell death. **Therapeutic Effects:** Bactericidal action; spectrum is broader than penicillins. **Spectrum:** Active against Streptococci, Pneumococci, Enterococci, *Haemophilus influenzae*, *Escherichia coli*, *Proteus mirabilis*, *Neisseria meningitidis*, *Neisseria gonorrhoeae*, *Shigella*, *Chlamydia trachomatis*, *Salmonella*, *Borrelia burgdorferi*, *H. pylori*.

Adverse Reactions/Side Effects

CNS: SEIZURES (HIGH DOSES). **GI:** PSEUDOMEMBRANOUS COLITIS, diarrhea, nausea, vomiting, elevated liver enzymes. **Derm:** rashes, urticaria. **Hemat:** blood dyscrasias. **Misc:** ALLERGIC REACTIONS, INCLUDING ANAPHYLAXIS, SERUM SICKNESS, superinfection.

PHYSICAL THERAPY IMPLICATIONS

Examination and Evaluation

- Watch for seizures; notify physician immediately if patient develops or increases seizure activity.
- Monitor signs of pseudomembranous colitis, including diarrhea, abdominal pain, fever, pus or mucus

in stool, and other severe or prolonged GI problems (nausea, vomiting, heartburn). Notify physician or nursing staff immediately of these signs.

- Monitor signs of allergic reactions and anaphylaxis, including pulmonary symptoms (tightness in the throat and chest, wheezing, cough dyspnea) or skin reactions (rash, pruritus, urticaria). Notify physician or nursing staff immediately if these reactions occur.
- Assess muscle aches and joint pain (arthralgia) that may be caused by serum sickness. Notify physician if these symptoms seem to be drug related rather than caused by musculoskeletal injury, or if muscle and joint pain are accompanied by allergic-like reactions (fever, rashes, etc.)
- Monitor signs of blood dyscrasias such as eosinophilia (fatigue, weakness, myalgia) and leukopenia (fever, sore throat, signs of infection). Report these signs to the physician.

Interventions

- Always wash hands thoroughly and disinfect equipment (whirlpools, electrotherapeutic devices, treatment tables, and so forth) to help prevent the spread of infection. Use universal precautions or isolation procedures as indicated for specific patients.

Patient/Client-Related Instruction

- Instruct patient to notify physician immediately of signs of superinfection, including black, furry overgrowth on tongue, vaginal itching or discharge, and loose or foul-smelling stools.
- Instruct patient and family/caregivers to report other troublesome side effects such as severe or prolonged skin problems (rash, itching) or GI problems (nausea, vomiting, diarrhea).

Pharmacokinetics

Absorption: Well absorbed from duodenum (75–90%). More resistant to acid inactivation than other penicillins.
Distribution: Diffuses readily into most body tissues and fluids. CSF penetration increased when meninges are inflamed. Crosses placenta; enters breast milk in small amounts.
Metabolism and Excretion: 70% excreted unchanged in the urine; 30% metabolized by the liver.
Half-life: Neonates: 3.7 hr; Infants and Children: 1–2 hr; Adults: 0.7–1.4 hr.

TIME/ACTION PROFILE (blood levels)

ROUTE	ONSET	PEAK	DURATION
PO	30 min	1–2 hr	8–12 hr

Contraindications/Precautions

Contraindicated in: Hypersensitivity to penicillins; Tablets for oral suspension (DisperMox) contain aspartame; avoid in patients with phenylketonuria.
Use Cautiously in: Severe renal insufficiency (↓ dose if CCr <30 mL/min); Infectious mononucleosis, acute lymphocytic leukemia, or cytomegalovirus infection (↑ risk of rash); Patients with a history of cephalosporin allergy; OB//Lactation: Has been used safely in pregnant and breast-feeding women.

Interactions

Drug-Drug: Probenecid ↓ renal excretion and ↑ blood levels of amoxicillin—therapy may be combined for this purpose. May ↑ effect of **warfarin**. May ↓ effectiveness of **oral contraceptives**. **Allopurinol** may ↑ frequency of rash.

Route/Dosage

Most Infections

PO (Adults): 250–500 mg q 8 hr *or* 500–875 mg q 12 hr (not to exceed 2–3 g/day).
PO (Adults and Children ≥12 yr): *Extended-release tablets (for strep throat)*—775 mg once daily for 10 days.
PO (Children >3 mo): 25–50 mg/kg/day in divided doses q 8 hr *or* 25–50 mg/kg/day individual doses q 12 hr; *Acute otitis media due to highly resistant strains of S. pneumoniae*—80–90 mg/kg/day divided q 12 hr; *Postexposure inhalational anthrax prophylaxis*—<40 kg: 45 mg/kg/day in divided doses q 8 hr; >40 kg: 500 mg q 8 hr.
PO (Infants ≤3 mo and neonates): 20–30 mg/kg/day in divided doses q 12 hr.

H. pylori

PO (Adults): *Triple therapy*—1000 mg amoxicillin twice daily with lansoprazole 30 mg twice daily and clarithromycin 500 mg twice daily for 14 days *or* 1000 mg amoxicillin twice daily with omeprazole 20 mg twice daily and clarithromycin 500 mg twice daily for 14 days *or* amoxicillin 1000 mg twice daily with esomeprazole 40 mg daily and clarithromycin 500 mg twice daily for 10 days. *Dual therapy*—1000 mg amoxicillin 3 times daily with lansoprazole 30 mg 3 times daily for 14 days.

Endocarditis Prophylaxis

PO (Adults): 2 g 1 hr prior to procedure.
PO (Children): 50 mg/kg 1 hr prior to procedure (not to exceed adult dose).

Gonorrhea

PO (Adults and Children ≥40 kg): single 3-g dose.
PO (Children >2 yr and <40 kg): 50 mg/kg with probenecid 25 mg/kg as a single dose.

Renal Impairment

PO (Adults CCr 10–30 mL/min): 250–500 mg q 12 hr.

Renal Impairment

PO (Adults CCr <10 mL/min): 250–500 mg q 24 hr.

Availability (generic available)

Chewable tablets (cherry, banana, peppermint flavors): 125 mg, 200 mg, 250 mg, 400 mg. **Tablets:** 500 mg, 875 mg. **Extended-release tablets:** 775 mg. **Capsules:** 250 mg, 500 mg. **Suspension (pediatric drops) (bubblegum flavor):** 50 mg/mL in 30-mL bottles. **Suspension (strawberry [125 mg/5 mL] and bubblegum [200 mg/5 mL, 250 mg/5 mL, 400 mg/5 mL] flavors):** 125 mg/5 mL, 200 mg/5 mL, 250 mg/5 mL, 400 mg/5 mL. **Tablets for oral suspension (strawberry):** 200 mg, 400 mg. ***In combination with:*** clarithromycin and lansoprazole in a compliance package (Prevpac). See Appendix B.

amphetamine mixtures

(am-**fet**-a-meen)

Amphetamine Salt, Adderall, Adderall XR

Classification

Therapeutic: central nervous system stimulants

Schedule II

Indications

Narcolepsy. Attention deficit–hyperactivity disorder (ADHD).

Action

Causes release of norepinephrine from nerve endings. Pharmacologic effects are: CNS and respiratory stimulation, Vasoconstriction, Mydriasis (pupillary dilation). **Therapeutic Effects:** Increased motor activity, mental alertness, and decreased fatigue in narcoleptic patients . Increased attention span in ADHD.

Adverse Reactions/Side Effects

CNS: hyperactivity, insomnia, restlessness, tremor, behavioral disturbances, dizziness, hallucinations, headache, mania, irritability, thought disorder. **CV:** palpitations, tachycardia, cardiomyopathy (increased with prolonged use, high doses), hypertension, hypotension. **GI:** anorexia, constipation, cramps, diarrhea, dry mouth, metallic taste, nausea, vomiting. **GU:** erectile dysfunction, increased libido. **Derm:** urticaria. **Endo:** growth inhibition (with long term use in children). **Misc:** psychologic dependence.

PHYSICAL THERAPY IMPLICATIONS

Examination and Evaluation

- Be alert for signs of excessive CNS stimulation, including hyperactivity, restlessness, tremor, hallucinations, mania, irritability, or disordered thoughts. Report these signs to the physician.
- Monitor attentiveness and behavior in patients with ADHD. Report any changes in attention and hyperactivity, and document whether this drug appears to be producing the desired effects.
- Monitor alertness in patients with narcolepsy; document the frequency and duration of sleeping episodes to help assess the effects of drug therapy.
- Assess heart rate, ECG, and heart sounds, especially during exercise (See Appendices G, H). Report fast heart rate (tachycardia), or symptoms of other arrhythmias, including palpitations, chest discomfort, shortness of breath, fainting, and fatigue/weakness.
- Assess blood pressure and compare to normal values (See Appendix F). Report changes in blood pressure, either a problematic decrease in BP (hypotension), or a sustained increase in BP (hypertension).
- Be alert for signs of cardiomyopathy, especially at high doses for prolonged periods. Signs include breathlessness with exertion, fatigue, dizziness, palpitations, and peripheral and pulmonary edema. Report these signs to the physician.
- Assess growth rate in children receiving chronic therapy; report delayed or stunted growth to the physician.

Interventions

- Because of the risk of arrhythmias, cardiomyopathy, and abnormal BP responses, use caution during aerobic exercise and other forms of therapeutic exercise. Assess exercise tolerance frequently (blood pressure, heart rate, fatigue levels), and terminate exercise immediately if any untoward responses occur (See Appendix L).

Patient/Client-related Instruction

- Instruct patient and family/caregivers to report other troublesome side effects including severe or prolonged headache, sleep loss, skin problems (hives, itching), sexual dysfunction (decreased libido, erectile dysfunction), or GI problems (nausea, vomiting, constipation, diarrhea, abdominal cramps, metallic taste, dry mouth).

Pharmacokinetics

Absorption: Well absorbed after oral administration.
Distribution: Widely distributed in body tissues, with high concentrations in the brain and CSF. Crosses placenta and enters breast milk.
Metabolism and Excretion: Some metabolism by the liver. Urinary excretion is pH-dependent. Alkaline urine promotes reabsorption and prolongs action.
Half-life: Children 6–12 yrs: 9–11 hr; Adults: 10–13 hr (depends on urine pH).

TIME/ACTION PROFILE (CNS stimulation)

ROUTE	ONSET	PEAK	DURATION
PO	tablet: 0.5–1 hr	tablet: 3 hr capsule: 7 hr	4–6 hr

Contraindications/Precautions

Contraindicated in: Hyperexcitable states including hyperthyroidism; Psychotic personalities; Suicidal or homicidal tendencies; Chemical dependence; Glaucoma; Structural cardiac abnormalities (may increase the risk of sudden death); OB/Pedi: Potentially embryotoxic.

Use Cautiously in: Cardiovascular disease (sudden death has occurred in children with structural cardiac abnormalities or other serious heart problems); History of substance abuse (misuse may result in serious cardiovascular events/sudden death); Hypertension; Diabetes mellitus; Tourette's syndrome (may exacerbate tics); Geri: Geriatric or debilitated patients may be more susceptible to side effects.

Interactions

Drug-Drug: Use with **MAO inhibitors** or **meperidine** can result in hypertensive crisis. ↑ adrenergic effects with other **adrenergics** or **thyroid preparations. Drugs that alkalinize urine (sodium bicarbonate, acetazolamide)** ↓ excretion, ↑ effects. **Drugs that acidify urine (ammonium chloride,** large doses of **ascorbic acid)** ↑ excretion, ↓ effects. ↑ risk of hypertension and bradycardia with **beta blockers**. ↑ risk of arrhythmias with **digoxin. Tricyclic antidepressants** may ↑ effect of amphetamine but may ↑ risk of arrhythmias, hypertension, or hyperpyrexia.

Drug-Natural: Use with **St. John's wort** may ↑ serious side effects (avoid concurrent use).

Drug-Food: Foods that alkalinize the urine (fruit juices) can ↑ effect of amphetamine.

Route/Dosage

Dose is expressed in total amphetamine content (amphetamine + dextroamphetamine).

Narcolepsy

PO (Adults and Children ≥12 yr): 10–60 mg/day in divided doses; start with 10 mg/day, increase by 10 mg/day at weekly intervals. Sustained-release capsules can be given once daily, tablets every 8–12 hr.

PO (Children 6–12 yr): 5 mg once daily; may increase by 5 mg/day at weekly intervals to a maximum of 60 mg/day.

ADHD

PO (Children ≥6 yr): 5 mg/day 1–2 times daily; increase daily dose by 5 mg at weekly intervals. Sustained-release capsules can be given once daily, tablets every 8–12 hr. If starting therapy with extended release capsules, start with 10 mg once daily and increase by 10 mg/day at weekly intervals (up to 40 mg/day).

PO (Adults): 20 mg/day initially (as extended-release product).

PO (Children 3–5 yr): 2.5 mg/day in the morning; increase daily dose by 2.5 mg at weekly intervals not to exceed 40 mg/day.

Availability (generic available)

Amount is expressed in total amphetamine content (amphetamine + dextroamphetamine. **Tablets:** 5 mg, 7.5 mg, 10 mg, 12.5 mg, 15 mg, 20 mg, 30 mg. **Extended-release capsules:** 5 mg, 10 mg, 15 mg, 20 mg, 25 mg, 30 mg.

amphotericin B deoxycholate

(am-foe-**ter**-i-sin)

Fungizone **amphotericin B cholesteryl sulfate,** Amphotec **amphotericin B lipid complex,** Abelcet **amphotericin B liposome,** AmBisome

Classification

Therapeutic: antifungals

Indications

IV: Treatment of progressive, potentially fatal fungal infections. The cholesteryl sulfate, lipid complex, and liposome formulations should be considered for patients who are intolerant (e.g., renal dysfunction) or refractory to amphotericin B deoxycholate. **Amphotericin B liposome:** Management of suspected fungal infections in febrile neutropenic patients: Treatment of visceral leishmaniasis, Treatment of cryptococcal meningitis in HIV patients.

Action

Binds to fungal cell membrane, allowing leakage of cellular contents. Toxicity (especially acute infusion reactions and nephrotoxicity) is less with lipid formulations. **Therapeutic Effects:** Can be fungistatic or fungicidal (depends on concentration achieved and susceptibility of organism). **Spectrum:** Active against *Aspergillus, Blastomyces, Candida, Coccidioides, Cryptococcus, Histoplasma, Leishmania* (liposomal formulation only), *Mucor*.

Adverse Reactions/Side Effects

CNS: anxiety, confusion, headache, insomnia. **Resp:** dyspnea, hypoxia, wheezing. **CV:** chest pain, hypotension, tachycardia, edema, hypertension. **GI:** diarrhea, hyperbilirubinemia, liver enzyme elevation, nausea, vomiting, abdominal pain. **GU:** nephrotoxicity, hematuria. **F and E:** hyperglycemia, hypocalcemia , hypokalemia, hypomagnesemia. **Hemat:** anemia, leukopenia, thrombocytopenia. **Derm:** pruritis, rashes. **Local:** phlebitis. **MS:** arthralgia, myalgia. **Misc:** HYPERSENSITIVITY REACTIONS, chills, fever, acute infusion reactions.

PHYSICAL THERAPY IMPLICATIONS

Examination and Evaluation

- Monitor signs of hypersensitivity reactions, including pulmonary symptoms (tightness in the throat and chest, wheezing, cough dyspnea) or skin reactions (rash, angioedema, pruritis, urticaria). Notify physician or nursing staff immediately if these reactions occur.
- Monitor signs of leukopenia (fever, sore throat, signs of infection), thrombocytopenia (bruising, nose bleeds, and bleeding gums), or unusual weakness and fatigue that might be due to anemia or other blood dyscrasias. Report these signs to the physician.
- Assess blood pressure (BP) and compare to normal values (See Appendix F). Report changes in BP, either a problematic decrease in BP (hypotension) or a sustained increase in BP (hypertension).
- Assess heart rate, ECG, and heart sounds, especially during exercise (See Appendices G, H). Report tachycardia or other rhythm disturbances, or symptoms of increased arrhythmias, including palpitations, chest pain, shortness of breath, fainting, and fatigue/weakness.
- Assess peripheral edema using girth measurements, volume displacement, and measurement of pitting edema (See Appendix N). Report increased swelling in feet and ankles or a sudden increase in body weight due to fluid retention.
- Assess any signs of thrombophlebitis, including localized pain, redness, or swelling in the affected area. Report these signs to the physician.
- Monitor any breathing problems, and report wheezing, shortness of breath, hypoxia, or labored/difficult breathing. Assess pulmonary function by measuring lung volumes, breath sounds, respiratory rate, and other symptoms (See Appendices I, J, K) to document changes in respiratory status.
- Monitor signs of hypoglycemia (weakness, malaise, irritability, fatigue) or hyperglycemia (drowsiness, fruity breath, increased urination, unusual thirst). Patients with diabetes mellitus should check blood glucose levels frequently.
- Monitor signs of low potassium levels (hypokalemia), such as muscle weakness, aches, and cramps, and low magnesium levels (hypomagnesemia), such as lethargy, irritability, insomnia, muscle tremors, and confusion. Notify physician of these signs.
- Assess any joint or muscle pain to rule out musculoskeletal pathology; that is, try to determine if pain is drug induced rather than caused by anatomic or biomechanical problems.
- Report allergic-like responses (wheezing, laryngeal edema, urticaria, other skin reactions) that occur during and after administration (infusion-related reactions).
- Monitor personality changes, including anxiety and confusion. Notify physician if these changes become problematic.

Interventions

- Always wash hands thoroughly and disinfect equipment (whirlpools, electrotherapeutic devices, treatment tables, and so forth) to help prevent the spread of infection. Use universal precautions or isolation procedures as indicated for specific patients.
- Because of the risk of arrhythmias and abnormal BP and respiratory responses, use caution during aerobic exercise and other forms of therapeutic exercise. Assess exercise tolerance frequently (BP, heart rate, respiratory function, fatigue levels), and terminate exercise immediately if any untoward responses occur (See Appendix L).

Patient/Client-Related Instruction

- Advise patient to report signs of kidney toxicity, including blood or pus in urine, decreased urine output, weight gain from fluid retention, and fatigue.
- Instruct patient and family/caregivers to report other troublesome side effects such as severe or prolonged headache, sleep loss, chills, fever, or GI problems (nausea, vomiting, diarrhea, abdominal pain).

Pharmacokinetics

Absorption: Not absorbed orally.
Distribution: Extensively distributed to body tissues and fluids. Poor penetration into CSF.
Metabolism and Excretion: Elimination is very prolonged. Detectable in urine up to 7 wk after discontinuation.
Half-life: Biphasic—initial phase, 24–48 hr; terminal phase, 15 days. *Cholesteryl sulfate*—28 hr. *Lipid complex*—174 hr. *Liposomal*—100–153 hr.

TIME/ACTION PROFILE (blood levels)

ROUTE	ONSET	PEAK	DURATION
IV	rapid	end of infusion	24 hr

Contraindications/Precautions

Contraindicated in: Hypersensitivity; Lactation: Potential for distribution into breast milk and toxicity in infant; discontinue nursing.
Use Cautiously in: Renal impairment or electrolyte abnormalities; Patients receiving concurrent leukocyte transfusions (increased risk of pulmonary toxicity); OB: Has been used safely.

Interactions

Drug-Drug: Increased risk of renal toxicity, bronchospasm, and hypotension with **antineoplastics.** Concurrent use with **corticosteroids** ↑ risk of hypokalemia. Concurrent use with **zidovudine** may increase the risk of myelotoxicity and nephrotoxicity. Combined use with **flucytosine** ↑ antifungal activity but may ↑ the risk of toxicity from flucytosine. Combined use with **azole antifungals** may induce fungal resistance. Increased risk of nephrotoxicity with other **nephrotoxic agents** such as **aminoglycosides, cyclosporine,** or **tacrolimus.** Hypokalemia from amphotericin ↑ the risk of **digoxin** toxicity. Hypokalemia may enhance the curariform effects of **neuromuscular blocking agents.**

Route/Dosage

Specific dosage and duration of therapy depend on nature of infection being treated.

Amphotericin Deoxycholate

IV (Adults): Give test dose of 1 mg. If test dose tolerated, initiate therapy with 0.25 mg/kg/day (doses up to 1.5 mg/kg/day may be used, depending on type of infection) (alternate-day dosing may also be used); *Bladder irrigation*—Instill 50 mcg/mL solution into bladder daily for 5–10 days.

IV (Infants and Children): Give test dose of 0.1 mg/kg (maximum dose 1 mg) or may administer initial dose of 0.25–1 mg/kg/day over 6 hr (without test dose) (some infections may require 1.5 mg/kg/day; alternate-day dosing may be used).

Intrathecal (Adults): 25–300 mcg q 48–72 hr, ↑ to 500 mcg—1 mg as tolerated (maximum total dose = 15 mg).

Intrathecal (Children): 25–100 mcg q 48–72 hr; ↑ to 500 mcg as tolerated.

Amphotericin B Cholesteryl Sulfate (Amphotec)

IV (Adults and Children): 3–4 mg/kg q 24 hr (no test dose needed).

Amphotericin B Lipid Complex (Abelcet)

IV (Adults and Children): 5 mg/kg q 24 hr (no test dose needed).

Amphotericin B Liposome (AmBisome)

IV (Adults and Children): *Empiric therapy*— 3 mg/kg q 24 hr; *Documented infections*— 3–5 mg/kg q 24 hr; *Visceral leishmaniasis (immunocompetent patients)*— 3 mg/kg q 24 hr on days 1–5, then 3 mg/kg q 24 hr on days 14 and 21; *Visceral leishmaniasis (immunosuppressed patients)*—4 mg/kg q 24 hr on days 1–5, then 4 mg/kg q 24 hr on days 10, 17, 24, 31, and 38; *Cryptococcal meningitis in HIV patients*—6 mg/kg q 24 hr.

Availability

Amphotericin Deoxycholate
Powder for injection: 50 mg/vial.
Amphotericin B Cholesteryl Sulfate
Powder for injection: 50 mg/vial, 100 mg/vial.
Amphotericin B Lipid Complex
Suspension for injection: 100 mg/20-mL vial.
Amphotericin B Liposome
Powder for injection: 50 mg/vial.

ampicillin (am-pi-sil-in)

Ampicin, Apo-Ampi, Marcillin, Nu-Ampi, Novo-Ampicillin, Omnipen, Penbritin, Principen, Polycillin, Totacillin

Classification
Therapeutic: anti-infectives
Pharmacologic: aminopenicillins

Indications

Treatment of the following infections: Skin and skin structure infections; Soft-tissue infections; Otitis media, Sinusitis; Respiratory infections; Genitourinary infections; Meningitis; Septicemia; Endocarditis prophylaxis. **Unlabeled Use:** Prevention of infection in certain high-risk patients undergoing cesarean section.

Action

Binds to bacterial cell wall, resulting in cell death. **Therapeutic Effects:** Bactericidal action; spectrum is broader than penicillin. **Spectrum:** Active against Streptococci, Nonpenicillinase-producing staphylococci, *Listeria*, Pneumococci, Enterococci, *Haemophilus influenzae*, *Escherichia coli*, *Enterobacter*, *Klebsiella*, *Proteus mirabilis*, *Neisseria meningitidis*, *N. gonorrhoeae*, *Shigella*, *Salmonella*.

Adverse Reactions/Side Effects

CNS: SEIZURES (HIGH DOSES). **GI:** PSEUDOMEMBRANOUS COLITIS, diarrhea, nausea, vomiting. **Derm:** rashes, urticaria. **Hemat:** blood dyscrasias. **Misc:** ALLERGIC REACTIONS, INCLUDING ANAPHYLAXIS AND SERUM SICKNESS, superinfection.

PHYSICAL THERAPY IMPLICATIONS

Examination and Evaluation

- Watch for seizures; notify physician immediately if patient develops or increases seizure activity.
- Monitor signs of pseudomembranous colitis, including diarrhea, abdominal pain, fever, pus or mucus in stool, and other severe or prolonged GI problems (nausea, vomiting, heartburn). Notify physician or nursing staff immediately of these signs.

- Monitor signs of allergic reactions and anaphylaxis, including pulmonary symptoms (tightness in the throat and chest, wheezing, cough dyspnea) or skin reactions (rash, pruritus, urticaria). Notify physician or nursing staff immediately if these reactions occur.
- Assess muscle aches and joint pain (arthralgia) that may be caused by serum sickness. Notify physician if these symptoms seem to be drug related rather than caused by musculoskeletal injury, or if muscle and joint pain are accompanied by allergic-like reactions (fever, rashes, etc.)
- Monitor signs of blood dyscrasias such as eosinophilia (fatigue, weakness, myalgia) and leukopenia (fever, sore throat, signs of infection). Report these signs to the physician.

Interventions

- Always wash hands thoroughly and disinfect equipment (whirlpools, electrotherapeutic devices, treatment tables, and so forth) to help prevent the spread of infection. Use universal precautions or isolation procedures as indicated for specific patients.

Patient/Client-Related Instruction

- Instruct patient to notify physician immediately of signs of superinfection, including black, furry overgrowth on tongue, vaginal itching or discharge, and loose or foul-smelling stools.
- Instruct patient and family/caregivers to report other troublesome side effects such as severe or prolonged skin problems (rash, itching) or GI problems (nausea, vomiting, diarrhea).

Pharmacokinetics

Absorption: Moderately absorbed from the duodenum (30–50%).

Distribution: Diffuses readily into body tissues and fluids. CSF penetration is increased in the presence of inflamed meninges. Crosses the placenta; enters breast milk in small amounts.

Metabolism and Excretion: Variably metabolized by the liver (12–50%). Renal excretion is variable (25–60% after oral dosing; 50–85% after IM administration).

Half-life: Neonates: 1.7–4 hr; Children and Adults: 1–1.5 hr (increased in renal impairment).

TIME/ACTION PROFILE (blood levels)

ROUTE	ONSET	PEAK	DURATION
PO	rapid	1.5–2 hr	4–6 hr
IM	rapid	1 hr	4–6 hr
IV	rapid	end of infusion	4–6 hr

Contraindications/Precautions

Contraindicated in: Hypersensitivity to penicillins.

Use Cautiously in: Severe renal insufficiency (dosage reduction required if CCr <10 mL/min); Infectious mononucleosis, acute lymphocytic leukemia or cytomegalovirus infection (increased incidence of rash); Patients allergic to cephalosporins; OB: Has been used during pregnancy; Lactation: Is distributed into breast milk. Can cause rash, diarrhea, and sensitization in the infant.

Interactions

Drug-Drug: Probenecid decreases renal excretion and increases blood levels of ampicillin—therapy may be combined for this purpose. Large doses may increase the risk of bleeding with **warfarin**. Incidence of rash increases with concurrent **allopurinol** therapy. May decrease the effectiveness of oral **hormonal contraceptives**.

Route/Dosage

Respiratory and Soft-Tissue Infections

PO (Adults and Children ≥20 kg): 250–500 mg q 6 hr.

PO (Children <20 kg): 50–100 mg/kg/day in divided doses q 6–8 hr (not to exceed 2–3 g/day).

IM, IV (Adults and Children ≥40 kg): 500 mg to 3 g q 6 hr (not to exceed 14 g/day).

IM, IV (Children <40 kg): 100–200 mg/kg/day in divided doses q 6–8 hr (not to exceed 12 g/day).

Bacterial Meningitis Caused by *H. influenzae*, *Streptococcus pneumoniae*, Group B streptococcus, or *N. meningitidis* or Septicemia

IM, IV (Adults): 500 mg to 3 g q 6 hr (not to exceed 14 g/day).

IM, IV (Children >1 mo): 200–400 mg/kg/day in divided doses q 6 hr (not to exceed 12 g/day).

IM, IV (Neonates ≤7 days): 200 mg/kg/day divided q 8 hr.

IM, IV (Neonates >7 days): 300 mg/kg/day divided q 6 hr.

GI/GU Infections Other Than *N. gonorrhoeae*

PO (Adults and Children >20 kg): 250–500 mg q 6 hr (larger doses for more serious/chronic infections).

PO (Children ≤20 kg): 50–100 mg/kg/day in divided doses q 6 hr.

N. gonorrhoeae

PO (Adults): 3 g with 1 g probenecid.

IM, IV (Adults and Children ≥40 kg): 500 mg q 6 hr.

IM, IV (Children <40 kg): 100–200 mg/kg/day in divided doses q 6–8 hr.

Urethritis Caused by *N. gonorrhoeae* in Men

IM, IV (Adults and Children ≥40 kg): 500 mg, repeated 8–12 hr later; additional doses may be necessary for more complicated infections (prostatitis, epididymitis).

Prevention of Bacterial Endocarditis

IM, IV (Adults): 2 g 30 min before procedure (gentamicin may be added for high-risk patients); additional 1 g may be given 6 hr later for high-risk patients.

IM, IV (Children): 50 mg/kg (not to exceed 2 g) 30 min before procedure (gentamicin may be added for high-risk patients); additional 25 mg/kg may be given 6 hr later for high-risk patients.

Renal Impairment

(Adults and Children): CCr ≤10 mL/min—Increase dosing interval to q 12 hr.

Availability

Capsules: 250 mg, 500 mg. **Suspension (wild cherry flavor):** 125 mg/5 mL, 250 mg/5 mL. **Powder for injection:** 125 mg, 250 mg, 500 mg, 1 g, 2 g, 10 g.

amyl nitrite (am-il nye-trite)

Classification

Therapeutic: antianginals, antidotes

Pharmacologic: nitrates

Indications

Acute treatment of angina pectoris. **Unlabeled Use:** Acute management of cyanide poisoning. Diagnosis of cardiac murmurs.

Action

Reduces systemic arterial pressure (reduces afterload). Forms methemoglobin, which combines with cyanide, forming a nontoxic compound (cyanmethemoglobin). **Therapeutic Effects:** Relief of angina pectoris. Prevention of fatal outcome in cyanide poisoning.

Adverse Reactions/Side Effects

CNS: headache, restlessness, dizziness, fainting, weakness. **EENT:** ↑ intraocular pressure. **Resp:** shortness of breath. **CV:** hypotension, tachycardia, flushing. **Derm:** cyanosis of lips, fingernails, or palms (indicates methemoglobinemia). **GI:** nausea. **Hemat:** HEMOLYTIC ANEMIA, METHEMOGLOBINEMIA.

PHYSICAL THERAPY IMPLICATIONS

Examination and Evaluation

- Monitor signs of hemolytic anemia (unusual weakness and fatigue, dizziness, jaundice, abdominal pain), or methemoglobinemia (bluish coloring of the skin, lips, fingernails; headache; shortness of breath; lack of energy). Notify physician immediately if these signs occur.
- Assess episodes of angina pectoris at rest and during exercise. Document whether drug therapy is helpful in reducing the frequency and severity of angina attacks.
- Assess dizziness and syncope that might affect gait, balance, and other functional activities (See Appendix C). Some dizziness is expected immediately after administration, but residual balance problems and functional limitations should be reported to the physician and nursing staff, and the patient and family/caregivers should guard against falls and trauma.
- Assess blood pressure periodically, and compare to normal values (See Appendix F). Report low blood pressure (hypotension), especially if patient experiences dizziness, fainting, or other symptoms.
- Assess heart rate, ECG, and heart sounds, especially during exercise (See Appendices G, H). Report fast heart rate (tachycardia) or symptoms of other arrhythmias, including palpitations, chest discomfort, shortness of breath, fainting, and fatigue/weakness.

Interventions

- Design and implement aerobic exercise and endurance-training programs to improve coronary perfusion, reduce angina, and improve myocardial pumping ability.
- Because of an increased risk of angina and arrhythmias, use caution during aerobic exercise and endurance conditioning. Terminate exercise if patient exhibits untoward symptoms (chest pain, shortness of breath, unusual fatigue), or displays other criteria for exercise termination (see Appendix L).
- Avoid physical therapy interventions that cause systemic vasodilation (large whirlpool, Hubbard tank). Additive effects of this drug and these interventions will cause a dangerous fall in blood pressure.
- To minimize hypotension, patient should lie down until after administration, and move slowly when resuming a more upright position after drug effects subside (approximately 10 min).
- Make sure patient brings amyl nitrate ampules to all physical therapy appointments, and that this drug is readily available during exercise and other interventions.

Patient/Client-Related Instruction

- Advise patient to sit or lie down and use medication at first sign of an angina attack. Relief should occur within 1–5 min. If pain is not relieved 5 min after 1 dose, call 911 or go to the nearest emergency room.
- Counsel patients about additional interventions to help control angina and cardiac dysfunction, including regular exercise, weight loss, sodium restriction, stress reduction, moderation of alcohol consumption, and smoking cessation.
- Inform patient that headache is a common side effect, especially after inhalation. Notify health care professional if headache is persistent or severe.
- Instruct patient or family/caregivers to report other troublesome side effects such as severe or prolonged restlessness, vision problems, shortness of breath, or nausea.

Pharmacokinetics

Absorption: Amyl nitrite is well absorbed through nasal mucosa.
Distribution: Widely distributed.
Metabolism and Excretion: Combines to form methemoglobin.
Half-life: Unknown.

TIME/ACTION PROFILE (antianginal)

ROUTE	ONSET	PEAK	DURATION
inhalation	30 sec	unknown	5–10 min

Contraindications/Precautions

Contraindicated in: Hypersensitivity; Patients taking **sildenafil**, **tadalafil**, or **vardenafil**; Severe anemia; Cerebral hemorrhage; Glaucoma; Recent head trauma; Pregnancy and lactation.
Use Cautiously in: Hypotension; Hypovolemia; Constrictive pericarditis or cardiac tamponade; Hyperthyroidism; Recent MI; Hypertrophic cardiomyopathy; Geriatric patients (increased risk of orthostatic hypotension).

Interactions

Drug-Drug: ↑ hypotension with **antihypertensives** or acute ingestion of **alcohol**. Decreases the effects of **norepinephrine**. Antianginal activity decreased by **epinephrine**, and **phenylephrine**.

Route/Dosage

Antianginal

Intranasal, Inhalation (Adults): 1 ampule crushed and inhaled; may be repeated in 3–5 min (1–6 inhalations).

Cyanide Poisoning

Inhalation (Adults and Children): Inhale for 15–30 sec of each minute until sodium nitrite infusion is prepared.

Availability (generic available)

Inhalant (ampules for inhalation): 0.3 mL.

anakinra (a-na-kin-ra)

Kineret

Classification
Therapeutic: antirheumatics (disease-modifying antirheumatic drugs [DMARDs])
Pharmacologic: interleukin antagonists

Indications

Reduction of the signs and symptoms of moderately to severely active rheumatoid arthritis in patients who have failed other DMARDs (may be used in combination with other DMARDs other than tumor necrosis factor [TNF]–blocking agents).

Action

Blocks the destructive effects of interleukin-1 on cartilage and bone resorption by inhibiting its binding at specific tissue receptor sites. **Therapeutic Effects:** Slowed progression of rheumatoid arthritis.
Adverse Reactions/Side Effects CNS: headache. **GI:** diarrhea, nausea. **Hemat:** neutropenia. **Local:** injection site reactions. **Misc:** INFECTIONS, hypersensitivity reactions (rare).

PHYSICAL THERAPY IMPLICATIONS

Examination and Evaluation

- Watch for signs of infection, especially respiratory infections as indicated by fatigue, chills, fever, night sweats, loss of appetite, and pulmonary pathology (persistent cough, coughing up blood, chest pain when breathing and coughing). Report these signs to the physician immediately.
- Although rare, be alert for signs of hypersensitivity reactions, including pulmonary symptoms (tightness in the throat and chest, wheezing, cough, dyspnea) or skin reactions (rash, pruritus, urticaria). Notify physician immediately if these reactions occur.
- Monitor and report signs of neutropenia such as fever, sore throat, and other signs of infection. Periodic blood tests may be needed to monitor WBC and RBC counts.
- If treating arthritic conditions, periodically assess impairments (pain, range of motion), functional ability, and disability to help document whether antirheumatic drug therapy is successful.
- Assess the subcutaneous injection site for pain, swelling, and irritation. Report prolonged or excessive injection-site reactions to the physician.

Interventions

- Implement appropriate manual therapy techniques, physical agents, therapeutic exercises, and orthotic/assistive devices to reduce pain, improve function, and augment the effects of antirheumatic drug therapy.
- Help patients with arthritis explore other nonpharmacologic methods to reduce chronic arthritis pain, such as relaxation techniques, exercise, counseling, and so forth.

Patient/Client-Related Instruction

- Advise patient to guard against infection (frequent hand washing, etc.) and to avoid crowds and contact with persons with contagious diseases.
- Instruct patient to report other troublesome side effects, including severe or prolonged headache or GI problems (diarrhea, nausea).

Pharmacokinetics

Absorption: Well absorbed (95%) following SC administration.
Distribution: Unknown.
Metabolism and Excretion: Unknown.
Half-life: 4–6 hr.

TIME/ACTION PROFILE (clinical response)

ROUTE	ONSET	PEAK	DURATION
SC	within 12 wk	unknown	unknown

Contraindications/Precautions

Contraindicated in: Active infections; Hypersensitivity; Hypersensitivity to other *Escherichia coli*–derived products.
Use Cautiously in: Other chronic debilitating illness; Underlying immunosuppression; Renal impairment; OB/Lactation/Pedi: Safety not established; Geri: May be more sensitive to toxicity due to age-related decline in renal function; increased incidence of infection in geriatric population.
Exercise Extreme Caution in: Concurrent use of TNF-blocking agents such as etanercept (higher risk of serious infections).

Interactions

Drug-Drug: ↑ risk of serious infection with **TNF-blocking agents**, such as **etanercept**. May ↓ antibody response to and increase the risk of adverse reactions from **vaccines**; avoid concurrent administration of **live vaccines**.

Route/Dosage

Subcut (Adults ≥18 yr): 100 mg/day.

Availability

Solution for injection: 100 mg/mL in 1-mL prefilled glass syringes.

anastrazole (a-nass-stra-zole)

Arimidex

Classification
Therapeutic: antineoplastics
Pharmacologic: aromatase inhibitors

Indications

Postmenopausal hormone receptor–positive or unknown, locally advanced, or metastatic breast cancer. Advanced postmenopausal breast cancer in with disease progression despite tamoxifen therapy.

Action

Inhibits the enzyme aromatase, which is partially responsible for conversion of precursors to estrogen.
Therapeutic Effects: Lowers levels of circulating estrogen, which may halt progression of estrogen-sensitive breast cancer.

Adverse Reactions/Side Effects

CNS: <u>headache</u>, <u>weakness</u>, dizziness. **EENT:** pharyngitis. **Resp:** dyspnea, increased cough. **CV:** peripheral edema. **GI:** <u>nausea</u>, abdominal pain, anorexia, constipation, diarrhea, dry mouth, vomiting. **GU:** pelvic pain, vaginal bleeding, vaginal dryness. **Derm:** rash, including mucocutaneous disorders, sweating. **Metab:** weight gain. **MS:** <u>back pain</u>, bone pain. **Neuro:** paresthesia. **Misc:** ALLERGIC REACTIONS, INCLUDING ANGIOEDEMA, URTICARIA, AND ANAPHYLAXIS, <u>hot flashes</u>, <u>pain</u>.

PHYSICAL THERAPY IMPLICATIONS

Examination and Evaluation

- Monitor signs of allergic reactions (angioedema, anaphylaxis, urticaria), including rashes, raised patches of red or white skin (welts), burning/itching skin, swelling in the face, tightness in the throat and chest, wheezing, dry cough, or difficult/labored breathing. Notify physician or nursing staff immediately if these reactions occur.
- Assess peripheral edema using girth measurements, volume displacement, and measurement of pitting edema (See Appendix N). Report increased swelling in feet and ankles or a sudden increase in body weight due to fluid retention.
- Assess any back pain, bone pain, or other musculoskeletal pain. Suggest additional tests (radiography, MRI) as needed to rule out fracture.
- Be alert for signs of paresthesia (numbness, tingling). Establish baseline electroneuromyographic values at the beginning of drug treatment whenever possible, and reexamine these values periodically to document drug-induced changes in peripheral nerve function.
- Assess dizziness that might affect gait, balance, and other functional activities (See Appendix C). Report balance problems and functional limitations to the physician and nursing staff, and caution the patient and family/caregivers to guard against falls and trauma.
- Periodically assess body weight and other anthropometric measures (body mass index, body composition). Report a rapid or unexplained weight gain.

Interventions

- For patients who are medically able to begin exercise, implement appropriate resistive exercises and aerobic training to maintain muscle strength and aerobic capacity during cancer chemotherapy, or to help restore function after chemotherapy.

Patient/Client-Related Instruction

- Advise patient and family/caregivers that fatigue and weakness are likely and may be severe. Functional abilities may be limited, and patient may need to use assistive devices during ambulation.
- Advise patient about the likelihood of GI reactions such as diarrhea, nausea, vomiting, constipation, abdominal pain, and loss of appetite. Instruct patient or family and caregivers to report severe or unexpected GI reactions.
- Advise patient that rashes and other skin reactions (sweating, inflammation of mucous membranes) are likely. Report severe or unexpected skin reactions to the physician.
- Advise women about possible pelvic pain and vaginal dryness or bleeding. Instruct patient to notify physician about any severe or prolonged pelvic or vaginal reactions.
- Instruct patient to report other troublesome side effects such as severe or prolonged headache, cough, difficulty breathing, upper respiratory tract irritation, or hot flashes.

Pharmacokinetics

Absorption: 83–85% absorbed following oral administration.
Distribution: Unknown.
Metabolism and Excretion: 85% metabolized by the liver; 11% excreted renally.
Half-life: 50 hr.

TIME/ACTION PROFILE (lowering of serum estradiol)

ROUTE	ONSET	PEAK	DURATION
PO	within 24 hr	14 days	6 days*

*Following cessation of therapy.

Contraindications/Precautions

Contraindicated in: OB: Potential harm to fetus or spontaneous abortion.
Use Cautiously in: Women with childbearing potential; Lactation/Pedi: Safety not established.

Interactions

Drug-Drug: None significant.

Route/Dosage

PO (Adults): 1 mg daily.

Availability

Tablets: 1 mg.

HIGH ALERT

anesthetics (topical/mucosal)

benzocaine (**ben**-zoe-kane)
Americaine, Americaine Anesthetic Lubricant, Americaine Hemorrhoidal, ✱Baby Orajel, Canker Pain Relief, Children's Chloraseptic Lozenges, ✱Dentocaine, Dent-Zel-Ite, DermaFlex, Endocaine, Hurricaine, Lagol, Lanacane, Orajel Mouth-Aid, Orabase Gel, Medicone, Maximum Strength Anbesol, Mycinettes, Numzident, Num-Zit Lotion, ✱Orajel Liquid, Shield Burnasept Spray, Spec-T Sore Throat Anesthetic

dibucaine (**dye**-byoo-kane)
Nupercainal

dyclonine (**dye**-klon-een)
Sucrets Children's Sore Throat, Dyclone, Sucrets Maximum Strength, Vapor Lemon Sucrets

pramoxine (pra-**mox**-een)
Fleet Relief, ProctoFoam NS, Tronolane, Tronothane

tetracaine (**tet**-ra-kane)
Pontocaine, Viractin

Classification
Therapeutic: anesthetics (topical/local)

Indications

Topical: Relief of pruritus or pain associated with minor skin disorders, including burns, abrasions, bruises, insect stings/bites, dermatitis, hemorrhoids, or other forms of skin irritation. **Mucosal:** Provide local anesthesia to mucosal surfaces before instrumentation, minor procedures, or endoscopy. Decrease irritation caused by minor mouth and throat conditions, including sore throat, gingivitis, stomatitis, or teething. Also used to suppress the gag reflex during endoscopy or intubation.

Action

Inhibit initiation and conduction of sensory nerve impulses. **Therapeutic Effects:** Local anesthesia with subsequent loss of sensation or relief of pain and/or pruritus.

Adverse Reactions/Side Effects

EENT: mucosal use: decreased or absent gag reflex.
Derm: topical use: burning, edema, irritation, stinging, tenderness, urticaria. **Misc:** ALLERGIC REACTIONS, INCLUDING ANAPHYLAXIS.

PHYSICAL THERAPY IMPLICATIONS

Examination and Evaluation

- Monitor signs of allergic reactions and anaphylaxis, including pulmonary symptoms (laryngeal edema, bronchospasm, wheezing, cough, dyspnea) or skin reactions (rash, pruritus, urticaria). Notify physician or nursing staff immediately if these reactions occur.
- When applied topically, assess the site of application and monitor any skin reactions such as tenderness, irritation, burning, swelling, or itching. Report severe or prolonged skin reactions to the physician.

Patient/Client-Related Instruction

- Instruct patient and family/caregivers to use the product as directed, and avoid excessive or unnecessary use.

Pharmacokinetics

Absorption: Benzocaine is poorly absorbed through intact skin. Other agents may be readily absorbed. Degree of absorption increases with surface area; presence of lesions, cuts, or abrasions; and amount of agent applied.
Distribution: Unknown.
Metabolism and Excretion: Ester-type agents (para-aminobenzoic acid [PABA] derivatives, benzocaine, tetracaine) are metabolized by plasma and liver cholinesterases. Small amounts of amide-type agents (dibucaine) that may be absorbed are mostly metabolized by the liver.
Half-life: Unknown.

TIME/ACTION PROFILE (mucosal anesthetic effects)

ROUTE	ONSET	PEAK	DURATION
Benzocaine	about 1 min	unknown	15–20 min
Dibucaine	within 15 min	unknown	2–4 hr
Dyclonine	up to 10 min	unknown	60 min
Pramoxine	3–5 min	unknown	unknown
Tetracaine	3–10 min	unknown	30–60 min

Contraindications/Precautions

Contraindicated in: Hypersensitivity. Cross-sensitivity may occur among related agents (amide types— dibucaine; ester types—benzocaine, tetracaine); Hypersensitivity to any components of preparations, including stabilizers, colorants, or bases; Active, untreated infection of affected area; Not to be used in the eye; Some products contain alcohol and should be avoided in patients with known alcohol intolerance; Pedi: Topical benzocaine products should not be used in children <2 yr.
Use Cautiously in: Debilitated patients; Large or severely abraded areas of skin or mucous membrane; Prolonged use (not recommended); Pedi: Increased risk of systemic toxicity, safety not established for some products; use smaller doses due to potential for methemoglobinemia; Geri: Increased risk of toxicity; use smaller doses.

Interactions

Drug-Drug: Toxicity of ester-type agents may be increased by concurrent use of **cholinesterase inhibitors**.

Route/Dosage

Benzocaine

Topical/Mucosal: (Adults and Children): Apply cream, ointment, topical solutions, or dental/oral products as needed. Lozenges may be used hourly (not to exceed 12 lozenges/day). Rectal products may be used twice daily.

Dibucaine

Topical (Adults and Children): Apply as needed (not to exceed 30 g/day in adults or 7.5 g/day in children). Can be used 3–4 times daily.

Dyclonine

Topical/Mucosal: (Adults): 2- or 3-mg lozenge may be dissolved in the mouth q 2 hr (not to exceed 10 lozenges/day), or solution may be used 4 times daily. *For anesthetizing mucosal surfaces*—up to 300 mg in solution may be used.
Topical/Mucosal: (Children ≥2 yr): 1.2-mg lozenge may be dissolved in mouth q 2 hr (not to exceed 10 lozenges/day).

Pramoxine

Topical/Mucosal: (Adults): Topical products may be used q 3 hr as needed. Rectal products may be used up to 5 times daily.

Tetracaine

Topical/Mucosal: (Adults): Apply cream as needed (not to exceed 28.35 g/day). Topical solutions may be used to anesthetize mucous membranes of the larynx, trachea, or esophagus.

Availability

Benzocaine

Dental gel: 7.5% OTC, 10% OTC, 20% OTC. **Film-forming gel:** 15% OTC. **Lozenges:** 10 mg OTC, 15mg OTC. **Dental ointment:** 20% OTC. **Dental paste:** 20% OTC. **Dental topical solution:** 0.2% OTC, 5% OTC, 20% OTC. **Rectal ointment:** 20% OTC. **Gel:** 20% OTC. **Aerosol:** 20% OTC. **Topical solution:** 20% OTC. ***In combination with:*** menthol (Dermoplast) OTC, butamben and tetracaine (Cetacaine), and phenol OTC. See Appendix B.

Dibucaine

Ointment: 1% OTC. **Rectal ointment:** 1% OTC.

Dyclonine
Lozenges: 1.2 mg OTC, 2 mg OTC, 3 mg OTC. **Topical oral solution:** 0.1% OTC.

Pramoxine
Cream: 1% OTC. **Rectal aerosol foam:** 1% OTC. **Rectal cream:** 1% OTC. **Rectal ointment:** 1% OTC. ***In combination with:*** menthol (PrameGel) OTC. See Appendix B.

Tetracaine
Cream: 1% OTC. **Topical solution:** 2%. **Topical aerosol solution:** 700 mcg/spray butamben and tetracaine (Supracaine) OTC. ***In combination with:*** menthol (Pontocaine Ointment), butamben and benzocaine (Cetacaine). See Appendix B.

anidulafungin
(a-**ni**-du-la-fun-gin)
Eraxis

Classification
Therapeutic: antifungals
Pharmacologic: echinocandins

Indications
Candidemia and other serious candidal infections including intra-abdominal abscess, peritonitis. Esophageal candidiasis.

Action
Inhibits the synthesis of fungal cell wall. **Therapeutic Effects:** Death of susceptible fungi. **Spectrum:** Active against *Candida albicans*, *C. glabrata*, *C. parapsilosis*, and *C. tropicalis*.

Adverse Reactions/Side Effects
Resp: dyspnea. **CV:** hypotension. **GI:** diarrhea, ↑ liver enzymes. **Derm:** flushing, rash, urticaria. **F and E:** hypokalemia.

PHYSICAL THERAPY IMPLICATIONS

Examination and Evaluation
- Assess blood pressure periodically, and compare to normal values (See Appendix F). Report low blood pressure (hypotension), especially if patient experiences dizziness, fatigue, or other symptoms.
- Monitor any muscle weakness, aches, or cramps that might indicate low potassium levels (hypokalemia). Report prolonged or excessive muscle problems to the physician.
- Monitor respiratory function at rest and during exercise. Report difficult or labored breathing (dyspnea) to the physician.

Interventions
- Always wash hands thoroughly and disinfect equipment (whirlpools, electrotherapeutic devices, treatment tables, and so forth) to help prevent the spread of infection. Use universal precautions or isolation procedures as indicated for specific patients.

Patient/Client-Related Instruction
- Instruct patient to report other troublesome side effects such as prolonged or severe diarrhea or skin reactions (rash, hives, itching, flushing).

Pharmacokinetics
Absorption: IV administration results in complete bioavailability.
Distribution: Crosses the placenta.
Metabolism and Excretion: Undergoes chemical degradation without hepatic metabolism; <1% excreted in urine.
Half-life: 40–50 hr.

TIME/ACTION PROFILE (blood levels)

ROUTE	ONSET	PEAK	DURATION
IV	rapid	end of infusion	24 hr

Contraindications/Precautions
Contraindicated in: Hypersensitivity.
Use Cautiously in: Underlying liver disease (may worsen); OB: Pregnancy or lactation (use only if benefits outweigh potential risk; Pedi: Safe use in children not established.

Interactions
Drug-Drug: None noted.

Route/Dosage
IV (Adults): *Esophageal candidiasis*—100 mg loading dose on day 1, then 50 mg daily. *Candidemia and other candidal infections*—200 mg loading dose on day 1, then 100 mg daily.

Availability
Lyophilized powder for IV use (requires reconstitution): 50 mg/vial

apomorphine (a-po-**mor**-feen)
Apokyn

Classification
Therapeutic: antiparkinson agents
Pharmacologic: dopamine agonists

Indications
Acute, intermittent treatment of hypomotility; "off" episodes due to advanced Parkinson's disease.

Action

Stimulation of specific dopamine receptors improves motor function. **Therapeutic Effects:** Improved motor function.

Adverse Reactions/Side Effects

CNS: dizziness, hallucinations, somnolence, confusion, sudden drowsiness, headache. **EENT:** rhinorrhea. **CV:** CARDIAC ARREST, chest pain, hypotension, angina, CHF, QTc prolongation. **GI:** nausea, vomiting. **GU:** priapism. **Derm:** flushing, pallor, sweating. **Local:** injection site pain. **MS:** arthralgia, back pain, limb pain. **Neuro:** aggravation of Parkinson's disease, dyskinesia. **Misc:** yawning.

PHYSICAL THERAPY IMPLICATIONS

Examination and Evaluation

- Be alert for signs of cardiac arrest, and seek immediate medical assistance if the patient collapses, loses consciousness, stops breathing, and lacks a pulse.
- Assess gait and motor function to help document anti-Parkinson effects, especially when treating severe hypomobility or akinetic episodes ("off" periods).
- Document increased side effects such as involuntary movements (dyskinesias) or fluctuations in response (on-off phenomenon, end-of-dose akinesia). Notify physician because increased side effects might require dose adjustment or a change in medication regimen.
- Monitor confusion, hallucinations, and other psychologic problems. Repeated or excessive symptoms may require change in dose or medication.
- Assess blood pressure periodically, and compare to normal values (See Appendix F). Report low blood pressure (hypotension), especially if patient experiences increased dizziness, fainting, or other symptoms.
- Assess signs of congestive heart failure, including dyspnea, rales/crackles, peripheral edema, jugular venous distention, and exercise intolerance. Report these signs to the physician.
- Assess dizziness and drowsiness that might affect gait, balance, and other functional activities (See Appendix C). Report balance problems and functional limitations to the physician and nursing staff, and caution the patient and family/caregivers to guard against falls and trauma.
- Assess any back, joint, or limb pain to rule out musculoskeletal pathology; that is, try to determine if pain is drug induced rather than caused by anatomic or biomechanical problems.
- Monitor injection site for pain, swelling, and irritation. Report prolonged or excessive injection site reactions to the physician.

Interventions

- Implement therapeutic exercises (coordination exercises, gait training, cardiovascular conditioning) to complement the effects of drug therapy and help achieve optimal function.
- Guard against falls and trauma (hip fractures, head injury, and so forth). Implement fall prevention strategies (See Appendix E), especially if patient exhibits Parkinson's symptoms (postural instability, rigidity) combined with drug side effects (dizziness, dyskinesias).
- Because of the risk of cardiac arrest and other cardiac involvement, use extreme caution during aerobic exercise and other forms of therapeutic exercise. Assess exercise tolerance frequently (blood pressure, heart rate, fatigue levels), and terminate exercise immediately if any untoward responses occur (See Appendix L).
- To minimize orthostatic hypotension, patient should move slowly when assuming a more upright position.

Patient/Client-Related Instruction

- Advise patient and family or caregiver about the signs of cardiac arrest (see above under Examination and Evaluation), and to seek immediate medical assistance if these signs develop.
- Advise patient to avoid alcohol because of the increased risk of sedation and adverse effects.
- Instruct patient to report other side effects such as severe or prolonged headache, nasal irritation, painful/prolonged erection (priapism), skin reactions (flushing, pallor, sweating), or GI problems (nausea, vomiting).

Pharmacokinetics

Absorption: Well absorbed (100%) following SC administration.

Distribution: Enters CSF.

Metabolism and Excretion: Unknown.

Half-life: 40 min.

TIME/ACTION PROFILE (blood levels)

ROUTE	ONSET	PEAK	DURATION
SC	rapid	10–60 min	2 hr

Contraindications/Precautions

Contraindicated in: Hypersensitivity to apomorphine or bisulfites; Concurrent use of 5-HT$_3$ antagonists (granisetron, ondansetron, palonosetron, alosetron, dolasetron); Lactation: May appear in human milk; discontinue medication or discontinue breast-feeding.

Use Cautiously in: Hypokalemia, hypomagnesemia, bradycardia, congenital QTc prolongation or concurrent use of drugs causing QTc prolongation (↑ risk of serious arrhythmias); Mild to moderate renal impairment (↓ starting dose); Mild to moderate hepatic impairment; OB: Use only if clearly needed; Pedi: Safety not established; Geri: Increased risk of confusion/ hallucinations, falls, and cardiac, respiratory, and gastrointestinal events.

Exercise Extreme Caution in: Cardiovascular or cerebrovascular disease (may exacerbate condition).

Interactions

Drug-Drug: Profound hypotension, loss of consciousness occurs with **5-HT_3 antagonists.** ↑ risk of hypotension with **alcohol, antihypertensives, vasodilators,** especially **nitrates.**

Route/Dosage

SC (Adults): *Test dose*—0.2 mL (2 mg); with further assessment and monitoring, doses should be titrated at 0.1 mL (1 mg) less than highest tolerated dose. Doses may be increased by 0.1 mL (1 mg) every few days as an outpatient or no more frequently than every 2 hr in a supervised setting. Only single doses should be used during a particular off period. If more than 1 wk passes between doses, titration should be restarted at the 0.2 mL (2 mg) level. Doses should not exceed 0.6 mL (6 mg).

Availability

Solution for injection (contains bisulfites): 10 mg/mL in 2-mL ampules and 3-mL glass cartridges.

arformoterol (ar-for-mo-te-rol)

Brovana

Classification

Therapeutic: bronchodilators
Pharmacologic: adrenergics

Indications

Long-term management of bronchospasm associated with chronic obstructive pulmonary disease (COPD).

Action

Produces accumulation of cyclic adenosine monophosphate (cAMP) at beta-adrenergic receptors, resulting in relaxation of airway smooth muscle. Relatively specific for $beta_2$ (pulmonary) receptors. **Therapeutic Effects:** bronchodilation.

Adverse Reactions/Side Effects

CNS: headache, insomnia, nervousness, weakness. **Resp:** PARADOXICAL BRONCHOSPASM. **CV:** ECG changes, tachycardia. **GI:** vomiting. **Derm:** rash. **F and E:** hypokalemia. **Hemat:** leukocytosis. **MS:** cramps. **Neuro:** tremor. **Misc:** hypersensitivity reactions including anaphylaxis, fever.

PHYSICAL THERAPY IMPLICATIONS

Examination and Evaluation

- Monitor signs of paradoxical bronchospasm (wheezing, cough, dyspnea, tightness in chest and throat), especially at higher or excessive doses. If condition occurs, advise patient to withhold medication and notify physician or other health care professional immediately.
- Assess pulmonary function at rest and during exercise (See Appendices I, J, K) to document effectiveness of medication in controlling bronchospasm.
- Monitor signs of hypersensitivity reactions and anaphylaxis, including pulmonary symptoms (bronchospasm, wheezing, cough, dyspnea) or skin reactions (rash, pruritus, urticaria). Notify physician immediately if these reactions occur.
- Assess heart rate, ECG, and heart sounds, especially during exercise (See Appendices G, H). Report tachycardia or symptoms of other arrhythmias, including palpitations, chest pain, shortness of breath, fainting, and fatigue/weakness.
- Monitor and report signs of CNS toxicity, including nervousness, sleep loss, or tremor. Sustained or severe CNS signs may indicate overdose or excessive use of this drug.
- Monitor and report any muscle weakness, aches, or cramps that might indicate low potassium levels (hypokalemia).

Interventions

- When implementing airway clearance techniques or respiratory muscle training, attempt to intervene when the airway is maximally bronchodilated. Peak responses typically occur 30 min after inhalation.
- Because of the risk of cardiovascular stimulation, use caution during aerobic exercise and endurance conditioning. Cardiac effects should be minimal at lower doses or occasional inhaled use. Cardiovascular effects such as arrhythmias, angina pectoris, or increased BP may occur at higher doses or during excessive use, and are caused by inadvertent stimulation of beta receptors on the heart.

Patient/Client-Related Instruction

- Advise patient to not exceed the recommended dose or frequency of inhalations. Contact physician immediately if bronchospasm is not relieved by medication or is accompanied by diaphoresis, dizziness, or other symptoms.
- Counsel patient on proper use of inhaler; observe use of this device whenever possible to ensure proper technique.
- Instruct patient and family/caregivers to report severe or prolonged headache, fatigue, vomiting, fever, or skin rash.

Pharmacokinetics
Absorption: Some systemic absorption occurs from pulmonary sites.
Distribution: Unknown.
Metabolism and Excretion: Mostly metabolized by the liver 1% excreted unchanged in urine.
Half-life: 26 hr.

TIME/ACTION PROFILE

ROUTE	ONSET	PEAK	DURATION
inhalation	unknown	30 min	12 hr

Contraindications/Precautions
Contraindicated in: Hypersensitivity; Acutely deteriorating COPD (onset of action is delayed); Pedi: Safe use not established; Concurrent use of other long-acting $beta_2$ agonist bronchodilators.
Use Cautiously in: Cardiovascular disorders, including coronary insufficiency, arrhythmias, and hypertension; Hepatic impairment; Geri: Elderly patients may be more sensitive to drug effects; OB: Safe use in pregnancy or lactation not established; use only when maternal benefit outweighs fetal risk, may interfere with uterine motility.

Interactions
Drug-Drug: Concurrent use with **MAO inhibitors**, **tricyclic antidepressants,** or other **agents that may prolong the QTc interval** may result in serious arrhythmias and should be undertaken with extreme caution. ↑ risk of hypokalemia with **theophylline**, **corticosteroids, potassium-losing diuretics. Beta blockers** may ↓ therapeutic effects. ↑ adrenergic effects may occur with concurrent use of **adrenergics.**

Route/Dosage
Inhaln (Adults): 15 mcg twice daily.

Availability
Inhalation solution: 15 mcg/2-mL vial.

argatroban (ar-gat-tro-ban)
Argatroban

Classification
Therapeutic: anticoagulants
Pharmacologic: thrombin inhibitors

Indications
Prophylaxis or treatment of thrombosis in patients with heparin-induced thrombocytopenia. As an anticoagulant in patients with or at risk for heparin-induced thrombocytopenia who are undergoing percutaneous coronary intervention (PCI).

Action
Inhibits thrombin by binding to its receptor sites. Inhibition of thrombin prevents activation of factors V, VIII, and XII; the conversion of fibrinogen to fibrin; platelet adhesion and aggregation. **Therapeutic Effects:** Decreased thrombus formation and extension with decreased sequelae of thrombosis (emboli, postphlebitic syndromes).

Adverse Reactions/Side Effects
CV: hypotension. **GI:** diarrhea, nausea, vomiting. **Hemat:** BLEEDING. **Misc:** ALLERGIC REACTIONS, INCLUDING ANAPHYLAXIS, fever.

PHYSICAL THERAPY IMPLICATIONS

Examination and Evaluation
- Assess for signs of bleeding and hemorrhage (bleeding gums; nosebleed; unusual bruising; black, tarry stools; hematuria; fall in hematocrit or blood pressure). Notify physician or nursing staff immediately if this drug causes excessive anticoagulation.
- Monitor signs of allergic reactions and anaphylaxis, including pulmonary symptoms (tightness in the throat and chest, wheezing, cough, dyspnea) or skin reactions (rash, pruritus, urticaria). Notify physician or nursing staff immediately if these reactions occur.
- Assess blood pressure periodically and compare to normal values (See Appendix F). Report low blood pressure (hypotension), especially if patient experiences dizziness, fatigue, or other symptoms.

Interventions
- Use caution with any physical interventions that could increase bleeding, including wound débridement, chest percussion, joint mobilization, and application of local heat.

Patient/Client-Related Instruction
- Instruct patient to immediately report signs of GI bleeding, including abdominal pain, vomiting blood, blood in stools, or black, tarry stools.
- Instruct patient to report other bothersome side effects such as severe or prolonged fever or GI problems (nausea, vomiting, diarrhea).

Pharmacokinetics
Absorption: IV administration results in complete bioavailability.
Distribution: Unknown.
Metabolism and Excretion: Mostly metabolized by the liver; excreted primarily in feces via biliary excretion. 16% excreted unchanged in urine, 14% excreted unchanged in feces.
Half-life: 39–51 min (increased in hepatic impairment).

TIME/ACTION PROFILE (anticoagulant effect)

ROUTE	ONSET	PEAK	DURATION
IV	immediate	1–3 hr	2–4 hr

Contraindications/Precautions

Contraindicated in: Major bleeding; Hypersensitivity; Lactation.

Use Cautiously in: Hepatic impairment (↓ initial infusion rate recommended); OB: Use only if clearly needed; Pedi: Safety not established in children <18 yr.

Interactions

Drug-Drug: Risk of bleeding may be ↑ by concurrent use of **antiplatelet agents, thrombolytic agents,** or **other anticoagulants.**

Drug-Natural: ↑ bleeding risk with **anise, arnica, chamomile, clove, feverfew, garlic, ginger, ginkgo,** ***Panax ginseng,*** and others.

Route/Dosage

IV (Adults): 2 mcg/kg/min as a continuous infusion; adjust infusion rate on the basis of activated partial thromboplastin time (aPTT). *Patients undergoing PCI*—350 mcg/kg bolus followed by infusion at 25 mcg/kg/min, activated clotting time (ACT) should be assessed 5–10 min later. If ACT is 300–450 sec, procedure may be started. If ACT <300 sec, give additional bolus of 150 mcg/kg and increase infusion rate to 30 mg/kg/min. If ACT is >450 sec. infusion rate should be decreased to 15 mcg/kg/min and ACT rechecked after 5–10 min. If thrombotic complications occur or ACT drops to <300 sec, an additional bolus of 150 mcg/kg may be given and the infusion rate increased to 40 mcg followed by ACT monitoring. If anticoagulation is required after surgery, lower infusion rates should be used.

Hepatic Impairment

IV (Adults): 0.5 mcg/kg/min as a continuous infusion; adjust infusion rate on the basis of aPTT.

Availability

Solution for injection (must be diluted 100-fold): 250 mg/2.5-mL vial.

aripiprazole (a-ri-pip-ra-zole)

Abilify

Classification

Therapeutic: antipsychotics, mood stabilizers

Pharmacologic: dihydrocarbostyril

Indications

Schizophrenia. Acute and maintenance therapy of manic and mixed episodes associated with bipolar disorder (as monotherapy or with lithium or valproate). Adjunct treatment of depression in adults. Agitation associated with schizophrenia or bipolar disorder.

Action

Psychotropic activity may be due to agonist activity at dopamine D_2 and serotonin 5-HT_{1A} receptors and antagonist activity at the 5-HT_{2A} receptor. Also has alpha$_1$-adrenergic blocking activity. **Therapeutic Effects:** Decreased manifestations of schizophrenia; Decreased mania in bipolar patients; Decreased symptoms of depression. Decreased agitation associated with schizophrenia or bipolar disorder.

Adverse Reactions/Side Effects

CNS: akathisia, confusion, depression, drowsiness, extrapyramidal reactions, fatigue, hostility, insomnia, lightheadedness, manic reactions, impaired cognitive function, nervousness, restlessness, seizures, suicidal thoughts, tardive dyskinesia. **Resp:** dyspnea. **CV:** bradycardia, chest pain, edema, hypertension, orthostatic hypotension, tachycardia. **EENT:** blurred vision, conjunctivitis, ear pain. **GI:** constipation, anorexia, ↑ salivation, nausea, vomiting, weight loss. **GU:** urinary incontinence. **Hemat:** anemia. **Derm:** dry skin, ecchymosis, skin ulcer, sweating. **MS:** muscle cramps, neck pain. **Metab:** hyperglycemia. **Neuro:** abnormal gait, tremor. **Misc:** NEUROLEPTIC MALIGNANT SYNDROME, ↓ heat regulation.

PHYSICAL THERAPY IMPLICATIONS

Examination and Evaluation

- Monitor and report signs of neuroleptic malignant syndrome, including hyperthermia, diaphoresis, generalized muscle rigidity, altered mental status, tachycardia, changes in blood pressure (BP), and incontinence. Symptoms typically occur within 4–14 days after initiation of drug therapy, but can occur at any time during drug use.
- Be alert for new seizures or increased seizure activity, especially at the onset of drug treatment. Document the number, duration, and severity of seizures, and report these findings immediately to the physician.
- Assess motor function, and be alert for extrapyramidal symptoms. Report these symptoms immediately, especially tardive dyskinesia, because this problem may be irreversible. Common extrapyramidal symptoms include:
  - Tardive dyskinesia (uncontrolled rhythmic movement of mouth, face, and extremities, lip smacking or puckering, puffing of cheeks, uncontrolled chewing, rapid or worm-like movements of tongue).
  - Pseudoparkinsonism (shuffling gait, rigidity, tremor, pill-rolling motion, loss of balance control, difficulty speaking or swallowing, mask-like face).

- Akathisia (restlessness or desire to keep moving).
- Other dystonias and dyskinesias (dystonic muscle spasms, twisting motions, twitching, inability to move eyes, weakness of arms or legs).

- Be alert for suicidal thoughts and ideology. Notify physician immediately if patient exhibits signs of depression or other changes in mood and behavior such as nervousness, restlessness, hostility, confusion, or manic reactions.
- Assess levels of drowsiness or lightheadedness, especially in older adults. Determine if these side effects might impair gait, balance, and other functional activities.
- Monitor signs of anemia, including unusual fatigue, shortness of breath with exertion, bruising, and pale skin. Notify physician immediately if these signs occur.
- Assess BP, and report a sustained increase in BP (hypertension) or a fall in BP when patient assumes a more upright position (lying to standing, sitting to standing, lying to sitting). Document orthostatic hypotension and contact physician when systolic BP falls >20 mmHg, or diastolic BP falls >10 mm Hg.
- Assess heart rate, ECG, and heart sounds, especially during exercise (See Appendices G, H). Report arrhythmias (tachycardia, bradycardia, others), or symptoms of rhythm disturbances including palpitations, chest discomfort, shortness of breath, fainting, and fatigue/weakness.
- Assess peripheral edema using girth measurements, volume displacement, and measurement of pitting edema (See Appendix N). Report increased swelling in feet and ankles or a sudden increase in body weight due to fluid retention.
- Be alert for signs of hyperglycemia, including confusion, drowsiness, flushed/dry skin, fruit-like breath odor, rapid/deep breathing, polyuria, loss of appetite, and unusual thirst. Patients with diabetes mellitus should check blood glucose levels frequently.
- Assess any muscle cramps, neck pain, tremor, or gait abnormalities. Try to determine if symptoms are drug induced rather than caused by neurologic or musculoskeletal pathology.
- Periodically assess body weight and other anthropometric measures (body mass index, body composition). Report a substantial weight loss or decreased body fat.

Interventions

- Guard against falls and trauma (hip fractures, head injury, and so forth) caused by drowsiness, dizziness, blurred vision, or extrapyramidal symptoms; implement fall- prevention strategies (See Appendix E).
- Because of the risk of arrhythmias and abnormal BP responses, use caution during aerobic exercise and other forms of therapeutic exercise. Assess exercise tolerance frequently (BP, heart rate, fatigue levels), and terminate exercise immediately if any untoward responses occur (See Appendix L).
- To minimize orthostatic hypotension, patient should move slowly when assuming a more upright position.
- This drug impairs body temperature regulation; use care during exercise and during other activities that increase body temperature (hot whirlpools, saunas, and so forth).
- Help patient and family/caregivers explore nonpharmacologic methods (exercise, counseling, support groups, and so forth) to reduce schizophrenic episodes and mood disorders.

Patient/Client-Related Instruction

- Advise patient to avoid alcohol and other CNS depressants because of the increased risk of sedation and adverse effects.
- Instruct patient to report other problematic side effects such as severe or prolonged ear pain, blurred vision, eye inflammation, labored breathing, urinary incontinence, skin reactions (sweating, ulceration, bruising, dry skin), or GI problems (constipation, nausea, vomiting, appetite loss).

Pharmacokinetics

Absorption: Well absorbed (87%) following oral administration; 100% following IM injection.
Distribution: Extensive extravascular distribution.
Protein Binding: *aripiprazole and dehydro-aripiprazole*—>99%.
Metabolism and Excretion: Mostly metabolized by the liver (CYP3A4 and CYP2D6 enzymes); one metabolite (dehydro-aripiprazole) has antipsychotic activity. 18% excreted unchanged in feces; <1% excreted unchanged in urine. A small percentage of patients are poor metabolizers and may need smaller doses.
Half-life: *Aripiprazole*—75 hr; *dehydro-aripiprazole—94 hr.*

TIME/ACTION PROFILE (antipsychotic effect)

ROUTE	ONSET	PEAK	DURATION
PO	unknown	2 wk	unknown
IM	unknown	1–3 hr	unknown

Contraindications/Precautions

Contraindicated in: Hypersensitivity; Lactation: Presumed to be excreted in breast milk; discontinue drug or bottle feed.

Use Cautiously in: Known cardiovascular or cerebrovascular disease; Conditions which cause hypotension (dehydration, treatment with antihypertensives or diuretics); Diabetes (may ↑ risk of hyperglycemia); Seizure disorders; Patients at risk for aspiration pneumonia; Concurrent ketoconazole or other potential CYP3A4 inhibitors (reduce aripiprazole dose by 50%); Concurrent quinidine, fluoxetine, paroxetine, or other potential CYP2D6 inhibitors; Concurrent carbamazepine or other potential CYP3A4 inducers; OB: Use only if benefit outweighs risk to fetus; Pedi: May ↑ risk of suicide attempt/ideation, especially during dose early treatment or dose adjustment; risk may be greater in children, adolescents, and young adults taking antidepressants (safe use in children/adolescents not established); Geri: ↑ risk of mortality in elderly patients treated for dementia-related psychosis.

Interactions

Drug-Drug: Ketoconazole or **other potential CYP3A4 inhibitors** decrease metabolism and increase effects (reduce aripiprazole dose by 50%). **Quinidine, fluoxetine, paroxetine,** or **other potential CYP2D6 inhibitors** decrease metabolism and increase effects (reduce aripiprazole dose by at least 50%). Concurrent **carbamazepine** or **other potential CYP3A4 inducers** (double aripiprazole dose; then decrease to 10–15 mg/day when interfering drug is withdrawn).

Route/Dosage

Schizophrenia

PO (Adults): 10 or 15 mg daily; doses up to 30 mg/day have been used; increments in dosing should not be made before 2 wk at a given dose.

PO (Children 13–17 yr): 2 mg daily; ↑ to 5 mg daily after 2 days, and then to target dose of 10 mg daily after another 2 days; may further ↑ dose in 5-mg increments if needed (max: 30 mg/day).

Bipolar mania

PO (Adults): 15 mg daily as monotherapy or with lithium or valproate; may ↑ to 30 mg daily, based on response.

PO (Children 10–17 yr): 2 mg daily; ↑ to 5 mg daily after 2 days, and then to target dose of 10 mg daily after another 2 days; may further ↑ dose in 5-mg increments if needed (max: 30 mg/day).

Depression

PO (Adults): 2–5 mg daily, may titrate upward at 1-wk intervals to 5–10 mg daily; not to exceed 15 mg/day.

Agitation Associated with Schizophrenia or Bipolar Disorder

IM (Adults): 9.75 mg/day, may use a dose of 5.25 mg based on clinical situation. May give additional doses up to a cumulative dose of 30 mg/day, if needed.

Availability

Tablets: 2 mg, 5 mg, 10 mg, 15 mg, 20 mg, 30 mg. **Tablets, orally disintegrating:** 10 mg, 15 mg. **Oral solution (orange cream):** 1 mg/mL. **Injection:** 7.5 mg/mL in ready-to-use vials.

armodafinil (ar-mo-daf-i-nil)

Nuvigil

Classification

Therapeutic: central nervous system stimulants

Schedule IV

Indications

To improve wakefulness in patients with excessive daytime drowsiness due to narcolepsy, obstructive sleep apnea/hypopnea syndrome, and shift work disorder.

Action

Produces CNS stimulation. **Therapeutic Effects:** Improved wakefulness.

Adverse Reactions/Side Effects

CNS: dizziness, headache, insomnia, anxiety, psychiatric reactions. **CV:** ↑ blood pressure. **GI:** nausea, dry mouth. **Derm:** STEVENS-JOHNSON SYNDROME, rash. **Misc:** MULTIORGAN HYPERSENSITIVITY, ALLERGIC REACTIONS, INCLUDING ANAPHYLACTOID REACTIONS AND ANGIOEDEMA.

PHYSICAL THERAPY IMPLICATIONS

Examination and Evaluation

- Monitor signs of allergic reactions, including anaphylaxis and angioedema. Signs include pulmonary symptoms (tightness in the throat and chest, wheezing, cough, dyspnea) and skin reactions (rash, pruritus, urticaria, swelling in the face, dermatitis, exfoliation). Be especially alert for skin reactions because certain skin reactions may indicate serious hypersensitivity reactions (Stevens-Johnson syndrome). Notify physician or nursing staff immediately if these reactions occur.
- Monitor alertness in patients with narcolepsy; document the frequency and duration of sleeping episodes to help assess the effects of drug therapy.
- Be alert for signs of CNS excitation, including sleep loss, anxiety, and other psychiatric reactions. Report these signs to the physician.
- Assess blood pressure and compare to normal values (See Appendix F). Report a sustained increase in blood pressure (BP) (hypertension).

Patient/Client-Related Instruction

- Instruct patient and family/caregivers to report other troublesome side effects, including severe or prolonged nausea or dry mouth.

Pharmacokinetics

Absorption: Readily absorbed following oral administration.
Distribution: Unknown.
Metabolism and Excretion: Mostly metabolized (partially by the CYP3A4 enzyme system; <10% excreted in urine).
Half-life: 15 hr.

TIME/ACTION PROFILE (blood levels)

ROUTE	ONSET	PEAK	DURATION
PO	unknown	2 hr	unknown

Contraindications/Precautions

Contraindicated in: Hypersensitivity to modafinil or armodafinil.
Use Cautiously in: Concurrent alcohol ingestion; History of drug abuse, especially history of stimulant abuse; Severe hepatic impairment (↓ dose recom mended); Recent MI or unstable angina; Geri: Blood levels may by ↑ due to ↓ clearance (lower dose may be necessary); Pedi: Safety and efficacy not established for children <17 yr.

Interactions

Drug-Drug: Since armodafinil is partially metabolized by the CPY3A4 enzyme system, concurrent use of **drugs that induce the CYP3A system**, including **carbamazepine**, **phenobarbital**, and **rifampin**, may ↓ levels and effectiveness. Concurrent use of **drugs that inhibit the CYP3A system**, including **ketonazole** and **erythromycin**, may ↑ levels and effectiveness. Armodafinil also induces the CYP3A system and may ↓ effectiveness of **hormonal contraceptives** (additional or alternative methods recommended), **cyclosporine** (dosage adjustment may be necessary), **midazolam** and **triazolam** (excess sedation may occur, dose reduction may be necessary). Armodafinil also inhibits the CYP2C19 system and may ↑ effects of **phenytoin**, **diazepam**, **propranolol**, **omeprazole**, and **clomipramine** (dose reduction and monitoring for toxicity recommended). Use cautiously with **MAO inhibitors** and other **CNS stimulants**.

Route/Dosage

Obstructive Sleep Apnea/Hypopnea Syndrome and Narcolepsy

PO (Adults): *Obstructive Sleep Apnea/Hypopnea Syndrome and Narcolepsy*—150 mg or 150 mg once daily in the morning; *Shift Work Sleep Disorder*—150 mg once daily one hour before start of work.

Availability

Tablets: 50 mg, 150 mg, 250 mg.

HIGH ALERT

arsenic trioxide

(ar-sen-ik trye-**ox**-ide)

Trisenox

Classification

Therapeutic: antineoplastics

Pharmacologic: heavy metals

Indications

Induction of remission and consolidation in patients with acute promyelocytic leukemia (APL) who do not respond to or tolerate retinoid and anthracycline chemotherapy and whose disease is associated with the presence of the t(15; 17) translocation or PML/RAR-alpha gene expression.

Action

Alters DNA and fusion proteins in leukemic cells.
Therapeutic Effects: Improved hematologic parameters in patients with APL.

Adverse Reactions/Side Effects

CNS: fatigue, headache, insomnia, weakness. **Resp:** hypoxia, dyspnea, pleural effusion. **CV:** QT PROLONGATION, COMPLETE AV BLOCK, atrial arrhythmias. **GI:** abdominal pain, constipation, increase liver enzymes. **GU:** renal failure. **Derm:** dermatitis. **Endo:** hyperglycemia, hypoglycemia. **F and E:** acidosis, hypocalcemia, hyperkalemia, hypokalemia, hypomagnesemia. **Hemat:** NEUTROPENIA, APL DIFFERENTIATION SYNDROME, DISSEMINATED INTRAVASCULAR COAGULATION, THROMBOCYTOPENIA, hyperleukocytosis, anemia, leukocytosis. **MS:** back pain, arthralgia, bone pain, neck pain, limb pain, myalgia. **Misc:** allergic reactions, fever, infection/sepsis.

PHYSICAL THERAPY IMPLICATIONS

Examination and Evaluation

- Assess heart rate, ECG, and heart sounds, especially during exercise (See Appendices G, H). Report any rhythm disturbances or symptoms of increased arrhythmias, including palpitations, chest discomfort, shortness of breath, fainting, and fatigue/weakness.
- Be alert for signs of neutropenia (fever, sore throat, signs of infection), thrombocytopenia (bruising, nose bleeds, bleeding gums), disseminated intravascular coagulation (excessive bleeding from surgical wounds or hemorrhage from the mouth, nose rectum, vagina), or unusual weakness and

fatigue that might be due to other anemias or leukemias, including acute promyelocytic leukemia (APL) differentiation syndrome. Report these signs to the physician or nursing staff immediately.

- Assess any breathing problems or signs of pleural effusion (chest pain, cough, shortness of breath, rapid shallow breathing) or hypoxia (pale or blue skin, confusion, fatigue, headache). Monitor pulse oximetry and perform pulmonary function tests (See Appendices I, J, K) to quantify suspected changes in ventilation and respiratory function.
- Monitor signs of allergic reactions, including pulmonary symptoms (tightness in the throat and chest, wheezing, cough, dyspnea) or skin reactions (rash, pruritus, urticaria). Notify physician or nursing staff immediately if these reactions occur.
- Monitor signs of renal failure, including decreased urine output, increased blood pressure, muscle cramps/twitching, edema/weight gain from fluid retention, yellowish brown skin, and confusion that progresses to seizures and coma. Report these signs to the physician immediately.
- Monitor neuromuscular signs of acid-base or electrolyte imbalances (acidosis, hypocalcemia, hypokalemia), including lethargy, weakness, cramping, and muscle hyperexcitability and tetany. Notify physician immediately if these signs occur.
- Monitor signs of hypoglycemia (weakness, malaise, irritability, fatigue) or hyperglycemia (drowsiness, fruity breath, increased urination, unusual thirst). Patients with diabetes mellitus should check blood glucose levels frequently.
- Assess any muscle, joint, or bone pain to rule out musculoskeletal pathology; that is, try to determine if pain is drug induced rather than caused by anatomic or biomechanical problems.

Interventions

- For patients who are medically able to begin exercise, implement appropriate resistive exercises and aerobic training to maintain muscle strength and aerobic capacity during cancer chemotherapy, or to help restore function after chemotherapy.
- Because of potential cardiac arrhythmias, blood dyscrasias, and pulmonary problems, use caution during aerobic exercise and endurance conditioning Terminate exercise if patient exhibits untoward symptoms (chest pain, shortness of breath, etc.), or displays other criteria for exercise termination (See Appendix L).

Patient/Client-Related Instruction

- Advise patient to guard against infection (frequent hand washing, etc.) and avoid crowds and contact with persons with contagious diseases.
- Advise patient and family/caregivers that fatigue and weakness are likely and may be severe. Functional abilities may be limited, and patient may need to use assistive devices during ambulation.
- Instruct patient or family/caregivers to report other bothersome side effects such as severe or prolonged headache, fever, sleep loss, dermatitis, or GI problems (constipation, abdominal pain).

Pharmacokinetics

Absorption: IV administration results in complete bioavailability.
Distribution: Arsenic is stored in liver, kidney, heart, lung, hair, and nails.
Metabolism and Excretion: Converted from pentavalent arsenic to trivalent arsenic by arsenate reductase and further concerted by methyltransferases in the liver. Methylated arsenic is excreted in urine.
Half-life: Unknown.

TIME/ACTION PROFILE (effect on hematologic parameters)

ROUTE	ONSET	PEAK	DURATION
IV	unknown	unknown	unknown

Contraindications/Precautions

Contraindicated in: Hypersensitivity to arsenic; OB: Can cause fetal injury; Lactation: Excreted in breast milk.
Use Cautiously in: Renal impairment.
Exercise Extreme Caution in: Preexisting electrolyte abnormalities (correct prior to administration); Concurrent use of drugs known to prolong QT interval; Concurrent use of potassium-wasting diuretics or amphotericin; Pedi: Safety not established in children <5 yr.

Interactions

Drug-Drug: Use cautiously with other agents known to cause QT prolongation, including some **antiarrhythmics** or **thioridazine**. Concurrent use of amphotericin B, potassium- or magnesium-wasting diuretics (increased risk of serious arrhythmias).

Route/Dosage

IV (Adults and Children ≥5 yr): *Induction*—0.15 mg/kg/day until bone marrow remission (not to exceed 60 doses); *consolidation*—starting 3–6 wk after completion of induction; 0.15 mg/kg/day for 25 doses over a period of 5 wk.

Availability

Solution for injection: 10/10-mL single-use ampules.

A

HIGH ALERT

asparaginase (a-spare-a-ji-nase)
Elspar, ✱Kidrolase

Classification
Therapeutic: antineoplastics
Pharmacologic: enzymes

Indications

Part of combination chemotherapy in the treatment of acute lymphocytic leukemia (ALL).

Action

Catalyst in the conversion of asparagine (an amino acid) to aspartic acid and ammonia. Depletes asparagine in leukemic cells. **Therapeutic Effects:** Death of leukemic cells.

Adverse Reactions/Side Effects

CNS: SEIZURES, agitation, coma, confusion, depression, dizziness, fatigue, hallucinations, headache, irritability, somnolence. **GI:** nausea, vomiting, anorexia, cramps, hepatotoxicity, pancreatitis, weight loss. **Derm:** rashes, urticaria. **Endo:** hyperglycemia. **Hemat:** coagulation abnormalities, transient bone marrow depression. **Metab:** hyperammonemia, hyperuricemia. **Misc:** HYPERSENSITIVITY REACTIONS, INCLUDING ANAPHYLAXIS.

PHYSICAL THERAPY IMPLICATIONS

Examination and Evaluation

- Monitor signs of hypersensitivity reactions or anaphylaxis, including pulmonary symptoms (tightness in the throat and chest, wheezing, cough, dyspnea) or skin reactions (rash, pruritus, urticaria). Notify physician or nursing staff immediately if these reactions occur.
- Be alert for new seizures or increased seizure activity, especially at the onset of drug treatment. Document the number, duration, and severity of seizures, and report these findings immediately to the physician.
- Watch for other signs of neurotoxicity or neurologic signs of increased ammonia levels (hyperammonemia), including agitation, confusion, headache, dizziness, mood changes, decreased alertness, and hallucinations. Notify physician if these signs occur.
- Report any abnormal bruising or bleeding or signs of bone marrow depression, including leukopenia (fever, sore throat, signs of infection), thrombocytopenia (nose bleeds, bleeding gums), or unusual weakness and fatigue that might be due to anemia.
- Be alert for signs of hyperglycemia, including confusion, drowsiness, flushed/dry skin, fruit-like breath odor, rapid/deep breathing, polyuria, loss of appetite, and unusual thirst. Patients with diabetes mellitus should check blood glucose levels frequently.
- Periodically assess body weight and report a rapid or unexplained weight loss.

Interventions

- For patients who are medically able to begin exercise, implement appropriate resistive exercises and aerobic training to maintain muscle strength and aerobic capacity during cancer chemotherapy or to help restore function after chemotherapy.

Patient/Client-Related Instruction

- Advise patient to guard against infection (frequent hand washing, etc.) and avoid crowds and contact with persons with contagious diseases.
- Advise patient and family/caregivers that fatigue and weakness are likely and may be severe. Functional abilities may be limited, and patient may need to use assistive devices during ambulation.
- Advise patient that rashes and other skin reactions are likely and to report severe or unexpected skin reactions to the physician.
- Advise patient about the likelihood of GI reactions such as nausea, vomiting, cramps, and abdominal pain. Instruct patient to report severe or prolonged GI problems, signs of liver toxicity (yellow skin or eyes, abdominal pain, severe nausea and vomiting, fever, sore throat, malaise, weakness, facial edema), or pancreatitis (upper abdominal pain after eating, indigestion, weight loss, oily stools).

Pharmacokinetics

Absorption: Is absorbed from IM sites.
Distribution: Remains in the intravascular space. Poor penetration into the CSF.
Metabolism and Excretion: Slowly sequestered in the reticuloendothelial system.
Half-life: IV: 8–30 hr; IM: 39–49 hr.

TIME/ACTION PROFILE (depletion of asparagine)

ROUTE	ONSET	PEAK†	DURATION
IM	immediate	14–24 hr	23–33 days
IV	immediate	unknown	23–33 days

†Plasma levels of asparaginase

Contraindications/Precautions

Contraindicated in: Previous hypersensitivity; Lactation: May cause unwanted effects in the nursing infant.
Use Cautiously in: History of hypersensitivity reactions; Severe liver disease; Renal or pancreatic disease; CNS depression; Clotting abnormalities; Chronic debilitating illnesses; OB: Use only if the potential benefit justifies the potential risk to the fetus.

Interactions

Drug-Drug: May negate the antineoplastic activity of **methotrexate**. May enhance the hepatotoxicity of other **hepatotoxic drugs**. Concurrent IV use with or immediately preceding **vincristine** and **prednisone** may result in ↑ neurotoxicity and hyperglycemia. May alter the response to **live vaccines** (↓ antibody response, ↑ risk of adverse reactions).

Route/Dosage

Various other regimens may be used.

Multiple-Agent Induction Regimen (in Combination with Vincristine and Prednisone)

IV (Children): 1000 IU/kg/day for 10 successive days beginning on day 22 of regimen.
IM (Children): 6000 IU/m^2 on days 4, 7, 10, 13, 16, 19, 22, 25, 28.

Single-Agent Therapy for Acute Lymphocytic Leukemia

IV (Adults and Children): 200 IU/kg daily for 28 days.

Desensitization Regimen

IV (Adults and Children): Administer 1 IU, then double dose every 10 min until total dose for that day has been given or reaction occurs.

Test Dose

Intradermal (Adults and Children): 2 IU.

Availability

Injection: 10,000-IU vial (with mannitol).

aspirin (as-pir-in)

Acuprin, *Apo-ASA, *Apo-ASEN, *Arthrinol, *Arthrisin, *Artria S.R, ASA, Aspergum, Aspir-Low, Aspirtab, *Astrin, Bayer Aspirin, Bayer Timed-Release Arthritic Pain Formula, *Coryphen, Easprin, Ecotrin, 8-Hour Bayer Timed-Release, Empirin, *Entrophen, Halfprin, *Headache Tablets, Healthprin, Norwich Aspirin, *Novasen, *PMS-ASA, Sloprin, St. Joseph Adult Chewable Aspirin, Therapy Bayer, ZORprin

Other Names:
Acetylsalicylic acid

Classification
Therapeutic: antipyretics, nonopioid analgesics
Pharmacologic: salicylates

Indications

Inflammatory disorders, including Rheumatoid arthritis, Osteoarthritis. Mild-to-moderate pain. Fever. Prophylaxis of transient ischemic attacks and MI. **Unlabeled Use:** Adjunctive treatment of Kawasaki's disease.

Action

Produce analgesia and reduce inflammation and fever by inhibiting the production of prostaglandins. Decreases platelet aggregation. **Therapeutic Effects:** Analgesia. Reduction of inflammation. Reduction of fever. Decreased incidence of transient ischemic attacks and MI.

Adverse Reactions/Side Effects

EENT: tinnitus. **GI:** GI BLEEDING, dyspepsia, epigastric distress, nausea, abdominal pain, anorexia, hepatotoxicity, vomiting. **Hemat:** anemia, hemolysis. **Derm:** rash, urticaria. **Misc:** ALLERGIC REACTIONS, INCLUDING ANAPHYLAXIS AND LARYNGEAL EDEMA.

PHYSICAL THERAPY IMPLICATIONS

Examination and Evaluation

- Monitor signs of allergic reactions and anaphylaxis, including pulmonary symptoms (laryngeal edema, wheezing, cough, dyspnea) or skin reactions (rash, pruritus, urticaria). Notify physician immediately if these reactions occur. Allergic reactions are more common in people with asthma, nasal polyps, or aspirin-induced allergies.
- Be alert for signs of GI bleeding, including abdominal pain, vomiting blood, blood in stools, or black, tarry stools. Report these signs to the physician immediately.
- Watch for signs of hemolysis and anemia, including unusual fatigue, shortness of breath, dizziness, headache, coldness in your hands and feet, pale skin, and chest pain. Report these signs to the physician.
- Assess pain and other variables (range of motion, muscle strength) to document whether this drug is successful in helping manage the patient's pain and decreasing impairments.
- Assess blood pressure periodically and compare to normal values (See Appendix F). Aspirin and other NSAIDs can increase blood pressure (BP) in certain patients.

Interventions

- Implement appropriate manual therapy techniques, physical agents, and therapeutic exercises to reduce pain and decrease the need for aspirin and other NSAIDs.
- Use caution with any physical interventions that could increase bleeding, including wound débridement, chest percussion, joint mobilization, and application of local heat.
- Help patient explore other nonpharmacologic methods to reduce chronic pain, such as relaxation techniques, exercise, counseling, and so forth.
- If used to prevent myocardial infarction or transient ischemic attacks, use caution during aerobic exercise

and other forms of therapeutic exercise. Assess exercise tolerance frequently (BP, heart rate, fatigue levels), and terminate exercise immediately if any untoward responses occur (See Appendix L).

Patient/Client-Related Instruction

- Advise patient that analgesics are usually more effective if given before pain becomes severe; emphasize that adequate pain control will allow better participation in physical therapy.
- Advise patient about the risks of gastric irritation. Instruct patient to notify health care professional of severe or prolonged GI effects such as nausea, vomiting, abdominal pain, indigestion, and heartburn.
- Advise patient to reduce alcohol intake because alcohol increases the risk of gastric toxicity.
- Instruct patient to report signs of liver dysfunction, including anorexia, abdominal pain, severe nausea and vomiting, yellow skin or eyes, skin rashes, flu-like symptoms, and muscle/joint pain.
- Inform patient that aspirin and other NSAIDs may impair bone and cartilage healing. Advise patient to consult physician about aspirin use, especially after fractures, spinal fusion, and other bone surgeries.
- Instruct patient to report excessive or prolonged headache or ringing/buzzing in the ears (tinnitus); these signs may indicate aspirin toxicity.
- Caution patient about the use of over-the-counter products that contain aspirin, other NSAIDs, or acetaminophen while taking high doses of aspirin. Use of multiple NSAIDs increases the risk of toxicity and overdose.

Pharmacokinetics

Absorption: Well absorbed from the upper small intestine; absorption from enteric-coated preparations may be unreliable; rectal absorption is slow and variable.
Distribution: Rapidly and widely distributed; crosses the placenta and enters breast milk.
Metabolism and Excretion: Extensively metabolized by the liver; inactive metabolites excreted by the kidneys. Amount excreted unchanged by the kidneys depends on urine pH; as pH increases, amount excreted unchanged increases from 2–3% up to 80%.
Half-life: 2–3 hr for low doses; up to 15–30 hr with larger doses because of saturation of liver metabolism.

TIME/ACTION PROFILE (analgesia/fever reduction)

ROUTE	ONSET	PEAK	DURATION
PO	5–30 min	1–3 hr	3–6 hr

Contraindications/Precautions

Contraindicated in: Hypersensitivity to aspirin or other salicylates; Cross-sensitivity with other NSAIDs may exist (less with nonaspirin salicylates); Bleeding disorders or thrombocytopenia; Pedi: May increase risk of Reye's syndrome in children or adolescents with viral infections.
Use Cautiously in: History of GI bleeding or ulcer disease; Chronic alcohol use/abuse; Severe hepatic or renal disease; OB: Salicylates may have adverse effects on fetus and mother and should be avoided during pregnancy, especially during the 3rd trimester; Lactation: Safety not established; Geri: ↑ risk of adverse reactions, especially GI bleeding; More sensitive to toxic levels.

Interactions

Drug-Drug: May ↑ the risk of bleeding with **warfarin, heparin, heparin-like agents, thrombolytic agents, dipyridamole, ticlopidine, clopidogrel, tirofiban**, or **eptifibatide**, although these agents are frequently used safely in combination and in sequence. **Ibuprofen:** may negate the cardioprotective antiplatelet effects of low-dose aspirin. May ↑ risk of bleeding with **cefoperazone, cefotetan**, and **valproic acid**. May ↑ activity of **penicillins, phenytoin, methotrexate, valproic acid, oral hypoglycemic agents**, and **sulfonamides**. May ↓ beneficial effects of **sulfinpyrazone**. **Urinary acidification** ↑ reabsorption and may ↑ serum salicylate levels. **Alkalinization of the urine** or the ingestion of large amounts of **antacids** ↑ excretion and ↓ serum salicylate levels. May blunt the therapeutic response to **diuretics** and **ACE inhibitors**. ↑ risk of GI irritation with **NSAIDs**.
Drug-Natural: ↑ anticoagulant effect and bleeding risk with **arnica, chamomile, clove, feverfew, garlic, ginger, ginkgo, *Panax ginseng***, and others.
Drug-Food: Foods capable of acidifying the urine (See Appendix L) may ↑ serum salicylate levels.

Route/Dosage

Pain/Fever

PO, Rect (Adults): 325–1000 mg q 4–6 hr (not to exceed 4 g/day). *Extended-release tablets*—650 mg q 8 hr or 800 mg q 12 hr.
PO, Rectal (Children 2–11 yr): 10–15 mg/kg/dose q 4–6 hr; maximum dose: 4 g/day.

Inflammation

PO (Adults): 2.4 g/day initially; increased to maintenance dose of 3.6–5.4 g/day in divided doses (up to 7.8 g/day for acute rheumatic fever).
PO (Children): 60–100 mg/kg/day in divided doses (up to 130 mg/kg/day for acute rheumatic fever).

Prevention of Transient Ischemic Attacks

PO (Adults): 50–325 mg once daily.

Prevention of Myocardial Infarction/Antiplatelet effects

PO (Adults): 80–325 mg once daily. *Suspected acute MI*—160 mg as soon as MI is suspected.

PO (Children): 3–10 mg/kg/day given once daily (round dose to a convenient amount).

Kawasaki's Disease

PO (Children): 80–100 mg/kg/day in 4 divided doses until fever resolves; may be followed by maintenance dose of 3–5 mg/kg/day as a single dose for up to 8 wk.

Availability (generic available)

Tablets: 81 mg OTC, 162.5 mg OTC, 325 mg OTC, 500 mg OTC, 650 mg OTC, 975 mg OTC. **Chewable tablets:** 80 mg OTC, 81 mg OTC. **Chewing gum:** 227 mg OTC. **Dispersible tablets:** 325 mg OTC, 500 mg OTC. **Enteric-coated (delayed-release) tablets:** 80 mg OTC, 165 mg OTC, 300 mg OTC, 325 mg OTC, 500 mg OTC, 600 mg OTC, 650 mg OTC, 975 mg OTC. **Extended-release tablets:** 325 mg OTC, 650 mg OTC, 800 mg. **Delayed-release capsules:** 325 mg OTC, 500 mg OTC. **Suppositories:** 60 mg OTC, 120 mg OTC, 125 mg OTC, 130 mg OTC, 150 mg OTC, 160 mg OTC, 195 mg OTC, 200 mg OTC, 300 mg OTC, 320 mg OTC, 325 mg OTC, 600 mg OTC, 640 mg OTC, 650 mg OTC, 1.2 g OTC. ***In combination with:*** antihistamines, decongestants, cough suppressants OTC, and opioids. See Appendix B.

atazanavir (a-ta-zan-a-vir)

Reyataz

Classification

Therapeutic: antiretrovirals

Pharmacologic: protease inhibitors

Indications

HIV infection (with other antiretrovirals).

Action

Inhibits the action of HIV protease, preventing maturation of virions. **Therapeutic Effects:** ↑ CD4 cell counts and ↓ viral load with subsequent slowed progression of HIV and its sequelae.

Adverse Reactions/Side Effects

When used in combination with other antiretrovirals

CNS: headache, depression, dizziness, insomnia. **CV:** ↑ PR interval, heart block. **GI:** nausea, abdominal pain, ↑ bilirubin, cholelithiasis, diarrhea, jaundice, vomiting, ↑ transaminases. **Derm:** rash. **Endo:** hyperglycemia. **Metab:** fat redistribution. **MS:** myalgia. **Misc:** fever.

PHYSICAL THERAPY IMPLICATIONS

Examination and Evaluation

- Assess heart rate, ECG, and heart sounds, especially during exercise (See Appendices G, H). Report any rhythm disturbances or symptoms of increased arrhythmias or heart block, including palpitations, chest discomfort, shortness of breath, fainting, and fatigue/weakness.
- Assess any muscle pain to rule out musculoskeletal pathology; that is, try to determine if pain is drug induced rather than caused by anatomic or biomechanical problems.
- Be alert for signs of hyperglycemia, including confusion, drowsiness, flushed/dry skin, fruit-like breath odor, rapid/deep breathing, polyuria, loss of appetite, and unusual thirst. Patients with diabetes mellitus should check blood glucose levels frequently.
- Assess dizziness that might affect gait, balance, and other functional activities (See Appendix C). Report balance problems and functional limitations to the physician and nursing staff, and caution the patient and family/caregivers to guard against falls and trauma.
- Monitor personality changes such as depression and increased thoughts of suicide. Notify physician if these changes become problematic.

Interventions

- Implement resistive exercises and other therapeutic exercises as needed to maintain muscle strength and function, and prevent muscle wasting associated with HIV infection and AIDS.
- Because of the risk of arrhythmias, use caution during aerobic exercise and other forms of therapeutic exercise. Assess exercise tolerance frequently (blood pressure, heart rate, fatigue levels), and terminate exercise immediately if any untoward responses occur (See Appendix L).

Patient/Client-Related Instruction

- Emphasize the importance of taking atazanavir as directed even if the patient is asymptomatic, and that this drug must always be used in combination with other antiretroviral drugs. Do not take more than prescribed amount and do not stop taking without consulting health care professional.
- Inform patient that atazanavir does not cure HIV or AIDS or prevent associated or opportunistic infections. Atazanavir does not reduce the risk of transmission of HIV to others through sexual contact or blood contamination. Caution patient to use a condom and avoid sharing needles or donating blood to prevent spreading the AIDS virus to others.
- Inform patient that redistribution and accumulation of body fat may occur, causing central obesity, thin arms and legs, dorsocervical fat enlargement

(buffalo hump), breast enlargement, and other symptoms that resemble Cushing's syndrome (moon face, striations on abdominal skin). Discuss possible effects on body image, and help patient explore coping mechanisms.

- Advise patient about the likelihood of GI reactions, including diarrhea, nausea, vomiting, abdominal pain, and gallstones. Instruct patient to report severe or prolonged GI problems.
- Instruct patient to report other troublesome side effects such as prolonged or severe headache, sleep loss, fever, or skin rash.

Pharmacokinetics

Absorption: Rapidly absorbed (↑ by food).
Distribution: Enters cerebrospinal fluid and semen.
Metabolism and Excretion: 80% metabolized (CYP3A); 13% excreted unchanged in urine.
Half-life: 7 hr.

TIME/ACTION PROFILE (blood levels)

ROUTE	ONSET	PEAK	DURATION
PO	rapid	2.5 hr	24 hr

Contraindications/Precautions

Contraindicated in: Hypersensitivity; Severe hepatic impairment; Concurrent use of ergotamine, ergonovine, dihydroergotamine, methylergonovine, midazolam, pimozide, triazolam, rifampin, irinotecan, lovastatin, simvastatin, indinavir, proton-pump inhibitors (for treatment-experienced patients), or St. John's wort; Pedi: ↑ risk of kernicterus in infants <3 mo.
Use Cautiously in: Mild to moderate hepatic impairment; Preexisting conduction system disease (marked first-degree AV block or second- or third-degree AV block) or concurrent use of other drugs that increase the PR interval (especially those metabolized by CYP3A4, including verapamil or diltiazem); Diabetes mellitus; Hemophilia (↑ risk of bleeding); Pedi: Children <6 yr (safety not established); OB: Use only if clearly needed; Breastfeeding is not recommended if HIV infected.

Interactions

Drug-Drug: Atazanavir is an inhibitor of CYP3A and UGT1A1 enzyme systems. It is also a substrate of CYP3A. ↑ levels of **ergotamine, ergonovine, dihydroergotamine, methylergonovine, midazolam, pimozide, triazolam, lovastatin, simvastatin, and irinotecan;** concurrent use may result in life- threatening CNS, cardiovascular, hematologic, or musculoskeletal toxicity and is contraindicated. Combination therapy with **tenofovir** may lead to ↓ virologic response and possible resistance (100 mg **ritonavir** should be added to boost blood levels and dose of atazanavir ↓ to 300 mg/day). Levels are significantly ↓ by **rifampin, proton-pump inhibitors**, and **St. John's wort**; may promote viral resistance, avoid concurrent use. Concurrent use with **indinavir** may ↑ risk of hyperbilirubinemia and should be avoided. Concurrent use with **didanosine** buffered tablets will ↓ absorption and levels; give atazanavir with food 2 hr before or 1 hr after **didanosine. Efavirenz** decreases levels and may promote viral resistance; 600 mg efavirenz should be given with 100 mg ritonavir to counteract this effect and ↓ dose of atazanavir to 300 mg/day. ↑ **saquinavir** levels. Levels are ↑ by **ritonavir**; ↓ atazanavir dose to 300 mg/day. **Nevirapine** may ↓ levels; avoid concurrent use. **Antacids** or **buffered medications** will ↓ absorption; atazanavir should be given 2 hr before or 1 hr after. ↑ levels of **lidocaine, amiodarone**, or **quinidine**; blood level monitoring is recommended. ↑ risk of bleeding with **warfarin**. ↑ of **tricyclic antidepressants**; blood level monitoring is recommended. ↑ levels of **rifabutin**; ↓ rifabutin dose by 75% (150 mg every other day or 3 times weekly). ↑ levels of **diltiazem** and its active metabolite; ↓ diltiazem dose by 50% and ECG monitoring recommended. Similar precautions may be needed with **felodipine, nifedipine, nicardipine**, and **verapamil**. ↑ levels of **fluticasone**; consider alternative therapy; should not be used when atazanavir used with ritonavir. ↓ levels of **voriconazole** when atazanavir is used with ritonavir; avoid concurrent use. **Voriconazole** may also ↑ levels of atazanavir (when used without ritonavir). ↑ levels of **ketoconazole** or **itraconazole** when atazanavir is used with ritonavir. ↑ levels of **trazodone**; ↓ dose of trazodone. ↑ levels of **sildenafil, vardenafil**, and **tadalafil**; ↓ **sildenafil** dose to 25 mg every 48 hr; ↓ **vardenafil** dose to 2.5 mg every 72 hr; ↓ **tadalafil** dose to 10 mg every 72 hr. Exercise caution and monitor for hypertension, visual changes and priapism. ↑ levels and risk of myopathy from **atorvastatin** or **rosuvastatin** (use lowest dose of these agents or consider fluvastatin or pravastatin). Levels may be ↓ by **histamine H_2 antagonists**, promoting viral resistance; separate doses by at least 12 hr. ↑ levels of **cyclosporine, sirolimus**, and **tacrolimus**; monitor immunosuppressant blood levels. ↑ levels of **clarithromycin**; ↓ clarithromycin dose by 50% or consider alternative therapy. May ↓ levels of some **estrogens** found in **hormonal contraceptives**; use alternative nonhormonal method of contraception. Concurrent use of other **drugs known to ↑ PR interval**.

Route/Dosage

PO (Adults): *Therapy-naive*—400 mg once daily; should be used at a dose of 300 mg once daily with ritonavir 100 mg once daily if used concomitantly with tenofovir, efavirenz, H_2 receptor antagonist, or proton pump inhibitor. *Therapy-experienced*—300 mg once daily with ritonavir 100 mg once daily; should be used at dose of 400 mg once daily with ritonavir 100 mg daily if used with tenofovir and a H_2 receptor antagonist.

PO (Children ≥6 yr and Therapy-Naive): *15–24 kg*—150 mg once daily with ritonavir 80 mg once daily; *25–31 kg*—200 mg once daily with ritonavir 100 mg once daily; *32–38 kg*—250 mg once daily with ritonavir 100 mg once daily; *6–12 yr and ≥39 kg*—300 mg once daily with ritonavir 100 mg once daily; *≥13 yr and ≥39 kg*—400 mg once daily.
PO (Children ≥6 yr and Therapy-Experienced): *25–31 kg*—200 mg once daily with ritonavir 100 mg once daily; *32–38 kg*—250 mg once daily with ritonavir 100 mg once daily; *≥39 kg*—300 mg once daily with ritonavir 100 mg once daily.

Renal Impairment

PO (Adults): *Therapy-Naive and Hodgkin's disease (HD)*—300 mg once daily with ritonavir 100 mg once daily; *Therapy-Experienced and HD*—contraindicated.

Hepatic Impairment

PO (Adults): *Moderate hepatic impairment*—300 mg once daily (do not use with ritonavir).

Availability

Capsules: 100 mg, 150 mg, 200 mg, 300 mg.

atenolol (a-**ten**-oh-lole)

Apo-Atenolol, Novo-Atenolol, Tenormin

Classification
Therapeutic: antianginals, antihypertensives
Pharmacologic: beta blockers

Indications

Management of hypertension. Management of angina pectoris. Prevention of MI.

Action

Blocks stimulation of $beta_1$ (myocardial)-adrenergic receptors. Does not usually affect $beta_2$ (pulmonary, vascular, uterine)-receptor sites. **Therapeutic Effects:** Decreased blood pressure and heart rate. Decreased frequency of attacks of angina pectoris. Prevention of MI.

Adverse Reactions/Side Effects

CNS: fatigue, weakness, anxiety, depression, dizziness, drowsiness, insomnia, memory loss, mental status changes, nervousness, nightmares. **EENT:** blurred vision, stuffy nose. **Resp:** bronchospasm, wheezing. **CV:** BRADYCARDIA, CHF, PULMONARY EDEMA, hypotension, peripheral vasoconstriction. **GI:** constipation, diarrhea, liver function abnormalities, nausea, vomiting. **GU:** erectile dysfunction, decreased libido, urinary frequency. **Derm:** rashes. **Endo:** hyperglycemia, hypoglycemia. **MS:** arthralgia, back pain, joint pain. **Misc:** drug-induced lupus syndrome.

PHYSICAL THERAPY IMPLICATIONS

Examination and Evaluation

- Assess routinely for signs of CHF and pulmonary edema, including dyspnea, rales/crackles, weight gain, peripheral edema, and jugular venous distention. Report these signs to the physician immediately.
- Assess heart rate, ECG, and heart sounds, especially during exercise (See Appendices G, H). Report an abnormally slow heart rate (bradycardia) or symptoms of other arrhythmias such as palpitations, chest discomfort, shortness of breath, fainting, and fatigue/weakness.
- Assess blood pressure (BP) periodically and compare to normal values (See Appendix F) to help document antihypertensive effects.
- Assess exercise tolerance and episodes of angina pectoris. Document improvements in these variables, but also report any decline in exercise tolerance or increased frequency/severity of anginal attacks.
- Monitor signs of peripheral vasoconstriction, such as extreme coldness in the hands and feet, cyanosis, and muscle cramping. Notify physician of severe or prolonged signs of vasoconstriction.
- Assess symptoms of bronchospasm (wheezing, coughing, tightness in chest). Perform pulmonary function tests to quantify suspected changes in ventilation and respiration (See Appendices I, J, K). Repeated or prolonged bronchoconstriction may require a change in dose or medication.
- Be alert for signs of hypoglycemia (weakness, malaise, irritability, fatigue) or hyperglycemia (drowsiness, fruity breath, increased urination, unusual thirst). Medication may mask some signs of hypoglycemia, but dizziness and sweating may still occur. Patients with diabetes mellitus should check blood glucose levels frequently.
- Assess any back, joint, or muscle pain to rule out musculoskeletal pathology; that is, try to determine if pain is drug induced rather than caused by anatomic or biomechanical problems.
- Assess dizziness and drowsiness that might affect gait, balance, and other functional activities (See Appendix C). Report balance problems and functional limitations to the physician, and caution the patient and family/caregivers to guard against falls and trauma.
- Monitor excessive fatigue or weakness. Beta blockers often cause some degree of fatigue and weakness, but any sudden or severe change in muscle strength or energy levels should be reported.
- Monitor mood and personality changes, including depression, anxiety, nervousness, memory loss, or other changes in behavior. Notify physician if these changes become problematic.

- Monitor signs of drug-induced lupus syndrome, including increased BP, fever, joint pain, skin rashes, and redness/irritation of the eye (uveitis). Notify physician promptly if these signs appear.

Interventions

- Because of an increased risk of cardiac arrhythmias and CHF, use caution during aerobic exercise and endurance conditioning. Likewise, monitor patients closely during treatment of other cardiac problems (angina, recent MI). Terminate exercise if patient exhibits untoward symptoms (chest pain, shortness of breath, unusual fatigue) or displays other criteria for exercise termination (see Appendix L).
- Establish aerobic exercise workloads that account for the effects of beta blockers on heart rate. Some heart rate guidelines may not be appropriate because beta blockers typically decrease maximal HR by 20–30 bpm. Use other guidelines such as rating of perceived exertion (RPE, modified Borg's scale) to determine exercise workloads.
- To minimize orthostatic hypotension, patient should move slowly when assuming a more upright position.

Patient/Client-Related Instruction

- Remind patients to take medication as directed to control hypertension and other cardiac conditions, even if they are asymptomatic.
- Counsel patients about additional interventions to help control BP and cardiac dysfunction such as regular exercise, weight loss, sodium restriction, stress reduction, moderation of alcohol consumption, and smoking cessation.
- Instruct patient or family/caregivers to report other troublesome side effects such as severe or prolonged insomnia, nightmares, dry eyes, sexual problems (decreased libido, erectile dysfunction), skin reactions (rash, itching), or GI problems (nausea, vomiting, constipation, diarrhea).

Pharmacokinetics

Absorption: 50–60% absorbed after oral administration.
Distribution: Minimal penetration of CNS. Crosses the placenta and enters breast milk.
Metabolism and Excretion: 40–50% excreted unchanged by the kidneys; remainder excreted in feces as unabsorbed drug.
Half-life: 6–9 hr.

TIME/ACTION PROFILE (cardiovascular effects)

ROUTE	ONSET	PEAK	DURATION
PO	1 hr	2–4 hr	24 hr

Contraindications/Precautions

Contraindicated in: Uncompensated CHF; Pulmonary edema; Cardiogenic shock; Bradycardia or heart block.
Use Cautiously in: Renal impairment (dosage reduction recommended if CCr ≤35 mL/min); Hepatic impairment; Geriatric patients (increased sensitivity to beta blockers; initial dosage reduction recommended); Pulmonary disease (including asthma; beta selectivity may be lost at higher doses); Diabetes mellitus (may mask signs of hypoglycemia); Thyrotoxicosis (may mask symptoms); Patients with a history of severe allergic reactions (intensity of reactions may be increased); OB: Crosses the placenta and may cause fetal/neonatal bradycardia, hypotension, hypoglycemia, or respiratory depression; Lactation/Pedi: Safety not established.

Interactions

Drug-Drug: General anesthesia, IV phenytoin, and **verapamil** may cause additive myocardial depression. Additive bradycardia may occur with **digoxin**. Additive hypotension may occur with other **antihypertensives**, acute ingestion of **alcohol**, or **nitrates**. Concurrent use with **amphetamine, cocaine, ephedrine, epinephrine, norepinephrine, phenylephrine,** or **pseudoephedrine** may result in unopposed alpha-adrenergic stimulation (excessive hypertension, bradycardia). Concurrent **thyroid** administration may decrease effectiveness. May alter the effectiveness of **insulins** or **oral hypoglycemic agents** (dosage adjustments may be necessary). May decrease the effectiveness of **theophylline**. May decrease the beneficial $beta_1$ cardiovascular effects of **dopamine** or **dobutamine**. Use cautiously within 14 days of **MAO inhibitor** therapy (may result in hypertension).

Route/Dosage

PO (Adults): *Antianginal*—50 mg once daily; may be increased after 1 wk to 100 mg/day (up to 200 mg/day). *Antihypertensive*—25–50 mg once daily; may be increased after 2 wk to 50–100 mg once daily. *MI*—50 mg, then 50 mg 12 hr later, then 100 mg/day as a single dose or in 2 divided doses for 6–9 days or until hospital discharge.

Renal Impairment

PO (Adults): *CCr 15–35 mL/min*—dosage should not exceed 50 mg/day; *CCr <15 mL/min*—dosage should not exceed 50 mg every other day.

Availability (generic available)

Tablets: 25 mg, 50 mg, 100 mg. ***In combination with:*** chlorthalidone (Tenoretic). See Appendix B.

atomoxetine (a-to-mox-e-teen)

Strattera

Classification

Therapeutic: agents for attention deficit disorder

Pharmacologic: selective norepinephrine reuptake inhibitors

Indications

Attention-Deficit/Hyperactivity Disorder (ADHD).

Action

Selectively inhibits the presynaptic transporter of norepinephrine. **Therapeutic Effects:** Increased attention span.

Adverse Reactions/Side Effects

CNS: SUICIDAL THOUGHTS, dizziness, fatigue, mood swings, behavioral disturbances, hallucinations, mania, thought disorder. **Adults:** insomnia. **CV:** hypertension, orthostatic hypotension, tachycardia. **GI:** dyspepsia, severe liver injury (rare), nausea, vomiting. **Adults:** dry mouth, constipation. **Derm:** rash, urticaria. **GU: Adults:** dysmenorrhea, ejaculatory problems, ↓ libido, erectile dysfunction, urinary hesitation, urinary retention. **Metab:** ↓ appetite, weight/growth loss. **Misc:** ALLERGIC REACTIONS, INCLUDING ANGIONEUROTIC EDEMA.

PHYSICAL THERAPY IMPLICATIONS

Examination and Evaluation

- Monitor signs of allergic reactions and angioneurotic edema. Signs include rashes, raised patches of red or white skin (welts), burning/itching skin, swelling in the face, and difficulty breathing. Notify physician of these signs immediately.
- Be alert for signs of suicidal thoughts, especially in the initial period of drug therapy, and in children and teenagers. Likewise, inform physician if patient demonstrates other thought disturbances or behavioral changes such as mania, moods swings, or hallucinations.
- Monitor attentiveness and behavior in patients with ADHD. Report any changes in attention and hyperactivity, and document whether this drug appears to be producing the desired effects.
- Assess heart rate, ECG, and heart sounds, especially during exercise (See Appendices G, H). Report fast heart rate (tachycardia) or symptoms of other arrhythmias, including palpitations, chest discomfort, shortness of breath, fainting, and fatigue/weakness.
- Assess blood pressure (BP) and compare to normal values (See Appendix F). Report changes in BP: either a problematic decrease in BP (hypotension) or a sustained increase in BP (hypertension).
- Assess dizziness that might affect gait, balance, and other functional activities (See Appendix C). Report balance problems and functional limitations to the physician, and caution the patient and family/caregivers to guard against falls and trauma.
- Periodically assess body weight, and monitor growth rate in children. Report a rapid or unexplained weight loss or stunted growth.

Interventions

- Because of the risk of arrhythmias and abnormal BP responses, use caution during aerobic exercise and other forms of therapeutic exercise. Assess exercise tolerance frequently (BP, heart rate, fatigue levels), and terminate exercise immediately if any untoward responses occur (See Appendix L).

Patient/Client-Related Instruction

- Instruct patient and family/caregivers to report other troublesome side effects, including severe or prolonged menstrual irregularities, sexual dysfunction, urinary dysfunction, skin reactions (rash, hives, itching), or GI problems (indigestion, nausea, vomiting, constipation, dry mouth).

Pharmacokinetics

Absorption: Well absorbed following oral administration.
Distribution: Unknown.
Protein Binding: 98%.
Metabolism and Excretion: Mostly metabolized by the liver (CYP2D6 enzyme pathway). A small percentage of the population are poor metabolizers and will have higher blood levels with ↑ effects).
Half-life: 5 hr.

TIME/ACTION PROFILE

ROUTE	ONSET	PEAK	DURATION
PO	unknown	1–2 hr	12–24 hr

Contraindications/Precautions

Contraindicated in: Concurrent or within 2 wk therapy with MAO inhibitors; Angle-closure glaucoma.
Use Cautiously in: Hypertension, tachycardia, cardiovascular or cerebrovascular disease; Preexisting psychiatric illness; May ↑ risk of suicide attempt/ideation, especially during dose early treatment or dose adjustment; risk may be greater in children or adolescents; Concurrent albuterol or vasopressors (↑ risk of adverse cardiovascular reactions); OB: Use only if benefits outweigh risks to fetus; Lactation/Pedi: Safety not established.

Interactions

Drug-Drug: Concurrent use with **MAO inhibitors** may result in serious, potentially fatal reactions (do not use within 2 wk of each other). ↑ risk of cardiovascular effects with **albuterol** or **vasopressors** (use cautiously).

Drugs which inhibit the CYP2D6 enzyme pathway (quinidine, fluoxetine, paroxetine) will ↑ blood levels and effects; dose ↓ recommended.

Route/Dosage

PO (Children and adolescents <70 kg): 0.5 mg/kg/day initially, may be ↑ every 3 days to a daily target dose of 1.2 mg/kg, given as a single dose in the morning or evenly divided doses in the morning and late afternoon/early evening (not to exceed 1.4 mg/kg/day or 100 mg/day whichever is less). *If taking concurrent CYP2D6 inhibitor (quinidine, fluoxetine, paroxetine)*—0.5 mg/kg/day initially, may ↑ if needed to 1.2 mg/kg/day after 4 wk.

PO (Adults, adolescents, and children >70 kg): 40 mg/day initially, may be ↑ every 3 days to a daily target dose of 80 mg/day given as a single dose in the morning or evenly divided doses in the morning and late afternoon/early evening; may be further ↑ after 2–4 wk up to 100 mg/day. *If taking concurrent CYP2D6 inhibitor (quinidine, fluoxetine, paroxetine)*—40 mg/day initially, may ↑ if needed to 80 mg/day after 4 wk.

Hepatic Impairment

PO (Adults and Children): *Moderate hepatic impairment (Child-Pugh Class B)*—↓ initial and target dose by 50%; *Severe hepatic impairment (Child-Pugh Class C)*—↓ initial and target dose to 25% of normal.

Availability

Capsules: 10 mg, 18 mg, 25 mg, 40 mg, 60 mg, 80 mg, 100 mg.

atorvastatin (a-tore-va-stat-in)

Lipitor

Classification

Therapeutic: lipid-lowering agents

Pharmacologic: HMG CoA reductase inhibitors

Indications

Adjunctive management of primary hypercholesterolemia and mixed dyslipidemia. Primary prevention of coronary heart disease (myocardial infarction, stroke, angina, and coronary revascularization) in asymptomatic patients with increased total and low-density lipoprotein (LDL) cholesterol and decreased high-density lipoprotein (HDL) cholesterol.

Action

Inhibits 3-hydroxy-3-methylglutaryl coenzyme A (HMG CoA) reductase, an enzyme which is responsible for catalyzing an early step in the synthesis of cholesterol. **Therapeutic Effects:** Lowering of total and LDL cholesterol and triglycerides. Slightly increases HDL cholesterol. Reduction of lipids/cholesterol reduces the risk of myocardial infarction and stroke sequelae. Slows the progression of coronary atherosclerosis with resultant decrease in coronary heart disease–related events.

Adverse Reactions/Side Effects

CNS: dizziness, headache, insomnia, weakness. **EENT:** rhinitis. **Resp:** bronchitis. **CV:** chest pain, peripheral edema. **GI:** abdominal cramps, constipation, diarrhea, flatus, heartburn, altered taste, drug-induced hepatitis, dyspepsia, elevated liver enzymes, nausea, pancreatitis. **GU:** erectile dysfunction. **Derm:** rashes, pruritus. **MS:** RHABDOMYOLYSIS, arthralgia, arthritis, myalgia, myositis. **Misc:** HYPERSENSITIVITY REACTIONS, INCLUDING ANGIONEUROTIC EDEMA.

PHYSICAL THERAPY IMPLICATIONS

Examination and Evaluation

- Assess any muscle pain, tenderness, or weakness, especially if accompanied by fever, malaise, and dark-colored urine. Advise patient that these symptoms may represent drug-induced myopathy, and that myopathy can progress to severe muscle damage (rhabdomyolysis). Report any unexplained musculoskeletal symptoms to the physician immediately, and suspend exercise and gait training until these symptoms can be evaluated.
- Monitor signs of angioneurotic edema and other hypersensitivity reactions, including rashes, raised patches of red or white skin (welts), burning/ itching skin, swelling in the face, and difficulty breathing. Notify physician of these signs immediately.
- Assess dizziness and weakness that might affect gait, balance, and other functional activities (see Appendix C). Report balance problems and functional limitations to the physician, and caution the patient and family/caregivers to guard against falls and trauma.
- Assess peripheral edema using girth measurements, volume displacement, and measurement of pitting edema (See Appendix N). Report increased swelling in feet and ankles or a sudden increase in body weight due to fluid retention.
- Monitor chest pain or symptoms of bronchitis (cough, production of sputum, shortness of breath, wheezing). Report prolonged or severe symptoms to the physician.

Interventions

- In patients with drug-induced myopathy, implement gradual strengthening and other therapeutic exercises to facilitate recovery from muscle pain and weakness. Use caution during early stages to

avoid fatigue of affected muscles, and implement assistive devices (walker, cane, crutches) as needed to prevent falls and assist mobility. Increase exercise intensity as tolerated; recovery from myopathy typically takes 4–6 wk, but can be longer in older patients or people with comorbidities.
- Design and implement aerobic exercise and endurance training programs to improve cardiovascular function and help reduce the risk of coronary heart disease.

Patient/Client-Related Instruction
- Remind patients to take medication as directed to control hyperlipidemia even though they are asymptomatic.
- Counsel patients about additional interventions to help control lipid disorders and improve cardiovascular health, including dietary modification, regular exercise, moderation of alcohol consumption, and smoking cessation.
- Instruct patient to report signs of drug-induced hepatitis (anorexia, abdominal pain, severe nausea and vomiting, yellow skin or eyes, skin rashes, flu-like symptoms) or pancreatitis (upper abdominal pain after eating, indigestion, weight loss, oily stools).
- Instruct patient to report other GI reactions, including prolonged or severe constipation, diarrhea, nausea, indigestion, heartburn, altered taste, abdominal cramps, or flatulence.
- Instruct patient to report other bothersome side effects such as severe or prolonged headache, sleep loss, nasal irritation, erectile dysfunction, or skin reactions (rash, itching).

Pharmacokinetics
Absorption: Rapidly absorbed but undergoes extensive gastrointestinal and hepatic metabolism resulting in 14% bioavailability (30% for lipid-lowering activity).
Distribution: Probably enters breast milk.
Protein Binding: ≥98%.
Metabolism and Excretion: Extensively metabolized by the liver, most during first pass; excreted in bile and feces. <2% excreted unchanged by the kidneys. Two metabolites have lipid-lowering activity.
Half-life: 14 hr (lipid-lowering activity due to atorvastatin and its metabolites—20–30 hr).

TIME/ACTION PROFILE (cholesterol-lowering effect)

ROUTE	ONSET	PEAK	DURATION
PO	unknown	unknown	20–30 hr*

*Following discontinuation.

Contraindications/Precautions
Contraindicated in: Hypersensitivity; Active liver disease or unexplained persistent elevations in AST & ALT; OB: Potential for fetal anomalies; Lactation: May appear in breast milk.

Use Cautiously in: History of liver disease; Alcoholism; Renal impairment; Concurrent use of gemfibrozil, azole antifungals, erythromycin, clarithromycin, protease inhibitors, niacin, or cyclosporine (higher risk of myopathy/rhabdomyolysis); OB: Women of childbearing age; Pedi: Safety not established.

Interactions
Drug-Drug: Metabolized by the hepatic CYP3A4 enzyme system. Cholesterol-lowering effect may be additive with **bile acid sequestrants (cholestyramine, colestipol)**. Bioavailability may be ↓ by **bile acid sequestrants**. ↑ risk of myopathy with concurrent use of **cyclosporine, gemfibrozil, erythromycin, clarithromycin, ritonavir/saquinavir, lopinavir/ritonavir** large doses of **niacin**, and **azole antifungals** (combined use with gemfibrozil not recommended; temporary discontinuation of atorvastatin recommended during azole antifungals). May slightly ↑ serum **digoxin** levels. May ↑ levels of **oral contraceptives**. May ↑ effects of **warfarin**.
Drug-Food: Grapefruit juice ↑ levels and risk of rhabdomyolysis.

Route/Dosage
PO (Adults): 10–20 mg once daily initially; (may start with 40 mg/day if LDL-C needs to be decreased by >45%); may be increased every 2–4 wk up to 80 mg/day.
PO (Children 10–17 yr): 10 mg/day initially, may be increased every 4 wk up to 20 mg/day.

Availability
Tablets: 10 mg, 20 mg, 40 mg, 80 mg. ***In combination with:*** amlodipine (Caduet); see Appendix B.

atovaquone (a-toe-va-kwone)
Mepron

Classification
Therapeutic: antiprotozoals

Indications
Treatment of mild-to-moderate *Pneumocystis carinii* pneumonia (PCP) in patients who are unable to tolerate trimethoprim-sulfamethoxazole. Prophylaxis of PCP.

Action
Inhibits the action of enzymes necessary to nucleic acid and ATP synthesis in protozoa. **Therapeutic Effects:** Antiprotozoal action against *P. carinii*.

Adverse Reactions/Side Effects
CNS: headache, insomnia. **Resp:** cough. **GI:** diarrhea, nausea, vomiting. **Derm:** rash. **Misc:** fever.

PHYSICAL THERAPY IMPLICATIONS

Examination and Evaluation

- Assess pulmonary function by measuring lung volumes, breath sounds, respiratory rate, and other symptoms (cough, dyspnea, shortness of breath) (See Appendices I, J, K). Report changes in pulmonary function to help document the effects of drug therapy in treating PCP infections.

Interventions

- Implement therapeutic exercises and airway clearance techniques as needed to maintain and improve pulmonary function in patients with respiratory infections.

Patient/Client-Related Instruction

- Remind patient to take this drug as directed for the full course of treatment even if feeling better.
- Instruct patient and family/caregivers to report other troublesome side effects such as severe or prolonged headache, sleep loss, skin rash, fever, or GI problems (diarrhea, nausea, vomiting).

Pharmacokinetics

Absorption: Absorption is poor but is increased by food, particularly fat.
Distribution: Enters CSF in very low concentrations (<1% of plasma levels).
Protein Binding: >99.9%.
Metabolism and Excretion: Undergoes enterohepatic recycling; elimination occurs in feces.
Half-life: 2.2–2.9 days.

TIME/ACTION PROFILE (blood levels)

ROUTE	ONSET	PEAK	DURATION
PO	unknown	1–8 hr; 24–96 hr*	12 hr

*Two peaks are due to enterohepatic recycling.

Contraindications/Precautions

Contraindicated in: Hypersensitivity; Lactation: May appear in breast milk.
Use Cautiously in: Decreased hepatic, renal, or cardiac function (dosage modification may be necessary); GI disorders (absorption may be limited); OB: Safety not established; Pedi: Safety not established.

Interactions

Drug-Drug: May interact with **drugs that are highly bound to plasma proteins** (does not appear to interact with phenytoin).
Drug-Food: **Food** enhances absorption.

Route/Dosage

Treatment

PO (Adults): 750 mg twice daily for 21 days.
PO (Children): 40 mg/kg/day (unlabeled).

Prevention

PO (Adults and Adolescents 13–16 yr): 1500 mg once daily.

Availability

Suspension: 750 mg/5 mL.

atropine (at-ro-peen)

Atro-Pen

Classification
Therapeutic: antiarrhythmics
Pharmacologic: anticholinergics, antimuscarinics

Indications

IM: Given preoperatively to decrease oral and respiratory secretions. **IV:** Treatment of sinus bradycardia and heart block. **PO:** Adjunctive therapy in the management of peptic ulcer and irritable bowel syndrome. **IV:** Reversal of adverse muscarinic effects of anticholinesterase agents (neostigmine, physostigmine, or pyridostigmine). **IM, IV:** Treatment of anticholinesterase (organophosphate pesticide) poisoning. **Inhalation:** Treatment of exercise-induced bronchospasm.

Action

Inhibits the action of acetylcholine at postganglionic sites located in Smooth muscle, Secretory glands, CNS (antimuscarinic activity). Low doses decrease Sweating, Salivation, Respiratory secretions. Intermediate doses result in Mydriasis (pupillary dilation), Cycloplegia (loss of visual accommodation), Increased heart rate. GI and GU tract motility are decreased at larger doses. **Therapeutic Effects:** Increased heart rate. Decreased GI and respiratory secretions. Reversal of muscarinic effects. May have a spasmolytic action on the biliary and genitourinary tracts.

Adverse Reactions/Side Effects

CNS: drowsiness, confusion, hyperpyrexia. **EENT:** blurred vision, cycloplegia, photophobia, dry eyes, mydriasis. **CV:** tachycardia, palpitations, arrhythmias. **GI:** dry mouth, constipation, impaired GI motility. **GU:** urinary hesitancy, retention, impotency. **Resp:** tachypnea, pulmonary edema. **Misc:** flushing, decreased sweating.

PHYSICAL THERAPY IMPLICATIONS

Examination and Evaluation

- Assess heart rate, ECG, and heart sounds, especially during exercise (See Appendices G, H). Although intended to treat certain arrhythmias, this drug can unmask or precipitate new arrhythmias (proarrhythmic effect). Report any rhythm disturbances or symptoms of increased arrhythmias, including palpitations, chest pain, shortness of breath, fainting, and fatigue/weakness.

- Watch for signs of pulmonary edema, including cough, shortness of breath, rapid breathing (tachypnea), chest pain, and labored breathing. Monitor pulse oximetry and perform pulmonary function tests (See Appendices I, J, K) to quantify suspected changes in ventilation and respiratory function.
- If treating inflammatory bowel diseases, monitor any changes in symptoms (decreased abdominal pain, decreased diarrhea, improved appetite) to help document whether drug therapy is successful.
- If treating exercise-induced bronchospasm, assess lung volumes, breath sounds, respiratory rate, and other symptoms (wheezing, dyspnea, shortness of breath) during exercise (See Appendices I, J, K). Report changes in pulmonary function to help document the effects of drug therapy in treating this problem.
- Be alert for decreased sweating and altered/increased body temperature (hyperpyrexia). Notify physician of a prolonged or persistent elevation in body temperature.

Interventions

- Because of the risk of arrhythmias, impaired thermoregulation, and pulmonary problems (edema, exercise-induced asthma), use caution during aerobic exercise and other forms of therapeutic exercise. Assess exercise tolerance frequently (blood pressure, heart rate, fatigue levels), and terminate exercise immediately if any untoward responses occur (See Appendix L).

Patient/Client-Related Instruction

- Instruct patient and family/caregivers to report other troublesome side effects such as severe or prolonged drowsiness, confusion, vision problems, skin flushing, problems with urination, sexual dysfunction, or GI problems (constipation, dry mouth).

Pharmacokinetics

Absorption: Well absorbed following oral, SC, or IM administration.
Distribution: Readily crosses the blood-brain barrier. Crosses the placenta and enters breast milk.
Metabolism and Excretion: Mostly metabolized by the liver; 30–50% excreted unchanged by the kidneys.
Half-life: Children <2 yr: 4–10 hr; Children >2 yr: 1.5–3.5 hr; Adults: 4–5 hr.

TIME/ACTION PROFILE (inhibition of salivation)

ROUTE	ONSET	PEAK	DURATION
PO	30 min	30–60 min	4–6 hr
IM, SC	rapid	15–50 min	4–6 hr
IV	immediate	2–4 min	4–6 hr

Contraindications/Precautions

Contraindicated in: Hypersensitivity; Angle-closure glaucoma; Acute hemorrhage; Tachycardia secondary to cardiac insufficiency or thyrotoxicosis; Obstructive disease of the GI tract.
Use Cautiously in: Intra-abdominal infections; Prostatic hyperplasia; Chronic renal, hepatic, pulmonary, or cardiac disease; OB/Lactation: Safety not established; IV administration may produce fetal tachycardia; Pedi: Infants with Down's syndrome have increased sensitivity to cardiac effects and mydriasis. Children may have increased susceptibility to adverse reactions. Exercise care when prescribing to children with spastic paralysis or brain damage; Geri: Increased susceptibility to adverse reactions.

Interactions

Drug-Drug: ↑ anticholinergic effects with other **anticholinergics**, including **antihistamines**, **tricyclic antidepressants**, **quinidine**, and **disopyramide**. Anticholinergics may alter the absorption of other **orally administered drugs** by slowing motility of the GI tract. **Antacids** ↓ absorption of **anticholinergics**. May ↑ GI mucosal lesions in patients taking oral **potassium chloride** tablets. May alter response to **beta blockers**.

Route/Dosage

Preanesthesia (to Decrease Salivation/Secretions)

IM, IV, SC, PO (Adults): 0.4–0.6 mg 30–60 min preop.
IM, IV, SC, PO (Children >5 kg): 0.01–0.02 mg/kg/dose 30–60 min preop to a maximum of 0.4 mg/dose; minimum: 0.1 mg/dose.
IM, IV, SC, PO (Children <5 kg): 0.02 mg/kg/dose 30–60 min preop then q 4–6 hr as needed.

Bradycardia

IV (Adults): 0.5–1 mg; may repeat as needed q 5 min, not to exceed a total of 2 mg (q 3–5 min in Advanced Cardiac Life Support guidelines) or 0.04 mg/kg (total vagolytic dose).
IV (Children): 0.02 mg/kg (maximum single dose is 0.5 mg in children and 1 mg in adolescents); may repeat q 5 min up to a total dose of 1 mg in children (2 mg in adolescents).
Endotracheal: (Children): use the IV dose and dilute before administration.

A

Reversal of Adverse Muscarinic Effects of Anticholinesterases

IV (Adults): 0.6–12 mg for each 0.5–2.5 mg of neostigmine methylsulfate or 10–20 mg of pyridostigmine bromide concurrently with anticholinesterase.

Organophosphate Poisoning

IM (Adults): 2 mg initially, then 2 mg q 10 min as needed up to 3 times total.
IV (Adults): 1–2 mg/dose q 10–20 min until atropinic effects observed then q 1–4 hr for 24 hr; up to 50 mg in first 24 hr and 2 g over several days may be given in severe intoxication.
IM (Children >10 yr >90 lb): 2 mg.
IM (Children 4–10 yr 40–90 lb): 1 mg.
IM (Children 6 mo–4 yr 15–40 lb): 0.5 mg.
IV (Children): 0.02–0.05 mg/kg q 10–20 min until atropinic effects observed then q 1–4 hr for 24 hr.

Bronchospasm

Inhalation (Adults): 0.025–0.05 mg/kg/dose q 4–6 hr as needed; maximum 2.5 mg/dose.
Inhalation (Children): 0.03–0.05 mg/kg/dose 3–4 times/day; maximum 2.5 mg/dose.

Availability (generic available)

Tablets: 0.4 mg. ***In combination with:*** phenobarbital oral solution (Antrocol). See Appendix B. **Injection:** 0.05 mg/mL, 0.1 mg/mL, 0.4 mg/mL, 1 mg/mL, 0.5 mg/0.7 mL Auto-injector, 1 mg/0.7 mL Auto-injector, 2 mg/0.7 mL Auto-injector.

auranofin (au-rane-oh-fin)

Ridaura

Classification

Therapeutic: antirheumatics (disease-modifying antirheumatic drugs [DMARDs]), gold compounds

Indications

Treatment of progressive rheumatoid arthritis resistant to conventional therapy.

Action

Inhibits inflammatory process. Modifies immune response (immunomodulating properties). **Therapeutic Effects:** Relief of pain and inflammation. Slowing of the disease process in rheumatoid arthritis.

Adverse Reactions/Side Effects

CNS: peripheral neuropathy. **EENT:** conjunctivitis, corneal gold deposition. **GU:** proteinuria, hematuria. **Resp:** bronchitis, pulmonary fibrosis, pneumonitis. **CV:** bradycardia. **GI:** GI BLEEDING, abdominal pain, cramping, diarrhea, gingivitis, glossitis, metallic taste, stomatitis, anorexia, difficulty swallowing, ↑ liver enzymes, dyspepsia, flatulence, nausea, vomiting. **Derm:** dermatitis, rash, alopecia, urticaria, photosensitivity reactions, pruritus. **Hemat:** AGRANULOCYTOSIS, APLASTIC ANEMIA, thrombocytopenia, anemia, eosinophilia, leukopenia. **Misc:** ALLERGIC REACTIONS, INCLUDING ANAPHYLAXIS, ANGIOEDEMA.

PHYSICAL THERAPY IMPLICATIONS

Examination and Evaluation

- Monitor signs of allergic reactions, including anaphylaxis and angioedema. Signs include pulmonary symptoms (tightness in the throat and chest, wheezing, cough, dyspnea) or skin reactions (rash, pruritus, urticaria, burning/itching skin, swelling in the face). Notify physician immediately if these reactions occur.
- Monitor and report signs of agranulocytosis (fever, sore throat, mucosal lesions, infection), aplastic anemia (unusual fatigue, shortness of breath with exertion), thrombocytopenia (bruising, nose bleeds, bleeding gums), or other weakness or coagulation problems that might indicate other blood dyscrasias. Periodic blood tests may be needed to monitor WBC and RBC counts.
- Assess any breathing problems or signs of pulmonary fibrosis, pneumonitis, or bronchitis such as dry cough, wheezing, rales, chest pain, shortness of breath, and difficult or labored breathing. Monitor pulse oximetry and perform pulmonary function tests (See Appendices I, J, K) to quantify suspected changes in ventilation and respiratory function.
- Be alert for signs of peripheral neuropathy (numbness, tingling, decreased muscle strength). Establish baseline electroneuromyographic values at the beginning of drug treatment whenever possible, and reexamine these values periodically to document drug-induced changes in peripheral nerve function.
- Periodically assess impairments (pain, range of motion), functional ability, and disability to help document whether antirheumatic drug therapy is successful.

Interventions

- Implement appropriate manual therapy techniques, physical agents, therapeutic exercises, and orthotic/assistive devices to reduce pain, improve function, and augment the effects of antirheumatic drug therapy.
- Help patients with arthritis explore other nonpharmacologic methods to reduce chronic arthritis pain,

such as relaxation techniques, exercise, counseling, and so forth.

- Causes photosensitivity; use care if administering UV treatments. Advise patient to avoid direct sunlight and use sunscreens and protective clothing.

Patient/Client-Related Instruction

- Instruct patient to immediately report signs of GI bleeding, including abdominal pain, vomiting blood, blood in stools, or black, tarry stools. Instruct patient to also report other GI problems such as severe or prolonged diarrhea, nausea, vomiting, flatulence, indigestion, abdominal cramps, loss of appetite, and inflammation in/around the mouth.
- Advise patient that rash and other skin reactions (dermatitis, pruritus, urticaria, hair loss) are likely. Report severe or unexpected skin reactions to the physician.
- Advise patient to guard against infection (frequent hand washing, etc.), and to avoid crowds and contact with persons with contagious diseases.
- Instruct patient to report other troublesome side effects, including severe or prolonged eye irritation (conjunctivitis) or blood in the urine.

Pharmacokinetics

Absorption: 20–25% absorbed from the GI tract.
Distribution: Widely distributed; appears to concentrate in arthritic joints more than in uninvolved joints. Enters breast milk.
Metabolism and Excretion: 60% of absorbed dose slowly excreted by the kidneys; 40% of absorbed dose excreted in the feces.
Half-life: 26 days in blood, 40–128 days in tissue.

TIME/ACTION PROFILE (anti-inflammatory activity)

ROUTE	ONSET	PEAK	DURATION
PO	3–6 mo	unknown	unknown

Contraindications/Precautions

Contraindicated in: Hypersensitivity; Previous gold toxicity (e.g., anaphylaxis, necrotizing enterocolitis, pulmonary fibrosis, exfoliative dermatitis, bone marrow aplasia, hematologic disorders); OB: Potential for congenital anomalies; Lactation: Appears in breast milk. Use formula or discontinue auranofin.
Use Cautiously in: History of blood dyscrasias; Rashes; Severe hepatic or renal dysfunction; Inflammatory bowel disease; Patients taking other immunosuppressant drugs; Pedi: Efficacy and safety not established.

Interactions

Drug-Drug: Bone marrow toxicity may be additive with other **myelosuppressive agents (antineoplastics, radiation therapy, azathioprine)** or high doses of **corticosteroids**. Concurrent use with **penicillamine** ↑ the risk of adverse hematologic or renal reactions. May ↑ blood levels of **phenytoin**.

Route/Dosage

PO (Adults): 6 mg/day in 1–2 doses; may increase to 9 mg/day in 3 divided doses if no improvement after 6 mo.

Availability

Capsules: 3 mg.

azacitidine (a-za-**sye**-ti-deen)

Vidaza

Classification
Therapeutic: antineoplastics
Pharmacologic: nucleoside analogues

Indications

Myelodysplastic syndromes, including some refractory anemias, chronic myelomonocytic leukemia.

Action

Inhibits DNA synthesis. **Therapeutic Effects:** Death of rapidly replicating cells, particularly malignant ones.

Adverse Reactions/Side Effects

CNS: fatigue. **GI:** HEPATOTOXICITY, constipation, diarrhea, nausea, vomiting. **GU:** nephrotoxicity, renal tubular acidosis. **Derm:** ecchymosis. **F and E:** hypokalemia. **Hemat:** anemia, neutropenia, thrombocytopenia. **Local:** injection-site erythema. **Misc:** ALLERGIC REACTIONS, INCLUDING ANAPHYLAXIS, fever.

PHYSICAL THERAPY IMPLICATIONS

Evaluation and Examination

- Be alert for signs of hepatotoxicity, including anorexia, abdominal pain, severe nausea and vomiting, yellow skin or eyes, fever, sore throat, malaise, weakness, facial edema, lethargy, and unusual bleeding or bruising. Report these signs to the physician immediately.
- Monitor signs of allergic reactions and anaphylaxis, including pulmonary symptoms (tightness in the throat and chest, wheezing, cough, dyspnea) or skin reactions (rash, pruritus, urticaria). Notify physician or nursing staff immediately if these reactions occur.
- Monitor signs of neutropenia (fever, sore throat, signs of infection), thrombocytopenia (bruising, nose bleeds, and bleeding gums), or unusual weakness and fatigue that might be due to anemia. Report these signs to the physician.
- Monitor signs of nephrotoxicity, including blood or pus in urine, decreased urine output, weight gain from fluid retention, and fatigue. Report these signs to the physician.

- Monitor and report any muscle weakness, aches, or cramps that might indicate low potassium levels (hypokalemia).
- Monitor injection site for redness and swelling. Report prolonged or excessive injection site reactions to the physician.

Interventions

- For patients who are medically able to begin exercise, implement appropriate resistive exercises and aerobic training to maintain muscle strength and aerobic capacity during cancer chemotherapy, or to help restore function after chemotherapy.

Patient/Client-related Instruction

- Instruct patient and family/caregivers to report other troublesome side effects such as severe or prolonged fever or GI problems (nausea, vomiting, diarrhea, constipation).

Pharmacokinetics

Absorption: Rapidly absorbed following subcutaneous administration; 89% bioavailable.
Distribution: Unknown.
Metabolism and Excretion: 85% excreted in urine; some hepatic metabolism may occur. Less than 1% fecal elimination.
Half-life: 4 hr.

TIME/ACTION PROFILE (effects on bone marrow)

ROUTE	ONSET	PEAK	DURATION
SC	unknown	unknown	unknown

Contraindications/Precautions

Contraindicated in: Hypersensitivity; Advanced malignant hepatic tumors; OB: Potential for congenital anomalies; Lactation: Potential for serious side effects in infants.
Use Cautiously in: Renal impairment; Liver disease; OB: Patients with childbearing potential (male and female) due to potential fetal harm; Pedi: Safety not established.

Interactions

Drug-Drug: Additive bone marrow depression may occur with other **antineoplastics**.

Route/Dosage

SC, IV (Adults): 75 mg/m²/day for 7 days every 4 wk; may be increased to 100 mg/m²/day for 7 days every 4 wk if no beneficial effect occurs after 2 cycles. Continue for as long as patient benefits.

Availability

Suspension for injection (requires reconstitution): 100 mg/vial.

azathioprine
(ay-za-**thye**-oh-preen)
Azasan, Imuran

Classification
Therapeutic: immunosuppressants
Pharmacologic: purine antagonists

Indications

Prevention of renal transplant rejection (with corticosteroids, local radiation, or other cytotoxic agents). Treatment of severe, active, erosive rheumatoid arthritis unresponsive to more conventional therapy. **Unlabeled Use:** Management of Crohn's disease.

Action

Antagonizes purine metabolism with subsequent inhibition of DNA and RNA synthesis. **Therapeutic Effects:** Suppression of cell-mediated immunity and altered antibody formation.

Adverse Reactions/Side Effects

EENT: retinopathy. **Resp:** pulmonary edema. **GI:** anorexia, hepatotoxicity, nausea, vomiting, diarrhea, mucositis, pancreatitis. **Derm:** alopecia, rash. **Hemat:** anemia, leukopenia, pancytopenia, thrombocytopenia. **MS:** arthralgia. **Misc:** SERUM SICKNESS, chills, fever, Raynaud's phenomenon.

PHYSICAL THERAPY IMPLICATIONS

Examination and Evaluation

- Monitor signs of hypersensitivity reactions, especially signs of serum sickness such as muscle aches, joint pains, fever, and skin rash. Notify physician or nursing staff immediately if these reactions occur.
- Watch for and report signs of leukopenia (fever, sore throat, signs of infection), thrombocytopenia (bruising, nose bleeds, and bleeding gums), or unusual weakness and fatigue that might be due to anemia or other blood dyscrasias. Periodic blood tests may be needed to monitor WBC and RBC counts.
- Assess any breathing problems or signs of pulmonary edema such as rales/crackles chest pain, shortness of breath, and difficult or labored breathing. Monitor pulse oximetry and perform pulmonary function tests (See Appendices I, J, K) to quantify suspected changes in ventilation and respiratory function.
- If treating rheumatoid arthritis, periodically assess patient's impairments (pain, range of motion), functional ability, and disability to help document whether antirheumatic drug therapy is successful.
- Assess any new or increased joint pain to rule out musculoskeletal pathology; that is, try to determine

if pain is drug induced rather than caused by arthritis or anatomic and biomechanical problems.

- Monitor signs of Raynaud's phenomenon as indicated by decreased circulation to the fingers and toes resulting in pain, numbness, swelling, and color changes in the affected digits. Report these signs to the physician, and educate patient about how to avoid the onset of symptoms (keep hands warm, avoid caffeine, stress, and other triggers).
- If treating inflammatory bowel diseases, monitor any changes in symptoms (decreased abdominal pain, decreased diarrhea, improved appetite) to help document whether drug therapy is successful.

Interventions

- Implement appropriate manual therapy techniques, physical agents, therapeutic exercises, and orthotic/assistive devices to reduce pain, improve function, and augment the effects of antirheumatic drug therapy.
- Help patient explore other nonpharmacologic methods to reduce chronic arthritis pain such as relaxation techniques, exercise, counseling, and so forth.

Patient/Client-Related Instruction

- Instruct patient to report signs of retinopathy such as blurred vision, loss of vision, and spots or dark strings floating in vision (floaters). Visual problems are more common at higher doses.
- Advise patient about the likelihood of GI reactions such as nausea, vomiting, diarrhea, and loss of appetite. Instruct patient to report severe or prolonged GI problems, or signs of liver toxicity (yellow skin or eyes, abdominal pain, severe nausea and vomiting, fever, sore throat, malaise, weakness, facial edema) or pancreatitis (upper abdominal pain after eating, indigestion, weight loss, oily stools).
- Because of immunosuppressant effects, advise patient to guard against infection (frequent hand washing, etc.) and to avoid crowds and contact with persons with contagious diseases.
- Instruct patient to report other untoward side effects such as severe or prolonged chills, fever, or skin reactions (rash, hair loss).

Pharmacokinetics

Absorption: Readily absorbed after oral administration.
Distribution: Crosses the placenta. Enters breast milk in low concentrations.
Metabolism and Excretion: Metabolized to mercaptopurine, which is further metabolized. Minimal renal excretion of unchanged drug.
Half-life: 3 hr.

TIME/ACTION PROFILE

ROUTE	ONSET	PEAK	DURATION
PO (anti-inflammatory)	6–8 wk	12 wk	unknown
IV (immunosuppression)	days–wk	unknown	days–wk

Contraindications/Precautions

Contraindicated in: Hypersensitivity; Concurrent use of mycophenolate; OB: Has been shown to cause fetal harm; Lactation: Appears in breast milk.
Use Cautiously in: Infections; Malignancies; Decreased bone marrow reserve; Previous or concurrent radiation therapy; Other chronic debilitating illnesses; Severe renal impairment/oliguria (increased sensitivity); OB: Patients with childbearing potential.

Interactions

Drug-Drug: Additive myelosuppression with **antineoplastics**, **cyclosporine**, and **myelosuppressive agents**. **Allopurinol** inhibits the metabolism of azathioprine, increasing toxicity. Dose of azathioprine should be decreased by 25–33% with concurrent allopurinol. May ↓ antibody response to **live-virus vaccines** and ↑ the risk of adverse reactions.
Drug-Natural: Concomitant use with **echinacea** and **melatonin** may interfere with immunosuppression.

Route/Dosage

Renal Allograft Rejection Prevention

PO, IV (Adults and Children): 3–5 mg/kg/day initially; maintenance dose 1–3 mg/kg/day.

Rheumatoid Arthritis

PO (Adults and Children): 1 mg/kg/day for 6–8 wk, increase by 0.5 mg/kg/day q 4 wk until response or up to 2.5 mg/kg/day, then decrease by 0.5 mg/kg/day q 4–8 wk to minimal effective dose.

Availability (generic available)

Tablets: 50 mg, 75 mg, 100 mg. **Injection:** 100-mg vial.

azelastine (a-**zel**-as-teen)

Astelin

Classification

Therapeutic: allergy, cold, and cough remedies, antihistamines

Indications

Management of the symptoms of seasonal allergic rhinitis in patients ≥5 yr. Management of vasomotor rhinitis in patients ≥12 yr.

Action

Locally antagonizes the effects of histamine at H_1 receptor sites; does not bind to or inactivate histamine. **Therapeutic Effects:** Decreased sneezing, nasal rhinitis, pruritus, and postnasal drip.

Adverse Reactions/Side Effects

CNS: drowsiness, dizziness, dysesthesia, fatigue, headache. **EENT:** epistaxis, nasal burning, pharyngitis, sinusitis, sneezing. **GI:** bitter taste, dry mouth, nausea. **Metab:** weight gain. **MS:** myalgia.

PHYSICAL THERAPY IMPLICATIONS

Examination and Evaluation

- Assess dizziness and drowsiness that might affect gait, balance, and other functional activities (See Appendix C). Report balance problems and functional limitations to the physician, and caution the patient and family/caregivers to guard against falls and trauma.
- Assess any muscle pain to rule out musculoskeletal pathology; that is, try to determine if pain is drug induced rather than caused by anatomic or biomechanical problems.
- Periodically assess body weight and other anthropometric measures (body mass index, body composition). Report a rapid or unexplained weight gain or increased body fat.

Interventions

- Guard against falls and trauma (hip fractures, head injury, and so forth). Implement fall prevention strategies, especially in older adults or if balance is impaired (See Appendix E).

Patient/Client-Related Instruction

- Advise patient about the risk of daytime drowsiness and decreased attention and mental focus. These problems can be severe in certain people. Use care if driving or in other activities that require quick reactions and strong concentration.
- Advise patient to avoid alcohol and other CNS depressants because of the increased risk of sedation and adverse effects.
- Instruct patient to report prolonged or severe nasal irritation, including excessive sneezing, nosebleeds, burning sensations, or other troublesome nasopharyngeal symptoms.
- Instruct patient and family/caregivers to report severe or prolonged headache, fatigue, or GI problems (nausea, dry mouth, bitter taste).

Pharmacokinetics

Absorption: 40% absorbed after intranasal administration.
Distribution: 14.5 L/kg.
Metabolism and Excretion: Most of absorbed azelastine is metabolized by the liver (converted to an active metabolite.
Half-life: 22 hr.

TIME/ACTION PROFILE (relief of symptoms)

ROUTE	ONSET	PEAK	DURATION
intranasal	rapid	2–3 hr*	12 hr

*Plasma concentration.

Contraindications/Precautions

Contraindicated in: Hypersensitivity.
Use Cautiously in: OB/Lactation: Safety not established; Pedi: Safety not established in children <5 yr.

Interactions

Drug-Drug: Additive CNS depression with **CNS depressants**, including **alcohol**, **sedative/hypnotics**, and **opioid analgesics**. Concurrent use of **cimetidine** increases blood levels.
Drug-Natural: Concomitant use of **kava**, **valerian**, **skullcap**, **chamomile**, or **hops** can increase CNS depression. Theoretically, **St. John's wort** could interfere with azelastine metabolism.

Route/Dosage

Intranasal (Adults and Children ≥12 yr): 2 sprays/nostril twice daily.
Intranasal (Children 5–11 yr): 1 spray/nostril twice daily.

Availability

Nasal spray: 137 mcg/spray in 30-mL bottle (200 sprays/bottle).

azithromycin
(aye-zith-row-my-sin)
Zithromax, Zmax

Classification
Therapeutic: agents for atypical mycobacterium, anti-infectives
Pharmacologic: macrolides

Indications

Treatment of the following infections due to susceptible organisms: Upper respiratory tract infections, including streptococcal pharyngitis, acute bacterial exacerbations of chronic bronchitis, and tonsillitis; Lower respiratory tract infections, including bronchitis and pneumonia; Acute otitis media; Skin and skin structure infections; Nongonococcal urethritis, cervicitis, gonorrhea, and chancroid. Prevention of disseminated *Mycobacterium avium* complex (MAC) infection in patients with advanced HIV infection. *Extended-release suspension (Zmax):* Acute bacterial sinusitis and community-acquired pneumonia in adults. **Unlabeled Use:** Prevention of bacterial endocarditis. Treatment of cystic fibrosis lung disease.

Action

Inhibits protein synthesis at the level of the 50S bacterial ribosome. **Therapeutic Effects:** Bacteriostatic action against susceptible bacteria. **Spectrum:** Active against the following gram-positive aerobic bacteria: *Staphylococcus aureus, Streptococcus pneumoniae, Streptococcus pyogenes* (group A strep). Active against these gram-negative aerobic bacteria: *Haemophilus influenzae, Moraxella catarrhali, Neisseria gonorrhoeae.* Also active against: *Mycoplasma, Legionella, Chlamydia pneumoniae, Ureaplasma urealyticum, Borrelia burgdorferi, M. avium.* Not active against methicillin-resistant *S. aureus.*

Adverse Reactions/Side Effects

CNS: dizziness, seizures, drowsiness, fatigue, headache. **CV:** chest pain, hypotension, palpitations, QT prolongation (rare). **GI:** PSEUDOMEMBRANOUS COLITIS, abdominal pain, diarrhea, nausea, cholestatic jaundice, elevated liver enzymes, dyspepsia, flatulence, melena, oral candidiasis. **GU:** nephritis, vaginitis. **Hemat:** anemia, leukopenia, thrombocytopenia. **Derm:** photosensitivity, Stevens-Johnson syndrome, rashes. **EENT:** ototoxicity. **F and E:** hyperkalemia. **Misc:** ANGIOEDEMA.

PHYSICAL THERAPY IMPLICATIONS

Examination and Evaluation

- Monitor signs of pseudomembranous colitis, including diarrhea, abdominal pain, fever, pus or mucus in stool, and other severe or prolonged GI problems (nausea, vomiting, heartburn). Notify physician or nursing staff immediately of these signs.
- Monitor patient for signs of angioedema, including rashes, raised patches of red or white skin (welts), burning/itching skin, swelling in the face, and difficulty breathing. Notify physician of these signs immediately.
- Monitor rashes or other skin reactions such as hives, acne, dermatitis, abnormal sweating, and exfoliation. Notify physician immediately because certain skin reactions may indicate serious hypersensitivity reactions (Stevens-Johnson syndrome).
- Monitor signs of leukopenia (fever, sore throat, signs of infection), thrombocytopenia (bruising, nose bleeds, bleeding gums), or unusual weakness and fatigue that might be due to anemia. Report these signs to the physician.
- Monitor symptoms of high plasma potassium levels (hyperkalemia), including bradycardia, fatigue, weakness, numbness, and tingling. Notify physician because severe cases can lead to life-threatening arrhythmias and paralysis.
- Be alert for new seizures or increased seizure activity, especially at the onset of drug treatment. Document the number, duration, and severity of seizures, and report these findings immediately to the physician.
- Monitor and report signs of nephritis, including blood in urine, decreased urine output, and weight gain from fluid retention.
- Assess heart rate, ECG, and heart sounds, especially during exercise (See Appendices G, H). Report any rhythm disturbances or symptoms of increased arrhythmias, including palpitations, chest pain, shortness of breath, fainting, and fatigue/weakness.
- Assess blood pressure periodically and compare to normal values (See Appendix F). Report low blood pressure (hypotension), especially if patient experiences dizziness, fatigue, or other symptoms.
- Monitor signs of ototoxicity such as hearing loss, tinnitus, disturbed balance, and vertigo. Report these signs to the physician.
- Assess dizziness or drowsiness that might affect gait, balance, and other functional activities (See Appendix C). Report balance problems and functional limitations to the physician and nursing staff, and caution the patient and family/caregivers to guard against falls and trauma.

Interventions

- Always wash hands thoroughly and disinfect equipment (whirlpools, electrotherapeutic devices, treatment tables, and so forth) to help prevent the spread of infection. Employ universal precautions or isolation procedures as indicated for specific patients.
- Because of the risk of arrhythmias and hypotension, use caution during aerobic exercise and other forms of therapeutic exercise. Assess exercise tolerance frequently (blood pressure, heart rate, fatigue levels), and terminate exercise immediately if any untoward responses occur (See Appendix L).
- Guard against falls and trauma (hip fractures, head injury, and so forth), especially if ototoxicity affects balance reactions. Implement fall prevention strategies, especially in older adults (See Appendix E).
- Causes photosensitivity; use care if administering UV treatments. Advise patient to avoid direct sunlight and use sunscreens and protective clothing.

Patient/Client-Related Instruction

- Advise patient about the likelihood of GI reactions such as nausea, indigestion, diarrhea, abdominal pain, and flatulence. Instruct patient to report severe or prolonged GI problems.
- Instruct patient and family/caregivers to report other troublesome side effects such as severe or prolonged headache, vaginal irritation, infections in/around the mouth, or skin rash.

Pharmacokinetics

Absorption: Rapidly absorbed (40%) after oral administration. IV administration results in complete bioavailability.

Distribution: Widely distributed to body tissues and fluids. Intracellular and tissue levels exceed those in serum; low CSF levels.
Metabolism and Excretion: Mostly excreted unchanged in bile; 4.5% excreted unchanged in urine.
Half-life: 11–14 hr after single dose; 2–4 days after several doses; 59 hr after extended release suspension.

TIME/ACTION PROFILE (serum)

ROUTE	ONSET	PEAK	DURATION
PO	rapid	2.5–3.2 hr	24 hr
IV	rapid	end of infusion	24 hr

Contraindications/Precautions
Contraindicated in: Hypersensitivity to azithromycin, erythromycin, or other macrolide anti-infectives.
Use Cautiously in: Severe liver impairment (dosage adjustment may be required); Severe renal impairment (CCr <10 mL/min); OB/Lactation: Safety not established; Pedi: Safety not established in children <5 yr.

Interactions
Drug-Drug: Aluminum- and **magnesium-containing antacids** decrease peak serum levels. **Nelfinavir** increases serum levels (monitor carefully). Other macrolide anti-infectives have been known to increase serum levels and effects of **digoxin, theophylline, ergotamine, dihydroergotamine, triazolam, carbamazepine, cyclosporine, tacrolimus,** and **phenytoin**; careful monitoring of concurrent use is recommended.

Route/Dosage
Most Respiratory and Skin Infections
PO (Adults): 500 mg on 1st day, then 250 mg/day for 4 more days (total dose of 1.5 g). *Acute bacterial sinusitis*—500 mg once daily for 3 days or single 2-g dose of extended-release suspension (Zmax).
PO (Children ≥6 months): 10 mg/kg (not >500 mg/dose) on 1st day, then 5 mg/kg (not >250 mg/dose) for 4 more days. *Pharyngitis/tonsilitis*—12 mg/kg once daily for 5 days (not >500 mg/dose). *Acute bacterial sinusitis*—10 mg/kg/day for 3 days.

Otitis media
PO (Children ≥6 mo): 30 mg/kg single dose (not >1500 mg/dose) *or* 10 mg/kg/day as a single dose (not >500 mg/dose) for 3 days *or* 10 mg/kg as a single dose (not >500 mg/dose) on 1st day, then 5 mg/kg as a single dose (not >250 mg/dose) daily for 4 more days.

Acute Bacterial Exacerbations of Chronic Bronchitis
PO (Adults): 500 mg on 1st day, then 250 mg/day for 4 more days (total dose of 1.5 g) *or* 500 mg daily for 3 days.

Community-Acquired Pneumonia
IV, PO (Adults): *More severe*—500 mg IV q 24 hr for at least 2 doses, then 500 mg PO q 24 hr for a total of 7–10 days; *less severe*—500 mg PO, then 250 mg/day PO for 4 more days or 2-g single dose as extended-release suspension (Zmax).
PO (Children >6 mo): 10 mg/kg on 1st day, then 5 mg/kg for 4 more days.

Pelvic Inflammatory Disease
IV, PO (Adults): 500 mg IV q 24 hr for 1–2 days, then 250 mg PO q 24 hr for a total of 7 days.

Endocarditis Prophylaxis
PO (Adults): 500 mg 1 hr before procedure.
PO (Children): 15 mg/kg 1 hr before procedure.

Nongonococcal Urethritis, Cervicitis, Chancroid, Chlamydia
PO (Adults): Single 1-g dose.
PO (Children): *Chancroid:* Single 20 mg/kg dose (not >1000 mg/dose). *Urethritis or cervicitis:* Single 10 mg/kg dose (not >1000 mg/dose).

Gonorrhea
PO (Adults): Single 2-g dose.

Prevention of Disseminated MAC Infection
PO (Adults): 1.2 g once weekly (alone or with rifabutin).
PO (Children): 5 mg/kg once daily (not >250 mg/dose) or 20 mg/kg (not >1200 mg/dose) once weekly (alone or with rifabutin).

Cystic Fibrosis
PO (Children ≥6 yr, weight ≥25 kg to <40 kg): 250 mg q MWF (Monday, Wednesday, Friday) ≥40 kg: 500 mg q MWF.

Availability (generic available)
Tablets: 250 mg, 500 mg, 600 mg. **Powder for oral suspension (cherry, creme de vanilla, and banana flavor):** 1 g/pkt. **Powder for oral suspension (cherry, creme de vanilla, and banana flavor):** 100 mg/5 mL in 15-mL bottles, 200 mg/5 mL in 15-mL, 22.5-mL, and 30-mL bottles. **Extended-release oral suspension (ZMax) (cherry-banana):** 2-g single-dose bottle. **Powder for injection:** 500 mg/vial.

aztreonam (az-tree-oh-nam)
Azactam

Classification
Therapeutic: anti-infectives
Pharmacologic: monobactams

Indications

Treatment of serious gram-negative infections including Septicemia; Skin and skin structure infections; Intra-abdominal infections; Gynecologic infections; Respiratory tract infections; Urinary tract infections. Useful for treatment of multiresistant strains of some bacteria, including aerobic gram-negative pathogens.

Action

Binds to the bacterial cell wall membrane, causing cell death. **Therapeutic Effects:** Bactericidal action against susceptible bacteria. **Spectrum:** Displays significant activity against gram-negative aerobic organisms only: *Escherichia coli*, *Serratia*, *Klebsiella oxytoca or K. pneumoniae*, *Citrobacter*, *Proteus mirabilis*, *Pseudomonas aeruginosa*, *Enterobacter*, *Haemophilus influenzae*. Not active against: *Staphylococcus aureus*, *Enterococcus*, *Bacteroides fragilis*, Streptococci.

Adverse Reactions/Side Effects

CNS: SEIZURES. **GI:** PSEUDOMEMBRANOUS COLITIS, altered taste, diarrhea, nausea, vomiting. **Derm:** rash. **Local:** pain at IM site, phlebitis at IV site. **Misc:** ALLERGIC REACTIONS, INCLUDING ANAPHYLAXIS, superinfection.

PHYSICAL THERAPY IMPLICATIONS

Examination and Evaluation

- Watch for seizures; notify physician immediately if patient develops or increases seizure activity.
- Monitor signs of pseudomembranous colitis, including diarrhea, abdominal pain, fever, pus or mucus in stool, and other severe or prolonged GI problems (nausea, vomiting, heartburn). Notify physician or nursing staff immediately of these signs.
- Monitor signs of allergic reactions and anaphylaxis, including pulmonary symptoms (tightness in the throat and chest, wheezing, cough dyspnea) or skin reactions (rash, pruritus, urticaria). Notify physician or nursing staff immediately if these reactions occur.
- Monitor injection site for pain, swelling, and irritation. Report prolonged or excessive injection-site reactions to the physician.

Interventions

- Always wash hands thoroughly and disinfect equipment (whirlpools, electrotherapeutic devices, treatment tables, and so forth) to help prevent the spread of infection. Use universal precautions or isolation procedures as indicated for specific patients.

Patient/Client-Related Instruction

- Instruct patient to notify physician immediately of signs of superinfection, including black, furry overgrowth on tongue, vaginal itching or discharge, and loose or foul-smelling stools.
- Instruct patient and family/caregivers to report other troublesome side effects such as severe or prolonged skin rash or GI problems (nausea, vomiting, diarrhea, altered taste).

Pharmacokinetics

Absorption: Well absorbed following IM administration.
Distribution: Widely distributed. Crosses the placenta and enters breast milk in low concentrations.
Metabolism and Excretion: 60–70% excreted unchanged by the kidneys. Small amounts metabolized by the liver.
Half-life: 1.5–2 hr (increased in renal impairment).

TIME/ACTION PROFILE (blood levels)

ROUTE	ONSET	PEAK	DURATION
IM	rapid	60 min	6–8 hr
IV	rapid	end of infusion	6–8 hr

Contraindications/Precautions

Contraindicated in: Hypersensitivity.
Use Cautiously in: Renal impairment (dosage reduction required if CCr 30 mL/min or less); Cross-sensitivity with penicillins or cephalosporins may occur rarely. Has been used safely in patients with a history of penicillin or cephalosporin allergy; OB/ Lactation: Safety not established; Pedi: Safety not established for children <9 mo; Geri: Geriatric patients have age-related decrease in renal function.

Interactions

Drug-Drug: Serum levels may be increased by **furosemide** or **probenecid**.

Route/Dosage

IM, IV (Adults): *Moderately severe infections*—1–2 g q 8–12 hr; *severe or life-threatening infections* (*including those due to* Pseudomonas aeruginosa)—2 g q 6–8 hr; *urinary tract infections*—0.5–1 g q 8–12 hr.
IV (Children 9 mo–16 yr): *Mild to moderate infections infections*—30 mg/kg q 8 hr; *moderate to severe infections infections*—30 mg/kg q 6–8 hr; *cystic fibrosis*—50 mg/kg q 6–8 hr.

Renal Impairment

IV (Adults): *CCr 10–30 mL/min*—1–2 g initially, then 50% of usual dosage at usual interval; *CCr <10 mL/min*—500 mg–2 g initially, then 25% of usual dosage at usual interval ($\frac{1}{8}$ of initial dose should also be given after each hemodialysis session).

Availability

Injection: 0.5-g, 1-g, 2-g vials, infusion bottles, and plastic containers.

B

baclofen (bak-loe-fen)

Kemstro, Lioresal

Classification

Therapeutic: antispasticity agents,
Pharmacologic: skeletal muscle relaxants (centrally acting)

Indications

PO: Treatment of reversible spasticity due to multiple sclerosis or spinal cord lesions. **Intrathecal:** Treatment of severe spasticity originating in the spinal cord. **Unlabeled Use:** Management of pain in trigeminal neuralgia.

Action

Inhibits reflexes at the spinal level. **Therapeutic Effects:** Decreased muscle spasticity; bowel and bladder function may also be improved.

Adverse Reactions/Side Effects

CNS: SEIZURES (IT), dizziness, drowsiness, fatigue, weakness, confusion, depression, headache, insomnia. **EENT:** nasal congestion, tinnitus. **CV:** edema, hypotension. **GI:** nausea, constipation. **GU:** frequency. **Derm:** pruritus, rash. **Metab:** hyperglycemia, weight gain. **Neuro:** ataxia. **Misc:** hypersensitivity reactions, sweating.

PHYSICAL THERAPY IMPLICATIONS

Examination and Evaluation

- Be alert for new seizures or increased seizure activity, especially during intrathecal (spinal) administration. Document the number, duration, and severity of seizures, and report these findings immediately to the physician.
- Assess patient's spasticity, ROM, functional ability, and posture (e.g., head control and trunk stability), especially when beginning baclofen treatment or during dose adjustments. Communicate with physician, family/caregivers, and other health professionals to determine if dosage is helping achieve desired functional outcomes.
- During intrathecal administration:
  - Monitor patient closely during initial (test) doses and titration. Resuscitative equipment should be immediately available for life-threatening or intolerable side effects.
  - Monitor sudden changes in spasticity, muscle strength, or CNS symptoms (confusion, somnolence, agitation, hallucinations) that might indicate pump malfunction.
  - Make sure patient and caregivers understand how to protect the pump and catheter, and adhere to an appropriate schedule for pump refills.
- Assess dizziness, drowsiness, and ataxia that might affect gait, balance, transfers, and other functional activities (See Appendix C). Report balance problems and functional limitations to the physician, and caution the patient and family/caregivers to guard against falls and trauma.
- Monitor signs of hypersensitivity reactions, including pulmonary symptoms (tightness in the throat and chest, wheezing, cough, dyspnea) or skin reactions (rash, pruritus, urticaria). Notify physician immediately if these reactions occur.
- Assess blood pressure periodically and compare to normal values (See Appendix F). Report low blood pressure (hypotension), especially if patient experiences dizziness, fatigue, or other symptoms.
- Assess peripheral edema using girth measurements, volume displacement, and measurement of pitting edema (See Appendix N). Report increased swelling in feet and ankles or a sudden increase in body weight due to fluid retention.
- Be alert for signs of hyperglycemia, including confusion, drowsiness, flushed/dry skin, fruit-like breath odor, rapid/deep breathing, polyuria, loss of appetite, and unusual thirst. Patients with diabetes mellitus should check blood glucose levels frequently.
- Monitor changes in mood and behavior including confusion and depression. Report these changes to the physician.
- If treating trigeminal neuralgia, use appropriate pain scales (visual analogue scales, others) to document whether this drug is successful in helping manage the patient's pain.
- Assess body weight periodically, and report a rapid or unexplained weight gain.

Interventions

- Implement aggressive therapeutic exercises (neuromuscular reeducation, postural stabilization, gait training, and/or other task-specific training) to help patient adjust to reduced spasticity and tone.
- Guard against falls and trauma due to sedation, dizziness, or abnormally low tone in the trunk and lower extremities.
- To minimize orthostatic hypotension, patient should move slowly when assuming a more upright position.

Patient/Client-Related Instruction

- Advise patient to avoid alcohol and other CNS depressants because of the increased risk of sedation and adverse effects.

- Caution patient and caregivers against abrupt baclofen withdrawal because it may precipitate an acute withdrawal reaction (hallucinations, increased spasticity, seizures, mental changes, restlessness). Baclofen should be discontinued gradually 2 wk or longer.
- Instruct patient or family/caregivers to report other bothersome side effects such as severe or prolonged headache, sleep loss, nasal congestion, ringing/buzzing in the ears (tinnitus), increased urination, skin reactions (rash, itching, sweating), or GI problems (nausea, constipation).

Pharmacokinetics

Absorption: Well absorbed after oral administration.
Distribution: Widely distributed; crosses the placenta.
Metabolism and Excretion: 70–80% eliminated unchanged by the kidneys.
Half-life: 2.5–4 hr.

TIME/ACTION PROFILE (effects on spasticity)

ROUTE	ONSET	PEAK	DURATION
PO	hrs–wks	unknown	unknown
IT	0.5–1 hr	4 hr	4–8 hr

Contraindications/Precautions

Contraindicated in: Hypersensitivity; Orally disintegrating tablets contain aspartame and should not be used in patients with phenylketonuria.
Use Cautiously in: Patients in whom spasticity maintains posture and balance; Patients with epilepsy (may ↓ seizure threshold); Renal impairment (↓ dose may be required); OB/Lactation/Pedi: Safety not established; Geri: Geriatric patients are at ↑ risk of CNS side effects.

Interactions

Drug-Drug: ↑ CNS depression with other **CNS depressants,** including **alcohol, antihistamines, opioid analgesics,** and **sedative/hypnotics**. Use with **MAO inhibitors** may lead to ↑ CNS depression or hypotension.
Drug-Natural: Concomitant use of **kava, valerian,** or **chamomile** can ↑ CNS depression.

Route/Dosage

PO (Adults): 5 mg 3 times daily. May increase q 3 days by 5 mg/dose up to 80 mg/day (some patients may have a better response to 4 divided doses).
Intrathecal (Adults): 100–800 mcg/day infusion; dose is determined by response during screening phase.
Intrathecal (Children): 25–1200 mcg/day infusion (average 275 mcg/day); dose is determined by response during screening phase.

Availability (generic available)

Tablets: 10 mg, 20 mg. **Orally disintegrating tablets (Kemstro) (orange):** 10 mg, 20 mg. **Intrathecal injection:** 50 mcg/mL, 500 mcg/mL, 2000 mcg/mL.

balsalazide (ba-sal-a-zide)

Colazal

Classification

Therapeutic: gastrointestinal anti-inflammatories—therapeutic
Pharmacologic: salicylates

Indications

Treatment of mild-to-moderately active ulcerative colitis.

Action

Drug is metabolized in the colon to mesalamine (5-aminosalicylic acid), which is a local anti-inflammatory. **Therapeutic Effects:** Reduction in the symptoms of ulcerative colitis.

Adverse Reactions/Side Effects

GI: HEPATOTOXICITY, abdominal pain, diarrhea.

PHYSICAL THERAPY IMPLICATIONS

Examination and Evaluation

- Be alert for signs of hepatotoxicity, including anorexia, abdominal pain, severe nausea and vomiting, yellow skin or eyes, fever, sore throat, malaise, weakness, facial edema, lethargy, and unusual bleeding or bruising. Notify physician of these signs immediately.

Patient/Client-Related Instruction

- Advise patient to avoid alcohol and foods that may cause an increase in GI irritation.
- Instruct patient to report troublesome GI effects such as diarrhea and abdominal pain.

Pharmacokinetics

Absorption: Absorption is low and variable; drug is delivered intact to the colon.
Distribution: Mostly delivered intact to the colon; remainder of distribution unknown.
Protein Binding: ≥99%.
Metabolism and Excretion: Following delivery to the colon, bacteria break balsalazide down into mesalamine (5-aminosalicylic acid) and an inactive metabolite; mostly excreted in feces.
Half-life: *Mesalamine*—12 hr (range 2–15 hr).

TIME/ACTION PROFILE (decreased symptoms)

ROUTE	ONSET	PEAK	DURATION
PO	unknown	up to 8 wk	unknown

B

Contraindications/Precautions

Contraindicated in: Hypersensitivity to salicylates or other metabolites.

Use Cautiously in: Pyloric stenosis (may have prolonged gastric retention of capsules); OB: Use only if clearly needed; Lactation/Pedi: Safety not established.

Interactions

Drug-Drug: None known.

Route/Dosage

PO (Adults): 3 750-mg capsules 3 times daily for 8–12 wk.

PO (Children 5–17 yr): 3 750-mg capsules 3 times daily for up to 8 wk *or* 1 750-mg capsule 3 times daily for up to 8 wk.

Availability

Capsules: 750 mg.

basiliximab (ba-sil-ix-i-mab)

Simulect

Classification

Therapeutic: immunosuppressants

Pharmacologic: monoclonal antibodies

Indications

Prevention of acute organ rejection in patients undergoing renal transplantation; used with corticosteroids and cyclosporine.

Action

Binds to and blocks specific interleukin-2 (IL-2) receptor sites on activated T lymphocytes. **Therapeutic Effects:** Prevention of acute organ rejection following renal transplantation.

Adverse Reactions/Side Effects

Noted for patients receiving corticosteroids and cyclosporine in addition to basiliximab

CNS: dizziness, headache, insomnia, weakness. **EENT:** abnormal vision, cataracts. **Resp:** coughing. **CV:** HEART FAILURE, edema, hypertension, angina, arrhythmias, hypotension. **GI:** abdominal pain, constipation, diarrhea, dyspepsia, moniliasis, nausea, vomiting, GI bleeding, gingival hyperplasia, stomatitis. **Derm:** acne, wound complications, hypertrichosis, pruritus. **Endo:** hyperglycemia, hypoglycemia. **F and E:** acidosis, hypercholesterolemia, hyperkalemia, hyperuricemia, hypocalcemia, hypokalemia, hypophosphatemia. **Hemat:** bleeding, coagulation abnormalities. **MS:** back pain, leg pain. **Neuro:** tremor, neuropathy, paresthesia. **Misc:** HYPERSENSITIVITY REACTIONS, INCLUDING ANAPHYLAXIS, infection, weight gain, chills.

PHYSICAL THERAPY IMPLICATIONS

Examination and Evaluation

- Be alert for signs of hypersensitivity reactions and anaphylaxis, including pulmonary symptoms (tightness in the throat and chest, wheezing, cough, dyspnea) or skin reactions (rash, pruritus, urticaria). Notify physician or nursing staff immediately if these reactions occur.
- Watch for signs of heart failure, including dyspnea, rales/crackles, peripheral edema, jugular venous distention, and exercise intolerance. Report these signs to the physician immediately.
- Monitor signs of GI bleeding (abdominal pain, vomiting blood, blood in stools, black/tarry stools) or other coagulation problems (bleeding gums, nosebleed, excessive bruising). Report these signs to the physician or nursing staff immediately.
- Assess blood pressure (BP) and compare to normal values (See Appendix F). Report changes in BP, either a problematic decrease in BP (hypotension) or a sustained increase in BP (hypertension).
- Assess heart rate, ECG, and heart sounds, especially during exercise (See Appendices G, H). Report any ECG abnormalities or signs of arrhythmias, including palpitations, chest discomfort, shortness of breath, fainting, and fatigue/weakness.
- Assess peripheral edema using girth measurements, volume displacement, and measurement of pitting edema (See Appendix N). Report increased swelling of feet and ankles or a sudden increase in body weight due to fluid retention.
- Monitor signs of hypoglycemia (weakness, malaise, irritability, fatigue) or hyperglycemia (drowsiness, fruity breath, increased urination, unusual thirst). Patients with diabetes mellitus should check blood glucose levels frequently.
- Be alert for signs of paresthesia and neuropathy, including numbness, tingling, and muscle weakness. Establish baseline electroneuromyographic values at the beginning of drug treatment whenever possible, and reexamine these values periodically to document drug-induced changes in peripheral nerve function.
- Monitor neuromuscular signs of acid-base imbalance (acidosis, alkalosis) or electrolyte imbalances (hypocalcemia, hypokalemia, hyperkalemia, hypomagnesemia, hypophosphatemia, hyponatremia), including headache, lethargy, irritability, insomnia, confusion, weakness, cramping, tremors, and changes in muscle excitability. Notify physician immediately if these signs occur.

- Assess any back or leg to rule out musculoskeletal pathology; that is, try to determine if pain is drug induced rather than caused by anatomic or biomechanical problems.
- Assess dizziness or weakness that might affect gait, balance, and other functional activities (See Appendix C). Report balance problems and functional limitations to the physician and nursing staff, and caution the patient and family/caregivers to guard against falls and trauma.
- Periodically assess body weight and other anthropometric measures (body mass index, body composition). Report a rapid or unexplained weight gain or increased body fat.

Interventions

- Implement appropriate strengthening, aerobic, and other therapeutic exercises to improve function and promote recovery following organ transplants.
- Because of the risk of arrhythmias and abnormal BP responses, use caution during aerobic exercise and other forms of therapeutic exercise. Assess exercise tolerance frequently (BP, heart rate, fatigue levels), and terminate exercise immediately if any untoward responses occur (See Appendix L).

Patient/Client-Related Instruction

- Because of immunosuppressant effects, advise patient to guard against infection (frequent hand washing, etc.) and to avoid crowds and contact with persons with contagious diseases.
- Advise patient that wound healing may be delayed; instruct patient to check skin regularly and report any nonhealing sores.
- Advise patient that this drug may cause problems in fat metabolism (hyperlipidemia). Remind patient that periodic blood tests may be needed to monitor plasma lipids.
- Instruct patient to report other bothersome side effects such as severe or prolonged headache, sleep loss, vision disturbances, cough, infections, chills, skin reactions (itching, acne), or GI problems (nausea, vomiting, diarrhea, constipation, indigestion, abdominal pain, infection/inflammation in or around the mouth).

Pharmacokinetics

Absorption: IV administration results in complete bioavailability.
Distribution: Unknown.
Metabolism and Excretion: Unknown.
Half-life: 7.2 days.

TIME/ACTION PROFILE (effect on immune function)

ROUTE	ONSET	PEAK	DURATION
IV	2 hr	unknown	36 days

Contraindications/Precautions

Contraindicated in: Hypersensitivity; OB: May affect fetal developing immune system; Lactation: May enter breast milk.
Use Cautiously in: Women with childbearing potential; Geri: Due to greater incidence of infection.

Interactions

Drug-Drug: Immunosuppression may be ↑ with other **immunosuppressants**.
Drug-Natural: Concomitant use with **echinacea** and **melatonin** may interfere with immunosuppression.

Route/Dosage

IV (Adults and Children ≥35 kg): 20 mg given 2 hr before transplantation; repeated 4 days after transplantation. Second dose should be withheld if complications or graft loss occurs.
IV (Children <35 kg): 10 mg given 2 hr before transplantation; repeated 4 days after transplantation. Second dose should be withheld if complications or graft loss occurs.

Availability

Powder for reconstitution: 20 mg/vial, 10 mg/vial.

becaplermin (be-**kap**-ler-min)

Regranex

Classification
Therapeutic: wound/ulcer/decubiti healing agent
Pharmacologic: platelet-derived growth factors

Indications

Treatment of lower extremity diabetic neuropathic ulcers extending to subcutaneous tissue or beyond and having adequate blood supply.

Action

Promotes chemotaxis of cells involved in wound repair and enhances formation of granulation tissue. **Therapeutic Effects:** Improved healing.

Adverse Reactions/Side Effects

Derm: erythematous rash at application site. **Misc:** MALIGNANCY (MAY LEAD TO ↑ MORTALITY, ESPECIALLY WITH USE OF ≥3 TUBES).

PHYSICAL THERAPY IMPLICATIONS

Examination and Evaluation

- Assess the size, depth, color, drainage, and periwound area to help document whether drug therapy is successful in promoting wound healing.
- Monitor any new or increased skin reactions at the site of application, including rash, redness, and irritation. Be especially alert for any abnormal growth

of tissues in/around the wound. Report any suspicious skin reactions to the physician.

Interventions

- Implement wound-care procedures (whirlpool, pulsed lavage, gentle débridement) as needed to cleanse ulcers. Make sure the drug is reapplied and dressings are changed according to the recommended procedures.
- When indicated, use appropriate physical agents (ultrasound, electric stimulation, ultraviolet light) to facilitate wound healing and augment drug effects.
- Use assistive devices (walker, crutches) as needed to minimize weight bearing and help protect foot ulcers.

Patient/Client-Related Instruction

- Check that the patient and family or caregivers understand topical application and wound-care procedures, and adhere to the recommended dosing schedule.
- Instruct patient and family/caregivers about proper footwear, hygiene, and visual inspection to prevent recurrence or development of new ulcers.

Pharmacokinetics

Absorption: Minimal absorption (<3%).
Distribution: Action is primarily local.
Metabolism and Excretion: Unknown.
Half-life: Unknown.

TIME/ACTION PROFILE (improvement in ulcer healing)

ROUTE	ONSET	PEAK	DURATION
topical	within 10 wk	unknown	unknown

Contraindications/Precautions

Contraindicated in: Known hypersensitivity to becaplermin or parabens; Known neoplasm at site of application; Wounds that close by primary intention.
Use Cautiously in: Known malignancy; OB/Lactation/Pedi: Safety not established.

Interactions

Drug-Drug: None known.

Route/Dosage

Topical (Adults): Length of gel *in inches* from 15- or 7.5-g tube = length × width of ulcer area × 0.6; from the 2-g tube = length × width of ulcer area × 1.3. Length of gel *in centimeters* from 15- or 7.5-g tube = length × width of ulcer area ÷ 4; from the 2-g tube = length × width of ulcer area ÷ 2; for 12 hr each day.

Availability

Gel: 100 mcg/g (0.01%) in 2-, 7.5-, and 15-g tubes Rx.

beclomethasone
(bek-low-**meth**-a-sone)
Qvar

Classification
Therapeutic: anti-inflammatories (steroidal)
Pharmacologic: corticosteroids

Indications

Maintenance treatment of asthma as prophylactic therapy. May decrease requirement for or eliminate use of systemic corticosteroids in patients with asthma.

Action

Potent, locally acting anti-inflammatory and immune modifier. **Therapeutic Effects:** Decreases frequency and severity of asthma attacks. Improves asthma symptoms.

Adverse Reactions/Side Effects

CNS: headache. **EENT:** cataracts, dysphonia, oropharyngeal fungal infections, pharyngitis, rhinitis, sinusitis. **Resp:** bronchospasm, cough, wheezing. **Endo:** adrenal suppression (increased dose, long-term therapy only), decreased growth (children). **MS:** back pain.

PHYSICAL THERAPY IMPLICATIONS

Examination and Evaluation

- Assess pulmonary function periodically by measuring lung volumes, breath sounds, respiratory rate, and other symptoms (wheezing, dyspnea, shortness of breath) (See Appendices I, J, K). Report changes in pulmonary function to help document the effects of drug therapy in treating asthma.
- Observe for paradoxical bronchospasm (cough, wheezing, dyspnea), especially at higher or excessive doses. If condition occurs, advise patient to withhold medication and notify physician immediately.
- Assess muscle strength periodically during long-term use. Although inhalation reduces the risk of systemic musculoskeletal damage, some degree of weakness and bone loss may still occur during prolonged, extensive use.
- Assess any back pain to rule out musculoskeletal pathology; that is, try to determine if pain is drug induced rather than caused by anatomic or biomechanical problems.
- Report signs of adrenal suppression, including hypotension, weight loss, weakness, nausea, vomiting, anorexia, lethargy, confusion, and restlessness.
- Assess growth rate in children receiving chronic therapy; report delayed or stunted growth to the physician.

Interventions

- Implement resistive exercises and weight-bearing activities to minimize muscle wasting and osteoporosis. Use caution to prevent musculoskeletal damage in patients with preexisting muscle and bone loss.
- Design and implement appropriate aerobic exercise and respiratory muscle–training programs to maintain optimal cardiovascular and pulmonary function. Work with patient and family/caregivers to find forms of exercise (e.g., swimming) that can help improve respiratory function without triggering asthma attacks.
- Protect skin from breakdown, especially over bony prominences.

Patient/Client-Related Instruction

- Counsel patient on proper use of metered-dose inhaler; observe use of this device whenever possible to ensure proper technique.
- Advise patient to not exceed the recommended dose or frequency of inhalations. Contact physician immediately if bronchospasm is not relieved by medication or is accompanied by severe headache or other symptoms.
- Caution patient not to use this drug to treat acute symptoms. A rapid-acting inhaled beta-adrenergic bronchodilator is typically used for relief of acute asthma attacks.
- Instruct patient to report any loss of vision that might indicate cataracts or increased intraocular pressure.
- Advise patient that corticosteroids cause immunosuppression and may mask symptoms of infection. Instruct patient to avoid people with known contagious illnesses and to report possible infections immediately.
- Advise patient about the likelihood of upper respiratory tract infection or irritation, including pharyngitis, sinusitis, rhinitis, and problems with vocalization (dysphonia). Instruct patient to report severe or prolonged upper respiratory problems to the physician.
- Advise patients on long-term treatment to consult physician before stopping this medication. Stopping the medication suddenly may result in adrenocortical shock (severe hypotension, hypoglycemia, weakness, vomiting). If these signs appear, notify health care professional immediately; may be life threatening.
- Instruct patient and family/caregivers to report other troublesome side effects such as severe or prolonged headache.

Pharmacokinetics

Absorption: 20%. Action is primarily local following inhalation.
Distribution: Crosses the placenta and enters breast milk in small amounts.
Metabolism and Excretion: Following inhalation, beclomethasone dipropionate is primarily converted to beclomethasone 17–monopropionate (active metabolite); primarily excreted in feces (<10% excreted in urine).
Half-life: 2.8 hr.

TIME/ACTION PROFILE (improvement in symptoms)

ROUTE	ONSET	PEAK	DURATION
inhalation	within 24 hr	1–4 wk*	unknown

*Improvement in pulmonary function; decreased airway responsiveness may take longer.

Contraindications/Precautions

Contraindicated in: Hypersensitivity (product contains alcohol); Acute attack of asthma/status asthmaticus.
Use Cautiously in: Active untreated infections; Diabetes or glaucoma; Underlying immunosuppression (due to disease or concurrent therapy); Systemic corticosteroid therapy (should not be abruptly discontinued when inhalable therapy is started; additional corticosteroids needed in stress or trauma); OB/Lactation: Safety not established; Pedi: Safety not established in children <5 yr; prolonged or high-dose therapy may lead to complications.

Interactions

Drug-Drug: None known.

Route/Dosage

Inhalation (Adults and Children ≥12 yr): *Previously on bronchodilators alone*—40–80 mcg twice daily (not to exceed 320 mcg twice daily). *Previously on inhaled corticosteroids*—40–160 mcg twice daily (not to exceed 320 mcg twice daily).
Inhaln (Children 5–11 yr): *Previously on bronchodilators alone*—40 mcg twice daily (not to exceed 80 mcg twice daily). *Previously on inhaled corticosteroids*—40 mcg twice daily (not to exceed 80 mcg twice daily).

Availability

Inhalation aerosol: 40 mcg/metered inhalation in 7.3-g canister (delivers 100 metered inhalations), 80 mcg/metered inhalation in 7.3-g canister (delivers 100 metered inhalations).

belimumab (be-li-moo-mab)

Benlysta

Classification
Therapeutic: immunosuppressants
Pharmacologic: monoclonal antibodies

Indications

Treatment of active autoantibody-positive systemic lupus erythematosus (SLE) in patients currently receiving standard therapy.

Action

A monoclonal antibody produced by recombinant DNA technique that specifically binds to B-lymphocyte stimulator protein (BLyS), thereby inactivating it.
Therapeutic Effects: ↓ survival of B cells, including autoreactive ones and ↓ differentiation into immunoglobulin-producing plasma cells. Result is ↓ disease activity with lessened damage/improvement in mucocutaneous, musculoskeletal, and immunologic manifestations of SLE.

Adverse Reactions/Side Effects

CNS: depression, insomnia, migraine. **GI:** nausea, diarrhea. **GU:** cystitis. **Hemat:** leukopenia. **MS:** extremity pain. **Misc:** allergic reactions including ANAPHYLAXIS, INFECTION, infusion reactions, fever.

PHYSICAL THERAPY IMPLICATIONS

Examination and Evaluation

- Monitor signs of allergic reactions and anaphylaxis, including pulmonary symptoms (tightness in the throat and chest, wheezing, cough, dyspnea) or skin reactions (rash, pruritus, urticaria, dermatitis). Be especially alert for responses that occur during and after administration (infusion-related reactions). Notify physician or nursing staff immediately if these reactions occur.
- Be alert for signs of leukopenia and infections, including fever, sore throat, mucosal lesions, chills, nausea, vomiting, diarrhea, and localized inflammation. Notify physician or nursing staff of these signs immediately.
- Periodically assess symptoms of SLE such as joint pain/stiffness, muscle weakness, fatigue, skin lesions (rashes, bruising), Raynaud-like symptoms (decreased circulation to the fingers and toes), and changes in mood and behavior (depression, anxiety, memory deficits). Document whether drug therapy is successful in reducing these symptoms.
- Monitor personality changes, including depression and increased thoughts of suicide. Notify physician if these changes become problematic.
- Assess any extremity pain to rule out musculoskeletal pathology; that is, try to determine if pain is drug induced rather than caused by anatomic or biomechanical problems.

Interventions

- Design and implement strengthening activities, cardiac conditioning, and other therapeutic exercises as tolerated to maintain function and complement drug effects in patients with SLE.

Patient/Client-Related Instruction

- Advise patient to guard against infection (frequent hand washing, etc.) and to avoid crowds and contact with persons with contagious diseases.
- Instruct patient to report other troublesome side effects such as prolonged or severe insomnia, migraine headaches, bladder pain/irritation, fever, or GI problems (nausea, diarrhea).

Pharmacokinetics

Absorption: IV administration results in complete bioavailability.
Distribution: Unknown
Metabolism and Excretion: Unknown
Half-life: 19.4 days

TIME/ACTION PROFILE (reduction in activated B cells)

ROUTE	ONSET	PEAK	DURATION
IV	8 wk	unknown	52 wk*

*With continuous treatment.

Contraindications/Precautions

Contraindicated in: Hypersensitivity; Concurrent use of other biologicals or cyclophosphamide; Concurrent use of live vaccines; Lactation: Breast-feeding not recommended.
Use Cautiously in: Infections (consider temporary withdrawal for acute infections, treat aggressively); Previous history of depression or suicidal ideation (may worsen); Geri: May be more sensitive to drug effects, consider age-related changes in renal, hepatic, and cardiac function, concurrent drug therapy, and chronic disease states; OB: Use during pregnancy only if potential maternal benefit outweighs potential fetal risk; women with childbearing potential should use adequate contraception during and for 4 mo following treatment.

Interactions

Drug-Drug: ↑ risk of adverse reactions and ↓ immune response to **live vaccines**; should not be given concurrently.

Route/Dosage

PO (Adults): 10 mg/kg every 2 wk for 3 doses, then every 4 wk.

Availability

Lyophilized powder for IV administration (requires reconstitution and dilution): 120 mg/vial, 400 mg/vial.

benazepril (ben-aye-ze-pril)

Lotensin

Classification

Therapeutic: antihypertensives

Pharmacologic: ACE inhibitors

Indications

Alone or with other agents in the management of hypertension.

Action

Angiotensin-converting enzyme (ACE) inhibitors block the conversion of angiotensin I to the vasoconstrictor angiotensin II. ACE inhibitors also prevent the degradation of bradykinin and other vasodilatory prostaglandins. ACE inhibitors also increase plasma renin levels and reduce aldosterone levels. Net result is systemic vasodilation. **Therapeutic Effects:** Lowering of blood pressure in patients with hypertension.

Adverse Reactions/Side Effects

CNS: dizziness, drowsiness, fatigue, headache. **Resp:** cough. **CV:** hypotension. **GI:** nausea. **GU:** impaired renal function. **Derm:** rashes. **F and E:** hyperkalemia. **Misc:** ANGIOEDEMA.

PHYSICAL THERAPY IMPLICATIONS

Examination and Evaluation

- Monitor signs of angioedema, including rashes, raised patches of red or white skin (welts), burning/itching skin, swelling in the face, and difficulty breathing. Notify physician of these signs immediately.
- Assess blood pressure periodically and compare to normal values (See Appendix F) to help determine antihypertensive effects. Report low blood pressure (hypotension), especially if patient experiences dizziness, fatigue, or other symptoms.
- Assess dizziness and drowsiness that might affect gait, balance, and other functional activities (See Appendix C). Report balance problems and functional limitations to the physician, and caution the patient and family/caregivers to guard against falls and trauma.
- Be alert for signs of high plasma potassium levels (hyperkalemia), including bradycardia, fatigue, weakness, numbness, and tingling. Notify physician because severe cases can lead to life-threatening arrhythmias and paralysis.

Interventions

- Avoid physical therapy interventions that cause systemic vasodilation (large whirlpool, Hubbard tank). Additive effects of this drug and the intervention may cause a dangerous fall in blood pressure.
- To minimize orthostatic hypotension, patient should move slowly when assuming a more upright position.

Patient/Client-Related Instruction

- Remind patients to take medication as directed to control hypertension and other cardiac conditions even if they are asymptomatic.
- Counsel patients about additional interventions to help control blood pressure, including regular exercise, weight loss, sodium restriction, stress reduction, moderation of alcohol consumption, and smoking cessation.
- Instruct patient to report signs of impaired renal function, including decreased urine output, cloudy urine, or sudden weight gain due to fluid retention.
- Instruct patient to notify physician of a prolonged dry cough; drug therapy may need to be altered to resolve this side effect.
- Instruct patient or family/caregivers to report other troublesome side effects such as severe or prolonged headache, nausea, or skin rash.

Pharmacokinetics

Absorption: 37% absorbed after oral administration.
Distribution: Crosses the placenta; enters breast milk in small amounts.
Protein Binding: 95%.
Metabolism and Excretion: Converted by the liver to benazeprilat, the active metabolite; 20% excreted in urine; 11–12% nonrenal (biliary) elimination.
Half-life: *Benazeprilat:* 10–11 hr.

TIME/ACTION PROFILE (antihypertensive effect)

ROUTE	ONSET	PEAK	DURATION
PO	within 1 hr*	1–2 wk†	24 hr†

*After single dose.
†Chronic dosing.

Contraindications/Precautions

Contraindicated in: Hypersensitivity; History of angioedema with previous use of ACE inhibitors; OB: Can cause injury or death of fetus—if pregnancy occurs, discontinue immediately; Lactation: Appears in breast milk; patient must discontinue benazepril or provide alternate to breast milk.
Use Cautiously in: Patients with renal impairment, hypovolemia, hyponatremia, and concurrent diuretic therapy; Black patients (monotherapy for hypertension less effective, may require additional therapy; higher risk of angioedema); Surgery/anesthesia (hypotension may be exaggerated); Lactation: Safety not established; Pedi: Safety not established children <6 yr; Geri: Initial dosage reduction recommended.
Exercise Extreme Caution in: Family history of angioedema.

Interactions

Drug-Drug: Excessive hypotension may occur with concurrent use of **diuretics**. Additive hypotension with other **antihypertensives**. Increased risk of hyperkalemia with concurrent use of **potassium supplements, potassium-sharing diuretics, potassium-containing salt substitutes**, or **angiotensin II receptor antagonists**. Antihypertensive response may be blunted by **NSAIDs**. Increases levels and may increase risk of **lithium** toxicity.

Route/Dosage

PO (Adults): 10 mg once daily, increased gradually to maintenance dose of 20–40 mg/day in 1–2 divided doses (initiate therapy at 5 mg once daily in patients receiving diuretics).
PO (Children ≥6 yr): 0.2 mg/kg once daily; may be titrated up to 0.6 mg/kg/day (or 40 mg/day).

Renal Impairment

PO (Adults): *CCr <30 mL/min*—Initiate therapy with 5 mg once daily.

Renal Impairment

PO (Children ≥6 yr): CCr *<30 mL/min*—Contraindicated.

Availability (generic available)

Tablets: 5 mg, 10 mg, 20 mg, 40 mg. ***In combination with:*** amlodipine (Lotrel) and hydrochlorothiazide (Lotensin HCT). See Appendix B.

bendamustine

(ben-da-**muss**-teen)
Treanda

Classification
Therapeutic: antineoplastics
Pharmacologic: benzimidazoles

Indications

Treatment of chronic lymphocytic leukemia.

Action

Damages DNA resulting in death of rapidly replicating cells. **Therapeutic Effects:** Decreased proliferation of leukemic cells.

Adverse Reactions/Side Effects

CNS: fatigue, weakness. **Resp:** cough. **GI:** nausea, vomiting, diarrhea. **Derm:** skin reactions. **Hemat:** anemia, LEUKOPENIA, NEUTROPENIA, THROMBOCYTOPENIA. **Metab:** hyperuricemia. **Misc:** TUMOR LYSIS SYNDROME, allergic reactions, including anaphylaxis, fever, infusion reactions.

PHYSICAL THERAPY IMPLICATIONS

Examination and Evaluation

- Monitor signs of leukopenia and neutropenia (fever, sore throat, signs of infection), thrombocytopenia (bruising, nose bleeds, bleeding gums), or unusual weakness and fatigue that might be due to anemia. Report these signs to the physician or nursing staff immediately.
- Be alert for signs of electrolyte imbalances that might indicate tumor lysis syndrome. Signs include severe muscle weakness or paralysis due to increased plasma potassium (hyperkalemia), or muscle hyperexcitability and tetany due to phosphate and calcium imbalances (hyperphosphatemia and hypocalcemia). Notify physician or nursing staff immediately if these signs occur.
- Monitor signs of allergic reactions and anaphylaxis, including pulmonary symptoms (tightness in the throat and chest, wheezing, cough, dyspnea) or skin reactions (rash, pruritus, urticaria). Reactions may be especially prevalent during or immediately after administration (infusion reactions). Notify physician or nursing staff immediately if these reactions occur.

Interventions

- For patients who are medically able to begin exercise, implement appropriate resistive exercises and aerobic training to maintain muscle strength and aerobic capacity during cancer chemotherapy or to help restore function after chemotherapy.

Patient/Client-Related Instruction

- Advise patient to guard against infection (frequent hand washing, etc.) and avoid crowds and contact with persons with contagious diseases.
- Advise patient that weakness and fatigue are likely, and may be severe. Implement assistive devices (walker, crutches, cane) and appropriate safety precautions to guard against falls due to weakness.
- Instruct patient to report other bothersome side effects, including severe or prolonged cough, fever, skin reactions, or GI problems (nausea, vomiting, diarrhea).

Pharmacokinetics

Absorption: IV administration results in complete bioavailability.
Distribution: Distributes freely into red blood cells.
Protein Binding: 94–96%.
Metabolism and Excretion: Mostly metabolized (partially by the CYP1A2 enzyme system; 90% excreted in feces; some renal elimination. Although metabolites have antineoplastic activity, levels are extremely low.
Half-life: approximately 40 minutes

TIME/ACTION PROFILE (blood levels)

ROUTE	ONSET	PEAK	DURATION
IV	rapid	end of infusion	unknown

Contraindications/Precautions
Contraindicated in: Hypersensitivity to bendamustine or mannitol; CCr <40 mL/min. Use with caution in lesser degrees of renal impairment; Moderate or severe hepatic impairment; OB: Pregnancy or lactation.
Use Cautiously in: Patients at risk for tumor lysis syndrome (concurrent allopurinol recommended); Mild hepatic impairment; Mild-to-moderate renal impairment; Patients with childbearing potential; Geri: Elderly patients may be more susceptible to adverse reactions; Pedi: Safe use in children not established.

Interactions
Drug-Drug: Concurrent use of **CYP1A2 inducers/inhibitors** can alter levels of bendamustine. **Inhibitors of CYP1A2,** including **fluvoxamine** and **ciprofloxacin** may ↑ levels of bendamustine and ↓ levels of active metabolites. **Inducers of CYP1A2,** including **omeprazole** and **smoking,** may ↓ levels of bendamustine and ↑ levels of its active metabolites. Consider alternative treatments.

Route/Dosage
IV (Adults): 100 mg/m^2 on days 1 and 2 of a 28-day cycle, up to 6 cycles; dose modification required for toxicity.

Availability
Lyophilized powder for injection (requires reconstitution): 100-mg vial.

benzonatate (ben-zoe-na-tate)
Tessalon

Classification
Therapeutic: allergy, cold, and cough remedies, antitussives (local anesthetic)

Indications
Relief of nonproductive cough due to minor throat or bronchial irritation from inhaled irritants or colds.

Action
Anesthetizes cough or stretch receptors in vagal nerve afferent fibers found in lungs, pleura, and respiratory passages. May also decrease transmission of the cough reflex centrally. **Therapeutic Effects:** Decrease in cough.

Adverse Reactions/Side Effects
CNS: headache, mild dizziness, sedation. **EENT:** burning sensation in eyes, nasal congestion. **GI:** constipation, GI upset, nausea. **Derm:** pruritus, skin eruptions. **Misc:** chest numbness, chilly sensation, hypersensitivity reactions.

PHYSICAL THERAPY IMPLICATIONS

Examination and Evaluation
- Assess frequency and nature of cough and lung sounds (See Appendix K) to help document whether this drug is effective in reducing cough.
- Monitor signs of hypersensitivity reactions, including pulmonary symptoms (tightness in the throat and chest, wheezing, cough, dyspnea) or skin reactions (rash, pruritus, urticaria). Notify physician immediately if these reactions occur.
- Assess dizziness that might affect gait, balance, and other functional activities (See Appendix C). Report balance problems and functional limitations to the physician, and caution the patient and family/caregivers to guard against falls and trauma.

Patient/Client-Related Instruction
- Advise patient to minimize cough by avoiding irritants, such as cigarette smoke, fumes, and dust. Humidification of environmental air, frequent sips of water, and sugarless hard candy may also decrease the frequency of dry, irritating cough.
- Advise patient that any cough lasting more than 1 wk or accompanied by fever, chest pain, persistent headache, or skin rash warrants medical attention.
- Instruct patient or family/caregivers to report other problematic side effects such as severe or prolonged headache, sedation, burning sensation in the eyes, nasal congestion, chills, chest numbness, skin reactions (itching, skin eruptions), or GI problems (nausea, upset stomach, constipation).

Pharmacokinetics
Absorption: Unknown.
Distribution: Unknown.
Metabolism and Excretion: Unknown.
Half-life: Unknown.

TIME/ACTION PROFILE (antitussive effect)

ROUTE	ONSET	PEAK	DURATION
PO	15–20 min	unknown	3–8 hr

Contraindications/Precautions
Contraindicated in: Hypersensitivity to benzonatate. Cross-sensitivity with other ester-type local anesthetics (tetracaine, procaine, and others) may occur.
Use Cautiously in: OB/Lactation: Safety not established; Pedi: Safety not established in children <10 yr.

Interactions
Drug-Drug: Additive CNS depression may occur with **antihistamines, alcohol, opioids,** and **sedative/hypnotics.**

Route/Dosage

PO (Adults and Children ≥10 yr): 100 mg 3 times daily (up to 600 mg/day).

Availability (generic available)

Capsules: 100 mg.

benztropine (benz-troe-peen)

✹Apo-Benztropine, Cogentin

Classification

Therapeutic: antiparkinson agents

Pharmacologic: anticholinergics

Indications

Adjunctive treatment of all forms of Parkinson's disease, including drug-induced extrapyramidal effects and acute dystonic reactions.

Action

Blocks cholinergic activity in the CNS, which is partially responsible for the symptoms of Parkinson's disease. Restores the natural balance of neurotransmitters in the CNS. **Therapeutic Effects:** Reduction of rigidity and tremors.

Adverse Reactions/Side Effects

CNS: confusion, depression, dizziness, hallucinations, headache, sedation, weakness. **EENT:** blurred vision, dry eyes, mydriasis. **CV:** arrhythmias, hypotension, palpitations, tachycardia. **GI:** constipation, dry mouth, ileus, nausea. **GU:** hesitancy, urinary retention. **Misc:** decreased sweating.

PHYSICAL THERAPY IMPLICATIONS

Examination and Evaluation

- Assess patient's gait and motor function to help document antiparkinson effects, especially when starting drug therapy, or during dosing changes or addition of other antiparkinson drugs. Motor function should be assessed at different times of the day, such as when drugs are reaching therapeutic levels (i.e., 1–2 hr after oral dose), as well as when drug effects are minimal (just before the next dose).
- Assess heart rate, ECG, and heart sounds, especially during exercise (See Appendices G, H). Report fast heart rate (tachycardia) or signs of other arrhythmias, including palpitations, chest discomfort, shortness of breath, fainting, and fatigue/weakness.
- Assess blood pressure (BP) periodically and compare to normal values (See Appendix F). Report low blood pressure (hypotension), especially if patient experiences dizziness, fatigue, or other symptoms.
- Assess dizziness and drowsiness that might affect gait, balance, and other functional activities (See Appendix C). Report balance problems and functional limitations to the physician and nursing staff, and caution the patient and family/caregivers to guard against falls and trauma.
- Monitor confusion, hallucinations, depression, and other psychologic problems. Repeated or excessive symptoms may require change in dose or medication.

Interventions

- Implement therapeutic exercises (coordination exercises, gait training, cardiovascular conditioning) to compliment the effects of drug therapy and help achieve optimal function.
- Because of the risk of arrhythmias and abnormal BP responses, use caution during aerobic exercise and other forms of therapeutic exercise. Assess exercise tolerance frequently (BP, heart rate, fatigue levels), and terminate exercise immediately if any untoward responses occur (See Appendix L).
- Guard against falls and trauma (hip fractures, head injury, and so forth). Implement fall-prevention strategies (see Appendix E), especially if patient exhibits Parkinson's symptoms (postural instability, rigidity) combined with drug side effects (dizziness, blurred vision, weakness).

Patient/Client-Related Instruction

- Instruct patient to report other bothersome side effects, including severe or prolonged headache, vision problems, decreased sweating, urinary problems (hesitancy, retention), or GI problems (nausea, constipation, dry mouth).

Pharmacokinetics

Absorption: Well absorbed following PO and IM administration.

Distribution: Unknown.

Metabolism and Excretion: Unknown.

Half-life: Unknown.

TIME/ACTION PROFILE (antidyskinetic activity)

ROUTE	ONSET	PEAK	DURATION
PO	1–2 hr	several days	24 hr
IM, IV	within min	unknown	24 hr

Contraindications/Precautions

Contraindicated in: Hypersensitivity; Children <3 yr; Angle-closure glaucoma; Tardive dyskinesia.

Use Cautiously in: Prostatic hyperplasia; Seizure disorders; Cardiac arrhythmias; OB/Lactation: Safety not established; Geri: ↑ risk of adverse reactions.

✹ = Canadian drug name; *CAPITALS indicate life-threatening; underlines indicate most frequent.

Interactions

Drug-Drug: Additive anticholinergic effects with **drugs sharing anticholinergic properties**, such as **antihistamines, phenothiazines, quinidine, disopyramide**, and **tricyclic antidepressants**. Counteracts the cholinergic effects of **bethanechol**. **Antacids** and **antidiarrheals** may ↓ absorption.
Drug-Natural: ↑ anticholinergic effect with **angel's trumpet, jimson weed**, and **scopolia**.

Route/Dosage

Parkinsonism

PO (Adults): 1–2 mg/day in 1–2 divided doses (range 0.5–6 mg/day).

Acute Dystonic Reactions

IM, IV (Adults): 1–2 mg, then 1–2 mg PO twice daily.

Drug-Induced Extrapyramidal Reactions

PO, IM, IV (Adults): 1–4 mg given once or twice daily (1–2 mg 2–3 times daily may also be used PO).

Availability (generic available)

Tablets: 0.5 mg, 1 mg, 2 mg. **Injection:** 1 mg/mL.

bepotastine (be-poe-**tass**-teen)

Bepreve

Classification
Therapeutic: ocular agents
Pharmacologic: antihistamines

Indications

Treatment of itching associated with allergic conjunctivitis.

Action

Acts as a histamine H_1 receptor antagonist; also inhibits the release of histamine from mast cells; does not bind to or inactivate histamine. **Therapeutic Effects:** Decreased ocular itching associated with allergic conjunctivitis.

Adverse Reactions/Side Effects

CNS: headache. **EENT:** nasopharyngitis. **GI:** taste in mouth following instillation.

PHYSICAL THERAPY IMPLICATIONS

Examination and Evaluation

- Monitor eye pain, itching, and inflammation to help document whether drug therapy is successful in resolving allergic conjunctivitis.

Patient/Client-Related Instruction

- Check that the patient and family or caregivers understand ophthalmic application procedures and adhere to the recommended dosing schedule.
- Instruct patient and family/caregivers to report other troublesome side effects such as severe or prolonged headache, altered taste, or inflammation of the nose and pharynx.

Pharmacokinetics

Absorption: Some systemic absorption follows ophthalmic administration.
Distribution: Unknown
Metabolism and Excretion: Minimally metabolized by the liver; 75–90% excreted unchanged in urine
Half-life: Unknown

TIME/ACTION PROFILE (antihistaminic activity)

ROUTE	ONSET	PEAK	DURATION
ophthalmic	within 15 min	1–2 hr*	12 hr

*Blood levels.

Contraindications/Precautions

Contraindicated in: Hypersensitivity.
Use Cautiously in: Contact lens use OB: Use during pregnancy if potential maternal benefit justifies the potential risk to fetus; Lactation: Use cautiously during breastfeeding; Pedi: Safe and effective use in children <2 yr has not been established.

Interactions

Drug-Drug: None noted

Route/Dosage

Ophthalmic (Adults): 1 drop in affected eye(s) twice daily.

Availability

Ophthalmic solution: 1.5%

beractant (be-**rak**-tant)

Survanta

Classification
Therapeutic: anti-RDS agents
Pharmacologic: pulmonary surfactants

Indications

Treatment and prophylaxis of respiratory distress syndrome (RDS, hyaline membrane disease) in premature infants.

Action

Replaces endogenous pulmonary surfactant in premature infants, allowing normal surface activity in alveoli. Consists of natural bovine lung extract. **Therapeutic Effects:** Decreased incidence, mortality, and complications from RDS.

Adverse Reactions/Side Effects

Resp: oxygen desaturation (as a result of administration process). **CV:** transient bradycardia.

PHYSICAL THERAPY IMPLICATIONS

Examination and Evaluation

- Monitor oxygen saturation levels following administration. Notify physician or nursing staff immediately about a sudden decrease is oxygen saturation.
- Assess heart rate, and report a sustained decrease in heart rate (bradycardia).

Interventions

- When indicated, implement chest physical therapy interventions such as positioning, suctioning, and chest percussion/vibration to maintain respiratory function and augment drug effects in premature infants.

Pharmacokinetics

Absorption: Administered directly to site of action. Systemic absorption not known.
Distribution: Rapidly distributes to lung tissue.
Metabolism and Excretion: Enters surfactant pathways in which recycling and reutilization occur.
Half-life: Unknown.

TIME/ACTION PROFILE (improved oxygenation)

ROUTE	ONSET	PEAK	DURATION
intratracheal	within min	unknown	unknown

Contraindications/Precautions

Contraindicated in: No known contraindications.
Use Cautiously in: No known cautions. Nosocomial infections may be more common.

Interactions

Drug-Drug: None known.

Route/Dosage

Intratracheal (Infants, Premature): 100 mg phospholipids/kg birth weight (4 mL/kg birth weight); 4 doses may be given in first 48 hr of life, no closer than q 6 hr apart.

Availability

Intratracheal suspension: 25 mg phospholipid/mL—4-mL and 8-mL vials.

besifloxacin (be-si-flox-a-sin)

Besivance

Classification
Therapeutic: anti-infectives
Pharmacologic: fluoroquinolones

Indications

Treatment of bacterial conjunctivitis.

Action

Inhibits bacterial DNA synthesis by inhibiting DNA gyrase. **Therapeutic Effects:** Death of susceptible bacteria with decreased symptoms and sequelae of bacterial conjunctivitis. **Spectrum:** Active against CDC coryneform group G, *Corynebacterium pseudodiphtheriticum*, *C. striatum*, *Haemophilus influenzae*, *Moraxella lacunata*, *Staphylococcus aureus*, *S. epidermidis*, *S. hominis*, *S. lugdunensis*, *Streptococcus mitis* group, *Str. oralis*, *Str. Pneumoniae*, and *Str. Salivarius*.

Adverse Reactions/Side Effects

CNS: headache. **EENT:** conjunctival redness, blurred vision, eye irritation, eye pain, eye pruritus.

PHYSICAL THERAPY IMPLICATIONS

Examination and Evaluation

- Monitor eye pain, itching, and inflammation to help document whether drug therapy is successful in resolving bacterial conjunctivitis.
- Watch for any new or increased eye reactions, including pain, redness, irritation, itching, or blurred vision. Report severe or worsening eye reactions to the physician.

Patient/Client-Related Instruction

- Check that the patient and family or caregivers understand ophthalmic application procedures and adhere to the recommended dosing schedule.
- Instruct patient and family/caregivers to report other troublesome side effects such as severe or prolonged headache.

Pharmacokinetics

Absorption: Minimal absorption follows ophthalmic use.
Distribution: Unknown
Metabolism and Excretion: Unknown
Half-life: 7 hr

TIME/ACTION PROFILE

ROUTE	ONSET	PEAK	DURATION
Ophthalmic	unknown	unknown	6–12 hr

Contraindications/Precautions

Contraindicated in: Contact lens use.
Use Cautiously in: OB: Use during pregnancy only if potential benefit justifies potential risk to fetus; Lactation: Use cautiously during lactation; Pedi: Safe use in children <1 yr not established.

Interactions

Drug-Drug: None noted

Route/Dosage

Ophth (Adults and Children ≥1 yr): 1 drop in affected eye(s) 3 times daily (4–12 hr apart) for 7 days.

Availability

Ophthalmic suspension: 0.6% 5 mL in 7.5-mL bottle.

betamethasone (systemic)

(bay-ta-**meth**-a-sone)

Betaject, Celestone

Classification

Therapeutic: anti-inflammatories (steroidal)
Pharmacologic: corticosteroids

Indications

Management of adrenocortical insufficiency; chronic use in other situations is limited because of mineralocorticoid activity. Used systemically and locally in a wide variety of chronic diseases, including Inflammatory; Allergic; Hematologic; Neoplastic; Autoimmune disorders. Replacement therapy in adrenal insufficiency. **Unlabeled Use:** Short-term administration to high-risk mothers before delivery to prevent respiratory distress syndrome in the newborn.

Action

In pharmacologic doses, suppresses inflammation and the normal immune response. Has numerous intense metabolic effects (see Adverse Reactions and Side Effects). Suppresses adrenal function at chronic doses of 0.6 mg/day. Has negligible mineralocorticoid activity. **Therapeutic Effects:** Suppression of inflammation and modification of the normal immune response. Replacement therapy in adrenal insufficiency.

Adverse Reactions/Side Effects

Adverse reactions/side effects are much more common with high-dose/long-term therapy

CNS: depression, euphoria, headache, increased intracranial pressure (children only), personality changes, psychoses, restlessness. **EENT:** cataracts, increased intraocular pressure. **CV:** hypertension. **GI:** PEPTIC ULCERATION, anorexia, nausea, vomiting. **Derm:** acne, decreased wound healing, ecchymoses, fragility, hirsutism, petechiae. **Endo:** adrenal suppression, hyperglycemia. **F and E:** fluid retention (long-term high doses), hypokalemia, hypokalemic alkalosis. **Hemat:** THROMBOEMBOLISM, thrombophlebitis. **Metab:** weight gain, weight loss. **MS:** muscle wasting, osteoporosis, aseptic necrosis of joints, muscle pain. **Misc:** cushingoid appearance (moon face, buffalo hump), increased susceptibility to infection.

PHYSICAL THERAPY IMPLICATIONS

Examination and Evaluation

- Monitor signs of thrombophlebitis (lower extremity swelling, warmth, erythema, tenderness) and thromboembolism (shortness of breath, chest pain, cough, bloody sputum). Notify physician immediately, and request objective tests (Doppler ultrasound, lung scan, others) if thrombosis is suspected.
- Monitor and report signs of peptic ulcer, including heartburn, nausea, vomiting blood, tarry stools, and loss of appetite.
- Assess any muscle or joint pain. Report persistent or increased musculoskeletal pain to determine presence of bone or joint pathology (aseptic necrosis, fracture).
- Assess muscle strength periodically to document the degree of muscle wasting during long-term use.
- Measure blood pressure periodically and compare to normal values (See Appendix F). Report a sustained increase in blood pressure (hypertension) to the physician.
- Assess peripheral edema using girth measurements, volume displacement, and measurement of pitting edema (See Appendix N). Report increased swelling in feet and ankles or a sudden increase in body weight due to fluid retention.
- Monitor personality changes, including depression, euphoria, restlessness, hallucinations, and psychosis. Notify physician if these changes become problematic.
- Assess signs of increased intracranial pressure in children, including changes in mood and behavior, decreased consciousness, headache, lethargy, seizures, and vomiting. Notify physician of these signs immediately.
- Be alert for signs of low potassium levels (hypokalemia) and metabolic acidosis, including hyperventilation, cardiac arrhythmias, dizziness, and confusion. Notify physician immediately if these signs occur.
- Report signs of adrenal suppression, including hypotension, weight loss, weakness, nausea, vomiting, anorexia, lethargy, confusion, and restlessness.
- Monitor signs of hyperglycemia (confusion; drowsiness; flushed, dry skin; fruit-like breath odor; rapid, deep breathing; polyuria; loss of appetite; unusual thirst). Insulin dosages may need to be adjusted to prevent repeated episodes of hyperglycemia.
- Periodically assess body weight and other anthropometric measures (body mass index, body composition). Report a rapid or unexplained weight gain or weight loss.

Interventions

- Implement resistive exercises and weight-bearing activities to minimize muscle wasting and osteoporosis. Use caution to prevent musculoskeletal damage in patients with preexisting muscle and bone loss.
- Protect skin from breakdown, especially over bony prominences.

Patient/Client-Related Instruction

- Advise patient that wound healing may be delayed; instruct patient to check skin regularly and report any nonhealing sores.
- Advise patient that corticosteroids cause immunosuppression and may mask symptoms of infection. Instruct patient to avoid people with known contagious illnesses and to report possible infections immediately.
- Advise patients on long-term treatment to consult physician before stopping this medication. Stopping the medication suddenly may result in adrenocortical shock (severe hypotension, hypoglycemia, weakness, vomiting). If these signs appear, notify the physician immediately; may be life threatening.
- Instruct patient to report any loss of vision that might indicate cataracts or increased intraocular pressure.
- Advise patient about possible "cushingoid" appearance, including puffiness in the face (moon face), increased fat in the torso, thin arms and legs, abdominal skin striations, bruising, and deposition of fat at the posterior base of the neck (buffalo hump). Discuss possible effects on body image, and help patient explore coping mechanisms.
- Instruct patient and family/caregivers to report other troublesome side effects such as severe or prolonged headache or skin reactions (acne, hair growth).

Pharmacokinetics

Absorption: Well absorbed after oral administration. Sodium phosphate salt is rapidly absorbed after IM administration. Acetate salt is slowly but completely absorbed after IM administration. Absorption from local sites (intra-articular, intralesional) is slow but complete.
Distribution: Widely distributed; crosses the placenta and probably enters breast milk.
Metabolism and Excretion: Metabolized mostly by the liver.
Half-life: 3–5 hr (plasma), 36–54 hr (tissue); adrenal suppression lasts 3.25 days.

TIME/ACTION PROFILE (anti-inflammatory activity)

ROUTE	ONSET	PEAK	DURATION
PO	unknown	1–2 hr	3.25 days
IM, IV (sodium phosphate)	rapid	unknown	unknown
IM (acetate/ sodium phosphate)	1–3 hr	unknown	1 wk

Contraindications/Precautions

Contraindicated in: Active untreated infections (may be used in patients being treated for tuberculous meningitis); Traumatic brain injury (high doses may ↑ mortality); Lactation: Avoid chronic use; Some products contain bisulfites and should be avoided in patients with known hypersensitivity.
Use Cautiously in: Chronic treatment (will lead to adrenal suppression; use lowest possible dose for shortest period of time); Hypothyroidism; Cirrhosis; Ulcerative colitis; Stress (surgery, infections); supplemental doses may be needed; Potential infections may mask signs (fever, inflammation); OB: Safety not established; Pedi: Chronic use will result in decreased growth; use lowest possible dose for shortest period of time.

Interactions

Drug-Drug: Additive hypokalemia with **thiazide** and **loop diuretics** or **amphotericin B**. Hypokalemia may ↑ risk of **digitalis glycoside** toxicity. May ↑ requirement for **insulins** or **oral hypoglycemic agents**. **Phenytoin**, **phenobarbital**, and **rifampin** stimulate metabolism; may ↓ effectiveness. **Oral contraceptives** may block metabolism. ↑ risk of adverse GI effects with **NSAIDs** (including aspirin). At chronic doses that suppress adrenal function, may ↓ antibody response to and ↑ risk of adverse reactions from **live-virus vaccines**.

Route/Dosage

PO (Adults): 0.6–7.2 mg/day as single daily dose or in divided doses.
PO (Children): *Adrenocortical insufficiency*—17.5 mcg/kg (500 mcg/m^2)/day in 3 divided doses. *Other uses*—62.5–250 mcg/kg (1.875–7.5 mg/m^2)/day in 3 divided doses.
IM, IV (Adults): 0.5–9 mg IM as betamethasone sodium phosphate/acetate suspension. *Prevention of respiratory distress syndrome in newborn*—12 mg IM daily for 2–3 days before delivery (unlabeled).
IM (Children): *Adrenocortical insufficiency*—17.5 mcg/kg (500 mcg/m^2)/day in 3 divided doses every 3rd day or 5.8–8.75 mcg/kg (166–250 mcg/m^2)/day as a

single dose. *Other uses*—20.8–125 mcg/kg (0.625–3.75 mg/m^2) of the base q 12–24 hr.

Availability (generic available)

Syrup: 0.6 mg/5 mL. **Suspension for injection (sodium phosphate and acetate):** 6 mg (total)/mL.

betaxolol (be-tax-oh-lol)

Kerlone

Classification

Therapeutic: antihypertensives

Pharmacologic: beta blockers

Indications

Management of hypertension.

Action

Blocks stimulation of $beta_1$ (myocardial)–adrenergic receptors. Does not usually affect $beta_2$ (pulmonary, vascular, uterine) receptor sites. **Therapeutic Effects:** Decreased blood pressure and heart rate.

Adverse Reactions/Side Effects

CNS: fatigue, weakness, anxiety, depression, dizziness, drowsiness, insomnia, memory loss, mental status changes, nightmares. **EENT:** blurred vision, stuffy nose. **Resp:** bronchospasm, wheezing. **CV:** BRADYCARDIA, CHF, PULMONARY EDEMA, hypotension, peripheral vasoconstriction. **GI:** constipation, diarrhea, liver function abnormalities, nausea, vomiting. **GU:** erectile dysfunction, decreased libido, urinary frequency. **Derm:** rashes. **Endo:** hyperglycemia, hypoglycemia. **MS:** arthralgia, back pain, joint pain. **Misc:** drug-induced lupus syndrome.

PHYSICAL THERAPY IMPLICATIONS

Examination and Evaluation

- Assess heart rate, ECG, and heart sounds, especially during exercise (See Appendices G, H). Report an abnormally slow heart rate (bradycardia) or symptoms of other arrhythmias, including palpitations, chest discomfort, shortness of breath, fainting, and fatigue/weakness.
- Assess routinely for signs of CHF and pulmonary edema, including dyspnea, rales/crackles, weight gain, peripheral edema, and jugular venous distention. Report these signs to the physician immediately.
- Assess blood pressure periodically and compare to normal values (See Appendix F) to help document antihypertensive effects.
- Assess symptoms of bronchospasm (wheezing, coughing, tightness in chest). Perform pulmonary function tests to quantify suspected changes in ventilation and respiration (See Appendices I, J, K). Repeated or prolonged bronchoconstriction may require a change in dose or medication.
- Monitor signs of peripheral vasoconstriction, such as extreme coldness in the hands and feet, cyanosis, and muscle cramping. Notify physician of severe or prolonged signs of vasoconstriction.
- Be alert for signs of hypoglycemia (weakness, malaise, irritability, fatigue) or hyperglycemia (drowsiness, fruity breath, increased urination, unusual thirst). Medication may mask some signs of hypoglycemia, but dizziness and sweating may still occur. Patients with diabetes mellitus should check blood glucose levels frequently.
- Assess any back, joint, or muscle pain to rule out musculoskeletal pathology; that is, try to determine if pain is drug induced rather than caused by anatomic or biomechanical problems.
- Monitor mood and personality changes, including depression, anxiety, nervousness, memory loss, or other changes in behavior. Notify physician if these changes become problematic.
- Assess dizziness and drowsiness that might affect gait, balance, and other functional activities (See Appendix C). Report balance problems and functional limitations to the physician, and caution the patient and family/caregivers to guard against falls and trauma.
- Monitor excessive fatigue or weakness. Beta blockers often cause some degree of fatigue and weakness, but any sudden or severe change in muscle strength or energy levels should be reported.
- Monitor signs of drug-induced lupus syndrome, including increased blood pressure (BP), fever, joint pain, skin rashes, and redness/irritation of the eye (uveitis). Notify physician promptly if these signs appear.

Interventions

- Because of an increased risk of CHF and cardiac arrhythmias, use caution during aerobic exercise and endurance conditioning. Terminate exercise if patient exhibits untoward symptoms (chest pain, shortness of breath, unusual fatigue) or displays other criteria for exercise termination (See Appendix L).
- Establish aerobic exercise workloads that account for the effects of beta blockers on heart rate. Some heart rate guidelines may not be appropriate because beta blockers typically decrease maximal HR by 20–30 bpm. Use other guidelines such as rating of perceived exertion (RPE, modified Borg scale) to determine exercise workloads.
- To minimize orthostatic hypotension, patient should move slowly when assuming a more upright position.

Patient/Client-Related Instruction

- Remind patients to take medication as directed to control hypertension even if they are asymptomatic.

- Counsel patients about additional interventions to help control BP, including regular exercise, weight loss, sodium restriction, stress reduction, moderation of alcohol consumption, and smoking cessation.
- Instruct patient or family/caregivers to report other troublesome side effects such as severe or prolonged insomnia, nightmares, blurred vision, stuffy nose, increased urinary frequency, decreased libido, erectile dysfunction, skin rash, or GI problems (nausea, vomiting, constipation, diarrhea).

Pharmacokinetics

Absorption: Well absorbed after oral administration.
Distribution: Widely distributed.
Metabolism and Excretion: Mostly metabolized by the liver, 20% excreted unchanged by the kidneys.
Half-life: 15–20 hr.

TIME/ACTION PROFILE (antihypertensive effect)

ROUTE	ONSET	PEAK	DURATION
PO	3–4 hr	3–4 hr	24 hr

Contraindications/Precautions

Contraindicated in: Uncompensated CHF; Pulmonary edema; Cardiogenic shock; Bradycardia or heart block.
Use Cautiously in: Renal or hepatic impairment; Pulmonary disease (including asthma; $beta_1$ selectivity may be lost at higher doses); avoid use if possible; Diabetes mellitus; Thyrotoxicosis; Patients with a history of severe allergic reactions (intensity of reactions may be increased); OB/Lactation/Pedi: Safety not established; all agents cross the placenta and may cause fetal/neonatal bradycardia, hypotension, hypoglycemia, or respiratory depression; Geri: ↑ sensitivity to beta blockers; initial dosage reduction recommended.

Interactions

Drug-Drug: General anesthetics, IV phenytoin, and **verapamil** may cause additive myocardial depression. Additive bradycardia may occur with **digoxin**. Additive hypotension may occur with other **antihypertensives**, acute ingestion of **alcohol**, or **nitrates**. Concurrent use with **amphetamine, cocaine, ephedrine, epinephrine, norepinephrine, phenylephrine**, or **pseudoephedrine** may result in unopposed alpha-adrenergic stimulation (excessive hypertension, bradycardia). Concurrent **thyroid preparation** administration may decrease effectiveness. May alter the effectiveness of **insulins** or **oral hypoglycemic agents** (dosage adjustments may be necessary). May decrease the effectiveness of **theophylline**. May decrease the beneficial $beta_1$-cardiovascular effects of **dopamine** or **dobutamine**. Use cautiously within 14 days of **MAO inhibitor** therapy (may result in hypertension).

Route/Dosage

PO (Adults): 10 mg once daily, may be increased to 20 mg after 7 days; start with 5 mg in geriatric patients.

Renal Impairment

PO (Adults): start with 5 mg once daily.

Availability (generic available)

Tablets: 10 mg, 20 mg.

bevacizumab

(be-va-**kiz**-oo-mab)
Avastin

Classification
Therapeutic: antineoplastics
Pharmacologic: monoclonal antibodies

Indications

Metastatic colon or rectal carcinoma (with IV 5-fluorouracil). First-line treatment of patients with unresectable, locally advanced, recurrent or metastatic nonsquamous, non–small cell lung cancer with carboplatin and paclitaxel.

Action

A monoclonal antibody that binds to vascular endothelial growth factor (VEGF), preventing its attachment to binding sites on vascular endothelium, thereby inhibiting growth of new blood vessels (angiogenesis). **Therapeutic Effects:** Decreased metastatic disease progression and microvascular growth.

Adverse Reactions/Side Effects

CNS: reversible posterior leukoencephalopathy syndrome (RPLS). **CV:** ARTERIAL THROMBOEMBOLIC EVENTS, CHF, hypertension, hypotension. **Resp:** HEMOPTYSIS, nongastrointestinal fistulas, nasal septum perforation. **GI:** GI PERFORATION. **GU:** nephrotic syndrome, proteinuria. **Hemat:** BLEEDING. **Misc:** WOUND DEHISCENCE, impaired wound healing, infusion reactions.

PHYSICAL THERAPY IMPLICATIONS

Examination and Evaluation

- Continually monitor for signs of arterial thrombosis that leads to MI (sudden chest pain, pain radiating into the arm or jaw, shortness of breath, dizziness, sweating, anxiety, nausea) or ischemic stroke (sudden severe headache, confusion, nausea, vomiting, paralysis, numbness, speech problems, visual disturbances). Seek immediate medical assistance if patient develops these signs.

- Monitor and immediately report any bleeding problems, including coughing up blood or other abnormal bleeding (nosebleeds, bleeding gums, excessive bruising).
- Be alert for signs of bowel perforation, including sudden severe abdominal pain accompanied by nausea, vomiting, chills, and fever. Report these signs immediately to the physician or nursing staff.
- Monitor signs of CHF (dyspnea, rales/crackles, peripheral edema, jugular venous distention, exercise intolerance); report these signs to the physician.
- Monitor signs of reversible posterior leukoencephalopathy syndrome, including headache, confusion, seizures, and loss of vision. Early recognition and adjustment of drug dosage is important in resolving this syndrome.
- Assess blood pressure periodically and compare to normal values (See Appendix F). Report a sustained increase in blood pressure (hypertension) or a problematic decrease in blood pressure (hypotension).
- Monitor and report signs of nephrotic syndrome, including edema and weight gain from fluid retention.

Interventions

- Protect suture lines and wounds to prevent reopening (dehiscence). Implement physical agents whenever possible to promote wound healing.
- For patients who are medically able to begin exercise, implement appropriate resistive exercises and aerobic training to maintain muscle strength and aerobic capacity during cancer chemotherapy or to help restore function after chemotherapy.
- Because of the risk of MI and stroke, use extreme caution during aerobic exercise and other forms of therapeutic exercise. Assess exercise tolerance frequently (blood pressure, heart rate, fatigue levels), and terminate exercise immediately if any untoward responses occur (See Appendix L).

Patient/Client-Related Instruction

- Advise patient and family or caregiver about the signs of MI and stroke (see signs above in Examination and Evaluation) and to seek immediate medical assistance if these signs develop.
- Instruct patient and family or caregiver to immediately report signs of bowel perforation or abnormal bleeding (see signs above in Examination and Evaluation).

Pharmacokinetics

Absorption: IV administration results in complete bioavailability.
Distribution: Unknown.
Metabolism and Excretion: Unknown.
Half-life: 20 days (range 11–50 days).

TIME/ACTION PROFILE

ROUTE	ONSET	PEAK	DURATION
IV	rapid	end of infusion	14 days

Contraindications/Precautions

Contraindicated in: Hypersensitivity; Recent hemoptysis or other serious recent bleeding episode; First 28 days after major surgery; OB: Angiogenesis is critical to the developing fetus. Contraindicated unless benefit to mother outweighs potential fetal harm; Lactation: Discontinue nursing during treatment and, due to long half-life, for several weeks following treatment.
Use Cautiously in: Cardiovascular disease; Pedi: Safety not established; Geri: ↑ risk of serious adverse reactions, including arterial thromboembolic events.

Interactions

Drug-Drug: ↑ blood levels of SN 38 (the active metabolite of **irinotecan**); significance is not known.

Route/Dosage

Colon Cancer

IV (Adults): 5 mg/kg infusion every 14 days.

Lung Cancer

IV (Adults): 15 mg/kg infusion every 3 wk.

Availability

Solution for injection (requires dilution): 100 mg/4 mL vial, 400 mg/16 mL vial.

bicalutamide
(bye-ka-**loot**-a-mide)
Casodex

Classification
Therapeutic: antineoplastics
Pharmacologic: antiandrogens

Indications

Treatment of metastatic prostate carcinoma in conjunction with luteinizing hormone–releasing hormone (LHRH) analogues (goserelin, leuprolide).

Action

Antagonizes the effects of androgen at the cellular level. **Therapeutic Effects:** Decreased spread of prostate carcinoma.

Adverse Reactions/Side Effects

CNS: weakness, dizziness, headache, insomnia. **Resp:** dyspnea. **CV:** chest pain, hypertension, peripheral edema. **GI:** constipation, diarrhea, nausea, abdominal pain, increased liver enzymes, vomiting. **GU:** hematuria, erectile dysfunction, incontinence, nocturia, urinary tract infections. **Derm:** alopecia, rashes, sweating. **Endo:** breast pain, gynecomastia. **Hemat:** anemia. **Metab:** hyperglycemia, weight loss. **MS:** back pain, pelvic pain, bone pain. **Neuro:** paresthesia. **Misc:** generalized pain, hot flashes, flu-like syndrome, infection.

PHYSICAL THERAPY IMPLICATIONS

Examination and Evaluation

- Assess blood pressure periodically and compare to normal values (See Appendix F). Report a sustained increase in blood pressure (hypertension) to the physician.
- Monitor cardiopulmonary symptoms such as chest pain or difficult, labored breathing. Report severe or unexpected cardiac and respiratory problems to the physician.
- Assess peripheral edema using girth measurements, volume displacement, and measurement of pitting edema (See Appendix N). Report increased swelling in feet and ankles or a sudden increase in body weight due to fluid retention.
- Monitor signs of anemia, including unusual fatigue, shortness of breath with exertion, bruising, and pale skin. Notify physician immediately if these signs occur.
- Be alert for signs of hyperglycemia, including confusion, drowsiness, flushed/dry skin, fruit-like breath odor, rapid/deep breathing, polyuria, loss of appetite, and unusual thirst. Patients with diabetes mellitus should check blood glucose levels frequently.
- Assess any back, pelvic, or other bone or generalized pain to rule out musculoskeletal pathology; that is, try to determine if pain is drug induced rather than caused by anatomic or biomechanical problems.
- Be alert for signs of paresthesia (numbness, tingling). Establish baseline electroneuromyographic values at the beginning of drug treatment whenever possible, and reexamine these values periodically to document drug-induced changes in peripheral nerve function.
- Assess dizziness and weakness that might affect gait, balance, and other functional activities (See Appendix C). Report balance problems and functional limitations to the physician and nursing staff, and caution the patient and family/caregivers to guard against falls and trauma.
- Periodically assess body weight and other anthropometric measures (body mass index, body composition). Report a rapid or unexplained weight loss.

Interventions

- For patients who are medically able to begin exercise, implement appropriate resistive exercises and aerobic training to maintain muscle strength and aerobic capacity during cancer chemotherapy or to help restore function after chemotherapy.
- Because of cardiopulmonary side effects, use caution during aerobic exercise and other forms of therapeutic exercise. Assess exercise tolerance frequently (respiratory symptoms, blood pressure, heart rate, fatigue levels), and terminate exercise immediately if any untoward responses occur (See Appendix L).

Patient/Client-Related Instruction

- Advise patient and family/caregivers that fatigue and weakness are likely and may be severe. Functional abilities may be limited, and patient may need to use assistive devices during ambulation.
- Advise patient about the likelihood of GI reactions such as diarrhea, nausea, vomiting, constipation, and abdominal pain. Instruct patient or family and caregivers to report severe or unexpected GI reactions.
- Advise patient that hair loss and other skin reactions (rashes, sweating) are likely. Report other severe or unexpected skin reactions to the physician.
- Instruct patient to report problems with urination, including blood in the urine, increased nighttime urination, incontinence, or pain and burning that might indicate a urinary tract infection.
- Instruct patient or family/caregivers to report other troublesome side effects including severe or prolonged headache, sleep loss, erectile dysfunction, breast pain/enlargement, hot flashes, or flu-like symptoms (fever, chills, body aches).

Pharmacokinetics

Absorption: Well absorbed after oral administration.
Distribution: Unknown.
Protein Binding: 96%.
Metabolism and Excretion: Mostly metabolized by the liver.
Half-life: 5.8 days.

TIME/ACTION PROFILE (blood levels)

ROUTE	ONSET	PEAK	DURATION
PO	unknown	31.3 hr	unknown

Contraindications/Precautions

Contraindicated in: Hypersensitivity; OB: Not for use in women.
Use Cautiously in: Moderate-to-severe liver impairment; Patients with childbearing potential; Lactation: Not for use in women; Pedi: Safety not established.

Interactions

Drug-Drug: May increase the effect of **warfarin**.

Route/Dosage

PO (Adults): 50 mg once daily (must be given concurrently with LHRH analogue or following surgical castration).

Availability (generic available)

Tablets: 50 mg.

biperiden (bye-per-i-den)

Akineton

Classification

Therapeutic: antiparkinson agents

Pharmacologic: anticholinergics

Indications

Adjunctive treatment of all forms of Parkinson's disease, including drug-induced extrapyramidal effects and acute dystonic reactions.

Action

Blocks cholinergic activity in the CNS, which is partially responsible for the symptoms of Parkinson's disease. Restores the natural balance of neurotransmitters in the CNS. **Therapeutic Effects:** Reduction of rigidity and tremors.

Adverse Reactions/Side Effects

CNS: confusion, depression, dizziness, hallucinations, headache, sedation, weakness. **EENT:** blurred vision, dry eyes, mydriasis. **CV:** arrhythmias, hypotension, palpitations, tachycardia. **GI:** constipation, dry mouth, ileus, nausea. **GU:** hesitancy, urinary retention. **Misc:** decreased sweating.

PHYSICAL THERAPY IMPLICATIONS

Examination and Evaluation

- Assess patient's gait and motor function to help document antiparkinson effects, especially when starting drug therapy, or during dosing changes or addition of other antiparkinson drugs. Motor function should be assessed at different times of the day, such as when drugs are reaching therapeutic levels (i.e., 1–2 hr after oral dose), as well as when drug effects are minimal (just before the next dose).
- Assess heart rate, ECG, and heart sounds, especially during exercise (See Appendices G, H). Report fast heart rate (tachycardia) or signs of other arrhythmias, including palpitations, chest discomfort, shortness of breath, fainting, and fatigue/weakness.
- Assess blood pressure (BP) periodically and compare to normal values (See Appendix F). Report low BP (hypotension), especially if patient experiences dizziness, fatigue, or other symptoms.
- Assess dizziness and drowsiness that might affect gait, balance, and other functional activities (See Appendix C). Report balance problems and functional limitations to the physician and nursing staff, and caution the patient and family/caregivers to guard against falls and trauma.
- Monitor confusion, hallucinations, depression, and other psychologic problems. Repeated or excessive symptoms may require change in dose or medication.

Interventions

- Implement therapeutic exercises (coordination exercises, gait training, cardiovascular conditioning) to complement the effects of drug therapy and help achieve optimal function.
- Because of the risk of arrhythmias and abnormal BP responses, use caution during aerobic exercise and other forms of therapeutic exercise. Assess exercise tolerance frequently (BP, heart rate, fatigue levels), and terminate exercise immediately if any untoward responses occur (See Appendix L).
- Guard against falls and trauma (hip fractures, head injury, and so forth). Implement fall-prevention strategies (See Appendix E), especially if patient exhibits Parkinson's symptoms (postural instability, rigidity) combined with drug side effects (dizziness, blurred vision, weakness).

Patient/Client-Related Instruction

- Instruct patient to report other bothersome side effects, including severe or prolonged headache, vision problems, decreased sweating, urinary problems (hesitancy, retention), or GI problems (nausea, constipation, dry mouth).

Pharmacokinetics

Absorption: Well absorbed after oral or IM administration.
Distribution: Unknown.
Metabolism and Excretion: Unknown.
Half-life: Unknown.

TIME/ACTION PROFILE (relief of symptoms)

ROUTE	ONSET	PEAK	DURATION
PO	unknown	unknown	unknown
IM	10–30 min	unknown	unknown
IV	unknown	unknown	1–8 hr

Contraindications/Precautions

Contraindicated in: Hypersensitivity; Angle-closure glaucoma; Bowel obstruction; Megacolon; Tardive dyskinesia.
Use Cautiously in: Prostatic enlargement; Seizure disorders; Cardiac arrhythmias; OB/Lactation: Safety not established; Geri: Increased risk of adverse reactions; lower doses may be necessary.

Interactions

Drug-Drug: Additive anticholinergic effects with **drugs sharing anticholinergic properties**, such as **antihistamines**, **phenothiazines**, **quinidine**,

disopyramide, and **tricyclic antidepressants**. Counteracts the cholinergic effects of **bethanechol**. **Antacids** or **antidiarrheals** may ↓ absorption.
Drug-Natural: ↑ anticholinergic effects with **angel's trumpet** and **jimson weed**, and **scopolia**.

Route/Dosage

Parkinsonism

PO (Adults): 2 mg 3–4 times daily initially (not to exceed 16 mg/day).

Extrapyramidal Reactions

PO (Adults): 2 mg 1–3 times daily.
IM, IV (Adults): 2 mg, may repeat q 30 min (not to exceed 8 mg or 4 doses/24 hr).
IM (Children): 40 mcg (0.04 mg)/kg or 1.2 mg/m^2, may repeat q 30 min (not to exceed 4 doses/24 hr).

Availability

Tablets: 2 mg. **Injection:** 5 mg/mL.

bisoprolol (bis-oh-proe-lol)

Monocor, Zebeta

Classification
Therapeutic: antihypertensives
Pharmacologic: beta blockers

Indications

Management of hypertension.

Action

Blocks stimulation of $beta_1$ (myocardial)–adrenergic receptors. Does not usually affect $beta_2$(pulmonary, vascular, uterine) receptor sites **Therapeutic Effects:** Decreased blood pressure and heart rate.

Adverse Reactions/Side Effects

CNS: fatigue, weakness, anxiety, depression, dizziness, drowsiness, insomnia, memory loss, mental status changes, nervousness, nightmares. **EENT:** blurred vision, stuffy nose. **Resp:** bronchospasm, wheezing. **CV:** BRADYCARDIA, CHF, PULMONARY EDEMA, hypotension, peripheral vasoconstriction. **GI:** constipation, diarrhea, liver function abnormalities, nausea, vomiting. **GU:** erectile dysfunction, decreased libido, urinary frequency. **Derm:** rashes. **Endo:** hyperglycemia, hypoglycemia. **MS:** arthralgia, back pain, joint pain. **Misc:** drug-induced lupus syndrome.

PHYSICAL THERAPY IMPLICATIONS

Examination and Evaluation

- Assess heart rate, ECG, and heart sounds, especially during exercise (See Appendices G, H). Report an abnormally slow heart rate (bradycardia) or symptoms of other arrhythmias, including palpitations, chest discomfort, shortness of breath, fainting, and fatigue/weakness.
- Assess routinely for signs of CHF and pulmonary edema, including dyspnea, rales/crackles, weight gain, peripheral edema, and jugular venous distention. Report these signs to the physician immediately.
- Assess blood pressure (BP) periodically and compare to normal values (See Appendix F) to help document antihypertensive effects. Report low BP (hypotension), especially if patient experiences dizziness, fatigue, or other symptoms.
- Assess symptoms of bronchospasm (wheezing, coughing, tightness in chest). Perform pulmonary function tests to quantify suspected changes in ventilation and respiration (See Appendices I, J, K). Repeated or prolonged bronchoconstriction may require a change in dose or medication.
- Monitor signs of peripheral vasoconstriction, such as extreme coldness in the hands and feet, cyanosis, and muscle cramping. Notify physician of severe or prolonged signs of vasoconstriction.
- Be alert for signs of hypoglycemia (weakness, malaise, irritability, fatigue) or hyperglycemia (drowsiness, fruity breath, increased urination, unusual thirst). Medication may mask some signs of hypoglycemia, but dizziness and sweating may still occur. Patients with diabetes mellitus should check blood glucose levels frequently.
- Assess any back, joint, or muscle pain to rule out musculoskeletal pathology; that is, try to determine if pain is drug induced rather than caused by anatomic or biomechanical problems.
- Monitor mood and personality changes, including depression, anxiety, nervousness, memory loss, or other changes in mental status and behavior. Notify physician if these changes become problematic.
- Assess dizziness and drowsiness that might affect gait, balance, and other functional activities (See Appendix C). Report balance problems and functional limitations to the physician, and caution the patient and family/caregivers to guard against falls and trauma.
- Monitor excessive fatigue or weakness. Beta blockers often cause some degree of fatigue and weakness, but any sudden or severe change in muscle strength or energy levels should be reported.
- Monitor signs of drug-induced lupus syndrome, including increased BP, fever, joint pain, skin rashes, and redness/irritation of the eye (uveitis). Notify physician promptly if these signs appear.

Interventions

- Because of an increased risk of CHF and cardiac arrhythmias, use caution during aerobic exercise and endurance conditioning. Terminate exercise if patient exhibits untoward symptoms (chest pain, shortness of breath, unusual fatigue.) or displays other criteria for exercise termination (See Appendix L).
- Establish aerobic exercise workloads that account for the effects of beta blockers on heart rate. Some heart rate guidelines may not be appropriate because beta blockers typically decrease maximal HR by 20–30 bpm. Use other guidelines such as rating of perceived exertion (RPE, modified Borg scale) to determine exercise workloads.
- To minimize orthostatic hypotension, patient should move slowly when assuming a more upright position.

Patient/Client-Related Instruction

- Remind patients to take medication as directed to control hypertension even if they are asymptomatic.
- Counsel patients about additional interventions to help control BP, including regular exercise, weight loss, sodium restriction, stress reduction, moderation of alcohol consumption, and smoking cessation.
- Instruct patient or family/caregivers to report other troublesome side effects such as severe or prolonged insomnia, nightmares, blurred vision, stuffy nose, increased urinary frequency, decreased libido, erectile dysfunction, skin rash, or GI problems (nausea, vomiting, constipation, and/or diarrhea).

Pharmacokinetics

Absorption: Well absorbed after oral administration, but 20% undergoes first-pass hepatic metabolism.
Distribution: Unknown.
Metabolism and Excretion: 50% excreted unchanged by the kidneys; remainder renally excreted as metabolites; 2% excreted in feces.
Half-life: 9–12 hr.

TIME/ACTION PROFILE (antihypertensive effect)

ROUTE	ONSET	PEAK	DURATION
PO	unknown	1–4 hr	24 hr

Contraindications/Precautions

Contraindicated in: Uncompensated CHF; Pulmonary edema; Cardiogenic shock; Bradycardia or heart block.
Use Cautiously in: Renal impairment (dosage reduction recommended); Hepatic impairment (dosage reduction recommended); Pulmonary disease (including asthma; $beta_1$ selectivity may be lost at higher doses); avoid use if possible; Diabetes mellitus (may mask signs of hypoglycemia); Thyrotoxicosis (may mask symptoms); Patients with a history of severe allergic reactions (intensity of reactions may be increased); OB/Lactation/Pedi: Safety not established; crosses the placenta and may cause fetal/neonatal bradycardia, hypotension, hypoglycemia, or respiratory depression; Geri: Increased sensitivity to beta blockers; initial dosage reduction recommended.

Interactions

Drug-Drug: General anesthetics, IV phenytoin, and **verapamil** may cause additive myocardial depression. Additive bradycardia may occur with **digoxin.** Additive hypotension may occur with other **antihypertensives**, acute ingestion of **alcohol**, or **nitrates**. Concurrent use with **amphetamine, cocaine, ephedrine, epinephrine, norepinephrine, phenylephrine,** or **pseudoephedrine** may result in unopposed alpha-adrenergic stimulation (excessive hypertension, bradycardia). Concurrent thyroid preparation administration may decrease effectiveness. May alter the effectiveness of **insulins** or **oral hypoglycemic agents** (dosage adjustments may be necessary). May decrease the effectiveness of **theophylline**. May decrease the beneficial $beta_1$-cardiovascular effects of **dopamine** or **dobutamine**. Use cautiously within 14 days of **MAO inhibitor** therapy (may result in hypertension).

Route/Dosage

PO (Adults): 5 mg once daily; may be increased to 10 mg once daily (range 2.5–20 mg/day).

Renal Impairment

Hepatic Impairment

PO (Adults): *CCr <40 mL/min*—Initiate therapy with 2.5 mg/day, titrate cautiously.

Availability (generic available)

Tablets: 5 mg, 10 mg. ***In combination with:*** hydrochlorothiazide (Ziac). See Appendix B.

bivalirudin (bye-val-i-roo-din)

Angiomax

Classification

Therapeutic: anticoagulants
Pharmacologic: thrombin inhibitors

Indications

Used in conjunction with aspirin to reduce the risk of acute ischemic complications in patients with unstable angina who are undergoing percutaneous transluminal angioplasty (PCTA) or percutaneous coronary intervention (PCI). Patients with or at risk of heparin-induced thrombocytopenia (HIT) and thrombosis syndrome (HITTS) who are undergoing PCI.

Action

Specifically and reversibly inhibits thrombin by binding to its receptor sites. Inhibition of thrombin prevents activation of factors V, VIII, and XII; the conversion of fibrinogen to fibrin; platelet adhesion and aggregation. **Therapeutic Effects:** Decreased acute ischemic complications in patients with unstable angina (death, MI, or the urgent need for revascularization procedures).

Adverse Reactions/Side Effects

CNS: headache, anxiety, insomnia, nervousness. **CV:** hypotension, bradycardia, hypertension. **GI:** nausea, abdominal pain, dyspepsia, vomiting. **Hemat:** BLEEDING. **Local:** injection site pain. **MS:** back pain. **Misc:** pain, fever, pelvic pain.

PHYSICAL THERAPY IMPLICATIONS

Examination and Evaluation

- Assess signs of bleeding and hemorrhage (bleeding gums; nosebleed; unusual bruising; black, tarry stools; hematuria; fall in hematocrit or blood pressure). Notify physician or nursing staff immediately of these signs.
- Assess blood pressure (BP) and compare to normal values (See Appendix F). Report changes in BP, either a problematic decrease in BP (hypotension) or a sustained increase in BP (hypertension).
- Assess heart rate, ECG, and heart sounds, especially during exercise (See Appendices G, H). Report an abnormally slow heart rate (bradycardia) or signs of other arrhythmias, including palpitations, chest discomfort, shortness of breath, fainting, and fatigue/weakness.
- Assess any back pain or pelvic pain to rule out musculoskeletal pathology; that is, try to determine if pain is drug induced rather than caused by anatomic or biomechanical problems. Be especially alert for sudden back pain that might indicate abdominal hemorrhage.
- Monitor and report anxiety, nervousness, or other problematic changes in mood and behavior.
- Monitor injection site for pain, swelling, and irritation. Report prolonged or excessive injection site reactions to the physician or nursing staff.

Interventions

- Use caution with any physical interventions that could increase bleeding, including wound débridement, chest percussion, joint mobilization, and application of local heat.

Patient/Client-Related Instruction

- Instruct patient to immediately report signs of GI bleeding, including abdominal pain, vomiting blood, blood in stools, or black, tarry stools.
- Instruct patient to report other bothersome side effects such as severe or prolonged fever, sleep loss, or GI problems (nausea, vomiting, indigestion, abdominal pain).

Pharmacokinetics

Absorption: IV administration results in complete bioavailability.
Distribution: Unknown.
Metabolism and Excretion: Cleared from plasma by a combination of renal mechanisms and proteolytic breakdown.
Half-life: 25 min (increased in renal impairment).

TIME/ACTION PROFILE (anticoagulant effect)

ROUTE	ONSET	PEAK	DURATION
IV	immediate	unknown	1–2 hr

Contraindications/Precautions

Contraindicated in: Active major bleeding; Hypersensitivity.
Use Cautiously in: Any disease state associated with an increased risk of bleeding; Heparin-induced thrombocytopenia or heparin-induced thrombocytopenia-thrombosis syndrome; Patients with unstable angina not undergoing PCTA; Patients with other acute coronary syndromes; Concurrent use with other platelet aggregation inhibitors (safety not established); Renal impairment (infusion rate reduction recommended if GFR <60 mL/min); Lactation/Pedi: Safety not established; OB: Use only if clearly needed.

Interactions

Drug-Drug: Risk of bleeding may be ↑ by concurrent use of **abciximab, heparin, low-molecular-weight heparins/heparinoids, ticlopidine, thrombolytics,** or any other **drugs that inhibit coagulation.**
Drug-Natural: ↑ risk of bleeding with **arnica, chamomile, clove, dong quai, feverfew, garlic, ginger, gingko, *Panax ginseng*,** and others.

Route/Dosage

IV (Adults): 0.75 mg/kg as a bolus injection, followed by an infusion at a rate of 1.75 mg/kg/hr for the duration of the PCI procedure. An activated clotting time (ACT) should be performed 5 min after bolus dose and an additional bolus dose of 0.3 mg/kg may be administered if needed. Continuation of the infusion (at a rate of 1.75 mg/kg/hr) for up to 4 hr postprocedure is optional. If needed, the infusion may be continued beyond this initial 4 hr at a rate of 0.2 mg/kg/hr for up to 20 hr. Therapy should be initiated prior to the procedure and given in conjunction with aspirin.

Renal Impairment

IV (Adults): No reduction in the bolus dose is needed in any patient with renal impairment. *GFR 10–29 mL/min*—Reduce infusion rate to

1 mg/kg/hr; *Dialysis-dependent patients (off dialysis)*—Reduce infusion rate to 0.25 mg/kg/hr. ACT should be monitored in all patients with renal impairment.

Availability

Powder for injection: 250 mg/vial.

HIGH ALERT

bleomycin (blee-oh-mye-sin)

Blenoxane

Classification

Therapeutic: antineoplastics

Pharmacologic: antitumor antibiotics

Indications

Treatment of Lymphomas, Squamous cell carcinoma, Testicular embryonal cell carcinoma, Choriocarcinoma, Teratocarcinoma. Intrapleural administration to prevent the reaccumulation of malignant effusions.

Action

Inhibits DNA and RNA synthesis. **Therapeutic Effects:** Death of rapidly replicating cells, particularly malignant ones.

Adverse Reactions/Side Effects

CNS: aggressive behavior, disorientation, weakness. **Resp:** PULMONARY FIBROSIS, pneumonitis. **CV:** hypotension, peripheral vasoconstriction. **GI:** anorexia, nausea, stomatitis, vomiting. **Derm:** hyperpigmentation, mucocutaneous toxicity, alopecia, erythema, rashes, urticaria, vesiculation. **Hemat:** anemia, leukopenia, thrombocytopenia. **Local:** pain at tumor site, phlebitis at IV site. **Metab:** weight loss. **Misc:** ANAPHYLACTOID REACTIONS, chills, fever.

PHYSICAL THERAPY IMPLICATIONS

Examination and Evaluation

- Assess pulmonary function periodically by measuring lung volumes, breath sounds, and respiratory rate (See Appendices I, J, K). Notify physician immediately if patient experiences signs of pulmonary fibrosis or pneumonitis such as dry cough, dyspnea, chest pain, shortness of breath, cyanosis, and fever.
- Monitor signs of anaphylactoid reactions, including pulmonary symptoms (tightness in the throat and chest, wheezing, cough, dyspnea) or skin reactions (rash, pruritus, urticaria). Notify physician or nursing staff immediately if these reactions occur.
- Be alert for disorientation, aggressive behavior, or other alterations in mental status (See Appendix D). Notify physician promptly if these symptoms develop.
- Assess blood pressure (BP) periodically and compare to normal values (See Appendix F). Report low BP (hypotension), especially if patient experiences dizziness, fainting, or other symptoms.
- Monitor signs of peripheral vasoconstriction, such as extreme coldness in the hands and feet, cyanosis, and muscle cramping. Notify physician of severe or prolonged signs of vasoconstriction.
- Watch for signs of leukopenia (fever, sore throat, signs of infection), thrombocytopenia (bruising, nose bleeds, bleeding gums) or unusual weakness and fatigue that might be due to anemia. Report these signs to the physician or nursing staff.
- Periodically assess body weight and other anthropometric measures (body mass index, body composition). Report a rapid or unexplained weight loss or decreased body fat.
- Monitor IV injection site for pain, swelling, and inflammation. Report prolonged or excessive injection site reactions to the physician.

Interventions

- For patients who are medically able to begin exercise, implement appropriate resistive exercises and aerobic training to maintain muscle strength and aerobic capacity during cancer chemotherapy or to help restore function after chemotherapy.
- Because of the risk of pulmonary fibrosis and abnormal BP responses, use caution during aerobic exercise and other forms of therapeutic exercise. Assess exercise tolerance frequently (BP, heart rate, breathing responses, fatigue levels), and terminate exercise immediately if any untoward responses occur (See Appendix L).

Patient/Client-Related Instruction

- Advise patient about the likelihood of GI reactions including nausea, vomiting, loss of appetite, and inflammation in/around the mouth. Instruct patient to report severe or unexpected GI reactions.
- Advise patient that hair loss and other skin reactions (rash, itching, hives, blistering, changes in pigmentation) are likely. Severe or unexpected skin reactions should be reported to the physician or nursing staff.
- Advise patient to guard against infection (frequent hand washing, etc.) and avoid crowds and contact with persons with contagious diseases.

Pharmacokinetics

Absorption: Well absorbed from IM and SC sites. Absorption follows intrapleural and intraperitoneal administration.

Distribution: Widely distributed, concentrates in skin, lungs, peritoneum, kidneys, and lymphatics.

Metabolism and Excretion: 60–70% excreted unchanged by the kidneys.

Half-life: 2 hr (increased in renal impairment).

TIME/ACTION PROFILE (tumor response)

ROUTE	ONSET	PEAK	DURATION
IV, IM, SC	2–3 wk	unknown	unknown

Contraindications/Precautions

Contraindicated in: Hypersensitivity; OB/Lactation: Potential for fetal, infant harm.

Use Cautiously in: Renal impairment (dose reduction required if <35 mL/min); Pulmonary impairment; Nonmalignant chronic debilitating illness; Patients with childbearing potential; Geri: Increased risk of pulmonary toxicity and related decrease in renal function.

Interactions

Drug-Drug: Hematologic toxicity ↑ with concurrent use of **radiation therapy** and other **antineoplastics**. Concurrent use with **cisplatin** ↓ elimination of bleomycin and may ↑ toxicity. ↑ risk of pulmonary toxicity with other **antineoplastics** or thoracic **radiation therapy**. **General anesthesia** ↑ the risk of pulmonary toxicity. ↑ risk of Raynaud's syndrome when used with **vinblastine**.

Route/Dosage

Lymphoma patients should receive initial test doses of 2 units or less for the first 2 doses.

IV, IM, SC (Adults and Children): 0.25–0.5 unit/kg (10–20 units/m^2) weekly or twice weekly initially. If favorable response, lower maintenance doses given (1 unit/day or 5 units/wk IM or IV). May also be given as continuous IV infusion at 0.25 unit/kg or 15 units/m^2/day for 4–5 days.

Intrapleural: (Adults): 15–20 units instilled for 4 hr, then removed.

Availability (generic available)

Injection: 15 units/vial, 30 units/vial.

bortezomib (bor-tez-o-mib)

Velcade

Classification

Therapeutic: antineoplastics

Pharmacologic: proteasome inhibitors

Indications

Multiple myeloma (as initial therapy or after progression); with melphalan and prednisone). Mantle cell lymphoma after at least one other therapy.

Action

Inhibits proteasome, a regulator of intracellular protein catabolism, resulting in disruption of various intracellular processes. Cytotoxic to a variety of cancerous cells. **Therapeutic Effects:** Death of rapidly replicating cells, particularly malignant ones.

Adverse Reactions/Side Effects

CNS: fatigue, malaise, weakness, dizziness, syncope. **EENT:** blurred vision, diplopia. **CV:** hypotension, CHF. **Resp:** pneumonia. **GI:** anorexia, constipation, diarrhea, nausea, vomiting. **Hemat:** BLEEDING, anemia, neutropenia, thrombocytopenia. **Neuro:** peripheral neuropathy. **Misc:** fever, tumor lysis syndrome.

PHYSICAL THERAPY IMPLICATIONS

Examination and Evaluation

- Be alert for any unusual bleeding and signs of thrombocytopenia (bruising, nose bleeds, bleeding gums), neutropenia (fever, sore throat, signs of infection), or any unusual weakness and fatigue that could be due to anemia. Report these signs to the physician or nursing staff immediately.
- Assess any breathing problems or signs of pneumonia such as cough, fever, chills, and chest pain during inspiration and expiration. Monitor pulse oximetry and perform pulmonary function tests (See Appendices I, J, K) to quantify suspected changes in ventilation and respiratory function.
- Assess blood pressure (BP) periodically and compare to normal values (See Appendix F). Report low BP (hypotension), especially if patient experiences dizziness, syncope, or other symptoms.
- Monitor signs of congestive heart failure, including dyspnea, rales/crackles, peripheral edema, jugular venous distention, and exercise intolerance. Report these signs to the physician.
- Monitor neuromuscular signs of electrolyte imbalances that might indicate tumor lysis syndrome. Signs include severe muscle weakness or paralysis due to increased plasma potassium (hyperkalemia) or muscle hyperexcitability and tetany due to phosphate and calcium imbalances (hyperphosphatemia and hypocalcemia). Notify physician immediately if these signs occur.
- Monitor signs of peripheral neuropathy (numbness, tingling, decreased muscle strength). Establish baseline electroneuromyographic values at the beginning of drug treatment whenever possible, and reexamine these values periodically to document drug-induced changes in peripheral nerve function.

Interventions

- For patients who are medically able to begin exercise, implement appropriate resistive exercises and

aerobic training to maintain muscle strength and aerobic capacity during cancer chemotherapy or to help restore function after chemotherapy.
- Because of possible heart failure and abnormal BP responses, use caution during aerobic exercise and endurance conditioning. Terminate exercise if patient exhibits untoward symptoms (chest pain, shortness of breath, etc.) or displays other criteria for exercise termination (See Appendix L).

Patient/Client-Related Instruction
- Advise patient to guard against infection (frequent hand washing, etc.) and avoid crowds and contact with persons with contagious diseases.
- Advise patient and family/caregivers that fatigue and weakness are likely and may be severe. Functional abilities may be limited, and patient may need to use assistive devices during ambulation.
- Advise patient about the likelihood of GI reactions (constipation, diarrhea, nausea, vomiting, loss of appetite). Instruct patient to report severe, prolonged GI problems.
- Instruct patient to report any vision disturbances, including blurred or double vision.

Pharmacokinetics
Absorption: IV administration results in complete bioavailability.
Distribution: Unknown.
Metabolism and Excretion: Mostly metabolized by the liver (P450 enzymes); excretion is unknown.
Half-life: 9–15 hr.

TIME/ACTION PROFILE

ROUTE	ONSET	PEAK	DURATION
IV	unknown	38 days*	Unknown

*Median time to response based on clinical parameters.

Contraindications/Precautions
Contraindicated in: Hypersensitivity to bortezomib, boron, or mannitol; OB: Potential fetal harm; Lactation: Potential for serious adverse reaction in nursing infants.
Use Cautiously in: OB: Women with childbearing potential; Hepatic impairment (may ↑ levels, risk of toxicity); History of or risk factors for CHF; Pedi: Safety not established.

Interactions
Drug-Drug: Concurrent neurotoxic medications, including **amiodarone**, some **antivirals, nitrofurantoin, isoniazid**, or **HMG CoA reductase inhibitors** may ↑ risk of peripheral neuropathy.

Route/Dosage
IV (Adults): 1.3 mg/m^2 twice weekly for 2 wk (days 1, 4, 8, and 11) followed by a 10-day rest; further cycles/doses depend on response and toxicity.

Availability
Lyophilized powder for injection (requires reconstitution): 3.5 mg/vial.

bosentan (boe-sen-tan)
Tracleer

Classification
Therapeutic: vasodilators
Pharmacologic: endothelin receptor antagonists

Indications
Primary pulmonary hypertension in patients with WHO class III or IV symptoms.

Action
Antagonizes the effects of the neurohormone endothelin by binding to its receptor sites in endothelium and vascular smooth muscle. **Therapeutic Effects:** Improved exercise capacity and decreased clinical deterioration.

Adverse Reactions/Side Effects
CNS: headache, fatigue. **EENT:** nasopharyngitis. **CV:** edema, hypotension, palpitations. **GI:** HEPATOTOXICITY, dyspepsia. **Derm:** flushing, pruritus. **Hemat:** anemia.

PHYSICAL THERAPY IMPLICATIONS

Examination and Evaluation
- Be alert for signs of hepatotoxicity, including anorexia, abdominal pain, severe nausea and vomiting, yellow skin or eyes, fever, sore throat, malaise, weakness, facial edema, lethargy, and unusual bleeding or bruising. Notify physician immediately if these signs occur.
- Assess exercise tolerance to help determine if drug therapy is successful in improving exercise capacity. Document any changes in exercise time, intensity, fatigue, and so forth.
- Assess blood pressure periodically, and compare to normal values (See Appendix F). Report low blood pressure (hypotension), especially if patient experiences dizziness, fatigue, or other symptoms.
- Monitor signs of anemia, including unusual fatigue, shortness of breath with exertion, and bruising. Notify physician immediately if these signs occur.
- Assess peripheral edema using girth measurements, volume displacement, and measurement of pitting edema (See Appendix N). Report increased swelling in feet and ankles or a sudden increase in body weight due to fluid retention.

Interventions
- Implement aerobic exercise and endurance training as tolerated to maintain or improve cardiovascular and pulmonary function.

B

Patient/Client-Related Instruction

- Instruct patient or family/caregivers to report other troublesome side effects such as severe or prolonged headache, indigestion, palpitations, irritation/inflammation in the nose and pharynx, and skin problems (itching, warmth, redness).

Pharmacokinetics

Absorption: 50% absorbed following oral administration in normal patients.
Distribution: 18 L; does not penetrate erythrocytes.
Protein Binding: >98%.
Metabolism and Excretion: Highly metabolized; one metabolite contributes to pharmacologic activity. Eliminated via biliary excretion; <3% excreted in urine.
Half-life: 5 hr.

TIME/ACTION PROFILE (blood levels)

ROUTE	ONSET	PEAK	DURATION
PO	unknown	3–5 hr	unknown

Contraindications/Precautions

Contraindicated in: Hypersensitivity; Concurrent use of cyclosporine or glyburide; Moderate-to-severe liver impairment; OB/High risk for fetal harm (malformation, stillbirth) if administered to pregnant women. Pregnancy must be ruled out before start of treatment and reliable contraception used throughout treatment. Hormonal contraceptives (all forms) cannot be the sole form of contraception (see drug-drug interactions). Monthly pregnancy tests for women with childbearing potential is recommended throughout course of therapy; Lactation: Not recommended.
Use Cautiously in: Mildly impaired liver function or history of liver disease; Women with childbearing potential; Pedi: Safety not established.

Interactions

Drug-Drug: Bosentan is metabolized by and induces the CYP3A4 and 2C9 enzyme systems. May ↓ effectiveness of **hormonal contraceptives** (additional method of contraception recommended). Significantly ↓ **cyclosporine** levels; **cyclosporine** significantly ↑ bosentan levels (concurrent use is contraindicated). ↑ risk of hepatotoxicity with **glyburide** (avoid concurrent use). **Ketoconazole** ↑ bosentan levels. ↓ levels of **simvastatin**, **lovastatin**, and **atorvastatin**. ↓ levels of warfarin. May ↓ levels of **tacrolimus** and **sirolimus**.

Route/Dosage

PO (Adults): 62.5 mg twice daily for 4 wk initially, then increased to maintenance dose of 125 mg twice daily.
PO (Adults <40 kg and >12 yr): 62.5 mg twice daily as initial and maintenance dose.

Availability

Tablets: 62.5 mg, 125 mg.

botulinum toxin (type A)

(bot-yoo-**lye**-num **toks**-in)
Botox Cosmetic

Classification
Therapeutic: cosmetic agents
Pharmacologic: neurotoxins

Indications

Temporary improvement in the appearance of moderate-to-severe glabellar lines (brow furrow) associated with corrugator and/or procerus muscle activity in adults ≤65 yr. **Unlabeled Use:** Treatment of spasticity in specific muscle groups.

Action

Produces partial chemical denervation by inhibiting the release of acetylcholine. Result is local decrease in muscle activity. **Therapeutic Effects:** Decreased brow furrow with improved appearance. Decreased muscle spasticity.

Adverse Reactions/Side Effects

CNS: headache. **EENT:** temporary eyelid droop. **GI:** nausea. **Local:** discomfort at injection sites. **MS:** local muscle weakness. **Misc:** ALLERGIC REACTIONS, INCLUDING ANAPHYLAXIS (RARE).

PHYSICAL THERAPY IMPLICATIONS*

*When injected intramuscularly to treat spasticity

Examination and Evaluation

- Monitor signs of allergic reactions and anaphylaxis, including pulmonary symptoms (laryngeal edema, wheezing, cough, dyspnea) or skin reactions (rash, pruritus, urticaria). Notify physician immediately if these reactions occur.
- Be alert for possible systemic effects that might occur if botulinum toxin spreads beyond the IM injection site. Systemic effects include difficulty swallowing (dysphagia), difficulty speaking (dysphonia), and respiratory distress (dyspnea, decreased pulse oximetry values, cyanosis). Report signs of systemic botulism to the physician immediately. Excessive respiratory depression requires emergency care.
- Assess spasticity, ROM, and functional ability as the drug begins to take effect. Document whether

changes in spasticity and tone are consistent with rehabilitation goals.

- Monitor IM injection site for redness and irritation. Report prolonged or excessive skin reactions to the physician.

Interventions

- Implement aggressive therapeutic exercises (neuromuscular reeducation, postural stabilization, gait training, other task-specific training) to facilitate voluntary motor function and help patient adjust to reduced spasticity and tone.
- Provide appropriate assistive devices (walker, cane, crutches) while patient adjusts to reduced levels of spasticity. Specifically, make sure patient can ambulate and transfer safely while adjusting to reduced tone in the lower extremities.
- When indicated, incorporate serial casting and similar techniques to capitalize on drug effects and achieve maximal soft tissue lengthening and help reduce contractures.

Patient/Client-Related Instruction

- Explain to patient and family/caregivers that results typically last 2–3 months. Periodic reinjection may be needed to sustain antispasticity effects.
- Instruct patient or family/caregivers to report severe or prolonged headache, nausea, or other untoward responses.

Pharmacokinetics

Absorption: Minimal systemic absorption; action is primarily local.
Distribution: Unknown.
Metabolism and Excretion: Unknown.
Half-life: Unknown.

TIME/ACTION PROFILE (cosmetic results)

ROUTE	ONSET	PEAK	DURATION
IM	24–48 hr	unknown	3–4 mo

Contraindications/Precautions

Contraindicated in: Hypersensitivity; Presence of infection at planned injection sites; OB: Potential for spontaneous abortion or fetal deformity.
Use Cautiously in: Peripheral motor neuropathic diseases (e.g., amyotrophic lateral sclerosis, motor neuropathy) or neuromuscular junctional disorders (e.g., myasthenia gravis, Lambert-Eaton syndrome) (increased risk of significant systemic effects such as dysphagia or respiratory compromise); Inflammation at planned injection site; Marked facial asymmetry, ptosis, excessive dermatochalasis, deep dermal scarring, thick sebaceous skin, inability to lessen glabellar lines by physical spreading; Excessive weakness or atrophy in target muscles; Cervical dystonia (increased risk of dysphagia); Lactation; Pedi: Safety not established for children under 12 yr; Geri: Use lowest effective dose.

Interactions

Drug-Drug: Neuromuscular effects may be potentiated by **aminoglycosides, quinidine,** and other **drugs that alter neuromuscular transmission.** Additive effects may occur with other forms of **botulinum toxin.**

Route/Dosage

IM (Adults): 0.1 mL into each of five sites (two in each corrugator muscle and one in the procerus muscle; total dose of 20 units); not more frequently than every 3 mo.

Availability

Powder for reconstitution: 100 units/vial.

bromocriptine
(broe-moe-**krip**-teen)
✱Alti-Bromocriptine,
✱Apo-Bromocriptine, Parlodel

Classification
Therapeutic: antiparkinson agents
Pharmacologic: dopamine agonists

Indications

Adjunct to levodopa in the treatment of parkinsonism. Treatment of hyperprolactinemia (amenorrhea/galactorrhea), including associated female infertility. Treatment of acromegaly. **Unlabeled Use:** Management of pituitary prolactinomas. Management of neuroleptic malignant syndrome.

Action

Activates dopamine receptors in the CNS. Decreases prolactin secretion. **Therapeutic Effects:** Relief of rigidity and tremor in parkinsonism. Restoration of fertility in hyperprolactinemia. Decreased growth hormone in acromegaly.

Adverse Reactions/Side Effects

CNS: dizziness, confusion, drowsiness, hallucinations, headache, insomnia, nightmares. **EENT:** burning eyes, nasal stuffiness, visual disturbances. **Resp:** effusions, pulmonary infiltrates. **CV:** MI, hypotension. **GI:** nausea, abdominal pain, anorexia, dry mouth, metallic taste, vomiting. **Derm:** urticaria. **MS:** leg cramps. **Misc:** digital vasospasm (acromegaly only).

PHYSICAL THERAPY IMPLICATIONS

Examination and Evaluation

- Monitor cardiac symptoms at rest and during exercise. Seek immediate medical assistance if symptoms of MI develop, including sudden chest pain, pain radiating into the arm or jaw, shortness of breath, dizziness, sweating, anxiety, and nausea.

- Assess patient's motor function to help determine antiparkinson effects, especially when starting drug therapy, or during dosing changes or addition of other antiparkinson drugs. Motor function should be assessed at different times of the day, such as when drugs are reaching peak therapeutic levels (i.e., 1–2 hr after oral dose), as well as when drug effects are minimal (just before the next dose).
- Document increased side effects such as involuntary movements (dyskinesias) or fluctuations in response (on-off phenomenon, end-of-dose akinesia). Notify physician because increased side effects might require dose adjustment or a change in medication regimen.
- Assess dizziness and drowsiness that might affect gait, balance, and other functional activities (See Appendix C). Report balance problems and functional limitations to the physician, and caution the patient and family/caregivers to guard against falls and trauma.
- Monitor confusion, hallucinations, and other psychologic problems. Repeated or excessive symptoms may require change in dose or medication.
- Assess blood pressure (BP) periodically and compare to normal values (See Appendix F). Report low BP (hypotension), especially if patient experiences increased dizziness, syncope, or other symptoms.
- Monitor respiratory function at rest and during exercise. Notify physician if patient experiences signs of pulmonary infiltrates or effusion, including cough, shortness of breath, chest pain, or labored breathing.
- If used to treat acromegaly, periodically assess body weight and other anthropometric measures (body mass index, limb circumferences) to help document whether drug therapy is effective in reducing the effects of increased growth hormone.
- If treating acromegaly, watch for signs of digital vasospasm as indicated by decreased circulation to the fingers and toes resulting in pain, numbness, swelling, and color changes in the affected digits. Report these signs to the physician, and educate patient about how to avoid the onset of symptoms (keep hands warm, avoid caffeine, stress, and other triggers).
- If used to treat neuroleptic malignant syndrome, assess symptoms such as muscle rigidity, altered mental status, tachycardia, and abnormal BP to help document whether drug therapy is effective in resolving this syndrome.
- If treating increased prolactin secretion (hyperprolactinemia), monitor symptoms in women such as menstrual irregularities and abnormal lactation, and monitor symptoms in men such as erectile dysfunction, breast enlargement, and decreased libido. Document whether drug therapy is successful in reducing these symptoms.

Interventions

- Because of the risk of MI, use extreme caution during aerobic exercise and other forms of therapeutic exercise. Assess exercise tolerance frequently (BP, heart rate, fatigue levels), and terminate exercise immediately if any untoward responses occur (See Appendix L).
- Implement fall prevention strategies (See appendix E) and attempt to reduce the risk of falls and trauma caused by a combination of Parkinson's symptoms (postural instability, rigidity) and drug side effects (dizziness, dyskinesias).
- Implement therapeutic exercises (coordination exercises, gait training, cardiovascular conditioning) to complement the effects of drug therapy and help achieve optimal function.
- To minimize orthostatic hypotension, patient should move slowly when assuming a more upright position.

Patient/Client-Related Instruction

- Advise patient and family/caregivers to seek immediate medical assistance if symptoms of MI develop (see above under Examination and Evaluation).
- Advise patient to avoid alcohol because of the increased risk of sedation and adverse effects.
- Instruct patient to report other troublesome side effects such as severe or prolonged nasal congestion, burning eyes, vision disturbances, hives, leg cramps, and GI problems (nausea, vomiting, abdominal pain, loss of appetite, dry mouth, metallic taste).

Pharmacokinetics

Absorption: Poorly absorbed (30%) from the GI tract.
Distribution: Unknown.
Metabolism and Excretion: Completely metabolized by the liver.
Half-life: Biphasic—initial phase 4–4.5 hr, terminal phase 45–50 hr.

TIME/ACTION PROFILE (suppression of various parameters)

ROUTE	ONSET	PEAK	DURATION
PO*	30–90 min	1–2 hr	8–12 hr
PO†	2 hr	8 hr	24 hr
PO‡§	1–2 hr	4–8 wk§	4–8 hr

*Effect on parkinsonian symptoms.
†Effect on serum prolactin levels.
‡Effect on growth hormone.
§During chronic therapy.

Contraindications/Precautions

Contraindicated in: Hypersensitivity to bromocriptine, ergot alkaloids, or bisulfites (capsules only); Severe cardiovascular disease or peripheral vascular disease; Lactation.

Use Cautiously in: Cardiac disease; Mental disturbances; May restore fertility (additional contraception may be required if pregnancy is undesirable); Severe liver impairment (dose reduction required); OB/Lactation/Pedi: Safety not established.

Interactions

Drug-Drug: Additive hypotension with **antihypertensives**. Additive CNS depression with **antihistamines**, **alcohol**, **opioid analgesics**, and **sedative/hypnotics**. Additive neurologic effects with **levodopa**. Effective on prolactin levels, may be antagonized by **phenothiazines**, **haloperidol**, **methyldopa**, **tricyclic antidepressants**, and **reserpine**.

Route/Dosage

Parkinsonism

PO (Adults): 1.25 mg 1–2 times daily, increased by 2.5 mg/day in 2- to 4-wk intervals (range is 2.5–100 mg/day in divided doses; up to 40 mg/day has been used).

Hyperprolactinemia

PO (Adults): 1.25–2.5 mg/day initially, may be gradually increased q 3–7 days up to 2.5 mg 2–3 times daily.

Acromegaly

PO (Adults): 1.25–2.5 mg/day for 3 days, increase by 1.25–2.5 mg q 3–7 days until optimal response is obtained (usual range 10–30 mg/day; up to 100 mg/day).

Pituitary Adenomas

PO (Adults): 1.25 mg 2–3 times daily, may be increased over several weeks (range 2.5–20 mg/day).

Neuroleptic Malignant Syndrome (Unlabeled)

PO (Adults): 5 mg once daily initially, dose increased as required up to 20 mg/day.

Availability (generic available)

Tablets: 2.5 mg, 5 mg. **Capsules:** 5 mg.

brompheniramine

(brome-fen-ir-a-meen)

Bromfenac, Dimetapp Allergy, Nasahist B, ✦ Dimetane

Classification

Therapeutic: allergy, cold, and cough remedies, antihistamines

Pharmacologic: alkylamine

Indications

Symptomatic relief of allergic symptoms (rhinitis, urticaria) caused by histamine release. Severe allergic or hypersensitivity reactions, including anaphylaxis and transfusion reactions.

Action

Antagonizes the effects of histamine at H_1-receptor sites; does not bind to or inactivate histamine.

Therapeutic Effects: Decreased symptoms of histamine excess (sneezing, rhinorrhea, nasal and ocular pruritus, ocular tearing and redness).

Adverse Reactions/Side Effects

CNS: <u>drowsiness</u>, <u>sedation</u>, dizziness, excitation (in children). **EENT:** <u>blurred vision</u>. **CV:** <u>hypertension</u>, arrhythmias, hypotension, palpitations. **GI:** <u>dry mouth</u>, constipation, obstruction. **GU:** retention, urinary hesitancy. **Derm:** sweating. **Misc:** hypersensitivity reaction (IV use).

PHYSICAL THERAPY IMPLICATIONS

Examination and Evaluation

- Assess blood pressure (BP) and compare to normal values (See Appendix F). Report changes in BP, either a problematic decrease in BP (hypotension) or a sustained increase in BP (hypertension).
- Assess heart rate, ECG, and heart sounds, especially during exercise (See Appendices G, H). Report any rhythm disturbances or symptoms of increased arrhythmias, including palpitations, chest discomfort, shortness of breath, fainting, and fatigue/weakness.
- Monitor signs of hypersensitivity reactions during and after IV administration. Signs include pulmonary symptoms (tightness in the throat and chest, wheezing, cough, dyspnea) or skin reactions (rash, pruritus, urticaria). Notify physician or nursing staff immediately if these reactions occur.
- Monitor symptoms of nasal allergies (sneezing, rhinitis, itching eyes, cough) or chronic urticaria (rash, hives, itching) to help document benefits of this drug in treating these disorders.
- When treating anaphylaxis: assess for signs of successful treatment, including decreased skin reactions (rash, urticaria) and increased airway patency and ventilation (decreased dyspnea, wheezing, and so forth).
- Assess dizziness and drowsiness that might affect gait, balance, and other functional activities (See Appendix C). Report balance problems and functional limitations to the physician, and caution the patient and family/caregivers to guard against falls and trauma.
- Monitor signs of increased excitation in children. Severe or problematic excitation may require a change in dose or drug.

B

Interventions

- Guard against falls and trauma (hip fractures, head injury, and so forth). Implement fall-prevention strategies, especially in older adults or if balance is impaired (See Appendix E).
- Because of an increased risk of arrhythmias and abnormal BP responses, use caution during aerobic exercise and other forms of therapeutic exercise Assess exercise tolerance frequently (BP, heart rate, fatigue levels), and terminate exercise immediately if any untoward responses occur (See Appendix L).

Patient/Client-Related Instruction

- Advise patient about the risk of daytime drowsiness and decreased attention and mental focus. These problems can be severe in certain people. Use care if driving or in other activities that require quick reactions and strong concentration.
- Advise patient to avoid alcohol and other CNS depressants because of the increased risk of sedation and adverse effects.
- Instruct patient to report severe or prolonged problems with urination, including difficulty initiating urination or urinary retention.
- Instruct patient to report other troublesome side effects, including constipation, dry mouth, or excessive sweating.

Pharmacokinetics

Absorption: Well absorbed following PO/IM administration.
Distribution: Widely distributed; minimal amounts excreted in breast milk; crosses the blood-brain barrier.
Metabolism and Excretion: Extensively metabolized by the liver.
Half-life: 12–35 hr.

TIME/ACTION PROFILE (relief of allergic symptoms)

ROUTE	ONSET	PEAK	DURATION
PO	15–30 min	1–2 hr	4–6 hr
IM, SC	20–30 min	unknown	8–12 hr
IV	rapid	unknown	8–12 hr

Contraindications/Precautions

Contraindicated in: Hypersensitivity; Acute attacks of asthma; Known alcohol intolerance (some elixirs); Lactation: Potential for adverse reaction in nursing infants.
Use Cautiously in: Angle-closure glaucoma; Liver disease; OB: Safety not established; Geri: More susceptible to adverse reactions; use lower initial dose.

Interactions

Drug-Drug: Additive CNS depression with other **CNS depressants,** including **alcohol**, **opioids**, and **sedative/hypnotics**. **MAO inhibitors** intensify and prolong the anticholinergic effects of antihistamines.

Route/Dosage

PO (Adults and Children ≥12 yr): 4 mg q 4–6 hr daily as needed (not to exceed 24 mg/day).
PO (Children 6–12 yr): 2 mg q 4–6 hr as needed (not to exceed 12 mg/day).
PO (Children 2–6 yr): 1 mg q 4–6 hr as needed (not to exceed 6 mg/day).
SC, IM, IV (Adults): 10 mg q 8–12 hr as needed (not to exceed 40 mg/day).
SC, IM, IV (Children): 125 mcg (0.125 mg)/kg or 3.75 mg/m^2 3–4 times daily as needed.

Availability (generic available)

Tablets: 4 mg OTC. **Capsules (liqui-gels):** 4 mg. **Elixir:** 2 mg/5 mL Rx, OTC. **Injection:** 10 mg/mL. ***In combination with:*** pseudoephedrine (Andehist, Touro Allergy) and pseudoephedrine with dextromethorphan (Andehist DM, Histinex DM). See Appendix B.

budesonide (byoo-**des**-oh-nide)

Pulmicort Respules, Pulmicort Turbuhaler

Classification
Therapeutic: anti-inflammatories (steroidal)
Pharmacologic: corticosteroids

Indications

Nebulization—Maintenance treatment and prophylactic therapy of asthma. *Oral inhalation*—Chronic control of persistent bronchial asthma. May decrease requirement for or eliminate use of systemic corticosteroids over time in patients with asthma. *Intranasal*—Management of allergic rhinitis. *Oral*—Treatment and maintenance of remission of mild to moderate Crohn's disease.

Action

Potent, locally acting anti-inflammatory and immune modifier. **Therapeutic Effects:** Decreases frequency/severity of asthma attacks. Improves asthma symptoms.

Adverse Reactions/Side Effects

CNS: headache. **Derm:** rash. **EENT:** otitis media, dysphonia, epistaxis, oropharyngeal fungal infections, pharyngitis, rhinitis, sinusitis. **Resp:** bronchospasm, cough. **GI:** abdominal pain, diarrhea, dyspepsia, gastroenteritis, nausea, vomiting. **Endo:** adrenal suppression (high-dose, long-term therapy only), decreased growth (children), weight gain. **MS:** back pain. **Misc:** flu-like syndrome.

PHYSICAL THERAPY IMPLICATIONS

Examination and Evaluation

- Assess pulmonary function periodically by measuring lung volumes, breath sounds, respiratory rate, and other symptoms (wheezing, dyspnea, shortness of breath) (See Appendices I, J, K). Report changes in pulmonary function to help document the effects of drug therapy in treating asthma.
- Observe for paradoxical bronchospasm (cough, wheezing, dyspnea), especially at higher or excessive doses. If condition occurs, advise patient to withhold medication and notify physician immediately.
- Assess muscle strength periodically during long-term use. Although inhalation reduces the risk of systemic musculoskeletal damage, some degree of weakness and bone loss may still occur during prolonged, extensive use.
- Assess any back pain to rule out musculoskeletal pathology; that is, try to determine if pain is drug induced rather than caused by anatomic or biomechanical problems.
- Report signs of adrenal suppression, including hypotension, weight loss, weakness, nausea, vomiting, anorexia, lethargy, confusion, and restlessness.
- Assess growth rate in children receiving chronic therapy; report delayed or stunted growth to the physician.
- If treating inflammatory bowel diseases, monitor any changes in symptoms (decreased abdominal pain, decreased diarrhea, improved appetite) to help document whether drug therapy is successful.

Interventions

- Implement resistive exercises and weight-bearing activities to minimize muscle wasting and osteoporosis. Use caution to prevent musculoskeletal damage in patients with preexisting muscle and bone loss.
- Design and implement appropriate aerobic exercise and respiratory muscle training programs to maintain optimal cardiovascular and pulmonary function. Work with patient and family/caregivers to find forms of exercise (e.g., swimming) that can help improve respiratory function without triggering asthma attacks.

Patient/Client-Related Instruction

- Counsel patient on proper use of inhalation techniques (nebulizer, powder inhalers, nasal sprays); observe administration whenever possible to ensure proper technique.
- Advise patient to not exceed the recommended dose or frequency of inhalations. Contact physician immediately if bronchospasm is not relieved by medication or is accompanied by severe headache or other symptoms.
- Caution patient not to use this drug to treat acute symptoms. A rapid-acting inhaled beta-adrenergic bronchodilator is typically used for relief of acute asthma attacks.
- Advise patient that corticosteroids cause immunosuppression and may mask symptoms of infection. Instruct patient to avoid people with known contagious illnesses and to report possible infections immediately.
- Advise patient about the likelihood of upper respiratory tract infection or irritation, including pharyngitis, sinusitis, rhinitis, nosebleeds, and problems with vocalization (dysphonia). Instruct patient to report severe or prolonged upper respiratory problems to the physician.
- Advise patient about the likelihood of GI reactions such as abdominal pain, nausea, vomiting, diarrhea, indigestion, and loss of appetite. Instruct patient to report severe or prolonged GI problems.
- Advise patients on long-term treatment to consult physician before stopping this medication. Stopping the medication suddenly may result in adrenocortical shock (severe hypotension, hypoglycemia, weakness, vomiting). If these signs appear, notify the physician immediately; may be life threatening.
- Instruct patient and family/caregivers to report other troublesome side effects such as severe or prolonged headache, flu-like symptoms, or ear infections.

Pharmacokinetics

Absorption: *Turbuhaler*—39%; *Intranasal spray*—34%; *Respules*—6%. Action is primarily local following inhalation.
Distribution: Crosses placenta; enters breast milk in small amounts.
Protein Binding: 85–90%.
Metabolism and Excretion: Metabolized by the liver following absorption from lungs; 60% excreted in urine, 40% in feces.
Half-life: *Adults*—2–3.6 hr; *Children 10–14 yrs*—1.5 hr; *Children 4–6 yrs*—2.3 hr (after nebulization).

TIME/ACTION PROFILE (improvement in symptoms)

ROUTE	ONSET	PEAK	DURATION
inhalation	within 24 hr	1–4 wk*	unknown
intranasal	within 10 hr	2 wk	unknown
nebulization	with 2–8 days	4–6 wk	unknown

*Improvement in pulmonary function; decreased airway responsiveness may take longer.

Contraindications/Precautions

Contraindicated in: Hypersensitivity to budesonide; Acute attack of asthma/status asthmaticus.

B

Use Cautiously in: Active untreated infections; Diabetes or glaucoma; Underlying immunosuppression (from disease or concurrent therapy); Systemic corticosteroid therapy (should not be abruptly discontinued when inhaled therapy is started; additional corticosteroids needed during stress or trauma); OB: Has been used safely but should be used only if clearly needed; Lactation: Effects on infant are not known; Pedi: Higher than recommended doses can lead to suppression of hypothalamic-pituitary-adrenal (HPA) function and suppression of linear growth.

Interactions

Drug-Drug: Ketoconazole, itraconazole, clarithromycin, erythromycin, ritonavir, and other CYP3A4 inhibitors ↓ metabolism and ↑ levels of budesonide.

Route/Dosage

Turbuhaler

Inhalation (Adults): *Previously on bronchodilators alone*—200–400 mcg (1–2 inhalations) twice daily (not to exceed 2 inhalations twice daily); *Previously on other inhaled corticosteroids*—200–400 mcg (1–2 inhalations) twice daily (not to exceed 4 inhalations twice daily); *Previously on oral corticosteroids*—400–800 mcg (2–4 inhalations) twice daily (not to exceed 4 inhalations twice daily).

Inhalation (Children ≥6 yr): *Previously on bronchodilators alone or other inhaled corticosteroids*—200 mcg (1 inhalation) twice daily (not to exceed 2 inhalations twice daily); *Previously on oral corticosteroids*—Not to exceed 400 mcg (2 inhalations) twice daily.

Respules

Inhalation (Children 1–8 yr): *Previously on bronchodilators alone*—0.5 mg once daily or 0.25 mg twice daily (not to exceed 0.5 mg/day); *Previously on other inhaled corticosteroids*—0.5 mg once daily or 0.25 mg twice daily (not to exceed 1 mg/day); *Previously on oral corticosteroids*—1 mg once daily or 0.5 mg twice daily (not to exceed 1 mg/day).

Intranasal Suspension

Intranasal (Adults and Children >6 yr): 2 sprays (1 spray/nostril) once daily; dose may be increased if needed to a maximum of 4 sprays once daily in children <12 yr and 8 sprays once daily in children >12 yr and adults.

Capsules

PO (Adults): *Active Crohn's disease*—9 mg once daily in the morning for ≤8 wk; may repeat 8-wk course for recurring episodes. *Maintenance of remission*—6 mg once daily for up to 3 mo; once symptoms are controlled, taper to complete cessation.

Availability

Inhalation powder (Turbuhaler): 200 mcg/metered inhalation (delivers 200 metered inhalations) Rx. **Inhalation powder (Flexhaler):** 90 mcg/metered inhalation (delivers 60 metered inhalations) Rx, 180 mcg/metered inhalation (delivers 120 metered inhalations) Rx. **Inhalation suspension (Respules):** 0.25 mg/2 mL in single-dose ampules (5 ampules/envelope) Rx, 0.5 mg/2 mL in single-dose ampules (5 ampules/envelope) Rx, 1 mg/2 mL in single-dose ampules (5 ampules/envelope). **Capsule, enteric coated (Entocort EC):** 3 mg. **Nasal suspension (Rhinocort Aqua):** 32 mcg/inhalation (8.6 g) (delivers 120 metered spray). ***In combination with:*** formoterol (Symbicort; see Appendix B).

bumetanide (byoo-met-a-nide)

Bumex, ✱Burinex

Classification

Therapeutic: diuretics

Pharmacologic: loop diuretics

Indications

Edema due to heart failure, hepatic disease, or renal impairment.

Action

Inhibits the reabsorption of sodium and chloride from the loop of Henle and distal renal tubule. Increases renal excretion of water, sodium chloride, magnesium, potassium, and calcium. Effectiveness persists in impaired renal function. **Therapeutic Effects:** Diuresis and subsequent mobilization of excess fluid (edema, pleural effusions).

Adverse Reactions/Side Effects

CNS: dizziness, encephalopathy, headache. **EENT:** hearing loss, tinnitus. **CV:** hypotension. **GI:** diarrhea, dry mouth, nausea, vomiting. **GU:** excessive urination. **Derm:** photosensitivity, pruritus, rash. **Endo:** hyperglycemia, hyperuricemia. **F and E:** dehydration, hypocalcemia, hypochloremia, hypokalemia, hypomagnesemia, hyponatremia, hypovolemia, metabolic alkalosis. **MS:** arthralgia, muscle cramps, myalgia. **Misc:** increased BUN.

PHYSICAL THERAPY IMPLICATIONS

Examination and Evaluation

- Monitor signs of fluid, electrolyte, or acid-base imbalances, including dizziness, drowsiness, blurred vision, confusion, hypotension, or muscle cramps and weakness. Report excessive or prolonged symptoms to the physician.

- Assess dizziness that might affect gait, balance, and other functional activities (See Appendix C). Report balance problems and functional limitations to the physician, and caution the patient and family/caregivers to guard against falls and trauma.
- Monitor drug effects by assessing peripheral edema using girth measurements, volume displacement, and measurement of pitting edema (See Appendix N). Also monitor signs of pulmonary edema such as dyspnea and rales/crackles (See Appendix K). Document whether peripheral and pulmonary symptoms are controlled adequately by diuretic therapy.
- Assess blood pressure periodically and compare to normal values (See Appendix F). Report low blood pressure (hypotension), especially if patient experiences dizziness or syncope.
- Be alert for signs of encephalopathy, including decreased alertness, lethargy, and incoordination. Notify physician of these signs before they progress to more severe changes in mental status such as dementia, seizures, and coma.
- Assess any joint pain, muscle pain, or muscle cramps to rule out musculoskeletal pathology; that is, try to determine if musculoskeletal symptoms are drug induced rather than caused by anatomic or biomechanical problems.
- Monitor signs of hyperglycemia such as drowsiness, fruity breath, increased urination, and unusual thirst. Patients with diabetes mellitus should check blood glucose levels frequently.

Interventions

- Implement fall prevention strategies, especially in older adults or if patient exhibits sedation, dizziness, blurred vision, or other impairments that affect gait and balance (See Appendix E).
- Use caution during aerobic exercise, especially in hot environments. Increased sweating will cause fluid and electrolyte loss, and may exaggerate diuretic side effects (dizziness, muscle cramps, and so forth).
- To minimize orthostatic hypotension, patient should move slowly when assuming a more upright position.
- Causes photosensitivity; use care if administering UV treatments.

Patient/Client-Related Instruction

- Remind patient and family/caregivers that diuretics typically increase urine output. Any unusual problems such as excessive or painful urination should be reported to the physician.
- Counsel patients about additional interventions to help control edema and improve circulation, including sodium restriction, regular exercise, weight loss, moderation of alcohol consumption, and smoking cessation.
- Instruct patient to report troublesome GI problems such as severe or prolonged nausea, vomiting, diarrhea, or dry mouth.
- Advise patient about photosensitivity, and to use sunscreens, protective clothing, and avoid prolonged sun exposure. Instruct patient to also report any rashes or other skin reactions.
- Instruct patient to report any hearing loss or ringing/buzzing in the ears (tinnitus).

Pharmacokinetics

Absorption: Well absorbed after oral or IM administration.
Distribution: Widely distributed.
Protein Binding: 72–96%.
Metabolism and Excretion: Partially metabolized by liver; 50% eliminated unchanged by kidneys and 20% excreted in feces.
Half-life: 60–90 min (6 hr in neonates).

TIME/ACTION PROFILE (diuretic effect)

ROUTE	ONSET	PEAK	DURATION
PO	30–60 min	1–2 hr	4–6 hr
IM	30–60 min	1–2 hr	4–6 hr
IV	2–3 min	15–45 min	2–3 hr

Contraindications/Precautions

Contraindicated in: Hypersensitivity; Cross-sensitivity with thiazides and sulfonamides may occur; Hepatic coma or anuria.
Use Cautiously in: Severe liver disease (may precipitate hepatic coma; concurrent use with potassium-sparing diuretics may be necessary); Electrolyte depletion; Diabetes mellitus; Increasing azotemia; Lactation/Pedi: Safety not established; bumetanide is a potent displacer of bilirubin and should be used cautiously in critically ill or jaundiced neonates because of risk of kernicterus. Injection contains benzyl alcohol, which may cause gasping syndrome in neonates; Geri: May have increased risk of side effects, especially hypotension and electrolyte imbalance, at usual doses.

Interactions

Drug-Drug: ↑ hypotension with **antihypertensives, nitrates**, or acute ingestion of **alcohol**. ↑ risk of hypokalemia with other **diuretics, amphotericin B, stimulant laxatives**, and **corticosteroids**. Hypokalemia may ↑ risk of **digoxin** toxicity and ↑ risk of arrhythmia in patients taking drugs that prolong the QT interval. ↓ **lithium** excretion, may cause **lithium** toxicity. ↑ **risk** of ototoxicity with **aminoglycosides. NSAIDS**↓ effects of bumetanide.

Route/Dosage

PO (Adults): 0.5–2 mg/day given in 1–2 doses; titrate to desired response (maximum daily dose = 10 mg/day).
IM, IV (Adults): 0.5–1 mg/dose, may repeat q 2–3 hr as needed (up to 10 mg/day).

Availability (generic available)

Tablets: 0.5 mg, 1 mg, 2 mg, 5 mg. **Injection:** 0.25 mg/mL.

bupivacaine (byoo-pi-vi-kane)

Marcaine, Sensorcaine

Classification
Therapeutic: epidural local anesthetics, anesthetics (topical/local)

Indications

Local or regional anesthesia or analgesia for surgical, obstetric, or diagnostic procedures.

Action

Local anesthetics inhibit initiation and conduction of sensory nerve impulses by altering the influx of sodium and efflux of potassium in neurons, slowing or stopping pain transmission. **Therapeutic Effects:** Decreased pain or induction of anesthesia; low doses have minimal effect on sensory or motor function; higher doses may produce complete motor blockade.

Adverse Reactions/Side Effects

CNS: SEIZURES, anxiety, dizziness, headache, irritability. **EENT:** blurred vision, tinnitus. **CV:** CARDIOVASCULAR COLLAPSE, arrhythmias, bradycardia, hypotension. **GI:** nausea, vomiting. **GU:** urinary retention. **Derm:** pruritus. **F and E:** metabolic acidosis. **Neuro:** circumoral tingling/numbness, tremor. **Misc:** allergic reactions, fever.

PHYSICAL THERAPY IMPLICATIONS

Examination and Evaluation

- Be alert for new seizures or increased seizure activity. Document the number, duration, and severity of seizures, and report these findings immediately to the physician.
- Monitor cardiac symptoms at rest and during exercise, and be alert for signs of severe cardiac insufficiency due to cardiac arrest (cardiovascular collapse). Seek immediate medical assistance if symptoms of cardiac arrest develop, including sudden chest pain, pain radiating into the arm or jaw, shortness of breath, dizziness, sweating, anxiety, and nausea.
- Monitor signs of allergic reactions, including pulmonary symptoms (laryngeal edema, bronchospasm, wheezing, cough, dyspnea) or skin reactions (rash, pruritus, urticaria). Notify physician or nursing staff immediately if these reactions occur.
- Assess heart rate, ECG, and heart sounds, especially during exercise (See Appendices G, H). Report an unusually slow heart rate (bradycardia) or signs of other arrhythmias, including palpitations, chest discomfort, shortness of breath, fainting, and fatigue/weakness.
- Be alert for other signs of systemic toxicity, including confusion, nervousness, tremor, headache, blurred or double vision, nausea, vomiting, slurred speech, ringing in ears, tremors, twitching, difficulty breathing, hypotension, severe dizziness or fainting, and unusually slow heart rate. Report these signs to the physician or nursing staff immediately.
- Monitor signs of metabolic acidosis, including headache, lethargy, stupor, seizures, vision disturbances, increased respiration, cardiac arrhythmias, weakness, and GI symptoms (nausea, vomiting, and/or abdominal pain). Notify physician or nursing staff immediately if these signs occur.
- If used postsurgically for continuous nerve block, use appropriate pain scales and sensory testing to document level of local anesthesia.
- Assess dizziness that might affect gait, balance, and other functional activities (See Appendix C). Report balance problems and functional limitations to the physician and nursing staff, and caution the patient and family/caregivers to guard against falls and trauma.

Interventions

- Because of the risk of arrhythmias and cardiac arrest, use extreme caution during aerobic exercise and other forms of therapeutic exercise. Assess exercise tolerance frequently (blood pressure, heart rate, fatigue levels), and terminate exercise immediately if any untoward responses occur (See Appendix L).
- Use caution when exercising patients receiving continuous nerve blocks to specific joints. Joint sensation will be diminished or absent, so care must be taken to avoid overstressing joint tissues.
- Be especially careful when ambulating patients with continuous femoral nerve block, because the knee may buckle if quadriceps motor function is impaired. Use splints or knee immobilizer to support the knee whenever necessary.

Patient/Client-Related Instruction

- Advise patient and family or caregivers about the signs of cardiac arrest (see above under

Examination and Evaluation), and to seek immediate medical assistance if these signs develop.

- Instruct patient and family/caregivers to report other severe or prolonged side effects such as urinary retention, skin problems (rash, itching), or GI reactions (nausea, vomiting).

Pharmacokinetics

Absorption: Systemic absorption follows epidural administration, but amount absorbed depends on dose.
Distribution: If systemic absorption occurs, this agent is widely distributed and crosses the placenta.
Metabolism and Excretion: Small amounts that may reach systemic circulation are mostly metabolized by the liver; 6% excreted unchanged in the urine.
Half-life: 1.5—5 hr (after epidural use).

TIME/ACTION PROFILE (analgesia)

ROUTE	ONSET	PEAK	DURATION
Epidural	10–30 min	unknown	2–8 hr*

*Duration of anesthetic block.

Contraindications/Precautions

Contraindicated in: Hypersensitivity; cross-sensitivity with other amide local anesthetics may occur (ropivacaine, lidocaine, mepivacaine, prilocaine); Contains bisulfites and should be avoided in patients with known intolerance; OB: Obstetric paracervical block anesthesia.
Use Cautiously in: Concurrent use of other local anesthetics; Liver disease; Concurrent use of anticoagulants (including low-dose heparin and low-molecular-weight heparins/heparinoids) ↑ the risk of spinal/epidural hematomas; Pedi: Safety not established in children <12 yr.

Interactions

Drug-Drug: Additive toxicity may occur with concurrent use of other **amide local anesthetics** (including **lidocaine**, **mepivacaine**, and **prilocaine**). Use of solution containing **epinephrine** with **MAO inhibitors** may cause hypertension.

Route/Dosage

Solutions containing preservatives should not be used for caudal or epidural blocks.
Epidural (Adults and Children >12 yr): 10–20 mL of 0.25% (partial to moderate block), 0.5% (moderate to complete block), or 0.75% (complete block) solution. Administer in increments of 3–5 mL allowing sufficient time to detect toxic signs/symptoms of inadvertent IV or IT administration. A test dose of 2–3 mL of 0.5% with epinephrine solution is recommended prior to epidural blocks.
Caudal block: (Adults and Children >12 yr): 15–30 mL of 0.25% or 0.5% solution. A test dose of 2–3 mL of 0.5% with epinephrine solution is recommended prior to caudal blocks.
Peripheral nerve block: (Adults and Children >12 yr): 5 mL of 0.25% or 0.5% solution (maximum dose = 400 mg).
Sympathetic nerve block: (Adults and Children >12 yr): 20–50 mL of 0.25% solution.
Dental block: (Adults and Children >12 yr): 1.8–3.6 mL per site of 0.5% with epinephrine solution.
Local Infiltration: (Adults and Children >12 yr): 0.25% solution infiltrated locally (maximum dose = 175 mg).

Availability

Solution for injection (with and without preservatives): 0.25%, 0.5%, 0.75%. ***In combination with:*** epinephrine 1:200,000.

HIGH ALERT

buprenorphine

(byoo-pre-**nor**-feen)
Buprenex, Subutex

Classification
Therapeutic: opioid analgesics
Pharmacologic: opioid agonists/antagonists

Schedule III

Indications

IM, IV: Management of moderate to severe acute pain. **SL:** Treatment of opioid dependence; suppresses withdrawal symptoms in opioid detoxification.

Action

Binds to opiate receptors in the CNS. Alters the perception of and response to painful stimuli while producing generalized CNS depression. Has partial antagonist properties that may result in opioid withdrawal in physically dependent patients when used as an analgesic. **Therapeutic Effects: IM, IV:** Decreased severity of pain. **SL:** Suppression of withdrawal symptoms during detoxification and maintenance from heroin or other opioids. Produces a relatively mild withdrawal compared to other agents.

Adverse Reactions/Side Effects

CNS: confusion, dysphoria, hallucinations, sedation, dizziness, euphoria, floating feeling, headache, unusual dreams. **EENT:** blurred vision, diplopia, miosis (high doses). **Resp:** respiratory depression. **CV:** hypertension, hypotension, palpitations. **GI:** nausea, constipation, dry mouth, ileus, vomiting. **GU:** urinary retention. **Derm:** sweating, clammy feeling. **Misc:** physical dependence, psychologic dependence, tolerance.

PHYSICAL THERAPY IMPLICATIONS

Examination and Evaluation

- Assess symptoms of respiratory depression, including decreased respiratory rate, confusion, bluish color of the skin and mucous membranes (cyanosis), and difficult, labored breathing (dyspnea). Monitor pulse oximetry and perform pulmonary function tests (See Appendix I) to quantify suspected changes in ventilation and respiratory function. Excessive respiratory depression requires emergency care.

- Be alert for excessive sedation or changes in mood and behavior (euphoria, dysphoria, confusion, hallucinations). Notify physician or nurse immediately if patient is unconscious or extremely difficult to arouse.
- Use appropriate pain scales (visual analogue scales, others) to document whether this drug is successful in helping manage the patient's pain.
- Assess blood pressure (BP) and compare to normal values (See Appendix F). Report changes in BP, either a problematic decrease in BP (hypotension) or a sustained increase in BP (hypertension).
- Assess dizziness that might affect gait, balance, and other functional activities (See Appendix C). Report balance problems and functional limitations to the physician and nursing staff, and caution the patient and family/caregivers to guard against falls and trauma.

Interventions

- Implement appropriate manual therapy techniques, physical agents, and therapeutic exercises to reduce pain and help wean patient off opioid analgesics as soon as possible.
- Because of the risk of respiratory depression and abnormal BP responses, use caution during aerobic exercise and other forms of therapeutic exercise. Assess exercise tolerance frequently (BP, heart rate, respiratory rate, fatigue levels), and terminate exercise immediately if any untoward responses occur (See Appendix L).
- Help patient explore other nonpharmacologic methods to reduce chronic pain, including relaxation techniques, exercise, counseling, and so forth.
- Guard against falls and trauma (hip fractures, head injury). Implement fall-prevention strategies (See Appendix E), especially if patient exhibits sedation, dizziness, or blurred vision.
- To minimize orthostatic hypotension, patient should move slowly when assuming a more upright position.
- If used to treat opioid dependence, administer massage, physical agents (heat, whirlpool), and therapeutic exercise to help decrease withdrawal symptoms and increase the chance of successful abstinence.

Patient/Client-Related Instruction

- Advise patient that opioid analgesics are usually more effective if given before pain becomes severe; emphasize that adequate pain control will allow better participation in physical therapy.
- Educate patient about the dangers of opioid overdose; encourage patient to adhere to proper dosing schedule.
- Emphasize that the risk of physical addiction (tolerance and dependence) is usually minimal during short-term treatment of pain. Advise patient that addiction is more likely during excessive or inappropriate use of opioid analgesics.
- Advise patient to avoid alcohol and other CNS depressants because of the increased risk of sedation and decreased CNS function.
- Advise patient to increase fluid intake and dietary fiber to avoid constipation. Laxatives may also be helpful in patients susceptible to fecal impaction (e.g., people with spinal cord injury).
- Instruct patient to report other troublesome side effects such as severe or prolonged headache, urinary retention, unusual dreams, vision disturbances, palpitations, increased sweating, or GI problems (nausea, vomiting, dry mouth).

Pharmacokinetics

Absorption: Well absorbed after IM and SL use; IV administration results in complete bioavailability.
Distribution: Crosses the placenta; enters breast milk. CNS concentration is 15–25% of plasma.
Protein Binding: 96%.
Metabolism and Excretion: Mostly metabolized by the liver mostly via the CYP3A4 enzyme system; one metabolite is active.
Half-life: 2–3 hr (parenteral).

TIME/ACTION PROFILE (analgesia)

ROUTE	ONSET	PEAK	DURATION
IM	15 min	60 min	6 hr*
IV	rapid	<60 min	6 hr*

*4–5 hr in children.

Contraindications/Precautions

Contraindicated in: Hypersensitivity; Lactation: Enters breast milk; avoid use or discontinue nursing.
Use Cautiously in: Increased intracranial pressure; Severe renal, hepatic, or pulmonary disease; Hypothyroidism; Adrenal insufficiency; Alcoholism; Debilitated patients (dose reduction required); Undiagnosed abdominal pain; Prostatic hyperplasia; OB: Safety not established; neonatal withdrawal may occur in infants born to patients receiving SL buprenorphine during pregnancy; Geri: Dose reduction required.

Interactions

Drug-Drug: Use with extreme caution in patients receiving **MAO inhibitors** (↑ CNS and respiratory depression and hypotension—↓ buprenorphine dose by 50%; may need to ↓ **MAO inhibitor** dose). ↑ CNS depression with **alcohol**, **antihistamines**, **antidepressants**, and **sedative/hypnotics**. May ↓ effectiveness of other **opioid analgesics**. Inhibitors of the CYP3A4 enzyme system, including **azole antifungals (itraconazole, ketoconazole)**, **erythromycin**, **protease inhibitor antiretrovirals (ritonavir, indinavir, saquinavir)**, ↑ blood levels and effects; dose reduction may be necessary during concurrent use. Inducers of the CYP3A4 enzyme system, including **carbamazepine**, **rifampin**, or **phenytoin**, ↓ blood levels and effects; dose modification may be necessary during concurrent use. Concurrent abuse of IV buprenorphine and **benzodiazepines** may result in coma and death.
Drug-Natural: Concomitant use of **kava**, **valerian**, **chamomile**, or **hops** can ↑ CNS depression.

Route/Dosage

Analgesia

IM, IV (Adults): 0.3 mg q 4–6 hr as needed. May repeat initial dose after 30 min (up to 0.3 mg q 4 hr or 0.6 mg q 6 hr); 0.6-mg doses should be given only IM.
IM, IV (Children 2–12 yr): 2–6 mcg (0.002–0.006 mg)/kg q 4–6 hr.

Treatment of opioid dependence

SL (Adults): 12–16 mg/day as a single dose.

Availability (generic available)

Sublingual tablets: 2 mg, 8 mg. ***In combination with:*** naloxone (Suboxone). See Appendix B. **Injection:** 300 mcg (0.3 mg)/mL.

bupropion (byoo-proe-pee-on)

Aplenzin, Budeprion SR, Budeprion XL, Wellbutrin, Wellbutrin SR, Wellbutrin XL, Zyban

Classification
Therapeutic: antidepressants, smoking deterrents
Pharmacologic: aminoketones

Indications

Treatment of depression (with psychotherapy). Depression in patients with seasonal affective disorder (XL only). Smoking cessation (Zyban only). **Unlabeled Use:** Treatment of ADHD in adults (SR only). To increase sexual desire in women.

Action

Decreases neuronal reuptake of dopamine in the CNS. Diminished neuronal uptake of serotonin and norepinephrine (less than tricyclic antidepressants).
Therapeutic Effects: Diminished depression. Decreased craving for cigarettes.

Adverse Reactions/Side Effects

CNS: SEIZURES, SUICIDAL THOUGHTS, agitation, headache, insomnia, mania, psychoses. **GI:** dry mouth, nausea, vomiting, change in appetite, weight gain, weight loss. **Derm:** photosensitivity. **Endo:** hyperglycemia, hypoglycemia, syndrome of inappropriate ADH secretion. **Neuro:** tremor.

PHYSICAL THERAPY IMPLICATIONS

Examination and Evaluation

- Be alert for new seizures or increased seizure activity, especially at the onset of drug treatment. Document the number, duration, and severity of seizures, and report these findings immediately to the physician.
- Be alert for increased depression or expression of suicidal thoughts, especially in the initial period of drug therapy, and in children and teenagers. Notify physician or other mental health professional immediately if patient exhibits worsening depression or suicidal ideology.
- Be alert for agitation, mania, psychosis, or other alterations in mental status. Notify physician promptly if these symptoms develop (See Appendix D).
- Watch for signs of hypoglycemia (weakness, malaise, irritability, fatigue) or hyperglycemia (drowsiness, fruity breath, increased urination, unusual thirst). Patients with diabetes mellitus should check blood glucose levels frequently.
- Monitor signs of fluid-electrolyte imbalance due to syndrome of inappropriate antidiuretic hormone (SIADH). SIADH causes increased water retention that leads to relatively low sodium concentration (hyponatremia). Symptoms include confusion, lethargy, weakness, myoclonus, and depressed reflexes. Severe or sudden onset may also cause seizures, ataxia, nystagmus, tremor, dysarthria, dysphagia, and coma. Notify physician if these signs occur.
- Periodically assess body weight and other anthropometric measures (body mass index, body composition). Report a rapid or unexplained weight gain or weight loss.

Interventions

- Help patient explore nonpharmacologic methods to reduce depression or quit smoking (exercise, counseling, support groups, etc.).
- Causes photosensitivity; use care if administering UV treatments. Advise patient to avoid direct sunlight and use sunscreens and protective clothing.

Patient/Client-Related Instruction

- Advise patient that antidepressant effects may not occur immediately; it may take 2 wk or more before an improvement in mood is observed.
- Advise patient to avoid alcohol and other CNS depressants because of the increased risk of sedation and adverse effects.
- Instruct patient to report other bothersome side effects such as severe or prolonged headache, sleep loss, or GI problems (nausea, vomiting, dry mouth).

Pharmacokinetics

Absorption: Although well absorbed, rapidly and extensively metabolized by the liver.
Distribution: Unknown.
Metabolism and Excretion: Extensively metabolized by the liver. Some conversion to active metabolites.
Half-life: 14 hr (active metabolites may have longer half-lives).

TIME/ACTION PROFILE (antidepressant effect)

ROUTE	ONSET	PEAK	DURATION
PO	1–3 wk	unknown	unknown

Contraindications/Precautions

Contraindicated in: Hypersensitivity; History of bulimia and anorexia nervosa; Concurrent MAO inhibitor or ritonavir therapy; Lactation: Potential for serious adverse reactions in nursing infants.
Use Cautiously in: Renal/hepatic impairment (↓ dose recommended); Recent history of MI; History of suicide attempt; Unstable cardiovascular status; May ↑ risk of suicide attempt/ideation, especially during early treatment or dose adjustment; this risk appears to be greater in adolescents or children; OB: Use only if benefit to patient outweighs potential risk to fetus; Geri: ↑ risk of drug accumulation; ↑ sensitivity to effects.
Exercise Extreme Caution in: History of seizures, head trauma, or concurrent medications that ↓ seizure threshold (theophylline, antipsychotics, antidepressants, systemic corticosteroids); Severe hepatic cirrhosis (↓ dose required); Pedi: ↑ risk of suicidal thinking and behavior. Observe carefully, especially at initiation of therapy and during ↑ or ↓ in dose.

Interactions

Drug-Drug: ↑ risk of adverse reactions when used with **amantadine**, **levodopa**, or **MAO inhibitors** (concurrent use of MAO inhibitors is contraindicated). ↑ risk of seizures with **phenothiazines**, **antidepressants**, **theophylline**, **corticosteroids**, **OTC stimulants/anorectics**, or cessation of **alcohol** or **benzodiazepines** (avoid or minimize alcohol use). Blood levels ↑ by **ritonavir** (avoid concurrent use). **Carbamazepine** may ↓ blood levels and effectiveness. Concurrent use with **nicotine** replacement may cause hypertension. ↑ risk of bleeding with **warfarin**. Bupropion and one of its metabolites inhibit the CYP2D6 enzyme system and may ↑ levels and risk of toxicity from **antidepressants** (SSRIs and tricyclic), some **beta blockers**, **antiarrhythmics**, and **antipsychotics**.

Route/Dosage

Depression

PO (Adults): *Immediate-release*—100 mg twice daily initially; after 3 days may ↑ to 100 mg 3 times daily; after at least 4 wk of therapy, may ↑ up to 450 mg/day in divided doses (not to exceed 150 mg/dose; wait at least 6 hr between doses at the 300 mg/day dose or at least 4 hr between doses at the 450 mg/day dose). *Sustained-release*—150 mg once daily in the morning; after 3 days, may ↑ to 150 mg twice daily with at least 8 hr between doses; after at least 4 wk of therapy, may ↑ to a maximum daily dose of 400 mg given as 200 mg twice daily. *Extended-release (Wellbutrin XL)*—150 mg once daily in the morning, may be ↑ after 4 days to 300 mg once daily; some patients may require up to 450 mg/day as a single daily dose. *Extended-release (Aplenzin)*—174 mg once daily in the morning, may be ↑ after 4 days to 348 mg once daily; some patients may require up to 522 mg/day as a single daily dose.

Seasonal Affective Disorder

PO (Adults): 150 mg/day in the morning; if dose is well tolerated, ↑ to 300 mg/day in 1 wk. Doses should be tapered to 150 mg/day for 2 wk before discontinuing.

Smoking cessation

PO (Adults): *Zyban*—150 mg once daily for 3 days, then 150 mg twice daily for 7–12 wk (doses should be at least 8 hr apart).

Availability (generic available)

Tablets: 75 mg, 100 mg. **Sustained-release tablets:** 100 mg, 150 mg, 200 mg. **Extended-release tablets (Wellbutrin XL):** 150 mg, 300 mg. **Extended-release tablets (Aplenzin):** 174 mg, 348 mg, 522 mg.

buspirone (byoo-**spye**-rone)

BuSpar

Classification

Therapeutic: antianxiety agents
Pharmacologic: azaspirodecanedione

Indications

Management of anxiety.

Action

Binds to serotonin and dopamine receptors in the brain. Increases norepinephrine metabolism in the brain. **Therapeutic Effects:** Relief of anxiety.

Adverse Reactions/Side Effects

CNS: dizziness, drowsiness, excitement, fatigue, headache, insomnia, nervousness, weakness, personality changes. **EENT:** blurred vision, nasal congestion, sore throat, tinnitus, altered taste or smell, conjunctivitis. **Resp:** chest congestion, hyperventilation, shortness of breath. **CV:** chest pain, palpitations, tachycardia, hypertension, hypotension, syncope. **GI:** nausea, abdominal pain, constipation, diarrhea, dry mouth, vomiting. **GU:** changes in libido, dysuria, urinary frequency, urinary hesitancy. **Derm:** rashes, alopecia, blisters, dry skin, easy bruising, edema, flushing, pruritus. **Endo:** irregular menses. **MS:** myalgia. **Neuro:** incoordination, numbness, paresthesia, tremor. **Misc:** clamminess, sweating, fever.

PHYSICAL THERAPY IMPLICATIONS

Examination and Evaluation

- Assess blood pressure (BP) and compare to normal values (See Appendix F). Report changes in BP, either a problematic decrease in BP (hypotension) or a sustained increase in BP (hypertension).
- Assess heart rate, ECG, and heart sounds, especially during exercise (See Appendices G, H). Report rapid heart rate (tachycardia) or symptoms of other arrhythmias, including palpitations, chest discomfort, shortness of breath, syncope, and fatigue/weakness.
- Monitor any breathing problems, and report shortness of breath, rapid shallow breathing, or abnormal breath sounds that might indicate pulmonary congestion (See Appendix K).
- Monitor personality changes, including excitement and nervousness. Notify physician if these changes become problematic.
- Assess any muscle aches or pain to rule out musculoskeletal pathology; that is, try to determine if pain is drug induced rather than caused by anatomic or biomechanical problems.
- Assess signs of paresthesia (numbness, tingling), tremors, or incoordination. Perform objective tests, including electroneuromyography and sensory testing to document any drug-related neuropathic changes.
- Assess dizziness and drowsiness that might affect gait, balance, and other functional activities (See Appendix C). Report balance problems and functional limitations to the physician and nursing staff, and caution the patient and family/caregivers to guard against falls and trauma.

Interventions

- Guard against falls and trauma (hip fractures, head injury, and so forth). Implement fall- prevention strategies, especially in older adults or if drowsiness and dizziness carry over into the daytime (See Appendix E).
- Because of the risk of arrhythmias and abnormal BP responses, use caution during aerobic exercise and other forms of therapeutic exercise. Assess exercise tolerance frequently (BP, heart rate, fatigue levels), and terminate exercise immediately if any untoward responses occur (See Appendix L).
- Help patient explore nonpharmacologic methods to reduce anxiety, such as relaxation techniques, exercise, counseling, support groups, and so forth.
- To minimize orthostatic hypotension, patient should move slowly when assuming a more upright position.

Patient/Client-Related Instruction

- Advise patient to avoid alcohol and other CNS depressants because of the increased risk of sedation and adverse effects.
- Advice patient about the likelihood of GI problems, including constipation, nausea, vomiting, diarrhea, abdominal pain, dry mouth, and altered taste. Severe or prolonged GI problems should be reported to the physician.
- Instruct patient to report other troublesome side effects, including severe or prolonged headache, sleep loss, urinary problems, vision disturbances, ringing/buzzing in the ears (tinnitus), fever, sweating, changes in libido, menstrual irregularities, or skin reactions (rash, itching, hair loss, blistering, bruising).

Pharmacokinetics

Absorption: Rapidly absorbed.
Distribution: Unknown.
Protein Binding: 95% bound to plasma proteins.
Metabolism and Excretion: Extensively metabolized by the liver (CYP3A4 enzyme system); 20–40% excreted in feces.
Half-life: 2–3 hr.

TIME/ACTION PROFILE (relief of anxiety)

ROUTE	ONSET	PEAK	DURATION
PO	7–10 days	3–4 wk	unknown

Contraindications/Precautions

Contraindicated in: Hypersensitivity; Severe hepatic or renal impairment; Concurrent use of MAO inhibitors; Ingestion of large amounts of grapefruit juice.
Use Cautiously in: Patients receiving other antianxiety agents (other agents should be slowly withdrawn to prevent withdrawal or rebound phenomenon); Patients receiving other psychotropics; Lactation/OB/Pedi: Safety not established.

Interactions

Drug-Drug: Use with **MAO inhibitors** may result in hypertension and is not recommended. **Erythromycin**, **nefazodone**, **ketoconazole**, **itraconazole**, **ritonavir**, and other **inhibitors of CYP3A4** ↑ blood levels and effects of buspirone; dose reduction is recommended (↓ to 2.5 mg twice daily with erythromycin, ↓ to 2.5 mg once daily with nefazodone). **Rifampin**, **dexamethasone**, **phenytoin**, **phenobarbital**, **carbamazepine**, and other **inducers of CYP3A4** ↓ blood levels and effects of buspirone; dose adjustment may be necessary. Avoid concurrent use with **alcohol**.
Drug-Natural: Concomitant use of **kava**, **valerian**, or **chamomile** can ↑ CNS depression.
Drug-Food: Grapefruit juice ↑ serum levels and effect; ingestion of large amounts of grapefruit juice is not recommended.

Route/Dosage

PO (Adults): 7.5 mg twice daily; increase by 5 mg/day q 2–4 days as needed (not to exceed 60 mg/day). Usual dose is 20–30 mg/day (in 2 divided doses).

Availability (generic available)

Tablets: 5 mg, 7.5 mg, 10 mg, 15 mg, 30 mg.

HIGH ALERT

busulfan (byoo-sul-fan)

Busulfex, Myleran

Classification
Therapeutic: antineoplastics
Pharmacologic: alkylating agents

Indications

PO: Treatment of chronic myelogenous leukemia (CML) and bone marrow disorders. **IV:** With cyclophosphamide as a conditioning regimen before allogenic hematopoietic progenitor cell transplantation for CML.

Action

Disrupts nucleic acid function and protein synthesis (cell-cycle phase–nonspecific). **Therapeutic Effects:** Death of rapidly growing cells, especially malignant ones.

Adverse Reactions/Side Effects

Incidence and severity of adverse reactions and side effects are increased with IV use

CNS: IV: SEIZURES, CEREBRAL HEMORRHAGE/COMA, anxiety, confusion, depression, dizziness, headache, encephalopathy, mental status changes, weakness. **EENT:** ***PO***—cataracts; ***IV***—epistaxis, pharyngitis, ear disorders. **CV:** hepatic veno-oclusive disease (↑ allogenic transplantation). **Resp:** ***PO***—PULMONARY FIBROSIS; ***IV***— alveolar hemorrhage, asthma, atelectasis, cough, hemoptysis, hypoxia, pleural effusion, pneumonia, rhinitis, sinusitis. **CV:** ***PO***—CARDIAC TAMPONADE (WITH HIGH-DOSE CYCLOPHOSPHAMIDE); ***IV***—chest pain, hypotension, tachycardia, thrombosis, arrhythmias, atrial fibrillation, cardiomegaly, ECG changes, edema, heart block, hypertension, left-sided heart failure, pericardial effusion, ventricular extrasystoles. **GI:** ***PO***—drug-induced hepatitis, nausea, vomiting; ***IV***—abdominal enlargement, anorexia, constipation, diarrhea, dry mouth, hematemesis, nausea, rectal discomfort, vomiting, abdominal pain, dyspepsia, hepatomegaly, pancreatitis, stomatitis. **GU:** oliguria, dysuria, hematuria. **Derm:** ***PO***—itching, rashes, acne, alopecia, erythema nodosum, exfoliative dermatitis, hyperpigmentation. **Endo:** ***PO***—sterility, gynecomastia. **F and E:** hypokalemia, hypomagnesemia, hypophosphatemia. **Hemat:** BONE MARROW DEPRESSION. **Local:** inflammation/pain at injection site. **Metab:** ***PO and IV***—hyperuricemia; ***IV***—hyperglycemia. **MS:** arthralgia, myalgia, back pain. **Misc:** allergic reactions, chills, fever, infection.

PHYSICAL THERAPY IMPLICATIONS

Examination and Evaluation

- Be alert for new seizures or increased seizure activity, especially at the onset of drug treatment. Document the number, duration, and severity of seizures, and report these findings to the physician immediately.
- Watch for signs of heart failure (dyspnea, rales/crackles, peripheral edema, jugular venous distention, exercise intolerance) or cardiac tamponade (accumulation of fluid around the heart that causes chest pain, difficulty breathing, and so forth). Report these signs to the physician immediately.
- Monitor signs of cerebral hemorrhage, including sudden severe headache, confusion, nausea, vomiting, paralysis, numbness, speech problems, visual disturbances, or loss of consciousness. These signs require immediate medical attention.
- Assess pulmonary function periodically by measuring lung volumes, breath sounds, and respiratory rate (See Appendices I, J, K). Notify physician immediately if patient experiences signs of pulmonary fibrosis (dry cough, dyspnea, shortness of breath, cyanosis) or breathing problems that might indicate other pulmonary impairments (alveolar hemorrhage, lung collapse, asthma, pneumonia).

- Assess heart rate, ECG, and heart sounds, especially during exercise (See Appendices G, H). Report any rhythm disturbances or symptoms of increased arrhythmias, including palpitations, chest discomfort, shortness of breath, fainting, and fatigue/weakness.
- Assess blood pressure (BP) periodically, and report a symptomatic decrease in BP (hypotension) or a sustained increase in BP (hypertension).
- Watch for signs of blood dyscrasias related to bone marrow suppression, including leukopenia (fever, sore throat, signs of infection), thrombocytopenia (bruising, nose bleeds and bleeding gums), or unusual weakness and fatigue that might be due to anemia. Report these signs to the physician or nursing staff.
- Assess any muscle, joint, or back pain to rule out musculoskeletal pathology; that is, try to determine if pain is drug induced rather than caused by anatomic or biomechanical problems.
- Be alert for signs of hyperglycemia, including confusion, drowsiness, flushed/dry skin, fruit-like breath odor, rapid/deep breathing, polyuria, loss of appetite, and unusual thirst. Patients with diabetes mellitus should check blood glucose levels frequently.
- Monitor neuromuscular signs of electrolyte imbalances (hypokalemia, hypomagnesemia, etc.), including headache, lethargy, weakness, cramping, and muscle hyperexcitability and tetany. Notify physician immediately if these signs occur.
- Monitor personality changes, including depression, anxiety, confusion, or changes in mental status. Notify physician if these changes become problematic.
- Monitor IV injection site for pain, swelling, and irritation. Report prolonged or excessive injection site reactions to the physician.

Interventions

- For patients who are medically able to begin exercise, implement appropriate resistive exercises and aerobic training to maintain muscle strength and aerobic capacity during cancer chemotherapy or to help restore function after chemotherapy.
- Because of the risk of cardiac and pulmonary dysfunction, use caution during aerobic exercise and other forms of therapeutic exercise. Assess exercise tolerance frequently (BP, heart rate, fatigue levels), and terminate exercise immediately if any untoward responses occur (See Appendix L).

Patient/Client-Related Instruction

- Advise patient about the likelihood of GI reactions such as nausea, vomiting, diarrhea, constipation, abdominal pain, indigestion, and inflammation in/around the mouth. Instruct patient to also report signs of drug-induced hepatitis (anorexia, severe nausea and vomiting, yellow skin or eyes, skin rashes, flu-like symptoms, muscle/joint pain) or pancreatitis (upper abdominal pain after eating, indigestion, weight loss, oily stools).
- Advise patient that hair loss and other skin reactions (rash, pruritus, acne, exfoliation, discoloration) are likely. Report severe or unexpected skin reactions to the physician.
- Advise patient to guard against infection (frequent hand washing, etc.) and avoid crowds and contact with persons with contagious diseases.
- Instruct patient or family/caregivers to report other bothersome side effects such as severe or prolonged headache, hearing problems, cataracts, upper respiratory tract irritation, problems with urination, allergic reactions, breast enlargement in men, or flu-like symptoms (fever, chills).

Pharmacokinetics

Absorption: Rapidly absorbed from the GI tract.
Distribution: Unknown.
Metabolism and Excretion: Extensively metabolized by the liver.
Half-life: 2.5 hr.

TIME/ACTION PROFILE (effects on blood counts)

ROUTE	ONSET	PEAK	DURATION
PO	1–2 wk	wk	up to 1 mo*
IV	unknown	unknown	13 days†

*Complete recovery may take up to 20 mo.
†After administration of last dose.

Contraindications/Precautions

Contraindicated in: Hypersensitivity; Failure to respond to previous courses; OB/Lactation: Potential for serious side effects in fetus or infant.
Use Cautiously in: Active infections; Decreased bone marrow reserve; Obese patients (base dose on ideal body weight); Other chronic debilitating diseases; Patients with childbearing potential; Geri: Begin therapy at lower end of dose range due to increased frequency of impaired cardiac, hepatic, or renal function.

Interactions

Drug-Drug: Concurrent or previous (within 72 hr) use of **acetaminophen** may ↓ elimination and ↑ toxicity. Concurrent use with high-dose **cyclophosphamide** in patients with thalassemia may result in cardiac tamponade. Concurrent use with **itraconazole** or **phenytoin** ↓ blood level effectiveness. Long-term continuous therapy with **thioguanine** may ↑ risk of hepatic toxicity. ↑ bone marrow suppression with other **antineoplastics** or **radiation therapy**. May ↓ the antibody response to and ↑ risk of adverse reactions from **live-virus vaccines**.

Route/Dosage

Many other regimens are used. See current protocols for up-to-date dosage.

B

PO (Adults): *Induction*—1.8 mg/m²/day or 60 mcg (0.06 mg)/kg/day until WBCs <15,000/mm³. Usual dose is 4–8 mg/day (range 1–12 mg/day). *Maintenance*—1–3 mg/day.
PO (Children): 0.06–0.12 mg/kg/day or 1.8–4.6 mg²/m²/day initially. Titrate dose to maintain WBC of approximately 20,000/mm³.
IV (Adults): 0.8 mg/kg q 6 hr (dose based on ideal body weight or actual weight, whichever is less; in obese patients, dosage should be based on adjusted ideal body weight) for 4 days (total of 16 doses); given in combination with cyclophosphamide.

Availability

Tablets: 2 mg. **Solution for injection:** 6 mg/mL in 10-mL ampules (60 mg).

BUTALBITAL

butalbital, acetaminophen
(byoo-**tal**-bi-tal & a-seet-a-**min**-oh-fen)
Bucet, Phrenilin, Phrenilin Forte, Tencon

butalbital, acetaminophen, caffeine (byoo-**tal**-bi-tal, a-seet-a-**min**-oh-fen, & **kaf**-een)
Esgic-Plus, Fioricet

butalbital, aspirin, caffeine
(byoo-**tal**-bi-tal, **as**-pir-in, & **kaf**-een)
Fiorinal, ✱Tecnal, ✱Trianal

Classification
Therapeutic: nonopioid analgesics (combination with barbiturate)
Pharmacologic: barbiturates

Indications

Relief of the symptom complex of tension (or muscle contraction) headaches (use should be short term only as the butalbital component may be habit forming).

Action

Contains a barbiturate (butalbital) for its sedative effect. Also contains an analgesic (aspirin or acetaminophen) for relief of pain. Caffeine may also be included in some formulations because it may be of benefit in tension headaches. **Therapeutic Effects:** Decreased severity of pain with some sedation.

Adverse Reactions/Side Effects

CNS: <u>drowsiness</u>, confusion, delirium, depression, dizziness, excitation, headache (with chronic use), irritability, lethargy, nervousness, numbness, tingling. **EENT:** earache, nasal congestion, tinnitus. **Resp:** respiratory depression. **CV:** tachycardia. **GI:** constipation, dry mouth, dysphagia, flatulence, heartburn. **Derm:** dermatitis, pruritus, rash, sweating. **MS:** leg pain, muscle weakness. **Misc:** fever, physical dependence, psychologic dependence, tolerance.

PHYSICAL THERAPY IMPLICATIONS

Implications refer to the butalbital (barbiturate) component. For information on the analgesic component in the formulation, see the aspirin or acetaminophen monograph.

Examination and Evaluation

- Assess the frequency and severity of headaches, and document whether drug therapy is successful in decreasing headache attacks.
- Monitor and report daytime drowsiness and other changes in mood or behavior, including confusion depression, lethargy, irritability, nervousness, excitation, or delirium. Repeated or excessive symptoms may require change in dose or medication.
- Assess heart rate, ECG, and heart sounds, especially during exercise (See Appendices G, H). Report increased heart rate (tachycardia) or symptoms of other arrhythmias, including palpitations, chest discomfort, shortness of breath, fainting, and fatigue/weakness.
- Assess any leg pain or muscle weakness to rule out musculoskeletal pathology; that is, try to determine if pain is drug induced rather than caused by anatomic or biomechanical problems.
- Assess dizziness that might affect gait, balance, and other functional activities (See Appendix C). Report balance problems and functional limitations to the physician, and caution the patient and family/caregivers to guard against falls and trauma.

Interventions

- Implement appropriate manual therapy techniques, physical agents, and therapeutic exercises to reduce headache pain and decrease the need for this drug.
- Because of the risk of tachycardia and other arrhythmias, use caution during aerobic exercise and other forms of therapeutic exercise. Assess exercise tolerance frequently (blood pressure, heart rate, fatigue levels), and terminate exercise immediately if any untoward responses occur (See Appendix L).

Patient/Client-Related Instruction

- Advise patient to avoid alcohol and other CNS depressants because of the increased risk of sedation and adverse effects.
- Instruct patient or family/caregivers to report other bothersome side effects such as severe or prolonged fever, earache, ringing/buzzing in the ears (tinnitus), nasal congestion, skin reactions (rash, dermatitis, itching, sweating), or GI problems (constipation, flatulence, heartburn, dry mouth, difficulty swallowing).

Pharmacokinetics

Absorption: Well absorbed.
Distribution: Widely distributed; crosses the placenta and enters breast milk.
Metabolism and Excretion: Butalbital primarily eliminated by kidneys as unchanged drug or metabolites (59–88% of dose); acetaminophen primarily metabolized by liver.
Half-life: Butalbital = 35 hr; acetaminophen = 1–3 hr.

TIME/ACTION PROFILE

ROUTE	ONSET	PEAK	DURATION
PO	15–30 min	1–2 hr	30 hr

Contraindications/Precautions

Contraindicated in: Hypersensitivity to individual components; Lactation; Porphyria.
Use Cautiously in: History of suicide attempt or drug addiction; Chronic alcohol use; Severe hepatic or renal disease; Patients concomitantly receiving other CNS depressants; Geri: Appears on Beers' list. Geriatric patients are at increased risk for side effects (dosage reduction recommended); Children <12 yr (safety not established).

Interactions

Drug-Drug: Additive CNS depression with other **CNS depressants**, including **alcohol**, **antihistamines**, **antidepressants**, **opioid analgesics**, and **sedative/hypnotics**. May ↑ liver metabolism and ↓ the effectiveness of other drugs, including **amiodarone**, **benzodiazepines**, **bupropion**, **calcium channel blockers**, **carbamazepine**, **citalopram**, **clarithromycin**, **cyclosporine**, **erythromycin**, **fluoxetine**, **fluvoxamine**, **glipizide**, **hormonal contraceptives**, **losartan**, **methadone**, **mirtazapine**, **nateglinide**, **nefazodone**, **nevirapine**, **phenytoin**, **pioglitazone**, **promethazine**, **propranolol**, **protease inhibitors**, **proton pump inhibitors**, **rifampin**, **ropinirole**, **rosiglitazone**, **selegiline**, **sertraline**, **tacrolimus**, **theophylline**, **venlafaxine**, **voriconazole**, **warfarin**, and **zafirlukast**. **MAO inhibitors**, **felbamate**, **primidone**, and **valproic acid** may prevent metabolism and ↑ the effectiveness of butalbital.
Drug-Natural: St. John's wort may ↓ barbiturate effect. Concurrent use of **kava kava**, **valerian**, **skullcap**, **chamomile**, or **hops** can ↑ CNS depression.

Route/Dosage

PO (Adults): 1–2 capsules or tablets (50–100 mg butalbital) every 4 hr as needed for pain (should not exceed 6 tablets or capsules/24 hr).

Availability (generic available)

Tablets: 50 mg butalbital/325 mg acetaminophen, 50 mg butalbital/650 mg acetaminophen. **Capsules:** 50 mg butalbital/650 mg acetaminophen.

butenafine (byoo-ten-a-feen)

Lotrimin Ultra, Mentax

Classification
Therapeutic: antifungals (topical)

Indications

Treatment of a variety of cutaneous fungal infections, including tinea pedis (athlete's foot), tinea cruris (jock itch), tinea corporis (ringworm), and tinea versicolor.

Action

Affects the synthesis of the fungal cell wall. **Therapeutic Effects:** Decrease in symptoms of fungal infection.

Adverse Reactions/Side Effects

Local: burning, itching, local hypersensitivity reactions, redness, stinging.

PHYSICAL THERAPY IMPLICATIONS

Examination and Evaluation

- Assess healing of skin lesions to help document drug effectiveness.

Interventions

- Avoid contact with cutaneous lesions when treating patient.
- Always wash hands thoroughly and disinfect equipment (whirlpools, electrotherapeutic devices, treatment tables, and so forth) to help prevent the spread of infection.

Patient/Client-Related Instruction

- Advise patient to report any increased local sensitivity to this drug (pain, burning, itching, swelling).
- Instruct patient about proper hygiene, e.g., thoroughly wash and dry the affected area, wear clean socks and ventilated shoes for tinea pedis, and so forth.
- Advise patient to apply the drug as directed for the full course of treatment even if feeling better.
- Inform patient that early relief of cutaneous symptoms may be seen in 2–3 days. Full therapeutic response may take 2 wk for tinea cruris, tinea corporis, and tinea versicolor and 4 weeks for tinea pedis.

B

- Advise patient to seek medical help if infections persist or recur after the full treatment. Recurrent fungal infections may be a sign of systemic illness.

Pharmacokinetics

Absorption: Absorption through intact skin is minimal.
Distribution: Distribution after topical administration is primarily local.
Metabolism and Excretion: Hepatic via hydroxylation.
Half-life: 35 hr.

TIME/ACTION PROFILE

ROUTE	ONSET	PEAK	DURATION
topical	unknown	up to 4 wk	unknown

Contraindications/Precautions

Contraindicated in: Hypersensitivity to active ingredients, additives, preservatives, or bases; Some products contain alcohol or bisulfites and should be avoided in patients with known intolerance.
Use Cautiously in: Nail and scalp infections (may require additional systemic therapy); OB/Lactation: Safety not established.

Interactions

Drug-Drug: None significant.

Route/Dosage

Topical (Adults and Children >12 yr): Apply once daily for 2 wk for patients with tinea corporis, tinea cruris, or tinea versicolor. Apply once daily for 4 wk or twice daily for 7 days for patients with tinea pedis.

Availability

Cream: 1% Rx, OTC.

HIGH ALERT

butorphanol (byoo-tor-fa-nole)

Stadol, Stadol NS

Classification
Therapeutic: opioid analgesics
Pharmacologic: opioid agonists/antagonists

Schedule IV

Indications

Management of moderate to severe pain. Analgesia during labor. Sedation before surgery. Supplement in balanced anesthesia.

Action

Binds to opiate receptors in the CNS. Alters the perception of and response to painful stimuli while producing generalized CNS depression. Has partial antagonist properties that may result in opioid withdrawal in physically dependent patients. **Therapeutic Effects:** Decreased severity of pain.

Adverse Reactions/Side Effects

CNS: confusion, dysphoria, hallucinations, sedation, euphoria, floating feeling, headache, unusual dreams. **EENT:** blurred vision, diplopia, miosis (high doses). **Resp:** respiratory depression. **CV:** hypertension, hypotension, palpitations. **GI:** nausea, constipation, dry mouth, ileus, vomiting. **GU:** urinary retention. **Derm:** sweating, clammy feeling. **Misc:** physical dependence, psychologic dependence, tolerance.

PHYSICAL THERAPY IMPLICATIONS

Examination and Evaluation

- Assess symptoms of respiratory depression, including decreased respiratory rate, confusion, bluish color of the skin and mucous membranes (cyanosis), and difficult, labored breathing (dyspnea). Monitor pulse oximetry and perform pulmonary function tests (See Appendix I) to quantify suspected changes in ventilation and respiratory function. Excessive respiratory depression requires emergency care.
- Be alert for excessive sedation or changes in mood and behavior (euphoria, dysphoria, confusion, hallucinations). Notify physician or nurse immediately if patient is unconscious or extremely difficult to arouse.
- Use appropriate pain scales (visual analogue scales, others) to document whether this drug is successful in helping manage the patient's pain.
- Assess blood pressure (BP) and compare to normal values (See Appendix F). Report changes in BP, either a problematic decrease in BP (hypotension) or a sustained increase in BP (hypertension).

Interventions

- Implement appropriate manual therapy techniques, physical agents, and therapeutic exercises to reduce pain and help wean patient off opioid analgesics as soon as possible.
- Because of the risk of abnormal BP responses, use caution during aerobic exercise and other forms of therapeutic exercise. Assess exercise tolerance frequently (BP, heart rate, fatigue levels), and terminate exercise immediately if any untoward responses occur (See Appendix L).
- Help patient explore other nonpharmacologic methods to reduce chronic pain, such as relaxation techniques, exercise, counseling, and so forth.
- Guard against falls and trauma (hip fractures, head injury). Implement fall-prevention strategies

(See Appendix E), especially if patient exhibits sedation, dizziness, or blurred vision.
- To minimize orthostatic hypotension, patient should move slowly when assuming a more upright position.

Patient/Client-Related Instruction

- Advise patient that opioid analgesics are usually more effective if given before pain becomes severe; emphasize that adequate pain control will allow better participation in physical therapy.
- Educate patient about the dangers of opioid overdose; encourage patient to adhere to proper dosing schedule.
- Emphasize that the risk of physical addiction (tolerance and dependence) is usually minimal during short-term treatment of pain. Advise patient that addiction is more likely during excessive or inappropriate use of opioid analgesics.
- Advise patient to avoid alcohol and other CNS depressants because of the increased risk of sedation and decreased CNS function.
- Advise patient to increase fluid intake and dietary fiber to avoid constipation. Laxatives may also be helpful in patients susceptible to fecal impaction (e.g., people with spinal cord injury).
- Instruct patient to report other troublesome side effects such as severe or prolonged headache, urinary retention, unusual dreams, heart palpitations, excessive sweating, vision disturbances, or GI problems (nausea, vomiting, dry mouth).

Pharmacokinetics

Absorption: Well absorbed from IM sites and nasal mucosa.
Distribution: Crosses the placenta and enters breast milk.
Metabolism and Excretion: Mostly metabolized by the liver; 11–14% excreted in the feces. Minimal renal excretion.
Half-life: 3–4 hr.

TIME/ACTION PROFILE (analgesia)

ROUTE	ONSET	PEAK	DURATION
IM	within 15 min	30–60 min	3–4 hr
IV	within mins	4–5 min	2–4 hr
intranasal	within 15 min	1–2 hr	4–5 hr

Contraindications/Precautions

Contraindicated in: Hypersensitivity; Patients physically dependent on opioids (may precipitate withdrawal).
Use Cautiously in: Head trauma; Increased intracranial pressure; Severe renal, hepatic, or pulmonary disease (increase interval to q 6–8 hr initially in hepatic/renal impairment); Hypothyroidism; Adrenal insufficiency; Alcoholism; Undiagnosed abdominal pain; Prostatic hyperplasia; OB/Lactation/Pedi: Safety not established but has been used during labor (may cause respiratory depression in the newborn); Geri: Decrease usual dose by 50%; give at twice the usual interval initially.

Interactions

Drug-Drug: Use with extreme caution in patients receiving **MAO inhibitors** (may produce severe, potentially fatal reactions—reduce initial dose of butorphanol to 25% of usual dose). Additive CNS depression with **alcohol**, **antidepressants**, **antihistamines**, and **sedative/hypnotics**. May precipitate withdrawal in patients who are physically dependent on **opioids** and have not been detoxified. May ↓ effects of concurrently administered **opioids**.
Drug-Natural: Concomitant use of **kava**, **valerian**, **chamomile**, or **hops** can ↑ CNS depression.

Route/Dosage

IM (Adults): 2 mg q 3–4 hr as needed (range 1–4 mg).
IV (Adults): 1 mg q 3–4 hr as needed (range 0.5–2 mg).
IM, IV (Geriatric Patients): 1 mg q 4–6 hr; increased as necessary.
Intranasal (Adults): 1 mg (1 spray in 1 nostril) initially. An additional dose may be given 60–90 min later. This sequence may be repeated in 3–4 hr. If pain is severe, an initial dose of 2 mg (1 spray in each nostril) may be given. May be repeated in 3–4 hr.
Intranasal (Geriatric Patients): 1 mg (1 spray in 1 nostril) initially. An additional dose may be given 90–120 min later. This sequence may be repeated in 3–4 hr.

Availability (generic available)

Injection: 1 mg/mL, 2 mg/mL. **Intranasal solution:** 10 mg/mL, in 2.5-mL metered-dose spray pump (14–15 doses; 1 mg/spray).

C

cabazitaxel (ka-ba-zi-**tax**-el)
Jevtana
Classification
Therapeutic: antineoplastics
Pharmacologic: taxoids, antimicrotubulars

Indications
Hormone-refractory metastatic prostate cancer previously treated with a regimen including docetaxel (used in combination with prednisone).

Action
Binds to intracellular tubulin and promotes its assembly into microtubules while inhibiting disassembly. Result is inhibition of mitosis and interphase. **Therapeutic Effects:** Death of rapidly replicating cells, particularly malignant ones, with ↓ spread of metastatic prostate cancer.

Adverse Reactions/Side Effects
CNS: weakness, fatigue. **Resp:** dyspnea. **CV:** arrhythmias, hypotension. **GI:** DIARRHEA, abdominal pain, abnormal taste, anorexia, constipation, nausea, vomiting, dyspepsia. **GU:** RENAL FAILURE, hematuria. **Derm:** alopecia. **F and E:** electrolyte imbalance. **Hemat:** NEUTROPENIA, THROMBOCYTOPENIA, anemia, leukopenia. **MS:** arthralgia, back pain, muscle spasms; **Neuro:** peripheral neuropathy; **Misc:** ALLERGIC REACTIONS, INCLUDING ANAPHYLAXIS, fever.

PHYSICAL THERAPY IMPLICATIONS

Examination and Evaluation
- Be alert for signs of allergic reactions and anaphylaxis, including pulmonary symptoms (tightness in the throat and chest, wheezing, cough, dyspnea) or skin reactions (rash, pruritus, urticaria). Notify physician or nursing staff immediately if these reactions occur.
- Watch for signs of renal failure, including decreased urine output, hematuria, increased blood pressure, muscle cramps/twitching, edema/weight gain from fluid retention, yellowish brown skin, and confusion that progresses to seizures and coma. Report these signs to the physician or nursing staff immediately.
- Watch for signs of leukopenia and neutropenia (fever, sore throat, other signs of infection), thrombocytopenia (bruising, nose bleeds, bleeding gums), or unusual weakness and fatigue that might be due to anemia. Report these signs to the physician or nursing staff immediately.
- Watch for untoward GI reactions, and immediately report severe or prolonged diarrhea.
- Assess heart rate, ECG, and heart sounds, especially during exercise (See Appendices G, H). Report any rhythm disturbances or symptoms of increased arrhythmias, including palpitations, chest discomfort, shortness of breath, fainting, and fatigue/weakness.
- Assess blood pressure periodically and compare to normal values (See Appendix F). Report low blood pressure (hypotension), especially if patient experiences dizziness or syncope.
- Monitor signs of electrolyte imbalances, including high plasma potassium levels (bradycardia, fatigue, weakness, numbness, tingling), high calcium levels (muscle pain and weakness, joint pain, confusion, lethargy), or high phosphate levels (ectopic calcification). Notify physician because severe cases can lead to life-threatening arrhythmias and paralysis.
- Be alert for signs of peripheral neuropathy, such as numbness, tingling, and decreased muscle strength. Establish baseline electroneuromyographic values using EMG and nerve conduction at the beginning of drug treatment whenever possible, and reexamine these values periodically to document drug-induced changes in peripheral nerve function.
- Assess any joint pain, back pain, or muscle spasms to rule out musculoskeletal pathology; that is, try to determine if pain is drug induced rather than caused by anatomic or biomechanical problems.

Interventions
- For patients who are medically able to begin exercise, implement appropriate resistive exercises and aerobic training to maintain muscle strength and aerobic capacity during cancer chemotherapy or to help restore function after chemotherapy.
- Because of the risk of arrhythmias and abnormal blood pressure responses, use caution during aerobic exercise and other forms of therapeutic exercise. Assess exercise tolerance frequently (blood pressure, heart rate, fatigue levels), and terminate exercise immediately if any untoward responses occur (See Appendix L).

Patient/Client-Related Instruction
- Advise patient to guard against infection (frequent hand washing, etc.) and to avoid crowds and contact with persons with contagious diseases.
- Advise patient and family/caregivers that fatigue and weakness are likely and may be severe. Functional abilities may be limited, and patient may need to use assistive devices during ambulation.
- Advise patient about the likelihood of GI reactions, including nausea, vomiting, diarrhea, constipation, abnormal taste, indigestion, loss of appetite, and abdominal pain. Instruct patient or family/caregivers to report severe or prolonged GI reactions.

- Advise patient that hair loss and other skin reactions are likely. Instruct patient to report severe or unexpected skin problems.
- Instruct patient and family/caregivers to report other troublesome side effects such as severe or prolonged fever or difficult, labored breathing.

Pharmacokinetics

Absorption: IV administration results in complete bioavailability.
Distribution: Equally distributed between blood and plasma.
Metabolism and Excretion: Extensively (>95%) metabolized by the liver, 80–90% by CYP3A4/5 enzyme system. Metabolites are excreted in urine and feces. Minimal renal excretion
Half-life: *Terminal elimination*—95 hr

TIME/ACTION PROFILE (blood levels)

ROUTE	ONSET	PEAK	DURATION
IV	rapid	end of infusion	unknown

Contraindications/Precautions

Contraindicated in: Severe hypersensitivity to cabazitaxel or polysorbate 80; Neutrophils ≤1,500/mm³; Hepatic impairment (total bilirubin ≥ upper limits of normal, or AST and/or ALT ≥1.5 × upper limits of normal); Concurrent use of strong CYP3A4 inhibitors, inducers, and St. John's wort; OB: Avoid use during pregnancy (may cause fetal harm); Lactation: Breast-feeding should be avoided.
Use Cautiously in: Concurrent use of moderate CYP3A4 inhibitors; OB: Patients with child-bearing potential (pregnancy should be avoided). Patients with severe renal impairment (CCr <30 mL/min) or end-stage renal disease; Geri: Patients >65 yr ↑ risk of adverse reactions; Pedi: Safe and effective use in children has not been established.

Interactions

Drug-Drug: Concomitant administration of **strong CYP3A inhibitors,** including **ketoconazole, itraconazole, clarithromycin, atazanavir, indinavir, nefazodone, nelfinavir, ritonavir, saquinavir, telithromycin,** and **voriconazole** ↑ levels and risk of toxicity and should be avoided; Concomitant administration of **strong CYP3A inducers,** including **phenytoin, carbamazepine, rifampin, rifabutin, rifapentine,** and **phenobarbital** may ↓ levels and effectiveness and should be avoided.
Drug-Natural: St. John's wort may ↓ levels and effectiveness and should be avoided.

Route/Dosage

PO (Adults): 25 mg/m² every 3 wk as a 1-hr infusion (with prednisone 10 mg PO daily).

Availability

Viscous solution for injection (requires 2 dilutions prior to IV administration): 60 mg/1.5 mL (contains polysorbate 80) comes with diluent (5.7 mL of 13% [w/w] ethanol in water for injection).

cabergoline (ka-ber-goe-leen)

Dostinex

Classification
Therapeutic: antihyperprolactinemics
Pharmacologic: dopamine agonists

Indications

Treatment of hyperprolactinemia (idiopathic or pituitary in origin). **Unlabeled Use:** Adjunctive treatment of Parkinson's disease.

Action

Inhibits secretion of prolactin by acting as a dopamine agonist. In Parkinson's disease, dopamine agonists directly stimulate neural dopamine receptors. **Therapeutic Effects:** Decreased secretion of prolactin in hyperprolactinemia. Reduced involuntary movements associated with Parkinson's disease.

Adverse Reactions/Side Effects

CNS: dizziness, headache, depression, drowsiness, fatigue, nervousness, vertigo, weakness. **Resp:** PULMONARY FIBROSIS, pleural effusion. **EENT:** abnormal vision. **CV:** VALVULAR DISORDERS, orthostatic hypotension, hot flashes. **GI:** constipation, nausea, abdominal pain, dyspepsia, vomiting. **GU:** dysmenorrhea. **Endo:** breast pain. **Neuro:** paresthesia.

PHYSICAL THERAPY IMPLICATIONS

Examination and Evaluation

- Assess any breathing problems, and report signs of pulmonary fibrosis or pleural effusion such as dry cough, wheezing, chest pain, shortness of breath, and difficult or labored breathing. Monitor pulse oximetry and perform pulmonary function tests (See Appendices I, J, K) to quantify suspected changes in ventilation and respiratory function.
- Assess heart sounds to monitor possible valvular disorders (See Appendices H). Report any abnormal sounds or symptoms of cardiac dysfunction, including palpitations, chest discomfort, shortness of breath, fainting, and fatigue/weakness.
- If treating increased prolactin secretion (hyperprolactinemia), monitor symptoms in women such as menstrual irregularities and abnormal lactation, and symptoms in men such as erectile dysfunction, breast enlargement, and decreased libido.

Document whether drug therapy is successful in reducing these symptoms.

- If treating Parkinson disease, assess gait and motor function to help determine antiparkinson effects, especially when starting drug therapy or during dosing changes or addition of other antiparkinson drugs. Motor function should be assessed at different times of the day, such as when drugs are reaching peak therapeutic levels (i.e., 30–60 min after oral dose), as well as when drug effects are minimal (just before the next dose).
- Assess blood pressure when patient assumes a more upright position (lying to standing, sitting to standing, lying to sitting). Document orthostatic hypotension and contact physician when systolic blood pressure (BP) falls >20 mm Hg or diastolic BP falls >10 mm Hg.
- Assess signs of paresthesia (numbness, tingling) or muscle twitching. Perform objective tests, including electroneuromyography and sensory testing to document any drug-related neuropathic changes.
- Monitor depression, nervousness, or other psychologic problems. Repeated or excessive symptoms may require change in dose or medication.
- Assess dizziness, drowsiness, or vertigo that might affect gait, balance, and other functional activities (See Appendix C). Report balance problems and functional limitations to the physician, and caution the patient and family/caregivers to guard against falls and trauma.

Interventions

- For patients with Parkinson disease, implement therapeutic exercises (coordination exercises, gait training, cardiovascular conditioning) to complement the effects of drug therapy and help achieve optimal function.
- Guard against falls and trauma (hip fractures, head injury, and so forth). Implement fall-prevention strategies (See Appendix E), especially if patient exhibits Parkinson's symptoms (postural instability, rigidity) combined with drug side effects (dizziness, blurred vision, dyskinesias).
- Because of the risk of valvular disorders and pulmonary fibrosis, use caution during aerobic exercise and other forms of therapeutic exercise. Assess exercise tolerance frequently (BP, heart rate, respiratory function, fatigue levels), and terminate exercise immediately if any untoward responses occur (See Appendix L).
- To minimize orthostatic hypotension, patient should move slowly when assuming a more upright position.

Patient/Client-Related Instruction

- Advise patient to avoid alcohol because of the increased risk of sedation and adverse effects.
- Advise patient about the likelihood of GI reactions such as nausea, vomiting, constipation, abdominal pain, and indigestion. Instruct patient to report severe or prolonged GI problems.
- Instruct patient to report other troublesome side effects such as severe or prolonged headaches, vision disturbances, breast pain, and menstrual irregularities.

Pharmacokinetics

Absorption: Well absorbed but undergoes extensive first-pass hepatic metabolism.
Distribution: Widely distributed; concentrates in pituitary.
Metabolism and Excretion: Extensively metabolized by the liver; <4% excreted unchanged in urine.
Protein Binding: 40–42%.
Half-life: 63–69 hr.

TIME/ACTION PROFILE (effect on serum prolactin levels)

ROUTE	ONSET	PEAK	DURATION
PO	unknown	2–3 hr	unknown

Contraindications/Precautions

Contraindicated in: Hypersensitivity to cabergoline or ergot alkaloids; Uncontrolled hypertension; History of pulmonary, pericardial, valvular, or retroperitoneal fibrotic disorders; Lactation: Has been associated with hypertension, stroke, and seizures. Not to be used for suppression of physiologic lactation.
Use Cautiously in: Hepatic impairment; OB: Use in pregnancy only if clearly needed; Pedi: Safety not established.

Interactions

Drug-Drug: ↑ risk of hypotension with **antihypertensives**. May ↑ the effects of **sibutramine**, **SSRIs**, and other **serotonin agonists** (induces serotonin syndrome). Effectiveness may be decreased by **phenothiazines**, **butyrophenones (haloperidol)**, **thioxanthenes**, or **metoclopramide** (avoid concurrent use).

Route/Dosage

PO (Adults): 0.25 mg twice weekly; may be increased at 4-wk intervals up to 1 mg twice weekly.

Availability (generic available)

Tablets: 0.5 mg.

calcitonin (kal-si-toe-nin)

calcitonin (salmon)

Miacalcin

calcitonin (rDNA)

Fortical

Classification

Therapeutic: hypocalcemics

Pharmacologic: hormones

Indications

IM, SC: Treatment of Paget's disease of bone. Adjunctive therapy for hypercalcemia. **IM, SC, Intranasal:** Management of postmenopausal osteoporosis.

Action

Inhibits osteoclastic bone resorption and promotes renal excretion of calcium. **Therapeutic Effects:** Decreased rate of bone turnover. Lowering of serum calcium.

Adverse Reactions/Side Effects

CNS: ***nasal only***—headaches. **EENT:** ***nasal only***—rhinitis, epistaxis, nasal irritation. **GI: IM, SC:** nausea, vomiting. **GU: IM, SC:** urinary frequency. **Derm:** rashes. **Local:** injection site reactions. **MS:** ***nasal***—arthralgia, back pain. **Misc:** ALLERGIC REACTIONS, INCLUDING ANAPHYLAXIS, facial flushing, swelling.

PHYSICAL THERAPY IMPLICATIONS

Examination and Evaluation

- Watch for signs of allergic reactions and anaphylaxis, including pulmonary symptoms (tightness in the throat and chest, wheezing, cough, dyspnea) or skin reactions (rash, pruritus, urticaria). Notify physician immediately if these reactions occur.
- Be alert for signs of hypocalcemic tetany, especially during the first several doses of calcitonin. Signs include nervousness, irritability, paresthesia, muscle twitching, tetanic spasms, and seizures. Report these signs to the physician immediately.
- Assess bone pain periodically to document whether drug therapy can help reduce symptoms of Paget's disease.
- Assess any new episodes of joint pain or back pain, especially during intranasal use. Attempt to determine if pain is drug related rather than caused by musculoskeletal lesions.
- Monitor IM or SC injection site for pain, swelling, and irritation. Report prolonged or excessive injection-site reactions to the physician.

Interventions

- Institute weight-bearing and resistance exercises as tolerated to maintain or increase bone mineral density. Start with low-impact or aquatic programs in patients with extensive demineralization or pre-existing lesions, and increase exercise intensity slowly to prevent fractures.
- Protect against falls and fractures (See Appendix E). Modify home environment (remove throw rugs, improve lighting, etc.), and provide assistive devices (cane, walker) or other protective devices as needed to improve balance and prevent falls.
- Do not apply physical agents (heat, cold, electrotherapeutic modalities) or massage at the injection site; these interventions can alter drug absorption from subcutaneous tissues.

Patient/Client-Related Instruction

- Advise patient about the benefits of proper diet in sustaining bone mineralization and plasma calcium levels. If necessary, refer patient for nutritional counseling about supplemental calcium and vitamin D.
- Encourage patient to modify behaviors that increase the risk of osteoporosis (stop smoking, reduce alcohol consumption).
- Instruct patient to report problems related to intranasal administration, including severe or prolonged headache, nasal irritation, or nosebleeds.
- Instruct patient to report other troublesome side effects, including facial swelling/flushing, urinary frequency, skin rash, or GI problems (nausea, vomiting).

Pharmacokinetics

Absorption: Completely absorbed from IM and SC sites. Rapidly absorbed from nasal mucosa; absorption is 3% compared with parenteral administration.

Distribution: Unknown.

Metabolism and Excretion: Rapidly metabolized in kidneys, blood, and tissues.

Half-life: 40–90 min.

TIME/ACTION PROFILE

ROUTE	ONSET	PEAK	DURATION
IM, SC*	unknown	2 hr	6–8 hr
intranasal†	rapid	31–39 min	unknown

*Effects on serum calcium; effects on serum alkaline phosphates and urinary hydroxyproline in Paget's disease may require 6–24 mo of continuous treatment.

†Serum levels of administered calcitonin.

Contraindications/Precautions

Contraindicated in: Hypersensitivity to calcitonin, salmon protein, or gelatin diluent (in some products); OB/Lactation: Use is not recommended.

Use Cautiously in: Pedi: Safety not established.

Interactions

Drug-Drug: Previous bisphosphonate therapy, including **alendronate**, **risedronate**, **etidronate**, **ibandronate**, or **pamidronate**, may ↓ response to calcitonin.

Route/Dosage

Postmenopausal osteoporosis

IM, SC (Adults): 100 IU every other day.
Intranasal (Adults): 1 spray (200 IU)/day in alternating nostrils.

Paget's disease

IM, SC (Adults): 100 IU/day initially, after titration, maintenance dose is usually 50 IU/day or every other day.

Hypercalcemia

IM, SC (Adults): 4 IU/kg q 12 hr; if adequate response not achieved, may increase dose after 1–2 days to 8 IU/kg q 12 hr, and if necessary after 2 more days may be increased to 8 IU/kg q 6 hr.

Availability

Injection: 200 IU/mL in 2-mL vials. **Nasal spray:** 200 IU/actuation in 3.7-mL bottles.

calcitriol (ointment)

(kal-si-**trye**-ole)
Vectical ointment

Classification
Therapeutic: antipsoriatics
Pharmacologic: vitamin D analogues

Indications

Mild-to-moderate plaque psoriasis.

Action

Exact mechanism is unknown, but may affect keratinocyte proliferation and differentiation and decrease the action of proinflammatory cytokines. **Therapeutic Effects:** Decreased severity of plaque psoriasis.

Adverse Reactions/Side Effects

GU: hypercalcuria. **Derm:** pruritus, skin discomfort.

PHYSICAL THERAPY IMPLICATIONS

Examination and Evaluation

- Assess the area being treated to help document whether drug therapy is successful in decreasing skin plaques and other psoriatic skin lesions.
- Monitor any new or increased reactions at the site of application, including pain, irritation, burning, swelling, and rash. Report severe or prolonged skin reactions to the physician.

Interventions

- Implement ultraviolet light therapy when indicated to help treat psoriasis and augment the effects of drug therapy.

Patient/Client-Related Instruction

- Check that the patient and family or caregivers understand topical application procedures and adhere to the recommended dosing schedule.
- Instruct patient to report signs of excess calcium in the urine (hypercalcuria). Signs include increased urination, painful urination, increased nighttime urination, and increased thirst.

Pharmacokinetics

Absorption: Although intended action is skin, some systemic absorption follows topical use.
Distribution: Unknown.
Metabolism and Excretion: Absorbed calcitriol undergoes enterohepatic recycling and is excreted in bile.
Half-life: 5–8 hr.

TIME/ACTION PROFILE: improvement in psoriatic lesions

ROUTE	ONSET	PEAK	DURATON
topical	unknown	within 8 wk	unknown

Contraindications/Precautions

Contraindicated in: No contraindications noted.
Use Cautiously in: Concurrent use of medications known to ↑ serum calcium levels, including thiazide diuretics, calcium supplements, or high doses of vitamin D; Exposure of the treated areas to natural or artificial sunlight, including tanning booths, sun lamps, or phototherapy; use should be limited or avoided; OB: Use during pregnancy only if potential benefit to patient justifies risk to fetus; Lactation: Use cautiously; Pedi: Safety and effectiveness in patients <18 yr has not been established.

Interactions

Drug-Drug: Concurrent use with **medications known to ↑ serum calcium levels**, including **thiazide diuretics**, **calcium supplements**, or **high doses of vitamin D** may additively ↑ serum calcium levels; use cautiously.

Route/Dosage

Topical (Adults 18 yr): Apply twice daily; use should not exceed 200 g/wk.

Availability

Ointment: 3 mcg/g in 5- and 100-g tubes.

canakinumab (kan-a-kin-u-mab)
Ilaris

Classification
Therapeutic: none assigned
Pharmacologic: interleukin antagonists

Indications
Treatment of cryopyrin-associated periodic syndromes (CAPS) including familial cold autoinflammatory syndrome (FCAS) an Muckle-Wells syndrome (MWS).

Action
Binds and neutralizes the activity of excess interleukin associated with CAPS. **Therapeutic Effects:** Decreased symptoms of CAPS, including fever, urticaria-like rash, arthralgia, myalgia, fatigue, and conjunctivitis.

Adverse Reactions/Side Effects
CNS: headache, vertigo. **EENT:** nasopharyngitis. **Resp:** bronchitis. **GI:** diarrhea, nausea, gastroenteritis. **Local:** injection site reactions. **Metab:** weight gain. **MS:** musculoskeletal pain. **Misc:** Increased risk of serious infections/reinfections, influenza.

PHYSICAL THERAPY IMPLICATIONS

Examination and Evaluation
- Report any signs of infection, especially pulmonary signs associated with pneumonia, influenza, and invasive fungal infections. Common pulmonary signs of infection include persistent cough, dyspnea, chest pain, coughing up blood, fatigue, fever, chills, and loss of appetite.
- Periodically assess impairments such as joint pain, muscle aches, fatigue, skin rash, and conjunctivitis to help document whether drug therapy is successful in treating CAPS and related syndromes.
- Assess any new bone or muscle pain to rule out musculoskeletal pathology; that is, try to determine if pain is drug induced rather than caused by anatomic and biomechanical problems.
- Periodically assess body weight and other anthropometric measures (body mass index, body composition). Report a rapid or unexplained weight gain or increased body fat.
- Monitor IV injection site for pain, swelling, and irritation. Report prolonged or excessive injection-site reactions to the physician.

Patient/Client-Related Instruction
- Instruct patient to guard against infection (frequent hand washing, etc.), and to avoid crowds and contact with persons with contagious diseases.
- Instruct patient to report other troublesome side effects including severe or prolonged headache, vertigo, irritation of the nose and pharynx, or GI problems (nausea, diarrhea, abdominal pain).

Pharmacokinetics
Absorption: 70% absorbed following SCs administration.
Distribution: Unknown.
Metabolism and Excretion: Unknown.
Half-life: 26 days.

TIME/ACTION PROFILE

ROUTE	ONSET	PEAK	DURATION
SC	within 8 days*,†	7 days‡	8 wk

*Noted as normalization of markers of inflammation.
‡Blood levels.

Contraindications/Precautions
Contraindicated in: None noted.
Use Cautiously in: Active untreated infection, history of recurrent infections or conditions increasing the propensity of infections; OB: Use during pregnancy only if clearly needed; Lactation: Use cautiously during lactation; Pedi: Safety and effectiveness in children <4 yr has not been established.

Interactions
Drug-Drug: Avoid concurrent use of **live vaccines**; all vaccinations should be completed prior to treatment; Concurrent use with **tumor necrosis factor (TNF) inhibitors** may ↑ risk of serious infections; May alter activity of **drugs metabolized by the CYP450 enzyme system,** including **warfarin**; careful monitoring of such drugs with narrow therapeutic indices should be undertaken.

Route/Dosage
SC (Adults ≥40 kg): 150 mg every 8 wk.
SC (Adults and Children 15–40 kg): 2 mg/kg; may be increased to 3 mg/kg q 8 wk.

Availability
Lyophilized powder for solution for SC injection: 180 mg/vial.

candesartan (kan-de-sar-tan)
Atacand

Classification
Therapeutic: antihypertensives
Pharmacologic: angiotensin II receptor antagonists

Indications
Alone or with other agents in the management of hypertension. Treatment of heart failure (New York Heart Association class II–IV) in patients with left

ventricular systolic dysfunction (ejection fraction ≤40%) (can be used with an ACE inhibitor and beta blocker).

Action

Blocks the vasoconstrictor and aldosterone-secreting effects of angiotensin II at various receptor sites, including vascular smooth muscle and the adrenal glands. **Therapeutic Effects:** Lowering of blood pressure in patients with hypertension. Reduced cardiovascular death and heart failure–related hospitalizations in patients with heart failure.

Adverse Reactions/Side Effects

CNS: dizziness, fatigue, headache. **CV:** hypotension, chest pain, edema. **F and E:** hyperkalemia. **GI:** abdominal pain, diarrhea, nausea. **GU:** impaired renal function. **MS:** arthralgia, back pain. **Misc:** ANGIOEDEMA.

PHYSICAL THERAPY IMPLICATIONS

Examination and Evaluation

- Watch for signs of angioedema, including rashes, raised patches of red or white skin (welts), burning/itching skin, swelling in the face, and difficulty breathing. Notify physician immediately if these signs occur.
- Assess blood pressure periodically and compare to normal values (See Appendix F) to help determine antihypertensive effects. Report low blood pressure (hypotension), especially if patient experiences dizziness, fatigue, or other symptoms.
- Assess signs and symptoms of CHF (dyspnea, rales/crackles, peripheral edema, jugular venous distention, exercise intolerance) to help document whether drug therapy is effective in reducing these symptoms.
- Assess peripheral edema using girth measurements, volume displacement, and measurement of pitting edema (See Appendix N). Report increased swelling in feet and ankles or a sudden increase in body weight due to vasodilation or fluid retention.
- Assess any back pain or joint pain to rule out musculoskeletal pathology; that is, try to determine if pain is drug induced rather than caused by anatomic or biomechanical problems.
- Monitor signs of high plasma potassium levels (hyperkalemia), including bradycardia, fatigue, weakness, numbness, and tingling. Notify physician because severe cases can lead to life-threatening arrhythmias and paralysis.
- Assess dizziness that might affect gait, balance, and other functional activities (See Appendix C). Report balance problems and functional limitations to the physician, and caution the patient and family/caregivers to guard against falls and trauma.

Interventions

- Implement aerobic exercise and cardiac conditioning programs to augment drug therapy and maintain or improve cardiovascular pump function in patients with heart failure and other cardiac conditions.
- Avoid physical therapy interventions that cause systemic vasodilation (large whirlpool, Hubbard tank). Additive effects of this drug and the intervention may cause a dangerous fall in blood pressure.
- To minimize orthostatic hypotension, patient should move slowly when assuming a more upright position.

Patient/Client-Related Instruction

- Remind patients to take medication as directed to control hypertension and other cardiac conditions even if they are asymptomatic.
- Instruct patients with heart failure to weigh themselves every day and to call their physician if they gain 3 lb or more in 1 day or more than 5 lb in 1 wk. Sudden weight gain may indicate fluid buildup due to worsening heart failure.
- Counsel patients about additional interventions to help control blood pressure and cardiac dysfunction such as regular exercise, weight loss, sodium restriction, stress reduction, moderation of alcohol consumption, and smoking cessation.
- Instruct patient to report signs of impaired renal function, including decreased urine output, cloudy urine, or sudden weight gain due to fluid retention.
- Instruct patient or family/caregivers to report other troublesome side effects such as severe or prolonged headache, fatigue, chest pain, or GI problems (nausea, diarrhea, abdominal pain).

Pharmacokinetics

Absorption: Candesartan cilexetil is a prodrug that is converted to candesartan (the active component); 15% bioavailability of candesartan.
Distribution: Crosses the placenta and enters breast milk.
Protein Binding: >99%.
Metabolism and Excretion: Minor metabolism by the liver; 33% excreted in urine; 67% in feces (via bile).
Half-life: 9 hr.

TIME/ACTION PROFILE (antihypertensive effect)

ROUTE	ONSET	PEAK	DURATION
PO	2–4 hr*	4 wk†	24 hr†

*After single dose.
†Chronic dosing.

Contraindications/Precautions

Contraindicated in: Hypersensitivity; Bilateral renal artery stenosis; OB: Can cause injury or death

of fetus. Lactation: Appears in breast milk; patient must discontinue candesartan or provide alternate to breast milk.
Use Cautiously in: Volume- or salt-depleted patients or patients receiving large doses of diuretics (correct deficits before initiating therapy or initiate at lower doses); Black patients (may not be as effective); Impaired renal function due to primary renal disease or congestive heart failure (may worsen renal function); Hepatic impairment; Women of childbearing potential—if pregnancy occurs, discontinue immediately; Pedi: Safety not established in children <18 yr.

Interactions
Drug-Drug: Antihypertensive effect may be blunted by **NSAIDs**. Additive hypotension with other **antihypertensives**. Excessive hypotension may occur with concurrent use of **diuretics**. Increased risk of hyperkalemia with concurrent use of **trimethoprim (high dose)**, **potassium supplements**, **potassium-containing salt substitutes**, **angiotensin-converting enzyme inhibitors**, or **potassium-sparing diuretics**. ↑ levels and may ↑ risk of **lithium** toxicity.

Route/Dosage
Hypertension
PO (Adults): 16 mg once daily; may be increased up to 32 mg/day in 1–2 divided doses (initiate therapy at a lower dose in patients who are receiving diuretics or are volume depleted).

Hepatic Impairment
(Adults): *Moderate hepatic impairment*—Initiate at lower doses.

Heart Failure
PO (Adults): 4 mg once daily initially; dose may be doubled at 2-wk intervals up to target dose of 32 mg once daily.

Availability
Tablets: 4 mg, 8 mg, 16 mg, 32 mg. ***In combination with:*** hydrochlorothiazide (Atacand HCT). See Appendix B.

HIGH ALERT

capecitabine (kap-pe-**site**-a-been)
Xeloda

Classification
Therapeutic: antineoplastics
Pharmacologic: antimetabolites

Indications
Metastatic colorectal cancer. Adjuvant treatment for Dukes' C colon cancer following primary resection. Metastatic breast cancer that has worsened despite prior therapy with anthracycline (daunorubicin, doxorubicin, idarubicin) (to be used in combination with docetaxel). Metastatic breast cancer that is resistant to both paclitaxel and an anthracycline (daunorubicin, doxorubicin, idarubicin) or is resistant to paclitaxel and further anthracycline therapy is contraindicated.

Action
Converted in tissue to 5-fluorouracil (5-FU), which inhibits DNA and RNA synthesis by preventing thymidine production. The enzyme responsible for the final step in the conversion to 5-FU may be found in higher concentrations in some tumors. **Therapeutic Effects:** Death of rapidly replicating cells, particularly malignant ones.

Adverse Reactions/Side Effects
CNS: fatigue, headache, dizziness, insomnia. **EENT:** eye irritation, epistaxis, rhinorrhea. **CV:** edema, chest pain. **GI:** DIARRHEA, NECROTIZING ENTEROCOLITIS, abdominal pain, anorexia, constipation, dysgeusia, hyperbilirubinemia, nausea, stomatitis, vomiting, dyspepsia, xerostomia. **Derm:** dermatitis, hand-and-foot syndrome, nail disorder, alopecia, erythema, rashes. **F and E:** dehydration. **Hemat:** anemia, leukopenia, thrombocytopenia. **MS:** arthralgia, myalgia. **Neuro:** peripheral neuropathy. **Resp:** cough, dyspnea. **Misc:** fever.

PHYSICAL THERAPY IMPLICATIONS
Examination and Evaluation
- Be alert for signs of severe intestinal infection and inflammation that might indicate necrotizing enterocolitis. Signs include vomiting, constipation, tarry or bloody stools, unstable body temperature, lack of appetite, and a swollen, red, tender, or shiny abdomen. Report these signs to the physician or nursing staff immediately.
- Monitor and report other GI reactions, including severe diarrhea.
- Monitor signs of leukopenia (fever, sore throat, signs of infection), thrombocytopenia (bruising, nose bleeds, and bleeding gums), or unusual weakness and fatigue that might be due to anemia. Report these signs to the physician immediately.
- Assess peripheral edema using girth measurements, volume displacement, and measurement of pitting edema (See Appendix N). Report increased swelling in feet and ankles or a sudden increase in body weight due to fluid retention.
- Assess any breathing problems, and report difficult/labored breathing or a persistent cough.
- Assess signs of peripheral neuropathy such as numbness, tingling, and decreased muscle strength. Establish baseline electroneuromyographic values

using EMG and nerve conduction at the beginning of drug treatment whenever possible, and reexamine these values periodically to document drug-induced changes in peripheral nerve function.

- Assess any muscle or joint pain to rule out musculoskeletal pathology; that is, try to determine if pain is drug induced rather than caused by anatomic or biomechanical problems.
- Assess dizziness that might affect gait, balance, and other functional activities (See Appendix C). Report balance problems and functional limitations to the physician and nursing staff, and caution the patient and family/caregivers to guard against falls and trauma.

Interventions

- For patients who are medically able to begin exercise, implement appropriate resistive exercises and aerobic training to maintain muscle strength and aerobic capacity during cancer chemotherapy or to help restore function after chemotherapy.

Patient/Client-Related Instruction

- Advise patient about the risk of pain, redness, and dry, scaly skin on the palms of the hands and soles of the feet (hand-and-foot syndrome). Instruct patient to protect the hands and feet from heat and friction, and to apply lotion to the affected areas. Superficial cold application can also temporarily reduce symptoms.
- Advise patient and family/caregivers about the likelihood of GI reactions such as nausea, vomiting, diarrhea, constipation, indigestion, abdominal pain, loss of appetite, difficulty swallowing, and irritation of the oral mucosa. Instruct patient to report severe or prolonged GI problems.
- Advise patient and family/caregivers about the risk of infections, to guard against infection (frequent hand washing, etc.), and to avoid crowds and contact with persons with contagious diseases.
- Instruct patient and family/caregivers to maintain adequate fluid intake and avoid dehydration.
- Instruct patient and family/caregivers to report other troublesome side effects such as severe or prolonged headache, sleep loss, eye irritation, nasal irritation, nosebleeds, fever, or skin reactions (rash, hair loss, redness, dermatitis).

Pharmacokinetics

Absorption: Well absorbed after oral administration.
Distribution: Unknown.
Metabolism and Excretion: Metabolized mostly in tissue and by the liver; inactive metabolites are excreted primarily in urine.
Half-life: 45 min.

TIME/ACTION PROFILE (blood levels)

ROUTE	ONSET	PEAK	DURATION
PO	Unknown*	1.5 hr (2 hr for 5-FU)†	unknown

*Onset of antineoplastic effect is 6 wk.
†Peak 5-FU levels occur at 2 hr.

Contraindications/Precautions

Contraindicated in: Hypersensitivity to capecitabine or 5-FU; Dihydropyrimidine dehydrogenase deficiency (enzyme metabolizes 5-FU to nontoxic compounds); Severe renal impairment (CCr <30 mL/min); OB: Potential for fetal harm or death; Lactation: Potential for serious adverse effects in nursing infants.
Use Cautiously in: Mild-moderate renal impairment (↓ starting dose to 75% in patients with CCr 30–50 mL/min); Hepatic dysfunction; Coronary artery disease; Pedi: Safety not established; Geri: ↓ risk of severe diarrhea in patients ≥80 yr).

Interactions

Drug-Drug: May ↑ risk of bleeding with **warfarin** (frequent monitoring of PT/INR recommended). Toxicity ↑ by concurrent **leucovorin**. **Antacids** may ↑ absorption. May ↑ blood levels and risk of toxicity from **phenytoin** (may need to ↓ phenytoin dose).
Drug-Food: Food ↑ absorption, although capecitabine should be given within 30 min after a meal.

Route/Dosage

PO (Adults): 1250 mg/m^2 twice daily for 14 days, followed by 7-day rest period; given as 3-wk cycles.

Renal Impairment

PO (Adults CCr 30-50 mL/min): Decrease initial dose to 75% of usual.

Availability

Tablets: 150 mg, 500 mg.

capsaicin (kap-**say**-sin)

Axsam, Capsin, Capzasin-P, Dolorac, No Pain-HP, Pain Doctor, Pain-X, R-Gel, Rid a Pain HP, Zostrix, Zostrix-HP

Classification
Therapeutic: nonopioid analgesics (topical)

Indications

Temporary management of pain due to rheumatoid arthritis and osteoarthritis. Treatment of pain associated with postherpetic neuralgia or diabetic neuropathy. **Unlabeled Use:** Treatment of postmastectomy pain syndrome. Treatment of complex regional pain syndrome.

Action

May deplete and prevent the reaccumulation of a chemical (substance P) responsible for transmitting painful impulses from peripheral sites to the CNS. **Therapeutic Effects:** Relief of discomfort associated with painful peripheral syndromes.

Adverse Reactions/Side Effects

Resp: cough. **Derm:** transient burning.

PHYSICAL THERAPY IMPLICATIONS

Examination and Evaluation

- Use appropriate pain scales (visual analogue scales, others) to document whether this drug is successful in helping manage the patient's pain.
- Monitor the application site, and report any prolonged burning sensations or other skin reactions.

Interventions

- Implement appropriate physical agents, therapeutic exercises, and manual techniques to reduce pain and complement the effects of this drug.
- Help patient explore other nonpharmacologic methods to reduce chronic pain, such as relaxation techniques, exercise, counseling, and so forth.

Patient/Client-Related Instruction

- Check that the patient and family or caregivers understand topical application procedures and adhere to the recommended dosing schedule.
- Instruct patient to report any troublesome side effects such as severe or prolonged cough.

Pharmacokinetics

Absorption: Unknown.
Distribution: Unknown.
Metabolism and Excretion: Unknown.
Half-life: Unknown.

TIME/ACTION PROFILE

ROUTE	ONSET	PEAK	DURATION
topical	1–2 wk	2–4 wk*	unknown

*May take up to 6 wk for head and neck neuralgias.

Contraindications/Precautions

Contraindicated in: Hypersensitivity to capsaicin or hot peppers; Not for use near eyes or on open or broken skin.
Use Cautiously in: OB/Lactation/Pedi: Safety not established for pregnant women, breast-feeding infants, or children <2 yr.

Interactions

Drug-Drug: None significant.

Route/Dosage

Topical (Adults and Children ≥2 yr): Apply to affected areas 3–4 times daily.

Availability

Cream: 0.025% OTC, 0.075% OTC. **Gel:** 0.05% OTC. **Lotion:** 0.025% OTC. **Roll-on:** 0.075% OTC. ***In combination with:*** methyl salicylate (Ziks OTC). See Appendix B.

captopril (kap-toe-pril)

Capoten

Classification
Therapeutic: antihypertensives
Pharmacologic: ACE inhibitors

Indications

Alone or with other agents in the management of hypertension. Management of heart failure. Reduction of risk of death, heart failure–related hospitalizations, and development of overt heart failure following myocardial infarction. Treatment of diabetic nephropathy in patients with type 1 diabetes mellitus and retinopathy.

Action

Angiotensin-converting enzyme (ACE) inhibitors block the conversion of angiotensin I to the vasoconstrictor angiotensin II. ACE inhibitors also prevent the degradation of bradykinin and other vasodilatory prostaglandins. ACE inhibitors also increase plasma renin levels and reduce aldosterone levels. Net result is systemic vasodilation. **Therapeutic Effects:** Lowering of blood pressure in patients with hypertension. Improved survival and reduced symptoms in patients with heart failure. Improved survival and reduced development of overt heart failure after myocardial infarction. Decreased progression of diabetic nephropathy with decreased need for transplantation or dialysis.

Adverse Reactions/Side Effects

CNS: dizziness, fatigue, headache, insomnia. **Resp:** cough, **CV:** hypotension, chest pain, palpitations, tachycardia. **GI:** taste disturbances, abdominal pain, anorexia, constipation, diarrhea, nausea, vomiting. **GU:** proteinuria, impaired renal function. **Derm:** ANGIOEDEMA, rashes, pruritus. **F and E:** hyperkalemia. **Hemat:** AGRANULOCYTOSIS, neutropenia. **Misc:** fever.

PHYSICAL THERAPY IMPLICATIONS

Examination and Evaluation

- Watch for signs of angioedema, including rashes, raised patches of red or white skin (welts), burning/itching skin, swelling in the face, and difficulty breathing. Notify physician immediately of these signs.
- Monitor signs of agranulocytosis and neutropenia (fever, sore throat, mucosal lesions, signs of

infection, bruising). Report these signs to the physician immediately.

- Assess blood pressure periodically and compare to normal values (See Appendix F) to help determine antihypertensive effects. Report low blood pressure (hypotension), especially if patient experiences dizziness, fatigue, or syncope.
- Assess signs and symptoms of CHF (dyspnea, rales/crackles, peripheral edema, jugular venous distention, exercise intolerance) to help document whether drug therapy is effective in reducing these symptoms.
- Assess heart rate, ECG, and heart sounds, especially during exercise (See Appendices G, H). Report any rhythm disturbances or symptoms of increased arrhythmias, including palpitations, chest discomfort, shortness of breath, fainting, and fatigue/weakness.
- Monitor signs of high plasma potassium levels (hyperkalemia), including bradycardia, fatigue, weakness, numbness, and tingling. Notify physician because severe cases can lead to life-threatening arrhythmias and paralysis.
- If treating diabetic neuropathy, establish baseline electroneuromyographic values using EMG and nerve conduction at the beginning of drug treatment whenever possible. Periodically reexamine these values to document progress and potential improvement in peripheral nerve function.
- Assess dizziness that might affect gait, balance, and other functional activities (See Appendix C). Report balance problems and functional limitations to the physician, and caution the patient and family/caregivers to guard against falls and trauma.

Interventions

- Implement aerobic exercise and cardiac conditioning programs to augment drug therapy and maintain or improve cardiovascular pump function in patients with heart failure and other cardiac conditions.
- Because of an increased risk of cardiac arrhythmias (tachycardia, others), use caution during aerobic exercise and endurance conditioning. Terminate exercise if patient exhibits untoward symptoms (chest pain, shortness of breath, unusual fatigue), or displays other criteria for exercise termination (See Appendix L).
- Avoid physical therapy interventions that cause systemic vasodilation (large whirlpool, Hubbard tank). Additive effects of this drug and the intervention may cause a dangerous fall in blood pressure.
- To minimize orthostatic hypotension, patient should move slowly when assuming a more upright position.

Patient/Client-Related Instruction

- Remind patients to take medication as directed to control hypertension and other cardiac conditions even if they are asymptomatic.
- Instruct patients with heart failure to weigh themselves every day, and call their physician if they gain 3 lb or more in 1 day or more than 5 lb in 1 week. Sudden weight gain may indicate fluid buildup due to worsening heart failure.
- Counsel patients about additional interventions to help control blood pressure and cardiac dysfunction, including regular exercise, weight loss, sodium restriction, stress reduction, moderation of alcohol consumption, and smoking cessation.
- Instruct patient to report signs of impaired renal function, including decreased urine output, cloudy urine, or sudden weight gain due to fluid retention.
- Instruct patient to notify physician of a prolonged dry cough; drug therapy may need to be altered to resolve this side effect.
- Instruct patient or family/caregivers to report other troublesome side effects such as severe or prolonged headache, insomnia, skin reactions (rash, itching), or GI problems (nausea, vomiting, constipation, diarrhea, loss of appetite, taste disturbances, abdominal pain).

Pharmacokinetics

Absorption: 60–75% absorbed following oral administration (decreased by food).
Distribution: Crosses the placenta; enters breast milk in small amounts.
Metabolism and Excretion: 50% metabolized by the liver to inactive compounds, 50% excreted unchanged in urine.
Half-life: Infants with CHF: 3.3 hr (range 1.2–12.4 hr); Children: 1.5 hr (range 0.98–2.3 hr); Adults: 1.9 hr (increased to 20–40 hr in renal impairment); Adults with CHF: 2.1 hr.

TIME/ACTION PROFILE (effect on blood pressure—single dose*)

ROUTE	ONSET	PEAK	DURATION
PO	15–60 min	60–90 min	6–12 hr

*Full effects may not be noted for several weeks.

Contraindications/Precautions

Contraindicated in: Hypersensitivity; History of angioedema with previous use of ACE inhibitors; OB: Can cause injury or death of fetus—if pregnancy occurs, discontinue immediately; Lactation: Appears in breast milk; patient must discontinue drug or provide alternate to breast milk.

Use Cautiously in: Patients with collagen vascular disease, renal impairment, hypovolemia, hyponatremia, and concurrent diuretic therapy; Surgery/anesthesia (hypotension may be exaggerated); Black patients (monotherapy for hypertension less effective, may require additional therapy; higher risk of angioedema); Women of childbearing potential; Geri: Initial dosage reduction recommended.
Exercise Extreme Caution in: History of angioedema.

Interactions

Drug-Drug: Excessive hypotension may occur with concurrent use of **diuretics**. Additive hypotension with other **antihypertensives**. ↑ risk of hyperkalemia with concurrent use of **potassium supplements, potassium-sparing diuretics, potassium-containing salt substitutes**, or **angiotensin II receptor antagonists**. Antihypertensive response may be blunted by **NSAIDs**. ↑ levels and may ↑ the risk of **lithium** toxicity.
Drug-Natural: Avoid natural licorice (causes sodium and water retention and ↑ potassium loss).
Drug-Food: Food significantly reduces absorption. Administer captopril 1 hr before meals.

Route/Dosage

Note: Use lower doses (½ of those listed) in patients who are sodium and water depleted due to diuretics.

Hypertension

PO (Adults and Adolescents): 12.5–25 mg 2–3 times daily; may be ↑ at 1- to 2-wk intervals up to 150 mg 3 times daily (initiate therapy with 6.25–12.5 mg 2–3 times daily in patients receiving diuretics).

Heart Failure

PO (Adults): 25 mg 3 times daily (6.25–12.5 mg 3 times daily in patients who have been vigorously diuresed); titrated up to target dose of 50 mg 3 times daily (max dose = 450 mg/day).
PO (Children): 0.3 mg/kg—0.5 mg/kg/dose 3 times daily, titrate up to a maximum of 6 mg/kg/day in 2–4 divided doses; *Older Children:* 6.25–12.5 mg/dose q 12–24 hr, titrate up to a maximum of 6 mg/kg/day in 2–4 divided doses.
PO (Infants): 0.15–0.3 mg/kg/dose, titrate up to a maximum of 6 mg/kg/day in 1–4 divided doses.
PO (Neonates): 0.05–0.1 mg/kg/dose q 8–24 hr, may ↑ as needed up to 0.5 mg/kg q 6–24 hr; *Premature neonates:* 0.01 mg/kg/dose q 8–12 hr.

Left Ventricular Dysfunction Post-MI

PO (Adults): 6.25-mg test dose, followed by 12.5 mg 3 times daily; may be ↑ up to 50 mg 3 times daily.

Diabetic Nephropathy

PO (Adults): 25 mg 3 times daily.

Renal Impairment

PO (Adults): ClCr 10–50 mL/min: Administer 75% of dose; ClCr <10 mL/min: Administer 50% of dose.

Availability (generic available)

Tablets: 12.5 mg, 25 mg, 50 mg, 100 mg. ***In combination with:*** hydrochlorothiazide (Capozide). See Appendix B.

carbamazepine

(kar-ba-**maz**-e-peen)

Apo-Carbamazepine, Carbatrol, Epitol, Equetro, Novo-Carbamaz, Tegretol, Tegretol CR, Tegretol-XR, Teril

Classification
Therapeutic: anticonvulsants, mood stabilizers
Pharmacologic: iminostilbenes

Indications

Treatment of tonic-clonic, mixed, and complex-partial seizures. Management of pain in trigeminal neuralgia or diabetic neuropathy. **Equetro only:** Acute mania and mixed mania. **Unlabeled Use:** Other forms of neurogenic pain.

Action

Decreases synaptic transmission in the CNS by affecting sodium channels in neurons. **Therapeutic Effects:** Prevention of seizures. Relief of pain in trigeminal neuralgia. Decreased mania.

Adverse Reactions/Side Effects

CNS: ataxia, drowsiness, fatigue, psychosis, sedation, suicidal behavior or ideation, vertigo. **EENT:** blurred vision, nystagmus, corneal opacities. **Resp:** pneumonitis. **CV:** CHF, edema, hypertension, hypotension, syncope. **GI:** hepatitis, pancreatitis, weight gain. **GU:** hesitancy, urinary retention. **Derm:** photosensitivity, RASHES, STEVENS-JOHNSON SYNDROME, TOXIC EPIDERMAL NECROLYSIS, urticaria. **Endo:** syndrome of inappropriate antidiuretic hormone (SIADH), hyponatremia. **Hemat:** AGRANULOCYTOSIS, APLASTIC ANEMIA, THROMBOCYTOPENIA, eosinophilia, leukopenia. **Misc:** chills, fever, lymphadenopathy, elevated liver enzymes, multiorgan hypersensitivity reactions, hepatic failure (rare).

PHYSICAL THERAPY IMPLICATIONS

Examination and Evaluation

- Monitor skin reactions such as rash, itching/burning skin, hives, exfoliation, and dermatitis. Notify physician immediately because certain skin reactions may indicate serious hypersensitivity reactions (Stevens-Johnson syndrome, toxic epidermal necrosis).
- Be alert for signs of agranulocytosis (fever, sore throat, mucosal lesions, signs of infection), aplastic

anemia (unusual fatigue, weakness, dizziness, pallor), thrombocytopenia (bruising, nose bleeds, bleeding gums), or fatigue and poor health that might be due to other anemias and blood dyscrasias. Report these signs to the physician immediately. Periodic blood tests may be needed to monitor WBC and RBC counts.

- Document the number, duration, and severity of seizures to help determine if this drug is effective in reducing seizure activity.
- If used to treat trigeminal neuralgia or other types of neurogenic pain, assess pain using visual analogue scales or other appropriate pain scales to document whether this drug is successful in helping manage the patient's pain.
- If treating acute or mixed mania, monitor the patient's mood and behavior and report changes in manic symptoms (excitement, agitation) to help determine drug effectiveness.
- Assess vertigo, ataxia, or syncope that might affect gait, balance, and other functional activities (See Appendix C). Report balance problems and functional limitations to the physician, and caution the patient and family/caregivers to guard against falls and trauma.
- Be alert for suicidal thoughts and ideology; notify physician immediately if patient exhibits signs of depression or other changes in mood and behavior.
- Monitor daytime drowsiness, confusion, agitation, or psychosis-like reactions. Repeated or excessive symptoms may require change in dose or medication.
- Assess blood pressure (BP) and compare to normal values (See Appendix F). Report changes in BP, either a problematic decrease in BP (hypotension) or a sustained increase in BP (hypertension).
- Assess signs of congestive heart failure such as dyspnea, rales/crackles, peripheral edema, jugular venous distention, and exercise intolerance. Report these signs to the physician.
- Assess peripheral edema using girth measurements, volume displacement, and measurement of pitting edema (See Appendix N). Report increased swelling in feet and ankles or a sudden increase in body weight due to fluid retention.
- Be alert for signs of pneumonitis, including dyspnea, cough, shortness of breath, fever, and rales. Report these signs to the physician.
- Monitor signs of fluid-electrolyte imbalance due to SIADH. SIADH causes increased water retention that leads to relatively low sodium concentration (hyponatremia). Symptoms include confusion, lethargy, weakness, myoclonus, and depressed reflexes. Severe or sudden onset may also cause seizures, ataxia, nystagmus, tremor, dysarthria, dysphagia, and coma. Notify physician if these signs occur.
- Periodically assess body weight and other anthropometric measures (body mass index, body composition). Report a rapid or unexplained weight gain or increased body fat.

Interventions

- Guard against falls and trauma (hip fractures, head injury, and so forth), especially if vertigo, syncope, or ataxia affects gait and balance. Implement fall-prevention strategies, especially if balance is impaired (See Appendix E).
- To minimize orthostatic hypotension, patient should move slowly when assuming a more upright position.
- Because of the risk of CHF and abnormal BP responses, use caution during aerobic exercise and other forms of therapeutic exercise. Assess exercise tolerance frequently (BP, heart rate, fatigue levels), and terminate exercise immediately if any untoward responses occur (See Appendix L).
- Causes photosensitivity; use care if administering UV treatments. Advise patient to avoid direct sunlight and use sunscreens and protective clothing.

Patient/Client-Related Instruction

- Advise patient to avoid alcohol and other CNS depressants because of the increased risk of sedation and adverse effects.
- Advise patients on prolonged antiseizure therapy not to discontinue medication without consulting their physician. Abrupt withdrawal may cause increased seizures.
- Advise patient about the risk of daytime drowsiness and decreased attention and mental focus. Use care if driving or in other activities that require strong concentration and fast responses.
- Advise patient about the likelihood of GI reactions, and to report signs of hepatotoxicity (anorexia, abdominal pain, severe nausea and vomiting, yellow skin or eyes, fever, sore throat, malaise, weakness, facial edema, lethargy, unusual bleeding or bruising) or pancreatitis (upper abdominal pain after eating, indigestion, weight loss, oily stools).
- Instruct patient and family/caregivers to report other troublesome side effects such as severe or prolonged chills, fever, swollen/tender lymph nodes, visual problems (double vision, nystagmus), or urinary problems (hesitancy, retention).

Pharmacokinetics

Absorption: Absorption is slow but complete. Suspension produces earlier, higher peak and lower trough levels.

Distribution: Widely distributed. Crosses the blood-brain barrier. Crosses the placenta rapidly and enters breast milk in high concentrations.
Protein Binding: *Carbamazepine*—75–90%; *epoxide*—50%.
Metabolism and Excretion: Extensively metabolized in the liver by cytochrome P450 3A4 to active epoxide metabolite; epoxide metabolite has anticonvulsant and antineuralgic activity.
Half-life: *Carbamazepine:* single dose—25–65 hr; chronic dosing—*Children*—8–14 hr; *Adults*—12–17 hr; *epoxide:* 34 ± 9 hr.

TIME/ACTION PROFILE (anticonvulsant activity)

ROUTE	ONSET	PEAK	DURATION
PO	up to one month*	4–5 hr†	6–12 hr
PO-ER	up to one month*	2–3–12 hr†	12 hr

*Onset of antineuralgic activity is 8–72 hr.
†Listed for tablets; peak level occurs 1.5 hr after a chronic dose of suspension.

Contraindications/Precautions

Contraindicated in: Hypersensitivity; Bone marrow suppression; Concomitant use or use within 14 days of MAO inhibitors; OB: Use only during pregnancy if potential benefits outweigh risks to the fetus; additional vitamin K during last weeks of pregnancy has been recommended; Lactation: Discontinue drug or bottle feed.
Use Cautiously in: All patients (may ↑ risk of suicidal thoughts/behaviors); Cardiac or hepatic disease; Renal failure (dosing adjustment required for ClCr <10 mL/min; Increased intraocular pressure; Geri: Older men with prostatic hyperplasia may be at increased risk for acute urinary retention or difficulty initiating stream.
Exercise Extreme Caution in: Patients positive for HLA-B*1502 allele (unless benefits clearly outweigh the risks).

Interactions

Drug-Drug: May ↑ metabolism of and therefore ↓ levels/effectiveness of **corticosteroids, doxycycline, felbamate, quinidine, warfarin, estrogen-containing contraceptives, barbiturates, cyclosporine, benzodiazepines, theophylline, lamotrigine, phenytoin, topiramate, valproic acid, bupropion,** and **haloperidol. Danazol** ↑ blood levels (avoid concurrent use if possible). Concurrent use (within 2 wk) of **MAO inhibitors** may result in hyperpyrexia, hypertension, seizures, and death. **Verapamil, diltiazem, propoxyphene, itraconazole, ketoconazole, erythromycin, clarithromycin, SSRIs, antidepressants,** or **cimetidine** may inhibit the hepatic metabolism or carbamazepine and ↑ levels; may cause toxicity. Enzyme inducers such as **rifampin, phenobarbital, phenytoin, primidone,** and **methsuximide** may ↓ serum concentration of carbamazepine. May ↑ risk of hepatotoxicity from **isoniazid. Felbamate** ↓ carbamazepine levels but ↑ levels of active metabolite. May ↓ effectiveness and ↑ risk of toxicity from **acetaminophen**. May ↑ risk of CNS toxicity from **lithium**. May ↓ duration of action of **nondepolarizing neuromuscular blocking agents**.
Drug-Food: Grapefruit juice ↑ serum levels and oral bioavailability by 40% and therefore may ↑ effects.

Route/Dosage

PO (Adults): *Anticonvulsant*—200 mg twice daily (tablets) or 100 mg 4 times daily (suspension); ↑ by 200 mg/day q 7 days until therapeutic levels are achieved (range is 600–1200 mg/day in divided doses q 6–8 hr; not to exceed 1 g/day in 12–15 yr olds. Extended-release products are given twice daily (XR, CR). *Antineuralgic*—100 mg twice daily or 50 mg 4 times daily (suspension); ↑ by up to 200 mg/day until pain is relieved, then maintenance dose of 200–1200 mg/day in divided doses (usual range, 400–800 mg/day).
PO (Children 6–12 yr): 100 mg twice daily (tablets) or 50 mg 4 times daily (suspension) ↑ by 100 mg weekly until therapeutic levels are obtained (usual range 400–800 mg/day; not to exceed 1 g/day). Extended-release products (XR, CR) are given twice daily.
PO (Children <6 yr): 10–20 mg/kg/day in 2–3 divided doses; may be ↑ at weekly intervals until optimal response and therapeutic levels are achieved. Usual maintenance dose is 250–350 mg/day (not to exceed 35 mg/kg/day).

Availability (generic available)

Tablets: 200 mg. **Chewable tablets:** 100 mg, 200 mg. **Extended-release capsules:** 100 mg, 200 mg, 300 mg. **Extended-release tablets:** 100 mg, 200 mg, 400 mg. **Oral suspension (citrus/vanilla flavor):** 100 mg/5 mL.

HIGH ALERT

carboplatin (kar-boe-pla-tin)

Paraplatin, Paraplatin-AQ

Classification
Therapeutic: antineoplastics
Pharmacologic: alkylating agents

Indications

Advanced ovarian carcinoma (with other agents). Palliative treatment of ovarian carcinoma unresponsive to other modalities.

Action

Inhibits DNA synthesis by producing cross-linking of parent DNA strands (cell-cycle phase–nonspecific).

Therapeutic Effects: Death of rapidly replicating cells, particularly malignant ones.

Adverse Reactions/Side Effects

CNS: weakness. **EENT:** ototoxicity. **GI:** abdominal pain, nausea, vomiting, constipation, diarrhea, hepatitis, stomatitis. **GU:** gonadal suppression, nephrotoxicity. **Derm:** alopecia, rash. **F and E:** hypocalcemia, hypokalemia, hypomagnesemia, hyponatremia. **Hemat:** ANEMIA, LEUKOPENIA, THROMBOCYTOPENIA. **Metab:** hyperuricemia. **Neuro:** peripheral neuropathy. **Misc:** HYPERSENSITIVITY REACTIONS, INCLUDING ANAPHYLAXIS-LIKE REACTIONS.

PHYSICAL THERAPY IMPLICATIONS

Examination and Evaluation

- Monitor signs of hypersensitivity reactions, including anaphylaxis. Reactions include pulmonary symptoms (tightness in the throat and chest, wheezing, cough, dyspnea) and skin reactions (rash, pruritus, urticaria, burning skin). Notify physician or nursing staff immediately if these reactions occur.
- Monitor signs of leukopenia (fever, sore throat, signs of infection), thrombocytopenia (bruising, nose bleeds, bleeding gums), or unusual weakness and fatigue that might be due to anemia or other blood dyscrasias. Notify physician of these signs immediately.
- Monitor neuromuscular signs of electrolyte imbalances (hypocalcemia, hypokalemia, hyponatremia, hypomagnesemia), including headache, lethargy, weakness, cramping, and muscle hyperexcitability and tetany. Notify physician immediately if these signs occur.
- Assess signs of peripheral neuropathy such as numbness, tingling, and decreased muscle strength. Establish baseline electroneuromyographic values using EMG and nerve conduction at the beginning of drug treatment whenever possible, and reexamine these values periodically to document drug-induced changes in peripheral nerve function.
- Monitor signs of ototoxicity such as hearing loss, tinnitus, disturbed balance, and vertigo. Report these signs to the physician.

Interventions

- For patients who are medically able to begin exercise, implement appropriate resistive exercises and aerobic training to maintain muscle strength and aerobic capacity during cancer chemotherapy, or to help restore function after chemotherapy.
- Guard against falls and trauma (hip fractures, head injury). Implement fall prevention strategies, especially if patient exhibits balance deficits related to ototoxicity (See Appendix E).

Patient/Client-Related Instruction

- Advise patient to guard against infection (frequent hand washing, etc.), and to avoid crowds and contact with persons with contagious diseases.
- Make sure patient and family or caregivers understand the need to immediately report allergic responses or signs of blood dyscrasias as listed above (see Examination and Evaluation).
- Advise patient about the likelihood of GI reactions such as nausea, vomiting, diarrhea, constipation, abdominal pain, and irritation of the oral mucosa. Instruct patient to report severe or prolonged GI problems, and to immediately report signs of drug-induced hepatitis, including anorexia, abdominal pain, severe nausea and vomiting, yellow skin or eyes, skin rashes, flu-like symptoms, and muscle/joint pain.
- Advise patient and family/caregivers that fatigue and weakness are likely and may be severe. Functional abilities may be limited, and patient may need to use assistive devices during ambulation.
- Instruct patient to report signs of nephrotoxicity, including hematuria, increased urinary frequency, cloudy urine, and decreased urine output.
- Advise patient that skin rash and hair loss are likely. Report severe or unexpected skin reactions to the physician.

Pharmacokinetics

Absorption: IV administration results in complete bioavailability.
Distribution: Unknown.
Protein Binding: Platinum is irreversibly bound to plasma proteins.
Metabolism and Excretion: Excreted mostly by the kidneys.
Half-life: *Carboplatin*—2.6–5.9 hr (increased in renal impairment); *platinum*—5 days.

TIME/ACTION PROFILE (effects on blood counts)

ROUTE	ONSET	PEAK	DURATION
IV	unknown	21 days	28 days

Contraindications/Precautions

Contraindicated in: Hypersensitivity to carboplatin, cisplatin, or mannitol; OB: Pregnancy or lactation.
Use Cautiously in: Hearing loss; Electrolyte abnormalities; Renal impairment (dose reduction recommended if creatinine <60 mL/min); Active infections; Diminished bone marrow reserve (dose reduction recommended); Other chronic debilitating illnesses; Geri: ↑ risk of thrombocytopenia, consider renal function in dose determination; Patients with child-bearing potential; Pedi: Safe use in children not established.

Interactions

Drug-Drug: ↑ nephrotoxicity and ototoxicity with other **nephrotoxic** and **ototoxic drugs (aminoglycosides, loop diuretics)**. ↑ bone marrow depression with other **bone marrow–depressing drugs** or **radiation therapy**. May ↓ antibody response to **live-virus vaccines** and ↑ risk of adverse reactions.

Route/Dosage

Other dosing formulas are used.

IV (Adults): *Initial treatment*—300 mg/m² with cyclophosphamide at 4-wk intervals. *Treatment of refractory tumors*—360 mg/m² as a single dose; may be repeated at 4-wk intervals, depending on response.

Renal Impairment

IV (Adults): *CCr 41–59 mL/min*—initial dose 250 mg/m²; *CCr 16–40 mL/min*—initial dose 200 mg/m².

Availability (generic available)

Lyophilized powder for injection: 50-mg vials, 150-mg vials, 450-mg vials. **Aqueous solution for injection:** 50 mg/5 mL vial, 150 mg/15 mL vial, 450 mg/45 mL vial, 600 mg/60 mL vial.

carisoprodol (kar-i-sop-roe-dole)

Soma, Vanadom

Classification

Therapeutic: skeletal muscle relaxants (centrally acting)

Pharmacologic: carbamate derivative

Indications

Adjunct to rest and physical therapy in the treatment of muscle spasm associated with acute painful musculoskeletal conditions.

Action

Skeletal muscle relaxation, probably due to CNS depression. **Therapeutic Effects:** Skeletal muscle relaxation.

Adverse Reactions/Side Effects

CNS: dizziness, drowsiness, agitation, ataxia, depression, headache, insomnia, irritability, syncope. **Resp:** asthma attacks. **CV:** hypotension, tachycardia. **GI:** epigastric distress, hiccups, nausea, vomiting. **Derm:** flushing, rashes. **Hemat:** eosinophilia, leukopenia. **Misc:** ANAPHYLACTIC SHOCK, fever, psychologic dependence, severe idiosyncratic reaction.

PHYSICAL THERAPY IMPLICATIONS

Examination and Evaluation

- Be alert for signs of anaphylactic shock, including pulmonary symptoms (tightness in the throat and chest, wheezing, cough, dyspnea), skin reactions (rash, pruritus, urticaria, flushed or pale skin), dizziness, fainting, tachycardia, and GI problems (nausea, vomiting, diarrhea). Seek immediate medical assistance if patient develops these signs.
- Assess patient's pain, stiffness, and ROM to help document antispasm effects.
- Assess heart rate, ECG, and heart sounds, especially during exercise (See Appendices G, H). Report any rhythm disturbances such as tachycardia or symptoms of increased arrhythmias, including palpitations, chest discomfort, shortness of breath, fainting, and fatigue/weakness.
- Assess blood pressure (BP) periodically and compare to normal values (See Appendix F). Report low BP (hypotension), especially if patient experiences dizziness, syncope, or other symptoms.
- Assess symptoms of asthma attacks and bronchospasm (wheezing, coughing, tightness in chest, dyspnea). Perform pulmonary function tests to quantify suspected changes in ventilation and respiration (See Appendices I, J, K).
- Monitor for signs of eosinophilia (fatigue, weakness, myalgia) or leukopenia (fever, sore throat, signs of infection). Report these signs to the physician.
- Assess dizziness and ataxia that might affect gait, balance, and other functional activities (See Appendix C). Report balance problems and functional limitations to the physician, and caution the patient and family/caregivers to guard against falls and trauma.
- Be alert for agitation, irritability, depression, or other alterations in mood and behavior. Notify physician promptly if these symptoms become problematic.

Interventions

- Implement appropriate manual therapy techniques, physical agents, and therapeutic exercises to reduce pain and wean patient off muscle relaxants as soon as possible.
- Help patient explore other nonpharmacologic methods to reduce chronic pain, such as relaxation techniques, exercise, counseling, and so forth.
- Implement fall-prevention strategies, especially if balance is impaired (See Appendix E).
- Because of the risk of cardiac arrhythmias and abnormal BP responses, use caution during aerobic exercise and other forms of therapeutic exercise. Terminate exercise if patient exhibits untoward symptoms (chest pain, shortness of breath, unusual fatigue), or displays other criteria for exercise termination (See Appendix L).
- To minimize orthostatic hypotension, patient should move slowly when assuming a more upright position.

C

Patient/Client-Related Instruction

- Advise patient and family or caregiver about the signs of anaphylactic shock (See above under Examination and Evaluation), and to seek immediate medical assistance if these signs develop, or if patient exhibits any other sudden, severe allergy-like responses (idiosyncratic reactions).
- Inform patient that long-term use can cause tolerance and physical/psychologic dependence; encourage adherence to physical therapy so that drug therapy can be discontinued as soon as possible.
- Inform patient that this drug may cause severe drowsiness, dizziness, and reduced psychomotor skills. Patients should avoid driving or other activities that require concentration and fast reactions.
- Advise patient to avoid alcohol and other CNS depressants because of the increased risk of sedation and adverse effects.
- Warn patient about anticholinergic effects such as dry mouth, constipation, urinary retention, sedation, and weakness; anticholinergic effects are often more severe in older adults.
- Instruct patient and family/caregivers to report other troublesome side effects such as severe or prolonged headache, fever, skin reactions (rash, flushing), or GI problems (nausea, vomiting, heartburn, hiccups).

Pharmacokinetics

Absorption: Well absorbed after oral administration.
Distribution: Crosses the placenta; high concentrations in breast milk.
Metabolism and Excretion: Mostly metabolized by the liver.
Half-life: 8 hr.

TIME/ACTION PROFILE (skeletal muscle relaxation)

ROUTE	ONSET	PEAK	DURATION
PO	30 min	unknown	4–6 hr

Contraindications/Precautions

Contraindicated in: Hypersensitivity to carisoprodol or to meprobamate; Porphyria or suspected porphyria.
Use Cautiously in: Severe liver or kidney disease; OB/Lactation/Pedi: Safety not established for pregnant women, breast-feeding infants, or children <16 yr; Geri: Poorly tolerated due to anticholinergic effects. Appears on Beers" list.

Interactions

Drug-Drug: Additive CNS depression with other **CNS depressants**, including **alcohol**, **antihistamines**, **opioid analgesics**, and **sedative/hypnotics**.
Drug-Natural: Concomitant use of **kava-kava**, **valerian**, **skullcap**, **chamomile**, or **hops** can increase CNS depression.

Route/Dosage

PO (Adults ≥16 yr): 250–350 mg 4 times daily for no >2–3 wk.

Availability (generic available)

Tablets: 250 mg, 350 mg. ***In combination with:*** aspirin (Soma compound) and codeine. See Appendix B.

HIGH ALERT

carmustine (kar-mus-teen)

BCNU, BiCNU, Gliadel

Classification
Therapeutic: antineoplastics
Pharmacologic: alkylating agents

Indications

Alone or with other treatments (surgery, radiation) in the management of: Brain tumors; Multiple myeloma; Hodgkin's disease; Other lymphomas.

Action

Inhibits DNA and RNA synthesis (cell-cycle phase–nonspecific). **Therapeutic Effects:** Death of rapidly replicating cells, especially malignant ones.

Adverse Reactions/Side Effects

Resp: PULMONARY FIBROSIS, pulmonary infiltrates. **GI:** hepatotoxicity, nausea, vomiting, anorexia, diarrhea, esophagitis. **GU:** renal failure. **Derm:** alopecia. **Hemat:** LEUKOPENIA, THROMBOCYTOPENIA, anemia. **Local:** pain at IV site.

PHYSICAL THERAPY IMPLICATIONS

Examination and Evaluation

- Assess pulmonary function periodically by measuring lung volumes, breath sounds, and respiratory rate (See Appendices I, J, K). Notify physician or nursing staff immediately if patient experiences signs of pulmonary fibrosis or pulmonary infiltrates (dry cough, dyspnea, chest pain, shortness of breath, cyanosis).
- Watch for signs of leukopenia (fever, sore throat, signs of infection), thrombocytopenia (bruising, nose bleeds, bleeding gums), or unusual weakness and fatigue that might be due to anemia. Report these signs to the physician or nursing staff immediately.
- Monitor signs of renal failure, including decreased urine output, increased blood pressure, muscle

cramps/twitching, edema/weight gain from fluid retention, yellowish brown skin, and confusion that progresses to seizures and coma. Report these signs to the physician or nursing staff immediately.

- Monitor IV injection site for pain, swelling, and irritation. Report prolonged or excessive injection site reactions to the physician.

Interventions

- For patients who are medically able to begin exercise, implement appropriate resistive exercises and aerobic training to maintain muscle strength and aerobic capacity during cancer chemotherapy or to help restore function after chemotherapy.
- Because of the risk of pulmonary fibrosis and blood dyscrasias, use caution during aerobic exercise and other forms of therapeutic exercise. Assess exercise tolerance frequently (blood pressure, heart rate, fatigue levels), and terminate exercise immediately if any untoward responses occur (See Appendix L).

Patient/Client-Related Instruction

- Advise patient about the likelihood of GI reactions (nausea, vomiting, diarrhea, heartburn, loss of appetite). Instruct patient to also report signs of hepatotoxicity, including abdominal pain, severe nausea and vomiting, yellow skin or eyes, fever, sore throat, malaise, weakness, facial edema, lethargy, and unusual bleeding or bruising.
- Advise patient that hair loss and other skin reactions (rash, pruritus) are likely. Report severe or unexpected skin reactions to the physician.
- Advise patient to guard against infection (frequent hand washing, etc.), and avoid crowds and contact with persons with contagious diseases.

Pharmacokinetics

Absorption: Following IV administration, absorption is complete. Following implantation, action is primarily local.
Distribution: Highly lipid soluble; readily penetrates CSF. Enters breast milk.
Metabolism and Excretion: Rapidly metabolized. Some metabolites have antineoplastic activity.
Half-life: *Biologic*—15–30 min; *chemical*—5 min.

TIME/ACTION PROFILE (effect on platelet counts)

ROUTE	ONSET	PEAK	DURATION
IV	days	4–5 wk	6 wk

Contraindications/Precautions

Contraindicated in: Hypersensitivity; Pregnancy or lactation.
Use Cautiously in: Infections; Depressed bone marrow reserve; Geriatric patients (consider age-related decrease in body mass, renal/hepatic/cardiovascular function, concurrent medications, and chronic illnesses); Impaired pulmonary, hepatic, or renal function; Other chronic debilitating illnesses; Patients with childbearing potential.

Interactions

Drug-Drug: ↑ bone marrow depression with other **antineoplastics** or **radiation therapy. Smoking** ↑ risk of pulmonary toxicity. May ↓ antibody response to **live-virus vaccines** and ↑ risk of adverse reactions. Myelosuppression may be ↑ by **cimetidine**.

Route/Dosage

IV (Adults and Children): 150–200 mg/m² single dose every 6–8 wk *or* 75–100 mg/m²/day for 2 days q 6 wk *or* 40 mg/m²/day for 5 days q 6 wk.
Intracavitary: (Adults): Up to 61.6 mg (8 implants) placed in cavity created during surgical resection of brain tumor.

Availability

Injection: 100-mg vial. **Intracavitary wafer:** 7.7 mg in packages of 8.

carvedilol (kar-ve-dil-ole)

Coreg, Coreg CR

Classification
Therapeutic: antihypertensives
Pharmacologic: beta blockers

Indications

Hypertension. CHF (ischemic or cardiomyopathic) with digoxin, diuretics, and ACE inhibitors. Left ventricular dysfunction after myocardial infarction.

Action

Blocks stimulation of $beta_1$ (myocardial) and $beta_2$ (pulmonary, vascular, and uterine)–adrenergic receptor sites. Also has alpha1 blocking activity, which may result in orthostatic hypotension. **Therapeutic Effects:** Decreased heart rate and blood pressure. Improved cardiac output, slowing of the progression of CHF and decreased risk of death.

Adverse Reactions/Side Effects

CNS: dizziness, fatigue, weakness, anxiety, depression, drowsiness, insomnia, memory loss, mental status changes, nervousness, nightmares. **EENT:** blurred vision, dry eyes, nasal stuffiness. **Resp:** bronchospasm, wheezing. **CV:** BRADYCARDIA, CHF, PULMONARY EDEMA. **GI:** diarrhea, constipation, nausea. **GU:** erectile dysfunction, decreased libido. **Derm:** itching, rashes. **Endo:** hyperglycemia, hypoglycemia. **MS:** arthralgia, back pain, muscle cramps. **Neuro:** paresthesia. **Misc:** drug-induced lupus syndrome.

PHYSICAL THERAPY IMPLICATIONS

Examination and Evaluation

- Assess signs and symptoms of CHF, including dyspnea, rales/crackles, peripheral edema, jugular venous distention, and exercise intolerance. Document changes in these symptoms to help determine whether drug therapy is effective in treating CHF.
- Assess any breathing problems or signs of pulmonary edema, including cough, shortness of breath, bronchospasm, chest pain, and labored breathing. Monitor pulse oximetry and perform pulmonary function tests (See Appendices I, J, K) to quantify suspected changes in ventilation and respiratory function. Repeated or prolonged bronchoconstriction may require a change in dose or medication (e.g., switch to a more cardioselective beta blocker).
- Assess heart rate, ECG, and heart sounds, especially during exercise (See Appendices G, H). Report an unusually slow heart rate (bradycardia) or signs of other arrhythmias, including palpitations, chest discomfort, shortness of breath, fainting, and fatigue/weakness.
- Be alert for signs of hypoglycemia (weakness, malaise, irritability, fatigue) or hyperglycemia (drowsiness, fruity breath, increased urination, unusual thirst). Medication may mask some signs of hypoglycemia, but dizziness and sweating may still occur. Patients with diabetes mellitus should check blood glucose levels frequently.
- Assess any back or joint pain to rule out musculoskeletal pathology; that is, try to determine if pain is drug induced rather than caused by anatomic or biomechanical problems.
- Assess signs of paresthesia (numbness, tingling) or muscle cramping. Perform objective tests, including electroneuromyography and sensory testing to document any drug-related neuropathic changes.
- Assess dizziness and drowsiness that might affect gait, balance, and other functional activities (See Appendix C). Report balance problems and functional limitations to the physician, and caution the patient and family/caregivers to guard against falls and trauma.
- Monitor mood and personality changes, including depression, anxiety, nervousness, memory loss, or other changes in mental status. Notify physician if these changes become problematic.
- Monitor excessive fatigue or weakness. Beta blockers often cause some degree of fatigue and weakness, but any sudden or severe change in muscle strength or energy levels should be reported.
- Monitor signs of drug-induced lupus syndrome, including increased blood pressure (BP), fever, joint pain, skin rashes, and redness/irritation of the eye (uveitis). Notify physician promptly if these signs appear.

Interventions

- Because of an increased risk of cardiac arrhythmias, CHF, and pulmonary edema, use extreme caution during aerobic exercise and endurance conditioning. Terminate exercise if patient exhibits untoward symptoms (chest pain, shortness of breath, unusual fatigue), or displays other criteria for exercise termination (See Appendix L).
- Establish aerobic exercise workloads that account for the effects of beta blockers on heart rate. Some heart rate (HR) guidelines may not be appropriate because beta blockers typically decrease maximal HR by 20–30 bpm. Use other guidelines such as rating of perceived exertion (RPE, modified Borg scale) to determine exercise workloads.
- To minimize orthostatic hypotension, patient should move slowly when assuming a more upright position.

Patient/Client-Related Instruction

- Remind patients to take medication as directed to control cardiac function even if they are asymptomatic.
- Instruct patients with heart failure to weigh themselves every day, and call their physician if they gain 3 lb or more in 1 day or more than 5 lb in 1 week. Sudden weight gain may indicate fluid buildup due to worsening heart failure.
- Counsel patients about additional interventions to help control cardiac arrhythmias, including regular exercise, caffeine restriction, stress reduction, moderation of alcohol consumption, and smoking cessation.
- Instruct patient or family/caregivers to report other troublesome side effects such as severe or prolonged insomnia, nightmares, blurred vision, dry eyes, stuffy nose, sexual problems (decreased libido, erectile dysfunction), skin reactions (rash, itching), or GI problems (nausea, constipation, diarrhea).

Pharmacokinetics

Absorption: Well absorbed but rapidly undergoes extensive first-pass hepatic metabolism, resulting in 25–35% bioavailability. Food slows absorption.
Distribution: Unknown.
Protein Binding: 98%.
Metabolism and Excretion: Extensively metabolized, excreted in feces via bile, <2% excreted unchanged in urine.
Half-life: 7–10 hr.

TIME/ACTION PROFILE (cardiovascular effects)

ROUTE	ONSET	PEAK	DURATION
PO	within 1 hr	1–2 hr	12 hr
PO-CR	unknown	5 hr	24 hr

Contraindications/Precautions

Contraindicated in: Pulmonary edema; Cardiogenic shock; Bradycardia, heart block, or sick sinus syndrome (unless a pacemaker is in place); Uncompensated CHF requiring IV inotropic agents (wean before starting carvedilol); Severe hepatic impairment; Asthma or other bronchospastic disorders.

Use Cautiously in: CHF (condition may deteriorate during initial therapy); Renal impairment; Hepatic impairment; Diabetes mellitus (may mask signs of hypoglycemia); Thyrotoxicosis (may mask symptoms); Peripheral vascular disease; History of severe allergic reactions (intensity of reactions may be increased); OB: Crosses placenta and may cause fetal/neonatal bradycardia, hypotension, hypoglycemia, or respiratory depression); Lactation/Pedi: Safety not established; Geri: Increased sensitivity to beta blockers; initial dosage reduction recommended.

Interactions

Drug-Drug: General anesthetics, IV phenytoin, diltiazem, and **verapamil** may cause ↑ myocardial depression. ↑ risk of bradycardia with **digoxin.** ↑ hypotension may occur with other **antihypertensives**, acute ingestion of **alcohol**, or **nitrates**. Concurrent use with **clonidine** ↑ hypotension and bradycardia. May ↑ withdrawal phenomenon from **clonidine** (discontinue carvedilol first). Concurrent administration of **thyroid preparations** may ↓ effectiveness. May alter the effectiveness of **insulins** or **oral hypoglycemic agents** (dose adjustments may be necessary). May ↓ effectiveness of **theophylline**. May ↓ beneficial $beta_1$-cardiovascular effects of **dopamine** or **dobutamine**. Use cautiously within 14 days of **MAO inhibitor** therapy (may result in hypotension/bradycardia). **Cimetidine** may ↑ toxicity from carvedilol. Concurrent **NSAIDs** may ↓ antihypertensive action. Effectiveness may be ↓ by **rifampin**. May ↑ serum **digoxin** levels. May ↑ blood levels of **cyclosporine** (monitor blood levels).

Route/Dosage

PO (Adults): *Hypertension*—6.25 mg twice daily, may be increased q 7–14 days up to 25 mg twice daily or *extended-release*—20 mg once daily, dose may be doubled every 7–14 days up to 80 mg once daily; *CHF*—3.125 mg twice daily for 2 wk; may be increased to 6.25 mg twice daily. Dose may be doubled q 2 wk as tolerated (not to exceed 25 mg twice daily in patients <85 kg or 50 mg twice daily in patients >85 kg *or extended-release*—10 mg once daily, dose may be doubled every 2 wks as tolerated up to 80 mg once daily; *Left ventricular dysfunction after MI*—6.25 mg twice daily, increase after 3–10 days to 12.5 twice daily, then to target dose of 25 mg twice daily; some patients may require lower initial doses and slower titration *or extended-release*—20 mg once daily, dose may be doubled every 3–10 days up to 80 mg once daily.

Availability (generic available)

Tablets: 3.125 mg, 6.25 mg, 12.5 mg, 25 mg. **Extended-release capsules:** 10 mg, 20 mg, 40 mg, 80 mg.

caspofungin (kas-po-fun-gin)

Cancidas

Classification

Therapeutic: antifungals (systemic)
Pharmacologic: echinocandins

Indications

Invasive aspergillosis refractory to, or intolerant of, other therapies. Candidemia and associated serious infections (intra-abdominal abscesses, peritonitis, pleural space infections). Esophageal candidiasis. Suspected fungal infections in febrile neutropenic patients.

Action

Inhibits the synthesis of β (1,3)-D-glucan, a necessary component of the fungal cell wall. **Therapeutic Effects:** Death of susceptible fungi.

Adverse Reactions/Side Effects

CNS: headache. **GI:** diarrhea, nausea, vomiting. **Derm:** flushing. **Local:** venous irritation at injection site. **Misc:** ALLERGIC REACTIONS, INCLUDING ANAPHYLAXIS, fever.

PHYSICAL THERAPY IMPLICATIONS

Examination and Evaluation

- Monitor signs of allergic reactions and anaphylaxis, including pulmonary symptoms (tightness in the throat and chest, wheezing, cough, dyspnea) or skin reactions (rash, pruritus, urticaria). Notify physician or nursing staff immediately if these reactions occur.
- Monitor IV injection site for pain, swelling, and irritation. Report prolonged or excessive injection-site reactions to the physician.

Interventions

- Always wash hands thoroughly and disinfect equipment (whirlpools, electrotherapeutic devices, treatment tables, and so forth) to help prevent the spread of infection. Employ universal precautions or isolation procedures as indicated for specific patients.

Patient/Client-Related Instruction

- Instruct patient to report other troublesome side effects such as prolonged or severe headache, fever, flushing, or GI reactions (diarrhea, nausea, vomiting).

Pharmacokinetics

Absorption: IV administration results in complete bioavailability.
Distribution: Widely distributed to tissues.
Protein Binding: 97%.
Metabolism and Excretion: Slowly and extensively metabolized; <1.5% excreted unchanged in urine.
Half-life: Polyphasic: β *phase*—9–11 hr; γ *phase*—40–50 hr.

TIME/ACTION PROFILE

ROUTE	ONSET	PEAK	DURATION
IV	unknown	end of infusion	24 hr

Contraindications/Precautions

Contraindicated in: Hypersensitivity; Concurrent use with cyclosporine.
Use Cautiously in: Moderate hepatic impairment (decreased maintenance dose recommended); Pedi: Children <3 mo (safety not established).

Interactions

Drug-Drug: Concurrent use with **cyclosporine** is not recommended due to ↑ risk of hepatic toxicity. May ↓ blood levels and effects of **tacrolimus**. Blood levels and effectiveness may be ↓ by **rifampin**; maintenance dose should be ↑ to 70 mg (in patients with normal liver function). Blood levels and effectiveness may be also be ↓ by **efavirenz, nelfinavir, nevirapine, phenytoin, dexamethasone,** or **carbamazepine.** An ↑ in the maintenance dose to 70 mg should be considered in patients who are not clinically responding.

Route/Dosage

IV (Adults): 70 mg initially followed by 50 mg daily, duration determined by clinical situation and response; *Esophageal candidiasis*—50 mg daily, duration determined by clinical situation and response.
IV (Children ≥3 mo): 70 mg/m^2 (max 70 mg) initially followed by 50 mg/m^2 daily (max 70 mg/day), duration determined by clinical situation and response.

Moderate Hepatic Impairment (Child-Pugh Score 5–6)

IV (Adults): 70 mg initially followed by 35 mg daily, duration determined by clinical situation and response.

Availability

Powder for injection: 50 mg/vial, 70 mg/vial.

cefaclor (sef-a-klor)

Raniclor, ✱Ceclor

Classification
Therapeutic: anti-infectives
Pharmacologic: second-generation cephalosporins

Indications

Treatment of the following infections caused by susceptible organisms: Respiratory tract infections; Skin and skin structure infections; Urinary tract infections; Otitis media.

Action

Binds to bacterial cell wall membrane, causing cell death. **Therapeutic Effects:** Bactericidal action against susceptible bacteria. **Spectrum:** Similar to that of first-generation cephalosporins but has increased activity against several other gram-negative pathogens, including *Haemophilus influenzae*, *Escherichia coli*, *Klebsiella pneumoniae*, *Proteus mirabilis*. Not active against methicillin-resistant staphylococci or enterococci.

Adverse Reactions/Side Effects

CNS: SEIZURES (VERY HIGH DOSES). **GI:** PSEUDOMEMBRANOUS COLITIS, diarrhea, nausea, vomiting. **Derm:** rashes, urticaria. **Hemat:** agranulocytosis, bleeding, eosinophilia, hemolytic anemia, neutropenia. **Misc:** ALLERGIC REACTIONS, INCLUDING ANAPHYLAXIS AND SERUM SICKNESS, superinfection.

PHYSICAL THERAPY IMPLICATIONS

Examination and Evaluation

- Watch for seizures; notify physician immediately if patient develops or increases seizure activity.
- Monitor signs of pseudomembranous colitis, including diarrhea, abdominal pain, fever, pus or mucus in stools, and other severe or prolonged GI problems (nausea, vomiting, heartburn). Notify physician or nursing staff immediately of these signs.
- Monitor signs of allergic reactions and anaphylaxis, including pulmonary symptoms (tightness in the throat and chest, wheezing, cough dyspnea) or skin reactions (rash, pruritus, urticaria). Notify physician or nursing staff immediately if these reactions occur.
- Assess muscle aches and joint pain (arthralgia) that may be caused by serum sickness. Notify physician if these symptoms seem to be drug related rather

than caused by musculoskeletal injury or if muscle and joint pain are accompanied by allergy-like reactions (fever, rashes, etc.)

- Monitor signs of blood dyscrasias, including eosinophilia (fatigue, weakness, myalgia), thrombocytopenia (bruising, nose bleeds, bleeding gums, other bleeding problems), hemolytic anemia (malaise, dizziness, jaundice, abdominal pain), and agranulocytosis or neutropenia (fever, sore throat, mucosal lesions, signs of infection, bruising). Report these signs to the physician.

Interventions

- Always wash hands thoroughly and disinfect equipment (whirlpools, electrotherapeutic devices, treatment tables, and so forth) to help prevent the spread of infection. Employ universal precautions or isolation procedures as indicated for specific patients.

Patient/Client-Related Instruction

- Instruct patient to notify physician immediately of signs of superinfection, including black, furry overgrowth on tongue, vaginal itching or discharge, and loose or foul-smelling stools.
- Instruct patient and family/caregivers to report other troublesome side effects such as severe or prolonged skin problems (rash, hives) or GI problems (nausea, vomiting, diarrhea).

Pharmacokinetics

Absorption: Well absorbed after oral administration.
Distribution: Widely distributed. Penetration into CSF is poor. Crosses the placenta and enters breast milk in low concentrations.
Metabolism and Excretion: Excreted primarily unchanged by the kidneys.
Half-life: 30–60 min (increased in renal impairment).

TIME/ACTION PROFILE

ROUTE	ONSET	PEAK	DURATION
PO	rapid	30–60 min	6–12 hr
PO-CD	unknown	unknown	12 hr

Contraindications/Precautions

Contraindicated in: Hypersensitivity to cephalosporins; Serious hypersensitivity to penicillins.
Use Cautiously in: Renal impairment; History of GI disease, especially colitis; Pregnancy and lactation (has been used safely).

Interactions

Drug-Drug: Probenecid ↓ excretion and ↑ blood levels. **Antacids** ↓ absorption.

Route/Dosage

PO (Adults): 250–500 mg q 8 hr or 375–500 mg q 12 hr as extended-release tablets.
PO (Children >1 mo): 6.7–13.4 mg/kg q 8 hr or 10–20 mg/kg q 12 hr (up to 1 g/day).

Availability (generic available)

Capsules: 250 mg, 500 mg. **Extended-release tablets (CD):** 375 mg, 500 mg. **Chewable tablet (fruity):** 125 mg, 187 mg, 250 mg, 375 mg. **Oral suspension (strawberry):** 125 mg/5 mL, 187 mg/5 mL, 250 mg/5 mL, 375 mg/5 mL.

cefadroxil (sef-a-drox-ill)

Duricef

Classification

Therapeutic: anti-infectives
Pharmacologic: first-generation cephalosporins

Indications

Treatment of the following infections due to susceptible organisms: Skin and skin structure infections (including burn wounds), Pharyngitis and/or tonsillitis, Urinary tract infections. Not suitable for the treatment of meningitis.

Action

Bind to bacterial cell wall membrane, causing cell death. **Therapeutic Effects:** Bactericidal action against susceptible bacteria. **Spectrum:** Active against many gram-positive cocci, including *Streptococcus pneumoniae*, group A beta-hemolytic streptococci, penicillinase-producing staphylococci. Not active against methicillin-resistant staphylococci, *Bacteroides fragilis*, *Enterococcus*. Active against some gram-negative rods, including *Klebsiella pneumoniae*, *Proteus mirabilis*, *Moraxella catarrhalis*, *Escherichia coli*.

Adverse Reactions/Side Effects

CNS: SEIZURES (VERY HIGH DOSES). **GI:** PSEUDOMEMBRANOUS COLITIS, diarrhea, nausea, vomiting, dyspepsia. **Derm:** rashes, pruritus, urticaria. **Hemat:** agranulocytosis, thrombocytopenia. **Misc:** allergic reactions, including anaphylaxis and serum sickness, superinfection.

PHYSICAL THERAPY IMPLICATIONS

Examination and Evaluation

- Watch for seizures; notify physician immediately if patient develops or increases seizure activity.
- Monitor signs of pseudomembranous colitis, including diarrhea, abdominal pain, fever, pus or mucus in stools, and other severe or prolonged GI problems (nausea, vomiting, heartburn). Notify physician or nursing staff immediately of these signs.
- Monitor signs of allergic reactions and anaphylaxis, including pulmonary symptoms (tightness in the

throat and chest, wheezing, cough dyspnea) or skin reactions (rash, pruritus, urticaria). Notify physician or nursing staff immediately if these reactions occur.

- Assess muscle aches and joint pain (arthralgia) that may be caused by serum sickness. Notify physician if these symptoms seem to be drug related rather than caused by musculoskeletal injury or if muscle and joint pain are accompanied by allergy-like reactions (fever, rashes, etc.)
- Monitor signs of agranulocytosis (fever, sore throat, mucosal lesions, signs of infection) or thrombocytopenia (bruising, nose bleeds, bleeding gums). Report these signs to the physician.

Interventions

- Always wash hands thoroughly and disinfect equipment (whirlpools, electrotherapeutic devices, treatment tables, and so forth) to help prevent the spread of infection. Employ universal precautions or isolation procedures as indicated for specific patients.

Patient/Client-Related Instruction

- Instruct patient to notify physician immediately of signs of superinfection, including black, furry overgrowth on tongue, vaginal itching or discharge, and loose or foul-smelling stools.
- Instruct patient and family/caregivers to report other troublesome side effects such as severe or prolonged skin problems (rash, hives, itching) or GI problems (nausea, vomiting, diarrhea, heartburn).

Pharmacokinetics

Absorption: Well absorbed after oral administration.
Distribution: Widely distributed. Crosses the placenta and enters breast milk in low concentrations. Minimal CSF penetration.
Metabolism and Excretion: Excreted almost entirely unchanged by the kidneys.
Half-life: 1–2 hr (increased in renal impairment).

TIME/ACTION PROFILE (blood levels)

ROUTE	ONSET	PEAK	DURATION
PO	rapid	1.5–2 hr	12–24 hr

Contraindications/Precautions

Contraindicated in: Hypersensitivity to cephalosporins; Serious hypersensitivity to penicillins.
Use Cautiously in: Renal impairment (dosage reduction and/or increased dosing interval recommended if CCr ≤50 mL/min); History of GI disease, especially colitis; Geriatric patients (dosage adjustment due to age-related decrease in renal function may be necessary); Pregnancy or lactation (half-life is shorter and blood levels lower during pregnancy; has been used safely).

Interactions

Drug-Drug: Probenecid decreases excretion and increases blood levels of renally excreted cephalosporins. Concurrent use of **loop diuretics** or **aminoglycosides** may increase the risk of renal toxicity.

Route/Dosage

PO (Adults): *Pharyngitis and/or tonisilitis*—500 mg q 12 hr or 1 g q 24 hr for 10 days. *Skin and soft tissue infections*—500 mg q 12 hr or 1 g q 24 hr. *Urinary tract infections*—500 mg–1 g q 12 hr or 1–2 g q 24 hr.
PO (Children): *Pharyngitis, tonsillitis, or impetigo*—15 mg/kg q 12 hr or 30 mg/kg q 24 hr for 10 days. *Skin and soft tissue infections*—15 mg/kg q 12 hr. *Urinary tract infections*—15 mg/kg q 12 hr.

Renal Impairment

PO (Adults): *CCr 25–50 mL/min*—500 mg q 12 hr; *CCr 10–25 mL/min*—500 mg q 24 hr; *CCr 0–10 mL/min*—500 mg q 36 hr.

Availability (generic available)

Capsules: 500 mg. **Tablets:** 1 g. **Oral suspension:** 250 mg/5 mL, 500 mg/5 mL.

cefazolin (sef-a-zoe-lin)

Ancef, Kefzol

Classification

Therapeutic: anti-infectives
Pharmacologic: first-generation cephalosporins

Indications

Treatment of the following infections due to susceptible organisms: Skin and skin structure infections (including burn wounds); Pneumonia; Urinary tract infections; Biliary tract infections; Genital infections; Bone and joint infections; Septicemia; Bacterial endocarditis prophylaxis for dental and upper respiratory procedures. Perioperative prophylaxis. Not suitable for the treatment of meningitis.

Action

Binds to bacterial cell wall membrane, causing cell death. **Therapeutic Effects:** Bactericidal action against susceptible bacteria. **Spectrum:** Active against many gram-positive cocci, including *Streptococcus pneumoniae*, group A beta-hemolytic streptococci, penicillinase-producing staphylococci. Not active against methicillin-resistant staphylococci, *Bacteroides fragilis*, *Enterococcus*. Active against some gram-negative rods, including *Proteus mirabilis*, *Escherichia coli*.

Adverse Reactions/Side Effects

CNS: SEIZURES (HIGH DOSES). **GI:** PSEUDOMEMBRANOUS COLITIS, diarrhea, nausea, vomiting, cramps. **Derm:** rash, pruritus, urticaria, Stevens-Johnson syndrome. **Hemat:** leukopenia, neutropenia, thrombocytopenia. **Local:** pain at IM site, phlebitis at IV site. **Misc:** allergic reactions, including anaphylaxis and serum sickness, superinfection.

PHYSICAL THERAPY IMPLICATIONS

Examination and Evaluation

- Watch for seizures; notify physician immediately if patient develops or increases seizure activity.
- Monitor signs of pseudomembranous colitis, including diarrhea, abdominal pain, fever, pus or mucus in stools, and other severe or prolonged GI problems (nausea, vomiting, heartburn). Notify physician or nursing staff immediately of these signs.
- Monitor signs of allergic reactions and anaphylaxis, including pulmonary symptoms (tightness in the throat and chest, wheezing, cough dyspnea) or skin reactions (rash, pruritus, urticaria). Skin reactions may indicate serious hypersensitivity reactions (Stevens-Johnson syndrome). Notify physician or nursing staff immediately if these reactions occur.
- Assess muscle aches and joint pain (arthralgia) that may be caused by serum sickness. Notify physician if these symptoms seem to be drug related rather than caused by musculoskeletal injury or if muscle and joint pain are accompanied by allergy-like reactions (fever, rashes, etc.).
- Instruct patient to report signs of leukopenia and neutropenia (fever, sore throat, signs of infection) or thrombocytopenia (bruising, nose bleeds, and bleeding gums). Report these signs to the physician.
- Monitor injection site for pain, swelling, and irritation. Report prolonged or excessive injection site reactions to the physician.

Interventions

- Always wash hands thoroughly and disinfect equipment (whirlpools, electrotherapeutic devices, treatment tables, and so forth) to help prevent the spread of infection. Employ universal precautions or isolation procedures as indicated for specific patients.

Patient/Client-Related Instruction

- Instruct patient to notify physician of signs of superinfection, including black, furry overgrowth on tongue, vaginal itching or discharge, and loose or foul-smelling stools.
- Instruct patient and family/caregivers to report other troublesome side effects such as severe or prolonged skin problems (rash, hives, itching) or GI problems (nausea, vomiting, diarrhea, cramps).

Pharmacokinetics

Absorption: Well absorbed after IM administration.
Distribution: Widely distributed. Penetrates bone and synovial fluid well. Crosses the placenta and enters breast milk in low concentrations. Minimal CSF penetration.
Protein Binding: 74–86%.
Metabolism and Excretion: Excreted almost entirely unchanged by the kidneys.
Half-life: Neonates: 3–5 hr; Adults: 90–150 min (increased in renal impairment).

TIME/ACTION PROFILE (blood levels)

ROUTE	ONSET	PEAK	DURATION
IM	rapid	0.5–2 hr	6–12 hr
IV	rapid	5 min	6–12 hr

Contraindications/Precautions

Contraindicated in: Hypersensitivity to cephalosporins; Serious hypersensitivity to penicillins.
Use Cautiously in: Renal impairment (dosage reduction and/or increased dosing interval recommended if CCr <30 mL/min); Hepatic impairment; History of GI disease, especially colitis; OB: Half-life is shorter and blood levels lower during pregnancy; has been used safely. Lactation: Low concentrations of drug appear in breast milk; Geri: Dosage adjustment due to age-related decrease in renal function may be necessary.

Interactions

Drug-Drug: Probenecid decreases excretion and increases blood levels of renally excreted cephalosporins.

Route/Dosage

IM, IV (Adults): *Moderate-to-severe infections*—500 mg–2 g q 6–8 hr; maximum 12 g/day. *Mild infections with gram-positive cocci*—250–500 mg q 8 hr. *Uncomplicated urinary tract infection*—1 g q 12 hr. *Pneumococcal pneumonia*—500 mg q 12 hr. *Infective endocarditis or septicemia*—1–1.5 g q 6 hr. *Perioperative prophylaxis*—1 g within 30–60 min prior to incision (an additional 500 mg–1 g should be given for surgeries ≥2 hr). 500 mg–1 g should then be given for all surgeries q 6–8 hr for 24 hr following the surgery.
IM, IV (Children and Infants >1 mo): 50–100 mg/kg/day divided q 8 hr; maximum: 6 g/day *Bacterial endocarditis prophylaxis in penicillin-allergic patients*—25 mg/kg 30 min prior to procedure; maximum dose: 1 g.
IM, IV (Neonates ≤7 days): 40 mg/kg/day divided q 12 hr.

IM, IV (Neonates >7 days and ≤2 kg): 40 mg/kg/day divided q 12 hr.
IM, IV (Neonates >7 days and >2 kg): 60 mg/kg/day divided q 8 hr.

Renal Impairment

IM, IV (Adults): *CCr 10–30 mL/min*—Administer dose q 12 hr; *CCr ≤10 mL/min*—Administer q 24 hr.

Availability (generic available)

Powder for injection: 500 mg Rx, 1 g Rx, 10 g Rx, 20 g Rx. **Premixed containers:** 500 mg/50 mL D_5W Rx, 1 g/50 mL D_5W Rx.

cefdinir (sef-di-nir)

Omnicef

Classification
Therapeutic: anti-infectives
Pharmacologic: third-generation cephalosporins

Indications

Treatment of the following infections caused by susceptible organisms: Community-acquired pneumonia (adults only); Acute exacerbations of chronic bronchitis (adults only); Acute maxillary sinusitis (adults only); Pharyngitis and tonsillitis; Uncomplicated skin and skin structure infections; Acute bacterial otitis media (children only).

Action

Binds to bacterial cell wall membrane, causing cell death. **Therapeutic Effects:** Bactericidal action against susceptible bacteria. **Spectrum:** Active against the following gram-positive organisms: *Staphylococcus aureus*, *Streptococcus pneumoniae*, *Streptococcus pyogenes*. Active against the following gram-negative organisms: *Haemophilus influenzae* (including β-lactamase–producing strains), *Haemophilus parainfluenzae* (including β-lactamase–producing strains), *Moraxella catarrhalis* (including β-lactamase–producing strains). Not active against methicillin-resistant staphylococci or enterococci.

Adverse Reactions/Side Effects

CNS: SEIZURES, headache. **GI:** PSEUDOMEMBRANOUS COLITIS, diarrhea, vomiting, abdominal pain, nausea. **GU:** vaginal moniliasis, vaginitis. **Derm:** rash, pruritus. **Misc:** ALLERGIC REACTIONS, INCLUDING ANAPHYLAXIS.

PHYSICAL THERAPY IMPLICATIONS

Examination and Evaluation

- Watch for seizures; notify physician immediately if patient develops or increases seizure activity.
- Monitor signs of pseudomembranous colitis, including diarrhea, abdominal pain, fever, pus or mucus in stools, and other severe or prolonged GI problems (nausea, vomiting, heartburn). Notify physician or nursing staff immediately of these signs.
- Monitor signs of allergic reactions and anaphylaxis, including pulmonary symptoms (tightness in the throat and chest, wheezing, cough dyspnea) or skin reactions (rash, pruritus, urticaria). Notify physician or nursing staff immediately if these reactions occur.

Interventions

- Always wash hands thoroughly and disinfect equipment (whirlpools, electrotherapeutic devices, treatment tables, and so forth) to help prevent the spread of infection. Use universal precautions or isolation procedures as indicated for specific patients.

Patient/Client-Related Instruction

- Instruct patient and family/caregivers to report other troublesome side effects such as severe or prolonged headache, skin problems (rash, itching), vaginal inflammation or infection, or GI problems (nausea, vomiting, diarrhea, abdominal pain).

Pharmacokinetics

Absorption: 16–25% absorbed after oral administration.
Distribution: Widely distributed.
Metabolism and Excretion: Mostly excreted unchanged in urine.
Half-life: 1.7 hr (increased in renal impairment).

TIME/ACTION PROFILE (blood levels)

ROUTE	ONSET	PEAK	DURATION
PO	rapid	2–4 hr	12–24 hr

Contraindications/Precautions

Contraindicated in: Hypersensitivity to cephalosporins; Serious hypersensitivity to penicillins.
Use Cautiously in: Renal impairment (dosage reduction recommended if CCr <30 mL/min); Diabetes (suspension contains sucrose); History of GI disease, especially colitis; Geriatric patients (dosage adjustment due to age-related decrease in renal function may be necessary); Pregnancy, lactation, or children <6 mo (safety not established).

Interactions

Drug-Drug: Antacids and **iron supplements** ↓ absorption (administer at least 2 hr before or 2 hr after). **Probenecid** ↓ excretion and ↑ blood levels.

Route/Dosage

PO (Adults and Children ≥13 yr): 300 mg q 12 hr or 600 mg q 24 hr (twice daily dosing must be used for community-acquired pneumonia or uncomplicated skin and skin structure infections).

Renal Impairment

(Adults and Children ≥13 yr): *CCr <30 mL/min*–300 mg q 24 hr.

PO (Children 6 mo–12 yr): 7 mg/kg q 12 hr or 14 mg/kg q 24 hr (not to exceed 600 mg/day). Twice daily dosing must be used for uncomplicated skin and skin structure infections.

Renal Impairment

(Children 6 mo–12 yr): *CCr <30 mL/min*–7 mg/kg q 24 hr.

Availability

Oral suspension (strawberry flavor): 125 mg/5 mL Rx, 250 mg/5 mL. **Capsules:** 300 mg.

cefditoren (sef-di-tore-en)

Spectracef

Classification

Therapeutic: anti-infectives

Pharmacologic: third-generation cephalosporins

Indications

Treatment of the following infections caused by susceptible organisms: Acute exacerbations of chronic bronchitis, Community-acquired pneumonia, Pharyngitis and tonsillitis, Uncomplicated skin and skin structure infections.

Action

Binds to bacterial cell wall membrane, causing cell death. **Therapeutic Effects:** Bactericidal action against susceptible bacteria. **Spectrum:** Active against the following gram-positive organisms: *Staphylococcus aureus* (methicillin-susceptible strains, including β-lactamase–producing strains), *Streptococcus pneumoniae* (penicillin-susceptible strains only), *Str. pyogenes*. Active against the following gram-negative organisms: *Haemophilus influenzae* (including β-lactamase–producing strains), *H. parainfluenzae* (including β-lactamase–producing strains), *Moraxella catarrhalis* (including β-lactamase–producing strains).

Adverse Reactions/Side Effects

CNS: SEIZURES (HIGH DOSES), headache. **GI:** PSEUDOMEMBRANOUS COLITIS, diarrhea, abdominal pain, dyspepsia, nausea, vomiting. **GU:** hematuria, vaginal moniliasis. **Hemat:** bleeding, eosinophilia, hemolytic anemia, lymphocytosis, neutropenia, thrombocytosis. **Misc:** allergic reactions. including anaphylaxis, superinfection.

PHYSICAL THERAPY IMPLICATIONS

Examination and Evaluation

- Watch for seizures; notify physician immediately if patient develops or increases seizure activity.
- Monitor signs of pseudomembranous colitis, including diarrhea, abdominal pain, fever, pus or mucus in stools, and other severe or prolonged GI problems (nausea, vomiting, heartburn). Notify physician or nursing staff immediately of these signs.
- Monitor signs of allergic reactions and anaphylaxis, including pulmonary symptoms (tightness in the throat and chest, wheezing, cough dyspnea) or skin reactions (rash, pruritus, urticaria). Notify physician or nursing staff immediately if these reactions occur.
- Monitor signs of blood dyscrasias, including eosinophilia (fatigue, weakness, myalgia), hemolytic anemia (malaise, dizziness, jaundice, abdominal pain), neutropenia (fever, sore throat, mucosal lesions, signs of infection), and thrombocytopenia (bruising, nose bleeds, bleeding gums, other unusual bleeding). Report these signs to the physician.
- Assess dizziness that might affect gait, balance, and other functional activities (See Appendix C). Report balance problems and functional limitations to the physician and nursing staff, and caution the patient and family/caregivers to guard against falls and trauma.

Interventions

- Always wash hands thoroughly and disinfect equipment (whirlpools, electrotherapeutic devices, treatment tables, and so forth) to help prevent the spread of infection. Use universal precautions or isolation procedures as indicated for specific patients.

Patient/Client-Related Instruction

- Instruct patient to notify physician immediately of signs of superinfection, including black, furry overgrowth on tongue, vaginal itching or discharge, and loose or foul-smelling stools.
- Instruct patient and family/caregivers to report other troublesome side effects such as severe or prolonged headache, skin problems (rash, hives), vaginal infections, blood in the urine, or GI problems (nausea, vomiting, diarrhea, abdominal pain, heartburn).

Pharmacokinetics

Absorption: Cefditoren pivoxil is a prodrug that is converted to cefditoren (the active component) in GI tract during absorption. Bioavailability 14% in fasting state, increased by high fat meal.

Distribution: Widely distributed.

Protein Binding: 88%.

C

Metabolism and Excretion: Mostly excreted unchanged by the kidneys.
Half-life: 1.6 hr (increased in renal impairment).

TIME/ACTION PROFILE (blood levels)

ROUTE	ONSET	PEAK	DURATION
PO	rapid	1.5–3 hr	12 hr

Contraindications/Precautions

Contraindicated in: Hypersensitivity to cephalosporins; Serious hypersensitivity to penicillins; Carnitine deficiency or inborn errors of metabolism resulting in significant carnitine deficiency (produces renal excretion of carnitine); Milk protein hypersensitivity (contains sodium caseinate).
Use Cautiously in: Renal impairment (dosage adjustment recommended if CCr <50 mL/min); Geri: Dose adjustment due to age-related decrease in renal function may be necessary; OB/Lactation/Pedi: Pregnancy, lactation or children <12 yr (safety not established).

Interactions

Drug-Drug: Antacids and **histamine H_2 receptor antagonists** ↓ absorption (avoid concurrent use). **Probenecid** ↓ excretion and ↑ blood levels.

Route/Dosage

PO (Adults and Children ≥12 yr): *Acute bacterial exacerbation of chronic bronchitis, community-acquired pneumonia*—400 mg twice daily; *Pharyngitis/tonsillitis, uncomplicated skin/skin structure infections*—200 mg twice daily.

Renal Impairment

PO (Adults and Children ≥12 yr): *CCr 30–49 mL/min*—dose should not exceed 200 mg twice daily; *CCr <30 mL/min*—dose should not exceed 200 mg once daily.

Availability

Tablets: 200 mg, 400 mg.

cefepime (sef-e-peem)
Maxipime

Classification
Therapeutic: anti-infectives
Pharmacologic: fourth-generation cephalosporins

Indications

Treatment of the following infections caused by susceptible organisms: Uncomplicated skin and skin structure infections, Bone and joint infections, Uncomplicated and complicated urinary tract infections, Respiratory tract infections, Complicated intra-abdominal infections (with metronidazole), Septicemia. Empiric treatment of febrile neutropenic patients.

Action

Binds to the bacterial cell wall membrane, causing cell death. **Therapeutic Effects:** Bactericidal action against susceptible bacteria. **Spectrum:** Similar to that of second- and third-generation cephalosporins, but activity against staphylococci is less, whereas activity against gram-negative pathogens is greater, even for organisms resistant to first-, second-, and third-generation agents. Notable is increased action against *Enterobacter*, *Haemophilus influenzae* (including β-lactamase–producing strains), *Escherichia coli*, *Klebsiella pneumoniae*, *Neisseria*, *Proteus*, *Providencia*, *Pseudomonas aeruginosa*, *Serratia*, *Moraxella catarrhalis* (including β-lactamase–producing strains). Not active against methicillin-resistant staphylococci or enterococci.

Adverse Reactions/Side Effects

CNS: SEIZURES (HIGH DOSES IN PATIENTS WITH RENAL IMPAIRMENT), encephalopathy, headache. **GI:** PSEUDOMEMBRANOUS COLITIS, diarrhea, nausea, vomiting. **Derm:** rashes, pruritus, urticaria. **Hemat:** bleeding, eosinophilia, hemolytic anemia, neutropenia, thrombocytopenia. **Local:** pain at IM site, phlebitis at IV site. **Misc:** ALLERGIC REACTIONS, INCLUDING ANAPHYLAXIS, superinfection, fever.

PHYSICAL THERAPY IMPLICATIONS

Examination and Evaluation

- Watch for seizures; notify physician immediately if patient develops or increases seizure activity.
- Monitor signs of pseudomembranous colitis, including diarrhea, abdominal pain, fever, pus or mucus in stools, and other severe or prolonged GI problems (nausea, vomiting, heartburn). Notify physician or nursing staff immediately of these signs.
- Monitor signs of allergic reactions and anaphylaxis, including pulmonary symptoms (tightness in the throat and chest, wheezing, cough dyspnea) or skin reactions (rash, pruritus, urticaria). Notify physician or nursing staff immediately if these reactions occur.
- Be alert for signs of encephalopathy, including decreased alertness, lethargy, and incoordination. Notify physician of these signs before they progress to more severe changes in mental status such as dementia, seizures, and coma.

- Monitor signs of blood dyscrasias, including eosinophilia (fatigue, weakness, myalgia), hemolytic anemia (malaise, dizziness, jaundice, abdominal pain), neutropenia (fever, sore throat, mucosal lesions, signs of infection), and thrombocytopenia (bruising, nose bleeds, bleeding gums, other unusual bleeding). Report these signs to the physician.
- Monitor injection site for pain, swelling, and irritation. Report prolonged or excessive injection-site reactions to the physician.

Interventions

- Always wash hands thoroughly and disinfect equipment (whirlpools, electrotherapeutic devices, treatment tables, and so forth) to help prevent the spread of infection. Employ universal precautions or isolation procedures as indicated for specific patients.

Patient/Client-Related Instruction

- Instruct patient to notify physician immediately of signs of superinfection, including black, furry overgrowth on tongue, vaginal itching or discharge, and loose or foul-smelling stools.
- Instruct patient and family/caregivers to report other troublesome side effects such as severe or prolonged headache, fever, skin problems (rash, hives, itching), or GI problems (nausea, vomiting, diarrhea).

Pharmacokinetics

Absorption: Well absorbed after IM administration; IV administration results in complete bioavailability.
Distribution: Widely distributed. Crosses the placenta; enters breast milk in low concentrations. Some CSF penetration.
Metabolism and Excretion: 85% excreted unchanged in urine.
Half-life: 2 hr (increased in renal impairment).

TIME/ACTION PROFILE

ROUTE	ONSET	PEAK	DURATION
IM	rapid	1–2 hr	12 hr
IV	rapid	end of infusion	12 hr

Contraindications/Precautions

Contraindicated in: Hypersensitivity to cephalosporins; Serious hypersensitivity to penicillins.
Use Cautiously in: Renal impairment (↓ dosing/↑ dosing interval recommended if CCr ≤60 mL/min); History of GI disease, especially colitis; Patients with hepatic dysfunction or poor nutritional status (may be at increased risk of bleeding); Geriatric patients (dose adjustment due to age-related decrease in renal function may be necessary); OB/Lactation/Pedi: Pregnancy, lactation, and children <2 mo (safety not established).

Interactions

Drug-Drug: Probenecid ↓ excretion and ↑ blood levels. Concurrent use of **loop diuretics** or **aminoglycosides** may ↑ risk of nephrotoxicity.

Route/Dosage

IM (Adults): *Mild-to-moderate uncomplicated or complicated urinary tract infections due to Escherichia coli*—0.5–1 g every 12 hr.
IV (Adults): *Moderate-to-severe pneumonia*—1–2 g every 12 hr. *Mild-to-moderate uncomplicated or complicated urinary tract infections*—0.5–1 g every 12 hr. *Severe uncomplicated or complicated urinary tract infections, moderate-to-severe uncomplicated skin and skin structure infections, complicated intra-abdominal infections*—2 g every 12 hr. *Empiric treatment of febrile neutropenia*—2 g every 8 hr.
IV (Children 2 mo–16 yr): *Uncomplicated and complicated urinary tract infections, uncomplicated skin and skin structure infections, pneumonia*—50 mg/kg every 12 hr (not to exceed 2 g/dose). *Febrile neutropenia*—50 mg/kg every 8 hr (not to exceed 2 g/dose).

Renal Impairment

IM, IV (Adults): (See manufacturer's specific recommendations) *CCr 30–60 mL/min*—0.5–1 g every 24 hr or 2 g every 12–24 hr; *CCr 11–29 mL/min*—0.5–2 g every 24 hr; *CCr <11 mL/min*—250 mg – 1 g every 24 hr.

Availability (generic available)

Powder for injection: 500 mg, 1 g, 2 g.

cefixime (se-fix-eem)

Suprax

Classification
Therapeutic: anti-infectives
Pharmacologic: third-generation cephalosporins

Indications

Treatment of Urinary and gynecologic infections, including gonorrhea, Respiratory tract infections, Otitis media.

Action

Binds to the bacterial cell wall membrane, causing cell death. **Therapeutic Effects:** Bactericidal action against susceptible bacteria. **Spectrum:** Similar to that of second-generation cephalosporins, but activity against staphylococci is less, while activity against gram-negative pathogens is greater, even for organisms resistant to first- and second-generation agents. Notable is increased action against *Enterobacter*, *Haemophilus influenzae*, *Escherichia coli*, *Klebsiella* *pneumoniae, Neisseria, Proteus, Providencia, Serratia, Moraxella catarrhalis, Borrelia burgdorferi.*

Adverse Reactions/Side Effects

CNS: SEIZURES (VERY HIGH DOSES). **GI:** PSEUDOMEMBRANOUS COLITIS, diarrhea, nausea, vomiting, cramps. **Derm:** rashes, urticaria. **Hemat:** bleeding, blood dyscrasias, hemolytic anemia. **Misc:** ALLERGIC REACTIONS, INCLUDING ANAPHYLAXIS AND SERUM SICKNESS, superinfection.

PHYSICAL THERAPY IMPLICATIONS

Examination and Evaluation

- Watch for seizures; notify physician immediately if patient develops or increases seizure activity.
- Monitor signs of pseudomembranous colitis, including diarrhea, abdominal pain, fever, pus or mucus in stools, and other severe or prolonged GI problems (nausea, vomiting, heartburn). Notify physician or nursing staff immediately of these signs.
- Monitor signs of allergic reactions and anaphylaxis, including pulmonary symptoms (tightness in the throat and chest, wheezing, cough dyspnea) or skin reactions (rash, pruritus, urticaria). Notify physician or nursing staff immediately if these reactions occur.
- Assess muscle aches and joint pain (arthralgia) that may be caused by serum sickness. Notify physician if these symptoms seem to be drug related rather than caused by musculoskeletal injury or if muscle and joint pain are accompanied by allergy-like reactions (fever, rashes, etc.)
- Monitor signs of blood dyscrasias, including hemolytic anemia (unusual weakness and fatigue, dizziness, jaundice, abdominal pain) and thrombocytopenia (bruising, nose bleeds, bleeding gums, other unusual bleeding). Report these signs to the physician.

Interventions

- Always wash hands thoroughly and disinfect equipment (whirlpools, electrotherapeutic devices, treatment tables, and so forth) to help prevent the spread of infection. Use universal precautions or isolation procedures as indicated for specific patients.

Patient/Client-Related Instruction

- Instruct patient to notify physician immediately of signs of superinfection, including black, furry overgrowth on tongue, vaginal itching or discharge, loose or foul-smelling stools.
- Instruct patient and family/caregivers to report other troublesome side effects such as severe or prolonged skin problems (rash, hives) or GI problems (nausea, vomiting, diarrhea, cramps).

Pharmacokinetics

Absorption: 40–50% absorbed following oral administration (oral suspension).
Distribution: Widely distributed. Crosses the placenta; enters breast milk in low concentrations. CSF penetration better than with first- and second-generation agents.
Metabolism and Excretion: 50% excreted unchanged in urine; ≥10% excreted in bile.
Half-life: 3–4 hr (increased in renal impairment).

TIME/ACTION PROFILE (blood levels)

ROUTE	ONSET	PEAK	DURATION
PO	rapid	2–6 hr	24 hr

Contraindications/Precautions

Contraindicated in: Hypersensitivity to cephalosporins; Serious hypersensitivity to penicillins.
Use Cautiously in: Renal impairment (↓ dosing/↑ dosing interval recommended if CCr ≤60 mL/min); History of GI disease, especially colitis; Geri: Geriatric patients (dose adjustment due to age-related decrease in renal function may be necessary); OB: Pregnancy and lactation (has been used safely).

Interactions

Drug-Drug: Probenecid ↓ excretion and ↑ serum levels. Concurrent use of large doses of cephalosporins and **NSAIDs** may ↑ the risk of bleeding. Concurrent use of **loop diuretics** or **nephrotoxic agents**, including **aminoglycosides**, may ↑ risk of nephrotoxicity. May ↑ **carbamazepine** levels.

Route/Dosage

PO (Adults and Children >12 yr or >50 kg): *Most infections*—400 mg once daily. *Gonorrhea*—400 mg single dose.
PO (Children): 8 mg/kg once daily or 4 mg/kg every 12 hr.

Renal Impairment

PO (Adults): *CCr 21–60 mL/min*—75% of standard dose; *CCr ≤20 mL/min*—50% of standard dose.

Availability

Oral suspension (strawberry flavor): 100 mg/5 mL. **Tables:** 400 mg.

cefoperazone
(sef-oh-**per**-a-zone)
Cefobid

Classification
Therapeutic: anti-infectives
Pharmacologic: third-generation cephalosporins

Indications
Treatment of the following infections caused by susceptible organisms: Skin and skin structure infections; Urinary tract infections; Gynecologic infections, including gonorrhea; Respiratory tract infections; Intra-abdominal infections; Septicemia.

Action
Binds to the bacterial cell wall membrane, causing cell death. **Therapeutic Effects:** Bactericidal action against susceptible bacteria. **Spectrum:** Similar to that of second-generation cephalosporins, but activity against staphylococci is less, while activity against gram-negative pathogens is greater, even for organisms resistant to first- and second-generation agents. Notable is increased action against *Citrobacter*, *Enterobacter*, *Haemophilus influenzae*, *Escherichia coli*, *Klebsiella pneumoniae*, *Morganella morganii*, *Neisseria gonorrhoeae*, *Proteus*, *Providencia*, *Pseudomonas aeruginosa*, *Serratia*. Has some activity against enterococci. Has some activity against anaerobes, including *Bacteroides fragilis*.

Adverse Reactions/Side Effects
CNS: SEIZURES (HIGH DOSES). **GI:** PSEUDOMEMBRANOUS COLITIS, diarrhea, nausea, vomiting. **Derm:** rashes, urticaria. **Hemat:** bleeding, eosinophilia, neutropenia. **Local:** pain at IM site, phlebitis at IV site. **Misc:** ALLERGIC REACTIONS, INCLUDING ANAPHYLAXIS, superinfection.

PHYSICAL THERAPY IMPLICATIONS

Examination and Evaluation
- Watch for seizures; notify physician immediately if patient develops or increases seizure activity.
- Monitor signs of pseudomembranous colitis, including diarrhea, abdominal pain, fever, pus or mucus in stools, and other severe or prolonged GI problems (nausea, vomiting, heartburn). Notify physician or nursing staff immediately of these signs.
- Monitor signs of allergic reactions and anaphylaxis, including pulmonary symptoms (tightness in the throat and chest, wheezing, cough dyspnea) or skin reactions (rash, pruritis, urticaria). Notify physician or nursing staff immediately if these reactions occur.
- Monitor signs of blood dyscrasias, including eosinophilia (fatigue, weakness, myalgia), neutropenia (fever, sore throat, mucosal lesions, signs of infection), and thrombocytopenia (bruising, nose bleeds, bleeding gums, other unusual bleeding). Report these signs to the physician.
- Monitor injection site for pain, swelling, and irritation. Report prolonged or excessive injection site reactions to the physician.

Interventions
- Always wash hands thoroughly and disinfect equipment (whirlpools, electrotherapeutic devices, treatment tables, and so forth) to help prevent the spread of infection. Employ universal precautions or isolation procedures as indicated for specific patients.

Patient/Client-Related Instruction
- Instruct patient to notify physician immediately of signs of superinfection, including black, furry overgrowth on tongue, vaginal itching or discharge, and loose or foul-smelling stools.
- Instruct patient and family/caregivers to report other troublesome side effects such as severe or prolonged skin problems (rash, hives) or GI problems (nausea, vomiting, diarrhea).

Pharmacokinetics
Absorption: Well absorbed following IM administration; IV administration results in complete bioavailability.
Distribution: Widely distributed. Crosses the placenta; enters breast milk in low concentrations. CSF penetration better than with first- and second-generation agents.
Protein Binding: ≥90%.
Metabolism and Excretion: Excreted in bile.
Half-life: 2 hr.

TIME/ACTION PROFILE (blood levels)

ROUTE	ONSET	PEAK	DURATION
IM	rapid	1–2 hr	12 hr
IV	rapid	end of infusion	12 hr

Contraindications/Precautions
Contraindicated in: Hypersensitivity to cephalosporins; Serious hypersensitivity to penicillins.
Use Cautiously in: Hepatic/biliary impairment or combined hepatic/biliary/renal impairment (dosage reduction/increased dosing interval recommended); Patients with poor nutritional status, malabsorption states, or alcoholism (may be at increased risk of bleeding); History of GI disease, especially colitis; Pregnancy and lactation (has been used safely).

Interactions
Drug-Drug: Ingestion of **alcohol** within 48–72 hr of cefoperazone may result in a disulfiram-like reaction. May potentiate the effects of **anticoagulants** and ↑ the risk of bleeding. Concurrent use of **loop**

diuretics or **aminoglycosides** may ↑ the risk of nephrotoxicity.

Route/Dosage

IM, IV (Adults): *Mild-to-moderate infections*—1–2 g every 12 hr. *Severe infections*—2–4 g q 8 hr or 1.5–3 g q 6 hr.

Hepatic Impairment

IV (Adults): *Impaired hepatic function/biliary obstruction*—daily dose should not exceed 4 g; *combined hepatic and renal impairment*—daily dose should not exceed 1–2 g.

Availability

Powder for injection: 1 g Rx, 2 g Rx, 10 g.
Premixed containers: 1 g/50 mL, 2 g/50 mL.

cefotaxime (sef-oh-**taks**-eem)

Claforan

Classification
Therapeutic: anti-infectives
Pharmacologic: third-generation cephalosporins

Indications

Treatment of the following infections caused by susceptible organisms: Skin and skin structure infections; Bone and joint infections; Urinary tract infections; Gynecologic infections, including gonorrhea; Lower respiratory tract infections; Intra-abdominal infections; Septicemia; Meningitis; Lyme disease. Perioperative prophylaxis.

Action

Binds to the bacterial cell wall membrane, causing cell death. **Therapeutic Effects:** Bactericidal action against susceptible bacteria. **Spectrum:** Similar to that of second-generation cephalosporins, but activity against staphylococci is less, whereas activity against gram-negative pathogens is greater, even for organisms resistant to first- and second-generation agents. Notable is increased action against: *Acinetobacter*, *Citrobacter*, *Enterobacter*, *Haemophilus influenzae* (including β-lactamase–producing strains), *Haemophilus parainfluenzae*, *Escherichia coli*, *Klebsiella pneumoniae*, *Morganella morganii*, *Neisseria gonorrhoeae and N. meningitidis*, *Proteus*, *Providencia*, *Serratia*, *Moraxella catarrhalis*, *Borrelia burgdorferi*. Has some activity against anaerobes, including *Bacteroides fragilis*. Not active against methicillin-resistant staphylococci.

Adverse Reactions/Side Effects

CNS: SEIZURES (HIGH DOSES). **GI:** PSEUDOMEMBRANOUS COLITIS, diarrhea, nausea, vomiting. **Derm:** rashes, pruritus, urticaria. **Hemat:** agranulocytosis, bleeding, eosinophilia, hemolytic anemia, neutropenia, thrombocytopenia. **Local:** pain at IM site, phlebitis at IV site. **Misc:** ALLERGIC REACTIONS, INCLUDING ANAPHYLAXIS, superinfection.

PHYSICAL THERAPY IMPLICATIONS

Examination and Evaluation

- Watch for seizures; notify physician immediately if patient develops or increases seizure activity.
- Monitor signs of pseudomembranous colitis, including diarrhea, abdominal pain, fever, pus or mucus in stools, and other severe or prolonged GI problems (nausea, vomiting, heartburn). Notify physician or nursing staff immediately of these signs.
- Monitor signs of allergic reactions and anaphylaxis, including pulmonary symptoms (tightness in the throat and chest, wheezing, cough dyspnea) or skin reactions (rash, pruritus, urticaria). Notify physician or nursing staff immediately if these reactions occur.
- Monitor signs of blood dyscrasias, including agranulocytosis and neutropenia (fever, sore throat, mucosal lesions, signs of infection), eosinophilia (fatigue, weakness, myalgia), hemolytic anemia (malaise, dizziness, jaundice, abdominal pain), and thrombocytopenia (bruising, nose bleeds, bleeding gums, other unusual bleeding). Report these signs to the physician.
- Monitor injection site for pain, swelling, and irritation. Report prolonged or excessive injection-site reactions to the physician.

Interventions

- Always wash hands thoroughly and disinfect equipment (whirlpools, electrotherapeutic devices, treatment tables, and so forth) to help prevent the spread of infection. Employ universal precautions or isolation procedures as indicated for specific patients.

Patient/Client-Related Instruction

- Instruct patient to notify physician immediately of signs of superinfection, including black, furry overgrowth on tongue, vaginal itching or discharge, and loose or foul-smelling stools.
- Instruct patient and family/caregivers to report other troublesome side effects such as severe or prolonged skin problems (rash, hives, itching) or GI problems (nausea, vomiting, diarrhea).

Pharmacokinetics

Absorption: Well absorbed following IM administration; IV administration results in complete bioavailability.
Distribution: Widely distributed. Crosses the placenta; enters breast milk in low concentrations. CSF penetration better than with first- and second-generation agents.
Metabolism and Excretion: Partly metabolized to active metabolite; 20–36% excreted unchanged in the urine.
Half-life: Premature neonates: 5–6 hr; Full-term neonates: 2–3.4 hr; Children: 1.5 hr; Adults: 1–1.5 hr (increased in renal impairment).

TIME/ACTION PROFILE (blood levels)

ROUTE	ONSET	PEAK	DURATION
IM	rapid	0.5 hr	4–12 hr
IV	rapid	end of infusion	4–12 hr

Contraindications/Precautions

Contraindicated in: Hypersensitivity to cephalosporins; Serious hypersensitivity to penicillins.
Use Cautiously in: Renal impairment (decreased dosing recommended if CCr <20 mL/min); History of GI disease, especially colitis; Geri: Dosage adjustment may be necessary due to age-related decrease in renal function.

Interactions

Drug-Drug: Probenecid ↓ excretion and ↑ serum levels. Concurrent use of **aminoglycosides** may ↑ the risk of nephrotoxicity.

Route/Dosage

IM, IV (Adults and Children >12 yr): *Most uncomplicated infections*—1 g every 12 hr. *Moderate or severe infections*—1–2 g every 6–8 hr. *Life-threatening infections*—2 g every 4 hr (maximum dose: 12 g/day). *Gonococcal urethritis/cervicitis or rectal gonorrhea in females*—500 mg IM (single dose). *Rectal gonorrhea in males*—1 g IM (single dose). *Perioperative prophylaxis*—1 g 30–90 min before initial incision (1-time dose).
IM, IV (Children 1 mo-12 yr): *<50 kg*—100–200 mg/kg/day divided q 6–8 hr. *Meningitis*—200 mg/kg/day divided q 6 hr. *Invasive pneumococcal meningitis*—225–300 mg/kg/day divided q 6–8 hr. *≥ 50 kg*— see adult dosing.
IV (Neonates 1–4 wk): 50 mg/kg every 6–8 hr.
IV (Neonates ≤1 wk): 50 mg/kg every 8–12 hr.

Renal Impairment

IM, IV (Adults): *CCr <20 mL/min*—decrease dose by 50%.

Availability

Powder for injection: 500 mg, 1 g, 2 g, 10 g, 20 g.
Premixed containers: 1 g/50 mL, 2 g/50 mL.

cefotetan (sef-oh-tee-tan)

Cefotan

Classification
Therapeutic: anti-infectives
Pharmacologic: second-generation cephalosporins

Indications

Treatment of the following infections caused by susceptible organisms: Lower respiratory tract infections, Skin and skin structure infections, Bone and joint infections, Urinary tract infections, Gynecologic infections, Intra-abdominal infections. Perioperative prophylaxis.

Action

Binds to bacterial cell wall membrane, causing cell death. **Therapeutic Effects:** Bactericidal action against susceptible bacteria. **Spectrum:** Similar to that of first-generation cephalosporins but has increased activity against several other gram-negative pathogens, including *Haemophilus influenzae* (including β-lactamase–producing strains), *Escherichia coli*, *Klebsiella pneumoniae*, *Morganella morganii*, *Neisseria gonorrhoeae*, *Proteus*, *Providencia*, *Serratia marcescens*, *Moraxella catarrhalis*. Also has activity against *Bacteroides fragilis*. Not active against methicillin-resistant staphylococci or enterococci.

Adverse Reactions/Side Effects

CNS: SEIZURES (HIGH DOSES). **GI:** PSEUDOMEMBRANOUS COLITIS, diarrhea, nausea. **Derm:** rashes, urticaria. **Hemat:** bleeding, eosinophilia, hemolytic anemia, leukopenia, thrombocytopenia. **Local:** pain at IM site, phlebitis at IV site. **Misc:** ALLERGIC REACTIONS, INCLUDING ANAPHYLAXIS, superinfection.

PHYSICAL THERAPY IMPLICATIONS

Examination and Evaluation

- Watch for seizures; notify physician immediately if patient develops or increases seizure activity.
- Monitor signs of pseudomembranous colitis, including diarrhea, abdominal pain, fever, pus or mucus in stools, and other severe or prolonged GI problems (nausea, vomiting, heartburn). Notify physician or nursing staff immediately of these signs.
- Monitor signs of allergic reactions and anaphylaxis, including pulmonary symptoms (tightness in the throat and chest, wheezing, cough dyspnea) or skin reactions (rash, pruritus, urticaria). Notify physician or nursing staff immediately if these reactions occur.
- Monitor signs of blood dyscrasias, including eosinophilia (fatigue, weakness, myalgia),

thrombocytopenia (bruising, nose bleeds, bleeding gums, other bleeding problems), hemolytic anemia (malaise, dizziness, jaundice, abdominal pain), and leukopenia (fever, sore throat, mucosal lesions, signs of infection). Report these signs to the physician.

- Monitor injection site for pain, swelling, and irritation. Report prolonged or excessive injection-site reactions to the physician.

Interventions

- Always wash hands thoroughly and disinfect equipment (whirlpools, electrotherapeutic devices, treatment tables, and so forth) to help prevent the spread of infection. Employ universal precautions or isolation procedures as indicated for specific patients.

Patient/Client-Related Instruction

- Instruct patient to notify physician immediately of signs of superinfection, including black, furry overgrowth on tongue, vaginal itching or discharge, and loose or foul-smelling stools.
- Instruct patient and family/caregivers to report other troublesome side effects such as severe or prolonged skin problems (rash, hives) or GI problems (nausea, diarrhea).

Pharmacokinetics

Absorption: Well absorbed following IM administration; IV administration results in complete bioavailability.
Distribution: Widely distributed. Penetration into CSF is poor. Crosses the placenta and enters breast milk in low concentrations.
Metabolism and Excretion: Excreted primarily unchanged by the kidneys.
Protein Binding: 88%.
Half-life: 3–4.6 hr.

TIME/ACTION PROFILE

ROUTE	ONSET	PEAK	DURATION
IM	rapid	1–3 hr	12 hr
IV	rapid	end of infusion	12 hr

Contraindications/Precautions

Contraindicated in: Hypersensitivity to cephalosporins; Serious hypersensitivity to penicillins.
Use Cautiously in: Renal impairment (dosage reduction/increased dosing interval recommended if CCr ≤30 mL/min); History of GI disease, especially colitis; Patients with hepatic dysfunction, poor nutritional state, or cancer (may be at increased risk of bleeding); Geriatric patients (dosage adjustment due to age-related decrease in renal function may be necessary; also may be at increased risk of bleeding); Pregnancy and lactation (has been used safely).

Interactions

Drug-Drug: Probenecid ↓ excretion and ↑ blood levels. If **alcohol** is ingested within 48–72 hr of cefotetan, a disulfiram-like reaction may occur. May potentiate the effects of **anticoagulants** and ↑ the risk of bleeding. Concurrent use of **aminoglycosides** may ↑ the risk of nephrotoxicity.

Route/Dosage

IM, IV (Adults): *Most infections*—1–2 g q 12 hr. *Severe/life-threatening infections*—2–3 g q 12 hr. *Urinary tract infections*—500 mg–2 g q 12 hr or 1–2 g q 24 hr. *Perioperative prophylaxis*—1–2 g 30–60 min before initial incision (1-time dose).

Renal Impairment

IM, IV (Adults): *CCr 10–30 mL/min*—Usual adult dose q 24 hr or ½ usual adult dose q 12 hr; *<CCr 10 mL/min*— Usual adult dose q 48 hr or ¼ usual adult dose q 12 hr.

Availability

Powder for injection: 1 g Rx, 2 g Rx, 10 g Rx. **Premixed containers:** 1 g/50 mL Rx, 2 g/50 mL Rx.

cefoxitin (se-fox-i-tin)

Mefoxin

Classification
Therapeutic: anti-infectives
Pharmacologic: second-generation cephalosporins

Indications

Treatment of the following infections caused by susceptible organisms: Lower respiratory tract infections, Skin and skin structure infections, Bone and joint infections, Urinary tract infections, Gynecologic infections, Intra-abdominal infections, Septicemia. Perioperative prophylaxis.

Action

Binds to bacterial cell wall membrane, causing cell death. **Therapeutic Effects:** Bactericidal action against susceptible bacteria. **Spectrum:** Similar to that of first-generation cephalosporins but has increased activity against several other gram-negative pathogens, including *Haemophilus influenzae*, *Escherichia coli*, *Klebsiella pneumoniae*, *Morganella morganii*, *Neisseria gonorrhoeae* (including penicillinase-producing strains), *Proteus*, *Providencia*,

Moraxella catarrhalis. Also active against *Bacteroides fragilis*. Not active against methicillin-resistant staphylococci or enterococci.

Adverse Reactions/Side Effects

CNS: SEIZURES (HIGH DOSES). **GI:** PSEUDOMEMBRANOUS COLITIS, diarrhea, nausea, vomiting. **Derm:** rashes, urticaria. **Hemat:** bleeding, eosinophilia, hemolytic anemia, leukopenia, thrombocytopenia. **Local:** pain at IM site, phlebitis at IV site. **Misc:** ALLERGIC REACTIONS, INCLUDING ANAPHYLAXIS, superinfection.

PHYSICAL THERAPY IMPLICATIONS

Examination and Evaluation

- Watch for seizures; notify physician immediately if patient develops or increases seizure activity.
- Monitor signs of pseudomembranous colitis, including diarrhea, abdominal pain, fever, pus or mucus in stools, and other severe or prolonged GI problems (nausea, vomiting, heartburn). Notify physician or nursing staff immediately of these signs.
- Monitor signs of allergic reactions and anaphylaxis, including pulmonary symptoms (tightness in the throat and chest, wheezing, cough dyspnea) or skin reactions (rash, pruritus, urticaria). Notify physician or nursing staff immediately if these reactions occur.
- Monitor signs of blood dyscrasias, including eosinophilia (fatigue, weakness, myalgia), thrombocytopenia (bruising, nose bleeds, bleeding gums, other bleeding problems), hemolytic anemia (malaise, dizziness, jaundice, abdominal pain), and leukopenia (fever, sore throat, mucosal lesions, signs of infection). Report these signs to the physician.
- Monitor injection site for pain, swelling, and irritation. Report prolonged or excessive injection-site reactions to the physician.

Interventions

- Always wash hands thoroughly and disinfect equipment (whirlpools, electrotherapeutic devices, treatment tables, and so forth) to help prevent the spread of infection. Employ universal precautions or isolation procedures as indicated for specific patients.

Patient/Client-Related Instruction

- Instruct patient to notify physician immediately of signs of superinfection, including black, furry overgrowth on tongue, vaginal itching or discharge, and loose or foul-smelling stools.
- Instruct patient and family/caregivers to report other troublesome side effects such as severe or prolonged skin problems (rash, hives) or GI problems (nausea, vomiting, diarrhea).

Pharmacokinetics

Absorption: Well absorbed following IM administration; IV administration results in complete bioavailability.
Distribution: Widely distributed. Penetration into CSF is poor. Crosses the placenta and enters breast milk in low concentrations.
Metabolism and Excretion: Excreted primarily unchanged by the kidneys.
Half-life: 40–60 min (increased in renal impairment).

TIME/ACTION PROFILE

ROUTE	ONSET	PEAK	DURATION
IM	rapid	30 min	4–8 hr
IV	rapid	end of infusion	4–8 hr

Contraindications/Precautions

Contraindicated in: Hypersensitivity to cephalosporins; Serious hypersensitivity to penicillins.
Use Cautiously in: Renal impairment (dosage reduction/increased dosing interval recommended if CCr ≤50 mL/min; History of GI disease, especially colitis; Geriatric patients (dosage adjustment due to age-related decrease in renal function may be necessary); Pregnancy and lactation (has been used safely).

Interactions

Drug-Drug: Probenecid ↓ excretion and ↑ blood levels. Concurrent use of **aminoglycosides** may ↑ the risk of nephrotoxicity.

Route/Dosage

IM, IV (Adults): *Most infections*—1 g q 6–8 hr. *Severe infections*—1 g q 4 hr or 2 g q 6–8 hr. *Life-threatening infections*—2 g q 4 hr or 3 g q 6 hr. *Perioperative prophylaxis*—2 g 30–60 min before initial incision, then 2 g q 6 hr for up to 24 hr.
IM, IV (Children and Infants >3 mo): *Most infections*—13.3–26.7 mg/kg q 4 hr or 20–40 mg/kg q 6 hr. *Perioperative prophylaxis*—30–40 mg/kg within 60 min of incision, then 30–40 mg/kg q 6 hr for up to 24 hr.

Renal Impairment

- ***IM, IV (Adults):*** *CCr 30–50 mL/min—1–2 g q 8–12 hr; CCr 10–29 mL/min—1–2 g q 12–24 hr; CCr 5–9 mL/min—0.5–1 g q 12–24 hr; CCr <5 mL/min—0.5–1 g q 24–48 hr.*

Availability

- ***Powder for injection:*** *1 g, 2 g, 10 g.* ***Premixed containers:*** *1 g/50 mL D_5W, 2 g/50 mL D_5W.*

cefpodoxime (sef-poe-**dox**-eem)

Banan, Vantin

Classification

Therapeutic: anti-infectives

Pharmacologic: third-generation cephalosporins

Indications

Treatment of the following infections caused by susceptible organisms: Skin and skin structure infections, Uncomplicated urinary tract infections, Uncomplicated gynecologic infections, including gonorrhea, Respiratory tract infections, Otitis media.

Action

Binds to the bacterial cell wall membrane, causing cell death. **Therapeutic Effects:** Bactericidal action against susceptible bacteria. **Spectrum:** Similar to that of second-generation cephalosporins, but activity against staphylococci is less, whereas activity against gram-negative pathogens is greater, even for organisms resistant to first- and second-generation agents. Notable is increased action against: *Haemophilus influenzae* (including β-lactamase–producing strains), *Escherichia coli*, *Klebsiella pneumoniae*, *Neisseria gonorrhoeae*, *Proteus*. Not active against methicillin-resistant staphylococci or enterococci.

Adverse Reactions/Side Effects

CNS: SEIZURES (VERY HIGH DOSES), headache. **GI:** PSEUDOMEMBRANOUS COLITIS, diarrhea, abdominal pain, nausea, vomiting. **Derm:** rashes, urticaria. **GU:** vaginal moniliasis. **Hemat:** bleeding, blood dyscrasias, hemolytic anemia. **Misc:** ALLERGIC REACTIONS, INCLUDING ANAPHYLAXIS, superinfection.

PHYSICAL THERAPY IMPLICATIONS

Examination and Evaluation

- Watch for seizures; notify physician immediately if patient develops or increases seizure activity.
- Monitor signs of pseudomembranous colitis, including diarrhea, abdominal pain, fever, pus or mucus in stools, and other severe or prolonged GI problems (nausea, vomiting, heartburn). Notify physician or nursing staff immediately of these signs.
- Monitor signs of allergic reactions and anaphylaxis, including pulmonary symptoms (tightness in the throat and chest, wheezing, cough dyspnea) or skin reactions (rash, pruritus, urticaria). Notify physician or nursing staff immediately if these reactions occur.
- Monitor signs of blood dyscrasias, including hemolytic anemia (unusual weakness and fatigue, dizziness, jaundice, abdominal pain) and thrombocytopenia (bruising, nose bleeds, bleeding gums, other unusual bleeding). Report these signs to the physician.

Interventions

- Always wash hands thoroughly and disinfect equipment (whirlpools, electrotherapeutic devices, treatment tables, and so forth) to help prevent the spread of infection. Employ universal precautions or isolation procedures as indicated for specific patients.

Patient/Client-Related Instruction

- Instruct patient to notify physician immediately of signs of superinfection, including black, furry overgrowth on tongue, vaginal itching or discharge, and loose or foul-smelling stools.
- Instruct patient and family/caregivers to report other troublesome side effects such as severe or prolonged headache, skin problems (rash, hives), vaginal infections, or GI problems (nausea, vomiting, diarrhea, abdominal pain).

Pharmacokinetics

Absorption: Cefpodoxime proxetil is a prodrug that is converted to cefpodoxime (the active component) in GI tract during absorption; 50% absorbed after oral administration; absorption of tablets increased with food.

Distribution: Widely distributed. Crosses the placenta; enters breast milk.

Metabolism and Excretion: 29–33% excreted unchanged in urine.

Half-life: 2–3 hr (increased in renal impairment).

TIME/ACTION PROFILE (blood levels)

ROUTE	ONSET	PEAK	DURATION
PO	unknown	2–3 hr	12 hr

Contraindications/Precautions

Contraindicated in: Hypersensitivity to cephalosporins; Serious hypersensitivity to penicillins; Lactation: Lactation.

Use Cautiously in: Renal impairment (↑ dosing interval recommended if CCr <30 mLmin); History of GI disease, especially colitis; Geri: Dose adjustment due to age-related ↓ in renal function may be necessary); OB/Pedi: Pregnancy and infants <2 mo (safety not established).

Interactions

Drug-Drug: Probenecid ↓ excretion and increases blood levels. Concurrent use of **loop diuretics** or

nephrotoxic agents, including **aminoglycosides** may ↑ risk of nephrotoxicity. **Antacids** or **histamine H_2 receptor antagonists** ↓ absorption of cefpodoxime (take 2 hr before or after).

Route/Dosage

PO (Adults and Children ≥12 yr): *Most infections*—200 mg q 12 hr; *Skin and skin structure infections*—400 mg q 12 hr; *Urinary tract infections/pharyngitis*—100 mg q 12 hr; *Gonorrhea*—200 mg single dose.

PO (Children 2 mo–12 yr): *Pharyngitis/tonsillitis/otitis media/acute maxillary sinusitis*—5 mg/kg q 12 hr (not to exceed 200 mg/dose).

Renal Impairment

PO (Adults): *CCr <30 mL/min*—Increase dosing interval to q 24 hr.

Availability (generic available)

Tablets: 100 mg, 200 mg. **Oral suspension (lemon creme flavor):** 50 mg/5 mL, 100 mg/5 mL.

cefprozil (sef-proe-zil)

Cefzil

Classification

Therapeutic: anti-infectives

Pharmacologic: second-generation cephalosporins

Indications

Treatment of the following infections caused by susceptible organisms: Respiratory tract infections, Uncomplicated skin and skin structure infections, Otitis media.

Action

Binds to bacterial cell wall membrane, causing cell death. **Therapeutic Effects:** Bactericidal action against susceptible bacteria. **Spectrum:** Similar to that of first-generation cephalosporins but has increased activity against several other gram-negative pathogens, including *Haemophilus influenzae* (including β-lactamase–producing strains), *Proteus*, *Moraxella catarrhalis* (including β-lactamase–producing strains). Not active against methicillin-resistant staphylococci or enterococci.

Adverse Reactions/Side Effects

CNS: SEIZURES (VERY HIGH DOSES), dizziness. **GI:** PSEUDOMEMBRANOUS COLITIS, abdominal pain, diarrhea, nausea, vomiting. **Derm:** rashes, urticaria. **GU:** vaginitis. **Hemat:** eosinophilia, hemolytic anemia, leukopenia. **Misc:** ALLERGIC REACTIONS, INCLUDING ANAPHYLAXIS, superinfection.

PHYSICAL THERAPY IMPLICATIONS

Examination and Evaluation

- Watch for seizures; notify physician immediately if patient develops or increases seizure activity.
- Monitor signs of pseudomembranous colitis, including diarrhea, abdominal pain, fever, pus or mucus in stools, and other severe or prolonged GI problems (nausea, vomiting, heartburn). Notify physician or nursing staff immediately of these signs.
- Monitor signs of allergic reactions and anaphylaxis, including pulmonary symptoms (tightness in the throat and chest, wheezing, cough dyspnea) or skin reactions (rash, pruritus, urticaria). Notify physician or nursing staff immediately if these reactions occur.
- Monitor signs of blood dyscrasias, including eosinophilia (fatigue, weakness, myalgia), hemolytic anemia (malaise, dizziness, jaundice, abdominal pain), and leukopenia (fever, sore throat, mucosal lesions, signs of infection). Report these signs to the physician.
- Assess dizziness that might affect gait, balance, and other functional activities (See Appendix C). Report balance problems and functional limitations to the physician and nursing staff, and caution the patient and family/caregivers to guard against falls and trauma.

Interventions

- Always wash hands thoroughly and disinfect equipment (whirlpools, electrotherapeutic devices, treatment tables, and so forth) to help prevent the spread of infection. Employ universal precautions or isolation procedures as indicated for specific patients.

Patient/Client-Related Instruction

- Instruct patient to notify physician immediately of signs of superinfection, including black, furry overgrowth on tongue, vaginal itching or discharge, and loose or foul-smelling stools.
- Instruct patient and family/caregivers to report other troublesome side effects such as severe or prolonged skin problems (rash, hives), vaginal inflammation, or GI problems (nausea, vomiting, diarrhea, abdominal pain).

Pharmacokinetics

Absorption: Well absorbed following oral administration.
Distribution: Widely distributed. Enters breast milk in low concentrations.
Metabolism and Excretion: Excreted primarily unchanged by the kidneys.
Half-life: 90 min (increased in renal impairment).

TIME/ACTION PROFILE

ROUTE	ONSET	PEAK	DURATION
PO	unknown	1–2 hr	12–24 hr

Contraindications/Precautions

Contraindicated in: Hypersensitivity to cephalosporins; Serious hypersensitivity to penicillins. **Use Cautiously in:** Renal impairment (dosage reduction recommended if CCr <30 mL/min); History of GI disease, especially colitis; Suspension contains aspartame and should be avoided in patients with phenylketonuria; Geriatric patients (dosage adjustment due to age-related decrease in renal function may be necessary); Pregnancy and lactation (has been used safely).

Interactions

Drug-Drug: Probenecid ↓ excretion and ↑ blood levels. Concurrent use of **aminoglycosides** may ↑ risk of nephrotoxicity.

Route/Dosage

PO (Adults and Children ≥13 yr): *Most infections*—250–500 mg q 12 hr or 500 mg q 24 hr.
PO (Children 6 mo–12 yr): *Otitis media*—15 mg/kg q 12 hr; *Acute sinusitis*—7.5–15 mg/kg q 12 hr (higher dose to be used for moderate-to-severe infections).
PO (Children 2–12 yr): *Pharyngitis/tonsillitis*—7.5 mg/kg q 12 hr; *Skin and skin structure infections*—20 mg/kg q 24 hr.

Renal Impairment

(Adults and Children ≥6 mo): *CCr <30 mL/min*—½ of usual dose at normal dosing interval.

Availability

Tablets: 250 mg, 500 mg. **Oral suspension (bubblegum flavor):** 125 mg/5 mL, 250 mg/5 mL.

ceftaroline (sef-tar-oh-leen)

Teflaro

Classification
Therapeutic: anti-infectives
Pharmacologic: cephalosporins (derivative)

Indications

Treatment of acute bacterial skin/skin structure infections and community-acquired pneumonia.

Action

Binds to bacterial cell wall membrane, causing cell death. **Therapeutic Effects:** Bactericidal action against susceptible bacteria. **Spectrum:** *Treatment of skin/skin structure infections*—Active against *Staphylococcus aureus* (including methicillin-susceptible and methicillin-resistant strains), *Streptococcus pyogenes*, *Str. agalactiae*, *Escherichia coli*, *Klebsiella pneumoniae*, and *K. oxytoca*; *Treatment of community-acquired pneumonia*—*Str. pneumoniae* (including pneumonia with bacteremia), *S. aureus* (methicillin-susceptible strains only), *Haemophilus influenzae*, *K. pneumoniae*, *K. oxytoca*, and *Escherichia coli*.

Adverse Reactions/Side Effects

GI: PSEUDOMEMBRANOUS COLITIS, diarrhea, nausea. **Derm:** rash. **Hemat:** hemolytic anemia. **Local:** phlebitis at injection site. **Misc:** HYPERSENSITIVITY REACTIONS, INCLUDING ANAPHYLAXIS.

PHYSICAL THERAPY IMPLICATIONS

Examination and Evaluation

- Monitor signs of pseudomembranous colitis, including diarrhea, abdominal pain, fever, pus or mucus in stools, and other severe or prolonged GI problems (nausea, vomiting, heartburn). Notify physician or nursing staff immediately of these signs.
- Monitor signs of hypersensitivity reactions and anaphylaxis, including pulmonary symptoms (tightness in the throat and chest, wheezing, cough dyspnea) or skin reactions (rash, pruritus, urticaria). Notify physician or nursing staff immediately if these reactions occur.
- Monitor signs of hemolytic anemia, including unusual fatigue, shortness of breath, dizziness, headache, coldness in your hands and feet, pale skin, and chest pain. Notify physician or nursing staff immediately if these signs occur.
- Monitor IV injection-site for pain, swelling, and inflammation (phlebitis). Report prolonged or excessive injection-site reactions to the physician.

Interventions

- Always wash hands thoroughly and disinfect equipment (whirlpools, electrotherapeutic devices, treatment tables, and so forth) to help prevent the spread of infection. Employ universal precautions or isolation procedures as indicated for specific patients.

Patient/Client-Related Instruction

- Instruct patient and family/caregivers to report other troublesome side effects such as severe or prolonged skin rash or GI problems (nausea, diarrhea).

Pharmacokinetics

Absorption: IV administration results in complete bioavailability of parent drug.

Distribution: Unknown.
Metabolism and Excretion: Ceftaroline fosamil is rapidly converted by plasma phosphatases to ceftaroline, the active metabolite; 88% excreted in urine, 6% in feces.
Half-life: 2.6 hr (after multiple doses)

TIME/ACTION PROFILE (blood levels)

ROUTE	ONSET	PEAK	DURATION
IV	rapid	end of infusion	12 hr

Contraindications/Precautions

Contraindicated in: Known serious hypersensitivity to cephalosporins.
Use Cautiously in: Known hypersensitivity to other beta-lactams; Renal impairment (dosage reduction required for CCr ≤50 mL/min); Geri: dose adjustment may be necessary for age-related ↓ in renal function; OB: Use in pregnancy only if potential benefit outweighs potential risk to fetus; Lactation: Use cautiously if breast-feeding; Pedi: Safe and effective use in children <18 yr not established.

Interactions

Drug-Drug: None noted.

Route/Dosage

IV (Adults 18 yr): *Skin/skin structure infections*—600 mg q 12 hr for 5–14 days; *Community-acquired pneumonia*—600 mg q 12 hr for 5–7 days.

Renal Impairment

IV (Adults >18 yr): *CCr >30 to ≤50 mL/min*—400 mg q 12 hr; *CCr ≥15 to ≤30 mL/min*—300 mg q 12 hr; *CCr <15 mL/min*—200 mg q 12 hr.

Availability

Powder for injection (requires reconstitution): 400 mg/vial, 600 mg/vial.

ceftazidime (sef-tay-zi-deem)

Fortaz, Tazicef

Classification
Therapeutic: anti-infectives
Pharmacologic: third-generation cephalosporins

Indications

Treatment of the following infections caused by susceptible organisms: Skin and skin structure infections, Bone and joint infections, Urinary tract infections, Gynecologic infections, Lower respiratory tract infections, Intra-abdominal infections, Septicemia, Febrile neutropenia, Meningitis.

Action

Binds to the bacterial cell wall membrane, causing cell death. **Therapeutic Effects:** Bactericidal action against susceptible bacteria. **Spectrum:** Similar to that of second-generation cephalosporins, but activity against staphylococci is less, while activity against gram-negative pathogens (particularly *Pseudomonas aeruginosa*) is greater, even for organisms resistant to first- and second-generation agents. Notable is increased action against *Citrobacter*, *Enterobacter*, *Haemophilus influenzae* (including β-lactamase–producing strains), *Escherichia coli*, *Klebsiella pneumoniae*, *Neisseria meningitidis*, *Proteus*, *Providencia*, *Pseudomonas aeruginosa*, *Serratia*, *Moraxella catarrhalis*. Not active against methicillin-resistant staphylococci or enterococci.

Adverse Reactions/Side Effects

CNS: SEIZURES (HIGH DOSES IN PATIENTS WITH RENAL IMPAIRMENT), encephalopathy. **GI:** PSEUDOMEMBRANOUS COLITIS, abdominal pain, diarrhea, nausea, vomiting. **Derm:** rashes, pruritus, urticaria. **Hemat:** bleeding, blood dyscrasias, hemolytic anemia. **Local:** pain at IM site, phlebitis at IV site. **Misc:** ALLERGIC REACTIONS, INCLUDING ANAPHYLAXIS, superinfection, fever.

PHYSICAL THERAPY IMPLICATIONS

Examination and Evaluation

- Watch for seizures; notify physician immediately if patient develops or increases seizure activity.
- Monitor signs of pseudomembranous colitis, including diarrhea, abdominal pain, fever, pus or mucus in stools, and other severe or prolonged GI problems (nausea, vomiting, heartburn). Notify physician or nursing staff immediately of these signs.
- Monitor signs of allergic reactions and anaphylaxis, including pulmonary symptoms (tightness in the throat and chest, wheezing, cough dyspnea) or skin reactions (rash, pruritus, urticaria). Notify physician or nursing staff immediately if these reactions occur.
- Be alert for signs of encephalopathy, including decreased alertness, lethargy, and incoordination. Notify physician of these signs before they progress to more severe changes in mental status such as dementia, seizures, and coma.
- Monitor signs of blood dyscrasias including hemolytic anemia (unusual weakness and fatigue, dizziness, jaundice, abdominal pain) and thrombocytopenia (bruising, nose bleeds, bleeding gums, other unusual bleeding). Report these signs to the physician.
- Monitor injection site for pain, swelling, and irritation. Report prolonged or excessive injection site reactions to the physician.

C

Interventions

- Always wash hands thoroughly and disinfect equipment (whirlpools, electrotherapeutic devices, treatment tables, and so forth) to help prevent the spread of infection. Employ universal precautions or isolation procedures as indicated for specific patients.

Patient/Client-Related Instruction

- Instruct patient to notify physician immediately of signs of superinfection, including black, furry overgrowth on tongue, vaginal itching or discharge, and loose or foul-smelling stools.
- Instruct patient and family/caregivers to report other troublesome side effects such as severe or prolonged fever, skin problems (rash, hives, itching), or GI problems (nausea, vomiting, diarrhea, abdominal pain).

Pharmacokinetics

Absorption: Well absorbed following IM administration; IV administration results in complete bioavailability.
Distribution: Widely distributed. Crosses the placenta; enters breast milk in low concentrations. CSF penetration better than with first- and second-generation agents.
Protein Binding: 17%.
Metabolism and Excretion: 80–90% excreted unchanged in urine.
Half-life: Neonates: 2.2–4.7 hr; Adults: 2 hr (increased in renal impairment).

TIME/ACTION PROFILE

ROUTE	ONSET	PEAK	DURATION
IV	rapid	end of infusion	6–12 hr

Contraindications/Precautions

Contraindicated in: Hypersensitivity to cephalosporins; Serious hypersensitivity to penicillins.
Use Cautiously in: Renal impairment (decreased dosing/increased dosing interval recommended if CCr ≤50 mL/min); History of GI disease, especially colitis; Lactation: Direct drug effects and modification of bowel flora may occur in the nursing infant; Geri: Dosage adjustment may be necessary due to age-related decrease in renal function.

Interactions

Drug-Drug: Concurrent use of **loop diuretics** or **nephrotoxic agents,** including **aminoglycosides,** may ↑ the risk of nephrotoxicity. Bactericidal activity ↓ by **chloramphenicol**.

Route/Dosage

IM, IV (Adults and Children ≥12 yr): *Pneumonia and skin/skin structure infections*—500 mg–1 g q 8 hr. *Bone and joint infections*—2 g q 12 hr. *Severe and life-threatening infections*—2 g q 8 hr. *Complicated urinary tract infections*—500 mg q 8–12 hr. *Uncomplicated urinary tract infections*—250 mg q 12 hr. *Cystic fibrosis lung infection caused by* Pseudomonas aeruginosa—30–50 mg/kg q 8 hr (max daily dose: 6 g).
IM, IV (Children 1 mo–12 yr): 100–150 mg/kg/day divided q 8 hr (maximum dose: 6 g/day).
IM, IV (Neonates ≤4 wk): 50 mg/kg q 8–12 hr.

Renal Impairment

IM, IV (Adults): *CCr 31–50 mL/min*—1 g q 12 hr; *CCr 16–30 mL/min*—1 g q 24 hr; *CCr 6–15 mLmin*—500 mg q 24 hr; *CCr < 5 mL/min*—500 mg q 48 hr.

Availability

Powder for injection: 500 mg Rx, 1 g Rx, 2 g Rx, 6 g Rx. **Premixed containers:** 1 g/50 mL Rx, 2 g/50 mL Rx.

ceftibuten (sef-tye-**byoo**-ten)

Cedax

Classification
Therapeutic: anti-infectives
Pharmacologic: third-generation cephalosporins

Indications

Treatment of the following infections caused by susceptible organisms: Acute exacerbations of chronic bronchitis, Otitis media, Pharyngitis and tonsillitis.

Action

Binds to the bacterial cell wall membrane, causing cell death. **Therapeutic Effects:** Bactericidal action against susceptible bacteria. **Spectrum:** Similar to that of second-generation cephalosporins, but activity against staphylococci is less, whereas activity against gram-negative pathogens is greater, even for organisms resistant to first- and second-generation agents. Notable is increased action against *Haemophilus influenzae* (including β-lactamase–producing strains), *Escherichia coli*, *Klebsiella pneumoniae*, *Proteus*, *Providencia*, *Moraxella catarrhalis* (including β-lactamase–producing strains).

Adverse Reactions/Side Effects

CNS: SEIZURES (VERY HIGH DOSES IN PATIENTS WITH RENAL IMPAIRMENT), dizziness, headache. **GI:** PSEUDOMEMBRANOUS COLITIS, abdominal pain, diarrhea, dyspepsia, nausea, vomiting. **Derm:** rashes, urticaria. **Hemat:** bleeding, eosinophilia, hemolytic anemia, leukopenia, thrombocytopenia, thrombocytosis. **Misc:** ALLERGIC REACTIONS, INCLUDING ANAPHYLAXIS, superinfection.

PHYSICAL THERAPY IMPLICATIONS

Examination and Evaluation

- Watch for seizures; notify physician immediately if patient develops or increases seizure activity.
- Monitor signs of pseudomembranous colitis, including diarrhea, abdominal pain, fever, pus or mucus in stools, and other severe or prolonged GI problems (nausea, vomiting, heartburn). Notify physician or nursing staff immediately of these signs.
- Monitor signs of allergic reactions and anaphylaxis, including pulmonary symptoms (tightness in the throat and chest, wheezing, cough dyspnea) or skin reactions (rash, pruritus, urticaria). Notify physician or nursing staff immediately if these reactions occur.
- Monitor signs of blood dyscrasias including eosinophilia (fatigue, weakness, myalgia), hemolytic anemia (malaise, dizziness, jaundice, abdominal pain), leukopenia (fever, sore throat, mucosal lesions, signs of infection), thrombocytopenia (bruising, nose bleeds, bleeding gums, other unusual bleeding), or thrombocytosis (headache, dizziness, chest pain, fainting, visual disturbances, numbness or tingling in the hands and feet). Report these signs to the physician.
- Assess dizziness that might affect gait, balance, and other functional activities (See Appendix C). Report balance problems and functional limitations to the physician and nursing staff, and caution the patient and family/caregivers to guard against falls and trauma.

Interventions

- Always wash hands thoroughly and disinfect equipment (whirlpools, electrotherapeutic devices, treatment tables, and so forth) to help prevent the spread of infection. Use universal precautions or isolation procedures as indicated for specific patients.

Patient/Client-Related Instruction

- Instruct patient to notify physician immediately of signs of superinfection, including black, furry overgrowth on tongue, vaginal itching or discharge, and loose or foul-smelling stools.
- Instruct patient and family/caregivers to report other troublesome side effects such as severe or prolonged headache, skin problems (rash, hives), or GI problems (nausea, vomiting, diarrhea, abdominal pain, heartburn).

Pharmacokinetics

Absorption: Well absorbed after oral administration; absorption decreased by food.
Distribution: Widely distributed. Crosses the placenta.
Metabolism and Excretion: 56% excreted in urine; 39% in feces.
Half-life: 120–144 min (increased in renal impairment).

TIME/ACTION PROFILE

ROUTE	ONSET	PEAK	DURATION
PO	rapid	3 hr	24 hr

Contraindications/Precautions

Contraindicated in: Hypersensitivity to cephalosporins; Serious hypersensitivity to penicillins.
Use Cautiously in: Renal impairment (decreased dosing recommended if CCr <50 mL/min; Diabetes (suspension contains sucrose); History of GI disease, especially colitis; Geriatric patients (dosage adjustment due to age-related decrease in renal function may be necessary); Pregnancy, lactation, and infants <6 mo (safety not established).

Interactions

Drug-Drug: None known.

Route/Dosage

PO (Adults and Children ≥12 yr): 400 mg once daily for 10 days.
PO (Children 6 mo–12 yr): 9 mg/kg once daily for 10 days (max daily dose: 400 mg).

Renal Impairment

PO (Adults): *CCr 30–49 mL/min*—200 mg or 4.5 mg/kg q 24 hr; *CCr 5–29 mL/min*— 100 mg or 2.25 mg/kg q 24 hr.

Availability

Capsules: 400 mg. **Oral suspension (cherry flavor):** 90 mg/5 mL.

ceftizoxime (sef-ti-zox-eem)

Cefizox

Classification
Therapeutic: anti-infectives
Pharmacologic: third-generation cephalosporins

Indications

Treatment of the following infections caused by susceptible organisms: Skin and skin structure infections, Bone and joint infections, Urinary tract infections, Gynecologic infections, including gonorrhea, Lower respiratory tract infections, Intra-abdominal infection, Septicemia, Meningitis.

Action

Binds to the bacterial cell wall membrane, causing cell death. **Therapeutic Effects:** Bactericidal action against susceptible bacteria. **Spectrum:** Similar to that of second-generation cephalosporins, but activity against staphylococci is less, whereas activity against gram-negative pathogens is greater, even for organisms resistant to first- and second-generation agents. Notable is increased action against *Enterobacter*, *Haemophilus influenzae*, *Escherichia coli*, *Klebsiella pneumoniae*, *Neisseria*, *Proteus*, *Providencia*, *Serratia*, *Moraxella catarrhalis*, *Morganella morganii*. Has some activity against anaerobes, including *Bacteroides fragilis*. Not active against methicillin-resistant staphylococci or enterococci.

Adverse Reactions/Side Effects

CNS: SEIZURES (HIGH DOSES). **GI:** PSEUDOMEMBRANOUS COLITIS, diarrhea, nausea, vomiting. **Derm:** pruritus, rashes, urticaria. **Hemat:** bleeding, eosinophilia, hemolytic anemia, leukopenia, neutropenia, thrombocytopenia, thrombocytosis. **Local:** pain at IM site, phlebitis at IV site. **Misc:** ALLERGIC REACTIONS, INCLUDING ANAPHYLAXIS, superinfection, fever.

PHYSICAL THERAPY IMPLICATIONS

Examination and Evaluation

- Watch for seizures; notify physician immediately if patient develops or increases seizure activity.
- Monitor signs of pseudomembranous colitis, including diarrhea, abdominal pain, fever, pus or mucus in stools, and other severe or prolonged GI problems (nausea, vomiting, heartburn). Notify physician or nursing staff immediately of these signs.
- Monitor signs of allergic reactions and anaphylaxis, including pulmonary symptoms (tightness in the throat and chest, wheezing, cough dyspnea) or skin reactions (rash, pruritus, urticaria). Notify physician or nursing staff immediately if these reactions occur.
- Monitor signs of blood dyscrasias including eosinophilia (fatigue, weakness, myalgia), hemolytic anemia (malaise, dizziness, jaundice, abdominal pain), leukopenia and neutropenia (fever, sore throat, mucosal lesions, signs of infection), thrombocytopenia (bruising, nose bleeds, bleeding gums, other unusual bleeding), or thrombocytosis (headache, dizziness, chest pain, fainting, visual disturbances, numbness or tingling in the hands and feet). Report these signs to the physician.
- Monitor injection site for pain, swelling, and irritation. Report prolonged or excessive injection-site reactions to the physician.

Interventions

- Always wash hands thoroughly and disinfect equipment (whirlpools, electrotherapeutic devices, treatment tables, and so forth) to help prevent the spread of infection. Employ universal precautions or isolation procedures as indicated for specific patients.

Patient/Client-related Instruction

- Instruct patient to notify physician immediately of signs of superinfection, including black, furry overgrowth on tongue, vaginal itching or discharge, and loose or foul-smelling stools.
- Instruct patient and family/caregivers to report other troublesome side effects such as severe or prolonged fever, skin problems (rash, hives, itching), or GI problems (nausea, vomiting, diarrhea).

Pharmacokinetics

Absorption: Well absorbed after IM administration; IV administration results in complete bioavailability.
Distribution: Widely distributed. Crosses the placenta; enters breast milk in low concentrations. CSF penetration better than with first- and second-generation agents.
Metabolism and Excretion: 70–100% excreted unchanged in urine.
Half-life: 84–114 min (increased in renal impairment).

TIME/ACTION PROFILE

ROUTE	ONSET	PEAK	DURATION
IM	rapid	0.5–1.5 hr	6–12 hr
IV	rapid	end of infusion	6–12 hr

Contraindications/Precautions

Contraindicated in: Hypersensitivity to cephalosporins; Serious hypersensitivity to penicillins.
Use Cautiously in: Renal impairment (decreased dosing/increased dosing interval recommended if CCr ≤80 mL/min); History of GI disease, especially colitis; Geriatric patients (dosage adjustment due to age-related decrease in renal function may be necessary); Pregnancy, lactation, and children < 6 mo (safety not established).

Interactions

Drug-Drug: Probenecid decreases excretion and increases blood levels. Concurrent use of **loop diuretics** or **nephrotoxic agents**, including **aminoglycosides,** may increase the risk of nephrotoxicity.

Route/Dosage

IM, IV (Adults): *Severe infections*—1–2 g q 8–12 hr. *Life-threatening infections*—3–4 g q 8 hr. *Uncomplicated urinary tract infections*—500 mg q 12 hr. *Gonococcal urethritis/cervicitis*—1 g IM (single dose).

IM, IV (Children ≥6 mo): 50 mg/kg q 6–8 hr (not to exceed 200 mg/kg/day).

Renal Impairment

IM, IV (Adults): *CCr 50–79 mL/min*—500 mg–1.5 g q 8 hr; *CCr 5–49 mL/min*—250 mg–1 g q 12 hr; *CCr 0–4 mL/min*—500 mg–1 g q 48 hr or 250–500 mg q 24 hr.

Availability

Powder for injection: 1 g, 2 g, 10 g. **Premixed containers:** 1 g/50 mL, 2 g/50 mL.

ceftriaxone (sef-try-**aks**-one)

Rocephin

Classification

Therapeutic: anti-infectives

Pharmacologic: third-generation cephalosporins

Indications

Treatment of Skin and skin structure infections, Bone and joint infections, Complicated and uncomplicated urinary tract infections, Uncomplicated gynecologic infections, including gonorrhea, Lower respiratory tract infections, Intra-abdominal infections, Septicemia, Meningitis, Otitis media. Perioperative prophylaxis.

Action

Binds to the bacterial cell wall membrane, causing cell death. **Therapeutic Effects:** Bactericidal action against susceptible bacteria. **Spectrum:** Similar to that of second-generation cephalosporins, but activity against staphylococci is less, while activity against gram-negative pathogens is greater, even for organisms resistant to first- and second-generation agents. Notable is increased action against: *Acinetobacter*, *Enterobacter*, *Haemophilus influenzae* (including β-lactamase–producing strains), *Haemophilus parainfluenzae*, *Escherichia coli*, *Klebsiella pneumoniae*, *Morganella morganii*, *Neisseria*, *Proteus*, *Providencia*, *Serratia*, *Moraxella catarrhalis*. Has some activity against anaerobes, including *Bacteroides fragilis*. Not active against methicillin-resistant staphylococci or enterococci.

Adverse Reactions/Side Effects

CNS: SEIZURES (HIGH DOSES). **GI:** PSEUDOMEMBRANOUS COLITIS, diarrhea, cholelithiasis, sludging in the gallbladder. **Derm:** rashes, urticaria. **Hemat:** bleeding, eosinophilia, hemolytic anemia, leukopenia, thrombocytosis. **Local:** pain at IM site, phlebitis at IV site. **Misc:** ALLERGIC REACTIONS, INCLUDING ANAPHYLAXIS, superinfection.

PHYSICAL THERAPY IMPLICATIONS

Examination and Evaluation

- Watch for seizures; notify physician immediately if patient develops or increases seizure activity.
- Monitor signs of pseudomembranous colitis, including diarrhea, abdominal pain, fever, pus or mucus in stools, and other severe or prolonged GI problems (nausea, vomiting, heartburn). Notify physician or nursing staff immediately of these signs.
- Monitor signs of allergic reactions and anaphylaxis, including pulmonary symptoms (tightness in the throat and chest, wheezing, cough dyspnea) or skin reactions (rash, pruritus, urticaria). Notify physician or nursing staff immediately if these reactions occur.
- Monitor signs of blood dyscrasias, including eosinophilia (fatigue, weakness, myalgia), hemolytic anemia (malaise, dizziness, jaundice, abdominal pain), leukopenia (fever, sore throat, mucosal lesions, signs of infection), thrombocytopenia (bruising, nose bleeds, bleeding gums, other unusual bleeding), or thrombocytosis (headache, dizziness, chest pain, fainting, visual disturbances, numbness or tingling in the hands and feet). Report these signs to the physician.
- Monitor injection site for pain, swelling, and irritation. Report prolonged or excessive injection site reactions to the physician.

Interventions

- Always wash hands thoroughly and disinfect equipment (whirlpools, electrotherapeutic devices, treatment tables, and so forth) to help prevent the spread of infection. Use universal precautions or isolation procedures as indicated for specific patients.

Patient/Client-Related Instruction

- Instruct patient to notify physician immediately of signs of superinfection, including black, furry overgrowth on tongue, vaginal itching or discharge, and loose or foul-smelling stools.
- Instruct patient and family/caregivers to report other troublesome side effects such as severe or prolonged fever, skin problems (rash, hives), diarrhea, or signs of gallstones (sudden intense pain in the abdomen or right side, jaundice, chills, fever).

Pharmacokinetics

Absorption: Well absorbed following IM administration; IV administration results in complete bioavailability.

Distribution: Widely distributed. CSF penetration better than with first- and second-generation agents. Crosses the placenta; enters breast milk in low concentrations.

C

Protein Binding: ≥90%.
Metabolism and Excretion: 33–67% excreted in urine as unchanged drug, remainder excreted in feces.
Half-life: 6–9 hr.

TIME/ACTION PROFILE

ROUTE	ONSET	PEAK	DURATION
IM	rapid	1–2 hr	12–24 hr
IV	rapid	end of infusion	12–24 hr

Contraindications/Precautions

Contraindicated in: Hypersensitivity to cephalosporins; Serious hypersensitivity to penicillins; Pedi: Neonates ≤28 days (use in hyperbilirubinemic neonates may lead to kernicterus).
Use Cautiously in: Combined severe hepatic and renal impairment (dosage reduction/increased dosing interval recommended); History of GI disease, especially colitis; OB/Lactation: Pregnancy and lactation.

Interactions

Drug-Drug: Should not be administered within 48 hr of calcium-containing solutions.

Route/Dosage

IM, IV (Adults): *Most infections*—1–2 g q 12–24 hr. *Gonorrhea*—250 mg IM (single dose). *Meningitis*—2 g q 12 hr. *Perioperative prophylaxis*—1 g 0.5–2 hr before surgery (single dose).
IM, IV (Children): *Most infections*—50–75 mg/kg/day (not to exceed 2 g/day) divided q 12–24 hr. *Meningitis*—100 mg/kg/day (not to exceed 4 g/day) divided q 12–24 hr. *Uncomplicated gonorrhea*—125 mg IM (single dose). *Acute otitis media*—50 mg/kg (not to exceed 1 g) IM single dose.

Availability (generic available)

Powder for injection: 250 mg, 500 mg, 1 g, 2 g, 10 g.
Premixed containers: 1 g/50 mL, 2 g/50 mL.

cefuroxime (se-fyoor-ox-eem)

Ceftin, Zinacef

Classification
Therapeutic: anti-infectives
Pharmacologic: second-generation cephalosporins

Indications

Treatment of Respiratory tract infections, Skin and skin structure infections, Bone and joint infections (IV), Urinary tract infections, Gynecologic infections, Septicemia (IV), Otitis media (PO), Meningitis (IV), Lyme disease (PO). Perioperative prophylaxis (IV).

Action

Binds to bacterial cell wall membrane, causing cell death. **Therapeutic Effects:** Bactericidal action against susceptible bacteria. **Spectrum:** Similar to that of first-generation cephalosporins but has increased activity against several other gram-negative pathogens, including *Haemophilus influenzae* (including β-lactamase–producing strains), *Haemophilus parainfluenzae, Escherichia coli, Klebsiella pneumoniae, Neisseria, Proteus, Moraxella catarrhalis, Borrelia burgdorferi*. Not active against methicillin-resistant staphylococci or enterococci.

Adverse Reactions/Side Effects

CNS: SEIZURES (HIGH DOSES). **GI:** PSEUDOMEMBRANOUS COLITIS, diarrhea, nausea, vomiting, cramps. **Derm:** rashes, urticaria, diaper dermatitis. **Hemat:** bleeding, eosinophilia, hemolytic anemia, leukopenia. **Local:** pain at IM site, phlebitis at IV site. **Misc:** ALLERGIC REACTIONS, INCLUDING ANAPHYLAXIS, superinfection.

PHYSICAL THERAPY IMPLICATIONS

Examination and Evaluation

- Watch for seizures; notify physician immediately if patient develops or increases seizure activity.
- Monitor signs of pseudomembranous colitis, including diarrhea, abdominal pain, fever, pus or mucus in stools, and other severe or prolonged GI problems (nausea, vomiting, heartburn). Notify physician or nursing staff immediately of these signs.
- Monitor signs of allergic reactions and anaphylaxis, including pulmonary symptoms (tightness in the throat and chest, wheezing, cough dyspnea) or skin reactions (rash, pruritus, urticaria). Notify physician or nursing staff immediately if these reactions occur.
- Monitor signs of blood dyscrasias, including eosinophilia (fatigue, weakness, myalgia), hemolytic anemia (malaise, dizziness, jaundice, abdominal pain), leukopenia (fever, sore throat, mucosal lesions, signs of infection), and thrombocytopenia (bruising, nose bleeds, bleeding gums, other bleeding problems). Report these signs to the physician.
- Monitor injection site for pain, swelling, and irritation. Report prolonged or excessive injection site reactions to the physician.

Interventions

Always wash hands thoroughly and disinfect equipment (whirlpools, electrotherapeutic devices, treatment tables, and so forth) to help prevent the spread of infection. Employ universal precautions or isolation procedures as indicated for specific patients.

Patient/Client-related Instruction

- Instruct patient to notify physician immediately of signs of superinfection, including black, furry overgrowth on tongue, vaginal itching or discharge, and loose or foul-smelling stools.
- Instruct patient and family/caregivers to report other troublesome side effects such as severe or prolonged skin problems (rash, hives, dermatitis) or GI problems (nausea, vomiting, diarrhea, cramps).

Pharmacokinetics

Absorption: Well absorbed after oral and IM administration; IV administration results in complete bioavailability.
Distribution: Widely distributed. Penetrates into CSF with IV administration. Crosses the placenta and enters breast milk in low concentrations.
Protein Binding: 50%.
Metabolism and Excretion: Excreted primarily unchanged in the urine.
Half-life: 1–2 hr (increased in renal impairment).

TIME/ACTION PROFILE

ROUTE	ONSET	PEAK	DURATION
PO	unknown	2–3 hr	8–12 hr
IM	rapid	15–60 min	6–12 hr
IV	rapid	end of infusion	6–12 hr

Contraindications/Precautions

Contraindicated in: Hypersensitivity to cephalosporins; Serious hypersensitivity to penicillins.
Use Cautiously in: Renal impairment (dosage reduction/increased dosing interval recommended if CCr ≤20 mL/min); History of GI disease, especially colitis; Geriatric patients (dosage adjustment may be required due to age-related decrease in renal function); Pregnancy and lactation (has been used safely).

Interactions

Drug-Drug: Probenecid ↓ excretion and ↑ blood levels. **Aminoglycosides** and **loop diuretics** may ↑ the risk of nephrotoxicity.

Route/Dosage

Note: Cefuroxime oral tablets and oral suspension are not bioequivalent and are not substitutable on a mg/mg basis.

PO (Adults and Children >12 yr): *Pharyngitis/tonsillitis, maxillary sinusitis, uncomplicated urinary tract infections*—250 mg q 12 hr. *Bronchitis, uncomplicated skin/skin structure infections*—250–500 mg q 12 hr. *Gonorrhea*—1-g single dose. *Lyme disease*—500 mg q 12 hr for 20 days.

PO (Children 3 mo–12 yr): *Otitis media, acute bacterial maxillary sinusitis, impetigo*—15 mg/kg q 12 hr as oral suspension (not to exceed 1 g/day) *or* 250 mg q 12 hr as tablets. *Pharyngitis/tonsillitis*—10 mg/kg q 12 hr as oral suspension, not to exceed 500 mg/day.

IM, IV (Adults): *Uncomplicated urinary tract infections, skin/skin structure infections, disseminated gonococcal infections, uncomplicated pneumonia*—750 mg q 8 hr. *Bone/joint infections, severe or complicated infections*—1.5 g q 8 hr. *Life-threatening infections*—1.5 g q 6 hr. *Meningitis*—3 g q 8 hr. *Perioperative prophylaxis*—1.5 g IV 30–60 min before initial incision; 750 mg IM/IV q 8 hr can be given when procedure prolonged. *Prophylaxis during open-heart surgery*—1.5 g IV at induction of anesthesia and then q 12 hr for 3 additional doses. *Gonorrhea*—1.5 g IM (750 mg in 2 sites) with 1 g probenecid PO.

IM, IV (Children and Infants >3 mo): *Most infections*—50–100 mg/kg/day divided q 6–8 hr (max dose: 6 g/day). *Bone and joint infections*—150 mg/kg/day divided q 8 hr (max dose: 6 g/day).

Renal Impairment

IM, IV (Adults): *CCr 10–20 mL/min*—750 mg q 12 hr; *CCr <10 mL/min*—750 mg q 24 hr.

Availability (generic available)

Tablets: 250 mg, 500 mg. **Oral suspension (tutti-frutti):** 125 mg/5 mL, 250 mg/5 mL. **Powder for injection:** 750 mg, 1.5 g, 7.5 g. **Premixed containers:** 750 mg/50 mL, 1.5 g/50 mL.

celecoxib (sel-e-kox-ib)

Celebrex

Classification
Therapeutic: antirheumatics, nonsteroidal anti-inflammatory agents
Pharmacologic: COX-2 inhibitors

Indications

Relief of signs and symptoms of osteoarthritis, rheumatoid arthritis, ankylosing spondylitis, and juvenile rheumatoid arthritis. Reduction of the number of adenomatous colorectal polyps in familial adenomatous polyposis (FAP), as an adjunct to usual care (endoscopic surveillance, surgery). Management of acute pain, including primary dysmenorrhea.

Action

Inhibits the enzyme COX-2. This enzyme is required for the synthesis of prostaglandins. Has analgesic, anti-inflammatory, and antipyretic properties. **Therapeutic Effects:** Decreased pain and inflammation caused by arthritis or spondylitis. Decreased number of colorectal polyps. Decreased pain.

Adverse Reactions/Side Effects
CNS: dizziness, headache, insomnia. **CV:** edema. **GI:** GI BLEEDING, abdominal pain, diarrhea, dyspepsia, flatulence,

nausea. **Derm:** EXFOLIATIVE DERMATITIS, STEVENS-JOHNSON SYNDROME, TOXIC EPIDERMAL NECROLYSIS, rash.

C

PHYSICAL THERAPY IMPLICATIONS

Examination and Evaluation

- Monitor rashes or other skin reactions (hives, itching, dermatitis, exfoliation). Notify physician immediately because certain skin reactions may indicate serious hypersensitivity reactions (Stevens-Johnson syndrome, toxic epidermal necrolysis).
- Watch for signs of GI bleeding, including abdominal pain, vomiting blood, blood in stools, or black, tarry stools. Although celecoxib may produce fewer GI side effects than other NSAIDs, some patients may still experience GI bleeding and other gastric problems (diarrhea, nausea, flatulence, heartburn). Report these signs to the physician immediately.
- Continually monitor for signs of MI (sudden chest pain, pain radiating into the arm or jaw, shortness of breath, dizziness, sweating, anxiety, nausea) and stroke (sudden severe headache, confusion, nausea, vomiting, paralysis, numbness, speech problems, visual disturbances). Although rare, celecoxib has been associated with coronary and cerebral thrombosis. Seek immediate medical assistance if patient develops these signs.
- Assess pain and other variables (range of motion, muscle strength) to document whether this drug is successful in helping manage the patient's pain and decreasing impairments.
- Assess dizziness that might affect gait, balance, and other functional activities (See Appendix C). Report balance problems and functional limitations to the physician, and caution the patient and family/caregivers to guard against falls and trauma.
- Assess peripheral edema using girth measurements, volume displacement, and measurement of pitting edema (See Appendix N). Report increased swelling in feet and ankles or a sudden increase in body weight due to vasodilation or fluid retention.

Interventions

- Implement appropriate manual therapy techniques, physical agents, and therapeutic exercises to reduce pain, improve function, and decrease the need for celecoxib and other analgesics.
- Because of the risk of MI and stroke, use caution during aerobic exercise and other forms of therapeutic exercise. Assess exercise tolerance frequently (blood pressure, heart rate, fatigue levels), and terminate exercise immediately if any untoward responses occur (See Appendix L).
- Help patient explore other nonpharmacologic methods to reduce chronic pain (relaxation techniques, exercise, counseling, etc.).

Patient/Client-Related Instruction

- Advise patient and family or caregivers about the signs of MI and stroke (See above under Examination and Evaluation), and to seek immediate medical assistance if these signs develop.
- Advise patient that analgesics are usually more effective if given before pain becomes severe; emphasize that adequate pain control will allow better participation in physical therapy.
- Advise patient to reduce alcohol intake because alcohol increases the risk of gastric toxicity.
- Caution patient about the use of over-the-counter products that contain NSAIDs or acetaminophen while taking prescription doses of celecoxib. Use of multiple analgesics increases the risk of toxicity and overdose.

Pharmacokinetics

Absorption: Bioavailability unknown.
Distribution: 97% bound to plasma proteins; extensive tissue distribution.
Metabolism and Excretion: Mostly metabolized by the liver; <3% excreted unchanged in urine and feces.
Half-life: 11 hr.

TIME/ACTION PROFILE (pain reduction)

ROUTE	ONSET	PEAK	DURATION
PO	24–48 hr	unknown	12–24 hr*

*After discontinuation.

Contraindications/Precautions

Contraindicated in: Hypersensitivity; Cross-sensitivity may exist with other NSAIDs, including aspirin; History of allergic-type reactions to sulfonamides; History of asthma, urticaria, or allergic-type reactions to aspirin or other NSAIDs, including the aspirin triad (asthma, nasal polyps, and severe hypersensitivity reactions to aspirin); Advanced renal disease; Perioperative pain from coronary artery bypass graft (CABG) surgery; OB: Should not be used in late pregnancy (may cause premature closure of the ductus arteriosus). Lactation: Potential for serious neonatal adverse effects. Discontinue drug or bottle feed.
Use Cautiously in: Cardiovascular disease or risk factors for cardiovascular disease (may ↑ risk of serious cardiovascular thrombotic events, myocardial infarction, and stroke, especially with

prolonged use); Preexisting renal disease, heart failure, liver dysfunction, concurrent diuretic or ACE inhibitor therapy (increased risk of renal impairment); Hypertension or fluid retention; Renal insufficiency (may precipitate acute renal failure); Serious dehydration (correct deficits before administering); Preexisting asthma; Pedi: Safety not established in children <2 yr or for longer than 6 mo; Geri: Concurrent therapy with corticosteroids or anticoagulants, long duration of NSAID therapy, history of smoking, alcoholism, geriatric patients, or poor general health status (increased risk of GI bleeding). **Exercise Extreme Caution in:** History of ulcer disease or GI bleeding.

Interactions

Drug-Drug: Significant interactions may occur when celecoxib is coadministered with other drugs that inhibit the CYP450 2C9 enzyme system. May ↓ effectiveness of **ACE inhibitors**, **thiazide diuretics**, and **furosemide**. **Fluconazole** ↑ celecoxib blood levels (dosage reduction recommended). May ↑ risk of bleeding with **warfarin**. May ↑ serum **lithium** levels. Does not inhibit the cardioprotective effect of low-dose **aspirin**.

Route/Dosage

PO (Adults): *Osteoarthritis*—200 mg/day as a single dose *or* 100 mg twice daily. *Rheumatoid arthritis*—100–200 mg twice daily. *Ankylosing spondylitis*—200 mg once daily *or* 100 mg twice daily; dose may be increased after 6 wk to 400 mg daily. *Familial adenomatous polyposis*—400 mg twice daily. *Acute pain, including dysmenorrhea*—400 mg initially, then a 200 mg dose if needed on the first day; then 200 mg twice daily as needed.

PO (Children2 yr and older, ≥10–≤25 kg): 50 mg capsule twice daily.

PO (Children 2 yr and older, >25 kg): 100 mg capsule twice daily.

Availability

Capsules: 50 mg, 100 mg, 200 mg, 400 mg.

cephalexin (sef-a-lex-in)

Apo-Cephalex, DOM-Cephalexin, Keflex, Nu-Cephalex, PMS Cephalexin

Classification

Therapeutic: anti-infectives

Pharmacologic: first-generation cephalosporins

Indications

Treatment of the following infections caused by susceptible organisms: Skin and skin structure infections, Respiratory tract infections, Otitis media, Urinary tract infections, Bone infections.

Action

Binds to bacterial cell wall membrane, causing cell death. **Therapeutic Effects:** Bactericidal action against susceptible bacteria. **Spectrum:** Active against many gram-positive cocci, including *Streptococcus pneumoniae*, group A beta-hemolytic streptococci, staphylococci (including penicillinase-producing strains). Active against the following gram-negative organisms: *Escherichia coli*, *Haemophilus influenzae*, *Klebsiella pneumoniae*, *Moraxella catarrhalis*, *Proteus*. Not active against methicillin-resistant staphylococci or enterococci: *Enterococcus*. Not active against anaerobes.

Adverse Reactions/Side Effects

CNS: SEIZURES (HIGH DOSES). **GI:** PSEUDOMEMBRANOUS COLITIS, diarrhea, abdominal pain, nausea, vomiting. **Derm:** rashes, urticaria. **Hemat:** eosinophilia, hemolytic anemia, neutropenia, thrombocytopenia. **Misc:** allergic reactions, including anaphylaxis, superinfection.

PHYSICAL THERAPY IMPLICATIONS

Examination and Evaluation

- Watch for seizures; notify physician immediately if patient develops or increases seizure activity.
- Monitor signs of pseudomembranous colitis, including diarrhea, abdominal pain, fever, pus or mucus in stools, and other severe or prolonged GI problems (nausea, vomiting, heartburn). Notify physician or nursing staff immediately of these signs.
- Monitor signs of allergic reactions and anaphylaxis, including pulmonary symptoms (tightness in the throat and chest, wheezing, cough dyspnea) or skin reactions (rash, pruritus, urticaria). Notify physician or nursing staff immediately if these reactions occur.
- Monitor signs of eosinophilia (fatigue, weakness, myalgia), neutropenia (fever, sore throat, signs of infection), thrombocytopenia (bruising, nose bleeds, bleeding gums), or hemolytic anemia (malaise, dizziness, jaundice, abdominal pain). Report these signs to the physician.

Interventions

- Always wash hands thoroughly and disinfect equipment (whirlpools, electrotherapeutic devices, treatment tables, and so forth) to help prevent the spread of infection. Use universal precautions or isolation procedures as indicated for specific patients.

C

Patient/Client-Related Instruction

- Instruct patient to notify physician immediately of signs of superinfection, including black, furry overgrowth on tongue, vaginal itching or discharge, and loose or foul-smelling stools.
- Instruct patient and family/caregivers to report other troublesome side effects such as severe or prolonged skin problems (rash, hives) or GI problems (nausea, vomiting, diarrhea, abdominal pain).

Pharmacokinetics

Absorption: Well absorbed after oral administration.
Distribution: Widely distributed. Crosses the placenta and enters breast milk in low concentrations. Poor CSF penetration.
Metabolism and Excretion: Excreted almost entirely unchanged in the urine.
Half-life: Neonates: 5 hr; Children: 2.5 hr; Adults: 50–80 min (increased in renal impairment).

TIME/ACTION PROFILE (blood levels)

ROUTE	ONSET	PEAK	DURATION
PO	rapid	1 hr	6–12 hr

Contraindications/Precautions

Contraindicated in: Hypersensitivity to cephalosporins; Serious hypersensitivity to penicillins.
Use Cautiously in: Renal impairment; History of GI disease, especially colitis; OB/Lactation: Pregnancy and lactation (has been used safely).

Interactions

Drug-Drug: Probenecid ↓ excretion and ↑ blood levels of renally excreted cephalosporins. Concurrent use of **loop diuretics** or **aminoglycosides** may ↑ risk of renal toxicity.

Route/Dosage

PO (Adults): *Most infections*—250–500 mg q 6 hr. *Uncomplicated cystitis, skin and soft tissue infections, streptococcal pharyngitis*—500 mg q 12 hr. Maximum dose: 4 g/day.
PO (Children): *Most infections*—25–50 mg/kg/day divided q 6–8 hr (can be administered q 12 hr in skin/skin structure infections or streptococcal pharyngitis). *Otitis media*—75–100 mg/kg/day divided q 6 hr. Maximum dose: 4 g/day.

Availability (generic available)

Capsules: 250 mg, 333 mg, 500 mg, 750 mg. **Tablets:** 250 mg, 500 mg. **Oral suspension:** 125 mg/5 mL, 250 mg/5 mL.

certolizumab pegol

(ser-toe-liz-u-mab **peg**-all)
Cimzia

Classification
Therapeutic: gastrointestinal anti-inflammatories—therapeutic
Pharmacologic: tumor necrosis factor blockers

Indications

Moderate-to-severe active Crohn's disease when response to conventional therapy has been inadequate.

Action

Neutralizes tumor necrosis factor (TNF), a prime mediator of inflammation; pegylation provides a long duration of action. **Therapeutic Effects:** Decreased signs/symptoms of Crohn's disease.

Adverse Reactions/Side Effects

Derm: skin reactions (rarely severe). **Hemat:** hematologic reactions. **MS:** arthralgia. **Misc:** ALLERGIC REACTIONS, INCLUDING ANAPHYALXIS, INFECTIONS, lupus-like syndrome.

PHYSICAL THERAPY IMPLICATIONS

Examination and Evaluation

- Monitor signs of allergic reactions and anaphylaxis, including pulmonary symptoms (tightness in the throat and chest, wheezing, cough, dyspnea) or skin reactions (rash, pruritus, urticaria). Notify physician or nursing staff immediately if these reactions occur.
- Be alert for signs of systemic infections, especially respiratory infections (fever, chills, cough, mucus production, shortness of breath, wheezing, chest discomfort, fatigue) and GI infections (nausea, vomiting, diarrhea, abdominal pain). Notify physician immediately of these signs.
- Monitor signs of hematologic reactions such as leukopenia (fever, sore throat, signs of infection), thrombocytopenia (bruising, nose bleeds, and bleeding gums), or unusual weakness and fatigue that might be due to anemia. Report any suspicious signs of blood disorders.
- Monitor any changes in GI symptoms (decreased abdominal pain, decreased diarrhea, improved appetite) to help document whether drug therapy is successful in managing Crohn's disease.
- Assess any joint pain to rule out musculoskeletal pathology; that is, try to determine if pain is drug

induced rather than caused by anatomic or biomechanical problems.

- Monitor signs of lupus-like syndrome, including increased blood pressure (BP), fever, joint pain, skin rashes, and redness/irritation of the eye (uveitis). Notify physician promptly if these signs appear.

Patient/Client-Related Instruction

- Advise patient to avoid alcohol and foods that may cause an increase in GI irritation.
- Instruct patient and family/caregivers to report other troublesome side effects such as severe or prolonged skin reactions (rash, dermatitis).

Pharmacokinetics

Absorption: 80% absorbed following SC administration.
Distribution: Unknown.
Metabolism and Excretion: Unknown.
Half-life: 14 days.

TIME/ACTION PROFILE (blood levels)

ROUTE	ONSET	PEAK	DURATION
SC	unknown	50–120 hr	2–4 wk

Contraindications/Precautions

Contraindicated in: Active untreated infection; Hepatitis B reactivation.
Use Cautiously in: History of recurrent infections, concurrent immunosuppressants, medical conditions associated with increased risk of infection, current residence in areas where tuberculosis or histoplasmosis are endemic, history of hepatitis B infection (may reactivate); History of demyelinating disorders (may exacerbate); History of heart failure; Geri: May increase risk of infections; OB: Use pregnancy only if clearly needed; avoid breast-feeding; Pedi: Safe use in children not established.

Interactions

Drug-Drug: Concurrent use with **anakinra** ↑ risk of serious infections. May ↓ antibody response to or ↑ risk of adverse reactions to **live vaccines**.

Route/Dosage

Subcut (Adults): 400 mg initially, repeat 2 and 4 wk later; may be followed by maintenance dose of 400 mg q 4 wk.

Availability

Lyophilized powder for subcutaneous injection (requires reconstitution): 200-mg vial, 100-mg vial.

cetirizine (se-ti-ra-zeen)

Zyrtec

Classification

Therapeutic: allergy, cold, and cough remedies, antihistamines
Pharmacologic: piperazines (peripherally selective)

Indications

Relief of allergic symptoms caused by histamine release, including Seasonal and perennial allergic rhinitis; Chronic urticaria.

Action

Antagonizes the effects of histamine at H_1 receptor sites; does not bind to or inactivate histamine. Anticholinergic effects are minimal and sedation is dose related. **Therapeutic Effects:** Decreased symptoms of histamine excess (sneezing, rhinorrhea, ocular tearing and redness, pruritus).

Adverse Reactions/Side Effects

CNS: dizziness, drowsiness (significant with doses >10 mg/day), fatigue. **EENT:** pharyngitis. **GI:** dry mouth.

PHYSICAL THERAPY IMPLICATIONS

Examination and Evaluation

- Monitor symptoms of seasonal allergies (sneezing, rhinitis, itching eyes, cough) or chronic idiopathic urticaria (rash, hives, itching) to help document benefits of this drug in treating these disorders.
- Assess dizziness and drowsiness that might affect gait, balance, and other functional activities (See Appendix C). Report balance problems and functional limitations to the physician, and caution the patient and family/caregivers to guard against falls and trauma.

Interventions

- Guard against falls and trauma (hip fractures, head injury, and so forth). Implement fall- prevention strategies, especially in older adults or if balance is impaired (See Appendix E).

Patient/Client-Related Instruction

- Advise patient about the risk of daytime drowsiness and decreased attention and mental focus. Although the risk of drowsiness is considerably lower with this drug compared to traditional antihistamines, patients should use care if driving or in other activities that require quick reactions and strong concentration.

- Advise patient to avoid alcohol and other CNS depressants because of the increased risk of sedation and adverse effects.
- Instruct patient to report other troublesome side effects, including severe or prolonged dry mouth or upper respiratory tract irritation.

Pharmacokinetics

Absorption: Well absorbed following oral administration.
Distribution: Unknown.
Protein Binding: 93%.
Metabolism and Excretion: Excreted primarily unchanged by the kidneys.
Half-life: 7.4–9 hr (decreased in children to 6.2 hr, increased in renal impairment up to 19–21 hr).

TIME/ACTION PROFILE (antihistaminic effects)

ROUTE	ONSET	PEAK	DURATION
PO	30 min	4–8 hr	24 hr

Contraindications/Precautions

Contraindicated in: Hypersensitivity to cetirizine, hydroxyzine, or any component; Lactation: Excreted in breast milk; not recommended for use.
Use Cautiously in: Patients with hepatic or renal impairment (dosage reduction recommended if CCr ≤31 mL/min or hepatic function is impaired); OB/Pedi: Safety not established for pregnant women or children <6 mo; Geri: Initiate at lower doses.

Interactions

Drug-Drug: Additive CNS depression may occur with **alcohol, opioid analgesics,** or **sedative/hypnotics. Theophylline** may ↓ clearance and increase toxicity.

Route/Dosage

PO (Adults and children >6 yr): 5–10 mg given once or divided twice daily.
PO (Children 2–5 yr): 2.5 mg once daily initially, may be increased to 5 mg once daily or 2.5 mg q 12 hr.
PO (Children 1–2 yr): 2.5 mg once daily; may be ↑ to 2.5 mg q 12 hr.
PO (Children 6–12 mo): 2.5 once daily.

Hepatic/Renal Impairment

PO (Adults and Children >12 yr): *CCr ≤31 mL/min, hepatic impairment or hemodialysis*—5 mg once daily.
PO (Children 6–11 yr): start therapy at <2.5 mg/day.
PO (Children <6 yr): use not recommended.

Availability (generic available)

Tablets: 5 mg OTC, 10 mg OTC. **Chewable tablets (grape):** 5 mg OTC, 10 mg OTC. **Syrup (banana-grape and bubblegum flavors):** 1 mg/mL in 120-mL and 480-mL bottles OTC. ***In combination with:*** pseudoephedrine (Zyrtec-D 12 Hour). See Appendix B.

C

cetuximab (se-tux-i-mab)

Erbitux

Classification
Therapeutic: antineoplastics
Pharmacologic: monoclonal antibodies

Indications

Locally or regionally advanced squamous cell carcinoma of the head and neck with radiation. Recurrent or metastatic squamous cell carcinoma of the head and neck progressing after platinum-based therapy. Epidermal growth factor receptor (EGFR)–expressing metastatic colorectal cancer in patients who have not responded to irinotecan and oxaliplatin. Metastatic colorectal cancer (with irinotecan) when tumors express EGFR and have not responded to or are intolerant of irinotecan alone.

Action

Binds specifically to EGFR, thereby preventing the binding of endogenous epidermal growth factor (EGF). This prevents cell growth and differentiation processes. Combination with irinotecan enhances antitumor effects of irinotecan. **Therapeutic Effects:** Decreased tumor growth and spread.

Adverse Reactions/Side Effects

Most adverse reactions reflect combination therapy with irinotecan
CNS: malaise, depression, headache, insomnia. **EENT:** conjunctivitis. **Resp:** dyspnea, ↑ cough, interstitial lung disease. **CV:** PULMONARY EMBOLISM. **GI:** abdominal pain, constipation, diarrhea, nausea, vomiting, anorexia, stomatitis. **GU:** renal failure. **Derm:** acneform dermatitis, alopecia, nail disorder, pruritus, skin desquamation. **F and E:** dehydration, hypomagnesemia, peripheral edema. **Hemat:** anemia, leukopenia. **MS:** back pain. **Metab:** weight loss. **Misc:** INFUSION REACTIONS, fever, desquamation of mucosal epithelium.

PHYSICAL THERAPY IMPLICATIONS

Examination and Evaluation

- Monitor signs of pulmonary embolism, including sudden shortness of breath, chest pain, cough, and bloody sputum. Notify physician immediately, and request objective tests (Doppler ultrasound, lung scan, others) if thromboembolism is suspected.

- Report allergy-like responses (wheezing, laryngeal edema, urticaria, other skin reactions) that occur during and after administration (infusion-related reactions).
- Assess any breathing problems or signs of interstitial lung disease such as dry cough, wheezing, chest pain, shortness of breath, and difficult or labored breathing. Monitor pulse oximetry and perform pulmonary function tests (See Appendices I, J, K) to quantify suspected changes in ventilation and respiratory function.
- Watch for signs of leukopenia (fever, sore throat, mucosal lesions, other signs of infection) and anemia (unusual fatigue, weakness, pallor). Report these signs to the physician immediately.
- Monitor signs of renal failure, including decreased urine output, increased blood pressure, muscle cramps/twitching, edema/weight gain from fluid retention, yellowish brown skin, and confusion that progresses to seizures and coma. Report these signs to the physician immediately.
- Watch for signs of low magnesium levels (hypomagnesemia), such as lethargy, irritability, insomnia, muscle tremors, and confusion. Notify physician of these signs.
- Assess peripheral edema using girth measurements, volume displacement, and measurement of pitting edema (See Appendix N). Report increased swelling in feet and ankles or a sudden increase in body weight due to fluid retention.
- Assess any back pain to rule out musculoskeletal pathology; that is, try to determine if pain is drug induced rather than caused by anatomic or biomechanical problems.
- Monitor and report depression, malaise, sleep loss, or other changes in mood and behavior.
- Periodically assess body weight and other anthropometric measures (body mass index, body composition). Report a rapid or unexplained weight loss or decreased body fat.

Interventions

- For patients who are medically able to begin exercise, implement appropriate resistive exercises and aerobic training to maintain muscle strength and aerobic capacity during cancer chemotherapy or to help restore function after chemotherapy.
- Use caution during aerobic exercise and endurance conditioning because of potential pulmonary toxicity. Terminate exercise if patient exhibits untoward symptoms (chest pain, shortness of breath, etc.), or displays other criteria for exercise termination (See Appendix L).
- Make sure patient maintains adequate fluid intake to avoid dehydration, especially during exercise.

Patient/Client-Related Instruction

- Advise patient to guard against infection (frequent hand washing, etc.), and to avoid crowds and contact with persons with contagious diseases.
- Advise patient that skin reactions are likely, including rash, acne, dermatitis, pruritus, and skin loss/peeling. Report severe or unexpected skin reactions to the physician.
- Advise patient about the likelihood of GI reactions such as abdominal pain, constipation, diarrhea, nausea, vomiting, loss of appetite, and inflammation in/around the mouth. Instruct patient to report severe or prolonged GI problems.
- Instruct patient to maintain adequate fluid intake and avoid dehydration.
- Instruct patient or family/caregivers to report other bothersome side effects such as severe or prolonged headache, fever, weight loss, or eye irritation (conjunctivitis).

Pharmacokinetics

Absorption: IV administration results in complete bioavailability.
Distribution: Unknown.
Metabolism and Excretion: Unknown.
Half-life: 97–114 hr.

TIME/ACTION PROFILE

ROUTE	ONSET	PEAK	DURATION
IV	unknown	unknown	unknown

Contraindications/Precautions

Contraindicated in: Hypersensitivity to cetuximab or murine (mouse) proteins; OB: Pregnancy or lactation.
Use Cautiously in: Exposure to sunlight (may exacerbate dermatologic toxicity); Pedi: Children (safety not established).

Interactions

Drug-Drug: None noted.

Route/Dosage

Head & Neck Cancer with Radiation

IV (Adults): 400 mg/m² administered 1 wk prior to initiation of radiation therapy, followed by weekly maintenance doses of 250 mg/m² for the duration of radiation therapy. Complete infusion 1 hr prior to radiation therapy; dose modification recommended for dermatologic toxicity.

Head and Neck Cancer Monotherapy

IV (Adults): 400 mg/m² initial loading dose, followed by weekly maintenance doses of 250 mg/m² until disease progression or unacceptable toxicity; dose modification recommended for dermatologic toxicity.

Colorectal Cancer

IV (Adults): 400 mg/m² initial loading dose, followed by weekly maintenance doses of 250 mg/m²; dose modification recommended for dermatologic toxicity.

Availability

Solution for injection: 2 mg/mL in 50-mL vials.

chloramphenicol

(klor-am-**fen**-i-kole)

Chloromycetin

Classification

Therapeutic: anti-infectives

Indications

IV: Management of the following serious infections when less toxic agents cannot be used: Skin and soft-tissue infections, Intra-abdominal infections, CNS infections (including meningitis), Bacteremia. **Ophth:** Management of local infections.

Action

Inhibits protein synthesis in susceptible bacteria at the level of the 50S ribosome. **Therapeutic Effects:** Bacteriostatic action. **Spectrum:** Wide variety of gram-positive aerobic organisms, including *Streptococcus pneumoniae* and other streptococci, Some enterococci (especially vancomycin-resistant). Gram-negative pathogens: *Haemophilus influenzae*, *Neisseria meningitidis*, *Salmonella*, *Shigella*. Anaerobes: *Bacteroides fragilis*, *Prevotella melaninogenica*. Other organisms inhibited: *Rickettsia*, *Chlamydia*, *Mycoplasma*.

Adverse Reactions/Side Effects

CNS: confusion, delirium, depression, headache. **EENT:** blurred vision, optic neuritis. **GI:** bitter taste (IV only), diarrhea, enterocolitis, glossitis, nausea, stomatitis, vomiting. **Derm:** rashes, urticaria. **Hemat:** APLASTIC ANEMIA, bone marrow depression, neutropenia, thrombocytopenia. **Neuro:** peripheral neuritis. **Misc:** ANGIOEDEMA, GRAY SYNDROME IN NEWBORNS, fever.

PHYSICAL THERAPY IMPLICATIONS

Examination and Evaluation

- Monitor signs of aplastic anemia, including unusual fatigue, shortness of breath with exertion, and bruising. Notify physician immediately if these signs occur.
- Monitor signs of angioedema, including rashes, raised patches of red or white skin (welts), burning/itching skin, swelling in the face, and difficulty breathing. Notify physician immediately of these signs.
- Monitor newborns for signs of gray syndrome (also called chloramphenicol toxicity in newborns), including gray/ashen skin color, cyanosis, respiratory distress, hypotension, vomiting, and hypothermia. Report these signs immediately to the physician or nursing staff.
- Report signs of neutropenia (fever, sore throat, signs of infection), thrombocytopenia (bruising, nose bleeds, bleeding gums), and fatigue that might be due to bone marrow depression or other blood dyscrasias.
- Be alert for signs of peripheral neuritis (numbness, tingling, decreased muscle strength). Establish baseline electroneuromyographic values at the beginning of drug treatment whenever possible, and reexamine these values periodically to document drug-induced changes in peripheral nerve function.
- Monitor signs of CNS toxicity, including confusion, delirium, depression, and headache. Report these signs to the physician.

Interventions

- Always wash hands thoroughly and disinfect equipment (whirlpools, electrotherapeutic devices, treatment tables, and so forth) to help prevent the spread of infection. Use universal precautions or isolation procedures as indicated for specific patients.

Patient/Client-Related Instruction

- Advise patient to report any signs of optic neuritis such as blurred vision or other vision disturbances.
- Advise patient about the likelihood of GI reactions, including nausea, vomiting, diarrhea, abdominal pain, inflammation in/around the mouth, and taste abnormalities. Instruct patient to report severe or prolonged GI problems.
- Instruct patient and family/caregivers to report other troublesome side effects such as severe or prolonged fever or skin problems (rash, hives).

Pharmacokinetics

Absorption: Some systemic and intraocular absorption follows ophthalmic administration.
Distribution: Widely distributed. Crosses the blood-brain barrier with CSF levels 60% of serum values. Crosses the placenta; enters breast milk.
Metabolism and Excretion: Mostly metabolized by the liver; <10% excreted unchanged by the kidneys.
Half-life: 1.5–3.5 hr.

TIME/ACTION PROFILE (blood levels)

ROUTE	ONSET	PEAK	DURATION
IV	rapid	end of infusion	6–12 hr

Contraindications/Precautions

Contraindicated in: Hypersensitivity; Previous toxic reaction to chloramphenicol.

Use Cautiously in: Patients with severe hepatic or renal disease (increased risk of reactions due to inability to metabolize and excrete chloramphenicol); OB/Lactation: Safety not established; Pedi/Geri: Increased risk of toxicity due to inability to metabolize and excrete chloramphenicol).

Interactions

Drug-Drug: May ↑ effects of the following drugs: **oral hypoglycemic agents**, **warfarin**, and **phenytoin**. **Phenobarbital** or **rifampin** may ↓ chloramphenicol blood levels. May delay response to **vitamin B** or **folic acid** therapy. Bone marrow depression may be additive with **bone marrow–depressing agents (antineoplastics)**.

Route/Dosage

IV (Adults): 12.5 mg/kg q 6 hr (up to 100 mg/kg/day).
IV (Children): *Most infections*—12.5 mg/kg q 6 hr (max daily dose: 4 g). *Bacteremia/meningitis*—up to 50–100 mg/kg/day.
IV (Infants >2 wk): 12.5 mg/kg q 6 hr (max daily dose: 4 g). *Bacteremia/meningitis*—up to 50–100 mg/kg/day.
IV (Neonates >–7 days and >2 kg): 25 mg/kg q 12 hr.
IV (Neonates birth–7 days or ≤2 kg): 25 mg/kg once daily.

Availability

Powder for injection: 1-g vials.

chlordiazepoxide

(klor-dye-az-e-**pox**-ide)

Apo-Chlordiazepoxide, Libritabs, Librium, Mitran, Novopoxide, Poxi

Classification

Therapeutic: antianxiety agents, sedative/hypnotics

Pharmacologic: benzodiazepines

Schedule IV

Indications

Adjunct management of anxiety. Treatment of alcohol withdrawal. Adjunct management of anxiety associated with acute myocardial infarction.

Action

Acts at many levels of the CNS to produce anxiolytic effect. Depresses the CNS, probably by potentiating gamma-aminobutyric acid (GABA), an inhibitory neurotransmitter. **Therapeutic Effects:** Sedation. Relief of anxiety.

Adverse Reactions/Side Effects

CNS: dizziness, drowsiness, hangover, headache, mental depression, paradoxical excitation, sedation. **EENT:** blurred vision. **GI:** constipation, diarrhea, nausea, vomiting, weight gain. **Derm:** rashes. **Local:** pain at IM site. **Misc:** physical dependence, psychologic dependence, tolerance.

PHYSICAL THERAPY IMPLICATIONS

Examination and Evaluation

- Monitor daytime drowsiness and ,"hangover" symptoms (headache, nausea, irritability, dysphoria). Repeated or excessive symptoms may require change in dose or medication.
- Assess dizziness that might affect gait, balance, and other functional activities (See Appendix C). Report balance problems and functional limitations to the physician, and caution the patient and family/caregivers to guard against falls and trauma.
- Report any behavioral or personality changes such as decreased mental acuity or excessive excitation.
- Periodically assess body weight and other anthropometric measures (body mass index, body composition). Report a rapid or unexplained weight gain or increased body fat.
- Monitor IM injection site for pain, swelling, and irritation. Report prolonged or excessive injection-site reactions to the physician.

Interventions

- Guard against falls and trauma (hip fractures, head injury, and so forth). Implement fall- prevention strategies, especially in older adults or if drowsiness and dizziness carry over into the daytime (See Appendix E).
- Help patient explore nonpharmacologic methods to reduce anxiety, such as relaxation techniques, exercise, counseling, support groups, and so forth.

Patient/Client-Related Instruction

- Instruct patients on prolonged treatment not to discontinue medication without consulting their physician. Prolonged use can cause tolerance and dependence, and abrupt withdrawal can cause insomnia, unusual irritability or nervousness, and seizures.
- Advise patient to avoid alcohol and other CNS depressants because of the increased risk of sedation and adverse effects.

- Instruct patient to report other bothersome side effects such as severe or prolonged headache, blurred vision, skin rash, or GI problems (nausea, vomiting, diarrhea, constipation).

Pharmacokinetics

Absorption: Well absorbed from the GI tract. IM absorption may be slow and unpredictable.
Distribution: Widely distributed. Crosses the blood-brain barrier. Crosses the placenta; enters breast milk. Recommend to discontinue drug or bottle feed.
Metabolism and Excretion: Highly metabolized by the liver. Some products of metabolism are active as CNS depressants.
Half-life: 5–30 hr.

TIME/ACTION PROFILE (sedation)

ROUTE	ONSET	PEAK	DURATION
PO	1–2 hr	0.5–4 hr	up to 24 hr
IM	15–30 min	unknown	unknown
IV	1–5 min	unknown	0.25–1 hr

Contraindications/Precautions

Contraindicated in: Hypersensitivity; Some products contain tartrazine and should be avoided in patients with known intolerance; Cross-sensitivity with other benzodiazepines may occur; Comatose patients or those with preexisting CNS depression; Uncontrolled severe pain; Pulmonary disease; Angle-closure glaucoma; Porphyria; OB/Lactation: May cause CNS depression, flaccidity, feeding difficulties, and weight loss in infants; Pedi: Not for use in children ≤6 yr.
Use Cautiously in: Hepatic dysfunction; Severe renal impairment; History of suicide attempt or substance abuse; Geri: Long-acting benzodiazepines cause prolonged sedation in the elderly. Appears on Beers' list and is associated with ↑ risk of falls (↓ dose required or consider short-acting benzodiazepine); Debilitated patients (initial dose reduction required).

Interactions

Drug-Drug: Alcohol, antidepressants, antihistamines, and **opioid analgesics**—concurrent use results in additive CNS depression. **Cimetidine, oral contraceptives, disulfiram, fluoxetine, isoniazid, ketoconazole, metoprolol, propoxyphene, propranolol,** or **valproic acid** may enhance effects. May ↓ efficacy of **levodopa. Rifampin** or **barbiturates** may ↓ effectiveness of chlordiazepoxide. Sedative effects may be ↓ by **theophylline.**
Drug-Natural: Concomitant use of **kava, valerian, chamomile,** or **hops** can ↑ CNS depression.

Route/Dosage

PO (Adults): *Alcohol withdrawal*—50–100 mg, repeated until agitation is controlled (up to 400 mg/day). *Anxiety*—5–25 mg 3–4 times daily.
PO (Geriatric Patients or Debilitated Patients): *Anxiety*—5 mg 2–4 times daily initially, increased as needed.
PO (Children >6 yr): *Anxiety*—5 mg 2–4 times daily, up to 10 mg 2–3 times daily.
IM, IV (Adults): *Alcohol withdrawal*—50–100 mg initially; may be repeated in 2–4 hr. *Anxiety*—50–100 mg initially, then 25–50 mg 3–4 times daily as required (25–50 mg initially in geriatric patients). *Preoperative sedation*—50–100 mg 1 hr preoperative.
IM, IV (Geriatric Patients or Debilitated Patients): *Anxiety/sedation*—25–50 mg/dose.
IM, IV (Children >12 yr): *Anxiety/sedation*—25–50 mg/dose.

Availability (generic available)

Capsules: 5 mg, 10 mg, 25 mg. **Tablets:** 5 mg, 10 mg, 25 mg. **Injection:** 100-mg ampule. ***In combination with:*** amitriptyline (Limbitrol DS), clidinium (Librax). See Appendix B.

chloroquine (klor-oh-kwin)

Aralen

Classification
Therapeutic: antimalarials, antirheumatics (disease-modifying antirheumatic drugs [DMARDs])

Indications

Prophylaxis and treatment of acute attacks of malaria. Treatment of extraintestinal amebiasis. **Unlabeled Use:** Treatment of severe rheumatoid arthritis. Treatment of systemic lupus erythematosus.

Action

Inhibits protein synthesis in susceptible organisms by inhibiting DNA and RNA polymerase. **Therapeutic Effects:** Death of plasmodia responsible for causing malaria. Death of ameba responsible for causing amebiasis. Improvement in inflammation in rheumatoid arthritis and systemic lupus erythematosus.

Adverse Reactions/Side Effects

CNS: SEIZURES, delirium, depression, headache, personality changes, psychosis. **EENT:** hearing impairment, retinopathy, tinnitus, visual disturbances. **CV:** cardiomyopathy, ECG changes (T-wave abnormalities, QRS prolongation), hypotension. **GI:** abdominal cramps, anorexia, diarrhea, nausea, vomiting. **Derm:** alopecia, dermatoses, photosensitivity, pigmentary changes, pruritus, skin eruptions. **Hemat:** AGRANULOCYTOSIS, APLASTIC ANEMIA, LEUKOPENIA, thrombocytopenia. **Neuro:** neuromyopathy, peripheral neuritis, weakness.

PHYSICAL THERAPY IMPLICATIONS

Examination and Evaluation

- Be alert for new seizures or increased seizure activity, especially at the onset of drug treatment. Document the number, duration, and severity of seizures, and report these findings immediately to the physician.
- Monitor signs of agranulocytosis and leukopenia (fever, sore throat, mucosal lesions, signs of infection, bruising), thrombocytopenia (bruising, nose bleeds, bleeding gums), or unusual weakness and fatigue that might be due to aplastic anemia. Periodic blood tests may be needed to monitor WBC and RBC counts.
- If treating rheumatoid arthritis or lupus erythematosus, periodically assess patient's impairments (pain, range of motion), functional ability, and disability to help document whether antirheumatic drug therapy is successful.
- Be alert for signs of peripheral neuromyopathy and neuritis (numbness, tingling, decreased muscle strength). Establish baseline electroneuromyographic values at the beginning of drug treatment whenever possible, and reexamine these values periodically to document drug-induced changes in peripheral nerve function.
- Monitor signs of cardiomyopathy, including dyspnea, shortness of breath, exercise intolerance, peripheral edema, and rales/crackles. Notify physician of these signs immediately.
- Assess heart rate, ECG, and heart sounds, especially during exercise (See Appendices G, H). Report any rhythm disturbances or symptoms of cardiac dysfunction, including palpitations, chest discomfort, shortness of breath, fainting, and fatigue/weakness.
- Assess blood pressure periodically, and compare to normal values (See Appendix F). Report low blood pressure (hypotension), especially if patient experiences dizziness, fatigue, or other symptoms.
- Monitor changes in personality, mood, and behavior, including depression, delirium, psychosis, and other personality changes. Notify physician if these changes become problematic.
- If treating malaria, monitor any changes in symptoms (decreased fever, chills, sweating) to help determine if antimalarial drug therapy is successful.

Interventions

- Because of the risk of ECG changes and cardiomyopathy, use caution during aerobic exercise and other forms of therapeutic exercise. Assess exercise tolerance frequently (blood pressure, heart rate, fatigue levels), and terminate exercise immediately if any untoward responses occur (See Appendix L).
- Implement appropriate manual therapy techniques, physical agents, therapeutic exercises, and orthotic/assistive devices to reduce pain, improve function, and augment the effects of antirheumatic drug therapy.
- Help patient explore other nonpharmacologic methods to reduce chronic pain, such as relaxation techniques, exercise, counseling, and so forth.
- Causes photosensitivity; use care if administering UV treatments. Advise patient to avoid direct sunlight and use sunscreens and protective clothing.

Patient/Client-related Instruction

- Instruct patient to report visual disturbances (blurred vision, double vision) or hearing problems (ringing in the ears, hearing loss). Visual and auditory problems are more common at higher doses.
- Remind patient to take this drug as directed when treating malaria even if patient is asymptomatic.
- Instruct patient to report other untoward side effects such as severe or prolonged headache, skin reactions (hyperpigmentation, pruritus, skin eruptions, hair loss), or GI problems (nausea, vomiting, diarrhea, cramps, loss of appetite).

Pharmacokinetics

Absorption: Well absorbed following oral administration.
Distribution: Widely distributed; high tissue concentrations achieved. Crosses the placenta, enters breast milk.
Metabolism and Excretion: 30% metabolized by the liver. Metabolite also has antiplasmodial activity; 70% excreted unchanged by the kidneys.
Half-life: 3–5 days.

TIME/ACTION PROFILE (antimalarial activity)

ROUTE	ONSET	PEAK	DURATION
PO	rapid	1–2 hr	days–wks

Contraindications/Precautions

Contraindicated in: Hypersensitivity; Hypersensitivity to other 4-aminoquinolones (hydroxychloroquine); Visual damage caused by chloroquine or other 4-aminoquinolones; Lactation: Potential for serious adverse reactions in nursing infants.
Use Cautiously in: Liver disease; Alcoholism; Patients receiving hepatotoxic drugs; Porphyria (may exacerbate condition); Psoriasis; G6PD deficiency; Bone marrow depression; Hearing impairment; Epilepsy; OB: Although safety not established, has been used; Pedi: Extremely sensitive to chloroquine effects; Geri: May be predisposed to adverse effects).

Interactions

Drug-Drug: Antacids may ↓ absorption. Blood levels may be ↑ by **cimetidine, fluconazole, ketoconazole, clarithromycin, erythromycin, fluoxetine,**

nefazodone, paroxetine, protease inhibitors, quinidine, ritonavir, and **verapamil**. May ↓ absorption of **ampicillin** (separate administration of these agents by at least 2 hr). May ↑ blood levels of **cyclosporine, fluoxetine, lidocaine, mirtazapine,nefazodone, paroxetine, risperidone, ritonavir, thioridazine, tricyclic antidepressants,** and **venlafaxine**. Blood levels may be decreased by **carbamazepine, nevirapine, phenobarbital, phenytoin,** and **rifampin**. May increase the risk of hepatotoxicity when administered with other **hepatotoxic agents**. **Urinary acidifiers** may increase renal excretion and decrease effectiveness.
Drug-Food: Foods that acidify urine (See Appendix L) may ↑ excretion and ↓ effectiveness.

Route/Dosage

Doses below expressed as chloroquine base: 1 mg of chloroquine base = 1.67 mg chloroquine phosphate or 1.25 mg chloroquine hydrochloride.

Suppression/Prophylaxis of Malaria

PO (Adults): 300 mg once weekly, starting 2 wk prior to entering endemic areas and for 8 wk afterward. If suppressive therapy is not initiated prior to entering endemic area, initial dose should be 300 mg followed by another 300-mg dose 6 hr later, followed by the usual dosage regimen.
PO (Children): 5 mg/kg once weekly, starting 2 wk prior to entering endemic areas and for 8 wk afterward (not to exceed 300 mg/day). If suppressive therapy is not initiated prior to entering endemic area, initial dose should be 5 mg/kg followed by another 5 mg/kg dose 6 hr later, followed by the usual dosage regimen.

Treatment of Acute Attack of Malaria

PO (Adults): 600 mg initially, then 300 mg at 6–8 hr, 24 hr, and 48 hr after initial dose.
PO (Children): 10 mg/kg initially (not to exceed 600 mg), then 5 mg/kg at 6 hr, 24 hr, and 48 hr after initial dose (not to exceed 300 mg/day).

Extraintestinal Amebiasis

PO (Adults): 600 mg daily for 2 days, then 300 mg daily for at least 2–3 wk (in combination with other antiprotozoals).
PO (Children): 10 mg/kg (not to exceed 300 mg/day for 2–3 wk).

Rheumatoid Arthritis/Systemic Lupus Erythematosus

PO (Adults): 150 mg once daily; reduce dosage following maximal response.

Availability

Chloroquine Phosphate

Tablets: 250 mg (150-mg base), 500 mg (300-mg base).

chlorothiazide

(klor-oh-**thye**-a-zide)
Diuril

Classification
Therapeutic: antihypertensives, diuretics
Pharmacologic: thiazide diuretics

Indications

Management of mild-to-moderate hypertension. Treatment of edema associated with Congestive heart failure, Renal dysfunction, Cirrhosis, Corticosteroid therapy, Estrogen therapy.

Action

Increases excretion of sodium and water by inhibiting sodium reabsorption in the distal tubule. Promotes excretion of sodium, chloride, potassium, magnesium, phosphate, water, and bicarbonate. May produce arteriolar dilation. **Therapeutic Effects:** Lowering of blood pressure in hypertensive patients and diuresis with mobilization of edema.

Adverse Reactions/Side Effects

CNS: dizziness, drowsiness, lethargy, weakness. **CV:** hypotension. **GI:** anorexia, cramping, hepatitis, nausea, vomiting, pancreatitis. **Derm:** photosensitivity, rashes. **Endo:** hyperglycemia. **F and E:** hypokalemia, dehydration, hypercalcemia, hypochloremic alkalosis, hypomagnesemia, hyponatremia, hypophosphatemia, hypovolemia. **Hemat:** rarely blood dyscrasias, thrombocytopenia. **Metab:** hyperuricemia, hypercholesterolemia. **MS:** muscle cramps. **Misc:** blurred vision.

PHYSICAL THERAPY IMPLICATIONS

Examination and Evaluation

- Assess blood pressure periodically and compare to normal values (See Appendix F) to help document antihypertensive effects. Report low blood pressure (hypotension), especially if patient experiences dizziness or syncope.
- Monitor signs of fluid, electrolyte, or acid-base imbalances, including lethargy, drowsiness, blurred vision, confusion, hypotension, and muscle cramps and weakness. Report excessive of prolonged symptoms to the physician.
- Assess dizziness that might affect gait, balance, and other functional activities (See Appendix C). Report balance problems and functional limitations to the physician, and caution the patient and family/caregivers to guard against falls and trauma.
- When used to treat edema, help determine drug effects by assessing peripheral edema using girth

measurements, volume displacement, and measurement of pitting edema (See Appendix N). Also monitor signs of pulmonary edema such as dyspnea and rales/crackles (See Appendix K). Document whether peripheral and pulmonary symptoms are controlled adequately by diuretic therapy.

- Be alert for signs of hyperglycemia, including confusion, drowsiness, flushed/dry skin, fruit-like breath odor, rapid/deep breathing, polyuria, loss of appetite, and unusual thirst. Patients with diabetes mellitus should check blood glucose levels frequently.
- Monitor and report signs of thrombocytopenia (bruising, nose bleeds, bleeding gums), or unusual weakness and fatigue that might be due to anemia or other blood dyscrasias.

Interventions

- Implement fall-prevention strategies, especially in older adults of if patient exhibits sedation, dizziness, blurred vision, or other impairments that affect gait and balance (See Appendix E).
- Use caution during aerobic exercise, especially in hot environments. Increased sweating will cause fluid and electrolyte loss, and may exaggerate diuretic side effects (dizziness, muscle cramps, and so forth).
- To minimize orthostatic hypotension, patient should move slowly when assuming a more upright position.
- Causes photosensitivity; use care if administering UV treatments. Advise patient to use sunscreens, protective clothing, and avoid prolonged sun exposure.

Patient/Client-Related Instruction

- Remind patients to take medication as directed to control hypertension and other cardiac conditions even if they are asymptomatic.
- Counsel patients about additional interventions to help control blood pressure and cardiac dysfunction, including regular exercise, weight loss, sodium restriction, stress reduction, moderation of alcohol consumption, and smoking cessation.
- Advise patient that this drug may cause problems in fat and uric acid metabolism (hypercholesterolemia and hyperuricemia, respectively). Remind patient that periodic blood tests may be needed to monitor plasma lipids and uric acid levels.
- Advise patient about the likelihood of GI reactions such as nausea, vomiting, loss of appetite, and abdominal cramps. Instruct patient to report severe or prolonged GI problems, signs of hepatitis (yellow skin or eyes, abdominal pain, severe nausea and vomiting, fever, sore throat, malaise, weakness, facial edema), or signs of pancreatitis (abdominal pain after eating, indigestion, weight loss, oily stools).

Pharmacokinetics

Absorption: Poor (10–20%) after oral administration.
Distribution: Distributed into extracellular space; crosses the placenta and enters breast milk.
Metabolism and Excretion: Excreted mainly unchanged by the kidneys.
Half-life: 1–2 hr.

TIME/ACTION PROFILE (diuretic effect)

ROUTE	ONSET	PEAK	DURATION
PO, IV	2 hr	4 hr	6–12 hr (PO); 2 hr (IV)

Contraindications/Precautions

Contraindicated in: Hypersensitivity (cross-sensitivity with other thiazides or sulfonamides may exist); Some products contain tartrazine and should be avoided in patients with known intolerance; Anuria; Lactation: Discontinue or bottle feed.
Use Cautiously in: Renal or hepatic impairment; OB: May cause jaundice or thrombocytopenia in newborn; Pedi: May cause jaundice or thrombocytopenia in newborn; Geri: May have increased risk of side effects due to age-related decrease in renal function.

Interactions

Drug-Drug: Additive hypotension with other **antihypertensives**, acute ingestion of **alcohol** or **nitrates**. Additive hypokalemia with **corticosteroids**, **amphotericin B**, **loop diuretics**, **piperacillin**, or **ticarcillin**. ↓ the excretion of **lithium**. **Cholestyramine** or **colestipol** ↓ absorption. Hypokalemia ↑ risk of **digoxin** toxicity. **NSAIDs** may decrease effectiveness.

Route/Dosage

When used as a diuretic in adults, generally given daily, but may be given every other day or 2–3 days/wk.
PO (Adults): 125 mg–2 g/day as a single dose or in 2 divided doses.
PO (Children >6 months): 20 mg/kg/day as a single dose or in 2 divided doses. Maximum dose: 1 g/day.
PO (Neonates up to 6 months): 20–40 mg/kg/day in 2 divided doses. Maximum dose: 375 mg/day.
IV (Adults): *Diuretic*—100–500 mg/day as a single dose or 2 divided doses.
IV (Children >6 months): 4 mg/kg/day in 1–2 divided doses. Maximum dose: 20 mg/kg/day.
IV (Neonates up to 6 months): 2–8 mg/kg/day in 2 divided doses. Maximum dose: 20 mg/kg/day.

Availability (generic available)

Tablets: 250 mg Rx, 500 mg Rx. **Oral suspension:** 250 mg/5 mL Rx. **Powder for injection:** 500 mg Rx. ***In combination with:*** methyldopa, reserpine Rx. See Appendix B.

C

chlorpheniramine

(klor-fen-ir-a-meen)

Aller-Chlor Allergy, Chlo-Amine, Chlorate, Chlor-Trimeton, Chlor-Trimeton Allergy 4 Hour, Chlor-Trimeton Allergy 8 Hour, Chlor-Trimeton Allergy 12 Hour, ✱ Chlor-Tripolon, Novo-Pheniram, PediaCare Allergy Formula, Phenetron, Telechlor, Teldrin

Classification

Therapeutic: allergy, cold, and cough remedies, antihistamines

Indications

Relief of allergic symptoms caused by histamine release, including Nasal allergies, Allergic dermatoses. Management of severe allergic or hypersensitivity reactions, including anaphylaxis and transfusion reactions.

Action

Antagonizes the effects of histamine at H_2 receptor sites; does not bind to or inactivate histamine. **Therapeutic Effects:** Decreased symptoms of histamine excess (sneezing, rhinorrhea, nasal and ocular pruritus, ocular tearing, and redness).

Adverse Reactions/Side Effects

CNS: drowsiness, dizziness, excitation (in children). **EENT:** blurred vision. **CV:** hypertension, arrhythmias, hypotension, palpitations. **GI:** dry mouth, constipation, obstruction. **GU:** retention, urinary hesitancy.

PHYSICAL THERAPY IMPLICATIONS

Examination and Evaluation

- Assess blood pressure (BP) and compare to normal values (See Appendix F). Report changes in BP, either a problematic decrease in BP (hypotension) or a sustained increase in BP (hypertension).
- Assess heart rate, ECG, and heart sounds, especially during exercise (See Appendices G, H). Report any rhythm disturbances or symptoms of increased arrhythmias, including palpitations, chest discomfort, shortness of breath, fainting, and fatigue/weakness.
- Monitor symptoms of nasal allergies (sneezing, rhinitis, itching eyes, cough) or allergic skin reactions (rash, hives, itching) to help document benefits of this drug in treating these disorders.
- When treating anaphylaxis: assess for signs of successful treatment, including decreased skin reactions (rash, urticaria) and increased airway patency and ventilation (decreased dyspnea, wheezing, and so forth).
- Assess dizziness and drowsiness that might affect gait, balance, and other functional activities (See Appendix C). Report balance problems and functional limitations to the physician, and caution the patient and family/caregivers to guard against falls and trauma.
- Monitor signs of increased excitation in children. Severe or problematic excitation may require a change in dose or drug.

Interventions

- Guard against falls and trauma (hip fractures, head injury, and so forth). Implement fall-prevention strategies, especially in older adults or if balance is impaired (See Appendix E).
- Because of an increased risk of arrhythmias and abnormal BP responses, use caution during aerobic exercise and other forms of therapeutic exercise. Assess exercise tolerance frequently (BP, heart rate, fatigue levels), and terminate exercise immediately if any untoward responses occur (See Appendix L).

Patient/Client-Related Instruction

- Advise patient about the risk of daytime drowsiness and decreased attention and mental focus. These problems can be severe in certain people. Use care if driving or in other activities that require quick reactions and strong concentration.
- Advise patient to avoid alcohol and other CNS depressants because of the increased risk of sedation and adverse effects.
- Instruct patient to report other troublesome side effects, including severe or prolonged constipation, dry mouth, blurred vision, or problems with urination (difficulty initiating urination, urinary retention).

Pharmacokinetics

Absorption: Well absorbed following oral and parenteral administration.
Distribution: Widely distributed. Minimal amounts excreted in breast milk. Crosses the blood-brain barrier.
Metabolism and Excretion: Extensively metabolized by the liver.
Half-life: 12–15 hr.

✱ = Canadian drug name; *CAPITALS indicate life-threatening; underlines indicate most frequent.

TIME/ACTION PROFILE (antihistaminic effects)

ROUTE	ONSET	PEAK	DURATION
PO	15–30 min	6 hr	4–12 hr
PO-ER	unknown	unknown	8–24 hr
SC	unknown	unknown	4–12 hr
IM	unknown	unknown	4–12 hr
IV	rapid	unknown	4–12 hr

Contraindications/Precautions

Contraindicated in: Hypersensitivity; Acute attacks of asthma; Lactation: Avoid use or use alternative feeding method; Known alcohol intolerance (some liquid forms).

Use Cautiously in: Angle-closure glaucoma; Liver disease; Geri: Appears on Beers' list. Geriatric patients are more susceptible to adverse reactions due to anticholinergic effects; OB: Pregnancy (safety not established).

Interactions

Drug-Drug: ↑ CNS depression with other **CNS depressants**, including **alcohol**, **opioid analgesics**, and **sedative/hypnotics**. **MAO inhibitors** intensify and prolong anticholinergic effects of antihistamines. ↑ anticholinergic effects with other **drugs possessing anticholinergic properties**, including **antidepressants**, **atropine**, **haloperidol**, **phenothiazines**, **quinidine**, and **disopyramide**.

Route/Dosage

PO (Adults): 4 mg q 4–6 hr *or* 8–12 mg of extended-release formulation q 8–12 hr (not to exceed 24 mg/day).

PO (Geriatric Patients): 4 mg twice daily *or* 8 mg of extended-release formulation at bedtime.

PO (Children 6–12 yr): 2 mg 3–4 times daily (not to exceed 12 mg/day).

Injectable Formulation is Available Only in Canada

SC, IM, IV (Adults): 5- to 40-mg single dose (not to exceed 40 mg/day).

SC (Children): 87.5 mcg (0.0875 mg)/kg or 2.5 mg/m^2 q 6 hr as needed.

Availability (generic available)

Tablets: 4 mg Rx, OTC, 8 mg Rx, OTC, 12 mg Rx, OTC. **Chewable tablets (orange flavor):** 2 mg Rx, OTC. **Timed-release tablets:** 8 mg Rx, OTC, 12 mg Rx, OTC. **Timed-release capsules:** 8 mg Rx, OTC, 12 mg Rx, OTC. **Syrup:** 1 mg/5 mL Rx, OTC, 2 mg/5 mL Rx, OTC, 2.5 mg/5 mL Rx, OTC. **Injection:** 10 mg/mL, 100 mg/mL. ***In combination with:*** Codeine (Codeprex), pseudoephedrine (Advil), and decongestants Rx, OTC. See Appendix B.

chlorpromazine

(klor-**proe**-ma-zeen)

Chlorpromanyl, Largactil, Novo-Chlorpromazine, Thorazine, Thor-Prom

Classification

Therapeutic: antiemetics, antipsychotics

Pharmacologic: phenothiazines

Indications

Second-line treatment for schizophrenia and psychoses after failure with atypical antipsychotics. Hyperexcitable, combative behavior in children. Nausea and vomiting. Intractable hiccups. Preoperative sedation. Acute intermittent porphyria. **Unlabeled Use:** Vascular headache. Bipolar disorder.

Action

Alters the effects of dopamine in the CNS. Has significant anticholinergic/alpha-adrenergic blocking activity. **Therapeutic Effects:** Diminished signs/symptoms of psychosis. Relief of nausea/vomiting/intractable hiccups. Decreased symptoms of porphyria.

Adverse Reactions/Side Effects

CNS: NEUROLEPTIC MALIGNANT SYNDROME, sedation, extrapyramidal reactions, tardive dyskinesia. **EENT:** blurred vision, dry eyes, lens opacities. **CV:** hypotension (↑ with IM, IV), tachycardia. **GI:** constipation, dry mouth, anorexia, hepatitis, ileus, priapism. **GU:** urinary retention. Derm: photosensitivity, pigment changes, rashes. **Endo:** galactorrhea, amenorrhea. **Hemat:** AGRANULOCYTOSIS, leukopenia. **Metab:** hyperthermia. **Misc:** allergic reactions.

PHYSICAL THERAPY IMPLICATIONS

Examination and Evaluation

- Monitor and report signs of neuroleptic malignant syndrome (hyperthermia, diaphoresis, generalized muscle rigidity, altered mental status, tachycardia, changes in blood pressure [BP], incontinence). Symptoms typically occur within 4–14 days after initiation of drug therapy, but can occur at any time during drug use.
- Watch for signs of agranulocytosis and leucopenia, including fever, sore throat, mucosal lesions, and other signs of infection. Report these signs to the physician immediately.
- Assess motor function, and be alert for extrapyramidal symptoms. Report these symptoms immediately, especially tardive dyskinesia, because this problem

C

may be irreversible. Common extrapyramidal symptoms include:
  - Tardive dyskinesia (uncontrolled rhythmic movement of mouth, face, and extremities, lip smacking or puckering, puffing of cheeks, uncontrolled chewing, rapid or worm-like movements of tongue).
  - Pseudoparkinsonism (shuffling gait, rigidity, tremor, pill-rolling motion, loss of balance control, difficulty speaking or swallowing, mask-like face).
  - Akathisia (restlessness or desire to keep moving).
  - Other dystonias and dyskinesias (dystonic muscle spasms, twisting motions, twitching, inability to move eyes, weakness of arms or legs).
- Assess BP periodically and compare to normal values (See Appendix F). Report low BP (hypotension), especially if patient experiences dizziness or syncope.
- Assess heart rate, ECG, and heart sounds, especially during exercise (See Appendices G, H). Report a rapid heart rate (tachycardia) or symptoms of other arrhythmias, including palpitations, chest discomfort, shortness of breath, fainting, and fatigue/weakness.
- Monitor signs of allergic reactions, including pulmonary symptoms (laryngeal edema, wheezing, dyspnea) or skin reactions (rash, pruritus, urticaria). Notify physician immediately if these reactions occur.
- If used to control behavioral problems in children, document any changes in combative or hyperactive behavior to help determine drug efficacy and appropriate dosing.
- If used to control vascular headache, monitor the frequency, severity, and duration of attacks to help document the effects of drug therapy.
- If used to control nausea and vomiting, monitor the frequency, severity, and duration of GI problems to help document drug effectiveness.

Interventions

- Guard against falls and trauma (hip fractures, head injury, and so forth) caused by drowsiness, blurred vision, or extrapyramidal symptoms; implement fall-prevention strategies (See Appendix E).
- Because of the risk of tachycardia and abnormal BP responses, use caution during aerobic exercise and other forms of therapeutic exercise. Assess exercise tolerance frequently (BP, heart rate, fatigue levels), and terminate exercise immediately if any untoward responses occur (See Appendix L).
- To minimize orthostatic hypotension, patient should move slowly when assuming a more upright position.
- This drug impairs body temperature regulation; use care during exercise, and during other activities that increase body temperature (hot whirlpools, saunas, and so forth).
- Causes photosensitivity; use care if administering UV treatments. Advise patient to avoid direct sunlight and use sunscreens and protective clothing.
- Help patient and family/caregivers explore non-pharmacologic methods (exercise, counseling, support groups, and so forth) to reduce schizophrenic episodes and behavioral problems.

Patient/Client-Related Instruction

- Advise patient to avoid alcohol and other CNS depressants because of the increased risk of sedation and adverse effects.
- Instruct patient to report GI problems (constipation, loss of appetite), or signs of drug-induced hepatitis (anorexia, abdominal pain, severe nausea and vomiting, yellow skin or eyes, flu-like symptoms, muscle/joint pain).
- Instruct patient to report other problematic side effects such as excessive or prolonged sedation, vision problems, dry eyes, dry mouth, skin rash, skin discoloration, urinary retention, painful/sustained erections, nipple discharge, or menstrual disturbances.

Pharmacokinetics

Absorption: Variable absorption from tablets/suppositories; better with oral liquid formulations. Well absorbed following IM administration.
Distribution: Widely distributed; high CNS concentrations. Crosses the placenta; enters breast milk.
Protein Binding: ≥90%.
Metabolism and Excretion: Highly metabolized by the liver and GI mucosa. Some metabolites are active.
Half-life: 30 hr.

TIME/ACTION PROFILE (antipsychotic activity, antiemetic activity, sedation)

ROUTE	ONSET	PEAK	DURATION
PO	30–60 min	unknown	4–6 hr
IM	unknown	unknown	4–8 hr
IV	rapid	unknown	unknown

Contraindications/Precautions

Contraindicated in: Hypersensitivity; Hypersensitivity to sulfites (injectable) or benzyl alcohol (sustained-release capsules); Cross-sensitivity with other phenothiazines may occur; Angle-closure glaucoma; Bone marrow depression; Severe liver/cardiovascular disease; Concurrent pimozide use.
Use Cautiously in: Geriatric/debilitated patients (↓ initial dose); Diabetes; Respiratory disease; Prostatic hyperplasia; CNS tumors; Epilepsy; Intestinal

obstruction; OB/Lactation: Safety not established. Discontinue drug or bottle feed; Pedi: Children with acute illnesses, infections, gastroenteritis, or dehydration (increased risk of extrapyramidal reactions); Geri: ↑ risk of mortality in elderly patients treated for dementia-related psychosis.

Interactions

Drug-Drug: Concurrent use with **pimozide** ↑ the risk of potentially serious cardiovascular reactions. May alter serum **phenytoin** levels. ↓ pressor effect of **norepinephrine** and eliminates bradycardia. Antagonizes peripheral vasoconstriction from **epinephrine** and may reverse some of its actions. May ↓ elimination and ↑ effects of **valproic acid**. May ↓ the pharmacologic effects of **amphetamine** and **related compounds**. May ↓ the effectiveness of **bromocriptine**. May ↑ blood levels and effects of **tricyclic antidepressants**. **Antacids** or **adsorbent antidiarrheals** may ↓ adsorption; administer 1 hr before or 2 hr after chlorpromazine. **Activated charcoal** ↓ absorption. ↑ risk of anticholinergic effects with **antihistamines, tricyclic antidepressants, quinidine**, or **disopyramide**. Premedication with chlorpromazine ↑ the risk of neuromuscular excitation and hypotension when followed by **barbiturate** anesthesia. **Barbiturates** may ↑ metabolism and ↓ effectiveness. Chlorpromazine may ↓ **barbiturate** blood levels. Additive hypotension with **antihypertensives**. Additive CNS depression with **alcohol, antidepressants, antihistamines, MAO inhibitors, opioid analgesics, sedative/hypnotics**, or **general anesthetics**. Concurrent use with **lithium** may produce disorientation, unconsciousness, or extrapyramidal symptoms. Concurrent use with **meperidine** may produce excessive sedation and hypotension. May ↑ the risk of seizures with subarachnoid **metrizamide**. Concurrent use with **propranolol** ↑ blood levels of both drugs.

Drug-Natural: Concomitant use of **kava, valerian, chamomile**, or **hops** can ↑ CNS depression. ↑ anticholinergic effects with **angel's trumpet, jimson weed**, and **scopolia**.

Route/Dosage

PO (Adults): *Psychoses*—10–25 mg 2–4 times daily; may increase every 3–4 days (usual dose is 200 mg/day; up to 1 g/day). *Nausea and vomiting*—10–25 mg q 4 hr as needed. *Preoperative sedation*—25–50 mg 2–3 hr before surgery. *Hiccups/porphyria* —25–50 mg 3–4 times daily.

PO (Children): *Psychoses/nausea and vomiting*—0.55 mg/kg (15 mg/m²) q 4–6 hr as needed. *Preoperative sedation*—0.55 mg/kg (15 mg/m²) 2–3 hr before surgery.

IM (Adults): *Severe psychoses*—25–50 mg initially, may be repeated in 1 hr; increase to maximum of 400 mg q 3–12 hr if needed (up to 1 g/day). *Nausea/vomiting*—25 mg initially, may repeat with 25–50 mg q 3–4 hr as needed. *Nausea/vomiting during surgery*—12.5 mg, may be repeated in 30 min as needed. *Preoperative sedation*—12.5–25 mg 1–2 hr prior to surgery. *Hiccups/tetanus*—25–50 mg 3–4 times daily. *Porphyria*—25 mg q 6–8 hr until patient can take PO.

IM (Children >6 mo): *Psychoses/nausea and vomiting*—0.55 mg/kg (15 mg/m²) q 6–8 hr (not to exceed 40 mg/day in children 6 mo–5 yr, or 75 mg/day in children 5–12 yr). *Nausea/vomiting during surgery*—0.275 mg/kg, may repeat in 30 min as needed. *Preoperative sedation*—0.55 mg/kg 1–2 hr prior to surgery. *Tetanus*—0.55 mg/kg q 6–8 hr.

IV (Adults): *Nausea/vomiting during surgery*—up to 25 mg. *Hiccups/tetanus*—25–50 mg. *Porphyria*—25 mg q 8 hr.

IV (Children): *Nausea/vomiting during surgery*—0.275 mg/kg. *Tetanus*—0.55 mg/kg.

Availability (generic available)

Tablets: 10 mg, 25 mg, 50 mg, 100 mg, 200 mg. **Injection:** 25 mg/mL.

chlorpropamide
(klor-**proe**-pa-mide)
Apo-Chlorpropamide, Diabinese, Novo-Propamide

Classification
Therapeutic: antidiabetics
Pharmacologic: sulfonylureas

Indications

Control of blood sugar in type 2 diabetes mellitus when diet therapy fails. Requires some pancreatic function. **Unlabeled Use:** Management of neurogenic diabetes insipidus.

Action

Lowers blood sugar by stimulating the release of insulin from the pancreas and increasing the sensitivity to insulin at receptor sites. May also decrease hepatic glucose production. **Therapeutic Effects:** Lowering of blood sugar in diabetic patients.

Adverse Reactions/Side Effects

CNS: anorexia, dizziness, headache. **GI:** constipation, diarrhea, drug-induced hepatitis, increased appetite, nausea, vomiting. **Derm:** photosensitivity, rash, pruritus, urticaria. **Endo:** hypoglycemia, syndrome of inappropriate antidiuretic hormone (SIADH) secretion. **F and E:** hyponatremia. **Hemat:** APLASTIC ANEMIA, agranulocytosis, eosinophilia, hemolytic anemia, leukopenia, pancytopenia, thrombocytopenia. **Misc:** disulfiram-like reaction.

C

PHYSICAL THERAPY IMPLICATIONS

Examination and Evaluation

- Monitor signs of aplastic anemia (fatigue, weakness, shortness of breath with exertion, tachycardia, dizziness, headache), agranulocytosis (fever, sore throat, mucosal lesions, signs of infection, bruising), thrombocytopenia (bruising, nose bleeds, and bleeding gums), or unusual weakness and fatigue that might be due to other blood dyscrasias. Report these signs to the physician immediately.
- Be alert for signs of hypoglycemia, especially during and after exercise. Common neuromuscular signs include anxiety; restlessness; tingling in hands, feet, lips, or tongue; chills; cold sweats; confusion; difficulty in concentration; drowsiness; excessive hunger; headache; irritability; nervousness; tremor; weakness; unsteady gait. Report persistent or repeated episodes of hypoglycemia to the physician.
- Monitor signs of fluid-electrolyte imbalance due to syndrome of inappropriate antidiuretic hormone (SIADH). SIADH causes increased water retention that leads to relatively low sodium concentration (hyponatremia). Symptoms include confusion, lethargy, weakness, myoclonus, and depressed reflexes. Severe or sudden onset may also cause seizures, ataxia, nystagmus, tremor, dysarthria, dysphagia, and coma. Notify physician if these signs occur.
- Monitor and report signs of disulfiram-like reaction (i.e., toxicity occurring when this drug is taken with alcohol). Signs include throbbing headache, difficulty breathing, nausea, vomiting, sweating, thirst, chest pain, palpitations, tachycardia, hypotension, syncope, agitation, confusion, weakness, vertigo, and blurred vision.
- Assess any dizziness (See Appendix C) that might impair gait, balance, and other complex motor tasks (driving a car). Report balance problems and functional limitations to the physician, and caution the patient and family/caregivers to guard against falls and trauma.
- Assess blood pressure periodically (See Appendix F). A sudden or sustained increase in blood pressure (hypertension) may indicate problems in diabetes management, and should be reported to the physician.

Interventions

- Implement aerobic exercise and endurance training programs to maintain optimal body weight, improve insulin sensitivity, and reduce the risk of macrovascular disease (heart attack, stroke) and microvascular problems (reduced blood flow to tissues and organs that causes poor wound healing, neuropathy, retinopathy, and nephropathy).
- Provide a source of oral glucose (fruit juice, glucose gels/tablets, etc.) to treat mild hypoglycemia. Call for emergency assistance if symptoms persist or in cases of severe hypoglycemia. Emergency treatment typically consists of IV glucose, glucagon, or epinephrine.
- Causes photosensitivity; use care if administering UV treatments.

Patient/Client-Related Instruction

- Encourage patient to monitor blood glucose before and after exercise, and to adjust food intake to maintain normal glycemic levels.
- Emphasize the importance of adhering to nutritional guidelines, and the need for periodic assessment of glycemic control (serum glucose and glycosylated hemoglobin levels) throughout the management of diabetes mellitus.
- Advise patient about symptoms of hyperglycemia (confusion, drowsiness; flushed, dry skin; fruit-like breath odor; rapid, deep breathing, polyuria; loss of appetite; unusual thirst). Drug dosages may need to be adjusted to prevent repeated episodes of hyperglycemia.
- Instruct patient to report severe or prolonged GI problems (diarrhea, constipation, cramps) or signs of drug-induced hepatitis (anorexia, abdominal pain, severe nausea and vomiting, yellow skin or eyes, skin rashes, flu-like symptoms, muscle/joint pain).
- Advise patient about photosensitivity and to use sunscreens, protective clothing, and avoid prolonged sun exposure. Advise patient also to report any rashes or other skin reactions.

Pharmacokinetics

Absorption: Well absorbed after oral administration.
Distribution: 0.13–0.23 L/kg; enters breast milk.
Metabolism and Excretion: Mostly metabolized by the liver; 10–30% excreted in urine as unchanged drug.
Protein Binding: 60–90%.
Half-life: 36 hr.

TIME/ACTION PROFILE (hypoglycemic activity)

ROUTE	ONSET	PEAK	DURATION
PO	60 min	3–6 hr	24 hr

Contraindications/Precautions

Contraindicated in: Hypersensitivity; Cross-sensitivity with sulfonamides (including thiazide diuretics) may occur; Type 1 diabetics; Diabetic coma or ketoacidosis; Severe renal or hepatic disease; Uncontrolled infection, serious burns, or trauma; Lactation: Discontinue or bottle feed.

Use Cautiously in: Severe cardiovascular disease; Hepatic or renal impairment (increased risk of hypoglycemia); Infection, stress, or changes in diet may alter requirements for control of blood sugar; Impaired thyroid, pituitary, or adrenal function; Malnutrition, high fever, prolonged nausea, or vomiting; OB: Safety not established; insulin recommended during pregnancy; Geri: Prolonged half-life in geriatric patients may cause hypoglycemia; dosage reduction may be required. Appears on Beers' list.

Interactions

Drug-Drug: Ingestion of **alcohol** may result in disulfiram-like reaction. Effectiveness may be decreased by concurrent use of **diuretics, calcium channel blockers, corticosteroids, phenothiazines, hormonal contraceptives, estrogens, thyroid agents, phenytoin, nicotinic acid, adrenergics,** and **isoniazid. Alcohol, androgens (testosterone), chloramphenicol, fluoroquinolones, MAO inhibitors, miconazole, NSAIDs, probenecid, salicylates, sulfonamides,** and **warfarin** may ↑ the risk of hypoglycemia. Concurrent use with **warfarin** may alter the response to both agents (may ↑ effects of both; close monitoring recommended during any changes in dosage). **Beta blockers** may alter the response to oral hypoglycemic agents (↑ or ↓ requirements; nonselective agents may cause prolonged hypoglycemia).

Drug-Natural: Glucosamine may worsen hypoglycemia. **Fenugreek, chromium,** and **coenzyme Q-10** may produce additive hypoglycemic effects.

Route/Dosage

PO (Adults): 250 mg once daily, initially; may increase dose by 50–125 mg/day at 3- to 5-day intervals. Maximum daily dose is 750 mg. *Older, debilitated, or malnourished patients*—initiate therapy with 100–125 mg once daily; may increase dose by 50–125 mg/day at 3- to 5-day intervals. Maximum daily dose is 750 mg. *Antidiuretic dose*—100–250 mg/day.

Hepatic Impairment

PO (Adults): initiate therapy with 100–125 mg/day.

Renal Impairment

PO (Adults CCr ≥50 mL/min): initiate therapy with 100–125 mg once daily.

Renal Impairment

PO (Adults CCr <50 mL/min): Avoid use.

Availability

Tablets: 100 mg, 250 mg.

chlorthalidone

(klor-**thal**-i-doan)

Apo-Chlorthalidone, Hygroton, Thalitone, ✱Uridon

Classification

Therapeutic: antihypertensives, diuretics

Pharmacologic: thiazide diuretics

Indications

Management of mild-to-moderate hypertension. Treatment of edema associated with Congestive heart failure, Renal dysfunction, Cirrhosis, Glucocorticoid therapy, Estrogen therapy.

Action

Increases excretion of sodium and water by inhibiting sodium reabsorption in the distal tubule. Promotes excretion of chloride, potassium, magnesium, and bicarbonate. May produce arteriolar dilation. **Therapeutic Effects:** Lowering of blood pressure in hypertensive patients and diuresis with mobilization of edema.

Adverse Reactions/Side Effects

CNS: dizziness, drowsiness, lethargy, weakness. **CV:** hypotension. **GI:** anorexia, cramping, hepatitis, nausea, vomiting. **Derm:** photosensitivity, rashes. **Endo:** hyperglycemia. **F and E:** hypokalemia, dehydration, hypercalcemia, hypochloremic alkalosis, hypomagnesemia, hyponatremia, hypophosphatemia, hypovolemia. **Hemat:** blood dyscrasias. **Metab:** hyperuricemia, hypercholesterolemia. **MS:** muscle cramps. **Misc:** pancreatitis.

PHYSICAL THERAPY IMPLICATIONS

Examination and Evaluation

- Monitor signs of fluid, electrolyte, or acid-base imbalances, including dizziness, drowsiness, blurred vision, confusion, hypotension, or muscle cramps and weakness. Report excessive or prolonged symptoms to the physician.
- Assess dizziness and weakness that might affect gait, balance, and other functional activities (See Appendix C). Report balance problems and functional limitations to the physician, and caution the patient and family/caregivers to guard against falls and trauma.
- Assess blood pressure periodically and compare to normal values (See Appendix F) to help document antihypertensive effects.
- When used to treat edema, help determine drug effects by assessing peripheral edema using girth measurements, volume displacement, and measurement of pitting edema (See Appendix N). Also monitor signs of pulmonary edema such as dyspnea and rales/crackles (See Appendix K). Document

whether peripheral and pulmonary symptoms are controlled adequately by diuretic therapy.

- Monitor signs of hyperglycemia such as drowsiness, fruity breath, increased urination, and unusual thirst. Patients with diabetes mellitus should check blood glucose levels frequently.

Interventions

- Implement fall prevention strategies, especially in older adults or if patient exhibits sedation, dizziness, blurred vision, or other impairments that affect gait and balance (See Appendix E).
- Use caution during aerobic exercise, especially in hot environments. Increased sweating will cause fluid and electrolyte loss, and may exaggerate diuretic side effects (dizziness, muscle cramps, and so forth).
- To minimize orthostatic hypotension, patient should move slowly when assuming a more upright position.
- Causes photosensitivity; use care if administering UV treatments.

Patient/Client-Related Instruction

- Remind patients to take medication as directed to control hypertension and other cardiac conditions even if they are asymptomatic.
- Counsel patients about additional interventions to help control blood pressure and cardiac dysfunction, including regular exercise, weight loss, sodium restriction, stress reduction, moderation of alcohol consumption, and smoking cessation.
- Instruct patient to report signs of thrombocytopenia (bruising, nose bleeds, and bleeding gums) or unusual weakness and fatigue that might be due to anemia or other blood dyscrasias.
- Advise patient about the possibility of GI reactions such as cramping, nausea, vomiting, and loss of appetite. Instruct patient or family and caregivers to report severe or prolonged GI symptoms or signs of hepatitis (abdominal pain, severe nausea and vomiting, yellow skin or eyes, fever, sore throat, malaise, weakness, facial edema, lethargy, unusual bleeding or bruising) or pancreatitis (upper abdominal pain after eating, indigestion, weight loss, oily stools).
- Advise patient about photosensitivity, and to use sunscreens, protective clothing, and avoid prolonged sun exposure. Instruct patient also to report any rashes or other skin reactions.
- Advise patient that this drug may cause problems in fat and uric acid metabolism (hypercholesterolemia and hyperuricemia, respectively). Remind patient that periodic blood tests may be needed to monitor plasma lipids and uric acid levels.

Pharmacokinetics

Absorption: Rapidly absorbed after administration.
Distribution: Distributed into extracellular space; crosses the placenta and enters breast milk.
Metabolism and Excretion: Excreted mainly unchanged by the kidneys.
Half-life: 35–50 hr.

TIME/ACTION PROFILE (diuretic effect)

ROUTE	ONSET	PEAK	DURATION
PO	2 hr	2 hr	48–72 hr

Contraindications/Precautions

Contraindicated in: Hypersensitivity (cross-sensitivity with other thiazides or sulfonamides may exist); Some products contain tartrazine and should be avoided in patients with known intolerance; Anuria; Lactation.
Use Cautiously in: Renal or hepatic impairment; OB: May cause jaundice or thrombocytopenia newborn.

Interactions

Drug-Drug: Additive hypotension with other **antihypertensive agents**, acute ingestion of **alcohol** or **nitrates**. Additive hypokalemia with **corticosteroids**, **amphotericin B**, **piperacillin**, or **ticarcillin**. ↓ the excretion of **lithium**. **Cholestyramine** or **colestipol** ↓ absorption. Hypokalemia ↑ risk of **digoxin** toxicity. **NSAIDs** may ↓ effectiveness.

Route/Dosage

When used as a diuretic in adults, generally given daily, but may be given every other day or 2–3 days/wk.
PO (Adults): 12.5–100 mg once daily (doses above 25 mg are associated with greater likelihood of electrolyte abnormalities).

Availability (generic available)

Tablets: 25 mg, 50 mg, 100 mg. ***In combination with:*** atenolol, clonidine, reserpine. See Appendix B.

chlorzoxazone

(klor-**zox**-a-zone)
EZE-DS, Paraflex, Parafon Forte DSC, Relaxazone, Remular, Remular-S, Strifon Forte DSC

Classification

Therapeutic: skeletal muscle relaxants (centrally acting)

Indications

Adjunct to rest and physical therapy in the treatment of muscle spasm associated with acute painful musculoskeletal conditions.

Action

Skeletal muscle relaxation, most likely due to CNS depression. **Therapeutic Effects:** Skeletal muscle relaxation with decreased discomfort.

Adverse Reactions/Side Effects

CNS: <u>dizziness</u>, <u>drowsiness</u>. **GI:** GI BLEEDING, constipation, diarrhea, heartburn, nausea, vomiting. **Derm:** allergic dermatitis. **Hemat:** AGRANULOCYTOSIS, anemia. **Misc:** ALLERGIC REACTIONS, INCLUDING ANGIOEDEMA.

PHYSICAL THERAPY IMPLICATIONS

Examination and Evaluation

- Monitor signs of allergic reactions and angioedema, including skin reactions, such as rash, itching, burning, welts, and swelling in the face, and pulmonary symptoms, such as tightness in the throat and chest, wheezing, cough, and dyspnea. Seek immediate medical assistance if these reactions occur.
- Monitor signs of GI bleeding, including abdominal pain, vomiting blood, blood in stools, or black, tarry stools. Notify physician immediately if of these signs occur.
- Be alert for signs of agranulocytosis (fever, sore throat, mucosal lesions, signs of infection, bruising) or unusual weakness and fatigue that might be due to anemia. Report these signs to the physician.
- Assess patient's pain, stiffness, and ROM to help document antispasm effects.
- Assess dizziness that might affect gait, balance, and other functional activities (See Appendix C). Report balance problems and functional limitations to the physician, and caution the patient and family/caregivers to guard against falls and trauma.

Interventions

- Implement appropriate manual therapy techniques, physical agents, and therapeutic exercises to reduce pain and wean patient off muscle relaxants as soon as possible.
- Help patient explore other nonpharmacologic methods to reduce chronic pain, such as relaxation techniques, exercise, counseling, and so forth.
- Implement fall-prevention strategies, especially if balance is impaired (See Appendix E).

Patient/Client-Related Instruction

- Advise patient and family or caregiver about the signs of allergic reactions, GI bleeding, and blood dyscrasias (see above under Examination and Evaluation), and to seek immediate medical assistance if these signs develop.
- Inform patient that long-term use can cause tolerance and physical/psychologic dependence; encourage adherence to physical therapy so that drug therapy can be discontinued as soon as possible.
- Inform patient that this drug may cause severe drowsiness, dizziness, and reduced psychomotor skills. Patients should avoid driving or other activities that require concentration and fast reactions.
- Advise patient to avoid alcohol and other CNS depressants because of the increased risk of sedation and adverse effects.
- Warn patient about anticholinergic effects such as dry mouth, constipation, urinary retention, sedation, and weakness; anticholinergic effects are often more severe in older adults.
- Instruct patient and family/caregivers to report other troublesome side effects such as severe or prolonged dermatitis or GI problems (nausea, vomiting, diarrhea, heartburn).

Pharmacokinetics

Absorption: Readily absorbed after oral administration.
Distribution: Unknown.
Metabolism and Excretion: Mostly metabolized by the liver; $<1\%$ excreted unchanged in urine.
Half-life: 1.1 hr.

TIME/ACTION PROFILE (skeletal muscle effects)

ROUTE	ONSET	PEAK	DURATION
PO	within 1 hr	1–2 hr	3–4 hr

Contraindications/Precautions

Contraindicated in: Hypersensitivity; Porphyria.
Use Cautiously in: Underlying cardiovascular disease; Impaired renal or hepatic function; OB/Lactation/Pedi: Safety not established; Geri: Appears on Beer' list. Poorly tolerated due to anticholinergic effects.

Interactions

Drug-Drug: ↑ risk of CNS depression with other **CNS depressants**, including **alcohol, antihistamines, antidepressants, sedative/hypnotics**, or **opioid analgesics**.
Drug-Natural: Concomitant use of **kava, valerian, skullcap, chamomile**, or **hops** can ↑ CNS depression.

Route/Dosage

PO (Adults): 250–750 mg 3–4 times daily.
PO (Children): 20 mg/kg or 600 mg/m^2/day in 3–4 divided doses.

Availability (generic available)

Tablets: 250 mg, 500 mg.

cholestyramine

(koe-less-**tear**-a-meen)

LoCHOLEST, LoCHOLEST Light, Prevalite, Questran, Questran Light

Classification

Therapeutic: lipid-lowering agents

Pharmacologic: bile acid sequestrants

Indications

Management of primary hypercholesterolemia. Pruritus associated with elevated levels of bile acids. **Unlabeled Use:** Diarrhea associated with excess bile acids.

Action

Bind bile acids in the GI tract, forming an insoluble complex. Result is increased clearance of cholesterol. **Therapeutic Effects:** Decreased plasma cholesterol and low-density lipoproteins (LDLs). Decreased pruritus.

Adverse Reactions/Side Effects

EENT: irritation of the tongue. **GI:** abdominal discomfort, constipation, nausea, fecal impaction, flatulence, hemorrhoids, perianal irritation, steatorrhea, vomiting. **Derm:** irritation, rashes. **F and E:** hyperchloremic acidosis. **Metab:** vitamin A, D, and K deficiency.

PHYSICAL THERAPY IMPLICATIONS

Examination and Evaluation

- Monitor signs of hyperchloremic acidosis, including headache, lethargy, stupor, seizures, vision disturbances, increased respiration, cardiac arrhythmias, weakness, and GI symptoms (nausea, vomiting, abdominal pain). Notify physician immediately if these signs occur.
- Monitor signs of vitamin deficiencies, including deficiencies of vitamin A (vision disturbances, poor night vision), vitamin D (bone pain, muscle weakness, hypertension), and vitamin K (bleeding gums, nosebleeds, bruising). Notify physician if these signs persist.

Interventions

- Design and implement aerobic exercise and endurance training programs to improve cardiovascular function and help reduce the risk of coronary heart disease.

Patient/Client-Related Instruction

- Remind patients to take medication as directed to control hyperlipidemia even though they are asymptomatic.
- Counsel patients about additional interventions to help control lipid disorders and improve cardiovascular health, including dietary modification, regular exercise, moderation of alcohol consumption, and smoking cessation.
- Advise patient about the likelihood of GI problems including nausea, constipation, abdominal pain, flatulence, oily/foul smelling stools, hemorrhoids, and fecal impaction. Instruct patient to report severe or prolonged GI problems.
- Instruct patient and family/caregivers to report other troublesome side effects such as severe or prolonged tongue irritation or skin reactions (rash, irritation).

Pharmacokinetics

Absorption: Action takes place in the GI tract. No absorption occurs.

Distribution: No distribution.

Metabolism and Excretion: After binding bile acids, insoluble complex is eliminated in the feces.

Half-life: Unknown.

TIME/ACTION PROFILE (hypocholesterolemic effects)

ROUTE	ONSET	PEAK	DURATION
PO	24–48 hr	1–3 wk	2–4 wk

Contraindications/Precautions

Contraindicated in: Hypersensitivity; Complete biliary obstruction; Some products contain aspartame and should be avoided in patients with phenylketonuria.

Use Cautiously in: History of constipation.

Exercise Extreme Caution in: Children (may cause intestinal obstruction; deaths have occurred).

Interactions

Drug-Drug: May ↓ absorption/effects of orally administered **acetaminophen, amiodarone, clindamycin, clofibrate, digoxin, diuretics, gemfibrozil, glipizide, corticosteroids, imipramine, mycophenolate, methotrexate, methyldopa, niacin, NSAIDs, penicillin, phenytoin, phosphates, propranolol, tetracyclines, tolbutamide, thyroid preparations, ursodiol, warfarin, and fat-soluble vitamins (A, D, E, and K).** May ↓ absorption of other **orally administered medications.**

Route/Dosage

PO (Adults): 4 g 1–2 times daily (initially, may be increased as needed/tolerated up to 24 g/day in 6 divided doses).

PO (Children): 240 mg/kg/day in 2–3 divided doses (not >8 g/day).

Availability (generic available)

Powder for suspension with aspartame (strawberry flavor [LoCHOLEST], unflavored [Prevalite, Questran Light]): 4 g cholestyramine/packet or scoop. **Powder for suspension (strawberry flavor [LoCHOLEST], unflavored [Questran, generic]):** 4 g cholestyramine/packet or scoop.

choline and magnesium salicylates (koe-leen mag-neez-ee-um sa-lis-i-lates)

Trilisate

Classification

Therapeutic: antipyretics, nonopioid analgesics
Pharmacologic: salicylates

Indications

Inflammatory disorders, including Rheumatoid arthritis, Osteoarthritis. Mild-to-moderate pain. Fever.

Action

Produce analgesia and reduce inflammation and fever by inhibiting the production of prostaglandins. **Therapeutic Effects:** Analgesia. Reduction of inflammation. Reduction of fever.

Adverse Reactions/Side Effects

EENT: tinnitus. **GI:** GI BLEEDING, dyspepsia, epigastric distress, nausea, abdominal pain, anorexia, hepatotoxicity, vomiting. **Misc:** ALLERGIC REACTIONS, INCLUDING ANAPHYLAXIS AND LARYNGEAL EDEMA.

PHYSICAL THERAPY IMPLICATIONS

Examination and Evaluation

- Monitor signs of allergic reactions and anaphylaxis, including pulmonary symptoms (tightness in the throat and chest, wheezing, cough, dyspnea) or skin reactions (rash, pruritus, urticaria). Report these signs to the physician immediately.
- Be alert for signs of GI bleeding, including abdominal pain, vomiting blood, blood in stools, or black, tarry stools. Report these signs to the physician immediately.
- Watch for other signs of increased bleeding, such as excessive bruising, bleeding gums, and nosebleeds. Notify physician of these signs immediately.
- Assess pain and other variables (range of motion, muscle strength) to document whether this drug is successful in helping manage the patient's pain and decreasing impairments.

Interventions

- Implement appropriate manual therapy techniques, physical agents, and therapeutic exercises to reduce pain and decrease the need for salicylates.
- Help patient explore other nonpharmacologic methods to reduce chronic pain, such as relaxation techniques, exercise, counseling, and so forth.

Patient/Client-Related Instruction

- Advise patient that analgesics are usually more effective if given before pain becomes severe; emphasize that adequate pain control will allow better participation in physical therapy.
- Advise patient about the likelihood of GI reactions (nausea, vomiting, indigestion, abdominal pain, loss of appetite). Instruct patient to report severe or prolonged GI problems or signs of liver toxicity (yellow skin or eyes, abdominal pain, severe nausea and vomiting, fever, sore throat, malaise, weakness, facial edema).
- Advise patient to reduce alcohol intake because alcohol increases the risk of gastric toxicity.
- Instruct patient to report excessive or prolonged headache or ringing/buzzing in the ears (tinnitus); these signs may indicate salicylate toxicity.
- Caution patient about the use of over-the-counter products that contain aspirin, other NSAIDs, or acetaminophen while taking high doses of salicylates. Use of multiple NSAIDs increases the risk of toxicity and overdose.

Pharmacokinetics

Absorption: Well absorbed after oral administration.
Distribution: Rapidly and widely distributed; crosses the placenta and enters breast milk.
Protein Binding: 90–95%.
Metabolism and Excretion: Extensively metabolized by the liver; inactive metabolites excreted by the kidneys. Amount excreted unchanged by the kidneys depends on urine pH; as pH increases, amount excreted unchanged increases from 2–3% up to 80%.
Half-life: 2–3 hr for low doses; up to 15–30 hr with larger doses because of saturation of liver metabolism.

TIME/ACTION PROFILE

ROUTE	ONSET	PEAK	DURATION
PO	5–30 min	1–3 hr	3–6 hr

Contraindications/Precautions

Contraindicated in: Hypersensitivity to aspirin or other salicylates; Cross-sensitivity with other NSAIDs may exist (less with nonaspirin salicylates).
Use Cautiously in: History of GI bleeding or ulcer disease; Chronic alcohol use/abuse; Severe renal disease (magnesium toxicity may occur); Severe hepatic disease; OB: Salicylates may have adverse effects on fetus and mother; should be avoided during pregnancy, especially during the 3rd trimester; Lactation: Safety not established; Pedi: May increase the risk of Reye's syndrome in children or adolescents recovering from chickenpox or flu symptoms; Geri: ↑ risk of adverse

reactions, especially GI bleeding; more sensitive to toxic levels.

Interactions

Drug-Drug: May ↑ activity of **penicillins, phenytoin, methotrexate, valproic acid, oral hypoglycemic agents**, and **sulfonamides**. May ↓ beneficial effects of **probenecid** or **sulfinpyrazone**. **Urinary acidification** ↑ reabsorption and may ↑ serum salicylate levels. **Alkalinization of the urine** or the ingestion of large amounts of **antacids** ↑ excretion and ↓ serum salicylate levels. May blunt the therapeutic response to **diuretics** or other **antihypertensives**. ↑ risk of GI irritation with **NSAIDs**. May increase hypoprothrombinemic effect of **warfarin**.
Drug-Food: Foods capable of acidifying the urine (see Appendix L) may ↑ serum salicylate levels.

Route/Dosage

5 mL of liquid equivalent to 500 mg salicylate or 650 mg of aspirin. Tablet strength expressed in milligrams (mg) of salicylate: 500-mg tablet equivalent to 650 mg of aspirin, 750-mg tablet equivalent to 975 mg of aspirin, 1000-mg tablet equivalent to 1.3 g of aspirin.
PO (Adults): *Analgesic/antipyretic*—2–3 g of salicylate/day in 2–3 divided doses. *Anti-inflammatory*—3 g/day at bedtime or in 2–3 divided doses.
PO (Children): 30–60 mg/kg/day given in 3–4 divided doses.

Availability

Tablets: 500 mg, 750 mg, 1000 mg. **Liquid:** 500 mg/5 mL.

ciclesonide (nasal)

(si-**kless**-o-nide)
Omnaris

Classification
Therapeutic: allergy, cold, and cough remedies
Pharmacologic: corticosteroids

Indications

Symptomatic management of seasonal/perennial allergic rhinitis.

Action

Acts as a potent, locally acting anti-inflammatory and immune modifier. **Therapeutic Effects:** Decreased symptoms of allergic rhinitis.

Adverse Reactions/Side Effects

CNS: headache. **EENT:** ear pain, epistaxis, local stinging, nasopharyngitis. **Endo:** adrenal suppression (↑ dose, long-term therapy only).

PHYSICAL THERAPY IMPLICATIONS

Examination and Evaluation

- Report signs of adrenal suppression, including hypotension, weight loss, weakness, nausea, vomiting, anorexia, lethargy, confusion, and restlessness.
- Monitor symptoms of allergic rhinitis (nasopharyngeal pain, inflammation, itching, mucous discharge) to help document whether this drug is successful in managing these symptoms.

Patient/Client-Related Instruction

- Advise patient not to exceed the recommended dose or frequency of intranasal applications.
- Advise patients on long-term treatment to consult physician before stopping this medication. Stopping the medication suddenly may result in adrenocortical shock (severe hypotension, hypoglycemia, weakness, vomiting). If these signs appear, notify physician immediately; may be life threatening.
- Instruct patient and family/caregivers to report other troublesome side effects such as severe or prolonged headache, ear pain, or nasal problems (inflammation, nosebleeds, local pain/stinging).

Pharmacokinetics

Absorption: <1% systemically absorbed following intranasal administration.
Distribution: Action is primarily local.
Protein Binding: >99%.
Metabolism and Excretion: Activated by enzymatic conversion to des-ciclesonide, which is the pharmacologically active drug. Small amounts absorbed are metabolized by the liver.
Half-life: Unknown.

TIME/ACTION PROFILE

ROUTE	ONSET	PEAK	DURATION
intranasal	24–48 hr	1–5 wk	unknown

Contraindications/Precautions

Contraindicated in: Hypersensitivity.
Use Cautiously in: Concurrent ketoconazole; OB/Lactation: Safe use in pregnancy or lactation not established; Pedi: Safe use in children <12 yr not established.

Interactions

Drug-Drug: Ketoconazole ↑ blood levels; use cautiously.

Route/Dosage

PO (Adults): 2 sprays (50 mcg/spray) in each nostril once daily.

Availability

Aqueous suspension spray for nasal use: 50 mcg/actuation in 12.5-g bottles.

ciclopirox (sye-kloe-peer-ox)

Loprox, Penlac, Stieprox

Classification

Therapeutic: antifungals (topical)

Pharmacologic: hydroxypyridone

Indications

Treatment of cutaneous fungal infections, including cutaneous candidiasis (lotion and cream only), tinea pedis (athlete's foot) (gel, lotion, and cream only), tinea cruris (jock itch) (lotion and cream only), tinea corporis (ringworm) (gel, lotion, and cream only), tinea versicolor (lotion and cream only), seborrheic dermatitis (shampoo and gel only), and onychomycosis of fingernails and toenails (nail lacquer only).

Action

Inhibits the transport of essential elements in fungal cell, disrupting the synthesis of DNA, RNA, and protein. **Therapeutic Effects:** Decrease in symptoms of fungal infection.

Adverse Reactions/Side Effects

Local: burning, itching, local hypersensitivity reactions, redness, stinging.

PHYSICAL THERAPY IMPLICATIONS

Examination and Evaluation

- Assess healing of skin lesions to help document drug effectiveness.

Interventions

- Avoid contact with cutaneous lesions when treating patient.
- Always wash hands thoroughly and disinfect equipment (whirlpools, electrotherapeutic devices, treatment tables, and so forth) to help prevent the spread of infection.

Patient/Client-Related Instruction

- Advise patient to report any increased local sensitivity to this drug (pain, burning, itching, redness, stinging).
- Instruct patient about proper hygiene; e.g., thoroughly wash and dry the affected area, wear clean socks and ventilated shoes for tinea pedis, and so forth.
- Advise patient to apply the drug as directed for the full course of treatment even if the patient feels better.
- Inform patient that early relief of cutaneous symptoms may be seen in 2–3 days. Full therapeutic response may take up to 4 wk.
- Advise patient to seek medical help if infections persist or recur after the full treatment. Recurrent fungal infections may be a sign of systemic illness.

Pharmacokinetics

Absorption: Absorption through intact skin is minimal (<5%).
Distribution: Distribution after topical administration is primarily local.
Metabolism and Excretion: Eliminated by kidneys (3–10% for gel).
Half-life: 5.5 hr (gel).

TIME/ACTION PROFILE

ROUTE	ONSET	PEAK	DURATION
topical	unknown	unknown	unknown

Contraindications/Precautions

Contraindicated in: Hypersensitivity to active ingredients, additives, preservatives, or bases; Some products contain alcohol (nail lacquer) and should be avoided in patients with known intolerance.
Use Cautiously in: OB/Lactation: Safety not established.

Interactions

Drug-Drug: Not known.

Route/Dosage

Topical (Adults and Children >10 yr): *Shampoo:* Apply 5 mL (10 mL may be used for long hair) to scalp and leave on for 3 min before rinsing off. Use twice weekly (wait at least 3 days between treatments) for 4 wk. *Cream/lotion:* Apply twice daily for 2–4 wk. *Gel:* Apply twice daily for 4 wk. *Topical solution (nail lacquer):* Apply to nails once daily (at bedtime or 8 hr before bathing) for up to 48 wk. Each daily application should be made over the previous coat and then removed with alcohol every 7 days.

Availability (generic available)

Cream: 0.77% Rx. **Gel:** 0.77% Rx. **Lotion:** 0.77% Rx. **Nail Lacquer Solution:** 8% Rx. **Shampoo:** 1% Rx, 1.5% Rx.

cidofovir (sye-doe-foe-veer)

Vistide

Classification

Therapeutic: antivirals

Pharmacologic: cytidine nucleotide analog

Indications

Management of cytomegalovirus (CMV) retinitis in HIV-infected patients (with probenecid).

C

Action

Suppresses replication of CMV by inhibiting viral DNA synthesis. **Therapeutic Effects:** Slows progression of CMV retinitis; may not be curative.

Adverse Reactions/Side Effects

CNS: headache, weakness. **EENT:** decreased intraocular pressure, hearing loss, iritis, ocular hypotony, uveitis. **Resp:** dyspnea, pneumonia. **GI:** HEPATIC DYSFUNCTION, PANCREATITIS, abdominal pain, nausea, vomiting, anorexia, diarrhea. **GU:** RENAL FAILURE, proteinuria. **Derm:** alopecia, rash. **F and E:** decreased serum bicarbonate. **Hemat:** neutropenia, anemia. **Metab:** METABOLIC ACIDOSIS. **Misc:** chills, fever, infection.

PHYSICAL THERAPY IMPLICATIONS

Examination and Evaluation

- Monitor signs of renal failure, including decreased urine output, increased blood pressure, muscle cramps/twitching, edema/weight gain from fluid retention, yellowish brown skin, and confusion that progresses to seizures and coma. Report these signs immediately to the physician.
- Be alert for signs of liver dysfunction (anorexia, abdominal pain, severe nausea and vomiting, yellow skin or eyes, fever, sore throat, malaise, weakness, facial edema, lethargy, unusual bleeding or bruising) or pancreatitis (upper abdominal pain after eating, indigestion, weight loss, oily stools). Report these signs to the physician immediately.
- Monitor signs of metabolic acidosis, including headache, lethargy, stupor, seizures, increased respiration, cardiac arrhythmias, weakness, and GI symptoms (nausea, vomiting, abdominal pain). Notify physician immediately if these signs occur.
- Monitor any breathing difficulties; notify physician immediately if patient experiences signs of pneumonia, including cough, fever, chills, dyspnea, and chest pain during inspiration and expiration.
- Be alert for any visual or hearing disturbances; report these problems for further evaluation.
- Monitor signs of neutropenia (fever, sore throat, signs of infection), or unusual weakness, fatigue, and pallor that might be due to anemia. Report these signs to the physician.

Interventions

- Always wash hands thoroughly and disinfect equipment (whirlpools, electrotherapeutic devices, treatment tables, and so forth) to help prevent the spread of infection. Use universal precautions as indicated for specific patients.

Patient/Client-Related Instruction

- Instruct patient and family/caregivers to report other troublesome side effects, including severe or prolonged headache, chills, fever, infection, skin problems (rash, hair loss), or GI problems (diarrhea, nausea, vomiting, loss of appetite, abdominal pain).

Pharmacokinetics

Absorption: IV administration results in complete bioavailability.
Distribution: Unknown.
Metabolism and Excretion: Excreted mostly unchanged by the kidneys.
Half-life: Unknown.

TIME/ACTION PROFILE

ROUTE	ONSET	PEAK	DURATION
IV	rapid	end of infusion	unknown

Contraindications/Precautions

Contraindicated in: Hypersensitivity to cidofovir, probenecid, or sulfonamides; Serum Cr >1.5 mg/dL, CCr ≤55 mL/min, or urine protein ≥100 mg/dL (≥2+ proteinuria); Concurrent use of foscarnet, amphotericin B, aminoglycoside anti-infectives, NSAIDs, or IV pentamidine.
Use Cautiously in: Pregnancy or children (safety not established); breast-feeding is not recommended in HIV-positive patients.
Exercise Extreme Caution in: Any condition or medication that increases the risk of dehydration.

Interactions

Drug-Drug: ↑ risk of nephrotoxicity with **aminoglycosides, amphotericin B, foscarnet,** and **pentamidine** and should be avoided; wait 7 days after giving other nephrotoxic agents. **Probenecid**, which is required concurrently, may interact with **acetaminophen, acyclovir, ACE inhibitors, barbiturates, benzodiazepines, bumetanide, methotrexate, famotidine, furosemide, NSAIDs, theophylline**, and **zidovudine**.

Route/Dosage

IV (Adults): 5 mg/kg once weekly for 2 wk, followed by 5 mg/kg every 2 wk (must be given with probenecid).

Renal Impairment

IV (Adults): *Increase in serum creatinine of 0.3–0.4 mg/dL*—decrease dose to 3 mg/kg; discontinue if serum creatinine increases ≥0.5 mg/dL over baseline.

Availability
Solution for injection: 75 mg/mL in 5-mL ampules.

cilostazol (sil-os-tah-zol)
Pletal

Classification
Therapeutic: antiplatelet agents
Pharmacologic: platelet aggregation inhibitors

Indications
Reduction of the symptoms of intermittent claudication as measured by increased walking distance.

Action
Inhibits the enzyme cyclic adenosine monophosphate (cAMP) phosphodiesterase III (PDE III), which results in increased cAMP in platelets and blood vessels, producing inhibition of platelet aggregation and vasodilation.
Therapeutic Effects: Reduced symptoms of intermittent claudication with improved walking distance.

Adverse Reactions/Side Effects
CNS: headache, dizziness. **CV:** palpitations, tachycardia. **GI:** diarrhea.

PHYSICAL THERAPY IMPLICATIONS

Examination and Evaluation
- Assess patient's walking distance and pain-free walking time. Document any increase in walking distance and time as an indication that this drug is helping reduce intermittent claudication.
- Assess heart rate, ECG, and heart sounds, especially during exercise (See Appendices G, H). Report fast heart rate (tachycardia) or signs of other arrhythmias, including palpitations, chest discomfort, shortness of breath, fainting, and fatigue/weakness.
- Assess dizziness that might affect gait, balance, and other functional activities (See Appendix C). Report balance problems and functional limitations to the physician, and caution the patient and family/caregivers to guard against falls and trauma.

Interventions
- Implement therapeutic exercises and ambulation activities to augment the effects of drug therapy and promote increased walking distance. Patients should attempt to walk as long as possible after the onset of leg pain, and progressively increase the time spent walking before stopping due to claudication.
- Because of the risk of tachycardia and other arrhythmias, use caution during aerobic exercise and other forms of therapeutic exercise. Assess exercise tolerance frequently (blood pressure, heart rate, fatigue levels), and terminate exercise immediately if any untoward responses occur (See Appendix L).

Patient/Client-Related Instruction
- Instruct patient to report other bothersome side effects, including severe or prolonged headache or diarrhea.

Pharmacokinetics
Absorption: Slowly absorbed after oral administration.
Distribution: Unknown.
Protein Binding: 95–98% bound to plasma proteins; one active metabolite is 97.4% bound, the other is 66% bound.
Metabolism and Excretion: Extensively metabolized by the liver, two metabolites have platelet aggregation inhibitory activity; metabolites are mostly excreted by the kidneys.
Half-life: *Cilostazol and its active metabolites*—11–13 hr.

TIME/ACTION PROFILE (symptom reduction)

ROUTE	ONSET	PEAK	DURATION
PO	2–4 wk	up to 12 wk	unknown

Contraindications/Precautions
Contraindicated in: Hypersensitivity; CHF; OB: Potential for congenital defects, stillbirth, and low birth weight; Lactation: Potential risk to nursing infants; discontinue or bottle feed.
Use Cautiously in: Pedi: Safety not established.

Interactions
Drug-Drug: Concurrent administration of **ketoconazole, itraconazole, erythromycin, diltiazem, fluconazole, miconazole, fluvoxamine, fluoxetine, nefazodone, sertraline,** or **omeprazole** ↓ metabolism and ↑ levels and activity of cilostazol (use lower doses). Concurrent use with **aspirin** has additive effects on platelet function.
Drug-Food: Grapefruit juice inhibits metabolism and ↑ effects; concurrent use should be avoided.

Route/Dosage
PO (Adults): 100 mg twice daily (50 mg twice daily if receiving inhibitors of cilostazol metabolism).

Availability (generic available)
Tablets: 50 mg, 100 mg.

cimetidine (sye-met-i-deen)
Apo-Cimetidine, Novocimetine, Peptol, Tagamet, Tagamet HB

Classification
Therapeutic: antiulcer agents
Pharmacologic: histamine H_2 antagonists

Indications

Short-term treatment of active duodenal ulcers and benign gastric ulcers. Maintenance therapy for duodenal ulcers after healing of active ulcer(s). Management of gastroesophageal reflux disease (GERD). Treatment of heartburn, acid indigestion, and sour stomach (OTC use). Management of gastric hypersecretory states (Zollinger-Ellison syndrome). IV: Prevention and treatment of stress-induced upper GI bleeding in critically ill patients. **Unlabeled Use:** Management of GI symptoms associated with the use of NSAIDs. Prevention of stress ulceration or aspiration pneumonitis. Prevention of acid inactivation of supplemental pancreatic enzymes in patients with pancreatic insufficiency. Management of urticaria.

Action

Inhibits the action of histamine at the H_2 receptor site located primarily in gastric parietal cells, resulting in inhibition of gastric acid secretion. **Therapeutic Effects:** Healing and prevention of ulcers. Decreased symptoms of gastroesophageal reflux. Decreased secretion of gastric acid.

Adverse Reactions/Side Effects

CNS: confusion, dizziness, drowsiness, hallucinations, headache. **CV:** ARRHYTHMIAS. **GI:** constipation, diarrhea, drug-induced hepatitis, nausea. **GU:** decreased sperm count, erectile dysfunction. **Endo:** gynecomastia. **Hemat:** AGRANULOCYTOSIS, APLASTIC ANEMIA, anemia, neutropenia, thrombocytopenia. **Local:** pain at IM site. **Misc:** hypersensitivity reactions.

PHYSICAL THERAPY IMPLICATIONS

Examination and Evaluation

- Assess heart rate, ECG, and heart sounds, especially during exercise (See Appendices G, H). Report any rhythm disturbances or symptoms of increased arrhythmias, including palpitations, chest discomfort, shortness of breath, fainting, and fatigue/weakness.
- Report signs of agranulocytosis and neutropenia (fever, sore throat, mucosal lesions, signs of infection, bruising), aplastic anemia (unusual fatigue, weakness), or thrombocytopenia (bruising, bleeding gums, nose bleeds).
- Monitor signs of hypersensitivity reactions, including pulmonary symptoms (tightness in the throat or chest, wheezing, cough, dyspnea) or skin reactions (rash, pruritus, urticaria). Notify physician or nursing staff immediately if these reactions occur.
- Assess dizziness and drowsiness that might affect gait, balance, and other functional activities (see Appendix C). Report balance problems and functional limitations to the physician and nursing staff, and caution the patient and family/caregivers to guard against falls and trauma.
- Monitor other CNS symptoms such as confusion, hallucinations, and headache. Excessive or prolonged CNS symptoms may require a reduction in dose.
- If treating allergic skin reactions (urticaria), assess degree of itching, skin rash, and inflammation to help determine effects of drug therapy.
- Monitor IM injection site for pain, swelling, and irritation. Report prolonged or excessive injection-site reactions to the physician.

Interventions

- Use caution during aerobic exercise and endurance conditioning because of an increased risk of cardiac arrhythmias. Terminate exercise if patient exhibits untoward symptoms (chest pain, shortness of breath, etc.) or displays other criteria for exercise termination (See Appendix L).

Patient/Client-Related Instruction

- Advise patient to avoid alcohol and foods that may cause an increase in GI irritation.
- Instruct patient to report troublesome GI effects (constipation, diarrhea, nausea) or signs of drug-induced hepatitis (anorexia, abdominal pain, severe nausea and vomiting, yellow skin or eyes, skin rashes, flu-like symptoms, muscle/joint pain).
- Advise men to consult their physician if they experience erectile dysfunction or breast enlargement (gynecomastia).

Pharmacokinetics

Absorption: Well absorbed following oral and IM administration.
Distribution: Enters breast milk and cerebrospinal fluid.
Metabolism and Excretion: 30% metabolized by the liver; remainder is eliminated unchanged by the kidneys.
Half-life: 2 hr.

TIME/ACTION PROFILE

ROUTE	ONSET	PEAK	DURATION
PO	30 min	45–90 min	4–5 hr
M, IV	10 min	30 min	4–5 hr

Contraindications/Precautions

Contraindicated in: Hypersensitivity; Oral liquid contains alcohol and should be avoided in patients with known intolerance.
Use Cautiously in: Renal impairment (more susceptible to adverse CNS reactions; increased dosage interval

recommended if renal impairment is severe); OB/Lactation: Safety not established; Geri: Appears on Beers' list. Geriatric patients are more susceptible to adverse CNS reactions (dosage reduction recommended).

Interactions

Drug-Drug: Cimetidine inhibits drug-metabolizing enzymes in the liver; may lead to increased blood levels and toxicity with the following—some **benzodiazepines** (especially **chlordiazepoxide, diazepam,** and **midazolam**), some **beta blockers (labetalol, metoprolol, propranolol), caffeine, calcium channel blockers, carbamazepine, chloroquine, lidocaine, metronidazole, moricizine, pentoxifylline, phenytoin, propafenone, quinidine, quinine, metformin, sulfonylureas, theophylline, triamterene, tricyclic antidepressants**, and **warfarin**. The effects of **succinylcholine, flecainide, procainamide, carmustine**, and **fluorouracil** are ↑ by cimetidine. ↓ the absorption of **ketoconazole**. **Antacids** and **sucralfate** ↓ absorption.
Drug-Natural: ↑ **caffeine** levels and side effects with caffeine-containing herbs (**cola nut, guarana, mate, tea, coffee**).

Route/Dosage

PO (Adults): *Short-term treatment of active ulcers*—300 mg 4 times daily or 800 mg at bedtime or 400–600 mg twice daily (not to exceed 2.4 g/day). *Duodenal ulcer prophylaxis*—300 mg twice daily or 400 mg at bedtime. *GERD*—800–1600 mg/day in divided doses. *Gastric hypersecretory conditions*—300–600 mg q 6 hr (up to 12 g/day have been used). *OTC use*—up to 200 mg may be taken twice daily (for no more than 2 wk).
PO (Children): *Short-term treatment of active ulcers*—20–40 mg/kg/day in 4 divided doses.
IM, IV (Adults): *Short-term treatment of active ulcers*—300 mg q 6 hr (not to exceed 2.4 g/day). *Continuous IV infusion*—900 mg infused over 24 hr (37.5 mg/hr); may be preceded by a 150-mg bolus dose. *Gastric hypersecretory conditions*—300–600 mg q 6 hr (up to 12 g/day have been used). *Prevention of aspiration pneumonitis*—300 mg IM 1 hr before anesthesia, then 300 mg IV q 4 hr until patient is conscious (unlabeled). *Prevention of upper GI bleeding in critically ill patients*—50 mg/hr (25 mg/hr if CCr <30 mL/min).
IM, IV (Children): *Short-term treatment of active ulcers*—5–10 mg/kg q 6–8 hr.

Renal Impairment

PO, IV (Adults): 300 mg q 8–12 hr; further adjustment may be required for concurrent hepatic impairment.
PO (Children): 10–15 mg/kg/day given in divided doses q 8–12 hr.

Availability (generic available)

Tablets: 100 mg OTC, 200 mg OTC, 300 mg, 400 mg, 600 mg, 800 mg. **Oral liquid (mint-peach):** 300 mg/5 mL, 200 mg/5 mL OTC. **Solution for injection:** 300 mg/2-mL vials, 300 mg/50 mL 0.9% NaCl.

ciprofloxacin (sip-roe-flox-a-sin)

Cipro, Cipro XR, Proquin XR

Classification
Therapeutic: anti-infectives
Pharmacologic: fluoroquinolones

Indications

PO, IV: Treatment of the following bacterial infections: Urinary tract and gynecologic infections, including cystitis, gonorrhea, and prostatitis; Respiratory tract infections, including acute sinusitis, acute exacerbations of chronic bronchitis, and pneumonia; Skin and skin structure infections: Bone and joint infections; Infectious diarrhea; Complicated intra-abdominal infections (with metronidazole); Typhoid fever. Postexposure prophylaxis of inhalational anthrax. Cutaneous anthrax. **Unlabeled Use:** Febrile neutropenia.

Action

Inhibits bacterial DNA synthesis by inhibiting DNA gyrase enzyme. **Therapeutic Effects:** Death of susceptible bacteria. **Spectrum:** Active against gram-positive pathogens, including *Staphylococcus aureus, S. epidermidis, S. saprophyticus, Streptococcus pyogenes, S. pneumoniae, Enterococcus faecalis, Bacillus anthracis* (anthrax). Gram-negative spectrum notable for activity against *Escherichia coli, Klebsiella pneumoniae, Enterobacter cloacae, Salmonella typhi, Shigella* spp., *Proteus mirabilis, P. vulgaris, Providencia stuartii, P. rettgeri, Morganella morganii, Pseudomonas aeruginosa, Serratia marcescens, Haemophilus influenzae, Neisseria gonorrhoeae, Moraxella catarrhalis, Campylobacter jejuni.*

Adverse Reactions/Side Effects

CNS: SEIZURES, dizziness, drowsiness, headache, insomnia, agitation, confusion. **GI:** PSEUDOMEMBRANOUS COLITIS, abdominal pain, diarrhea, abnormal liver enzymes , nausea. **GU:** vaginitis. **Derm:** photosensitivity, rash. **Endo:** hyperglycemia, hypoglycemia. **Hemat:** eosinophilia . **Local:** phlebitis at IV site. **MS:** tendinitis, tendon rupture. **Neuro:** peripheral neuropathy. **Misc:** hypersensitivity reactions, including ANAPHYLAXIS.

PHYSICAL THERAPY IMPLICATIONS

Examination and Evaluation

- Be alert for new seizures or increased seizure activity, especially at the onset of drug treatment. Document the number, duration, and severity of

seizures, and report these findings immediately to the physician or nursing staff.

- Monitor signs of hypersensitivity reactions and anaphylaxis, including pulmonary symptoms (tightness in the throat and chest, wheezing, cough, dyspnea) or skin reactions (rash, pruritus, urticaria). Notify physician or nursing staff immediately if these reactions occur.
- Watch for signs of pseudomembranous colitis, including diarrhea, abdominal pain, fever, pus or mucus in stools, or other severe or prolonged GI problems (nausea, cramps, vomiting). Report these signs to the physician or nursing staff immediately.
- Assess any tendon pain. Tendinopathy and rupture can occur, especially in large, weight-bearing tendons (Achilles', patellar tendons). Risk of tendon damage is greater in patients >65 yr old, transplant recipients (i.e., kidney, heart, lung), patients with preexisting tendon damage, and patients taking corticosteroids concurrently.
- Assess signs of peripheral neuropathy such as numbness, tingling, and decreased muscle strength. Establish baseline electroneuromyographic values using EMG and nerve conduction at the beginning of drug treatment whenever possible, and reexamine these values periodically to document drug-induced changes in peripheral nerve function.
- Assess dizziness and drowsiness that might affect gait, balance, and other functional activities (See Appendix C). Report balance problems and functional limitations to the physician and nursing staff, and caution the patient and family/caregivers to guard against falls and trauma.
- Be alert for confusion, agitation, or other alterations in mental status (See Appendix D). Notify physician promptly if these symptoms develop.
- Monitor signs of hypoglycemia (weakness, malaise, irritability, fatigue) or hyperglycemia (drowsiness, fruity breath, increased urination, unusual thirst). Patients with diabetes mellitus should check blood glucose levels frequently.
- Monitor for signs of eosinophilia (fatigue, weakness, myalgia); report these signs to the physician.
- Assess IV site during and after IV administration, and report signs of phlebitis and venous thrombosis (local pain, swelling, inflammation).

Interventions

- If tendon symptoms occur, notify the physician and protect the affected area to avoid tendon ruptures. Do not stretch or exercise the affected tendon, and provide crutches, walker, or other assistive devices if lower extremities are involved.
- Always wash hands thoroughly and disinfect equipment (whirlpools, electrotherapeutic devices, treatment tables, and so forth) to help prevent the spread of infection. Use universal precautions or isolation procedures as indicated for specific patients.
- Causes photosensitivity; use care if administering UV treatments. Advise patient to avoid direct sunlight and use sunscreens and protective clothing.

Patient/Client-Related Instruction

- Instruct patient to report other troublesome side effects such as severe or prolonged headache, sleep loss, vaginal irritation, skin rash, or GI problems (nausea, diarrhea, abdominal pain).

Pharmacokinetics

Absorption: 70% absorbed after oral administration; IV administration results in complete bioavailability.
Distribution: Widely distributed. High tissue and urinary levels are achieved. Crosses the placenta; enters breast milk.
Metabolism and Excretion: 15% metabolized by the liver, 40–50% excreted unchanged by the kidneys.
Half-life: 4 hr.

TIME/ACTION PROFILE (blood levels)

ROUTE	ONSET	PEAK	DURATION
PO	rapid	1–2 hr	12 hr
PO-ER	rapid	1–4 hr	24 hr
IV	rapid	end of infusion	12 hr

Contraindications/Precautions

Contraindicated in: Hypersensitivity (cross-sensitivity within class may exist); OB: Do not use unless potential benefit outweighs potential fetal risk; Pedi: Use only for treatment of anthrax and complicated urinary tract infections in children 1–17 yr due to possible arthropathy.
Use Cautiously in: Known or suspected CNS disorder; Renal impairment (dose reduction if CCr ≤50 mL/min); Concurrent use of corticosteroids (↑ risk of tendinitis/tendon rupture); Kidney, heart, or lung transplant patients (↑ risk of tendinitis/tendon rupture); Lactation: Safety not established except for treatment of anthrax; Geri: ↑ risk of adverse reactions.

Interactions

Drug-Drug: Concurrent use with **theophylline** may result in ↑ **theophylline** concentrations and therefore serious and potentially fatal reactions due to theophylline toxicity; if concurrent use cannot be avoided, serum theophylline levels should be monitored. Administration with **antacids, iron salts, bismuth subsalicylate, sucralfate**, and **zinc salts**

↓ absorption. May alter the effects of **warfarin**. May ↓ blood levels and effectiveness of **phenytoin**. Serum levels may be ↓ by **antineoplastics**. **Cimetidine** may interfere with elimination. Beneficial effects may be antagonized by **nitrofurantoin**. **Probenecid** ↓ renal elimination. May ↑ risk of nephrotoxicity from **cyclosporine**. Concurrent use with **foscarnet** may ↑ risk of seizures. Concurrent therapy with **corticosteroids** may ↑ risk of tendon rupture.
Drug-Natural: Fennel ↓ bioavailability.
Drug-Food: Absorption is impaired by **concurrent enteral feeding** (because of metal cations). Absorption of norfloxacin is ↓ by **food** and/or **dairy products** (take 1 hr before or 2 hr after).

Route/Dosage

Most infections

PO (Adults): 500–750 mg q 12 hr.
IV (Adults): 400 mg q 12 hr.

Urinary tract infections

PO (Adults): 250–500 mg q 12 hr; *or* 1000 mg q 24 hr for 10–14 days as extended-release tablets. *Uncomplicated urinary tract infections*—100 mg q 12 hr for 3 days *or* 500 mg q 24 hr for 3 days as extended-release tablets.
PO (Children 1–17 yr): *Complicated urinary tract infections*—10–20 mg/kg q 12 hr (not to exceed 750 mg/dose) for 10–21 days.
IV (Adults): 200 mg q 12 hr.
IV (Children 1–17 yr): *Complicated urinary tract infections*—6–10 mg/kg q 8 hr (not to exceed 400 mg/dose) for 10–21 days.

Gonorrhea

PO (Adults): 250-mg single dose.

Inhalational Anthrax

PO, IV (Adults): 400 mg q 12 hr IV, change to 500 mg PO twice daily when clinically appropriate for a total of 60 days; 1 or 2 other anti-infectives may be added initially, depending on clinical situation.
PO, IV (Children): 10–15 mg/kg q 12 hr IV, change to 10–15 mg/kg PO q 12 hr when clinically appropriate for a total of 60 days; 1 or 2 other anti-infectives may be added initially, depending on clinical situation.

Cutaneous anthrax

PO (Adults): 500 mg twice daily for 60 days; some patients may require intravenous therapy initially depending on clinical situation (for IV dose see inhalational anthrax above).
PO (Children): 10–15 mg/kg q 12 hr for 60 days; some patients may require intravenous therapy initially depending on clinical situation (for IV dose see inhalational anthrax above).

Availability (generic available)

Tablets: 100 mg, 250 mg, 500 mg, 750 mg. **Extended-release tablets:** 500 mg, 1000 mg. **Oral suspension (strawberry flavor):** 250 mg/5 mL in 100 mL bottle, 500 mg/5 mL in 100 mL bottle. **Injection:** 200 mg/20 mL, 400 mg/40 mL, 200 mg/100 mL premixed in D_5W, 400 mg/200 mL premixed in D_5W, 1200 mg/120 mL bulk package.

HIGH ALERT

cisplatin (sis-plat-in)

Platinol, Platinol-AQ

Classification
Therapeutic: antineoplastics
Pharmacologic: alkylating agents

Indications

Metastatic testicular and ovarian carcinoma. Advanced bladder cancer. Head and neck cancer. Cervical cancer. Lung cancer. Other tumors.

Action

Inhibits DNA synthesis by producing cross-linking of parent DNA strands (cell-cycle phase–nonspecific).
Therapeutic Effects: Death of rapidly replicating cells, particularly malignant ones.

Adverse Reactions/Side Effects

CNS: SEIZURES, malaise, weakness. **EENT:** ototoxicity, tinnitus. **GI:** severe nausea, vomiting, diarrhea, hepatotoxicity. **GU:** nephrotoxicity, sterility. **Derm:** alopecia. **F and E:** hypocalcemia, hypokalemia, hypomagnesemia. **Hemat:** LEUKOPENIA, THROMBOCYTOPENIA, anemia. **Local:** phlebitis at IV site. **Metab:** hyperuricemia. **Neuro:** peripheral neuropathy. **Misc:** anaphylactoid reactions.

PHYSICAL THERAPY IMPLICATIONS

Examination and Evaluation

- Be alert for new seizures or increased seizure activity, especially at the onset of drug treatment. Document the number, duration, and severity of seizures, and report these findings to the physician immediately.
- Monitor signs of leukopenia (fever, sore throat, signs of infection), thrombocytopenia (bruising, nose bleeds, bleeding gums), or unusual weakness and fatigue that might be due to anemia or other blood dyscrasias. Notify physician of these signs immediately.

C

- Monitor signs of allergic reactions, including anaphylaxis. Reactions include pulmonary symptoms (tightness in the throat and chest, wheezing, cough, dyspnea) and skin reactions (rash, pruritus, urticaria, burning skin). Notify physician or nursing staff immediately if these reactions occur.
- Assess signs of peripheral neuropathy such as numbness, tingling, and decreased muscle strength. Establish baseline electroneuromyographic values using EMG and nerve conduction at the beginning of drug treatment whenever possible, and reexamine these values periodically to document drug-induced changes in peripheral nerve function.
- Monitor neuromuscular signs of electrolyte imbalances (hypocalcemia, hypokalemia, hypomagnesemia), including headache, lethargy, weakness, cramping, and muscle hyperexcitability and tetany. Notify physician immediately if these signs occur.
- Monitor signs of ototoxicity such as hearing loss, tinnitus, disturbed balance, and vertigo. Report these signs to the physician.
- Assess IV site during and after IV administration, and report signs of phlebitis (local pain, swelling, inflammation).

Interventions

- For patients who are medically able to begin exercise, implement appropriate resistive exercises and aerobic training to maintain muscle strength and aerobic capacity during cancer chemotherapy or to help restore function after chemotherapy.
- Guard against falls and trauma (hip fractures, head injury). Implement fall-prevention strategies, especially if patient exhibits balance deficits related to ototoxicity (See Appendix E).

Patient/Client-Related Instruction

- Advise patient to guard against infection (frequent hand washing, etc.), and to avoid crowds and contact with persons with contagious diseases.
- Make sure patient and family or caregivers understand the need to report immediately allergic responses or signs of blood dyscrasias as listed above (see Examination and Evaluation).
- Advise patient about the likelihood of GI reactions (nausea, vomiting, diarrhea). Instruct patient to report severe or prolonged GI problems, and to report immediately signs of hepatic toxicity, including anorexia, abdominal pain, severe nausea and vomiting, yellow skin or eyes, skin rashes, flu-like symptoms, and muscle/joint pain.
- Advise patient and family/caregivers that fatigue and weakness are likely and may be severe. Functional abilities may be limited, and patient may need to use assistive devices during ambulation.
- Instruct patient to report signs of nephrotoxicity, including hematuria, increased urinary frequency, cloudy urine, and decreased urine output.
- Advise patient that hair loss is likely. Report severe or unexpected skin reactions to the physician.

Pharmacokinetics

Absorption: IV administration results in complete bioavailability.
Distribution: Widely distributed; accumulates for months; enters breast milk.
Metabolism and Excretion: Excreted mainly by the kidneys.
Half-life: 30–100 hr.

TIME/ACTION PROFILE (effects on blood counts)

ROUTE	ONSET	PEAK	DURATION
IV	unknown	18–23 days	39 days

Contraindications/Precautions

Contraindicated in: Hypersensitivity; Pregnancy or lactation.
Use Cautiously in: Hearing loss; Renal impairment (dosage ↓ recommended); CHF; Electrolyte abnormalities; Active infections; Bone marrow depression; Geriatric patients (↑ risk of nephrotoxicity, peripheral neuropathy); Chronic debilitating illnesses; Patients with childbearing potential.

Interactions

Drug-Drug: ↑ nephrotoxicity and ototoxicity with other **nephrotoxic** and **ototoxic drugs (aminoglycosides, loop diuretics)**. ↑ risk of hypokalemia and hypomagnesemia with **loop diuretics** and **amphotericin B**. May ↓ **phenytoin** levels. ↑ bone marrow depression with other **antineoplastics** or **radiation therapy**. May ↓ antibody response to **live-virus vaccines** and ↑ adverse reactions.

Route/Dosage

Other regimens are used.
IV (Adults): *Metastatic testicular tumors*—20 mg/m^2 daily for 5 days repeated q 3–4 wk. *Metastatic ovarian cancer*—75–100 mg/m^2; repeat q 4 wk in combination cyclophosphamide *or* 100 mg/m^2 q 3 wk if used as a single agent. *Advanced bladder cancer*—50–70 mg/m^2 q 3–4 wk as a single agent.

Availability (generic available)

Powder for injection: 10-mg, 50-mg vials.
Injection: 1 mg/mL in 50- and 100-mg vials.

citalopram (si-tal-oh-pram)
Celexa

Classification
Therapeutic: antidepressants
Pharmacologic: selective serotonin reuptake inhibitors (SSRIs)

Indications
Depression. **Unlabeled Use:** Premenstrual dysphoric disorder (PMDD). Obsessive-compulsive disorder (OCD). Panic disorder. Generalized anxiety disorder (GAD). Posttraumatic stress disorder (PTSD). Social anxiety disorder (social phobia).

Action
Selectively inhibits the reuptake of serotonin in the CNS. **Therapeutic Effects:** Antidepressant action.

Adverse Reactions/Side Effects
CNS: apathy, confusion, drowsiness, insomnia, weakness, agitation, amnesia, anxiety, decreased libido, dizziness, fatigue, impaired concentration, increased depression, migraine headache, suicide attempt. **EENT:** abnormal accommodation. **Resp:** cough. **CV:** postural hypotension, tachycardia. **GI:** abdominal pain, anorexia, diarrhea, dry mouth, dyspepsia, flatulence, increased saliva, nausea, altered taste, increased appetite, vomiting. **GU:** amenorrhea, dysmenorrhea, ejaculatory delay, erectile dysfunction, polyuria. **Derm:** increased sweating, photosensitivity, pruritus, rash. **Metab:** decreased weight, increased weight. **F and E:** hyponatremia. **MS:** arthralgia, myalgia. **Neuro:** tremor, paresthesia. **Misc:** fever, yawning.

PHYSICAL THERAPY IMPLICATIONS

Examination and Evaluation
- Be alert for increased depression and suicidal thoughts and ideology, especially when initiating drug treatment or in children and teenagers. Notify physician or mental health professional immediately if patient exhibits worsening depression or other changes in mood and behavior.
- Watch for confusion, apathy, sedation, agitation, anxiety, or other alterations in cognitive status (See Appendix D). Notify physician promptly if these symptoms develop.
- Assess blood pressure (BP) when patient assumes a more upright position (lying to standing, sitting to standing, lying to sitting). Document orthostatic hypotension and contact physician when systolic BP falls >20 mm Hg or diastolic BP falls >10 mm Hg.
- Assess heart rate, ECG, and heart sounds, especially during exercise (See Appendices G, H). Report a rapid heart rate (tachycardia) or signs of other arrhythmias, including palpitations, chest discomfort, shortness of breath, fainting, and fatigue/weakness.
- Assess dizziness and drowsiness that might affect gait, balance, and other functional activities (See Appendix C). Report balance problems and functional limitations to the physician, and caution the patient and family/caregivers to guard against falls and trauma.
- Assess any joint of muscle pain to rule out musculoskeletal pathology; that is, try to determine if pain is drug induced rather than caused by anatomic or biomechanical problems.
- Assess paresthesias (numbness, tingling) or tremor. Perform objective tests, including electroneuromyography and sensory testing to document any drug-related neuropathic changes.
- Report signs of low sodium levels (hyponatremia), including headache, confusion, lethargy, fatigue, decreased consciousness, or muscle abnormalities (weakness, spasms, cramps).
- Periodically assess body weight and other anthropometric measures (body mass index, body composition). Report a rapid or unexplained weight gain or weight loss.

Interventions
- Guard against falls and trauma (hip fractures, head injury, and so forth), and implement fall-prevention strategies (See Appendix E).
- Because of the risk of arrhythmias and hypotension, use caution during aerobic exercise and other forms of therapeutic exercise. Assess exercise tolerance frequently (BP, heart rate, fatigue levels), and terminate exercise immediately if any untoward responses occur (See Appendix L).
- To minimize orthostatic hypotension, patient should move slowly when assuming a more upright position.
- Help patient explore nonpharmacologic methods to reduce depression (exercise, counseling, support groups, and so forth).
- Causes photosensitivity; use care if administering UV treatments. Advise patient to avoid direct sunlight and use sunscreens and protective clothing.

Patient/Client-Related Instruction
- Advise patient that antidepressant effects may not occur immediately; it may take 2 wk or more before an improvement in mood is observed.
- Advise patient to avoid alcohol and other CNS depressants because of the increased risk of sedation and adverse effects.
- Instruct patient to report other troublesome side effects such as severe or prolonged headache, sleep loss, blurred vision, cough, increased urination, increased sweating, rash, fever, erectile dysfunction,

C

menstrual abnormalities, or GI problems (nausea, vomiting, diarrhea, flatulence, indigestion, dry mouth, altered taste, abdominal pain).

Pharmacokinetics

Absorption: 80% absorbed after oral administration.
Distribution: Enters breast milk.
Metabolism and Excretion: Mostly metabolized by the liver (10% by CYP3A4 and 2C19 enzymes); excreted unchanged in urine.
Half-life: 35 hr.

TIME/ACTION PROFILE (antidepressant effect)

ROUTE	ONSET	PEAK	DURATION
PO	1–4 wk	unknown	unknown

Contraindications/Precautions

Contraindicated in: Hypersensitivity; Concurrent MAO inhibitor or pimozide therapy.
Use Cautiously in: History of mania; History of suicide attempt/ideation (↑ risk during early therapy and during dose adjustment); History of seizure disorder; Illnesses or conditions that are likely to result in altered metabolism or hemodynamic responses; Severe renal or hepatic impairment; OB: Use during third trimester may result in neonatal serotonin syndrome requiring prolonged hospitalization, respiratory and nutritional support; Lactation: Present in breast milk and may result in lethargy with ↓ feeding in infants; weigh risk/benefits; Pedi: May ↑ risk of suicide attempt/ideation, especially during early treatment or dose adjustment in children/adolescents (unlabeled for pediatric use); Geri: ↓ doses recommended.

Interactions

Drug-Drug: May cause serious, potentially fatal reactions when used with **MAO inhibitors**; allow at least 14 days between citalopram and **MAO inhibitors.** Concurrent use with **pimozide** may result in prolongation of the QTc interval and is contraindicated. Use cautiously with other **centrally acting drugs** (including **alcohol, antihistamines, opioid analgesics,** and **sedative/hypnotics**; concurrent use with **alcohol** is not recommended). **Cimetidine** ↑ blood levels of citalopram. Serotonergic effects may be ↑ by **lithium** (concurrent use should be carefully monitored). **Ketoconazole, itraconazole, erythromycin,** and **omeprazole** may ↑ blood levels. **Carbamazepine** may ↓ blood levels. May ↑ blood levels of **metoprolol.** Concurrent use with **tricyclic antidepressants** should be undertaken with caution because of altered pharmacokinetics. Concurrent use with **5-HT$_1$ agonists** used for migraine headaches may ↑ risk of adverse reactions (weakness, hyperreflexia, incoordination). Use cautiously with **tricyclic antidepressants** due to unpredictable effects on serotonin and norepinephrine reuptake. ↑ risk of bleeding with **aspirin, NSAIDs, clopidogrel,** or **warfarin.**
Drug-Natural: ↑ risk of serotonergic side effects including serotonin syndrome with **St. John's wort** and **SAMe.**

Route/Dosage

PO (Adults): 20 mg once daily initially; may be increased by 20 mg/day at weekly intervals, up to 60 mg/day (usual dose is 40 mg/day).
PO (Geriatric Patients): 20 mg once daily initially; may be increased to 40 mg/day only in nonresponding patients.

Hepatic Impairment

PO (Adults): 20 mg once daily initially; may be increased to 40 mg/day only in nonresponding patients.

Availability (generic available)

Tablets: 10 mg, 20 mg, 40 mg. **Oral solution (peppermint flavor):** 10 mg/5 mL.

HIGH ALERT

cladribine (klad-ri-been)

Leustatin

Classification
Therapeutic: antineoplastics
Pharmacologic: antimetabolites

Indications

Management of active hairy cell leukemia manifested as anemia, leukopenia, thrombocytopenia, or clinical symptoms. **Unlabeled Use:** chronic lymphocytic leukemia, chronic myelogenous leukemia, non-Hodgkin's lymphomas, progressive multiple sclerosis.

Action

Inhibits DNA synthesis. **Therapeutic Effects:** Death of rapidly replicating cells, particularly malignant ones.

Adverse Reactions/Side Effects

CNS: fatigue, headache, dizziness, insomnia, malaise, weakness. **EENT:** epistaxis. **Resp:** abnormal breath sounds, cough, dyspnea. **CV:** edema, tachycardia. **GI:** anorexia, diarrhea, nausea, vomiting, abdominal pain, constipation. **Derm:** rash, erythema, petechiae, pruritus, sweating. **Hemat:** NEUTROPENIA, anemia, thrombocytopenia. **Local:** injection site reactions, phlebitis, thrombosis. **MS:** arthralgia, myalgia. **Misc:** chills, fever, infection, trunk pain.

PHYSICAL THERAPY IMPLICATIONS

Examination and Evaluation

- Monitor signs of neutropenia (fever, sore throat, signs of infection), thrombocytopenia (bruising, nose bleeds, and bleeding gums), or unusual weakness and fatigue that might be due to anemia. Report these signs to the physician immediately.
- Assess heart rate, ECG, and heart sounds, especially during exercise (See Appendices G, H). Report a rapid heart rate (tachycardia) or signs of other arrhythmias, including palpitations, chest discomfort, shortness of breath, fainting, and fatigue/weakness.
- Assess peripheral edema using girth measurements, volume displacement, and measurement of pitting edema (See Appendix N). Report increased swelling in feet and ankles or a sudden increase in body weight due to fluid retention.
- Assess any breathing problems, and report difficult/labored breathing, persistent cough, or abnormal breath sounds (See Appendix K).
- Assess any muscle, trunk, or joint pain to rule out musculoskeletal pathology; that is, try to determine if pain is drug induced rather than caused by anatomic or biomechanical problems.
- Assess dizziness and weakness that might affect gait, balance, and other functional activities (See Appendix C). Report balance problems and functional limitations to the physician and nursing staff, and caution the patient and family/caregivers to guard against falls and trauma.
- Monitor injection site for pain and irritation. Report prolonged or excessive injection-site reactions or signs of phlebitis (redness, warmth, swelling) to the physician.

Interventions

- For patients who are medically able to begin exercise, implement appropriate resistive exercises and aerobic training to maintain muscle strength and aerobic capacity during cancer chemotherapy or to help restore function after chemotherapy.
- Because of the risk of arrhythmias, use extreme caution during aerobic exercise and other forms of therapeutic exercise. Assess exercise tolerance frequently (blood pressure, heart rate, fatigue levels), and terminate exercise immediately if any untoward responses occur (See Appendix L).

Patient/Client-related Instruction

- Advise patient and family/caregivers about the risk of infections, and to guard against infection (frequent hand washing, etc.), and to avoid crowds and contact with persons with contagious diseases.
- Advise patient and family/caregivers that fatigue and weakness are likely and may be severe. Functional abilities may be limited, and patient may need to use assistive devices during ambulation.
- Advise patient and family/caregivers about the likelihood of GI reactions such as nausea, vomiting, diarrhea, constipation, abdominal pain, and loss of appetite. Instruct patient to report severe or prolonged GI problems.
- Instruct patient and family/caregivers to report other troublesome side effects such as severe or prolonged headache, sleep loss, nosebleeds, chills, fever, or skin reactions (rash, itching, bruising, redness, excessive sweating).

Pharmacokinetics

Absorption: IV administration results in complete bioavailability.
Distribution: Extensively distributed to body tissues; penetrates into cerebrospinal fluid.
Metabolism and Excretion: Unknown.
Half-life: 3–22 hr.

TIME/ACTION PROFILE (noted as effect on peripheral counts)

ROUTE	ONSET	PEAK	DURATION*
platelets	unknown	unknown	12 days
absolute neutrophil count	unknown	unknown	5 wk
hemoglobin	unknown	unknown	8 wk

*Time to normalization of counts.

Contraindications/Precautions

Contraindicated in: Hypersensitivity; Diluent contains benzyl alcohol and should be avoided in patients with known intolerance; Pregnant or lactating patients.
Use Cautiously in: Patients with active infections; Patients taking medications that cause immunosuppression or bone marrow depression; Impaired hepatic or renal function (increased risk of toxicity); Patients with childbearing potential; Children (safety not established).

Interactions

Drug-Drug: Additive bone marrow depression may occur with other **antineoplastics** or **radiation therapy**.

Route/Dosage

IV (Adults): *Hairy cell leukemia*—0.09 mg/kg/day for 7 days.

Availability

Injection: 1 mg/mL.

C

clarithromycin

(kla-rith-roe-mye-sin)

Biaxin, Biaxin XL

Classification

Therapeutic: agents for atypical mycobacterium, anti-infectives, antiulcer agents

Pharmacologic: macrolides

Indications

Respiratory tract infections including streptococcal pharyngitis, sinusitis, bronchitis, and pneumonia. Treatment (with ethambutol) and prevention of disseminated *Mycobacterium avium* complex (MAC). Treatment of following pediatric infections: Otitis media, Sinusitis, Pharyngitis, Skin/skin structure infections. Part of a combination regimen for ulcer disease due to *Helicobacter pylori*. Endocarditis prophylaxis.

Action

Inhibits protein synthesis at the level of the 50S bacterial ribosome. **Therapeutic Effects:** Bacteriostatic action. **Spectrum:** Active against these gram-positive aerobic bacteria: *Staphylococcus aureus*, *Streptococcus pneumoniae*, *S.s pyogenes* (group A strep). Active against these gram-negative aerobic bacteria: *Haemophilus influenzae*, *Moraxella catarrhalis*. Also active against *Mycoplasma*, *Legionella*, *H. pylori*, *M. avium*.

Adverse Reactions/Side Effects

CNS: headache. **Derm:** pruritus, rash, Stevens-Johnson syndrome. **GI:** PSEUDOMEMBRANOUS COLITIS, abdominal pain/discomfort, abnormal taste, diarrhea, dyspepsia, nausea.

PHYSICAL THERAPY IMPLICATIONS

Examination and Evaluation

- Be alert for signs of pseudomembranous colitis, including diarrhea, abdominal pain, fever, pus or mucus in stools, and other severe or prolonged GI problems (nausea, vomiting, heartburn). Notify physician or nursing staff immediately of these signs.
- Monitor rashes or other skin reactions (pruritus, hives, acne, abnormal sweating, exfoliation). Notify physician immediately because certain skin reactions may indicate serious hypersensitivity reactions (Stevens-Johnson syndrome).

Interventions

- Always wash hands thoroughly and disinfect equipment (whirlpools, electrotherapeutic devices, treatment tables, and so forth) to help prevent the spread of infection. Employ universal precautions or isolation procedures as indicated for specific patients.

Patient/Client-Related Instruction

- Advise patient about the likelihood of GI reactions, including nausea, diarrhea, indigestion, abnormal taste, and abdominal pain. Instruct patient to report severe or prolonged GI problems.

Pharmacokinetics

Absorption: Rapidly absorbed (50%) after oral administration.
Distribution: Widely distributed; tissue levels may exceed those in serum.
Protein Binding: 65–70%.
Metabolism and Excretion: 10–15% converted by the liver to 14-hydroxyclarithromycin, which has anti-infective activity; 20–30% excreted unchanged in urine. Metabolized by and also inhibits the CYP3A enzyme system.
Half-life: Dose dependent and prolonged with renal dysfunction: *250-mg dose*—3–4 hr; *500-mg dose*—5–7 hr.

TIME/ACTION PROFILE (serum levels)

ROUTE	ONSET	PEAK	DURATION
PO	unknown	2 hr	12 hr
PO-XL	unknown	4 hr	24 hr

Contraindications/Precautions

Contraindicated in: Hypersensitivity to clarithromycin, erythromycin, or other macrolide anti-infectives; Concurrent use of pimozide; OB: Avoid use during pregnancy unless no alternatives are available; Lactation: Not recommend for breast-feeding women.
Use Cautiously in: Severe liver or renal impairment (dose adjustment required if CCr <30 mL/min); Myasthenia gravis.

Interactions

Drug-Drug: Clarithromycin is an inhibitor of the CYP3A enzyme system. Concurrent use with other agents metabolized by this system can ↑ levels and risk of toxicity. May prolong the QT interval and ↑ risk of arrhythmias with **pimozide**; concurrent use is contraindicated. Similar effects may occur with antiarrhythmics; ECG should be monitored for QTc prolongation and serum levels monitored. May ↑ serum levels and the risk of toxicity from **carbamazepine, some benzodiazepines (midazolam, triazolam, alprazolam), cyclosporine, buspirone, disopyramide, ergot alkaloids, felodipine, omeprazole, tacrolimus, digoxin**, or **theophylline**. **Ritonavir**

↑ blood levels (↓ clarithromycin dose in patients with CC <60 mL/min). ↑ levels of **HMG CoA reductase inhibitors** and may ↑ risk of rhabdomyolysis. May ↑ effect of **warfarin** and **sildenafil** (dose reduction may be warranted). May ↑ or ↓ effects of **zidovudine.** Blood levels are ↑ by **delavirdine** and **fluconazole**. Blood levels may be ↓ by **rifampin** and **rifabutin**. ↑ risk of colchicine toxicity when administered with **colchicine**, especially in the elderly.

Route/Dosage

PO (Adults): *Pharyngitis/tonsillitis*—250 mg q 12 hr for 10 days; *Acute maxillary sinusitis*—500 mg q 12 hr for 14 days or 1000 mg once daily for 14 days as XL tablets; *Acute exacerbation of chronic bronchitis*—250–500 mg q 12 hr for 7–14 days or 1000 mg once daily for 7 days as XL tablets; *Community-acquired pneumonia*—250 mg q 12 hr for 7–14 days or 1000 mg once daily for 7 days as XL tablets; *skin/skin structure infections*—250 mg q 12 hr for 7–14 days; *H. pylori*—500 mg 2–3 times daily with a proton pump inhibitor (lansoprazole or omeprazole) or ranitidine with or without amoxicillin for 10–14 days; *Endocarditis prophylaxis*—500 mg 1 hr before procedure; *MAC prophylaxis/treatment*—500 mg twice daily, for active infection another antimycobacterial is required.
PO (Children): *Most infections*—15 mg/kg/day divided q 12 hr for 7–14 days (up to 500 mg/dose for MAC). *Endocarditis prophylaxis*—15 mg/kg 1 hr before procedure.

Renal Impairment

PO (Adults): *CCr <30 mL/min*—250 mg 1–2 times daily, a 500-mg initial dose may be used.
PO (Children): *CCr <30 mL/min*—decrease dose by 50% or double dosing interval.

Availability (generic available)

Tablets: 250 mg, 500 mg. **Extended-release tablets:** 500 mg. **Oral suspension (fruit punch and vanilla flavors):** 125 mg/5 mL, 250 mg/5 mL. ***In combination with:*** amoxicillin and lansoprazole as part of a compliance package (Prevpac). See Appendix B.

clemastine (klem-as-teen)

Dayhist Allergy, Tavist Allergy

Classification
Therapeutic: allergy, cold, and cough remedies, antihistamines

Indications

Relief of allergic symptoms caused by histamine release, including Allergic rhinitis, Urticaria.

Action

Antagonizes the effects of histamine at H_1 receptor sites; does not bind to or inactivate histamine. **Therapeutic Effects:** Decreased symptoms of histamine excess (sneezing, rhinorrhea, nasal and ocular pruritus, ocular tearing, and redness).

Adverse Reactions/Side Effects

CNS: drowsiness, confusion, dizziness, paradoxical excitation (children). **EENT:** blurred vision. **CV:** hypertension, arrhythmias, hypotension, palpitations, tachycardia. **GI:** dry mouth, constipation, nausea, obstruction, vomiting. **GU:** urinary retention. **Derm:** rash. **Resp:** thick mucus.

PHYSICAL THERAPY IMPLICATIONS

Examination and Evaluation

- Assess blood pressure (BP) and compare to normal values (See Appendix F). Report changes in BP, either a problematic decrease in BP (hypotension) or a sustained increase in BP (hypertension).
- Assess heart rate, ECG, and heart sounds, especially during exercise (See Appendices G, H). Report any rhythm disturbances or symptoms of increased arrhythmias, including palpitations, chest discomfort, shortness of breath, fainting, and fatigue/weakness.
- Monitor symptoms of allergic rhinitis (sneezing, rhinitis, itching eyes, cough) or urticaria (rash, hives, itching) to help document benefits of this drug in treating these disorders.
- Assess dizziness and drowsiness that might affect gait, balance, and other functional activities (See Appendix C). Report balance problems and functional limitations to the physician, and caution the patient and family/caregivers to guard against falls and trauma.
- Assess confusion or other alterations in cognitive function (See Appendix D). Notify the physician if these symptoms become problematic.
- Monitor signs of increased excitation in children. Severe or problematic excitation may require a change in dose or drug.

Interventions

- Guard against falls and trauma (hip fractures, head injury, and so forth). Implement fall-prevention strategies, especially in older adults or if balance is impaired (See Appendix E).
- Because of an increased risk of arrhythmias and abnormal BP responses, use caution during aerobic exercise and other forms of therapeutic exercise. Assess exercise tolerance frequently (BP, heart rate, fatigue levels), and terminate exercise immediately if any untoward responses occur (See Appendix L).

Patient/Client-Related Instruction

- Advise patient about the risk of daytime drowsiness and decreased attention and mental focus. These problems can be severe in certain people. Use care if driving or in other activities that require quick reactions and strong concentration.

- Advise patient to avoid alcohol and other CNS depressants because of the increased risk of sedation and adverse effects.
- Instruct patient to report other troublesome side effects, including severe or prolonged skin rash, blurred vision, thickened mucus, urinary retention, or GI problems (nausea, vomiting, constipation, dry mouth).

Pharmacokinetics

Absorption: Well absorbed following oral administration.
Distribution: Enters breast milk in high concentrations.
Metabolism and Excretion: Extensively metabolized by the liver.
Half-life: Unknown.

TIME/ACTION PROFILE (antihistaminic effects)

ROUTE	ONSET	PEAK	DURATION
PO	15–60 min	1–2 hr	8–16 hr

Contraindications/Precautions

Contraindicated in: Hypersensitivity; Angle-closure glaucoma; Lactation (avoid use); Known alcohol intolerance (liquid form).
Use Cautiously in: Acute asthma attacks; Liver disease; Prostatic hyperplasia; Hyperthyroidism; Hypertension; Geriatric patients (more susceptible to adverse reactions); Pregnancy or children <6 yr (safety not established).

Interactions

Drug-Drug: Additive CNS depression with other **CNS depressants**, including **alcohol**, **opioid analgesics**, and **sedative/hypnotics**. May antagonize effects of **cholinergic agonists** (e.g., **tacrine**, **donepezil**).
Drug-Natural: Concomitant use of **kava**, **valerian**, **skullcap**, **chamomile**, or **hops** can increase CNS depression.

Route/Dosage

PO (Adults): *OTC labeling*—1.34 mg (1 mg base) twice daily. *Rx labeling*—1.34 mg (1 mg base) twice daily; may increase up to 2.68 mg (2 mg base) 3 times daily.
PO (Children 6–12 yr): 0.67–1.34 mg (0.5–1 mg base) twice daily. Not to exceed 4.02 mg/day (3 mg/day base).

Availability (generic available)

Tablets: 1 mg OTC, 1.34 mg (1 mg base) OTC, 2.68 mg (2 mg base). **Syrup (citrus flavor):** 0.67 mg/5 mL Rx (0.67 mg clemastine fumarate = 0.5 mg base) (contains 5.5% alcohol).

clevidipine (kle-vid-i-peen)

Cleviprex

Classification
Therapeutic: antihypertensives
Pharmacologic: calcium channel blockers (dihydropyridine)

Indications

Reduction of blood pressure when oral therapy is not feasible/desirable.

Action

Inhibits calcium transport into vascular smooth muscle, resulting in inhibition of excitation-contraction coupling and subsequent contraction. Decreases systemic vascular resistance; does not reduce cardiac filling pressure (preload). Has no effect on venous capacitance vessels.
Therapeutic Effects: Decreases blood pressure.

Adverse Reactions/Side Effects

CNS: headache. **CV:** CHF, hypotension, rebound hypertension, reflex tachycardia. **GI:** nausea, vomiting. **MS:** arthralgia.

PHYSICAL THERAPY IMPLICATIONS

Examination and Evaluation

- Assess blood pressure periodically and compare to normal values (See Appendix F) to help document antihypertensive effects.
- Assess signs of congestive heart failure, including dyspnea, rales/crackles, peripheral edema, jugular venous distention, and exercise intolerance. Report these signs to the physician immediately.
- Assess heart rate and ECG during and after IV administration (See Appendices G, H). Report an increase in heart rate, especially if BP decreases substantially (reflex tachycardia).
- Assess any joint pain to rule out musculoskeletal pathology; that is, try to determine if pain is drug induced rather than caused by anatomic or biomechanical problems.

Interventions

- Because of an increased risk of hypotension and reflex tachycardia, use caution during aerobic exercise and endurance conditioning. Terminate exercise if patient exhibits untoward symptoms (chest pain, shortness of breath, excessive fatigue) or displays other criteria for exercise termination (See Appendix L).
- Avoid physical therapy interventions that cause systemic vasodilation (large whirlpool, Hubbard tank).

Additive effects of this drug and the intervention may cause a dangerous fall in blood pressure.
- To minimize orthostatic hypotension, patient should move slowly when assuming a more upright position.

Patient/Client-Related Instruction

- Counsel patients about additional interventions to help control blood pressure, including regular exercise, weight loss, sodium restriction, stress reduction, moderation of alcohol consumption, and smoking cessation.
- Instruct patient or family/caregivers to report other troublesome side effects such as severe or prolonged headache or GI problems (nausea, vomiting).

Pharmacokinetics

Absorption: IV administration results in complete bioavailability.
Distribution: Unknown.
Protein Binding: >99.5%.
Metabolism and Excretion: Rapidly metabolized by esterases in plasma and tissue to inactive metabolites; metabolites are excreted in urine (63–74%) and feces (7–22%).
Half-life: *Initial phase*—1 min; *terminal phase*—15 min.

TIME/ACTION PROFILE

ROUTE	ONSET	PEAK	DURATION
IV	2–4 min	30 min*	end of infusion

*Time to target blood pressure.

Contraindications/Precautions

Contraindicated in: Hypersensitivity; Allergy to soybeans, eggs/egg products, defective lipid metabolism, including pathologic hyperlipidemia, lipoid nephrosis, or acute pancreatitis; severe aortic stenosis.
Use Cautiously in: Geri: Titrate dose cautiously, initiate therapy at low end of dose range; consider age-related decrease in hepatic, renal or cardiac function, concomitant diseases or other drug therapy; OB: Use only if maternal benefit outweighs potential risk to fetus; Lactation: Consider possible infant exposure; Pedi: Safety not established for patients <18 yr.

Interactions

Drug-Drug: ↑ risk of excess hypotension with other **antihypertensives**. Does not protect against effects of abrupt **beta blocker** withdrawal.

Route/Dosage

IV (Adults): *Initial dose:* 1–2 mg/hr; *Dose titration:* Double dose every 90 sec initially; as blood pressure approaches goal, increase dose by less than doubling and lengthen the time between dose adjustments to every 5–10 min. Usual dose required is 4–6 mg/hr. Severe hypertensive patients may require higher doses with a maximum of 16 mg/hr or less. Doses up to 32 mg/hr have been used, but generally should not exceed 21 mg/hr in a 24-hr period due to lipid load.

Availability

Emulsion for injection 0.5 mg/mL: 50-mL vial, 100-mL vial.

clindamycin (klin-da-mye-sin)

Cleocin, Cleocin T, Clinda-Derm, Clindagel, Clindesse, ClindaMax, Clindets, C/T/S, ✱ Dalacin C, ✱ Dalacin T, Evoclin

Classification
Therapeutic: anti-infectives
Pharmacologic: lincosamides

Indications

PO, IM, IV: Treatment of Skin and skin structure infections, Respiratory tract infections, Septicemia, Intra-abdominal infections, Gynecologic infections, Osteomyelitis, Endocarditis prophylaxis. **Topical:** Severe acne. **Vag:** Bacterial vaginosis. **Unlabeled Use: PO, IM, IV:** Treatment of *Pneumocystis carinii* pneumonia, CNS toxoplasmosis, and babesiosis.

Action

Inhibits protein synthesis in susceptible bacteria at the level of the 50S ribosome. **Therapeutic Effects:** Bactericidal or bacteriostatic, depending on susceptibility and concentration. **Spectrum:** Active against most gram-positive aerobic cocci, including Staphylococci, *Streptococcus pneumoniae*, Other streptococci, but not enterococci. Has good activity against those anaerobic bacteria that cause bacterial vaginosis, including *Bacteroides fragilis*, *Gardnerella vaginalis*, *Mobiluncus* spp., *Mycoplasma hominis*, and *Corynebacterium*. Also active against *P. carinii* and *Toxoplasma gondii*.

Adverse Reactions/Side Effects

CNS: dizziness, headache, vertigo. **CV:** arrhythmias, hypotension. **GI:** PSEUDOMEMBRANOUS COLITIS, diarrhea, bitter taste (IV only), nausea, vomiting. **Derm:** rashes. **Local:** phlebitis at IV site.

PHYSICAL THERAPY IMPLICATIONS

Examination and Evaluation

- Monitor signs of pseudomembranous colitis, including diarrhea, abdominal pain, fever, pus or mucus in stools, and other severe or prolonged GI problems (nausea, vomiting, heartburn). Notify physician or nursing staff immediately of these signs.

- Assess dizziness or vertigo that might affect gait, balance, and other functional activities (See Appendix C). Report balance problems and functional limitations to the physician and nursing staff, and caution the patient and family/caregivers to guard against falls and trauma.
- Assess heart rate, ECG, and heart sounds, especially during exercise (See Appendices G, H). Report any rhythm disturbances or symptoms of increased arrhythmias, including palpitations, chest discomfort, shortness of breath, fainting, and fatigue/weakness.
- Assess blood pressure periodically, and compare to normal values (See Appendix F). Report low blood pressure (hypotension), especially if patient experiences dizziness, fatigue, or other symptoms.
- Monitor injection site for pain, swelling, and irritation. Report prolonged or excessive injection-site reactions to the physician.

Interventions

- Always wash hands thoroughly and disinfect equipment (whirlpools, electrotherapeutic devices, treatment tables, and so forth) to help prevent the spread of infection. Employ universal precautions or isolation procedures as indicated for specific patients.
- Because of the risk of arrhythmias and hypotension, use caution during aerobic exercise and other forms of therapeutic exercise. Assess exercise tolerance frequently (blood pressure, heart rate, fatigue levels), and terminate exercise immediately if any untoward responses occur See Appendix L).

Patient/Client-Related Instruction

- Advise patient about the likelihood of GI reactions such as nausea, vomiting, diarrhea, and taste abnormalities. Instruct patient to report severe or prolonged GI problems.
- Instruct patient and family/caregivers to report other troublesome side effects such as severe or prolonged headache or skin rash.

Pharmacokinetics

Absorption: Well absorbed following PO/IM administration. Minimal absorption following topical/vaginal use.
Distribution: Widely distributed. Does not significantly cross blood-brain barrier. Crosses the placenta; enters breast milk.
Protein Binding: 94%.
Metabolism and Excretion: Mostly metabolized by the liver.
Half-life: Neonates: 3.6–8.7 hr; Infants up to 1 yr: 3 hr; Children and adults: 2–3 hr.

TIME/ACTION PROFILE (blood levels)

ROUTE	ONSET	PEAK	DURATION
PO	rapid	60 min	6–8 hr
IM	rapid	1–3 hr	6–8 hr
IV	rapid	end of infusion	6–8 hr

Contraindications/Precautions

Contraindicated in: Hypersensitivity; Previous pseudomembranous colitis; Severe liver impairment; Diarrhea; Known alcohol intolerance (topical solution, suspension).
Use Cautiously in: OB: Safety not established for systemic and topical; vaginal approved for use in 3rd trimester of pregnancy; Lactation: Has been used safely but does appear in breast milk and exposes infant to drug and its side effects.

Interactions

Drug-Drug: Kaolin/pectin may ↓ GI absorption. May enhance the neuromuscular blocking action of other **neuromuscular blocking agents**. **Topical:** Concurrent use with **irritants**, **abrasives**, or **desquamating agents** may result in additive irritation.

Route/Dosage

PO (Adults): *Most infections*—150–450 mg q 6 hr. P. carinii *pneumonia*—1200–1800 mg/day in divided doses with 15–30 mg primaquine/day (unlabeled). *CNS toxoplasmosis*—1200–2400 mg/day in divided doses with pyrimethamine 50–100 mg/day (unlabeled); *Bacterial endocarditis prophylaxis*—600 mg 1 hr before procedure.
PO (Children >1 mo): 10–30 mg/kg/day divided q 6–8 hr; maximum dose 1.8 g/day. *Bacterial endocarditis prophylaxis*—20 mg/kg 1 hr before procedure.
IM, IV (Adults): *Most infections*—300–600 mg q 6–8 hr *or* 900 mg q 8 hr (up to 4.8 g/day IV has been used; single IM doses of >600 mg are not recommended). P. carinii *pneumonia*—2400–2700 mg/day in divided doses with primaquine (unlabeled). *Toxoplasmosis*—1200–4800 mg/day in divided doses with pyrimethamine. *Bacterial endocarditis prophylaxis*—600 mg 30 min before procedure.
IM, IV (Children >1 mo): 25–40 mg/kg/day divided q 6–8 hr; maximum dose: 4.8 g/day. *Bacterial endocarditis prophylaxis*—20 mg/kg 30 min before procedure; maximum dose: 600 mg.
IM, IV (Infants <1 mo and <2 kg): 5 mg/kg q 8–12 hr *≥2 kg*— 20–30 mg/kg/day divided q 6–8 hr.
Vaginal (Adults and Adolescents): *Cleocin, Clindamax*—1 applicator full (5 g) q hs for 3 or 7 days

(7 days in pregnant patients); *Clindesse*—one applicator full (5 g) single dose *or* 1 suppository (100 mg) at bedtime for 3 nights.
Topical (Adults and Adolescents): *Solution*—1% solution/suspension applied twice daily (range 1–4 times daily). *Foam, gel*—1% foam or gel applied once daily.

Availability (generic available)

Capsules: 75 mg, 150 mg, 300 mg. **Oral suspension:** 75 mg/5 mL. **Injection:** 150 mg/mL. **Premixed infusion:** 300 mg/50 mL, 600 mg/50 mL, 900 mg/50 mL. **Topical:** 1% lotion, gel, foam, solution, suspension, single-use applicators. ***In combination with:*** benzoyl peroxide (BenzaClin) (see Appendix B). **Vaginal cream:** 2% cream. **Vaginal suppositories (ovules):** 100 mg. ***In combination with:*** tretinoin (Ziana) (see Appendix B).

clobetasol (kloe-bay-ta-sol)

Clobex, ✱Dermovate, Temovate, Temovate E

Classification
Therapeutic: anti-inflammatories (steroidal)
Pharmacologic: corticosteroids

Indications

Management of inflammation and pruritus associated with various allergic/immunologic skin problems.

Action

Suppresses normal immune response and inflammation. **Therapeutic Effects:** Suppression of dermatologic inflammation and immune processes.

Adverse Reactions/Side Effects

Derm: allergic contact dermatitis, atrophy, burning, dryness, edema, folliculitis, hypersensitivity reactions, hypertrichosis, hypopigmentation, irritation, maceration, miliaria, perioral dermatitis, secondary infection, striae. **Misc:** adrenal suppression (use of occlusive dressings, long-term therapy).

PHYSICAL THERAPY IMPLICATIONS

Examination and Evaluation

- Assess the area being treated to help document whether drug therapy is successful in resolving skin conditions.
- Monitor any new or increased reactions at the site of application, including inflammation, irritation, infection, burning, swelling, exfoliation, and rash. Report severe or prolonged skin reactions to the physician.
- Report signs of adrenal suppression, including hypotension, weight loss, weakness, nausea, vomiting, anorexia, lethargy, confusion, and restlessness.

Interventions

- Protect skin from breakdown, especially over bony prominences.

Patient/client-Related Instruction

- Advise patients on long-term treatment to consult physician before stopping this medication. Stopping the medication suddenly may result in adrenocortical shock (severe hypotension, hypoglycemia, weakness, vomiting). If these signs appear, notify physician immediately; may be life threatening.
- Check that the patient and family or caregivers understand topical application procedures and adhere to the recommended dosing schedule.

Pharmacokinetics

Absorption: Minimal. Prolonged use on large surface areas or large amounts applied or use of occlusive dressings may increase systemic absorption.
Distribution: Remains primarily at site of action.
Metabolism and Excretion: Usually metabolized in skin; may be modified to resist local metabolism and have a prolonged local effect.
Half-life: Unknown.

TIME/ACTION PROFILE (response depends on condition being treated)

ROUTE	ONSET	PEAK	DURATION
topical	mins–hrs	hrs–days	hrs–days

Contraindications/Precautions

Contraindicated in: Hypersensitivity or known intolerance to corticosteroid or components of vehicles (ointment or cream base, preservative, alcohol); Untreated bacterial or viral infections.
Use Cautiously in: Hepatic dysfunction; Diabetes mellitus, cataracts, glaucoma, or tuberculosis (use of large amounts of high-potency agents may worsen condition); Patients with preexisting skin atrophy; OB/Lactation/Pedi: Pregnancy, lactation, or children (chronic high-dose use may result in adrenal suppression in mother, growth suppression in children; children may be more susceptible to adrenal and growth suppression); Not recommended for use in children <12 yr.

Interactions

Drug-Drug: None significant.

Route/Dosage

Topical (Adults and Children): Apply to affected area(s) 1–3 times daily (depends on preparation and condition being treated).

Availability (generic available)

Cream: 0.05%. **Emollient cream:** 0.05%. **Foam:** 005%. **Gel:** 0.05%. **Lotion:** 0.05%. **Ointment:** 0.05%. **Scalp solution:** 0.05%. **Shampoo:** 0.05%. **Spray:** 0.05%.

C

clocortolone (kloe-kore-toe-lone)

Cloderm

Classification

Therapeutic: anti-inflammatories (steroidal)

Pharmacologic: corticosteroids

Indications

Management of inflammation and pruritus associated with various allergic/immunologic skin problems.

Action

Suppresses normal immune response and inflammation. **Therapeutic Effects:** Suppression of dermatologic inflammation and immune processes.

Adverse Reactions/Side Effects

Derm: allergic contact dermatitis, atrophy, burning, dryness, edema, folliculitis, hypersensitivity reactions, hypertrichosis, hypopigmentation, irritation, maceration, miliaria, perioral dermatitis, secondary infection, striae. **Misc:** adrenal suppression (use of occlusive dressings, long-term therapy).

PHYSICAL THERAPY IMPLICATIONS

Examination and Evaluation

- Assess the area being treated to help document whether drug therapy is successful in resolving skin conditions.
- Monitor any new or increased reactions at the site of application, including inflammation, irritation, infection, burning, swelling, exfoliation, and rash. Report severe or prolonged skin reactions to the physician.
- Report signs of adrenal suppression, including hypotension, weight loss, weakness, nausea, vomiting, anorexia, lethargy, confusion, and restlessness.

Interventions

- Protect skin from breakdown, especially over bony prominences.

Patient/Client-Related Instruction

- Advise patients on long-term treatment to consult physician before stopping this medication. Stopping the medication suddenly may result in adrenocortical shock (severe hypotension, hypoglycemia, weakness, vomiting). If these signs appear, notify physician immediately; may be life threatening.
- Check that the patient and family or caregivers understand topical application procedures, and adhere to the recommended dosing schedule.

Pharmacokinetics

Absorption: Minimal. Prolonged use on large surface areas or large amounts applied or use of occlusive dressings may increase systemic absorption.
Distribution: Remains primarily at site of action.
Metabolism and Excretion: Usually metabolized in skin.
Half-life: Unknown.

TIME/ACTION PROFILE (response depends on condition being treated)

ROUTE	ONSET	PEAK	DURATION
topical	mins–hrs	hrs–days	hrs–days

Contraindications/Precautions

Contraindicated in: Hypersensitivity or known intolerance to corticosteroids or components of vehicles (ointment or cream base, preservative, alcohol); Untreated bacterial or viral infections.
Use Cautiously in: Hepatic dysfunction; Diabetes mellitus, cataracts, glaucoma, or tuberculosis (use of large amounts of high-potency agents may worsen condition); Patients with preexisting skin atrophy; Pregnancy, lactation, or children (chronic high-dose usage may result in adrenal suppression in mother, growth suppression in children; children may be more susceptible to adrenal and growth suppression).

Interactions

Drug-Drug: None significant.

Route/Dosage

Topical (Adults and Children ≥12 yr): Apply to affected area(s) 3 times daily.

Availability

Cream: 0.1% Rx.

clofarabine (klo-far-a-been)

Clolar

Classification

Therapeutic: antineoplastics

Pharmacologic: antimetabolites

Indications

Refractory/relapsed acute lymphoblastic leukemia in children and young people aged 1–21 yr.

Action

Converted intracellularly to the active 5′-triphosphate metabolite which acts as a purine nucleoside antimetabolite; net result is inhibition of DNA synthesis. Produces

🍁 = Canadian drug name; *CAPITALS indicate life-threatening; underlines indicate most frequent.

a rapid reduction of peripheral leukemia cells.
Therapeutic Effects: Death of rapidly replicating cells, particularly malignant ones.

Adverse Reactions/Side Effects

CNS: fatigue. **Resp:** pharyngitis. **CV:** pericardial effusion, tachycardia, edema. **GI:** diarrhea, hepatic toxicity, nausea, abdominal pain, constipation, mucositis, vomiting. **F and E:** dehydration. **Hemat:** NEUTROPENIA, anemia, thrombocytopenia. **Local:** injection site pain. **Misc:** SYSTEMIC INFLAMMATORY RESPONSE SYNDROME, TUMOR LYSIS SYNDROME, infections, fever, chills.

PHYSICAL THERAPY IMPLICATIONS

Examination and Evaluation

- Monitor neuromuscular signs of electrolyte imbalances that might indicate tumor lysis syndrome. Signs include severe muscle weakness or paralysis due to increased plasma potassium (hyperkalemia) or muscle hyperexcitability and tetany due to phosphate and calcium imbalances (hyperphosphatemia and hypocalcemia). Notify physician immediately if these signs occur.
- Be alert for signs of systemic inflammatory response syndrome. Signs include abnormal body temperature (>38C or <36C), tachycardia (heart rate of >90 bpm) and a respiratory rate of >20 breaths/min. Notify physician immediately; additional diagnostic tests can confirm this syndrome (e.g., a white blood cell count >12,000/μL or <4000/μL or >10% bands).
- Monitor signs of neutropenia (fever, sore throat, signs of infection), thrombocytopenia (bruising, nose bleeds, and bleeding gums) or unusual weakness and fatigue that might be due to anemia. Report these signs to the physician immediately.
- Assess peripheral edema using girth measurements, volume displacement, and measurement of pitting edema (see Appendix N). Report increased swelling in feet and ankles or a sudden increase in body weight due to fluid retention.
- Monitor IV injection site for pain, swelling, and irritation. Report prolonged or excessive injection site reactions to the physician.

Interventions

- For patients who are medically able to begin exercise, implement appropriate resistive exercises and aerobic training to maintain muscle strength and aerobic capacity during cancer chemotherapy or to help restore function after chemotherapy.
- Because of the risk of tachycardia and pericardial effusion, use caution during aerobic exercise and other forms of therapeutic exercise. Assess exercise tolerance frequently (blood pressure, heart rate, fatigue levels), and terminate exercise immediately if any untoward responses occur (See Appendix L).

Patient/Client-Related Instruction

- Advise patient and family/caregivers about the likelihood of GI reactions (nausea, vomiting, diarrhea, constipation, abdominal pain, irritation of the oral mucosa). Instruct patient to report severe or prolonged GI problems or signs of liver toxicity (yellow skin or eyes, abdominal pain, severe nausea and vomiting, fever, sore throat, malaise, weakness, facial edema).
- Advise patient and family/caregivers about the risk of infections, to guard against infection (frequent hand washing, etc.), and to avoid crowds and contact with persons with contagious diseases.
- Instruct patient and family/caregivers to maintain adequate fluid intake and avoid dehydration.
- Instruct patient and family/caregivers to report other troublesome side effects such as severe or prolonged chills, fever, or pharyngitis.

Pharmacokinetics

Absorption: IV administration results in complete bioavailability.
Distribution: Unknown.
Metabolism and Excretion: 46–60% excreted unchanged in urine.
Half-life: 5.2 hr.

TIME/ACTION PROFILE (effect on WBCs)

ROUTE	ONSET	PEAK	DURATION
IV	rapid	unknown	2–6 wk

Contraindications/Precautions

Contraindicated in: None; Pregnancy or lactation.
Use Cautiously in: Hepatic or renal impairment; Concurrent use of nephrotoxic or hepatotoxic drugs.

Interactions

Drug-Drug: Concurrent use of **hepatotoxic or nephrotoxic drugs** ↑ risk of hepatotoxicity and nephrotoxicity and should be avoided for the 5-day treatment period.

Route/Dosage

IV (Children and young people aged 1–21 yr): 52 mg/m^2 ≤ daily for 5 days; cycle may be repeated every 2–6 wk.

Availability

Solution for IV administration: 20 mg/mL vials.

clomipramine

(kloe-**mip**-ra-meen)
Anafranil

Classification
Therapeutic: antiobsessive agents
Pharmacologic: tricyclic antidepressants

C

Indications

Obsessive-Compulsive Disorder (OCD). **Unlabeled Use:** Depression, neuropathic pain/chronic pain.

Action

Potentiates the effect of serotonin (antiobsessional effect) and norepinephrine in the CNS. Has moderate anticholinergic effects. **Therapeutic Effects:** Diminished obsessive-compulsive behavior.

Adverse Reactions/Side Effects

CNS: SEIZURES, lethargy, sedation, weakness, aggressive behavior. **EENT:** blurred vision, dry eyes, dry mouth, vestibular disorder. **CV:** ARRHYTHMIAS, ECG changes, orthostatic hypotension. **GI:** constipation, nausea, vomiting, weight gain, eructation. **GU:** male sexual dysfunction, urinary retention. **Derm:** dry skin, photosensitivity. **Endo:** gynecomastia. **Hemat:** anemia. **MS:** muscle weakness. **Neuro:** extrapyramidal reactions. **Misc:** hyperthermia.

PHYSICAL THERAPY IMPLICATIONS

Examination and Evaluation

- Be alert for new seizures or increased seizure activity, especially at the onset of drug treatment. Document the number, duration, and severity of seizures, and report these findings to the physician immediately.
- Assess heart rate, ECG, and heart sounds, especially during exercise (See Appendices G, H). Report any rhythm disturbances or symptoms of increased arrhythmias, including palpitations, chest discomfort, shortness of breath, fainting, and fatigue/weakness.
- Assess blood pressure (BP) when patient assumes a more upright position (lying to standing, sitting to standing, lying to sitting). Document orthostatic hypotension and contact physician when systolic BP falls >20 mm Hg or diastolic BP falls >10 mm Hg.
- Monitor signs of anemia, including unusual fatigue, shortness of breath with exertion, and bruising, and pale skin. Notify physician immediately if these signs occur.
- Be alert for sedation, lethargy, aggressive behavior, or other alterations in mental status. Notify physician or mental health professional if these side effects become problematic.
- Be alert for increased depression and suicidal thoughts and ideology, especially when initiating drug treatment or in children and teenagers. Notify physician or mental health professional immediately if patient exhibits worsening depression or other changes in mood and behavior.
- Assess motor function, and be alert for extrapyramidal reactions, including Parkinson-like symptoms, dyskinesias, dystonias, or other motor abnormalities. Report any motor problems that might affect gait, balance, and other functional activities.
- Monitor muscle strength and vestibular function. Report unexplained strength loss or balance problems, especially if these problems affect gait and functional activities.
- If used to treat chronic pain, assess pain levels periodically to help determine drug efficacy.
- Periodically assess body weight and other anthropometric measures (body mass index, body composition). Report a rapid or unexplained weight gain or increased body fat.

Interventions

- Guard against falls and trauma (hip fractures, head injury, and so forth), and implement fall-prevention strategies (See Appendix E).
- Because of the risk of cardiac arrhythmias and hypotension, use caution during aerobic exercise and other forms of therapeutic exercise. Assess exercise tolerance frequently (BP, heart rate, fatigue levels), and terminate exercise immediately if any untoward responses occur (See Appendix L).
- To minimize orthostatic hypotension, patient should move slowly when assuming a more upright position.
- Because of an increased risk of hyperthermia, use caution during aerobic exercise in hot environments. Monitor the patient's exercise tolerance and terminate exercise if patient appears overheated or any untoward effects occur (See Appendix L).
- Help patient explore nonpharmacologic methods to reduce depression (exercise, counseling, support groups, and so forth).
- If treating neuropathic pain or other pain syndromes, implement appropriate interventions (physical agents, manual techniques, therapeutic exercise) to manage pain and reduce the need for drug therapy. Help patient also explore other nonpharmacological methods to reduce chronic pain (relaxation techniques, imagery, counseling, and so forth).
- Causes photosensitivity; use care if administering UV treatments. Advise patient to avoid direct sunlight and to use sunscreens and protective clothing.

Patient/Client-Related Instruction

- Advise patient that antidepressant effects may not occur immediately; it may take 2 wk or more before an improvement in mood is observed.
- Advise patient to avoid alcohol and other CNS depressants because of the increased risk of sedation and adverse effects.
- Advise patient that this medication should be tapered at the completion of long-term therapy. Abrupt discontinuation may cause nausea, vomiting, diarrhea,

headache, trouble sleeping with vivid dreams, and irritability

- Instruct patient to report other troublesome side effects such as severe or prolonged blurred vision, dry eyes, dry skin, urinary retention, sexual dysfunction, increased breast growth in men (gynecomastia), or GI problems (nausea, vomiting, constipation, dry mouth).

Pharmacokinetics

Absorption: Well absorbed from the GI tract.
Distribution: Widely distributed; enters breast milk.
Protein Binding: ≥90%.
Metabolism and Excretion: Extensively metabolized by the liver. Some conversion to a pharmacologically active metabolite (desmethylclomipramine). Undergoes enterohepatic recirculation and secretion into gastric juices.
Half-life: 21–31 hr.

TIME/ACTION PROFILE

ROUTE	ONSET	PEAK	DURATION
PO	1–6 wk	unknown	unknown

Contraindications/Precautions

Contraindicated in: Hypersensitivity; Angle-closure glaucoma; Recent myocardial infarction; History of QTc prolongation; Cardiac arrythmias; Heart failure; Concurrent MAO inhibitor or clonidine use (avoid if possible); OB: Potential for fetal harm or neonatal withdrawal syndrome; Lactation: Discontinue drug or bottle feed.
Use Cautiously in: History of seizures (threshold may be lowered); Patients with preexisting cardiovascular disease; Older men with prostatic hyperplasia (may be more susceptible to urinary retention); Hyperthyroidism (↑ risk of arrhythmias); May ↑ risk of suicide attempt/ideation, especially during dose early treatment or dose adjustment; risk may be greater in children or adolescents; Pedi: Safety not established in children <10 yr; Geri: ↑ risk of arrhythmias.

Interactions

Drug-Drug: May cause hypotension and tachycardia when used with **MAO inhibitors** (concurrent use not recommended). Wait 2 wk before initiating clomipramine after **MAO Inhibitors** are stopped. Wait 2 wk before initiating **MAO inhibitors** after clomipramine is stopped . May prevent the therapeutic response to **antihypertensives**. Use with **clonidine** may result in hypertensive crisis (avoid concurrent use). ↑ CNS depression with other **CNS depressants**, including **alcohol**, **antihistamines**, **opioids**, and **sedative/hypnotics**. Adrenergic and anticholinergic side effects may be ↑ with other **agents having adrenergic/anticholinergic properties**. Effects and toxicity may be ↑ by concurrent use with **SSRI antidepressants** (wait several weeks after stopping SSRIs to start clomipramine; up to 5 wk for fluoxetine), **phenothiazines**, **cimetidine**, or **oral contraceptives**. **Nicotine** may ↑ metabolism and ↓ effectiveness. Transient delirium may occur with **disulfiram**.
Drug-Natural: ↑ risk of serotonergic side effects, including serotonin syndrome with **St. John's wort** and **SAMe**. **Kava**, **valerian**, or **chamomile** can increase CNS depression.
Drug-Food: Grapefruit juice ↑ serum levels and effect.

Route/Dosage

PO (Adults): *Antiobsessive*—25 mg/day, increased over 2-wk period to 100 mg/day in divided doses. May be further increased over several weeks up to 250–300 mg/day in divided doses. Once stabilizing dose is reached, entire daily dose may be given at bedtime. *Antidepressant*—25 mg 3 times daily; may be increased as needed (unlabeled).
PO (Geriatric Patients): 20–30 mg/day initially; may be increased as needed.
PO (Children >10–17 yr): 25 mg/day initially, increased over 2-wk period to 3 mg/kg/day or 100 mg/day (whichever is smaller) in divided doses. May be further increased to 3 mg/kg/day or 200 mg/day (whichever is smaller) in divided doses. Once stabilizing dose is reached, entire daily dose may be given at bedtime.

Availability (generic available)

Capsules: 10 mg, 25 mg, 50 mg, 75 mg.

clonazepam (kloe-**naz**-e-pam)

Klonopin, Rivotril, Syn-Clonazepam

Classification
Therapeutic: anticonvulsants
Pharmacologic: benzodiazepines

Schedule IV

Indications

Prophylaxis of Petit mal, Petit mal variant, Akinetic, Myoclonic seizures. Panic disorder with or without agoraphobia. **Unlabeled Use:** Uncontrolled leg movements during sleep. Neuralgias. Sedation. Adjunct management of acute mania, acute psychosis, or insomnia.

Action

Anticonvulsant effects may be due to presynaptic inhibition. Produces sedative effects in the CNS, probably by stimulating inhibitory gamma-aminobutyric acid (GABA) receptors. **Therapeutic Effects:** Prevention of seizures. Decreased manifestations of panic disorder.

Adverse Reactions/Side Effects

CNS: behavioral changes, drowsiness, fatigue, slurred speech, sedation, abnormal eye movements, diplopia, nystagmus. **Resp:** increased secretions. **CV:** palpitations. **GI:** constipation, diarrhea, hepatitis, weight gain. **GU:** dysuria, nocturia, urinary retention. **Hemat:** anemia, eosinophilia, leukopenia, thrombocytopenia. **Neuro:** ataxia, hypotonia. **Misc:** fever, physical dependence, psychologic dependence, tolerance.

PHYSICAL THERAPY IMPLICATIONS

Examination and Evaluation

- In patients with seizures, document the number, duration, and severity of seizures to help determine drug efficacy.
- Monitor daytime drowsiness, short-term memory deficits, behavioral changes, slurred speech, and "hangover" symptoms (headache, nausea, malaise, irritability, dysphoria). Repeated or excessive symptoms may require change in dose or medication.
- Assess balance and risk of falls (See Appendix E), especially in older adults, or in patients exhibiting sedation, dizziness, ataxia, or visual disturbances.
- Monitor signs of eosinophilia (fatigue, weakness, myalgia), leukopenia (fever, sore throat, signs of infection), thrombocytopenia (bruising, nose bleeds, bleeding gums), or unusual weakness and fatigue that might be due to anemia. Report these signs to the physician.
- If treating neuralgia, use visual analog scales and other appropriate pain scales to assess the patient's pain and help document effects of drug therapy.
- Monitor motor function and report an excessive decrease in muscle tone (hypotonia) or problems with coordination (ataxia).
- Periodically assess body weight and other anthropometric measures (body mass index, body composition). Report a rapid or unexplained weight gain or increased body fat.

Interventions

- Guard against falls and trauma (hip fractures, head injury, and so forth). Implement fall-prevention strategies, especially in older adults or if drowsiness, ataxia, or visual disturbances affect gait and balance (See Appendix E).
- Help patient explore nonpharmacologic methods to decrease anxiety and reduce panic attacks, such as relaxation techniques, regular exercise, avoid caffeine, and so forth.

Patient/Client-Related Instruction

- Instruct patients on prolonged treatment not to discontinue medication without consulting their physician. Long-term use can cause tolerance and physical/psychologic dependence, and abrupt withdrawal can cause insomnia, unusual irritability or nervousness, and seizures.
- Advise patient to avoid alcohol and other CNS depressants because of the increased risk of sedation and adverse effects.
- Instruct patient to report severe or prolonged GI problems (constipation, diarrhea), and to watch for signs of drug-induced hepatitis such as anorexia, abdominal pain, severe nausea and vomiting, yellow skin or eyes, skin rashes, flu-like symptoms, and muscle/joint pain.
- Instruct patient to report other bothersome side effects, including severe or prolonged fatigue, palpitations, pulmonary congestion, visual disturbances, fever, or problems with urination.

Pharmacokinetics

Absorption: Well absorbed from the GI tract.
Distribution: Probably crosses the blood-brain barrier and the placenta.
Metabolism and Excretion: Mostly metabolized by the liver.
Half-life: 18–50 hr.

TIME/ACTION PROFILE (anticonvulsant activity)

ROUTE	ONSET	PEAK	DURATION
PO	20–60 min	1–2 hr	6–12 hr

Contraindications/Precautions

Contraindicated in: Hypersensitivity to clonazepam or other benzodiazepines; Severe liver disease.
Use Cautiously in: All patients (may ↑ risk of suicidal thoughts/behaviors); Angle-closure glaucoma; Obstructive sleep apnea; Chronic respiratory disease; History of porphyria; Do not discontinue abruptly; OB: Safety not established; chronic use during pregnancy may result in withdrawal in the neonate; Lactation: May enter breast milk; discontinue drug or bottle feed; Pedi: Safety not established; Geri: May experience excessive sedation at usual doses; decreased dosage recommended.

Interactions

Drug-Drug: Alcohol, **antidepressants**, **antihistamines**, other **benzodiazepines**, and **opioid analgesics**—concurrent use results in ↑ CNS depression. **Cimetidine**, **hormonal contraceptives**, **disulfiram**, **fluoxetine**, **isoniazid**, **ketoconazole**, **metoprolol**, **propoxyphene**, **propranolol**, or **valproic acid** may ↓ metabolism of clonazepam and ↑ its actions. May ↓ efficacy of **levodopa**. **Rifampin** or **barbiturates** may ↑ metabolism and ↓ effectiveness of clonazepam. Sedative effects may be ↓ by **theophylline**.

May ↑ serum **phenytoin** levels. **Phenytoin** may ↓ serum clonazepam levels.
Drug-Natural: Concomitant use of **kava, valerian**, or **chamomile** can ↑ CNS depression.

Route/Dosage

PO (Adults): 0.5 mg 3 times daily; may ↑ by 0.5–1 mg q 3 days. Total daily maintenance dose not to exceed 20 mg. *Panic disorder*—0.125 mg twice daily; ↑ after 3 days toward target dose of 1 mg/day (some patients may require up to 4 mg/day).
PO (Children <10 yr or 30 kg): Initial daily dose 0.01–0.03 mg/kg/day (not to exceed 0.05 mg/kg/day) given in 2–3 equally divided doses; ↑ by no more than 0.25–0.5 mg q 3 days until therapeutic blood levels are reached (not to exceed 0.2 mg/kg/day).

Availability (generic available)

Tablets: 0.5 mg, 1 mg, 2 mg. **Orally-disintegrating tablets:** 0.125 mg, 0.25 mg, 0.5 mg, 1 mg, 2 mg.

clonidine (klon-i-deen)

Catapres, Catapres-TTS, Dixarit, Duraclon

Classification
Therapeutic: antihypertensives
Pharmacologic: adrenergics (centrally acting)

Indications

PO, Transdermal: Management of mild-to-moderate hypertension. **Epidural:** Management of cancer pain unresponsive to opioids alone. **Unlabeled Use:** Management of opioid withdrawal.

Action

Stimulates alpha-adrenergic receptors in the CNS; which results in decreased sympathetic outflow inhibiting cardioacceleration and vasoconstriction centers. Prevents pain signal transmission to the CNS by stimulating alpha-adrenergic receptors in the spinal cord. **Therapeutic Effects:** Decreased blood pressure. Decreased pain.

Adverse Reactions/Side Effects

CNS: drowsiness, depression, dizziness, nervousness, nightmares. **CV:** bradycardia, hypotension (increased with epidural), palpitations. **GI:** dry mouth, constipation, nausea, vomiting. **GU:** erectile dysfunction. **Derm:** rash, sweating. **F and E:** sodium retention. **Metab:** weight gain. **Misc:** withdrawal phenomenon.

PHYSICAL THERAPY IMPLICATIONS

Examination and Evaluation

- Assess blood pressure periodically and compare to normal values (See Appendix F). Document whether drug therapy is successful in controlling hypertension. Also report low blood pressure (BP), especially if patient experiences dizziness or syncope.
- If used to treat cancer pain, use appropriate pain scales (visual analogue scales, others) to document whether this drug is successful in helping manage the patient's pain.
- Assess heart rate, ECG, and heart sounds, especially during exercise (See Appendices G, H). Report an unusually slow heart rate (HR) (bradycardia) or signs of other arrhythmias, including palpitations, chest discomfort, shortness of breath, fainting, and fatigue/weakness.
- Assess dizziness and drowsiness that might affect gait, balance, and other functional activities (See Appendix C). Report balance problems and functional limitations to the physician, and caution the patient and family/caregivers to guard against falls and trauma.
- Be alert for signs of depression, nervousness, or other changes in mood and behavior. Notify physician if these changes become problematic.
- Assess peripheral edema using girth measurements, volume displacement, and measurement of pitting edema (See Appendix N). Report increased swelling in feet and ankles or a sudden increase in body weight due to sodium and water retention.
- Be alert for a rapid increase in BP and HR if clonidine is suddenly discontinued (withdrawal phenomenon). Report these increases to the physician immediately.

Interventions

- Because of the risk of arrhythmias and abnormal BP responses, use caution during aerobic exercise and other forms of therapeutic exercise. Assess exercise tolerance frequently (BP, HR, fatigue levels), and terminate exercise immediately if any untoward responses occur (See Appendix L).
- Avoid physical therapy interventions that cause systemic vasodilation (large whirlpool, Hubbard tank). Additive effects of this drug and the intervention may cause a dangerous fall in BP.
- If treating cancer pain, implement appropriate interventions (physical agents, manual techniques, therapeutic exercise) as tolerated to manage pain and reduce the need for drug therapy. Help patient also explore other nonpharmacologic methods to reduce pain such as relaxation techniques, imagery, counseling, and so forth.
- To minimize orthostatic hypotension, advise patient to move slowly when assuming a more upright position.

Patient/Client-Related Instruction

- Remind patients to take medication as directed to control hypertension even if they are asymptomatic.

- Counsel patients about additional interventions to help control BP, such as regular exercise, weight loss, sodium restriction, stress reduction, moderation of alcohol consumption, and smoking cessation.
- Instruct patient or family/caregivers to report other bothersome side effects such as severe or prolonged nightmares, sexual dysfunction, skin reactions (rash, excessive sweating), or GI problems (constipation, nausea, vomiting, dry mouth).

Pharmacokinetics

Absorption: Well absorbed from the GI tract and skin. Enters systemic circulation following epidural use. Some absorption follows sublingual administration.
Distribution: Widely distributed; enters CNS. Crosses the placenta readily; enters breast milk in high concentrations.
Metabolism and Excretion: Mostly metabolized by the liver; 40–50% eliminated unchanged in urine.
Half-life: *Plasma*—12–22 hr; *CNS*—1.3 hr.

TIME/ACTION PROFILE (PO, TD = antihypertensive effect; epidural = analgesia)

ROUTE	ONSET	PEAK	DURATION
PO	30–60 min	2–4 hr	8–12 hr
TD	2–3 days	unknown	7 days*
Epidural	unknown	unknown	unknown

*8 hr following removal of patch.

Contraindications/Precautions

Contraindicated in: Hypersensitivity; *Epidural*—injection-site infection, anticoagulant therapy, or bleeding problems.
Use Cautiously in: Serious cardiac or cerebrovascular disease; Renal insufficiency; Geri: Appears on Beers' list due to increased risk of orthostatic hypotension and adverse CNS effects in geriatric patients (↓ dose recommended); Pregnancy or lactation (safety not established).

Interactions

Drug-Drug: Additive sedation with **CNS depressants**, including **alcohol**, **antihistamines**, **opioid analgesics**, and **sedative/hypnotics**. Additive hypotension with other **antihypertensives** and **nitrates**. Additive bradycardia with **myocardial depressants**, including **beta blockers**. **MAO inhibitors**, **amphetamines**, **beta blockers**, **prazosin**, or **tricyclic antidepressants** may ↓ antihypertensive effect. Withdrawal phenomenon may be ↑ by discontinuation of **beta blockers**. Epidural clonidine prolongs the effects of epidurally administered **local anesthetics**. May ↓ effectiveness of **levodopa**. ↑ risk of adverse cardiovascular reactions with **verapamil**.

Route/Dosage

PO (Adults): *Hypertension (initial dose)*—100 mcg (0.1 mg) bid, increase by 100–200 mcg (0.1–0.2 mg)/day q 2–4 days. *Usual maintenance dose* is 200–600 mcg (0.2–0.6 mg)/day in 2–3 divided doses (up to 2.4 mg/day). *Urgent treatment*—200 mcg (0.2 mg) loading dose, then 100 mcg (0.1 mg) q hr until blood pressure is controlled or 800 mcg (0.8 mg) total has been administered; follow with maintenance dosing. *Opioid withdrawal*—300 mcg (0.3 mg)–1.2 mg/day, may be decreased by 50%/day for 3 days, then discontinued or decreased by 100–200 mcg (0.1–0.2 mg)/day.
PO (Geriatric Patients): 100 mcg (0.1 mg) at bedtime initially, increased as needed.
PO (Children): 50–400 mcg (0.05–0.4 mg) twice daily.
TD (Adults): *Hypertension*—TD system delivering 100–300 mcg (0.1–0.3 mg)/24 hr applied every 7 days. Initiate with 100 mcg (0.1 mg)/24 hr system; dosage increments may be made q 1–2 wk when system is changed.
Epidural (Adults): 30 mcg/hr initially; titrated according to need.
Epidural (Children): 0.5 mcg/kg/hr initially; titrated according to need.

Availability (generic available)

Tablets: 25 mcg (0.025 mg), 100 mcg (0.1 mg), 200 mcg (0.2 mg), 300 mcg (0.3 mg). **TD systems:** Catapres-TTS 1, releases 0.1 mg/24 hr, Catapres-TTS 2, releases 0.2 mg/24 hr, Catapres-TTS 3, releases 0.3 mg/24 hr. **Solution for epidural injection:** 100 mcg/mL in 10-mL vials, 500 mcg/mL in 10-mL vials. ***In combination with:*** chlorthalidone (Clorpress). See Appendix B.

clopidogrel (kloe-pid-oh-grel)

Plavix

Classification

Therapeutic: antiplatelet agents
Pharmacologic: platelet aggregation inhibitors

Indications

Reduction of atherosclerotic events (MI, stroke, vascular death) in patients at risk for such events, including recent MI, acute coronary syndrome (unstable angina/non–Q-wave MI), stroke, or peripheral vascular disease.

Action

Inhibits platelet aggregation by irreversibly inhibiting the binding of ATP to platelet receptors. **Therapeutic**

Effects: Decreased occurrence of atherosclerotic events in patients at risk.

Adverse Reactions/Side Effects

Incidence of adverse reactions similar to that of aspirin

CNS: depression, dizziness, fatigue, headache. **EENT:** epistaxis. **Resp:** cough, dyspnea. **CV:** chest pain, edema, hypertension. **GI:** GI BLEEDING, abdominal pain, diarrhea, dyspepsia, gastritis. **Derm:** pruritus, purpura, rash. **Hemat:** BLEEDING, NEUTROPENIA, THROMBOTIC THROMBOCYTOPENIC PURPURA. **Metab:** hypercholesterolemia. **MS:** arthralgia, back pain. **Misc:** fever, hypersensitivity reactions.

PHYSICAL THERAPY IMPLICATIONS

Examination and Evaluation

- Be alert for signs of GI bleeding signs (abdominal pain, vomiting blood, blood in stools, black/tarry stools) or other signs of bleeds (bleeding gums, nosebleeds, unusual bruising, hematuria; fall in hematocrit or blood pressure). Notify physician or nursing staff immediately if these signs occur.
- Monitor signs of thrombotic thrombocytopenic purpura, such as purplish spots on the skin, decreased consciousness, fatigue, weakness, shortness of breath on exertion, and tachycardia. Report these signs to the physician or nursing staff immediately.
- Assess blood pressure periodically and compare to normal values (See Appendix F). Report a sustained increase in blood pressure (hypertension) to the physician.
- Assess peripheral edema using girth measurements, volume displacement, and measurement of pitting edema (See Appendix N). Report increased swelling in feet and ankles or a sudden increase in body weight due to fluid retention.
- Monitor excessive coughing, chest pain, or difficult, labored breathing. Report severe or prolonged respiratory symptoms.
- Monitor signs of hypersensitivity reactions, including pulmonary symptoms (tightness in the throat and chest, wheezing, cough, dyspnea) or skin reactions (rash, pruritus, urticaria). Notify physician or nursing staff immediately if these reactions occur.
- Monitor and report signs of neutropenia including fever, sore throat, and other signs of infection.
- Assess dizziness and drowsiness that might affect gait, balance, and other functional activities (See Appendix C). Report balance problems and functional limitations to the physician and nursing staff, and caution the patient and family/caregivers to guard against falls and trauma.
- Assess any back pain or joint pain to rule out musculoskeletal pathology; that is, try to determine if pain is drug induced rather than caused by anatomic or biomechanical problems.

Interventions

- Use caution with any physical interventions that could increase bleeding, including wound débridement, chest percussion, joint mobilization, and application of local heat.
- Use caution during aerobic exercise in patients at risk for MI, stroke, or other cardiovascular events. Assess exercise tolerance frequently (blood pressure, heart rate, fatigue levels), and terminate exercise immediately if any untoward responses occur (See Appendix L).

Patient/Client-Related Instruction

- Remind patients to take medication as directed to reduce the risk of heart attack and stroke even if they are asymptomatic.
- Counsel patients about additional interventions to help reduce the risk of cardiovascular pathology, including regular exercise, weight loss, sodium restriction, stress reduction, moderation of alcohol consumption, and smoking cessation.
- Advise patient that this drug may cause problems in fat metabolism, including increased cholesterol. Remind patient that periodic blood tests may be needed to monitor plasma lipids.
- Instruct patient or family/caregivers to report other bothersome side effects such as severe or prolonged headache, fatigue, depression, fever, skin reactions (rash, itching), or GI problems (diarrhea, abdominal pain, indigestion).

Pharmacokinetics

Absorption: Well absorbed following oral administration; rapidly metabolized to an active antiplatelet compound. Parent drug has no antiplatelet activity.
Distribution: Unknown.
Protein Binding: *Clopidogrel*—98%; *active metabolite*— 94%.
Metabolism and Excretion: Rapidly and extensively converted by the liver to its active metabolite, which is then eliminated 50% in urine and 45% in feces.
Half-life: 8 hr (active metabolite).

TIME/ACTION PROFILE (effects on platelet function)

ROUTE	ONSET	PEAK	DURATION
PO	within 24 hr	3–7 days	5 days*

*Following discontinuation.

Contraindications/Precautions

Contraindicated in: Hypersensitivity; Pathologic bleeding (peptic ulcer, intracranial hemorrhage); Lactation.
Use Cautiously in: Patients at risk for bleeding (trauma, surgery, or other pathologic conditions); History of GI bleeding/ulcer disease; Severe hepatic impairment; OB/Lactation/Pedi: Safety not established; use in pregnancy only if clearly indicated.

Interactions

Drug-Drug: Concurrent **abciximab, eptifibatide, tirofiban, aspirin, NSAIDs, heparin, heparinoids, thrombolytic agents, ticlopidine,** or **warfarin** may ↑ risk of bleeding. May ↓ metabolism and ↑ effects of **phenytoin, tolbutamide, tamoxifen, torsemide, fluvastatin,** and many **NSAIDs**.
Drug-Natural: ↑ bleeding risk with **anise, arnica, chamomile, clove, fenugreek, feverfew, garlic, ginger, ginkgo, *Panax ginseng*,** and others.

Route/Dosage

Recent MI, Stroke, or Peripheral Vascular Disease

PO (Adults): 75 mg once daily.

Acute Coronary Syndrome

PO (Adults): 300 mg initially, then 75 mg once daily; aspirin 75–325 mg once daily should be given concurrently.

Availability

Tablets: 75 mg, 300 mg.

clorazepate (klor-az-e-pate)

Apo-Clorazepate, Gen-XENE, Novo-Clopate, Tranxene, Tranxene-SD

Classification
Therapeutic: anticonvulsants, sedative/hypnotics
Pharmacologic: benzodiazepines

Schedule IV

Indications

Management of simple partial seizures. Anxiety disorder, symptoms of anxiety. Acute alcohol withdrawal. **Unlabeled Use:** Anxiety associated with acute myocardial infarction.

Action

Acts at many levels in the CNS to produce anxiolytic effect and CNS depression (by stimulating inhibitory ammaaminobutyric acid [GABA] receptors). Produces skeletal muscle relaxation (by inhibiting spinal polysynaptic afferent pathways). Also has anticonvulsant effect (enhances presynaptic inhibition). **Therapeutic Effects:** Relief of anxiety. Sedation. Prevention of seizures.

Adverse Reactions/Side Effects

CNS: <u>dizziness</u>, <u>drowsiness</u>, <u>lethargy</u>, hangover, headache, mental depression, slurred speech, ataxia, paradoxical excitation. **EENT:** blurred vision. **Resp:** respiratory depression. **GI:** constipation, diarrhea, nausea, vomiting, weight gain (unusual). **Derm:** rashes. **Misc:** physical dependence, psychologic dependence, tolerance.

PHYSICAL THERAPY IMPLICATIONS

Examination and Evaluation

- In patients with seizures, document the number, duration, and severity of seizures to help determine drug efficacy.
- Monitor daytime drowsiness and "hangover," symptoms such as headache, nausea, irritability, lethargy, dysphoria, and slurred speech. Repeated or excessive symptoms may require change in dose or medication.
- Assess confusion (See Appendix D) or other changes in behavior or cognition (decreased mental acuity, excessive excitation). Report problematic changes in cognitive function.
- Assess symptoms of respiratory depression such as dyspnea and cyanosis. Monitor pulse oximetry and perform pulmonary function tests (See Appendices I, J, K) to quantify suspected changes in ventilation and respiratory function.
- Assess dizziness and ataxia that might affect gait, balance, and other functional activities (See Appendix C). Report balance problems and functional limitations to the physician, and caution the patient and family/caregivers to guard against falls and trauma.

Interventions

- Guard against falls and trauma (hip fractures, head injury, and so forth). Implement fall-prevention strategies, especially in older adults or if drowsiness and dizziness carry over into the daytime (See Appendix E).
- Help patient explore nonpharmacologic methods to reduce anxiety such as relaxation techniques, exercise, counseling, support groups, and so forth.

Patient/Client-Related Instruction

- Instruct patients on prolonged treatment not to discontinue medication without consulting their physician. Prolonged use can cause tolerance and dependence, and abrupt withdrawal can cause insomnia, unusual irritability or nervousness, and seizures.
- Advise patient to avoid alcohol and other CNS depressants because of the increased risk of sedation and adverse effects.
- Instruct patient to report other bothersome side effects such as severe or prolonged headache, blurred vision, skin rash, weight gain, or GI problems (nausea, vomiting, diarrhea, constipation).

Pharmacokinetics

Absorption: Well absorbed from the GI tract as desmethyldiazepam.
Distribution: Widely distributed. Crosses the placenta; enters breast milk.
Metabolism and Excretion: Metabolized by the liver; some conversion to active compounds.
Half-life: 48 hr.

TIME/ACTION PROFILE (sedation)

ROUTE	ONSET	PEAK	DURATION
PO	1–2 hr	1–2 hr	up to 24 hr*

*May last longer in geriatric patients.

Contraindications/Precautions

Contraindicated in: Hypersensitivity; Cross-sensitivity with other benzodiazepines may occur; Preexisting CNS depression; Severe uncontrolled pain; Angle-closure glaucoma; OB/Lactation: May cause CNS depression, flaccidity, feeding difficulties, and seizures in infant. In lactation, discontinue drug or bottle feed.
Use Cautiously in: Preexisting hepatic dysfunction; Patients who may be suicidal or have been addicted to drugs in the past; Debilitated patients (dosage reduction required); Severe pulmonary disease; Geri: Long-acting benzodiazepines cause prolonged sedation in the elderly. Appears on Beers' list and is associated with increased risk of falls (↓ dose required or consider short-acting benzodiazepine).

Interactions

Drug-Drug: Alcohol, antidepressants, antihistamines, and **opioid analgesics**—concurrent use results in ↑ CNS depression. **Cimetidine, hormonal contraceptives, disulfiram, fluoxetine, isoniazid, ketoconazole, metoprolol, propoxyphene, propranolol,** or **valproic acid** may ↓ the metabolism of clorazepate, ↑ its actions. May ↓ efficacy of **levodopa**. **Rifampin** or **barbiturates** may ↓ the metabolism and ↓ effectiveness of clorazepate. Sedative effects may be ↓ by **theophylline**.
Drug-Natural: Concomitant use of **kava, valerian,** or **chamomile** ↑ CNS depression.

Route/Dosage

Prescribe largest dose at bedtime to avoid daytime sedation. Can be used on prn basis for anxiety.
PO (Adults): *Anxiety*—7.5–15 mg 2–4 times daily *or* 15 mg at bedtime initially. May also be given in a single dose of 11.25–22.5 mg at bedtime. *Alcohol withdrawal*—30 mg initially, then 15 mg 2–4 times daily on 1st day, then gradually decreased over subsequent days. *Anticonvulsant*—7.5 mg 3 times daily; can increase by no more than 7.5 mg/day at weekly intervals (daily dose not to exceed 90 mg).
PO (Geriatric Patients or Debilitated Patients): *Anxiety*—3.75–15 mg/day; may be increased.
PO (Children 9–12 yr): *Anticonvulsant*—7.5 mg twice daily initially; may increase by 7.5 mg/wk (not to exceed 60 mg/day).

Availability

Tablets: 3.75 mg, 7.5 mg, 11.25 mg, 15 mg, 22.5 mg.
Capsules: 3.75 mg, 7.5 mg, 15 mg.

clotrimazole (topical)
(kloe-**try**-ma-zole)
✱Canesten, ✱Clotrimaderm, Cruex, ✱Lotriderm, Lotrimin

clotrimazole (vaginal)
(kloe-**try**-ma-zole)
✱Canesten, ✱Clotrimaderm, Gyne-Lotrimin-3, Mycelex-7, ✱Trivagizole-3

Classification
Therapeutic: antifungals (topical, vaginal)

Indications

Treatment of a variety of cutaneous fungal infections, including cutaneous candidiasis, tinea pedis (athlete's foot), tinea cruris (jock itch), tinea corporis (ringworm), and tinea versicolor. Treatment of vulvovaginal candidiasis.

Action

Affects the permeability of the fungal cell wall, allowing leakage of cellular contents. **Therapeutic Effects:** Decrease in symptoms of fungal infection.

Adverse Reactions/Side Effects

Local: burning, itching, local hypersensitivity reactions, redness, stinging.

PHYSICAL THERAPY IMPLICATIONS

Examination and Evaluation

- Monitor symptoms and healing of skin lesions to help document drug effectiveness.

Interventions

- Avoid contact with cutaneous lesions when treating patient.
- Always wash hands thoroughly and disinfect equipment (whirlpools, electrotherapeutic devices, treatment tables, and so forth) to help prevent the spread of infection.

Patient/Client-Related Instruction

- Advise patient to report any increased local sensitivity to this drug (pain, burning, swelling).
- Instruct patient about proper hygiene; e.g., thoroughly wash and dry the affected area, wear clean socks and ventilated shoes for tinea pedis, and so forth.

- Advise patient to apply the drug as directed for the full course of treatment even if feeling better.
- Inform patient that early relief of cutaneous symptoms may be seen in 2–3 days. Full therapeutic response may take 2 wk for cutaneous candidiasis, tinea cruris, and tinea corporis and 3–4 wk for tinea pedis.
- Vaginal infections: therapeutic response is usually seen after 1 wk. Therapy should be continued during menstrual period.
- Advise patient to seek medical help if infections persist or recur after the full treatment. Recurrent fungal infections may be a sign of systemic illness.

Pharmacokinetics

Absorption: Absorption through intact skin is minimal.
Distribution: Distribution after topical administration is primarily local.
Metabolism and Excretion: Systemic metabolism and excretion is negligible with local application.
Half-life: Not applicable.

TIME/ACTION PROFILE

ROUTE	ONSET	PEAK	DURATION
topical	unknown	unknown	unknown
vaginal cream	unknown	8–24 hr	unknown
vaginal tablet	unknown	1–2 days	unknown

Contraindications/Precautions

Contraindicated in: Hypersensitivity to active ingredients, additives, preservatives, or bases.
Use Cautiously in: Nail and scalp infections (may require additional systemic therapy); patients with recurrent vulvovaginal yeast infections. OB/Lactation: Safety not established.

Interactions

Drug-Drug: Not known.

Route/Dosage

Topical (Adults and Children >3 yr): Apply cream or solution twice daily for 1–4 wk.
Vag (Adults and Children >12 yr): *Vaginal tablets*—100 mg at bedtime for 7 nights (preferred regimen for pregnancy) *or* 200 mg at bedtime for 3 nights. *Vaginal cream*—1 applicator full (5 g) of 1% cream at bedtime for 7 days *or* 1 applicator full (5 g) of 2% cream at bedtime for 3 days.

Availability (generic available)

Cream: 1% OTC. **Solution:** 1% OTC. ***In combination with:*** betamethasone (Lotrisone) Rx. See Appendix B. **Vaginal tablets:** 100 mg OTC, 200 mg OTC. **Vaginal cream:** 1% OTC, 2% OTC.

C

cloxacillin (klox-a-sill-in)

Apo-Cloxi, Cloxapen, Novo-Cloxin, Nu-Cloxi, Orbenin

Classification
Therapeutic: anti-infectives
Pharmacologic: penicillinase-resistant penicillins

Indications

Treatment of the following infections due to penicillinase-producing staphylococci: Respiratory tract infections, Sinusitis, Skin and skin structure infections.

Action

Bind to bacterial cell wall, leading to cell death. Not inactivated by penicillinase enzymes. **Therapeutic Effects:** Bactericidal action. **Spectrum:** Active against most gram-positive aerobic cocci. Spectrum is notable for activity against Penicillinase-producing strains of *Staphylococcus aureus*, *S. epidermidis*. Not active against methicillin-resistant bacteria.

Adverse Reactions/Side Effects

CNS: SEIZURES. **GI:** diarrhea, epigastric distress, nausea, vomiting, pseudomembranous colitis. **GU:** interstitial nephritis. **Derm:** rash, urticaria. **Hemat:** eosinophilia, leukopenia. **Misc:** ALLERGIC REACTIONS, INCLUDING ANAPHYLAXIS AND SERUM SICKNESS, superinfection.

PHYSICAL THERAPY IMPLICATIONS

Examination and Evaluation

- Watch for seizures; notify physician immediately if patient develops or increases seizure activity.
- Monitor signs of allergic reactions and anaphylaxis, including pulmonary symptoms (tightness in the throat and chest, wheezing, cough dyspnea) or skin reactions (rash, pruritus, urticaria). Notify physician or nursing staff immediately if these reactions occur.
- Assess muscle aches and joint pain (arthralgia) that may be caused by serum sickness. Notify physician if these symptoms seem to be drug related rather than caused by musculoskeletal injury, or if muscle and joint pain are accompanied by allergy-like reactions (fever, rashes, etc.)
- Monitor signs of eosinophilia (fatigue, weakness, myalgia) or leukopenia (fever, sore throat, signs of infection); report these signs to the physician.

Interventions

- Always wash hands thoroughly and disinfect equipment (whirlpools, electrotherapeutic devices, treatment tables, and so forth) to help prevent the spread of infection. Employ universal precautions or isolation procedures as indicated for specific patients.

Patient/Client-Related Instruction

- Instruct patient to notify physician immediately if signs of the following occur:
  - Pseudomembranous colitis (diarrhea, abdominal pain, fever, pus or mucus in stools) or other severe or prolonged GI problems (nausea, vomiting, heartburn).
  - Superinfection (black, furry overgrowth on tongue; vaginal itching or discharge; loose or foul-smelling stools).
  - Interstitial nephritis (blood in urine, decreased urine output, weight gain from fluid retention).
- Instruct patient and family/caregivers to report other troublesome side effects such as severe or prolonged skin problems (rash, itching) or GI problems (nausea, vomiting, diarrhea, heartburn).

Pharmacokinetics

Absorption: Moderately absorbed (50%) following oral administration.
Distribution: Widely distributed; penetration into CSF is minimal but sufficient in the presence of inflamed meninges; crosses the placenta and enters breast milk.
Metabolism and Excretion: Some metabolism by the liver (9–22%) and some renal excretion of unchanged drug (30–45%).
Half-life: 0.5–1.1 hr (increased in severe hepatic, in renal dysfunction, and in neonates).

TIME/ACTION PROFILE

ROUTE	ONSET	PEAK	DURATION
cloxacillin PO	30 min	30–120 min	6 hr

Contraindications/Precautions

Contraindicated in: Previous hypersensitivity to penicillins (cross-sensitivity exists with cephalosporins and other beta-lactam antibiotics).
Use Cautiously in: Severe renal or hepatic impairment.

Interactions

Drug-Drug: Cloxacillin may ↓ effectiveness of oral contraceptive agents. **Probenecid** ↓ renal excretion and ↑ blood levels of cloxacillin (therapy may be combined for this purpose). **Neomycin** may ↓ absorption of cloxacillin. Concurrent use with **methotrexate** ↓ methotrexate elimination and ↑ risk of serious toxicity.

Route/Dosage

PO (Adults): 250–500 mg q 6 hr.
PO (Children >1 mo): 50–100 mg/kg/day divided q 6 hr up to a maximum of 4 g/day.

Availability (generic available)

Capsules: 250 mg, 500 mg. **Oral solution:** 125 mg/5 mL. **Powder for injection:** 250-mg, 500-mg, and 2-g vials.

clozapine (kloe-za-peen)

Clozaril, FazaClo

Classification
Therapeutic: antipsychotics
Pharmacologic: tricyclic dibenzodiazepines

Indications

Schizophrenia unresponsive to or intolerant of standard therapy with other antipsychotics (treatment refractory). To reduce recurrent suicidal behavior in schizophrenic patients.

Action

Binds to dopamine receptors in the CNS. Also has anticholinergic and alpha-adrenergic blocking activity. Produces fewer extrapyramidal reactions and less tardive dyskinesia than standard antipsychotics but carries high risk of hematologic abnormalities. **Therapeutic Effects:** Diminished schizophrenic behavior. Diminished suicidal behavior.

Adverse Reactions/Side Effects

CNS: NEUROLEPTIC MALIGNANT SYNDROME, SEIZURES, dizziness, sedation. **EENT:** visual disturbances. **CV:** MYOCARDITIS, hypotension, tachycardia, ECG changes, hypertension. **GI:** constipation, abdominal discomfort, dry mouth, ↑ salivation, nausea, vomiting, weight gain. **Derm:** rash, sweating. **Endo:** hyperglycemia. **Hemat:** AGRANULOCYTOSIS, LEUKOPENIA. **Neuro:** extrapyramidal reactions. **Misc:** fever.

PHYSICAL THERAPY IMPLICATIONS

Examination and Evaluation

- Watch for and report signs of neuroleptic malignant syndrome, including hyperthermia, diaphoresis, generalized muscle rigidity, altered mental status, tachycardia, changes in blood pressure (BP), and incontinence. Symptoms typically occur within 4–14 days after initiation of drug therapy, but can occur at any time during drug use.
- Be alert for new seizures or increased seizure activity, especially at the onset of drug treatment. Document the number, duration, and severity of seizures, and report these findings immediately to the physician.
- Monitor and report signs of myocarditis, including unexplained fatigue, dyspnea, tachypnea, fever, chest pain, palpitations, ECG changes (ST-T wave abnormalities), tachycardia, and other arrhythmias.

Clozapine is usually discontinued if these symptoms occur.

- Be alert for signs of agranulocytosis and leukopenia, including fever, sore throat, mucosal lesions, and signs of infection. Report these signs to the physician immediately.
- Assess motor function, and be alert for extrapyramidal symptoms. Report these symptoms immediately, especially tardive dyskinesia, as this problem may be irreversible. Common extrapyramidal symptoms include:
  - Tardive dyskinesia (uncontrolled rhythmic movement of mouth, face, and extremities, lip smacking or puckering, puffing of cheeks, uncontrolled chewing, rapid or worm-like movements of tongue).
  - Pseudoparkinsonism (shuffling gait, rigidity, tremor, pill-rolling motion, loss of balance control, difficulty speaking or swallowing, mask-like face).
  - Akathisia (restlessness or desire to keep moving).
  - Other dystonias and dyskinesias (dystonic muscle spasms, twisting motions, twitching, inability to move eyes, weakness of arms or legs).
- Assess BP and compare to normal values (See Appendix F). Report changes in BP, either a problematic decrease in BP (hypotension) or a sustained increase in BP (hypertension).
- Assess heart rate, ECG, and heart sounds, especially during exercise (See Appendices G, H). Report a rapid heart rate (tachycardia) or signs of other arrhythmias, including palpitations, chest discomfort, shortness of breath, fainting, and fatigue/weakness.
- Assess dizziness and sedation that might affect gait, balance, and other functional activities (See Appendix C). Report balance problems and functional limitations to the physician, and caution the patient and family/caregivers to guard against falls and trauma.
- Be alert for signs of hyperglycemia, including confusion, drowsiness, flushed/dry skin, fruit-like breath odor, rapid/deep breathing, polyuria, loss of appetite, and unusual thirst. Patients with diabetes mellitus should check blood glucose levels frequently.
- Periodically assess body weight and other anthropometric measures (body mass index, body composition). Report a substantial weight gain or increased body fat.

Interventions

- Guard against falls and trauma (hip fractures, head injury, and so forth) caused by drowsiness, dizziness, or extrapyramidal symptoms; implement fall-prevention strategies (See Appendix E).
- To minimize orthostatic hypotension, patient should move slowly when assuming a more upright position.
- Because of possible myocarditis and cardiac arrhythmias, use caution during aerobic exercise and endurance conditioning. Assess exercise tolerance frequently (BP, heart rate, fatigue levels), and terminate exercise immediately if any untoward responses occur (See Appendix L).
- Help patient and family/caregivers explore non-pharmacologic methods (exercise, counseling, support groups, and so forth) to reduce schizophrenic episodes and suicidal thoughts.

Patient/Client-Related Instruction

- Advise patient to avoid alcohol and other CNS depressants because of the increased risk of sedation and adverse effects.
- Instruct patient to report other problematic side effects such as severe or prolonged vision disturbances, skin reactions (rash, excessive sweating), or GI problems (nausea, vomiting, constipation, abdominal pain, dry mouth, excessive salivation).

Pharmacokinetics

Absorption: Well absorbed after oral administration.
Distribution: Rapid and extensive distribution; crosses blood-brain barrier and placenta.
Protein Binding: 95%.
Metabolism and Excretion: Mostly metabolized on first pass through the liver.
Half-life: 8–12 hr.

TIME/ACTION PROFILE (antipsychotic effect)

ROUTE	ONSET	PEAK	DURATION
PO	unknown	wks	4–12 hr

Contraindications/Precautions

Contraindicated in: Hypersensitivity; Bone marrow depression; Severe CNS depression/coma; Uncontrolled epilepsy; Granulocytopenia; Lactation: Discontinue drug or bottle feed.
Use Cautiously in: Prostatic enlargement; Angle-closure glaucoma; Malnourished patients or patients with cardiovascular, hepatic, or renal disease (use lower initial dose, titrate more slowly); Diabetes; Seizure disorder; Pedi: Children <16 yr (safety not established); Geri: ↑ risk of mortality in elderly patients treated for dementia-related psychosis.

Interactions

Drug-Drug: ↑ anticholinergic effects with other **agents having anticholinergic properties**, including **antihistamines, quinidine, disopyramide**, and **antidepressants**. Concurrent use with **SSRI antidepressants**

(especially **fluvoxamine**), **cimetidine**, **ciprofloxacin**, and **erythromycin** ↑ blood levels and risk of toxicity. ↑ CNS depression with **alcohol**, **antidepressants**, **antihistamines**, **opioid analgesics**, or **sedative/hypnotics**. ↑ hypotension with **nitrates**, acute ingestion of **alcohol**, or **antihypertensives**. ↑ risk of bone marrow suppression with **antihypertensives** or **radiation therapy**. Use with **lithium** ↑ risk of adverse CNS reactions, including seizures. **Phenytoin**, **nicotine**, and **rifampin** may ↓ levels and lead to ↓ efficacy. **Drug-Natural:** Caffeine-containing herbs (**cola nut**, **tea**, **coffee**) may ↑ serum levels and side effects. **St. John's wort** may ↓ blood levels and efficacy.

Route/Dosage

PO (Adults): 25 mg 1–2 times daily initially; ↑ by 25–50 mg/day over a period of 2 wk up to target dose of 300–450 mg/day. May ↑ by up to 100 mg/day once or twice further (not to exceed 900 mg/day). Treatment should be continued for at least 2 yr in patients with suicidal behavior.

Availability (generic available)

Tablets: 25 mg, 100 mg. **Orally disintegrating tablets (mint):** 25 mg, 100 mg.

HIGH ALERT

codeine (koe-deen)

Paveral

Classification

Therapeutic: allergy, cold, and cough remedies, antitussives, opioid analgesics
Pharmacologic: opioid agonists

Schedule II, III, IV, V (depends on content)

Indications

Management of mild-to-moderate pain. Antitussive (in smaller doses). **Unlabeled Use:** Management of diarrhea.

Action

Binds to opiate receptors in the CNS. Alters the perception of and response to painful stimuli while producing generalized CNS depression. Decreases cough reflex. Decreases GI motility. **Therapeutic Effects:** Decreased severity of pain. Suppression of the cough reflex. Relief of diarrhea.

Adverse Reactions/Side Effects

CNS: confusion, sedation, dysphoria, euphoria, floating feeling, hallucinations, headache, unusual dreams. **EENT:** blurred vision, diplopia, miosis. **Resp:** respiratory depression. **CV:** hypotension, bradycardia. **GI:** constipation, nausea, vomiting. **GU:** urinary retention. **Derm:** flushing, sweating. **Misc:** physical dependence, psychologic dependence, tolerance.

PHYSICAL THERAPY IMPLICATIONS

Examination and Evaluation

- Assess symptoms of respiratory depression, including decreased respiratory rate, confusion, bluish color of the skin and mucous membranes (cyanosis), and difficult, labored breathing (dyspnea). Monitor pulse oximetry and perform pulmonary function tests (See Appendix I) to quantify suspected changes in ventilation and respiratory function. Excessive respiratory depression requires emergency care.
- Be alert for excessive sedation or changes in mood and behavior (euphoria, dysphoria, confusion, hallucinations). Notify physician or nurse immediately if patient is unconscious or extremely difficult to arouse.
- Use appropriate pain scales (visual analogue scales, others) to document whether this drug is successful in helping manage the patient's pain.
- Assess blood pressure periodically and compare to normal values (See Appendix F). Report low blood pressure (hypotension), especially if patient experiences dizziness, fainting, or other symptoms.
- Assess heart rate, ECG, and heart sounds, especially during exercise (see Appendices G, H). Report slow heart rate (bradycardia) or symptoms of other arrhythmias, including palpitations, chest discomfort, shortness of breath, fainting, and fatigue/weakness.
- If used as a cough suppressant, assess cough and lung sounds (See Appendix K) and monitor sputum production. Document whether this drug is effective as a cough suppressant.
- If used as an antidiarrheal, monitor improvements in GI symptoms (decreased diarrhea, cramping, etc.) to help determine if drug therapy is successful.

Interventions

- Implement appropriate manual therapy techniques, physical agents, and therapeutic exercises to reduce pain and help wean patient off opioid analgesics as soon as possible.
- Because of the risk of respiratory depression, bradycardia, and hypotension, use caution during aerobic exercise and other forms of therapeutic exercise. Assess exercise tolerance frequently (blood pressure, heart rate, respiratory rate, fatigue levels), and terminate exercise immediately if any untoward responses occur (See Appendix L).
- Help patient explore other nonpharmacologic methods to reduce chronic pain, such as relaxation techniques, exercise, counseling, and so forth.
- Guard against falls and trauma (hip fractures, head injury). Implement fall-prevention strategies

(See Appendix E), especially if patient exhibits sedation, dizziness, or blurred vision.

- To minimize orthostatic hypotension, patient should move slowly when assuming a more upright position.

Patient/Client-Related Instruction

- Advise patient that opioid analgesics are usually more effective if given before pain becomes severe; emphasize that adequate pain control will allow better participation in physical therapy.
- Educate patient about the dangers of opioid overdose; encourage patient to adhere to proper dosing schedule.
- Emphasize that the risk of physical addiction (tolerance and dependence) is usually minimal during short-term treatment of pain. Advise patient that addiction is more likely during excessive or inappropriate use of opioid analgesics.
- Advise patient to avoid alcohol and other CNS depressants because of the increased risk of sedation and decreased CNS function.
- Advise patient to increase fluid intake and dietary fiber to avoid constipation. Laxatives may also be helpful in patients susceptible to fecal impaction (e.g., people with spinal cord injury).
- Instruct patient to report other troublesome side effects such as severe or prolonged headache, urinary retention, unusual dreams, excessive sweating, vision disturbances, or GI problems (nausea, vomiting).

Pharmacokinetics

Absorption: 50% absorbed from the GI tract. Completely absorbed from IM sites. Oral and parenteral doses are not equal.
Distribution: Widely distributed. Crosses the placenta; enters breast milk.
Metabolism and Excretion: Mostly metabolized by the liver; 10% converted to morphine, 5–15% excreted unchanged in urine.
Half-life: 2.5–4 hr.

TIME/ACTION PROFILE (analgesia)

ROUTE	ONSET	PEAK	DURATION
PO	30–45 min	60–120 min	4 hr
IM	10–30 min	30–60 min	4 hr
SC	10–30 min	unknown	4 hr

Contraindications/Precautions

Contraindicated in: Hypersensitivity.
Use Cautiously in: Head trauma; Increased intracranial pressure; Severe renal, hepatic, or pulmonary disease; Hypothyroidism; Adrenal insufficiency; Alcoholism; Geri: Geriatric or debilitated patients (dose reduction required; more susceptible to CNS depression, constipation); Undiagnosed abdominal pain; Prostatic hyperplasia; OB: Has been used during labor; respiratory depression may occur in the newborn; Pregnancy or lactation (avoid chronic use).

Interactions

Drug-Drug: Use with extreme caution in patients receiving **MAO inhibitors** (reduce initial dose to 25% of usual dose). Additive CNS depression with **alcohol, antidepressants, antihistamines,** and **sedative/hypnotics**. Administration of **partial antagonists (buprenorphine, butorphanol, nalbuphine,** or **pentazocine)** may precipitate opioid withdrawal in physically dependent patients. **Nalbuphine** or **pentazocine** may ↓ analgesia.
Drug-Natural: Concomitant use of **kava, valerian, skullcap, chamomile,** or **hops** can ↑ CNS depression.

Route/Dosage

PO (Adults): *Analgesic*—15–60 mg q 3–6 hr prn. *Antitussive*—10–20 mg q 4–6 hr prn (not to exceed 120 mg/day). *Antidiarrheal*—30 mg up to 4 times daily.
PO (Children 6–12 yr): *Analgesic*—0.5 mg/kg (15 mg/m^2) q 4–6 hr (up to 4 times daily) prn. *Antitussive*—5–10 mg q 4–6 hr prn (not to exceed 60 mg/day). *Antidiarrheal*—0.5 mg/kg up to 4 times daily.
PO (Children 2–5 yr): *Analgesic*—0.5 mg/kg (15 mg/m^2) q 4–6 hr (up to 4 times daily) prn. *Antitussive*—0.25 mg/kg up to 4 times daily. *Antidiarrheal*—0.5 mg/kg up to 4 times daily.
IM, IV, SC (Adults): *Analgesic*—15–60 mg q 4–6 hr prn.
IM, IV, SC (Infants and Children): *Analgesic*—0.5 mg/kg (15 mg/m^2) q 4–6 hr prn.

Availability (generic available)

Tablets: 15 mg, 30 mg, 60 mg. **Oral solution:** 10 mg/5 mL, 15 mg/5 mL. **Injection:** 30 mg/mL, 60 mg/mL. ***In combination with:*** antihistamines, decongestants, antipyretics, caffeine, butalbital, and nonopioid analgesics. See Appendix B.

HIGH ALERT

colchicine (kol-chi-seen)

Classification
Therapeutic: antigout agents

Indications

Acute attacks of gouty arthritis (larger doses). Prevention of recurrences of gout (smaller doses). **Unlabeled**

Use: Treatment of hepatic cirrhosis and familial Mediterranean fever.

Action

Interferes with the functions of WBCs in initiating and perpetuating the inflammatory response to monosodium urate crystals. **Therapeutic Effects:** Decreased pain and inflammation in acute attacks of gout. Prevention of recurrent attacks of gout.

Adverse Reactions/Side Effects

GI: diarrhea, nausea, vomiting, abdominal pain. **GU:** anuria, hematuria, renal damage. **Derm:** alopecia. **Hemat:** AGRANULOCYTOSIS, APLASTIC ANEMIA, leukopenia, thrombocytopenia. **Local:** phlebitis at IV site. **Neuro:** peripheral neuritis.

PHYSICAL THERAPY IMPLICATIONS

Examination and Evaluation

- Monitor and report signs of agranulocytosis (fever, sore throat, mucosal lesions, signs of infection, bruising) or any unusual weakness and fatigue that might be due to aplastic anemia or other anemias. Also report signs of other blood dyscrasias such as thrombocytopenia (bruising, nose bleeds, bleeding gums). Periodic blood tests may be needed to monitor WBC and RBC counts.
- Be alert for signs of kidney damage, including bloody urine (hematuria) and decreased or absent urine output. Report these signs to the physician immediately.
- Periodically assess patient's impairments (pain, range of motion), functional ability, and disability to help determine if gout symptoms are reduced by drug therapy.
- Be alert for signs of peripheral neuritis (numbness, tingling, decreased muscle strength). Establish baseline electroneuromyographic values at the beginning of drug treatment whenever possible, and reexamine these values periodically to document drug-induced changes in peripheral nerve function.
- Assess injection site during and after IV administration, and report signs of phlebitis (local pain, swelling, inflammation).

Interventions

- Implement appropriate manual therapy techniques, physical agents, therapeutic exercises, and orthotic/assistive devices to reduce pain, improve function, and augment the effects of antigout drug therapy.

Patient/Client-Related Instruction

- Instruct patient to report other untoward side effects such as problems with hair loss (alopecia) or severe or prolonged GI reactions (nausea, vomiting, diarrhea, abdominal pain).

Pharmacokinetics

Absorption: Absorbed from the GI tract, then reenters GI tract from biliary secretions, when more absorption may occur.
Distribution: Concentrates in WBCs.
Metabolism and Excretion: Partially metabolized by the liver. Secreted in bile back into GI tract; eliminated in the feces. Small amount excreted in the urine.
Half-life: 20 min (plasma), 60 hr (WBCs).

TIME/ACTION PROFILE (anti-inflammatory activity)

ROUTE	ONSET	PEAK	DURATION
PO	12 hr	24–72 hr	unknown
IV	within 6–12 hr	unknown	unknown

Contraindications/Precautions

Contraindicated in: Hypersensitivity; Pregnancy; Severe renal (CCr <10 mL/min) or GI disease.
Use Cautiously in: Elderly or debilitated patients (toxicity may be cumulative); Renal impairment (dose reduction suggested if CCr <50 mL/min; total IV dose not >2 mg); Lactation or children (safety not established).

Interactions

Drug-Drug: Additive bone marrow depression may occur with **bone marrow depressants** or **radiation therapy**. Additive adverse GI effects with **NSAIDs**. May cause reversible malabsorption of **vitamin B_1** and **vitamin B_2**. ↑ toxicity with **clarithromycin**, especially in the elderly.

Route/Dosage

PO (Adults): *Treatment of acute attacks*—0.6–1.2 mg, then 0.6 mg q 1–2 hr *or* 1–1.2 mg q 2 hr until relief, GI side effects, or a total cumulative dose of 8 mg is achieved. *Prophylaxis*—0.6 mg daily (may be used up to 3 times daily or as little as 1–4 times weekly). If surgery is planned, give 3 times daily for 3 days before and 3 days after procedure.
IV (Adults): *Treatment of acute attack*—2 mg initially, then 0.5 mg q 6 hr *or* 1 mg q 6–12 hr, until relief or cumulative dose of 4 mg has been given. Other regimens may use lower doses. *Prophylaxis*—0.5–1 mg 1–2 times daily. Other regimens may use lower doses.

Availability (generic available)

Tablets: 0.6 mg, 1 mg. **Injection:** 0.5 mg/mL in 2-mL ampules.

colesevelam (koe-le-**sev**-e-lam)

Welchol

Classification
Therapeutic: lipid-lowering agents
Pharmacologic: bile acid sequestrants

C

Indications

Adjunctive therapy to diet and exercise for the reduction of LDL cholesterol in patients with primary hypercholesterolemia; may be used alone or in combination with hepatic hydroxymethylglutaryl coenzyme A (HMG CoA) reductase inhibitor. Adjunctive therapy to diet and exercise to improve glycemic control in patients with type 2 diabetes.

Action

Binds bile acids in the GI tract. Result in increased clearance of cholesterol. Mechanism for lowering blood glucose unknown. **Therapeutic Effects:** Decreased cholesterol and blood glucose.

Adverse Reactions/Side Effects

GI: constipation, dyspepsia.

PHYSICAL THERAPY IMPLICATIONS

Examination and Evaluation

- Monitor any untoward GI responses such as constipation and indigestion. Notify physician if these responses become problematic.

Interventions

- Design and implement aerobic exercise and endurance training programs to improve cardiovascular function and glycemic control and help to reduce the risk of coronary heart disease.

Patient/Client-Related Instruction

- Remind patients to take medication as directed to control hyperlipidemia even though they are asymptomatic.
- Counsel patients about additional interventions to help control lipid disorders and improve cardiovascular health, including dietary modification, regular exercise, moderation of alcohol consumption, and smoking cessation.

Pharmacokinetics

Absorption: Not absorbed; action is primarily local in the GI tract.
Distribution: Unknown.
Metabolism and Excretion: Unknown.
Half-life: Unknown.

TIME/ACTION PROFILE (cholesterol-lowering effect)

ROUTE	ONSET	PEAK	DURATION
PO	24–48 hr	2 wk	unknown

Contraindications/Precautions

Contraindicated in: Hypersensitivity; Bowel obstruction; Triglycerides >500 mg/dL; History of pancreatitis due to hypertriglyceridemia.

Use Cautiously in: Triglycerides >300 mg/dL; Dysphagia, swallowing disorders, severe GI motility disorders, or major GI tract surgery; Pregnancy, lactation, or children (safety not established).

Interactions

Drug-Drug: May ↓ absorption of **glyburide, levothyroxine, phenytoin, estrogen-containing oral contraceptives** (give ≥4 hr before colesevelam).

Route/Dosage

PO (Adults): 3 tablets twice daily or 6 tablets once daily.

Availability

Tablets: 625 mg.

colestipol (koe-**les**-ti-pole)

Colestid

Classification
Therapeutic: lipid-lowering agents
Pharmacologic: bile acid sequestrants

Indications

Management of primary hypercholesterolemia. Pruritus associated with elevated levels of bile acids. **Unlabeled Use:** Diarrhea associated with excess bile acids.

Action

Binds bile acids in the GI tract, forming an insoluble complex. Result is increased clearance of cholesterol. **Therapeutic Effects:** Decreased plasma cholesterol and LDL. Decreased pruritus.

Adverse Reactions/Side Effects

EENT: irritation of the tongue. **GI:** abdominal discomfort, constipation, nausea, fecal impaction, flatulence, hemorrhoids, perianal irritation, steatorrhea, vomiting. **Derm:** irritation, rashes. **F and E:** hyperchloremic acidosis. **Metab:** vitamins A, D, and K deficiency.

PHYSICAL THERAPY IMPLICATIONS

Examination and Evaluation

- Monitor signs of hyperchloremic acidosis, including headache, lethargy, stupor, seizures, vision disturbances, increased respiration, cardiac arrhythmias, weakness, and GI symptoms (nausea, vomiting, abdominal pain). Notify physician immediately if these signs occur.
- Monitor signs of vitamin deficiencies, including deficiencies of vitamin A (vision disturbances, poor night vision), vitamin D (bone pain, muscle weakness, hypertension), and vitamin K (bleeding

gums, nosebleeds, bruising). Notify physician if these signs persist.

Interventions

- Design and implement aerobic exercise and endurance training programs to improve cardiovascular function and help reduce the risk of coronary heart disease.

Patient/Client-Related Instruction

- Remind patients to take medication as directed to control hyperlipidemia even though they are asymptomatic.
- Counsel patients about additional interventions to help control lipid disorders and improve cardiovascular health, including dietary modification, regular exercise, moderation of alcohol consumption, and smoking cessation.
- Advise patient about the likelihood of GI problems, including nausea, constipation, abdominal pain, flatulence, oily/foul-smelling stools, hemorrhoids, and fecal impaction. Instruct patient to report severe or prolonged GI reactions.
- Instruct patient and family/caregivers to report other troublesome side effects such as severe or prolonged tongue irritation or skin reactions (rash, irritation).

Pharmacokinetics

Absorption: Action takes place in the GI tract. No absorption occurs.
Distribution: No distribution.
Metabolism and Excretion: After binding bile acids, insoluble complex is eliminated in the feces.
Half-life: Unknown.

TIME/ACTION PROFILE (hypocholesterolemic effects)

ROUTE	ONSET	PEAK	DURATION
PO	24–48 hr	1 mo	1 mo

Contraindications/Precautions

Contraindicated in: Hypersensitivity; Complete biliary obstruction; Some products contain aspartame and should be avoided in patients with phenylketonuria.
Use Cautiously in: History of constipation.
Exercise Extreme Caution in: Pedi: May cause potentially fatal intestinal obstruction in children.

Interactions

Drug-Drug: May decrease absorption/effects of orally administered **acetaminophen, amiodarone, clindamycin, clofibrate, digoxin, diuretics, gemfibrozil, glipizide, corticosteroids, imipramine, mycophenolate, methotrexate, methyldopa, niacin, NSAIDs, penicillin, phenytoin, phosphates, propranolol, tetracyclines, tolbutamide, thyroid preparations, ursodiol, warfarin,** and **fat-soluble vitamins (A, D, E, and K)**. May decrease absorption of other **orally administered medications**.

Route/Dosage

PO (Adults): *Granules*—5 g 1–2 times daily; may be increased q 1–2 mo up to 30 g/day in 1–2 doses. *Tablets*—2 g 1–2 times daily; may be increased q 1–2 mo up to 16 g/day in 1–2 doses.

Availability

Granules for suspension (unflavored): 5 g/packet or scoop. **Flavored granules for suspension with aspartame (orange flavor):** 5 g/packet or scoop. **Tablets:** 1 g.

collagenase clostridium histolyticum (kol-**laj**-en-ase kloss-**trid**-ee-yum **his**-toe-**lit**-i-cum)

Xiaflex

Classification
Therapeutic: none assigned

Indications

Treatment of Dupuytren's contracture with a palpable cord in adults.

Action

Lysis of collagen deposits present in Dupuytren's cord. **Therapeutic Effects:** Enzymatic disruption of Dupuytren's cord.

Adverse Reactions/Side Effects

CV: vasovagal syncope. **MS:** ligament injury, complex regional pain syndrome (CRPS), sensory abnormality of hand, tendon rupture. **Local:** contusion, hemorrhage, injection site reaction, pain, pruritus, swelling. **Misc:** ALLERGIC REACTIONS, INCLUDING ANAPHYLAXIS, axillary pain, lymphadenopathy.

PHYSICAL THERAPY IMPLICATIONS

Examination and Evaluation

- Watch for signs of allergic reactions and anaphylaxis, including pulmonary symptoms (tightness in the throat and chest, wheezing, cough, dyspnea), or skin reactions (rash, pruritus, urticaria). Notify physician immediately if these reactions occur.
- Be alert for fainting (vasovagal syncope) that occurs after injection or during treatment of the affected hand. Be ready to protect the patient from falls and trauma that might occur because of syncope during treatment sessions.
- Assess injection site for pain, swelling, itching, inflammation, or signs of contusion and hemorrhage. Report prolonged or excessive injection site reactions to the physician.

Interventions

- Implement appropriate therapeutic exercises to increase ROM and strength in the affected tendon.

Use caution, however, and monitor continually for any increased tendon symptoms, localized pain, or sensory loss in the hand. If symptoms increase, notify the physician and protect the affected area to avoid tendon ruptures. Do not stretch or exercise the affected tendon until the hand has been reexamined.

Patient/Client-Related Instruction

- Instruct patient to report other troublesome side effects such as severe or prolonged axillary pain or swollen lymph nodes.

Pharmacokinetics

Absorption: Unknown.
Distribution: Unknown.
Metabolism and Excretion: Unknown.
Half-life: Unknown.

TIME/ACTION PROFILE (cord disruption)

ROUTE	ONSET	PEAK	DURATION
Intralesional	within 24 hr	unknown	unknown

Contraindications/Precautions

Contraindicated in: None known.
Use Cautiously in: Abnormal coagulation, including concurrent anticoagulants other than low-dose aspirin within 7 days of treatment; OB: Use only if clearly needed; Lactation: Use cautiously; Pedi: Safety and effectiveness not established.

Interactions

Drug-Drug: Concurrent use of **anticoagulants** may ↑ risk of local bleeding.

Route/Dosage

IL (Adults): 0.58 mg into a palpable cord with a contracture of a metacarpophalangeal (MP) joint or a proximal interphalangeal (PIP) joint.

Availability

Lyophilized powder for injection (requires reconstitution): 0.9 mg/vial (delivers 0.58 mg/dose).

conivaptan (con-i-vap-tan)

Vaprisol

Classification
Therapeutic: electrolyte modifiers
Pharmacologic: vasopressin receptor antagonists

Indications

Euvolemic hyponatremia, which may be due to inappropriate secretion of antidiuretic hormone, hypothyroidism, adrenal insufficiency, or pulmonary disorders. Treatment of hypervolemic hyponatremia in hospitalized patients.

Action

Antagonizes vasopressin at V_2 receptor sites in renal collecting ducts, resulting in excretion of free water. **Therapeutic Effects:** Restoration of normal fluid and electrolyte status.

Adverse Reactions/Side Effects

CNS: headache, confusion, insomnia. **CV:** hypertension, hypotension. **GI:** diarrhea. **GU:** polyuria. **F and E:** dehydration, hypokalemia, hypomagnesemia, hyponatremia. **Local:** injections site reactions. **Misc:** fever, thirst.

PHYSICAL THERAPY IMPLICATIONS

Examination and Evaluation

- Monitor neuromuscular signs of fluid and electrolyte imbalances, including low levels of sodium (hyponatremia), potassium (hypokalemia), and magnesium (hypomagnesemia). Signs of imbalances include headache, confusion, lethargy, irritability, weakness, muscle cramping, and muscle hyperexcitability and tetany. Notify physician immediately if these signs occur.
- Assess blood pressure (BP) and compare to normal values (See Appendix F). Report changes in BP, either a problematic decrease in BP (hypotension) or a sustained increase in BP (hypertension).
- Monitor IV injection site for pain, swelling, and irritation. Report prolonged or excessive injection site reactions to the physician.

Interventions

- Make sure patient maintains adequate fluid intake to avoid dehydration, especially during exercise.

Patient/Client-Related Instruction

- Instruct patient and family/caregivers to maintain adequate fluid intake and avoid dehydration.
- Instruct patient and family/caregivers to report other troublesome side effects such as severe or prolonged headache, sleep loss, fever, increased urination, or diarrhea.

Pharmacokinetics

Absorption: IV administration results in complete bioavailability.
Distribution: Unknown.
Protein Binding: 99% protein bound.
Metabolism and Excretion: Metabolized solely by the CYP3A4 enzyme system. 83% excreted in feces as metabolites, 12% in urine (as metabolites).
Half-life: 5 hr.

TIME/ACTION PROFILE

ROUTE	ONSET	PEAK	DURATION
IV	unknown	12 hr	end of infusion

Contraindications/Precautions

Contraindicated in: Hypersensitivity; Hypovolemic hyponatremia; Concurrent use of ketoconazole, itraconazole, clarithromycin, ritonavir, or indinavir.

Use Cautiously in: Impaired hepatic or renal function; OB: Pregnancy and lactation (safety not established); Pedi: Children (safety not established).

Interactions

Drug-Drug: Blood levels and effects are ↑ by **ketoconazole**, **itraconazole**, **clarithromycin**, **ritonavir**, or **indinavir** (concurrent use is contraindicated). ↑ blood levels and may ↑ effects of **midazolam**, **simvastatin**, **amlodipine**, and **other drugs metabolized by CYP3A4**; careful monitoring recommended. May also ↑ **digoxin** levels.

Route/Dosage

IV (Adults): 20 mg loading dose initially, followed by 20 mg/day as a continuous infusion.

Availability

Solution for IV administration (must be diluted): 20 mg/4-mL ampule.

CONTRACEPTIVES, HORMONAL

MONOPHASIC ORAL CONTRACEPTIVES

ethinyl estradiol/desogestrel
(**eth**-in-il es-tra-**dye**-ole/dess-oh-**jes**-trel)
Apri 28, Desogen, Ortho-Cept, Reclipsen, Solia

ethinyl estradiol/drospirenone
(**eth**-in-il es-tra-**dye**-ole/droe-**spy**-re-nown)
Yasmin, Yaz

ethinyl estradiol/ethynodiol
(**eth**-in-il es-tra-**dye**-ole/eth-e-noe-**dye**-ole)
Kelnor 1/35, Zovia 1/35, Zovia 1/50

ethinyl estradiol/levonorgestrel
(**eth**-in-il es-tra-**dye**-ole/lee-voe-nor-**jes**-trel)
Alesse-28, Aviane-28, Lessina-28, Levlen-28, Levlite-28, Levora-28, Lutera, Nordette-28, Portia-28, Sronyx

ethinyl estradiol/norethindrone
(**eth**-in-il es-tra-**dye**-ole/nor-eth-**in**-drone)
Balziva, Brevicon, Femcon Fe, Junel 21 1/20, Junel 21 1.5/20, Junel Fe 1/20, Junel Fe 1.5/30, Loestrin 21 1/20, Loestrin 21 1.5/30, Loestrin Fe 1/20, Loestrin Fe 1.5/30, Microgestin Fe 1/20, Modicon, Necon 0.5/35, Necon 1/35, Norethin 1/35E, Norinyl 1+35, Nortrel 0.5/35, Nortrel 1/35, Ortho-Novum 1/35, Ovcon 35, Ovcon 50, Zenchant

ethinyl estradiol/norgestimate
(**eth**-in-il es-tra-**dye**-ole/nor-**jest**-i-mate)
MonoNessa, Ortho-Cyclen, Previfem, Sprintec

ethinyl estradiol/norgestrel
(**eth**-in-il es-tra-**dye**-ole/nor-**jess**-trel)
Cryselle, Lo/Ovral 28, Low-Ogestrel 28, Ogestrel 28

mestranol/norethindrone
(**mes**-tra-nole/nor-eth-**in**-drone)
Necon 1/50, Norethin 1/50M, Norinyl 1+50, Ortho-Novum 1/50

BIPHASIC ORAL CONTRACEPTIVES

ethinyl estradiol/desogestrel
(**eth**-in-il es-tra-**dye**-ole/dess-oh-**jes**-trel)
Kariva, Mircette

ethinyl estradiol/norethindrone
(**eth**-in-il es-tra-**dye**-ole/nor-eth-**in**-drone)
Necon 10/11, Ortho-Novum 10/11

TRIPHASIC ORAL CONTRACEPTIVES

ethinyl estradiol/desogestrel
(**eth**-in-il es-tra-**dye**-ole/dess-oh-**jes**-trel)
Cesia, Cyclessa, Velivet

ethinyl estradiol/levonorgestrel
(**eth**-in-il es-tra-**dye**-ole/lee-voe-nor-**jes**-trel)
Enpresse, Tri-Levlen, Triphasil 28, Trivora 28

ethinyl estradiol/norethindrone
(**eth**-in-il es-tra-**dye**-ole/nor-eth-**in**-drone)
Aranelle, Leena, Necon 7/7/7, Nortrel 7/7/7, Ortho-Novum 7/7/7, Tri-Norinyl

C

ethinyl estradiol/norgestimate
(**eth**-in-il es-tra-**dye**-ole/nor-**jes**-ti-mate)
Ortho Tri-Cyclen, Ortho Tri-Cyclen Lo, Tri-Nessa, Tri-Previfem, Tri-Sprintec

EXTENDED-CYCLE ORAL CONTRACEPTIVE
ethinyl estradiol/levonorgestrel
(**eth**-in-il es-tra-**dye**-ole/lee-voe-nor-**jes**-trel)
Lybrel, Seasonale, Seasonique

PROGESTIN-ONLY ORAL CONTRACEPTIVES
norethindrone (nor-eth-**in**-drone)
Errin, Camila, Jolivette, Micronor, Nor-Q D

PROGRESSIVE ESTROGEN ORAL CONTRACEPTIVES
norethindrone/ethinyl acetate
(nor-eth-**in**-drone/**eth**-in-il **as**-e-tate)
Estrostep, Estrostep Fe

CONTRACEPTIVE IMPLANT
etonogestrel (e-toe-noe-**jes**-trel)
Implanon

EMERGENCY CONTRACEPTIVE
levonorgestrel (**lee**-voe-nor-jes-trel)
Plan B

INJECTABLE CONTRACEPTIVE
medroxyprogesterone
(**me-drox**-ee-proe-jes-te-rone)
Depo-Provera, Depo-subQ Provera 104

INTRAUTERINE CONTRACEPTIVE
levonorgestrel (**lee**-voe-nor-jes-trel)
Mirena

Vaginal Ring Contraceptive
ethinyl estradiol/etonogestrel
(**eth**-in-il es-tra-**dye**-ole/e-toe-noe-**jes**-trel)
NuvaRing

Transdermal Contraceptive
ethinyl estradiol/norelgestromin
(**eth**-in-il es-tra-**dye**-ole/nor-el-**jes**-troe-min)
Ortho Evra

Classification
Therapeutic: contraceptive hormones

Indications

Prevention of pregnancy. Regulation of menstrual cycle. Emergency contraception (some products). Treatment of premenstrual dysphoric disorder (Yaz, Yasmin). Management of acne in women >14 yr who desire contraception, have no health problems, and have failed topical treatment.

Action

Monophasic Oral Contraceptives: Provide a fixed dosage of estrogen/progestin over a 21-day cycle. Ovulation is inhibited by suppression of follicle-stimulating hormone (FSH) and luteinizing hormone (LH). May alter cervical mucus and the endometrial environment, preventing penetration by sperm and implantation of the egg. **Biphasic Oral Contraceptives:** Ovulation is inhibited by suppression of FSH and LH. May alter cervical mucus and the endometrial environment, preventing penetration by sperm and implantation of the egg. In addition, smaller dose of progestin in phase 1 allows for proliferation of endometrium. Larger amount in phase 2 allows for adequate secretory development. **Triphasic Oral Contraceptives:** Ovulation is inhibited by suppression of FSH and LH. May alter cervical mucus and the endometrial environment, preventing penetration by sperm and implantation of the egg. Varying doses of estrogen/progestin may more closely mimic natural hormonal fluctuations. **Extended-cycle:** Provides continuous estrogen/progestin for 84 days (365 days for Lybrel), then off for 7 days, resulting in 4 menstrual periods/year (no periods/year for Lybrel). **Progressive Estrogen:** Contains constant amount of progestin with 3 progressive doses of estrogen. **Progestin-Only Contraceptives/Contraceptive Implant/Intrauterine Levonorgestrel/ Medroxyprogesterone Injection:** Mechanism not clearly known. May alter cervical mucus and the endometrial environment, preventing penetration by sperm and implantation of the egg. Ovulation may also be suppressed. **Emergency Contraceptive Pills (ECPs):** Inhibit ovulation/fertilization; may also alter tubal transport of sperm/egg and prevent implantation. **Vaginal Ring, Transdermal Patch:** Inhibits ovulation, decreases sperm entry into uterus, and decreases likelihood of implantation. **Antiacne effect:** Combination of estrogen/progestin may increase sex hormone binding globulin (SHBG) resulting in decreased unbound testosterone, which may be a cause of acne. **Therapeutic Effects:** Prevention of pregnancy. Decreased severity of acne. Decrease in premenstrual dysphoric disorder.

Adverse Reactions/Side Effects

CNS: depression, migraine headache. **EENT:** contact lens intolerance, optic neuritis, retinal thrombosis. **CV:** CEREBRAL HEMORRHAGE, CEREBRAL THROMBOSIS, CORONARY THROMBOSIS, PULMONARY EMBOLISM, edema, hypertension, Raynaud's phenomenon, thromboembolic phenomena, thrombophlebitis. **GI:** abdominal cramps, bloating, cholestatic jaundice, gallbladder disease, liver tumors, nausea, vomiting. **GU:** amenorrhea, breakthrough bleeding, dysmenorrhea, spotting, *Intrauterine levonorgestrel only*—uterine embedment/uterine rupture. **Derm:** melasma, rash. **Endo:** hyperglycemia. **MS:** *Injectable medroxyprogesterone only*—bone loss. **Misc:** weight change.

PHYSICAL THERAPY IMPLICATIONS

Examination and Evaluation

- Monitor continually, and seek immediate medical assistance if patient develops any of the following signs or syndromes:
  - Cerebral hemorrhage or thrombosis, as indicated by severe headache, confusion, nausea, vomiting, paralysis, numbness, speech problems, and visual disturbances.
  - Coronary thrombosis, as indicated by sudden chest pain, pain radiating into the arm or jaw, shortness of breath, dizziness, sweating, anxiety, and nausea.
  - Pulmonary embolism, as indicated by shortness of breath, chest pain, cough, and bloody sputum.
- Assess any signs of thrombophlebitis, including localized pain, redness, or swelling in the affected area. Report these signs to the physician.
- Assess blood pressure periodically. Report a sustained increase in blood pressure (hypertension) to the physician.
- Assess peripheral edema using girth measurements, volume displacement, and measurement of pitting edema (See Appendix N). Report increased swelling in feet and ankles or a sudden increase in body weight due to fluid retention.
- Be alert for signs of hyperglycemia, including confusion, drowsiness, flushed/dry skin, fruit-like breath odor, rapid/deep breathing, polyuria, loss of appetite, and unusual thirst. Patients with diabetes mellitus should check blood glucose levels frequently.
- Monitor signs of Raynaud's phenomenon as indicated by decreased circulation to the fingers and toes resulting in pain, numbness, swelling, and color changes in the affected digits. Report these signs to the physician, and educate patient about how to avoid the onset of symptoms (keep hands warm, avoid caffeine, stress, and other triggers).
- Periodically assess body weight and other anthropometric measures (body mass index, body composition). Report any rapid or unexplained changes in body weight gain or percentage body fat.

Interventions

- Because of the risk of thrombosis and thromboembolism, use caution during aerobic exercise and other forms of therapeutic exercise. Assess exercise tolerance frequently (blood pressure, heart rate, fatigue levels), and terminate exercise immediately if any untoward responses occur (See Appendix L).
- If administered via local injection, implant, or patches, do not apply massage or physical agents (heat, cold, electrotherapeutic modalities) at or near the application site.

Patient/Client-Related Instruction

- Caution patient and family/caregivers about risks of coronary thrombosis, stroke, and thromboembolism, and review warning signs of these problems (see above under Evaluation and Examination).
- Caution patient that cigarette smoking while taking contraceptives may increase the risk of infarction and thromboembolic disease, especially for women older than age 35.
- Advise women about possible changes in menstrual function. Instruct patient to notify health care professional about any abnormal bleeding or unexpected disruption of menstrual cycles.
- Advise patient about the likelihood of GI reactions, including nausea, vomiting, bloating, and abdominal cramps. Instruct patient to report severe or prolonged GI problems.
- Instruct patient to report other troublesome side effects such as severe or prolonged depression, vision disturbances, migraine headaches, or skin disorders (rash, discoloration).

Pharmacokinetics

Absorption: *Ethinyl estradiol*—rapidly absorbed; *norethindrone*—65% absorbed; *Desogestrel and levonorgestrel*—100% absorbed. Others are well absorbed after oral administration. Slowly absorbed from implant, subcutaneous or IM injection. Some absorption follows intrauterine implantation.
Distribution: Unknown.
Protein Binding: *Ethinyl estradiol*—97–98%. *Drospirenone*—97%.
Metabolism and Excretion: *Ethinyl estradiol and norethindrone*—undergo extensive first-pass hepatic

metabolism. *Mestranol*—is rapidly converted to ethinyl estradiol. *Desogestrel*—is rapidly metabolized to 3-keto-desogestgrel, the active metabolite. Most agents are metabolized by the liver.
Half-life: *Ethinyl estradiol*—6–20 hr; *Levonorgestrel*—45 hr; *Norethindrone*—5–14 hr; *Desogestrel (metabolite)*—38 ± 20 hr; *Drospirenone*—30 hr; *Norgestimate (metabolite)*—12–20 hr; *others*—unknown.

TIME/ACTION PROFILE (prevention of pregnancy)

ROUTE	ONSET	PEAK	DURATION
PO	1 mo	1 mo	1 mo*
implant	1 mo	1 mo	5 yr
intrauterine system	1 mo	1 mo	3 yr
IM	1 mo	1 mo	3 mo
SC	unknown	1 wk	3 mo

*Only during month of taking contraceptive.

Contraindications/Precautions

Contraindicated in: Pregnancy; History of thromboembolic disease (e.g., DVT, PE, MI, stroke); Valvular heart disease; Major surgery with extended periods of immobility; Diabetes with vascular involvement; Headache with focal neurologic symptoms; Uncontrolled hypertension; History of breast, endometrial, or estrogen-dependent cancer; Abnormal genital bleeding; Liver disease; Hypersensitivity to parabens (injectable only); *Intrauterine levonorgestrel only*—Intrauterine anomaly, postpartum endometriosis, multiple sexual partners, pelvic inflammatory disease, liver disease, genital actinomycosis, immunosuppression, IV drug abuse, untreated genitourinary infection, history of ectopic pregnancy; Some products contain tartrazine and should be avoided in patients with known hypersensitivity intolerance; Lactation: Avoid use.
Use Cautiously in: History of cigarette smoking or age >30–35 yr (increased risk of cardiovascular or thromboembolic phenomenon); Presence of other cardiovascular risk factors (obesity, hyperglycemia, elevated lipids, hypertension); History of diabetes mellitus, bleeding disorders, concurrent anticoagulant therapy or headaches; Pedi: Should not be used before menarche.

Interactions

Drug-Drug: Oral contraceptive efficacy may be ↓ by **penicillins**, **chloramphenicol**, **barbiturates**, chronic **alcohol** use, **carbamazepine**, **oxcarbazepine**, **felbamate**, systemic **corticosteroids**, **phenytoin**, **topiramate**, **primidone**, **modafinil**, **rifampin**, **rifabutin**, some **protease inhibitor antiretrovirals** (including **ritonavir**), or **tetracyclines**. May ↑ effects/risk of toxicity of some **benzodiazepines**, **beta blockers**, **corticosteroids**, **cyclosporine**, and **theophylline**. ↑ risk of hepatic toxicity with **dantrolene** (estrogen only). **Indinavir**, **itraconazole**, **ketoconazole**, **fluconazole**, and **atorvastatin** may ↑ effects/risk of toxicity. **Smoking** ↑ risk of thromboembolic phenomena (estrogen only). May ↓ levels of **acetaminophen**, **temazepam**, **lamotrigine**, **lorazepam**, **oxazepam**, or **morphine**. *Drospirenone—containing products only*—concurrent use with **NSAIDs**, **potassium-sparing diuretics**, **potassium supplements**, **ACE inhibitors**, or **angiotensin II receptor antagonists** may result in hyperkalemia.
Drug-Natural: Concomitant use with **St. John's wort** may ↓ contraceptive efficacy and cause breakthrough bleeding and irregular menses.

Route/Dosage

Monophasic Oral Contraceptives

PO (Adults): On 21-day regimen, take first tablet on first Sunday after menses begin (take on Sunday if menses begin on Sunday) for 21 days, then skip 7 days and begin again. Regimen may also be started on first day of menses, continue for 21 days, then skip 7 days and begin again. Some regimens contain 7 placebo tablets, so that 1 tablet is taken every day for 28 days.

Biphasic Oral Contraceptives

PO (Adults): Given in 2 phases. First phase is 10 days of smaller amount of progestin. Second phase is larger amount of progestin. Amount of estrogen remains constant for same length of time (total of 21 days), then skip 7 days and begin again. Some regimens contain 7 placebo tablets for 28-day regimen.

Triphasic Oral Contraceptives

PO (Adults): Progestin amount varies throughout 21-day cycle. Estrogen component stays the same or may vary. Some regimens contain 7 placebo tablets for 28-day regimen.

Extended-Cycle Contraceptive

PO (Adults): *Seasonale and Seasonique*—Start taking first active pill on first Sunday after menses start (if first day is Sunday, start then), continue for 84 days of active pill, followed by 7 days of placebo tablets, then resume 84/7 cycle again. *Lybre*—Begin taking the first pill during the first day of the menstrual cycle and start the next pack the day after the previous pack ends.

Progestin-Only Oral Contraceptives

PO (Adults): Start on first day of menses. Taken daily and continuously.

Progressive Estrogen Oral Contraceptives
PO (Adults): Estrogen amount increases q 7 days throughout 21-day cycle. Progestin component stays the same. Some regimens contain 7 placebo tablets for 28-day regimen.

Emergency Contraceptive
PO (Adults and Adolescents): Given within 72 hr of unprotected intercourse and repeated 12 hr later. *Plan B*—1 tablet followed by 1 more tablet 12 hr later; *Ovral*—2 white tablets followed by 2 more white tablets 12 hr later; *Lo/Ovral*—4 white tablets followed by 4 more white tablets 12 hr later; *Levlen, Nordette*—4 light orange tablets followed by 4 more light orange tablets 12 hr later; *Triphasil, Tri-Levlen*—4 yellow tablets followed by 4 more yellow tablets 12 hr later.

Injectable Contraceptive
medroxyprogesterone (Depo-Provera)
IM (Adults): 150 mg within first 5 days of menses or within 5 days postpartum, if not breast-feeding. If breast-feeding, give 6 wk postpartum; repeat q 3 mo.

medroxyprogesterone (Depo-Sub Q Provera 104)
SC (Adults): 104 mg within first 5 days of menses or within 5 days postpartum if not breast-feeding. If breast-feeding, give 6 wk postpartum; repeat q 12–14 wk.

Vaginal Ring Contraceptive
Vaginal (Adults): 1 ring inserted on or prior to day 5 of menstrual cycle. Ring is left in place for 3 wk, then removed for 1 wk, then a new ring is inserted.

Transdermal Patch
Transdermal (Adults): Patch is applied on day 1 of menstrual cycle (or convenient day in first week), changed weekly thereafter for 3 weeks. Week 4 is patch-free. Cycle is then repeated.

Acne
PO (Adults): Ortho Tri-Cyclen only, taken daily for 21 days, off for 7 days.

Availability
Combination Estrogen/Progestin Oral Contraceptives (generic available)
Oral contraceptive tablets: Usually in monthly packs with enough (21) active tablets to complete a 28-day cycle. Some contain 7 inert tablets to complete the cycle with or without supplemental iron.

Extended-Cycle Contraceptive
Tablets: Seasonale—84 active tablets containing 0.03 mg ethinyl estradiol and 0.15 mg levonorgestrel and 7 inactive tablets. Seasonique—active tablets containing 0.03 mg ethinyl estradiol, 0.15 mg levonorgestrel, and 7 inactive tablets containing 0.01 mg ethinyl estradiol. Lybrel—28 active tablets containing 0.09 mg levonorgestrel and 0.02 mg ethinyl estradiol.

Levonorgestrel
Emergency contraceptives: 2 tablets containing 0.75 mg levonorgestrel (Plan B). **Implant:** Rod contains 68 mg etonogestrel. **Intrauterine system:** contains 52 mg levonorgestrel (releases 20 mcg/day).

Medroxyprogesterone
Injectable IM: 150 mg/mL. **Injectable Subcutaneous:** 104 mg/0.65 mL (in prefilled syringes).

Vaginal Ring Contraceptive
Ring: delivers 0.015 mg ethinyl estradiol and 0.120 mg etonogestrel/day.

Transdermal Patch
Patch: contains 0.75 mg ethinyl estradiol and 6 mg of norelgestromin; releases 20 mg ethinyl estradiol/150 mg norelgestromin per 24 hr.

cortisone (kor-ti-sone)
✱Cortone

Classification
Therapeutic: anti-inflammatories (steroidal)
Pharmacologic: corticosteroids

Indications
Management of adrenocortical insufficiency; chronic use in other situations is limited because of mineralocorticoid activity. Replacement therapy in adrenal insufficiency.

Action
In pharmacologic doses, suppresses inflammation and the normal immune response. Numerous intense metabolic effects (see Adverse Reactions/Side Effects). Suppresses adrenal function at chronic doses of 20 mg/day. Replaces endogenous cortisol in deficiency states. Also has potent mineralocorticoid (sodium-retaining) activity. **Therapeutic Effects:** Suppression of inflammation and modification of the normal immune response. Replacement therapy in adrenal insufficiency.

Adverse Reactions/Side Effects
Adverse reactions/side effects are much more common with high-dose/long-term therapy
CNS: depression, euphoria, headache, increased intracranial pressure (children only), personality changes, psychoses, restlessness. **EENT:** cataracts, increased intraocular pressure. **CV:** hypertension. **GI:** PEPTIC ULCERATION, anorexia, nausea, vomiting. **Derm:** acne, decreased wound healing, ecchymoses, fragility, hirsutism, petechiae. **Endo:** adrenal suppression, hyperglycemia. **F and E:** fluid retention (long-term

high doses), hypokalemia, hypokalemic alkalosis. **Hemat:** THROMBOEMBOLISM, thrombophlebitis. **Metab:** weight gain, weight loss. **MS:** muscle wasting, osteoporosis, aseptic necrosis of joints, muscle pain. **Misc:** cushingoid appearance (moon face, buffalo hump), increased susceptibility to infection.

PHYSICAL THERAPY IMPLICATIONS

Examination and Evaluation

- Monitor signs of thrombophlebitis (lower extremity swelling, warmth, erythema, tenderness) and thromboembolism (shortness of breath, chest pain, cough, bloody sputum). Notify physician immediately, and request objective tests (Doppler ultrasound, lung scan, others) if thrombosis is suspected.
- Monitor and report signs of peptic ulcer, including heartburn, nausea, vomiting blood, tarry stools, and loss of appetite.
- Assess any muscle or joint pain. Report persistent or increased musculoskeletal pain to determine presence of bone or joint pathology (aseptic necrosis, fracture).
- Assess muscle strength periodically to determine degree of muscle wasting during long-term use.
- Measure blood pressure periodically and compare to normal values (See Appendix F). Report a sustained increase in blood pressure (hypertension) to the physician.
- Assess peripheral edema using girth measurements, volume displacement, and measurement of pitting edema (See Appendix N). Report increased swelling in feet and ankles or a sudden increase in body weight due to fluid retention.
- Monitor personality changes, including depression, euphoria, hallucinations, and psychosis. Notify physician if these changes become problematic.
- Be alert for signs of low potassium levels (hypokalemia) and metabolic acidosis, including hyperventilation, cardiac arrhythmias, dizziness, and confusion. Notify physician immediately if these signs occur.
- Report signs of adrenal suppression, including hypotension, weight loss, weakness, nausea, vomiting, anorexia, lethargy, confusion, and restlessness.
- Monitor signs of hyperglycemia (confusion; drowsiness; flushed, dry skin; fruit-like breath odor; rapid, deep breathing; polyuria; loss of appetite; unusual thirst). Insulin dosages may need to be adjusted to prevent repeated episodes of hyperglycemia.
- Periodically assess body weight and other anthropometric measures (body mass index, body composition). Report a rapid or unexplained weight gain or weight loss.

Interventions

- Implement resistive exercises and weight-bearing activities to minimize muscle wasting and osteoporosis. Use caution to prevent musculoskeletal damage in patients with preexisting muscle and bone loss.
- Protect skin from breakdown, especially over bony prominences.

Patient/Client-Related Instruction

- Advise patient that wound healing may be delayed; instruct patient to check skin regularly and report any nonhealing sores.
- Advise patient that corticosteroids cause immunosuppression and may mask symptoms of infection. Instruct patient to avoid people with known contagious illnesses and to report possible infections immediately.
- Advise patients on long-term treatment to consult physician before stopping this medication. Stopping the medication suddenly may result in adrenocortical shock (severe hypotension, hypoglycemia, weakness, vomiting). If these signs appear, notify health care professional immediately; may be life threatening.
- Instruct patient to report any loss of vision that might indicate cataracts or increased intraocular pressure.
- Advise patient about possible cushingoid appearance, including puffiness in the face (moon face), increased fat in the torso, thin arms and legs, abdominal skin striations, bruising, and deposition of fat at the posterior base of the neck (buffalo hump). Discuss possible effects on body image, and help patient explore coping mechanisms.
- Instruct patient and family/caregivers to report other troublesome side effects such as severe or prolonged headache or skin reactions (acne, hair growth).

Pharmacokinetics

Absorption: Well absorbed after oral administration.
Distribution: Widely distributed; crosses the placenta and enters breast milk.
Metabolism and Excretion: Metabolized mostly by the liver to inactive metabolites.
Half-life: 0.5–2 hr (plasma), 8–12 hr (tissue).

TIME/ACTION PROFILE (anti-inflammatory activity)

ROUTE	ONSET	PEAK	DURATION
PO	rapid	2 hr	1.25–1.5 days

Contraindications/Precautions

Contraindicated in: Active untreated infections (may be used in patients being treated for tuberculous meningitis); Lactation (avoid chronic use).

Use Cautiously in: Chronic treatment (will lead to adrenal suppression; use lowest possible dose for shortest period of time), unless being used to treat adrenal insufficiency; Stress (surgery, infections); supplemental doses may be needed; Hypothyroidism; Cirrhosis; Ulcerative colitis; Potential infections may mask signs (fever, inflammation); OB: Safety not established; Pedi: Chronic use will result in decreased growth; use lowest possible dose for shortest period of time.

Interactions

Drug-Drug: Additive hypokalemia with **thiazide, loop diuretics**, or **amphotericin B**. Hypokalemia may ↑ risk of **digitalis glycoside** toxicity. May ↑ requirement for **insulins** or **oral hypoglycemic agents**. **Phenytoin, phenobarbital**, and **rifampin** stimulate metabolism; may ↓ effectiveness. **Oral contraceptives** may block metabolism. ↑ risk of adverse GI effects with **NSAIDs** (including aspirin). At chronic doses that suppress adrenal function, may ↓ antibody response to and ↑ the risk of adverse reactions from **live-virus vaccines**.

Route/Dosage

PO (Adults): 25–300 mg/day in divided doses q 12–24 hr.

PO (Children): *Adrenocortical insufficiency*—0.7 mg/kg/day (20–25 mg/m²/day) in divided doses q 8 hr. *Other uses*—2.5–10 mg/kg/day (75–300 mg/m²/day) in divided doses q 6–8 hr.

Availability (generic available)

Tablets: 25 mg.

cromolyn (kroe-moe-lin)

✱ Apo-Cromolyn, Intal, Gastrocrom, NasalCrom

Classification

Therapeutic: antiasthmatics, allergy, cold, and cough remedies

Pharmacologic: mast cell stabilizers

Indications

Inhalation: Prophylaxis (long-term control) of bronchial asthma. Prevention of exercise-induced bronchospasm. **Intranasal:** Prevention and treatment of seasonal and perennial allergic rhinitis. **PO:** Mastocytosis. Treatment of food allergy. Treatment of inflammatory bowel disease.

Action

Prevents the release of histamine and slow-reacting substance of anaphylaxis (SRS-A) from sensitized mast cells. **Therapeutic Effects:** Decreased frequency and intensity of asthmatic episodes or allergic reactions.

Adverse Reactions/Side Effects

CNS: dizziness, headache. **Derm:** rash, urticaria, angioedema. **EENT: intranasal:** nasal irritation, nasal congestion, sneezing. **Resp: inhalation:** irritation of the throat and trachea, cough, wheezing, bronchospasm. **GI:** nausea, unpleasant taste. **Misc:** ALLERGIC REACTIONS, INCLUDING ANAPHYLAXIS OR WORSENING OF CONDITIONS BEING TREATED.

PHYSICAL THERAPY IMPLICATIONS

Examination and Evaluation

- Monitor signs of allergic reactions and anaphylaxis, including pulmonary symptoms (tightness in the throat and chest, wheezing, cough, dyspnea) or skin reactions (rash, pruritus, urticaria). Notify physician immediately if these reactions occur.
- Assess symptoms of bronchospasm, including wheezing, coughing, and tightness in the throat and chest. Perform pulmonary function tests to quantify suspected changes in ventilation and respiration (See Appendices I, J, K). Notify physician immediately if symptoms increase.
- If treating inflammatory bowel disease, monitor any changes in GI symptoms (decreased abdominal pain, decreased diarrhea, improved appetite) to help document whether drug therapy is successful.
- Assess dizziness that might affect gait, balance, and other functional activities (See Appendix C). Report balance problems and functional limitations to the physician, and caution the patient and family/caregivers to guard against falls and trauma.

Interventions

- For patients with asthma, design and implement appropriate aerobic exercise and respiratory muscle training programs to maintain optimal pulmonary function. Work with patient and family/caregivers to find forms of exercise (e.g., swimming) that can help improve respiratory function without triggering exercise-induced asthma attacks.

Patient/Client-Related Instruction

- Advise patient to not exceed the recommended dose or frequency of inhalation or intranasal applications.
- Instruct patient and family/caregivers to report other troublesome side effects such as severe or prolonged headache, nausea, unpleasant taste, skin reactions (rash, itching, welts, swelling of the face), or nasal problems (rhinitis, sneezing, congestion).

Pharmacokinetics

Absorption: Oral: 0.5–2 %; Inhalation: Poorly absorbed systemically (total bioavailability is 8%); action is local. Small amounts may reach systemic circulation after inhalation.

Distribution: Because only small amounts are absorbed, distribution is not known.

Metabolism and Excretion: Small amounts absorbed are excreted unchanged in bile and urine.
Half-life: 80–90 min.

TIME/ACTION PROFILE

ROUTE	ONSET	PEAK	DURATION
inhalation	1–2 wk	2–4 wk	unknown
nasal	1–2 wk	2–4 wk	unknown

Contraindications/Precautions

Contraindicated in: Hypersensitivity; Acute attacks of asthma (inhalation products).
Use Cautiously in: Renal or hepatic dysfunction; Bronchospasm—Will not relieve and may worsen acute attacks (inhalation); OB/Lactation: Safety not established; Pedi: Safety not established in children <2 yr.

Interactions

Drug-Drug: Not known.

Route/Dosage

Inhaln (Adults and Children ≥2 yr): *Nebulized solution*—One ampule (20 mg) of the nebulizer solution or 2 inhalations (0.8 mg/inhalation) as aerosol 4 times daily (inhaler for children ≥5 yr). For prevention of bronchospasm, use 2 inhalations or one nebulized ampule (20 mg) 10–15 min before exposure to known precipitating situation.
Inhalation (Adults and Children >12 yr): *Metered spray*—2–4 inhalations 3–4 times daily.
Inhalation (Children 5–12 yr): *Metered spray*—1–2 inhalations 3–4 times daily.
Intranasal (Adults and Children ≥2 yr): 1 spray (5.2 mg/spray) into each nostril 3–4 times daily (up to 6 times daily).
PO (Adults and Children >12 yr): 200 mg 4 times a day.
PO (Children 2–12 yr): 100 mg 4 times a day; not to exceed 40 mg/kg/day.

Availability

Solution for nebulization: 10 mg/mL Rx. **Aerosol inhalation:** 800 mcg/actuation in 8.1-g (112 actuations) or 14.2-g (200 actuations) containers Rx. **Nasal solution:** 40 mg/m (5.2 mg/spray) in 13-mL (≥100 sprays) or 26-mL (≥200 sprays) containers OTC.
Oral solution: 100 mg/5 mL Rx.

cyclobenzaprine

(sye-kloe-**ben**-za-preen)
Amrix, Flexeril

Classification
Therapeutic: skeletal muscle relaxants (centrally acting)

Indications

Management of acute painful musculoskeletal conditions associated with muscle spasm. **Unlabeled Use:** Management of fibromyalgia.

Action

Reduces tonic somatic muscle activity at the level of the brainstem. Structurally similar to tricyclic antidepressants. **Therapeutic Effects:** Reduction in muscle spasm and hyperactivity without loss of function.

Adverse Reactions/Side Effects

CNS: dizziness, drowsiness, confusion, fatigue, headache, nervousness. **EENT:** dry mouth, blurred vision. **CV:** arrhythmias. **GI:** constipation, dyspepsia, nausea, unpleasant taste. **GU:** urinary retention.

PHYSICAL THERAPY IMPLICATIONS

Examination and Evaluation

- Assess patient's pain, stiffness, and ROM to help document antispasm effects.
- If treating fibromyalgia, use visual analogue scales and other appropriate pain scales to assess the patient's pain and help document effects of drug therapy.
- Assess heart rate, ECG, and heart sounds, especially during exercise (See Appendices G, H). Report any rhythm disturbances or symptoms of increased arrhythmias, including palpitations, chest discomfort, shortness of breath, fainting, and fatigue/weakness.
- Assess dizziness that might affect gait, balance, and other functional activities (See Appendix C). Report balance problems and functional limitations to the physician, and caution the patient and family/caregivers to guard against falls and trauma.
- Be alert for confusion, nervousness, or other alterations in mental status (See Appendix D). Notify physician promptly if these symptoms become problematic.

Interventions

- Implement appropriate manual therapy techniques, physical agents, and therapeutic exercises to reduce pain and wean patient off muscle relaxants as soon as possible.
- Help patient explore other nonpharmacologic methods to reduce chronic pain, such as relaxation techniques, exercise, counseling, and so forth.
- Implement fall prevention strategies, especially if balance is impaired (See Appendix E).
- Because of the risk of cardiac arrhythmias, use caution during aerobic exercise and other forms of therapeutic exercise. Terminate exercise if patient exhibits untoward symptoms (chest pain, shortness

of breath, unusual fatigue) or displays other criteria for exercise termination (See Appendix L).
- To minimize orthostatic hypotension, patient should move slowly when assuming a more upright position.

Patient/Client-Related Instruction
- Inform patient that long-term use can cause tolerance and dependence; encourage adherence to physical therapy so that drug therapy can be discontinued as soon as possible.
- Inform patient that this drug may cause severe drowsiness, dizziness, and reduced psychomotor skills. Patients should avoid driving or other activities that require concentration and fast reactions.
- Advise patient to avoid alcohol and other CNS depressants because of the increased risk of sedation and adverse effects.
- Warn patient about anticholinergic effects such as dry mouth, constipation, urinary retention, sedation, and weakness; anticholinergic effects are often more severe in older adults.
- Instruct patient and family/caregivers to report other severe or prolonged GI problems, including nausea, indigestion, and altered taste.

Pharmacokinetics
Absorption: Well absorbed from the GI tract.
Distribution: Unknown.
Protein Binding: 93%.
Metabolism and Excretion: Mostly metabolized by the liver.
Half-life: 1–3 days.

TIME/ACTION PROFILE (skeletal muscle relaxation)

ROUTE	ONSET	PEAK*	DURATION
PO	within 1 hr	3–8 hr	12–24 hr
Extended release	unknown	unknown	24 hr

*Full effects may not occur for 1–2 wk.

Contraindications/Precautions
Contraindicated in: Hypersensitivity; Should not be used within 14 days of MAO inhibitor therapy; Immediate period after MI; Severe or symptomatic cardiovascular disease; Cardiac conduction disturbances; Hyperthyroidism.
Use Cautiously in: Cardiovascular disease; Geri: Appears on Beers' list. Poorly tolerated due to anticholinergic effects; Pregnancy, lactation, and children <15 yr (safety not established).

Interactions
Drug-Drug: Additive CNS depression with other **CNS depressants**, including **alcohol, antihistamines, opioid analgesics**, and **sedative/hypnotics**. Additive anticholinergic effects with **drugs possessing anticholinergic properties**, including **antihistamines, antidepressants, atropine, disopyramide, haloperidol**, and **phenothiazines**. Avoid use within 14 days of **MAO inhibitors** (hyperpyretic crisis, seizures, and death may occur). May blunt the response to **guanadrel**.
Drug-Natural: Concomitant use of **kava, valerian, chamomile**, or **hops** can ↑ CNS depression.

Route/Dosage
PO (Adults): *Acute painful musculoskeletal conditions*—10 mg 3 times daily (range 20–40 mg/day in 2–4 divided doses; not to exceed 60 mg/day) *or* extended-release—15–30 mg once daily. *Fibromyalgia*—5–40 mg at bedtime (unlabeled).

Availability (generic available)
Tablets: 5 mg, 10 mg. **Extended-release capsules:** 15 mg, 30 mg.

HIGH ALERT

cyclophosphamide
(sye-kloe-**fos**-fa-mide)
Cytoxan, Neosar, Procytox

Classification
Therapeutic: antineoplastics, immunosuppressants
Pharmacologic: alkylating agents

Indications
Alone or with other modalities in the management of Hodgkin's disease, Malignant lymphomas, Multiple myeloma, Leukemias, Mycosis fungoides, Neuroblastoma, Ovarian carcinoma, Breast carcinoma and a variety of other tumors. Minimal change nephrotic syndrome in children. **Unlabeled Use:** Severe active rheumatoid arthritis or Wegener's granulomatosis.

Action
Interferes with DNA replication and RNA transcription, ultimately disrupting protein synthesis (cell-cycle phase–nonspecific). **Therapeutic Effects:** Death of rapidly replicating cells, particularly malignant ones. Also has immunosuppressant action in smaller doses.

Adverse Reactions/Side Effects
Resp: PULMONARY FIBROSIS. **CV:** MYOCARDIAL FIBROSIS, hypotension. **GI:** anorexia, nausea, vomiting. **GU:** HEMORRHAGIC CYSTITIS, hematuria. **Derm:** alopecia. **Endo:** gonadal suppression, syndrome of inappropriate antidiuretic hormone (SIADH). **Hemat:** LEUKOPENIA, thrombocytopenia, anemia. **Metab:** hyperuricemia. **Misc:** secondary neoplasms.

PHYSICAL THERAPY IMPLICATIONS

Examination and Evaluation
- Assess pulmonary function periodically by measuring lung volumes, breath sounds, and respiratory

C

rate (See Appendices I, J, K). Notify physician or nursing staff immediately if patient experiences signs of pulmonary fibrosis (dry cough, dyspnea, shortness of breath, cyanosis).

- Assess heart rate and ECG, especially during exercise. Report any abnormal cardiac responses or signs of myocardial fibrosis such as cardiac arrhythmias, chest discomfort, shortness of breath, fainting, fatigue, or weakness.
- Watch for signs of leukopenia (fever, sore throat, signs of infection), thrombocytopenia (bruising, nose bleeds, and bleeding gums), or unusual weakness and fatigue that might be due to anemia. Report these signs to the physician or nursing staff immediately.
- Monitor signs of bladder inflammation (hemorrhagic cystitis), including blood in the urine, increased frequency, and painful or difficult urination. Report these signs to the physician or nursing staff immediately.
- Assess blood pressure periodically, and compare to normal values (See Appendix F). Report low blood pressure (hypotension), especially if patient experiences dizziness or syncope.
- Monitor and report neurologic signs of water and electrolyte imbalances due to syndrome of inappropriate antidiuretic hormone (SIADH). Excess ADH can cause increased water retention and a relative sodium deficiency (hyponatremia). Symptoms include confusion, lethargy, weakness, myoclonus, decreased reflexes, tremor, nystagmus, dysarthria, seizures, and coma.
- Watch for signs of secondary neoplasms, including a change in bowel or bladder habits, nonhealing sores, unusual bleeding or discharge, a lump in the breast or other parts of the body, chronic indigestion or difficulty in swallowing, obvious changes in a wart or mole, and persistent coughing or hoarseness. Report these signs to the physician immediately.

Interventions

- For patients who are medically able to begin exercise, implement appropriate resistive exercises and aerobic training to maintain muscle strength and aerobic capacity during cancer chemotherapy or to help restore function after chemotherapy.
- Because of the risk of pulmonary and myocardial fibrosis, use caution during aerobic exercise and other forms of therapeutic exercise. Assess exercise tolerance frequently (blood pressure, heart rate, fatigue levels), and terminate exercise immediately if any untoward responses occur (See Appendix L).

Patient/Client-Related Instruction

- Instruct patient to guard against infection (frequent hand washing, etc.), and to avoid crowds and contact with persons with contagious diseases.
- Advise patient about the likelihood of GI reactions (nausea, vomiting, diarrhea, loss of appetite). Instruct patient to report severe or prolonged GI problems.
- Advise patient that hair loss and other skin reactions (rash, pruritus) are likely. Report severe or unexpected skin reactions to the physician.

Pharmacokinetics

Absorption: Inactive parent drug is well absorbed from the GI tract. Converted to active drug by the liver.
Distribution: Widely distributed. Limited penetration of the blood-brain barrier. Crosses the placenta; enters breast milk.
Metabolism and Excretion: Converted to active drug by the liver; 30% eliminated unchanged by the kidneys.
Half-life: 4–6.5 hr.

TIME/ACTION PROFILE (effects on blood counts)

ROUTE	ONSET	PEAK	DURATION
PO, IV	7 days	7–15 days	21 days

Contraindications/Precautions

Contraindicated in: Hypersensitivity; Pregnancy or lactation.
Use Cautiously in: Active infections; Bone marrow depression; Other chronic debilitating illnesses; Patients with childbearing potential.

Interactions

Drug-Drug: Phenobarbital or **rifampin** may ↑ toxicity of cyclophosphamide. Concurrent **allopurinol** or **thiazide diuretics** may exaggerate bone marrow depression. May prolong neuromuscular blockade from **succinylcholine**. Cardiotoxicity may be additive with other **cardiotoxic agents (cytarabine, daunorubicin, doxorubicin)**. May ↓ serum **digoxin** levels. Additive bone marrow depression with other **antineoplastics** or **radiation therapy**. May potentiate the effects of **warfarin**. May ↓ antibody response to **live-virus vaccines** and ↑ risk of adverse reactions. Prolongs the effects of **cocaine**.

Route/Dosage

Many regimens are used.
PO (Adults): 1–5 mg/kg/day.
PO (Children): *Induction*—2–8 mg/kg/day (60–250 mg/m²/day) in divided doses for 6 days or longer. *Maintenance* —2–5 mg/kg (50–150 mg/m²/day) twice weekly.

IV (Adults): 40–50 mg/kg in divided doses over 2–5 days *or* 10–15 mg/kg q 7–10 days *or* 3–5 mg/kg twice weekly *or* 1.5–3 mg/kg/day. Other regimens may use larger doses.
IV (Children): *Induction*—2–8 mg/kg/day (60–250 mg/m^2/day) in divided doses for 6 days or longer. Total dose for 7 days may be given as a single weekly dose. *Maintenance*—10–15 mg/kg every 7–10 days or 30 mg/kg q 3–4 wk.

Availability (generic available)

Tablets: 25 mg, 50 mg. **Injection:** 100 mg, 200 mg, 500 mg, 750 mg, 1 g, 2 g.

cyclosporine (sye-kloe-**spor**-een)

Neoral, Sandimmune, Gengraf

Classification
Therapeutic: immunosuppressants, antirheumatics (disease-modifying antirheumatic drugs [DMARDs])
Pharmacologic: polypeptides (cyclic)

Indications

PO, IV: Prevention and treatment of rejection in renal, cardiac, and hepatic transplantation (with corticosteroids). **PO:** Treatment of severe active rheumatoid arthritis (Neoral only). Treatment of severe recalcitrant psoriasis in adult nonimmunocompromised patients (Neoral only). **Unlabeled Use:** Management of recalcitrant ulcerative colitis. Treatment of steroid-resistant nephrotic syndrome. Treatment of severe steroid-resistant autoimmune disease. Prevention and treatment of graft-versus-host disease in bone marrow transplant patients.

Action

Inhibits normal immune responses (cellular and humoral) by inhibiting interleukin-2, a factor necessary for initiation of T-cell activity. **Therapeutic Effects:** Prevention of rejection reactions. Slowed progression of rheumatoid arthritis or psoriasis.

Adverse Reactions/Side Effects

CNS: SEIZURES, tremor, confusion, flushing, headache, psychiatric problems. **CV:** hypertension. **GI:** diarrhea, hepatotoxicity, nausea, vomiting, abdominal discomfort, anorexia, pancreatitis. **GU:** nephrotoxicity. **Derm:** hirsutism, acne. **F and E:** hyperkalemia, hypomagnesemia. **Hemat:** anemia, leukopenia, thrombocytopenia. **Metab:** hyperlipidemia, hyperuricemia. **Neuro:** hyperesthesia, paresthesia. **Misc:** gingival hyperplasia, hypersensitivity reactions, infections.

PHYSICAL THERAPY IMPLICATIONS

Examination and Evaluation

- Be alert for new seizures or increased seizure activity, especially at the onset of drug treatment. Document the number, duration, and severity of seizures, and report these findings immediately to the physician.
- Monitor other signs of CNS toxicity, including tremor, confusion, and psychiatric disturbances. Notify physician if these changes become problematic.
- If treating rheumatoid arthritis, periodically assess patient's impairments (pain, range of motion), functional ability, and disability to help document whether antirheumatic drug therapy is successful.
- If treating psoriasis, monitor skin responses to help document whether drug therapy is successful in resolving this condition.
- Monitor signs of hypersensitivity reactions, including pulmonary symptoms (tightness in the throat and chest, wheezing, cough, dyspnea) or skin reactions (rash, pruritus, urticaria). Notify physician immediately if these reactions occur.
- Monitor signs of leukopenia (fever, sore throat, mucosal lesions, signs of infection, bruising), thrombocytopenia (bruising, nose bleeds, bleeding gums), or unusual weakness and fatigue that might be due to anemia. Periodic blood tests may be needed to monitor WBC and RBC counts.
- Be alert for signs of paresthesia (numbness, tingling) or hyperesthesia (increased sensitivity to touch, pain). Establish baseline electroneuromyographic values at the beginning of drug treatment whenever possible, and reexamine these values periodically to document drug-induced changes in peripheral nerve function.
- Assess blood pressure periodically and compare to normal values (See Appendix F). Report a sustained increase in blood pressure (hypertension) to the physician.
- Monitor signs of high plasma potassium levels (hyperkalemia), including bradycardia, fatigue, weakness, numbness, and tingling. Likewise, monitor signs of low magnesium levels (hypomagnesemia), such as lethargy, irritability, insomnia, muscle tremors, and confusion. Notify physician of these signs.

Interventions

- Implement appropriate manual therapy techniques, physical agents, therapeutic exercises, and orthotic/assistive devices to reduce pain, improve function, and augment the effects of antirheumatic drug therapy.
- Help patient explore other nonpharmacologic methods to reduce chronic arthritis pain, such as relaxation techniques, exercise, counseling, and so forth.

Patient/Client-Related Instruction

- Advise patient about the likelihood of GI reactions such as nausea, vomiting, diarrhea, abdominal pain, and loss of appetite. Instruct patient to report severe or prolonged GI problems, signs of liver toxicity (yellow skin or eyes, abdominal pain, severe nausea and vomiting, fever, sore throat, malaise, weakness, facial edema), or pancreatitis (upper abdominal pain after eating, indigestion, weight loss, oily stools).

- Advise patient to report signs of nephrotoxicity, including blood or pus in urine, decreased urine output, weight gain from fluid retention, and fatigue.
- Because of immunosuppressant effects, advise patient to guard against infection (frequent hand washing, etc.), and to avoid crowds and contact with persons with contagious diseases.
- Advise patient that this drug may cause problems in fat and uric acid metabolism (hyperlipidemia and hyperuricemia, respectively). Remind patient that periodic blood tests may be needed to monitor plasma lipids and uric acid levels.
- Instruct patient to report other bothersome side effects such as severe or prolonged headache, infections, or skin reactions (acne, unusual hair growth).

Pharmacokinetics

Absorption: Erratically absorbed (range 10–60%) after oral administration, with significant first-pass metabolism by the liver. Microemulsion (Neoral) has better bioavailability.
Distribution: Widely distributed, mainly into extracellular fluid and blood cells. Crosses the placenta; enters breast milk.
Protein Binding: 90–98%.
Metabolism and Excretion: Extensively metabolized by the liver (first pass); excreted in bile, small amounts excreted unchanged in urine.
Half-life: Children—7 hr; adults—19 hr.

TIME/ACTION PROFILE (blood levels)

ROUTE	ONSET	PEAK	DURATION
PO	Unknown*	2–6 hr	Unknown
IV	unknown	end of infusion	Unknown

*Onset of action in rheumatoid arthritis is 4–8 wk and may last 4 wk after discontinuation; for psoriasis, onset is 2–6 wk and lasts 6 wk following discontinuation.

Contraindications/Precautions

Contraindicated in: Hypersensitivity to cyclosporine or polyoxyethylated castor oil (vehicle for IV form); Should not be given to pregnant or lactating women unless benefits outweigh risks; Disulfiram therapy or known alcohol intolerance (IV and oral liquid dosage forms contain alcohol); Psoriasis patients receiving immunosuppressants or radiation; Uncontrolled hypertension.
Use Cautiously in: Severe hepatic impairment (dose reduction recommended); Renal impairment (frequent dose changes may be necessary); Active infection; Children (larger or more frequent doses may be required).

Interactions

Drug-Drug: ↑ blood levels and/or risk of toxicity with **azithromycin, clarithromycin, amphotericin B, aminoglycosides, amiodarone, anabolic steroids,** some **calcium channel blockers, cimetidine, colchicine, danazol, erythromycin, fluconazole, fluoroquinolones, ketoconazole, itraconazole, metoclopramide, methotrexate, miconazole, NSAIDs, melphalan,** or **hormonal contraceptives.** ↑ nephrotoxicity with **acyclovir, amphotericin B, aminoglycosides, NSAIDs, trimethoprim, ciprofloxacin** and **vancomycin.** ↑ immunosuppression with other **immunosuppressants** (cyclophosphamide, azathioprine, corticosteroids). **Quinupristin/dalfopristin** ↑ cyclosporine levels. **Barbiturates, phenytoin, rifampin, rifabutin, carbamazepine,** or **sulfonamides** may ↓ effect of cyclosporine. ↑ risk of hyperkalemia with **potassium-sparing diuretics, potassium supplements,** or **ACE inhibitors.** ↑ serum levels/risk of toxicity from **digoxin** (↓ digoxin dose by 50%). Prolongs the action of **neuromuscular blocking agents.** ↑ risk of seizures with **imipenem/cilastatin.** May ↓ antibody response to **live-virus vaccines** and ↑ risk of adverse reactions. ↑ risk of rhabdomyolysis with **HMG CoA reductase inhibitors.** Concurrent use with **tacrolimus** should be avoided. **Orlistat** ↓ absorption; avoid concurrent use.
Drug-Natural: Concomitant use with **echinacea** and **melatonin** may interfere with immunosuppression. Use with **St. John's wort** may cause ↓ serum levels and organ rejection for transplant patients. Some **HIV protease inhibitors** may ↑ blood levels and the risk of toxicity.
Drug-Food: Concurrent ingestion of **grapefruit or grapefruit juice** ↑ absorption and should be avoided. **Food** ↓ absorption of microemulsion products (Neoral).

Route/Dosage

Doses are adjusted on the basis of serum level monitoring.

Prevention of Transplant Rejection (Sandimmune)

PO (Adults and Children): 14–18 mg/kg/dose 4–12 hr before transplant then 5–15 mg/kg/day

divided q 12–24 hr postoperatively, taper by 5% weekly to maintenance dose of 3–10 mg/kg/day.
IV (Adults and Children): 5–6 mg/kg/dose 4–12 hr before transplant, then 2–10 mg/kg/day in divided doses q 8–24 hr; change to PO as soon as possible.
Prevention of Transplant Rejection (Neoral)
PO (Adults and Children): 4–12 mg/kg/day divided q 12 hr (dose varies depending on organ transplanted).
Rheumatoid Arthritis (Neoral only)
PO (Adults and Children): 2.5 mg/kg/day given in 2 divided doses; may increase by 0.5–0.75 mg/kg/day after 8 and 12 wk, up to 4 mg/kg/day. Decrease dose by 25–50% if adverse reactions occur.
Severe Psoriasis (Neoral only)
PO (Adults): 2.5 mg/kg/day given in 2 divided doses, for at least 4 wk; then may increase by 0.5 mg/kg/day q 2 wk, up to 4 mg/kg/day. Decrease dose by 25–50% if adverse reactions occur.
Autoimmune Diseases (Neoral only)
PO (Adults and Children): 1–3 mg/kg/day.

Availability (generic available)

Microemulsion soft gelatin capsules (Gengraf, Neoral): 25 mg, 100 mg. **Microemulsion oral solution (Gengraf, Neoral):** 100 mg/mL. **Soft gelatin capsules (Sandimmune):** 25 mg, 100 mg. **Oral solution (Sandimmune):** 100 mg/mL. **Injection (Sandimmune):** 50 mg/mL in 5-mL ampules.

cyproheptadine

(sye-proe-**hep**-ta-deen)
Periactin, PMS-Cyproheptadine

Classification
Therapeutic: allergy, cold, and cough remedies, antihistamines
Pharmacologic: piperidines

Indications

Relief of allergic symptoms caused by histamine release including Seasonal and perennial allergic rhinitis; Chronic urticaria, Cold urticaria. **Unlabeled Use:** Stimulation of appetite.

Action

Antagonizes the effects of histamine at H_1 receptor sites; does not bind to or inactivate histamine. Also blocks the effects of serotonin, which may result in increased appetite. **Therapeutic Effects:** Decreased symptoms of histamine excess (sneezing, rhinorrhea, nasal and ocular pruritus, ocular tearing and redness). Decreased cold urticaria.

Adverse Reactions/Side Effects

CNS: drowsiness, excitation (increased in children). **EENT:** blurred vision. **CV:** arrhythmias, hypotension, palpitations. **GI:** dry mouth, constipation. **GU:** hesitancy, retention. **Derm:** photosensitivity, rashes. **Misc:** weight gain.

PHYSICAL THERAPY IMPLICATIONS

Examination and Evaluation

- Assess blood pressure (BP) periodically and compare to normal values (See Appendix F). Report low BP (hypotension), especially if patient experiences dizziness or syncope.
- Assess heart rate, ECG, and heart sounds, especially during exercise (See Appendices G, H). Report any rhythm disturbances or symptoms of increased arrhythmias, including palpitations, chest discomfort, shortness of breath, fainting, and fatigue/weakness.
- Monitor symptoms of seasonal allergies (sneezing, rhinitis, itching eyes, cough) or chronic urticaria (rash, hives, itching) to help document benefits of this drug in treating these disorders.
- Monitor signs of increased excitation in children. Severe or problematic excitation may require a change in dose or drug.
- Periodically assess body weight and other anthropometric measures (body mass index, body composition). Report a rapid or unexplained weight gain or increased body fat.

Interventions

- Guard against falls and trauma (hip fractures, head injury, and so forth). Implement fall- prevention strategies, especially in older adults or if balance is impaired (See Appendix E).
- Because of an increased risk of arrhythmias and abnormal BP responses, use caution during aerobic exercise and other forms of therapeutic exercise. Assess exercise tolerance frequently (BP, heart rate, fatigue levels), and terminate exercise immediately if any untoward responses occur (See Appendix L).
- Causes photosensitivity; use care if administering UV treatments. Advise patient to avoid direct sunlight and use sunscreens and protective clothing.

Patient/Client-Related Instruction

- Advise patient about the risk of daytime drowsiness and decreased attention and mental focus. These problems can be severe in certain people. Use care if driving or in other activities that require quick reactions and strong concentration.
- Advise patient to avoid alcohol and other CNS depressants because of the increased risk of sedation and adverse effects.
- Instruct patient to report other troublesome side effects such as severe or prolonged skin rash, blurred vision, problems with urination, or GI problems (constipation, dry mouth).

C

Pharmacokinetics

Absorption: Apparently well absorbed after oral dosing.
Distribution: Unknown.
Metabolism and Excretion: Mostly metabolized by the liver.
Half-life: Unknown.

TIME/ACTION PROFILE (antihistaminic effects)

ROUTE	ONSET	PEAK	DURATION
PO	15–60 min	1–2 hr	8 hr

Contraindications/Precautions

Contraindicated in: Hypersensitivity; Acute attacks of asthma; Lactation; Known alcohol intolerance (syrup only).
Use Cautiously in: Geri: Appears on Beers' list. Geriatric patients are sensitive to anticholinergic effects and have increased risk for side effects, Angle-closure glaucoma, Liver disease, Pregnancy (safety not established).

Interactions

Drug-Drug: Additive CNS depression with other **CNS depressants**, including **alcohol**, **opioid analgesics**, and **sedative/hypnotics. MAO inhibitors** may intensify and prolong the anticholinergic effects of **antihistamines**.

Route/Dosage

PO (Adults): 4 mg q 8 hr (range 4–20 mg/day in 3 divided doses; up to 0.5 mg/kg/day).
PO (Children 6–14 yr): 2–4 mg q 8–12 hr (not to exceed 16 mg/day).
PO (Children 2–6 yr): 2 mg q 8–12 hr (not to exceed 12 mg/day).

Availability (generic available)

Tablets: 4 mg, 4 mg OTC. **Syrup:** 2 mg/5 mL, 2 mg/5 mL OTC.

HIGH ALERT

cytarabine (sye-tare-a-been)

Ara-C, ✱Cytosar, Cytosar-U, DepoCyt
OTHER NAMES:
Cytosine arabinoside

Classification
Therapeutic: antineoplastics
Pharmacologic: antimetabolites

Indications

IV: Used mainly in combination chemotherapeutic regimens for the treatment of leukemias and non-Hodgkin's lymphomas. **Intrathecal:** Treatment of lymphomatous meningitis.

Action

Inhibits DNA synthesis by inhibiting DNA polymerase (cell-cycle S-phase–specific). **Therapeutic Effects:** Death of rapidly replicating cells, particularly malignant ones.

Adverse Reactions/Side Effects

CNS: CNS dysfunction (high dose), confusion, drowsiness, headache. **EENT:** corneal toxicity (high dose), hemorrhagic conjunctivitis (high dose). **Resp:** PULMONARY EDEMA (HIGH DOSE). **CV:** edema. **GI:** <u>nausea</u>, <u>vomiting</u>, hepatitis, hepatotoxicity, severe GI ulceration (high dose), stomatitis. **GU:** urinary incontinence. **Derm:** alopecia, rash. **Endo:** sterility. **Hemat: (less with IT use):** <u>anemia</u>, <u>leukopenia</u>, <u>thrombocytopenia</u>. **Metab:** hyperuricemia. **Neuro: Intrathecal only:** CHEMICAL ARACHNOIDITIS, abnormal gait. **Misc:** cytarabine syndrome, fever.

PHYSICAL THERAPY IMPLICATIONS

Examination and Evaluation

- Assess any breathing problems or signs of pulmonary edema, including cough, shortness of breath, chest pain, and labored breathing. Monitor pulse oximetry and perform pulmonary function tests (See Appendices I, J, K) to quantify suspected changes in ventilation and respiratory function.
- Watch for signs of chemical arachnoiditis, such as numbness, tingling, pain in the extremities, difficulty controlling the limbs, and an inability to sit for long periods. Notify physician immediately if these signs occur.
- Monitor and report other signs of CNS dysfunction, including confusion, anxiety, and psychosis-like symptoms.
- Monitor signs of leukopenia (fever, sore throat, signs of infection), thrombocytopenia (bruising, nose bleeds, and bleeding gums) or unusual weakness and fatigue that might be due to anemia. Report these signs to the physician immediately.
- Assess peripheral edema using girth measurements, volume displacement, and measurement of pitting edema (See Appendix N). Report increased swelling in feet and ankles or a sudden increase in body weight due to fluid retention.
- Monitor any muscle or bone pain. These symptoms accompanied by fever, rash, and malaise may indicate cytarabine syndrome, and the physician should be notified.

- Assess gait and report the appearance of any abnormal gait patterns, especially after intrathecal administration.

Interventions

- For patients who are medically able to begin exercise, implement appropriate resistive exercises and aerobic training to maintain muscle strength and aerobic capacity during cancer chemotherapy or to help restore function after chemotherapy.
- Guard against falls and trauma such hip fractures and head injury (See Appendix E). Implement fall-prevention strategies, especially if patient exhibits gait abnormalities.
- Do not apply physical agents (heat, cold, electrotherapeutic modalities) or massage at the subcutaneous injection site; these interventions can alter drug absorption from subcutaneous tissues.

Patient/Client-Related Instruction

- Advise patient and family/caregivers about the risk of infections, to guard against infection (frequent hand washing, etc.), and to avoid crowds and contact with persons with contagious diseases.
- Instruct patient to report bleeding around the eyes (hemorrhagic conjunctivitis) or visual disturbances that might indicate corneal toxicity.
- Advise patient about the likelihood of GI reactions such as nausea, vomiting, diarrhea, loss of appetite, and irritation of the mouth. Instruct patient to report severe or prolonged GI problems, signs of ulceration (abdominal pain, vomiting blood, blood in the stools), or signs of liver toxicity (yellow skin or eyes, severe nausea and vomiting, fever, sore throat, malaise, weakness, facial edema).
- Instruct patient and family/caregivers to report other troublesome side effects such as severe or prolonged headache, urinary incontinence, fever, or skin reactions (rash, hair loss).

Pharmacokinetics

Absorption: Absorption occurs from SC sites, but blood levels are lower than with IV administration; IT administration results in negligible systemic exposure.
Distribution: Widely distributed; IV- and SC-administered cytarabine crosses the blood-brain barrier but not in sufficient quantities. Crosses the placenta.
Metabolism and Excretion: Metabolized mostly by the liver; <10% excreted unchanged by the kidneys. Metabolism to inactive drug in the CSF is negligible because the enzyme that metabolizes it is present in very low concentrations in the CSF.
Half-life: *IV, SC*—1–3 hr; *IT*—100–236 hr.

TIME/ACTION PROFILE (IV, SC—effects on WBCs; IT—levels in CSF)

ROUTE	ONSET	PEAK	DURATION
SC, IV (1st phase)	24 hr	7–9 days	12 days
SC, IV (2nd phase)	15–24 days	15–24 days	25–34 days
IT	rapid	5 hr	14–28 days

Contraindications/Precautions

Contraindicated in: Hypersensitivity; OB: Pregnancy or lactation; Active meningeal infection (IT only).
Use Cautiously in: Active infections; Decreased bone marrow reserve; Renal/hepatic disease; Other chronic debilitating illnesses; OB: Patients with childbearing potential.

Interactions

Drug-Drug: ⊠ bone marrow depression with other **antineoplastics** or **radiation therapy**. ⊠ risk of cardiomyopathy when used in high-dose regimens with **cyclophosphamide**. May ⊠ antibody response to **live-virus vaccines** and ⊠ risk of adverse reactions. May ⊠ absorption of **digoxin** tablets. May ⊠ the efficacy of **gentamicin** when used to treat *Klebsiella pneumoniae* infections. Recent treatment with **asparaginase** may ⊠ risk of pancreatitis. ⊠ neurotoxicity with concurrently administered **IT antineoplastics** (IT only).

Route/Dosage

Dose regimens vary widely.
IV (Adults): *Induction dose*—200 mg/m²/day for 5 days q 2 wk as a single agent or 2–6 mg/kg/day (100–200 mg/m²/day) as a single daily dose *or* in 2–3 divided doses for 5–10 days or until remission occurs as part of combination chemotherapy. *Maintenance*—70–200 mg/m²/day for 2–5 days monthly. *Refractory leukemias/lymphomas*—3 g/m² q 12 hr for up to 12 doses.
Subcut, IM (Adults): *Maintenance*—1–1.5 mg/kg q 1–4 wk.
Intrathecal (Adults): *DepoCyt Induction*— 50 mg (intraventricular or lumbar puncture) every 14 days for 2 doses (weeks 1 and 3); *consolidation*— 50 mg (intraventricular or lumbar puncture) every 14 days for 3 doses (weeks 5, 7 and 9), followed by 1 additional dose at week 13; *maintenance*—50 mg (intraventricular or lumbar puncture) every 28 days for 4 doses (weeks 17, 21, 25, and 29). If drug-related neurotoxicity occurs, dose should be reduced to 25 mg or discontinued (dexamethasone 4 mg PO/IV twice daily for 5 days should be started concurrently with IT cytarabine).

Availability (generic available)

Powder for injection: 100 mg, 500 mg, 1 g, 2 g.
Sustained-release liposome injection for IT use: 50 mL/5-mL vial.

D

dabigatran (da-bye-gat-ran)

Pradaxa

Classification

Therapeutic: anticoagulants

Pharmacologic: thrombin inhibitors

Indications

To ↓ risk of stroke/systemic embolization associated with nonvalvular atrial fibrillation

Action

Acts as a direct inhibitor of thrombin. **Therapeutic Effects:** Lowered risk of thrombotic sequelae (stroke and systemic embolization) of nonvalvular atrial fibrillation.

Adverse Reactions/Side Effects

GI: abdominal pain, diarrhea, dyspepsia, gastritis, nausea. **Hemat:** BLEEDING. **Misc:** HYPERSENSITIVITY REACTIONS, INCLUDING ANAPHYLAXIS.

PHYSICAL THERAPY IMPLICATIONS

Examination and Evaluation

- Watch for signs of bleeding and hemorrhage, including bleeding gums, nosebleeds, unusual bruising, black/tarry stools, hematuria, and a fall in hematocrit or blood pressure. Notify physician or nursing staff immediately of these signs.
- Monitor signs of hypersensitivity reactions and anaphylaxis, including pulmonary symptoms (tightness in the throat and chest, wheezing, cough, dyspnea) or skin reactions (rash, pruritus, urticaria). Notify physician or nursing staff immediately if these reactions occur.

Interventions

- Use caution with any physical interventions that could increase bleeding, including wound débridement, chest percussion, joint mobilization, and application of local heat.

Patient/Client-Related Instruction

- Instruct patient to report immediately signs of GI bleeding, including abdominal pain, vomiting blood, blood in stools, or black, tarry stools.
- Instruct patient to report other GI problems such as severe or prolonged nausea, diarrhea, indigestion, and stomach pain.

Pharmacokinetics

Absorption: 3–7% absorbed following oral administration.

Distribution: Unknown.

Metabolism and Excretion: Of the amount absorbed, mostly excreted by kidneys (80%); 86% of ingested dose is eliminated in feces due to poor bioavailability.

Half-life: 12–17 hr.

TIME/ACTION PROFILE (effects on coagulation)

ROUTE	ONSET	PEAK	DURATION
PO	within hrs	unknown	2 days*

*Following discontinuation, 3–5 days in renal impairment.

Contraindications/Precautions

Contraindicated in: Hypersensitivity; Active pathologic bleeding; Concurrent use of Pg-P inducers.

Use Cautiously in: Concurrent medications/preexisting conditions that ↑ bleeding risk (other anticoagulants, antiplatelet agents, antifibrinolytics, heparins, chronic NSAID use, labor and delivery); Surgical procedures (discontinue 1–2 days prior if CCr ≥50 mL/min or 3–4 days prior if CCr <50 mL/min); Geri: ↑ risk of bleeding; Lactation: Use cautiously during breastfeeding; Pedi: Safety and effectiveness not established.

Interactions

Drug-Drug: Concurrent use of other **anticoagulants, antiplatelet agents, antifibrinolytics, heparins, prasugrel, clopidogrel**, or chronic use of **NSAIDs** ↑ risk of bleeding; Concurrent use of **P-gp inducers,** including **rifampin,** ↓ blood levels and effectiveness and should be avoided.

Route/Dosage

PO (Adults): 150 mg twice daily; *CCr 15–30 mL/min*—75 mg twice daily.

Availability

Capsules: 75 mg, 150 mg

HIGH ALERT

dacarbazine (da-kar-ba-zeen)

DTIC, DTIC-Dome

Classification

Therapeutic: antineoplastics

Pharmacologic: alkylating agents

Indications

Treatment of metastatic malignant melanoma (single agent). Treatment of Hodgkin's disease as second-line therapy (with other agents).

Action

Disrupts DNA and RNA synthesis (cell-cycle phase–nonspecific). **Therapeutic Effects:** Death of rapidly growing tissue cells, especially malignant ones.

Adverse Reactions/Side Effects

GI: HEPATIC NECROSIS, anorexia, nausea, vomiting, diarrhea, hepatic vein thrombosis. **Derm:** alopecia, facial flushing, photosensitivity, rash. **Endo:** gonadal suppression. **Hemat:** anemia, leukopenia, thrombocytopenia. **Local:** pain at IV site, phlebitis at IV site, tissue necrosis. **MS:** myalgia. **Neuro:** facial paresthesia. **Misc:** ANAPHYLAXIS, fever, flu-like syndrome, malaise.

PHYSICAL THERAPY IMPLICATIONS

Examination and Evaluation

- Be alert for signs of hepatotoxicity and hepatic necrosis, including anorexia, abdominal pain, severe nausea and vomiting, yellow skin or eyes, fever, sore throat, malaise, weakness, facial edema, lethargy, and unusual bleeding or bruising. Report these signs to the physician or nursing staff immediately.
- Watch for signs of allergic reactions and anaphylaxis, including pulmonary symptoms (tightness in the throat and chest, wheezing, cough, dyspnea) or skin reactions (rash, pruritus, urticaria). Notify physician or nursing staff immediately if these reactions occur.
- Monitor signs of leukopenia (fever, sore throat, signs of infection), thrombocytopenia (bruising, nose bleeds, bleeding gums), or unusual weakness and fatigue that might be due to anemia. Report these signs to the physician or nursing staff.
- Assess any muscle pain to rule out musculoskeletal pathology; that is, try to determine if pain is drug induced rather than caused by anatomic or biomechanical problems.
- Assess signs of parasthesia (numbness, tingling) in the face or elsewhere. Perform objective tests including electroneuromyography and sensory testing to document any drug-related neuropathic changes.
- Monitor IV injection site for pain, swelling, and tissue necrosis. Report prolonged or excessive injection site reactions to the physician.

Interventions

- For patients who are medically able to begin exercise, implement appropriate resistive exercises and aerobic training to maintain muscle strength and aerobic capacity during cancer chemotherapy or to help restore function after chemotherapy.
- Causes photosensitivity; use care if administering UV treatments. Advise patient to avoid direct sunlight and use sunscreens and protective clothing.

Patient/Client-Related Instruction

- Instruct patient to guard against infection (frequent hand washing, etc.), and to avoid crowds and contact with persons with contagious diseases.
- Advise patient about the likelihood of GI reactions such as nausea, vomiting, diarrhea, and loss of appetite. Instruct patient to report severe or prolonged GI problems.
- Advise patient that hair loss and other skin reactions (rash, pruritus) are likely. Report severe or unexpected skin reactions to the physician.

Pharmacokinetics

Absorption: IV administration results in complete bioavailability.
Distribution: Large volume of distribution; probably concentrates in liver; some CNS penetration.
Metabolism and Excretion: 50% metabolized by the liver, 50% excreted unchanged by the kidneys.
Half-life: 5 hr (increased in renal and hepatic dysfunction).

TIME/ACTION PROFILE (effects on blood counts)

ROUTE	ONSET	PEAK	DURATION
IV (WBCs)	16–20 days	21–25 days	3–5 days
IV (platelets)	unknown	16 days	3–5 days

Contraindications/Precautions

Contraindicated in: Hypersensitivity; Pregnancy or lactation.
Use Cautiously in: Active infections; Bone marrow depression; Children (safety not established); Renal dysfunction; Hepatic dysfunction.

Interactions

Drug-Drug: Additive bone marrow depression with other **antineoplastics**. **Carbamazepine, phenobarbital, rifampin**, and **aminoglutethimide** may increase metabolism and decrease effectiveness. Blood levels may be increased with **amiodarone, ciprofloxacin, fluvoxamine, ketoconazole, norfloxacin, ofloxacin, isoniazid**, or **miconazole**. May decrease antibody response to **live-virus vaccines** and increase the risk of adverse reactions.

Route/Dosage

Other regimens are used.
IV (Adults): *Malignant melanoma*—2–4.5 mg/kg/day for 10 days administered q 4 wk *or* 250 mg/m^2/day for 5 days administered every 3 wk. *Hodgkin's disease*—150 mg/m^2/day for 5 days (in combination with other agents) administered q 4 wk *or* 375 mg/m^2 (in combination with other agents) administered every 15 days.

Availability

Powder for injection: 200 mg.

D

daclizumab (da-kliz-yoo-mab)

Zenapax

Classification

Therapeutic: immunosuppressants

Pharmacologic: monoclonal antibodies

Indications

Prevention of acute organ rejection during renal transplantation (with cyclosporine and corticosteroids).

Action

Binds specifically to interleukin-2 (IL-2) receptor sites on activated lymphocytes, acting as an IL-2 receptor antagonist. This prevents further activation of lymphocytes and allograft rejection. **Therapeutic Effects:** Prevention of renal allograft rejection.

Adverse Reactions/Side Effects

CNS: dizziness, fatigue, headache, insomnia. **Resp:** PULMONARY EDEMA, coughing, dyspnea. **CV:** chest pain, edema, hypertension (↑ in children), hypotension, tachycardia. **GI:** abdominal discomfort, constipation, diarrhea (↑ in children), dyspepsia, epigastric pain, nausea, pyrosis, vomiting (↑ in children). **GU:** dysuria, oliguria, renal tubular necrosis. **Derm:** acne, impaired wound healing, pruritus (↑ in children). **Hemat:** thrombosis. **MS:** arthralgia, back pain, musculoskeletal pain. **Neuro:** tremor. **Misc:** Allergic reactions, including anaphylaxis, fever (↑ in children), postoperative pain (↑ in children), urinary and respiratory tract infections (↑ in children).

PHYSICAL THERAPY IMPLICATIONS

Examination and Evaluation

- Assess any breathing problems or signs of pulmonary edema, including cough, shortness of breath, chest pain, and labored breathing. Monitor pulse oximetry and perform pulmonary function tests (See Appendices I, J, K) to quantify suspected changes in ventilation and respiratory function.
- Be alert for signs of allergic reactions and anaphylaxis, including pulmonary symptoms (tightness in the throat and chest, wheezing, cough, dyspnea) or skin reactions (rash, pruritus, urticaria). Notify physician or nursing staff immediately if these reactions occur.
- Assess blood pressure (BP) and compare to normal values (See Appendix F). Report changes in BP, either a problematic decrease in BP (hypotension) or a sustained increase in BP (hypertension).
- Assess heart rate, ECG, and heart sounds, especially during exercise (See Appendixes G, H). Report a rapid heart rate (tachycardia) or signs of other arrhythmias, including palpitations, chest discomfort, shortness of breath, fainting, and fatigue/weakness.
- Monitor abnormal blood coagulation, including venous thrombosis (lower extremity swelling, warmth, erythema, tenderness) and arterial thrombosis (extreme coldness in the hands and feet, cyanosis, muscle cramping). Notify physician immediately, and request objective tests (Doppler ultrasound, others) if thrombosis is suspected.
- Assess peripheral edema using girth measurements, volume displacement, and measurement of pitting edema (See Appendix N). Report increased swelling in feet and ankles or a sudden increase in body weight due to fluid retention.
- Monitor signs of hypoglycemia (weakness, malaise, irritability, fatigue) or hyperglycemia (drowsiness, fruity breath, increased urination, unusual thirst). Patients with diabetes mellitus should check blood glucose levels frequently.
- Be alert for signs of paresthesia and neuropathy, including numbness, tingling, and muscle weakness. Establish baseline electroneuromyographic values at the beginning of drug treatment whenever possible, and reexamine these values periodically to document drug-induced changes in peripheral nerve function.
- Assess any joint, back, or other musculoskeletal pain to rule out musculoskeletal pathology; that is, try to determine if pain is drug induced rather than caused by anatomic or biomechanical problems.
- Assess dizziness that might affect gait, balance, and other functional activities (See Appendix C). Report balance problems and functional limitations to the physician and nursing staff, and caution the patient and family/caregivers to guard against falls and trauma.

Interventions

- Implement appropriate strengthening, aerobic, and other therapeutic exercises to improve function and promote recovery following organ transplants.
- Because of the risk of arrhythmias and abnormal BP responses, use caution during aerobic exercise and other forms of therapeutic exercise. Assess exercise tolerance frequently (BP, heart rate, fatigue levels), and terminate exercise immediately if any untoward responses occur (See Appendix L).

Patient/Client-Related Instruction

- Because of immunosuppressant effects, advise patient to guard against infection (frequent hand washing, etc.), and to avoid crowds and contact with persons with contagious diseases.
- Advise patient that wound healing may be delayed; instruct patient to check skin regularly and report any nonhealing sores.
- Instruct patient to report other bothersome side effects such as severe or prolonged headache, sleep

loss, infections, fever, problems with urination, skin reactions (itching, acne), or GI problems (nausea, vomiting, diarrhea, constipation, indigestion, heartburn, abdominal pain).

Pharmacokinetics

Absorption: IV administration results in complete bioavailability.
Distribution: Crosses the placenta.
Metabolism and Excretion: Binds to lymphocytes.
Half-life: 20 days.

TIME/ACTION PROFILE (saturation of IL-2 receptors)

ROUTE	ONSET	PEAK	DURATION
IV	rapid	after 5th dose	120 days*

*Posttransplantation.

Contraindications/Precautions

Contraindicated in: Hypersensitivity.
Use Cautiously in: Geriatric patients; Pregnancy, lactation, or children (has been used in children; ↑ risk of hypertension and dehydration).

Interactions

Drug-Drug: None known.
Drug-Natural: Concomitant use with **astragalus, echinacea,** and **melatonin** may interfere with immunosuppression.

Route/Dosage

IV (Adults and Children): 1 mg/kg, with 1st dose given no more than 24 hr before transplantation, then q 2 wk for a total of 5 doses.

Availability

Concentrate for injection (must be diluted): 25 mg/5 mL in 5-mL vials.

HIGH ALERT

dactinomycin

(dak-ti-noe-**mye**-sin)
Cosmegan

OTHER NAMES
actinomycin-D

Classification
Therapeutic: antineoplastics
Pharmacologic: antitumor antibiotics

Indications

Alone or with other treatment modalities in the management of: Wilms' tumor, Rhabdomyosarcoma, Ewing's sarcoma, Trophoblastic neoplasms, Testicular carcinoma, Metastatic nonseminomatous testicular cancer, Gestational trophoblastic neoplasia. As a component of regional perfusion for treatment of locally recurrent solid malignancies.

Action

Inhibits RNA synthesis by forming a complex with DNA (cell-cycle phase–nonspecific). **Therapeutic Effects:** Death of rapidly replicating cells, particularly malignant ones. Also has immunosuppressive properties.

Adverse Reactions/Side Effects

CNS: lethargy, malaise. **GI:** anorexia, nausea, stomatitis, vomiting, abdominal pain, ascites, diarrhea, dysphagia, esophagitis, hepatotoxicity, ulceration. **Derm:** acne, alopecia, erythema (especially of previously irradiated skin), hyperpigmentation (especially of previously irradiated skin), skin eruptions, photosensitivity, rash. **EENT:** pharyngitis. **Endo:** hypocalcemia, gonadal suppression. **Hemat:** anemia, leukopenia, thrombocytopenia. **Local:** phlebitis at IV site. **MS:** myalgia. **Resp:** pneumonitis. **Misc:** fever.

PHYSICAL THERAPY IMPLICATIONS

Examination and Evaluation

- Monitor respiratory function and report signs of pneumonitis, including dry cough, dyspnea, chest pain, shortness of breath, and fever. Report these signs, especially if patient begins to show acute respiratory distress.
- Watch for signs of leukopenia (fever, sore throat, signs of infection), thrombocytopenia (bruising, nose bleeds, bleeding gums), or unusual weakness and fatigue that might be due to anemia. Report these signs to the physician or nursing staff.
- Assess any muscle pain or neuromuscular signs of low calcium levels (hypocalcemia), including headache, lethargy, weakness, cramping, and muscle hyperexcitability and tetany. Notify physician immediately if these signs become problematic.
- Monitor IV injection site for pain, swelling, and inflammation (phlebitis). Report signs of phlebitis or other prolonged or excessive injection site reactions to the physician.

Interventions

- For patients who are medically able to begin exercise, implement appropriate resistive exercises and aerobic training to maintain muscle strength and aerobic capacity during cancer chemotherapy or to help restore function after chemotherapy.
- Use caution during exercise, especially if patient has any respiratory problems (pneumonitis) or severe fatigue due to anemia of other blood dyscrasias. Assess exercise tolerance frequently (blood pressure, heart rate, breathing responses, fatigue levels), and terminate exercise immediately if any untoward responses occur (See Appendix L).
- Causes photosensitivity; use care if administering UV treatments. Advise patient to avoid direct sunlight and use sunscreens and protective clothing.

Patient/Client-Related Instruction

- Instruct patient to guard against infection (frequent hand washing, etc.), and to avoid crowds and contact with persons with contagious diseases.
- Advise patient about the likelihood of GI reactions, including nausea, vomiting, diarrhea, difficulty swallowing, heartburn, loss of appetite, and inflammation in or around the mouth. Instruct patient to report severe or unexpected GI reactions or signs of hepatotoxicity (abdominal pain/swelling, severe nausea and vomiting, yellow skin or eyes, fever, sore throat, malaise, weakness, facial edema, lethargy, unusual bleeding or bruising).
- Advise patient that hair loss and other skin reactions (rash, pruritus, acne, blistering, change in pigmentation) are likely. Report severe or unexpected skin reactions to the physician.
- Instruct patient to report other troublesome side effects such as severe or prolonged fever or irritation of the throat and pharynx.

Pharmacokinetics

Absorption: IV administration results in complete bioavailability.
Distribution: Widely distributed, with extensive tissue binding; does not cross the blood-brain barrier. Crosses the placenta.
Metabolism and Excretion: Excreted in bile (50%) and feces (14%) as unchanged drug; small amounts excreted unchanged by the kidneys (10%).
Half-life: 36 hr.

TIME/ACTION PROFILE (effects on blood counts)

ROUTE	ONSET	PEAK	DURATION
IV	7 days	14–21 days	21–28 days

Contraindications/Precautions

Contraindicated in: Hypersensitivity; Pregnant or lactating women; Patients with concurrent or recent chickenpox or herpes zoster infection; Children <6 mo.
Use Cautiously in: Active infections; Immunosuppressed patients; Concurrent radiation therapy; Hepatic dysfunction; Patients with childbearing potential.

Interactions

Drug-Drug: ↑ bone marrow depression with other **antineoplastics** or **radiation therapy**. May ↓ antibody response to **live-virus vaccines** and ↑ risk of adverse reactions (avoid concurrent use).

Route/Dosage

Dose in obese or edematous patients should be based on body surface area.

Wilms' Tumor, Rhabdomyosarcoma, Ewing's Sarcoma

IV (Adults and Children >6 mo): 15 mcg/kg/day for 5 days administered in various combinations and schedules.

Metastatic Nonseminomatous Testicular Cancer

IV (Adults): 1000 mcg/m^2≤ as single dose in combination with other agents.

Gestational Trophoblastic Neoplasms

IV (Adults): 12 mcg/kg/day for 5 days as a single agent *or* 500 mcg /day for 2 days in combination with other agents.

Regional Perfusion in Locally Recurrent Solid Malignancies

Regional perfusion: (Adults): *Lower extremity/pelvis*—50 mcg/kg; *upper extremity*—35 mcg/kg.

Availability

Powder for injection: 0.5-mg vials.

dalfampridine

(dal-fam-pri-deen)
Ampyra

Other Names:
4-aminopyridine, 4-AP, fampridine

Classification
Therapeutic: anti–multiple sclerosis agents
Pharmacologic: potassium channel blocker

Indications

Treatment of multiple sclerosis (MS); to improve walking speed.

Action

Acts as a potassium channel blocker, which may increase conduction of action potentials. **Therapeutic Effects:** Increased walking speed in patients with MS.

Adverse Reactions/Side Effects

CNS: SEIZURES, dizziness, headache, insomnia, weakness. **EENT:** nasopharyngitis, pharyngolaryngeal pain. **GI:** constipation, dyspepsia, nausea. **GU:** urinary tract infection. **MS:** back pain. **Neuro:** balance disorder, MS relapse, paresthesia.

PHYSICAL THERAPY IMPLICATIONS

- Be alert for new seizures or increased seizure activity, especially at the onset of drug treatment. Document the number, duration, and severity of

seizures, and report these findings to the physician immediately.

- Periodically assess balance, coordination, spasticity, gait, and other aspects of neuromuscular function. Document any improvement in function, but also report worsening of impairments or a relapse of MS symptoms.
- Assess any back pain to rule out musculoskeletal pathology; that is, try to determine if pain is drug induced rather than caused by anatomic or biomechanical problems.
- Assess signs of paresthesia (numbness, tingling) or muscle weakness. Perform objective tests, including electroneuromyography and sensory testing to document any drug-related neuropathic changes.
- Assess dizziness that might affect gait, balance, and other functional activities (See Appendix C). Report balance problems and functional limitations to the physician and nursing staff, and caution the patient and family/caregivers to guard against falls and trauma.

Interventions

- Design and implement coordination, balance, gait training, and other therapeutic exercises to maintain function, and complement drug effects in patients with MS.

Patient/Client-Related Instruction

- Instruct patient to report other troublesome side effects such as prolonged or severe headache, sleep loss, upper respiratory tract irritation, urinary tract infection, or GI problems (nausea, indigestion, constipation).

Pharmacokinetics

Absorption: Rapidly and completely absorbed (96%).
Distribution: Unknown
Metabolism and Excretion: 96% eliminated in urine, 0.5% in feces
Half-life: 5.2–6.5 hr

TIME/ACTION PROFILE (improvement in walking speed)

ROUTE	ONSET	PEAK	DURATION
PO	unknown	3–4 hr	24 hr

Contraindications/Precautions

Contraindicated in: History of seizures; Moderate/severe renal impairment (↑ risk of seizures); Lactation: Avoid use.
Use Cautiously in: Geri: Consider age-related ↓ in renal function; OB: Use only if potential benefit justifies potential risk to fetus; Pedi: Safety and effectiveness not established.

Interactions

Drug-Drug: None noted.

Route/Dosage

PO (Adults): 10 mg twice daily.

Availability

Extended-release tablets: 10 mg

HIGH ALERT

dalteparin (dal-te-pa-rin)

Fragmin

Classification
Therapeutic: anticoagulants
Pharmacologic: antithrombotics

Indications

Prevention of deep vein thrombosis (DVT) and pulmonary embolism (PE) in surgical or medical patients. Prevention of ischemic complications (with aspirin) in patients with unstable angina, non–Q-wave MI. **Unlabeled Use:** Systemic anticoagulation for other diagnoses.

Action

Potentiates the inhibitory effect of antithrombin on factor Xa and thrombin. **Therapeutic Effects:** Prevention of thrombus formation. Decreased incidence of death or recurrent MI.

Adverse Reactions/Side Effects

CNS: dizziness. **GI:** reversible increase in liver enzymes. **Hemat:** BLEEDING, thrombocytopenia.

PHYSICAL THERAPY IMPLICATIONS

Examination and Evaluation

- Assess for signs of bleeding and hemorrhage, including bleeding gums, nosebleeds, unusual bruising, black/tarry stools, hematuria, and a fall in hematocrit or blood pressure. Notify physician or nursing staff immediately if dalteparin causes excessive anticoagulation.
- Monitor symptoms of DVT (pain, swelling, warmth, redness) to determine if drug therapy is effective in preventing or reducing venous thrombosis. Request or administer objective tests (Doppler ultrasound) if symptoms increase.
- In patients with DVT, watch for signs of pulmonary embolism (shortness of breath, chest pain, cough, bloody sputum). Notify physician or nursing staff immediately if these signs occur.
- Be alert for acute arterial or venous thrombosis caused by heparin-induced thrombocytopenia (HIT). Although the risk of HIT is lower compared with traditional heparin, dalteparin may initiate an immune reaction in certain patients where antibodies attack circulating platelets. Although most cases of HIT are minor and asymptomatic, some patients

may experience life- or limb-threatening platelet clots, resulting in MI, ischemic stroke, acute leg ischemia, or venous thromboembolism. HIT can occur during and up to several weeks after heparin therapy. Any signs of increased clotting should be reported immediately.

- Assess dizziness that might affect gait, balance, and other functional activities (See Appendix C). Report balance problems and functional limitations to the physician and nursing staff, and caution the patient and family/caregivers to guard against falls and trauma.
- Assess injection site for pain, swelling, and irritation. Report prolonged or excessive injection-site reactions to the physician or nursing staff.

Interventions

- Use caution with any physical interventions that could increase bleeding, including wound débridement, chest percussion, joint mobilization, and application of local heat.
- Recommend or implement other physical methods to decrease DVT and prevent thromboembolism, including graduated compression stockings and intermittent pneumatic compression pumps.
- Implement early mobilization and ambulation to reduce the risk of new or increased DVT. Early ambulation appears to be safe in patients with DVT if the patient is adequately heparinized (INR values in acceptable range), does not have an active pulmonary embolism, or have other risk factors that contraindicate ambulation.
- Use caution during aerobic exercise and other forms of therapeutic exercise in patients with unstable angina or MI. Assess exercise tolerance frequently (blood pressure, heart rate, fatigue levels), and terminate exercise immediately if any untoward responses occur (See Appendix L).
- Do not apply physical agents (heat, cold, electrotherapeutic modalities) or massage over the injection site; these interventions can alter drug absorption from subcutaneous tissues.

Patient/Client-Related Instruction

- Instruct patient to immediately report signs of GI bleeding, including abdominal pain, vomiting blood, blood in stools, or black, tarry stools.

Pharmacokinetics

Absorption: Well absorbed (87%) after administration.
Distribution: Unknown.
Metabolism and Excretion: Unknown.
Half-life: 2.1–2.3 hr.

TIME/ACTION PROFILE (antithrombotic effect)

ROUTE	ONSET	PEAK	DURATION
SC	rapid	4 hr	up to 24 hr

Contraindications/Precautions

Contraindicated in: Hypersensitivity to dalteparin, heparin, or pork products; Active major bleeding; Thrombocytopenia related to previous dalteparin therapy.
Use Cautiously in: Patients with severe renal or hepatic impairment; Retinopathy (hypertensive or diabetic); Spinal or epidural anesthesia; **Geri:** Geriatric patients (risk of bleeding may be ↑, consider age-related ↓ in renal function and body weight); **OB, Pedi:** Pregnancy, lactation, or children (safety not established; products containing benzyl alcohol should not be used in neonates).
Exercise Extreme Caution in: Spinal/epidural anesthesia or spinal puncture (↑ risk of spinal/epidural hematoma that may lead to long-term or permanent paralysis); Severe uncontrolled hypertension; Bacterial endocarditis, bleeding disorders; GI bleeding/ulceration/pathology; Hemorrhagic stroke; Recent CNS or ophthalmologic surgery; Active GI bleeding/ulceration; History of thrombocytopenia related to heparin.

Interactions

Drug-Drug: Risk of bleeding ↑ by concurrent use of **thrombolytics, anticoagulants, or agents that affect platelet function,** including **NSAIDS, ticlopidine, clopidogrel, tirofiban,** or **eptifibatide.**

Route/Dosage

DVT Prophylaxis

SC (Adults): *Abdominal surgery*—2500 IU 1–2 hr before surgery, then once daily for 5–10 days; *high-risk patients undergoing abdominal surgery*—5000 IU evening before surgery, then once daily for 5–10 days or 2500 IU 1–2 hr before surgery, another 2500 IU 12 hr later, then 5000 IU daily for 5–10 days; *hip replacement surgery*—2500 IU within 2 hr before surgery, another 2500 IU evening of the day of surgery ≥6 hr after first dose, then 5000 IU daily for 5–10 days (if surgery is in the evening omit 2nd dose day of surgery) or 5000 IU evening before surgery, then 5000 IU daily for 5–10 days. *Medical patients with severely restricted mobility*—5000 IU for 12–14 days.

Angina/Non–Q-wave MI

SC (Adults): 120 IU/kg (not to exceed 10,000 IU) q 12 hr with concurrent aspirin.

Systemic Anticoagulation (Unlabeled)

SC (Adults): 200 IU/kg once daily or 100 IU/kg twice daily.

Availability

Injection: 2500 anti–factor Xa IU /0.2 mL (single-use syringe) Rx, 5000 anti–actor Xa IU/0.2 mL (single-use syringe) Rx, 10,000 anti–factor Xa IU/ mL (9.5 mL multiuse vial) Rx.

danazol (da-na-zole)

Cyclomen, Danocrine

Classification

Therapeutic: hormones
Pharmacologic: androgens

Indications

Treatment of moderate endometriosis that is unresponsive to conventional therapy. Palliative therapy of fibrocystic breast disease. Prophylaxis of hereditary angioedema.

Action

Inhibits pituitary output of gonadotropins, resulting in suppression of ovarian function. Has weak androgenic-anabolic activity. **Therapeutic Effects:** Atrophy of ectopic endometrial tissue in endometriosis. Decreased pain and nodularity in fibrocystic breast disease. Correction of biochemical abnormalities in hereditary angioedema.

Adverse Reactions/Side Effects

CNS: emotional lability. **EENT:** deepening of voice. **CV:** edema. **GI:** hepatitis (cholestatic jaundice). **GU:** amenorrhea, clitoral enlargement, testicular atrophy. **Derm:** acne, hirsutism, oiliness. **Endo:** amenorrhea, anovulation, decreased breast size (women), decreased libido. **Metab:** weight gain.

PHYSICAL THERAPY IMPLICATIONS

Examination and Evaluation

- Monitor symptoms of endometriosis (painful periods, pain during sexual intercourse, excessive menstrual bleeding, GI problems), or breast pain and tenderness associated with benign fibrocystic breast disease. Report any changes in these symptoms to help document the effects of drug therapy.
- For patients with hereditary angioedema, monitor symptoms such as laryngeal edema, swelling in the face and extremities, and GI problems (diarrhea, vomiting, abdominal cramping). Document any changes in these symptoms to help assess the effects of drug therapy.
- Be alert for signs of drug-induced hepatitis, including anorexia, abdominal pain, severe nausea and vomiting, yellow skin or eyes, skin rashes, flu-like symptoms, and muscle/joint pain. Report these signs to the physician immediately.
- Assess peripheral edema using girth measurements, volume displacement, and measurement of pitting edema (See Appendix N). Report increased swelling in feet and ankles or a sudden increase in body weight due to fluid retention.
- Monitor and report emotional lability or other changes in mood and behavior.
- Periodically assess body weight and report a sustained or substantial weight gain.

Patient/Client-related Instruction

- Instruct patient to report signs of drug-induced hepatitis, including anorexia, abdominal pain, severe nausea and vomiting, yellow skin or eyes, skin rashes, flu-like symptoms, and muscle/joint pain.
- Instruct patient to report severe or troublesome changes in sexual function or characteristics, including decreased libido, testicular atrophy in men, and clitoral enlargement and decreased breast size in women.
- Instruct women to notify health care professional about decreased or absent menstruation.
- Instruct patient to report other troublesome side effects such as severe or prolonged skin reactions (acne, oiliness, increased hair growth) or deepening of the voice.

Pharmacokinetics

Absorption: Absorbed from the GI tract.
Distribution: Unknown.
Metabolism and Excretion: Metabolized by the liver.
Half-life: 4.5 hr.

TIME/ACTION PROFILE (disease response)

ROUTE	ONSET	PEAK	DURATION
PO (endometriosis)	unknown	6–8 wk	60–90 days
PO (fibrocystic disease)	1 mo	2–6 mo	1 yr
PO (angioedema)	unknown	1–3 mo	unknown

Contraindications/Precautions

Contraindicated in: Hypersensitivity; Male patients with breast or prostate cancer; Hypercalcemia; Severe hepatic, renal, or cardiac disease; Pregnancy or lactation.
Use Cautiously in: Previous history of liver disease; History of porphyria; Coronary artery disease; Prepubertal boys.

Interactions

Drug-Drug: May potentiate **warfarin, oral hypoglycemic agents, insulins**, or **corticosteroids.** May increase **cyclosporine** or **carbamazepine** levels and risk of toxicity. May increase the requirement for **insulin** in patients with diabetes.

Route/Dosage

PO (Adults and Adolescents): *Endometriosis*—400 mg twice daily (for milder cases may initiate therapy with 100–200 mg twice daily). *Fibrocystic breast disease*—50–200 mg twice daily. *Hereditary* *angioedema*—200 mg 2–3 times daily. Attempt to decrease dosage by 50% or less q 1–3 mo. If acute attack occurs, increase dose by up to 200 mg/day.

Availability

Capsules: 50 mg, 100 mg, 200 mg.

dantrolene (dan-troe-leen)

Dantrium

Classification

Therapeutic: skeletal muscle relaxants (direct acting)

Indications

PO: Treatment of spasticity associated with Spinal cord injury, Stroke, Cerebral palsy, Multiple sclerosis. Prophylaxis of malignant hyperthermia. **IV:** Emergency treatment of malignant hyperthermia. **Unlabeled Use:** Management of neuroleptic malignant syndrome.

Action

Acts directly on skeletal muscle, causing relaxation by decreasing calcium release from sarcoplasmic reticulum in muscle cells. Prevents intense catabolic process associated with malignant hyperthermia. **Therapeutic Effects:** Reduction of muscle spasticity. Prevention of malignant hyperthermia.

Adverse Reactions/Side Effects

CNS: drowsiness, muscle weakness, confusion, dizziness, headache, insomnia, malaise, nervousness. **EENT:** excessive lacrimation, visual disturbances. **Resp:** pleural effusions. **CV:** changes in blood pressure, tachycardia. **GI:** HEPATOTOXICITY, diarrhea, anorexia, cramps, dysphagia, GI bleeding, vomiting. **GU:** crystalluria, dysuria, frequency, erectile dysfunction, incontinence, nocturia. **Derm:** pruritus, sweating, urticaria. **Hemat:** eosinophilia. **Local:** irritation at IV site, phlebitis. **MS:** myalgia. **Misc:** chills, drooling, fever.

PHYSICAL THERAPY IMPLICATIONS

Examination and Evaluation

- Be alert for signs of hepatotoxicity, including anorexia, abdominal pain, severe nausea and vomiting, yellow skin or eyes, fever, sore throat, malaise, weakness, facial edema, lethargy, and unusual bleeding or bruising. Report these signs to the physician immediately.
- Assess patient's spasticity, ROM, functional ability, and posture (e.g., head control and trunk stability), especially when beginning Dantrium treatment or during dose adjustments. Communicate with physician, family/caregivers, and other health professionals to determine if dosage is helping achieve desired functional outcomes.
- Assess dizziness or drowsiness that might affect gait, balance, and other functional activities (See Appendix C). Report balance problems and functional limitations to the physician, and caution the patient and family/caregivers to guard against falls and trauma.
- Monitor symptoms such as confusion, nervousness, insomnia, or malaise. Report these problems; excessive or prolonged CNS symptoms may require a reduction in dose.
- Monitor signs of eosinophilia such as fatigue, weakness, and muscle pain (myalgia); report these signs to the physician.
- Assess blood pressure (BP) and compare to normal values (See Appendix F). Report changes in BP, either a problematic decrease in BP (hypotension) or a sustained increase in BP (hypertension).
- Assess heart rate, ECG, and heart sounds, especially during exercise (see Appendixes G, H). Report a rapid heart rate (tachycardia) or symptoms of other arrhythmias, including palpitations, chest discomfort, shortness of breath, fainting, and fatigue/weakness.
- Assess any breathing problems or signs of pleural effusion, including shortness of breath, chest pain, cough, and labored breathing. Monitor pulse oximetry and perform pulmonary function tests (See Appendices I, J, K) to quantify suspected changes in ventilation and respiratory function.
- Assess injection site during and after IV administration, and report signs of phlebitis (local pain, swelling, inflammation).

Interventions

- Implement aggressive therapeutic exercises (neuromuscular reeducation, postural stabilization, gait training, other task-specific training) to help patient adjust to reduced spasticity and tone.
- Because of the risk of bradycardia and abnormal BP responses, use caution during aerobic exercise and other forms of therapeutic exercise. Assess exercise tolerance frequently (BP, heart rate, fatigue levels), and terminate exercise immediately if any untoward responses occur (See Appendix L).
- Guard against falls and trauma due to sedation, dizziness, or abnormally low tone in the trunk and lower extremities. Implement fall-prevention strategies, especially if patient exhibits excessive sedation, dizziness, or other impairments that affect gait and balance (See Appendix E).
- To minimize orthostatic hypotension, patient should move slowly when assuming a more upright position.

Patient/Client-Related Instruction

- Advise patient to avoid alcohol and other CNS depressants because of the increased risk of sedation, liver toxicity, and other adverse effects.
- Instruct patient or family/caregivers to report other troublesome side effects such as severe or prolonged vision disturbances, urinary problems, erectile dysfunction, flu-like symptoms (fever, chills), skin reactions (hives, itching, increased sweating), or GI problems (vomiting, diarrhea, cramps, problems swallowing, excessive drooling, loss of appetite, blood in the stools).

Pharmacokinetics

Absorption: 35% absorbed after oral administration.
Distribution: Unknown.
Metabolism and Excretion: Almost entirely metabolized by the liver.
Half-life: 8.7 hr.

TIME/ACTION PROFILE (effects on spasticity)

ROUTE	ONSET	PEAK	DURATION
PO	1 wk	unknown	6–12 hr
IV	rapid	rapid	unknown

Contraindications/Precautions

Contraindicated in: No contraindications to IV form in treatment of hyperthermia; Pregnancy and lactation; Situations in which spasticity is used to maintain posture or balance.
Use Cautiously in: Cardiac, pulmonary, or previous liver disease; Women, patients >35 yr (increased risk of hepatotoxicity).

Interactions

Drug-Drug: Additive CNS depression with **CNS depressants**, including **alcohol**, **antihistamines**, **opioid analgesics**, **sedative/hypnotics**, and parenteral **magnesium sulfate**. ↑ risk of hepatotoxicity with other **hepatotoxic agents** or **estrogens**. ↑ risk of arrhythmias with **verapamil**.
Drug-Natural: Concomitant use of **kava**, **valerian**, **chamomile**, or **hops** can ↑ CNS depression.

Route/Dosage

PO (Adults): *Spasticity*—25 mg/day initially; increase by 25 mg/day q 4–7 days until desired response or total of 100 mg 4 times daily is reached. *Prevention of malignant hyperthermia*—4–8 mg/kg/day in 3–4 divided doses for 1–2 days before procedure; last dose 3–4 hr preoperatively. *Post–hyperthermic crisis follow-up*—4–8 mg/kg/day in 3–4 divided doses for 1–3 days after IV treatment.
PO (Children >5 yr): *Spasticity*—0.5 mg/kg twice daily; increase by 0.5 mg/kg/day q 4–7 days until desired response is obtained or dosage of 3 mg/kg 4 times daily is reached (not to exceed 400 mg/day). *Prevention of malignant hyperthermia*—4–8 mg/kg/day in 3–4 divided doses for 1–2 days before procedure; last dose 3–4 hr preoperatively. *Post–hyperthermic crisis follow-up*—4–8 mg/kg/day in 3–4 divided doses for 1–3 days after IV treatment.
IV (Adults and Children): *Treatment of malignant hyperthermia*—at least 1 mg/kg (up to 3 mg/kg), continued until symptoms decrease or a cumulative dose of 10 mg/kg has been given. If symptoms reappear, dose may be repeated. *Prevention of malignant hyperthermia*—2.5 mg/kg before anesthesia.

Availability (generic available)

Capsules: 25 mg, 50 mg, 100 mg. **Powder for injection:** 20 mg/vial.

dapsone (dap-sohn)

Aczone, ✦Avlosulfon

Classification
Therapeutic: leprostatic agents

Indications

Treatment of leprosy (in combination with other agents). Treatment of dermatitis herpetiformis. Treatment of acne vulgaris (topical). **Unlabeled Use:** Prevention (as monotherapy) and treatment of *Pneumocystis carinii* pneumonia (with trimethoprim or other agents).

Action

Interferes with folate synthesis in susceptible organisms. **Therapeutic Effects:** Bacteriostatic action.
Spectrum: Active against *Mycobacterium leprae*, *Pneumocystis carinii*.

Adverse Reactions/Side Effects

CNS: headache, insomnia, mood changes, tonic-clonic movements (topical), vertigo. **EENT:** blurred vision, tinnitus, pharyngitis (topical). **GI:** HEPATOTOXICITY, abdominal pain, nausea, pancreatitis, vomiting.
Derm: exfoliative dermatitis, hypersensitivity reactions, including erythema nodosum leprosum, photosensitivity, Stevens-Johnson syndrome, systemic lupus erythematosus. **Hemat:** AGRANULOCYTOSIS, METHEMOGLOBINEMIA, hemolytic anemia, reticulocytosis.
Neuro: peripheral neuropathy.

PHYSICAL THERAPY IMPLICATIONS

Examination and Evaluation

- Be alert for signs of liver toxicity, including anorexia, abdominal pain, severe nausea and vomiting, yellow skin or eyes, fever, sore throat, malaise, weakness, facial edema, lethargy, and unusual bleeding or bruising. Report these signs to the physician immediately.
- Monitor signs of agranulocytosis (fever, sore throat, mucosal lesions, signs of infection), methemoglobinemia (bluish coloring of skin, headache, shortness of breath, lack of energy), or other unusual

weakness and fatigue that might be due to other anemias and blood dyscrasias. Report these signs to the physician immediately.

- Monitor signs of hypersensitivity reactions, including skin reactions (rash, hives, itching) and Stevens-Johnson syndrome (severe dermatitis and exfoliation). Notify physician immediately because these signs may indicate serious hypersensitivity reactions.
- Monitor signs of peripheral neuropathy (numbness, tingling). Perform objective tests (nerve conduction, monofilaments) to document any neuropathic changes.
- Determine if vertigo or abnormal movements affects gait and balance and if patient is at an increased risk of falls (See Appendices C, E).

Interventions

- Always wash hands thoroughly and disinfect equipment (whirlpools, electrotherapeutic devices, treatment tables, and so forth) to help prevent the spread of infection. Use universal precautions or isolation procedures as indicated for specific patients.
- Causes photosensitivity; use care if administering UV treatments.

Patient/Client-Related Instruction

- Advise patient about photosensitivity, and to use sunscreens, protective clothing, and avoid prolonged sun exposure. Advise patient to also report any rashes or other skin reactions.
- Advise patient about the likelihood of GI reactions such as nausea, vomiting, and abdominal pain. Instruct patient to report severe or prolonged GI problems or signs of pancreatitis (upper abdominal pain after eating, indigestion, weight loss, oily stools).
- Instruct patient and family/caregivers to report other troublesome side effects such as severe or prolonged headache, sleep loss, mood changes, blurred vision, ringing/buzzing in the ears (tinnitus), or throat irritation.

Pharmacokinetics

Absorption: Slowly absorbed (70–80%) following oral administration; acidic environment promotes absorption.
Distribution: Widely distributed; crosses the placenta and enters breast milk in significant concentrations.
Protein Binding: *Dapsone*—70–90%; *monacetyl dapsone (MADDS)*—99%.
Metabolism and Excretion: Mostly metabolized by the liver to MADDS, its major metabolite, which is then metabolized back to dapsone.
Half-life: 10–50 hr.

TIME/ACTION PROFILE (blood levels)

ROUTE	ONSET	PEAK	DURATION
PO	unknown	unknown	unknown
topical	unknown	unknown	unknown

Contraindications/Precautions

Contraindicated in: Hypersensitivity (cross-sensitivity with sulfonamides may occur); Lactation: Lactation.
Use Cautiously in: Severe anemia; G6PD deficiency; Impaired hepatic function; OB: Pregnancy.

Interactions

Drug-Drug: Concurrent administration with **didanosine** or **antacids** may ↓ absorption of dapsone (separate administration times by 2 hr). Blood levels may be ↑ by **amiodarone, fluconazole, ketoconazole, itraconazole, clarithromycin, erythromycin, quinidine, verapamil,** or **diltiazem**. Blood levels may be ↓ by **rifampin, phenytoin, phenobarbital,** or **carbamazepine**. Coadministration with **trimethoprim** results in ↑ levels of both agents. Concurrent use with **agents causing blood dyscrasias or hemolytic anemia** may ↑ the risk of these adverse effects.
Drug-Natural: St. John's wort may ↓ blood levels of dapsone.

Route/Dosage

Leprosy

PO (Adults): 50–100 mg/day for 3–10 yrs.
PO (Children): 1–2 mg/kg/day, up to 100 mg/day.

Dermatitis Herpetiformis

PO (Adults): Initiate therapy with 50 mg/day, up to 300 mg/day may be required.

Acne Vulgaris

Topical (Adults and Children ≥12 yr): Apply small amount twice daily.

Pneumocystis carinii Pneumonia

PO (Adults): *Prophylaxis*—100 mg/day; *Treatment*—100 mg/day (in combination with trimethoprim) for 21 days.
PO (Children >1 mo): *Prophylaxis*—2 mg/kg/day (up to 100 mg/day) once daily, or 4 mg/kg once weekly (up to 200 mg/dose).

Availability

Tablets: 25 mg, 100 mg. **Topical Gel:** 5% Rx.

daptomycin (dap-toe-mye-sin)

Cubicin

Classification
Therapeutic: anti-infectives
Pharmacologic: cyclic lipopeptide antibacterial agents

Indications

Complicated skin and skin structure infections caused by aerobic gram-positive bacteria.

Action

Causes rapid depolarization of membrane potential following binding to bacterial membrane; this results in inhibition of protein, DNA, and RNA synthesis. **Therapeutic Effects:** Death of bacteria with resolution of infection. **Spectrum:** Active against *Staphylococcus aureus* (including methicillin-resistant strains), *Streptococcus pyogenes*, *S. agalactiae*, some *S. dysgalactiae*, and *Enterococcus faecalis* (vancomycin-susceptible strains).

Adverse Reactions/Side Effects

CNS: dizziness. **Resp:** dyspnea. **CV:** hypertension, hypotension. **GI:** PSEUDOMEMBRANOUS COLITIS, constipation, diarrhea, nausea, vomiting, ↑ liver function tests. **GU:** renal failure. **Derm:** pruritus, rash. **Hemat:** anemia. **Local:** injection site reactions. **MS:** ↑ CPK. **Misc:** fever.

PHYSICAL THERAPY IMPLICATIONS

Examination and Evaluation

- Monitor signs of pseudomembranous colitis, including diarrhea, abdominal pain, fever, pus or mucus in stools, and other severe or prolonged GI problems (nausea, vomiting, heartburn). Notify physician or nursing staff immediately of these signs.
- Monitor signs of renal failure, including decreased urine output, increased blood pressure (BP), muscle cramps/twitching, edema/weight gain from fluid retention, yellowish brown skin, and confusion that progresses to seizures and coma. Report these signs to the physician immediately.
- Assess BP and compare to normal values (See Appendix F). Report changes in BP, either a problematic decrease in BP (hypotension) or a sustained increase in BP (hypertension).
- Monitor signs of anemia, including unusual fatigue, shortness of breath with exertion, and bruising. Notify physician immediately if these signs occur.
- Assess any breathing problems, and report signs of difficult of labored breathing.
- Assess dizziness that might affect gait, balance, and other functional activities (See Appendix C). Report balance problems and functional limitations to the physician and nursing staff, and caution the patient and family/caregivers to guard against falls and trauma.
- Monitor IV injection site for pain, swelling, and irritation. Report prolonged or excessive injection site reactions to the physician.

Interventions

- Always wash hands thoroughly and disinfect equipment (whirlpools, electrotherapeutic devices, treatment tables, and so forth) to help prevent the spread of infection. Employ universal precautions or isolation procedures as indicated for specific patients.

Patient/Client-Related Instruction

- Instruct patient to notify physician immediately of signs of superinfection, including black, furry overgrowth on tongue, vaginal itching or discharge, and loose or foul-smelling stools.
- Instruct patient and family/caregivers to report other troublesome side effects such as severe or prolonged fever, skin problems (rash, itching), or GI problems (nausea, vomiting, diarrhea, constipation).

Pharmacokinetics

Absorption: IV administration results in complete bioavailability.
Distribution: Unknown.
Protein Binding: 92%.
Metabolism and Excretion: Metabolism not known; mostly excreted by kidneys.
Half-life: 8.1 hr.

TIME/ACTION PROFILE

ROUTE	ONSET	PEAK	DURATION
IV	rapid	end of infusion	24 hr

Contraindications/Precautions

Contraindicated in: Hypersensitivity.
Use Cautiously in: CCr <30 mL/min (dose reduction required); Geriatric patients (may have ↓ clinical response with ↑ risk of adverse reactions); Pregnancy (use only if clearly needed); Lactation; Children <18 yr (safety not established).

Interactions

Drug-Drug: Tobramycin ↑ blood levels. Concurrent **HMG CoA reductase inhibitors** may ↑ the risk of myopathy.

Route/Dosage

IV (Adults): 4 mg/kg q 24 hr.

Renal Impairment

IV (Adults): *CCr <30 mL/min*—4 mg/kg every 48 hr.

Availability

Powder for injection: 500 mg/vial.

darbepoetin (dar-be-poe-e-tin)

Aranesp

Classification

Therapeutic: antianemics
Pharmacologic: hormones (rDNA)

Indications

Anemia associated with chronic renal failure. Chemotherapy-induced anemia in patients with nonmyeloid malignancies.

Action

Stimulates erythropoiesis (production of red blood cells). **Therapeutic Effects:** Maintains and may elevate red blood cell counts, decreasing the need for transfusions.

Adverse Reactions/Side Effects

CNS: SEIZURES, dizziness, fatigue, headache, weakness. **Resp:** cough, dyspnea, bronchitis. **CV:** CHF, MI, STROKE, THROMBOTIC EVENTS (ESPECIALLY WITH HEMOGLOBIN >12 G/DL), edema, hypertension, hypotension, chest pain. **GI:** abdominal pain, nausea, diarrhea, vomiting, constipation. **Derm:** pruritus. **Hemat:** pure red cell aplasia. **MS:** myalgia, arthralgia, back pain, limb pain. **Misc:** fever, allergic reactions, flu-like syndrome, sepsis, ↑ mortality and ↑ tumor growth (with hemoglobin ≥12 g/dL).

PHYSICAL THERAPY IMPLICATIONS

Examination and Evaluation

- Be alert for new seizures or increased seizure activity, especially at the onset of drug treatment. Document the number, duration, and severity of seizures, and report these findings immediately to the physician.
- Monitor continually, and seek immediate medical assistance if patient develops any of the following signs or syndromes:
  - Stroke, as indicated by severe headache, confusion, nausea, vomiting, paralysis, numbness, speech problems, and visual disturbances.
  - Myocardial infarction, as indicated by sudden chest pain, pain radiating into the arm or jaw, shortness of breath, dizziness, sweating, anxiety, and nausea.
  - Congestive heart failure, as indicated by dyspnea, rales/crackles, peripheral edema, jugular venous distention, and exercise intolerance.
- Assess blood pressure (BP) and compare to normal values (See Appendix F). Report changes in BP, either a problematic decrease in BP (hypotension) or a sustained increase in BP (hypertension).
- Assess any difficult or labored breathing problems or signs of cough or bronchitis. Monitor pulse oximetry and perform pulmonary function tests (See Appendices I, J, K) to quantify suspected changes in ventilation and respiratory function.
- Assess peripheral edema using girth measurements, volume displacement, and measurement of pitting edema (See Appendix N). Report increased swelling in feet and ankles or a sudden increase in body weight due to fluid retention.
- Monitor signs of allergic reactions, including pulmonary symptoms (tightness in the throat and chest, wheezing, cough, dyspnea) or skin reactions (rash, pruritus, urticaria). Notify physician or nursing staff immediately if these reactions occur.
- Assess any muscle, joint, back, or limb pain to rule out musculoskeletal pathology; that is, try to determine if pain is drug induced rather than caused by anatomic or biomechanical problems.
- Assess dizziness that might affect gait, balance, and other functional activities (See Appendix C). Report balance problems and functional limitations to the physician and nursing staff, and caution the patient and family/caregivers to guard against falls and trauma.

Interventions

- Because of the risk of thrombotic events and heart failure, use caution during aerobic exercise and other forms of therapeutic exercise. Assess exercise tolerance frequently (BP, heart rate, fatigue levels), and terminate exercise immediately if any untoward responses occur (See Appendix L).
- If administered via subcutaneous injection, do not apply massage or physical agents (heat, cold, electrotherapeutic modalities) at or near the application site. These interventions can alter drug absorption from subcutaneous tissues.

Patient/Client-Related Instruction

- Caution patient and family/caregivers about risks of myocardial infarction, stroke, and heart failure, and review warning signs of these problems (see above under Evaluation and Examination).
- Instruct patient to report other troublesome side effects such as severe or prolonged headache, itching skin, signs of infection, flu-like symptoms (chills, fever, body aches) or GI problems (nausea, vomiting, constipation, diarrhea, abdominal pain).

Pharmacokinetics

Absorption: 30–50% following SC administration; IV administration results in complete bioavailability.
Distribution: Confined to the intravascular space.
Metabolism and Excretion: Unknown.
Half-life: *SC*—49 hr; *IV*—21 hr.

TIME/ACTION PROFILE (increase in RBCs)

ROUTE	ONSET	PEAK	DURATION
IV, SC	2–6 wk	unknown	unknown

Contraindications/Precautions

Contraindicated in: Hypersensitivity; Uncontrolled hypertension.
Use Cautiously in: History of hypertension; Underlying hematologic diseases, including hemolytic anemia, sickle-cell anemia, thalassemia and porphyria (safety not established); OB/Lactation/Pedi: Safety not established.

Interactions
Drug-Drug: None reported.

Route/Dosage

Anemia due to Chronic Renal Failure
(Use lowest dose that will gradually increase hemoglobin level and avoid RBC transfusion)
IV, SC (Adults): *Starting treatment with darbepoetin (no previous epoetin)*—0.45 mcg/kg once weekly (may start with 0.75 mcg/kg q 2 wk in patients not on dialysis); adjust dose to attain target Hgb of 10–12 g/dl; if Hgb ↑ by >1 g/dL in 2 wk or if the Hgb is ↑ and nearing 12 g/dL, ↓ dose by 25%; if Hgb ↑ by <1 g/dL after 4 wk of therapy (with adequate iron stores), ↑ dose by 25%; do not ↑ dose more frequently than q 4 wk. *Conversion from epoetin to darbepoetin*—weekly epoetin dose <2500 units = 6.25 mcg/week darbepoetin, weekly epoetin dose 2500-4999 units = 12.5 mcg/week darbepoetin, weekly epoetin dose 5000–10,999 units = 25 mcg/week darbepoetin, weekly epoetin dose 11,000–17,999 units = 40 mcg/week darbepoetin, weekly epoetin dose 18,000–33,999 units = 60 mcg/week darbepoetin, weekly epoetin dose 34,000–89,999 units = 100 mcg/week darbepoetin, weekly epoetin dose >90,000 units = 200 mcg/week darbepoetin.

Anemia due to Chemotherapy
(Use only for chemotherapy-related anemia and discontinue when chemotherapy course is completed)
SC (Adults): 2.25 mcg/kg weekly or 500 mcg q 3 wk; target Hgb should not exceed 12 g/dL. If Hgb ↑ by >1 g/dL in 2 wk or if the Hgb >12 g/dL or Hgb reaches level to avoid transfusion, ↓ dose by 40%; if Hgb ↑ by <1 g/dL after 6 wk of therapy, ↑ dose to 4.5 mcg/kg.

Availability
Albumin solution for injection: 25 mcg/mL 1-mL vial, 40 mcg/mL 1-mL vial, 60 mcg/mL 1-mL vial, 100 mcg/mL 1-mL vial, 150 mcg/mL 0.75-mL vial, 200 mcg/mL 1-mL vial, 300 mcg/mL 1-mL vial, 500 mcg/mL 1-mL vial. **Prefilled syringes:** 60 mcg/0.3 mL, 100 mcg/0.5 mL, 200 mcg/0.4 mL.

darifenacin (dar-i-fen-a-sin)
Enablex

Classification
Therapeutic: urinary tract antispasmodics
Pharmacologic: anticholinergics

Indications
Overactive bladder with symptoms (urge incontinence, urgency, frequency).

Action
Acts as a muscarinic (cholinergic) receptor antagonist; antagonizes bladder smooth muscle contraction. **Therapeutic Effects:** Decreased symptoms of overactive bladder.

Adverse Reactions/Side Effects
CNS: dizziness. **EENT:** blurred vision. **GI:** constipation, dry mouth, dyspepsia, nausea. **Metab:** heat intolerance.

PHYSICAL THERAPY IMPLICATIONS

Examination and Evaluation
- Monitor the frequency and urgency of urination to help document whether this drug is successful in controlling overactive bladder.
- Assess dizziness and blurred vision that might affect gait, balance, and other functional activities (See Appendix C). Report balance problems and functional limitations to the physician, and caution the patient and family/caregivers to guard against falls and trauma.

Interventions
- Implement pelvic floor strengthening and other therapeutic exercises to help maintain adequate sphincter control and prevent urine leakage during coughing, sneezing, and so forth.
- Because of heat intolerance, use care during aerobic exercises. Exercises should be done in a cool environment to prevent hyperthermia.

Patient/Client-Related Instruction
- Instruct patient to report other bothersome side effects such as severe or prolonged nausea, constipation, dry mouth, or indigestion.

Pharmacokinetics
Absorption: 15–19% absorbed.
Distribution: Unknown.
Protein Binding: 98%.
Metabolism and Excretion: Extensively metabolized by the CYP2D6 enzyme system in most individuals; poor metabolizers (7% of whites, 2% of African Americans) have less CYP2D6 activity with less metabolism occurring. Some metabolism via CYP3A4 enzyme system. 60% excreted renally as metabolites, 40% in feces as metabolites.
Half-life: 13–19 hr.

TIME/ACTION PROFILE

ROUTE	ONSET	PEAK	DURATION
PO	unknown	7 hr	24 hr

Contraindications/Precautions
Contraindicated in: Hypersensitivity; Urinary retention; Gastric retention; Uncontrolled angle-closure glaucoma; Severe hepatic impairment.
Use Cautiously in: Concurrent use of CYP3A4 inhibitors (use lower dose/clinical monitoring may be necessary); Moderate hepatic impairment (lower dose recommended); Bladder outflow obstruction; GI obstructive disorders, ↓ GI motility, Severe constipation or ulcerative colitis; Myasthenia gravis; Angle-closure glaucoma; Lactation or children (safety not established);

Pregnancy (use only if maternal benefit outweighs fetal risk).

Interactions

Drug-Drug: Blood levels and risk of toxicity are ↑ by concurrent use of strong CYP3A4 inhibitors, including **ketoconazole, itraconazole, ritonavir, nelfinavir, clarithromycin,** and **nefazodone**; daily dose should not exceed 7.5 mg. Concurrent use of moderate inhibitors of CYP3A4, especially those with narrow therapeutic indices, including **flecainide, thioridazine,** and **tricyclic antidepressants** should be undertaken with caution.

Route/Dosage

PO (Adults): 7.5 mg once daily; may be ↑ after 2 wk to 15 mg once daily.

Availability

Extended-release tablets: 7.5 mg, 15 mg.

darunavir (da-run-a-veer)

Prezista

Classification

Therapeutic: antiretrovirals

Pharmacologic: protease inhibitors

Indications

HIV infection (with other antiretrovirals) in adults who have already received and progressed on other antiretroviral combinations.

Action

Inhibits HIV-1 protease, selectively inhibiting the cleavage of HIV-encoded specific polyproteins in infected cells. This prevents the formation of mature viral particles. **Therapeutic Effects:** Increased CD4 cell counts and decreased viral load with subsequent slowed progression of HIV infection and its sequelae.

Adverse Reactions/Side Effects

Based on concurrent use with ritonavir

GI: HEPATOTOXICITY, constipation, diarrhea, nausea, vomiting. **Endo:** hyperglycemia. **Metab:** body fat redistribution. **Derm:** rash.

PHYSICAL THERAPY IMPLICATIONS

Examination and Evaluation

- Be alert for signs of hepatotoxicity, including anorexia, abdominal pain, severe nausea and vomiting, yellow skin or eyes, fever, sore throat, malaise, weakness, facial edema, lethargy, and unusual bleeding or bruising. Notify physician immediately if these signs occur.
- Monitor and report signs of hyperglycemia, including confusion, drowsiness, fatigue, weakness, rapid breathing, fruity or pungent breath, excessive thirst, frequent urination, nausea, vomiting, and abdominal pain.

Interventions

- Implement resistive exercises and other therapeutic exercises as tolerated to maintain muscle strength and function and prevent muscle wasting associated with HIV infection and AIDS.

Patient/Client-Related Instruction

- Emphasize the importance of taking darunavir as directed even if the patient is asymptomatic, and that this drug must always be used in combination with other antiretroviral drugs. Do not take more than prescribed amount and do not stop taking without consulting health care professional.
- Inform patient that darunavir does not cure HIV or AIDS or prevent associated or opportunistic infections. Darunavir does not reduce the risk of transmission of HIV to others through sexual contact or blood contamination. Caution patient to use a condom, and to avoid sharing needles or donating blood to prevent spreading the AIDS virus to others.
- Inform patient that redistribution and accumulation of body fat may occur, causing central obesity, thin arms and legs, dorsocervical fat enlargement (buffalo hump), breast enlargement, and other symptoms that resemble Cushing's syndrome (moon face, striations on abdominal skin). Discuss possible effects on body image, and help patient explore coping mechanisms.
- Instruct patient to report other troublesome side effects such as prolonged or severe skin rash or GI problems (diarrhea, nausea, vomiting, constipation).

Pharmacokinetics

Absorption: *Without ritonavir*—37% absorbed following oral administration; *with ritonavir*—82%. Food increases absorption by 30%.
Distribution: Unknown.
Protein Binding: 95% bound to plasma proteins.
Metabolism and Excretion: Extensively metabolized by CYP3A enzyme system. 41% eliminated unchanged in feces, 8% in urine.
Half-life: 15 hr.

TIME/ACTION PROFILE

ROUTE	ONSET	PEAK	DURATION
PO	unknown	2.5–4 hr	12 hr

Contraindications/Precautions

Contraindicated in: Concurrent dihydroergotamine, ergonovine, ergotamine, methylergonovine, midazolam, pimozide, or triazolam; OB: Lactation; HIV may be transmitted in human milk; Pedi: Safety not established.

Use Cautiously in: Hepatic impairment; Sulfa allergy; Geri: Consider age-related impairment in hepatic function, concurrent chronic disease states and drug therapy; OB: Use in pregnancy only if maternal benefit outweighs fetal risk.

Interactions

Drug-Drug: Darunavir and ritonavir are both inhibitors of CYP3A and are metabolized by CYP3A. Multiple drug-drug interactions can be expected with drugs that share, inhibit, or induce these pathways. Consult product information for more specific details. **Carbamazepine**, **phenobarbital**, **rifampin**, and **phenytoin** ↑ metabolism and may ↓ antiretroviral effectiveness; concurrent use is contraindicated. ↓ metabolism of and may ↑ risk of ergot toxicity with **dihydroergotamine**, **ergonovine**, **ergotamine**, **methylergonovine**; concurrent use is contraindicated. ↓ metabolism of and may ↑ risk of serious myopathy with **lovastatin** and simvastatin; concurrent use is contraindicated. ↑ levels and risk of cardiotoxicity with **pimozide**; concurrent use is contraindicated. ↑ levels and risk of excess CNS depression with **midazolam** or **triazolam**; concurrent use is contraindicated. ↑ levels and risk of myopathy from **atorvastatin**, **rosuvastatin**, or **pravastatin** (use lowest dose of these agents or consider fluvastatin). Concurrent use with **efavirenz** results in ↓ darunavir levels and ↑ efavirenz levels; use combination cautiously. Concurrent use with **lopinavir/ritonavir** ↓ darunavir levels and may ↓ antiretroviral effectiveness; although concurrent use is not recommended, additional ritonavir may be required. Concurrent use with **saquinavir** ↓ darunavir levels and may ↓ antiretroviral effectiveness; concurrent use is not recommended. ↑ levels and risk of toxicity with **lidocaine, quinidine**, and **amiodarone;** use cautiously and with available blood level monitoring. ↓ levels and may ↓ anticoagulant effect of **warfarin**; monitor INR. ↑ levels and risk of adverse reactions to **trazodone**; use cautiously and decrease dose if necessary. ↑ levels of **clarithromycin**, especially in patients with renal impairment (CCr <60 mL/min); ↓ dose of clarithromycin required. **Ketoconazole** and **itraconazole** may ↑ darunavir levels. Darunavir ↑ levels of **ketoconazole** and **itraconazole**; daily dose of itraconazole or ketoconazole should not be >200 mg. ↓ blood levels and may ↓ antifungal effectiveness of **voriconazole**; avoid concurrent use if possible. Concurrent use with **rifabutin** ↑ rifabutin levels and ↓ darunavir levels; (may be due to ritonavir); rifabutin dose should be decreased to 150 mg every other day. ↑ levels and may ↑ risk of adverse cardiovascular side effects of **felodipine**, **nifedipine**, or **nicardipine**; monitor clinical response carefully. **Dexamethasone** ↓ levels and may ↓ antiretroviral effectiveness. May ↑ systemic levels of **inhaled fluticasone**; choose alternative inhaled corticosteroid. ↑ levels of, and may ↑ risk of toxicity with, **cyclosporine**, **tacrolimus**, or **sirolimus**; blood level monitoring recommended. ↓ levels and may precipitate opiate abstinence syndrome from **methadone**. ↑ levels of, and ↑ risk of serious toxicity from, **sildenafil**, **tadalafil**, or **vardenafil**; dose reduction required. ↓ levels and may ↓ antidepressant effectiveness of **sertraline** and **paroxetine**; adjust dose by clinical response.
Drug-Natural: St. John's wort ↑ metabolism and may ↓ antiretroviral effectiveness.

Route/Dosage

PO (Adults): 600 mg with ritonavir 100 mg twice daily.

Availability

Tablets: 300 mg, 600 mg.

dasatinib (da-sat-i-nib)

Sprycel

Classification
Therapeutic: antineoplastics
Pharmacologic: enzyme inhibitors

Indications

Chronic, accelerated, or myeloid or lymphoid blast phase chronic myeloid leukemia (CML)–resistant/intolerant to prior therapy. Philadelphia chromosome–positive acute lymphoblastic leukemia–resistant/intolerant to prior therapy.

Action

Inhibits tyrosine kinases resulting in inhibition of leukemic cell lines, including those resistant to imatinib. **Therapeutic Effects:** Decreased progression of leukemias.

Adverse Reactions/Side Effects

CNS: SEIZURES, altered affect, anxiety, confusion, depression, drowsiness, insomnia, malaise, syncope, vertigo. **EENT:** conjunctivitis, dry eye, tinnitus. **Resp:** asthma, pneumonitis. **CV:** CHF, MI, PULMONARY EDEMA, QTC PROLONGATION, hypertension, hypotension, palpitations. **GI:** abdominal pain, altered appetite, dysgeusia, dyspepsia, ileus, mucositis, nausea, vomiting. **GU:** RENAL FAILURE, urinary frequency. **Derm:** acne, alopecia, dry skin, flushing, nail disorder, photosensitivity, pigment disorder, rash, sweating, urticaria. **Endo:** gynecomastia. **F and E:** fluid retention, hypocalcemia. **Hemat:** BLEEDING EVENTS, anemia, neutropenia, pancytopenia, thrombocytopenia. **Metab:** hyperuricemia. **MS:** muscle inflammation/weakness. **Neuro:** tremor. **Misc:** INFECTIONS, PALMAR-PLANTAR ERYTHRODYSESTHESIA, TUMOR LYSIS SYNDROME.

PHYSICAL THERAPY IMPLICATIONS

Examination and Evaluation

- Be alert for new seizures or increased seizure activity, especially at the onset of drug treatment. Document the number, duration, and severity of seizures, and report these findings to the physician immediately.

- Monitor continually for signs of MI, including sudden chest pain, pain radiating into the arm or jaw, shortness of breath, dizziness, sweating, anxiety, and nausea. Seek immediate medical assistance if patient develops these signs.
- Assess signs of congestive heart failure, including dyspnea, rales/crackles, peripheral edema, jugular venous distention, and exercise intolerance. Report these signs to the physician.
- Assess any breathing problems or signs of pulmonary edema, including cough, shortness of breath, chest pain, and labored breathing. Monitor pulse oximetry and perform pulmonary function tests (See Appendices I, J, K) to quantify suspected changes in ventilation and respiratory function.
- Assess heart rate, ECG, and heart sounds, especially during exercise (See Appendices G, H). Report any rhythm disturbances or symptoms of increased arrhythmias, including palpitations, chest discomfort, shortness of breath, fainting, and fatigue/weakness.
- Assess blood pressure (BP) and compare to normal values (See Appendix F). Report changes in BP, either a problematic decrease in BP (hypotension) or a sustained increase in BP (hypertension).
- Monitor signs of renal failure, including decreased urine output, increased BP, muscle cramps/twitching, edema/weight gain from fluid retention, yellowish brown skin, and confusion that progresses to seizures and coma. Report these signs to the physician immediately.
- Assess for signs of bleeding and hemorrhage such as bleeding gums, nosebleed, unusual bruising, black/tarry stools, hematuria, and a fall in hematocrit or BP. Notify physician immediately if these signs occur.
- Be alert for palmer-planter erythrodysesthesia, as indicated by pain, redness, and dry, scaly skin on the palms of the hands and soles of the feet. Report these signs immediately to the physician. Instruct patient also to protect the hands and feet from heat and friction and to apply lotion to the affected areas. Superficial cold application can also temporarily reduce symptoms.
- Monitor neuromuscular signs of electrolyte imbalances that might indicate tumor lysis syndrome. Signs include severe muscle weakness or paralysis due to increased plasma potassium (hyperkalemia) or muscle hyperexcitability and tetany due to phosphate and calcium imbalances (hyperphosphatemia and hypocalcemia). Notify physician immediately if these signs occur.
- Monitor signs of neutropenia (fever, sore throat, signs of infection), thrombocytopenia (bruising, nose bleeds, bleeding gums), or unusual weakness and fatigue that might be caused by anemia or other blood dyscrasias. Report these signs to the physician or nursing staff immediately.
- Assess balance and risk of falls, especially if patient exhibits vertigo or syncope (See Appendix E). Report balance deficits to the physician and nursing staff.
- Assess any muscle pain, weakness, or tremor to rule out musculoskeletal pathology; that is, try to determine if pain is drug induced rather than caused by anatomic or biomechanical problems.
- Be alert for anxiety, confusion, depression, or other alterations in mental status or behavioral affect. Notify health care professional these symptoms become problematic.

Interventions

- For patients who are medically able to begin exercise, implement appropriate resistive exercises and aerobic training to maintain muscle strength and aerobic capacity during cancer chemotherapy or to help restore function after chemotherapy.
- Because of potential cardiac and pulmonary toxicity, use caution during aerobic exercise and endurance conditioning. Terminate exercise if patient exhibits untoward symptoms (chest pain, shortness of breath, unusual fatigue) or displays other criteria for exercise termination (See Appendix L).

Patient/Client-Related Instruction

- Advise patient to guard against infection (frequent hand washing, etc.), and to avoid crowds and contact with persons with contagious diseases.
- Advise patient that skin reactions are likely, including rash, hives, hair loss, acne, increased sweating, and changes in pigmentation. Report severe or unexpected skin reactions to the physician.
- Advise patient about the likelihood of GI reactions such as abdominal pain, constipation, nausea, vomiting, loss of appetite, and heartburn. Instruct patient to report severe or prolonged GI problems.
- Instruct patient to report other bothersome side effects such as severe or prolonged vertigo, eye inflammation, ringing/buzzing in the ears (tinnitus), increased breast size in men (gynecomastia), increased urinary frequency, or fluid retention.

Pharmacokinetics

Absorption: Well absorbed following oral administration. Absorption is pH dependent.
Distribution: Extensively distributed into extravascular space.
Protein Binding: 96%.
Metabolism and Excretion: Extensively metabolized, mostly by the CYP3A4 enzyme system. 85% eliminated

in feces, mostly as metabolites; 4% eliminated in urine, mostly as metabolites.
Half-life: 3–5 hr.

TIME/ACTION PROFILE

ROUTE	ONSET	PEAK	DURATION
PO	unknown	0.5–6 hr	12 hr

Contraindications/Precautions

Contraindicated in: Lactation: OB: Pregnancy or lactation.
Use Cautiously in: Risk of QTc prolongation, including hypokalemia, hypomagnesemia congenital prolonged QT syndrome, concurrent antiarrhythmic drugs or other drugs that prolong QT interval, including cumulative high-dose anthracycline therapy (correct electrolyte abnormalities prior to use); Concurrent use of anticoagulants or agents that inhibit platelet function; Pedi: Safety not established.

Interactions

Drug-Drug: The following drugs may ↑ dasatinib levels and risk of toxicity by inhibiting CYP3A4: **ketoconazole, itraconazole, erythromycin, clarithromycin, ritonavir, atazanavir, indinavir, nefazodone, nelfinavir, saquinavir**, and **telithromycin**; concurrent use should be avoided. If concurrent use is required, reduced dose of dasatinib may be required. The following drugs may ↓ dasatinib levels by inducing CYP3A4: **dexamethasone, phenytoin, carbamazepine, rifampin** and **phenobarbital**; alternative agents should be chosen. **Antacids** may alter absorption; simultaneous use should be avoided (dose at least 2 hr prior to or 2 hr after dasatinib). **Histamine H_2 blockers** and **proton pump inhibitors** may also ↓ absorption and should be avoided; consider antacids as an alternative. **Alfentanil, cyclosporine, fentanyl, pimozide, quinidine, sirolimus, tacrolimus**, or **ergot alkaloids (ergotamine, dihydroergotamine)** should be administered with caution because of their narrow therapeutic indices and the unpredictability of enzyme induction/inhibition.
Drug-Natural: St. John's wort may alter levels and effectiveness; avoid concurrent use.

Route/Dosage

Accelerated or myeloid or lymphoid blast phase CML

PO (Adults): 70 mg twice daily.

Chronic phase CML

PO (Adults): 100 mg twice daily.

Availability

Tablets: 20 mg, 50 mg, 70 mg, 100 mg.

HIGH ALERT

daunorubicin hydrochloride
(daw-noe-**roo**-bi-sin **hye**-droe-**klor**-ide)
Cerubidine

daunorubicin citrate liposome
(daw-noe-**roo**-bi-sin **sy**-trate **lye**-poe-sohm)
DaunoXome

Classification
Therapeutic: antineoplastics
Pharmacologic: anthracyclines

Indications

Daunorubicin hydrochloride: In combination with other antineoplastics in the treatment of leukemias. **Daunorubicin citrate liposome:** Management of advanced Kaposi's sarcoma in HIV-infected patients.

Action

Forms a complex with DNA, which subsequently inhibits DNA and RNA synthesis (cell-cycle phase–nonspecific). **Therapeutic Effects:** Death of rapidly replicating cells, particularly malignant ones. Also has immunosuppressive properties.

Adverse Reactions/Side Effects

CNS: DaunoXome: fatigue, headache, depression, dizziness, insomnia, malaise. **EENT:** rhinitis, abnormal vision, sinusitis. **CV:** CARDIOTOXICITY, arrhythmias. **GI:** nausea, vomiting, esophagitis, hepatoxicity, stomatitis. **GU:** red urine, gonadal suppression. **Derm:** alopecia, increased sweating, pruritus. **Hemat:** anemia, leukopenia, thrombocytopenia. **Local:** phlebitis at IV site. **Metab:** hyperuricemia. **MS: DaunoXome:** back pain, arthralgia, myalgia. **Neuro: DaunoXome:** neuropathy. **Misc:** allergic reactions, chills, fever, flushing, chest tightness, influenza-like symptoms.

PHYSICAL THERAPY IMPLICATIONS

Examination and Evaluation

- Assess heart rate, ECG, and blood pressure, especially during exercise. Report any arrhythmias or other signs of cardiac toxicity, including chest discomfort, shortness of breath, dyspnea, rales/crackles, peripheral edema, jugular venous distention, fainting, or severe fatigue and weakness.
- Monitor signs of leukopenia (fever, sore throat, signs of infection), thrombocytopenia (bruising, nose bleeds, bleeding gums), or unusual weakness and fatigue that might be due to anemia. Report these signs to the physician or nursing staff.
- Be alert for signs of peripheral neuropathy (numbness, tingling, decreased muscle strength). Establish

baseline electroneuromyographic values using EMG and nerve conduction at the beginning of drug treatment whenever possible, and reexamine these values periodically to document drug-induced changes in peripheral nerve function.

- Assess any back, joint, or muscle pain, especially with the liposomal form of this drug. Attempt to rule out musculoskeletal pathology; that is, determine if pain is drug induced rather than caused by anatomic or biomechanical problems.
- Monitor signs of allergic reactions, including pulmonary symptoms (tightness in the throat and chest, wheezing, cough, dyspnea) or skin reactions (rash, pruritus, urticaria). Notify physician or nursing staff immediately if these reactions occur.
- Assess dizziness that might affect gait, balance, and other functional activities (See Appendix C). Report balance problems and functional limitations to the physician and nursing staff, and caution the patient and family/caregivers to guard against falls and trauma.
- Monitor IV injection site for pain, swelling, and inflammation (phlebitis). Report signs of phlebitis or other prolonged or excessive injection site reactions to the physician.

Interventions

- For patients who are medically able to begin exercise, implement appropriate resistive exercises and aerobic training to maintain muscle strength and aerobic capacity during cancer chemotherapy or to help restore function after chemotherapy.
- Because of the risk of cardiotoxicity, use caution during aerobic exercise and other forms of therapeutic exercise. Assess exercise tolerance frequently (blood pressure, heart rate, fatigue levels), and terminate exercise immediately if any untoward responses occur (See Appendix L).

Patient/Client-Related Instruction

- Instruct patient to guard against infection (frequent hand washing, etc.), and to avoid crowds and contact with persons with contagious diseases.
- Advise patient about the likelihood of GI reactions such as nausea, vomiting, heartburn, and irritation in or around the mouth. Instruct patient or family and caregivers also to report signs of hepatotoxicity, including loss of appetite, abdominal pain, severe nausea and vomiting, yellow skin or eyes, fever, sore throat, malaise, weakness, facial edema, lethargy, and unusual bleeding or bruising.
- Advise patient that hair loss and other skin reactions (pruritus, increased sweating) are likely. Other severe or unexpected skin reactions should be reported to the physician.
- Instruct patient or family/caregivers to report other bothersome side effects such as severe or prolonged headache, sleep loss, depression, malaise, inflammation in sinuses/nasal passages, vision disturbances, fever, or flu-like symptoms.

D

Pharmacokinetics

Absorption: Administered IV only, resulting in complete bioavailability.
Distribution: Widely distributed. Crosses the placenta.
Metabolism and Excretion: Extensively metabolized by the liver. Converted partially to a compound that also has antineoplastic activity (daunorubicinol); 40% eliminated by biliary excretion.
Half-life: *Daunorubicin*—18.5 hr. *Daunorubicinol*—26.7 hr.

TIME/ACTION PROFILE (effects on blood counts)

ROUTE	ONSET	PEAK	DURATION
IV	7–10 days	10–14 days	21 days
IV (liposome)	unknown	unknown	unknown

Contraindications/Precautions

Contraindicated in: Hypersensitivity to daunorubucin or any other components in the formulation; Symptomatic CHF/arrhythmias; Pregnant or lactating women.
Use Cautiously in: Active infections or decreased bone marrow reserve; Geriatric patients or patients with other chronic debilitating illnesses (dosage reduction recommended for patients ≥60 yr); May reactivate skin lesions produced by previous radiation therapy; Hepatic or renal impairment (dosage reduction recommended if serum creatinine >3 mg/dL or serum bilirubin >1.2 mg/dL); Patients who have received previous anthracycline therapy or who have underlying cardiovascular disease (increased risk of cardiotoxicity); Patients with childbearing potential.

Interactions

Drug-Drug: Additive myelosuppression with other **antineoplastics**. May ↓ antibody response to **live-virus vaccines** and ↑ risk of adverse reactions. **Cyclophosphamide** ↑ the risk of cardiotoxicity. ↑ risk of hepatic toxicity with other **hepatotoxic agents**.

Route/Dosage

Daunorubicin hydrochloride:

Other dose regimens are used. In adults, cumulative dose should not exceed 550 mg/m^2 (450 mg/m^2 if previous chest radiation).
IV (Adults <60 yr): 45 mg/m^2/day for 3 days in first course, then for 2 days of second course (as part of combination regimen).
IV (Adults ≥60 yr): 30 mg/m^2/day for 3 days in first course, then for 2 days of second course (as part of combination regimen).

IV (Children >2 yr): 25 mg/m^2 once weekly (as part of combination regimen). In children <2 yr or BSA <0.5 m^2, dosage should be determined on a mg/kg basis.

Other dose regimens are used. In adults, cumulative dose should not exceed 550 mg/m^2 (450 mg/m^2 if previous chest radiation).

Daunorubicin citrate liposome:

IV (Adults): 40 mg/m^2 q 2 wk.

Renal Impairment

IV (Adults): *Serum creatinine >3 mg/dL*—reduce dose by 50%.

Hepatic Impairment

IV (Adults): *Serum bilirubin 1.2–3 mg/dL*—reduce dose by 25%; *serum bilirubin >3 mg/dL*—reduce dose by 50%.

Availability (generic available)

Powder for injection: 20 mg/vial. **Solution for injection:** 5 mg/mL in 4-mL vials (20 mg). **Liposomal dispersion for injection:** 2 mg/mL in 25-mL vial.

HIGH ALERT

decitabine (de-sit-a-been)

Dacogen

Classification

Therapeutic: antineoplastics

Pharmacologic: antimetabolites

Indications

Treatment of various myelodysplastic syndromes (MDSs).

Action

Inhibits DNA methyltransferase, causing apoptosis. Has more effect on rapidly replicating cells. **Therapeutic Effects:** Improved hematologic and clinical manifestations of MDSs.

Adverse Reactions/Side Effects

CNS: confusion, fatigue, insomnia, depression, lethargy. **EENT:** blurred vision. **Resp:** cough. **CV:** atrial fibrillation, pulmonary edema, tachycardia. **GI:** abdominal pain, constipation, diarrhea, stomatitis, vomiting, abnormal liver function tests. **Derm:** petechiae, rash. **F and E** edema, hypokalemia, hypomagnesemia, ascites. **Hemat:** BLEEDING, anemia, neutropenia, thrombocytopenia. **Local:** injection site irritation. **Metab:** hyperglycemia. **MS:** arthralgia, myalgia. **Misc:** INFECTION, fever, lymphadenopathy.

PHYSICAL THERAPY IMPLICATIONS

Examination and Evaluation

- Assess signs of bleeding and hemorrhage, such as bleeding gums, nosebleed, unusual bruising, black/tarry stools, hematuria, and a fall in hematocrit or blood pressure. Notify physician immediately if these signs occur.
- Assess any breathing problems or signs of pulmonary edema, including cough, shortness of breath, chest pain, and labored breathing. Monitor pulse oximetry and perform pulmonary function tests (See Appendices I, J, K) to quantify suspected changes in ventilation and respiratory function.
- Assess heart rate, ECG, and heart sounds, especially during exercise (See Appendices G, H). Report any rhythm disturbances or symptoms of increased arrhythmias, including palpitations, chest discomfort, shortness of breath, fainting, and fatigue/weakness.
- Monitor signs of neutropenia (fever, sore throat, signs of infection), thrombocytopenia (bruising, nose bleeds, bleeding gums), or unusual weakness and fatigue that might be caused by anemia or other blood dyscrasias. Report these signs to the physician or nursing staff immediately.
- Assess peripheral edema using girth measurements, volume displacement, and measurement of pitting edema (see Appendix N). Report increased swelling in feet and ankles, abdominal swelling (ascites), and/or a sudden increase in body weight due to fluid retention.
- Be alert for signs of hyperglycemia, including confusion, drowsiness, flushed/dry skin, fruit-like breath odor, rapid/deep breathing, polyuria, loss of appetite, and unusual thirst. Patients with diabetes mellitus should check blood glucose levels frequently.
- Assess any muscle or joint pain to rule out musculoskeletal pathology; that is, try to determine if pain is drug induced rather than caused by anatomic or biomechanical problems.
- Monitor any muscle weakness, aches, or cramps that might indicate low potassium levels (hypokalemia), or lethargy, irritability, insomnia, muscle tremors, and confusion associated with low magnesium levels (hypomagnesemia). Notify physician of these signs.
- Be alert for confusion, depression, lethargy, or other alterations in mental status or behavioral affect. Notify physician if these symptoms become problematic.
- Monitor IV injection site for pain, swelling, and irritation. Report prolonged or excessive injection site reactions to the physician.

Interventions

- For patients who are medically able to begin exercise, implement appropriate resistive exercises and aerobic training to maintain muscle strength and aerobic capacity during cancer chemotherapy or to help restore function after chemotherapy.
- Because of potential pulmonary toxicity, use caution during aerobic exercise and endurance conditioning. Terminate exercise if patient exhibits

untoward symptoms (chest pain, shortness of breath, etc.) or displays other criteria for exercise termination (See Appendix L).

Patient/Client-Related Instruction

- Advise patient to guard against infection (frequent hand washing, etc.), and to avoid crowds and contact with persons with contagious diseases.
- Advise patient that skin reactions are likely, including rash and small, hemorrhagic spots on the skin (petechiae). Report severe or unexpected skin reactions to the physician.
- Advise patient about the likelihood of GI reactions such as abdominal pain, constipation, diarrhea, vomiting, and inflammation in/around the mouth. Instruct patient to report severe or prolonged GI problems.
- Instruct patient to report other bothersome side effects such as severe or prolonged fever, sleep loss, or blurred vision.

Pharmacokinetics

Absorption: IV administration results in complete bioavailability.
Distribution: Unknown.
Metabolism and Excretion: Mostly metabolized by the liver.
Half-life: 0.5 hr.

TIME/ACTION PROFILE (blood levels)

ROUTE	ONSET	PEAK	DURATION
IV	Rapid	end of infusion	unknown

Contraindications/Precautions

Contraindicated in: Hypersensitivity; OB: Pregnancy or lactation.
Use Cautiously in: Patients with childbearing potential (males and females); Impaired hepatic/renal function; Geri: Elderly patients may be more sensitive to effects; Pedi: Safety in children not established.

Interactions

Drug-Drug: ↑ risk of myelosuppression with other **antineoplastics immunosuppressants** or **radiation therapy**. May ↓ antibody response to and ↑ risk of adverse reactions from **live-virus vaccines**.

Route/Dosage

IV (Adults): *First treatment cycle*—15 mg/m^2 as a continuous infusion over 3 hr repeated q 8 hr for 3 days. *Subsequent cycles*—cycle should be repeated every 6 wk for a minimum of 4 cycles; treatment may be continued as long as the patient continues to benefit. Dose adjustment/delay may be required for hematologic toxicity, renal or hepatic impairment or infection.

Availability

Lyophilized powder for injection (requires reconstitution): 50 mg/vial.

D

delavirdine (de-la-**veer**-deen)

Rescriptor

Classification
Therapeutic: antiretrovirals
Pharmacologic: nonnucleoside reverse transcriptase inhibitors

Indications

Treatment of HIV infection in combination with other antiretrovirals.

Action

Binds to reverse transcriptase, inhibiting viral DNA synthesis. **Therapeutic Effects:** Decreased viral load and increased CD4 cell count. Slowed progression of HIV infection and decreased severity of its sequelae.

Adverse Reactions/Side Effects

CNS: fatigue, headache. **GI:** diarrhea, increased amylase, increased liver enzymes, nausea, vomiting.
Derm: rash, pruritus. **Misc:** fat redistribution.

PHYSICAL THERAPY IMPLICATIONS

Examination and Evaluation

- Monitor excessive headache or fatigue. Some fatigue is expected, but any sudden or severe change in muscle strength or energy levels should be reported.

Interventions

- Implement resistive exercises and other therapeutic exercises as tolerated to maintain muscle strength and function and prevent muscle wasting associated with HIV infection and AIDS.

Patient/Client-Related Instruction

- Emphasize the importance of taking delavirdine as directed even if the patient is asymptomatic, and that this drug must always be used in combination with other antiretroviral drugs. Do not take more than prescribed amount and do not stop taking without consulting health care professional.
- Inform patient that delavirdine does not cure HIV or AIDS or prevent associated or opportunistic infections. Delavirdine does not reduce the risk of transmission of HIV to others through sexual contact or blood contamination. Caution patient to use a condom, and to avoid sharing needles or donating blood to prevent spreading the AIDS virus to others.

- Advise patient about possible fat redistribution, characterized by increased fat in the torso and thin arms and legs. Discuss possible effects on body image, and help patient explore coping mechanisms.
- Advise patient about the likelihood of GI reactions (nausea, vomiting, diarrhea) and skin problems (rash, itching). Instruct patient to report severe or prolonged GI or skin reactions.

Pharmacokinetics

Absorption: 85% absorbed after oral administration; increased when tablet is dispersed in water.
Distribution: Unknown.
Protein Binding: 98%.
Metabolism and Excretion: Extensively metabolized by the liver; <5% excreted unchanged in urine.
Half-life: 5.8 hr.

TIME/ACTION PROFILE (blood levels)

ROUTE	ONSET	PEAK	DURATION
PO	Rapid	1 hr	8 hr

Contraindications/Precautions

Contraindicated in: Hypersensitivity; Concurrent use of astemizole, benzodiazepines and antiarrhythmics, dihydropyridine, calcium channel blockers (nifedipine), ergot alkaloids, amphetamines, and sildenafil (may result in excessive sedation, vasoconstriction, or arrhythmias).
Use Cautiously in: Impaired hepatic function; Achlorhydria (requires acidic environment for absorption); Pregnancy, lactation, or children (safety not established; HIV-infected patients should not breast-feed).

Interactions

Drug-Drug: Delavirdine inhibits the hepatic drug-metabolizing enzyme CYPP3A4 and ↑ blood levels of **sedative/hypnotics antiarrhythmics, calcium channel blockers, ergot alkaloids, sildenafil**, and **pimozide**; this may result in potentially life-threatening adverse reactions (avoid concurrent use). Concurrent administration of **clarithromycin** significantly ↑ levels of both agents. Concurrent administration with **didanosine** ↓ levels of both agents (separate doses by 1 hr). **Fluoxetine** and **ketoconazole** ↑ delavirdine levels. **Antacids** ↓ absorption (do not use within 1 hr of each other). **Histamine blockers** ↓ absorption (avoid chronic use). Levels are ↓ by **rifabutin, rifampin, phenytoin, phenobarbital**, and **carbamazepine** (avoid concurrent use). ↑ levels of **amprenavir, indinavir**, and **saquinavir** (dosage reductions may be necessary). Concurrent use with **saquinavir** may ↑ risk of liver dysfunction.
Drug-Natural: Use with **St. John's wort** may ↓ levels and effectiveness, including development of drug resistance.

Route/Dosage

PO (Adults): 400 mg 3 times daily.

Availability

Tablets: 100 mg, 200 mg.

HIGH ALERT

denileukin diftitox

(den-i-**loo**-kin **dif**-ti-tox)
Ontak

Classification
Therapeutic: antineoplastics
Pharmacologic: cytotoxic proteins

Indications

Persistent or recurrent cutaneous T-cell lymphoma whose malignant cells express the CD25 component of the interleukin-2 (IL-2) receptor.

Action

A fusion protein that contains parts of diphtheria toxin fused to IL-2. Directs cytocidal action of diphtheria toxin to cells with IL-2 receptors. **Therapeutic Effects:** Regression of cutaneous T-cell lymphoma.

Adverse Reactions/Side Effects

CNS: dizziness, headache, confusion, insomnia, nervousness, weakness. **EENT:** loss of visual acuity, loss of color vision. **Resp:** cough, dyspnea, pharyngitis, rhinitis. **CV:** chest pain, edema, hypotension, tachycardia, arrhythmia, thrombotic events. **Derm:** rash, pruritus, sweating. **GI:** anorexia, diarrhea, nausea, vomiting, constipation, dyspepsia, dysphagia, increased transaminases. **GU:** albuminuria, hematuria. **F and E:** hypocalcemia, dehydration, hypokalemia. **Hemat:** anemia, leukopenia, thrombocytopenia. **Local:** injection site reactions. **Metab:** hypoalbuminemia, weight loss. **MS:** myalgia, arthralgia. **Neuro:** paresthesia. **Misc:** ACUTE HYPERSENSITIVITY REACTIONS, chills, fever, flu-like syndrome, infection.

PHYSICAL THERAPY IMPLICATIONS

Examination and Evaluation

- Monitor signs of acute hypersensitivity reactions, including pulmonary symptoms (tightness in the throat and chest, wheezing, cough, dyspnea) or skin reactions (rash, pruritus, urticaria). Notify physician or nursing staff immediately if these reactions occur.
- Monitor continually for signs of thrombotic events, including MI (sudden chest pain, pain radiating into the arm or jaw, shortness of breath, dizziness, sweating, anxiety, nausea), or ischemic stroke (sudden severe headache, confusion, nausea, vomiting, paralysis, numbness, speech problems, visual disturbances). Seek immediate medical assistance if patient develops these signs.

- Assess heart rate, ECG, and heart sounds, especially during exercise (See Appendices G, H). Report any rhythm disturbances (tachycardia, others) or symptoms of increased arrhythmias, including palpitations, chest discomfort, shortness of breath, fainting, and fatigue/weakness.
- Assess blood pressure periodically, and compare to normal values (See Appendix F). Report low blood pressure (hypotension), especially if patient experiences dizziness, chest pain, or other symptoms.
- Be alert for signs of neutropenia (fever, sore throat, signs of infection), thrombocytopenia (bruising, nose bleeds, bleeding gums), or unusual weakness and fatigue that might be due to other anemias. Report these signs immediately to the physician or nursing staff.
- Assess peripheral edema using girth measurements, volume displacement, and measurement of pitting edema (See Appendix N). Report increased swelling in feet and ankles or a sudden increase in body weight due to fluid retention.
- Monitor signs of CNS toxicity, including dizziness, confusion, headache, nervousness, or sleep loss. Notify physician if these signs become problematic.
- Monitor neuromuscular signs of electrolyte imbalances (hypocalcemia, hypokalemia), including lethargy, weakness, cramping, and muscle hyperexcitability and tetany. Notify physician immediately if these signs occur.
- Assess any muscle or joint pain to rule out musculoskeletal pathology; that is, try to determine if pain is drug induced rather than caused by anatomic or biomechanical problems.
- Monitor IV injection site for pain, swelling, and irritation. Report prolonged or excessive injection site reactions to the physician.
- Periodically assess body weight and report a rapid or unexplained weight loss.

Interventions

- For patients who are medically able to begin exercise, implement appropriate resistive exercises and aerobic training to maintain muscle strength and aerobic capacity during cancer chemotherapy or to help restore function after chemotherapy.
- Because of potential cardiac problems (arrhythmias, hypotension, thrombotic events), use caution during aerobic exercise and endurance conditioning. Terminate exercise if patient exhibits untoward symptoms (chest pain, shortness of breath, etc.) or displays other criteria for exercise termination (See Appendix L).
- Make sure patient maintains adequate fluid intake to avoid dehydration, especially during exercise.

Patient/Client-Related Instruction

- Advise patient to guard against infection (frequent hand washing, etc.), and to avoid crowds and contact with persons with contagious diseases.
- Advise patient and family/caregivers that fatigue and weakness are likely and may be severe. Functional abilities may be limited, and patient may need to use assistive devices during ambulation.
- Instruct patient to report any vision disturbances or loss of color vision.
- Advise patient that rashes and other skin reactions (itching, increased sweating) are likely. Severe or unexpected skin reactions should be reported to the physician.
- Advise patient about the likelihood of GI reactions such as diarrhea, nausea, vomiting, constipation, indigestion, and loss of appetite. Instruct patient to report severe or prolonged GI problems.
- Instruct patient to report signs of kidney dysfunction, including blood in the urine and increased urinary frequency.
- Instruct patient or family/caregivers to report other bothersome side effects such as severe or prolonged rhinitis, sinusitis, or flu-like symptoms (chills, fever, body aches).

Pharmacokinetics

Absorption: IV administration results in complete bioavailability.
Distribution: 0.06–0.08 L/kg.
Metabolism and Excretion: Metabolized by proteolytic breakdown.
Half-life: 70–80 min.

TIME/ACTION PROFILE

ROUTE	ONSET	PEAK	DURATION
IV	unknown	unknown	21 days

Contraindications/Precautions

Contraindicated in: Hypersensitivity to denileukin, diphtheria toxin, or interleukin-2; Lactation.
Use Cautiously in: Geriatric patients (increased risk of adverse reactions); Preexisting cardiovascular disease (increased risk of vascular leak syndrome); Pregnancy or children (safety not established).

Interactions

Drug-Drug: None noted.

Route/Dosage

IV (Adults): 9 or 18 mcg/kg/day for 5 consecutive days q 21 days.

Availability

Solution for injection (frozen): 150 mcg/mL.

denosumab (de-no-su-mab)
Prolia

Classification
Therapeutic: bone resorption inhibitors
Pharmacologic: monoclonal antibodies

Indications
Treatment of osteoporosis postmenopausal women who are at high risk for fracture or those who have failed/are intolerant of conventional osteoporosis therapy.

Action
A monoclonal antibody that binds specifically to the human receptor activator of nuclear factor kappa-B-ligand (RANKL), which is required for formation, function, and survival of osteoclasts. Binding inhibits osteoclast formation, function, and survival;
Therapeutic Effects: ↓ bone resorption with ↓ occurrence of fractures (vertebral, nonvertebral, hip).

Adverse Reactions/Side Effects
GI: PANCREATITIS. **GU:** cystitis. **Derm:** dermatitis, eczema, rashes. **F and E:** hypocalcemia. **Metab:** hypercholesterolemia. **MS:** back pain, extremity pain, musculoskeletal pain, osteonecrosis of the jaw, suppression of bone turnover. **Misc:** infection.

PHYSICAL THERAPY IMPLICATIONS

Examination and Evaluation
- Watch for signs of pancreatitis, including upper abdominal pain (especially after eating), indigestion, weight loss, and oily stools. Report these signs to the physician immediately.
- Assess any pain in the back or extremities. Report persistent or increased musculoskeletal pain to determine presence of bone or joint pathology, including fracture. Be especially aware of possible mouth and jaw pain due to osteonecrosis of the jaw.
- Watch for signs of low calcium levels (hypocalcemia), including tingling sensations in the fingers toes and around the mouth, and for signs of muscle hyperexcitability (cramping, twitching, spasms, tetany). Notify physician immediately if these signs occur.
- Be alert for signs of infection, including fever, sore throat, chills, nausea, vomiting, diarrhea, and localized inflammation. Report these signs to the physician immediately.

Interventions
- Institute weight-bearing and resistance exercises as tolerated to maintain or increase bone mineral density. Start with low-impact or aquatic programs in patients with extensive demineralization, and increase exercise intensity slowly to prevent fractures.
- Protect against falls and fractures (See Appendix E). Modify home environment (remove throw rugs, improve lighting, etc.) and provide assistive devices (cane, walker) or other protective devices as needed to improve balance and prevent falls.

Patient/Client-Related Instruction
- Advise patient about the benefits of proper diet in sustaining bone mineralization. If necessary, refer patient for nutritional counseling about supplemental calcium and vitamin D.
- Encourage patient to modify behaviors that increase the risk of osteoporosis (stop smoking, reduce alcohol consumption).
- Advise patient that this drug may cause problems in fat metabolism (hypercholesterolemia). Remind patient that periodic blood tests may be needed to monitor plasma lipids.
- Instruct patient to report other troublesome side effects such as severe or prolonged bladder pain or skin reactions (rash, dermatitis, eczema).

Pharmacokinetics
Absorption: Well absorbed following subcutaneous administration.
Distribution: Unknown.
Metabolism and Excretion: Unknown.
Half-life: 25.4 days

TIME/ACTION PROFILE (effects on bone resorption)

ROUTE	ONSET	PEAK	DURATION
SC	1 mo	Unknown*	12 mo†

*Maximum ↓ in serum calcium occurs at 10 days.
†Following discontinuation.

Contraindications/Precautions
Contraindicated in: Hypocalcemia (correct before administering); adequate supplemental calcium and vitamin D required; Lactation: Avoid use; ↓ mammary gland development and lactation.
Use Cautiously in: Conditions associated with hypocalcemia, including hypoparathyroidism, previous thyroid/parathyroid surgery, malabsorption syndromes, history of small intestinal excision, renal impairment/hemodialysis (CCr <30 mL/min); monitoring of calcium and other minerals recommended; Concurrent use of immunosuppressants or diseases resulting in immunosuppression (↑ risk of infection); Geri: May be more sensitive to drug effects; OB: Use in pregnancy only when potential benefit justifies potential risk to fetus; Pedi: Safe and effective use not established.

Interactions
Drug-Drug: Concurrent use of **immunosuppressants** ↑ risk of infection.

Route/Dosage
SC (Adults females): 60 mg q 6 mo.

Availability
Solution for injection: 60 mg/1 mL in 1-mL prefilled syringes and vials.

desipramine (des-ip-ra-meen)

Norpramin, Pertofrane

Classification

Therapeutic: antidepressants

Pharmacologic: tricyclic antidepressants

Indications

Depression. **Unlabeled Use:** Chronic pain syndromes. Anxiety. Insomnia.

Action

Potentiates the effect of serotonin and norepinephrine in the CNS. Has significant anticholinergic properties. **Therapeutic Effects:** Antidepressant action (may develop only over several weeks).

Adverse Reactions/Side Effects

CNS: drowsiness, fatigue. **EENT:** blurred vision, dry eyes, dry mouth. **CV:** ARRHYTHMIAS, hypotension, ECG changes. **GI:** constipation, drug-induced hepatitis, paralytic ileus, increased appetite, weight gain. **GU:** urinary retention, decreased libido. **Derm:** photosensitivity. **Endo:** changes in blood glucose, gynecomastia. **Hemat:** blood dyscrasias.

PHYSICAL THERAPY IMPLICATIONS

Examination and Evaluation

- Assess heart rate, ECG, and heart sounds, especially during exercise (See Appendices G, H). Immediately report any rhythm disturbances or symptoms of increased arrhythmias, including palpitations, chest discomfort, shortness of breath, fainting, and fatigue/weakness.
- Be alert for increased depression and suicidal thoughts and ideology, especially when initiating drug treatment or in children and teenagers. Notify physician or mental health professional immediately if patient exhibits worsening depression or other changes in mood and behavior.
- Assess blood pressure periodically and compare to normal values (See Appendix F). Report low blood pressure (hypotension), especially if patient experiences dizziness or syncope.
- Be alert for signs of leukopenia (fever, sore throat, signs of infection), thrombocytopenia (bruising, nose bleeds, and bleeding gums), or unusual weakness and fatigue that might be due to anemia or other blood dyscrasias. Report these signs to the physician.
- Be alert for sedation and fatigue, especially in older adults. Report excessive or prolonged symptoms that could affect balance, gait, and functional activities.
- Monitor signs of hypoglycemia (weakness, malaise, irritability, fatigue) or hyperglycemia (drowsiness, fruity breath, increased urination, unusual thirst). Patients with diabetes mellitus should check blood glucose levels frequently.
- If used to treat chronic pain, assess pain levels periodically to help determine drug efficacy.
- Periodically assess body weight and other anthropometric measures (body mass index, body composition). Report a rapid or unexplained weight gain or increased body fat.

Interventions

- Guard against falls and trauma (hip fractures, head injury, and so forth), and implement fall-prevention strategies (See Appendix E).
- Because of the risk of cardiac arrhythmias, use caution during aerobic exercise and endurance conditioning. Assess exercise tolerance frequently (blood pressure, heart rate, fatigue levels), and terminate exercise immediately if any untoward responses occur (see Appendix L).
- To minimize orthostatic hypotension, patient should move slowly when assuming a more upright position.
- Help patient explore nonpharmacologic methods to reduce depression and anxiety, including exercise, counseling, support groups, and so forth.
- If treating neuropathic pain or other pain syndromes, implement appropriate interventions (physical agents, manual techniques, therapeutic exercise) to manage pain and reduce the need for drug therapy. Help patient also explore other nonpharmacologic methods to reduce chronic pain (relaxation techniques, imagery, counseling, and so forth).
- Causes photosensitivity; use care if administering UV treatments. Advise patient to avoid direct sunlight and use sunscreens and protective clothing.

Patient/Client-Related Instruction

- Advise patient that antidepressant effects may not occur immediately; it may take 2 wk or longer before an improvement in mood is observed.
- Advise patient to avoid alcohol and other CNS depressants because of the increased risk of sedation and adverse effects.
- Advise patient that this medication should be tapered at the completion of long-term therapy. Abrupt discontinuation may cause nausea, vomiting, diarrhea, headache, trouble sleeping with vivid dreams, and irritability.
- Instruct patient to report severe or prolonged constipation or signs of liver dysfunction and hepatitis

(yellow skin or eyes, abdominal pain, severe nausea and vomiting, fever, sore throat, malaise, weakness, facial edema).

- Instruct patient to report other bothersome side effects such as severe or prolonged dry eyes/mouth, blurred vision, urinary retention, decreased libido, or increased breast growth in men (gynecomastia).

Pharmacokinetics

Absorption: Well absorbed from the GI tract.
Distribution: Widely distributed.
Protein Binding: 90–92%.
Metabolism and Excretion: Extensively metabolized by the liver. One metabolite is pharmacologically active (2-hydroxydesipramine). Undergoes enterohepatic recirculation and secretion into gastric juices. Small amounts enter breast milk.
Half-life: 12–27 hr.

TIME/ACTION PROFILE (antidepressant effect)

ROUTE	ONSET	PEAK	DURATION
PO	2–3 wk	2–6 wk	days–wks

Contraindications/Precautions

Contraindicated in: Angle-closure glaucoma; Recent MI, heart failure, known history of QTc prolongation.
Use Cautiously in: Patients with preexisting cardiovascular disease; Prostatic hyperplasia (↑ susceptibility to urinary retention); History of seizures (threshold may be ↓); May ↑ risk of suicide attempt/ideation especially during early treatment or dose adjustment; risk may be greater in children or adolescents; OB: Use during pregnancy only if potential maternal benefit outweighs risks to fetus; use during lactation may result in neonatal sedation; Pedi: Safety not established in children <12 yr; Geri: ↑ sensitivity to effects.

Interactions

Drug-Drug: Desipramine is metabolized in the liver by the cytochrome P4502D6 enzyme, and its action may be affected by drugs which compete for metabolism by or alter the activity of this enzyme, including other **antidepressants, phenothiazines, carbamazepine, class 1C antiarrhythmics (propafenone, flecainide, encainide)**; when used concurrently, dose reduction of one or the other or both may be necessary. Concurrent use of other drugs that inhibit the activity of the enzyme, including **cimetidine, quinidine, amiodarone**, and **ritonavir**, may result in ↑ effects. May cause hypotension, tachycardia, and potentially fatal reactions when used with **MAO inhibitors** (avoid concurrent use—discontinue 2 wk prior to). Concurrent use with **SSRI antidepressants** may result in ↑ toxicity and should be avoided (fluoxetine should be stopped 5 wk before). Concurrent use with **clonidine** may result in hypertensive crisis and should be avoided. **Phenytoin** may ↓ levels and effectiveness; ↑ doses of desipramine may be required to treat depression. Concurrent use with **levodopa** may result in delayed/↓ absorption of levodopa or hypertension. Blood levels and effects may be ↓ by **rifamycins, carbamazepine**, and **barbiturates**. Concurrent use with **moxifloxacin** ↑ risk of adverse cardiovascular reactions. ↑ CNS depression with other **CNS depressants,** including **alcohol, antihistamines, clonidine, opioid analgesics**, and **sedative/hypnotics. Barbiturates** may alter blood levels and effects. **Adrenergic** and **anticholinergic** side effects may be ↑ with other **agents having these properties. Hormonal contraceptives** ↑ levels and may cause toxicity. **Cigarette smoking** may ↑ metabolism and alter effects.
Drug-Natural: Concomitant use of **kava, valerian**, or **chamomile** can ↑ CNS depression. ↑ anticholinergic effects with **jimson weed** and **scopolia**.

Route/Dosage

PO (Adults): 100–200 mg/day as a single dose or in divided doses (up to 300 mg/day).
PO (Geriatric Patients): 25–50 mg/day in divided doses (up to 150 mg/day).
PO (Children >12 yr): 25–50 mg/day in divided doses; increased as needed up to 100 mg/day.
PO (Children 6–12 yr): 10–30 mg/day (1–5 mg/kg/day) in divided doses.

Availability (generic available)

Tablets: 10 mg, 25 mg, 50 mg, 75 mg, 100 mg, 150 mg.

desirudin (des-i-rude-in)

Iprivask

Classification
Therapeutic: anticoagulants
Pharmacologic: thrombin inhibitors

Indications

Prevention of deep vein thrombosis (DVT) after hip-replacement surgery.

Action

Selectively inhibits free and clot-bound thrombin. Inhibition of thrombin prevents activation of factors V, VIII, and XII; conversion of fibrinogen to fibrin; platelet adhesion and aggregation. **Therapeutic Effects:** Decreased incidence of DVT and subsequent pulmonary embolism after hip-replacement surgery.

Adverse Reactions/Side Effects

GI: nausea. **Hemat:** BLEEDING, anemia. **Local:** injection site reactions, wound secretion.

PHYSICAL THERAPY IMPLICATIONS

Examination and Evaluation

- Assess signs of bleeding and hemorrhage (bleeding gums; nosebleed; unusual bruising; black, tarry stools; hematuria; fall in hematocrit or blood pressure). Notify physician or nursing staff immediately of these signs.

- To help monitor drug effects, be alert for signs of DVTs (lower extremity swelling, warmth, erythema, tenderness) and thromboembolism (shortness of breath, chest pain, cough, bloody sputum). Notify physician or nursing staff immediately if these signs occur, and request objective tests (Doppler ultrasound, lung scan, others) if thrombosis is suspected.
- Monitor signs of anemia, including unusual fatigue, shortness of breath with exertion, pallor, and cyanosis. Notify physician or nursing staff immediately if these signs occur.
- Assess any wounds or suture lines for possible secretion and bleeding. Report any suspicious wound drainage to the physician or nursing staff.
- Monitor injection site for pain, swelling, and irritation. Report prolonged or excessive injection-site reactions to the physician or nursing staff.

Interventions

- Use caution with any physical interventions that could increase bleeding, including wound débridement, chest percussion, joint mobilization, and application of local heat.

Patient/Client-Related Instruction

- Instruct patient to report other bothersome side effects such as severe or prolonged nausea.

Pharmacokinetics

Absorption: Completely absorbed following subcutaneous administration.
Distribution: Binds specifically and directly to thrombin.
Metabolism and Excretion: 40–50% excreted unchanged by kidneys; some metabolism in kidneys and pancreas.
Half-life: 2 hr.

TIME/ACTION PROFILE (effect on aPTT)

ROUTE	ONSET	PEAK	DURATION
SC	rapid	1–3 hr	12 hr

Contraindications/Precautions

Contraindicated in: Hypersensitivity to natural or recombinant hirudins; Active bleeding; Coagulation disorders.
Use Cautiously in: Renal impairment (dosage change recommended if CCr ≤60 mL/min); Geriatric patients (due to age-related renal impairment); Hepatic impairment; Pregnancy (use only if benefits to mother outweigh fetal risk); Lactation, children (safety not established).
Exercise Extreme Caution in: Spinal/epidural anesthesia (increased risk of spinal/epidural hematomas and their sequelae, especially when used with NSAIDs, platelet inhibitors, or other anticoagulants).

Interactions

Drug-Drug: Dextran 40, systemic corticosteroids, thrombolytics, and other **anticoagulants** ↑ risk of bleeding (discontinue if possible; if not, monitor laboratory and clinical status closely). Agents altering platelet function, including **salicylates, NSAIDs, clopidogrel, ticlopidine, dipyridamole**, and **glycoprotein IIb/IIIa antagonists**, also ↑ risk of bleeding.

Route/Dosage

SC (Adults): 15 mg q 12 hr, start 5–15 min prior to surgery, but after regional block (if used), for up to 12 days.

Renal Impairment

SC (Adults): *CCr 31–60 mL/min*—start with 5 mg q 12 hr; further doses determined by daily aPTT; *CCr <31 mL/min*— start with 1.7 mg q 12 hr; further doses determined by daily aPTT.

Availability

Lyophilized powder for injection (requires reconstitution with specific diluent): 15.75 mg/vial with 0.6-mL ampule of diluent (contains mannitol, delivers 15-mg dose).

desloratadine

(des-lor-**at**-a-deen)
Clarinex

Classification
Therapeutic: allergy, cold, and cough remedies, antihistamines
Pharmacologic: piperidines

Indications

Symptoms of allergic rhinitis (seasonal and perennial). Chronic idiopathic urticaria.

Action

Blocks peripheral effects of histamine released during allergic reactions. **Therapeutic Effects:** Decreased symptoms of allergic reactions (nasal stuffiness, red swollen eyes). Decreased pruritus, reduction in number and size of hives in chronic idiopathic urticaria.

Adverse Reactions/Side Effects

CNS: drowsiness (rare). **EENT:** pharyngitis. **GI:** dry mouth. **Misc:** ALLERGIC REACTIONS, INCLUDING ANAPHYLAXIS.

PHYSICAL THERAPY IMPLICATIONS

Examination and Evaluation

- Monitor signs of allergic reactions and anaphylaxis, including pulmonary symptoms (tightness in the throat and chest, wheezing, cough, dyspnea) or skin reactions (rash, pruritus, urticaria). Notify physician immediately if these reactions occur.

- Monitor symptoms of seasonal allergies (sneezing, rhinitis, itching eyes, cough) or chronic idiopathic urticaria (rash, hives, itching) to help document benefits of this drug in treating these disorders.

Interventions

- Guard against falls and trauma (hip fractures, head injury, and so forth). Implement fall- prevention strategies, especially in older adults or if balance is impaired (See Appendix E).

Patient/Client-Related Instruction

- Advise patient about the risk of daytime drowsiness and decreased attention and mental focus. Although the risk of drowsiness is considerably lower with this drug compared to traditional antihistamines, patients should use care if driving or in other activities that require quick reactions and strong concentration.
- Advise patient to avoid alcohol and other CNS depressants because of the increased risk of sedation and adverse effects.
- Instruct patient to report other troublesome side effects, including dry mouth or upper respiratory tract irritation.

Pharmacokinetics

Absorption: Well absorbed; absorption for orally disintegrating tablets and oral tablets is identical.
Distribution: Enters breast milk.
Metabolism and Excretion: Extensively metabolized to 3-hydroxydesloratadine, an active metabolite; small percentage of patients may be slow metabolizers.
Half-life: 27 hr.

TIME/ACTION PROFILE (antihistaminic effects)

ROUTE	ONSET	PEAK	DURATION
PO	unknown	3 hr	24 hr

Contraindications/Precautions

Contraindicated in: Hypersensitivity; OB: Lactation.
Use Cautiously in: Patients with hepatic or renal impairment (↓ dose to 5 mg every other day); Geri: Dosing for the elderly should consider ↓ hepatic, renal, or cardiac function, concomitant diseases, other drug therapy, and ↑ risk of adverse reactions; Pedi: Children <6 mo (safety not established).

Interactions

Drug-Drug: The following interactions may occur, but are less likely to occur with desloratadine than with more sedating antihistamines. **MAO inhibitors** may ↑ and prolong effects of antihistamines. ↑ CNS depression may occur with other **CNS depressants,** including **alcohol, antidepressants, opioids,** and **sedative/hypnotics.**

Route/Dosage

PO (Adults and Children ≥12 yr): 5 mg once daily.

Hepatic Impairment
Renal Impairment

PO (Adults and Children ≥12 yr): 5 mg every other day.
PO (Children 6–11 yr): 2.5 mg once daily.
PO (Children 12 mo–5 yr): 1.25 mg once daily.
PO (Children 6–12 mo): 1 mg once daily.

Availability

Tablets: 5 mg. **Orally disintegrating tablets (RediTabs) (tutti frutti):** 2.5 mg, 5 mg. **Syrup (bubblegum):** 0.5 mg/mL. ***In combination with:*** pseudoephedrine (Clarinex-D 12 Hour, Clarinex-D 24 Hour; See Appendix B).

desmopressin

(des-moe-**pres**-sin)

DDAVP, DDAVP Rhinal Tube, DDAVP Rhinyle Drops, Octostim, Stimate

Classification

Therapeutic: hormones
Pharmacologic: antidiuretic hormones

Indications

PO, SC, IV, Intranasal: Treatment of diabetes insipidus caused by a deficiency of vasopressin. **Intranasal:** Controls bleeding in certain types of hemophilia and von Willebrand's disease.

Action

An analogue of naturally occurring vasopressin (antidiuretic hormone). Primary action is enhanced reabsorption of water in the kidneys. **Therapeutic Effects:** Prevention of nocturnal enuresis. Maintenance of appropriate body water content in diabetes insipidus. Control of bleeding in certain types of hemophilia or von Willebrand's disease.

Adverse Reactions/Side Effects

CNS: drowsiness, headache, listlessness. **EENT:** **intranasal:** nasal congestion, rhinitis. **Resp:** dyspnea. **CV:** hypertension, hypotension, tachycardia (large IV doses only). **GI:** mild abdominal cramps, nausea. **GU:** vulval pain. **Derm:** flushing. **F and E:** water intoxication/hyponatremia. **Local:** phlebitis at IV site.

PHYSICAL THERAPY IMPLICATIONS

Examination and Evaluation

- Be alert for an imbalance in body water and electrolytes that results in low sodium levels (hyponatremia). Signs include headache, confusion, listlessness, fatigue, irritability, muscle abnormalities (weakness, cramps, spasms), and decreased consciousness that can progress to coma and seizures. Notify physician if these signs occur.

- Assess blood pressure and compare to normal values (See Appendix F). Report changes in blood pressure, either a problematic decrease in BP (hypotension) or a sustained increase in BP (hypertension).
- Assess heart rate, ECG, and heart sounds, especially during administration of high IV doses (See Appendices G, H). Report a rapid heart rate (tachycardia) or symptoms of other such as palpitations, chest discomfort, shortness of breath, fainting, and fatigue/weakness.
- Assess any breathing problems, and report difficult or labored breathing (dyspnea).
- Assess administration site during and after IV administration, and report signs of phlebitis and venous thrombosis (local pain, swelling, inflammation).

Interventions

- Because of the risk of arrhythmias, abnormal BP responses, and pulmonary problems, use caution during aerobic exercise and other forms of therapeutic exercise. Assess exercise tolerance frequently (blood pressure, heart rate, fatigue levels), and terminate exercise immediately if any untoward responses occur (See Appendix L).

Patient/Client-Related Instruction

- Instruct patient to report other bothersome side effects such as severe or prolonged nasal congestion (when administered intranasally), skin reactions (flushing), or GI problems (nausea, abdominal cramps).

Pharmacokinetics

Absorption: 5% absorbed following oral administration; some 10–20% absorbed from nasal mucosa.
Distribution: Distribution not fully known. Enters breast milk.
Metabolism and Excretion: Unknown.
Half-life: 75 min.

TIME/ACTION PROFILE (PO, intranasal = antidiuretic effect; IV = effect on factor VIII activity)

ROUTE	ONSET	PEAK	DURATION
PO	1 hr	4–7 hr	unknown
intranasal	1 hr	1–5 hr	8–20 hr
IV	within mins	15–30 min	3 hr*

*4–24 hr in mild hemophilia A.

Contraindications/Precautions

Contraindicated in: Hypersensitivity; Hypersensitivity to chlorobutanol; Patients with type IIB or platelet-type (pseudo) von Willebrand's disease.
Use Cautiously in: Angina pectoris; Hypertension; OB/Lactation: Safety not established.

Interactions

Drug-Drug: Chlorpropamide, clofibrate, or **carbamazepine** may enhance the antidiuretic response to desmopressin. **Demeclocycline, lithium,** or **norepinephrine** may diminish the antidiuretic response to desmopressin. Large doses may enhance the effects of **vasopressors.**

Route/Dosage

Primary Nocturnal Enuresis

PO (Adults and Children ≥6 yr): 0.2 mg at bedtime; may be titrated up to 0.6 mg at bedtime to achieve desired response.

Diabetes Insipidus

PO (Adults and Children): 0.05 mg twice daily; adjusted as needed (usual range: 0.1–1.2 mg/day in 2–3 divided doses).
Intranasal (Adults): *DDAVP*–0.1–0.4 ml/day in 1–3 divided doses.
Intranasal (Children 3 mo–12 yr): *DDAVP*–0.05–0.3 mL/day in 1–2 divided doses.
Subcut, IV (Adults): 2–4 mcg/day in 2 divided doses.

Hemophilia A/von Willebrand's disease

Intranasal (Adults and Children ≥50 kg): *Stimate*–1 spray (150 mcg) in each nostril.
Intranasal (Adults and Children <50 kg): *Stimate*–1 spray (150 mcg) in one nostril.
IV (Adults and Children >3 mo): 0.3 mcg/kg, repeated as needed.

Availability (generic available)

Tablets: 0.1 mg, 0.2 mg. **Nasal spray (DDAVP):** 10 mcg/spray—5-mL bottle (0.1 mg/mL contains 50 doses). **Nasal spray (Stimate):** 150 mcg/spray. **Rhinal tube delivery system–nasal solution:** 2.5-mL vials with applicator tubes (0.1 mg/mL). **Injection:** 4 mcg/mL.

desonide (des-oh-nide)

Desonate, DesOwen, Verdeso

Classification
Therapeutic: anti-inflammatories (steroidal)
Pharmacologic: corticosteroids

Indications

Management of inflammation and pruritus associated with various allergic/immunologic skin problems.

Action

Suppresses normal immune response and inflammation. **Therapeutic Effects:** Suppression of dermatologic inflammation and immune processes.

Adverse Reactions/Side Effects

Derm: allergic contact dermatitis, atrophy, burning, dryness, edema, folliculitis, hypersensitivity reactions, hypertrichosis, hypopigmentation, irritation, maceration, miliaria, perioral dermatitis, secondary infection, striae. **Misc:** adrenal suppression (use of occlusive dressings, long-term therapy).

PHYSICAL THERAPY IMPLICATIONS

Examination and Evaluation

- Assess the area being treated to help document whether drug therapy is successful in resolving skin conditions.
- Monitor any new or increased reactions at the site of application, including inflammation, irritation, infection, burning, swelling, exfoliation, and rash. Report severe or prolonged skin reactions to the physician.
- Report signs of adrenal suppression, including hypotension, weight loss, weakness, nausea, vomiting, anorexia, lethargy, confusion, and restlessness.

Interventions

- Protect skin from breakdown, especially over bony prominences.

Patient/Client-Related Instruction

- Advise patients on long-term treatment to consult physician before stopping this medication. Stopping the medication suddenly may result in adrenocortical shock (severe hypotension, hypoglycemia, weakness, vomiting). If these signs appear, notify physician immediately; may be life threatening.
- Check that the patient and family or caregivers understand topical application procedures, and that they adhere to the recommended dosing schedule.

Pharmacokinetics

Absorption: Minimal. Prolonged use on large surface areas or large amounts applied or use of occlusive dressings may increase systemic absorption.
Distribution: Remains primarily at site of action.
Metabolism and Excretion: Usually metabolized in skin; may have been modified to resist local metabolism and have a prolonged local effect.
Half-life: Unknown.

TIME/ACTION PROFILE (response depends on condition being treated)

ROUTE	ONSET	PEAK	DURATION
topical	mins–hrs	hrs–days	hrs–days

Contraindications/Precautions

Contraindicated in: Hypersensitivity or known intolerance to corticosteroids or components of vehicles (ointment or cream base, preservative, alcohol); Untreated bacterial or viral infections.
Use Cautiously in: Hepatic dysfunction; Diabetes mellitus, cataracts, glaucoma, or tuberculosis (use of large amounts of high-potency agents may worsen condition); Patients with preexisting skin atrophy; Pregnancy, lactation, or children (chronic high-dose usage may result in adrenal suppression in mother, growth suppression in children; children may be more susceptible to adrenal and growth suppression).

Interactions

Drug-Drug: None significant.

Route/Dosage

Topical (Adults and Children ≥12 yr): Apply to affected area(s) 2–4 times daily (depends on preparation and condition being treated).
Topical (Children ≥3 mo): Apply to affected area(s) once daily.

Availability

Cream: 0.05%. **Gel:** 0.05%. **Ointment:** 0.05%. **Lotion:** 0.05%. **Foam:** 0.05%.

desoximetasone

(des-ox-i-**met**-a-sone)
Topicort

Classification
Therapeutic: anti-inflammatories (steroidal)
Pharmacologic: corticosteroids

Indications

Management of inflammation and pruritus associated with various allergic/immunologic skin problems.

Action

Suppresses normal immune response and inflammation. **Therapeutic Effects:** Suppression of dermatologic inflammation and immune processes.

Adverse Reactions/Side Effects

Derm: allergic contact dermatitis, atrophy, burning, dryness, edema, folliculitis, hypersensitivity reactions, hypertrichosis, hypopigmentation, irritation, maceration, miliaria, perioral dermatitis, secondary infection, striae. **Misc:** adrenal suppression (use of occlusive dressings, long-term therapy).

PHYSICAL THERAPY IMPLICATIONS

Examination and Evaluation

- Assess the area being treated to help document whether drug therapy is successful in resolving skin conditions.
- Monitor any new or increased reactions at the site of application, including inflammation, irritation, infection, burning, swelling, exfoliation, and rash. Report severe or prolonged skin reactions to the physician.
- Report signs of adrenal suppression, including hypotension, weight loss, weakness, nausea, vomiting, anorexia, lethargy, confusion, and restlessness.

Interventions

- Protect skin from breakdown, especially over bony prominences.

Patient/Client-Related Instruction

- Advise patients on long-term treatment to consult physician before stopping this medication. Stopping the medication suddenly may result in adrenocortical shock (severe hypotension, hypoglycemia, weakness, vomiting). If these signs appear, notify physician immediately; may be life threatening.
- Check that the patient and family or caregivers understand topical application procedures, and adhere to the recommended dosing schedule.

Pharmacokinetics

Absorption: Minimal. Prolonged use on large surface areas or large amounts applied or use of occlusive dressings may increase systemic absorption.
Distribution: Remains primarily at site of action.
Metabolism and Excretion: Usually metabolized in skin.
Half-life: Unknown.

TIME/ACTION PROFILE (response depends on condition being treated)

ROUTE	ONSET	PEAK	DURATION
topical	mins–hrs	hrs–days	hrs–days

Contraindications/Precautions

Contraindicated in: Hypersensitivity or known intolerance to corticosteroids or components of vehicles (ointment or cream base, preservative, alcohol); Untreated bacterial or viral infections.
Use Cautiously in: Hepatic dysfunction; Diabetes mellitus, cataracts, glaucoma, or tuberculosis (use of large amounts of high-potency agents may worsen condition); Patients with preexisting skin atrophy; Pregnancy, lactation, or children (chronic high-dose usage may result in adrenal suppression in mother, growth suppression in children; children may be more susceptible to adrenal and growth suppression); Children (should not be used in children <10 yr).

Interactions

Drug-Drug: None significant.

Route/Dosage

Topical (Adults): Apply to affected area(s) twice daily.
Topical (Children ≥10 yr): Apply to affected area(s) once daily.

Availability

Cream: 0.25% Rx, 0.05% Rx. **Gel:** 0.05% Rx.
Ointment: 0.25% Rx.

desvenlafaxine

(des-ven-la-**fax**-een)
Pristiq

D

Classification
Therapeutic: antidepressants
Pharmacologic: selective serotonin/norepinephrine reuptake inhibitors

Indications

Treatment of major depressive disorder, often in conjunction with psychotherapy.

Action

Inhibits serotonin and norepinephrine reuptake in the CNS. **Therapeutic Effects:** Decrease in depressive symptomatology, with fewer relapses/recurrences.

Adverse Reactions/Side Effects

CNS: SEIZURES, anxiety, dizziness, drowsiness, insomnia, headache. **EENT:** ↑ intraocular pressure, mydriasis. **Resp:** eosinophilic pneumonia, interstitial lung disease. **CV:** hypertension. **GI:** ↓ appetite, constipation, nausea. **GU:** male sexual dysfunction. **Derm:** sweating. **F and E:** hyponatremia. **Hemat:** ↑ risk of bleeding. **Metab:** hypercholesterolemia, hyperlipidemia. **Misc:** serotonin syndrome.

PHYSICAL THERAPY IMPLICATIONS

Examination and Evaluation

- Be alert for new seizures or increased seizure activity, especially at the onset of drug treatment. Document the number, duration, and severity of seizures, and report these findings immediately to the physician.
- Be alert for increased depression and suicidal thoughts, especially in the initial period of drug therapy, and in children and teenagers. Likewise, inform physician or mental health care professional if patient demonstrates other mood changes such as increased anxiety, nervousness, agitation, confusion, and emotional lability.
- Monitor and report signs of serotonin syndrome, including hyperthermia, rigidity, myoclonus, and autonomic instability with fluctuating vital signs and extreme agitation which may proceed to delirium and coma. Patients should not take desvenlafaxine with other drugs that increase serotonin levels (e.g., MAO inhibitors).
- Assess any breathing problems or signs of interstitial lung disease or eosinophilic pneumonia. Signs include cough, wheezing, chest pain, shortness of breath, fever, chills, and difficult or labored breathing. Monitor pulse oximetry and perform pulmonary function tests (See Appendices I, J, K) to

🍁 = Canadian drug name; *CAPITALS indicate life-threatening; underlines indicate most frequent.

quantify suspected changes in ventilation and respiratory function.

- Assess blood pressure (BP) and compare to normal values (See Appendix F). Report a sustained increase in BP (hypertension).
- Be alert for signs of prolonged bleeding time such as bleeding gums, nosebleeds, and unusual or excessive bruising. Report these signs to the physician.
- Monitor signs of low sodium levels (hyponatremia), including headache, confusion, lethargy, irritability, decreased consciousness, and neuromuscular abnormalities (muscle weakness and cramps). Report severe or prolonged signs to the physician.
- Assess dizziness and drowsiness that might affect gait, balance, and other functional activities (See Appendix C). Report balance problems and functional limitations to the physician, and caution the patient and family/caregivers to guard against falls and trauma.

Interventions

- Guard against falls and trauma (hip fractures, head injury, and so forth), and implement fall prevention strategies (See Appendix E).
- Help patient explore nonpharmacologic methods (exercise, counseling, support groups, and so forth) to reduce depression and anxiety.

Patient/Client-Related Instruction

- Advise patient that antidepressant effects may not occur immediately; it may take 2 weeks or more before an improvement in mood is observed.
- Advise patient to avoid alcohol and other CNS depressants because of the increased risk of sedation and adverse effects.
- Advise patient that this drug may cause problems in fat metabolism (hyperlipidemia, hypercholesterolemia). Remind patient that periodic blood tests may be needed to monitor plasma lipids.
- Instruct patient to report other problematic side effects such as severe or prolonged headache, sleep loss, vision disturbances, increased sweating, sexual dysfunction, or GI problems (nausea, constipation, loss of appetite).

Pharmacokinetics

Absorption: 80% absorbed following oral administration.
Distribution: Enters breast milk.
Metabolism and Excretion: 55% metabolized by the liver, 45% excreted unchanged in urine.
Half-life: **10 hr.**

TIME/ACTION PROFILE (blood levels)

ROUTE	ONSET	PEAK	DURATION
PO	unknown	7.5 hr	24 hr

Contraindications/Precautions

Contraindicated in: Hypersensitivity to venlafaxine or desvenlafaxine; Concurrent MAO inhibitors or within 14 days of stopping an MAO inhibitor; after desvenlafaxine is stopped, wait 7 days until starting an MAO inhibitor; Should not be use concurrently with venlafaxine.
Use Cautiously in: Untreated cerebrovascular or cardiovascular disease, including untreated hypertension (control BP before initiating therapy); Bipolar disorder (may activate mania/hypomania); History of increased intraocular pressure/angle-closure glaucoma; Renal impairment (consider modifications, dose should exceed 50 mg/day, especially in moderate-to-severe renal impairment); History of seizures or neurologic impairment; Hepatic impairment (dose should not exceed 100 mg/day); History of suicide attempt (may increase suicidal ideation during initiation or dose change, especially in children, adolescents, and young adults); Geri: Consider age-related decrease in renal function, decreased body mass, concurrent disease states and mediations; OB: Use in pregnancy or lactation only if maternal benefit outweighs fetal/infant risk; Pedi: Safety and effectiveness unknown.

Interactions

Drug-Drug: Concurrent use with **MAO inhibitors** may result in serious and potentially fatal interactions; avoid within 14 days of stopping an MAO inhibitor; after desvenlafaxine is stopped, wait 7 days until starting an MAO inhibitor. ↑ risk of bleeding with other **drugs that ↑ bleeding risk,** including **anticoagulants**, **antithrombotics**, **platelet aggregation inhibitors**, and **NSAIDs**. Use cautiously with other **CNS-active drugs**, including **alcohol** and **sedative/hypnotics** or **drugs that affect the serotonergic system**; effects of combination are unknown.

Route/Dosage

PO (Adults): 50 mg once daily.

Renal Impairment

PO (Adults): *Moderate renal impairment*—50 mg/day; *CCR <30 mL/min*—50 mg every other day.

Availability

Extended-release tablets: 50 mg, 100 mg.

dexamethasone

(deks-a-**meth**-a-sone)
DexPak

Classification
Therapeutic: anti-inflammatories (steroidal)
Pharmacologic: corticosteroids

Indications

Used systemically and locally in a wide variety of chronic diseases, including Inflammatory, Allergic, Hematologic,

Endocrine, Neoplastic, Dermatologic, and Autoimmune disorders. Management of cerebral edema. Diagnostic agent in adrenal disorders. **Unlabeled Use:** Short-term administration to high-risk mothers before delivery to prevent respiratory distress syndrome in the newborn. Adjunctive management of nausea and vomiting from chemotherapy. Treatment of airway edema prior to extubation. Used in neonates with bronchopulmonary dysplasia to facilitate ventilator weaning.

Action

In pharmacologic doses, suppresses inflammation and the normal immune response. Has numerous intense metabolic effects (see Adverse Reactions and Side Effects). Suppresses adrenal function at chronic doses of 0.75 mg/day. Has negligible mineralocorticoid activity. **Therapeutic Effects:** Suppression of inflammation and modification of the normal immune response.

Adverse Reactions/Side Effects

Adverse reactions/side effects are much more common with high-dose/long-term therapy

CNS: depression, euphoria, hallucinations, headache, increased intracranial pressure (children only), insomnia, personality changes, psychoses, restlessness. **EENT:** cataracts, increased intraocular pressure. **CV:** hypertension, edema. **GI:** PEPTIC ULCERATION, anorexia, nausea, increased appetite, vomiting. **Derm:** acne, decreased wound healing, ecchymoses, hirsutism, petechiae. **Endo:** adrenal suppression, hyperglycemia. **F and E:** amenorrhea, hypokalemia, alkalosis. **Hemat:** THROMBOEMBOLISM, thrombophlebitis. **Metab:** weight gain. **MS:** muscle wasting, osteoporosis, aseptic necrosis of joints, muscle pain. **Misc:** ALLERGIC REACTIONS, cushingoid appearance (moon face, buffalo hump), increased susceptibility to infection.

PHYSICAL THERAPY IMPLICATIONS

Examination and Evaluation

- Monitor signs of thrombophlebitis (lower extremity swelling, warmth, erythema, tenderness) and thromboembolism (shortness of breath, chest pain, cough, bloody sputum). Notify physician or nursing staff immediately, and request objective tests (Doppler ultrasound, lung scan, others) if thrombosis is suspected.
- Monitor and report signs of peptic ulcer, including heartburn, nausea, vomiting blood, tarry stools, and loss of appetite.
- Monitor signs of allergic reactions, including pulmonary symptoms (tightness in the throat and chest, wheezing, cough, dyspnea) or skin reactions (rash, pruritus, urticaria). Notify physician or nursing staff immediately if these reactions occur.
- Assess any muscle or joint pain. Report persistent or increased musculoskeletal pain to determine presence of bone or joint pathology (aseptic necrosis, fracture).
- Assess muscle strength periodically to determine degree of muscle wasting during long-term use.
- Measure blood pressure periodically and compare to normal values (See Appendix F). Report a sustained increase in blood pressure (hypertension) to the physician.
- Assess peripheral edema using girth measurements, volume displacement, and measurement of pitting edema (See Appendix N). Report increased swelling in feet and ankles or a sudden increase in body weight due to fluid retention.
- Monitor personality changes, including depression, euphoria, restlessness, hallucinations, and psychosis. Notify physician if these changes become problematic.
- Be alert for signs of low potassium levels (hypokalemia) and metabolic acidosis, including hyperventilation, cardiac arrhythmias, dizziness, and confusion. Notify physician immediately if these signs occur.
- Report signs of adrenal suppression, including hypotension, weight loss, weakness, nausea, vomiting, anorexia, lethargy, confusion, and restlessness.
- Monitor signs of hyperglycemia (confusion; drowsiness; flushed, dry skin; fruit-like breath odor; rapid, deep breathing; polyuria; loss of appetite; unusual thirst). Insulin dosages may need to be adjusted to prevent repeated episodes of hyperglycemia.
- Periodically assess body weight and other anthropometric measures (body mass index, body composition). Report a rapid or unexplained weight gain or weight loss.

Interventions

- Implement resistive exercises and weight-bearing activities to minimize muscle wasting and osteoporosis. Use caution to prevent musculoskeletal damage in patients with preexisting muscle and bone loss.
- Protect skin from breakdown, especially over bony prominences.

Patient/Client-Related Instruction

- Advise patient that wound healing may be delayed; instruct patient to check skin regularly and report any nonhealing sores.
- Advise patient that corticosteroids cause immunosuppression and may mask symptoms of infection. Instruct patient to avoid people with known contagious illnesses and to report possible infections immediately.

- Advise patients on long-term treatment to consult physician before stopping this medication. Stopping the medication suddenly may result in adrenocortical shock (severe hypotension, hypoglycemia, weakness, vomiting). If these signs appear, notify physician immediately; may be life threatening.
- Instruct patient to report any loss of vision that might indicate cataracts or increased intraocular pressure.
- Advise patient about possible cushingoid appearance, including puffiness in the face (moon face), increased fat in the torso, thin arms and legs, abdominal skin striations, bruising, and deposition of fat at the posterior base of the neck (buffalo hump). Discuss possible effects on body image, and help patient explore coping mechanisms.
- Instruct patient and family/caregivers to report other troublesome side effects such as severe or prolonged headache, menstrual problems, GI reactions (nausea, vomiting, loss of appetite), or skin reactions (acne, hair growth).

Pharmacokinetics

Absorption: Well absorbed after oral administration. Sodium phosphate salt is rapidly absorbed after IM administration. Absorption from local sites (intra-articular, intralesional) is slow but complete.
Distribution: Widely distributed, crosses the placenta, and appears to enter breast milk.
Metabolism and Excretion: Mostly metabolized by the liver.
Half-life: Low-birth-weight infants with bronchopulmonary dysplasia (BPD): 9.3 hr; children 3 mo–16 yr: 4.3 hr; Adults: 3–4.5 hr (plasma), 36–54 hr (tissue); adrenal suppression lasts 2.75 days.

TIME/ACTION PROFILE (anti-inflammatory activity)

ROUTE	ONSET	PEAK	DURATION
PO	unknown	1–2 hr	72 hr
IM, IV (phosphate)	Rapid	unknown	72 hr

Contraindications/Precautions

Contraindicated in: Active untreated infections (may be used in patients being treated for tuberculous meningitis); Known alcohol or bisulfite hypersensitivity or intolerance (some products contain these and should be avoided in susceptible patients); Lactation (avoid chronic use).
Use Cautiously in: Chronic treatment (will lead to adrenal suppression; use lowest possible dose for shortest period of time); Stress (surgery, infections); supplemental doses may be needed; Potential infections (may mask signs); OB: Safety not established; Pedi: Early postnatal administration of high doses can cause significant and persistent reductions in neuromotor and cognitive functioning; results in decreased growth; use lowest possible dose for shortest period of time.

Interactions

Drug-Drug: ↑ risk of hypokalemia with **thiazide** and **loop diuretics**, **amphotericin B**, **piperacillin**, or **ticarcillin**. Hypokalemia may ↑ risk of **digoxin** toxicity. May ↑ requirement for **insulin** or **oral hypoglycemic agents**. May ↓ levels of **phenytoin** and **isoniazid**. Levels may be ↑ with **oral contraceptives**. ↑ risk of adverse GI effects with **NSAIDs** (including **aspirin**), **alcohol**, and **caffeine**. At chronic doses that suppress adrenal function, may ↓ the antibody response to and ↑ risk of adverse reactions from **live-virus vaccines**. May ↑ or ↓ the effects of **warfarin**. Levels may be ↓ when used with **phenytoin**, **phenobarbital**, or **rifampin**. May ↑ risk of tendon rupture when used with **fluoroquinolones**.

Route/Dosage

PO, IM, IV (Adults): *Anti-inflammatory*—0.75–9 mg daily in divided doses q 6–12 hr. *Airway edema or extubation*—0.5–2 mg/kg/day divided q 6 hr; begin 24 hr prior to extubation and continue for 24 hr postextubation. *Cerebral edema*—10 mg IV, then 4 mg IM or IV q 6 hr until maximal response achieved, then switch to PO regimen and taper over 5–7 days.
PO, IM, IV (Children): *Airway edema or extubation*—0.5–2 mg/kg/day divided q 6 hr; begin 24 hr prior to extubation and continue for 24 hr postextubation. *Anti-inflammatory*—0.08–0.3 mg/kg/day or 2.5–10 mg/m²/day divided q 6–12 hr. *Physiologic replacement*—0.03–0.15 mg/kg/day or 0.6–0.75 mg/m²/day divided q 6–12 hr.
PO (Adults): *Suppression test*—1 mg at 11 PM or 0.5 mg q 6 hr for 48 hr.
IV (Children): *Chemotherapy induced emesis*—5–20 mg given 15–30 min before treatment. *Cerebral edema*—Loading dose 1–2 mg/kg followed by 1–1.5 mg/kg/day divided q 4–6 hr for 5 days (not to exceed 16 mg/day); then taper over 1–6 wk. *Bacterial meningitis*—0.6 mg/kg/day divided q 6 hr for 4 days (start at time of first antibiotic dose).
IV, PO (Adults): *Chemotherapy induced emesis*—10–20 mg given 15–30 min before each treatment or 10 mg q 12 hr on each treatment day. *Delayed nausea/vomiting*—4–10 mg PO 1–2 times/day for 2–4 days *or* 8 mg PO q 12 hr for 2 days, then 4 mg PO q 12 hr for 2 days *or* 20 mg PO 1 hr before chemotherapy, then 10 mg PO q 12 hr after chemotherapy, then 8 mg PO q 12 hr for 2 days, then 4 mg PO q 12 hr for 2 days.
IS (intrasynovial) (Adults): 0.4–6 mg/day.

Availability (generic available)

Tablets: 0.5 mg, 0.75 mg, 1 mg, 1.5 mg, 2 mg, 4 mg, 6 mg. **Elixir (raspberry flavor):** 0.5 mg/5 mL. **Oral solution (cherry flavor):** 0.5 mg/5 mL, 1 mg/mL. **Solution for injection (sodium phosphate):** 4 mg/mL, 10 mg/mL.

dexlansoprazole
(deks-lan-**soe**-pra-zole)
Kapidex

Classification
Therapeutic: antiulcer agents
Pharmacologic: proton-pump inhibitors

Indications
Healing/maintenance of healing of erosive esophagitis (EE). Treatment of heartburn from nonerosive gastroesophageal reflux disease (GERD).

Action
Binds to an enzyme in the presence of acidic gastric pH, preventing the final transport of hydrogen ions into the gastric lumen. **Therapeutic Effects:** Diminished accumulation of acid in the gastric lumen, with lessened acid reflux.

Adverse Reactions/Side Effects
GI: abdominal pain, diarrhea, flatulence, nausea, vomiting.

PHYSICAL THERAPY IMPLICATIONS

Examination and Evaluation
- Monitor improvements in GI symptoms (gastritis, heartburn, and so forth) to help determine if drug therapy is successful.

Interventions
- In cases of NSAID-induced gastritis, implement appropriate manual therapy techniques, physical agents, and therapeutic exercises to reduce pain and decrease the need for aspirin and other NSAIDs.

Patient/Client-Related Instruction
- Advise patient to avoid alcohol and foods that may cause an increase in GI irritation.
- Instruct patient to report bothersome or prolonged GI side effects such as nausea, vomiting, diarrhea, flatulence, and abdominal pain.

Pharmacokinetics
Absorption: Well absorbed following oral administration.
Distribution: Unknown.
Protein Binding: 96–99%.
Metabolism and Excretion: Extensively metabolized by the liver (CYP2C19 and CYP3A4 enzyme systems are involved); patients who are poor metabolizers may have higher blood levels; no active metabolites. No renal elimination.
Half-life: 1–2 hr.

TIME/ACTION PROFILE (blood levels)

ROUTE	ONSET	PEAK*	DURATION
PO	unknown	1–2 hr (1st); 4–5 hr (2nd)	24 hr

*Reflects effects of delayed release capsule.

Contraindications/Precautions
Contraindicated in: Hypersensitivity; Severe hepatic impairment; Geri: Avoid nursing.
Use Cautiously in: Moderate hepatic impairment (daily dose should not exceed 30 mg); Safe use in children <18 yr not established.

Interactions
Drug-Drug: ↓ levels of **atazanavir**; do not administer concurrently. May ↓ absorption of drugs requiring acid pH for absorption, including **ampicillin**, **digoxin**, **iron salts**, and **ketoconazole**. May ↑ effect of **warfarin**.

Route/Dosage
PO (Adults): *Healing of EE*—60 mg once daily for up to 8 wk; *maintenance of healing of EE*—30 mg once daily for up to 6 mo; *GERD*—30 mg once daily for 4 wk.

Hepatic Impairment
PO (Adults): *Moderate hepatic impairment*—daily dose should not exceed 30 mg.

Availability
Delayed-release capsules: 30 mg, 60 mg.

dexmedetomidine
(deks-med-e-**toe**-mi-deen)
Precedex

Classification
Therapeutic: sedative/hypnotics

Indications
Sedation of initially intubated and mechanically ventilated patients during treatment in an intensive care setting; should not be used for >24 hr.

Action
Acts as a relatively selective alpha-adrenergic agonist with sedative properties. **Therapeutic Effects:** Sedation.

Adverse Reactions/Side Effects
Resp: hypoxia. **CV:** BRADYCARDIA, SINUS ARREST, hypotension, transient hypertension. **GI:** nausea, vomiting. **Hemat:** anemia. **Misc:** fever.

PHYSICAL THERAPY IMPLICATIONS

Examination and Evaluation

- Assess heart rate, ECG, and heart sounds (See Appendices G, H). Report slow heart rate (bradycardia) or symptoms of other arrhythmias, including palpitations, chest discomfort, fainting, and fatigue/weakness.
- Assess blood pressure (BP) and compare to normal values (See Appendix F). Report changes in BP, either a problematic decrease in BP (hypotension) or a sustained increase in BP (hypertension).
- Monitor signs of low oxygen levels (hypoxia) or anemia, including pallor and cyanosis. Monitor pulse oximetry to quantify suspected problems with mechanical ventilation or blood delivery to tissues.

Patient/Client-Related Instruction

- Instruct patient or family/caregivers to report other troublesome side effects such as severe or prolonged fever or GI problems (nausea, vomiting).

Pharmacokinetics

Absorption: IV administration results in complete bioavailability.
Distribution: Unknown.
Protein Binding: 94%.
Metabolism and Excretion: Mostly metabolized by the liver, some metabolism by P450 enzyme system. Metabolites are mostly excreted in urine.
Half-life: 2 hr.

TIME/ACTION PROFILE (sedation)

ROUTE	ONSET	PEAK	DURATION
IV	rapid	unknown	unknown

Contraindications/Precautions

Contraindicated in: Hypersensitivity.
Use Cautiously in: Hepatic impairment (lower doses may be required); Advanced heart block; Geriatric patients (increased risk of bradycardia and hypotension in patients ≥65 yr; Pregnancy, lactation or children (safety not established).

Interactions

Drug-Drug: Sedation is enhanced by **anesthetics,** other **sedative/hypnotics,** and **opioid analgesics.**
Drug-Natural: Concomitant use of **kava, valerian, skullcap, chamomile,** or **hops** can ↑ CNS depression.

Route/Dosage

IV (Adults): *Loading infusion*—1 mcg/kg over 10 min followed by *maintenance infusion* of 0.2–0.7 mcg/kg/hr for maximum of 24 hr; rate is adjusted to achieve desired level of sedation.

Availability

Injection: 100 mcg/mL in 2-mL ampules and vials.

dexmethylphenidate
(deks-meth-il-**fen**-i-date)
Focalin, Focalin XR

Classification
Therapeutic: central nervous system stimulants
Pharmacologic: amphetamines

Schedule II

Indications

Adjunctive treatment of attention deficit hyperactivity disorder (ADHD).

Action

Produces CNS and respiratory stimulation with weak sympathomimetic activity. **Therapeutic Effects:** Increased attention span in ADHD.

Adverse Reactions/Side Effects

CNS: behavioral disturbances, hallucinations, insomnia, mania, nervousness, thought disorder. **EENT:** visual disturbances. **CV:** tachycardia. **GI:** abdominal pain, anorexia, nausea. **Metab:** growth suppression, weight loss (may occur with prolonged use). **Neuro:** twitching. **Misc:** fever.

PHYSICAL THERAPY IMPLICATIONS

Examination and Evaluation

- Hallucinations, disordered thoughts, or other behavioral disturbances. Report these signs to the physician.
- Assess heart rate, ECG, and heart sounds, especially during exercise (See Appendices G, H). Report fast heart rate (tachycardia) or symptoms of other arrhythmias, including palpitations, chest discomfort, shortness of breath, fainting, and fatigue/weakness.
- Monitor attentiveness and behavior in patients with ADHD. Report any changes in attention and hyperactivity, and document whether this drug appears to be producing the desired effects.
- Assess growth rate and body weight in children receiving chronic therapy; report a substantial weight loss or delayed/stunted growth to the physician.

Interventions

- Because of the risk of arrhythmias, use caution during aerobic exercise and other forms of therapeutic exercise. Assess exercise tolerance frequently (blood pressure, heart rate, fatigue levels), and terminate exercise immediately if any untoward responses occur (see Appendix L).

D

Patient/Client-related Instruction

- Instruct patient and family/caregivers to report other troublesome side effects such as severe or prolonged fever, sleep loss, and vision disturbances.

Pharmacokinetics

Absorption: Readily absorbed following oral administration.
Distribution: Unknown.
Metabolism and Excretion: Mostly metabolized by the liver; inactive metabolites are renally excreted.
Half-life: 2.2 hr.

TIME/ACTION PROFILE (improvement in symptoms)

ROUTE	ONSET	PEAK	DURATION
PO	7 days	1 mo	unknown

Contraindications/Precautions

Contraindicated in: Hypersensitivity; Hyperexcitable states (marked anxiety, agitation, or tension); Hyperthyroidism; Psychotic personalities, suicidal or homicidal tendencies; Glaucoma; Motor tics, family history or diagnosis of Tourette's syndrome; Concurrent use of MAO inhibitors; Should not be used to treat depression or prevent/treat normal fatigue; Psychoses (may exacerbate symptoms).
Use Cautiously in: History of cardiovascular disease; Hyperthyroidism; Hypertension; Diabetes mellitus; Geri: Geriatric/debilitated patients; Continual use (may result in psychologic or physical dependence); Seizure disorders (may lower seizure threshold); OB: Lactation: Pedi: Pregnancy, lactation, or children <6 yr (safety not established; use in pregnancy only if clearly needed).

Interactions

Drug-Drug: Concurrent use with or use within 14 days following discontinuation of **MAO inhibitors** may result in hypertensive crisis and is contraindicated. May ↓ effects of **antihypertensives**. May ↑ effects of **vasopressors**. May cause serious adverse reactions with **clonidine**. May ↑ effects of **warfarin, phenobarbital, phenytoin,** some **antidepressants**; dose adjustments may be necessary.

Route/Dosage

Tablets

PO (Adults and Children ≥6 yr): *Patients not previously taking methylphenidate*—2.5 mg twice daily, may be increased weekly as needed up to 10 mg twice daily; *Patients currently taking methylphenidate*—starting dose is $\frac{1}{2}$ of the methylphenidate dose, up to 10 mg twice daily.

Extended-release capsules

PO (Adults): *Patients not previously taking methylphenidate*—10 mg once daily, may be increased by 10 mg after 1 wk to 20 mg/day; *Patients currently taking methylphenidate*—starting dose is $\frac{1}{2}$ of the methylphenidate dose, up to 20 mg/day given as a single daily dose; *Patients currently taking dexmethylphenidate*—give same daily dose as a single dose.
PO (Children ≥6 yr): *Patients not previously taking methylphenidate*—5 mg once daily, may be increased by 5 mg weekly up to 20 mg/day; *Patients currently taking methylphenidate*—starting dose is $\frac{1}{2}$ of the methylphenidate dose, up to 20 mg/day, given as a single daily dose; *Patients currently taking dexmethylphenidate*—give same daily dose as a single dose.

Availability (generic available)

Tablets: 2.5 mg, 5 mg, 10 mg. **Extended-release capsules:** 5 mg, 10 mg, 15 mg, 20 mg.

dexrazoxane (deks-ra-**zoks**-ane)

Totect, Zinecard

Classification
Therapeutic: cardioprotective agents
Pharmacologic: chelating agents

Indications

Reduce incidence and severity of cardiomyopathy from doxorubicin in women with metastatic breast cancer who have already received a cumulative dose of doxorubicin >300 mg/m^2. Treatment of extravasation resulting from IV anthracycline chemotherapy.

Action

Acts as an intracellular chelating agent. **Therapeutic Effects:** Diminishes the cardiotoxic effects of doxorubicin. Decreased damage from extravasation of anthracyclines.

Adverse Reactions/Side Effects

Hemat: myelosuppression. **Local:** pain at injection site.

PHYSICAL THERAPY IMPLICATIONS

Examination and Evaluation

- Monitor signs of cardiomyopathy such as shortness of breath, dizziness, fatigue, fainting, palpitations, and peripheral/abdominal edema due to fluid accumulation. Increased signs may indicate a lack of drug effects in protecting the heart; notify the physician or nursing staff immediately.

- Monitor IV injection site for pain, swelling, and irritation. Report prolonged or excessive injection-site reactions to the physician.

Interventions

- For patients who are medically able to begin exercise, implement appropriate resistive exercises and aerobic training to maintain muscle strength and aerobic capacity during cancer chemotherapy or to help restore function after chemotherapy.

Patient/Client-Related Instruction

- Because of myelosuppression, advise patient to guard against infection (frequent hand washing, etc.), and to avoid crowds and contact with persons with contagious diseases.

Pharmacokinetics

Absorption: IV administration results in complete bioavailability.
Distribution: Unknown.
Metabolism and Excretion: Some metabolism occurs; 42% eliminated in urine.
Half-life: 2.1–2.5 hr.

TIME/ACTION PROFILE (cardioprotective effect)

ROUTE	ONSET	PEAK	DURATION
IV	rapid	unknown	unknown

Contraindications/Precautions

Contraindicated in: Any other type of chemotherapy except other anthracyclines (doxorubicin-like agents).
Use Cautiously in: CCr <40 mL/min (dose reduction required); OB: Pregnancy, lactation, or children (safety not established).

Interactions

Drug-Drug: Myelosuppression may be ↑ by **antineoplastics** or **radiation therapy**. Antitumor effects of concurrent combination chemotherapy with **fluorouracil** and **cyclophosphamide** may be ↓ by dexrazoxane.

Route/Dosage

Cardioprotective

IV (Adults): 10 mg of dexrazoxane/1 mg doxorubicin.

Renal Impairment

IV (Adults): decrease dose by 50%.

Extravasation protection

IV (Adults): 1000 mg/m^2 (maximum 2000 mg) given on days 1 and 2, and followed by a dose of 500 mg/m^2 (maximum 1000 mg) on day 3.

Renal Impairment

IV (Adults CCr <40 mL/min): decrease dose by 50%.

Availability (generic available)

Injection (Zinecard): 250-mg vial, 500-mg vial.
Injection (Totect): 500 mg vial.

dextroamphetamine

(deks-troe-am-**fet**-a-meen)
Dexedrine, Dextrostat

Classification
Therapeutic: central nervous system stimulants
Pharmacologic: amphetamines

Schedule II

Indications

Narcolepsy. Adjunct management of attention deficit hyperactivity disorder (ADHD). **Unlabeled Use:** Exogenous obesity.

Action

Produces CNS stimulation by releasing norepinephrine from nerve endings. Pharmacologic effects: CNS and respiratory stimulation, Vasoconstriction, Mydriasis (pupillary dilation), Contraction of the urinary bladder sphincter. **Therapeutic Effects:** Increased motor activity and mental alertness and decreased fatigue in narcoleptic patients. Increased attention span in ADHD.

Adverse Reactions/Side Effects

CNS: hyperactivity, insomnia, restlessness, tremor, behavioral disturbances, depression, dizziness, hallucinations, headache, irritability, mania, thought disorder. **CV:** palpitations, tachycardia, arrhythmias, hypertension. **GI:** anorexia, constipation, cramps, diarrhea, dry mouth, metallic taste, nausea, vomiting. **GU:** erectile dysfunction, increased libido. **Derm:** urticaria. **Misc:** physical dependence, psychologic dependence.

PHYSICAL THERAPY IMPLICATIONS

Examination and Evaluation

- Monitor attentiveness and behavior in patients with ADHD. Report any changes in attention and hyperactivity, and document whether this drug appears to be producing the desired effects.
- Monitor alertness in patients with narcolepsy; document the frequency and duration of sleeping episodes to help document the effects of drug therapy
- Be alert for signs of excessive CNS stimulation, including hyperactivity, restlessness, tremor, hallucinations, mania, irritability, or disordered thoughts. Report these signs to the physician.
- Assess heart rate, ECG, and heart sounds, especially during exercise (See Appendices G, H). Report fast heart rate (tachycardia) or symptoms of other arrhythmias, including palpitations, chest discomfort, shortness of breath, fainting, and fatigue/weakness.

- Assess blood pressure (BP) and compare to normal values (See Appendix F). Report a sustained increase in BP (hypertension).
- Assess dizziness that might affect gait, balance, and other functional activities (See Appendix C). Report balance problems and functional limitations to the physician and nursing staff, and caution the patient and family/caregivers to guard against falls and trauma.

Interventions

- Because of the risk of arrhythmias and abnormal BP responses, use caution during aerobic exercise and other forms of therapeutic exercise. Assess exercise tolerance frequently (BP, heart rate, fatigue levels), and terminate exercise immediately if any untoward responses occur (See Appendix L).

Patient/Client-Related Instruction

- If used to promote weight loss, make sure patient has discussed this use with his/her physician. Advise patient about the potential cardiac and CNS risks of amphetamines, and counsel patient about safer methods for weight loss such as diet and exercise.
- Instruct patient and family/caregivers to report other troublesome side effects, including severe or prolonged headache, sleep loss, skin problems (hives, itching), sexual changes (increased libido, erectile dysfunction), or GI problems (nausea, vomiting, constipation, diarrhea, abdominal cramps, metallic taste, dry mouth).

Pharmacokinetics

Absorption: Well absorbed.
Distribution: Widely distributed; high concentrations in brain and CSF. Crosses the placenta; enters breast milk; potentially embryotoxic.
Metabolism and Excretion: Some metabolism by the liver. Urinary excretion is pH dependent. Alkaline urine promotes reabsorption and prolongs action.
Half-life: 10–12 hr (6.8 hr in children).

TIME/ACTION PROFILE (CNS stimulation)

ROUTE	ONSET	PEAK	DURATION
PO	1–2 hr	3 hr	2–10 hr
PO-ER	unknown	unknown	up to 24 hr

Contraindications/Precautions

Contraindicated in: OB/Lactation: Pregnancy or lactation; Hyperexcitable states, including hyperthyroidism; Psychotic personalities; Suicidal or homicidal tendencies; Glaucoma; Some products contain tartrazine; avoid in patients with known hypersensitivity.

Use Cautiously in: Cardiovascular disease (sudden death has occurred in children with structural cardiac abnormalities or other serious heart problems); Hypertension; Diabetes mellitus; History of substance abuse; Debilitated patients; Continual use (may produce psychologic dependence or physical addiction); Geri: Appears on Beers' list. Elderly are at increased risk for cardiovascular side effects.

Interactions

Drug-Drug: ↑ adrenergic effects with other **adrenergics**. Use with **MAO inhibitors** can result in hypertensive crisis. Alkalinizing the urine **(sodium bicarbonate, acetazolamide)** prolongs effect. Acidification of urine (**ammonium chloride**, large doses of **ascorbic acid**) ↓ effect. **Phenothiazines** may ↓ effect of dextroamphetamine. May antagonize the response to **antihypertensives**. ↑ risk of cardiovascular side effects with **beta blockers** or **tricyclic antidepressants**.
Drug-Natural: St. John's wort may ↑ serious side effects; concurrent use is not recommended. Use with caffeine-containing herbs **(guarana, tea, coffee)** ↑ stimulant effect. **St. John's wort** may ↑ serious side effects; concurrent use is not recommended.

Route/Dosage

Attention Deficit Hyperactivity Disorder

PO (Adults): 5–40 mg/day in divided doses. Sustained-release capsules should not be used as initial therapy.
PO (Children ≥ 6 yr): 5 mg 1–2 times daily; increase by 5 mg daily at weekly intervals (maximum: 40 mg/day). Sustained-release capsules should not be used as initial therapy.
PO (Children 3–5 yr): 2.5 mg/day; increase by 2.5 mg daily at weekly intervals (maximum: 40 mg/day).

Narcolepsy

PO (Adults): 5–60 mg/day single dose or in divided doses. Sustained-release capsules should not be used as initial therapy.
PO (Children ≥12 yr): 10 mg/day; increase by 10 mg/day at weekly intervals until response is obtained 60 mg is reached.
PO (Children 6–12 yr): 5 mg/day, increase by 5 mg/day at weekly intervals until response is obtained or 60 mg is reached.

Exogenous obesity

PO (Adults and Children >12 yr): 5–30 mg/day in divided doses of 5–10 mg given 30–60 min before meals.

Availability (generic available)

Tablets: 5 mg. **Sustained-release capsules:** 5 mg, 10 mg, 15 mg.

dextromethorphan
(deks-troe-meth-**or**-fan)

Balminil DM, Benylin Adult, Benylin Pediatric, Broncho-Grippol-DM, Calmylin #1, Children's Hold, Creo-Terpin, Delsym, DexAlone, DM Syrup, Drixoral Liquid Cough Caps, ElixSure Children's Cough Syrup, Hold, Koffex, Little Colds Cough Formula Drops, Mediquell, Neo-DM, Ornex-DM, PediCare Infant's Long Acting Cough Drops, Pertussin Cough Suppressant, Pertussin CS, Pertussin ES, Robidex, Robitussin Cough Calmers, Robitussin CoughGels, Robitussin Maximum Strength Cough Suppressant, Robitussin Pediatric, Sedatuss, Simply Cough, Sucrets Cough Control Formula, TheraFlu Thin Strips Long Acting Cough, Triaminic Thin Strips Long Acting Cough, Vicks 44 Cough Relief, Vicks Formula 44 Pediatric Formula

Classification

Therapeutic: allergy, cold, and cough remedies, antitussives

Indications

Symptomatic relief of coughs caused by minor viral upper respiratory tract infections or inhaled irritants. Most effective for chronic nonproductive cough. A common ingredient in nonprescription cough and cold preparations.

Action

Suppresses the cough reflex by a direct effect on the cough center in the medulla. Related to opioids structurally but has no analgesic properties. **Therapeutic Effects:** Relief of irritating nonproductive cough.

Adverse Reactions/Side Effects

CNS: *high dose*—dizziness, sedation. **GI:** nausea.

PHYSICAL THERAPY IMPLICATIONS

Examination and Evaluation

- Assess frequency and nature of cough, lung sounds (See Appendix K), and amount and type of sputum produced. Document whether this drug is effective in reducing cough.
- Assess dizziness that might affect gait, balance, and other functional activities (See Appendix C). Report balance problems and functional limitations to the physician, and caution the patient and family/caregivers to guard against falls and trauma.

Patient/Client-Related Instruction

- Caution patient to avoid taking more than the recommended dose or taking alcohol or other CNS depressants concurrently with this medication; fatalities have occurred.
- Instruct patient to cough effectively: sit upright and take several deep breaths before attempting to cough.
- Advise patient to minimize cough by avoiding irritants, such as cigarette smoke, fumes, and dust. Humidification of environmental air, frequent sips of water, and sugarless hard candy may also decrease the frequency of dry, irritating cough.
- Advise patient that any cough lasting more than 1 wk or accompanied by fever, chest pain, persistent headache, or skin rash warrants medical attention.
- Instruct patient or family/caregivers to report other problematic side effects such as severe or prolonged nausea or sedation.

Pharmacokinetics

Absorption: Rapidly absorbed from the GI tract. Extended-release product is slowly absorbed.
Distribution: Unknown. Probably crosses the placenta and enters breast milk.
Metabolism and Excretion: Metabolized to dextrorphan, an active metabolite. Dextromethorphan and dextrorphan are renally excreted.
Half-life: Unknown.

TIME/ACTION PROFILE (cough suppression)

ROUTE	ONSET	PEAK	DURATION
PO	15–30 min	unknown	3–6 hr*
PO-ER	unknown	unknown	9–12 hr

*Up to 8 hr for Gelcaps.

Contraindications/Precautions

Contraindicated in: Hypersensitivity; Patients taking MAO inhibitors or SSRIs; Should not be used for chronic productive coughs; Some products contain alcohol and should be avoided in patients with known intolerance.

Use Cautiously in: Cough that lasts more than 1 wk or is accompanied by fever, rash, or headache—health care professional should be consulted; History of drug abuse or drug-seeking behavior (capsules have been abused resulting in deaths); Diabetes (some products contain sucrose); OB: Pregnancy (has been used safely); Pedi: Lactation or children <2 yr (safety not established).

Interactions

Drug-Drug: Use with **MAO inhibitors** may result in serotonin syndrome (nausea, confusion, changes in blood pressure); concurrent use should be avoided. ↑ CNS depression with **antihistamines, alcohol,**

antidepressants, sedative/hypnotics, or **opioids. Amiodarone, fluoxetine**, or **quinidine** may ↑ blood levels and adverse reactions from dextromethorphan.

Route/Dosage

PO (Adults and Children >12 yr): 10–20 mg q 4 hr *or* 30 mg q 6–8 hr *or* 60 mg of extended-release preparation bid (not to exceed 120 mg/day).
PO (Children 6–12 yr): 5–10 mg q 4 hr *or* 15 mg q 6–8 hr *or* 30 mg of extended-release preparation q 12 hr (not to exceed 60 mg/day).
PO (Children 2–6 yr): 2.5–5 mg q 4 hr *or* 7.5 mg q 6–8 hr *or* 15 mg of extended-release preparation q 12 hr (not to exceed 30 mg/day).

Availability

Gelcaps: 30 mg OTC. **Lozenges (cherry):** 2.5 mg OTC, 5 mg OTC. **Liquid (cherry, grape):** 3.5 mg/ 5 mL OTC, 5 mg/5 mL, 7.5 mg/5 mL OTC, 15 mg/5 mL OTC, 30 mg/ 5 mL OTC. **Syrup (cherry, cherry bubblegum):** 7.5 mg/5 mL OTC, 15 mg/15 mL OTC, 10 mg/5 mL OTC. **Extended-release suspension (orange):** 30 mg/5 mL OTC. **Drops (Grape):** 7.5 mg/0.8 mL OTC, 7.5 mg/1 mL OTC. **Orally disintegrating strips (cherry, grape):** 7.5 mg OTC, 15 mg OTC. ***In combination with:*** antihistamines, decongestants, and expectorants in cough and cold preparations OTC. See Appendix B.

dextromethorphan/quinidine

(deks-troe-meth-**or**-fan/ **kwin**-i-deen)
Neudexta

Classification
Therapeutic: none assigned

Indications

Management of Pseudobulbar Affect (PSA), a mood disorder consisting of extremes of emotional lability (such as laughing fits followed by crying jags) seen in association with amyotrophic lateral sclerosis (ALS) and multiple sclerosis (MS). Not effective for other forms of emotional lability.

Action

Dextromethorphan acts as an *N*-Methyl-D-aspartic acid (NMDA) receptor antagonist and sigma-1 agonist. Quinidine acts as an inhibitor of the CYP2D6 enzyme system, producing a marked ↑ in dextromethorphan blood levels. **Therapeutic Effects:** ↓ emotional lability.

Adverse Reactions/Side Effects

CNS: dizziness, weakness. **Resp:** cough. **CV:** peripheral edema, QT prolongation. **GI:** diarrhea, flatulence, hepatitis, ↑ liver enzymes, vomiting. **Hemat:** thrombocytopenia. **Misc:** hypersensitivity reactions including lupus-like syndrome.

D

PHYSICAL THERAPY IMPLICATIONS

Examination and Evaluation

- Monitor signs of hypersensitivity reactions, including lupus-like syndrome. Signs include increased blood pressure (BP), fever, joint pain, skin rashes, pulmonary symptoms (tightness in the throat and chest, wheezing, cough, dyspnea), and redness/irritation of the eye (uveitis). Notify physician promptly if these signs appear.
- Assess heart rate, ECG, and heart sounds, especially during exercise (See Appendices G, H). Report any rhythm disturbances (QT prolongation) or symptoms of increased arrhythmias, including palpitations, chest discomfort, shortness of breath, fainting, and fatigue/weakness.
- Assess peripheral edema using girth measurements, volume displacement, and measurement of pitting edema (See Appendix N). Report increased swelling in feet and ankles or a sudden increase in body weight due to fluid retention.
- Watch for signs of thrombocytopenia, including bruising, nose bleeds, and bleeding gums. Report these signs to the physician.
- Assess dizziness and weakness that might affect gait, balance, and other functional activities (See Appendix C). Report balance problems and functional limitations to the physician and nursing staff, and caution the patient and family/caregivers to guard against falls and trauma.

Interventions

- Guard against falls and trauma (hip fractures, head injury, and so forth) caused by dizziness and weakness; implement fall prevention strategies (See Appendix E).
- Help patient explore nonpharmacologic methods to reduce emotional lability, such as counseling, support groups, cognitive behavioral therapies, and so forth).

Patient/Client-Related Instruction

- Advise patient about the likelihood of GI reactions such as vomiting, diarrhea, and flatulence. Instruct patient to report severe or prolonged GI problems, and also to report signs of liver toxicity, including yellow skin or eyes, abdominal pain, severe nausea and vomiting, fever, sore throat, malaise, weakness, and facial edema.
- Instruct patient to report other problematic side effects such as severe or prolonged cough.

Pharmacokinetics

Absorption: *Dextromethorphan*—well absorbed following oral administration; *quinidine*—70–80% absorbed following oral administration.
Distribution: *quinidine*—widely distributed, crosses placenta, enters breast milk.
Metabolism and Excretion: Both extensively metabolized by the liver (*dextromethorphan* by CYP2D6, *quinidine* by CYP3A4); some metabolites of quinidine have antiarrhythmic activity. 5–20% of quinidine excreted unchanged by the kidneys; some renal elimination is pH dependent
Half-life: *Dextromethorphan*—13 hr; *quinidine*—7 hr (↑ in CHF and liver impairment).

TIME/ACTION PROFILE (blood levels)

ROUTE	ONSET	PEAK	DURATION
dextromethorphan PO	15–30 min	unknown	unknown
quinidine PO	30 min	1–1.5 hr	unknown

Contraindications/Precautions

Contraindicated in: Known hypersensitivity to dextromethorphan; Known hypersensitivity to quinidine, quinine, or mefloquine, including previous hepatitis, bone marrow depression, lupus-like syndrome, or other hypersensitivity reactions; Concurrent use of quinidine, quinine, or mefloquine; use within 14 days of MAOIs; Prolonged/congenital long QT interval, history suggestive of torsades de pointes, or CHF; Concurrent use of drugs that prolong the QT interval and are metabolized by the CYP2D6 enzyme system, including thioridazine and pimozide; Complete AV block (without implanted pacemaker) or risk of AV block.
Use Cautiously in: CYP2D6 Poor metabolizers (quinidine component will not contribute to effectiveness, seen in 7–10% of Caucasians and 3–8% of African Americans, consider genotyping those at ↑ risk of quinidine toxicity); Patients with left ventricular hypertrophy (LVH) or left ventricular dysfunction (LVD); History of hypertension, stroke, or coronary artery disease (↑ risk of QT prolongation); Electrolyte abnormalities, especially hypokalemia and hypomagnesemia (↑ risk of QT prolongation; correct before use); Myasthenia gravis (quinidine may worsen condition); Severe hepatic/renal impairment (increased blood levels likely); Other underlying neurologic diseases; OB: Use in pregnancy only if potential benefit outweighs potential risk to the fetus; Lactation: Use cautiously; Pedi: Safe and effective use in children <18 yr has not been established.

Interactions

Drug-Drug: Concurrent use with **MAOIs** ↑ risk of serious adverse reactions, including serotonin syndrome; MAOI use should be discontinued at least 14 days before—allow 14 days after discontinuing to start MAOIs;↑ blood levels and risk of adverse reactions from **desipramine** and **paroxetine**; ↓ dose of antidepressant and determine dose by clinical response; Concurrent therapy with strong or moderate inhibitors of the CYP3A4 enzyme system, including **aprepitant, atazanavir, clarithromycin, diltiazem, erythromycin, fluconazole, fosamprenavir, indinavir, itraconazole, ketoconazole, nefazodone, nelfinavir, ritonavir, saquinavir, telithromycin,** and **verapamil;** ↑ risk of QT prolongation, careful monitoring recommended; Concurrent use with **SSRIs** or **tricyclic antidepressants** may result in serotonin syndrome; Avoid concurrent use with **drugs that prolong QT interval** together with **drugs that are metabolized by CYP2D6**, including **thioridazine** and **pimozide;** When using with **drugs that prolong QT interval** and **drugs that are moderate/strong inhibitors of CYP3A4,** ECG monitoring is recommended; Concurrent use of **drugs that are metabolized by CYP2D6**, especially those with narrow therapeutic indices should be undertaken with caution, dose modifications or choosing an alternative agent may be necessary, including **codeine** and **hydrocodone;** ↑ blood levels and risk of toxicity/adverse reactions from **desipramine** (daily dose should not exceed 40 mg/day) or **paroxetine** (dose should not exceed 35 mg/day); ↑ blood levels and the risk of toxicity from **digoxin**, careful monitoring recommended;↑ CNS depressant with other **CNS depressants**, including **antihistamines**, some **antidepressants, sedative/hypnotics,** and **alcohol.**

Route/Dosage

PO (Adults): 1 capsule (dextromethorphan 30 mg/quinidine 10 mg) daily for 7 days, then increase to one capsule every 12 hr.

Availability

Capsules: dextromethorphan 30 mg/quinidine 10 mg/capsule

diazepam (dye-az-e-pam)

Apo-Diazepam, Diastat, Diazemuls, Novodipam, PMS-Diazepam, Valium, Vivol

Classification
Therapeutic: antianxiety agents, anticonvulsants, sedative/hypnotics, skeletal muscle relaxants (centrally acting)
Pharmacologic: benzodiazepines

Schedule IV

Indications

Adjunct in the management of Anxiety Disorder, Athetosis, Anxiety relief prior to cardioversion (injection), Stiff man syndrome, Preoperative sedation, Conscious sedation (provides light anesthesia and anterograde amnesia). Treatment of status epilepticus/uncontrolled seizures (injection). Skeletal muscle relaxant. Management of the symptoms of alcohol withdrawal. **Unlabeled Use:** Anxiety associated with acute myocardial infarction, insomnia.

Action

Depresses the CNS, probably by potentiating gamma-aminobutyric acid (GABA), an inhibitory neurotransmitter. Produces skeletal muscle relaxation by inhibiting spinal polysynaptic afferent pathways. Has anticonvulsant properties due to enhanced presynaptic inhibition. **Therapeutic Effects:** Relief of anxiety. Sedation. Amnesia. Skeletal muscle relaxation. Decreased seizure activity.

Adverse Reactions/Side Effects

CNS: dizziness, drowsiness, lethargy, depression, hangover, ataxia, slurred speech, headache, paradoxical excitation. **EENT:** blurred vision. **Resp:** respiratory depression. **CV:** hypotension (IV only). **GI:** constipation, diarrhea (may be caused by propylene glycol content in oral solution), nausea, vomiting, weight gain. **Derm:** rashes. **Local:** pain (IM), phlebitis (IV), venous thrombosis. **Misc:** physical dependence, psychologic dependence, tolerance.

PHYSICAL THERAPY IMPLICATIONS

Examination and Evaluation

- When used as a muscle relaxant, assess patient's muscle spasms, associated pain, and range of motion to help document drug efficacy.
- In patients with seizures, document changes in seizure activity to help determine drug efficacy.
- Assess dizziness, drowsiness, and ataxia that might affect gait, balance, and other functional activities (See Appendix C). Report balance problems and functional limitations to the physician, and caution the patient and family/caregivers to guard against falls and trauma.
- Monitor daytime drowsiness and "hangover" symptoms (headache, nausea, irritability, dysphoria, slurred speech). Repeated or excessive symptoms may require change in dose or medication.
- Be alert for a possible increase in excitation or worsening anxiety and agitation. Severe or problematic excitation may require a change in dose or drug.
- Measure blood pressure (sitting, standing, lying) and pulse rate, especially when patient begins drug therapy or when administered IV for severe or uncontrolled seizures. Report low blood pressure (hypotension), especially if patient experiences dizziness or syncope.
- Monitor any breathing problems, and report signs of respiratory depression such as shortness of breath, cyanosis, and labored or difficult breathing.
- Periodically assess body weight and other anthropometric measures (body mass index, body composition). Report a rapid or unexplained weight gain or increased body fat.
- Assess injection site during and after IV or IM administration. Report any localized pain or signs of phlebitis and venous thrombosis (swelling, inflammation).

Interventions

- In patients with muscle spasms, implement appropriate manual therapy techniques, physical agents, and therapeutic exercises to help resolve the spasms and reduce the need for long-term drug treatment and the risk of physical/psychologic dependence.
- Guard against falls and trauma (hip fractures, head injury, and so forth). Implement fall-prevention strategies, especially in older adults or if drowsiness and dizziness carry over into the daytime (See Appendix E).
- Help patient explore nonpharmacologic methods to reduce anxiety, such as relaxation techniques, exercise, counseling, support groups, and so forth.
- To minimize orthostatic hypotension, patient should move slowly when assuming a more upright position.

Patient/Client-Related Instruction

- Advise patients on prolonged treatment not to discontinue medication without consulting their physician. Long-term use can cause tolerance and physical/psychologic dependence, and abrupt withdrawal may cause insomnia, irritability, nervousness, and seizures.
- Advise patient to avoid alcohol and other CNS depressants because of the increased risk of sedation and adverse effects.
- Instruct patient to report other bothersome side effects such as severe or prolonged headache, skin rash, or GI problems (nausea, vomiting, diarrhea, constipation).

Pharmacokinetics

Absorption: Rapidly absorbed from the GI tract. Absorption from IM sites may be slow and unpredictable. Well absorbed (90%) from rectal mucosa. **Distribution:** Widely distributed. Crosses the blood-brain barrier. Crosses the placenta; enters breast milk.

Metabolism and Excretion: Highly metabolized by the liver. Some products of metabolism are active as CNS depressants.

Half-life: Neonates: 50–95 hr; infants 1 mo–2 yr: 40–50 hr; children 2–12 yr: 15–21 hr; children 12–16 yr: 18–20 hr; adults: 20–50 hr (up to 100 hr for metabolites).

TIME/ACTION PROFILE (sedation)

ROUTE	ONSET	PEAK	DURATION
PO	30–60 min	1–2 hr	up to 24 hr
IM	within 20 min	0.5–1.5 hr	unknown
IV	1–5 min	15–30 min	15–60 min*
rectal	2–10 min	1–2 hr	4–12 hr

*In status epilepticus, anticonvulsant duration is 15–20 min.

Contraindications/Precautions

Contraindicated in: Hypersensitivity; Cross-sensitivity with other benzodiazepines may occur; Comatose patients; Myasthenia gravis; Severe pulmonary impairment; Sleep apnea; Severe hepatic dysfunction; Preexisting CNS depression; Uncontrolled severe pain; Angle-closure glaucoma; Some products contain alcohol, propylene glycol, or tartrazine and should be avoided in patients with known hypersensitivity or intolerance; OB: ↑ risk of congenital malformations; Pedi: Children <6 mo (for oral; safety not established); Lactation: Recommend to discontinue drug or bottle feed.

Use Cautiously in: Severe renal impairment; History of suicide attempt or drug dependence; Debilitated patients (dose reduction required); Patients with low albumin; Pedi: Metabolites can accumulate in neonates. Injection contains benzyl alcohol, which can cause potentially fatal gasping syndrome in neonates; Geri: Long-acting benzodiazepines cause prolonged sedation in the elderly. Appears on Beers' list and is associated with ↑ risk of falls (↓ dose required or consider short-acting benzodiazepine).

Interactions

Drug-Drug: Alcohol, antidepressants, antihistamines, and **opioid analgesics**—concurrent use results in additive CNS depression. **Cimetidine, hormonal contraceptives, disulfiram, fluoxetine, isoniazid, ketoconazole, metoprolol, propoxyphene, propranolol,** or **valproic acid** may ↓ the metabolism of diazepam, enhancing its actions. May ↓ the efficacy of **levodopa. Rifampin** or **barbiturates** may ↑ the metabolism of diazepam and ↓ its effectiveness.. Sedative effects may be ↓ by **theophylline**. Concurrent use of **ritonavir** is not recommended.

Drug-Natural: Concomitant use of **kava, valerian,** or **chamomile** can ↑ CNS depression.

Route/Dosage

Antianxiety

PO (Adults): 2–10 mg 2–4 times daily.

IM, IV (Adults): 2–10 mg; may repeat in 3–4 hr as needed.

PO (Children >6 mo): 1–2.5 mg 3–4 times daily.

IM, IV (Children >1 mo): 0.04–0.3 mg/kg/dose q 2–4 hr to a maximum of 0.6 mg/kg within an 8-hr period if necessary.

Precardioversion

IV (Adults): 5–15 mg 5–10 min precardioversion.

Preendoscopy

IV (Adults): 2.5–20 mg.

IM (Adults): 5–10 mg 30 min preendoscopy.

Pediatric Conscious Sedation for Procedures

PO (Children >6 mo): 0.2–0.3 mg/kg (not to exceed 10 mg/dose) 45–60 min prior to procedure.

Status Epilepticus/Acute Seizure Activity

IV (Adults): 5–10 mg; may repeat q 10–15 min to a total of 30 mg; may repeat regimen again in 2–4 hr (IM route may be used if IV route unavailable); larger doses may be required.

IM, IV (Children ≥5 yr): 0.05–0.3 mg/kg/dose given over 3–5 min q 15–30 min to a total dose of 10 mg; repeat q 2–4 hr.

IM, IV (Children 1 mo–5 yr): 0.05–0.3 mg/kg/dose given over 3–5 min q 15–30 min to maximum dose of 5 mg; repeat in 2–4 hr if needed.

IV (Neonates): 0.1–0.3 mg/kg/dose given over 3–5 min q 15–30 min to maximum dose of 2 mg.

Rectal (Adults and Children >12 yr): 0.2 mg/kg; may repeat 4–12 hr later.

Rectal (Children 6–11 yr): 0.3 mg/kg; may repeat 4–12 hr later.

Rectal (Children 2–5 yr): 0.5 mg/kg; may repeat 4–12 hr later.

Febrile Seizure Prophylaxis

PO (Children >1 mo): 1 mg/kg/day divided q 8 hr at first sign of fever and continue for 24 hr after fever is gone.

Skeletal Muscle Relaxation

PO (Adults): 2–10 mg 3–4 times daily.

PO (Geriatric Patients or Debilitated Patients): 2–2.5 mg 1–2 times daily initially.

PO (Children >6 mo): 1–2.5 mg 3–4 times daily.

IM, IV (Adults): 5–10 mg; may repeat in 2–4 hr (larger doses may be required for tetanus).

IM, IV (Geriatric Patients or Debilitated Patients): 2–5 mg; may repeat in 2–4 hr (larger doses may be required for tetanus).

IM, IV (Children ≥5 yr): *Tetanus*—5–10 mg q 3–4 hr.

IM, IV (Children >1 mo): *Tetanus*—1–2 mg q 3–4 hr.

Alcohol Withdrawal

PO (Adults): 10 mg 3–4 times in first 24 hr; decrease to 5 mg 3–4 times daily.
IM, IV (Adults): 10 mg initially, then 5–10 mg in 3–4 hr as needed; larger or more frequent doses have been used.

Psychoneurotic Reactions

IM, IV (Adults): 2–10 mg; may be repeated in 3–4 hr.

Availability (generic available)

Tablets: 2 mg, 5 mg, 10 mg. **Oral solution:** 5 mg/mL (Intensol), 1 mg/mL. **Solution for injection:** 5 mg/mL (contains 10% alcohol and 40% propylene glycol). **Rectal gel delivery system:** 2.5 mg, 10 mg, 20 mg.

diazoxide (dye-az-**ox**-ide)

Hyperstat, Proglycem

Classification
Therapeutic: antihypertensives, hyperglycemic
Pharmacologic: vasodilators

Indications

IV: Treatment of hypertensive emergency. **PO:** Treatment of hypoglycemia associated with hyperinsulinism due to islet cell carcinoma or other causes.

Action

Directly relaxes vascular smooth muscle in peripheral arterioles. Produces ↓ in blood pressure (BP), reflex tachycardia, and increased cardiac output. Inhibits insulin release from the pancreas and ↓ peripheral utilization of glucose. **Therapeutic Effects:** Lowering of blood pressure. ↑ blood glucose.

Adverse Reactions/Side Effects

CNS: dizziness, headache. **CV:** hypotension, tachycardia, angina, edema, flushing. **Derm:** hirsutism. **Endo:** hyperglycemia, hyperuricemia. **F and E:** sodium and water retention. **GI:** nausea, vomiting, constipation. **Local:** phlebitis at IV site. **MS:** weakness.

PHYSICAL THERAPY IMPLICATIONS

Examination and Evaluation

- Assess BP, and determine if BP is maintained in the normal range (See Appendix F). Report low BP (hypotension), especially if patient experiences dizziness or syncope.
- Assess heart rate, ECG, and heart sounds, especially during exercise (See Appendices G, H). Report a rapid heart rate (tachycardia) or signs of other arrhythmias, including palpitation s, chest discomfort, shortness of breath, fainting, and fatigue/weakness.
- Monitor and report any episodes of angina pectoris at rest or during exercise.
- Assess peripheral edema using girth measurements, volume displacement, and measurement of pitting edema (See Appendix N). Report increased swelling in feet and ankles or a sudden increase in body weight due to sodium and water retention.
- Be alert for signs of hyperglycemia, including confusion, drowsiness, flushed/dry skin, fruit-like breath odor, rapid/deep breathing, polyuria, loss of appetite, and unusual thirst. Patients with diabetes mellitus should check blood glucose levels frequently.
- Assess dizziness that might affect gait, balance, and other functional activities (See Appendix C). Report balance problems and functional limitations to the physician and nursing staff, and caution the patient and family/caregivers to guard against falls and trauma.
- Assess IV site during and after IV administration, and report signs of phlebitis (local pain, swelling, inflammation).

Interventions

- Because of an increased risk of cardiac arrhythmias and abnormal BP responses, use caution during aerobic exercise and endurance conditioning. Terminate exercise if patient exhibits untoward symptoms (chest pain, shortness of breath, unusual fatigue), or displays other criteria for exercise termination (See Appendix L).
- Avoid physical therapy interventions that cause systemic vasodilation (large whirlpool, Hubbard tank). Additive effects of this drug and the intervention may cause a dangerous fall in BP.
- To minimize orthostatic hypotension, patient should move slowly when assuming a more upright position.

Patient/Client-Related Instruction

- Remind patients to take medication as directed to control hypertension even if they are asymptomatic.
- Counsel patients about additional interventions to help with the long-term control of BP, including regular exercise, weight loss, sodium restriction, stress reduction, moderation of alcohol consumption, and smoking cessation.
- Instruct patient or family/caregivers to report other troublesome side effects such as severe or prolonged headache, excessive body hair, or GI problems (nausea, vomiting, constipation).

Pharmacokinetics

Absorption: Well absorbed following oral administration.

Distribution: Crosses the blood-brain barrier and placenta.
Protein Binding: >90%.
Metabolism and Excretion: 50% metabolized by the liver; 50% excreted unchanged by the kidneys.
Half-life: 20–36 hr (prolonged in renal impairment).

TIME/ACTION PROFILE

ROUTE	ONSET	PEAK	DURATION
PO*	1 hr	8–12 hr	8 hr
IV†	immediate	5 min	3–12 hr

*Blood sugar.
†Blood pressure.

Contraindications/Precautions

Contraindicated in: Hypersensitivity; Hypersensitivity to bisulfites (IV only). Cross-sensitivity with sulfonamides may occur; Hypertension associated with pheochromocytoma or aortic dissection.
Use Cautiously in: Diabetics (hyperglycemia accompanies use); Cardiovascular disease; Renal or hepatic impairment; Pregnancy and lactation (safety not established; may inhibit labor).

Interactions

Drug-Drug: Concurrent **diuretic** therapy may potentiate hyperglycemic, hyperuricemic, and hypotensive effects. May ↑ the metabolism and ↓ the effectiveness of **phenytoin**. **Corticosteroids** may ↑ hyperglycemia. May ↑ the effects of **warfarin**. May alter the effects of **insulins** or **oral hypoglycemic agents**.
Drug-Natural: Glucosamine may worsen hyperglycemia. **Fenugreek**, **chromium**, and **coenzyme Q10** may produce additive hypoglycemic effects.

Route/Dosage

Hypertension

IV (Adults and Children): 1–3 mg/kg (not to exceed 150 mg/dose); may repeat dose in 5–15 min until BP is lowered to desired level; repeat administration every 4–24 hr may be used to maintain BP until oral antihypertensives are started.

Hyperinsulinemic Hypoglycemia

PO (Adults and Children): 1 mg/kg q 8 hr initially; further adjustments made on the basis of response. Usual maintenance dose is 3–8 mg/kg/day given in divided doses every 8–12 hr.
PO (Infants and Newborns): 2.7 mg/kg q 8 hr initially; further adjustments made on the basis of response. Usual maintenance dose is 8–15 mg/kg/day in divided doses every 8–12 hr.

Availability (generic available)

Capsules: 100 mg. **Oral suspension:** 50 mg/mL (contains 7.5% alcohol). **Injection:** 15 mg/mL.

diclofenac (dye-**kloe**-fen-ak)
diclofenac potassium
Cataflam, Apo–Diclo Rapide
diclofenac sodium
🍁 Apo-Diclo, Voltaren
diclofenac topical
Solaraze
diclofenac (topical patch)
Flector

Classification
Therapeutic: nonopioid analgesics, nonsteroidal anti-inflammatory agents
Pharmacologic: phenylacetic acid derivative

Indications

PO: Management of inflammatory disorders, including Rheumatoid arthritis, Osteoarthritis, Ankylosing spondylitis. Primary dysmenorrhea. Relief of mild-to-moderate pain. **Topical:** Treatment of actinic keratoses. **Topical patch:** treatment of acute pain due to minor strains, sprains, and contusions.

Action

Inhibits prostaglandin synthesis. **Therapeutic Effects:** Suppression of pain and inflammation. **Topical:** Clearance of actinic keratosis lesions.

Adverse Reactions/Side Effects

For oral diclofenac unless noted
CNS: dizziness, headache. **CV:** hypertension. **EENT:** tinnitus. **GI:** GI BLEEDING, abdominal pain, constipation, diarrhea, dyspepsia, flatulence, heartburn, liver enzyme elevation, nausea, vomiting. **GU:** acute renal failure, hematuria. **Derm:** EXFOLIATIVE DERMATITIS, STEVENS-JOHNSON SYNDROME, TOXIC EPIDERMAL NECROLYSIS, pruritus, rashes, eczema, photosensitivity. **F and E:** edema. **Hemat:** anemia, prolonged bleeding time. **Local: Topical only:** contact dermatitis, dry skin, exfoliation. **Misc:** ALLERGIC REACTIONS, INCLUDING ANAPHYLAXIS.

PHYSICAL THERAPY IMPLICATIONS

Examination and Evaluation

- Monitor signs of GI bleeding, including abdominal pain, vomiting blood, blood in stools, or black, tarry stools. Report these signs to the physician immediately.
- Monitor signs of allergic reactions and anaphylaxis, including pulmonary symptoms (laryngeal edema, wheezing, cough, dyspnea) or skin reactions (rash, pruritus, urticaria). Be especially alert for exfoliation, dermatitis, and other severe skin reactions that might indicate serious hypersensitivity reactions (Stevens-Johnson syndrome, toxic epidermal

necrolysis). Notify physician immediately if these reactions occur.

- Assess pain and other variables (range of motion, muscle strength) to document whether this drug is successful in helping manage the patient's pain and decrease impairments.
- Assess blood pressure (BP) periodically and compare to normal values (See Appendix F). NSAIDs can increase BP and promote hypertension in certain patients.
- Be alert for signs of prolonged bleeding time such as bleeding gums, nosebleeds, and unusual or excessive bruising. Report these signs to the physician.
- Assess peripheral edema using girth measurements, volume displacement, and measurement of pitting edema (See Appendix N). Report increased swelling in feet and ankles or a sudden increase in body weight due to fluid retention.
- Monitor signs of kidney dysfunction such as painful urination or blood in the urine. Report signs of renal failure immediately, including decreased urine output, increased BP, muscle cramps/twitching, edema/weight gain from fluid retention, yellowish brown skin, and confusion that progresses to seizures and coma.
- Monitor unusual weakness, fatigue, and pallor that might be due to anemia. Notify physician if these signs occur.
- Assess dizziness that might affect gait, balance, and other functional activities (See Appendix C). Report balance problems and functional limitations to the physician, and caution the patient and family/caregivers to guard against falls and trauma.
- If applied topically, monitor the application site for skin reactions such as dermatitis, exfoliation, and excessive dryness. Report severe or prolonged skin reactions to the physician.

Interventions

- Implement appropriate manual therapy techniques, physical agents, and therapeutic exercises to reduce pain and decrease the need for diclofenac and other NSAIDs.
- If treating arthritic conditions, recommend orthotic and assistive devices as needed to reduce pain, improve function, and augment the effects of drug therapy.
- Use caution with any physical interventions that could increase bleeding, including wound débridement, chest percussion, joint mobilization, and application of local heat.
- Help patient explore other nonpharmacologic methods to reduce chronic pain, such as relaxation techniques, exercise, counseling, and so forth.
- Causes photosensitivity; use care if administering UV treatments. Advise patient to avoid direct sunlight and use sunscreens and protective clothing, and to report any untoward skin reactions such as rash, itching, or eczema.

Patient/Client-Related Instruction

- Advise patient that analgesics are usually more effective if given before pain becomes severe; emphasize that adequate pain control will allow better participation in physical therapy.
- Inform patient that NSAIDs may impair bone and cartilage healing. Advise patient to consult physician about NSAID use, especially after fractures, spinal fusion, and other bone surgeries.
- Caution patient about the use of over-the-counter products that contain NSAIDs or acetaminophen while taking prescription doses of diclofenac. Use of multiple NSAIDs increases the risk of toxicity and overdose.
- Instruct patient to report excessive or prolonged headache or ringing/buzzing in the ears (tinnitus); these signs may indicate drug toxicity.
- Advise patient about the risks of gastric irritation. Instruct patient to notify physician of GI reactions such as severe or prolonged nausea, vomiting, diarrhea, constipation, indigestion, heartburn, flatulence, and abdominal pain.
- Advise patient to reduce alcohol intake because alcohol increases the risk of gastric toxicity.

Pharmacokinetics

Absorption: Undergoes first-pass metabolism by liver which results in 50% bioavailability. Oral diclofenac sodium is a delayed-release dosage form. Diclofenac potassium is an immediate-release dosage form. 10% of topically applied diclofenac is systemically absorbed.
Distribution: Crosses the placenta.
Protein Binding: >99%.
Metabolism and Excretion: Metabolized by the liver to several metabolites; 65% excreted in urine, 35% in bile.
Half-life: 2 hr.

TIME/ACTION PROFILE

ROUTE	ONSET	PEAK	DURATION
PO (inflammation)	few days–1 wk	2 wk or more	unknown
PO (pain)	30 min	unknown	up to 8 hr
topical	unknown	30 days*	unknown
topical patch	unknown	10–20 hr	unknown

*Complete healing of lesions following cessation of therapy.

Contraindications/Precautions

Contraindicated in: Hypersensitivity to diclofenac or other components of formulation; Cross-sensitivity may occur with other NSAIDs, including aspirin; Active GI bleeding/ulcer disease; Patients undergoing coronary artery bypass graft surgery.

Use Cautiously in: Severe renal/hepatic disease; Cardiovascular disease or risk factors for cardiovascular disease (may ↑ risk of serious cardiovascular thrombotic events, myocardial infarction, and stroke, especially with prolonged use); History of porphyria; History of peptic ulcer disease and/or GI bleeding; Geri: Geriatric patients (dosage reduction recommended; more susceptible to adverse reactions, including GI bleeding); Bleeding tendency or concurrent anticoagulant therapy; OB/Lactation: Pregnancy and lactation (not recommended for use during second half of pregnancy); Pedi: Pregnancy, lactation, and children (safety not established).

Interactions

Primarily noted for oral administration

Drug-Drug: ↑ adverse GI effects with **aspirin**, other **NSAIDs**, or **corticosteroids**. May ↓ effectiveness of **diuretics**, or **antihypertensives**. May ↑ levels/risk of toxicity from **cyclosporine**, **lithium**, or **methotrexate**. ↑ risk of bleeding with some **cephalosporins**, **thrombolytic agents**, **antiplatelet agents**, or **warfarin**. Concurrent use of oral **NSAIDs** during topical diclofenac therapy should be minimized.

Drug-Natural: ↑ bleeding risk with **arnica**, **chamomile**, **clove**, **dong quai**, **feverfew**, **garlic**, **ginger**, **ginkgo**, **Panax ginseng**, and others.

Route/Dosage

Different formulations of oral diclofenac (diclofenac sodium—enteric-coated tablets; diclofenac sodium—extended-release tablets; and diclofenac potassium—immediate-release tablets) are not bioequivalent and should not be substituted on a milligram-to-milligram basis.

Diclofenac Potassium

PO (Adults): *Analgesic/antidysmenorrheal*—100 mg initially, then 50 mg 3 times daily as needed; *Rheumatoid arthritis*—50 mg 3–4 times daily, after initial response reduce to lowest dose that controls symptoms; *Osteoarthritis*—50 mg 2–3 times daily, after initial response reduce to lowest dose that controls symptoms.

Diclofenac Sodium

PO (Adults): *Rheumatoid arthritis (delayed-release [enteric-coated] tablets)*—50 mg 3–4 times daily *or* 75 mg twice daily; after initial response reduce to lowest dose that controls symptoms (usual maintenance dose 25 mg 3 times daily). *Rheumatoid arthritis (extended-release tablets)*—100 mg once daily; if unsatisfactory response, dose may be ↑ to 100 mg twice daily. *Osteoarthritis (delayed-release [enteric-coated] tablets)*—50 mg 2–3 times daily *or* 75 mg twice daily; after initial response, ↓ to lowest dose that controls symptoms. *Osteoarthritis (extended-release tablets)*—100 mg once daily. *Ankylosing spondylitis (delayed-release [enteric-coated] tablets*—25 mg 4 times daily, with an additional 25 mg given at bedtime, if necessary.

Topical (Adults): Apply to lesions twice daily for 60–90 days.

Topical patch (Adults): 1 patch applied to most painful area twice daily.

Availability (generic available)

Diclofenac potassium immediate-release tablets: 50 mg. **Diclofenac sodium delayed-release (enteric-coated) tablets:** 25 mg, 50 mg, 75 mg. **Diclofenac sodium extended-release tablets:** 75 mg, 100 mg. **Gel:** 3% in 50- and 100-g tubes. **Topical patch:** 180 mg/patch. ***In combination with:*** 200 mcg misoprostol (Arthrotec). See Appendix B.

dicloxacillin (dye-klox-a-**sill**-in)

Dycill, Dynapen, Pathocil

Classification

Therapeutic: anti-infectives

Pharmacologic: penicillinase-resistant penicillins

Indications

Treatment of the following infections due to penicillinase-producing staphylococci: Respiratory tract infections, Sinusitis, Osteomyelitis, Skin and skin structure infections.

Action

Bind to bacterial cell wall, leading to cell death. Not inactivated by penicillinase enzymes. **Therapeutic Effects:** Bactericidal action. **Spectrum:** Active against most gram-positive aerobic cocci. Spectrum is notable for activity against Penicillinase-producing strains of *Staphylococcus aureus*, *S. epidermidis*. Not active against methicillin-resistant bacteria.

Adverse Reactions/Side Effects

NS: SEIZURES. **GI:** diarrhea, epigastric distress, nausea, vomiting, pseudomembranous colitis, ↑ liver enzymes. **GU:** interstitial nephritis. **Derm:** rash, urticaria. **Hemat:** eosinophilia, leukopenia. **Misc:** ALLERGIC REACTIONS, INCLUDING ANAPHYLAXIS AND SERUM SICKNESS, superinfection.

PHYSICAL THERAPY IMPLICATIONS

Examination and Evaluation

- Watch for seizures; notify physician immediately if patient develops or increases seizure activity.

- Monitor signs of allergic reactions and anaphylaxis, including pulmonary symptoms (tightness in the throat and chest, wheezing, cough dyspnea) or skin reactions (rash, pruritus, urticaria). Notify physician or nursing staff immediately if these reactions occur.
- Assess muscle aches and joint pain (arthralgia) that may be caused by serum sickness. Notify physician if these symptoms seem to be drug-related rather than caused by musculoskeletal injury, or if muscle and joint pain are accompanied by allergy-like reactions (fever, rashes, etc.)
- Monitor signs of eosinophilia (fatigue, weakness, myalgia) or leukopenia (fever, sore throat, signs of infection); report these signs to the physician.

Interventions

- Always wash hands thoroughly and disinfect equipment (whirlpools, electrotherapeutic devices, treatment tables, and so forth) to help prevent the spread of infection. Employ universal precautions or isolation procedures as indicated for specific patients.

Patient/Client-Related Instruction

- Instruct patient to notify physician immediately if signs of the following occur:
  - Pseudomembranous colitis (diarrhea, abdominal pain, fever, pus or mucus in stools) or other severe or prolonged GI problems (nausea, vomiting, heartburn).
  - Superinfection (black, furry overgrowth on tongue; vaginal itching or discharge; loose or foul-smelling stools).
  - Interstitial nephritis (blood in urine, decreased urine output, weight gain from fluid retention).
- Instruct patient and family/caregivers to report other troublesome side effects such as severe or prolonged skin problems (rash, itching) or GI problems (nausea, vomiting, diarrhea, heartburn).

Pharmacokinetics

Absorption: Rapidly but incompletely (35–76%) absorbed from the GI tract.
Distribution: Widely distributed; penetration into CSF is minimal but sufficient in the presence of inflamed meninges; crosses the placenta and enters breast milk.
Protein Binding: 96–98%.
Metabolism and Excretion: Some metabolism by the liver (6–10%) and some renal excretion of unchanged drug (60%); small amounts eliminated in the feces via the bile.
Half-life: 0.5–1 hr (increased in severe hepatic and renal dysfunction).

TIME/ACTION PROFILE

ROUTE	ONSET	PEAK	DURATION
PO	30 min	30–120 min	6 hr

Contraindications/Precautions

Contraindicated in: Previous hypersensitivity to penicillins (cross-sensitivity exists with cephalosporins and other beta-lactam antibiotics).
Use Cautiously in: Severe renal or hepatic impairment.

Interactions

Drug-Drug: Dicloxacillin may ↓ effectiveness of oral contraceptive agents. **Probenecid** ↓ renal excretion and ↑ blood levels of dicloxacillin (therapy may be combined for this purpose). **Neomycin** may ↓ absorption of dicloxacillin. Concurrent use with **methotrexate** ↓ methotrexate elimination and ↑ risk of serious toxicity.

Route/Dosage

PO (Adults and Children ≥40 kg): 125–250 mg q 6 hr (up to 2 g/day).
PO (Children <40 kg): 25–50 mg/kg/day divided q 6 hr; (up to 50–100 mg/kg/day divided q 6 hr has been used for osteomyelitis), maximum: 2 g/day.

Availability (generic available)

Capsules: 250 mg, 500 mg. **Oral suspension:** 62.5 mg/5 mL.

dicyclomine

(dye-**sye**-kloe-meen)
Bentyl, ✱ Bentylol, ✱ Formulex, Spasmoban

Classification
Therapeutic: antispasmodics
Pharmacologic: anticholinergics

Indications

Management of irritable bowel syndrome in patients who do not respond to usual interventions (sedation/change in diet).

Action

May have a direct and local effect on GI smooth muscle, reducing motility and tone. **Therapeutic Effects:** Decreased GI motility.

Adverse Reactions/Side Effects

CNS: confusion (increased in geriatric patients), drowsiness, light-headedness (IM only). **EENT:** blurred vision, increased intraocular pressure. **CV:** palpitations, tachycardia. **GI:** PARALYTIC ILEUS, constipation, heartburn, decreased salivation, dry mouth, nausea, vomiting. **GU:** erectile dysfunction, urinary hesitancy, urinary retention. **Derm:** decreased sweating. **Endo:** decreased lactation. **Local:** pain/redness at IM site. **Misc:** ALLERGIC REACTIONS, INCLUDING ANAPHYLAXIS.

PHYSICAL THERAPY IMPLICATIONS

Examination and Evaluation

- Be alert for signs of allergic reactions and anaphylaxis, including pulmonary symptoms (tightness in the throat and chest, wheezing, cough, dyspnea) or skin reactions (rash, pruritus, urticaria). Notify physician immediately if these reactions occur.
- Monitor signs of intestinal paralysis (paralytic ileus), including nausea, lack of bowel sounds or movements, abdominal bloating/distention, and vomiting. Report these signs to the physician immediately.
- Assess heart rate, ECG, and heart sounds, especially during exercise (See Appendices G, H). Report a rapid heart rate (tachycardia) or signs of other arrhythmias, including palpitations, chest discomfort, shortness of breath, fainting, and fatigue/weakness.
- Monitor any changes in irritable bowel symptoms (decreased abdominal pain, decreased diarrhea, improved appetite) to help document whether drug therapy is successful.
- Be alert for decreased sweating and altered/increased body temperature (hyperpyrexia). Notify physician of a prolonged or persistent elevation in body temperature.
- Monitor IM injection site for pain and redness. Report prolonged or excessive injection- site reactions to the physician.

Interventions

- Because of the risk of arrhythmias and impaired thermoregulation, use caution during aerobic exercise and other forms of therapeutic exercise. Assess exercise tolerance frequently (blood pressure, heart rate, fatigue levels), and terminate exercise immediately if any untoward responses occur (See Appendix L).

Patient/Client-Related Instruction

- Instruct patient and family/caregivers to report other troublesome side effects such as severe or prolonged drowsiness, light-headedness, confusion, vision problems, problems with urination, sexual dysfunction, or GI problems (nausea, vomiting, constipation, heartburn, dry mouth).

Pharmacokinetics

Absorption: Well absorbed after oral and IM administration.
Distribution: Unknown.
Metabolism and Excretion: 80% eliminated in urine, 10% in feces.
Half-life: 1.8 hr (initial phase), 9–10 hr (terminal phase).

TIME/ACTION PROFILE (antispasmodic effect)

ROUTE	ONSET	PEAK	DURATION
PO, IM	unknown	unknown	unknown

Contraindications/Precautions

Contraindicated in: Hypersensitivity; Obstruction of the GI or GU tract; Reflux esophagitis; Severe ulcerative colitis (risk of paralytic ileus); Unstable cardiovascular status; Glaucoma; Myasthenia gravis; Infants <6 mo; Lactation.
Use Cautiously in: High environmental temperatures (risk of heat prostration); Hepatic/renal impairment; Autonomic neuropathy; Cardiovascular disease; Prostatic hyperplasia; Geri: Appears on Beers' list. Geriatric patients have ↑ sensitivity to anticholinergics; Pregnancy (safety not established).

Interactions

Drug-Drug: Additive anticholinergic effects with other **anticholinergics**, including **antihistamines**, **quinidine**, and **disopyramide**. May alter the absorption of **other orally administered drugs** by slowing motility of the GI tract. **Antacids** or **adsorbent antidiarrheals** ↓ the absorption of anticholinergics. May ↑ GI mucosal lesions in patients taking oral **potassium chloride** tablets. ↑ risk of adverse cardiovascular reactions with **cyclopropane** anesthesia.

Route/Dosage

PO (Adults): 10–20 mg 3–4 times daily (up to 160 mg/day).
PO (Children ≥2 yr): 10 mg 3–4 times daily; adjusted as tolerated.
PO (Children 6 mo–2 yr): 5–10 mg 3–4 times daily; adjusted as tolerated.
IM (Adults): 20 mg q 4–6 hr; adjusted as tolerated.

Availability

Tablets: 10 mg, 20 mg. **Capsules:** 10 mg, 20 mg. **Syrup:** 10 mg/5 mL. **Solution for injection:** 10 mg/mL.

didanosine (dye-dan-oh-seen)

Videx, Videx EC

Other Names:
ddI, dideoxyinosine

Classification
Therapeutic: antiretrovirals
Pharmacologic: nucleoside reverse transcriptase inhibitors

Indications

HIV infection (with other antiretrovirals).

D

Action

Inhibits viral replication by interfering with viral RNA-directed DNA polymerase (reverse transcriptase). Converted intracellularly by the phosphorylation process to its active form. **Therapeutic Effects:** Increase in CD4 cell counts and decreased viral load, with decreased incidence of opportunistic infections and slowed progression in HIV-infected patients.

Adverse Reactions/Side Effects

CNS: SEIZURES, headache, dizziness, insomnia, lethargy, pain, weakness. **EENT:** rhinitis, ear pain, epistaxis, optic neuritis, parotid gland enlargement, photophobia, retinal depigmentation, sialoadenitis. **Resp:** cough, asthma. **CV:** arrhythmias, edema, hypertension, vasodilation. **GI:** LIVER FAILURE, PANCREATITIS, anorexia, diarrhea, liver function abnormalities, nausea, vomiting, abdominal pain, constipation, dry mouth, dyspepsia, flatulence, hepatic steatosis, stomatitis. **GU:** urinary frequency. **Derm:** alopecia, ecchymoses, rash. **Endo:** fat redistribution, hyperglycemia. **Hemat:** granulocytopenia, anemia, bleeding, leukopenia. **Metab:** LACTIC ACIDOSIS, hyperlipidemia, hyperuricemia, weight loss. **MS:** RHABDOMYOLYSIS, arthritis, myalgia. **Neuro:** peripheral neuropathy, poor coordination. **Misc:** chills, fever, anaphylactoid reactions.

PHYSICAL THERAPY IMPLICATIONS

Examination and Evaluation

- Be alert for new seizures or increased seizure activity, especially at the onset of drug treatment. Document the number, duration, and severity of seizures, and report these findings to the physician immediately.
- Be alert for signs of liver failure (anorexia, abdominal pain, severe nausea and vomiting, yellow skin or eyes, fever, sore throat, malaise, weakness, facial edema, lethargy, unusual bleeding or bruising) or pancreatitis (upper abdominal pain after eating, indigestion, weight loss, oily stools). Report these signs to the physician immediately.
- Monitor signs of lactic acidosis, including confusion, lethargy, stupor, shallow rapid breathing, tachycardia, hypotension, nausea, and vomiting. Notify physician immediately if these signs occur.
- Assess any musculoskeletal pain, muscle tenderness, or weakness, especially if accompanied by fever, malaise, and dark-colored urine. These symptoms may represent drug-induced myopathy, and that myopathy can progress to severe muscle damage (rhabdomyolysis). Report any unexplained musculoskeletal symptoms to the physician immediately.
- Be alert for signs of peripheral neuropathy (numbness, tingling, decreased muscle strength). Establish baseline electroneuromyographic values using EMG and nerve conduction at the beginning of drug treatment whenever possible, and reexamine these values periodically to document drug-induced changes in peripheral nerve function.
- Assess heart rate, ECG, and heart sounds, especially during exercise (See Appendices G, H). Report any rhythm disturbances or symptoms of increased arrhythmias, including palpitations, chest discomfort, shortness of breath, fainting, and fatigue/weakness.
- Assess blood pressure (BP) and compare to normal values (See Appendix F). Report a sustained increase in BP (hypertension).
- Assess peripheral edema using girth measurements, volume displacement, and measurement of pitting edema (See Appendix N). Report increased swelling in feet and ankles due to vasodilation.
- Monitor signs of asthma, including wheezing, cough, dyspnea, and shortness of breath. Assess pulmonary function by measuring lung volumes, breath sounds, and respiratory rate (See Appendices I, J, K), and report increased asthmatic responses.
- Monitor signs of granulocytopenia and leukopenia (fever, sore throat, mucosal lesions, signs of infection, bruising, bleeding) or unusual weakness and fatigue that might be due to anemia and other blood dyscrasias. Report these signs to the physician.
- Monitor signs of hypersensitivity and anaphylactoid reactions, including pulmonary symptoms (tightness in the throat and chest, wheezing, dyspnea) or skin reactions (rash, pruritus, urticaria). Notify physician or nursing staff immediately if these reactions occur.
- Assess dizziness that might affect gait, balance, and other functional activities (See Appendix C). Report balance problems and functional limitations to the physician and nursing staff, and caution the patient and family/caregivers to guard against falls and trauma.
- Monitor signs of hyperglycemia (confusion, drowsiness; flushed, dry skin; fruit-like breath odor; rapid, deep breathing; polyuria; loss of appetite; unusual thirst). Insulin dosages may need to be adjusted to prevent repeated episodes of hyperglycemia.
- Periodically assess body weight and other anthropometric measures (body mass index, body composition). Report a rapid or unexplained weight loss or decreased body fat.

Interventions

- Implement resistive exercises and other therapeutic exercises as tolerated to maintain muscle strength and function, and to prevent muscle wasting associated with HIV infection and AIDS.
- Because of the risk of lactic acidosis and arrhythmias, use caution during aerobic exercise and other forms of therapeutic exercise. Assess exercise tolerance frequently (BP, heart rate, fatigue levels), and terminate exercise immediately if any untoward responses occur (See Appendix L).

Patient/Client-Related Instruction

- Advise patient that this drug may cause problems in fat and glucose metabolism (hyperlipidemia and hyperglycemia, respectively). Remind patient that periodic blood tests may be needed to monitor plasma lipids and blood glucose.
- Emphasize the importance of taking didanosine as directed even if the patient is asymptomatic, and that this drug must always be used in combination with other antiretroviral drugs. Do not take more than prescribed amount and do not stop taking without consulting the physician.
- Inform patient that didanosine does not cure HIV or AIDS or prevent associated or opportunistic infections. Didanosine does not reduce the risk of transmission of HIV to others through sexual contact or blood contamination. Caution patient to use a condom, and avoid sharing needles or donating blood to prevent spreading the AIDS virus to others.
- Instruct patient to report other troublesome side effects such as prolonged or severe headache, sleep loss, vision or hearing disturbances, chills, fever, increased urinary frequency, skin problems (rash, bruising, hair loss), or GI problems (diarrhea, nausea, vomiting, constipation, abdominal pain, loss of appetite, flatulence).

Pharmacokinetics

Absorption: Rapidly degrades at gastric pH.
Distribution: CSF levels are 21% of plasma levels in adults.
Metabolism and Excretion: Metabolized as a purine; 55% eliminated by the kidneys (18% as unchanged drug; urinary excretion is less in children).
Half-life: 1.6 hr (0.8 hr in children).

TIME/ACTION PROFILE (retroviral plasma levels)

ROUTE	ONSET	PEAK	DURATION
PO	unknown	0.25–1.5 hr	12 hr

Contraindications/Precautions

Contraindicated in: Hypersensitivity; OB: Lactation; Concurrent use of ribavirin or allopurinol.
Use Cautiously in: History of gout; Renal impairment (dosage modification required if CCr <60 mL/min; ↑ risk of pancreatitis); History of seizures; Diabetes mellitus; Pedi: ↑ risk of pancreatitis.

Interactions

Drug-Drug: Ribavirin and **allopurinol** ↑ levels and risk of toxicity (concurrent use not recommended). Levels are ↑ by **tenofovir** (dose reduction recommended). Concurrent use with **ganciclovir** ↑ levels (dose adjustments may be necessary). **Methadone** ↓ levels of didanosine (dose adjustments may be necessary). Buffers in didanosine ↑ absorption of **ketoconazole, itraconazole, dapsone, tetracyclines,** and **fluoroquinolones** (do not administer within 2 hr of didanosine). ↑ risk of peripheral neuropathy with **isoniazid, phenytoin, zalcitabine, stavudine, ethambutol,** and **chloramphenicol** (use cautiously). ↑ risk of pancreatitis with other **alcohol, thiazide diuretics, IV pentamidine, tetracyclines** (use with extreme caution). ↑ risk of bone marrow depression with other **drugs causing bone marrow depression.** Concurrent **stavudine** during pregnancy ↑ the risk of fetal lactic acidosis.
Drug-Food: Administration with **food** ↓ absorption by 50%.

Route/Dosage

PO (Adults ≥60 kg): *Oral solution*—200 mg bid; *Videx EC capsules*—400 mg once daily; ***with tenofovir*** —250 mg once daily.
PO (Adults <60 kg): *Oral solution*—125 mg bid; *Videx EC Capsules*—250 mg once daily; ***with tenofovir*** —200 mg once daily.
PO (Children 2 wk–8 mo): *Oral solution*—100 mg/m^2 q 12 hr.
PO (Children >8 mo): *Oral solution*—120 mg q 12 hr.

Renal Impairment

PO (Adults >60 kg): *CCr 30–59 mL/min—Oral solution*—100 mg q 12 hr or 200 mg once daily; *Videx EC Capsules*—200 mg once daily; *CCr 10–29 mL/min—Oral solution*—150 mg once daily; *Videx EC Capsules*—125 mg once daily; *CCr <10 mL/min—Oral solution*—100 mg once daily *Videx EC Capsules*—125 mg once daily.
PO (Adults <60 kg): *CCr 30–59 mL/min—Oral solution*—75 mg q 12 hr or 150 mg once daily; *Videx EC Capsules*—125 mg once daily; *CCr 10–29 mL/min—Oral solution*—100 mg once daily; *Videx EC Capsules*—125 mg once daily; *CCr <10 mL/min—Oral solution*—75 mg once daily; *Videx EC Capsules*—not to be used.

Availability (generic available)

Delayed-release capsules (with enteric-coated beadlets): 125 mg, 200 mg, 250 mg, 400 mg. **Pediatric powder for oral solution (requires reconstitution):** 10 mg/mL, 20 mg/mL.

diflorasone (dye-flor-a-sone)
Florone, Florone E, Psorcon, Psorcon E

Classification
Therapeutic: anti-inflammatories (steroidal)
Pharmacologic: corticosteroids

Indications
Management of inflammation and pruritus associated with various allergic/immunologic skin problems.

Action
Suppresses normal immune response and inflammation. **Therapeutic Effects:** Suppression of dermatologic inflammation and immune processes.

Adverse Reactions/Side Effects
Derm: allergic contact dermatitis, atrophy, burning, dryness, edema, folliculitis, hypersensitivity reactions, hypertrichosis, hypopigmentation, irritation, maceration, miliaria, perioral dermatitis, secondary infection, striae. **Misc:** adrenal suppression (use of occlusive dressings, long-term therapy).

PHYSICAL THERAPY IMPLICATIONS

Examination and Evaluation
- Assess the area being treated to help document whether drug therapy is successful in resolving skin conditions.
- Monitor any new or increased reactions at the site of application, including inflammation, irritation, infection, burning, swelling, exfoliation, and rash. Report severe or prolonged skin reactions to the physician.
- Report signs of adrenal suppression, including hypotension, weight loss, weakness, nausea, vomiting, anorexia, lethargy, confusion, and restlessness.

Interventions
- Protect skin from breakdown, especially over bony prominences.

Patient/Client-Related Instruction
- Advise patients on long-term treatment to consult physician before stopping this medication. Stopping the medication suddenly may result in adrenocortical shock (severe hypotension, hypoglycemia, weakness, vomiting). If these signs appear, physician immediately; may be life threatening.
- Check that the patient and family or caregivers understand topical application procedures, and that they adhere to the recommended dosing schedule.

Pharmacokinetics
Absorption: Minimal. Prolonged use on large surface areas, application of large amounts, or use of occlusive dressings may increase systemic absorption.
Distribution: Remains primarily at site of action.
Metabolism and Excretion: Usually metabolized in skin.
Half-life: Unknown.

TIME/ACTION PROFILE (response depends on condition being treated)

ROUTE	ONSET	PEAK	DURATION
topical	mins–hrs	hrs–days	hrs–days

Contraindications/Precautions
Contraindicated in: Hypersensitivity or known intolerance to corticosteroids or components of vehicles (ointment or cream base, preservative, alcohol); Untreated bacterial or viral infections.
Use Cautiously in: Hepatic dysfunction; Diabetes mellitus, cataracts, glaucoma, or tuberculosis (use of large amounts of high-potency agents may worsen condition); Patients with preexisting skin atrophy; Pregnancy, lactation, or children (chronic high-dose usage may result in adrenal suppression in mother, growth suppression in children; children may be more susceptible to adrenal and growth suppression).

Interactions
Drug-Drug: None significant.

Route/Dosage
Topical (Adults): Apply to affected area(s) 1–4 times daily (depends on condition being treated).
Topical (Children): Apply to affected area(s) once daily.

Availability
Cream: 0.05% Rx. **Ointment:** 0.05% Rx.

diflunisal (dye-floo-ni-sal)
🍁 Apo-Diflunisal, Dolobid, 🍁 Novo-Diflunisal, 🍁 Nu-Diflunisal

Classification
Therapeutic: nonopioid analgesics, nonsteroidal anti-inflammatory agents
Pharmacologic: salicylic acid derivatives

Indications
Inflammatory disorders, including Rheumatoid arthritis, Osteoarthritis. Treatment of mild-to-moderate pain.

Action
Inhibits prostaglandin synthesis. Diflunisal is an NSAID chemically related to aspirin. **Therapeutic Effects:** Suppression of pain and inflammation.

Adverse Reactions/Side Effects

CNS: dizziness, drowsiness, headache. **EENT:** tinnitus. **CV:** arrhythmias, ↑ in blood pressure, chest pain, edema. **GI:** GI BLEEDING, abdominal discomfort, nausea, constipation, diarrhea, dyspepsia, vomiting. **GU:** renal failure. **Derm:** rash. **Hemat:** blood dyscrasias, prolonged bleeding time. **Misc:** ALLERGIC REACTIONS, INCLUDING ANAPHYLAXIS, chills.

PHYSICAL THERAPY IMPLICATIONS

Examination and Evaluation

- Monitor signs of GI bleeding, including abdominal pain, vomiting blood, blood in stools, or black, tarry stools. Report these signs to the physician immediately.
- Monitor signs of allergic reactions and anaphylaxis, including pulmonary symptoms (laryngeal edema, wheezing, cough, dyspnea) or skin reactions (rash, pruritus, urticaria). Notify physician immediately if these reactions occur.
- Assess pain and other variables (range of motion, muscle strength) to document whether this drug is successful in helping manage the patient's pain and decreasing impairments.
- Assess blood pressure (BP) periodically and compare to normal values (See Appendix F). NSAIDs can increase BP in certain patients.
- Assess heart rate, ECG, and heart sounds, especially during exercise (See Appendices G, H). Report any rhythm disturbances or symptoms of increased arrhythmias, including palpitations, chest discomfort, shortness of breath, fainting, and fatigue/weakness.
- Assess for signs of prolonged bleeding time such as bleeding gums, nosebleeds, and unusual or excessive bruising. Notify physician if these signs occur.
- Monitor unusual weakness and fatigue that might be due to anemia or other symptoms such as fever, sore throat, mucosal lesions, or signs of infection that might be due to other blood dyscrasias. Notify physician if these signs occur.
- Assess peripheral edema using girth measurements, volume displacement, and measurement of pitting edema (See Appendix N). Report increased swelling in feet and ankles or a sudden increase in body weight due to fluid retention.
- Monitor signs of kidney dysfunction such as painful urination or blood in the urine. Report signs of renal failure immediately, including decreased urine output, increased blood pressure, muscle cramps/twitching, edema/weight gain from fluid retention, yellowish brown skin, and confusion that progresses to seizures and coma.
- Assess dizziness and drowsiness that might affect gait, balance, and other functional activities (See Appendix C). Report balance problems and functional limitations to the physician, and caution the patient and family/caregivers to guard against falls and trauma.

Interventions

- Implement appropriate manual therapy techniques, physical agents, and therapeutic exercises to reduce pain and decrease the need for diflunisal and other NSAIDs.
- Because of the risk of arrhythmias, use caution during aerobic exercise and other forms of therapeutic exercise. Assess exercise tolerance frequently (BP, heart rate, fatigue levels), and terminate exercise immediately if any untoward responses occur (See Appendix L).
- If treating arthritic conditions, recommend orthotic and assistive devices as needed to reduce pain, improve function, and augment the effects of drug therapy.
- Use caution with any physical interventions that could increase bleeding, including wound débridement, chest percussion, joint mobilization, and application of local heat.
- Help patient explore other nonpharmacologic methods to reduce chronic pain, such as relaxation techniques, exercise, counseling, and so forth.

Patient/Client-Related Instruction

- Advise patient that analgesics are usually more effective if given before pain becomes severe; emphasize that adequate pain control will allow better participation in physical therapy.
- Inform patient that NSAIDs may impair bone and cartilage healing. Advise patient to consult physician about NSAID use, especially after fractures, spinal fusion, and other bone surgeries.
- Caution patient about the use of over-the-counter products that contain NSAIDs or acetaminophen while taking prescription doses of diflunisal. Use of multiple NSAIDs increases the risk of toxicity and overdose.
- Instruct patient to report excessive or prolonged headache or ringing/buzzing in the ears (tinnitus); these signs may indicate drug toxicity.
- Advise patient about the risks of gastric irritation. Instruct patient to notify physician of GI reactions such as severe or prolonged nausea, vomiting, diarrhea, constipation, indigestion, and abdominal pain.
- Advise patient to reduce alcohol intake because alcohol increases the risk of gastric toxicity.
- Instruct patient and family/caregivers to report other troublesome side effects such as severe or prolonged headache, chills, or skin rash.

Pharmacokinetics

Absorption: Well absorbed from the GI tract.
Distribution: Crosses the placenta; enters breast milk.
Protein Binding: >99%.

Metabolism and Excretion: Metabolized by the liver; excreted in urine as unchanged drug (3%) and as inactive metabolites.
Half-life: 8–12 hr.

TIME/ACTION PROFILE

ROUTE	ONSET	PEAK	DURATION
PO (analgesic)	1 hr	2–3 hr	8–12 hr
PO (anti-inflammatory)	few days–1 wk	2 wk	unknown

Contraindications/Precautions

Contraindicated in: Hypersensitivity; Cross-sensitivity may exist with other NSAIDs and aspirin; Active GI bleeding or ulcer disease; Patients with recent history of coronary artery bypass surgery; Pregnancy (3rd trimester); Lactation.
Use Cautiously in: Severe renal or hepatic disease; History of cardiovascular disease; History of ulcer disease; Adolescents (may ↑ the risk of Reye's syndrome if used during viral illness); Alcohol use; Elderly (↑ risk of adverse effects); Pregnancy (1st and 2nd trimesters); Children <12 yr (safety not established).

Interactions

Drug-Drug: Concurrent use with **aspirin** may ↓ effectiveness. Additive adverse GI effects with **aspirin, other NSAIDs, colchicine, corticosteroids**, or **alcohol**. Chronic use with **acetaminophen** may ↑ the risk of adverse renal and hepatic reactions ↑ acetaminophen blood levels by 50%). May ↓ the effectiveness of **diuretics** or **antihypertensives;** but ↑ levels of **hydrochlorothiazide**. May ↑ the hypoglycemic effects of **sulfonylureas. Probenecid** ↑ risk of toxicity from diflunisal. ↑ risk of bleeding with some **cephalosporins** or **anticoagulants**. May ↑ levels and ↑ the risk of toxicity from **cyclosporine, digoxin, lithium**, or **methotrexate**. ↑ risk of adverse hematologic reactions with **antineoplastics** or **radiation therapy**. Administration with **antacids** ↓ absorption of diflunisal. May ↑ the risk of adverse renal reactions when used with **gold compounds**.
Drug-Natural: ↑ bleeding risk with **anise, arnica, chamomile, clove, feverfew, garlic, ginger, ginkgo, ginseng**, and others.

Route/Dosage

PO (Adults): *Anti-inflammatory*—250–500 mg twice daily (maximum daily dose = 1.5 g). *Analgesic*—500 mg–1 g initially, then 250–500 mg q 8–12 hr (maximum daily dose = 1.5 g).

Availability (generic available)

Tablets: 250 mg, 500 mg.

difluprednate (ophthalmic)

(dye-floo-**pred**-nate)
Durezol

Classification
Therapeutic: ocular agents
Pharmacologic: corticosteroids

Indications

Treatment of inflammation and pain associated with ocular surgery.

Action

Decreases inflammation. **Therapeutic Effects:** Decreased pain and inflammation following ocular surgery.

Adverse Reactions/Side Effects

(CAPITALS indicate life-threatening; underlines indicate most frequent.)
EENT: ↑ intraocular pressure, blepharitis, cataracts, conjunctival hyperemia, corneal edema, delayed healing, eye pain, infections, iritis, photophobia.

PHYSICAL THERAPY IMPLICATIONS

Examination and Evaluation

- Assess the eye to help document whether drug therapy is successful in resolving ocular pain and inflammation.
- Monitor any new or increased reactions at the site of application such as pain, infection, swelling, redness, cloudy/blurry vision, and increased sensitivity to light (photophobia). Report increased ocular reactions to the physician.

Patient/Client-related Instruction

- Check that the patient and family or caregivers understand proper use of eye drops, and adhere to the recommended dosing schedule.

Pharmacokinetics

Absorption: Limited systemic absorption.
Distribution: Unknown.
Metabolism and Excretion: Unknown.
Half-life: Unknown.

TIME/ACTION PROFILE

ROUTE	ONSET	PEAK	DURATION
Ophth	unknown	unknown	unknown

Contraindications/Precautions

Contraindicated in: Active viral, mycobacterial or fungal infection of eyes and surrounding structures.
Use Cautiously in: OB: Use in pregnancy only if potential benefit justifies potential risk to the fetus; Lactation: Use cautiously during lactation;

Pedi: Safety and effectiveness in children have not been established.

Interactions

Drug-Drug: None noted.

Route/Dosage

Ophth (Adults): 1 drop four times daily, starting 24 hr after surgery for 2 wk, then twice daily for 1 week, then further tapered based on response.

Availability

Ophthalmic emulsion: 0.05% in 5 mL bottle.

HIGH ALERT

digoxin (di-jox-in)

Digitek, Lanoxicaps, Lanoxin

Classification

Therapeutic: antiarrhythmics, inotropics

Pharmacologic: digitalis glycosides

Indications

Treatment of congestive heart failure (CHF). Tachyarrhythmias: Atrial fibrillation and atrial flutter (slows ventricular rate), Paroxysmal atrial tachycardia.

Action

Increases the force of myocardial contraction. Prolongs refractory period of the AV node. Decreases conduction through the SA and AV nodes. **Therapeutic Effects:** Increased cardiac output (positive inotropic effect) and slowing of the heart rate (negative chronotropic effect).

Adverse Reactions/Side Effects

CNS: fatigue, headache, weakness. **EENT:** blurred vision, yellow or green vision. **CV:** ARRHYTHMIAS, bradycardia, ECG changes, AV block, SA block. **GI:** anorexia, nausea, vomiting, diarrhea. **Endo:** gynecomastia. **Hemat:** thrombocytopenia. **Metab:** electrolyte imbalances with acute digoxin toxicity.

PHYSICAL THERAPY IMPLICATIONS

Examination and Evaluation

- Assess heart rate, ECG, and heart sounds, especially during exercise (See Appendices G, H). Although intended to treat certain atrial arrhythmias, digoxin can precipitate new and potentially serious arrhythmias (proarrhythmic effect). Report any rhythm disturbances or symptoms of increased arrhythmias, including palpitations, chest pain, shortness of breath, fainting, and fatigue/weakness.
- Assess signs and symptoms of CHF (dyspnea, rales/crackles, peripheral edema, jugular venous distention, exercise intolerance) to help document whether drug therapy is effective in reducing these symptoms.
- Be alert for signs of digitalis toxicity. In adults and older children, the first signs of toxicity usually include abdominal pain, anorexia, nausea, vomiting, visual disturbances, bradycardia, and other arrhythmias. In infants and small children, the first symptoms of overdose are usually cardiac arrhythmias. If these appear, notify physician immediately. Blood tests may be needed to monitor digoxin levels, and adjustments in dosage may be indicated.
- Assess balance and risk of falls (See Appendix E), especially in older patients or in patients with weakness, fatigue, or blurred vision.
- Monitor and report signs of thrombocytopenia, including bruising, nose bleeds, and bleeding gums.

Interventions

- Design and implement aerobic exercise and endurance training programs to improve myocardial pumping ability and reduce symptoms of CHF.
- Use caution during aerobic exercise and endurance conditioning because of an increased risk of cardiac arrhythmias (bradycardia, tachycardia, others). Terminate exercise if patient exhibits untoward symptoms (chest pain, shortness of breath, etc.) or displays other criteria for exercise termination (See Appendix L).

Patient/Client-Related Instruction

- Remind patients to take medication as directed to control CHF or atrial arrhythmias, even if they are asymptomatic.
- Instruct patients to weigh themselves every day, and call their physician if they gain 3 or more lbs in 1 day or more than 5 lb in 1 week. Sudden weight gain may indicate fluid buildup due to worsening heart failure.
- Counsel patients about additional interventions to help control cardiac dysfunction, including regular exercise, weight loss, sodium restriction, stress reduction, moderation of alcohol consumption, and smoking cessation.
- Instruct patient or family/caregivers to report other troublesome side effects such as severe or prolonged headache, breast enlargement in men, or GI problems (nausea, vomiting, diarrhea, loss of appetite).

Pharmacokinetics

Absorption: 60–80% absorbed after oral administration of tablets; 70–85% absorbed after administration of elixir. Absorption from liquid-filled capsules is 90–100%; 80% absorbed from IM sites (IM route not recommended due to pain/irritation).

Distribution: Widely distributed; crosses placenta and enters breast milk.

Metabolism and Excretion: Excreted almost entirely unchanged by the kidneys.
Half-life: 36–48 hr (increased in renal impairment).
TIME/ACTION PROFILE (antiarrhythmic or inotropic effects, provided that a loading dose has been given)

ROUTE	ONSET	PEAK	DURATION
PO	30–120 min	2–8 hr	2–4 days*
IM	30 min	4–6 hr	2–4 days*
IV	5–30 min	1–4 hr	2–4 days*

*Duration listed is that for normal renal function; in impaired renal function, duration will be longer.

Contraindications/Precautions

Contraindicated in: Hypersensitivity; Uncontrolled ventricular arrhythmias; AV block; Idiopathic hypertrophic subaortic stenosis; Constrictive pericarditis; Known alcohol intolerance (elixir only).
Use Cautiously in: Hypokalemia (greatly ↑ risk of digoxin toxicity); Hypercalcemia (↑ risk of toxicity, especially with mild hypokalemia); Hypomagnesemia (may potentiate digoxin toxicity); Diuretic use (may cause electrolyte abnormalities, including hypokalemia and hypomagnesemia); Hypothyroidism; Geri: Geriatric patients (very sensitive to toxic effects, dose adjustments required for age-related decrease in renal function and body weight); MI; Renal impairment (dose reduction required); Obesity (dose should be based on ideal body weight); OB: Pregnancy (although safety has not been established, has been used during pregnancy without adverse effects on the fetus); Lactation: Similar concentrations in serum and breast milk result in subtherapeutic levels in infant; use with caution).

Interactions

Drug-Drug: Thiazide and **loop diuretics, piperacillin, ticarcillin, amphotericin B,** and **corticosteroids,** and excessive use of **laxatives** may cause hypokalemia, which may ↑ risk of toxicity. **Amiodarone,** some **benzodiazepines, cyclosporine, diphenoxylate, indomethacin, itraconazole, propafenone, propantheline, quinidine, quinine, spironolactone,** and **verapamil** may ↑ serum levels and may lead to toxicity (serum level monitoring/dose reduction may be required). Blood levels may be ↓ by oral **aminoglycosides,** some **antineoplastics (bleomycin, carmustine, cyclophosphamide, cytarabine, doxorubicin, methotrexate, procarbazine, vincristine), activated charcoal, cholestyramine, colestipol, kaolin/pectin, metoclopramide, penicillamine, rifampin,** or **sulfasalazine.** In a small percentage (10%) of patients, gut bacteria metabolize digoxin to inactive compounds; **macrolide anti-infectives (erythromycin, azithromycin, clarithromycin)** and **tetracyclines,** by killing these bacteria, will cause ↑ digoxin levels and toxicity; dose may need to be ↓ for up to 9 wk. Additive bradycardia may occur with **beta blockers** and other **antiarrhythmics (quinidine, disopyramide).** Concurrent use of **sympathomimetics** may ↑ risk of arrhythmias. **Thyroid hormones** may ↓ therapeutic effects.
Drug-Natural: Licorice and stimulant natural products (**aloe**) may ↑ risk of potassium depletion. **St. John's wort** may ↓ digoxin levels and effect.
Drug-Food: Concurrent ingestion of a **high-fiber meal** may ↓ absorption. Administer digoxin 1 hr before or 2 hr after such a meal.

Route/Dosage

For rapid effect, a larger initial loading/digitalizing dose should be given in several divided doses over 12–24 hr. Maintenance doses are determined for digoxin by renal function. All dosing must be evaluated by individual response. In general, doses required for atrial arrhythmias are higher than those for inotropic effect. When determining dose, consider that bioavailability of gelatin capsules (Lanoxicaps) is greater than that of tablets.
IV (Adults): *Digitalizing dose*—0.5–1 mg given as 50% of the dose initially and ¼ of the initial dose in each of 2 subsequent doses at 6- to 12-hr intervals.
IV (Children >10 yr): *Digitalizing dose*—8–12 mcg/kg given as 50% of the dose initially and ¼ of the initial dose in each of 2 subsequent doses at 6- to 12-hr intervals.
IV (Children 5–10 yr): *Digitalizing dose*—15–30 mcg/kg given as 50% of the dose initially and ¼ of the initial dose in each of 2 subsequent doses at 6- to 12-hr intervals.
IV (Children 2–5 yr): *Digitalizing dose*—25–35 mcg/kg given as 50% of the dose initially and ¼ of the initial dose in each of 2 subsequent doses at 6- to 12-hr intervals.
IV (Children 1–24 mo): *Digitalizing dose*—30–50 mcg/kg given as 50% of the dose initially and ¼ of the initial dose in each of 2 subsequent doses at 6- to 12-hr intervals.
IV (Infants full term): 20–30 mcg/kg given as 50% of the dose initially and ¼ ne quarter of the initial dose in each of 2 subsequent doses at 6- to 12-hr intervals.
IV (Infants—premature): *Digitalizing dose*—15–25 mcg/kg given as 50% of the dose initially and ¼ of the initial dose in each of 2 subsequent doses at 6- to 12-hr intervals.
PO (Adults): *Digitalizing dose*—0.75–1.5 mg given as 50% of the dose initially and ¼ of the initial dose in each of 2 subsequent doses at 6–12 hr intervals.

Maintenance dose—0.125–0.5 mg/day as tablets or 0.350–0.5 mg/day as gelatin capsules, depending on patient's lean body weight, renal function, and serum level.
PO (Geriatric Patients): Daily dosage should not exceed 0.125 mg except when treating atrial fibrillation.
PO (Children >10 yr): *Digitalizing dose*—10–15 mcg/kg given as 50% of the dose initially and ¼ of the initial dose in each of 2 subsequent doses at 6- to 12-hr intervals. *Maintenance dose*—2.5–5 mcg/kg given daily as a single dose.
PO (Children 5–10 yr): *Digitalizing dose*—20–35 mcg/kg given as 50% of the dose initially and ¼ of the initial dose in each of 2 subsequent doses at 6- to 12-hr intervals. *Maintenance dose*—5–10 mcg/kg given daily in 2 divided doses.
PO (Children 2–5 yr): *Digitalizing dose*—30–40 mcg/kg given as 50% of the dose initially and ¼ of the initial dose in each of 2 subsequent doses at 6- to 12-hr intervals. *Maintenance dose*—7.5–10 mcg/kg given daily in 2 divided doses.
PO (Children 1–24 mo): *Digitalizing dose*—35–60 mcg/kg given as 50% of the dose initially and ¼ of the initial dose in each of 2 subsequent doses at 6- to 12-hr intervals. *Maintenance dose*—10–15 mcg/kg given daily in 2 divided doses.
PO (Infants full term): *Digitalizing dose*—25–35 mcg/kg given as 50% of the dose initially and ¼ of the initial dose in each of 2 subsequent doses at 6- to 12-hr intervals. *Maintenance dose*—6–10 mcg/kg given daily in 2 divided doses.
PO (Infants premature): *Digitalizing dose*—20–30 mcg/kg given as 50% of the dose initially and ¼ of the initial dose in each of 2 subsequent doses at 6- to 12-hr intervals. *Maintenance dose*—5–7.5 mcg/kg given daily in 2 divided doses.

Availability (generic available)

Tablets: 0.125 mg, 0.25 mg. **Capsules:** 0.05 mg, 0.1 mg, 0.2 mg. **Pediatric elixir (lime flavor):** 0.05 mg/mL. **Injection:** 0.25 mg/mL. **Pediatric injection:** 0.1 mg/mL.

dihydroergotamine

(dye-hye-droe-er-**got**-a-meen)

D.H.E. 45, ✱ Dihydroergotamine-Sandoz, Migranal

Classification
Therapeutic: vascular headache suppressants
Pharmacologic: ergot alkaloids

Indications

Vascular headaches, including Migraine, Cluster headaches.

Action

Vasoconstriction of dilated blood vessels by stimulating alpha-adrenergic and serotonergic (5-HT) receptors. Larger doses may produce alpha-adrenergic blockade and vasodilation. **Therapeutic Effects:** Constriction of dilated carotid artery bed with resolution of vascular headache.

Adverse Reactions/Side Effects

CNS: dizziness. **EENT:** rhinitis. **CV:** MYOCARDIAL INFARCTION, hypertension, angina pectoris, arterial spasm, intermittent claudication. **GI:** abdominal pain, nausea, vomiting, altered taste, diarrhea, polydipsia. **MS:** extremity stiffness, muscle pain, stiff neck, stiff shoulders. **Neuro:** leg weakness, numbness or tingling in fingers or toes. **Misc:** fatigue.

PHYSICAL THERAPY IMPLICATIONS

Examination and Evaluation

- Continually monitor for signs of coronary artery vasospasm and MI, including sudden chest pain, pain radiating into the arm or jaw, shortness of breath, dizziness, sweating, anxiety, and nausea. Seek immediate medical assistance if patient develops these signs.
- Assess the frequency and severity of headaches, and document whether drug therapy is successful in decreasing migraine or cluster headache attacks.
- Assess blood pressure (BP) and compare to normal values (See Appendix F). Report a sustained increase in BP (hypertension).
- Assess any muscle pain, stiffness, or weakness to rule out musculoskeletal pathology; that is, try to determine if pain is drug induced rather than caused by anatomic or biomechanical problems.
- Be alert for sudden, intense leg pain during ambulation and other lower extremity exercises (intermittent claudication). Report the frequency and severity of these symptoms to the physician.
- Assess signs of numbness and tingling in the fingers and toes. Perform objective tests including electroneuromyography and sensory testing to document any drug-related neuropathic changes.
- Watch for dizziness that affects gait, balance, and other functional activities (See Appendix C). Report balance problems and functional limitations to the physician, and caution the patient and family/caregivers to guard against falls and trauma.

Interventions

- Because of the risk of MI and claudication, use extreme caution during aerobic exercise and other forms of therapeutic exercise. Assess exercise tolerance frequently (BP, heart rate, respiration, fatigue levels), and terminate exercise immediately if any untoward responses occur (See Appendix L).
- If a headache occurs and drug treatment is needed during a rehabilitation session, allow patient to

recover in a quiet, darkened room to allow the drug to achieve maximal effects.

Patient/Client-Related Instruction

- Advise patient and family or caregiver about the signs of MI (see above under Examination and Evaluation), and to seek immediate medical assistance if these signs develop.
- Advise the patient to bring this drug to each therapy session; this drug is most effective when taken at the first signs of a migraine attack. Make sure patients understand the correct administration techniques for intranasal inhalation or subcutaneous and IM injection.
- Advise patient to adhere to the correct dosing schedule, and not to exceed the recommended frequency and number of doses.
- Instruct patient to report other troublesome side effects such as severe or prolonged fatigue, nasal irritation, or GI problems (abdominal pain, nausea, vomiting, diarrhea, altered taste).

Pharmacokinetics

Absorption: Rapidly absorbed following IM and SC administration and 32% absorbed from nasal mucosa.
Distribution: Unknown.
Protein Binding: 90%.
Metabolism and Excretion: Highly metabolized (90%) by the liver. Some metabolites are active.
Half-life: 10 hr.

TIME/ACTION PROFILE (relief of headache)

ROUTE	ONSET	PEAK	DURATION
intranasal	within 30 min	unknown	unknown
IM, SC	15–30 min	15 min–2 hr	8 hr
IV	<5 min	15 min–2 hr	8 hr

Contraindications/Precautions

Contraindicated in: Peripheral vascular disease; Ischemic heart disease; Uncontrolled hypertension; Severe renal or liver disease; Malnutrition; Known alcohol intolerance (injection only); Pregnancy; Lactation; Concurrent use of CYP3A4 enzyme inhibitors (macrolide anti-infectives and protease inhibitors).
Use Cautiously in: Illnesses associated with peripheral vascular pathology such as diabetes mellitus; Concurrent administration of other vasoconstricting agents; Children <6 yr (safety not established).

Interactions

Drug-Drug: Concurrent use of CYP3A4 enzyme inhibitors (**macrolide anti-infectives** and **protease inhibitors**) may produce serious, life-threatening peripheral ischemia and is contraindicated. Concurrent use with **beta blockers**, **oral contraceptives**, or **nicotine** (heavy smoking) may ↑ risk of peripheral vasoconstriction. Dihydroergotamine antagonizes the antianginal effects of **nitrates**. Concurrent use with **vasoconstrictors** may have ↑ effects (avoid concurrent use). Concurrent use with **sumatriptan** may result in prolonged vasoconstriction (allow 24 hr between use).

Route/Dosage

IM, SC (Adults): 1 mg; may repeat in 1 hr to a total of 3 mg (not to exceed 3 mg/day or 6 mg/wk).
IM, SC (Children ≥6 yr): 0.5 mg; may be repeated in 1 hr.
IV (Adults): 0.5 mg; may repeat in 1 hr (not to exceed 2 mg/day or 6 mg/wk). For chronic intractable headache, 0.5–1 mg q 8 hr may be given until relief (not to exceed 6 mg/wk).
IV (Children ≥6 yr): 0.25 mg; may be repeated in 1 hr.
IV (Children and Adolescents 12–16 yr): *Severe, acute migraine*—0.25–0.5 mg; 1–2 more doses may be given q 20 min.
IV (Children 9–12 yr): *Severe, acute migraine*—0.2 mg; 1–2 more doses may be given q 20 min.
IV (Children 6–9 yr): *Severe, acute migraine*—0.1–0.15 mg; 1–2 more doses may be given q 20 min.
Intranasal (Adults): 1 spray (0.5 mg) in each nostril, repeat after 15 min (2 mg total dose); not to exceed 3 mg/24 hr or 4 mg/wk.

Availability

Injection: 1 mg/mL (contains alcohol). **Nasal spray:** 4 mg/1 mL in 1-mL ampules with nasal spray applicator.

diltiazem (dil-tye-a-zem)

Apo-Diltiaz, Cardizem, Cardizem CD, Cardizem LA, Cardizem SR, Cartia XT, Dilacor XR, Diltia XT, Novo-Diltazem, Nu-Diltiaz, Ratio-Diltiazem CD, Syn-Diltiazem, Taztia XT, Tiazac

Classification
Therapeutic: antianginals, antiarrhythmics (class IV), antihypertensives
Pharmacologic: calcium channel blockers

Indications

Hypertension. Angina pectoris and vasospastic (Prinzmetal's) angina. Supraventricular tachyarrhythmias and rapid ventricular rates in atrial flutter or fibrillation. **Unlabeled Use:** Management of Raynaud's syndrome.

Action

Inhibits transport of calcium into myocardial and vascular smooth muscle cells, resulting in inhibition of excitation-contraction coupling and subsequent contraction. **Therapeutic Effects:** Systemic vasodilation resulting in decreased blood pressure. Coronary vasodilation resulting in decreased frequency and severity of attacks of angina. Suppression of arrhythmias.

Adverse Reactions/Side Effects

CNS: abnormal dreams, anxiety, confusion, dizziness, drowsiness, headache, nervousness, psychiatric disturbances, weakness. **EENT:** blurred vision, disturbed equilibrium, epistaxis, tinnitus. **Resp:** cough, dyspnea. **CV:** ARRHYTHMIAS, CHF, peripheral edema, bradycardia, chest pain, hypotension, palpitations, syncope, tachycardia. **GI:** abnormal liver function studies, anorexia, constipation, diarrhea, dry mouth, dysgeusia, dyspepsia, nausea, vomiting. **GU:** dysuria, nocturia, polyuria, sexual dysfunction, urinary frequency. **Derm:** dermatitis, erythema multiforme, flushing, increased sweating, photosensitivity, pruritus/urticaria, rash. **Endo:** gynecomastia, hyperglycemia. **Hemat:** anemia, leukopenia, thrombocytopenia. **Metab:** weight gain. **MS:** joint stiffness, muscle cramps. **Neuro:** paresthesia, tremor. **Misc:** STEVENS-JOHNSON SYNDROME, gingival hyperplasia.

PHYSICAL THERAPY IMPLICATIONS

Examination and Evaluation

- Assess heart rate, ECG, and heart sounds, especially during exercise (See Appendices G, H). Although intended to treat certain arrhythmias, this drug can unmask or precipitate new arrhythmias (proarrhythmic effect). Report any rhythm disturbances or symptoms of increased arrhythmias, including palpitations, chest pain, shortness of breath, fainting, and fatigue/weakness.
- Monitor rashes or other skin reactions (hives, abnormal sweating, itching/burning, exfoliation). Notify physician immediately because certain skin reactions may indicate serious hypersensitivity reactions (Stevens-Johnson syndrome).
- Assess routinely for signs of CHF and pulmonary edema (dyspnea, cough, shortness of breath, rales/crackles, jugular venous distention). Report these signs to the physician.
- Assess blood pressure periodically and compare to normal values (see Appendix F) to help document antihypertensive effects.
- Assess episodes of angina pectoris at rest and during exercise. Document whether drug therapy is helpful in reducing the frequency and severity of anginal attacks.
- If used to treat Raynaud's syndrome, monitor the incidence and severity of vasospastic attacks to document whether diltiazem is successful in helping manage this condition.
- Assess peripheral edema using girth measurements, volume displacement, and measurement of pitting edema (See Appendix N). Report increased swelling in feet and ankles or a sudden increase in body weight due to peripheral vasodilation.
- Assess signs of paresthesia (numbness, tingling) or muscle twitching. Perform objective tests, including electroneuromyography and sensory testing to document any drug-related neuropathic changes.
- Watch for signs of hyperglycemia, including confusion, drowsiness, flushed/dry skin, fruit-like breath odor, rapid/deep breathing, polyuria, loss of appetite, and unusual thirst. Insulin dosages may need to be adjusted to prevent repeated episodes of hyperglycemia.
- Monitor and report signs of leukopenia (fever, sore throat, signs of infection), thrombocytopenia (bruising, nose bleeds, and bleeding gums), or unusual weakness and fatigue that might be due to anemia.
- Assess any joint pain or muscle cramping to rule out musculoskeletal pathology; that is, try to determine if pain is drug induced rather than caused by anatomic or biomechanical problems.
- Assess dizziness and weakness that might affect gait, balance, and other functional activities (See Appendix C). Report balance problems and functional limitations to the physician, and caution the patient and family/caregivers to guard against falls and trauma.
- Monitor mood and personality changes, including anxiety, nervousness, confusion, memory loss, or other changes in behavior. Notify physician if these changes become problematic.

Interventions

- Design and implement aerobic exercise and endurance training programs to normalize blood pressure, improve coronary perfusion, reduce angina, and improve myocardial pumping ability.
- Because of the risk of cardiac arrhythmias and CHF, use caution during aerobic exercise and other forms of therapeutic exercise. Assess exercise tolerance frequently (blood pressure, heart rate, fatigue levels), and terminate exercise immediately if any untoward responses occur (See Appendix L).
- Guard against falls and trauma (hip fractures, head injury). Implement fall-prevention strategies, especially if patient exhibits dizziness or disturbed equilibrium (See Appendix E).
- To minimize orthostatic hypotension, patient should move slowly when assuming a more upright position.
- Causes photosensitivity; use care if administering UV treatments.

D

Patient/Client-Related Instruction

- Remind patients to take medication as directed to control hypertension and other cardiac conditions even if they are asymptomatic.
- Counsel patients about additional interventions to help control blood pressure and cardiac dysfunction, including regular exercise, weight loss, sodium restriction, stress reduction, moderation of alcohol consumption, and smoking cessation.
- Advise patient about photosensitivity, and to use sunscreens, protective clothing, and avoid prolonged sun exposure. Advise patient to also report any rashes or other skin reactions.
- Instruct patient or family/caregivers to report other troublesome side effects such as severe or prolonged headache, nightmares, tremor, problems with urination, sexual problems (decreased libido, erectile dysfunction), breast enlargement in men (gynecomastia), or GI problems (nausea, vomiting, constipation, diarrhea, loss of appetite).

Pharmacokinetics

Absorption: Well absorbed, but rapidly metabolized after oral administration.
Distribution: Unknown.
Protein Binding: 70–80%.
Metabolism and Excretion: Mostly metabolized by the liver (CYP3A4 enzyme system).
Half-life: 3.5–9 hr.

TIME/ACTION PROFILE

ROUTE	ONSET	PEAK	DURATION
PO	30 min	2–3 hr	6–8 hr
PO–SR	unknown	unknown	12 hr
PO–CD, XR, LA	unknown	14 days*	up to 24 hr
IV	2–5 min	2–4 hr	unknown

*Maximum antihypertensive effect with chronic therapy.

Contraindications/Precautions

Contraindicated in: Hypersensitivity; Sick sinus syndrome; 2nd- or 3rd-degree AV block (unless an artificial pacemaker is in place); Blood pressure <90 mm Hg; Recent MI or pulmonary congestion; Concurrent use of rifampin.
Use Cautiously in: Severe hepatic impairment (↓ dose recommended); Geri: Geriatric patients (↓ dose/slower IV infusion rate recommended; ↑ risk of hypotension; consider age-related decrease in body mass, decreased hepatic/renal/cardiac function, concurrent drug therapy and other disease states); Severe renal impairment; Serious ventricular arrhythmias or CHF; OB/Lactation/Pedi: Pregnancy, lactation, or children (safety not established).

Interactions

Drug-Drug: ↑ hypotension may occur when used with **fentanyl**, other **antihypertensives**, **nitrates**, acute ingestion of **alcohol**, or **quinidine**. Antihypertensive effects may be ↓ by **NSAIDs**. Serum **digoxin** levels may be increased. Concurrent use with **beta blockers**, **digoxin**, **disopyramide**, or **phenytoin** may result in bradycardia, conduction defects, or CHF. **Phenobarbital** and **phenytoin** may ↑ metabolism and ↓ effectiveness. May ↓ metabolism of and ↑ risk of toxicity from **cyclosporine**, **quinidine**, or **carbamazepine**. **Cimetidine** and **ranitidine** ↑ blood levels and effects. May ↑ or ↓ the effects of **lithium** or **theophylline**.
Drug-Food: Grapefruit juice ↑ serum levels and effect.

Route/Dosage

PO (Adults): 30–120 mg 3–4 times daily or 60–120 mg twice daily as SR capsules or 180–240 mg once daily as CD or XR capsules or LA tablets (up to 360 mg/day).
IV (Adults): 0.25 mg/kg; may repeat in 15 min with a dose of 0.35 mg/kg. May follow with continuous infusion at 10 mg/hr (range 5–15 mg/hr) for up to 24 hr.

Availability (generic available)

Tablets: 30 mg, 60 mg, 90 mg, 120 mg. **Sustained-release capsules:** 60 mg, 90 mg, 120 mg. **Extended-release capsules (Cardizem CD, Dilacor XR, Tiazac, Cartia XT, Taztia XT):** 120 mg, 180 mg, 240 mg, 300 mg, 360 mg, 420 mg. **Extended-release tablets (Cardizem LA):** 120 mg, 180 mg, 240 mg, 300 mg, 360 mg, 420 mg. **Injection:** 5 mg/mL in 5-, 10-, and 25-mL vials.

dimenhydrinate

(dye-men-**hye**-dri-nate)
✱ Apo-Dimenhydrinate, Calm X, Dimetabs, Dinate, Dramamine, Dramanate, ✱ Gravol, Hydrate, ✱ PMS-Dimenhydrinate, ✱ Traveltabs, Triptone Caplets

Classification
Therapeutic: antiemetics, antihistamines

Indications

Nausea, vomiting, dizziness, and vertigo accompanying motion sickness.

Action

Inhibits vestibular stimulation. Has significant CNS depressant, anticholinergic, antihistaminic, and antiemetic properties. **Therapeutic Effects:** Decreased vestibular stimulation, which may prevent motion sickness.

Adverse Reactions/Side Effects

CNS: drowsiness, dizziness, headache, paradoxical excitation (children). **EENT:** blurred vision, tinnitus. **CV:** hypotension, palpitations. **GI:** anorexia, constipation, diarrhea, dry mouth. **GU:** dysuria, frequency. **Derm:** photosensitivity. **Local:** pain at IM site.

PHYSICAL THERAPY IMPLICATIONS

Examination and Evaluation

- Assess blood pressure periodically, and compare to normal values (see Appendix F). Report a sustained or symptomatic decrease in blood pressure (hypotension) or other cardiac symptoms (palpitations).
- Watch for signs of increased excitation and hyperactivity in children. Severe or problematic excitation may require a change in dose or drug.
- Monitor any improvements in symptoms (nausea, vomiting, dizziness, vertigo) to help document the effects of this drug.
- Assess dizziness and drowsiness that might affect gait, balance, and other functional activities (See Appendix C). Report balance problems and functional limitations to the physician, and caution the patient and family/caregivers to guard against falls and trauma.
- Assess IM injection site for excessive or prolonged pain and swelling.

Interventions

- Guard against falls and trauma (hip fractures, head injury, and so forth). Implement fall prevention strategies, especially in older adults or if balance is impaired (See Appendix E).
- In patients with chronic vestibular problems, implement therapeutic exercises and vestibular training activities to help reduce symptoms.
- Causes photosensitivity; use care if administering UV treatments. Advise patient to avoid direct sunlight and use sunscreens and protective clothing.

Patient/Client-related Instruction

- Advise patient about the risk of daytime drowsiness and decreased attention and mental focus. These problems can be severe in certain people. Use care if driving or in other activities that require quick reactions and strong concentration.
- Advise patient to avoid alcohol and other CNS depressants because of the increased risk of sedation and adverse effects.
- Instruct patient to report other bothersome side effects including severe or prolonged headache blurred vision, buzzing/ringing in the ears (tinnitus), problems with urination, or GI problems (constipation, diarrhea, dry mouth, loss of appetite).

Pharmacokinetics

Absorption: Well absorbed after oral or IM administration.

Distribution: Probably crosses the placenta and enters breast milk.

Metabolism and Excretion: Metabolized by the liver.

Half-life: Unknown.

TIME/ACTION PROFILE (anti–motion sickness, antiemetic activity)

ROUTE	ONSET	PEAK	DURATION
PO	15–60 min	1–2 hr	3–6 hr
rectal	30–45 min	unknown	6–12 hr
IM	20–30 min	1–2 hr	3–6 hr
IV	rapid	unknown	3–6 hr

Contraindications/Precautions

Contraindicated in: Hypersensitivity; Some products contain alcohol or tartrazine; in patients with known intolerance.

Use Cautiously in: Angle-closure glaucoma; Seizure disorders; Prostatic hyperplasia.

Interactions

Drug-Drug: ↑ CNS depression with other **antihistamines**, **alcohol**, **opioid analgesics**, and **sedative/hypnotics**. May mask signs or symptoms of ototoxicity in patients receiving **ototoxic drugs** (**aminoglycosides**, **ethacrynic acid**). ↑ anticholinergic properties with **tricyclic antidepressants**, **quinidine**, or **disopyramide**. **MAO inhibitors** intensify and prolong the anticholinergic effects of antihistamines.

Route/Dosage

PO (Adults): 50–100 mg q 4 hr (not to exceed 400 mg/day).

PO (Children 6–12 yr): 25–50 mg q 6–8 hr (not to exceed 300 mg/day).

Rect (Adults): 50–100 mg q 6–8 hr.

Rect (Children 8–12 yr): 25–50 mg q 8–12 hr.

Rect (Children 6–8 yr): 12.5–25 mg q 8–12 hr.

IM, IV (Adults): 50 mg q 4 hr as needed.

IM, IV (Children): 1.25 mg/kg (37.5 mg/m^2) q 6 hr as needed (not to exceed 300 mg/day).

Availability (generic available)

Tablets: 50 mg OTC. **Chewable tablets (orange flavor):** 50 mg OTC. **Capsules:** 50 mg OTC. **Extended-release capsules:** 25 mg OTC. **Elixir (cherry flavor):** 12.5 mg/5 mL OTC, 15 mg/5 mL OTC. **Liquid:** 12.5 mg/4 mL OTC. **Suppositories:** 50 mg OTC, 100 mg OTC. **Injection:** 50 mg/mL.

dinoprostone

(dye-noe-**prost**-one)

Cervidil Vaginal Insert, Prepidil Endocervical Gel, Prostin E Vaginal Suppository

Classification

Therapeutic: cervical ripening agent

Pharmacologic: oxytocics, prostaglandins

Indications

Endocervical Gel, Vaginal Insert: Used to "ripen" the cervix in pregnancy at or near term when induction of labor is indicated. Vaginal Suppository: Induction of midtrimester abortion, Management of missed abortion up to 28 wk, Management of nonmetastatic gestational trophoblastic disease (benign hydatidiform mole).

Action

Produces contractions similar to those occurring during labor at term by stimulating the myometrium (oxytocic effect). Initiates softening, effacement, and dilation of the cervix ("ripening"). Also stimulates GI smooth muscle. **Therapeutic Effects:** Initiation of labor. Expulsion of fetus.

Adverse Reactions/Side Effects

Endocervical Gel, Vaginal Insert

GU: uterine contractile abnormalities, warm feeling in vagina. **MS:** back pain. **Misc:** fever.

Suppository

CNS: <u>headache</u>, drowsiness, syncope. **Resp:** coughing, dyspnea, wheezing. **CV:** <u>hypotension</u>, hypertension. **GI:** <u>diarrhea</u>, <u>nausea</u>, <u>vomiting</u>. **GU:** UTERINE RUPTURE, urinary tract infection, uterine hyperstimulation, vaginal/uterine pain. **Misc:** ALLERGIC REACTIONS, INCLUDING ANAPHYLAXIS, <u>chills</u>, fever.

PHYSICAL THERAPY IMPLICATIONS

Examination and Evaluation

- Monitor signs of allergic reactions and anaphylaxis, including pulmonary symptoms (tightness in the throat and chest, wheezing, cough, dyspnea) or skin reactions (rash, pruritus, urticaria). Notify physician or nursing staff immediately if these reactions occur.
- Be alert for signs of uterine rupture. Signs include increased bleeding, sudden abdominal pain, and changes in fetal heart rate. Notify physician or nursing staff immediately if these signs occur.
- Assess blood pressure (BP) and compare to normal values (See Appendix F). Report changes in BP, either a problematic decrease in BP (hypotension resulting in syncope) or a sustained increase in BP (hypertension).

Interventions

- Provide massage, other manual techniques, or relaxation techniques as needed to relieve back pain and pain associated with childbirth.

Patient/Client-Related Instruction

- Instruct patient to report other bothersome side effects such as severe or prolonged headache, chills, fever, or GI problems (diarrhea, nausea, vomiting).

Pharmacokinetics

Absorption: Rapidly absorbed.
Distribution: Unknown. Action is mostly local.
Metabolism and Excretion: Metabolized by enzymes in lung, kidneys, spleen, and liver tissue.
Half-life: Unknown.

TIME/ACTION PROFILE

ROUTE	ONSET	PEAK	DURATION
cervical ripening (gel)	rapid	30–45 min	unknown
cervical ripening (insert)	rapid	unknown	12 hr
abortion time (suppository)	10 min	12–24 hr	2–3 hr

Contraindications/Precautions

Contraindicated in: Hypersensitivity to prostaglandins or additives in the gel or suppository; The gel/insert should be avoided in situations in which prolonged uterine contractions should be avoided, including: Previous cesarean section or uterine surgery, Cephalopelvic disproportion, Traumatic delivery or difficult labor, Multiparity (≥6 term pregnancies), Hyperactive or hypertonic uterus, Fetal distress (if delivery is not imminent), Unexplained vaginal bleeding, Placenta previa, Vasa previa, Active herpes genitalis, Obstetric emergency requiring surgical intervention, Situations in which vaginal delivery is contraindicated; Presence of acute pelvic inflammatory disease or ruptured membranes; Concurrent oxytocic therapy (wait for 30 min after removing insert before using oxytocin).
Use Cautiously in: Uterine scarring; Asthma; Hypotension; Cardiac disease; Adrenal disorders; Anemia; Jaundice; Diabetes mellitus; Epilepsy; Glaucoma; Pulmonary, renal, or hepatic disease; Multiparity (up to 5 previous term pregnancies).

Interactions

Drug-Drug: Augments the effects of other **oxytocics**.

Route/Dosage

Cervical Ripening

Vaginal (Adults, Cervical): *Endocervical gel*—0.5 mg; if response is unfavorable, may repeat in 6 hr (not to exceed 1.5 mg/24 hr). *Vaginal insert*—1 10-mg insert.

Abortifacient

Vaginal (Adults): 1 20-mg suppository, repeat q 3–5 hr (not to exceed 240 mg total or longer than 48 hr).

Availability

Endocervical gel (Prepidil): 0.5 mg dinoprostone in 3 g of gel vehicle in a prefilled syringe with catheters. **Vaginal insert (Cervidil):** 10 mg. **Vaginal suppository (Prostin E Vaginal):** 20 mg.

diphenhydramine (oral, parenteral), (dye-fen-**hye**-dra-meen)

✱ Allerdryl, Allergy Medication, AllerMax, Banophen, Benadryl Dye-Free Allergy, Benadryl Allergy, Benadryl, Compoz, Compoz Nighttime Sleep Aid, Diphen AF, Diphen Cough, ✱ Diphenhist, Dormin, Genahist, 40 Winks, Hyrexin-50, ✱ Insomnal, Maximum Strength Nytol, Maximum Strength Sleepinal, Midol PM, Miles Nervine, Nighttime Sleep Aid, Nytol, Scot-Tussin Allergy DM, Siladril, Silphen, Sleep-Eze 3, Sleepwell 2-night, Snooze Fast, Sominex, Tusstat, Twilite, Unisom Nighttime Sleep-Aid

Classification

Therapeutic: allergy, cold, and cough remedies, antihistamines, antitussives

Indications

Relief of allergic symptoms caused by histamine release, including Anaphylaxis, Seasonal and perennial allergic rhinitis, Allergic dermatoses. Parkinson's disease, and dystonic reactions from medications. Mild nighttime sedation. Prevention of motion sickness. Antitussive (syrup only).

Action

Antagonizes the effects of histamine at H_1-receptor sites; does not bind to or inactivate histamine. Significant CNS depressant and anticholinergic properties. **Therapeutic Effects:** Decreased symptoms of histamine excess (sneezing, rhinorrhea, nasal and ocular pruritus, ocular tearing and redness, urticaria). Relief of acute dystonic reactions. Prevention of motion sickness. Suppression of cough.

Adverse Reactions/Side Effects

CNS: drowsiness, dizziness, headache, paradoxical excitation (increased in children). **EENT:** blurred vision, tinnitus. **CV:** hypotension, palpitations. **GI:** anorexia, dry mouth, constipation, nausea. **GU:** dysuria, frequency, urinary retention. **Derm:** photosensitivity. **Resp:** chest tightness, thickened bronchial secretions, wheezing. **Local:** pain at IM site.

PHYSICAL THERAPY IMPLICATIONS

Examination and Evaluation

- Assess blood pressure periodically and compare to normal values (See Appendix F). Report a sustained or symptomatic decrease in blood pressure (hypotension) or other cardiac symptoms (palpitations).
- Monitor respiratory function at rest and during exercise. Notify physician if patient experiences any troublesome wheezing, tightness in the throat or chest, or abnormal bronchial secretions.
- Monitor symptoms of seasonal allergies (sneezing, rhinitis, itching eyes, cough) or allergic skin reactions (rash, hives, itching) to help document benefits of this drug in treating these disorders.
- If used as a cough suppressant, assess frequency and nature of cough, lung sounds, and amount and type of sputum produced. Document whether this drug is effective as a cough suppressant.
- If used to treat Parkinson's disease, assess patient's motor function, especially when starting drug therapy, or during dosing changes or addition of other antiparkinson drugs. Motor function should be assessed at different times of the day, such as when drugs are reaching peak therapeutic levels (i.e., 2–4 hr after oral dose), as well as when drug effects are minimal (just before the next dose).
- When treating anaphylaxis, assess for signs of successful treatment, including decreased skin reactions (rash, urticaria) and increased airway patency and ventilation (decreased dyspnea, wheezing, shortness of breath).
- Assess dizziness and drowsiness that might affect gait, balance, and other functional activities (See Appendix C). Report balance problems and functional limitations to the physician, and caution the patient and family/caregivers to guard against falls and trauma.
- Watch for signs of increased excitation and hyperactivity in children. Severe or problematic excitation may require a change in dose or drug.
- Monitor IM injection site for pain, swelling, and irritation. Report prolonged or excessive injection-site reactions to the physician.

Interventions

- Guard against falls and trauma (hip fractures, head injury, and so forth). Implement fall-prevention strategies, especially in older adults or if balance is impaired (See Appendix E).
- If used as a sedative-hypnotic, help patient explore nonpharmacologic methods to induce sleep such as relaxation techniques, avoiding caffeine, and so forth.
- Causes photosensitivity; use care if administering UV treatments. Advise patient to avoid direct sunlight and use sunscreens and protective clothing.

Patient/Client-Related Instruction

- Advise patient about the risk of daytime drowsiness and decreased attention and mental focus. These problems can be severe in certain people. Use care if driving or in other activities that require quick reactions and strong concentration.
- When treating cough:
  - Instruct patient to cough effectively: sit upright and take several deep breaths before attempting to cough.
  - Advise patient to minimize cough by avoiding irritants, such as cigarette smoke, fumes, and dust. Humidification of environmental air, frequent sips of water, and sugarless hard candy may also decrease the frequency of dry, irritating cough.
  - Advise patient that any cough lasting more than 1 wk or accompanied by fever, chest pain, persistent headache, or skin rash warrants medical attention.
- Advise patient to avoid alcohol and other CNS depressants because of the increased risk of sedation and adverse effects.
- Instruct patient and family/caregivers to report other bothersome side effects such as severe or prolonged headache, buzzing/ringing in the ears (tinnitus), problems with urination, or GI problems (nausea, constipation).

Pharmacokinetics

Absorption: Well absorbed after oral or IM administration but 40–60% of an oral dose reaches systemic circulation due to first-pass metabolism.
Distribution: Widely distributed. Crosses the placenta; enters breast milk.
Metabolism and Excretion: 95% metabolized by the liver.
Half-life: 2.4–7 hr.

TIME/ACTION PROFILE (antihistaminic effects)

ROUTE	ONSET	PEAK	DURATION
PO	15–60 min	2–4 hr	4–8 hr
IM	20–30 min	2–4 hr	4–8 hr
IV	rapid	unknown	4–8 hr

Contraindications/Precautions

Contraindicated in: Hypersensitivity; Acute attacks of asthma; Lactation; Known alcohol intolerance (some liquid products).
Use Cautiously in: Severe liver disease; Angle-closure glaucoma; Seizure disorders; Prostatic hyperplasia; Peptic ulcer; May cause paradoxical excitation in young children; Hyperthyroidism; OB: Safety not established; Lactation: Discontinue drug or bottle feed; Geri: Appears on Beers' list. Geriatric patients are more susceptible to adverse drug reactions and anticholinergic effects (delirium, acute confusion, dizziness, dry mouth, blurred vision, urinary retention, constipation, tachycardia); dosage reduction or nonanticholinergic antihistamine recommended.

Interactions

Drug-Drug: ↑ risk of CNS depression with other **antihistamines**, **alcohol**, **opioid analgesics**, and **sedative/hypnotics**. ↑ anticholinergic effects with **tricyclic antidepressants**, **quinidine**, or **disopyramide**. **MAO inhibitors** intensify and prolong the anticholinergic effects of antihistamines.
Drug-Natural: Concomitant use of **kava**, **valerian**, or **chamomile** can ↑ CNS depression.

Route/Dosage

PO (Adults and Children >12 yr): *Antihistaminic/antiemetic/antivertiginic*—25–50 mg q 4–6 hr, not to exceed 300 mg/day. *Antitussive*—25 mg q 4 hr as needed, not to exceed 150 mg/day. *Antidyskinetic*—25–50 mg q 4 hr (not to exceed 400 mg/day). *Sedative/hypnotic*—50 mg 20–30 min before bedtime.
PO (Children 6–12 yr): *Antihistaminic/antiemetic/antivertiginic*—12.5–25 mg q 4–6 hr (not to exceed 150 mg/day). *Antidyskinetic*—1–1.5 mg/kg q 6–8 hr as needed (not to exceed 300 mg/day). *Antitussive*—12.5 mg q 4 hr (not to exceed 75 mg/day). *Sedative/hypnotic*—1 mg/kg/dose 20–30 min before bedtime (not to exceed 50 mg).
PO (Children 2–6 yr): *Antihistaminic/antiemetic/antivertiginic*—6.25–12.5 mg q 4–6 hr (not to exceed 37.5 mg/day). *Antidyskinetic*—1–1.5 mg/kg q 4–6 hr as needed (not to exceed 300 mg/day). *Antitussive*—6.25 mg q 4 hr (not to exceed 37.5 mg/24 hr).

Sedative/hypnotic—1 mg/kg/dose 20–30 min before bedtime (not to exceed 50 mg).
IM, IV (Adults): 25–50 mg q 4 hr as needed (may need up to 100 mg dose, not to exceed 400 mg/day).
IM, IV (Children): 1.25 mg/kg (37.5 mg/m^2) 4 times daily (not to exceed 300 mg/day).

Availability (generic available)

Capsules: 25 mg Rx, OTC, 50 mg Rx, OTC. **Tablets:** 25 mg Rx, OTC, 50 mg Rx, OTC. **Chewable tablets (grape flavor):** 25 mg Rx, OTC. **Elixir (cherry and other flavors):** 12.5 mg/5 mL Rx, OTC. **Syrup (cherry and raspberry flavor):** 12.5 mg/5 mL Rx, OTC. **Injection:** 10 mg/mL, 50 mg/mL. ***In combination with:*** analgesics, decongestants, and expectorants, in OTC pain, sleep, cough, and cold preparations. See Appendix B.

diphenoxylate/atropine
(dye-fen-**ox**-i-late/**a**-troe-peen)
Logen, Lomanate, Lomotil, Lonox

difenoxin/atropine
(dye-fen-**ox**-in/**a**-troe-peen)
Motofen

Classification
Therapeutic: antidiarrheals
Pharmacologic: anticholinergics

Schedule V (diphenoxylate/atropine), IV (difenoxin/atropine)

Indications

Adjunctive therapy in the treatment of diarrhea.

Action

Inhibits excess GI motility. Structurally related to opioid analgesics but has no analgesic properties. Atropine added to discourage abuse. **Therapeutic Effects:** Decreased GI motility with subsequent decrease in diarrhea.

Adverse Reactions/Side Effects

CNS: dizziness, confusion, drowsiness, headache, insomnia, nervousness. **EENT:** blurred vision, dry eyes. **CV:** tachycardia. **GI:** constipation, dry mouth, epigastric distress, ileus, nausea, vomiting. **GU:** urinary retention. **Derm:** flushing.

PHYSICAL THERAPY IMPLICATIONS

Examination and Evaluation

- Monitor improvements in GI symptoms (decreased diarrhea) to help document whether drug therapy is successful.
- Assess dizziness that might affect gait, balance, and other functional activities (See Appendix C). Report balance problems and functional limitations to the physician, and caution the patient and family/caregivers to guard against falls and trauma.
- Monitor other CNS side effects such as confusion, drowsiness, blurred vision, headache, nervousness, or insomnia. Report severe or prolonged CNS symptoms to the physician.
- Assess heart rate, ECG, and heart sounds, especially during exercise (See Appendices G, H). Report increased heart rate (tachycardia) or symptoms of other arrhythmias such as palpitations, chest discomfort, shortness of breath, fainting, and fatigue/weakness.

Interventions

- Because of the tachycardia, use caution during aerobic exercise and other forms of therapeutic exercise. Assess exercise tolerance frequently (blood pressure, heart rate, fatigue levels), and terminate exercise immediately if any untoward responses occur (See Appendix L).

Patient/Client-Related Instruction

- Advise patient to avoid alcohol and foods that may increase GI irritation and diarrhea.
- Instruct patient to report other bothersome side effects such as severe or prolonged urinary retention, skin redness/warmth, or GI problems (constipation, nausea, vomiting, heartburn, dry mouth).

Pharmacokinetics

Absorption: Well absorbed from the GI tract.
Distribution: Enters breast milk.
Metabolism and Excretion: *Diphenoxylate*—mostly metabolized by the liver with some conversion to an active antidiarrheal compound (difenoxin). *Difenoxin*—metabolized by the liver. Minimal excretion in urine.
Half-life: *Diphenoxylate*—2.5 hr; *difenoxin*—4.5 hr.

TIME/ACTION PROFILE (antidiarrheal action)

ROUTE	ONSET	PEAK	DURATION
Difenoxin–PO	45–60 min	2 hr	3–4 hr
Diphenoxylate–PO	45–60 min	2 hr	3–4 hr

Contraindications/Precautions

Contraindicated in: Hypersensitivity; Severe liver disease; Infectious diarrhea (due to *Escherichia coli*, *Salmonella*, or *Shigella*); Diarrhea associated with pseudomembranous colitis; Dehydrated patients; Angle-closure glaucoma; Children <2 yr; Known alcohol intolerance (some liquid diphenoxylate/atropine products only).
Use Cautiously in: Patients physically dependent on opioids; Inflammatory bowel disease; Geriatric patients (more sensitive to effects); Children (more sensitive to effects, especially Down's syndrome patients); Prostatic hyperplasia; Pregnancy, lactation, or children <12 yr

(safety not established for difenoxin/atropine in children <12 yr; diphenoxylate/atropine should not be used in children <2 yr).

Interactions

Drug-Drug: Additive CNS depression with other **CNS depressants,** including **alcohol, antihistamines, opioid analgesics,** and **sedative/hypnotics.** Additive anticholinergic properties with other **drugs having anticholinergic properties,** including **tricyclic antidepressants** and **disopyramide.** Use with **MAO inhibitors** may result in hypertensive crisis.
Drug-Natural: Increased anticholinergic effects with **angel's trumpet, jimson weed,** and **scopolia.**

Route/Dosage

Difenoxin/Atropine

Doses given are in terms of difenoxin—each tablet contains 1 mg difenoxin with 0.025 mg of atropine
PO (Adults): 2 tablets initially, then 1 tablet after each loose stool or every 3–4 hr as needed (not to exceed 8 tablets/day).

Diphenoxylate/Atropine

Adult doses given are in terms of diphenoxylate—each tablet contains 2.5 mg diphenoxylate with 0.025 mg of atropine; pediatric doses are given in mg of diphenoxylate and in milliliters of diphenoxylate/atropine liquid; each 5 mL of liquid contains 2.5 mg diphenoxylate with 0.025 mg of atropine.
PO (Adults): 5 mg 3–4 times daily initially, then 5 mg once daily as needed (not to exceed 20 mg/day).
PO (Children): *Use liquid only*—0.3–0.4 mg/kg/day in 4 divided doses.

Availability

Difenoxin/Atropine

Tablets: 1 mg difenoxin/0.025 mg atropine.

Diphenoxylate/Atropine (generic available)

Tablets: 2.5 mg diphenoxylate/0.025 mg atropine.
Liquid (cherry flavor): 2.5 mg diphenoxylate/0.025 mg atropine per 5 mL.

dipyridamole

(dye-pir-**id**-a-mole)
♣ Apo-Dipyridamole, Dipridacot, ♣ Novo-Dipiradol, Persantine, Persantine IV

Classification
Therapeutic: antiplatelet agents, diagnostic agents (coronary vasodilators)
Pharmacologic: platelet adhesion inhibitors

Indications

PO: Prevention of thromboembolism in patients with prosthetic heart valves (with warfarin). Maintains patency after surgical grafting procedures, including coronary artery bypass (with aspirin). **IV:** As an alternative to exercise in myocardial perfusion scintigraphy (cardiac stress testing with radiotracer imaging).

Action

PO: Decreases platelet aggregation by inhibiting the enzyme phosphodiesterase. **IV:** Produces coronary vasodilation by inhibiting adenosine uptake. **Therapeutic Effects: PO:** Inhibition of platelet aggregation and subsequent thromboembolic events. **IV:** In diagnostic thallium imaging, dipyridamole dilates normal coronary arteries, reducing flow to vessels that are narrowed and causing abnormal thallium distribution.

Adverse Reactions/Side Effects

CNS: dizziness, headache, syncope **IV only:** transient cerebral ischemia, weakness. **Resp: IV only:** bronchospasm. **CV: IV only:** MI, hypotension, arrhythmias, flushing. **GI:** nausea, diarrhea, GI upset, vomiting. **Derm:** rash.

PHYSICAL THERAPY IMPLICATIONS

Examination and Evaluation

- Be alert for signs of transient cerebral ischemia, including sudden weakness/numbness on one side of the body, slurred speech, loss of vision, dizziness, and loss of balance and coordination. Report these signs to the physician immediately.
- Watch for symptoms of bronchospasm (wheezing, coughing, tightness in chest), especially after IV administration. Perform pulmonary function tests to quantify suspected changes in ventilation and respiration (See Appendices I, J, K).
- Assess heart rate, ECG, and heart sounds, especially during exercise (See Appendices G, H). Report any rhythm disturbances or symptoms of increased arrhythmias, including palpitations, chest discomfort, shortness of breath, fainting, and fatigue/weakness.
- Assess blood pressure periodically and compare to normal values (See Appendix F). Report low blood pressure (BP) (hypotension), especially if patient experiences dizziness or syncope.
- Assess dizziness that might affect gait, balance, and other functional activities (See Appendix C). Report balance problems and functional limitations to the physician, and caution the patient and family/caregivers to guard against falls and trauma.

Interventions

- Because of the risk of arrhythmias and abnormal BP responses, use caution during aerobic exercise and endurance conditioning. Assess exercise tolerance frequently (BP, heart rate, fatigue levels), and terminate exercise immediately if any untoward responses occur (See Appendix L).

Patient/Client-Related Instruction

- Remind patients to take medication as directed to reduce the risk of thromboembolism or graft occlusion even if they are asymptomatic.
- Counsel patients about additional interventions to help reduce the risk of heart disease, including regular exercise, weight loss, sodium restriction, stress reduction, moderation of alcohol consumption, and smoking cessation.

Pharmacokinetics

Absorption: Moderately absorbed (30–60%) after oral administration.
Distribution: Widely distributed. Crosses the placenta; enters breast milk.
Metabolism and Excretion: Metabolized by the liver; excreted in the bile.
Half-life: 10 hr.
TIME/ACTION PROFILE (PO = antiplatelet activity, IV = coronary vasodilation)

ROUTE	ONSET	PEAK	DURATION
PO	unknown	unknown	unknown
IV	unknown	6.5 min*	30 min

*From start of infusion.

Contraindications/Precautions

Contraindicated in: Hypersensitivity.
Use Cautiously in: Hypotensive patients; Geri: Appears on Beers' list. Geriatric patients may be more susceptible to orthostatic hypotension; Patients with platelet defects; Pregnancy (although safety not established, has been used without harm during pregnancy); Lactation or children <12 yr (safety not established).

Interactions

Drug-Drug: Additive effects with **aspirin** on platelet aggregation. Risk of bleeding may be ↑when used with **anticoagulants, thrombolytic agents, NSAIDs, cefoperazone, cefotetan, valproic acid**, or **sulfinpyrazone**. ↑ risk of hypotension with **alcohol**. **Theophylline** may negate the effects of dipyridamole during diagnostic thallium imaging.

Route/Dosage

PO (Adults): 225–400 mg/day in 3–4 divided doses.
IV (Adults): 570 mcg/kg; maximum dose 60 mg.

Availability (generic available)

Tablets: 25 mg, 50 mg, 75 mg, 100 mg. **Injection:** 5 mg/mL in 2-ml and 10-mL vials. ***In combination with:*** aspirin (Aggrenox). See Appendix B.

dirithromycin
(di-rith-roe-**mye**-sin)
Dynabac

Classification
Therapeutic: anti-infectives
Pharmacologic: macrolides

Indications

Treatment of the following infections: Acute bacterial exacerbations of chronic bronchitis due to *Haemophilus influenzae, Moraxella catarrhalis*, or *Streptococcus pneumoniae*, Secondary bacterial infections of acute bronchitis due to *M. catarrhalis* or *S. pneumoniae*, Community-acquired pneumonia due to *Legionella pneumophila, Mycoplasma pneumoniae*, or *S. pneumoniae*, Pharyngitis/tonsillitis due to *S. pyogenes*, Uncomplicated skin/skin structure infections due to methicillin-susceptible strains of *Staphylococcus aureus* or *S. pyogenes*.

Action

Suppresses protein synthesis at the level of the 50S bacterial ribosome. **Therapeutic Effects:** Bacteriostatic action against susceptible bacteria. **Spectrum:** Active against gram-positive aerobes, including *S. aureus* (methicillin-susceptible), *S. pneumoniae*, and *S. pyogenes*. Active against gram-negative aerobes, including *H. influenzae, L. pneumophila, M. catarrhalis*. Also active against *M. pneumoniae*.

Adverse Reactions/Side Effects

CNS: dizziness/vertigo, headache, insomnia, weakness. **Resp:** dyspnea, increased cough. **GI:** PSEUDOMEMBRANOUS COLITIS, abdominal pain, diarrhea, dyspepsia, flatulence, nausea, vomiting. **GU:** vaginitis. **Derm:** pruritus/urticaria, rash.

PHYSICAL THERAPY IMPLICATIONS

Examination and Evaluation

- Monitor signs of pseudomembranous colitis, including diarrhea, abdominal pain, fever, pus or mucus in stools, and other severe or prolonged GI problems (nausea, vomiting, heartburn). Notify physician or nursing staff of these signs immediately.
- Assess any breathing problems, and report increased cough or difficult, labored breathing.
- Assess dizziness and vertigo that might affect gait, balance, and other functional activities (See Appendix C). Report balance problems and functional limitations to the physician and nursing staff, and caution the patient and family/caregivers to guard against falls and trauma.

Interventions

- Always wash hands thoroughly and disinfect equipment (whirlpools, electrotherapeutic devices, treatment tables, and so forth) to help prevent the spread of infection. Employ universal precautions or isolation procedures as indicated for specific patients.

Patient/Client-related Instruction

- Instruct patient to report other troublesome side effects such as severe or prolonged headache, sleep loss, vaginal irritation, skin reactions (rash, itching, hives), or GI problems (diarrhea, nausea, vomiting, indigestion, abdominal pain).

Pharmacokinetics

Absorption: Dirithromycin is a prodrug. It is converted to erythromycylamine, the active compound, during intestinal absorption, resulting in bioavailability of 10%.
Distribution: *Erythromycylamine*—rapidly and widely distributed, resulting in high tissue concentrations.
Metabolism and Excretion: *Erythromycylamine*—81–97% eliminated in bile (fecal/hepatic route); 2% eliminated in urine.
Half-life: *Erythromycylamine*—2–36 hr.

TIME/ACTION PROFILE (blood levels*)

ROUTE	ONSET	PEAK	DURATION
PO	unknown	4 hr	24 hr

*Of erythromycylamine.

Contraindications/Precautions

Contraindicated in: Hypersensitivity to dirithromycin, erythromycin, or other macrolide anti-infectives; Known, suspected, or potential bacteremia (serum levels are inadequate).
Use Cautiously in: Moderate or severe hepatic impairment; Pregnancy, lactation, or children <12 yr (safety not established).

Interactions

Drug-Drug: Absorption slightly ↑ when used with **antacids** or **H_2-receptor antagonists**. May ↑ blood levels of **triazolam, digoxin, warfarin, ergotamine, cyclosporine, carbamazepine, alfentanil, disopyramide, phenytoin, bromocriptine, valproic acid, lovastatin,** and **simvastatin**.
Drug-Food: Food increases absorption.

Route/Dosage

PO (Adults and Children >12 yr): 500 mg/day as a single dose for 5–14 days (duration depends upon the indication).

Availability

Tablets: 250 mg.

disopyramide
(dye-soe-**peer**-a-mide)
Norpace, Norpace CR, ✱ Rythmodan, Rythmodan-LA

Classification
Therapeutic: antiarrhythmics (class I)

Indications

Suppression/prevention of unifocal and multifocal premature ventricular contractions (PVCs), paired PVCs, and ventricular tachycardia. **Unlabeled Use:** Treatment/prevention of supraventricular tachyarrhythmias.

Action

Decreases myocardial excitability and conduction velocity. Has anticholinergic properties. Little effect on heart rate but has a direct negative inotropic effect.
Therapeutic Effects: Suppression of ventricular arrhythmias.

Adverse Reactions/Side Effects

CNS: dizziness, fatigue, headache. **EENT:** blurred vision, dry eyes, dry throat. **CV:** CHF, arrhythmias, AV block, dyspnea, edema, hypotension. **GI:** constipation, dry mouth, abdominal pain, flatulence, nausea. **GU:** urinary hesitancy, urinary retention. **Endo:** hypoglycemia. **Misc:** impaired temperature regulation.

PHYSICAL THERAPY IMPLICATIONS

Examination and Evaluation

- Watch for signs of congestive heart failure (CHF), including dyspnea, rales/crackles, peripheral edema, jugular venous distention, and exercise intolerance. Report these signs to the physician immediately.
- Assess heart rate, ECG, and heart sounds, especially during exercise (See Appendices G, H). Although intended to treat certain arrhythmias, this drug can unmask or precipitate new arrhythmias (proarrhythmic effect). Report any rhythm disturbances or symptoms of increased arrhythmias, including palpitations, chest pain, shortness of breath, fainting, and fatigue/weakness.
- Assess blood pressure periodically and compare to normal values (See Appendix F). Report low blood pressure (hypotension), especially if patient experiences dizziness or syncope.
- Assess peripheral edema using girth measurements, volume displacement, and measurement of pitting edema (See Appendix N). Report increased swelling in feet and ankles or a sudden increase in body weight due to fluid retention.

- Monitor signs of hypoglycemia, especially during and after exercise. Common neuromuscular symptoms include anxiety, restlessness, tingling in hands/feet/lips/tongue, chills, cold sweats, confusion, difficulty in concentration, drowsiness, nightmares or trouble sleeping, excessive hunger, headache, irritability, nervousness, tremor, weakness, and unsteady gait. Report persistent or repeated episodes of hypoglycemia to the physician.
- Assess dizziness and fatigue that might affect gait, balance, and other functional activities (See Appendix C). Report balance problems and functional limitations to the physician, and caution the patient and family/caregivers to guard against falls and trauma.

Interventions

- Because of the risk of CHF and arrhythmias, use extreme caution during aerobic exercise and other forms of therapeutic exercise. Assess exercise tolerance frequently (blood pressure, heart rate, fatigue levels), and terminate exercise immediately if any untoward responses occur (See Appendix L).
- This drug impairs temperature regulation; use caution during aerobic exercise, especially in hot environments.

Patient/Client-Related Instruction

- Advise patient and family or caregivers about the signs of arrhythmias and CHF (see above under Examination and Evaluation), and to seek immediate medical assistance if these signs develop.
- Instruct patient and family/caregivers to report other side effects such as severe or prolonged headache, vision problems, difficult/labored breathing, urinary hesitancy/retention, or GI problems (nausea, constipation, abdominal pain, dry throat/mouth, flatulence).

Pharmacokinetics

Absorption: Well absorbed from the GI tract.
Distribution: Widely distributed; enters breast milk.
Metabolism and Excretion: Metabolized by the liver; 10% excreted unchanged in the feces, 50% excreted unchanged by the kidneys.
Half-life: 8–18 hr (increased in hepatic or renal impairment).

TIME/ACTION PROFILE (antiarrhythmic effects)

ROUTE	ONSET	PEAK	DURATION
PO	0.5–3.5 hr	2.5 hr	1.5–8.5 hr
PO-CR	0.5–3.5 hr	4.9 hr	12 hr

Contraindications/Precautions

Contraindicated in: Hypersensitivity; Cardiogenic shock; 2nd-degree and 3rd-degree heart block; Sick sinus syndrome (without a pacemaker).
Use Cautiously in: CHF or left ventricular dysfunction (dosage reduction recommended); Hepatic or renal insufficiency (dosage reduction recommended if CCr, ≤40 mL/min); Prostatic enlargement; Myasthenia gravis; Glaucoma; Geri: Appears on Beer' list. May induce heart failure in elderly patients; Children, pregnancy, or lactation (safety not established).

Interactions

Drug-Drug: May potentiate anticoagulant effect of **warfarin**. **Rifampin, phenobarbital**, and **phenytoin** may ↓ blood levels and effectiveness. **Cimetidine** or **erythromycin** may ↓ metabolism and ↑ blood levels. May have additive toxic cardiac effects when used with other **antiarrhythmics** (prolonged conduction and ↓ cardiac output), especially **verapamil**—avoid using disopyramide for 48 hr before or 24 hr after. Anticholinergic side effects may be additive with other **drugs having anticholinergic properties**, including **antihistamines** and **tricyclic antidepressants**. ↑ risk of arrhythmias with **pimozide**.
Drug-Natural: ↑ anticholinergic effects with **angel's trumpet**, **jimson weed**, and **scopolia**.

Route/Dosage

PO (Adults >50 kg): 150 mg q 6 hr (as immediate-release capsules) or 300 mg q 12 hr (as CR or LA dosage form; not to exceed 800 mg/day).
PO (Adults <50 kg or Patients with Poor Left Ventricular Function): 100 mg q 6–8 hr (as immediate-release capsules) or 200 mg q 12 hr (as CR or LA dosage form).
PO (Children 12–18 yr): 6–15 mg/kg daily, in divided doses q 6 hr.
PO (Children 4–12 yr): 10–15 mg/kg daily in divided doses q 6 hr.
PO (Children 1–4 yr): 10–20 mg/kg daily in divided doses q 6 hr.
PO (Children <1 yr): 10–30 mg/kg daily in divided doses q 6 hr.

Renal Impairment

PO (Adults): *CCr >40 mL/min or patients with hepatic impairment*—100 mg q 6 hr; *CCr 30–40 mL/min*—100 mg q 8 hr; *CCr 15–30 mL/min*—100 mg q 12 hr; *CCr <15 mL/min*—100 mg q 24 hr as immediate-release dosage form.

Availability (generic available)

Capsules: 100 mg, 150 mg. **Extended-release capsules:** 100 mg, 150 mg. **Extended-release tablets:** 150 mg. **Injection:** 10 mg/mL.

HIGH ALERT

dobutamine (doe-byoo-ta-meen)

Dobutrex

Classification

Therapeutic: inotropics
Pharmacologic: adrenergics

D

Indications

Short-term (<48 hr) management of heart failure caused by depressed contractility from organic heart disease or surgical procedures.

Action

Stimulates $beta_1$(myocardial)–adrenergic receptors with relatively minor effect on heart rate or peripheral blood vessels. **Therapeutic Effects:** Increased cardiac output without significantly increased heart rate.

Adverse Reactions/Side Effects

CNS: headache. **Resp:** shortness of breath. **CV:** hypertension, increased heart rate, premature ventricular contractions, angina pectoris, arrhythmias, hypotension, palpitations. **GI:** nausea, vomiting. **Local:** phlebitis. **Misc:** hypersensitivity reactions, including skin rash, fever, bronchospasm, or eosinophilia; nonanginal chest pain.

PHYSICAL THERAPY IMPLICATIONS

Examination and Evaluation

- Assess heart rate, ECG, and heart sounds, especially during exercise (See Appendices G, H). Report any rhythm disturbances or symptoms of increased arrhythmias, including palpitations, chest discomfort, shortness of breath, fainting, and fatigue/weakness.
- Assess signs and symptoms of CHF (dyspnea, rales/crackles, peripheral edema, jugular venous distention, exercise intolerance) to help document whether drug therapy is effective in reducing these symptoms.
- Monitor signs of hypersensitivity reactions, including pulmonary symptoms (tightness in the throat and chest, wheezing, cough, dyspnea, chest pain) or skin reactions (rash, pruritus, urticaria). Notify physician or nursing staff immediately if these reactions occur.
- Assess blood pressure (BP) and compare to normal values (See Appendix F). Report changes in BP, either a problematic decrease in BP (hypotension) or a sustained increase in BP (hypertension).
- Assess any signs of phlebitis, including localized pain, redness, or swelling in the affected area. Report these signs to the physician or nursing staff. Avoid ambulation and exercise to the affected extremity while awaiting further tests and evaluation.

Interventions

- Design and implement aerobic exercise and endurance training programs to improve myocardial pumping ability and reduce symptoms of CHF.
- Because of an increased risk of cardiac arrhythmias, use caution during aerobic exercise and endurance conditioning Terminate exercise if patient exhibits untoward symptoms (chest pain, shortness of breath, etc.), or displays other criteria for exercise termination (See Appendix L).

Patient/Client-Related Instruction

- Remind patients to take medication as directed to control CHF even if they are asymptomatic.
- Instruct patients to weigh themselves every day, and call their physician if they gain 3 or more lb in 1 day or more than 5 lb in 1 week. Sudden weight gain may indicate fluid buildup due to worsening heart failure.
- Counsel patients about additional interventions to help control cardiac dysfunction, including regular exercise, weight loss, sodium restriction, stress reduction, moderation of alcohol consumption, and smoking cessation.
- Instruct patient and family/caregivers to report other troublesome side effects such as severe or prolonged headache or GI problems (nausea, vomiting).

Pharmacokinetics

Absorption: Administered by IV infusion only, resulting in complete bioavailability.
Distribution: Unknown.
Metabolism and Excretion: Metabolized by the liver and other tissues.
Half-life: 2 min.

TIME/ACTION PROFILE (inotropic effects)

ROUTE	ONSET	PEAK	DURATION
IV	1–2 min	10 min	brief (min)

Contraindications/Precautions

Contraindicated in: Hypersensitivity to dobutamine or bisulfites; Idiopathic hypertrophic subaortic stenosis.
Use Cautiously in: History of hypertension (increased risk of exaggerated pressor response); MI; Atrial fibrillation (pretreatment with digitalis glycosides recommended); History of ventricular atopic activity (may be exacerbated); Hypovolemia (correct before administration); Pregnancy or lactation (safety not established); Children (has been used safely in children, although risk of tachycardia is increased).

Interactions

Drug-Drug: Use with **nitroprusside** may have a synergistic effect on ↑ cardiac output. **Beta blockers** may negate the effect of dobutamine. ↑ risk of arrhythmias or hypertension with some **anesthetics (cyclopropane, halothane), MAO inhibitors, oxytocics,** or **tricyclic antidepressants.**

Route/Dosage

IV (Adults and Children): Start with low infusion rates (0.5–1 mcg/kg/min), titrated at intervals of a few minutes, guided by the patient's response (range 2–20 mcg/kg/min, up to 40 mcg/kg/min).

Availability

Injection: 12.5 mg/mL in 20-, 40-, and 100-mL vials. **Premixed infusion:** 250 mg/250 mL, 500 mg/500 mL, 500 mg/250 mL, 1000 mg/250 mL.

HIGH ALERT

docetaxel (doe-se-tax-el)

Taxotere

Classification

Therapeutic: antineoplastics
Pharmacologic: taxoids

Indications

Breast cancer (locally advanced/metastatic breast cancer or with doxorubicin and cyclophosphamide as adjuvant treatment of node-positive disease). Non–small-cell lung cancer (locally advanced/metastatic) after failure on platinum regimen or with platinum as initial therapy). Advanced metastatic hormone-refractory prostate cancer (with prednisone). Squamous cell carcinoma of the head and neck (inoperable, locally advanced) with cisplatin and fluorouracil.

Action

Interferes with normal cellular microtubule function required for interphase and mitosis. **Therapeutic Effects:** Death of rapidly replicating cells, particularly malignant ones.

Adverse Reactions/Side Effects

CNS: fatigue, weakness. **Resp:** bronchospasm. **CV:** ASCITES, CARDIAC TAMPONADE, PERICARDIAL EFFUSION, PULMONARY EDEMA, peripheral edema. **GI:** diarrhea, nausea, stomatitis, vomiting. **Derm:** alopecia, rashes, dermatitis, desquamation, edema, erythema, nail disorders. **Hemat:** anemia, thrombocytopenia, leukopenia. **Local:** injection-site reactions. **MS:** myalgia, arthralgia. **Neuro:** neurosensory deficits, peripheral neuropathy. **Misc:** HYPERSENSITIVITY REACTIONS, INCLUDING ANAPHYLAXIS.

PHYSICAL THERAPY IMPLICATIONS

Examination and Evaluation

- Be alert for signs of pericardial effusion and cardiac tamponade, including chest pain, dyspnea, shortness of breath when reclining, dry cough, low-grade fever, fainting, dizziness, tachycardia, and a feeling of anxiety. Report these signs to the physician or nursing staff immediately.
- Assess any breathing problems, bronchospasm, or signs of pulmonary edema, including cough, shortness of breath, chest pain, and labored breathing. Monitor pulse oximetry and perform pulmonary function tests (See Appendices I, J, K) to quantify suspected changes in ventilation and respiratory function.
- Monitor signs of hypersensitivity reactions and anaphylaxis, including pulmonary symptoms (tightness in the throat and chest, wheezing, cough, dyspnea) or skin reactions (rash, pruritus, urticaria). Notify physician or nursing staff immediately if these reactions occur.
- Assess peripheral edema using girth measurements, volume displacement, and measurement of pitting edema (See Appendix N). Report increased swelling in feet and ankles or a sudden increase in body weight due to fluid retention.
- Monitor signs of leukopenia (fever, sore throat, signs of infection), thrombocytopenia (bruising, nose bleeds, bleeding gums), or unusual weakness and fatigue that might be due to anemia. Report these signs to the physician or nursing staff.
- Be alert for signs of peripheral neuropathy (numbness, tingling, decreased muscle strength). Establish baseline electroneuromyographic values using EMG and nerve conduction at the beginning of drug treatment whenever possible, and reexamine these values periodically to document drug-induced changes in peripheral nerve function.
- Assess any muscle or joint pain to rule out musculoskeletal pathology; that is, try to determine if pain is drug-induced rather than caused by anatomic or biomechanical problems.
- Monitor IV injection site for pain, swelling, and inflammation. Report prolonged or excessive injection site reactions to the physician.

Interventions

- For patients who are medically able to begin exercise, implement appropriate resistive exercises and aerobic training to maintain muscle strength and aerobic capacity during cancer chemotherapy or to help restore function after chemotherapy.
- Because of the risk of pericardial and pulmonary effusion, use caution during aerobic exercise and other forms of therapeutic exercise. Assess exercise tolerance frequently (blood pressure, heart rate, respiratory symptoms, fatigue levels), and terminate exercise immediately if any untoward responses occur (See Appendix L).

Patient/Client-Related Instruction

- Advise patient to guard against infection (frequent hand washing, etc.), and to avoid crowds and contact with persons with contagious diseases.
- Advise patient and family/caregivers that fatigue and weakness are likely and may be severe. Functional

abilities may be limited, and patient may need to use assistive devices during ambulation.

- Advise patient about the likelihood of GI reactions (nausea, vomiting, diarrhea, irritation in/around the mouth). Instruct patient or family and caregivers to report other severe or unexpected GI problems.
- Advise patient that hair loss and other skin reactions (rashes, inflammation, peeling/shedding of skin) are likely. Instruct patient to report severe or unexpected skin problems.

Pharmacokinetics

Absorption: IV administration results in complete bioavailability.
Distribution: Unknown.
Metabolism and Excretion: Extensively metabolized by the liver; metabolites undergo fecal elimination.
Half-life: 11.1 hr.

TIME/ACTION PROFILE (effect on blood counts)

ROUTE	ONSET	PEAK	DURATION
IV	rapid	5–9 days	7 days

Contraindications/Precautions

Contraindicated in: Hypersensitivity; Hypersensitivity to polysorbate 80; Known alcohol intolerance; Neutrophil count <1500/mm³; Liver impairment (serum bilirubin > upper limit of normal, ALT and/or AST >1.5 times upper limit of normal, with alkaline phosphatase >2.5 times upper limit of normal); OB: Pregnancy or lactation.
Use Cautiously in: OB: Patients with childbearing potential.

Interactions

Drug-Drug: ↑ bone marrow depression may occur with other **antineoplastics** or **radiation therapy**. **Cyclosporine**, **ketoconazole**, **erythromycin**, or **troleandomycin** may significantly alter the effects of docetaxel.

Route/Dosage

IV (Adults): *Breast cancer*—60–100 mg/m² every 3 wk; *Breast cancer adjuvant therapy*—75 mg/m² every 3 wk for 6 cycles (with doxorubicin and cyclophosphamide); *Non–small-cell lung cancer*—75 mg/m² every 3 wk (alone or with platinum); *Prostate cancer*—75 mg/m² every 3 wk (with oral prednisone); *Squamous cell cancer*—75 mg/m² every 3 wks for 4 cycles (with cisplatin and fluorouracil).

Availability

Injection concentrate: 20 mg/0.5 mL polysorbate 80 with diluent (13% ethanol), 80 mg/2 mL polysorbate 80 with diluent (13% ethanol).

docosanol (doe-koe-sa-nole)

Abreva

Classification
Therapeutic: antivirals (topical)

Indications

Treatment of recurrent oral-facial herpes simplex (cold sores, fever blisters).

Action

Prevents herpes simplex virus from entering cells by preventing viral particles from fusing with cell membranes. **Therapeutic Effects:** Reduced healing time. Decreased duration of symptoms (pain, burning, itching, tingling).

Adverse Reactions/Side Effects

All local reactions occurred at site of application
Local: acne, skin, itching, rash.

PHYSICAL THERAPY IMPLICATIONS

Examination and Evaluation

- Assess skin and mucosal lesions to help determine if drug therapy is successful in controlling infection. Report any local irritation or skin reactions (rash, itching, acne) at the application site.

Interventions

- Avoid contact with cutaneous or mucosal lesions when treating patient.
- Always wash hands thoroughly and disinfect equipment (whirlpools, electrotherapeutic devices, treatment tables, and so forth) to help prevent the spread of infection. Use universal precautions as indicated for specific patients.

Patient/Client-Related Instruction

- Advise patient to apply medication as directed. Docosanol should not be used more frequently or longer than prescribed.
- Remind patient that docosanol does not cure herpes infections. The virus lies dormant in nerve cells, and this drug will not prevent the spread of infection to others.

Pharmacokinetics

Absorption: Unknown.
Distribution: Unknown.
Metabolism and Excretion: Unknown.
Half-life: Unknown.

TIME/ACTION PROFILE

ROUTE	ONSET	PEAK	DURATION
Topical	unknown	unknown	unknown

Contraindications/Precautions

Contraindicated in: Hypersensitivity to docosanol or any other components of the formulation (benzyl alcohol, mineral oil, propylene glycol, or sucrose).
Use Cautiously in: Children <12 yr (safety not established); Pregnancy (use only if clearly needed).

Interactions

Drug-Drug: None significant.

Route/Dosage

Topical (Adults and Children ≥12 yr): Apply small amount 5 times daily to sores on lips or face until healed.

Availability

Cream: 10% cream in 2-g tubes OTC.

docusate (dok-yoo-sate)

docusate calcium

DC Softgels, Dioctocal, Pro-Cal-Sof, Sulfolax, Surfak

docusate sodium

Colace, Correctol Stool Softener Soft Gels, Diocto, Docu, Docusoft S, DOK, DOS Softgels, DOS, DOSS, DSS, Dulcolax Stool Softener, Ex-Lax Stool Softener, Fleet Sof-Lax, Modane Soft, Philliips Liqui-Gels, Regulax-SS, Regulex, Silace, ✱ Soflax, Stool Softener, Therevac SB

Classification
Therapeutic: laxatives
Pharmacologic: stool softeners

Indications

PO: Prevention of constipation (in patients who should avoid straining, such as after MI or rectal surgery).
Rectal: Used as enema to soften fecal impaction.

Action

Promotes incorporation of water into stool, resulting in softer fecal mass. May also promote electrolyte and water secretion into the colon. **Therapeutic Effects:** Softening and passage of stool.

Adverse Reactions/Side Effects

EENT: throat irritation. **GI:** mild cramps. **Derm:** rashes.

PHYSICAL THERAPY IMPLICATIONS

Examination and Evaluation

- Monitor any rashes or other abnormal skin responses. Report excessive or prolonged skin reactions to the physician.

Interventions

- Instruct patient how to breathe and avoid straining during bowel movements to prevent a Valsalva maneuver.

Patient/Client-Related Instruction

- Advise patient to avoid overuse of laxatives. Encourage patient to use other forms of bowel regulation, such as increasing fiber and bulk in the diet, increasing fluid intake, and regular exercise.
- Advise patient to report other troublesome side effects such as prolonged or severe throat irritation or abdominal cramps.

Pharmacokinetics

Absorption: Small amounts may be absorbed from the small intestine after oral administration. Absorption from the rectum is not known.
Distribution: Unknown.
Metabolism and Excretion: Amounts absorbed after oral administration are eliminated in bile.
Half-life: Unknown.

TIME/ACTION PROFILE (softening of stool)

ROUTE	ONSET	PEAK	DURATION
PO	24–48 hr (up to 3–5 days)	unknown	unknown
Rectal	2–15 min	unknown	unknown

Contraindications/Precautions

Contraindicated in: Hypersensitivity; Abdominal pain, nausea, or vomiting, especially when associated with fever or other signs of an acute abdomen.
Use Cautiously in: Excessive or prolonged use may lead to dependence; Should not be used if prompt results are desired; OB/Lactation: Has been used safely.

Interactions

Drug-Drug: None significant.

Route/Dosage

Docusate Calcium

PO (Adults): 240 mg once daily.

Docusate Sodium

PO (Adults and Children >12 yr): 50–400 mg in 1–4 divided doses.
PO (Children 6–12 yr): 40–150 mg in 1–4 divided doses.
PO (Children 3–6 yr): 20–60 mg in 1–4 divided doses.
PO (Children <3 yr): 10–40 mg in 1–4 divided doses.
Rect (Adults): 50–100 mg or 1 unit containing 283 mg docusate sodium, soft soap, and glycerin.

Availability (generic available)

Docusate Calcium

Capsules: 240 mg OTC.

Docusate Sodium (generic available)

Tablets: 100 mg OTC. **Capsules:** 50 mg OTC, 100 mg OTC, 120 mg OTC, 240 mg OTC, 250 mg OTC.

Syrup: 20 mg/5 mL OTC. **Liquid:** 150 mg/15 mL OTC. **Enema:** 283 mg/5 mL OTC. ***In combination with:*** stimulant laxatives OTC. See Appendix B.

dofetilide (doe-fet-i-lide)

Tikosyn

Classification

Therapeutic: antiarrhythmics (class III)

Pharmacologic: methanesulfonanilides

Indications

Maintenance of normal sinus rhythm (delay in time to recurrence of atrial fibrillation/atrial flutter [AF/AFl]) in patients with AF/AFl lasting more than 1 wk, and who have been converted to normal sinus rhythm. For the conversion of atrial fibrillation and atrial flutter to normal sinus rhythm.

Action

Blocks cardiac ion channels responsible for transport of potassium. Increases monophasic action potential duration. Increases effective refractory period. **Therapeutic Effects:** Prevention of recurrent AF/AFl. Conversion of AF/AFl to normal sinus rhythm.

Adverse Reactions/Side Effects

CNS: dizziness, headache. **CV:** VENTRICULAR ARRHYTHMIAS, chest pain, QT interval prolongation.

PHYSICAL THERAPY IMPLICATIONS

Examination and Evaluation

- Assess heart rate, ECG, and heart sounds, especially during exercise (See Appendices G, H). Although intended to treat certain arrhythmias, this drug can unmask or precipitate new arrhythmias (proarrhythmic effect). Report any rhythm disturbances or symptoms of increased arrhythmias, including palpitations, chest pain, shortness of breath, fainting, and fatigue/weakness.
- Assess dizziness that might affect gait, balance, and other functional activities (See Appendix C). Report balance problems and functional limitations to the physician, and caution the patient and family /caregivers to guard against falls and trauma.

Interventions

- Because of the risk of arrhythmias, use extreme caution during aerobic exercise and other forms of therapeutic exercise. Assess exercise tolerance frequently (blood pressure, heart rate, fatigue levels), and terminate exercise immediately if any untoward responses occur (See Appendix L).

Patient/Client-Related Instruction

- Advise patient and family or caregivers about the signs of arrhythmias (see above under Examination and Evaluation), and to seek immediate medical assistance if these signs develop.
- Instruct patient and family/caregivers to report other side effects such as severe or prolonged headache or chest pain.

Pharmacokinetics

Absorption: Well absorbed (>90%) following oral administration.

Distribution: Unknown.

Metabolism and Excretion: 80% excreted by kidneys via cationic renal secretion, mostly as unchanged drug; 20% excreted as inactive metabolites; some metabolism in the liver via cytochrome P450 system (CYP3A4 isoenzyme).

Half-life: 10 hr.

TIME/ACTION PROFILE (blood levels)

ROUTE	ONSET	PEAK	DURATION
PO	within hours	2–3 hr*	12–24 hr

*Steady-state levels are achieved after 2–3 days.

Contraindications/Precautions

Contraindicated in: Hypersensitivity; Congenital or acquired prolonged QT syndromes; Baseline QT interval or QTc of >440 msec (500 msec in patients with ventricular conduction abnormalities); Creatinine clearance (CCr) <20 mL/min; Concurrent use of verapamil or agents which inhibit the renal cation transport system, including cimetidine, ketoconazole, trimethoprim, megestrol, or prochlorperazine; Concurrent use of hydrochlorothiazide; OB: Lactation (use should be avoided).

Use Cautiously in: Underlying electrolyte abnormalities (increased risk of serious arrhythmias; correct prior to administration); CCr 20–60 mL/min (dosage reduction recommended); Severe hepatic impairment; OB: Pregnancy (use only when benefit to patient outweighs potential risk to fetus); Pedi: Children <18 yr (safety not established).

Interactions

Drug-Drug: Hydrochlorothiazide ↑ dofetilide levels and the risk of QT prolongation with arrhythmias; concurrent use in contraindicated. Concurrent use of renal cation transport inhibitors, including **cimetidine, trimethoprim,** and **ketoconazole,** ↑ blood levels and the risk of serious arrhythmias and is contraindicated. **Amiloride, metformin, megestrol, prochlorperazine,** and **triamterene** may have similar effects. **Phenothiazines, tricyclic**

antidepressants, some **macrolides** (including **erythromycin and telithromycin**), and **fluoroquinolones** may prolong QT interval and ↑ risk of arrhythmias; concurrent use is not recommended. Blood levels and risk of arrhythmias is also ↑ by **verapamil**; concurrent use is contraindicated and a 2-day washout period is recommended). Inhibitors of the cytochrome P450 system (CY P4503A4 isoenzyme), including **macrolide anti-infectives, azole antifungals, protease inhibitor antiretrovirals, SSRI antidepressants, amiodarone, cannabinoids, diltiazem, nefazodone, quinine**, and **zafirlukast**, may also ↑ blood levels and the risk of arrhythmias and concurrent use should be undertaken with caution. Should not be used concurrently with other **class I** or **III antiarrhythmics** due to ↑ risk of arrhythmias. **Phenothiazines** and **tricyclic antidepressants** also prolong QT interval and should not be used concurrently with dofetilide. Hypokalemia or hypomagnesemia from **potassium-depleting diuretics** ↑ the risk of arrhythmias; correct abnormalities prior to administration. Concurrent use of **digoxin** may also ↑ the risk of arrhythmias.

Drug-Food: Grapefruit juice may ↑ levels; avoid concurrent use.

Route/Dosage

Dosing should be adjusted according to renal function and assessment of QT interval.

PO (Adults): *Starting dose*—500 mcg twice daily; *maintenance dose*—250 mcg twice daily (not to exceed 500 mcg twice daily).

Renal Impairment

PO (Adults): *CCr 40–60 mL/min Starting dose*—250 mcg twice daily; *maintenance dose*—125 mcg twice daily; *CCr 20–40 mL/min Starting dose*—125 mcg twice daily; *maintenance dose*—125 mcg once daily.

Availability

Capsules: 125 mcg, 250 mcg, 500 mcg.

dolasetron (doe-**las**-e-tron)

Anzemet

Classification

Therapeutic: antiemetics

Pharmacologic: 5-HT_3 antagonists

Indications

Prevention of nausea and vomiting associated with emetogenic chemotherapy. Prevention and treatment of postoperative nausea/vomiting.

Action

Blocks the effects of serotonin at receptor sites (selective antagonist) located in vagal nerve terminals and in the chemoreceptor trigger zone in the CNS. **Therapeutic Effects:** Decreased incidence and severity of nausea/vomiting associated with emetogenic chemotherapy or surgery.

Adverse Reactions/Side Effects

CNS: headache (increased in cancer patients), dizziness, fatigue, syncope. **CV:** bradycardia, ECG changes, hypertension, hypotension, tachycardia. **GI:** diarrhea, dyspepsia. **GU:** oliguria. **Derm:** pruritus. **Misc:** chills, fever, pain.

PHYSICAL THERAPY IMPLICATIONS

Examination and Evaluation

- Monitor improvements in GI symptoms (nausea, vomiting) to help document whether drug therapy is successful.
- Assess heart rate, ECG, and heart sounds, especially during exercise (See Appendices G, H). Report any rhythm disturbances or symptoms of increased arrhythmias, including palpitations, chest discomfort, shortness of breath, fainting, and fatigue/weakness.
- Assess blood pressure (BP) and compare to normal values (See Appendix F). Report changes in BP, either a problematic decrease in BP (hypotension) or a sustained increase in BP (hypertension).
- Assess any unexplained or unusual pain to rule out musculoskeletal pathology; that is, try to determine if pain is drug-induced rather than caused by anatomic or biomechanical problems.
- Assess dizziness or syncope that affects gait, balance, and other functional activities (See Appendix C). Report balance problems and functional limitations to the physician and nursing staff, and caution the patient and family/caregivers to guard against falls and trauma.

Interventions

- Because of the risk of arrhythmias and abnormal BP responses, use caution during aerobic exercise and other forms of therapeutic exercise. Assess exercise tolerance frequently (BP, heart rate, fatigue levels), and terminate exercise immediately if any untoward responses occur (See Appendix L).

Patient/Client-Related Instruction

- Instruct patient to report bothersome or prolonged side effects, including headache, itching skin, problems with urination, chills, fever, or GI effects (diarrhea, indigestion).

Pharmacokinetics

Absorption: Well absorbed but rapidly metabolized to hydrodolasetron, the active metabolite.
Distribution: Unknown.
Metabolism and Excretion: 61% of hydrodolasetron is excreted unchanged by the kidneys.
Half-life: *Hydrodolasetron*—8.1 hr (shorter in children).

TIME/ACTION PROFILE (antiemetic effect)

ROUTE	ONSET	PEAK	DURATION
PO	unknown	1–2 hr	up to 24 hr
IV	unknown	15–30 min	up to 24 hr

Contraindications/Precautions

Contraindicated in: Hypersensitivity.
Use Cautiously in: Patients with risk factors for prolongation of cardiac conduction intervals (hypokalemia, hypomagnesemia, concurrent diuretic or antiarrhythmic therapy, congenital QT syndrome, cumulative high-dose anthracycline therapy); Pregnancy or lactation (safety not established).

Interactions

Drug-Drug: Concurrent **diuretic** or **antiarrhythmic** therapy or cumulative **high-dose anthracycline therapy** may ↑ risk of conduction abnormalities. Blood levels and effects of hydrodolasteron are ↑ by **atenolol** and **cimetidine**. Blood levels and effects of hydrodolasetron are ↓ by **rifampin**.

Route/Dosage

Prevention of Chemotherapy-Induced Nausea/Vomiting

PO (Adults): 100 mg given within 1 hr before chemotherapy.
PO (Children 2–16 yr): 1.8 mg/kg given within 1 hr before chemotherapy (not to exceed 100 mg).
IV (Adults and Children ≥2 yr): 1.8 mg/kg given 30 min before chemotherapy (usual dose in adults is 100 mg; not to exceed 100 mg in children).

Prevention/Treatment of Postoperative Nausea/Vomiting

PO (Adults): 100 mg given within 2 hr before surgery.
PO (Children 2–16 yr): 1.2 mg/kg (up to 100 mg/dose) given within 2 hr before surgery.
IV (Adults): 12.5 mg given 15 min before cessation of anesthesia (prevention) or as soon as nausea or vomiting begins (treatment).
IV (Children 2–16 yr): 0.35 mg/kg (up to 12.5 mg) given 15 min before cessation of anesthesia (prevention) or as soon as nausea or vomiting begins (treatment).

Availability

Tablets: 50 mg, 100 mg. **Injection:** 12.5 mg/0.625–mL ampules, 20 mg/mL in 5-mL vials.

D

HIGH ALERT

dopamine (dope-a-meen)

Intropin, ✱ Revimine

Classification
Therapeutic: inotropics, vasopressors
Pharmacologic: adrenergics

Indications

Adjunct to standard measures to improve: Blood pressure, Cardiac output, Urine output in treatment of shock unresponsive to fluid replacement.

Action

Small doses (0.5–3 mcg/kg/min) stimulate dopaminergic receptors, producing renal vasodilation. Larger doses (2–10 mcg/kg/min) stimulate dopaminergic and beta1-adrenergic receptors, producing cardiac stimulation and renal vasodilation. Doses >10 mcg/kg/min stimulate alpha-adrenergic receptors and may cause renal vasoconstriction. **Therapeutic Effects:** Increased cardiac output, increased blood pressure, and improved renal blood flow.

Adverse Reactions/Side Effects

CNS: headache. **EENT:** mydriasis (high dose). **Resp:** dyspnea. **CV:** arrhythmias, hypotension, angina, ECG change, palpitations, vasoconstriction. **GI:** nausea, vomiting. **Derm:** piloerection. **Local:** irritation at IV site.

PHYSICAL THERAPY IMPLICATIONS

Examination and Evaluation

- Assess blood pressure (BP) and compare to normal values (See Appendix F). Report whether drug therapy is successful in normalizing BP in patients with shock and other cardiac conditions.
- Assess heart rate, ECG, and heart sounds, especially during exercise (See Appendices G, H). Report any rhythm disturbances or symptoms of increased arrhythmias, including palpitations, chest discomfort, shortness of breath, fainting, and fatigue/weakness.
- Monitor urine output whenever possible, and report decreased urine output, cloudy urine, or sudden weight gain due to fluid retention.
- Monitor signs of peripheral vasoconstriction, such as extreme coldness in the hands and feet, cyanosis, and muscle cramping. Notify physician of severe or prolonged signs of vasoconstriction.

- Monitor IV injection site for pain, swelling, and irritation. Report prolonged or excessive injection-site reactions to the physician.

Interventions

- Because of an increased risk of cardiac arrhythmias and compromised cardiac output, use caution during aerobic exercise and endurance conditioning. Terminate exercise if patient exhibits untoward symptoms (chest pain, shortness of breath, etc.) or displays other criteria for exercise termination (see Appendix L).

Patient/Client-Related Instruction

- Instruct patient or family/caregivers to report other troublesome side effects such as severe or prolonged headache, dilated pupils (mydriasis), or GI problems (nausea, vomiting).

Pharmacokinetics

Absorption: Administered IV only, resulting in complete bioavailability.
Distribution: Widely distributed but does not cross the blood-brain barrier.
Metabolism and Excretion: Metabolized in liver, kidneys, and plasma.
Half-life: 2 min.

TIME/ACTION PROFILE (hemodynamic effects)

ROUTE	ONSET	PEAK	DURATION
IV	1–2 min	up to 10 min	<10 min

Contraindications/Precautions

Contraindicated in: Tachyarrhythmias; Pheochromocytoma; Hypersensitivity to bisulfites (some products).
Use Cautiously in: Hypovolemia; Myocardial infarction; Occlusive vascular diseases; Geri: Older patients may be more susceptible to adverse effects; OB/Pedi: Pregnancy, lactation, and children (safety not established).

Interactions

Drug-Drug: Use with **MAO inhibitors, ergot alkaloids (ergotamine), doxapram, guanadrel,** or some **antidepressants** results in severe hypertension. Use with IV **phenytoin** may cause hypotension and bradycardia. Use with **general anesthetics** may result in arrhythmias. **Beta blockers** may antagonize cardiac effects.

Route/Dosage

IV (Adults): *Dopaminergic (renal vasodilation) effects*—0.5–3 mcg/kg/min. *Beta-adrenergic (cardiac stimulation) effects*—2–10 mcg/kg/min. *Alpha-adrenergic (increased peripheral vascular resistance) effects*—10 mcg/kg/min; infusion rate may be ↑ as needed.
IV (Children): 5–20 mcg/kg/min, depending on desired response (0.5–3 mcg/kg/min has been used to improve renal blood flow).

Availability (generic available)

Injection for dilution: 40 mg/mL, 80 mg/mL, 160 mg/mL. **Premixed injection:** 200 mg/250 mL, 400 mg/250 mL, 800 mg/250 mL, 800 mg/500 mL.

doripenem (doe-ri-pen-em)

Doribax

Classification
Therapeutic: anti-infectives
Pharmacologic: carbapenems

Indications

Infections caused by susceptible organisms, including complicated intra-abdominal infections, complicated urinary tract infections, including pyelonephritis.

Action

Inhibits bacterial cell wall formation. **Therapeutic Effects:** Bactericidal action against susceptible bacteria.
Spectrum: Active against the following gram-positive organisms: *Acinetobacter baumannii*, *Escherichia coli*, *Klebsiella pneumonia*, *Proteus mirabilis*, and *Pseudomonas aeruginosa*. Also active against the following gram-negative organisms: *Streptococcus constellatus* and *S. intermedius*. Anaerobic spectrum includes *Bacteroides caccae*, *B. fragilis*, *B. thetaiotaomicron*, *B. uniformis*, *B. vulgatus*, and *Peptostreptococcus micros*.

Adverse Reactions/Side Effects

CV: headache. **GI:** PSEUDOMEMBRANOUS COLITIS, diarrhea, nausea, ↑ liver enzymes. **Hemat:** anemia. **Local:** phlebitis. **Misc:** ALLERGIC REACTIONS, INCLUDING ANAPHYLAXIS, infection with resistant organisms, superinfection.

PHYSICAL THERAPY IMPLICATIONS

Examination and Evaluation

- Monitor signs of pseudomembranous colitis, including diarrhea, abdominal pain, fever, pus or mucus in stools, and other severe or prolonged GI problems (nausea, vomiting, heartburn). Notify physician or nursing staff immediately of these signs.
- Monitor signs of allergic reactions and anaphylaxis, including pulmonary symptoms (tightness in the throat and chest, wheezing, cough dyspnea) or skin reactions (rash, pruritus, urticaria). Notify physician or nursing staff immediately if these reactions occur.
- Monitor signs of anemia, including unusual fatigue, shortness of breath with exertion, and bruising. Report these signs to the physician or nursing staff.
- Assess injection site during and after IV administration, and report signs of phlebitis such as local pain, swelling, and inflammation.

Interventions

- Always wash hands thoroughly and disinfect equipment (whirlpools, electrotherapeutic devices, treatment tables, and so forth) to help prevent the spread of infection. Use universal precautions or isolation procedures as indicated for specific patients.

Patient/Client-Related Instruction

- Instruct patient to notify physician immediately of signs of superinfection, including black, furry overgrowth on tongue, vaginal itching or discharge, and loose or foul-smelling stools.
- Instruct patient and family/caregivers to report other troublesome side effects such as severe or prolonged headache or GI problems (nausea, diarrhea).

Pharmacokinetics

Absorption: IV administration results in complete bioavailability.
Distribution: Penetrates renal and peritoneal and retroperitoneal tissues and fluids.
Metabolism and Excretion: Mostly excreted unchanged in urine; minimal metabolism.
Half-life: 1 hr.

TIME/ACTION PROFILE (blood levels)

ROUTE	ONSET	PEAK	DURATION
IV	unknown	end of infusion	8 hr*

*Normal renal function.

Contraindications/Precautions

Contraindicated in: Hypersensitivity to doripenem, other carbapenems, or beta-lactams.
Use Cautiously in: Geri: Consider age-related decrease in renal function when choosing dose; OB: Use cautiously during lactation; Pedi: Safe use in children has not been established.

Interactions

Drug-Drug: None noted.
Drug-Natural: May ↓ blood levels of **valproic acid**; this may result in loss of seizure control. **Probenecid** ↓ renal clearance and ↑ blood levels.

Route/Dosage

IV (Adults): 500 mg every 8 hr.

Renal Impairment

IV (Adults): *CCr 30–50 mL/min*—250 mg every 8 hr; *CCr >10–<30 mL/min*—250 mg every 12 hr.

Availability

Powder for injection (requires reconstitution): 500 mg/vial.

dornase alfa (dor-nase al-fa)

Pulmozyme

Classification
Therapeutic: cystic fibrosis therapy adjuncts
Pharmacologic: pulmonary enzymes

D

Indications

Adjunct management (with standard therapy) of cystic fibrosis.

Action

Breaks down excessive amounts of DNA found in the respiratory tract of patients with cystic fibrosis. Excessive DNA contributes to increased sputum viscosity and risk of infection. **Therapeutic Effects:** Decreased infection rates and requirement for parenteral anti-infectives. Improved pulmonary function.

Adverse Reactions/Side Effects

EENT: sore throat, voice alteration, conjunctivitis, hoarseness, rhinitis. **Resp:** cough, dyspnea. **CV:** chest pain. **Derm:** rash. **Misc:** fever.

PHYSICAL THERAPY IMPLICATIONS

Examination and Evaluation

- Assess the quantity and consistency of sputum to help document whether this drug is successful in reducing the viscosity of respiratory secretions.
- Monitor any chest pain and attempt to determine if pain is drug-induced or caused by cardiovascular dysfunction (e.g., angina that occurs during exercise).
- Assess any breathing problems, and report severe or persistent cough or difficult, labored breathing.

Interventions

- When implementing airway clearance techniques or other pulmonary interventions, attempt to intervene when the drug has produced mucolytic effects. Effects typically begin 15 min after inhalation.
- Design and implement breathing exercises to maximize ventilation and help prevent infections caused by pulmonary congestion.

Patient/Client-Related Instruction

- Counsel patient and family/caregivers on proper inhalation techniques. Emphasize the need to adhere to the recommended dose and frequency of inhalations.
- Instruct patient and family/caregivers to report other troublesome side effects such as severe or prolonged headache, skin rash, fever, nasal inflammation, eye irritation, sore throat, hoarseness, or voice changes.

Pharmacokinetics
Absorption: Negligible absorption following inhalation.
Distribution: Action is primarily local.
Metabolism and Excretion: Unknown.
Half-life: Unknown.

TIME/ACTION PROFILE (effect on noted parameters)

ROUTE	ONSET	PEAK	DURATION
Inhalation	within 15 min*	3 days–1 wk† weeks–months‡	48 hr

*Significant concentrations in sputum.

†Improvement in respiratory function.

‡Decreased incidence of respiratory tract infections.

Contraindications/Precautions
Contraindicated in: Hypersensitivity to dornase alfa or Chinese Hamster Ovary cell products.
Use Cautiously in: Children (incidence of cough, rhinitis, and rash is increased); Pregnancy or lactation (safety not established).

Interactions
Drug-Drug: None significant.

Route/Dosage
Inhaln (Adults and Children): 2.5 mg 1–2 times daily.

Availability
Solution for inhalation: 1 mg/mL in 2.5-mL single-use ampules.

doxapram (dox-a-pram)
Dopram

Classification
Therapeutic: central nervous system stimulants
Pharmacologic: pyrrolidinones

Indications
Used in carefully selected short-term situations with other supportive measures to treat postoperative patients with respiratory depression secondary to anesthesia. Prevention of acute hypercapnia during administration of oxygen to patients with acute respiratory insufficiency due to COPD (short-term only—less than 2 hr). Treatment of mild-to-moderate respiratory and CNS depression due to drug overdosage.

Action
In low doses, stimulates breathing by activating carotid receptors. Larger doses directly stimulate the respiratory center in medulla as well as produce generalized CNS stimulation. **Therapeutic Effects:** Transient increase in tidal volume, small increase in respiratory rate. Oxygenation is not increased.

Adverse Reactions/Side Effects
CNS: SEIZURES, apprehension, disorientation, dizziness, headache. **EENT:** gagging, mydriasis. **Resp:** LARYNGOSPASM, bronchospasm, cough, dyspnea, hiccups, rebound hypoventilation, tachypnea. **CV:** arrhythmias, changes in heart rate, chest pain, hypertension, T-wave inversion. **GI:** diarrhea, nausea, vomiting. **GU:** albuminuria, perineal/genital burning sensation, spontaneous voiding, urinary retention. **Derm:** flushing, pruritus, sweating. **Hemat:** hemolysis. **Local:** phlebitis. **MS:** involuntary movement, muscle spasticity, skeletal muscle hyperactivity. **Neuro:** generalized clonus, paresthesia, positive bilateral Babinski's sign. **Misc:** fever.

PHYSICAL THERAPY IMPLICATIONS

Examination and Evaluation
- Be alert for new seizures or increased seizure activity, especially at the onset of drug treatment. Document the number, duration, and severity of seizures, and report these findings immediately to the physician or nursing staff.
- Monitor signs of laryngeal spasm and bronchospasm such as wheezing, cough, dyspnea, and tightness in chest and throat. Notify physician or nursing staff immediately.
- Assess respiratory function using pulse oximetry and pulmonary function tests (see Appendix I) to help determine if drug therapy is successful in improving respiratory depression and normalizing blood gases.
- Assess heart rate, ECG, and heart sounds (See Appendices G, H). Report any rhythm disturbances or symptoms of increased arrhythmias, including palpitations, chest pain, shortness of breath, fainting, and fatigue/weakness.
- Assess blood pressure (BP) and compare to normal values (See Appendix F). Report a sustained increase in BP (hypertension).
- Assess dizziness that might affect gait, balance, and other functional activities (See Appendix C). Report balance problems and functional limitations to the physician and nursing staff, and caution the patient and family/caregivers to guard against falls and trauma.
- Monitor and report other changes in mood and behavior, including apprehension or disorientation.
- Assess any muscle hyperactivity, spasticity, involuntary movements, or numbness and tingling. Report severe or prolonged neuromuscular symptoms.

- Assess injection site during and after IV administration, and report signs of phlebitis (local pain, swelling, inflammation).

Interventions

- Because of the risk of cardiac effects (arrhythmias, hypertension) and residual respiratory depression, use caution during therapeutic exercise. Assess exercise tolerance frequently (BP, heart rate, fatigue levels), and terminate exercise immediately if any untoward responses occur (See Appendix L).

Patient/Client-Related Instruction

- Instruct patient to report severe or prolonged headache, fever, urinary problems, skin reactions (itching flushing, increased sweating), or GI problems (nausea, diarrhea, vomiting).

Pharmacokinetics

Absorption: Administered IV only; results in complete bioavailability.
Distribution: Unknown.
Metabolism and Excretion: Rapidly metabolized; metabolites mostly excreted by the kidneys.
Half-life: 2.4–4 hr.

TIME/ACTION PROFILE (increases in minute volume)

ROUTE	ONSET	PEAK	DURATION
IV	20–40 sec	1–2 min	5–12 min

Contraindications/Precautions

Contraindicated in: Hypersensitivity; Patients on mechanical ventilation; Head trauma; Seizures; Flail chest; Pulmonary embolism; Pneumothorax; Pulmonary fibrosis; Acute asthma; Extreme dyspnea; Cardiovascular or cerebrovascular disease; Newborns (contains benzyl alcohol).
Use Cautiously in: Patients with a history of asthma or arrhythmias; Hyperthyroidism; Pheochromocytoma; Serious uncorrected metabolic disorders; Hepatic or renal impairment; Pregnancy, lactation, or children <12 yr (safety not established).

Interactions

Drug-Drug: Pressor effects may be ↑ by concurrent use of **adrenergic amines** (sympathomimetics) or **MAO inhibitors**. May mask residual effects of **skeletal muscle relaxants**. Initial release of epinephrine caused by doxapram may cause adverse reactions when given concurrently with **anesthetics** known to sensitize the myocardium to the effects of catecholamines (wait 10 min following discontinuation of anesthetic to administer doxapram). Concurrent use with **aminophylline** or **theophylline** may worsen skeletal muscle hyperactivity.

Route/Dosage

Respiratory Depression Following Anesthesia

IV (Adults): *Intermittent injection*—0.5–1 mg/kg (not to exceed 1.5 mg/kg) initially; may repeat every 5 min to a total of 2 mg/kg. *Infusion*—Initiate at 5 mg/min until response is obtained; then decrease infusion rate to 1–3 mg/min (total dose by infusion method should not exceed 4 mg/kg).

Drug-Induced CNS Depression

IV (Adults): *Intermittent injection*—Give priming dose of 1–2 mg/kg; repeat in 5 min. May repeat at 1- to 2-hr intervals until sustained consciousness or total of 3 g/24 hr given. *Infusion*—Give priming dose of 1–2 mg/kg by direct injection; repeat in 5 min. If no response, continue supportive measures for 1–2 hr and repeat priming dose. If some respiratory stimulation occurs, initiate infusion at 1–3 mg/min. Discontinue infusion if patient begins to awaken or after 2 hr. Infusion may be restarted (along with priming dose) after rest interval of 30–120 min. Do not exceed 3 g/24 hr.

Acute Hypercapnia Secondary to COPD

IV (Adults): *Infusion*—1–2 mg/min (up to 3 mg/min). Should not be used for more than 2 hr.

Availability

Injection: 20 mg/mL.

doxazosin (dox-ay-zoe-sin)

Cardura

Classification
Therapeutic: antihypertensives
Pharmacologic: peripherally-acting antiadrenergics

Indications

Hypertension (alone or with other agents). Symptomatic benign prostatic hyperplasia (BPH).

Action

Dilates both arteries and veins by blocking postsynaptic alpha$_1$-adrenergic receptors. **Therapeutic Effects:** Lowering of blood pressure.

Adverse Reactions/Side Effects

CNS: dizziness, headache, depression, drowsiness, fatigue, nervousness, weakness. **EENT:** abnormal vision, blurred vision, conjunctivitis, epistaxis. **Resp:** dyspnea. **CV:** first-dose orthostatic hypotension, arrhythmias, chest pain, edema, palpitations. **GI:** abdominal discomfort, constipation, diarrhea, dry mouth, flatulence, nausea, vomiting. **GU:** decreased libido, sexual dysfunction. **Derm:** flushing, rash, urticaria. **MS:** arthralgia, arthritis, gout, myalgia.

PHYSICAL THERAPY IMPLICATIONS

Examination and Evaluation

- Assess blood pressure periodically and compare to normal values (see Appendix F). Document whether drug therapy is successful in controlling hypertension. Also, be alert for a fall in blood pressure (BP) and related symptoms (dizziness, syncope) that occur when the patient changes position (orthostatic hypotension), especially after the initial doses. Document orthostatic hypotension and contact physician when systolic BP falls >20 mm Hg or diastolic BP falls >10 mm Hg.
- If treating BPH, monitor signs such as difficulty starting a urine stream, painful urination, weak urine flow, feeling that the bladder is not completely empty, frequent nighttime urination, and an urge to urinate again soon after urinating. Document any change in BPH symptoms to help determine the effects of drug therapy.
- Assess heart rate, ECG, and heart sounds, especially during exercise (See Appendices G, H). Report any rhythm disturbances or symptoms of increased arrhythmias, including palpitations, chest discomfort, shortness of breath, fainting, and fatigue/weakness.
- Assess dizziness and weakness that might affect gait, balance, and other functional activities (See Appendix C). Report balance problems and functional limitations to the physician, and caution the patient and family/caregivers to guard against falls and trauma.
- Be alert for signs of depression, nervousness, or other changes in mood and behavior. Notify physician if these changes become problematic.
- Assess peripheral edema using girth measurements, volume displacement, and measurement of pitting edema (See Appendix N). Report increased swelling in feet and ankles or a sudden increase in body weight due to fluid retention.
- Assess any breathing problems, and report signs of difficult or labored breathing.
- Assess any back or joint pain to rule out musculoskeletal pathology; that is, try to determine if pain is drug induced rather than caused by anatomic or biomechanical problems.

Interventions

- Because of the risk of arrhythmias and abnormal BP responses, use caution during aerobic exercise and other forms of therapeutic exercise. Assess exercise tolerance frequently (BP, heart rate, fatigue levels), and terminate exercise immediately if any untoward responses occur (See Appendix L).
- Avoid physical therapy interventions that cause systemic vasodilation (large whirlpool, Hubbard tank). Additive effects of this drug and the intervention may cause a dangerous fall in BP.
- To minimize orthostatic hypotension, advise patient to move slowly when assuming a more upright position.

Patient/Client-Related Instruction

- Remind patients to take medication as directed to control hypertension even if they are asymptomatic.
- Counsel patients about additional interventions to help control BP, such as regular exercise, weight loss, sodium restriction, stress reduction, moderation of alcohol consumption, and smoking cessation.
- When treating BPH, advise patient that urinary symptoms (retention, dribbling, hesitancy, urgency) should improve, and to contact the physician if these symptoms continue to worsen.
- Instruct patient or family/caregivers to report other bothersome side effects such as severe or prolonged headache, drowsiness, vision disturbances, nosebleeds, sexual dysfunction, skin reactions (rash, hives, flushing), or GI problems (constipation, diarrhea, nausea, vomiting, flatulence, dry mouth).

Pharmacokinetics

Absorption: Well absorbed following oral administration.
Distribution: Probably enters breast milk; rest of distribution unknown.
Protein Binding: 98–99%.
Metabolism and Excretion: Extensively metabolized by the liver.
Half-life: 22 hr.

TIME/ACTION PROFILE (antihypertensive effect)

ROUTE	ONSET	PEAK	DURATION
PO	1–2 hr	2–6 hr	24 hr

Contraindications/Precautions

Contraindicated in: Hypersensitivity.
Use Cautiously in: Hepatic dysfunction and impaired renal function; Geri: Appears on Beers' list. Geriatric patients are at increased risk for hypotension and renal impairment; Pregnancy, lactation, or children (safety not established).

Interactions

Drug-Drug: ↑ risk of hypotension with acute ingestion of **alcohol, sildenafil, vardenafil,** other **antihypertensives**, or **nitrates**. May ↓ antihypertensive effect of **clonidine**.

Route/Dosage

PO (Adults): *Hypertension*—1 mg once daily, may be gradually increased at 2-wk intervals to 2–16 mg/day; incidence of postural hypotension greatly increased at doses >4 mg/day. *BPH*—1 mg once daily, may be gradually increased to 8 mg/day.

Availability (generic available)

Tablets: 1 mg, 2 mg, 4 mg, 8 mg.

doxepin (dox-e-pin)

Sinequan, Triadapin, Zonalon

Classification

Therapeutic: antianxiety agents, antidepressants, antihistamines (topical)

Pharmacologic: tricyclic antidepressants

Indications

PO: Depression. **Topical:** Short-term control of pruritus associated with Eczematous dermatitis, Lichen simplex chronicus. **Unlabeled Use: PO:** Chronic pain syndromes: Pruritus, Dermatitis, Anxiety, Insomnia.

Action

PO: Prevents the reuptake of norepinephrine and serotonin by presynaptic neurons; resultant accumulation of neurotransmitters potentiates their activity. Also possesses significant anticholinergic properties. **Topical:** Antipruritic action due to antihistaminic properties. **Therapeutic Effects: PO:** Relief of depression. Decreased anxiety. **Topical:** Decreased pruritus.

Adverse Reactions/Side Effects

CNS: fatigue, sedation, agitation, confusion, hallucinations. **EENT:** blurred vision, increased intraocular pressure. **CV:** hypotension, arrhythmias, ECG abnormalities. **GI:** constipation, dry mouth, hepatitis, increased appetite, weight gain, nausea, paralytic ileus. **GU:** urinary retention, decreased libido. **Derm:** photosensitivity, rashes. **Hemat:** blood dyscrasias. **Misc:** hypersensitivity reactions.

PHYSICAL THERAPY IMPLICATIONS

Examination and Evaluation

- Measure blood pressure periodically and compare to normal values (See Appendix F). Report low blood pressure (hypotension), especially if patient experiences dizziness or syncope.
- Assess heart rate, ECG, and heart sounds, especially during exercise (see Appendixes G, H). Report any rhythm disturbances or symptoms of increased arrhythmias, including palpitations, chest discomfort, shortness of breath, fainting, and fatigue/weakness.
- Monitor signs of hypersensitivity reactions, including pulmonary symptoms (tightness in the throat and chest, wheezing, cough, dyspnea) or skin reactions (rash, pruritus, urticaria). Notify physician immediately if these reactions occur.
- Watch for signs of leukopenia (fever, sore throat, signs of infection), thrombocytopenia (bruising, nose bleeds, bleeding gums), or unusual weakness and fatigue that might be due to anemia or other blood dyscrasias. Report these signs to the physician.
- Be alert for increased depression and suicidal thoughts and ideology, especially when initiating drug treatment or in children and teenagers. Notify physician or mental health professional immediately if patient exhibits worsening depression or other changes in mood and behavior.
- Monitor any confusion, agitation, hallucinations, or other alterations in cognitive function (See Appendix D). Notify physician promptly if these symptoms develop.
- If used to treat chronic pain, assess pain levels periodically to help document drug efficacy.
- If treating skin disorders, monitor skin lesions and related symptoms (redness, burning, itching) to help assess drug efficacy.
- Periodically assess body weight and other anthropometric measures (body mass index, body composition). Report a rapid or unexplained weight gain or increased body fat.

Interventions

- Guard against falls and trauma (hip fractures, head injury, and so forth), and implement fall-prevention strategies (See Appendix E).
- Because of the risk of cardiac arrhythmias and hypotension, use caution during aerobic exercise and endurance conditioning. Assess exercise tolerance frequently (blood pressure, heart rate, fatigue levels), and terminate exercise immediately if any untoward responses occur (See Appendix L).
- To minimize orthostatic hypotension, patient should move slowly when assuming a more upright position.
- Help patient explore nonpharmacologic methods to reduce depression and anxiety (exercise, counseling, support groups, and so forth).
- If treating neuropathic pain or other pain syndromes, implement appropriate interventions (physical agents, manual techniques, therapeutic exercise) to manage pain and reduce the need for drug therapy. Help patient also explore other nonpharmacologic methods to reduce chronic pain (relaxation techniques, imagery, counseling, and so forth).
- Causes photosensitivity; use care if administering UV treatments. Advise patient to avoid direct

sunlight and use sunscreens and protective clothing.

Patient/Client-Related Instruction

- Advise patient that antidepressant effects may not occur immediately; it may take 2 wk or more before an improvement in mood is observed.
- Advise patient to avoid alcohol and other CNS depressants because of the increased risk of sedation and adverse effects.
- Instruct patient to report GI problems such as nausea and constipation, and also to report signs of drug-induced hepatitis, including anorexia, abdominal pain, severe nausea and vomiting, yellow skin or eyes, skin rashes, flu-like symptoms, and muscle/joint pain.
- Instruct patient to report other troublesome side effects such as severe or prolonged headache, dry eyes/mouth, blurred vision, urinary retention, and decreased libido.

Pharmacokinetics

Absorption: Well absorbed from the GI tract, although much is metabolized on first pass through the liver. Some systemic absorption follows topical application.
Distribution: Widely distributed. Enters breast milk; probably crosses the placenta.
Metabolism and Excretion: Metabolized by the liver. Some conversion to active antidepressant compound. May reenter gastric juice via secretion from enterohepatic circulation, where more absorption may occur.
Half-life: 8–25 hr.

TIME/ACTION PROFILE (antidepressant activity)

ROUTE	ONSET	PEAK	DURATION
PO	2–3 wk	up to 6 wk	days–weeks

Contraindications/Precautions

Contraindicated in: Hypersensitivity; Some products contain bisulfites and should be avoided in patients with known intolerance; Untreated angle-closure glaucoma; Period immediately after myocardial infarction; history of QTc prolongation, heart failure, cardiac arrhythmia.
Use Cautiously in: Geri: Preexisting cardiovascular disease (↑ risk of adverse reactions); Prostatic enlargement (more susceptible to urinary retention); Seizures; OB: Use during pregnancy only if potential maternal benefit outweighs risks to fetus; use during lactation may result in neonatal sedation. Recommend discontinue drug or bottle feed; Pedi: May ↑ risk of suicide attempt/ideation especially during dose early treatment or dose adjustment; risk may be greater in children or adolescents; Pedi: Safety not established in children <12 yr); Geri: Appears on Beers' list and is associated with ↑ falls risk secondary to anticholinergic and sedative effects. Geriatric patients should have initial dosage reduction.

Interactions

Apply to both topical and oral uses
Drug-Drug: Doxepin is metabolized in the liver by the cytochrome P450 2D6 enzyme and its action may be affected by drugs that compete for metabolism by this enzyme, including other **antidepressants, phenothiazines, carbamazepine, class 1C antiarrhythmics (propafenone, flecainide)**; when used concurrently, dosage ↓ of one or the other or both may be necessary. Concurrent use of other drugs that inhibit the activity of the enzyme, including **cimetidine, quinidine, amiodarone**, and **ritonavir**, may result in ↑ effects of doxepin. May cause hypotension, tachycardia, and potentially fatal reactions when used with **MAO inhibitors** (avoid concurrent use—discontinue 2 wk prior to doxepin). Concurrent use with **SSRI antidepressants** may result in ↑ toxicity and should be avoided (fluoxetine should be stopped 5 wk before). Concurrent use with **clonidine** may result in hypertensive crisis and should be avoided. Concurrent use with **levodopa** may result in delayed/↓ absorption of levodopa or hypertension. Blood levels and effects may be ↓ by **rifamycins**. ↑ CNS depression with other **CNS depressants**, including **alcohol, antihistamines, clonidine, opioid analgesics**, and **sedative/hypnotics. Barbiturates** may alter blood levels and effects. **Adrenergic** and **anticholinergic** side effects may be ↑ with other **agents having these properties. Phenothiazines** or **hormonal contraceptives** ↑ levels and may cause toxicity. **Smoking** may ↑ metabolism and alter effects.
Drug-Natural: Concomitant use of **kava, valerian**, or **chamomile** can ↑ CNS depression. ↑ anticholinergic effects with **jimson weed** and **scopolia**.

Route/Dosage

PO (Adults): *Antidepressant/anti-anxiety*—25 mg 3 times daily, may be ↑ as needed (up to 150 mg/day in outpatients or 300 mg/day in inpatients; some patients may require only 25–50 mg/day). Once stabilized, entire daily dose may be given at bedtime. *Antipruritic*—10 mg at bedtime initially, may be ↑ up to 25 mg.
PO (Geriatric Patients): *Antidepressant*—25–50 mg/day initially, may be ↑ as needed.
Topical (Adults): Apply 4 times daily (wait 3–4 hr between applications) for up to 8 days.

Availability (generic available)

Capsules: 10 mg, 25 mg, 50 mg, 75 mg, 100 mg, 150 mg. **Oral concentrate:** 10 mg/mL. **Topical cream:** 5%.

HIGH ALERT

doxorubicin hydrochloride (dox-oh-**roo**-bi-sin hye-droe-**klor**-ide)
Adriamycin PFS, Adriamycin RDF, Rubex

doxorubicin, liposomal (dox-oh-**roo**-bi-sin **lye**-poe-sohm-al)
Doxil

Classification
Therapeutic: antineoplastics
Pharmacologic: anthracyclines

Indications
Doxorubicin hydrochloride: Alone or with other modalities in the treatment of various solid tumors, including Breast, Ovarian, Bladder, Bronchogenic carcinoma, Malignant lymphomas and leukemias. Doxorubicin, liposomal: AIDS-related Kaposi's sarcoma (KS) in patients who cannot tolerate or fail conventional therapy. Ovarian carcinoma. Multiple myeloma with bortezomib in patients who have not previously received bortezomib and have received at least one prior therapy.

Action
Inhibits DNA and RNA synthesis by forming a complex with DNA; action is cell-cycle S-phase–specific. Also has immunosuppressive properties. **Therapeutic Effects:** Death of rapidly replicating cells, particularly malignant ones.

Adverse Reactions/Side Effects
CNS: weakness. **Resp:** recall pneumonitis. **CV:** CARDIOMYOPATHY, ECG changes. **GI:** diarrhea, esophagitis, nausea, stomatitis, vomiting. **GU:** red urine. **Derm:** alopecia, palmar-plantar erythrodysesthesia (liposomal), photosensitivity. **Endo:** sterility, prepubertal growth failure with temporary gonadal impairment (children only). **Hemat:** anemia, leukopenia, thrombocytopenia. **Local:** phlebitis at IV site, tissue necrosis. **Metab:** hyperuricemia. **Misc:** ANAPHYLACTOID ALLERGIC REACTIONS, acute infusion-related reactions, fever.

PHYSICAL THERAPY IMPLICATIONS

Examination and Evaluation
- Be alert for signs of cardiomyopathy, including fatigue, dizziness, palpitations, breathlessness with exertion, and peripheral and pulmonary edema. Report these signs to the physician or nursing staff immediately.
- Monitor signs of allergic reactions and anaphylaxis, including pulmonary symptoms (tightness in the throat and chest, wheezing, cough, dyspnea) or skin reactions (rash, pruritus, urticaria). Be especially alert for allergy-like responses that occur during and immediately after administration (acute infusion-related events). Notify physician or nursing staff immediately if these reactions occur.
- Assess heart rate, ECG, and heart sounds, especially during exercise (See Appendices G, H). Report any rhythm disturbances or symptoms of increased arrhythmias, including palpitations, chest discomfort, shortness of breath, fainting, and fatigue/weakness.
- Be alert for signs of respiratory distress (dyspnea, cough, shortness of breath, fever, rales), in patients that received radiation treatments to the chest (recall pneumonitis). Report these signs to the physician immediately.
- Watch for signs of leukopenia (fever, sore throat, signs of infection), thrombocytopenia (bruising, nose bleeds, bleeding gums), or unusual weakness and fatigue that might be due to anemia. Report these signs to the physician or nursing staff.
- Monitor IV injection site for pain, swelling, and inflammation (phlebitis). Report signs of phlebitis, tissue necrosis, or other prolonged or excessive injection site reactions to the physician.

Interventions
- For patients who are medically able to begin exercise, implement appropriate resistive exercises and aerobic training to maintain muscle strength and aerobic capacity during cancer chemotherapy, or to help restore function after chemotherapy.
- Because of the risk of cardiomyopathy and arrhythmias, use caution during aerobic exercise and other forms of therapeutic exercise. Assess exercise tolerance frequently (blood pressure, heart rate, respiratory symptoms, fatigue levels), and terminate exercise immediately if any untoward responses occur (See Appendix L).
- Causes photosensitivity; use care if administering UV treatments. Advise patient to avoid direct sunlight and use sunscreens and protective clothing.

Patient/Client-Related Instruction
- Advise patient about the likelihood of GI reactions such as nausea, vomiting, diarrhea, heartburn, and irritation in or around the mouth. Instruct patient or family and caregivers to report other severe or unexpected GI problems.

- Advise patient that hair loss and other skin reactions are likely. Patients and family/caregivers should also be alert for palmar-plantar erythrodysesthesia (foot-hand syndrome), which causes pain, redness, and dry, scaly skin on the palms of the hands and soles of the feet. Instruct patient to protect the hands and feet from heat and friction, and to apply lotion to the affected areas. Superficial cold application can also temporarily reduce symptoms.
- Advise patient to guard against infection (frequent hand washing, etc.), and to avoid crowds and contact with persons with contagious diseases.

Pharmacokinetics

Absorption: Administered IV only, resulting in complete bioavailability.
Distribution: Widely distributed; does not cross the blood-brain barrier; extensively bound to tissues.
Metabolism and Excretion: Mostly metabolized by the liver. Converted by liver to an active compound. Excreted predominantly in the bile, 50% as unchanged drug. Less than 5% eliminated unchanged in the urine.
Half-life: 16.7 hr.

TIME/ACTION PROFILE (effect on blood counts)

ROUTE	ONSET	PEAK	DURATION
IV	10 days	14 days	21–24 days
IV (liposomal)	10 days	14 days	21–24 days

Contraindications/Precautions

Contraindicated in: Hypersensitivity; Pregnancy or lactation.
Use Cautiously in: History of cardiac disease or high cumulative doses of anthracyclines; Depressed bone marrow reserve; Liver impairment (reduce dose if serum bilirubin >1.2 mg/dL); Children, geriatric patients, mediastinal radiation, concurrent cyclophosphamide (risk of cardiotoxicity); Patients with childbearing potential.

Interactions

Drug-Drug: ↑ bone marrow depression with other **antineoplastics** or **radiation therapy**. Pediatric patients who have received concurrent doxorubicin and **dactinomycin** have an ↑ risk of recall pneumonitis at variable times following local radiation therapy. May ↑ skin reactions at previous **radiation therapy** sites. If **paclitaxel** is administered first, clearance of doxorubicin is ↓ and the incidence and severity of neutropenia and stomatitis are ↑ (problem is diminished if doxorubicin is administered first). Hematologic toxicity is ↑ and prolonged by concurrent use of **cyclosporine**; risk of coma and seizures is also ↑. Incidence and severity of neutropenia and thrombocytopenia are ↑ by concurrent **progesterone**. **Phenobarbital** may ↑ clearance and decrease effects of doxorubicin. Doxorubicin may ↓ metabolism and ↑ effects of **phenytoin**. **Streptozocin** may ↑ the half-life of doxorubicin (dosage ↓ of doxorubicin recommended). May ↑ risk of hemorrhagic cystitis from **cyclophosphamide** or hepatitis from **mercaptopurine**. Cardiac toxicity may be ↑ by **radiation therapy** or **cyclophosphamide**. May ↓ antibody response to **live-virus vaccines** and ↑ risk of adverse reactions.

Route/Dosage

Doxorubicin hydrochloride: Other regimens are used.
IV (Adults): 60–75 mg/m² daily, repeat q 21 days; or 25–30 mg/m² daily for 2–3 days, repeat q 3–4 wk or 20 mg/m²/wk. Total cumulative dose should not exceed 550 mg/m² without monitoring of cardiac function or 400 mg/m² in patients with previous chest radiation or other cardiotoxic chemotherapy.
IV (Children): 30 mg/m²/day for 3 days every 4 wk.

Hepatic Impairment

IV (Adults): Serum bilirubin 1.2–3 mg/dL—50% of usual dose; serum bilirubin 3.1–5 mg/dL—25% of usual dose.

Doxorubicin, liposomal: Other regimens are used.
IV (Adults): *AIDS-related KS*—20 mg/m² every 3 wk; *Metastatic ovarian cancer*—40–50 mg/m² every 4 wk; *Multiple myeloma*—30 mg/m² on day 4 after following bortezomib for up to 8 cycles.

Availability (generic available)

Powder for injection: 10-mg, 20-mg, 50-mg, 100-mg, 150-mg vials. **Injection:** 2 mg/mL.
Liposomal dispersion for injection: 20 mg/10 mL in 10-mL and 2-mL vials.

doxycycline* (dox-i-**sye**-kleen)

Apo-Doxy, Doryx, Doxy, Doxy Caps, ✱Doxycin, Monodox, Novo-Doxylin, Oracea, Periostat, Vibramycin, Vibra-Tabs

Classification
Therapeutic: anti-infectives
Pharmacologic: tetracyclines

*As the recommendations for treating/preventing anthrax are still evolving, all health care professionals are urged to check the most current recommendations at the Centers for Disease Control and Prevention Web site (www.bt.cdc.gov).

Indications

Treatment of various infections caused by unusual organisms, including *Mycoplasma*, *Chlamydia*, *Rickettsia*, *Borrelia burgdorferi*. Treatment of inhalational anthrax (postexposure) and cutaneous anthrax. Treatment of gonorrhea and syphilis in penicillin-allergic patients. Prevention of exacerbations of chronic bronchitis. Treatment of acne. Treatment of inflammatory lesions associated with rosacea (Oracea only). Malaria prophylaxis.

Action

Inhibits bacterial protein synthesis at the level of the 30S bacterial ribosome. Low-dose products used in the management of periodontitis inhibit collagenase. **Therapeutic Effects:** Bacteriostatic action against susceptible bacteria. **Spectrum:** Includes activity against some gram-positive pathogens: *Bacillus anthracis* (anthrax), *Clostridium perfringens*, *C. tetani*, *Listeria monocytogenes*, *Nocardia*, *Propionibacterium acnes*, *Actinomyces israelii*. Active against some gram-negative pathogens: *Haemophilus influenzae*, *Legionella pneumophila*, *Yersinia enterocolitica*, *Y. pestis*, *Neisseria gonorrhoeae*, *N. meningitidis*. Also active against several other pathogens, including *Mycoplasma*, *Treponema pallidum*, *Chlamydia*, *Rickettsia*, *Borrelia burgdorferi*.

Adverse Reactions/Side Effects

CNS: benign intracranial hypertension (higher in children). **GI:** PSEUDOMEMBRANOUS COLITIS, diarrhea, nausea, vomiting, esophagitis, hepatotoxicity, pancreatitis. **Derm:** photosensitivity, rashes. **Hemat:** blood dyscrasias. **Local:** phlebitis at IV site. **Misc:** hypersensitivity reactions, superinfection.

PHYSICAL THERAPY IMPLICATIONS

Examination and Evaluation

- Monitor signs of pseudomembranous colitis, including diarrhea, abdominal pain, fever, pus or mucus in stools, and other severe or prolonged GI problems (nausea, vomiting, heartburn). Notify physician or nursing staff immediately of these signs.
- Monitor signs of hypersensitivity reactions or anaphylaxis, including pulmonary symptoms (tightness in the throat and chest, wheezing, cough dyspnea) or skin reactions (rash, angioedema, pruritus, urticaria). Notify physician or nursing staff immediately if these reactions occur.
- Monitor signs of leukopenia (fever, sore throat, signs of infection), thrombocytopenia (bruising, nose bleeds, and bleeding gums), or unusual weakness and fatigue that might be due to anemia or other blood dyscrasias. Report these signs to physician or nursing staff.
- Monitor and report signs of benign intracranial hypertension, especially in children. Signs include dizziness, headache, tinnitus, nausea, and disturbed vision (e.g., blurry or double vision).
- Monitor IV injection site for pain, swelling, and irritation. Report prolonged or excessive injection-site reactions to the physician.

Interventions

- Always wash hands thoroughly and disinfect equipment (whirlpools, electrotherapeutic devices, treatment tables, and so forth) to help prevent the spread of infection. Employ universal precautions or isolation procedures as indicated for specific patients.
- Because of the risk of intracranial hypertension, avoid activities that might increase intracranial pressure such as elevating the feet above the head (Trendelenburg's position) or holding breath and straining during a bowel movement (Valsalva's maneuver).
- Causes photosensitivity; use care if administering UV treatments.

Patient/Client-Related Instruction

- Instruct patient to notify physician immediately of signs of superinfection, including black, furry overgrowth on tongue, vaginal itching or discharge, and loose or foul-smelling stools.
- Advise patient about the likelihood of GI reactions (nausea, vomiting, diarrhea, heartburn). Instruct patient to report severe or prolonged GI problems, signs of liver toxicity (yellow skin or eyes, abdominal pain, severe nausea and vomiting, fever, sore throat, malaise, weakness, facial edema), or pancreatitis (upper abdominal pain after eating, indigestion, weight loss, oily stools).
- Advise patient about photosensitivity, and to use sunscreens, protective clothing, and avoid prolonged sun exposure. Advise patient to also report any rashes or other skin reactions.

Pharmacokinetics

Absorption: Well absorbed from the GI tract.
Distribution: Widely distributed, some CSF and good bone penetration; crosses placenta and enters breast milk.
Metabolism and Excretion: 20–40% excreted unchanged in urine; some inactivation in intestine and some enterohepatic circulation with excretion in bile and feces.
Half-life: 14–17 hr (↑ in severe renal impairment).

TIME/ACTION PROFILE (blood levels)

ROUTE	ONSET	PEAK	DURATION
PO	1–2 hr	1.5–4 hr	12 hr
IV	rapid	end of infusion	12 hr

Contraindications/Precautions

Contraindicated in: Hypersensitivity; Some products contain alcohol or bisulfites and should be avoided in patients with known hypersensitivity or intolerance.
Use Cautiously in: Cachectic or debilitated patients; Renal disease; Hepatic impairment; Nephrogenic diabetes insipidus; OB: Pregnancy—risk of permanent staining of teeth in infant if used during last half of pregnancy; Lactation/Pedi: Lactation or children <8 yr—permanent staining of teeth (unless used for anthrax; doxycycline may be used to treat anthrax in pregnant women and children due to the seriousness of the disease).

Interactions

Drug-Drug: May ↑ effect of **warfarin.** May ↓ effectiveness of **estrogen-containing oral contraceptives. Antacids, calcium, iron,** and **magnesium** form insoluble compounds (chelates) and ↓ absorption of tetracyclines; this effect is least with doxycycline. **Cholestyramine** or **colestipol** ↓ absorption of tetracyclines. **Adsorbent antidiarrheals** may ↓ absorption. **Barbiturates, carbamazepine,** or **phenytoin** may ↓ the activity of doxycycline.
Drug-Food: Calcium in foods or **dairy products** ↓ absorption by forming insoluble compounds (chelates); this effect is minimal with doxycycline.

Route/Dosage

More common infections

PO (Adults and Children >45 kg): *Most infections*—100 mg q 12 hr on the 1st day, then 100–200 mg once daily or 50–100 mg q 12 hr; *Gonorrhea*—100 mg q 12 hr for 7 days or 300 mg followed 1 hr later by another 300-mg dose; *Malaria prophylaxis*—100 mg once daily; *Lyme disease*—100 mg twice daily; *Periodontitis*—20 mg twice daily; *Rosacea*—40 mg once daily in morning.

Inhalational anthrax

PO, IV (Adults): 100 mg q 12 hr IV change to 100 mg PO twice daily when clinically appropriate for a total of 60 days; 1 or 2 other anti-infectives may be added initially, depending on clinical situation.
PO, IV (Children >8 yr and >45 kg): 100 mg q 12 hr IV change to 100 mg twice daily PO when clinically appropriate for a total of 60 days; 1 or 2 other anti-infectives may be added initially, depending on clinical situation.
PO, IV (Children >8 yr ≤45 kg): 2.2 mg/kg q 12 hr IV change to 2.2 mg/kg twice daily PO when clinically appropriate for a total of 60 days; 1 or 2 other anti-infectives may be added initially, depending on clinical situation.
PO, IV (Children ≤8 yr): 2.2 mg/kg q 12 hr IV change to 2.2 mg/kg twice daily PO when clinically appropriate for a total of 60 days; 1 or 2 other anti-infectives may be added initially, depending on clinical situation.

Cutaneous anthrax

PO (Adults): 100 mg twice daily for 60 days; some patients may require intravenous therapy initially, depending on clinical situation.
PO (Children >8 yr and >45 kg): 100 mg q 12 hr; some patients may require intravenous therapy initially, depending on clinical situation.
PO (Children >8 yr and ≤45 kg): 2.2 mg/kg q 12 hr; some patients may require intravenous therapy initially, depending on clinical situation.
PO (Children ≤8 yr): 2.2 mg/kg q 12 hr; some patients may require intravenous therapy initially, depending on clinical situation.

Availability (generic available)

Tablets: 20 mg, 50 mg, 75 mg, 100 mg, 150 mg. **Capsules:** 50 mg, 75 mg, 100 mg. **Delayed-release capsules:** 100 mg. **Variable-release capsules (Oracea):** 40 mg. **Delayed-release tablets:** 75 mg, 100 mg, 150 mg. **Oral suspension (raspberry flavor):** 25 mg/5 mL. **Syrup (raspberry-apple flavor):** 50 mg/5 mL. **Powder for injection:** 100 mg.

dronabinol (droe-**nab**-i-nol)

Marinol

Other Names:
delta-9-tetrahydrocannabinol, THC

Classification
Therapeutic: antiemetics
Pharmacologic: cannabinoids

Schedule III

Indications

Prevention of serious nausea and vomiting from cancer chemotherapy when other more conventional agents have failed. Management of anorexia associated with weight loss in patients with AIDS.

Action

Active ingredient in marijuana. Has a wide variety of CNS effects, including inhibition of the vomiting control mechanism in the medulla oblongata. **Therapeutic Effects:** Suppression of nausea and vomiting. Increased appetite in patients with AIDS.

Adverse Reactions/Side Effects

CNS: <u>anxiety</u>, <u>concentration difficulty</u>, <u>confusion</u>, <u>dizziness</u>, <u>drowsiness</u>, <u>mood change</u>, abnormal thinking, depression, disorientation, hallucinations, headache, impaired judgment, memory lapse, paranoia. **EENT:** <u>dry mouth</u>. **CV:** palpitations, syncope, tachycardia. **GI:** abdominal pain, nausea, vomiting. **Derm:** facial flushing. **Neuro:** ataxia, paresthesia. **Misc:** physical dependence, psychologic dependence (high doses or prolonged therapy).

PHYSICAL THERAPY IMPLICATIONS

Examination and Evaluation

- Monitor improvements in GI symptoms (decreased nausea and vomiting, increased appetite) to help determine if drug therapy is successful.
- Assess dizziness, drowsiness, or ataxia that might affect gait, balance, and other functional activities (See Appendix C). Report balance problems and functional limitations to the physician and nursing staff, and caution the patient and family/caregivers to guard against falls and trauma.
- Assess heart rate, ECG, and heart sounds, especially during exercise (See Appendices G, H). Report fast heart rate (tachycardia) and symptoms of other arrhythmias, including palpitations, chest discomfort, shortness of breath, fainting, and fatigue/weakness.
- Monitor changes in mood and behavior such as anxiety, confusion, depression, disorientation, paranoia, memory lapses, impaired concentration, and hallucinations. Notify physician if these changes become problematic.
- Assess signs of paresthesia, including numbness, tingling, and muscle weakness. Perform objective tests, including electroneuromyography and sensory testing to document any drug-related neuropathic changes.

Interventions

- Because of the risk of arrhythmias, use caution during aerobic exercise and other forms of therapeutic exercise. Assess exercise tolerance frequently (blood pressure, heart rate, fatigue levels), and terminate exercise immediately if any untoward responses occur (See Appendix L).

Patient/Client-Related Instruction

- Advise patient about the risk of daytime drowsiness and decreased attention and mental focus. Use care if driving or in other activities that require strong concentration.
- Educate patient about the risk of physical and psychologic dependence during excessive or prolonged use; encourage patient to adhere to proper dosing schedule.
- Instruct patient to report bothersome GI side effects such as severe or prolonged nausea, vomiting, abdominal pain, or dry mouth.

Pharmacokinetics

Absorption: Extensively metabolized following absorption, resulting in poor bioavailability (10–20%).
Distribution: Enters breast milk in high concentrations. Highly lipid soluble. Persists in tissues for prolonged period of time.
Protein Binding: 97%.
Metabolism and Excretion: Extensively metabolized; 50% excreted via biliary elimination. At least 1 metabolite is psychoactive.
Half-life: 25–36 hr.

TIME/ACTION PROFILE (antiemetic effect)

ROUTE	ONSET	PEAK	DURATION
PO	unknown	2–4 hr	4–6 hr*

*Appetite stimulation lasts 24 hr or longer.

Contraindications/Precautions

Contraindicated in: Hypersensitivity to dronabinol, marijuana, or sesame oil; Nausea and vomiting due to any other causes; Lactation: Lactation.
Use Cautiously in: Patients with history of substance abuse; Cardiovascular disease (due to potential adverse effects); Mania, depression, or schizophrenia (use may worsen these conditions); Patients taking sedatives, hypnotics, or other psychoactive drugs (increased risk of adverse effects); Geri: ↑ risk of adverse effects; OB/Pedi: Safety and efficacy not established.

Interactions

Drug-Drug: Additive CNS depression with **alcohol, antihistamines, barbiturates, benzodiazepines, atropine, scopolamine, lithium, buspirone, muscle relaxants, opioid analgesics, tricyclic antidepressants,** and **sedative/hypnotics.** ↑ risk of tachycardia with **amphetamine, atropine, scopolamine, cocaine, sympathomimetics, antihistamines,** and **tricyclic antidepressants.** May ↑ blood levels of **theophylline.**
Drug-Natural: ↑ risk of tachycardia with **caffeine**-containing herbs (**cola nut, guarana, mate, tea, coffee**). Concomitant use of **kava, valerian, skullcap, chamomile,** or **hops** can ↑ CNS depression.

Route/Dosage

PO (Adults): *Antiemetic*—5 mg/m² 1–3 hr prior to chemotherapy; may repeat every 2–4 hr after chemotherapy to a total of 4–6 doses/day. If 5 mg/m² dose is ineffective and no significant adverse reactions have occurred, dosage may be increased by 2.5 mg/m² to a maximum of 15 mg/m²/dose. *Appetite stimulant*—2.5 mg twice daily initially; may be gradually increased as needed (up to 20 mg/day). Reduce dose to 2.5 mg/day in the evening or at bedtime if unable to tolerate 5 mg/day dose.

Availability (generic available)

Gelatin capsules: 2.5 mg, 5 mg, 10 mg.

dronedarone (droe-ned-a-rone)

Multaq

Classification

Therapeutic: antiarrhythmics

Pharmacologic: benzofurans

Indications

Reduces the risk of hospitalization in patients with paroxysmal or persistent atrial fibrillation (AF) or atrial flutter (AFl), who have had a recent episode of AF/AFl and have other cardiovascular risk factors and are currently in sinus rhythm or plan to be cardioverted.

Action

Has several antiarrhythmic properties; prolongs PR and QTc intervals. **Therapeutic Effects:** Suppression of AF/AFl.

Adverse Reactions/Side Effects

CNS: weakness. **CV:** CHF, QTc prolongation. **GI:** abdominal pain, diarrhea, nausea, taste abnormality, vomiting. **Derm:** photosensitivity.

PHYSICAL THERAPY IMPLICATIONS

Examination and Evaluation

- Watch for signs of congestive heart failure, including dyspnea, rales/crackles, peripheral edema, jugular venous distention, and exercise intolerance. Report these signs to the physician immediately.
- Assess heart rate, ECG, and heart sounds, especially during exercise (See Appendices G, H). Although intended to treat certain arrhythmias, this drug can unmask or precipitate new arrhythmias (proarrhythmic effect). Report any rhythm disturbances (QTc prolongation) or symptoms of increased arrhythmias, including palpitations, chest pain, shortness of breath, fainting, and fatigue/weakness.

Interventions

- Because of the risk of CHF and cardiac rhythm disturbances, use caution during aerobic exercise and other forms of therapeutic exercise. Assess exercise tolerance frequently (blood pressure, heart rate, fatigue levels), and terminate exercise immediately if any untoward responses occur (See Appendix L).
- Causes photosensitivity; use care if administering UV treatments. Advise patient to avoid direct sunlight and use sunscreens and protective clothing.

Patient/Client-Related Instruction

- Advise patient and family or caregivers about the signs of arrhythmias and CHF (See above under Examination and Evaluation), and to seek immediate medical assistance if these signs develop.
- Instruct patient and family/caregivers to report other side effects such as severe or prolonged weakness or GI problems (nausea, vomiting, diarrhea, abnormal taste, abdominal pain).

Pharmacokinetics

Absorption: Poor bioavailability (4%) due to extensive first pass hepatic metabolism (4%); food ↑ bioavailability (15%).

Distribution: Unknown

Protein Binding: >98%.

Metabolism and Excretion: Undergoes extensive first-pass hepatic metabolism; mostly by the CYP3A enzyme system. 6% excreted in urine as metabolites; 84% was excreted in feces as metabolites. Minimal elimination as unchanged drug.

Half-life: 13–19 hr.

TIME/ACTION PROFILE (antiarrhythmic effect)

ROUTE	ONSET	PEAK	DURATION
PO	unknown*	3–6 hr†‡	12 hr

*Steady-state blood levels are attained at 4–8 days.
†Peak levels after individual doses.

Contraindications/Precautions

Contraindicated in: Class IV heart failure or class II–III heart failure with recent decompensation; 2nd- or 3rd-degree atrioventricular (AV) block or sick sinus syndrome (unless a pacemaker is present); Heart rate <50 bpm; Concurrent use of strong CYP3A inhibitors or drugs/herbal products that prolong the QT interval; QTc interval ≥500 msec; Concurrent use of class I or III antiarrhythmics, including amiodarone, flecainide, propafenone, quinidine, disopyramide, dofetilide, and sotalol; must be discontinued prior to treatment. Severe hepatic impairment; OB: May cause fetal harm; Lactation: Avoid use.

Use Cautiously in: New/worsening heart failure; Hypokalemia or hypomagnesemia (may ↑ risk of arrhythmias); Mild or moderate hepatic impairment; OB: Women with childbearing potential; contraception should be used; Pedi: Safety and effectiveness not established.

Interactions

Drug-Drug: Dronedarone is metabolized by CYP3A and is a moderate inhibitor of CYP3A and CYP2D6 enzyme systems; interactions may occur with other drugs that are substrates for or are metabolized by theses systems; Dronedarone also inhibits P-gp, which can result in ↑ absorption of certain drugs; concurrent use of **strong CYP3A inhibitors,** including **ketoconazole, itraconazole, voriconazole, cyclosporine, telithromycin, clarithromycin,**

nefazodone, and ritonavir, or **drugs that prolong the QT interval,** including **phenothiazine antipsychotics, tricyclic antidepressants**, some oral **macrolide antibiotics**, and other **class I and III antiarrhythmics,** ↑ risk of serious adverse cardiovascular reactions and should be avoided. Concurrent use of CYP3A4 inducers, including **rifampin, phenobarbital, carbamazepine**, or **phenytoin,** ↓ blood levels and effectiveness and should be avoided. ↑ **digoxin** levels and the risk of toxicity (discontinue or ↓ dose by 50% before treatment and monitor carefully). Avoid concurrent use of other **antiarrhythmics**, including **amiodarone, flecainide, propafenone, quinidine, disopyramide, dofetilide**, and **sotalol,** due to ↑ risk of adverse cardiovascular reactions; discontinue prior to dronedarone therapy (concurrent use is contraindicated); concurrent use of **calcium channel blockers** ↑ risk of adverse cardiovascular reactions (initiate at lower dose and increase only after ECG evaluation); concurrent use of **beta blockers** ↑ risk of bradycardia (initiate at lower dose and increase only after ECG evaluation); may also ↑ levels and effects of **tricyclic antidepressants** and **selective serotonin reuptake inhibitors (SSRIs)**; may ↑ levels and risk of toxicity of some **HMG CoA reductase inhibitors (statins)**—see recommendations for specific agents; concurrent use with **CYP3A substrates,** including **sirolimus** and **tacrolimus,** may ↑ risk of serious adverse reactions; monitor and adjust dosage carefully.
Drug-Natural: St. John's wort ↓ blood levels and may ↓ effectiveness; avoid concurrent use.
Drug-Food: Grapefruit juice may ↑ levels and the risk of toxicity; avoid concurrent ingestion.

Route/Dosage
PO (Adults): 400 mg twice daily.

Availability
Tablets: 400 mg.

droperidol (droe-per-i-dole)
Inapsine

Classification
Therapeutic: sedative/hypnotics
Pharmacologic: butyrophenones

Indications
Used to produce tranquilization and as an adjunct to general and regional anesthesia. **Unlabeled Use:** Useful in decreasing postoperative or postprocedure nausea and vomiting.

Action
Similar to haloperidol—alters the action of dopamine in the CNS. **Therapeutic Effects:** Tranquilization. Suppression of nausea and vomiting in selected situations.

Adverse Reactions/Side Effects
CNS: SEIZURES, extrapyramidal reactions, abnormal EEG, anxiety, confusion, dizziness, excessive sedation, hallucinations, hyperactivity, mental depression, nightmares, restlessness, tardive dyskinesia. **CV:** ARRHYTHMIAS (INCLUDING TORSADES DE POINTES), QT prolongation. **EENT:** blurred vision, dry eyes. **Resp:** bronchospasm, laryngospasm. **CV:** hypotension, tachycardia. **GI:** constipation, dry mouth. **Misc:** chills, facial sweating, shivering.

PHYSICAL THERAPY IMPLICATIONS

Examination and Evaluation
- Be alert for new seizures or increased seizure activity. Document the number, duration, and severity of seizures, and report these findings immediately to the physician.
- Assess heart rate, ECG, and heart sounds, especially during exercise (See Appendices G, H). Report any rhythm disturbances or symptoms of increased arrhythmias, including palpitations, chest discomfort, shortness of breath, fainting, and fatigue/weakness.
- Assess motor function, and be alert for extrapyramidal symptoms. Report these symptoms immediately, especially tardive dyskinesia, because this problem may be irreversible. Common extrapyramidal symptoms include:
  - Tardive dyskinesia (uncontrolled rhythmic movement of mouth, face, and extremities, lip smacking or puckering, puffing of cheeks, uncontrolled chewing, rapid or worm-like movements of tongue).
  - Pseudoparkinsonism (shuffling gait, rigidity, tremor, pill-rolling motion, loss of balance control, difficulty speaking or swallowing, mask-like face).
  - Akathisia (restlessness or desire to keep moving).
  - Other dystonias and dyskinesias (dystonic muscle spasms, twisting motions, twitching, inability to move eyes, weakness of arms or legs).
- Assess blood pressure (BP) and report a symptomatic decrease in BP; that is, hypotension that results in dizziness and syncope.
- Assess symptoms of bronchospasm and laryngeal spasm, including wheezing, coughing, and tightness in the throat and chest. Perform pulmonary function tests as needed to quantify suspected changes in ventilation and respiration (See Appendices I, J, K).

- Monitor excessive sedation or changes in mood and behavior such as anxiety, confusion, restlessness, mental depression, nightmares, and hallucinations. Notify physician or nurse immediately if these changes become problematic.
- If used to control postoperative nausea and vomiting, monitor the frequency, severity, and duration of GI problems to help document drug effectiveness.

Interventions

- Guard against falls and trauma (hip fractures, head injury, and so forth) caused by drowsiness, blurred vision, or extrapyramidal symptoms; implement fall-prevention strategies (See Appendix E).
- Because of the risk of arrhythmias and abnormal BP responses, use caution during aerobic exercise and other forms of therapeutic exercise. Assess exercise tolerance frequently (BP, heart rate, fatigue levels), and terminate exercise immediately if any untoward responses occur (See Appendix L).
- To minimize orthostatic hypotension, patient should move slowly when assuming a more upright position.

Patient/Client-Related Instruction

- Instruct patient to report other problematic side effects such as prolonged or severe blurred vision, dry eyes, dry mouth, constipation, chills, shivering, or facial sweating.

Pharmacokinetics

Absorption: Well absorbed following IM administration.
Distribution: Appears to cross the blood-brain barrier and placenta.
Metabolism and Excretion: Mainly metabolized by the liver. Only 10% excreted unchanged by the kidneys.
Half-life: 2.2 hr.

TIME/ACTION PROFILE (sedation)

ROUTE	ONSET	PEAK	DURATION*
IM, IV	3–10 min	30 min	2–4 hr

*Listed as duration of tranquilization; alterations in consciousness may last up to 12 hr.

Contraindications/Precautions

Contraindicated in: Hypersensitivity; Known intolerance; Angle-closure glaucoma; Bone marrow depression; CNS depression; Severe liver or cardiac disease; Known or suspected QT prolongation.
Use Cautiously in: Geriatric, debilitated, or severely ill patients (smaller doses should be used); Diabetic patients; Respiratory insufficiency; Prostatic hyperplasia; CNS tumors; Intestinal obstruction; Seizures (may lower seizure threshold); Severe liver disease; Pregnancy, lactation, and children <2 yr (although safety not established, droperidol has been used during cesarean section without respiratory depression in the newborn); Age >65 yr, concurrent benzodiazepines, volatile anesthetics, IV opioids (may increase risk of serious arrhythmias); use lower initial doses.
Exercise Extreme Caution in: Patients with risk factors for prolonged QT syndrome (CHF, bradycardia, diuretic use, cardiac hypertrophy, hypokalemia, hypomagnesemia) or other drugs known to prolong QT interval.

Interactions

Drug-Drug: Additive hypotension with **antihypertensives** or **nitrates**. Additive CNS depression with other **CNS depressants**, including **alcohol**, **antihistamines**, **antidepressants**, **opioid analgesics**, and other **sedatives**. Concurrent use of **drugs known to prolong QT interval** (↑ risk of potentially life-threatening arrhythmias).
Drug-Natural: Concomitant use of **kava**, **valerian**, **chamomile**, or **hops** can ↑ CNS depression.

Route/Dosage

Premedication/Use Without Premedication in Diagnostic Procedures

IV, IM (Adults): 2.5–initially, 30–60 min prior to induction of anesthesia; additional doses of 1.25 mg IV may be needed, but should be undertaken with caution.
IM, IV (Children 2–12 yr): 0.1 mg/kg maximum initial dose.

Adjunct to General Anesthesia

IV (Adults): 2.5 mg additional doses of 1.25 mg IV may be needed, but should be undertaken with caution.
IM, IV (Children 2–12 yr): 0.1 mg/kg maximum initial dose.

Adjunct in Regional Anesthesia

IM, IV (Adults): 2.5 mg.

Antiemetic

IV (Adults): 0.5–1.25 mg q 4 hr as needed (unlabeled).

Availability (generic available)

Injection: 2.5 mg/mL.

drotrecogin (droe-tre-koe-jin)

Xigris

Classification
Therapeutic: anti-infectives
Pharmacologic: activated protein C, human

Indications

To reduce mortality in adult patients with sepsis.

Action

Probably acts by suppressing widespread inflammation associated with sepsis. **Therapeutic Effects:** Decrease mortality due to sepsis.

Adverse Reactions/Side Effects

Hemat: BLEEDING.

PHYSICAL THERAPY IMPLICATIONS

Examination and Evaluation

- Assess signs of bleeding and hemorrhage (bleeding gums; nosebleed; unusual bruising; black, tarry stools; hematuria; fall in hematocrit or blood pressure). Notify physician or nursing staff immediately if this drug causes excessive anticoagulation.

Interventions

Use caution with any physical interventions that could increase bleeding, including wound débridement, chest percussion, joint mobilization, and application of local heat.

Patient/Client-Related Instruction

- Instruct patient to immediately report signs of GI bleeding, including abdominal pain, vomiting blood, blood in stools, or black, tarry stools.

Pharmacokinetics

Absorption: IV administration results in complete bioavailability.
Distribution: Unknown.
Metabolism and Excretion: Unknown.
Half-life: Unknown.

TIME/ACTION PROFILE (activity)

ROUTE	ONSET	PEAK	DURATION
IV	unknown	end of infusion	unknown

Contraindications/Precautions

Contraindicated in: Hypersensitivity; Patients with a high risk of bleeding, including those with active internal bleeding, recent (within 3 mo) stroke, recent (within 2 mo) intracranial or intraspinal injury or severe head trauma, any trauma associated with an increased risk of life-threatening bleeding, presence of an epidural catheter, intracranial neoplasm/mass lesion/cerebral herniation; Patients not expected to survive due to preexisting medical condition(s); HIV-positive patients with CD4 cell counts ≤50/mm^3; Chronic dialysis patients; Patients who have undergone bone marrow, lung, liver, pancreas, or small bowel transplantation; OB: Lactation.
Use Cautiously in: Concurrent therapeutic heparin therapy (≥15 units/kg/hr), recent (within 3 days) thrombolytic therapy, recent (within 7 days) oral anticoagulants or glycoprotein IIb/IIIa inhibitors, recent (within 7 days) aspirin therapy >650 mg/day or other platelet inhibitors; Platelet count <30,000 × 10^6/L; Prothrombin time—INR >3; Recent (within 6 wk) GI bleeding; Recent (within 3 mo) ischemic stroke; Intracranial arteriovenous malformation or aneurysm; Known bleeding diathesis; Chronic severe hepatic disease; Any other serious bleeding risk; Surgical procedures (discontinue 2 hr before; resume 12 hr after if hemostasis is achieved); OB: Pregnancy (use only if clearly needed); Pedi: Children (safety not established).

Interactions

Drug-Drug: Risk of serious bleeding may be ↑ by **antiplatelet agents, anticoagulants, thrombolytic agents,** or **other agents that may affect coagulation**.
Drug-Natural: Risk of bleeding may be ↑ by **arnica, chamomile, clove, dong quai, feverfew, garlic, ginger, gingko, *Panax ginseng***, and others.

Route/Dosage

IV (Adults): 24 mcg/kg/hr for 96 hr.

Availability

Powder for intravenous infusion (requires reconstitution): 5-mg vial, 20-mg vial.

duloxetine (do-lox-e-teen)

Cymbalta

Classification
Therapeutic: antidepressants
Pharmacologic: selective serotonin/norepinephrine reuptake inhibitors

Indications

Major depressive disorder. Diabetic peripheral neuropathic pain. Generalized anxiety disorder. Fibromyalgia. **Unlabeled Use:** Stress urinary incontinence.

Action

Inhibits serotonin and norepinephrine reuptake in the CNS. Both antidepressant and pain inhibition are centrally mediated. **Therapeutic Effects:** Decreased depressive symptomatology. Decreased neuropathic pain. Decreased symptoms of anxiety. Decreased pain.

Adverse Reactions/Side Effects

CNS: NEUROLEPTIC MALIGNANT SYNDROME, SEIZURES, SUICIDAL THOUGHTS, fatigue, drowsiness, insomnia, activation of mania, dizziness, nightmares. **EENT:** blurred vision, ↑ intraocular pressure. **CV:** ↑ blood pressure. **GI:** HEPATOTOXICITY, ↓ appetite, constipation, dry mouth, nausea, diarrhea, ↑ liver enzymes, gastritis, vomiting. **F and E:** hyponatremia. **GU:** dysuria, abnormal orgasm, erectile dysfunction, ↓ libido, urinary retention. **Derm:** ↑ sweating, pruritus, rash. **Neuro:** tremor. **Misc:** SEROTONIN SYNDROME.

PHYSICAL THERAPY IMPLICATIONS

Examination and Evaluation

- Be alert for increased depression and suicidal thoughts and ideology, especially when initiating drug treatment, and in children and teenagers. Notify physician or other mental health care professional immediately if patient exhibits worsening depression or expresses thoughts of suicide.
- Watch for signs of neuroleptic malignant syndrome, including hyperthermia, diaphoresis, generalized muscle rigidity, altered mental status, tachycardia, changes in blood pressure (BP), and incontinence. Symptoms typically occur within 4–14 days after initiation of drug therapy, but can occur at any time during drug use. Report these signs to the physician immediately.
- Monitor and immediately report signs of serotonin syndrome, including hyperthermia, rigidity, myoclonus, and autonomic instability with fluctuating vital signs and extreme agitation that may proceed to delirium and coma. Patients should not take duloxetine with other drugs that increase serotonin levels (e.g., MAO inhibitors).
- Be alert for new seizures or increased seizure activity, especially at the onset of drug treatment. Document the number, duration, and severity of seizures, and report these findings immediately to the physician.
- Be alert for signs of hepatotoxicity, including anorexia, abdominal pain, severe nausea and vomiting, yellow skin or eyes, fever, sore throat, malaise, weakness, facial edema, lethargy, and unusual bleeding or bruising. Report these signs to the physician immediately.
- Inform physician if patient demonstrates other mood changes such as anxiety, nervousness, restlessness, or other signs of increased mania.
- When used to treat fibromyalgia, diabetic neuropathy, or other chronic pain syndromes, assess pain levels periodically to help document drug efficacy.
- Assess levels of drowsiness and dizziness (See Appendix C), especially in older adults. Determine if these side effects might impair gait, balance, and other functional activities.
- Assess BP and compare to normal values (See Appendix F). Report a sustained increase in BP (hypertension).
- Monitor signs of low sodium levels (hyponatremia), including headache, confusion, lethargy, irritability, decreased consciousness, and neuromuscular abnormalities (muscle weakness and cramps). Report severe or prolonged signs to the physician.

Interventions

- Guard against falls and trauma (hip fractures, head injury, and so forth), and implement fall-prevention strategies (See Appendix E).
- Help patient explore nonpharmacologic methods (exercise, counseling, support groups, and so forth) to reduce depression and other psychologic disorders.

Patient/Client-Related Instruction

- Advise patient that antidepressant effects may not occur immediately; it may take 2 wk or longer before an improvement in mood is observed.
- Advise patient to avoid alcohol and other CNS depressants because of the increased risk of sedation and adverse effects.
- Advise patient that this medication should be tapered at the completion of long-term therapy. Abrupt withdrawal may cause dizziness, sensory disturbances, agitation, anxiety, nausea, and sweating.
- Instruct patient to report severe or prolonged GI problems, including nausea, vomiting, diarrhea, constipation, abdominal pain, and loss of appetite.
- Instruct patient to report other problematic side effects such as severe or prolonged tremor, blurred vision, nightmares, sleep loss, urinary problems, sexual dysfunction, or skin reactions (rash, itching, increased sweating).

Pharmacokinetics

Absorption: Well absorbed following oral administration.
Distribution: Unknown.
Protein Binding: Highly (>90%) protein bound.
Metabolism and Excretion: Mostly metabolized, primarily by the CYP2D6 and CYP1A2 enzyme pathways.
Half-life: 12 hr.

TIME/ACTION PROFILE (blood levels)

ROUTE	ONSET	PEAK	DURATION
PO	unknown	6 hr	12 hr

Contraindications/Precautions

Contraindicated in: Hypersensitivity; Concurrent MAO inhibitor therapy; Uncontrolled angle-closure glaucoma; End stage renal disease; Chronic hepatic impairment or substantial alcohol use (increased risk of hepatitis); Lactation: May enter breast milk; discontinue or bottle feed.
Use Cautiously in: History of suicide attempt or ideation; History of mania (may activate mania/hypomania); Concurrent use of other centrally acting drugs (↑ risk of adverse reactions); History of seizure disorder; Controlled angle-closure glaucoma; Diabetic patients and those with renal impairment (consider lower initial dose with gradual increase); OB: Use during third trimester may result in neonatal serotonin syndrome requiring prolonged hospitalization, respiratory and nutritional support; Pedi: May ↑ risk of suicide attempt/ideation, especially during dose early treatment or dose adjustment; risk may be greater in

children or adolescents (safe use in children/adolescents not established).

Interactions

Drug-Drug: Concurrent use with **MAO inhibitors** may result in serious potentially fatal reactions (do not use within 14 days of discontinuing MAOI. Wait at least 5 days after stopping duloxetine to start MAOI). ↑ risk of hepatotoxicity with chronic **alcohol** abuse. Drugs that affect serotonergic neurotransmitter systems, including **linezolid**, **tramadol**, and **triptans** ↑ risk of serotonin syndrome.. **Drugs that inhibit CYP1A2**, including **fluvoxamine** and some **fluoroquinolones**, ↑ levels of duloxetine and should be avoided. **Drugs that inhibit CYP2D6**, including **paroxetine**, **fluoxetine**, and **quinidine**, ↑ levels of duloxetine and may increase the risk of adverse reactions. Duloxetine also inhibits CYP2D6 and may ↑ levels of drugs metabolized by CYP2D6, including **tricyclic antidepressants**, **phenothiazines**, and **class 1C antiarrhythmics** (**propafenone** and **flecainide**); concurrent use should be undertaken with caution. ↑ risk of serious arrhythmias with **thioridazine**; avoid concurrent use. ↑ risk of bleeding with **aspirin**, **NSAIDs**, or **warfarin**. **Drug-Natural:** Use with **St. John's wort** ↑of serotonin syndrome.

Route/Dosage

PO (Adults): *Antidepressant*—20–30 mg twice daily; *Neuropathic pain or generalized anxiety disorder*—60 mg once daily; *Fibromyalgia*—30 mg once daily for 1 wk, then ↑ to 60 mg once daily.

Renal Impairment

PO (Adults): start with lower dose and ↑ gradually.

Availability

Capsules: 20 mg, 30 mg, 60 mg.

dutasteride (doo-**tas**-te-ride)

Avodart

Classification

Therapeutic: benign prostatic hyperplasia (BPH) agents
Pharmacologic: androgen inhibitors

Indications

Management of the symptoms of BPH in men with an enlarged prostate gland (alone or with tamsulosin).

Action

Inhibits the enzyme 5-alpha-reductase, which is responsible for converting testosterone to its potent metabolite 5-alpha-dihydrotestosterone in the prostate gland and other tissues. 5-Alpha-dihydrotestosterone is partly responsible for prostatic hyperplasia. **Therapeutic Effects:** Reduced prostate size with associated decrease in urinary symptoms.

Adverse Reactions/Side Effects

GU: decreased libido, ejaculation disorders, erectile dysfunction. **Endo:** gynecomastia. **Derm:** rash, urticaria. **Misc:** ALLERGIC REACTIONS, ANGIOEDEMA.

PHYSICAL THERAPY IMPLICATIONS

Examination and Evaluation

- Monitor signs of allergic reactions and angioedema, including pulmonary symptoms (tightness in the throat and chest, wheezing, cough, dyspnea), skin reactions (rash, pruritus, urticaria, swelling in the face). Notify physician immediately of these signs.
- Monitor signs of BPH such as difficulty starting a urine stream, painful urination, weak urine flow, feeling that the bladder is not completely empty, frequent nighttime urination, and an urge to urinate again soon after urinating. Document any change in BPH symptoms to help assess the effects of drug therapy.

Patient/Client-Related Instruction

- When treating BPH, advise patient that urinary symptoms (retention, dribbling, hesitancy, urgency) should improve, and to contact the physician if these symptoms continue to worsen.
- Instruct patient or family/caregivers to report other bothersome side effects such as breast enlargement (gynecomastia), severe or prolonged skin reactions (rash, hives), or sexual dysfunction (decreased libido, ejaculation disorders, erectile dysfunction).

Pharmacokinetics

Absorption: Well absorbed (60%) following oral administration; also absorbed through skin.
Distribution: 11.5% of serum concentration partitions into semen.
Protein Binding: 99% bound to albumin; 96.6% bound to alpha-1 glycoprotein.
Metabolism and Excretion: Mostly metabolized by the liver via the CYP3A4 metabolic pathway; metabolites are excreted in feces.
Half-life: 5 wk.

TIME/ACTION PROFILE (reduction in dihydrotestosterone levels†)

ROUTE	ONSET	PEAK	DURATION
PO	unknown*	1–2 wk	unknown

*Symptoms may only improve over 3–12 mo.

Contraindications/Precautions

Contraindicated in: Hypersensitivity; Cross-sensitivity with other 5-alpha-reductase inhibitors may occur; Women; Pedi: Children.

Use Cautiously in: Hepatic impairment.

Interactions

Drug-Drug: Blood levels and effects may be increased by **ritonavir, ketoconazole, verapamil, diltiazem, cimetidine, ciprofloxacin,** or other **CYP3A4 enzyme inhibitors**.

Route/Dosage

PO (Adults): 0.5 mg once daily (with or without tamsulosin).

Availability

Soft gelatin capsules: 0.5 mg.

ecallantide (ee-kal-lan-tide)

Kalbitor

Classification

Therapeutic: antiangioedema agents

Pharmacologic: kallikrein inhibitors

Indications

Treatment of acute attacks of hereditary angioedema (HAE) in patients ≥16 yr.

Action

Acts as a selective, reversible inhibitor of kallikrein, thereby inhibiting its action in initiating bradykinin production, part of the cascade of events in HAE. **Therapeutic Effects:** Decreased severity of attack of HAE.

Adverse Reactions/Side Effects

CNS: headache, fatigue. **EENT:** nasopharyngitis. **GI:** nausea, abdominal pain, diarrhea. **Derm:** pruritus, rash, urticaria. **Local:** injection-site reactions. **Misc:** HYPERSENSITIVITY REACTIONS, INCLUDING ANAPHYLAXIS, fever.

PHYSICAL THERAPY IMPLICATIONS

Examination and Evaluation

- Watch for signs of hypersensitivity reactions and anaphylaxis, including pulmonary symptoms (tightness in the throat and chest, wheezing, cough, dyspnea) or skin reactions (rash, pruritus, urticaria, dermatitis, welts, burning/itching skin, swelling in the face). Notify physician or nursing staff immediately if these reactions occur.
- Monitor subcutaneous injection site for pain, swelling, and irritation. Report prolonged or excessive injection site reactions to the physician.

Patient/Client-Related Instruction

- Instruct patient to report other troublesome side effects such as prolonged or severe headache, fatigue, fever, upper respiratory tract irritation, skin reactions (rash, itching, hives), or GI problems (nausea, diarrhea, abdominal pain).

Pharmacokinetics

Absorption: Well absorbed following subcutaneous administration.
Distribution: Unknown.
Metabolism and Excretion: Renally eliminated.
Half-life: 2 hr.

TIME/ACTION PROFILE (symptom improvement)

ROUTE	ONSET	PEAK	DURATION
SC	unknown	2–4 hr	up to 24 hr

Contraindications/Precautions

Contraindicated in: Hypersensitivity.
Use Cautiously in: Geri: Consider age-related ↓ in hepatic, renal, or cardiac function, concomitant diseases or other drug therapy; lower initial dose may be considered; Lactation: Use cautiously; OB: Use only if clearly needed.

Interactions

Drug-Drug: None noted.

Route/Dosage

Subcut (Adults ≥16 yr): 30 mg given as 3 10-mg injections; an additional dose of 30 mg may be given within 24 hr.

Availability

Injection for subcutaneous use: 10 mg/mL.

econazole (ee-kon-a-zole)

Spectazole

Classification

Therapeutic: antifungals (topical)

Pharmacologic: azoles

Indications

Treatment of a variety of cutaneous fungal infections, including cutaneous candidiasis, tinea pedis (athlete's foot), tinea cruris (jock itch), tinea corporis (ringworm), and tinea versicolor.

Action

Affects the permeability of the fungal cell wall, allowing leakage of cellular contents. **Therapeutic Effects:** Decrease in symptoms of fungal infection.

Adverse Reactions/Side Effects

Local: burning, itching, local hypersensitivity reactions, redness, stinging.

PHYSICAL THERAPY IMPLICATIONS

Examination and Evaluation

- Assess healing of skin lesions to help document drug effectiveness.

Interventions

- Avoid contact with cutaneous lesions when treating patient.
- Always wash hands thoroughly and disinfect equipment (whirlpools, electrotherapeutic devices, treatment tables, and so forth) to help prevent the spread of infection.

Patient/Client-Related Instruction

- Advise patient to report any increased local sensitivity to this drug (pain, burning, itching, swelling).
- Instruct patient about proper hygiene; e.g., thoroughly wash and dry the affected area, wear clean socks and ventilated shoes for tinea pedis, and so forth.
- Advise patient to apply the drug as directed for the full course of treatment even if feeling better.
- Inform patient that early relief of cutaneous symptoms may be seen in 2–3 days. Full therapeutic response may take 2 wk for candidiasis, tinea cruris, tinea corporis, and tinea versicolor and 4 wk for tinea pedis.
- Advise patient to seek medical help if infections persist or recur after the full treatment. Recurrent fungal infections may be a sign of systemic illness.

Pharmacokinetics

Absorption: Absorption through intact skin is minimal.
Distribution: Distribution after topical administration is primarily local.
Metabolism and Excretion: Metabolism in the liver and <1% excreted in the urine and feces.
Half-life: Not applicable.

TIME/ACTION PROFILE

ROUTE	ONSET	PEAK	DURATION
topical	unknown	unknown	unknown

Contraindications/Precautions

Contraindicated in: Hypersensitivity to active ingredients, additives, preservatives, or bases.
Use Cautiously in: Nail and scalp infections (may require additional systemic therapy); OB/Lactation: Safety not established.

Interactions

Drug-Drug: Not known.

Route/Dosage

Topical (Adults and Children): Apply once daily in patients with tinea pedis (for 1 mo), tinea cruris (for 2 wk), tinea corporis (for 2 wk), and tinea versicolor (for 2 wk). Apply twice daily in patients with cutaneous candidiasis (for 2 wk).

Availability (generic available)

Cream: 1% Rx.

efalizumab (ef-a-liz-oo-mab)

Raptiva

Classification

Therapeutic: antipsoriatics
Pharmacologic: monoclonal antibodies

Indications

Moderate-to-severe plaque psoriasis in adults who are candidates for systemic therapy or phototherapy.

Action

Inhibits fusion of leukocytes to other cell types resulting in decreased migration of leukocytes to psoriatic areas. **Therapeutic Effects:** Decreased area and severity of plaque psoriasis.

Adverse Reactions/Side Effects

CNS: headache. **Derm:** photosensitivity, toxic epidermal necrolysis, worsening of psoriasis.
Hemat: hemolytic anemia, thrombocytopenia.
MS: arthralgia, arthritis, pain. **Misc:** MALIGNANCIES, SERIOUS INFECTIONS, fever, first dose reactions, hypersensitivity reactions, inflammatory/immune–mediated reactions.

PHYSICAL THERAPY IMPLICATIONS

Examination and Evaluation

- Monitor signs of malignancy, including a change in bowel or bladder habits, nonhealing sores, unusual bleeding or discharge, a lump in the breast or other parts of the body, chronic indigestion or difficulty in swallowing, obvious changes in a wart or mole, and persistent coughing or hoarseness. Report these signs to the physician immediately.
- Monitor signs of respiratory tract infection (dyspnea, fever, bronchitis, flu-like symptoms), GI infection (nausea, vomiting, diarrhea), or other severe systemic infections. Notify physician immediately because these infections may be severe or fatal, especially in patients taking immunosuppressive therapy.
- Periodically assess the size and appearance of skin lesions to help document whether antipsoriatic drug therapy is successful. Report a worsening of psoriasis or signs of toxic epidermal necrolysis (severe rash, dermatitis, exfoliation).
- Monitor signs of allergic or hypersensitivity reactions, including pulmonary symptoms (laryngeal edema, wheezing, cough, dyspnea) or skin reactions (rash, pruritus, urticaria). Notify physician if severe allergic reactions occur.
- Monitor signs of thrombocytopenia (bruising, nose bleeds, bleeding gums) or hemolytic anemia (unusual fatigue, shortness of breath, dizziness, headache, coldness in hands and feet, pale skin, chest pain). Report these signs to the physician immediately.
- Assess any back pain, joint pain, or signs of systemic inflammation. Attempt to differentiate whether pain is drug induced or caused by musculoskeletal or biomechanical problems.

Interventions

- Implement phototherapy (UV light) as indicated to augment drug effects in treating psoriasis. Be especially careful because this drug increases sensitivity to UV light, and a decrease in UV dosage may be necessary.

Patient/Client-Related Instruction

- Advise patient about photosensitivity, and to use sunscreens, protective clothing, and avoid prolonged sun exposure. Advise patient to also report any rashes or other skin reactions.
- Instruct patient to report other side effects such as severe or prolonged headache.

Pharmacokinetics

Absorption: 50% absorbed following SC administration.
Distribution: Unknown.
Metabolism and Excretion: Unknown.
Half-life: Unknown.

TIME/ACTION PROFILE

ROUTE	ONSET	PEAK	DURATION
SC	unknown	unknown	1 wk*

*25 days following discontinuation.

Contraindications/Precautions

Contraindicated in: Hypersensitivity; Active infection; Concurrent immunosuppressants; OB: Pregnancy, lactation.
Use Cautiously in: Chronic/recurrent infections; High risk/history of malignancy; Geri: May be more sensitive to effects; Pedi: Children (safety not established).

Interactions

Drug-Drug: ↑ risk of infections with other **immunosuppressants**. May ↓ antibody response to and ↑ risk of adverse reactions from **vaccinations**; acellular, live, and live-attenuated vaccines should be avoided.

Route/Dosage

Subcut (Adults): 0.7 mg/kg conditioning dose followed by 1 mg/kg once weekly (no single dose should exceed 200 mg).

Availability

Lyophilized powder for injection (requires reconstitution): 125 mg/vial.

efavirenz (e-fav-i-renz)

Sustiva

Classification
Therapeutic: antiretrovirals
Pharmacologic: nonnucleoside reverse transcriptase inhibitors

Indications

HIV infection (in combination with one or more other antiretroviral agents).

Action

Inhibits HIV reverse transcriptase, which results in disruption of DNA synthesis. **Therapeutic Effects:** Slowed progression of HIV infection and decreased occurrence of sequelae. Increases CD4 cell counts and decreases viral load.

Adverse Reactions/Side Effects

CNS: abnormal dreams, depression, dizziness, drowsiness, fatigue, headache, impaired concentration, insomnia, nervousness, psychiatric symptomatology. **GI:** nausea, abdominal pain, anorexia, diarrhea, dyspepsia, flatulence. **GU:** hematuria, renal calculi. **Derm:** RASH, increased sweating, pruritus. **Neuro:** hypoesthesia.

PHYSICAL THERAPY IMPLICATIONS

Examination and Evaluation

- Monitor skin rash and other skin reactions (sweating, pruritus). Report severe or unexpected skin reactions to the physician immediately.
- Monitor excessive headache or fatigue. Some fatigue is expected, but any sudden or severe change in muscle strength or energy levels should be reported.
- Assess dizziness that might affect gait, balance, and other functional activities (See Appendix C). Report balance problems and functional limitations to the physician and nursing staff, and caution the patient and family/caregivers to guard against falls and trauma.
- Be alert for nervousness, depression, impaired concentration, excessive drowsiness, or other alterations in behavior or mental status. Notify health care professional promptly if these symptoms develop.

Interventions

- Implement resistive exercises and other therapeutic exercises as tolerated to maintain muscle strength and function and to prevent muscle wasting associated with HIV infection and AIDS.

Patient/Client-Related Instruction

- Emphasize the importance of taking efavirenz as directed even if the patient is asymptomatic, and that this drug must always be used in combination with other antiretroviral drugs. Do not take more than prescribed amount and do not stop taking without consulting health care professional.
- Inform patient that efavirenz does not cure HIV or AIDS or prevent associated or opportunistic infections. Efavirenz does not reduce the risk of transmission of HIV to others through sexual contact or blood contamination. Caution patient to use a condom, and to avoid sharing needles or donating blood to prevent spreading the AIDS virus to others.
- Instruct patient to report signs of kidney stones (renal calculi), including bloody urine, severe pain in the side and back, pain on urination, and a persistent urge to urinate.
- Advise patient about the likelihood of GI reactions, including nausea, vomiting, diarrhea, abdominal pain, heartburn, and loss of appetite. Instruct patient to report severe or prolonged GI reactions.
- Instruct patient to report other troublesome side effects such as prolonged or severe headache, sleep loss, abnormal dreams, or a decreased sense of touch (hypoesthesia).

Pharmacokinetics

Absorption: 50% absorbed when ingested following a high-fat meal.
Distribution: 99.5–99.75% bound to plasma proteins; enters CSF.
Metabolism and Excretion: Mostly metabolized by the liver.
Half-life: *Following single dose*—52–76 hr. *Following multiple doses*—40–55 hr.

TIME/ACTION PROFILE (blood levels)

ROUTE	ONSET	PEAK	DURATION
PO	rapid	3–5 hr	24 hr

Contraindications/Precautions

Contraindicated in: Hypersensitivity; Concurrent pimozide, midazolam, triazolam, voriconazole (standard doses), or ergot derivatives.
Use Cautiously in: History of mental illness or substance abuse (↑ risk of psychiatric symptomatology); History of hepatic impairment (including hepatitis B or C infection or concurrent therapy with hepatotoxic agents); Pedi: Children (increased incidence of rash); OB: Pregnancy or lactation (use in pregnancy only if other options have been exhausted; breast-feeding not recommended in HIV-infected patients).

Interactions

Drug-Drug: ↑ levels of **pimozide, midazolam, triazolam, or ergot alkaloids** when used concurrently; may result in potentially serious adverse reactions, including arrhythmias, CNS, and respiratory depression. Induces (stimulates) the hepatic cytochrome P450 3A4 enzyme system and would be expected to influence the effects of other drugs that are metabolized by this system; efavirenz itself is also metabolized by this system. ↑ risk of CNS depression with other **CNS depressants**, including **alcohol**, **antidepressants**, **antihistamines**, and **opioid analgesics**. Concurrent use with **ritonavir** ↑ levels of both agents and the likelihood of adverse reactions, especially hepatotoxicity. May alter the effectiveness of **hormonal contraceptives**. Use with **voriconazole** significantly ↓ voriconazole levels and ↑ efavirenz levels; concurrent use with standard doses of voriconazole is contraindicated; if used together, ↑ dose of voriconazole to 400 mg q 12 hr and ↓ dose of efavirenz to 300 mg daily. ↓ **indinavir** blood levels (indinavir dosage ↑ recommended). ↓ **saquinavir** blood levels (avoid using saquinavir as the only protease inhibitor with efavirenz). May alter the effects of **warfarin**.
Drug-Natural: Use with **St. John's wort** may cause ↓ levels and effectiveness, including development of drug resistance.
Drug-Food: Ingestion following a high-fat meal ↑ absorption by 50%.

Route/Dosage

PO (Adults and Children >40 kg): 600 mg once daily.
PO (Children 32.5–40 kg): 400 mg once daily.
PO (Children 25–32.5 kg): 350 mg once daily.
PO (Children 20–25 kg): 300 mg once daily.
PO (Children 15–20 kg): 250 mg once daily.
PO (Children 10–15 kg): 200 mg once daily.

Availability

Capsules: 50 mg, 200 mg. **Tablets:** 600 mg. ***In combination with:*** emtricitabine and tenofovir (Atripla). See Appendix B.

eltrombopag (el-trom-boe-pag)

Promacta

Classification
Therapeutic: antithrombocytopenics
Pharmacologic: thrombopoietin receptor agonists

Indications
Treatment of chronic immune (idiopathic) thrombocytopenic purpura in patients who have had an inadequate response to corticosteroids, immunoglobulins, or splenectomy.

Action
Increases platelet production by initiating proliferation and differentiation of megakaryocytes from bone marrow progenitor cells. **Therapeutic Effects:** Increased platelet count with reduced risk of bleeding.

Adverse Reactions/Side Effects
EENT: development/worsening of cataracts.
GI: HEPATOTOXICITY. **Hemat:** bone marrow changes.

PHYSICAL THERAPY IMPLICATIONS

Examination and Evaluation
- Be alert for signs of hepatotoxicity, including anorexia, abdominal pain, severe nausea and vomiting, yellow skin or eyes, fever, sore throat, malaise, weakness, facial edema, lethargy, and unusual bleeding or bruising. Report these signs to the physician immediately.
- Assess skin periodically for red and purple patches (purpura). If successful, drug therapy should result in a decrease in the frequency and severity of these reactions.
- Monitor signs of anemia (unusual fatigue, shortness of breath with exertion, bruising) that might indicate bone marrow changes. Notify physician if these signs occur.

Patient/Client-Related Instruction
- Instruct patient to report any vision disturbances or cloudy, blurred vision.

Pharmacokinetics
Absorption: 52% absorbed following oral administration.
Distribution: Unknown.
Protein Binding: >99%.
Metabolism and Excretion: Extensively metabolized; 59% eliminated in feces, 20% as unchanged drug; 31% excreted in urine as metabolites.
Half-life: 21–35 hr.

TIME/ACTION PROFILE (effect on platelet count)

ROUTE	ONSET	PEAK	DURATION
PO	1 wk	2 wk	1 wk

Contraindications/Precautions
Contraindicated in: Lactation: Lactation.
Use Cautiously in: Myelodysplastic syndromes (may ↑ risk of hematologic malignancy); Hepatic impairment (lower initial dose may be required); Patients with East Asian ancestry (may require lower doses); Geri: Elderly patients may be more sensitive to drug effects; increase dose cautiously, consider age-related decrease in renal and hepatic function, concurrent disease states, and drug therapy; OB: Use in pregnancy only when potential maternal benefit outweighs potential risk to fetus.

Interactions
Drug-Drug: ↓ availability and absorption of **iron, calcium, aluminum, magnesium, selenium,** and **zinc** by chelation; do not administer within 4 hr of medications containing these and other polyvalent cations.
Drug-Food: ↓ availability and absorption of **iron, calcium, aluminum, magnesium, selenium,** and **zinc** by chelation; do not administer within 4 hr of foods containing these and other polyvalent cations.

Route/Dosage
PO (Adults): 50 mg once daily, may be increased to achieve a platelet count of ≥50 × 10^9/L (not to exceed 75 mg/day); *patient of East Asian ancestry or moderate-to-severe hepatic impairment*—25 mg once daily initially; may be increased to achieve a platelet count of ≥50 × 10^9/L (not to exceed 75 mg/day).

Availability
Tablets: 25 mg, 50 mg

emtricitabine (em-tri-sit-i-been)
Emtriva

Classification
Therapeutic: antiretrovirals
Pharmacologic: nucleoside reverse transcriptase inhibitors

Indications
HIV infection (with other antiretrovirals).

Action
Phosphorylated intracellularly where it inhibits HIV reverse transcriptase, resulting in viral DNA chain termination. **Therapeutic Effects:** Slowed progression of HIV infection and decreased occurrence of sequelae. Increases CD4 cell counts and decreases viral load.

Adverse Reactions/Side Effects
CNS: dizziness, headache, insomnia, weakness, depression, nightmares. **GI:** abdominal pain, diarrhea, nausea, SEVERE HEPATOMEGALY WITH STEATOSIS, dyspepsia, vomiting. **Derm:** rash, skin discoloration.
F and E: LACTIC ACIDOSIS. **MS:** arthralgia, myalgia.

Neuro: neuropathy, paresthesia. **Resp:** cough, rhinitis. **Misc:** fat redistribution.

PHYSICAL THERAPY IMPLICATIONS

Examination and Evaluation

- Be alert for signs of enlarged, fatty liver (hepatomegaly with steatosis) that can progress to liver dysfunction and liver failure. Signs of liver disease include anorexia, abdominal pain, abdominal swelling (ascites), severe nausea and vomiting, yellow skin or eyes, fever, sore throat, malaise, weakness, facial edema, lethargy, and unusual bleeding or bruising. Notify physician of these signs immediately.
- Monitor signs of lactic acidosis, including confusion, lethargy, stupor, shallow rapid breathing, tachycardia, hypotension, nausea, and vomiting. Notify physician immediately if these signs occur.
- Assess any muscle pain or joint pain to rule out musculoskeletal pathology; that is, try to determine if pain is drug induced rather than caused by anatomic or biomechanical problems.
- Be alert for signs of peripheral neuropathy (numbness, tingling, muscle weakness). Establish baseline electroneuromyographic values using EMG and nerve conduction at the beginning of drug treatment whenever possible, and reexamine these values periodically to document drug-induced changes in peripheral nerve function.
- Assess dizziness that might affect gait, balance, and other functional activities (See Appendix C). Report balance problems and functional limitations to the physician and nursing staff, and caution the patient and family/caregivers to guard against falls and trauma.

Interventions

- Implement resistive exercises and other therapeutic exercises as tolerated to maintain muscle strength and function and to prevent muscle wasting associated with HIV infection and AIDS.
- Because of the risk of lactic acidosis, use caution during aerobic exercise and other forms of therapeutic exercise. Assess exercise tolerance frequently (blood pressure, heart rate, fatigue levels), and terminate exercise immediately if any untoward responses occur (See Appendix L).

Patient/Client-Related Instruction

- Emphasize the importance of taking emtricitabine as directed even if the patient is asymptomatic, and that this drug must always be used in combination with other antiretroviral drugs. Do not take more than prescribed amount, and do not stop taking without consulting health care professional.
- Inform patient that emtricitabine does not cure HIV or AIDS or prevent associated or opportunistic infections. Emtricitabine does not reduce the risk of transmission of HIV to others through sexual contact or blood contamination. Caution patient to use a condom, and to avoid sharing needles or donating blood to prevent spreading the AIDS virus to others.
- Advise patient about possible fat redistribution, including increased fat in the torso with thin arms and legs. Discuss possible effects on body image, and help patient explore coping mechanisms.
- Instruct patient to report other troublesome side effects such as prolonged or severe headache, sleep loss, nightmares, depression, cough, nasal inflammation, skin reactions (rash, discoloration), or GI problems (diarrhea, nausea, vomiting, abdominal pain, indigestion).

Pharmacokinetics

Absorption: Rapidly and extensively absorbed; 93% bioavailable.
Distribution: Unknown.
Metabolism and Excretion: Some metabolism, 86% renally excreted, 14% fecal excretion.
Half-life: 10 hr.

TIME/ACTION PROFILE (blood levels*)

ROUTE	ONSET	PEAK	DURATION
PO	rapid	1–2 hr	24 hr

*Normal renal function.

Contraindications/Precautions

Contraindicated in: Hypersensitivity; Lactation: Lactation (breast-feeding is not recommended in HIV-infected patients); Pedi: Children <18 yr (safety not established).

Use Cautiously in: Geri: Elderly (may be at ↑ risk for adverse effects); Hepatitis B infection (may exacerbate following discontinuation); Renal impairment; OB: Pregnancy (use only if clearly needed).

Interactions

Drug-Drug: None noted.

Route/Dosage

PO (Adults ≥18 yr): 200 mg once daily.

Renal Impairment

PO (Adults ≥18 yr): *CCr 30–49 mL/min*—200 mg every 48 hr; *CCr 15–29 mL/min*—200 mg every 72 hr; *CCr <15 mL/min*—200 mg every 96 hr.

Availability

Capsules: 200 mg. **Oral solution (cotton candy flavor):** 10 mg/mL in 270-mL bottles. ***In combination with:*** efavirenz and emtricitabine (Atripla); tenofovir (Truvada). See Appendix B.

enalapril, enalaprilat

(e-**nal**-a-pril, e-**nal**-a-pril-at)
Vasotec, Vasotec IV

Classification
Therapeutic: antihypertensives
Pharmacologic: angiotensin-converting enzyme (ACE) inhibitors

Indications

Alone or with other agents in the management of hypertension. Management of symptomatic heart failure. Slowed progression of asymptomatic left ventricular dysfunction to overt heart failure. **Unlabeled Use:** Treatment of proteinuria in steroid-resistant nephrotic syndrome patients.

Action

ACE inhibitors block the conversion of angiotensin I to the vasoconstrictor angiotensin II. ACE inhibitors also prevent the degradation of bradykinin and other vasodilatory prostaglandins. ACE inhibitors also ↑ plasma renin levels and ↓ aldosterone levels. Net result is systemic vasodilation. **Therapeutic Effects:** Lowering of blood pressure in patients with hypertension. Increased survival and reduction of symptoms in patients with symptomatic heart failure. ↓ development of overt heart failure.

Adverse Reactions/Side Effects

CNS: dizziness, fatigue, headache, vertigo, weakness. **Resp:** cough. **CV:** hypotension, chest pain. **GI:** abdominal pain, diarrhea, nausea, vomiting. **GU:** proteinuria, impaired renal function. **Derm:** rashes. **F and E:** hyperkalemia. **Resp:** dyspnea. **Misc:** ANGIOEDEMA.

PHYSICAL THERAPY IMPLICATIONS

Examination and Evaluation

- Watch for signs of angioedema, including rashes, raised patches of red or white skin (welts), burning/itching skin, swelling in the face, and difficulty breathing. Notify physician immediately of these signs.
- Assess blood pressure periodically and compare to normal values (See Appendix F) to help determine antihypertensive effects. Report low blood pressure (hypotension), especially if patient experiences dizziness or syncope.
- Assess signs and symptoms of CHF (dyspnea, rales/crackles, peripheral edema, jugular venous distention, exercise intolerance) to help document whether drug therapy is effective in reducing these symptoms.
- Monitor symptoms of high plasma potassium levels (hyperkalemia), including bradycardia, fatigue, weakness, numbness, and tingling. Notify physician because severe cases can lead to life-threatening arrhythmias and paralysis.
- Assess dizziness and vertigo that might affect gait, balance, and other functional activities (see Appendix C). Report balance problems and functional limitations to the physician, and caution the patient and family/caregivers to guard against falls and trauma.

Interventions

- Implement aerobic exercise and cardiac-conditioning programs to augment drug therapy and maintain or improve cardiovascular pump function in patients with heart failure and other cardiac conditions.
- Avoid physical therapy interventions that cause systemic vasodilation (large whirlpool, Hubbard tank). Additive effects of this drug and the intervention may cause a dangerous fall in blood pressure.
- To minimize orthostatic hypotension, patient should move slowly when assuming a more upright position.

Patient/Client-Related Instruction

- Remind patients to take medication as directed to control hypertension and other cardiac conditions even if they are asymptomatic.
- Instruct patients with heart failure to weigh themselves every day, and call their physician if they gain 3 lb or more in 1 day or more than 5 lb in 1 week. Sudden weight gain may indicate fluid buildup due to worsening heart failure.
- Counsel patients about additional interventions to help control blood pressure and cardiac dysfunction, including regular exercise, weight loss, sodium restriction, stress reduction, moderation of alcohol consumption, and smoking cessation.
- Instruct patient to report signs of impaired renal function, including decreased urine output, cloudy urine, or sudden weight gain due to fluid retention.
- Instruct patient to notify physician of a prolonged dry cough or difficult, labored breathing; drug therapy may need to be altered to resolve this side effect.
- Instruct patient or family/caregivers to report other troublesome side effects such as severe or prolonged headache, fatigue, weakness, skin rash, or GI problems (nausea, vomiting, diarrhea, abdominal pain).

Pharmacokinetics

Absorption: *Enalapril:* 55–75% absorbed following oral administration. *Enalaprilat:* IV administration results in complete bioavailability.
Distribution: Crosses the placenta; small amounts enter breast milk.

Metabolism and Excretion: Converted by the liver to enalaprilat, the active metabolite; primarily eliminated by kidneys.

Half-life: *Enalapril:* Adults: 2 hr; Adults with CHF: 3.4–5.8 hr; Children and infants with CHF: 2.7 hr; Neonates with CHF: 10.3 hr; *Enalaprilat:* Adults: 35–38 hr; Children and infants with CHF: 11.1 hr; Infants 6 wk–8 mo: 6–10 hr; Neonates with CHF: 11.9 hr.

TIME/ACTION PROFILE (effect on blood pressure—single dose*)

ROUTE	ONSET	PEAK	DURATION
enalapril PO	1 hr	4–8 hr	12–24 hr
enalaprilat IV	15 min	1–4 hr	4–6 hr

*Full effects may not be noted for several weeks.

Contraindications/Precautions

Contraindicated in: Hypersensitivity; History of angioedema (either idiopathic or with previous use of ACE inhibitors); OB: Can cause injury or death of fetus—if pregnancy occurs, discontinue immediately; Lactation: Appears in breast milk; patient must discontinue enalapril or provide alternate to breast milk.

Use Cautiously in: Patients with renal impairment, hypovolemia, hyponatremia, and concurrent diuretic therapy; Black patients (monotherapy of hypertension less effective, may require additional therapy; higher risk of angioedema); Surgery/anesthesia (hypotension may be exaggerated); Women of childbearing potential; Pedi: Injectable product contains benzyl alcohol which is associated with gasping syndrome in neonates; Geri: Initial dose reduction recommended.

Exercise Extreme Caution in: Family history of angioedema.

Interactions

Drug-Drug: Excessive hypotension may occur with concurrent use of **diuretics**. Additive hypotension with other **antihypertensives**. ↑ risk of hyperkalemia with concurrent use of **potassium supplements, potassium-sparing diuretics, potassium-containing salt substitutes**, or **angiotensin II receptor antagonists**. Antihypertensive response may be blunted by **NSAIDs**. ↑ levels and may ↑ the risk of **lithium** toxicity.

Drug-Natural: Avoid natural licorice; causes sodium and water retention and ↑ potassium loss.

Route/Dosage

Hypertension

PO (Adults): 2.5–5 mg once daily, ↑ as required up to 40 mg/day in 1–2 divided doses (initiate therapy at 2.5 mg once daily in patients receiving diuretics).

PO (Children and Neonates): 0.1 mg/kg/day q 12–24 hr (once a day in neonates); may be slowly titrated up to a maximum of 0.5 mg/kg/day.

IV (Adults): 0.625–1.25 mg (0.625 mg if receiving diuretics) q 6 hr; can be titrated up to 5 mg q 6 hr.

IV (Children and Neonates): 5–10 mcg/kg/dose given q 8–24 hr.

Renal Impairment

PO, IV (Adults): *CCr 10–50 mL/min*—75% of dose; *CCr <10 mL/min*—50% of dose.

Renal Impairment

PO, IV (Children and Neonates): *CCr <30 mL/min*—Contraindicated.

Heart Failure

PO (Adults): 2.5 mg 1–2 times daily, titrated up to target dose of 10 mg bid; initiate therapy at 2.5 mg once daily in patients with hyponatremia (serum sodium <130 mEq/L).

Asymptomatic Left Ventricular Dysfunction

PO (Adults): 2.5 mg bid, titrated upward to a target dose of 10 mg bid.

Availability (generic available)

Enalapril

Tablets: 2.5 mg, 5 mg, 10 mg, 20 mg. ***In combination with:*** hydrochlorothiazide (Vaseretic). See Appendix B.

Enalaprilat

Injection: 1.25 mg/mL.

enfuvirtide (en-foo-veer-tide)

Fuzeon

Classification

Therapeutic: antiretrovirals

Pharmacologic: fusion inhibitors

Indications

Management of HIV infection in combination with other antiretrovirals in patients with evidence of progressive HIV-1 replication despite ongoing treatment.

Action

Prevents entry of HIV-1 into cells by interfering with the fusion of the virus with cellular membranes.

Therapeutic Effects: Decreased replication of the HIV virus. Slowed progression of HIV infection with decreased occurrence of sequelae. Improved CD4 cell count.

Adverse Reactions/Side Effects

CNS: fatigue. **EENT:** conjunctivitis. **Resp:** cough, pneumonia, sinusitis. **GI:** diarrhea, nausea, abdominal pain, anorexia, dry mouth, pancreatitis, weight loss.

Local: injection site reactions. **MS:** myalgia, limb pain. **Misc:** hypersensitivity reactions, herpes simplex.

PHYSICAL THERAPY IMPLICATIONS

Examination and Evaluation

- Monitor signs of hypersensitivity reactions, including pulmonary symptoms (tightness in the throat and chest, wheezing, cough, dyspnea) or skin reactions (rash, pruritus, urticaria). Notify physician or nursing staff immediately if these reactions occur.
- Monitor any breathing difficulties; notify physician immediately if patient experiences signs of pneumonia (cough, fever, chills, chest pain during inspiration and expiration).
- Assess any muscle or limb pain to rule out musculoskeletal pathology; that is, try to determine if pain is drug induced rather than caused by anatomic or biomechanical problems.
- Monitor fatigue and weakness. Some degree of fatigue is expected, but excessive or unusual fatigue should be reported.
- Monitor subcutaneous injection site for pain, swelling, and irritation. Report prolonged or excessive injection site reactions to the physician.

Interventions

- Implement resistive exercises and other therapeutic exercises as needed to maintain muscle strength and function and to prevent muscle wasting associated with HIV infection and AIDS.

Patient/Client-Related Instruction

- Emphasize the importance of taking enfuvirtide as directed even if the patient is asymptomatic and that this drug must always be used in combination with other antiretroviral drugs. Do not take more than prescribed amount and do not stop taking without consulting health care professional.
- Inform patient that enfuvirtide does not cure HIV or AIDS or prevent associated or opportunistic infections. Enfuvirtide does not reduce the risk of transmission of HIV to others through sexual contact or blood contamination. Caution patient to use a condom, and to avoid sharing needles or donating blood to prevent spreading the AIDS virus to others.
- Advise patient about the likelihood of GI reactions (nausea, diarrhea, dry mouth). Instruct patient to report severe or prolonged GI problems or signs of pancreatitis such as upper abdominal pain (especially after eating), indigestion, weight loss, and oily stools.
- Instruct patient to report other troublesome side effects such as prolonged or severe sinus inflammation, eye irritation, or aggravation of herpes simplex infections.

Pharmacokinetics

Absorption: 84% absorbed following subcutaneous administration.
Distribution: 5.5 L **Protein Binding:** 92% bound to plasma proteins.
Metabolism and Excretion: Broken down into component amino acids and then recycled in body pool.
Half-life: 3.8 hr.

TIME/ACTION PROFILE (blood levels)

ROUTE	ONSET	PEAK	DURATION
SC	unknown	8 hr	12 hr

Contraindications/Precautions

Contraindicated in: Hypersensitivity; Lactation (breast-feeding not recommended in HIV-infected patients).
Use Cautiously in: Pregnancy (use only if clearly indicated); Children <6 yr (safety not established).

Interactions

Drug-Drug: None noted.

Route/Dosage

Subcut (Adults): 90 mg bid.
Subcut (Children 6–16 yr): 2 mg/kg bid (not to exceed 90 mg/dose).

Availability

Lyophilized powder for SC administration: 108 mg/vial (to deliver a 90 mg/1 mL concentration).

HIGH ALERT

enoxaparin (e-nox-a-**pa**-rin)

Lovenox

Classification
Therapeutic: anticoagulants
Pharmacologic: antithrombotics

Indications

Prevention of deep vein thrombosis (DVT) and pulmonary embolism (PE) in surgical and medical patients. Treatment of DVT (with warfarin). Prevention of ischemic complications (with aspirin) from unstable angina, non–Q-wave MI. **Unlabeled Use:** Systemic anticoagulation for other diagnoses.

Action

Potentiates the inhibitory effect of antithrombin on factor Xa and thrombin. **Therapeutic Effects:** Prevention of thrombus formation.

Adverse Reactions/Side Effects

CNS: dizziness, headache, insomnia. **CV:** edema. **GI:** constipation, nausea, reversible increase in liver enzymes, vomiting. **GU:** urinary retention. **Derm:** ecchymoses, pruritus, rash, urticaria. **F and E:** hyperkalemia. **Hemat:** bleeding, anemia, thrombocytopenia. **Local:** erythema at injection site, hematoma, irritation, pain. **Misc:** fever.

PHYSICAL THERAPY IMPLICATIONS

Examination and Evaluation

- Monitor symptoms of DVT (pain, swelling, warmth, redness) to determine if drug therapy is effective in preventing or reducing venous thrombosis. Request or administer objective tests (Doppler ultrasound) if symptoms increase.
- In patients with DVT, watch for signs of pulmonary embolism (shortness of breath, chest pain, cough, bloody sputum). Notify physician or nursing staff immediately if these signs occur.
- Assess for signs of bleeding and hemorrhage, including bleeding gums, nosebleeds, unusual bruising, black/tarry stools, hematuria, and a fall in hematocrit or blood pressure. Notify physician or nursing staff immediately if enoxaparin causes excessive anticoagulation.
- Assess peripheral edema using girth measurements, volume displacement, and measurement of pitting edema (See Appendix N). Report increased swelling in feet and ankles or a sudden increase in body weight due to fluid retention or vasodilation.
- Monitor signs of anemia, including unusual fatigue, shortness of breath with exertion, bruising, and pale skin. Notify physician or nursing staff immediately if these signs occur.
- Monitor signs of high plasma potassium levels (hyperkalemia), including bradycardia, fatigue, weakness, numbness, and tingling. Notify physician or nursing staff because severe cases can lead to life-threatening arrhythmias and paralysis.
- Assess dizziness that might affect gait, balance, and other functional activities (See Appendix C). Report balance problems and functional limitations to the physician and nursing staff, and caution the patient and family/caregivers to guard against falls and trauma.
- Be alert for acute arterial or venous thrombosis caused by heparin-induced thrombocytopenia (HIT). Although the risk of HIT is lower compared with traditional heparin, enoxaparin may initiate an immune reaction in certain patients where antibodies attack circulating platelets. Although most cases of HIT are minor and asymptomatic, some patients may experience life- or limb-threatening platelet clots, resulting in myocardial infarction, ischemic stroke, acute leg ischemia, or venous thromboembolism. HIT can occur during and up to several weeks after heparin therapy. Any signs of increased clotting should be reported immediately.
- Assess injection site for pain, swelling, irritation, or bruising. Report prolonged or excessive injection-site reactions to the physician or nursing staff.

Interventions

- Use caution with any physical interventions that could increase bleeding, including wound débridement, chest percussion, joint mobilization, and application of local heat.
- Recommend or implement other physical methods to decrease DVT and prevent thromboembolism, including graduated compression stockings and intermittent pneumatic compression pumps.
- Implement early mobilization and ambulation to reduce the risk of new or increased DVT. Early ambulation appears to be safe in patients with DVT if the patient is adequately heparinized (INR values in acceptable range), does not have an active pulmonary embolism, or have other risk factors that contraindicate ambulation.
- Use caution during aerobic exercise and other forms of therapeutic exercise in patients with unstable angina or MI. Assess exercise tolerance frequently (blood pressure, heart rate, fatigue levels), and terminate exercise immediately if any untoward responses occur (See Appendix L).
- Do not apply physical agents (heat, cold, electrotherapeutic modalities) or massage over the injection site; these interventions can alter drug absorption from subcutaneous tissues.

Patient/client-related Instruction

- Instruct patient to report immediately signs of GI bleeding, including abdominal pain, vomiting blood, blood in stools, or black, tarry stools.
- Advise patient that rash and other skin reactions (itching, hives, discoloration) are likely. Severe or unexpected skin reactions should be reported to the physician.
- Instruct patient or family/caregivers to report other bothersome side effects such as severe or prolonged headache, sleep loss, fever, urinary retention, or GI problems (nausea, vomiting, constipation).

Pharmacokinetics

Absorption: 92% absorbed after SC administration.
Distribution: Unknown.
Metabolism and Excretion: Primarily renally eliminated.
Half-life: 3–6 hr.

TIME/ACTION PROFILE (anticoagulant effect)

ROUTE	ONSET	PEAK	DURATION
SC	unknown	unknown	12 hr

Contraindications/Precautions

Contraindicated in: Hypersensitivity; Hypersensitivity to benzyl alcohol (multidose vial); Positive in vitro test for antiplatelet antibody in the presence of enoxaparin; Active, major bleeding.
Use Cautiously in: Severe liver or kidney disease (adjust dose if CCr <30 mL/min); Retinopathy (hypertensive or diabetic); Uncontrolled hypertension; Recent history of ulcer disease; History of congenital or acquired bleeding disorder; Women <45 kg and men <57 kg (↑ exposure to enoxaparin with ↑ risk of bleeding; weight-adjusted dosing recommended); Geri: Enoxaparin elimination prolonged; Malignancy; OB/Lactation/Pedi: Safety not established; should not be used in pregnant patients with prosthetic heart valves without careful monitoring.
Exercise Extreme Caution in: Severe uncontrolled hypertension; Bacterial endocarditis, bleeding disorders; GI bleeding/ulceration/pathology; Hemorrhagic stroke; Recent CNS or ophthalmologic surgery; Active GI bleeding/ulceration; History of thrombocytopenia related to heparin; Spinal/epidural anesthesia or spinal puncture (increased risk of spinal/epidural hematoma that may lead to long-term or permanent paralysis).

Interactions

Drug-Drug: Risk of bleeding may be ↑ by concurrent use of **drugs that affect platelet function and coagulation,** including **warfarin, aspirin, thrombolytic agents, NSAIDs, dipyridamole,** some **penicillins, clopidogrel, abciximab, eptifibatide, tirofiban, ticlopidine,** and **dextran.**

Route/Dosage

DVT Prophylaxis

SC (Adults): *Knee replacement surgery*—30 mg q 12 hr starting 12–24 hr after surgery; *Hip replacement*—40 mg 12 hr before surgery then once daily; may be continued for up to 3 wk after hospital discharge; *Abdominal surgery*—40 mg 2 hr prior to surgery, then q 24 hr postop for 7–12 days or until ambulatory (up to 14 days); *Medical patients with acute illness*—40 mg once daily.

Treatment of DVT/PE

SC (Adults): *Outpatient*—1 mg/kg q 12 hr; *Inpatien* —1 mg/kg q 12 hr or 1.5 mg/kg q 24 hr. Warfarin should be started within 72 hr; enoxaparin may be continued for 5–17 days or until therapeutic anticoagulation with warfarin is achieved (INR >2 for 2 consecutive days).

Angina/Non–Q-wave MI

SC (Adults): 1 mg/kg q 12 hr for 2–8 days (up to 12.5 days).

Renal Impairment

SC (Adults CCr < 30 ml/min): *DVT prophylaxis for abdominal, knee, or hip surgery*—↓ 30 mg once daily; *Angina/Non–Q-wave MI, treatment of DVT*—1 mg/kg once daily.

Availability

Solution for injection (prefilled syringes): 30 mg/0.3 mL, 40 mg/0.4 mL, 60 mg/0.6 mL, 80 mg/0.8 mL, 100 mg/1 mL, 120mg/0.8 mL, 150 mg/1 mL.
Solution for injection: 300 mg/3-mL multidose vial.

entacapone (en-tak-a-pone)

Comtan

Classification
Therapeutic: antiparkinson agents
Pharmacologic: catechol-O-methyltransferase inhibitors

Indications

With levodopa/carbidopa to treat idiopathic Parkinson's disease when signs and symptoms of end-of-dose "wearing-off" (so-called fluctuating patients) occur.

Action

Acts as a selective and reversible inhibitor of the enzyme catechol-*O*-methyltransferase (COMT). Inhibition of this enzyme prevents the breakdown of levodopa, increasing availability to the CNS. **Therapeutic Effects:** Prolongs duration of response to levodopa with end-of-dose motor fluctuations. Decreased signs and symptoms of Parkinson's disease.

Adverse Reactions/Side Effects

CNS: NEUROLEPTIC MALIGNANT SYNDROME, dizziness, hallucinations, syncope. **Resp:** pulmonary infiltrates, pleural effusion, pleural thickening. **CV:** hypotension. **GI:** abdominal pain, diarrhea, nausea (during initiation), retroperitoneal fibrosis. **GU:** brownish orange discoloration of urine. **MS:** RHABDOMYOLYSIS. **Neuro:** dyskinesia.

PHYSICAL THERAPY IMPLICATIONS

Examination and Evaluation

- Be alert for signs of neuroleptic malignant syndrome, including hyperthermia, diaphoresis, generalized muscle rigidity, hallucinations, altered mental status, tachycardia, changes in blood pressure (BP), and incontinence. Symptoms typically occur within 4–14 days after initiation of drug therapy, but can occur at any time during drug use. Report these signs to the physician immediately.

- Assess any muscle pain, tenderness, or weakness, especially if accompanied by fever, malaise, and dark-colored urine. Advise patient that these symptoms may represent drug-induced myopathy, and that myopathy can progress to severe muscle damage (rhabdomyolysis). Report any unexplained musculoskeletal symptoms to the physician immediately.
- Assess gait and motor function to help determine antiparkinson effects, especially when starting drug therapy or during dosing changes or addition of other antiparkinson drugs. Motor function should be assessed at different times of the day, such as when drugs are reaching peak therapeutic levels (i.e., 30–60 min after oral dose), as well as when drug effects are minimal (just before the next dose).
- Document increased side effects such as involuntary movements (dyskinesias) or fluctuations in response (on-off phenomenon, end-of-dose akinesia). Notify physician because increased side effects might require dose adjustment or a change in medication regimen.
- Assess BP periodically and compare to normal values (See Appendix F). Report low BP (hypotension), especially if patient experiences increased dizziness, fainting, or other symptoms.
- Monitor respiratory function at rest and during exercise. Notify physician if patient experiences signs of pulmonary infiltrates or pleural effusion, including cough, shortness of breath, chest pain, or labored breathing.
- Assess dizziness and syncope that might affect gait, balance, and other functional activities (See Appendix C). Report balance problems and functional limitations to the physician, and caution the patient and family/caregivers to guard against falls and trauma.

Interventions

- Implement therapeutic exercises (coordination exercises, gait training, cardiovascular conditioning) to complement the effects of drug therapy and help achieve optimal function.
- Guard against falls and trauma (hip fractures, head injury, and so forth). Implement fall-prevention strategies (See Appendix E), especially if patient exhibits parkinsonian symptoms (postural instability, rigidity) combined with drug side effects (dizziness, syncope).
- To minimize orthostatic hypotension, patient should move slowly when assuming a more upright position.

Patient/Client-Related Instruction

- Advise patient to avoid alcohol because of the increased risk of sedation and adverse effects.
- Advise patient about the likelihood of GI reactions (diarrhea, nausea, abdominal pain). Instruct patient to report severe or prolonged GI problems.

Pharmacokinetics

Absorption: 35% absorbed following oral administration; absorption is rapid.
Distribution: Unknown.
Protein Binding: 98%.
Metabolism and Excretion: Minimal amounts excreted unchanged; highly metabolized followed by biliary excretion.
Half-life: *Initial phase*—0.4–0.7 hr; *second phase*—2.4 hr.

TIME/ACTION PROFILE (inhibition of COMT)

ROUTE	ONSET	PEAK	DURATION
PO	unknown	unknown	up to 8 hr

Contraindications/Precautions

Contraindicated in: Hypersensitivity; Concurrent nonselective MAO inhibitor therapy.
Use Cautiously in: Hepatic impairment; Concurrent use of drugs that are metabolized by COMT; Pregnancy, lactation, or children (safety not established).

Interactions

Drug-Drug: Concurrent use with selective **MAO inhibitors** is not recommended; both agents inhibit the metabolic pathways of catecholamines. Concurrent use of drugs that are metabolized by COMT, such as **isoproterenol, epinephrine, norepinephrine, dopamine, dobutamine,** and **methyldopa,** may ↑ risk of tachycardia, ↑ BP, and arrhythmias. **Probenecid, cholestyramine, erythromycin, rifampin, ampicillin,** and **chloramphenicol** may interfere with biliary elimination of entacapone; concurrent use should be undertaken with caution.

Route/Dosage

PO (Adults): 200 mg with each dose of levodopa/carbidopa up to a maximum of 8 times daily.

Availability

Tablets: 200 mg. ***In combination with:*** levodopa/carbidopa (Stalevo). See Appendix B.

entecavir (en-tek-a-veer)

Baraclude

Classification
Therapeutic: antivirals
Pharmacologic: nucleoside analogues

Indications

Chronic hepatitis B infection with evidence of active disease.

E

Action

Phosphorylated intracellularly to active form which acts as an analogue of guanosine, interfering with viral DNA synthesis. **Therapeutic Effects:** Decreased hepatic damage due to chronic hepatitis B infection.

Adverse Reactions/Side Effects

CNS: dizziness, fatigue, headache. **GI:** HEPATOMEGALY (WITH STEATOSIS), dyspepsia, nausea. **F and E:** LACTIC ACIDOSIS. **Derm:** rash.

PHYSICAL THERAPY IMPLICATIONS

Examination and Evaluation

- Be alert for signs of enlarged, fatty liver (hepatomegaly with steatosis) that can progress to liver dysfunction and liver failure. Signs of liver disease include anorexia, abdominal pain, abdominal swelling (ascites), severe nausea and vomiting, yellow skin or eyes, fever, sore throat, malaise, weakness, facial edema, lethargy, and unusual bleeding or bruising. Notify physician of these signs immediately.
- Monitor signs of lactic acidosis, including confusion, lethargy, stupor, shallow rapid breathing, tachycardia, hypotension, nausea, and vomiting. Notify physician immediately if these signs occur.
- Assess dizziness that might affect gait, balance, and other functional activities (See Appendix C). Report balance problems and functional limitations to the physician, and caution the patient and family/caregivers to guard against falls and trauma.

Interventions

- Because of the risk of lactic acidosis, use caution during aerobic exercise and other forms of therapeutic exercise. Assess exercise tolerance frequently (blood pressure, heart rate, fatigue levels), and terminate exercise immediately if any untoward responses occur (See Appendix L).

Patient/Client-Related Instruction

- Inform patient that entecavir does not cure hepatitis B virus (HBV), but may lower the amount of HBV in the body, may lower the ability of HBV to multiply and infect new liver cells, and may improve the condition of the liver. Entecavir does not reduce the risk of transmission of HBV to others through sexual contact or blood contamination. Caution patient to use a condom during sexual contact and to avoid sharing needles or donating blood to prevent spreading HBV to others.
- Instruct patient to report other troublesome side effects such as prolonged or severe headache, fatigue, skin rash, or GI problems (nausea, indigestion).

Pharmacokinetics

Absorption: Well absorbed following oral administration.
Distribution: Extensive tissue distribution.
Metabolism and Excretion: 62–73% excreted unchanged by kidneys.
Half-life: Plasma—128–149 hr; intracellular—15 hr.

TIME/ACTION PROFILE (blood levels)

ROUTE	ONSET	PEAK	DURATION
PO	rapid	0.5–1 hr	24 hr

Contraindications/Precautions

Contraindicated in: Hypersensitivity; Lactation: Lactation.
Use Cautiously in: Renal impairment (dose reduction recommended if CCr <50 mL/min; Liver transplant recipients (careful monitoring of renal function recommended); Patients coinfected with HIV (unless receiving highly active antiretroviral therapy; at ↑ risk for resistance); Geri: May have age-related ↓ in renal function; Pedi: Children <16 yr (safety not established); OB: Use only if clearly needed, considering benefits and risks.

Interactions

Drug-Drug: Concurrent use of drugs which may impair renal function may ↑ blood levels and risk of toxicity.

Route/Dosage

PO (Adults and Children >16 yr): 0.5 mg once daily; *history of lamivudine resistance*—1 mg once daily.

Renal Impairment

PO (Adults and Children >16 yr): *CCr 30–50 mL/min*—0.25 mg once daily, *history of lamivudine resistance*—0.5 mg once daily; *CCr 10– <30 mL/min*—0.15 mg once daily, *history of lamivudine resistance*—0.3 mg once daily; *CCr <10 mL/min*—0.05 mg once daily, *history of lamivudine resistance*—0.1 mg once daily.

Availability

Tablets: 0.5 mg, 1 mg. **Oral solution (orange):** 0.05 mg/mL.

HIGH ALERT

epinephrine (e-pi-nef-rin)

Adrenalin, Ana-Guard, AsthmaHaler Mist, AsthmaNefrin (racepinephrine), EpiPen, microNefrin, Nephron, Primatene, Sus-Phrine, S-2

Classification

Therapeutic: antiasthmatics, bronchodilators, vasopressors

Pharmacologic: adrenergics

Indications

SCbcut, IV, Inhalation: Management of reversible airway disease due to asthma or COPD. **SC, IV:** Management of severe allergic reactions. **IV, Intracardiac, Intratracheal, Intraosseous (part of advanced cardiac life support [ACLS] and pediatric advanced life support [PALS] guidelines):** Management of cardiac arrest (unlabeled). **Inhalation:** Management of upper airway obstruction and croup (racemic epinephrine). **Local/Spinal:** Adjunct in the localization/prolongation of anesthesia.

Action

Results in the accumulation of cyclic adenosine monophosphate (cAMP) at beta-adrenergic receptors. Affects both beta$_1$ (cardiac)–adrenergic receptors and beta$_2$ (pulmonary)–adrenergic receptor sites. Produces bronchodilation. Also has alpha-adrenergic agonist properties, which result in vasoconstriction. Inhibits the release of mediators of immediate hypersensitivity reactions from mast cells. **Therapeutic Effects:** Bronchodilation. Maintenance of heart rate and blood pressure (BP). Localization/prolongation of local/spinal anesthetic.

Adverse Reactions/Side Effects

CNS: nervousness, restlessness, tremor, headache, insomnia. **Resp:** paradoxical bronchospasm (excessive use of inhalers). **CV:** angina, arrhythmias, hypertension, tachycardia. **GI:** nausea, vomiting. **Endo:** hyperglycemia.

PHYSICAL THERAPY IMPLICATIONS

Examination and Evaluation

- In patients with airway disease, assess pulmonary function at rest and during exercise (See Appendices I, J, K) to document effectiveness of medication in controlling bronchospasm.
- Monitor signs of increased (paradoxical) bronchospasm such as wheezing, cough, dyspnea, and tightness in chest and throat. These signs are more common at high or excessive inhaled doses. If condition occurs, advise patient to withhold medication and notify physician or other health care professional immediately.
- Assess BP periodically and compare to normal values (See Appendix F). Report a sustained increase in BP (hypertension) to the physician.
- Assess heart rate, ECG, and heart sounds, especially during exercise (see Appendices G, H). Report any rhythm disturbances or symptoms of increased arrhythmias, including angina, palpitations, shortness of breath, fainting, and fatigue/weakness.
- Monitor and report signs of CNS toxicity, including nervousness, restlessness, insomnia, or tremor. Sustained or severe CNS signs may indicate overdose or excessive use of this drug.
- Monitor signs of hyperglycemia (drowsiness, fruity breath, increased urination, unusual thirst). Patients with diabetes mellitus should check blood glucose levels frequently.

Interventions

- When implementing airway clearance techniques or respiratory muscle training, attempt to intervene when the airway is maximally bronchodilated. Drug effect is usually very rapid (within 1 min) after inhalation, so chest physical therapy interventions can begin soon after drug administration.
- Because of the risk of cardiovascular stimulation, use extreme caution during aerobic exercise and endurance conditioning. Cardiovascular effects such as arrhythmias, angina pectoris, or increased BP occur more commonly with epinephrine compared to other bronchodilators because epinephrine stimulates beta$_1$ receptors on the heart and alpha$_1$ receptors on the vasculature as well as beta$_2$ receptors on the lungs.

Patient/Client-Related Instruction

- Advise patient not to exceed the recommended dose or frequency of inhalations for treating airway disease. Contact physician immediately if bronchospasm is not relieved by medication or is accompanied by diaphoresis, dizziness, or other symptoms.
- If injected to treat severe allergic reactions, make sure patient and family or caregivers understand proper administration techniques. Emphasize the need to always have the injectable form of this drug nearby.
- Counsel patient on proper use of inhaler; observe use of this device whenever possible to ensure proper technique.
- Instruct patient and family/caregivers to report severe or prolonged headache, sleep loss, or GI problems (nausea, vomiting, dry mouth).

Pharmacokinetics

Absorption: Well absorbed following SC administration; some absorption may occur following repeated inhalation of large doses.

Distribution: Does not cross the blood-brain barrier; crosses the placenta and enters breast milk.
Metabolism and Excretion: Action is rapidly terminated by metabolism and uptake by nerve endings.
Half-life: Unknown.

TIME/ACTION PROFILE (bronchodilation)

ROUTE	ONSET	PEAK	DURATION
inhalation	1 min	unknown	1–3 hr
SC	5–10 min	20 min	<1–4 hr
IM	6–12 min	unknown	<1–4 hr
IV	rapid	20 min	20–30 min

Contraindications/Precautions

Contraindicated in: Hypersensitivity to adrenergic amines; Cardiac arrhythmias; Some products may contain bisulfites or fluorocarbons (in some inhalers) and should be avoided in patients with known hypersensitivity or intolerance.
Use Cautiously in: Cardiac disease (angina, tachycardia, MI); Hypertension; Hyperthyroidism; Diabetes; Cerebral arteriosclerosis; Glaucoma (except for ophthalmic use); Elderly patients (more susceptible to adverse reactions; may require dosage reduction); Pregnancy (near term) and lactation; Excessive use may lead to tolerance and paradoxical bronchospasm (inhaler).

Interactions

Drug-Drug: Concurrent use with other **adrenergic agents** will have additive adrenergic side effects. Use with **MAO inhibitors** may lead to hypertensive crisis. **Beta blockers** may negate therapeutic effect. **Tricyclic antidepressants** enhance pressor response to epinephrine.
Drug-Natural: Use with caffeine-containing herbs **(cola nut, guarana, mate, tea, coffee)** ↑ stimulant effect.

Route/Dosage

SC, IM (Adults): *Anaphylactic reactions/asthma*—0.1–0.5 mg (single dose not to exceed 1 mg); may repeat q 10–15 min for anaphylactic shock or q 20 min–4 hr for asthma.
SC (Children >1 mo): *Anaphylactic reactions/asthma*—0.01 mg/kg (not to exceed 0.5 mg/dose) q 15 min for 2 doses, then q 4 hr.
IV (Adults): *Severe anaphylaxis*—0.1–0.25 mg q 5–15 min; may be followed by 1–4 mcg/min continuous infusion; *cardiopulmonary resuscitation (ACLS guidelines)*—1 mg q 3–5 min; *bradycardia (ACLS guidelines)*—2–10 mcg/min).
IV (Children): *Severe anaphylaxis*—0.1 mg (less in younger children); may be followed by 0.1 mcg/kg/min continuous infusion (may be increased up to 1.5 mcg/kg/min); *symptomatic bradycardia/pulseless arrest (PALS guidelines)*—0.01 mg/kg, may be repeated q 3–5 min higher doses (up to 0.1–0.2 mg/kg) may be considered; may also be given by the intraosseous route. May also be given by the endotracheal route in doses of 0.1–0.2 mg/kg diluted to a volume of 3–5 mL with normal saline followed by several positive pressure ventilations.
Inhalation (Adults): *Metered-dose inhaler*—1 inhalation (160–250 mcg), may be repeated after 1–2 min; additional doses may be repeated q 3 hr; *inhalation solution*—1 inhalation of 1% solution; may be repeated after 1–2 min; additional doses may be given q 3 hr; *racepinephrine*—Via hand nebulizer, 2–3 inhalations of 2.25% solution, may repeat in 5 min with 2–3 more inhalations, up to 4–6 times daily.
Inhalation (Children >1 mo): 0.25–0.5 mL of 2.25% racemic epinephrine solution diluted in 3 mL normal saline.
IV, Intratracheal (Neonates): 0.01–0.03 mg/kg q 3–5 min as needed.
IM (Children >1 mo < 30 kg): 0.15 mg (EpiPen Jr); > 30 kg: 0.3 mg (EpiPen).
Intracardiac (Adults): 0.3–0.5 mg.
Endotracheal: (Adults): *Cardiopulmonary resuscitation (ACLS guidelines)*—2–2.5 mg.
Topical (Adults and Children ≥6 yr): *Nasal decongestant*—Apply 1% solution as drops, spray, or with a swab.
Intraspinal: (Adults and Children): 0.2–0.4 mL of 1:1000 solution.
With Local Anesthetics: (Adults and Children): Use 1:200,000 solution with local anesthetic.

Availability (generic available)

Inhalation aerosol: 0.125% (≥300 inhalations/15 mL) OTC, 0.5% (≥300 inhalations/15 mL) OTC, 300 mcg/spray (≥300 inhalations/15 mL) OTC. **Inhalation solution:** 1% OTC. **Injection:** 0.1 mg/mL (1:10,000), 1 mg/mL (1:1000). **Autoinjector (EpiPen):** 0.15 mg/0.3 mL (1:2000), 0.3 mg/0.3 mL (1:1000). **Topical solution:** 0.1%.

HIGH ALERT

epirubicin (ep-i-roo-bi-sin)

Ellence

Classification
Therapeutic: antineoplastics
Pharmacologic: anthracyclines

Indications

A component of adjuvant therapy for evidence of axillary tumor involvement following resection of primary breast cancer.

Action

Inhibits DNA and RNA synthesis by forming a complex with DNA. **Therapeutic Effects:** Death of rapidly replicating cells, particularly malignant ones.

Adverse Reactions/Side Effects

CNS: lethargy. **CV:** CARDIOTOXICITY (DOSE-RELATED).
GI: nausea, vomiting, anorexia, diarrhea, mucositis. **Derm:** alopecia, flushing, itching, photosensitivity, radiation-recall reaction, rash, skin/nail hyperpigmentation. **Endo:** gonadal suppression. **Hemat:** LEUKOPENIA, anemia, thrombocytopenia, treatment-related leukemia/myelodysplastic syndromes. **Local:** injection site reactions, phlebitis at IV site, tissue necrosis. **Metab:** hot flashes, hyperuricemia. **Misc:** ANAPHYLAXIS, INFECTION.

PHYSICAL THERAPY IMPLICATIONS

Examination and Evaluation

- Assess heart rate, ECG, and blood pressure, especially during exercise. Report any arrhythmias or signs of cardiotoxicity, including chest discomfort, shortness of breath, dyspnea, rales/crackles, peripheral edema, jugular venous distention, fainting, or severe fatigue and weakness.
- Be alert for signs of leukopenia (fever, sore throat, signs of infection), thrombocytopenia (bruising, nose bleeds, bleeding gums), or unusual weakness and fatigue that might be due to anemia or other blood dyscrasias. Report these signs to the physician or nursing staff immediately.
- Monitor signs of allergic reactions or anaphylaxis, including pulmonary symptoms (tightness in the throat and chest, wheezing, cough, dyspnea) or skin reactions (rash, pruritus, urticaria). Notify physician or nursing staff immediately if these reactions occur.
- Monitor IV injection site for pain, swelling, and inflammation (phlebitis). Report signs of phlebitis, tissue necrosis, or other prolonged or excessive injection site reactions to the physician.

Interventions

- For patients who are medically able to begin exercise, implement appropriate resistive exercises and aerobic training to maintain muscle strength and aerobic capacity during cancer chemotherapy, or to help restore function after chemotherapy.
- Because of the risk of cardiotoxicity and blood dyscrasias, use caution during aerobic exercise and other forms of therapeutic exercise. Assess exercise tolerance frequently (blood pressure, heart rate, respiratory symptoms, fatigue levels), and terminate exercise immediately if any untoward responses occur (See Appendix L).
- Causes photosensitivity; use care if administering UV treatments. Advise patient to avoid direct sunlight and use sunscreens and protective clothing.

Patient/Client-Related Instruction

- Advise patient to guard against infection (frequent hand washing, etc.), and to avoid crowds and contact with persons with contagious diseases.
- Advise patient about the likelihood of GI reactions including diarrhea, nausea, vomiting, loss of appetite, and irritation in/around the mouth. Instruct patient or family and caregivers to report other severe or unexpected GI problems.
- Advise patient that rash, itching, hair loss and other skin reactions are likely. Patients and family/caregivers should be especially alert for severe skin reactions that occur when this drug is given after radiation treatments (radiation-recall reactions). Instruct patient to report severe or unexpected skin reactions.

Pharmacokinetics

Absorption: IV administration results in complete bioavailability.
Distribution: Rapidly and widely distributed; concentrates in RBCs.
Metabolism and Excretion: Extensively and rapidly metabolized by the liver and other tissues.
Half-life: 35 hr.

TIME/ACTION PROFILE (effect on WBCs)

ROUTE	ONSET	PEAK	DURATION
IV	unknown	10–14 days	21 days

Contraindications/Precautions

Contraindicated in: Hypersensitivity to epirubicin, other anthracyclines, or related compounds; Baseline neutrophil count <1500 cells/mm^3; Severe myocardial insufficiency or recent MI; Previous anthracyclines up to the maximum cumulative dose; Severe hepatic dysfunction; OB: Pregnancy or lactation; Concurrent cimetidine therapy.
Use Cautiously in: Severe renal impairment (serum creatinine >5 mg/dL); lower doses should be considered; Hepatic impairment (dose reduction recommended for bilirubin >1.2 mg/dL or AST >2–4 times upper limit of normal); Female patients ≥70 yr (increased risk of toxicity); Depressed bone marrow reserve; OB: Patients with childbearing potential; Pedi: Pediatric patients (safety not established; increased risk of acute cardiotoxicity and chronic CHF).

Interactions

Drug-Drug: Cimetidine ↑ blood levels and the risk of serious toxicity; concurrent use should be avoided.

Additive hematologic and gastrointestinal toxicity with other **antineoplastics** or **radiation therapy**. May ↓ the antibody response to **live-virus vaccines** and increase the risk of adverse reactions.

Route/Dosage

IV (Adults): 100–120 mg/m² repeated in 3–4 wk cycles (total dose may be given on day 1 or split and given in equally divided doses on day 1 and day 8 of each cycle (combination regimens may employ concurrent 5-fluorouracil and cyclophosphamide).

Hepatic Impairment

IV (Adults): *Bilirubin 1.2—3 mg/dL or AST 2–4 times upper limit of normal*—use 50% of recommended starting dose; *bilirubin >3 mg/dL or AST >4 times upper limit of normal*—use 25% of recommended starting dose.

Availability

Solution for injection (red): 50-mg/25-mL single-use vial, 200-mg/100-mL single-use vial.

eplerenone (e-ple-re-none)

Inspra

Classification

Therapeutic: antihypertensives

Pharmacologic: aldosterone antagonists

Indications

Hypertension (alone or with other agents). LV systolic dysfunction and evidence of HF post-MI.

Action

Blocks the effects of aldosterone by attaching to mineralocorticoid receptors. **Therapeutic Effects:** Lowering of blood pressure. Improves survival in patients with evidence of HF post-MI.

Adverse Reactions/Side Effects

CNS: dizziness, fatigue. **GI:** abnormal liver function tests, abdominal pain, diarrhea. **GU:** albuminuria. **Endo:** abnormal vaginal bleeding, gynecomastia. **F and E:** HYPERKALEMIA. **Metab:** hypercholesterolemia, hypertriglyceridemia. **Misc:** flu-like symptoms.

PHYSICAL THERAPY IMPLICATIONS

Examination and Evaluation

- Monitor signs of high plasma potassium levels (hyperkalemia), including bradycardia, fatigue, weakness, numbness, and tingling. Notify physician because severe cases can lead to life-threatening arrhythmias and paralysis.
- Assess blood pressure periodically and compare to normal values (See Appendix F) to help document antihypertensive effects.
- Assess dizziness and fatigue that might affect gait, balance, and other functional activities (See Appendix C). Report balance problems and functional limitations to the physician, and caution the patient and family/caregivers to guard against falls and trauma.

Interventions

- Implement fall prevention strategies, especially in older adults or if patient exhibits sedation, dizziness, clumsiness, or other impairments that affect gait and balance (See Appendix E).
- Use caution during aerobic exercise, especially after recent MI or in hot environments. Increased sweating will cause fluid and electrolyte loss and may exaggerate arrhythmias and diuretic side effects (dizziness, muscle cramps, and so forth).
- To minimize orthostatic hypotension, patient should move slowly when assuming a more upright position.

Patient/Client-Related Instruction

- Remind patients to take medication as directed to control hypertension and other cardiac conditions even if they are asymptomatic.
- Counsel patients about additional interventions to help control blood pressure and cardiac dysfunction, such as regular exercise, weight loss, sodium restriction, stress reduction, moderation of alcohol consumption, and smoking cessation.
- Advise patient that this drug may cause problems in fat metabolism, including hypercholesterolemia and hypertriglyceridemia. Remind patient that periodic blood tests may be needed to monitor plasma lipids.
- Instruct patient or family and caregivers to report other troublesome side effects such as severe flu-like symptoms, breast growth in men (gynecomastia), abnormal vaginal bleeding, or GI problems (diarrhea, abdominal pain).

Pharmacokinetics

Absorption: Well absorbed following oral administration.

Distribution: Unknown.

Metabolism and Excretion: Mostly metabolized by the liver (CYP3A4 enzyme system); <5% excreted unchanged by the kidneys.

Half-life: 4–6 hr.

TIME/ACTION PROFILE (antihypertensive effect)

ROUTE	ONSET	PEAK	DURATION
PO	unknown	4 wk	unknown

Contraindications/Precautions

Contraindicated in: Serum potassium >5.5 mEq/L; Type 2 diabetes with microalbuminuria (for patients with HTN; ↑ risk of hyperkalemia); Serum creatinine >2 mg/dL in males or >1.8 mg/dL in females (for patients with HTN); CCr ≤30 mL/min (for all patients); CCr <50 mL/min (for patients with HTN); Concurrent use of potassium supplements or potassium-sparing diuretics (for patients with HTN); Concurrent use of strong inhibitors of the CYP3A4 enzyme system (ketoconazole, itraconazole, nefazodone, clarithromycin, ritonavir, or nelfinavir); Lactation: Lactation.
Use Cautiously in: Severe hepatic impairment; OB: Use only if clearly needed; Pedi: Safety not established.

Interactions

Drug-Drug: Concurrent use of strong inhibitors of the CYP3A4 enzyme system (**ketoconazole, itraconazole, nefazodone, clarithromycin, ritonavir,** or **nelfinavir**) significantly ↑ effects of eplerenone; concurrent use contraindicated. Concurrent use of weak inhibitors of the CYP3A4 enzyme system (**erythromycin, saquinavir, fluconazole, verapamil**) may ↑ effects of eplerenone; initial dose of eplerenone should be ↓ by 50%. **NSAIDs** may ↓ antihypertensive effects. Concurrent use of **ACE inhibitors** or **angiotensin II receptor blockers** may ↑ risk of hyperkalemia.

Route/Dosage

Hypertension

PO (Adults): 50 mg daily initially; may be increased to 50 mg bid; *Patients receiving concurrent moderate CYP3A4 inhibitors (erythromycin, saquinavir, verapamil, fluconazole)*—25 mg once daily initially.

HF Post-MI

PO (Adults): 25 mg daily initially; increase in 4 wk to 50 mg daily; subsequent dose adjustments may need to be made based on serum potassium concentrations.

Availability

Tablets: 25 mg, 50 mg.

epoetin (e-poe-e-tin)

Epogen, EPO, ✱Eprex, Procrit

OTHER NAMES:
Erythropoietin

Classification
Therapeutic: antianemics
Pharmacologic: hormones

Indications

Anemia associated with chronic renal failure. Anemia secondary to zidovudine (AZT) therapy in HIV-infected patients. Anemia from chemotherapy in patients with nonmyeloid malignancies. Reduction of need for transfusions after surgery.

Action

Stimulates erythropoiesis (production of red blood cells). **Therapeutic Effects:** Maintains and may elevate RBCs, decreasing the need for transfusions.

Adverse Reactions/Side Effects

CNS: SEIZURES, headache. **CV:** CHF, MI, STROKE, THROMBOTIC EVENTS (ESPECIALLY WITH HEMOGLOBIN >12 G/DL), hypertension. **Derm:** transient rashes. **Endo:** restored fertility, resumption of menses. **Misc:** ↑ mortality and ↑ tumor growth (with hemoglobin ≥12 g/dL).

PHYSICAL THERAPY IMPLICATIONS

Examination and Evaluation

- Monitor continually and seek immediate medical assistance if patient develops any of the following signs or syndromes:
  - Myocardial infarction, as indicated by sudden chest pain, pain radiating into the arm or jaw, shortness of breath, dizziness, sweating, anxiety, and nausea.
  - Stroke as indicated by severe headache, confusion, nausea, vomiting, paralysis, numbness, speech problems, and visual disturbances.
  - Seizures as indicated by various symptoms depending on the type of seizure, such as decreased consciousness, changes in muscle tone, muscle twitches/jerking, convulsions, automatisms (lip smacking, chewing), and strange auditory, visual, and other sensations.
- Assess signs of congestive heart failure such as dyspnea, rales/crackles, peripheral edema, jugular venous distention, and exercise intolerance. Report these signs to the physician.
- Assess blood pressure periodically. Report a sustained increase in blood pressure (hypertension) to the physician.
- Monitor signs of increased tumor growth, including a change in bowel or bladder habits, unusual bleeding or discharge, a lump in the breast or other parts of the body, chronic indigestion or difficulty in swallowing, obvious changes in a wart or mole, and persistent coughing or hoarseness. Report these signs to the physician immediately.

Interventions

- Because of the risk of thrombosis, use caution during aerobic exercise and other forms of therapeutic exercise. Assess exercise tolerance frequently (blood pressure, heart rate, fatigue levels), and terminate exercise immediately if any untoward responses occur (See Appendix L).
- If administered via subcutaneous injection, do not apply massage or physical agents (heat, cold,

electrotherapeutic modalities) at or near the application site. These interventions can alter drug absorption from subcutaneous tissues.

Patient/Client-Related Instruction

- Caution patient and family/caregivers about risks of coronary thrombosis, stroke, and other thrombotic events, and review warning signs of these problems (see above under Evaluation and Examination).
- Instruct patient to report other troublesome side effects such as severe or prolonged headache or skin rash.

Pharmacokinetics

Absorption: Well absorbed after SC administration.
Distribution: Unknown.
Metabolism and Excretion: Unknown.
Half-life: 4–13 hr.

TIME/ACTION PROFILE (increase in RBCs)

ROUTE	ONSET*	PEAK	DURATION
IV, SC	7–10 days	within 2 mo	2 wk†

*Increase in reticulocytes.
†After discontinuation.

Contraindications/Precautions

Contraindicated in: Hypersensitivity to albumin or mammalian cell–derived products; Uncontrolled hypertension; Patients with erythropoietin levels >200 munits/mL; Patients receiving chemotherapy when anticipated outcome is cure.
Use Cautiously in: History of seizures; History of porphyria; OB/Lactation: Pregnancy or lactation.

Interactions

Drug-Drug: May ↑ requirement for **heparin** anticoagulation during hemodialysis.

Route/Dosage

(Use lowest dose that will gradually increase hemoglobin level and avoid RBC transfusion.)

Anemia of Chronic Renal Failure

SC, IV (Adults): 50–100 units/kg 3 times weekly initially; adjust dose to attain target hemoglobin of 10–12 g/dL.
SC, IV (Children): 50 units/kg 3 times weekly initially; adjust dose to attain target hemoglobin of 10–12 g/dL.

Anemia Secondary to AZT Therapy

SC, IV (Adults): 100 units/kg 3 times weekly for 8 wk; if inadequate response, may increase by 50–100 units/kg q 4–8 wk (max: 300 units/kg 3 times weekly).

Anemia from Chemotherapy

(Use only for chemotherapy-related anemia and discontinue when chemotherapy course is completed; do not initiate if hemoglobin ≥10 g/dL.)
SC (Adults): 150 units/kg 3 times weekly or 40,000 units weekly; adjust dose to maintain lowest hemoglobin level sufficient to avoid blood transfusions (do not exceed hemoglobin of 12 g/dL).
IV (Children): 600 units/kg 3 times weekly; adjust dose to maintain lowest hemoglobin level sufficient to avoid blood transfusions (do not exceed hemoglobin of 12 g/dL).

Surgery

SC (Adults): 300 units/kg/day for 10 days before surgery, day of surgery, and 4 days after *or* 600 units/kg 21, 14, and 7 days before surgery and on day of surgery.

Availability

Injection: 2000 units/mL, 3000 units/mL, 4000 units/mL, 10,000 units/mL, 20,000 units/mL, 40,000 units/mL.

epoprostenol

(e-poe-**pros**-te-nole)
Flolan, Prostacyclin, Prostaglandin I2 (PGI2), Prostaglandin X (PGX)

Classification
Therapeutic: vasodilators
Pharmacologic: prostaglandins, vasodilators

Indications

Management of primary pulmonary hypertension (PPH) and secondary pulmonary hypertension associated with scleroderma in New York Heart Association (NYHA) class III and IV patients who are no longer responding to standard therapy.

Action

A prostaglandin that directly dilates pulmonary and systemic arterial vasculature. Also inhibits platelet aggregation. **Therapeutic Effects:** Provides symptomatic improvement in patients with PPH and pulmonary hypertension secondary to scleroderma and increases survival in patients with PPH.

Adverse Reactions/Side Effects

CNS: anxiety, headache, dizziness. **Resp:** dyspnea. **CV:** tachycardia, bradycardia, chest pain, hypotension. **GI:** nausea, vomiting, abdominal pain, diarrhea. **Derm:** flushing. **MS:** myalgia, jaw pain. **Neuro:** hypesthesia/hyperesthesia/paresthesia. **Misc:** flu-like symptoms, injection-site reactions.

PHYSICAL THERAPY IMPLICATIONS

Examination and Evaluation

- Assess heart rate, ECG, and heart sounds, especially during exercise (See Appendices G, H). Report any rhythm disturbances or symptoms of increased arrhythmias, including palpitations, chest pain, shortness of breath, dyspnea, fainting, and fatigue/weakness.
- Assess blood pressure (BP) periodically and compare to normal values (See Appendix F). Report low BP (hypotension), especially if patient experiences dizziness, fatigue, or other symptoms.
- Assess dizziness and drowsiness that might affect gait, balance, and other functional activities (see Appendix C). Report balance problems and functional limitations to the physician and nursing staff, and caution the patient and family/caregivers to guard against falls and trauma.
- Assess any muscle or jaw pain to rule out musculoskeletal pathology; that is, try to determine if pain is drug induced rather than caused by anatomic or biomechanical problems.
- Assess signs of parasthesia (numbness, tingling) or increased/abnormal sensation. Perform objective tests, including electroneuromyography and sensory testing to document any drug-related neuropathic changes.
- Assess IV site during and after IV administration, and report any pain, swelling, inflammation, or other injection-site reactions.

Interventions

- Because of the risk of arrhythmias and abnormal BP responses, use caution during aerobic exercise and other forms of therapeutic exercise. Assess exercise tolerance frequently (BP, heart rate, fatigue levels), and terminate exercise immediately if any untoward responses occur (See Appendix L).
- Avoid physical therapy interventions that cause systemic vasodilation (large whirlpool, Hubbard tank). Additive effects of this drug and the intervention may cause a dangerous fall in BP.
- To minimize orthostatic hypotension, patient should move slowly when assuming a more upright position.

Patient/Client-Related Instruction

- Instruct patient or family/caregivers to report other troublesome side effects such as severe or prolonged headache, anxiety, skin flushing, flu-like symptoms, or GI problems (nausea, vomiting, diarrhea, abdominal pain).

Pharmacokinetics

Absorption: IV administration results in complete bioavailability.
Distribution: Unknown.
Metabolism and Excretion: Rapidly and extensively degraded in plasma; some metabolites are pharmacologically active.
Half-life: ≤6 min.

TIME/ACTION PROFILE (hemodynamic effects)

ROUTE	ONSET	PEAK	DURATION
IV	rapid (within min)	unknown	2–3 min*

*Following discontinuation.

Contraindications/Precautions

Contraindicated in: Hypersensitivity to epoprostenol or similar compounds; CHF due to severe left ventricular systolic dysfunction; Patients who develop pulmonary edema during dose initiation.
Use Cautiously in: Geri: Dose adjustments may be necessary; OB/Lactation/Pedi: Safety not established.

Interactions

Drug-Drug: Additive hypotension may occur with **antihypertensives**, **diuretics**, or other **vasodilators**. Although concurrent use is common and accepted, risk of bleeding may be increased by **anticoagulants** or other **agents affecting platelet function**. May increase levels of **digoxin**.

Route/Dosage

IV (Adults): Initiate at 2 ng/kg/min; may ↑ by 2 ng/kg/min q 15 min or more until dose-limiting adverse effects (e.g., nausea, vomiting, headache, abdominal pain, flushing, or dyspnea) are noted. If dose-limiting adverse effects occur, infusion rate may be decreased in decrements of 2 ng/kg/min at intervals of at least 15 min. Changes in infusion rate should be based upon persistence, recurrence, or worsening of symptoms and/or emergence of adverse reactions. Abrupt withdrawal or large reductions in infusion rate should be avoided.

Availability (generic available)

Powder for injection: 0.5-mg vials, 1.5-mg vials.
Sterile diluent for epoprostenol: 50-mL vials.

eprosartan (ep-roe-sar-tan)

Teveten

Classification

Therapeutic: antihypertensives
Pharmacologic: angiotensin II receptor antagonists

Indications

Alone or with other agents in the management of hypertension.

Action

Blocks the vasoconstrictor and aldosterone-secreting effects of angiotensin II at various receptor sites, including vascular smooth muscle and the adrenal glands. **Therapeutic Effects:** Lowering of blood pressure in patients with hypertension.

Adverse Reactions/Side Effects

CNS: depression, fatigue. **CV:** hypotension. **EENT:** pharyngitis, rhinitis. **F and E:** hyperkalemia. **GI:** abdominal pain. **GU:** impaired renal function. **MS:** pain. **Misc:** ANGIOEDEMA.

PHYSICAL THERAPY IMPLICATIONS

Examination and Evaluation

- Watch for signs of angioedema, including rashes, raised patches of red or white skin (welts), burning/itching skin, swelling in the face, and difficulty breathing. Notify physician immediately if these signs occur.
- Assess blood pressure periodically and compare to normal values (See Appendix F) to help determine antihypertensive effects. Report low blood pressure (hypotension), especially if patient experiences dizziness, fatigue, or other symptoms.
- Watch for signs of impaired kidney function, including hematuria, increased urinary frequency, cloudy urine, decreased urine output, and sudden weight gain due to fluid retention. Report these signs to the physician immediately.
- Monitor signs of high plasma potassium levels (hyperkalemia), including bradycardia, fatigue, weakness, numbness, and tingling. Notify physician because severe cases can lead to life-threatening arrhythmias and paralysis.
- Assess any back pain or joint pain to rule out musculoskeletal pathology; that is, try to determine if pain is drug induced rather than caused by anatomic or biomechanical problems.

Interventions

- Implement aerobic exercise and cardiac-conditioning programs to augment drug therapy and maintain or improve cardiovascular pump function in patients with hypertension and other cardiac conditions.
- Avoid physical therapy interventions that cause systemic vasodilation (large whirlpool, Hubbard tank). Additive effects of this drug and the intervention may cause a dangerous fall in blood pressure.
- To minimize orthostatic hypotension, patient should move slowly when assuming a more upright position.

Patient/Client-Related Instruction

- Remind patients to take medication as directed to control hypertension and other cardiac conditions even if they are asymptomatic.
- Counsel patients about additional interventions to help control blood pressure and cardiac dysfunction such as regular exercise, weight loss, sodium restriction, stress reduction, moderation of alcohol consumption, and smoking cessation.
- Instruct patient or family/caregivers to report other troublesome side effects such as severe or prolonged fatigue, depression, upper respiratory irritation, or abdominal pain.

Pharmacokinetics

Absorption: 13% absorbed following oral administration.
Distribution: Crosses the placenta.
Protein Binding: 98%.
Metabolism and Excretion: Excreted mostly unchanged in feces via biliary excretion.
Half-life: 20 hr.

TIME/ACTION PROFILE (antihypertensive effect with chronic dosing)

ROUTE	ONSET	PEAK	DURATION
PO	within 1–2 hr	2–3 wk	24 hr

Contraindications/Precautions

Contraindicated in: Hypersensitivity; Pregnancy or lactation.
Use Cautiously in: Volume- or salt-depleted patients or patients receiving large doses of diuretics (correct deficits before initiating therapy); Black patients (may not be as effective); Impaired renal function caused by primary renal disease or heart failure (may worsen renal function); Women of childbearing potential; Children <18 yr (safety not established).

Interactions

Drug-Drug: Additive hypotension with other **antihypertensives**. Excessive hypotension may occur with concurrent use of **diuretics**. ↑ risk of hyperkalemia with concurrent use of **potassium supplements, potassium-containing salt substitutes, angiotensin-converting enzyme inhibitors,** or **potassium-sparing diuretics.** Antihypertensive effect may be blunted by **NSAIDs.**

Route/Dosage

PO (Adults): 600 mg once daily when used as monotherapy in patients who are not volume depleted; may be increased to 800 mg/day (in 1–2 divided doses).

Renal Impairment

PO (Adults): *CCr < 60 mL/min*—Do not exceed 600 mg/day.

Availability

Tablets: 400 mg, 600 mg. ***In combination with:*** hydrochlorothiazide (Teveten HCT). See Appendix B.

HIGH ALERT

eptifibatide (ep-ti-fib-a-tide)

Integrilin

Classification

Therapeutic: antiplatelet agents
Pharmacologic: glycoprotein IIb/IIIa inhibitors

Indications

Acute coronary syndrome (unstable angina/non–Q-wave MI), including patients who will be managed medically and those who will undergo percutaneous coronary intervention (PCI) that may consist of percutaneous transluminal angioplasty (PCTA) or atherectomy. Treatment of patients undergoing PCI. Usually used concurrently with aspirin and heparin.

Action

Decreases platelet aggregation by reversibly antagonizing the binding of fibrinogen to the glycoprotein IIb/IIIa binding site on platelet surfaces. **Therapeutic Effects:** Inhibition of platelet aggregation resulting in decreased incidence of new MI, death, or refractory ischemia, reducing the need for repeat urgent cardiac intervention.

Adverse Reactions/Side Effects

Noted for patients receiving heparin and aspirin in addition to eptifibatide

CV: hypotension. **Hemat:** BLEEDING (INCLUDING GI AND INTRACRANIAL BLEEDING, HEMATURIA, AND HEMATOMAS).

PHYSICAL THERAPY IMPLICATIONS

Examination and Evaluation

- Watch for signs of bleeding and hemorrhage, including bleeding gums, nosebleeds, unusual bruising, black/tarry stools, hematuria, or a fall in hematocrit or blood pressure (BP). Report these signs to the physician or nursing staff immediately.
- Be especially alert for signs of intracranial bleeds, including sudden severe headache, confusion, nausea, vomiting, paralysis, numbness, speech problems, and visual disturbances. Notify physician or nursing staff immediately if these signs occur.
- Assess BP periodically, and compare to normal values (See Appendix F). Report low BP (hypotension), especially if patient experiences dizziness or syncope.

Interventions

- Use caution with any physical interventions that could increase bleeding, including wound débridement, chest percussion, joint mobilization, and application of local heat.
- Use caution during aerobic exercise and endurance conditioning in patients being treated for unstable angina and coronary artery disease. Assess exercise tolerance frequently (BP, heart rate, fatigue levels), and terminate exercise immediately if any untoward responses occur (See Appendix L).

Patient/Client-Related Instruction

- Instruct patient to report immediately signs of GI bleeding, including abdominal pain, vomiting blood, blood in stools, or black, tarry stools.
- Remind patients to take medication as directed to reduce the risk of coronary infarction even if they are asymptomatic.
- Counsel patients about additional interventions to help reduce the risk of heart disease, including regular exercise, weight loss, sodium restriction, stress reduction, moderation of alcohol consumption, and smoking cessation.

Pharmacokinetics

Absorption: IV administration results in complete bioavailability.
Distribution: Unknown.
Metabolism and Excretion: 50% excreted by the kidneys.
Half-life: 2.5 hr.

TIME/ACTION PROFILE (effects on platelet function)

ROUTE	ONSET	PEAK	DURATION
IV	immediate	following bolus	brief*

*Inhibition is reversible following cessation of infusion.

Contraindications/Precautions

Contraindicated in: Hypersensitivity; Active internal bleeding or history of bleeding within previous 30 days; Severe uncontrolled hypertension (systolic BP >200 mm Hg and/or diastolic BP >110 mm Hg); Major surgical procedure within 6 wk; History of hemorrhagic stroke or other stroke within 30 days; Concurrent use of other glycoprotein IIb/IIIa receptor antagonists; Platelet count <100,000/mm^3; Severe renal insufficiency (serum creatinine ≥4 mg/dL) or dependency on renal dialysis.
Use Cautiously in: Geri: ↑ risk of bleeding; Renal insufficiency (↓ infusion rate if CCr <50 mL/min); OB/Pedi: Pregnancy, lactation, or children (safety not established; use in pregnancy only if clearly needed).

Interactions

Drug-Drug: ↑ risk of bleeding with other drugs that affect hemostasis (**heparins, warfarin, NSAIDs, thrombolytic agents, abciximab, dipyridamole,**

ticlopidine, clopidogrel, some **cephalosporins, valproates**).
Drug-Natural: ↑ bleeding risk with **arnica, chamomile, clove, dong quai, feverfew, garlic, ginger, ginkgo,** and ***Panax ginseng***.

Route/Dosage

Acute Coronary Syndrome

IV (Adults ≤121 kg): 180 mcg/kg as a bolus dose, followed by 2 mcg/kg/min until hospital discharge or surgical intervention (up to 72 hr).

Percutaneous Coronary Intervention

IV (Adults): 180 mcg/kg as a bolus dose, immediately before PCI, followed by 2 mcg/kg/min infusion; a second bolus of 180 mcg/kg is given 10 min after first bolus; infusion should continue for 18–24 or hospital discharge (minimum of 12 hr).

Renal Impairment

(Adults CCr <50 mL/min): 180 mcg/kg bolus followed by 1 mcg/kg/min infusion; second bolus of 180 mcg/kg is given 10 min after first bolus for patients undergoing PCI.

Availability

Solution for injection: 20 mg/10 mL, 75 mg/100 mL, 200 mg/100 mL.

ergonovine (er-goe-**noe**-veen)

Ergometrine, Ergotrate

Classification

Therapeutic: none assigned

Pharmacologic: oxytocics

Indications

Prevention and treatment of postpartum or postabortion hemorrhage caused by uterine atony or involution. **Unlabeled Use:** As a diagnostic agent to provoke coronary artery spasm.

Action

Directly stimulates uterine and vascular smooth muscle. **Therapeutic Effects:** Uterine contraction.

Adverse Reactions/Side Effects

CNS: dizziness, headache. **EENT:** tinnitus. **Resp:** dyspnea. **CV:** arrhythmias, chest pain, hypertension, palpitations. **GI:** nausea, vomiting. **Derm:** sweating. **Misc:** allergic reactions.

PHYSICAL THERAPY IMPLICATIONS

Examination and Evaluation

- Assess heart rate, ECG, and heart sounds, especially during exercise (See Appendices G, H). Report any rhythm disturbances or symptoms of increased arrhythmias, including palpitations, chest pain, shortness of breath, dyspnea, fainting, and fatigue/weakness.
- Assess blood pressure (BP) and compare to normal values (See Appendix F). Report a sustained increase in BP (hypertension).
- Monitor signs of allergic reactions, including pulmonary symptoms (tightness in the throat and chest, wheezing, cough, dyspnea) or skin reactions (rash, pruritus, urticaria). Notify physician or nursing staff immediately if these reactions occur.
- Assess dizziness that might affect gait, balance, and other functional activities (See Appendix C). Report balance problems and functional limitations to the physician and nursing staff, and caution the patient and family/caregivers to guard against falls and trauma.

Interventions

- Because of the risk of arrhythmias and abnormal BP responses, use caution during aerobic exercise and other forms of therapeutic exercise. Assess exercise tolerance frequently (BP, heart rate, fatigue levels), and terminate exercise immediately if any untoward responses occur (See Appendix L).

Patient/Client-Related Instruction

- Instruct patient or family/caregivers to report other troublesome side effects such as severe or prolonged headache, ringing/buzzing in the ears (tinnitus), increased sweating, or GI problems (nausea, vomiting).

Pharmacokinetics

Absorption: Well absorbed after oral or IM administration.
Distribution: Unknown.
Metabolism and Excretion: Unknown. Probably metabolized by the liver.
Half-life: Unknown.

TIME/ACTION PROFILE (uterine contractions)

ROUTE	ONSET	PEAK	DURATION
PO	5–15 min	unknown	≥3 hr
IM	2–5 min	unknown	≥3 hr
IV	immediate	unknown	45 min

Contraindications/Precautions

Contraindicated in: Hypersensitivity; Avoid chronic use; Should not be used to induce labor.
Use Cautiously in: Hypertensive or eclamptic patients (increased susceptibility to hypertensive and arrhythmogenic side effects); Severe hepatic or renal disease; Sepsis; Third stage of labor.

Interactions

Drug-Drug: Excessive vasoconstriction may result when used with other **vasopressors**, such as **dopamine** or **nicotine**. May ↑ the risk of adverse reactions with **bromocriptine**.

Route/Dosage

Oxytocic

PO, SL (Adults): 0.2–0.4 mg q 6–12 hr (usual course is 48 hr).

IM, IV (Adults): 200 mcg (0.2 mg) q 2–4 hr for up to 5 doses.

Provocative Agent for Coronary Artery Spasm

IV (Adults): 50 mcg (0.05 mg) q 5 min until chest pain occurs or a total dose of 400 mcg (0.4 mg) has been given (unlabeled).

Availability

Tablets: 0.2 mg. **Injection:** 0.2 mg/mL, 0.25 mg/mL.

ergotamine (er-got-a-meen)

Ergomar, Ergostat, Gynergen

Classification

Therapeutic: vascular headache suppressants
Pharmacologic: ergot alkaloids

Indications

Treatment of vascular headaches, including Migraine with or without aura, Cluster headaches.

Action

Vasoconstriction of dilated blood vessels by stimulating alpha-adrenergic and serotonergic (5-HT) receptors. Larger doses may produce alpha-adrenergic blockade and vasodilation. **Therapeutic Effects:** Constriction of dilated carotid artery bed with resolution of vascular headache.

Adverse Reactions/Side Effects

CNS: dizziness. **CV:** MYOCARDIAL INFARCTION, hypertension, angina pectoris, arterial spasm, intermittent claudication. **GI:** abdominal pain, nausea, vomiting, diarrhea, polydipsia. **MS:** extremity stiffness, muscle pain, stiff neck, stiff shoulders. **Neuro:** leg weakness, numbness or tingling in fingers or toes. **Misc:** fatigue.

PHYSICAL THERAPY IMPLICATIONS

Examination and Evaluation

- Continually monitor for signs of MI, including sudden chest pain, pain radiating into the arm or jaw, shortness of breath, dizziness, sweating, anxiety, and nausea. Seek immediate medical assistance if patient develops these signs.
- Assess the frequency and severity of headaches, and document whether drug therapy is successful in decreasing migraine or cluster headache attacks.
- Assess blood pressure (BP) and compare to normal values (See Appendix F). Report a sustained increase in BP (hypertension).
- Monitor any chest pain (angina pectoris) or transient leg pain and cramping that occurs when walking (intermittent claudication). Document the frequency and severity of chest or leg pain and report these findings to the physician.
- Assess any leg weakness or coldness and numbness in the fingers and toes. Document peripheral blood flow and skin temperature whenever possible to determine if these symptoms are caused by peripheral vasoconstriction. Report these findings to the physician.
- Assess any back pain or stiffness to rule out musculoskeletal pathology; that is, try to determine if musculoskeletal problems are drug induced rather than caused by anatomic or biomechanical problems.
- Assess dizziness that might affect gait, balance, and other functional activities (See Appendix C). Report balance problems and functional limitations to the physician, and caution the patient and family/caregivers to guard against falls and trauma.

Interventions

- Because of the risk of MI, use extreme caution during aerobic exercise and other forms of therapeutic exercise. Assess exercise tolerance frequently (BP, heart rate, fatigue levels), and terminate exercise immediately if any untoward responses occur (See Appendix L).
- Implement appropriate interventions (manual techniques, physical agents, therapeutic exercise) to manage headache pain and reduce the need for drug therapy. Help patient also explore other nonpharmacologic methods to reduce chronic headache pain (relaxation techniques, imagery, and so forth).
- If a headache occurs and drug treatment is needed during a rehabilitation session, allow patient to recover in a quiet, darkened room to allow the drug to achieve maximal effects.

Patient/Client-Related Instruction

- Advise patient and family or caregiver about the signs of MI (see above under Examination and Evaluation), and to seek immediate medical assistance if these signs develop.
- Advise patient to adhere to the correct dosing schedule and not to exceed the recommended frequency and number of doses.
- Instruct patient or family/caregivers to report other bothersome side effects such as severe or prolonged

fatigue or GI problems (diarrhea, nausea, vomiting, abdominal pain).

Pharmacokinetics

Absorption: Unpredictably absorbed (60%) from the GI tract. Oral absorption may be enhanced by caffeine. Sublingual absorption is very poor.
Distribution: Crosses the blood-brain barrier and enters breast milk.
Protein Binding: 93–98%.
Metabolism and Excretion: Highly metabolized (90%) by the liver. Some metabolites are active.
Half-life: 1.5–2.5 hours.

TIME/ACTION PROFILE (relief of headache)

ROUTE	ONSET	PEAK	DURATION
PO	1–2 hr (variable)	1–5 hr	unknown
SL	unknown	unknown	unknown

Contraindications/Precautions

Contraindicated in: Peripheral vascular disease; Ischemic heart disease; Uncontrolled hypertension; Severe renal or liver disease; Malnutrition; Pregnancy; Lactation.
Use Cautiously in: Illnesses associated with peripheral vascular pathology such as diabetes mellitus; Concurrent administration of other vasoconstricting agents; Children <6 yr (safety not established).

Interactions

Drug-Drug: Concurrent use with **beta blockers, oral contraceptives, macrolide anti-infectives (erythromycin, troleandomycin)**, or **nicotine** (heavy smoking) may ↑ risk of peripheral vasoconstriction. Dihydroergotamine antagonizes the antianginal effects of **nitrates**. Concurrent use with **vasoconstrictors** may have additive effects (avoid concurrent use). Concurrent use with **almotriptan, naratriptan, rizatriptan, sumatriptan**, or **zolmitriptan** may result in prolonged vasoconstriction (allow 24 hr between use).

Route/Dosage

PO, SL (Adults): 1–2 mg initially, then 1–2 mg q 30 min until attack subsides or a total of 6 mg has been given. Should not be used more than twice weekly, with at least 5 days between courses; 1–2 mg PO at bedtime daily for 10–14 days have been used to terminate series of cluster headaches.

Availability

Sublingual tablets: 2 mg. **Tablets:** 1 mg. ***In combination with:*** caffeine in preparations for vascular headaches. See Appendix B.

eribulin (e-rib-yoo-lin)
Halaven

Classification
Therapeutic: antineoplastics
Pharmacologic: microtubule inhibitors

Indications

Metastatic breast cancer that has progressed despite at least two previous regimens which included an anthracycline and a taxane in either regimen.

Action

Inhibits intracellular microtubule growth phase, causing G_2/M cell-cycle block resulting in apoptotic cell death.
Therapeutic Effects: Death of rapidly replicating cells, particularly malignant ones, ↓ spread of breast cancer.

Adverse Reactions/Side Effects

CNS: fatigue, weakness, depression, dizziness, headache, insomnia. **EENT:** ↑ lacrimation. **CV:** QTC PROLONGATION, peripheral edema. **Resp:** cough, dyspnea, upper respiratory tract infection. **GI:** anorexia, constipation, nausea, abdominal pain, abnormal taste, dry mouth, dyspepsia, mucositis, diarrhea, vomiting. **Derm:** alopecia, rash. **F and E:** hypokalemia. **Hemat:** ANEMIA, NEUTROPENIA. **MS:** arthralgia, myalgia. **Neuro:** peripheral neuropathy. **Misc:** fever, urinary tract infection.

PHYSICAL THERAPY IMPLICATIONS

Examination and Evaluation

- Assess heart rate, ECG, and heart sounds, especially during exercise (See Appendices G, H). Report any rhythm disturbances such as QTc prolongation or symptoms of increased arrhythmias, including palpitations, chest discomfort, shortness of breath, fainting, and fatigue/weakness.
- Monitor signs of neutropenia (fever, sore throat, mucosal lesions, other signs of infection) and unusual weakness and fatigue that might be due to anemia. Report these signs to the physician or nursing staff immediately.
- Assess peripheral edema using girth measurements, volume displacement, and measurement of pitting edema (See Appendix N). Report increased swelling in feet and ankles or a sudden increase in body weight due to fluid retention.
- Assess any breathing problems, and watch for signs of upper respiratory tract infection such as cough, sneezing, dyspnea, shortness of breath, mucous production, fatigue, and a low-grade fever. Notify physician or nursing staff if these signs occur.

- Assess any joint or muscle pain to rule out musculoskeletal pathology; that is, try to determine if pain is drug induced rather than caused by anatomic or biomechanical problems.
- Be alert for signs of peripheral neuropathy (numbness, tingling, decreased muscle strength). Establish baseline electroneuromyographic values using EMG and nerve conduction at the beginning of drug treatment whenever possible, and reexamine these values periodically to document drug-induced changes in peripheral nerve function.
- Monitor and report any muscle weakness, aches, or cramps that might indicate low potassium levels (hypokalemia).
- Assess dizziness that might affect gait, balance, and other functional activities (See Appendix C). Report balance problems and functional limitations to the physician and nursing staff, and caution the patient and family/caregivers to guard against falls and trauma.

Interventions

- For patients who are medically able to begin exercise, implement appropriate resistive exercises and aerobic training to maintain muscle strength and aerobic capacity during cancer chemotherapy or to help restore function after chemotherapy.
- Because of the risk of cardiac arrhythmias, use caution during aerobic exercise and other forms of therapeutic exercise. Assess exercise tolerance frequently (blood pressure, heart rate, fatigue levels), and terminate exercise immediately if any untoward responses occur (See Appendix L).

Patient/Client-related Instruction

- Instruct patient to guard against infection (frequent hand washing, etc.), and to avoid crowds and contact with persons with contagious diseases.
- Advise patient and family/caregivers that fatigue and weakness are likely and may be severe. Functional abilities may be limited, and patient may need to use assistive devices during ambulation.
- Advise patient about the likelihood of GI reactions such as nausea, vomiting, diarrhea, constipation, abdominal pain, abnormal taste, dry mouth, indigestion, loss of appetite, and inflammation of the GI mucous membranes. Instruct patient or family and caregivers to report other severe or unexpected GI problems.
- Advise patient that hair loss and other skin reactions (rashes, itching) are likely. Instruct patient to report severe or unusual skin problems.
- Instruct patient and family/caregivers to report other troublesome side effects such as severe or prolonged headache, sleep loss, depression, increased tears, fever, or urinary tract infection.

Pharmacokinetics

Absorption: IV administration results in complete bioavailability.
Distribution: Unknown.
Metabolism and Excretion: Minimal metabolism, mostly excreted unchanged in feces (82%) and less in urine (9%).
Half-life: 40 hr.

TIME/ACTION PROFILE (effects on blood counts)

ROUTE	ONSET	PEAK	DURATION
IV	within days	7–14 days	up to 2 wk

Contraindications/Precautions

Contraindicated in: Severe hepatic impairment; Severe renal impairment (CCr <30mL/min); Congenital long QT syndrome; OB: Pregnancy; may cause fetal harm; Lactation: Avoid breast-feeding.
Use Cautiously in: CHF, bradyarrhythmias, concurrent use of drugs known to prolong the QT interval (including class Ia and III antiarrhythmics), electrolyte abnormalities (↑ risk of arrhythmias); Moderate renal impairment; lower initial dose recommended for CCr 30–50 mL/min; Mild-to-moderate hepatic impairment; lower initial dose recommended; OB: Women with childbearing potential; Pedi: Safe and effective use in children <18 yr has not been established.

Interactions

Drug-Drug: ↑ risk of bone marrow depression with other **antineoplastics** or **radiation therapy.** ↓ antibody response and ↑ risk of adverse reactions with **live-virus vaccines.**

Route/Dosage

IV (Adults): 1.4 mg/m^2 on days 1 and 8 of a 21-day cycle; dose modifications required for hepatic impairment, moderate renal impairment, neutropenia, thrombocytopenia, or peripheral neuropathy.

Renal Impairment

IV (Adults): *Mild hepatic impairment (Child-Pugh A)*—1.1 mg/m^2 on days 1 and 8 of a 21-day cycle *Moderate hepatic impairment (Child-Pugh B*—0.7 mg/m^2 on days 1 and 8 of a 21-day cycle.

Renal Impairment

IV (Adults): *Moderate renal impairment (CCr 30–50 mL/min)*—1.1 mg/m^2 on days 1 and 8 of a 21-day cycle.

Availability

Solution for IV administration: 0.5 mg/mL in 2-mL vials.

erlotinib (er-loe-ti-nib)
Tarceva

Classification
Therapeutic: antineoplastics
Pharmacologic: enzyme inhibitors

Indications
Locally advanced/metastatic non–small-cell lung cancer which has not responded to previous chemotherapy.

Action
Inhibits the enzyme tyrosine kinase which is associated with human epidermal growth factor receptor (EGFR); blocks growth stimulation signals in cancer cells.
Therapeutic Effects: Decreased spread of lung cancer with increased survival.

Adverse Reactions/Side Effects
CNS: fatigue. **EENT:** conjunctivitis, corneal ulceration.
Resp: INTERSTITIAL LUNG DISEASE, dyspnea, cough.
GI: diarrhea, abdominal pain, anorexia, nausea, stomatitis, vomiting, ↑ liver transaminases.
Derm: rash, dry skin, pruritus.

PHYSICAL THERAPY IMPLICATIONS

Examination and Evaluation
- Assess any breathing problems or signs of interstitial lung disease such as dry cough, wheezing, chest pain, shortness of breath, and difficult or labored breathing. Monitor pulse oximetry and perform pulmonary function tests (See Appendices I, J, K) to quantify suspected changes in ventilation and respiratory function.
- Monitor any vision disturbances or eye pain and inflammation. Report these signs to the physician.

Interventions
- For patients who are medically able to begin exercise, implement appropriate resistive exercises and aerobic training to maintain muscle strength and aerobic capacity during cancer chemotherapy or to help restore function after chemotherapy.
- Use caution during aerobic exercise and endurance conditioning because of potential pulmonary toxicity. Terminate exercise if patient exhibits untoward symptoms (chest pain, shortness of breath, unusual fatigue) or displays other criteria for exercise termination (See Appendix L).

Patient/Client-Related Instruction
- Advise patient and family/caregivers that fatigue and weakness are likely and may be severe. Functional abilities may be limited, and patient may need to use assistive devices during ambulation.
- Advise patient that skin reactions are likely, including rash, dry skin, and pruritus. Report severe or unexpected skin reactions to the physician.
- Advise patient about the likelihood of GI reactions (abdominal pain, diarrhea, nausea, vomiting, loss of appetite, inflammation in/around mouth). Instruct patient to report severe or prolonged GI problems.

Pharmacokinetics
Absorption: 60% absorbed; bioavailability increased to 100% with food.
Distribution: Unknown.
Protein Binding: 93% protein bound.
Metabolism and Excretion: Mostly metabolized by the liver (CYP3A4 enzyme system).
Half-life: 36 hr.

TIME/ACTION PROFILE (blood levels)

ROUTE	ONSET	PEAK	DURATION
Oral	unknown	4 hr	24 hr

Contraindications/Precautions
Contraindicated in: Pregnancy or lactation.
Use Cautiously in: Hepatic impairment; Previous chemotherapy/radiation, preexisting lung disease, metastatic lung disease (may ↑ risk of interstitial lung disease); Patients with childbearing potential; Children (safety not established).

Interactions
Drug-Drug: Strong inhibitors of CYP3A4, including **atazanavir, clarithromycin, indinavir, itraconazole, ketoconazole, nefazodone, nelfinavir, ritonavir, saquinavir, telithromycin,** or **voriconazole,** ↑ erlotinib levels and the risk of toxicity; dosage reduction should be considered. Strong inducers of CYP3A4, including **rifampin.** ↓ levels of erlotinib and may ↓ response; alternative therapy or ↑ dose should be considered. May ↑ risk of bleeding with **warfarin.**

Route/Dosage
PO (Adults): 150 mg daily taken at least 1 hr before or 2 hr after food.

Availability
Tablets: 25 mg, 100 mg, 150 mg.

ertapenem (er-ta-pen-em)

Invanz

Classification

Therapeutic: anti-infectives

Pharmacologic: carbapenems

Indications

Moderate-to-severe: complicated intra-abdominal infections, complicated skin and skin structure infections, community-acquired pneumonia, complicated urinary tract infections (including pyelonephritis), acute pelvic infections including postpartum endomyometritis, septic abortion, and postsurgical gynecologic infections. Prophylaxis of surgical site infection following elective colorectal surgery.

Action

Therapeutic Effects: Bactericidal action against susceptible bacteria. **Spectrum:** Active against the following aerobic gram-positive organisms: *Staphylococcus aureus* (methicillin-susceptible strains only), *S. epidermidis Streptococcus agalactiae*, *S. pneumoniae* (penicillin-susceptible strains only), and *S. pyogenes*. Also active against the following gram-negative aerobic organisms: *Escherichia coli*, *Haemophilus influenzae* (beta-lactamase–negative strains), *Klebsiella pneumonia*, *Moraxella catarrhalis, and Providencia rettgeri.* Additional anaerobic spectra include: *Bacteroides fragilis*, *B. distasonis*, *B. ovatus*, *B. thetaiotamicron*, *B. uniformis*, *B. vulgatis Clostridium clostrioforme*, *Eubacterium lentum*, *Peptostreptococcus*, *Porphyromonas asaccharolytica*, and *Prevotella bivia*.

Adverse Reactions/Side Effects

CNS: SEIZURES, headache. **GI:** PSEUDOMEMBRANOUS COLITIS, diarrhea, nausea, vomiting. **GU:** vaginitis. **Local:** phlebitis at IV site, pain at IM site. **Misc:** HYPERSENSITIVITY REACTION, INCLUDING ANAPHYLAXIS.

PHYSICAL THERAPY IMPLICATIONS

Examination and Evaluation

- Be alert for new seizures or increased seizure activity, especially at the onset of drug treatment. Document the number, duration, and severity of seizures, and report these findings immediately to the physician.
- Monitor signs of pseudomembranous colitis, including diarrhea, abdominal pain, fever, pus or mucus in stools, and other severe or prolonged GI problems (nausea, vomiting, heartburn). Notify physician or nursing staff immediately of these signs.
- Monitor signs of hypersensitivity reactions and anaphylaxis, including pulmonary symptoms (tightness in the throat and chest, wheezing, cough dyspnea) or skin reactions (rash, pruritus, urticaria). Notify physician or nursing staff immediately if these reactions occur.
- Assess injection site during and after IV administration, and report signs of phlebitis such as local pain, swelling, and inflammation.

Interventions

- Always wash hands thoroughly and disinfect equipment (whirlpools, electrotherapeutic devices, treatment tables, and so forth) to help prevent the spread of infection. Use universal precautions or isolation procedures as indicated for specific patients.

Patient/Client-Related Instruction

- Instruct patient to notify physician immediately of signs of superinfection, including black, furry overgrowth on tongue, vaginal itching or discharge, and loose or foul-smelling stools.
- Instruct patient and family/caregivers to report other troublesome side effects such as severe or prolonged headache, vaginal irritation, or GI problems (nausea, vomiting, diarrhea).

Pharmacokinetics

Absorption: 90% after IM administration; IV administration results in complete bioavailability.

Distribution: Enters breast milk.

Metabolism and Excretion: Mostly excreted by the kidneys.

Half-life: 1.8 hr (increased in renal impairment).

TIME/ACTION PROFILE (blood levels)

ROUTE	ONSET	PEAK	DURATION
IM	rapid	2 hr	24 hr
IV	rapid	end of infusion	24 hr

Contraindications/Precautions

Contraindicated in: Hypersensitivity; Cross-sensitivity may occur with penicillins, cephalosporins, and other carbapenems; Hypersensitivity to lidocaine (may be used as a diluent for IM administration).

Use Cautiously in: History of multiple hypersensitivity reactions; Seizure disorders; Geri: ↑ sensitivity due to age-related ↓ in renal function; Renal impairment; OB/Lactation/Pedi: Pregnancy, lactation, or children <18 yr (safety not established; use during lactation only when benefits outweigh risks, use in pregnancy only if clearly needed).

Interactions

Drug-Drug: Probenecid ↓ excretion and ↑ blood levels. May ↓ serum **valproate** levels (↑ risk of seizures).

Route/Dosage

IV, IM (Adults and Children 13 yr or older): 1 g once daily for up to 14 days (IV) or 7 days (IM).

IV, IM (Children 3 mo–12 yrs): 15 mg/kg bid (not to exceed 1 g/day) for up to 14 days (IV) or 7 days (IM).

Renal Impairment

IM, IV (Adults): *CCr ≤30 mL/min/1.73m²*—500 mg once daily.

Availability

Powder for injection: 1 g/vial.

erythromycin (oral)

(e-rith-roe-**mye**-sin)

erythromycin base

Apo-Erythro-EC, E-Base, E-Mycin, ✱Erybid, Eryc, Ery-Tab, Erythromid, Novo-rythro, PCE

erythromycin estolate

(e-rith-roe-**mye**-sines-toe-late)

Ilosone, Novo-rythro

erythromycin ethylsuccinate

(e-rith-roe-**mye**-sin eth-il-**suk**-si-nate)

Apo-Erythro-ES, E.E.S, EryPed

erythromycin stearate

(e-rith-roe-**mye**-sin **stee**-a-rate)

Erythrocin, Novo-rythro

Classification

Therapeutic: anti-infectives

Pharmacologic: macrolides

Indications

PO: Infections caused by susceptible organisms, including Upper and lower respiratory tract infections, Otitis media (with sulfonamides), Skin and skin structure infections, Pertussis, Diphtheria, Erythrasma, Intestinal amebiasis, Pelvic inflammatory disease, Nongonococcal urethritis, Syphilis, Legionnaires' disease, Rheumatic fever. Useful when penicillin is the most appropriate drug but cannot be used because of hypersensitivity, including Streptococcal infections, Treatment of syphilis or gonorrhea.

Action

Suppresses protein synthesis at the level of the 50S bacterial ribosome. **Therapeutic Effects:** Bacteriostatic action against susceptible bacteria. **Spectrum:** Active against many gram-positive cocci, including Streptococci, Staphylococci. Gram-positive bacilli, including *Clostridium*, *Corynebacterium*. Several gram-negative pathogens, notably: *Neisseria*, *Legionella pneumophila*. *Mycoplasma* and *Chlamydia* are also usually susceptible.

Adverse Reactions/Side Effects

CNS: seizures (rare). **CV:** QTC PROLONGATION (MAY RESULT IN TORSADES DE POINTES), VENTRICULAR ARRHYTHMIAS. **GI:** PSEUDOMEMBRANOUS COLITIS, nausea, vomiting, abdominal pain, cramping, diarrhea, drug-induced hepatitis, infantile hypertrophic pyloric stenosis, drug-induced pancreatitis (rare). **Derm:** rashes. **Misc:** allergic reactions, superinfection.

PHYSICAL THERAPY IMPLICATIONS

Examination and Evaluation

- Assess heart rate, ECG, and heart sounds, especially during exercise (See Appendices G, H). Report any ventricular arrhythmias or symptoms of increased arrhythmias, including palpitations, chest discomfort, shortness of breath, fainting, and fatigue/weakness.
- Monitor signs of pseudomembranous colitis, including diarrhea, abdominal pain, fever, pus or mucus in stools, and other severe or prolonged GI problems (nausea, vomiting, heartburn). Notify physician or nursing staff immediately of these signs.
- Be alert for new seizures or increased seizure activity, especially at the onset of drug treatment. Document the number, duration, and severity of seizures, and report these findings immediately to the physician.
- Monitor signs of allergic reactions, including rash and other skin reactions (pruritus, urticaria), and pulmonary symptoms (tightness in the throat and chest, wheezing, cough, dyspnea). Notify physician or nursing staff immediately if these reactions occur.

Interventions

- Always wash hands thoroughly and disinfect equipment (whirlpools, electrotherapeutic devices, treatment tables, and so forth) to help prevent the spread of infection. Employ universal precautions or isolation procedures as indicated for specific patients.
- Because of the risk of serious ventricular arrhythmias, use extreme caution during aerobic exercise and other forms of therapeutic exercise. Assess exercise tolerance frequently (blood pressure, heart rate, fatigue levels), and terminate exercise immediately if any untoward responses occur (See Appendix L).

Patient/Client-Related Instruction

- Instruct patient to notify physician immediately of signs of superinfection, including black, furry overgrowth on tongue, vaginal itching or discharge, and loose or foul-smelling stools.
- Advise patient about the likelihood of GI reactions, including nausea, vomiting, and abdominal pain. Instruct patient to report severe or prolonged GI problems, signs of liver toxicity (yellow skin or eyes, abdominal pain, severe nausea and vomiting, fever, sore throat, malaise, weakness, facial edema), or signs of pancreatitis (upper abdominal pain after eating, indigestion, weight loss, oily stools).

Pharmacokinetics

Absorption: Variable absorption from the duodenum after oral administration (dependent on salt form). Absorption of enteric-coated products is delayed.
Distribution: Widely distributed. Minimal CNS penetration. Crosses placenta; enters breast milk.
Protein Binding: 70–80%; 96% for estolate.
Metabolism and Excretion: Partially metabolized by the liver, excreted mainly unchanged in the bile; small amounts excreted unchanged in the urine.
Half-life: Neonates: 2.1 hr; Adults: 1.4–2 hr.

TIME/ACTION PROFILE (blood levels)

ROUTE	ONSET	PEAK	DURATION
PO	1 hr	1–4 hr	6–12 hr

Contraindications/Precautions

Contraindicated in: Hypersensitivity; Hepatic dysfunction (estolate salt); Concurrent pimozide; Tartrazine sensitivity (some products contain tartrazine—FDC yellow dye #5); OB: Pregnancy (estolate salt).
Use Cautiously in: Liver/renal disease; Myasthenia gravis; Geri: ↑ risk of ototoxicity if parenteral dose >4 g/day, ↑ risk of QTc prolongation; OB: Salts other than the estolate may be used in pregnancy to treat chlamydial infections or syphilis.

Interactions

Drug-Drug: Concurrent use with **pimozide** ↑ risk of serious arrhythmias (concurrent use contraindicated); similar effects may occur with **diltiazem, verapamil, ketoconazole, itraconazole, nefazodone,** and **protease inhibitors**; avoid concurrent use. ↑ blood levels and effects of **sildenafil, tadalafil,** and **vardenafil**; use lower doses. Concurrent **rifabutin** or **rifampin** may ↓ effect of erythromycin and ↑ risk of adverse GI reactions. ↑ levels and risk of toxicity from **alfentanil, alprazolam, buspirone, clozapine, bromocriptine, theophylline, carbamazepine, cyclosporine, cilostazol, diazepam, disopyramide, ergot alkaloids, felodipine, warfarin, methylprednisolone, midazolam, quinidine, rifabutin, tacrolimus, triazolam,** or **vinblastine**. Concurrent **HMG CoA reductase inhibitors** ↑ risk of myopathy/rhabdomyolysis. May ↑ serum **digoxin** levels in a few patients. **Theophylline** may ↓ blood levels. Beneficial effects may be ↓ by **clindamycin**.

Route/Dosage

250 mg of erythromycin base, estolate, or stearate = 400 mg of erythromycin ethylsuccinate.

Most Infections

PO (Adults): *Base, estolate, stearate*—250 mg q 6 hr, *or* 333 mg q 8 hr, *or* 500 mg q 12 hr. *Ethylsuccinate*—400 mg q 6 hr *or* 800 mg q 12 hr.
PO (Children >1 mo): *Base and ethylsuccinate* 30—50 mg/kg/day divided q 6–8 hr (maximum 2 g/day as base or 3.2 g/day as ethylsuccinate). *Estolate*—30–50 mg/kg/day divided q 6–12 hr (maximum 2 g/day). *Stearate*—30–50 mg/kg/day divided q 6 hr (maximum 2 g/day).
PO (Neonates): *Ethylsuccinate*—20–50 mg/kg/day divided q 6–12 hr.

Availability (generic available)

Erythromycin Base

Enteric-coated tablets: 250 mg, 333 mg. **Tablets with polymer-coated particles:** 333 mg, 500 mg. **Film-coated tablets:** 500 mg. **Delayed-release capsules:** 250 mg.

Erythromycin Estolate

Tablets: 500 mg. **Capsules:** 250 mg. **Oral suspension (orange flavor):** 125 mg/5 mL. **Oral suspension (cherry flavor):** 250 mg/5 mL.

Erythromycin Ethylsuccinate

Chewable tablets (fruit flavor): 200 mg. **Tablets:** 400 mg. **Oral suspension (fruit flavor, cherry):** 200 mg/5 mL. **Oral suspension (orange, banana flavors):** 400 mg/5 mL. **Drops (fruit flavor):** 100 mg/2.5 mL.

Erythromycin Stearate

Film-coated tablets: 250 mg. ***In combination with:*** sulfisoxazole (Eryzole, Pediazole). See Appendix B.

escitalopram (es-sit-al-oh-pram)

Lexapro

Classification
Therapeutic: antidepressants
Pharmacologic: selective serotonin reuptake inhibitors (SSRIs)

Indications

Major depressive disorder. Generalized anxiety disorder (GAD). **Unlabeled Use:** Panic disorder. Obsessive-compulsive disorder (OCD). Posttraumatic stress disorder (PTSD). Social anxiety disorder (social phobia). Premenstrual dysphoric disorder (PMDD).

Action

Selectively inhibits the reuptake of serotonin in the CNS. **Therapeutic Effects:** Antidepressant action.

Adverse Reactions/Side Effects

CNS: insomnia, dizziness, drowsiness, fatigue. **GI:** diarrhea, nausea, abdominal pain, constipation, dry mouth, indigestion. **GU:** anorgasmia, decreased libido, ejaculatory delay, erectile dysfunction. **Derm:** increased sweating. **Endo:** syndrome of inappropriate secretion of antidiuretic hormone (SIADH). **F and E:** hyponatremia. **Metab:** increased appetite.

PHYSICAL THERAPY IMPLICATIONS

Examination and Evaluation

- Be alert for increased depression and suicidal thoughts and ideology, especially when initiating drug treatment, or in children and teenagers. Notify physician or mental health professional immediately if patient exhibits worsening depression or other changes in mood and behavior.
- Assess dizziness and drowsiness that might affect gait, balance, and other functional activities (See Appendix C). Report balance problems and functional limitations to the physician, and caution the patient and family/caregivers to guard against falls and trauma.
- Monitor signs of fluid-electrolyte imbalance due to SIADH and hyponatremia. SIADH causes increased water retention that leads to relatively low sodium concentration (hyponatremia). Symptoms include confusion, lethargy, weakness, myoclonus, and depressed reflexes. Severe or sudden onset may also cause seizures, ataxia, nystagmus, tremor, dysarthria, dysphagia, and coma. Notify physician if these signs occur.
- Periodically assess body weight and other anthropometric measures (body mass index, body composition), especially if appetite is increased. Report a rapid or unexplained weight gain.

Interventions

- Help patient explore nonpharmacologic methods such as exercise, counseling, and support groups to help reduce depression, anxiety, and other mood disorders

Patient/Client-Related Instruction

- Advise patient that antidepressant effects may not occur immediately; it may take 2 wk or more before an improvement in mood is observed.
- Advise patient to avoid alcohol and other CNS depressants because of the increased risk of sedation and adverse effects.
- Advise patient that GI problems may occur, and to report severe or prolonged nausea, diarrhea, constipation, abdominal pain, dry mouth, or indigestion.
- Instruct patient to report other troublesome side effects such as severe or prolonged sleep loss, increased sweating, or changes in sexual function (decreased libido, erectile dysfunction, ejaculatory problems).

Pharmacokinetics

Absorption: 80% absorbed following oral administration.
Distribution: Enters breast milk.
Metabolism and Excretion: Mostly metabolized by the liver (primarily CYP3A4 and CYP2C19 isoenzymes); 7% excreted unchanged by kidneys.
Half-life: Increased in geriatric patients and patients with hepatic impairment.

TIME/ACTION PROFILE (antidepressant effect)

ROUTE	ONSET	PEAK	DURATION
PO	within 1–4 wk	unknown	unknown

Contraindications/Precautions

Contraindicated in: Hypersensitivity; Concurrent MAO inhibitors; Concurrent use of citalopram.
Use Cautiously in: History of mania (may activate mania/hypomania); History of seizures; Patients at risk for suicide; Hepatic impairment (dose reduction recommended); Geri: Hepatic impairment or geriatric patients (↓ doses recommended); Severe renal impairment; OB: Neonates exposed to SSRI in 3rd trimester may develop drug discontinuation syndrome, including respiratory distress, feeding difficulty, and irritability. Weigh risks and benefits; Lactation: May cause adverse effects in infant; consider risk/benefit; Pedi: May ↑ risk of suicide attempt/ideation, especially during early treatment or dose adjustment in children/adolescents (unlabeled for pediatric use).

Interactions

Drug-Drug: May cause serious, potentially fatal reactions when used with **MAO inhibitors**; allow at least 14 days between escitalopram and **MAO inhibitors**. Use cautiously with other **centrally acting drugs** (including **alcohol**, **antihistamines**, **opioid analgesics**, and **sedative/hypnotics**; concurrent use with **alcohol** is not recommended). Concurrent use with **sumatriptan** or other **5-HT$_3$ agonist vascular headache suppressants** may result in weakness, hyperreflexia, and incoordination. **Cimetidine** ↑ blood levels of escitalopram. Serotonergic effects may be ↑ by **lithium** (concurrent use should be carefully monitored). **Carbamazepine** may ↓ blood levels. May ↑ blood levels of **metoprolol**. Concurrent use with **tricyclic antidepressants** should be undertaken with caution because of altered pharmacokinetics. ↑ risk of bleeding with **aspirin, NSAIDs, clopidogrel**, or **warfarin**.
Drug-Natural: ↑ risk of serotonin syndrome with **St. John's wort** and **SAMe**.

Route/Dosage

PO (Adults): 10 mg once daily; may be increased to 20 mg once daily after 1 week.

Hepatic Impairment

PO (Adults): 10 mg once daily.
PO (Geriatric Patients): 10 mg once daily.

Availability

Tablets: 5 mg, 10 mg, 20 mg. **Oral solution (peppermint):** 1 mg/mL in 240-mL bottles.

HIGH ALERT

esmolol (es-moe-lole)

Brevibloc

Classification

Therapeutic: antiarrhythmics (class II)

Pharmacologic: beta blockers

Indications

Management of sinus tachycardia and supraventricular arrhythmias.

Action

Blocks stimulation of $beta_1$ (myocardial)-adrenergic receptors. Does not usually affect $beta_2$ (pulmonary, vascular, or uterine)–receptor sites. **Therapeutic Effects:** Decreased heart rate. Decreased AV conduction.

Adverse Reactions/Side Effects

CNS: fatigue, agitation, confusion, dizziness, drowsiness, weakness. **CV:** hypotension, peripheral ischemia. **GI:** nausea, vomiting. **Derm:** sweating. **Local:** injection-site reactions.

PHYSICAL THERAPY IMPLICATIONS

Examination and Evaluation

- Assess heart rate, ECG, and heart sounds, especially during exercise (See Appendices G, H). Although intended to treat certain arrhythmias, this drug can unmask or precipitate new arrhythmias (proarrhythmic effect). Report immediately an abnormally slow heart rate (bradycardia) or symptoms of other arrhythmias, including palpitations, chest pain, shortness of breath, fainting, and fatigue/weakness.
- Assess blood pressure periodically and compare to normal values (See Appendix F). Report low blood pressure (hypotension), especially if patient experiences dizziness or syncope.
- Monitor signs of peripheral ischemia, such as extreme coldness in the hands and feet, cyanosis, and muscle cramping. Notify physician of severe or prolonged signs of vasoconstriction.
- Assess dizziness and drowsiness that might affect gait, balance, and other functional activities (See Appendix C). Report balance problems and functional limitations to the physician and nursing staff, and caution the patient and family/caregivers to guard against falls and trauma.
- Monitor mood and personality changes, including agitation, confusion, or other changes in behavior. Notify physician if these changes become problematic.
- Monitor excessive fatigue or weakness. Beta blockers often cause some degree of fatigue and weakness, but any sudden or severe change in muscle strength or energy levels should be reported.
- Monitor IV injection site for pain, swelling, and irritation. Report prolonged or excessive injection-site reactions to the physician.

Interventions

- Because of possible effects on cardiac excitation, use caution during aerobic exercise and endurance conditioning. Terminate exercise if patient exhibits untoward symptoms (chest pain, shortness of breath, unusual fatigue) or displays other criteria for exercise termination (See Appendix L).
- Establish aerobic exercise workloads that account for the effects of beta blockers on heart rate (HR). Some HR guidelines may not be appropriate because beta blockers typically decrease maximal HR by 20–30 bpm. Use other guidelines such as rating of perceived exertion (RPE, modified Borg scale) to determine exercise workloads.
- To minimize orthostatic hypotension, patient should move slowly when assuming a more upright position.

Patient/Client-Related Instruction

- Counsel patients about additional interventions to help control cardiac arrhythmias, including regular exercise, caffeine restriction, stress reduction, moderation of alcohol consumption, and smoking cessation.
- Instruct patient or family/caregivers to report other troublesome side effects such as severe or prolonged sweating or GI problems (nausea, vomiting).

Pharmacokinetics

Absorption: IV administration results in complete bioavailability.

Distribution: Rapidly and widely distributed.

Metabolism and Excretion: Metabolized by enzymes in RBCs and liver.

Half-life: 9 min.

TIME/ACTION PROFILE (antiarrhythmic effect)

ROUTE	ONSET	PEAK	DURATION
IV	within mins	unknown	1–20 min

Contraindications/Precautions

Contraindicated in: Uncompensated CHF; Pulmonary edema; Cardiogenic shock; Bradycardia or heart block; Known alcohol intolerance.

Use Cautiously in: Geri: Geriatric patients (increased sensitivity to the effects of beta blockers); Thyrotoxicosis (may mask symptoms); Diabetes mellitus (may mask symptoms of hypoglycemia); Patients with a history of severe allergic reactions (intensity of reactions may be increased); OB/Pedi: Pregnancy, lactation, or children (safety not established; neonatal bradycardia, hypotension, hypoglycemia, and respiratory depression may occur rarely).

Interactions

Drug-Drug: General anesthesia, IV **phenytoin**, and **verapamil** may cause additive myocardial depression. Additive bradycardia may occur with **digoxin**. Additive hypotension may occur with other **antihypertensives**, acute ingestion of **alcohol**, or **nitrates**. Concurrent use with **amphetamine, cocaine, ephedrine, epinephrine, norepinephrine, phenylephrine**, or **pseudoephedrine** may result in unopposed alpha-adrenergic stimulation (excessive hypertension, bradycardia). Concurrent **thyroid** administration may decrease effectiveness. May alter the effectiveness of **insulins** or **oral hypoglycemic agents** (dosage adjustments may be necessary). May ↓ effectiveness of **theophylline**. May ↓ beneficial beta cardiovascular effects of **dopamine** or **dobutamine**. Use cautiously within 14 days of **MAO inhibitor** therapy (may result in hypertension).

Route/Dosage

IV (Adults): *Antiarrhythmic*—500-mcg/kg loading dose over 1 min initially, followed by 50-mcg/kg/min infusion for 4 min; if no response within 5 min, give 2nd loading dose of 500 mcg/kg over 1 min, then increase infusion to 100 mcg/kg/min for 4 min. If no response, repeat loading dose of 500 mcg/kg over 1 min and increase infusion rate by 50-mcg/kg/min increments (not to exceed 200 mcg/kg/min for 48 hr). As therapeutic end point is achieved, eliminate loading doses and decrease dose increments to 25 mg/kg/min. *Intraoperative antihypertensive/antiarrhythmic*—250–500-mcg/kg loading dose over 1 min initially, followed by 50-mcg/kg/min infusion for 4 min; if no response within 5 min, give 2nd loading dose of 250–500 mcg/kg over 1 min, then increase infusion to 100 mcg/kg/min for 4 min. If no response, repeat loading dose of 250–500 mcg/kg over 1 min and increase infusion rate by 50-mcg/kg/min increments (not to exceed 200 mcg/kg/min for 48 hr).

IV (Children): *Antiarrhythmic*—50 mcg/kg/min; may be increased q 10 min up to 300 mcg/kg/min.

Availability

Solution for injection (prediluted for use as loading dose): 10 mg/mL in 10-mL vials, 20 mg/mL in 5-mL vials. **Solution for injection (must be diluted to prepare continuous infusion):** 250 mg/mL in 10-mL ampules. **Premixed infusion:** 2000 mg/100 mL, 2500 mg/250 mL.

esomeprazole
(es-oh-**mep**-ra-zole)
Nexium

Classification
Therapeutic: antiulcer agents
Pharmacologic: proton-pump inhibitors

Indications

GERD/erosive esophagitis. Hypersecretory conditions, including Zollinger-Ellison syndrome. With amoxicillin and clarithromycin to eradicate *Helicobacter pylori* in duodenal ulcer disease or history of duodenal ulcer disease. Decrease risk of gastric ulcer during continuous NSAID therapy.

Action

Binds to an enzyme on gastric parietal cells in the presence of acidic gastric pH, preventing the final transport of hydrogen ions into the gastric lumen. **Therapeutic Effects:** Diminished accumulation of acid in the gastric lumen with lessened gastroesophageal reflux. Healing of duodenal ulcers. Decreased incidence of gastric ulcer during continuous NSAID therapy.

Adverse Reactions/Side Effects

CNS: headache. **GI:** abdominal pain, constipation, diarrhea, dry mouth, flatulence, nausea.

PHYSICAL THERAPY IMPLICATIONS

Examination and Evaluation

- Monitor improvements in GI symptoms (gastritis, heartburn, and so forth) to help determine if drug therapy is successful.

Interventions

- In cases of NSAID-induced gastritis, implement appropriate manual therapy techniques, physical agents, and therapeutic exercises to reduce pain and decrease the need for aspirin and other NSAIDs.

Patient/Client-Related Instruction

- Advise patient to avoid alcohol and foods that may cause an increase in GI irritation.
- Instruct patient to report bothersome or prolonged side effects, including headache or GI effects (nausea, constipation, diarrhea flatulence, abdominal pain, dry mouth).

Pharmacokinetics

Absorption: 90% absorbed following oral administration; food decreases absorption.
Distribution: Unknown.
Protein Binding: 97%.

Metabolism and Excretion: Extensively metabolized by the liver (cytochrome P450 [CY P450] system, primarily CYP2C19 isoenzyme); <1% excreted unchanged in urine.
Half-life: 1.0–1.5 hr.

TIME/ACTION PROFILE (blood levels*)

ROUTE	ONSET	PEAK	DURATION
PO	rapid	1.6 hr	24 hr
IV	rapid	end of infusion	24 hr

*Resolution of symptoms takes 5–8 days.

Contraindications/Precautions

Contraindicated in: Hypersensitivity; OB: Lactation (not recommended).
Use Cautiously in: Severe hepatic impairment (daily dose should not exceed 20 mg); Geri: Increased risk of hip fractures in patients using high doses for >1 year; OB: Pregnancy (use only if clearly needed); Pedi: Children <1 yr (safety not established).

Interactions

Drug-Drug: May ↓ absorption of drugs requiring acid pH, including **ketoconazole**, **itraconazole**, **atazanavir**, **ampicillin**, **iron salts**, and **digoxin**. May ↑ risk of bleeding with **warfarin** (monitor INR and PT).

Route/Dosage

Gastroesophageal Reflux Disease

PO (Adults): *Healing of erosive esophagitis*—20 or 40 mg once daily for 4–8 wk; *maintenance of healing of erosive esophagitis*—20 mg once daily; *symptomatic GERD*—20 mg once daily for 4 wk (additional 4 wk may be considered for nonresponders).
PO (Children 12–17 yrs): *Short-term treatment of GERD*—20–40 mg once daily up to 8 wk.
PO (Children 1–11 yr): *Short-term treatment of GERD*—10 mg once daily up to 8 wk; *Healing of erosive esophagitis*—<20 kg: 10 mg once daily for 8 wk; ≥20 kg: 10–20 mg once daily for 8 wk.
IV (Adults): 20 or 40 mg once daily.

H. pylori Eradication to Reduce the Risk of Duodenal Ulcer Recurrence (Triple Therapy)

PO (Adults): 40 mg once daily for 10 days with amoxicillin 1000 mg twice daily for 10 days and clarithromycin 500 mg twice daily for 10 days.

Decrease Gastric Ulcer During Continuous NSAID Therapy

PO (Adults): 20 or 40 mg once daily for up to 6 mo.

Pathologic Hypersecretory Conditions Including Zollinger-Ellison Syndrome

PO (Adults): 40 mg twice daily.

Hepatic Impairment

PO, IV (Adults): *Severe hepatic impairment*—Dose should not exceed 20 mg/day.

Availability

Delayed-release capsules: 20 mg, 40 mg. **Delayed-release oral suspension packets:** 10 mg, 20 mg, 40 mg. **Powder for injection (requires reconstitution):** 20 mg/vial, 40 mg/vial.

estazolam (es-taz-oh-lam)

ProSom

Classification
Therapeutic: sedative/hypnotics
Pharmacologic: benzodiazepines

Schedule IV

Indications

Short-term management of insomnia.

Action

Depresses the CNS, probably by potentiating gamma-aminobutyric acid (GABA), an inhibitory neurotransmitter. **Therapeutic Effects:** Relief of insomnia.

Adverse Reactions/Side Effects

CNS: abnormal thinking, behavior changes, drowsiness, hallucinations, headache, weakness, abnormal dreams, sleep-driving, confusion, depression, dizziness, hangover, malaise, nervousness. **Resp:** cold symptoms, pharyngitis. **CV:** chest pain. **GI:** abdominal pain, dyspepsia, nausea. **MS:** back pain, lower extremity pain, stiffness. **Neuro:** abnormal coordination, hypokinesia. **Misc:** body pain, physical dependence, psychologic dependence.

PHYSICAL THERAPY IMPLICATIONS

Examination and Evaluation

- Monitor daytime drowsiness, short-term memory deficits, and ,"hangover" symptoms (headache, nausea, malaise, irritability, dysphoria). Repeated or excessive symptoms may require change in dose or medication.
- Be alert for confusion, depression, nervousness, abnormal thoughts, hallucinations, or other alterations in cognitive function (See Appendix D). Notify physician promptly if these symptoms develop.
- Assess dizziness that might affect gait, balance, and other functional activities (See Appendix C). Report balance problems and functional limitations to the physician, and caution the patient and family/caregivers to guard against falls and trauma.
- Report any coordination problems or decreased bodily movements (hypokinesia) that are consistent with onset of drug therapy or changes in drug dose.
- Assess any back pain, lower extremity pain, weakness, or stiffness to rule out musculoskeletal pathology; that is, try to determine if symptoms are drug induced rather than caused by anatomic or biomechanical problems.

Interventions

- Guard against falls and trauma (hip fractures, head injury, and so forth). Implement fall-prevention strategies, especially in older adults or if drowsiness and dizziness carry over into the daytime (see Appendix E).
- Help patient explore nonpharmacologic methods to improve sleep, such as relaxation techniques, regular exercise, avoidance of caffeine, and so forth.

Patient/Client-Related Instruction

- Instruct patients on prolonged treatment not to discontinue medication without consulting their physician. Long-term use can cause tolerance and physical/psychologic dependence, and increased sleep problems (rebound insomnia) can occur when the drug is suddenly discontinued.
- Advise patient to avoid alcohol and other CNS depressants because of the increased risk of sedation and adverse effects.
- Caution patient and family/caregivers to guard against complex motor behaviors that can occur while asleep, including driving a car.
- Instruct patient to report other bothersome side effects, including severe or prolonged headache, cold symptoms, irritation of the throat and pharynx, chest pain, or GI problems (nausea, abdominal pain, indigestion).

Pharmacokinetics

Absorption: Well absorbed following oral administration.
Distribution: Highly lipid soluble. Crosses the blood-brain barrier and placenta; enters breast milk.
Protein Binding: 93%.
Metabolism and Excretion: Mostly metabolized by the liver; metabolites do not have CNS-depressant activity.
Half-life: 10–24 hr.

TIME/ACTION PROFILE (hypnotic activity)

ROUTE	ONSET	PEAK*	DURATION
PO	15–30 min	2 hr	6–8 hr

*Plasma level.

Contraindications/Precautions

Contraindicated in: Hypersensitivity to estazolam or other benzodiazepines; OB/Pedi: Pregnancy, lactation, or children.
Use Cautiously in: Hepatic or renal dysfunction; Geriatric or debilitated patients (initial dose reduction may be necessary); History of depression; History of drug abuse or suicide attempt.

Interactions

Drug-Drug: Additive CNS depression with **alcohol, antihistamines, antidepressants, MAO inhibitors,** other **sedative/hypnotics** (including benzodiazepines), or **opioid analgesics. Cimetidine** or **hormonal contraceptives** may ↓ metabolism and increase effects of estazolam. May ↓ efficacy of **levodopa. Rifampin** or cigarette smoking ↑ metabolism and ↓ effectiveness. **Theophylline** may antagonize the effectiveness of estazolam.
Drug-Natural: Concomitant use of **kava, valerian, chamomile,** or **hops** can ↑ CNS depression. See **sedative** drug-drug interactions. **St. John's wort** may affect estazolam levels and effectiveness; avoid use.

Route/Dosage

PO (Adults): 1 mg at bedtime; some patients may require 2 mg (range 0.5–2 mg). *Debilitated or small elderly patients*—may initiate at 0.5 mg; increase as needed.

Availability (generic available)

Tablets: 1 mg, 2 mg.

ESTRADIOL (es-tra-**dye**-ole)
Estrace, Gynodiol
estradiol acetate (es-tra-**dye**-ole **as**-e-tate)
Femtrace
estradiol cypionate (es-tra-**dye**-ole **sip**-ee-oh-nate)
depGynogen, Depo-Estradiol, Depogen, Dura-Estrin, E-Cypionate, Estragyn LA 5, Estro-Cyp, Estrofem, Estroject-LA, Estro-L.A
estradiol valerate (es-tra-**dye**-ole **val**-er-ate)
Clinagen LA, Delestrogen, Dioval, Duragen, Estra-L, Estro-Span, Femogex, Gynogen L.A, Menaval, Valergen
estradiol topical emulsion
Estrasorb
estradiol topical gel
Divigel, Elestrin, EstroGel
estradiol transdermal spray
EvaMist
estradiol transdermal system
Alora, Climara, Esclim, Estraderm, FemPatch, Menostar, Vivelle
estradiol vaginal tablet
Vagifem
estradiol vaginal ring
Femring, Estring

Classification
Therapeutic: hormones
Pharmacologic: estrogens

Indications

PO, IM, Topical, Transdermal: Replacement of estrogen (hormone replacement therapy, HRT) to diminish moderate-to-severe vasomotor symptoms of menopause and of various estrogen-deficiency states, including Female hypogonadism, Ovariectomy, Primary ovarian failure. Treatment and prevention of postmenopausal osteoporosis (not vaginal dose forms). **PO:** Inoperable metastatic postmenopausal breast or prostate carcinoma. **Vaginal:** Management of atrophic vaginitis that may occur with menopause (low dose), bothersome systemic symptoms of menopause (higher dose). Concurrent use of progestin is recommended during cyclical therapy to decrease the risk of endometrial carcinoma in patients with an intact uterus.

Action

Estrogens promote growth and development of female sex organs and the maintenance of secondary sex characteristics in women. Metabolic effects include reduced blood cholesterol, protein synthesis, and sodium and water retention. **Therapeutic Effects:** Restoration of hormonal balance in various deficiency states, including menopause. Treatment of hormone-sensitive tumors.

Adverse Reactions/Side Effects

CNS: headache, dizziness, lethargy. **EENT:** intolerance to contact lenses, worsening of myopia or astigmatism. **CV:** MI, THROMBOEMBOLISM, edema, hypertension. **GI:** nausea, weight changes, anorexia, increased appetite, jaundice, vomiting. **GU:** **women**—amenorrhea, dysmenorrhea, breakthrough bleeding, cervical erosions, loss of libido, vaginal candidiasis; **men**—erectile dysfunction, testicular atrophy. **Derm:** oily skin, acne, pigmentation, urticaria. **Endo:** gynecomastia (men), hyperglycemia. **F and E:** hypercalcemia, sodium and water retention. **MS:** leg cramps. **Misc:** breast tenderness.

PHYSICAL THERAPY IMPLICATIONS

Examination and Evaluation

- Be alert for signs of myocardial infarction, especially during exercise. Seek immediate medical assistance if symptoms of MI develop, including sudden chest pain, pain radiating into the arm or jaw, shortness of breath, dizziness, sweating, anxiety, and nausea.
- Monitor signs of venous thrombosis (lower extremity swelling, warmth, erythema, tenderness) and thromboembolism (shortness of breath, chest pain, cough, bloody sputum). Notify physician immediately, and request objective tests (Doppler ultrasound, lung scan, others) if thromboembolism is suspected.
- Assess blood pressure (BP) and compare to normal values (See Appendix F). Report a sustained increase in BP (hypertension) to the physician.
- Assess peripheral edema using girth measurements, volume displacement, and measurement of pitting edema (see Appendix N). Report increased swelling in feet and ankles or a sudden increase in body weight due to fluid retention.
- Monitor signs of high calcium levels (hypercalcemia), including muscle pain, cramps, weakness, joint pain, confusion, and lethargy. Notify physician because severe cases can lead to stupor and coma.
- Be alert for signs of hyperglycemia, including confusion, drowsiness, flushed/dry skin, fruit-like breath odor, rapid/deep breathing, polyuria, loss of appetite, and unusual thirst. Patients with diabetes mellitus should check blood glucose levels frequently.
- If treating menopausal symptoms, monitor severity and frequency of vasomotor symptoms (hot flashes) and other symptoms (vaginal/vulvular itching and irritation) to help document drug efficacy.
- Assess dizziness that might affect gait, balance, and other functional activities (See Appendix C). Report balance problems and functional limitations to the physician, and caution the patient and family/caregivers to guard against falls and trauma.
- Periodically assess body weight and other anthropometric measures (body mass index, body composition). Report a rapid or sustained change in body weight or lean body mass.

Interventions

- Because of the risk of MI and thromboembolism, use caution during aerobic exercise and other forms of therapeutic exercise. Assess exercise tolerance frequently (BP, heart rate, fatigue levels), and terminate exercise immediately if any untoward responses occur (See Appendix L).
- If treating osteoporosis, implement resistance and weight-bearing exercises to help increase bone mineral density.
- If administered transdermally (patches, gels), avoid touching the transdermal application site. Do not apply massage or physical agents (heat, cold, electrotherapeutic modalities) at or near the application site.

Patient/Client-Related Instruction

- Caution patient and family/caregivers about risks of myocardial infarction, and review warning signs of a heart attack.
- Caution patient that cigarette smoking during estrogen therapy may increase the risk of infarction and thromboembolic disease, especially for women older than 35.
- If applied transdermally, advise patient to follow instructions for application.
- Advise women about possible changes in menstrual function. Instruct patient to notify physician about any abnormal bleeding or about persistent vaginal infections (candidiasis).

- Emphasize importance of regular breast exams, especially in women on continuous, long-term estrogen treatment.
- If treating prostate cancer, advise men about possible side effects, including decreased libido, erectile dysfunction, testicular atrophy, and breast enlargement (gynecomastia).
- Advise patient to use sunscreen and protective clothing to decrease hyperpigmentation.
- Instruct patient to report other troublesome side effects such as severe or prolonged headache, visual disturbances, skin disorders (acne, hives, oily skin), or GI problems (nausea, vomiting, loss of appetite).

Pharmacokinetics

Absorption: Well absorbed after oral administration. Readily absorbed through skin and mucous membranes.
Distribution: Widely distributed. Crosses the placenta and enters breast milk.
Metabolism and Excretion: Mostly metabolized by the liver and other tissues. Enterohepatic recirculation occurs, and more absorption may occur from the GI tract.
Half-life: Gel: 36 hr.

TIME/ACTION PROFILE (estrogenic effects)

ROUTE	ONSET	PEAK	DURATION
PO	unknown	unknown	unknown
IM	unknown	unknown	unknown
TD	unknown	unknown	3–4 days (Estraderm), 7 days (Climara)
Topical	unknown	unknown	unknown
Vaginal ring	unknown	unknown	90 days
Vaginal tablet	unknown	unknown	3–4 days

Contraindications/Precautions

Contraindicated in: Thromboembolic disease; Undiagnosed vaginal bleeding; OB: Pregnancy (may result in harm to the fetus); Lactation.
Use Cautiously in: Underlying cardiovascular disease; Severe hepatic or renal disease; May increase the risk of endometrial carcinoma; History of porphyria.

Interactions

Drug-Drug: May alter requirement for **warfarin, oral hypoglycemic agents,** or **insulins. Barbiturates** or **rifampin** may ↓ effectiveness. **Smoking** ↑ risk of adverse CV reactions.

Route/Dosage

Estrogens should be used in the lowest doses for the shortest period of time consistent with desired therapeutic outcome.

Symptoms of Menopause, Atrophic Vaginitis, Female Hypogonadism, Ovarian Failure/Osteoporosis

PO (Adults): 0.45–2 mg daily or in a cycle.
IM (Adults): 1–5 mg monthly (estradiol cypionate) *or* 10–20 mg (estradiol valerate) monthly.
Topical Emulsion *(Estrasorb)*: (Adults): Apply 2 1.74-g pouches (4.35 mg estradiol) daily.
Gel: (Adults): Apply contents of one packet *(Divigel)* or one actuation from pump *(EstroGel, Elestrin)* daily.
Spray *EvaMist*: (Adults): 1 spray daily; may be increased to 2–3 sprays daily.
Transdermal (Adults): *Alora, Estraderm*—50- or 100-mcg/24-hr transdermal patch applied twice weekly. *Climara*—50–100-mcg/24-hr patch applied weekly. *FemPatch*—25-mcg/24-hr patch applied q 7 days. *Vivelle*—37.5–100-mcg/24-hr transdermal patch applied twice weekly. *Menostar*—14-mcg/24-hr patch applied q 7 days. Progestin may be administered for 10–14 days of each month.
Vaginal (Adults): *Cream*—2–4 g (0.2–0.4 mg estradiol) daily for 1–2 wk, then decrease to 1–2 g/day for 1–2 wk; then maintenance dose of 1 g 1–3 times weekly for 3 wk, then off for 1 wk; then repeat cycle once vaginal mucosa has been restored; *Vaginal ring (Estring)*—2-mg (releases 7.5 mcg estradiol/24 hr) q 3 mo; *Vaginal ring (Femring)*—12.4 mg (releases 50 mcg estradiol/24 hr) q 3 mo or 24.8 mg (releases 100 mcg estradiol/24 hr) q 3 mo (*Femring* requires concurrent progesterone); *Vaginal tablet*—25-mcg once daily for 2 wk, then twice weekly.

Postmenopausal Breast Carcinoma

PO (Adults): 10 mg 3 times daily.

Prostate Carcinoma

PO (Adults): 1–2 mg 3 times daily.
IM (Adults): 30 mg q 1–2 wk (estradiol valerate).

Availability

Tablets: 0.45 mg, 0.5 mg, 0.9 mg, 1 mg, 1.8 mg, 2 mg. **Injection (valerate in oil):** 10 mg/mL, 20 mg/mL, 40 mg/mL. **Injection (cypionate in oil):** 5 mg/mL. **Topical emulsion:** 4.35 mg/1.74-g pouch in boxes of 14 pouches in a 1-mo supply carton of 56 pouches. **Topical gel packet:** 0.25 g packet, 0.5-g packet, 1-g packet. **Topical gel pump (0.06%):** 0.87 g/actuation, 1.25 g/actuation. **Transdermal Spray:** metered-dose pump contains 8.1 mL, delivers 56 sprays of 1.53 mg each. **Transdermal system:** 14 mcg/24-hr release rate, 25 mcg/24-hr release rate, 37.5 mcg /24-hr release rate, 50 mcg/24-hr release rate, 60 mcg/24–hr release rate, 75 mcg/24-hr release rate, 100 mcg/24-hr release rate. **Vaginal cream:** 100 mcg/g. **Vaginal ring (Estring):** 2 mg (releases 7.5 mcg/day over 90 days). **Vaginal ring (Femring):** 12.4 mg (releases 50 mcg/day over 90 days), 24.8 mg (releases 100 mcg/day over 90 days). **Vaginal tablet:** 25 mcg.

estramustine (es-tra-mus-teen)

Emcyt

Classification

Therapeutic: antineoplastics, hormones
Pharmacologic: alkylating agents

Indications

Palliative treatment of advanced metastatic prostate cancer.

Action

Consists of combination of mechlorethamine, an alkylating agent, and estradiol, an estrogenic compound. Antineoplastic activity may be due to either component or the combination. Also decreases serum testosterone levels. **Therapeutic Effects:** Decreased spread of prostate cancer.

Adverse Reactions/Side Effects

CNS: insomnia. **CV:** THROMBOEMBOLISM, edema, hypertension. **GI:** diarrhea, nausea, anorexia, flatulence, vomiting. **Derm:** bruising, dry skin, pruritus, rashes. **Endo:** decreased libido, gynecomastia, gonadal suppression (azoospermia), hyperglycemia. **Hemat:** leukopenia, thrombocytopenia. **MS:** leg cramps. **Resp:** dyspnea. **Misc:** ANGIOEDEMA, allergic reactions.

PHYSICAL THERAPY IMPLICATIONS

Examination and Evaluation

- Monitor signs of allergic reactions and angioedema, including pulmonary symptoms (tightness in the throat and chest, wheezing, cough, dyspnea) or skin reactions (rashes, raised patches of red or white skin, burning/itching skin, swelling in the face). Notify physician or nursing staff immediately if these reactions occur.
- Monitor signs of venous thrombosis (lower extremity swelling, warmth, erythema, tenderness) and thromboembolism (shortness of breath, chest pain, cough, bloody sputum). Notify physician immediately, and request objective tests (Doppler ultrasound, lung scan, others) if thrombosis is suspected.
- Assess blood pressure periodically and compare to normal values (See Appendix F). Report a sustained increase in blood pressure (hypertension) to the physician.
- Be alert for signs of leukopenia (fever, sore throat, signs of infection) or thrombocytopenia (bruising, nose bleeds, bleeding gums). Report these signs immediately to the physician or nursing staff.
- Be alert for signs of hyperglycemia, including confusion, drowsiness, flushed/dry skin, fruit-like breath odor, rapid/deep breathing, polyuria, loss of appetite, and unusual thirst. Patients with diabetes mellitus should check blood glucose levels frequently.
- Assess peripheral edema using girth measurements, volume displacement, and measurement of pitting edema (See Appendix N). Report increased swelling in feet and ankles or a sudden increase in body weight due to fluid retention.
- Assess any leg cramps or other musculoskeletal impairments to rule out musculoskeletal pathology; that is, try to determine if pain is drug-induced rather than caused by anatomic or physiologic problems.

Interventions

- For patients who are medically able to begin exercise, implement appropriate resistive exercises and aerobic training to maintain muscle strength and aerobic capacity during cancer chemotherapy or to help restore function after chemotherapy.
- Because of potential cardiac problems (hypertension, thromboembolism), use caution during aerobic exercise and endurance conditioning. Terminate exercise if patient exhibits untoward symptoms (chest pain, shortness of breath, etc.) or displays other criteria for exercise termination (See Appendix L).

Patient/Client-Related Instruction

- Advise patient to guard against infection (frequent hand washing, etc.), and to avoid crowds and contact with persons with contagious diseases.
- Advise patient that rashes and other skin reactions (itching, dry skin, bruising) are likely. Severe or unexpected skin reactions should be reported to the physician.
- Advise patient about the likelihood of GI reactions such as diarrhea, nausea, vomiting, intestinal gas, and loss of appetite. Instruct patient to report severe or prolonged GI problems.
- Instruct patient or family/caregivers to report other bothersome side effects such as severe or prolonged sleep loss, decreased sex drive, or breast enlargement.

Pharmacokinetics

Absorption: Well absorbed (75%) after oral administration. During absorption, converted to estramustine, estramustine and then to estrogenic compounds (estrone and estradiol).
Distribution: Concentrates in prostatic tissue.
Metabolism and Excretion: Eliminated primarily by biliary and fecal excretion. Small amounts excreted by kidneys.
Half-life: 20–24 hr.

TIME/ACTION PROFILE (effect on tumor spread)

ROUTE	ONSET	PEAK	DURATION
PO	30–90 days	unknown	6 wk*

*Persistence of hematologic effects.

Contraindications/Precautions

Contraindicated in: Active thrombophlebitis or thromboembolic disorder; Known hypersensitivity to estradiol or mechlorethamine.

Use Cautiously in: History of thrombophlebitis or thromboembolic disorders; Hypercalcemia; Renal or hepatic impairment; Coronary artery disease; Hypertension; Heart failure; Diabetes mellitus; Cerebrovascular disease; Migraine headaches; Metabolic bone disease; Epilepsy; Patients with childbearing potential.

Interactions

Drug-Drug: Calcium supplements form an insoluble complex with estramustine that cannot be absorbed.

Drug-Food: Calcium in dairy foods forms an insoluble complex with estramustine that cannot be absorbed.

Route/Dosage

PO (Adults): 14 mg/kg/day in 3–4 divided doses (range 10–16 mg/kg/day).

Availability

Capsules: 140 mg.

estrogens, conjugated (equine) (es-troe-jenz)

C.E.S, Congest, Premarin

estrogens, conjugated (synthetic, A)

Cenestin

estrogens, conjugated (synthetic, B)

Enjuvia

Classification

Therapeutic: hormones

Pharmacologic: estrogens

Indications

PO: Treatment of moderate to severe vasomotor symptoms of menopause. Estrogen deficiency states, including Female hypogonadism, Ovariectomy, Primary ovarian failure. Prevention of postmenopausal osteoporosis. Advanced inoperable metastatic breast and prostatic carcinoma. **IM, IV:** Uterine bleeding resulting from hormonal imbalance. **Vaginal:** Management of atrophic vaginitis. Concurrent use of progestin is recommended during cyclical therapy to decrease the risk of endometrial carcinoma in patients with an intact uterus.

Action

Estrogens promote the growth and development of female sex organs and the maintenance of secondary sex characteristics in women. **Therapeutic Effects:** Restoration of hormonal balance in various deficiency states and treatment of hormone-sensitive tumors.

Adverse Reactions/Side Effects

(systemic use)

CNS: headache, dizziness, insomnia, lethargy, mental depression. **CV:** MI, THROMBOEMBOLISM, edema, hypertension. **GI:** nausea, weight changes, anorexia, increased appetite, jaundice, vomiting. **GU: women**—amenorrhea, breakthrough bleeding, dysmenorrhea, cervical erosion, loss of libido, vaginal candidiasis; **men**—erectile dysfunction, testicular atrophy. **Derm:** acne, oily skin, pigmentation, urticaria. **Endo:** gynecomastia (men), hyperglycemia. **F and E:** hypercalcemia, sodium and water retention. **MS:** leg cramps. **Misc:** breast tenderness.

PHYSICAL THERAPY IMPLICATIONS

Examination and Evaluation

- Be alert for signs of myocardial infarction, especially during exercise. Seek immediate medical assistance if symptoms of MI develop, including sudden chest pain, pain radiating into the arm or jaw, shortness of breath, dizziness, sweating, anxiety, and nausea.
- Monitor signs of venous thrombosis (lower extremity swelling, warmth, erythema, tenderness) and thromboembolism (shortness of breath, chest pain, cough, bloody sputum). Notify physician immediately, and request objective tests (Doppler ultrasound, lung scan, others) if thromboembolism is suspected.
- Assess blood pressure (BP) and compare to normal values (See Appendix F). Report a sustained increase in BP (hypertension) to the physician.
- Assess peripheral edema using girth measurements, volume displacement, and measurement of pitting edema (See Appendix N). Report increased swelling in feet and ankles or a sudden increase in body weight due to fluid retention.
- Monitor signs of high calcium levels (hypercalcemia), including muscle pain, cramps, weakness, joint pain, confusion, and lethargy. Notify physician because severe cases can lead to stupor and coma.
- Be alert for signs of hyperglycemia, including confusion, drowsiness, flushed/dry skin, fruit-like breath odor, rapid/deep breathing, polyuria, loss of appetite, and unusual thirst. Patients with diabetes mellitus should check blood glucose levels frequently.

- If treating menopausal symptoms, monitor severity and frequency of vasomotor symptoms (hot flashes) and other symptoms (vaginal/vulvular itching and irritation) to help document drug efficacy.
- Assess dizziness that might affect gait, balance, and other functional activities (See Appendix C). Report balance problems and functional limitations to the physician, and caution the patient and family/caregivers to guard against falls and trauma.
- Periodically assess body weight and other anthropometric measures (body mass index, body composition). Report a rapid or sustained change in body weight or lean body mass.

Interventions

- Because of the risk of MI and thromboembolism, use caution during aerobic exercise and other forms of therapeutic exercise. Assess exercise tolerance frequently (BP, heart rate, fatigue levels), and terminate exercise immediately if any untoward responses occur (See Appendix L).
- If treating osteoporosis, implement resistance and weight-bearing exercises to help increase bone mineral density.

Patient/Client-Related Instruction

- Caution patient and family/caregivers about risks of myocardial infarction, and review warning signs of a heart attack.
- Caution patient that cigarette smoking during estrogen therapy may increase the risk of infarction and thromboembolic disease, especially for women older than 35.
- Advise women about possible changes in menstrual function. Instruct patient to notify health care professional about any abnormal bleeding or about persistent vaginal infections (candidiasis).
- Emphasize importance of regular breast exams, especially in women on continuous, long-term estrogen treatment.
- If treating prostate cancer, advise men about possible side effects, including decreased libido, erectile dysfunction, testicular atrophy, and breast enlargement (gynecomastia).
- Advise patient to use sunscreen and protective clothing to decrease hyperpigmentation.
- Instruct patient to report other troublesome side effects such as severe or prolonged headache, insomnia, mental depression, visual disturbances, skin disorders (acne, hives, oily skin), or GI problems (nausea, vomiting, loss of appetite).

Pharmacokinetics

Absorption: Well absorbed after oral administration. Readily absorbed through skin and mucous membranes.

Distribution: Widely distributed. Crosses placenta and enters breast milk.

Metabolism and Excretion: Mostly metabolized by liver and other tissues. Enterohepatic recirculation occurs, with more absorption from GI tract.

Half-life: Unknown.

TIME/ACTION PROFILE (estrogenic effects†)

ROUTE	ONSET	PEAK	DURATION
PO*	rapid	unknown	24 hr
IM	delayed	unknown	6–12 hr
IV	rapid	unknown	6–12 hr

*Tumor response may take several weeks.

Contraindications/Precautions

Contraindicated in: Thromboembolic disease (e.g., DVT, PE, MI, stroke); Undiagnosed vaginal bleeding; History of breast cancer; History of estrogen-dependent cancer; Liver dysfunction; OB: Pregnancy (may result in harm to the fetus); OB: Lactation.

Use Cautiously in: Long-term use (more than 4–5 yr); may increase risk of myocardial infarction, stroke, invasive breast cancer, pulmonary emboli, deep vein thrombosis and dementia in postmenopausal women; Underlying cardiovascular disease; Hypertriglyceridemia; May increase the risk of endometrial carcinoma.

Interactions

Drug-Drug: May alter requirement for **warfarin, oral hypoglycemic agents,** or **insulins. Barbiturates, carbamazepine,** or **rifampin** may ↓ effectiveness. **Smoking** ↑ risk of adverse CV reactions. **Erythromycin, clarithromycin, itraconazole, ketoconazole,** and **ritonavir** may ↑ risk of adverse effects.

Drug-Natural: Grapefruit juice may ↑ risk of adverse effects.

Route/Dosage

Estrogens should be used in the lowest doses for the shortest period of time consistent with desired therapeutic outcome.

Ovariectomy, Primary Ovarian Failure

PO (Adults): 1.25 mg daily administered cyclically (3 wk on, 1 wk off).

Osteoporosis/Menopausal Symptoms

PO (Adults): 0.3–1.25 mg daily or in a cycle.

Female Hypogonadism

PO (Adults): 0.3–0.625 mg daily administered cyclically (3 wk on, 1 wk off).

Inoperable Breast Carcinoma—Men and Postmenopausal Women

PO (Adults): 10 mg 3 times daily.

Inoperable Prostate Carcinoma

PO (Adults): 1.25–2.5 mg 3 times daily.

Uterine Bleeding

IM, IV (Adults): 25 mg, may repeat in 6–12 hr if necessary.

Atrophic Vaginitis

PO (Adults): 0.3–1.25 mg daily.
Vaginal (Adults): 1.25–2.5 mg (2–4 g cream) daily for 3 wk, off for 1 wk, then repeat.

Availability (generic available)

Tablets: 0.3 mg, 0.45 mg, 0.625 mg, 0.9 mg, 1.25 mg. **Powder for injection:** 25 mg/vial. **Vaginal cream:** 0.625 mg/g. ***In combination with:*** medroxyprogesterone (Prempro and Premphase [compliance package]). See Appendix B.

estropipate (es-troe-pi-pate)

Ogen, Ortho-Est

OTHER NAMES:
piperazine estrone sulfate

Classification
Therapeutic: hormones
Pharmacologic: estrogens

Indications

PO: As part of HRT in the treatment of vasomotor symptoms of menopause. Treatment of various estrogen-deficiency states, including Female hypogonadism, Ovariectomy, Primary ovarian failure. Adjunctive therapy of postmenopausal osteoporosis. **Vaginal:** Management of atrophic vaginitis. Concurrent use of progestin is recommended during cyclical therapy to decrease the risk of endometrial carcinoma in patients with an intact uterus.

Action

Estrogens promote the growth and development of female sex organs and the maintenance of secondary sex characteristics in women. Metabolic effects include reduced blood cholesterol, protein synthesis, and sodium and water retention. **Therapeutic Effects:** Restoration of hormonal balance in various deficiency states.

Adverse Reactions/Side Effects

(systemic use)
CNS: headache, dizziness, lethargy, mental depression. **EENT:** intolerance to contact lenses, worsening of myopia or astigmatism. **CV:** MI, THROMBOEMBOLISM, edema, hypertension. **GI:** nausea, weight changes, anorexia, increased appetite, jaundice, vomiting. **GU:** **women**—amenorrhea, breakthrough bleeding, dysmenorrhea, cervical erosion, loss of libido, vaginal candidiasis; **men**—erectile dysfunction, testicular atrophy. **Derm:** acne, oily skin, pigmentation, urticaria. **Endo:** gynecomastia (men), hyperglycemia. **F and E:** hypercalcemia, sodium and water retention. **MS:** leg cramps. **Misc:** breast tenderness.

PHYSICAL THERAPY IMPLICATIONS

Examination and Evaluation

- Be alert for signs of myocardial infarction (MI), especially during exercise. Seek immediate medical assistance if symptoms of MI develop, including sudden chest pain, pain radiating into the arm or jaw, shortness of breath, dizziness, sweating, anxiety, and nausea.
- Monitor signs of venous thrombosis (lower extremity swelling, warmth, erythema, tenderness) and thromboembolism (shortness of breath, chest pain, cough, bloody sputum). Notify physician immediately, and request objective tests (Doppler ultrasound, lung scan, others) if thromboembolism is suspected.
- Assess blood pressure (BP) and compare to normal values (See Appendix F). Report a sustained increase in BP (hypertension) to the physician.
- Assess peripheral edema using girth measurements, volume displacement, and measurement of pitting edema (See Appendix N). Report increased swelling in feet and ankles or a sudden increase in body weight due to fluid retention.
- Monitor signs of high calcium levels (hypercalcemia), including muscle pain, cramps, weakness, joint pain, confusion, and lethargy. Notify physician because severe cases can lead to stupor and coma.
- Be alert for signs of hyperglycemia, including confusion, drowsiness, flushed/dry skin, fruit-like breath odor, rapid/deep breathing, polyuria, loss of appetite, and unusual thirst. Patients with diabetes mellitus should check blood glucose levels frequently.
- If treating menopausal symptoms, monitor severity and frequency of vasomotor symptoms (hot flashes) and other symptoms (vaginal/vulvular itching and irritation) to help determine drug efficacy.
- Assess dizziness that might affect gait, balance, and other functional activities (See Appendix C). Report balance problems and functional limitations to the physician, and caution the patient and family/caregivers to guard against falls and trauma.
- Periodically assess body weight and other anthropometric measures (body mass index, body composition). Report a rapid or sustained change in body weight or lean body mass.

Interventions

- Because of the risk of MI and thromboembolism, use caution during aerobic exercise and other forms of therapeutic exercise. Assess exercise tolerance frequently (BP, heart rate, fatigue levels), and terminate exercise immediately if any untoward responses occur (See Appendix L).

- If treating osteoporosis, implement resistance and weight-bearing exercises to help increase bone mineral density.

Patient/Client-Related Instruction

- Caution patient and family/caregivers about risks of myocardial infarction, and review warning signs of a heart attack.
- Caution patient that cigarette smoking during estrogen therapy may increase the risk of infarction and thromboembolic disease, especially for women older than 35.
- Advise women about possible changes in menstrual function. Instruct patient to notify health care professional about any abnormal bleeding or about persistent vaginal infections (candidiasis).
- Emphasize importance of regular breast exams, especially in women on continuous, long-term estrogen treatment.
- If treating prostate cancer, advise men about possible side effects, including decreased libido, erectile dysfunction, testicular atrophy, and breast enlargement (gynecomastia).
- Advise patient to use sunscreen and protective clothing to decrease hyperpigmentation.
- Instruct patient to report other troublesome side effects such as severe or prolonged headache, mental depression, visual disturbances, skin disorders (acne, hives, oily skin), or GI problems (nausea, vomiting, loss of appetite).

Pharmacokinetics

Absorption: Well absorbed after oral administration. Readily absorbed through skin and mucous membranes.
Distribution: Widely distributed. Crosses the placenta and enters breast milk.
Metabolism and Excretion: Mostly metabolized by the liver and other tissues. Enterohepatic recirculation occurs, and more absorption may occur from the GI tract.
Half-life: Unknown.

TIME/ACTION PROFILE (estrogenic effects)

ROUTE	ONSET	PEAK	DURATION
PO	unknown	unknown	24 hr

Contraindications/Precautions

Contraindicated in: Thromboembolic disease; Undiagnosed vaginal bleeding; Pregnancy (may result in harm to the fetus); Lactation.
Use Cautiously in: Underlying cardiovascular disease; Severe hepatic or renal disease; May increase the risk of endometrial carcinoma.

Interactions

Drug-Drug: May alter requirement for **warfarin, oral hypoglycemic agents**, or **insulins**. **Barbiturates** or **rifampin** may ↓ effectiveness. **Smoking** ↑ the risk of adverse cardiovascular reactions.

Route/Dosage

Vasomotor Symptoms of Menopause/Atrophic Vaginitis/Osteoporosis

PO (Adults): 0.75–6 mg daily or in a cycle.
Vag (Adults): 3–6 mg (2–4 g of 0.15% cream) daily for 3 wk, then off for 1 wk, then repeat cycle.

Female Hypogonadism/Ovarian Failure

PO (Adults): 1.5–9 mg daily or in a cycle.

Availability (generic available)

Tablets: 0.75 mg, 1.5 mg, 3 mg, 6 mg estropipate.
Vaginal cream: 1.5 mg/g.

eszopiclone (es-zop-i-klone)

Lunesta

Classification
Therapeutic: sedative/hypnotics
Pharmacologic: cyclopyrrolones

Schedule IV

Indications

Insomnia.

Action

Interacts with gamma-aminobutyric acid (GABA)–receptor complexes; not a benzodiazepine. **Therapeutic Effects:** Improved sleep with decreased latency and increased maintenance of sleep.

Adverse Reactions/Side Effects

CNS: abnormal thinking, behavior changes, depression, hallucinations, headache, sleep-driving. **CV:** chest pain, peripheral edema. **GI:** dry mouth, unpleasant taste. **Derm:** rash.

PHYSICAL THERAPY IMPLICATIONS

Examination and Evaluation

- Monitor and report daytime drowsiness, depression, behavior changes, hallucinations, and "drugged" feelings. Repeated or excessive symptoms may require change in dose or medication.
- Assess peripheral edema using girth measurements, volume displacement, and measurement of pitting edema (See Appendix N). Report increased swelling in feet and ankles or a sudden increase in body weight due to fluid retention.
- Monitor any chest pain and attempt to determine if pain is drug induced or caused by cardiovascular dysfunction (e.g., angina that occurs during exercise).

Interventions

- Guard against falls and trauma (hip fractures, head injury, and so forth). Implement fall-prevention strategies, especially in older adults or if drowsiness and dizziness carry over into the daytime (See Appendix E).
- Help patient explore non pharmacologic methods to improve sleep, including relaxation techniques, regular exercise, avoiding caffeine, and so forth.

Patient/Client-Related Instruction

- Instruct patients on prolonged treatment not to discontinue medication without consulting a health care professional. Long-term use can cause tolerance and physical/psychologic dependence, and abrupt withdrawal after 2 or more weeks of use may cause increased sleep loss (rebound insomnia).
- Advise patient about the risk of daytime drowsiness and decreased attention and mental focus. Use care if driving or in other activities that require strong concentration.
- Caution patient and family/caregivers that "sleep-walking" and other complex activities including driving a car (sleep-driving) may occur while completely asleep. Care should be taken to monitor such activities and prevent access to motor vehicles while under the influence of this drug.
- Advise patient to avoid alcohol and other CNS depressants because of the increased risk of sedation and adverse effects.
- Instruct patient and family/caregivers to report other troublesome side effects such as severe or prolonged skin rash, abnormal thoughts, dry mouth, or unpleasant taste.

Pharmacokinetics

Absorption: Rapidly absorbed after oral administration.
Distribution: Unknown.
Metabolism and Excretion: Extensively metabolized by the liver (CYP3A4 and CYP2E1 enzyme systems); metabolites are renally excreted, <10% excreted unchanged in urine.
Half-life: 6 hr.

TIME/ACTION PROFILE (blood levels)

ROUTE	ONSET	PEAK	DURATION
PO	rapid	1 hr	6 hr

Contraindications/Precautions

Contraindicated in: No known contraindications.
Use Cautiously in: Geri: Geriatric/debilitated patients (may have ↓ metabolism or increased sensitivity; use lower initial dose); Conditions that may alter metabolic or hemodynamic function; Severe hepatic impairment (use lower initial dose); OB/Pedi: Lactation and children <18 yr (safety not established); Pregnancy (safety not established; use only if maternal benefit justifies fetal risk).

Interactions

Drug-Drug: ↑ risk of CNS depression with other **CNS depressants**, including **antihistamines, antidepressants, opioids, sedative/hypnotics**, and **antipsychotics**. ↑ levels and risk of CNS depression with **drugs that inhibit the CYP3A4 enzyme system,** including **ketoconazole, itraconazole, clarithromycin, nefazodone, ritonavir,** and **nelfinavir**. Levels and effectiveness may be ↓ by **drugs that induce the CYP3A4 enzyme system,** including **rifampicin**.

Route/Dosage

PO (Adults): 2 mg immediately before bedtime, may be raised to 3 mg if needed (3 mg dose is more effective for sleep maintenance); *geriatric patients*—1 mg immediately before bedtime for patients with difficulty falling asleep; 2 mg for patients who difficulty staying asleep.

Hepatic Impairment

PO (Adults): *Severe hepatic impairment*—1 mg immediately before bedtime.
PO (Adults receiving concurrent CYP3A4 inhibitors): 1 mg immediately before bedtime; may be raised to 2 mg if needed.

Availability

Tablets: 1 mg, 2 mg, 3 mg.

etanercept (ee-tan-er-sept)

Enbrel

Classification

Therapeutic: antirheumatics (disease-modifying antirheumatic drugs, DMARDs)
Pharmacologic: anti-TNF agents

Indications

To decrease progression, signs and symptoms of rheumatoid arthritis, juvenile arthritis, ankylosing spondylitis, psoriatic arthritis. or plaque psoriasis when response has been inadequate to other disease-modifying agents. May be used with other agents.

Action

Binds to tumor necrosis factor (TNF), making it inactive. TNF is a mediator of inflammatory response.

Therapeutic Effects: Decreased inflammation and slowed progression of arthritis, spondylitis, or psoriasis.

Adverse Reactions/Side Effects

CNS: headache, dizziness, weakness. **EENT:** rhinitis, pharyngitis, sinusitis. **Resp:** upper respiratory tract infection, cough, respiratory disorder. **GI:** abdominal pain, dyspepsia. **Derm:** rash. **Hemat:** pancytopenia. **Local:** injection site reactions. **Misc:** INFECTIONS, ↑ risk of malignancies.

PHYSICAL THERAPY IMPLICATIONS

Examination and Evaluation

- Watch for any signs of infection, including upper respiratory tract infections. Signs of respiratory infection include cough, fever, nasal congestion, sneezing, runny nose, and sore throat. Report these signs to the physician immediately.
- Monitor and report signs of red and white blood cell deficiencies (pancytopenia), including leukopenia (fever, sore throat, signs of infection), thrombocytopenia (bruising, nose bleeds, and bleeding gums), or unusual weakness and fatigue that might be due to anemias. Periodic blood tests may be needed to monitor WBC and RBC counts.
- Assess dizziness or weakness that might affect gait, balance, and other functional activities (See Appendix C). Report balance problems and functional limitations to the physician, and caution the patient and family/caregivers to guard against falls and trauma.
- If treating arthritic conditions, periodically assess impairments (pain, range of motion), functional ability, and disability to help document whether antirheumatic drug therapy is successful.
- If treating psoriasis, monitor skin responses to help document whether drug therapy is successful in resolving this condition.
- Assess the subcutaneous injection site for pain, swelling, and irritation. Report prolonged or excessive injection-site reactions to the physician.

Interventions

- If treating arthritic conditions, implement appropriate manual therapy techniques, physical agents, therapeutic exercises, and orthotic/assistive devices to reduce pain, improve function, and augment the effects of antirheumatic drug therapy.
- Help patients with arthritis explore other nonpharmacologic methods to reduce chronic arthritis pain, such as relaxation techniques, exercise, counseling, and so forth.

Patient/Client-Related Instruction

- Advise patient to guard against infection (frequent hand washing, etc.), and to avoid crowds and contact with persons who have contagious diseases.
- Instruct patient to report other troublesome side effects, including severe or prolonged headache, upper respiratory tract inflammation/irritation, or GI problems (abdominal pain, indigestion).

Pharmacokinetics

Absorption: 60% absorbed after SC administration.
Distribution: Unknown.
Metabolism and Excretion: Unknown.
Half-life: 115 hr (range 98–300 hr).

TIME/ACTION PROFILE (symptom reduction)

ROUTE	ONSET	PEAK	DURATION
SC	2–4 wk	unknown	unknown

Contraindications/Precautions

Contraindicated in: Hypersensitivity; Sepsis; OB: Lactation; Untreated infections; Wegener's granulomatosis (receiving immunosuppressive agents); Concurrent cyclophosphamide or anakinra.
Use Cautiously in: Preexisting or recent demyelinating disorders (multiple sclerosis, myelitis, optic neuritis); History of tuberculosis (increased risk of reactivation); Underlying chronic diseases which may predispose to infections (advanced or poorly controlled diabetes mellitus); Latex allergy (needle cover of diluent syringe contains latex); Geri: May have ↑ risk of infection; Pedi: Children with significant exposure to varicella virus (temporarily discontinue etanercept; consider varicella zoster immune globulin); OB: Pregnancy (use only if needed).

Interactions

Drug-Drug: Concurrent use with **anakinra** ↑ risk of serious infections (not recommended). Concurrent use of **cyclophosphamide** may ↑ risk of malignancies. May ↓ the antibody response to **live-virus vaccine** and ↑ the risk of adverse reactions (do not administer concurrently).

Route/Dosage

SC (Adults): *Adult rheumatoid arthritis, ankylosing spondylitis, psoriatic arthritis*—50 mg once weekly; *adult plaque psoriasis*—50 mg twice weekly for 3 mo, then 50 mg once weekly; may also be given as 25–50 mg once weekly as an initial dose.
SC (Children 4–17 yr): *>63 kg*—0.8 mg/kg/wk (up to 50 mg) as a single injection; *31–62 kg*—0.8 mg/kg/wk either as 2 injections on the same day or divided and given on two separate days 3–4 days apart; *<31 kg*—0.8 mg/kg/wk as a single injection.

Availability

Prefilled syringes: 50 mg/mL. **Powder for injection:** 25 mg/vial.

ethacrynic acid

(eth-a-**krin**-ik **as**-id)

Edecrin

Classification

Therapeutic: diuretics

Pharmacologic: loop diuretics

Indications

Edema due to heart failure, hepatic impairment, or renal disease. Short-term management of ascites due to malignancy, idiopathic edema, and lymphedema. Alternative diuretic in patients with an allergy to sulfonamides.

Action

Inhibits the reabsorption of sodium and chloride from the loop of Henle and distal renal tubule. Increases renal excretion of water, sodium, chloride, magnesium, hydrogen, and calcium. Effectiveness persists in impaired renal function. **Therapeutic Effects:** Diuresis and subsequent mobilization of excess fluid (edema, pleural effusions).

Adverse Reactions/Side Effects

CNS: confusion, fatigue, headache, nervousness, vertigo. **EENT:** hearing loss, tinnitus. **CV:** hypotension. **GI:** abdominal pain, anorexia, diarrhea, dry mouth, dysphagia, nausea, vomiting. **GU:** excessive urination, hematuria. **Derm:** rash. **Endo:** hyperglycemia, hyperuricemia. **F and E:** dehydration, hypocalcemia, hypochloremia, hypokalemia, hypomagnesemia, hyponatremia, hypovolemia, metabolic alkalosis. **Hemat:** AGRANULOCYTOSIS, neutropenia, thrombocytopenia. **Misc:** fever, increased BUN.

PHYSICAL THERAPY IMPLICATIONS

Examination and Evaluation

- Monitor signs of agranulocytosis and neutropenia (fever, sore throat, mucosal lesions, signs of infection) or thrombocytopenia (bruising, nose bleeds, bleeding gums). Report these signs immediately to the physician.
- Monitor signs of fluid, electrolyte, or acid-base imbalances, including dizziness, drowsiness, blurred vision, confusion, hypotension, or muscle cramps and weakness. Report excessive or prolonged symptoms to the physician.
- Assess dizziness and vertigo that might affect gait, balance, and other functional activities (See Appendix C). Report balance problems and functional limitations to the physician, and caution the patient and family/caregivers to guard against falls and trauma.
- Monitor drug effects by assessing peripheral edema using girth measurements, volume displacement, and measurement of pitting edema (See Appendix N). Also monitor signs of pulmonary edema such as dyspnea and rales/crackles (See Appendix K). Document whether peripheral and pulmonary symptoms are controlled adequately by diuretic therapy.
- Assess blood pressure periodically and compare to normal values (See Appendix F). Report low blood pressure (hypotension), especially if patient experiences dizziness or syncope.
- Monitor signs of hyperglycemia such as drowsiness, fruity breath, increased urination, and unusual thirst. Patients with diabetes mellitus should check blood glucose levels frequently.

Interventions

- Implement fall-prevention strategies, especially in older adults or if patient exhibits sedation, dizziness, vertigo, or other impairments that affect gait and balance (See Appendix E).
- Use caution during aerobic exercise, especially in hot environments. Increased sweating will cause fluid and electrolyte loss and may exaggerate diuretic side effects (dizziness, muscle cramps, and so forth).
- To minimize orthostatic hypotension, patient should move slowly when assuming a more upright position.

Patient/Client-Related Instruction

- Remind patient and family/caregivers that diuretics typically increase urine output. Any unusual problems such as excessive urination or bloody urine should be reported to the physician.
- Counsel patients about additional interventions to help control edema and improve circulation, including sodium restriction, regular exercise, weight loss, moderation of alcohol consumption, and smoking cessation.
- Instruct patient to report troublesome GI problems such as severe or prolonged nausea, vomiting, diarrhea, abdominal pain, or loss of appetite.
- Instruct patient to report any hearing loss or ringing/buzzing in the ears (tinnitus).
- Instruct patient and family/caregivers to report other troublesome side effects such as severe or prolonged headache, nervousness, or skin rashes.

Pharmacokinetics

Absorption: Well absorbed after oral administration.
Distribution: Unknown.
Protein Binding: >90%.
Metabolism and Excretion: 35–40% metabolized by liver; 60% eliminated unchanged by kidneys.
Half-life: 2–4 hr.

TIME/ACTION PROFILE (diuretic effect)

ROUTE	ONSET	PEAK	DURATION
PO	30 min	2 hr	6–8 hr
IV	5 min	30 min	2 hr

Contraindications/Precautions

Contraindicated in: Hypersensitivity; Hepatic coma or anuria.
Use Cautiously in: Severe liver disease (may precipitate hepatic coma; concurrent use with potassium-sparing diuretics may be necessary); Electrolyte depletion; Diabetes mellitus; Increasing azotemia; OB/Lactation: Safety not established; Geri: Possible increased risk of side effects at usual doses, especially hypotension and electrolyte imbalance.

Interactions

Drug-Drug: ↑ hypotension with **antihypertensives, nitrates**, or acute ingestion of **alcohol**. ↑ risk of hypokalemia with other **diuretics, amphotericin B, stimulant laxatives**, and **corticosteroids**. Hypokalemia may ↑ risk of **digoxin** toxicity and ↑ risk of arrhythmia in patients taking drugs that prolong the QT interval. ↓ **lithium** excretion, may cause **lithium** toxicity. ↑ risk of ototoxicity with **aminoglycosides**. May ↑ the effectiveness of **warfarin**. **NSAIDS** ↓ effects of ethacrynic acid.

Route/Dosage

PO (Adults): 50–100 mg/day in 1–2 divided doses; may increase dose by 25–50 mg every few days until desired response (maximum dose = 400 mg/day).
PO (Children >1 mo): 1 mg/kg/dose once daily; may be increased every 2–3 days to a maximum of 3 mg/kg/day.
IV (Adults): 0.5–1 mg/kg/dose (maximum = 100 mg/dose); may repeat dose every 8–12 hr if needed.
IV (Children >1 mo): 1 mg/kg/dose, may repeat dose if indicated q 8–12 hr.

Availability

Tablet: 25 mg RX. **Injection:** 50 mg/vial Rx.

ethambutol (e-tham-byoo-tole)

✱Etibi, Myambutol

Classification
Therapeutic: antituberculars

Indications

Active tuberculosis or other mycobacterial diseases (with at least 1 other drug).

Action

Inhibits the growth of mycobacteria. **Therapeutic Effects:** Tuberculostatic effect against susceptible organisms.

Adverse Reactions/Side Effects

CNS: confusion, dizziness, hallucinations, headache, malaise. **EENT:** optic neuritis. **GI:** HEPATITIS, abdominal pain, anorexia, nausea, vomiting. **Metab:** hyperuricemia. **MS:** joint pain. **Neuro:** peripheral neuritis. **Misc:** anaphylactoid reactions, fever.

PHYSICAL THERAPY IMPLICATIONS

Examination and Evaluation

- Be alert for signs of hepatitis, including anorexia, abdominal pain, severe nausea and vomiting, yellow skin or eyes, fever, sore throat, malaise, weakness, facial edema, lethargy, and unusual bleeding or bruising. Report these signs to the physician immediately.
- Monitor signs of agranulocytosis (fever, sore throat, mucosal lesions, signs of infection), methemoglobinemia (bluish coloring of skin, headache, shortness of breath, lack of energy), or other unusual weakness and fatigue that might be due to other anemias and blood dyscrasias. Report these signs to the physician immediately.
- Monitor signs of hypersensitivity or anaphylactoid reactions, including pulmonary symptoms (tightness in the throat and chest, wheezing, cough, dyspnea) or skin reactions (rash, pruritus, urticaria). Notify physician or nursing staff immediately if these reactions occur.
- Monitor signs of peripheral neuritis (numbness, tingling). Perform objective tests (nerve conduction, monofilaments) to document any neuropathic changes.
- Assess any joint pain to rule out musculoskeletal pathology; that is, try to determine if pain is drug induced rather than caused by anatomic or biomechanical problems.
- Assess dizziness that might affect gait, balance, and other functional activities (See Appendix C). Report balance problems and functional limitations to the physician and nursing staff, and caution the patient and family/caregivers to guard against falls and trauma.
- Be alert for confusion, hallucinations, or other alterations in mental status. Notify the physician promptly if these symptoms develop.

Interventions

- Always wash hands thoroughly and disinfect equipment (whirlpools, electrotherapeutic devices, treatment tables, and so forth) to help prevent the spread of infection. Use universal precautions or isolation procedures as indicated for specific patients.

Patient/Client-Related Instruction

- Instruct patient to report any vision disturbances or eye pain and inflammation that might indicate optic neuritis.

- Instruct patient and family/caregivers to report other troublesome side effects such as severe or prolonged headache, fever, or GI problems (nausea, vomiting, loss of appetite, abdominal pain).

Pharmacokinetics

Absorption: Rapidly and well absorbed (80%) from the GI tract.
Distribution: Widely distributed; crosses blood-brain barrier in small amounts; crosses placenta and enters breast milk.
Metabolism and Excretion: 50% metabolized by the live; 50% eliminated unchanged by the kidneys.
Half-life: 3.3 hr (increased in renal or hepatic impairment).

TIME/ACTION PROFILE (blood levels)

ROUTE	ONSET	PEAK	DURATION
PO	rapid	2–4 hr	24 hr

Contraindications/Precautions

Contraindicated in: Hypersensitivity; Optic neuritis.
Use Cautiously in: Renal and severe hepatic impairment (dosage reduction required); Children <13 yr (safety not established); Pregnancy (although safety not established, ethambutol has been used with isoniazid in pregnant women without adverse effects on the fetus); Lactation.

Interactions

Drug-Drug: Neurotoxicity may be ↑ with other **neurotoxic agents**.

Route/Dosage

PO (Adults and Children >13 yr): 15–25 mg/kg/day (maximum 2.5 g/day) *or* 50 mg/kg (up to 2.5 g) twice weekly *or* 25–30 mg/kg (up to 2.5 g) 3 times weekly.

Availability (generic available)

Tablets: 100 mg, 400 mg.

ethosuximide

(eth-oh-**sux**-i-mide)
Zarontin

Classification
Therapeutic: anticonvulsants
Pharmacologic: succinimides

Indications

Absence seizures (petit mal).

Action

Elevates the seizure threshold. Suppresses abnormal wave and spike activity associated with absence (petit mal) seizures. **Therapeutic Effects:** Prevention of absence (petit mal) seizures.

Adverse Reactions/Side Effects

CNS: INCREASED FREQUENCY OF TONIC-CLONIC (GRAND MAL) SEIZURES, dizziness, drowsiness, euphoria, fatigue, headache, hyperactivity, irritability, psychiatric disturbances. **EENT:** myopia. **GI:** abdominal pain, anorexia, cramping, diarrhea, nausea, vomiting, weight loss, hiccups. **GU:** pink/brown discoloration of urine, vaginal bleeding. **Derm:** STEVENS-JOHNSON SYNDROME, hirsutism, rashes, urticaria. **Hemat:** agranulocytosis, eosinophilia, leukopenia, pancytopenia. **Neuro:** ataxia. **Misc:** systemic lupus erythematosus.

PHYSICAL THERAPY IMPLICATIONS

Examination and Evaluation

- Document the number, duration, and severity of seizures to help determine if this drug is effective in reducing seizure activity. Be especially alert for tonic-clonic seizure activity, and report an increase in the frequency of these seizures to the physician immediately.
- Monitor skin reactions such as rash, itching/burning skin, hives, exfoliation, and dermatitis. Notify physician immediately about because certain skin reactions may indicate serious hypersensitivity reactions (Stevens-Johnson syndrome).
- Be alert for signs of agranulocytosis and leukopenia (fever, sore throat, mucosal lesions, signs of infection), eosinophilia (fatigue, weakness, myalgia), or fatigue and poor health that might be due to other blood dyscrasias. Report these signs to the physician immediately. Periodic blood tests may be needed to monitor WBC and RBC counts.
- Assess dizziness or ataxia that might affect gait, balance, and other functional activities (See Appendix C). Report balance problems and functional limitations to the physician, and caution the patient and family/caregivers to guard against falls and trauma.
- Monitor daytime drowsiness, euphoria, irritability, or other psychiatric disturbances. Repeated or excessive symptoms may require change in dose or medication.
- Monitor signs of drug-induced lupus syndrome, including increased blood pressure (BP), fever, joint pain, skin rashes, and redness/irritation of the eye (uveitis). Notify physician promptly if these signs appear.
- Periodically assess body weight and other anthropometric measures (body mass index, body composition). Report a rapid or unexplained weight loss or decreased body fat.

Interventions

- Guard against falls and trauma (hip fractures, head injury, and so forth), especially if dizziness or ataxia affects gait and balance. Implement fall prevention strategies, especially if balance is impaired (See Appendix E).

Patient/Client-Related Instruction

- Advise patient to avoid alcohol and other CNS depressants because of the increased risk of sedation and adverse effects.
- Advise patients on prolonged antiseizure therapy not to discontinue medication without consulting their physician. Abrupt withdrawal may cause increased seizures.
- Advise patient about the risk of daytime drowsiness and decreased attention and mental focus. Use care if driving or in other activities that require strong concentration and fast responses.
- Advise patient about the likelihood of GI reactions such as nausea, vomiting, diarrhea, loss of appetite, abdominal pain, and hiccups. Instruct patient to report severe or prolonged GI problems.
- Instruct patient and family/caregivers to report other troublesome side effects such as severe or prolonged headache, vision problems, vaginal bleeding, or skin reactions (rash, itching, abnormal hair growth).

Pharmacokinetics

Absorption: Rapidly and completely absorbed from the GI tract following oral administration.
Distribution: Freely distributed throughout body water.
Metabolism and Excretion: Mostly metabolized by the liver. 10% excreted unchanged by the kidneys.
Half-life: 50–60 hr (adults); 30 hr (children).

TIME/ACTION PROFILE (anticonvulsant activity)

ROUTE	ONSET	PEAK	DURATION
PO	hrs–days	days	days

Contraindications/Precautions

Contraindicated in: Hypersensitivity; Pedi: Children <3 yr (safety not established).
Use Cautiously in: Hepatic or renal disease; Mixed seizure disorders (may increase risk of grand mal seizures); Bone marrow suppression; OB/Lactation: Safety not established.

Interactions

Drug-Drug: Seizure threshold may be lowered by **phenothiazines, antidepressants,** or **MAO inhibitors.** Additive CNS depression with other **CNS depressants,** including **alcohol, antihistamines, antidepressants, opioid analgesics,** and **sedative/hypnotics.** May ↑ **phenytoin** levels. May ↓ **phenobarbital** or **primidone** levels. Blood levels may be ↑ or ↓ by **valproic acid.**
Drug-Natural: See **sedative** interactions. **St. John's wort** may affect ethosuximide levels and effectiveness; avoid use. Concomitant use of **kava, valerian, skullcap, chamomile,** or **hops** can ↑ CNS depression.

Route/Dosage

PO (Adults and Children >6 yr): 250 mg bid initially; may increase by 250 mg/day every 4–7 days until control achieved (usual maintenance dose 20–40 mg/kg/day in 2 divided doses).
PO (Children 3–6 yr): 250 mg once daily initially; increase by 250 mg/day every 4–7 days until control achieved (optimal dose for most children is 20 mg/kg/day in 2 divided doses).

Availability (generic available)

Capsules: 250 mg. **Syrup:** 250 mg/5 mL.

etidronate (ee-ti-droe-nate)

Didrocal, Didronel

Classification
Therapeutic: bone resorption inhibitors, hypocalcemics
Pharmacologic: biphosphonates

Indications

Treatment of Paget's disease of bone. Treatment and prophylaxis of heterotopic calcification associated with total hip replacement or spinal cord injury. Used with other agents (saline diuresis) in the management of hypercalcemia associated with malignancies.

Action

Blocks the growth of calcium hydroxyapatite crystals by binding to calcium phosphate. **Therapeutic Effects:** Decreased bone resorption and turnover.

Adverse Reactions/Side Effects

GI: diarrhea, nausea **IV:** loss of taste, metallic taste.
GU: nephrotoxicity. **Derm:** rash. **MS:** musculoskeletal pain, microfractures, osteonecrosis (primarily of jaw).

PHYSICAL THERAPY IMPLICATIONS

Examination and Evaluation

- Assess any muscle or joint pain. Report persistent or increased musculoskeletal pain to determine presence of bone or joint pathology, including fracture. Be especially aware of possible mouth and jaw pain due to osteonecrosis of the jaw. Bone pain may persist or increase in patients with Paget's disease, but usually subsides days to months after therapy is discontinued.
- Assess changes in pain and inflammation at heterotopic ossification site(s) to help document drug effectiveness. Assess range of motion if ossification occurs near a joint, and document any changes in joint function.

- Monitor and report signs of abnormal calcium levels. Signs of high calcium levels (hypercalcemia) include nausea, vomiting, anorexia, weakness, constipation, thirst, and cardiac arrhythmias. Low calcium levels (hypocalcemia) are indicated by paresthesia, muscle twitching, laryngospasm, colic, cardiac arrhythmias, Chvostek's sign (facial muscle twitching when the facial nerve is tapped), or Trousseau's sign (finger and wrist flexion during temporary occlusion of the brachial artery).
- Watch for signs of nephrotoxicity, including hematuria, increased urinary frequency, cloudy urine, and decreased urine output. Report these signs to the physician.

Interventions

- Protect against falls and fractures (See Appendix E). Modify home environment (remove throw rugs, improve lighting, etc.), and provide assistive devices (cane, walker) or other protective devices as needed to improve balance and prevent falls.

Patient/Client-Related Instruction

- Advise patient about the benefits of proper diet in sustaining bone mineralization. If necessary, refer patient for nutritional counseling about supplemental calcium and vitamin D.
- Instruct patient to report other troublesome side effects such as severe or prolonged skin rash, change in taste, or GI problems (diarrhea, nausea).

Pharmacokinetics

Absorption: Absorption is generally poor (1–6%) after oral administration.
Distribution: Half of the absorbed dose is bound to hydroxyapatite crystals in areas of increased osteogenesis.
Metabolism and Excretion: Unabsorbed drug is eliminated in the feces; 50% of the absorbed dose is excreted unchanged by the kidneys.
Half-life: 5–7 hr.

TIME/ACTION PROFILE

ROUTE	ONSET	PEAK	DURATION
PO (Paget's disease)	1 mo*	unknown	1 yr
PO (heterotopic calcification)	unknown	unknown	several months
IV† (hypercalcemia)	24 hr	3 days	11 days

*As measured by decreased urinary hydroxyproline.
†As measured by decreased urinary calcium excretion.

Contraindications/Precautions

Contraindicated in: Hypersensitivity; Severe renal impairment (serum creatinine >5 mg/dL); Hypercalcemia due to hyperparathyroidism.
Use Cautiously in: Long bone fractures; CHF; Hypocalcemia; Hypovitaminosis D; Moderate renal impairment (dosage reduction recommended if serum creatinine 2.5–4.9 mg/dL); Dental surgery (may ↑ risk of jaw osteonecrosis); OB/Lactation/Pedi: Safety not established).

Interactions

Drug-Drug: Antacids, mineral supplements, or **buffers** (as in **didanosine**) containing **calcium, aluminum, iron,** or **magnesium** may ↓ absorption of etidronate. Hypocalcemic effect may be additive with **calcitonin**.
Drug-Food: Foods containing large amounts of **calcium, aluminum, iron,** or **magnesium** may ↓ absorption of etidronate.

Route/Dosage

Paget's Disease

PO (Adults): 5–10 mg/kg/day single dose for up to 6 mo *or* 11–20 mg/kg/day for not more than 3 mo.

Heterotopic Ossification (Hip Replacement)

PO (Adults): 20 mg/kg/day for 1 mo before and 3 mo after surgery.

Heterotopic Ossification (Spinal Cord Injury)

PO (Adults): 20 mg/kg/day for 2 wk, then decreased to 10 mg/kg/day for 10 wk.

Hypercalcemia

PO (Adults): 20 mg/kg/day for 30–90 days.
IV (Adults): 7.5 mg/kg/day for 3 days; has also been given as a single dose of 25–30 mg/kg over 24 hr. May be followed by oral therapy.

Availability

Tablets: 200 mg, 400 mg. **Injection:** 50 mg/mL in 6-mL ampules.

Desired Medication Outcomes

- Lowered serum calcium levels.
- Decreased bone pain and fractures in Paget's disease.
- Prevention or treatment of heterotopic ossification. Normal serum calcium levels are usually attained in 2–8 days in hypercalcemia associated with bony metastasis. Therapy may be repeated once after 1 wk.

etodolac (ee-toe-doe-lak)

Lodine, Lodine XL

Classification

Therapeutic: antirheumatics, nonopioid analgesics

Pharmacologic: pyranocarboxylic acid

Indications

Osteoarthritis. Rheumatoid arthritis. Mild-to-moderate pain (not XL tablets).

Action

Inhibits prostaglandin synthesis. Also has uricosuric action. **Therapeutic Effects:** Suppression of inflammation. Decreased severity of pain.

Adverse Reactions/Side Effects

CNS: depression, dizziness, drowsiness, insomnia, malaise, nervousness, syncope, weakness. **EENT:** blurred vision, photophobia, tinnitus. **Resp:** asthma. **CV:** CHF, edema, hypertension, palpitations. **GI:** GI BLEEDING, dyspepsia, abdominal pain, constipation, diarrhea, drug-induced hepatitis, dry mouth, flatulence, gastritis, nausea, stomatitis, thirst, vomiting. **GU:** dysuria, renal failure, urinary frequency. **Derm:** EXFOLIATIVE DERMATITIS, STEVENS-JOHNSON SYNDROME, TOXIC EPIDERMAL NECROLYSIS, ecchymoses, flushing, hyperpigmentation, pruritus, rashes, sweating. **Hemat:** anemia, prolonged bleeding time, thrombocytopenia. **Misc:** ALLERGIC REACTIONS, INCLUDING ANAPHYLAXIS, ANGIOEDEMA, chills, fever.

PHYSICAL THERAPY IMPLICATIONS

Examination and Evaluation

- Monitor signs of GI bleeding, including abdominal pain, vomiting blood, blood in stools, or black, tarry stools. Report these signs to the physician immediately.
- Monitor signs of allergic reactions such as anaphylaxis and angioedema, including pulmonary symptoms (laryngeal edema, wheezing, cough, dyspnea), or skin reactions (rash, pruritus, urticaria, swelling in the face). Be especially alert for exfoliation, dermatitis, and other severe skin reactions that might indicate serious hypersensitivity reactions (Stevens-Johnson syndrome, toxic epidermal necrolysis). Notify physician immediately if these reactions occur.
- Assess signs of congestive heart failure (dyspnea, rales/crackles, peripheral edema, jugular venous distention, exercise intolerance). Report these signs to the physician immediately.
- Assess pain and other variables (range of motion, muscle strength) to document whether this drug is successful in helping manage the patient's pain and decreasing impairments.
- Assess blood pressure (BP) periodically, and compare to normal values (See Appendix F). NSAIDs can increase BP and promote hypertension in certain patients.
- Be alert for signs of prolonged bleeding time such as bleeding gums, nosebleeds, and unusual or excessive bruising. Report these signs to the physician.
- Assess peripheral edema using girth measurements, volume displacement, and measurement of pitting edema (See Appendix N). Report increased swelling in feet and ankles or a sudden increase in body weight due to fluid retention.
- Assess symptoms of bronchospasm and asthma, including wheezing, coughing, dyspnea, and tightness in chest. Perform pulmonary function tests to quantify suspected changes in ventilation and respiration (See Appendices I, J, K).
- Monitor signs of kidney dysfunction such as painful urination or blood in the urine. Report signs of renal failure immediately, including decreased urine output, increased BP, muscle cramps/twitching, edema/weight gain from fluid retention, yellowish brown skin, and confusion that progresses to seizures and coma.
- Monitor signs of thrombocytopenia (bruising, nose bleeds, and bleeding gums) or unusual weakness and fatigue that might be due to anemia. Notify physician if these signs occur.
- Assess dizziness, drowsiness, and syncope that might affect gait, balance, and other functional activities (see Appendix C). Report balance problems and functional limitations to the physician, and caution the patient and family/caregivers to guard against falls and trauma.
- Monitor and report nervousness, depression, or other psychic disturbances.

Interventions

- Implement appropriate manual therapy techniques, physical agents, and therapeutic exercises to reduce pain and decrease the need for etodolac and other NSAIDs.
- Because of the risk of heart failure, use caution during aerobic exercise and other forms of therapeutic exercise. Assess exercise tolerance frequently (BP, heart rate, fatigue levels), and terminate exercise immediately if any untoward responses occur (see Appendix L).
- If treating arthritic conditions, recommend orthotic and assistive devices as needed to reduce pain, improve function, and augment the effects of drug therapy.
- Use caution with any physical interventions that could increase bleeding, including wound débridement, chest percussion, joint mobilization, and application of local heat.

- Help patient explore other nonpharmacologic methods to reduce chronic pain, such as relaxation techniques, exercise, counseling, and so forth.

Patient/Client-Related Instruction

- Advise patient that analgesics are usually more effective if given before pain becomes severe; emphasize that adequate pain control will allow better participation in physical therapy.
- Inform patient that NSAIDs may impair bone and cartilage healing. Advise patient to consult physician about NSAID use, especially after fractures, spinal fusion, and other bone surgeries.
- Caution patient about the use of over-the-counter products that contain NSAIDs or acetaminophen while taking prescription doses of etodolac. Use of multiple NSAIDs increases the risk of toxicity and overdose.
- Instruct patient to report excessive or prolonged headache or ringing/buzzing in the ears (tinnitus); these signs may indicate drug toxicity.
- Advise patient about the likelihood of GI reactions including nausea, vomiting, diarrhea, constipation, flatulence, indigestion, abdominal pain, and inflammation in/around the mouth. Instruct patient to report severe or prolonged GI problems or signs of drug-induced hepatitis such as yellow skin or eyes, abdominal pain, severe nausea and vomiting, fever, sore throat, malaise, weakness, and facial edema.
- Advise patient to reduce alcohol intake because alcohol increases the risk of gastric toxicity.
- Instruct patient and family/caregivers to report other troublesome side effects such as severe or prolonged chills, fever, sleep loss, heart palpitations, blurred vision, or skin reactions (rash, itching, bruising, increased sweating).

Pharmacokinetics

Absorption: Well absorbed after oral administration.
Distribution: Widely distributed.
Protein Binding: >99%.
Metabolism and Excretion: Mostly metabolized by the liver; <1% excreted unchanged in urine.
Half-life: 6–7 hr (single dose); 7.3 hr (chronic dosing).

TIME/ACTION PROFILE (analgesic effect)

ROUTE	ONSET	PEAK	DURATION
PO (analgesic)	0.5 hr	1–2 hr	4–12 hr
PO (anti-inflammatory)	days–wks	unknown	6–12 hr*

*Up to 24 hr as XL (extended-release) tablet.

Contraindications/Precautions

Contraindicated in: Hypersensitivity; Active GI bleeding or ulcer disease; Cross-sensitivity may exist with other NSAIDs, including aspirin.
Use Cautiously in: Cardiovascular disease or risk factors for cardiovascular disease (may ↑ risk of serious cardiovascular thrombotic events, myocardial infarction, and stroke, especially with prolonged use); Renal, or hepatic disease; Geri: Geriatric patients (increased risk of GI bleeding); History of ulcer disease; OB: Pregnancy (not recommended for use during second half of pregnancy); OB/Pedi: Lactation or children (safety not established).

Interactions

Drug-Drug: Concurrent use with **aspirin** may ↓ effectiveness. ↑ adverse GI effects with **aspirin,** other **NSAIDs, potassium supplements, corticosteroids, antiplatelet agents,** or **alcohol**. Chronic use with **acetaminophen** may ↑ risk of adverse renal reactions. May ↓ effectiveness of **diuretic** or **antihypertensive** therapy. May ↑ serum **lithium** levels and ↑ risk of toxicity. ↑ risk of toxicity from **methotrexate.** ↑ risk of bleeding with **cefotetan, cefoperazone, valproic acid, thrombolytics, antiplatelet agents,** or **anticoagulants**. Increased risk of adverse hematologic reactions with **antineoplastics** or **radiation therapy**. May increase the risk of nephrotoxicity from **cyclosporine**.
Drug-Natural: ↑ risk of bleeding with **arnica, chamomile, clove, dong quai, fever few, garlic, ginko,** and ***Panax ginseng***.

Route/Dosage

PO (Adults): *Analgesia*—200–400 mg q 6–8 hr (not to exceed 1200 mg/day). *Osteoarthritis/rheumatoid arthritis*—300 mg 2–3 times daily, 400 mg twice daily, or 500 mg twice daily; may also be given as 400–1200 mg once daily as XL tablets.

Availability (generic available)

Capsules: 200 mg, 300 mg. **Tablets:** 400 mg, 500 mg. **Extended-release tablets (XL):** 400 mg, 600 mg.

HIGH ALERT

etomidate (e-tom-i-date)

Amidate

Classification

Therapeutic: general anesthetics
Pharmacologic: **imidazoles**

Indications
Induction of general anesthesia. Supplemental anesthesia with other agents (nitrous oxide) for short procedures.

Action
Hypnotic CNS depressant without analgesic activity.
Therapeutic Effects: Induction/supplementation of general anesthesia.

Adverse Reactions/Side Effects
CV: arrhythmias, hypertension, hypotension. **Resp:** APNEA, LARYNGOSPASM, hyperventilation, hypoventilation. **GI:** postoperative nausea/vomiting. **Local:** transient injection site pain. **MS:** transient skeletal muscle movements.

PHYSICAL THERAPY IMPLICATIONS

Examination and Evaluation
- Monitor postoperative respiration, and notify physician or nursing staff immediately if patient exhibits any interruption in respiratory rate (apnea) or wheezing, coughing, tightness in chest, or shortness of breath that might indicate laryngospasm. Monitor pulse oximetry and perform pulmonary function tests (See Appendices I, J, K) to quantify suspected changes in ventilation, respiratory rate, and respiratory function.
- Assess heart rate, ECG, and heart sounds, especially during exercise (See Appendices G, H). Report any rhythm disturbances or symptoms of increased ↓ arrhythmias, including palpitations, chest discomfort, shortness of breath, fainting, and fatigue/weakness.
- Assess blood pressure (BP) and compare to normal values (See Appendix F). Report changes in BP, either a problematic decrease in BP (hypotension) or a sustained increase in BP (hypertension).
- Be alert for abnormal or involuntary muscle movements. Document the location, frequency, and severity of these movements, and report these findings to the physician or nursing staff.

Interventions
- Implement breathing activities and other therapeutic exercises to encourage ventilation and help overcome any residual effects of the anesthetic.
- Because of the risk of arrhythmias and abnormal BP responses, use caution during aerobic exercise and other forms of therapeutic exercise. Assess exercise tolerance frequently (BP, heart rate, fatigue levels), and terminate exercise immediately if any untoward responses occur (See Appendix L).
- Guard against falls and trauma (hip fractures, head injury) during the immediate postoperative period. Implement fall prevention strategies (See Appendix E), especially if patient exhibits sedation, dizziness, or blurred vision.

Patient/Client-Related Instruction
- Instruct patient to report other troublesome postoperative effects such as severe or prolonged injection site pain or GI problems (nausea, vomiting).

Pharmacokinetics
Absorption: IV administration results in complete bioavailability.
Distribution: Distributes rapidly from blood into CNS, followed by rapid clearance and tissue distribution.
Metabolism and Excretion: Mostly metabolized by the liver. 75% excreted in urine as inactive metabolite; 10–13% excreted in bile and feces.
Half-life: 1.25–5 hr.

TIME/ACTION PROFILE (hypnosis)

ROUTE	ONSET	PEAK	DURATION
IV	within 1 min	unknown	3–5 min

Contraindications/Precautions
Contraindicated in: Hypersensitivity; Prolonged infusion not recommended (suppresses cortisol production); Pregnancy, labor, delivery (including cesarean section).
Use Cautiously in: Patients undergoing severe stress (may require supplemental corticosteroids); Geriatric patients; Lactation or children <10 yr (safety not established).

Interactions
Drug-Drug: ↑ Increased CNS depression with other CNS depressants, including **antihistamines, antidepressants, sedative/hypnotics, antipsychotics** and **opioids**; ↓ dosage of other CNS depressants if necessary. **Verapamil** may ↑ anesthetic effect, which may ↑ risk of respiratory depression and apnea.

Route/Dosage
IV (Adults and Children >10 yr): 0.2–0.6 mg/kg (usual dose is 0.3 mg/kg) for induction. Smaller increments may be used during short procedures to supplement other agents.

Availability
Solution for injection: 2 mg/mL in 10- and 20-mL ampules and 20-mL Abbojects.

etonorgestgrel (implant)
(e-to-nor-**jes**-trel)
Implanon

Classification
Therapeutic: contraceptive hormones
Pharmacologic: progestins

Indications
Prevention of pregnancy.

Action
Suppresses ovulation, increases viscosity of cervical mucosa, and alters endometrium. **Therapeutic Effects:** Prevention of pregnancy.

Adverse Reactions/Side Effects
CNS: depression, dizziness, emotional lability, headache, nervousness. **CV:** THROMBOEMBOLIC EVENTS, hypertension. **GI:** hepatic adenomas. **GU:** dysmenorrhea, irregular/unpredictable menses, ↑ risk of ectopic pregnancy, ovarian cysts. **Derm:** acne. **Endo:** breast pain, leukorrhea. **Local:** implant-site reactions. **Metab:** weight gain. **MS:** back pain.

PHYSICAL THERAPY IMPLICATIONS

Examination and Evaluation
- Monitor signs of thrombophlebitis (localized pain, swelling, warmth, erythema, tenderness) and pulmonary embolism (shortness of breath, chest pain, cough, bloody sputum). Notify physician immediately, and request objective tests (Doppler ultrasound, lung scan, others) if thromboembolism is suspected.
- Assess blood pressure (BP) and compare to normal values (See Appendix F). Report a sustained increase in BP (hypertension).
- Report signs of liver dysfunction, including anorexia, abdominal pain, severe nausea and vomiting, yellow skin or eyes, skin rashes, flu-like symptoms, and muscle/joint pain.
- Monitor and report depression, nervousness, emotional lability, or other changes in mood and behavior.
- Assess any back pain to rule out musculoskeletal pathology; that is, try to determine if pain is drug induced rather than caused by anatomical or biomechanical problems.
- Assess dizziness and drowsiness that might affect gait, balance, and other functional activities (See Appendix C). Report balance problems and functional limitations to the physician, and caution the patient and family/caregivers to guard against falls and trauma.
- Periodically assess body weight and other anthropometric measures (body mass index, body composition). Report a rapid or sustained weight gain or a substantial change in lean body mass.
- Monitor subdermal implantation site for pain, swelling, and irritation. Report prolonged or excessive implant site reactions to the physician.

Interventions
- Because of the risk of thromboembolism, use caution during aerobic exercise and other forms of therapeutic exercise. Assess exercise tolerance frequently (BP, heart rate, fatigue levels), and terminate exercise immediately if any untoward responses occur (See Appendix L).
- Do not apply physical agents (heat, cold, electrotherapeutic modalities) or massage over the implantation site; these interventions can alter drug absorption from subcutaneous tissues.

Patient/Client-Related Instruction
- Caution patient and family/caregivers about risks of thromboembolism, and review warning signs of a pulmonary embolism (sudden shortness of breath, dyspnea, bloody sputum, cough).
- Caution patient that cigarette smoking may increase the risk of infarction and thromboembolic disease, especially for women older than 35.
- Advise women about possible changes in menstrual function. Instruct patient to notify the physician about any abnormal bleeding.
- Instruct patient to report other troublesome side effects such as prolonged or severe headache, acne, breast pain, or vaginal discharge.

Pharmacokinetics
Absorption: Reliably, constantly and slowly absorbed (100% bioavailable).
Distribution: Crosses the placenta and enters breast milk.
Metabolism and Excretion: Mostly metabolized by the liver.
Half-life: 25 hr.

TIME/ACTION PROFILE

ROUTE	ONSET	PEAK	DURATION
Subdermal	1 mo	unknown	3 yr

Contraindications/Precautions
Contraindicated in: Hypersensitivity; Known or suspected pregnancy; Active liver disease; Current/past history of thromboembolism; Active liver disease or hepatic tumors; Chronic use of drugs that induce liver

enzymes; Undiagnosed abnormal genital bleeding; Known/suspected breast cancer.
Use Cautiously in: OB: Lactation (may be used after 4th postpartum week); Obesity (contraceptive may be less effective); Conditions associated with fluid retention; Hypertension; Cigarette smoking or age >35 (↑ risk of thromboembolic events); Pedi: Safe use in children <18 yr is not established; should not be used before menarche.

Interactions

Drug-Drug: Barbiturates, griseofulvin, rifampin, phenytoin, carbamazepine, oxcarbazepine, topiramate, and **modafinil** induce liver enzymes and may ↓ contraceptive effectiveness. **Protease inhibitors** may alter blood levels and effects. Inhibitors of liver enzymes, including **itraconazole** and **ketoconazole,** may ↑ blood levels.
Drug-Natural: St. John's wort induces liver enzymes and may ↓ contraceptive effectiveness.

Route/Dosage

Subdermal: (Adults): 1 68-mg implant, contraceptive effect lasts for 3 yr.

Availability

Subdermally implantable rod: 68 mg.

etravirine (ee-tra-veer-een)

Intelence

Classification
Therapeutic: antiretrovirals
Pharmacologic: nonnucleoside reverse transcriptase inhibitors

Indications

HIV infection (with other antiretrovirals).

Action

Binds to the enzyme reverse transcriptase which results in disrupted viral DNA synthesis. **Therapeutic Effects:** Evidence of decreased viral replication and reduced viral load with slowed progression of HIV and its sequelae.

Adverse Reactions/Side Effects

CNS: SEIZURES, anxiety, confusion, fatigue, headache, insomnia, sleep disorders. **EENT:** blurred vision, vertigo. **CV:** MYOCARDIAL INFARCTION, angina pectoris, atrial fibrillation, hypertension. **GI:** nausea, abdominal pain, anorexia, dry mouth, hepatitis, stomatitis, vomiting. **GU:** renal failure. **Endo:** gynecomastia, hyperglycemia, hyperlipidemia. **Hemat:** anemia, hemolytic anemia. **Derm:** rash. **Metab:** fat redistribution. **Neuro:** peripheral neuropathy. **MS:** hemarthrosis. **Misc:** allergic reactions, including STEVENS-JOHNSON SYNDROME, IMMUNE RECONSTITUTION SYNDROME.

PHYSICAL THERAPY IMPLICATIONS

Examination and Evaluation

- Monitor continually for signs of MI such as sudden chest pain, pain radiating into the arm or jaw, shortness of breath, dizziness, sweating, anxiety, and nausea. Seek immediate medical assistance if patient develops these signs.
- Be alert for new seizures or increased seizure activity, especially at the onset of drug treatment. Document the number, duration, and severity of seizures, and report these findings immediately to the physician.
- Monitor skin rash and other skin reactions (dermatitis, exfoliation). Report skin problems immediately because they may represent serious hypersensitivity reactions (Stevens-Johnson syndrome).
- Be alert for signs of an unusually aggressive immune reaction to opportunistic infection (immune reconstitution syndrome). Signs include fever, pain, warmth and redness, and swelling at the site of infection. Notify physician of these signs immediately.
- Assess heart rate, ECG, and heart sounds, especially during exercise (See Appendices G, H). Report any rhythm disturbances or symptoms of increased arrhythmias, including palpitations, angina pectoris, shortness of breath, fainting, and fatigue/weakness.
- Assess blood pressure (BP) and compare to normal values (See Appendix F). Report a sustained increase in BP (hypertension).
- Monitor signs of anemia and hemolytic anemia, including unusual fatigue, shortness of breath, dizziness, headache, coldness in your hands and feet, pale skin, and chest pain. Report these signs to the physician.
- Monitor signs of renal failure, including decreased urine output, increased BP, muscle cramps/twitching, edema/weight gain from fluid retention, yellowishbrown skin, and confusion that progresses to seizures and coma. Report these signs to the physician immediately.
- Be alert for signs of peripheral neuropathy (numbness, tingling, decreased muscle strength). Establish baseline electroneuromyographic values using EMG and nerve conduction at the beginning of drug treatment whenever possible, and reexamine these values periodically to document drug-induced changes in peripheral nerve function.
- Assess any joint pain and attempt to determine if pain is caused by bleeding into the joint (hemarthrosis). Notify physician of suspected hemarthrosis.

Interventions

- Implement resistive exercises and other therapeutic exercises as tolerated to maintain muscle strength and function and prevent muscle wasting associated with HIV infection and AIDS.

Patient/Client-Related Instruction

- Caution patient and family/caregivers about risk of myocardial infarction, and review warning signs of MI (see above under Evaluation and Examination).
- Emphasize the importance of taking etravirine as directed even if the patient is asymptomatic and that this drug must always be used in combination with other antiretroviral drugs. Do not take more than prescribed amount and do not stop taking without consulting health care professional.
- Inform patient that etravirine does not cure HIV or AIDS or prevent associated or opportunistic infections. Etravirine does not reduce the risk of transmission of HIV to others through sexual contact or blood contamination. Caution patient to use a condom, and to avoid sharing needles or donating blood to prevent spreading the AIDS virus to others.
- Advise patient that this drug may cause problems in fat and glucose metabolism (hyperlipidemia and hyperglycemia, respectively). Remind patient that periodic blood tests may be needed to monitor plasma lipids and blood glucose.
- Advise patient about possible changes in body composition such as increased abdominal fat with thin arms and legs. Discuss possible effects on body image, and help patient explore coping mechanisms.
- Advise patient about the likelihood of GI reactions (nausea, vomiting, diarrhea, abdominal pain, irritation of the oral mucosa). Instruct patient to report severe or prolonged GI problems or signs of drug-induced hepatitis (yellow skin or eyes, abdominal pain, severe nausea and vomiting, fever, sore throat, malaise, weakness, facial edema).
- Instruct patient to report other troublesome side effects such as prolonged or severe headache, blurred vision, vertigo, increased breast size in men (gynecomastia), or changes in behavior or sleep patterns (anxiety, confusion, sleep loss).

Pharmacokinetics

Absorption: Well absorbed following oral administration. Food enhances absorption.
Distribution: Unknown.
Protein Binding: 99.9%.
Metabolism and Excretion: Mostly metabolized by the liver (CYP3A4, CYP2C9, and CYP2C19 enzyme systems); minimal renal excretion; mostly eliminated in feces as unchanged drug and metabolites.
Half-life: 41 hr.

TIME/ACTION PROFILE (blood levels)

ROUTE	ONSET	PEAK	DURATION
PO	unknown	2.5–4 hr	12 hr

E

Contraindications/Precautions

Contraindicated in: Concurrent use with other non-nucleoside reverse transcriptase inhibitors (NNRTIs), rifampin, rifapentine, St. John's wort.
Use Cautiously in: Concurrent use of antiarrhythmics, anticonvulsants, antifungals, clarithromycin, rifabutin, diazepam, dexamethasone, HMG CoA reductase inhibitors (statins), immunosuppressants; Geri: Consider age-related ↓ in organ function and body mass, concurrent disease states and medications; Pedi/OB/Lactation: Safety not established, breastfeeding not recommended in HIV-infected women.

Interactions

Drug-Drug: Etravirine is a substrate of the **CYP3A4**, **CYP2C9**, and **CYP2C19** enzyme systems; other medications that induce or inhibit these systems may be expected to alter the response to etravirine. Etravirine is an inducer of **CYP3A4** and an inhibitor of **CYP2C9** and **CYP2C19**. The effects of medications that are substrates of these enzyme systems may be altered by concurrent use. Concurrent use with other **NNRTIs**, including **efavirenz**, **nevirapine**, and **delavirdine**, may lead to ↓ effectiveness and should be avoided. Concurrent use with **protease inhibitors (PIs)**, including **atazanavir**, **fosamprenavir**, **nelfinavir**, and **indinavir**, may lead to altered plasma levels and should be undertaken with concurrent low-dose **ritonavir**. Concurrent use with higher dose **ritonavir**, combination **tipranavir/ritonavir**, **fosamprenavir/ritonavir**, and **atazanavir/ritonavir** alters levels and effectiveness of etravirine and should be avoided. Concurrent use of the combination **saquinavir/ritonavir** should be undertaken cautiously. ↓ blood levels and effectiveness of **antiarrhythmics**, including **amiodarone**, **bepridil**, **disopyramide**, **flecainide**, **lidocaine**, **mexiletine**, **quinidine**, **propafenone**, and **quinidine**; blood- level monitoring recommended. Blood levels and effects may be ↓ by anticonvulsants, including **carbamazepine**, **phenobarbital**, and **phenytoin**. Concurrent use with **voriconazole** may ↑ levels of both drugs; ↓ levels of **itraconazole** and **ketoconazole** (dose adjustments may be necessary). May alter levels and response to **clarithromycin**; other agents should be considered. **Rifampin** and **rifapentine** ↓ blood levels and effectiveness and should be avoided; **rifabutin** should only be used without a protease inhibitor/ritonavir combination.

May ↑ blood levels and sedation from **diazepam;** monitor for effects. Levels and effectiveness may be ↓ by **dexamethasone;** use cautiously and consider alternatives. May alter blood levels and effects of **fluvastatin, lovastatin,** and **simvastatin** (dose adjustments may be necessary). May alter blood levels and effects of **cyclosporine, sirolimus,** and **tacrolimus**; careful monitoring required.
Drug-Natural: St. John's wort may ↓ blood levels and effectiveness; avoid concurrent use.

Route/Dosage

PO (Adults): 200 mg twice daily.

Availability

Tablets: 100 mg.

everolimus (ee-ver-oh-li-mus)

Afinitor

Classification
Therapeutic: antineoplastics
Pharmacologic: mTOR inhibitors

Indications

Advanced renal cell carcinoma which has failed treatment with sunitinib or sorafenib.

Action

Acts as a kinase inhibitor, decreasing cell proliferation. **Therapeutic Effects:** Decreased spread of renal cell carcinoma.

Adverse Reactions/Side Effects

CNS: fatigue, weakness, headache. **Resp:** PNEUMONITIS, cough, dyspnea. **GI:** anorexia, diarrhea, mucositis, mouth ulcers, nausea, stomatitis, vomiting, dysgeusia. **F and E:** peripheral edema. **Derm:** dry skin, pruritus, rash. **Hemat:** anemia, leukopenia, thrombocytopenia. **Metab:** hyperglycemia, hyperlipidemia, hypertriglyceridemia. **MS:** extremity pain. **Misc:** INFECTIONS, hypersensitivity reactions, including anaphylaxis, fever.

PHYSICAL THERAPY IMPLICATIONS

Examination and Evaluation

- Assess for signs of pulmonary inflammation (pneumonitis), including difficulty breathing, cough, shortness of breath, fatigue, and a low-grade fever. Notify physician or nursing staff immediately if these signs occur.
- Be alert for signs of infection, including fever, sore throat, chills, nausea, vomiting, diarrhea, and localized inflammation. Notify physician or nursing staff of these signs immediately.
- Be alert for signs of leukopenia (fever, sore throat, signs of infection), thrombocytopenia (bruising, nose bleeds, bleeding gums), or unusual weakness and fatigue that might be due to anemia or other blood dyscrasias. Report these signs to the physician or nursing staff immediately.
- Assess peripheral edema using girth measurements, volume displacement, and measurement of pitting edema (See Appendix N). Report increased swelling in feet and ankles or a sudden increase in body weight due to fluid retention.
- Monitor signs of allergic reactions or anaphylaxis, including pulmonary symptoms (tightness in the throat and chest, wheezing, cough, dyspnea) or skin reactions (rash, pruritus, urticaria). Notify physician or nursing staff immediately if these reactions occur.
- Monitor fatigue and weakness. Some degree of fatigue is expected, but excessive or unusual fatigue should be reported.
- Assess any extremity pain to rule out musculoskeletal pathology; that is, try to determine if pain is drug induced rather than caused by anatomic or biomechanical problems.

Interventions

- For patients who are medically able to begin exercise, implement appropriate resistive exercises and aerobic training to maintain muscle strength and aerobic capacity during cancer chemotherapy or to help restore function after chemotherapy.
- Because of the risk of pulmonary toxicity and blood dyscrasias, use caution during aerobic exercise and other forms of therapeutic exercise. Assess exercise tolerance frequently (blood pressure, heart rate, respiratory symptoms, fatigue levels), and terminate exercise immediately if any untoward responses occur (See Appendix L).

Patient/Client-Related Instruction

- Instruct patient to guard against infection (frequent hand washing, etc.), and to avoid crowds and contact with persons with contagious diseases.
- Advise patient about the likelihood of GI reactions, including diarrhea, nausea, vomiting, loss of appetite, and irritation in/around the mouth. Instruct patient or family and caregivers to report other severe or unexpected GI problems.
- Advise patient that this drug may cause problems in fat and glucose metabolism (hyperlipidemia and hyperglycemia, respectively). Remind patient that periodic blood tests may be needed to monitor plasma lipids and blood glucose.
- Instruct patient to report other troublesome side effects such as prolonged or severe headache, or skin reactions (rash, itching, dry skin).

Pharmacokinetics

Absorption: Well absorbed following oral administration.

Distribution: 20% confined to plasma.
Metabolism and Excretion: Mostly metabolized by liver and other systems (CYP3A4 and PgP; metabolites are mostly excreted in feces [80%] and urine [5%]).
Half-life: 30 hr.

TIME/ACTION PROFILE (blood levels))

ROUTE	ONSET	PEAK	DURATION
PO	unknown	1–2 hr	24 hr

Contraindications/Precautions

Contraindicated in: Hypersensitivity to everolimus or other rapamycins; Severe hepatic impairment (Child-Pugh class C); OB: May cause fetal harm, avoid use during pregnancy; Lactation: Avoid breastfeeding.
Use Cautiously in: Moderate hepatic impairment (Child-Pugh class B); dose reduction required; Geri: Elderly patients may be more sensitive to drug effects; consider age-related decrease in hepatic function, concurrent disease states, and drug therapy; Pedi: Safe use in children has not been established.

Interactions

Drug-Drug: ↑ blood levels and risk of toxicity with **moderate and strong inhibitors of CYP 3A4 enzyme system and PgP,** including **amprenavir, aprepitant, atazanavir, clarithromycin, delavirdine, diltiazem, erythromycin, fluconazole, fosamprenavir, indinavir, itraconazole, ketoconazole, nefazodone, nelfinavir, ritonavir, saquinavir, telithromycin, verapamil,** and **voriconazole**; avoid concurrent use. Avoid concurrent use with **CYP3A4 inducers,** including **carbamazepine, dexamethasone, phenobarbital, phenytoin, rifabutin,** and **rifampin**; ↑ dose of everolimus may be required. May ↓ antibody formation and ↑ risk of adverse reactions from **live-virus vaccines.**
Natural-Food: ↑ blood levels and risk of toxicity with **grapefruit juice**; avoid concurrent use.

Route/Dosage

PO (Adults): 10 mg once daily; *Concurrent use of strong inducers of CYP3A4*—↑ dose in 5-mg increments up to 20 mg/daily.

Hepatic Impairment

PO (Adults): *Moderate hepatic impairment*—5 mg once daily.

Availability

Tablets: 5 mg, 10 mg.

exenatide (eks-en-a-tide)

Byetta

Classification
Therapeutic: antidiabetics
Pharmacologic: incretin mimetic agents

E

Indications

Type 2 diabetes uncontrolled by metformin, a sulfonylurea, or a thiazolidinedione (or a combination of these agents).

Action

Mimics the action of incretin which promotes endogenous insulin secretion and promotes other mechanisms of glucose lowering. **Therapeutic Effects:** Improved control of blood glucose.

Adverse Reactions/Side Effects

CV: dizziness, headache, jitteriness, weakness. **GI:** PANCREATITIS, diarrhea, nausea, vomiting, dyspepsia, gastrointestinal reflux. **Derm:** hyperhydrosis. **Metab:** ↓ appetite, weight loss.

PHYSICAL THERAPY IMPLICATIONS

Examination and Evaluation

- Monitor signs of pancreatitis, including upper abdominal pain (especially after eating), indigestion, weight loss, and oily stools. Report these signs immediately to the physician.
- Be alert for signs of hypoglycemia, especially during and after exercise. Common neuromuscular signs include anxiety; restlessness; tingling in hands, feet, lips, or tongue; chills; cold sweats; confusion; difficulty in concentration; drowsiness; excessive hunger; headache; irritability; nervousness; tremor; weakness; unsteady gait. Report persistent or repeated episodes of hypoglycemia to the physician.
- Assess dizziness that might affect gait, balance, and other functional activities (See Appendix C). Report balance problems to the physician, and caution the patient and family/caregivers to guard against falls and trauma.
- Assess blood pressure periodically (See Appendix F). A sudden or sustained increase in blood pressure (hypertension) may indicate problems in diabetes management and should be reported to the physician.
- Periodically assess body weight and report a substantial or sudden weight loss.

Interventions

- Implement aerobic exercise and endurance training programs to maintain optimal body weight, improve insulin sensitivity, and reduce the risk of macrovascular disease (heart attack, stroke) and microvascular problems (reduced blood flow to tissues and organs that causes poor wound healing, neuropathy, retinopathy, and nephropathy).

Patient/Client-Related Instruction

- Encourage patient to monitor blood glucose before and after exercise, and to adjust food intake to maintain normal glycemic levels.
- Emphasize the importance of adhering to nutritional guidelines, and the need for periodic assessment of glycemic control (serum glucose and glycosylated hemoglobin levels) throughout the management of diabetes mellitus.
- Advise patient about symptoms of hyperglycemia (confusion, drowsiness; flushed, dry skin; fruit-like breath odor; rapid, deep breathing, polyuria; loss of appetite; unusual thirst). Drug dosages may need to be adjusted to prevent repeated episodes of hyperglycemia.
- Instruct patient to report other troublesome side effects such as severe or prolonged headache, jitteriness, weakness, increased sweating, or GI problems (nausea, vomiting, diarrhea, heartburn).

Pharmacokinetics

Absorption: Well absorbed following SC administration.
Distribution: Unknown.
Metabolism and Excretion: Excreted mostly by glomerular filtration followed by degradation.
Half-life: 2.4 hr.

TIME/ACTION PROFILE (effects on postprandial blood glucose)

ROUTE	ONSET	PEAK	DURATION
SC	within 30 min	2.1 hr	8 hr

Contraindications/Precautions

Contraindicated in: Hypersensitivity; Type 1 diabetes or diabetic ketoacidosis; End-stage renal disease (CCr <30 mL/min); Severe gastrointestinal disease; OB: Lactation.
Use Cautiously in: OB: Use in pregnancy only if potential maternal benefit outweighs fetal risk; Pedi: Safety not established.

Interactions

Drug-Drug: Concurrent use with **sulfonylureas** may ↑ risk of hypoglycemia (↓ dose of **sulfonylurea** if hypoglycemia occurs). Due to slowed gastric emptying, may decrease absorption of **orally administered medications**, especially those requiring rapid GI absorption or require a specific level for efficacy (**anti-infectives, oral contraceptives**).

Route/Dosage

Subcut (Adults): 5 mcg within 60 min before morning and evening meal; after 1 mo, dose may be increased to 10 mcg depending on response.

Availability

Solution for SC injection: 250 mcg/mL in prefilled pen-injector that delivers either 5 mcg/dose (1.2-mL pen) or 10 mcg/dose (2.4-mL pen) for 60 doses (30 days of twice daily dosing).

ezetimibe (e-zet-i-mibe)

✱ Ezetrol, Zetia

Classification
Therapeutic: lipid-lowering agents
Pharmacologic: cholesterol absorption inhibitors

Indications

Alone or with other agents (HMG CoA reductase inhibitors) in the management of dyslipidemias, including primary hypercholesterolemia, homozygous familial hypercholesterolemia, and homozygous sitosterolemia.

Action

Inhibits absorption of cholesterol in the small intestine. **Therapeutic Effects:** Lowering of cholesterol, a known risk factor for atherosclerosis.

Adverse Reactions/Side Effects

GI: cholecystitis, cholelithiasis, ↑ hepatic transaminases (with HMG CoA reductase inhibitors), nausea, pancreatitis. **Derm:** rash. **Misc:** ANGIOEDEMA.

PHYSICAL THERAPY IMPLICATIONS

Examination and Evaluation

- Monitor signs of angioedema, including rashes, raised patches of red or white skin (welts), burning/itching skin, swelling in the face, and difficulty breathing. Notify physician immediately of these signs.
- Report signs of gallbladder inflammation (cholecystitis) and gallstones (cholelithiasis), including sudden intense pain in the abdomen or right side, bloating, jaundice, loss of appetite, nausea, vomiting, chills, and fever. Report these signs to the physician.
- Be alert for signs of pancreatitis, including upper abdominal pain (especially after eating), indigestion, weight loss, and oily stools. Report these signs to the physician.

Interventions

- Design and implement aerobic exercise and endurance training programs to improve cardiovascular function and help reduce the risk of coronary heart disease.

Patient/Client-Related Instruction

- Remind patients to take medication as directed to control hyperlipidemia even though they are asymptomatic.
- Counsel patients about additional interventions to help control lipid disorders and improve cardiovascular health, including dietary modification, regular exercise, moderation of alcohol consumption, and smoking cessation.
- Instruct patient and family/caregivers to report other troublesome side effects such as severe or prolonged nausea or skin rash.

Pharmacokinetics

Absorption: Following absorption, rapidly converted to ezetimibe-glucuronide, which is active. Bioavailability is variable.
Distribution: Unknown.
Metabolism and Excretion: Undergoes enterohepatic recycling, mostly eliminated in feces, minimal renal excretion.
Half-life: 22 hr.

TIME/ACTION PROFILE

ROUTE	ONSET	PEAK	DURATION
PO	unknown	unknown	unknown

Contraindications/Precautions

Contraindicated in: Hypersensitivity; Acute liver disease or unexplained laboratory evidence of liver disease (when used with HMG CoA reductase inhibitor); Moderate or severe hepatic insufficiency; Concurrent use of fibrates.
Use Cautiously in: OB: Lactation (use only if benefit to mother outweighs possible risks to infant); OB/Pedi: Pregnancy or children <10 yr (safety not established).

Interactions

Drug-Drug: Effects may be ↓ by **cholestyramine** or other **bile acid sequestrants**. Concurrent use of **fibrates** may ↑ blood levels of ezetimibe and also ↑ the risk of cholelithiasis. **Cyclosporine** may ↑ ezetimibe levels. May ↑ risk of rhabdomyolysis when used with **HMG CoA reductase inhibitors**.

Route/Dosage

PO (Adults): 10 mg once daily.

Availability

Tablets: 10 mg. ***In combination with:*** simvastatin (Vytorin). See Appendix B.

famciclovir (fam-sye-kloe-veer)

Famvir

Classification

Therapeutic: antivirals

Pharmacologic: purine nucleosides

Indications

Acute herpes zoster infections (shingles). Treatment/ suppression of recurrent herpes genitalis in immunocompetent patients. Treatment of recurrent mucocutaneous herpes simplex virus (HSV) infection in HIV-infected patients.

Action

Inhibits viral DNA synthesis in herpes-infected cells only. **Therapeutic Effects:** Decreased duration of herpes zoster infection with decreased duration of viral shedding. Decreased lesion formation and improved healing in recurrent HSV infection.

Adverse Reactions/Side Effects

CNS: headache, dizziness, fatigue. **GI:** diarrhea, nausea, vomiting.

PHYSICAL THERAPY IMPLICATIONS

Examination and Evaluation

- Assess skin and mucosal lesions to help document whether drug therapy is successful in controlling infection.
- Assess dizziness or fatigue that might affect gait, balance, or other functional activities (See Appendix C). Report balance problems and functional limitations to the physician and nursing staff, and caution the patient and family/caregivers to guard against falls and trauma.

Interventions

- Avoid contact with cutaneous or mucosal lesions when treating patients.
- Always wash hands thoroughly and disinfect equipment (whirlpools, electrotherapeutic devices, treatment tables, and so forth) to help prevent the spread of infection. Use universal precautions as indicated for specific patients.

Patient/Client-Related Instruction

- Advise patient to take or apply medication as directed. Famciclovir should not be used more frequently or longer than prescribed.
- Remind patient that famciclovir does not cure herpes infections. The virus lies dormant in the ganglia, and this drug will not prevent the spread of infection to others.
- Instruct patient and family/caregivers to report other troublesome side effects, including severe or prolonged headache or GI problems (diarrhea, nausea, vomiting).

Pharmacokinetics

Absorption: Following absorption, famciclovir is rapidly converted in the intestinal wall to penciclovir, the active compound.
Distribution: Unknown.
Metabolism and Excretion: Penciclovir is mostly excreted by the kidneys.
Half-life: *Penciclovir*—2.1–3 hr (increased in renal impairment).

TIME/ACTION PROFILE (penciclovir blood levels)

ROUTE	ONSET	PEAK	DURATION
PO	rapid	0.9 hr	8–12 hr

Contraindications/Precautions

Contraindicated in: Hypersensitivity.
Use Cautiously in: Patients with impaired renal function (increased dosage interval/decreased dose recommended if CCr <40–60 mL/min); Geri: Geriatric patients (because of age-related decrease in renal function); OB/Pedi: Pregnancy, lactation, or children <18 yr (safety not established).

Interactions

Drug-Drug: Probenecid ↑ plasma concentration of penciclovir.

Route/Dosage

Herpes Zoster

PO (Adults): 500 mg q 8 hr for 7 days.

Renal Impairment

PO (Adults): *CCr 40–59 mL/min*—500 mg q 12 hr; *CCr 20–39mL/min*—500 mg q 24 hr; *CCr <20 mL/min*—250 mg q 24 hr; *Hemodialysis*—250 mg after each dialysis.

Recurrent Genital Herpes Simplex Infections

PO (Adults): 1000 mg twice daily for one day.

Renal Impairment

PO (Adults): *CCr 40–59 mL/min*—500 mg bid for 1 day; *CCr 20–39 mL/min*—500 mg as a single dose; *CCr <20 mL/min*—250 mg as a single dose; *Hemodialysis*—250 mg as a single dose after dialysis.

Suppression of Recurrent Herpes Simplex Infections

PO (Adults): 250 mg q 12 hr for up to 1 yr.

Renal Impairment

PO (Adults): *CCr 20–39 mL/min*—125 mg q 12 hr for 5 days; *CCr <20 mL/min*—125 mg q 24 hr for 5 days; *Hemodialysis*—125 mg after each dialysis.

Recurrent Herpes Labialis Infections (cold sores)

PO (Adults): 1500 mg as a single dose.

Renal Impairment

PO (Adults): *CCr 40–59 mL/min*—750 mg as a single dose; *CCr 20–39 mL/min*—500 mg as a single dose; *CCr <20 mL/min*—250 mg as a single dose; *Hemodialysis*—250 mg as a single dose after dialysis.

Herpes Simplex in HIV-Infected Patients

PO (Adults): 500 mg q 12 hr for 7 days.

Renal Impairment

PO (Adults): *CCr 20–39 mL/min*—500 mg q 24 hr for 7 days; *CCr <20 mL/min*—250 mg q 24 hr for 7 days; *Hemodialysis*—250 mg after each dialysis.

Availability

Tablets: 125 mg, 250 mg, 500 mg.

famotidine (fa-moe-ti-deen)

Apo-Famotidine, Acid Control, Dyspep HB, Gen-Famotidine, Mylanta AR, Novo-Famotidine, Nu-Famotodine, Pepcid, Pepcid AC Maximum Strength, Pepcid RPD, Pepcid AC, Ulcidine

Classification

Therapeutic: antiulcer agents

Pharmacologic: histamine H_2 antagonists

Indications

Short-term treatment of active duodenal ulcers and benign gastric ulcers. Maintenance therapy for duodenal ulcers after healing of active ulcer(s). Management of gastroesophageal reflux disease (GERD). Treatment of heartburn, acid indigestion, and sour stomach (OTC use). Management of gastric hypersecretory states (Zollinger-Ellison syndrome). Prevention and treatment of stress-induced upper GI bleeding in critically ill patients. **Unlabeled Use:** Management of GI symptoms associated with the use of NSAIDs. Prevention of stress ulceration or aspiration pneumonitis. Prevention of acid inactivation of supplemental pancreatic enzymes in patients with pancreatic insufficiency. Management of urticaria.

Action

Inhibits the action of histamine at the H_2 receptor site located primarily in gastric parietal cells, resulting in inhibition of gastric acid secretion. **Therapeutic Effects:** Healing and prevention of ulcers. Decreased symptoms of gastroesophageal reflux. Decreased secretion of gastric acid.

Adverse Reactions/Side Effects

CNS: confusion, dizziness, drowsiness, hallucinations, headache. **CV:** ARRHYTHMIAS. **GI:** constipation, diarrhea, nausea. **GU:** decreased sperm count, erectile dysfunction. **Endo:** gynecomastia. **Hemat:** AGRANULOCYTOSIS, APLASTIC ANEMIA, anemia, neutropenia, thrombocytopenia. **Local:** pain at IV site. **Misc:** hypersensitivity reactions.

PHYSICAL THERAPY IMPLICATIONS

Examination and Evaluation

- Assess heart rate, ECG, and heart sounds, especially during exercise (see Appendices G, H). Report any rhythm disturbances or symptoms of increased arrhythmias, including palpitations, chest discomfort, shortness of breath, fainting, and fatigue/weakness.
- Report signs of agranulocytosis and neutropenia (fever, sore throat, mucosal lesions, signs of infection, bruising), aplastic anemia (unusual fatigue, weakness), or thrombocytopenia (bruising, bleeding gums, nose bleeds).
- Monitor signs of hypersensitivity reactions, including pulmonary symptoms (tightness in the throat or chest, wheezing, cough, dyspnea) or skin reactions (rash, pruritus, urticaria). Notify physician or nursing staff immediately if these reactions occur.
- Assess dizziness and drowsiness that might affect gait, balance, and other functional activities (See Appendix C). Report balance problems and functional limitations to the physician and nursing staff, and caution the patient and family/caregivers to guard against falls and trauma.
- Monitor other CNS symptoms such as confusion, hallucinations, and headache. Excessive or prolonged CNS symptoms may require a reduction in dose.
- If treating allergic skin reactions (urticaria), assess degree of itching, skin rash, and inflammation to help determine effects of drug therapy.
- Monitor IV injection site for pain, swelling, and irritation. Report prolonged or excessive injection site reactions to the physician.

Interventions

- Use caution during aerobic exercise and endurance conditioning because of an increased risk of cardiac arrhythmias. Terminate exercise if patient exhibits untoward symptoms (chest pain, shortness of breath, etc.) or displays other criteria for exercise termination (See Appendix L).

Patient/Client-Related Instruction

- Advise patient to avoid alcohol and foods that may cause an increase in GI irritation.
- Instruct patient to report troublesome GI effects such as severe or prolonged constipation, diarrhea, or nausea.
- Advise men to consult their physician if they experience erectile dysfunction or breast enlargement (gynecomastia).

Pharmacokinetics

Absorption: 40–45% absorbed following oral administration.
Distribution: Enters breast milk and cerebrospinal fluid.
Protein Binding: 15–20%.
Metabolism and Excretion: Up to 70% excreted unchanged by the kidneys; 30–35% metabolized by the liver.
Half-life: Infants: 4.5–15 hr; Children: 3.3–5.7 hr; Adults: 2.5–3.5 hr.

TIME/ACTION PROFILE

ROUTE	ONSET	PEAK	DURATION
PO	within 60 min	1–4 hr	6–12 hr
IV	within 60 min	0.5–3 hr	8–15 hr

Contraindications/Precautions

Contraindicated in: Hypersensitivity; Phenylketonuria (chewable tablets only); OB: Crosses placenta; no adequate human studies; Lactation: Discontinue breast-feeding to avoid exposure of infant to serious side effects.
Use Cautiously in: Renal impairment (more susceptible to adverse CNS reactions; increased dosage interval recommended if CCr <10 mL/min); Geri: More susceptible to adverse CNS reactions; dose reduction recommended. Pedi: Injection contains benzyl alcohol, which has been associated with gasping.

Interactions

Drug-Drug: ↓ the absorption of **ketoconazole**.

Route/Dosage

PO (Adults): *Short-term treatment of active ulcers*—40 mg/day at bedtime or 20 mg twice daily for up to 8 wk. *Duodenal ulcer prophylaxis*—20 mg once daily at bedtime. *GERD*—20 mg bid for up to 6 wk; up to 40 mg bid for up to 12 wk for esophagitis with erosions, ulcerations, and continuing symptoms. *Gastric hypersecretory conditions*—20 mg q 6 hr initially, up to 160 mg q 6 hr. *OTC use*—10 mg for relief of symptoms; for prevention,10 mg 60 min before eating or take 10 mg as chewable tablet 15 min before heartburn-inducing foods or beverages (not to exceed 20 mg/24 hr for up to 2 wk).
PO, IV (Children 1–12 yr): *Peptic ulcer*—0.5 mg/kg/day as a single bedtime dose or in divided doses bid (maximum: 40 mg daily); *GERD*—1 mg/kg/day in divided doses bid (maximum: 80 mg daily).
PO (Infants >3 mo—1 yr): *GERD*—0.5 mg/kg/dose bid.
PO (Infants and neonates <3 mo): *GERD*—0.5 mg/kg/dose once daily.
IV (Adults): 20 mg q 12 hr.

Renal Impairment

PO (Adults): *CCR 10–50 mL/min*—administer normal dose q 24 hr or 50% dose at normal dosing interval; *CCR <10 mL/min*—20 mg at bedtime; interval may need to be increased to every 36–48 hr.

Availability (generic available)

Tablets: 10 mg OTC, 20 mg Rx, OTC, 40 mg. **Chewable tablets with aspartame (mint flavor):** 10 mg OTC. **Orally disintegrating tablets with aspartame (mint flavor):** 20 mg, 40 mg. **Gelcaps:** 10 mg OTC. **Oral suspension (cherry-banana-mint flavor):** 40 mg/5 mL. **Solution for injection:** 10 mg/mL, 20 mg/50 mL 0.9% NaCl. ***In combination with:*** Antacids (Pepcid Complete). See Appendix B.

febuxostat (fe-bux-oh-stat)

Uloric

Classification
Therapeutic: antigout agents
Pharmacologic: xanthine oxidase inhibitors

Indications

Chronic management of hyperuricemia in patients with a history of gout.

Action

Decreases production of uric acid by inhibiting xanthine oxidase. **Therapeutic Effects:** Lowering of serum uric acid levels with resultant decrease in gouty attacks.

Adverse Reactions/Side Effects

GI: liver function abnormalities, nausea. **Derm:** rash. **MS:** gout flare, arthralgia.

PHYSICAL THERAPY IMPLICATIONS

Examination and Evaluation

- Be alert for signs of abnormal liver function, including anorexia, abdominal pain, severe nausea and vomiting, yellow skin or eyes, fever, sore throat, malaise, weakness, facial edema, lethargy, and unusual bleeding or bruising. Notify physician of these signs immediately.
- Assess joints affected by gout, and monitor pain and other variables (range of motion, muscle strength) to document whether this drug is successful in helping manage the patient's gout. Report any increased pain in joints (arthralgia) or gout flare-ups that might be related to drug treatment.

Interventions

- Implement appropriate manual therapy techniques, physical agents, and therapeutic exercises to decrease pain and help reduce the frequency and severity of gout attacks.

Patient/Client-Related Instruction

- Instruct patient and family/caregivers about the signs of liver toxicity (see above in Examination and Evaluation). Encourage early recognition and notification of the physician or other health care professional about these signs.
- Instruct patient and family/caregivers to report severe or prolonged nausea or skin rash.

Pharmacokinetics

Absorption: Well absorbed (49%) following oral administration.
Distribution: Unknown.
Protein Binding: 99.2%.
Metabolism and Excretion: Extensively metabolized by the liver; minimal renal excretion of unchanged drug; 45% eliminated in feces as unchanged drug, remainder is eliminated in urine and feces as inactive metabolites.
Half-life: 5–8 hr.

TIME/ACTION PROFILE (blood levels)

ROUTE	ONSET	PEAK	DURATION
PO	rapid	1–1.5 hr*	24 hr

*Maximum lowering of uric acid may take 2 wk.

Contraindications/Precautions

Contraindicated in: Concurrent azathioprine, mercaptopurine, or theophylline.
Use Cautiously in: Severe renal impairment (CCr <30 mL/min); Severe hepatic impairment; OB: Use in pregnancy only when potential maternal benefit outweighs potential fetal risk; Pedi: Safety in children <18 yr not established.

Interactions

Drug-Drug: Significantly ↑ blood levels of, and risk of serious toxicity from, **azathioprine**, **mercaptopurine**, and **theophylline**; concurrent use is contraindicated.

Route/Dosage

PO (Adults): 40 mg once daily initially; if serum uric acid does not drop to <6 mg/dL, dose should be increased to 80 mg daily.

Availability

Tablets: 40 mg, 80 mg.

felbamate (fel-ba-mate)

Felbatol

Classification
Therapeutic: anticonvulsants
Pharmacologic: carbamates

Indications

Used alone (monotherapy) or as adjunctive therapy with other anticonvulsants in treatment of partial seizures. Adjunctive therapy with other anticonvulsants in children (2–14 yr) who have partial or generalized seizures associated with Lennox-Gastaut syndrome. Because of deaths due to aplastic anemia and acute liver failure, felbamate should never be used as a first-line therapy, but should be reserved for patients whose epilepsy is so severe that these risks are considered acceptable given the drug's benefit.

Action

Probably acts by raising seizure threshold and preventing seizure spread. **Therapeutic Effects:** Decreased incidence of seizures.

Adverse Reactions/Side Effects

CNS: dizziness, drowsiness, fatigue, headache, insomnia, anxiety, psychologic disturbances. **EENT:** diplopia, pharyngitis, rhinitis, sinusitis. **GI:** ACUTE LIVER FAILURE, anorexia, constipation, dyspepsia, nausea, vomiting, altered taste, diarrhea, hiccups. **Derm:** acne, rashes. **Hemat:** APLASTIC ANEMIA. **MS:** myalgia. **Neuro:** ataxia. **Misc:** flu-like syndrome, weight loss.

PHYSICAL THERAPY IMPLICATIONS

Examination and Evaluation

- Be alert for signs of liver failure, including severe nausea and vomiting, anorexia, abdominal pain, yellow skin or eyes, fever, sore throat, malaise, weakness, facial edema, lethargy, and unusual bleeding or bruising. Report these signs to the physician immediately.

- Monitor signs of aplastic anemia, including unusual fatigue, weakness, dizziness, and pallor. Report these signs to the physician immediately. Periodic blood tests may be needed to monitor WBC and RBC counts.
- Document the number, duration, and severity of seizures to help determine if this drug is effective in reducing seizure activity.
- Assess dizziness or ataxia that might affect gait, balance, and other functional activities (See Appendix C). Report balance problems and functional limitations to the physician, and caution the patient and family/caregivers to guard against falls and trauma.
- Monitor daytime drowsiness, anxiety, or other psychologic disturbances. Repeated or excessive symptoms may require change in dose or medication.
- Assess any muscle pain to rule out musculoskeletal pathology; that is, try to determine if pain is drug induced rather than caused by anatomic or biomechanical problems.
- Periodically assess body weight and other anthropometric measures (body mass index, body composition). Report a rapid or unexplained weight loss or decreased body fat.

Interventions

- Guard against falls and trauma (hip fractures, head injury, and so forth), especially if dizziness or ataxia affect gait and balance. Implement fall-prevention strategies, especially if balance is impaired (See Appendix E).

Patient/Client-Related Instruction

- Advise patient to avoid alcohol and other CNS depressants because of the increased risk of sedation and adverse effects.
- Advise patients on prolonged antiseizure therapy not to discontinue medication without consulting their physician. Abrupt withdrawal may cause increased seizures.
- Advise patient about the risk of daytime drowsiness and decreased attention and mental focus. Use care if driving or in other activities that require strong concentration and fast responses.
- Advise patient about the likelihood of GI reactions such as nausea, vomiting, diarrhea, constipation, indigestion, loss of appetite, altered taste, and hiccups. Instruct patient to report severe or prolonged GI problems.
- Instruct patient and family/caregivers to report other troublesome side effects such as severe or prolonged headache, double vision, sleep loss, nasopharyngeal irritation, flu-like symptoms, or skin reactions (rash, acne).

Pharmacokinetics

Absorption: Well absorbed following oral administration.
Distribution: 0.7 L/kg.
Metabolism and Excretion: 40–50% excreted unchanged in urine; 40% metabolized by the liver.
Half-life: 20–23 hr.

TIME/ACTION PROFILE (blood levels)

ROUTE	ONSET	PEAK	DURATION
PO	Unknown	1–6 hr	unknown

Contraindications/Precautions

Contraindicated in: Hypersensitivity to felbamate or other carbamates (e.g., meprobamate); History of hepatic dysfunction; History of blood dyscrasias.
Use Cautiously in: Renal dysfunction.

Interactions

Drug-Drug: ↑ blood levels and risk of toxicity from **phenytoin, valproic acid,** and **phenobarbital.** ↓ **carbamazepine** blood levels but ↑ levels of **carbamazepine epoxide,** an active metabolite. Because of potential interactions, doses of **carbamazepine, phenytoin, valproic acid,** and **phenobarbital** should be ↓ by 20–33% when initiating felbamate therapy. Further reductions may be required. Concurrent use of other **hepatotoxic agents or drugs which may cause aplastic anemia** may ↑ the risk of these serious adverse reactions.
Drug-Natural: St. John's wort may affect felbamate levels and effectiveness; avoid use. Concomitant use of **kava, valerian, skullcap, chamomile,** or **hops** can ↑ CNS depression.

Route/Dosage

PO (Adults and Children >14 yr): *If used alone,* start with 1200 mg/day in 3–4 divided doses. May be ↑ by 600 mg/day at 2-wk intervals up to a total of 3600 mg. *If converting from other agents,* start with 1200 mg/day in 3–4 divided doses and ↓ other anticonvulsants by, 1/3. At week 2, ↑ felbamate to 2400 mg/day in 3–4 divided doses and ↓ other anticonvulsants by up to, 1/3 of their original dosage. At week 3, ↑ felbamate to 3600 mg/day in 3–4 divided doses while continuing to ↓ doses of other anticonvulsants. *If using as adjunctive therapy (with other agents),* start with 1200 mg/day in 3–4 divided doses, ↓ doses of other anticonvulsants by 20%. ↑ dose at weekly intervals by 1200 mg/day to 3600 mg/day. ↓ doses of other anticonvulsants as necessary.

PO (Children): *As adjunctive therapy,* start at 15 mg/kg/day in 3–4 divided doses, ↓ the dose of other anticonvulsants by 20%. ↑ dosage by 15 mg/kg/day (not to exceed 3600 mg/day) at weekly intervals to 45 mg/kg/day. ↓ doses of other anticonvulsants as necessary.

Availability

Tablets: 400 mg, 600 mg. **Oral suspension:** 600 mg/5 mL.

felodipine (fe-loe-di-peen)

Plendil, ✱Renedil

Classification

Therapeutic: antianginals, antihypertensives

Pharmacologic: calcium channel blockers

Indications

Management of hypertension, angina pectoris, and vasospastic (Prinzmetal's) angina.

Action

Inhibits the transport of calcium into myocardial and vascular smooth muscle cells, resulting in inhibition of excitation-contraction coupling and subsequent contraction. **Therapeutic Effects:** Systemic vasodilation resulting in decreased blood pressure. Coronary vasodilation resulting in decreased frequency and severity of attacks of angina.

Adverse Reactions/Side Effects

CNS: headache, abnormal dreams, anxiety, confusion, dizziness, drowsiness, nervousness, psychiatric disturbances, weakness. **EENT:** blurred vision, disturbed equilibrium, epistaxis, tinnitus. **Resp:** cough, dyspnea. **CV:** ARRHYTHMIAS, CHF, peripheral edema, bradycardia, chest pain, hypotension, palpitations, syncope, tachycardia. **GI:** abnormal liver function studies, anorexia, constipation, diarrhea, dry mouth, dysgeusia, dyspepsia, nausea, vomiting. **GU:** dysuria, nocturia, polyuria, sexual dysfunction, urinary frequency. **Derm:** dermatitis, erythema multiforme, flushing, increased sweating, photosensitivity, pruritus/urticaria, rash. **Endo:** gynecomastia, hyperglycemia. **Hemat:** anemia, leukopenia, thrombocytopenia. **Metab:** weight gain. **MS:** joint stiffness, muscle cramps. **Neuro:** paresthesia, tremor. **Misc:** STEVENS-JOHNSON SYNDROME, gingival hyperplasia.

PHYSICAL THERAPY IMPLICATIONS

Examination and Evaluation

- Assess heart rate, ECG, and heart sounds, especially during exercise (See Appendices G, H). Report any rhythm disturbances or symptoms of increased arrhythmias, including palpitations, chest pain, shortness of breath, fainting, and fatigue/weakness.
- Monitor rashes or other skin reactions (hives, abnormal sweating, itching/burning, exfoliation). Notify physician immediately because certain skin reactions may indicate serious hypersensitivity reactions (Stevens-Johnson syndrome).
- Assess routinely for signs of CHF and pulmonary edema (dyspnea, cough, shortness of breath, rales/crackles, jugular venous distention). Report these signs to the physician.
- Assess blood pressure periodically and compare to normal values (See Appendix F) to help document antihypertensive effects.
- Assess episodes of angina pectoris at rest and during exercise. Document whether drug therapy is helpful in reducing the frequency and severity of anginal attacks.
- Assess peripheral edema using girth measurements, volume displacement, and measurement of pitting edema (see Appendix N). Report increased swelling in feet and ankles due to peripheral vasodilation.
- Assess signs of paresthesia (numbness, tingling) or muscle twitching. Perform objective tests, including electroneuromyography and sensory testing to document any drug-related neuropathic changes.
- Monitor and report signs of leukopenia (fever, sore throat, signs of infection), thrombocytopenia (bruising, nose bleeds, and bleeding gums), or unusual weakness and fatigue that might be due to anemia. Periodic blood tests may be needed to monitor WBC and RBC counts.
- Watch for signs of hyperglycemia, including confusion, drowsiness, flushed/dry skin, fruit-like breath odor, rapid/deep breathing, polyuria, loss of appetite, and unusual thirst. Insulin dosages may need to be adjusted to prevent repeated episodes of hyperglycemia.
- Assess any joint stiffness or muscle cramping to rule out musculoskeletal pathology; that is, try to determine if pain is drug induced rather than caused by anatomic or biomechanical problems.
- Assess dizziness and weakness that might affect gait, balance, and other functional activities (See Appendix C). Report balance problems and functional limitations to the physician, and caution the patient and family/caregivers to guard against falls and trauma.
- Monitor mood and personality changes, including anxiety, nervousness, confusion, or other psychiatric disturbances. Notify physician if these changes become problematic.

Interventions

- Design and implement aerobic exercise and endurance training programs to normalize blood pressure, improve coronary perfusion, reduce angina, and improve myocardial pumping ability.

- Because of the risk of cardiac arrhythmias and CHF, use caution during aerobic exercise and other forms of therapeutic exercise. Assess exercise tolerance frequently (blood pressure, heart rate, fatigue levels), and terminate exercise immediately if any untoward responses occur (See Appendix L).
- Guard against falls and trauma (hip fractures, head injury). Implement fall-prevention strategies, especially if patient exhibits dizziness or disturbed equilibrium (See Appendix E).
- To minimize orthostatic hypotension, patient should move slowly when assuming a more upright position.
- Causes photosensitivity; use care if administering UV treatments.

Patient/Client-Related Instruction

- Remind patients to take medication as directed to control hypertension and other cardiac conditions even if they are asymptomatic.
- Counsel patients about additional interventions to help control blood pressure and cardiac dysfunction, including regular exercise, weight loss, sodium restriction, stress reduction, moderation of alcohol consumption, and smoking cessation.
- Advise patient about photosensitivity and to use sunscreens, protective clothing, and avoid prolonged sun exposure. Advise patient to also report any rashes or other skin reactions.
- Instruct patient or family/caregivers to report other troublesome side effects such as severe or prolonged headache, tinnitus, nightmares, tremor, weight gain, problems with urination, sexual dysfunction, breast enlargement in men (gynecomastia), or GI problems (nausea, vomiting, constipation, diarrhea, indigestion, loss of appetite).

Pharmacokinetics

Absorption: Well absorbed after oral administration, but extensively metabolized, resulting in decreased bioavailability.
Distribution: Unknown.
Protein Binding: >99%.
Metabolism and Excretion: Mostly metabolized; minimal amounts excreted unchanged by kidneys.
Half-life: 11–16 hr.

TIME/ACTION PROFILE (antihypertensive effect)

ROUTE	ONSET	PEAK	DURATION
PO	1 hr	2–4 hr	up to 24 hr

Contraindications/Precautions

Contraindicated in: Hypersensitivity (cross-sensitivity may occur); Sick sinus syndrome; 2nd- or 3rd-degree AV block (unless an artificial pacemaker is in place); Blood pressure <90 mm Hg.
Use Cautiously in: Severe hepatic impairment (dose reduction recommended); Geri: Dose reduction recommended; increased risk of hypotension; Severe renal impairment; History of serious ventricular arrhythmias or CHF; OB/Lactation/Pedi: Safety not established.

Interactions

Drug-Drug: Additive hypotension may occur when used concurrently with **fentanyl**, other **antihypertensives**, **nitrates**, acute ingestion of **alcohol**, or **quinidine**. Antihypertensive effects may be ↓ by concurrent use of **NSAIDs**. Concurrent use with **beta blockers**, **digoxin**, **disopyramide**, or **phenytoin** may result in bradycardia, conduction defects, or CHF. **Ketoconazole**, **itraconazole**, **propranolol** and **erythromycin** ↓ metabolism, ↑ blood levels and the risk of toxicity (dose reduction may be necessary).
Drug-Food: Grapefruit and **Grapefruit juice** ↑ serum levels and effect.

Route/Dosage

PO (Adults): 5 mg/day (2.5 mg/day in geriatric patients); may ↑ q 2 wk (range 5–10 mg/day; not to exceed 10 mg/day).

Availability (generic available)

Extended-release tablets: 2.5 mg, 5 mg, 10 mg.

fenofibrate (fen-o-fi-brate)

Antara, Fenoglide, Lipofen, ✱Lipidil Micro, ✱Lipidil Supra, Lofibra, Tricor, Triglide

Classification
Therapeutic: lipid-lowering agents
Pharmacologic: fibric acid derivatives

Indications

With dietary therapy to decrease LDL cholesterol, total cholesterol, triglycerides, and apolipoprotein B in adult patients with hypercholesterolemia or mixed dyslipidemia. With dietary management in the treatment of hypertriglyceridemia (types IV and V hyperlipidemia) in patients who are at risk for pancreatitis and do not respond to nondrug therapy.

Action

Fenofibric acid primarily inhibits triglyceride synthesis. **Therapeutic Effects:** Lowering of cholesterol and triglycerides with subsequent decreased risk of pancreatitis.

Adverse Reactions/Side Effects

CNS: fatigue/weakness, headache. **CV:** arrhythmias. **GI:** cholelithiasis, pancreatitis. **Derm:** rash, urticaria. **MS:** rhabdomyolysis. **Misc:** hypersensitivity reactions.

PHYSICAL THERAPY IMPLICATIONS

Examination and Evaluation

- Assess any muscle pain, tenderness, or weakness, especially if accompanied by fever, malaise, and dark-colored urine. Advise patient that these symptoms may represent drug-induced myopathy, and that myopathy can progress to severe muscle damage (rhabdomyolysis). Report any unexplained musculoskeletal symptoms to the physician immediately.
- Monitor signs of hypersensitivity reactions, including pulmonary symptoms (tightness in the throat and chest, wheezing, cough, dyspnea) or skin reactions (rash, pruritus, urticaria). Notify physician immediately if these reactions occur.
- Assess heart rate, ECG, and heart sounds, especially during exercise (See Appendices G, H). Report any rhythm disturbances or symptoms of increased arrhythmias, including palpitations, chest discomfort, shortness of breath, fainting, and fatigue/weakness.
- Report signs of gallstones (cholelithiasis), including sudden intense pain in the abdomen or right side, jaundice, chills, and fever.

Interventions

- In patients with drug-induced myopathy, implement gradual strengthening and other therapeutic exercises to facilitate recovery from muscle pain and weakness. Use caution during early stages to avoid fatigue of affected muscles, and implement assistive devices (walker, cane, crutches) as needed to prevent falls and assist mobility. Increase exercise intensity as tolerated; recovery from myopathy typically takes 4–6 wk, but can be longer in older patients or people with comorbidities.
- Design and implement aerobic exercise and endurance training programs to improve cardiovascular function and help reduce the risk of coronary heart disease.
- Because of the risk of arrhythmias, use caution during aerobic exercise and other forms of therapeutic exercise. Assess exercise tolerance frequently (blood pressure, heart rate, fatigue levels), and terminate exercise immediately if any untoward responses occur (See Appendix L).

Patient/Client-Related Instruction

- Remind patients to take medication as directed to control hyperlipidemia even though they are asymptomatic.
- Counsel patients about additional interventions to help control lipid disorders and improve cardiovascular health, including dietary modification, regular exercise, moderation of alcohol consumption, and smoking cessation.
- Advise patient to report signs of pancreatitis, including upper abdominal pain (especially after eating), indigestion, weight loss, and oily stools.
- Instruct patient to report other side effects such as prolonged or severe fatigue, weakness, or skin reactions (rash, hives).

Pharmacokinetics

Absorption: Well absorbed (60%) after oral administration; absorption is increased by food.
Distribution: Unknown.
Protein Binding: 99%.
Metabolism and Excretion: Rapidly converted to fenofibric acid, which is the active metabolite; fenofibric acid is metabolized by the liver. Fenofibric acid and its metabolites are primarily excreted in urine (60%).
Half-life: 20 hr.

TIME/ACTION PROFILE (lowering of triglycerides)

ROUTE	ONSET	PEAK	DURATION
PO	unknown	2 wk	unknown

Contraindications/Precautions

Contraindicated in: Hypersensitivity; Hepatic impairment (including primary biliary cirrhosis); Preexisting gallbladder disease; Severe renal impairment; Concurrent use of HMG CoA reductase inhibitors; Lactation: Lactation.
Use Cautiously in: Concurrent warfarin therapy; OB/Pedi: Pregnancy or children (use in pregnancy only if benefits outweigh risks to the fetus; safety not established).

Interactions

Drug-Drug: ↑ anticoagulant effects of **warfarin.** Concurrent use with **HMG CoA reductase inhibitors** ↑ risk of rhabdomyolysis (combined use should be avoided). Absorption is ↓ by **bile acid sequestrants** (fenofibrate should be given 1 hr before or 4–6 hr after). ↑ risk of nephrotoxicity with **cyclosporine.**

Route/Dosage

Primary hypercholesterolemia/mixed dyslipidemia

PO (Adults): *Antara*—130 mg/day initially; *Fenoglide*—120 mg/day; *Lofibra*—200 mg/day initially; *Tricor*—145 mg/day initially; *Triglide*—160 mg/day initially; *Lipofen*—50 mg daily; *Lipidil Supra*—160 mg daily.

Hypertriglyceridemia

PO (Adults): *Antara*—43–130 mg/day; *Fenoglide*—40–120 mg/day; *Lofibra*—67–200 mg/day initially;

Tricor—48–145 mg/day initially; *Triglide*—50–160 mg/day initially; *Lipofen*—50 mg daily; *Lipidil Supra*—160 mg daily.

Renal impairment/Geriatric patients

PO (Adults): *Antara*—43 mg/day; *Fenoglide*—start at 40 mg/day; *Lofibra*—67 mg/day; *Tricor*—48 mg/day.

Availability

Tablets (TriCor): 48 mg, 145 mg. **Tablets (Fenoglide):** 40 mg, 120 mg. **Tablets (Triglide):** 50 mg, 160 mg. **Micronized tablets (Lofibra):** 54 mg, 160 mg. **Microcoated tablets (Lipidil Supra):** 100 mg, 160 mg. **Micronized capsules (Antara):** 43 mg, 130 mg. **Capsules (Lipofen):** 50 mg, 100 mg, 150 mg. **Micronized capsules (Lofibra):** 67 mg, 134 mg, 200 mg. **Micronized capsules (Lipidil Micro):** 67 mg, 200 mg.

fenoldopam (fen-ole-doe-pam)

Corlopam

Classification

Therapeutic: antihypertensives

Pharmacologic: vasodilators

Indications

Short-term (<48 hr), in-hospital management of hypertensive emergencies, including malignant hypertension with end-organ deterioration.

Action

Acts as an agonist at dopamine D_1–like receptors. Also binds to alpha-adrenergic receptors. Acts as a vasodilator. **Therapeutic Effects:** Rapid lowering of blood pressure.

Adverse Reactions/Side Effects

CNS: headache, nervousness/anxiety, dizziness. **CV:** hypotension, tachycardia, ECG changes, peripheral edema. **GI:** nausea, abdominal pain, constipation, diarrhea, vomiting. **Derm:** flushing, sweating. **F and E:** hypokalemia. **Local:** injection site reactions. **MS:** back pain.

PHYSICAL THERAPY IMPLICATIONS

Examination and Evaluation

- Assess blood pressure periodically and compare to normal values (See Appendix F) to help document antihypertensive effects.
- Assess heart rate, ECG, and heart sounds, especially during exercise (See Appendices G, H). Report increased heart rate (tachycardia) or symptoms of other arrhythmias, including palpitations, chest pain, shortness of breath, fainting, and fatigue/weakness.
- Assess peripheral edema using girth measurements, volume displacement, and measurement of pitting edema (See Appendix N). Report increased swelling in feet and ankles due to peripheral vasodilation.
- Assess any back pain to rule out musculoskeletal pathology; that is, try to determine if pain is drug induced rather than caused by anatomic or biomechanical problems.
- Monitor and report any muscle weakness, aches, or cramps that might indicate low potassium levels (hypokalemia).
- Assess dizziness that might affect gait, balance, and other functional activities (See Appendix C). Report balance problems and functional limitations to the physician and nursing staff, and caution the patient and family/caregivers to guard against falls and trauma.
- Monitor IV injection site for pain, swelling, and irritation. Report prolonged or excessive injection site reactions to the physician.

Interventions

- After the emergency hypertensive episode has been controlled, design and implement aerobic exercise and endurance training programs to reduce hypertension.
- Because of an increased risk of tachycardia and other cardiac arrhythmias, use caution during aerobic exercise and endurance conditioning. Terminate exercise if patient exhibits untoward symptoms (chest pain, shortness of breath, etc.) or displays other criteria for exercise termination (See Appendix L).
- Avoid physical therapy interventions that cause systemic vasodilation (large whirlpool, Hubbard tank). Additive effects of this drug and the intervention may cause a dangerous fall in blood pressure.
- To minimize orthostatic hypotension, patient should move slowly when assuming a more upright position.

Patient/Client-Related Instruction

- Counsel patients about additional interventions to help control blood pressure, such as regular exercise, weight loss, sodium restriction, stress reduction, moderation of alcohol consumption, and smoking cessation.
- Instruct patient or family/caregivers to report other troublesome side effects such as severe or prolonged headache, nervousness, anxiety, skin reactions (flushing, sweating), or GI problems (nausea, vomiting, diarrhea, constipation, abdominal pain).

Pharmacokinetics

Absorption: IV administration results in complete bioavailability.

Distribution: Unknown.

Metabolism and Excretion: Mostly metabolized by the liver; 90% of metabolites are excreted in urine, 10% in feces.

Half-life: 5–10 min.

TIME/ACTION PROFILE (effect on blood pressure)

ROUTE	ONSET	PEAK	DURATION
IV	rapid	15 min	1–4 hr

Contraindications/Precautions

Contraindicated in: Hypersensitivity to fenoldopam or sulfites; Concurrent beta blocker therapy (will prevent reflex tachycardia).

Use Cautiously in: Glaucoma or intraocular hypertension; Pregnancy, lactation, or children (safety not established).

Interactions

Drug-Drug: Concurrent use with **beta blockers** may result in excessive hypotension (concurrent use should be avoided).

Route/Dosage

IV (Adults): 0.01–1.6 mcg/kg/min.

Availability

Concentrate for injection: 10 mg/mL in 1- and 2-mL single-use ampules (with sodium meta-bisulfite).

Misc: ALLERGIC REACTIONS, INCLUDING ANAPHYLAXIS.

fenoprofen (fen-oh-proe-fen)

Nalfon

Classification

Therapeutic: nonopioid analgesics

Pharmacologic: propionic acid derivatives

Indications

Rheumatoid arthritis. Osteoarthritis. Mild-to-moderate pain.

Action

Inhibits prostaglandin synthesis. **Therapeutic Effects:** Suppression of pain and inflammation.

Adverse Reactions/Side Effects

CNS: confusion, dizziness, drowsiness, headache. **EENT:** blurred vision, hearing loss, tinnitus. **CV:** edema, palpitations. **GI:** GI BLEEDING, HEPATITIS, dyspepsia, abdominal pain, constipation, diarrhea, discomfort, nausea, vomiting. **GU:** cystitis, dysuria, hematuria, renal failure. **Derm:** pruritus, rashes, sweating. **Hemat:** prolonged bleeding time. **Neuro:** tremor. **Misc:** ALLERGIC REACTIONS, INCLUDING ANAPHYLAXIS.

PHYSICAL THERAPY IMPLICATIONS

Examination and Evaluation

- Monitor signs of GI bleeding, including abdominal pain, vomiting blood, blood in stools, or black, tarry stools. Report these signs to the physician immediately.
- Be alert for signs of drug-induced hepatitis, including anorexia, abdominal pain, severe nausea and vomiting, yellow skin or eyes, skin rashes, flu-like symptoms, and muscle/joint pain. Report these signs to the physician immediately.
- Monitor signs of allergic reactions and anaphylaxis, including pulmonary symptoms (laryngeal edema, wheezing, cough, dyspnea) or skin reactions (rash, pruritus, urticaria). Notify physician immediately if these reactions occur.
- Assess pain and other variables (range of motion, muscle strength) to document whether this drug is successful in helping manage the patient's pain and decreasing impairments.
- Assess blood pressure (BP) periodically and compare to normal values (See Appendix F). NSAIDs can increase BP in certain patients.
- Assess for signs of prolonged bleeding time such as bleeding gums, nosebleeds, and unusual or excessive bruising. Notify physician if these signs occur.
- Assess peripheral edema using girth measurements, volume displacement, and measurement of pitting edema (See Appendix N). Report increased swelling in feet and ankles or a sudden increase in body weight due to fluid retention.
- Monitor signs of kidney dysfunction such as painful urination or blood in the urine. Report signs of renal failure immediately, including decreased urine output, increased BP, muscle cramps/twitching, edema/weight gain from fluid retention, yellowish brown skin, and confusion that progresses to seizures and coma.
- Assess dizziness and drowsiness that might affect gait, balance, and other functional activities (see Appendix C). Report balance problems and functional limitations to the physician, and caution the patient and family/caregivers to guard against falls and trauma.
- Monitor and report confusion, agitation, or other psychic disturbances.

Interventions

- Implement appropriate manual therapy techniques, physical agents, and therapeutic exercises to reduce pain and decrease the need for fenoprofen and other NSAIDs.

- If treating arthritic conditions, recommend orthotic and assistive devices as needed to reduce pain, improve function, and augment the effects of drug therapy.
- Use caution with any physical interventions that could increase bleeding, including wound débridement, chest percussion, joint mobilization, and application of local heat.
- Help patient explore other nonpharmacologic methods to reduce chronic pain such as relaxation techniques, exercise, counseling, and so forth.

Patient/Client-Related Instruction

- Advise patient that analgesics are usually more effective if given before pain becomes severe; emphasize that adequate pain control will allow better participation in physical therapy.
- Inform patient that NSAIDs may impair bone and cartilage healing. Advise patient to consult physician about NSAID use, especially after fractures, spinal fusion, and other bone surgeries.
- Caution patient about the use of over-the-counter products that contain NSAIDs or acetaminophen while taking prescription doses of fenoprofen. Use of multiple NSAIDs increases the risk of toxicity and overdose.
- Instruct patient to report excessive or prolonged headache or ringing/buzzing in the ears (tinnitus); these signs may indicate drug toxicity.
- Advise patient about the risks of gastric irritation. Instruct patient to notify physician of GI reactions such as severe or prolonged nausea, vomiting, diarrhea, constipation, indigestion, and abdominal pain.
- Advise patient to reduce alcohol intake because alcohol increases the risk of gastric toxicity.
- Instruct patient and family/caregivers to report other troublesome side effects such as severe or prolonged tremor, heart palpitations, vision disturbances, or skin reactions (rash, itching, increased sweating).

Pharmacokinetics

Absorption: Well absorbed from the GI tract.
Distribution: Enters breast milk in low concentrations.
Protein Binding: >99%.
Metabolism and Excretion: Mostly metabolized by the liver. 2–5% excreted unchanged by the kidneys.
Half-life: 3 hr.

TIME/ACTION PROFILE

ROUTE	ONSET	PEAK	DURATION
PO (analgesic activity)	15–30 min	1–2 hr	4–6 hr
PO (anti-inflammatory activity)	several days	2–3 wk	unknown

Contraindications/Precautions

Contraindicated in: Hypersensitivity to fenoprofen, aspirin, or other NSAIDS; Active GI bleeding or ulcer disease; Severe renal dysfunction; Perioperative pain in setting of coronary artery bypass surgery.
Use Cautiously in: Cardiovascular, renal, or hepatic disease; History of ulcer disease; Pregnancy (not recommended for use during third trimester); Elderly (increased risk of adverse events); Lactation or children (safety not established).

Interactions

Drug-Drug: Concurrent use with **aspirin** or **antacids** may ↓ effectiveness. Additive adverse GI effects with **aspirin**, other **NSAIDs, potassium supplements, corticosteroids,** or **alcohol.** May ↓ the effectiveness of **diuretics** or **antihypertensives.** May ↑ serum **lithium** levels and ↑ the risk of toxicity. ↑ the risk of toxicity from **methotrexate.** ↑ risk of bleeding with **cefotetan, heparin, thrombolytic agents, antiplatelet agents,** or **warfarin.** ↑ risk of adverse hematologic reactions with **antineoplastics** or **radiation therapy. Phenobarbital** may ↑ increase metabolism and ↓ effectiveness of fenoprofen. May ↑ the risk of nephrotoxicity with **cyclosporine.**
Drug-Natural: ↑ bleeding risk with **anise, arnica, chamomile, clove, feverfew, garlic, ginger, ginkgo, *Panax ginseng*,** and others.

Route/Dosage

Rheumatoid Arthritis/Osteoarthritis

PO (Adults): 300–600 mg 3–4 times daily (not to exceed 3.2 g/day).

Mild-to-Moderate Pain

PO (Adults): 200 mg q 4–6 hr.

Availability (generic available)

Capsules: 200 mg, 300 mg. **Tablets:** 600 mg.

fentanyl iontophoretic transdermal system (fen-ta-nil)

Ionsys

Classification

Therapeutic: opioid analgesics
Pharmacologic: opioid agonists

Schedule II

Indications

Short-term management of acute postoperative pain in hospitalized patients.

Action

Binds to opiate receptors in the CNS, altering the response to and perception of pain. **Therapeutic Effects:** Decreased pain.

Adverse Reactions/Side Effects

CNS: headache, anxiety, dizziness, insomnia, somnolence. **Resp:** RESPIRATORY DEPRESSION, hypoxia, pharyngitis. **CV:** bradycardia, hypertension, hypotension, tachycardia. **GI:** nausea, vomiting, abdominal pain, constipation, dyspepsia, flatulence, ileus. **GU:** urinary retention. **Derm:** application site reactions, itching. **F and E:** hypokalemia. **Hemat:** anemia. **MS:** back pain. **Neuro:** hypertonia. **Misc:** fever.

PHYSICAL THERAPY IMPLICATIONS

Examination and Evaluation

- Assess symptoms of respiratory depression, including decreased respiratory rate, confusion, bluish color of the skin and mucous membranes (cyanosis), and difficult, labored breathing (dyspnea). Monitor pulse oximetry and perform pulmonary function tests (See Appendix I) to quantify suspected changes in ventilation and respiratory function. Excessive respiratory depression requires emergency care.
- Be alert for excessive sedation or changes in mood and behavior (anxiety, confusion). Notify physician or nurse immediately if patient is unconscious or extremely difficult to arouse.
- Use appropriate pain scales (visual analogue scales, others) to document whether this drug is successful in helping manage the patient's pain.
- Assess blood pressure (BP) and compare to normal values (See Appendix F). Report changes in BP, either a problematic decrease in BP (hypotension) or a sustained increase in BP (hypertension).
- Assess heart rate, ECG, and heart sounds, especially during exercise (See Appendices G, H). Report rapid or slow heart rate (tachycardia or bradycardia, respectively), or symptoms of other arrhythmias, including palpitations, chest discomfort, shortness of breath, fainting, and fatigue/weakness.
- Assess dizziness that might affect gait, balance, and other functional activities (See Appendix C). Report balance problems and functional limitations to the physician and nursing staff, and caution the patient and family/caregivers to guard against falls and trauma.
- Monitor signs of anemia, including unusual fatigue, shortness of breath with exertion, pallor, and bruising. Notify physician if these signs occur.
- Monitor any muscle weakness, aches, back pain, cramps, or increased muscle tone that might indicate low potassium levels (hypokalemia). Report suspicious neuromuscular symptoms to the physician.
- Monitor application site for pain, swelling, and irritation. Report prolonged or excessive application-site reactions to the physician.

Interventions

- Implement appropriate manual therapy techniques, physical agents, and therapeutic exercises to reduce pain and help wean patient off opioid analgesics as soon as possible.
- Avoid contact with the transdermal application site, and do not apply massage or physical agents (heat, cold, electrotherapeutic modalities) at or near the application site.
- Because of the risk of respiratory depression and arrhythmias, use caution during aerobic exercise and other forms of therapeutic exercise. Assess exercise tolerance frequently (BP, heart rate, respiratory rate, fatigue levels), and terminate exercise immediately if any untoward responses occur (See Appendix L).
- Help patient explore other nonpharmacologic methods to reduce chronic pain, such as relaxation techniques, exercise, counseling, and so forth.
- Guard against falls and trauma (hip fractures, head injury). Implement fall-prevention strategies (See Appendix E), especially if patient exhibits sedation, dizziness, or blurred vision.
- To minimize orthostatic hypotension, patient should move slowly when assuming a more upright position.

Patient/Client-Related Instruction

- Advise patient that opioid analgesics are usually more effective if given before pain becomes severe; emphasize that adequate pain control will allow better participation in physical therapy.
- Make sure patient understands how to activate the iontophoretic device, and encourage patient to use the device as directed.
- Emphasize that the risk of physical addiction (tolerance and dependence) is usually minimal during short-term treatment of pain. Advise patient that addiction is more likely during excessive or inappropriate use of opioid analgesics.
- Advise patient to avoid alcohol and other CNS depressants because of the increased risk of sedation and decreased CNS function.
- Advise patient to increase fluid intake and dietary fiber to avoid constipation. Laxatives may also be

helpful in patients susceptible to fecal impaction (e.g., people with spinal cord injury).

- Instruct patient to report other troublesome side effects such as severe or prolonged headache, urinary retention, fever, sleep loss, or GI problems (nausea, vomiting, flatulence, indigestion, abdominal pain).

Pharmacokinetics

Absorption: Following activation, a single 40-mcg dose is delivered for dermal absorption; fentanyl is well absorbed from dermal sites on upper outer arm or chest.
Distribution: Crosses the placenta; enters breast milk.
Metabolism and Excretion: Mostly metabolized by the liver (CYP3A4 enzyme system); <10% excreted unchanged in urine.
Half-life: 11 hr (elimination half-life).

TIME/ACTION PROFILE

ROUTE	ONSET	PEAK	DURATION
transdermal	rapid (within min)	5 min	10 min

Contraindications/Precautions

Contraindicated in: Hypersensitivity to fentanyl or any components of the iontophoretic system (including cetylpyridinium); Children <18 yr.
Use Cautiously in: Pulmonary conditions that may predispose to hypoventilation; Bradyarrhythmias (may ↑ risk of bradycardia); Hepatic disease (impaired clearance may ↑ effects); Renal impairment; Geri: Elderly patients may be more sensitive to effects; consider altered drug disposition factors; High-frequency hearing impairment; X-ray imaging or CT scanning (contains radiopaque parts); MRI procedures, cardioversion, defibrillation (may damage system and should be removed prior); OB: Not recommended for use during pregnancy (crosses the placenta) or breast-feeding (enters breast milk; may cause CNS depression in the newborn).

Interactions

Drug-Drug: Drugs that induce the CYP3A4 enzyme system, including **rifampin, carbamazepine,** and **phenytoin** ↑ clearance and may ↓ analgesia. Concurrent use with CYP3A4 inhibitors, including **clarithromycin, erythromycin, itraconazole, ketoconazole nelfinavir, ritonavir, nefazodone, diltiazem, aprepitant, fluconazole, fosamprenavir,** and **verapamil,** may ↑ effects and ↑ risk of respiratory depression. ↑ risk of CNS depression, hypotension, and respiratory depression with **alcohol,** other **opioids,** or **CNS depressants,** including **sedatives, hypnotics, general anesthetics, phenothiazines, tranquilizers, skeletal muscle relaxants,** or **sedating antihistamines.**
Drug-Natural: St. John's wort ↑ metabolism and may ↓ analgesia.
Drug-Food: Grapefruit juice is a moderate inhibitor of the CYP3A4 enzyme system; concurrent use may ↑ blood levels and the risk of respiratory and CNS depression. Careful monitoring and dose adjustment is recommended.

Route/Dosage

Transdermal (Adults): Assure adequate analgesia before initiating iontophoretic system. System delivers 40 mcg every 10 min as needed; system can deliver maximum of 6 doses per hour and total of 80 doses in 24 hr. 3 systems may be applied sequentially for 72 hr.

Availability

Iontophoretic patch: Contains fentanyl 10.8 mg designed to deliver 40 mcg over 10 min/activation of dose button.

F

HIGH ALERT

fentanyl (transdermal)

(fen-ta-nil)

Duragesic

Classification

Therapeutic: opioid analgesics, analgesic adjuncts
Pharmacologic: opioid agonists

Schedule II

Indications

Moderate-to-severe chronic pain requiring continuous opioid analgesic therapy for an extended time at a dose of 25 mcg/hr or more of the transdermal system. Transdermal fentanyl is not recommended for the control of postoperative, mild, or intermittent pain, nor should it be used for short-term pain relief.

Action

Binds to opiate receptors in the CNS, altering the response to and perception of pain. **Therapeutic Effects:** Decrease in severity of chronic pain.

Adverse Reactions/Side Effects

CNS: confusion, sedation, weakness, dizziness, restlessness. **Resp:** APNEA, bronchoconstriction, laryngospasm, respiratory depression. **CV:** bradycardia. **GI:** anorexia, constipation, dry mouth, nausea, vomiting. **Derm:** sweating, erythema. **Local:** application site reactions. **MS:** skeletal and thoracic muscle rigidity. **Misc:** physical dependence, psychologic dependence.

PHYSICAL THERAPY IMPLICATIONS

Examination and Evaluation

- Assess respiration, and notify physician immediately if patient exhibits any interruption in respiratory rate (apnea) or signs of respiratory depression, including decreased respiratory rate, confusion, bluish color of the skin and mucous membranes (cyanosis), and difficult, labored breathing (dyspnea). Monitor pulse oximetry and perform pulmonary function tests (See Appendix I) to quantify suspected changes in ventilation and respiratory function. Apnea or excessive respiratory depression requires emergency care.
- Monitor signs of laryngeal spasm and bronchospasm, including tightness in the throat and chest, wheezing, cough, and severe shortness of breath. Notify physician or nursing staff immediately if these reactions occur.
- Be alert for excessive sedation or changes in mood and behavior (confusion, restlessness). Notify physician or nurse immediately if patient is unconscious or extremely difficult to arouse.
- Use appropriate pain scales (visual analogue scales, others) to document whether this drug is successful in helping manage the patient's pain.
- Assess heart rate, ECG, and heart sounds, especially during exercise (See Appendices G, H). Report slow heart rate (bradycardia) or symptoms of other arrhythmias, including palpitations, chest discomfort, shortness of breath, fainting, and fatigue/weakness.
- Assess dizziness that might affect gait, balance, and other functional activities (See Appendix C). Report balance problems and functional limitations to the physician and nursing staff, and caution the patient and family/caregivers to guard against falls and trauma.
- Be alert for residual muscle rigidity and decreased thoracic and limb movements. Report a prolonged or sustained increase in muscle tone.
- Monitor patch application site for pain, swelling, and irritation. Report prolonged or excessive application site reactions to the physician.

Interventions

- Implement appropriate manual therapy techniques, physical agents, and therapeutic exercises to reduce pain and help wean patient off opioid analgesics as soon as possible.
- Avoid contact with the transdermal application site, and do not apply massage or physical agents (heat, cold, electrotherapeutic modalities) at or near the application site.
- Because of the risk of respiratory depression and arrhythmias, use caution during aerobic exercise and other forms of therapeutic exercise. Assess exercise tolerance frequently (blood pressure, heart rate, respiratory rate, fatigue levels), and terminate exercise immediately if any untoward responses occur (See Appendix L).
- Help patient explore other nonpharmacologic methods to reduce chronic pain, such as relaxation techniques, exercise, counseling, and so forth.
- Guard against falls and trauma (hip fractures, head injury). Implement fall-prevention strategies (See Appendix E), especially if patient exhibits sedation, dizziness, or blurred vision.
- To minimize orthostatic hypotension, patient should move slowly when assuming a more upright position.

Patient/Client-Related Instruction

- Advise patient that opioid analgesics are usually more effective if given before pain becomes severe; emphasize that adequate pain control will allow better participation in physical therapy.
- Make sure patient and family/caregivers understand how to apply the patch; encourage adherence to proper application procedures and dosing schedule.
- Emphasize that the risk of physical addiction (tolerance and dependence) is usually minimal during short-term treatment of pain. Advise patient that addiction is more likely during excessive or inappropriate use of opioid analgesics.
- Advise patient to avoid alcohol and other CNS depressants because of the increased risk of sedation and decreased CNS function.
- Advise patient to increase fluid intake and dietary fiber to avoid constipation. Laxatives may also be helpful in patients susceptible to fecal impaction (e.g., people with spinal cord injury).
- Instruct patient to report other troublesome side effects such as severe or prolonged skin reactions (warmth, redness, increased sweating) or GI problems (nausea, vomiting, dry mouth, loss of appetite).

Pharmacokinetics

Absorption: Well absorbed (92% of dose) through skin surface under transdermal patch, creating a depot in the upper skin layers. Release from transdermal system into systemic circulation increases gradually to a constant rate, providing continuous delivery for 72 hr.
Distribution: Crosses the placenta; enters breast milk.
Metabolism and Excretion: Mostly metabolized by the liver (CYP3A4 enzyme system); 10–25% excreted unchanged by the kidneys.
Half-life: 17 hr after removal of a single application patch, increases to 21 hr after removal of multiple patches (because of continued release from deposition of drug in skin layers).

TIME/ACTION PROFILE (decreased pain)

ROUTE	ONSET	PEAK	DURATION
Transdermal	6 hr*	12–24 hr	72 hr†

*Achievement of blood levels associated with analgesia. Maximal response and dose titration may take up to 6 days.
†While patch is worn.

Contraindications/Precautions

Contraindicated in: Hypersensitivity to fentanyl or adhesives; Known intolerance; Acute pain (onset not rapid enough); Postoperative pain; Mild or intermittent pain; Alcohol intolerance (small amounts of alcohol released into skin); OB/Lactation: Not recommended during labor and delivery, avoid during lactation.
Use Cautiously in: Geri: Patients >60 yr, cachectic or debilitated patients (dose reduction suggested because of altered drug disposition); Diabetes; Patients with severe pulmonary or hepatic disease; CNS tumors; Increased intracranial pressure; Head trauma; Adrenal insufficiency; Undiagnosed abdominal pain; Hypothyroidism; Alcoholism; Cardiac disease (particularly bradyarrhythmias); Fever or situations that increase body temperature (increases release of fentanyl from delivery system); Titration period (additional analgesics may be required); Pedi: Safety not established for children <2 yr; pediatric patients initiating therapy at 25 mcg/hr should be opioid tolerant and receiving at least 60 mg oral morphine equivalents per day.

Interactions

Drug-Drug: Avoid use in patients who have received **MAO inhibitors** within the previous 14 days (may produce unpredictable, potentially fatal reactions). Concomitant use of **CYP3A4 inhibitors,** including **ritonavir, ketoconazole, itraconazole, clarithromycin, nelfinavir, nefazodone, diltiazem, aprepitant, fluconazole, fosamprenavir, verapamil,** and **erythromycin,** may result in ↑ plasma levels and ↑ risk of CNS and respiratory depression. Levels and effectiveness may be ↓ by **drugs that induce the CYP3A4 enzyme.** ↑ CNS and respiratory depression with other **CNS depressants,** including **alcohol, antihistamines, antidepressants, sedative/hypnotics,** and other **opioids.**
Drug-Natural: Concomitant use of **kava, valerian,** or **chamomile** can ↑ CNS depression.
Drug-Food: Grapefruit juice is a moderate inhibitor of the CYP3A4 enzyme system; concurrent use may ↑ blood levels and the risk of respiratory and CNS depression. Careful monitoring and dose adjustment is recommended.

Route/Dosage

Transdermal (Adults): 25 mcg/hr is the initial dose; patients who have not been receiving opioids should receive not more that 25 mcg/hr. During dose titration, additional short-acting opioids should be available for any breakthrough pain that may occur. Morphine 10 mg IM or 60 mg PO q 4 hr (60 mg/24 hr IM or 360 mg/24 hr PO) is considered to be approximately equivalent to transdermal fentanyl 100 mcg/hr. Transdermal patch lasts 72 hr in most patients. Some patients require a new patch every 48 hr.
Transdermal (Adults >60 yr, Debilitated, or Cachectic Patients): Initial dose should be 25 mcg/hr unless previous opioid use was >135 mg morphine PO/day (or other opioid equivalent).

Availability (generic available)

Transdermal systems: 12 mcg/hr, 25 mcg/hr, 50 mcg/hr, 75 mcg/hr, 100 mcg/hr.

ferumoxytol (fer-u-mox-y-tole)

Feraheme

Classification
Therapeutic: antianemics
Pharmacologic: iron supplements

Pregnancy Category C

Indications

Treatment of iron deficiency anemia in adult patients with chronic kidney disease (CKD).

Action

Consists of a superparamagnetic iron oxide coated with a carbohydrate shell; when the iron-carbohydrate complex enters the reticuloendothelial system (RES), iron is released from the iron-carbohydrate complex within macrophages. This iron can either enter the intracellular storage iron pool or be transferred to erythroid precursor cells for incorporation into hemoglobin. **Therapeutic Effects:** Improvement in anemia in patients with chronic kidney disease.

Adverse Reactions/Side Effects

CNS: dizziness. **CV:** hypertension, hypotension, peripheral edema. **GI:** constipation, diarrhea, nausea. **Hemat:** iron overload. **Misc:** HYPERSENSITIVITY REACTIONS, INCLUDING ANAPHYLAXIS AND ANAPHYLACTOID REACTIONS.

PHYSICAL THERAPY IMPLICATIONS

Examination and Evaluation

- Monitor signs of hypersensitivity reactions and anaphylaxis, including pulmonary symptoms (tightness

= Canadian drug name; *CAPITALS indicate life-threatening; underlines indicate most frequent.

in the throat and chest, wheezing, cough, dyspnea) or skin reactions (rash, pruritus, urticaria). Notify physician immediately if these reactions occur.

- Assess blood pressure (BP) and compare to normal values (See Appendix F). Report changes in BP, either a problematic decrease in BP (hypotension) or a sustained increase in BP (hypertension).
- Assess peripheral edema using girth measurements, volume displacement, and measurement of pitting edema (See Appendix N). Report increased swelling in feet and ankles or a sudden increase in body weight due to fluid retention.
- Assess any join pain, muscle pain, or unusual fatigue that might indicate iron overload. Attempt to rule out musculoskeletal pathology; that is, try to determine if pain is drug induced rather than caused by anatomic or biomechanical problems.
- Assess dizziness that might affect gait, balance, and other functional activities (See Appendix C). Report balance problems and functional limitations to the physician, and caution the patient and family/caregivers to guard against falls and trauma.

Patient/Client-Related Instruction

- Instruct patient and family/caregivers to report severe or prolonged GI problems, such as nausea, diarrhea, and constipation.

Pharmacokinetics

Absorption: IV administration results in complete bioavailability of iron-carbohydrate complex; however, iron is not liberated until incorporation into RES.
Distribution: Taken up by RES.
Metabolism and Excretion: Iron can either become part of intracellular ferritin or be transferred to erythroid precursor cells.
Half-life: 15 hr.

TIME/ACTION PROFILE (effect on anemia)

ROUTE	ONSET	PEAK	DURATION
IV	unknown	unknown	up to 1 mo

Contraindications/Precautions

Contraindicated in: Hypersensitivity; Evidence of iron overload; Anemia not due to iron deficiency; Lactation: Avoid use during breast-feeding.
Use Cautiously in: MRI; Geri: Consider age-related decrease in hepatic, renal, or cardiac function, and concurrent diseases or other drug therapy; dose cautiously; OB: Use during pregnancy only if potential benefit justifies potential risk to the fetus; Pedi: Safe and effective use in patients <18 yr not established.

Interactions

Drug-Drug: May ↓ absorption of concurrently administered **oral iron preparations.**

Route/Dosage

IV (Adults ≥18 yr): 510 mg initially, followed by a second 510-mg IV injection 3–8 days later. Course may be repeated after 1 mo.

Availability

Aqueous colloid for intravenous injection: 510-mg elemental iron/17 mL (30 mg/mL) vials.

fesoterodine
(fee-soe-**ter**-oh-deen)
Toviaz

Classification
Therapeutic: urinary tract antispasmodics
Pharmacologic: anticholinergics

Indications

Treatment of overactive bladder function that results in urinary frequency, urgency, or urge incontinence.

Action

Acts as a competitive muscarinic receptor antagonist resulting in inhibition of cholinergically mediated bladder contraction. **Therapeutic Effects:** Decreased urinary frequency, urgency, and urge incontinence.

Adverse Reactions/Side Effects

CV: tachycardia (dose related). **GI:** dry mouth, constipation, nausea, upper abdominal pain. **GU:** dysuria, urinary retention. **MS:** back pain.

PHYSICAL THERAPY IMPLICATIONS

Examination and Evaluation

- Assess heart rate, ECG, and heart sounds, especially during exercise (See Appendices G, H). Report an increased heart rate (tachycardia) or symptoms of other arrhythmias, including palpitations, chest discomfort, shortness of breath, fainting, and fatigue/weakness.
- Monitor signs of urine retention (difficult urination, painful or distended abdomen). Excessive urinary retention may require dose adjustment by physician.
- Assess any back pain to rule out musculoskeletal pathology; that is, try to determine if pain is drug induced rather than caused by anatomic or biomechanical problems.

Interventions

- When appropriate, implement pelvic floor muscle-strengthening activities and other therapeutic exercises to help maintain bladder control.

Patient/Client-Related Instruction

- Advise patient to increase fluid intake and dietary fiber to avoid constipation. Laxatives may also be helpful in patients susceptible to fecal impaction.
- Instruct patient and family/caregivers to report other troublesome side effects such as severe or prolonged headache, blurred vision, dry eyes, or GI problems (nausea, dry mouth, abdominal pain).

Pharmacokinetics

Absorption: Rapidly absorbed following oral administration, but is rapidly converted to its active metabolite (bioavailability of metabolite 52%; further metabolism occurs in the liver via CYP2D6 and CYP3A4 enzyme systems. 16% of active metabolite is excreted in urine, most of the remainder of inactive metabolites are renally excreted. 7% excreted in feces.
Distribution: Unknown.
Metabolism and Excretion: Rapidly converted by esterases to active metabolite.
Half-life: 7 hr (following oral administration).

TIME/ACTION PROFILE (active metabolite)

ROUTE	ONSET	PEAK	DURATION
PO	rapid	5 hr	24 hr

Contraindications/Precautions

Contraindicated in: Hypersensitivity; Urinary retention; Gastric retention; Severe hepatic impairment; Uncontrolled narrow-angle glaucoma.
Use Cautiously in: Significant bladder outlet obstruction (↑ risk of retention); Severe renal insufficiency (dose adjustment required); Decreased GI motility, including severe constipation; Treated narrow-angle glaucoma (use only if benefits outweigh risks); Myasthenia gravis; Severe renal impairment (dose should not exceed 4 mg/day); Geri: ↑ risk of anticholinergic side effects in patients >75 yr; OB/Lactation: Avoid using unless potential benefits outweighs potential risk to fetus/neonate; Pedi: Safety in children not established.

Interactions

Drug-Drug: Concurrent use of **potent CYP3A4 enzyme inhibitors,** including **ketoconazole, itraconazole,** and **clarithromycin** ↑ blood levels and risk of toxicity; daily dose should not exceed 4 mg. Use **less potent inhibitors of CYP3A4** (such as **erythromycin**) with caution; escalate dose carefully. Anticholinergic effects may alter the GI absorption of other drugs.

Route/Dosage

PO (Adults): 4 mg once daily initially may be ↑ to 8 mg/daily; *concurrent potent CYP3A4 inhibitors or CCr <30 mL/min*—dose should not exceed 4 mg/day.

Availability

Extended-release tablets: 4 mg, 8 mg.

fexofenadine

(fex-oh-**fen**-a-deen)
Allegra

Classification
Therapeutic: allergy, cold, and cough remedies, antihistamines
Pharmacologic: piperidines

Indications

Relief of symptoms of seasonal allergic rhinitis. Management of chronic idiopathic urticaria.

Action

Antagonizes the effects of histamine at peripheral histamine-1 (H_1) receptors, including pruritus and urticaria. Also has a drying effect on the nasal mucosa. **Therapeutic Effects:** Decreased sneezing, rhinorrhea, itchy eyes, nose, and throat associated with seasonal allergies. Decreased urticaria.

Adverse Reactions/Side Effects

CNS: drowsiness, fatigue. **GI:** dyspepsia. **Endo:** dysmenorrhea.

PHYSICAL THERAPY IMPLICATIONS

Examination and Evaluation

- Monitor symptoms of seasonal allergies (sneezing, rhinitis, itching eyes, cough) or chronic idiopathic urticaria (rash, hives, itching) to help document benefits of this drug in treating these disorders.

Interventions

- Guard against falls and trauma (hip fractures, head injury, and so forth). Implement fall-prevention strategies, especially in older adults or if balance is impaired (see Appendix E).

Patient/Client-Related Instruction

- Advise patient about the risk of daytime drowsiness and decreased attention and mental focus. Although the risk of drowsiness is lower with this drug compared to traditional antihistamines, patients should use care if driving or in other activities that require quick reactions and strong concentration.
- Advise patient to avoid alcohol and other CNS depressants because of the increased risk of sedation and adverse effects.
- Instruct patient to report other troublesome side effects, including menstrual irregularities or upset stomach.

Pharmacokinetics

Absorption: Rapidly absorbed after oral administration.
Distribution: Unknown.
Metabolism and Excretion: 80% excreted in urine, 11% excreted in feces.
Half-life: 14.4 hr (increased in renal impairment).

TIME/ACTION PROFILE (antihistaminic effect)

ROUTE	ONSET	PEAK	DURATION
PO	within 1 hr	2–3 hr	12–24 hr

Contraindications/Precautions

Contraindicated in: Hypersensitivity.
Use Cautiously in: Impaired renal function (increased dosing interval recommended); **OB, Pedi:** Pregnancy or lactation (safety not established).

Interactions

Drug-Drug: Magnesium and aluminum-containing antacids ↓ absorption and may decrease effectiveness.
Drug-Food: Apple, orange, and **grapefruit juice** ↓ absorption and may decrease effectiveness.

Route/Dosage

PO (Adults and Children ≥12 yr): 60 mg twice daily; or 180 mg once daily.
PO (Children 2–11 yr): 30 mg twice daily.
PO (Children 6 months–2 yr): 15 mg twice daily.

Renal Impairment

PO (Adults): 60 mg once daily as a starting dose.
PO (Children 6–11 yr): 30 mg once daily as a starting dose.

Availability (generic available)

Tablets: 30 mg, 60 mg, 180 mg. **Suspension (raspberry–cream):** 30 mg/5 mL in 30-ml and 300-ml bottles. ***In combination with:*** pseudoephedrine (Allegra-D). See Appendix B.

filgrastim (fil-gra-stim)

Neupogen

Other Names:
Granulocyte colony-stimulating factor (G-CSF)

Classification
Therapeutic: colony-stimulating factors
Pharmacologic: hematopoietic growth factors

Indications

Prevention of febrile neutropenia and associated infection in patients who have received bone marrow–depressing antineoplastics for the treatment of nonmyeloid malignancies. Reduction of time for neutrophil recovery and duration of fever in patients undergoing induction and consolidation chemotherapy for acute myelogenous leukemia. Reduction of time to neutrophil recovery and sequelae of neutropenia in patients with nonmyeloid malignancies undergoing myeloablative chemotherapy followed by bone marrow transplantation. Mobilization of hematopoietic progenitor cells into peripheral blood for collection by leukapheresis. Management of severe chronic neutropenia. **Unlabeled Use:** Neutropenia associated with HIV infection.

Action

A glycoprotein, filgrastim binds to and stimulates immature neutrophils to divide and differentiate. Also activates mature neutrophils. **Therapeutic Effects:** Decreased incidence of infection in patients who are neutropenic from chemotherapy or other causes. Improved harvest of progenitor cells for bone marrow transplantation.

Adverse Reactions/Side Effects

Hemat: excessive leukocytosis. **Local:** pain, redness at SC site. **MS:** medullary bone pain.

PHYSICAL THERAPY IMPLICATIONS

Examination and Evaluation

- Be alert for signs of increased white blood cell counts (leukocytosis), including fever, weakness, weight loss, loss of appetite, dizziness, fainting, dyspnea, bleeding/bruising, or pain or tingling in the arms, legs, or abdomen. Report these signs to the physician or nursing staff immediately.
- Assess any bone pain to rule out musculoskeletal pathology; that is, try to determine if pain is drug induced rather than caused by fracture or biomechanical problems.
- Monitor subcutaneous injection site for pain, swelling, and inflammation. Report prolonged or excessive injection-site reactions to the physician.

Interventions

- For patients who are medically able to begin exercise, implement appropriate resistive exercises and aerobic training to maintain muscle strength and aerobic capacity during cancer chemotherapy or to help restore function after chemotherapy.

Patient/Client-Related Instruction

- Instruct patient to guard against infection (frequent hand washing, etc.), and to avoid crowds and contact with persons with contagious diseases.

Pharmacokinetics

Absorption: Well absorbed after SC administration.
Distribution: Unknown.
Metabolism and Excretion: Unknown.
Half-life: 3.5 hr.

TIME/ACTION PROFILE

ROUTE	ONSET	PEAK	DURATION
IV, SC	unknown	unknown	4 days*

*Return of neutrophil count to baseline.

Contraindications/Precautions

Contraindicated in: Hypersensitivity to filgrastim or *Escherichia coli*–derived proteins.
Use Cautiously in: Malignancy with myeloid characteristics; Preexisting cardiac disease; Pregnancy, lactation, or children (safety not established).

Interactions

Drug-Drug: Simultaneous use with **antineoplastics** may have adverse effects on rapidly proliferating neutrophils—avoid use for 24 hr before and 24 hr after chemotherapy. **Lithium** may potentiate the release of neutrophils; concurrent use should be undertaken cautiously.

Route/Dosage

After Myelosuppressive Chemotherapy

IV, SC (Adults): 5 mcg/kg/day as a single injection daily for up to 2 wk. Dosage may be increased by 5 mcg/kg during each cycle of chemotherapy, depending on blood counts.

After Bone Marrow Transplantation

IV, SC (Adults): 10 mcg/kg/day as a 4- or 24-hr IV infusion or as a continuous SC infusion; initiate at least 24 hr after chemotherapy and at least 24 hr after bone marrow transplantation. Subsequent dosage is adjusted according to blood counts.

Peripheral Blood Progenitor Cell Collection and Therapy

SC (Adults): 10 mcg/kg/day as a bolus or continuous infusion for at least 4 days before first leukapheresis and continued until last leukapheresis; dosage modification suggested if WBC >100,000 cells/mm^3.

Severe Chronic Neutropenia

SC (Adults): *Congenital neutropenia*—6 mcg/kg twice daily. *Idiopathic/cyclical neutropenia*—5 mcg/kg daily (decrease if ANC remains >10,000/mm^3).

Availability

Injection: 300 mcg/mL in 1- and 1.6-mL vials.

finasteride (fi-nas-teer-ide)

Propecia, Proscar

Classification
Therapeutic: hair regrowth stimulants
Pharmacologic: androgen inhibitors

Indications

Benign prostatic hyperplasia (BPH); can be used with doxazosin. Androgenetic alopecia (male pattern baldness) in men only.

Action

Inhibits the enzyme 5-alpha-reductase, which is responsible for converting testosterone to its potent metabolite 5-alpha-dihydrotestosterone in prostate, liver, and skin; 5-alpha-dihydrotestosterone is partially responsible for prostatic hyperplasia and hair loss.
Therapeutic Effects: Reduced prostate size with associated decrease in urinary symptoms. Decreases hair loss; promotes hair regrowth.

Adverse Reactions/Side Effects

GU: decreased libido, decreased volume of ejaculate, erectile dysfunction.

PHYSICAL THERAPY IMPLICATIONS

Examination and Evaluation

- When treating BPH, monitor signs such as difficulty starting a urine stream, painful urination, weak urine flow, feeling that the bladder is not completely empty, frequent nighttime urination, and an urge to urinate again soon after urinating. Document any change in BPH symptoms to help assess the effects of drug therapy.

Interventions

- When appropriate, design and implement resistive exercise programs to help maintain muscle strength and bone integrity to offset the musculoskeletal effects of diminished 5-alpha-dihydrotestosterone biosynthesis.

Patient/Client-Related Instruction

- When treating BPH, advise patient that urinary symptoms (retention, dribbling, hesitancy, urgency) should improve, and to contact the physician if these symptoms continue to worsen.
- Instruct patient to report other bothersome side effects such as decreased libido or erectile dysfunction.

Pharmacokinetics

Absorption: Well absorbed after oral administration (63%).
Distribution: Enters prostatic tissue and crosses the blood-brain barrier. Remainder of distribution not known.
Protein Binding: 90%.
Metabolism and Excretion: Mostly metabolized; 39% excreted in urine as metabolites; 57% excreted in feces.
Half-life: 6 hr (range 6–15 hr; slightly increased in patients >70 yr).

TIME/ACTION PROFILE (reduction in dihydrotestosterone levels*)

ROUTE	ONSET	PEAK	DURATION
PO	rapid	8 hr	2 wk

*Clinical effects as noted by urinary tract symptoms and hair regrowth may not be evident for several months and remain for 4 mo after discontinuation.

Contraindications/Precautions

Contraindicated in: Hypersensitivity; Women.
Use Cautiously in: Patients with hepatic impairment or obstructive uropathy.

Interactions

Drug-Drug: None noted.

Route/Dosage

PO (Adults): *BPH*—5 mg once daily (Proscar); *androgenetic alopecia*—1 mg/day (Propecia).

Availability (generic available)

Tablets: 1 mg (Propecia), 5 mg (Proscar).

fingolimod (fin-**goe**-li-mod)

Gilenyna

Classification
Therapeutic: anti–multiple sclerosis agents
Pharmacologic: receptor modulators

Indications

Treatment of relapsing forms of multiple sclerosis.

Action

Converted by sphingosine kinase to the active metabolite fingolimod-phosphate, which binds to sphingosin-1 phosphate receptors, resulting in ↓ migration of lymphocytes into peripheral blood. This may ↓ lymphocyte migration into the CNS.
Therapeutic Effects: ↓ frequency of relapses/delayed accumulation of disability.

Adverse Reactions/Side Effects

CNS: headache. **EENT:** blurred vision, eye pain, macular edema. **Resp:** cough, ↓ pulmonary function. **CV:** BRADYCARDIA, HEART BLOCK. **GI:** diarrhea, ↑ hepatic transaminases. **Hemat:** leukopenia, lymphopenia. **MS:** back pain. **Misc:** ↑ risk of infection.

PHYSICAL THERAPY IMPLICATIONS

- Assess heart rate, ECG, and heart sounds, especially during exercise (see Appendixes G, H). Report an unusually slow heart rate (bradycardia) or signs of heart block and other arrhythmias, including palpitations, chest discomfort, shortness of breath, fainting, and fatigue/weakness.
- Periodically assess balance, coordination, spasticity, gait, and other aspects of neuromuscular function. Document any improvement in function, but also report worsening of impairments or a relapse of multiple sclerosis symptoms.
- Assess any breathing problems, and document signs of decreased pulmonary function such as shortness of breath, labored or difficult breathing, reduced pulse oximetry values, and cyanosis. Report severe or problematic respiratory impairments.
- Watch for signs of leukopenia and lymphopenia, including fever, sore throat, mucosal lesions, and other signs of infection. Report these signs to the physician.
- Assess any back pain to rule out musculoskeletal pathology; that is, try to determine if pain is drug induced rather than caused by anatomic or biomechanical problems.

Interventions

- Design and implement coordination, balance, gait training, and other therapeutic exercises to maintain function and complement drug effects in patients with MS.

Patient/Client-Related Instruction

- Instruct patient to guard against infection (frequent hand washing, etc.), and to avoid crowds and contact with persons with contagious diseases.
- Instruct patient to report other troublesome side effects such as prolonged or severe headache, blurred vision, eye pain, cough, or diarrhea.

Pharmacokinetics

Absorption: Well absorbed (93%) following oral administration.
Distribution: Extensively distributed to body tissues; 86% of parent drug distributes into red blood cells; active metabolite uptake 17%.
Metabolism and Excretion: Converted to its active metabolite, then metabolized mostly by the CYP4504F2 enzyme system, with further degradation by other enzyme systems. Most inactive metabolites excreted in urine (81%); <2.5% excreted as fingolimod and fingolimod-phosphate in feces.
Protein Binding: >99.7%.
Half-life: 6–9 hr.

TIME/ACTION PROFILE

ROUTE	ONSET	PEAK	DURATION
PO	unknown	1–2 mos*	2 mos†

*Time to steady-state blood levels, peak blood levels after a single dose at 12–16 hr.
†Time for complete elimination.

Contraindications/Precautions

Contraindicated in: Active acute/chronic untreated infections; OB: Pregnancy; may cause fetal harm; Lactation: Breast-feeding should be avoided.
Use Cautiously in: Concurrent class Ia or class III antiarrhythmics, beta blockers, calcium channel blockers, bradycardia, history of syncope, ischemic heart disease, or congestive heart failure (↑ risk of bradycardia/heart block); Severe hepatic impairment (↑ blood levels and risk of adverse reactions); Diabetes mellitus/history of uveitis (↑ risk of macular edema); Negative history for chickenpox or vaccination against varicella zoster virus vaccination; Geri: Use cautiously in patients >65 yr; risk of adverse reactions may be ↑, consider age-related ↓ in cardiac/renal/hepatic function, chronic illnesses, and concurrent drug therapy; Pedi: Safety and effectiveness not established for patients <18 yr.

Interactions

Drug-Drug: Concurrent use of **class Ia or class III antiarrhythmics** ↑ risk of serious arrhythmias; careful monitoring recommended. Concurrent use of **beta blockers** or **diltiazem** ↑ risk of bradycardia; careful monitoring recommended. Concurrent use of **ketoconazole** ↑ blood levels and of adverse reactions ↑ risk of immunosuppression with **antineoplastics, immunosuppressants**, or **immune-modulating therapies; Live attenuated vaccines** ↑ risk of infection.

Route/Dosage

PO (Adults): 0.5 mg once daily.

Availability

Hard capsules: 0.5 mg.

flecainide (flek-a-nide)

Tambocor

Classification

Therapeutic: antiarrhythmics (class IC)

Indications

Life-threatening ventricular arrhythmias, including ventricular tachycardia. Supraventricular tachyarrhythmias, including Paroxysmal supraventricular tachycardia (PSVT), Paroxysmal atrial fibrillation/flutter (PAF). **Unlabeled Use:** Single-dose treatment of atrial fibrillation.

Action

Slows conduction in cardiac tissue by altering transport of ions across cell membranes. **Therapeutic Effects:** Suppression of arrhythmias.

Adverse Reactions/Side Effects

CNS: dizziness, anxiety, fatigue, headache, mental depression. **EENT:** blurred vision, visual disturbances. **CV:** ARRHYTHMIAS, CHEST PAIN, CHF. **GI:** anorexia, constipation, drug-induced hepatitis, nausea, stomach pain, vomiting. **Derm:** rashes. **Neuro:** tremor.

PHYSICAL THERAPY IMPLICATIONS

Examination and Evaluation

- Assess heart rate, ECG, and heart sounds, especially during exercise (See Appendices G, H). Although intended to treat certain arrhythmias, this drug can unmask or precipitate new arrhythmias (proarrhythmic effect). Report any rhythm disturbances or symptoms of increased arrhythmias, including palpitations, chest pain, shortness of breath, fainting, and fatigue/weakness.
- Watch for signs of congestive heart failure (CHF), including dyspnea, rales/crackles, peripheral edema, jugular venous distention, and exercise intolerance. Report these signs to the physician immediately.
- Assess dizziness that might affect gait, balance, and other functional activities (See Appendix C). Report balance problems and functional limitations to the physician, and caution the patient and family/caregivers to guard against falls and trauma.

Interventions

- Because of the risk of CHF and serious cardiac arrhythmias, use extreme caution during aerobic exercise and other forms of therapeutic exercise. Assess exercise tolerance frequently (blood pressure, heart rate, fatigue levels), and terminate exercise immediately if any untoward responses occur (See Appendix L).

Patient/Client-Related Instruction

- Advise patient and family/caregivers about the signs of CHF and cardiac arrhythmias (See above under Examination and Evaluation), and to seek immediate medical assistance if these signs develop.
- Advise patient about the likelihood of GI reactions such as nausea, vomiting, constipation, stomach pain, and loss of appetite. Instruct patient to report severe or prolonged GI problems or signs of drug-induced hepatitis (yellow skin or eyes, abdominal pain, severe nausea and vomiting, fever, sore throat, malaise, weakness, facial edema).
- Instruct patient and family/caregivers to report other side effects such as severe or prolonged headache, vision problems, tremor, fatigue, or skin rash.

Pharmacokinetics

Absorption: Well absorbed from the GI tract following oral administration.
Distribution: Widely distributed.
Metabolism and Excretion: Mostly metabolized by liver; 30% excreted unchanged by kidneys.
Half-life: 11–14 hr.

TIME/ACTION PROFILE (antiarrhythmic effects)

ROUTE	ONSET	PEAK	DURATION
PO	days	days–wks	12 hr

Contraindications/Precautions

Contraindicated in: Hypersensitivity; Cardiogenic shock.
Use Cautiously in: CHF (dosage reduction may be required); Preexisting sinus node dysfunction or 2nd- or 3rd-degree heart block (without a pacemaker); Renal impairment (dosage reduction required if CCr <35 mL/min); Pregnancy, lactation, or children (safety not established).

Interactions

Drug-Drug: ↑ risk of arrhythmias with other **antiarrhythmics**, including **calcium channel blockers. Disopyramide, beta blockers,** or **verapamil** may have ↑ myocardial depressant effects; combination use should be undertaken cautiously. **Amiodarone** doubles serum flecainide levels (↓ flecainide dose by 50%). Increases serum **digoxin** levels by a small amount (15–25%). Concurrent **beta blocker** therapy may cause ↑ levels of beta blocker and flecainide. **Alkalinizing agents** promote reabsorption, ↑ blood levels, and may cause toxicity. **Acidifying agents** ↑ renal elimination and may ↓ effectiveness of flecainide (if urine pH <5).
Drug-Food: Foods that ↑ **urine pH** to >7 result in ↑ levels (strict **vegetarian diet**). **Foods or beverages that** ↓ **urine pH** to <5 ↑ renal elimination and may ↓ effectiveness of flecainide **(acidic juices)**.

Route/Dosage

Ventricular Tachycardia

PO (Adults): 100 mg q 12 hr initially, increased by 50 mg bid until response is obtained or maximum total daily dose of 400 mg is reached. Some patients may require q 8 hr dosing.

Renal Impairment

PO (Adults): *CCr <35 mL/min*—100 mg once a day or 50 mg q 12 hr initially; further dosing on the basis of frequent blood level monitoring.

PSVT/PAF

PO (Adults): 50 mg q 12 hr initially, increased by 50 mg bid until response is obtained or maximum total daily dose of 300 mg is reached. Some patients may require q 8 hr dosing.

Atrial Fibrillation (unlabeled)

PO (Adults): 200 mg or 300-mg single dose.

Availability (generic available)

Tablets: 50 mg, 100 mg, 150 mg.

HIGH ALERT

floxuridine (flox-yoor-i-deen)

FUDR

Classification
Therapeutic: antineoplastics
Pharmacologic: antimetabolites

Indications

Treatment of hepatic metastases of gastrointestinal carcinoma.

Action

Inhibits DNA and RNA synthesis by preventing thymidine production (cell-cycle S phase–specific). **Therapeutic Effects:** Death of rapidly replicating cells, particularly malignant ones.

Adverse Reactions/Side Effects

CNS: headache, fatigue. **GI:** bleeding, diarrhea, gastritis, nausea, stomatitis, vomiting, anorexia, ulcer. **Derm:** alopecia, erythema, maculopapular rash. **Endo:** gonadal suppression. **Hemat:** anemia, leukopenia, thrombocytopenia. **Misc:** fever.

PHYSICAL THERAPY IMPLICATIONS

Examination and Evaluation

- Monitor signs of leukopenia (fever, sore throat, signs of infection), thrombocytopenia (bruising, nose bleeds, and bleeding gums), or unusual weakness and fatigue that might be due to anemia. Report these signs to the physician immediately.

Interventions

- For patients who are medically able to begin exercise, implement appropriate resistive exercises and aerobic training to maintain muscle strength and aerobic capacity during cancer chemotherapy or to help restore function after chemotherapy.

Patient/Client-Related Instruction

- Advise patient and family/caregivers about the risk of infections, to guard against infection (frequent hand washing, etc.), and to avoid crowds and contact with persons with contagious diseases.
- Advise patient and family/caregivers that fatigue and weakness are likely and may be severe. Functional abilities may be limited, and patient may need to use assistive devices during ambulation.

- Advise patient about the likelihood of GI reactions such as nausea, vomiting, diarrhea, stomach pain, loss of appetite, and irritation of the mouth. Instruct patient to report severe or prolonged GI problems or signs of ulceration and GI bleeding (abdominal pain, vomiting blood, blood in the stools, black/tarry stools).
- Instruct patient and family/caregivers to report other troublesome side effects such as severe or prolonged headache, fever, or skin reactions (rash, warmth, redness, hair loss).

Pharmacokinetics

Absorption: Administered intra-arterially only, resulting in direct delivery to tumor sites.
Distribution: Distributes mostly to tumor site as a result of elective intra-arterial administration.
Metabolism and Excretion: Rapidly converted to floxuridine monophosphate (an active metabolite) and fluorouracil; 60–80% excreted by the lungs as respiratory CO. Small amounts of fluorouracil (<10–15%) excreted unchanged by the kidneys.
Half-life: *Fluorouracil*—20 hr.

TIME/ACTION PROFILE (effects on blood counts*)

ROUTE	ONSET	PEAK	DURATION
Intra-arterial	1–9 days	9–21 days	30 days

*Noted as effects due to conversion to fluorouracil.

Contraindications/Precautions

Contraindicated in: Hypersensitivity; Pregnancy or lactation.
Use Cautiously in: Patients with childbearing potential; Hepatic or renal dysfunction; History of high-dose pelvic irradiation or previous use of alkylating agents; Infections; Depressed bone marrow reserve.

Interactions

Drug-Drug: Additive bone marrow depression with other **bone marrow depressants** (other **antineoplastics** and **radiation therapy**). Concomitant use of pentostatin may cause fatal pulmonary toxicity (avoid concurrent use). May decrease antibody response to **live-virus vaccines** and increase risk of adverse reactions.

Route/Dosage

IA (Adults): 0.1–0.6 mg/kg/day as a continuous infusion for 14 days, followed by a 2-wk rest (only heparinized saline administered during this rest period).

Availability (generic available)

Powder for injection: 500 mg in 5- or 10-mL vials.

fluconazole (floo-kon-a-zole)

Diflucan

Classification
Therapeutic: antifungals (systemic)
Pharmacologic: azoles

F

Indications

PO, IV: Fungal infections caused by susceptible organisms, including Oropharyngeal or esophageal candidiasis, Serious systemic candidal infections, Urinary tract infections, Peritonitis, Cryptococcal meningitis. Prevention of candidiasis in patients who have undergone bone marrow transplantation. **PO:** Single-dose oral treatment of vaginal candidiasis. **Unlabeled Use:** Prevention of recurrent vaginal yeast infections.

Action

Inhibits synthesis of fungal sterols, a necessary component of the cell membrane. **Therapeutic Effects:** Fungistatic action against susceptible organisms. May be fungicidal in higher concentrations. **Spectrum:** *Cryptococcus neoformans*. *Candida* spp.

Adverse Reactions/Side Effects

Incidence of adverse reactions is increased in HIV patients

CNS: headache, dizziness, seizures. **GI:** HEPATOTOXICITY, abdominal discomfort, diarrhea, nausea, vomiting. **Derm:** EXFOLIATIVE SKIN DISORDERS, INCLUDING STEVENS-JOHNSON SYNDROME. **Endo:** hypokalemia, hypertriglyceridemia. **Misc:** allergic reactions, including anaphylaxis.

PHYSICAL THERAPY IMPLICATIONS

Examination and Evaluation

- Be alert for signs of hepatotoxicity, including anorexia, abdominal pain, severe nausea and vomiting, yellow skin or eyes, fever, sore throat, malaise, weakness, facial edema, lethargy, and unusual bleeding or bruising. Notify physician of these signs immediately.
- Monitor rashes or other skin reactions such as exfoliation, hives, itching, raised patches of red or white skin (welts), burning, acne, and abnormal sweating. Notify physician immediately because certain skin responses may indicate serious allergic reactions such as Stevens-Johnson syndrome.
- Monitor other signs of allergic reactions and anaphylaxis, including pulmonary symptoms such

as tightness in the throat and chest, wheezing, cough, and dyspnea. Notify physician immediately if these reactions occur.

- Be alert for new seizures or increased seizure activity, especially at the onset of drug treatment. Document the number, duration, and severity of seizures, and report these findings to the physician immediately.
- Monitor any muscle weakness, aches, or cramps that might indicate low potassium levels (hypokalemia). Notify physician immediately if these signs occur.
- Assess dizziness that might affect gait, balance, and other functional activities (See Appendix C). Report balance problems and functional limitations to the physician and nursing staff, and caution the patient and family/caregivers to guard against falls and trauma.

Interventions

- Always wash hands thoroughly and disinfect equipment (whirlpools, electrotherapeutic devices, treatment tables, and so forth) to help prevent the spread of infection. Employ universal precautions or isolation procedures as indicated for specific patients.

Patient/Client-Related Instruction

- Advise patient to take this drug as directed for the full course of treatment even if feeling better.
- Advise patient that this drug may cause problems in fat metabolism, including increased triglycerides. Remind patient that periodic blood tests may be needed to monitor plasma lipids.
- Instruct patient to report other troublesome side effects such as prolonged or severe headache or GI reactions (diarrhea, nausea, vomiting, abdominal pain).

Pharmacokinetics

Absorption: Well absorbed after oral administration.
Distribution: Widely distributed, good penetration into CSF, saliva, sputum, vaginal fluid, skin, eye, and peritoneum. Excreted in breast milk.
Metabolism and Excretion: >80% excreted unchanged by the kidneys; <10% metabolized by the liver.
Half-life: Premature neonates: 46–74 hr; Children: 19–25 hr (PO) and 15–17 hr (IV); Adults: 30 hr (increased in renal impairment).

TIME/ACTION PROFILE (blood levels)

ROUTE	ONSET	PEAK	DURATION
PO	unknown	2–4 hr	24 hr
IV	rapid	end of infusion	24 hr

Contraindications/Precautions

Contraindicated in: Hypersensitivity to fluconazole or other azole antifungals; Concurrent use with pimozide.

Use Cautiously in: Renal impairment (dose reduction required if CCr <50 mL/min); Geri: Increased risk of adverse reactions (rash, vomiting, diarrhea, seizures); consider age-related decrease in renal function in determining dose; Underlying liver disease; OB/Pedi: Pregnancy, lactation, or children (safety not established).

Interactions

Drug-Drug: ↑ activity of **warfarin**. **Rifampin, rifabutin**, and **isoniazid** ↓ levels. Fluconazole at doses >200 mg/day may inhibit the CYP3A4 enzyme system and affect the activity of drugs metabolized by this system. ↑ hypoglycemic effects of **tolbutamide, glyburide**, or **glipizide**. ↑ levels and risk of toxicity from **cyclosporine, rifabutin, tacrolimus, theophylline, zidovudine, alfentanil**, and **phenytoin**. ↑ levels and effects of **benzodiazepines, zolpidem, buspirone, nisoldipine, tricyclic antidepressants**, and **losartan**. May ↑ risk of bleeding with **warfarin**. May antagonize effects of **amphotericin B**.

Route/Dosage

Oropharyngeal Candidiasis

PO, IV (Adults): 200 mg initially, then 100 mg daily for at least 2 wk.
PO, IV (Children >14 days): 6 mg/kg initially, then 3 mg/kg/day for at least 2 wk.
PO, IV (Neonates <14 days, 30–36 wk gestation): same dose as older children except frequency is q 48 hr; Premature neonates <29 weeks gestation: 5–6 mg/kg/dose q 48–72 hr.

Esophageal Candidiasis

PO, IV (Adults): 200 mg initially, then 100 mg once daily for at least 3 wk (up to 400 mg/day).
PO, IV (Children >14 days): 6 mg/kg initially, then 3–12 mg/kg/day for at least 3 wk.
PO, IV (Neonates <14 days, 30–36 wk gestation): same dose as older children except frequency is q 48 hr; Premature neonates <29 wk gestation: 5–6 mg/kg/dose q 48–72 hr.

Vaginal Candidiasis

PO (Adults): 150-mg single dose; prevention of recurrence (unlabeled)—150 mg daily for 3 days then weekly for 6 mo.

Systemic Candidiasis

PO, IV (Adults): 400 mg/day initially, then 200–800 mg/day for 28 days.
PO, IV (Children >14 days): 6–12 mg/kg/day for 28 days.
PO, IV (Neonates <14 days, 30–36 wk gestation): same dose as older children except frequency is q 48 hr; Premature neonates <29 weeks gestation: 5–6 mg/kg/dose q 48–72 hr.

Cryptococcal Meningitis

PO, IV (Adults): *Treatment*—400 mg once daily until favorable clinical response, then 200–800 mg once daily for at least 10–12 wk after clearing of CSF; change to oral therapy as soon as possible. *Suppressive therapy*—200 mg once daily.
PO, IV (Children >14 days): 12 mg/kg/day initially, then 6–12 mg/kg/day for at least 10–12 wk after clearing of CSF; change to oral therapy as soon as possible. *Suppressive therapy*—6 mg/kg/day.
PO, IV (Neonates <14 days, 30–36 wk gestation): same dose as older children except frequency is q 48 hr; Premature neonates <29 weeks gestation: 5–6 mg/kg/dose q 48–72 hr.

Prevention of Candidiasis After Bone Marrow Transplant

PO, IV (Adults): 400 mg once daily; begin several days before procedure if severe neutropenia is expected, and continue for 7 days after ANC >1000 /mm^3.
PO, IV (Children >14 days): 10–12 mg/kg/day, not to exceed 600 mg/day.

Renal Impairment

PO, IV (Adults): *CCr 11–50 mL/min*—50% of the usual dose.

Availability (generic available)

Tablets: 50 mg, 100 mg, 150 mg, 200 mg. **Oral suspension (orange flavor):** 10 mg/mL in 35-mL bottle, 40 mg/mL in 35-mL bottle. **Premixed infusion:** 2 mg/mL in 100- or 200-mL bottles/containers.

flucytosine (floo-sye-toe-seen)

Ancobon, Ancotil, 5-FC

Classification
Therapeutic: antifungals
Pharmacologic: fluorinated pyrimidine analogs

Indications

Treatment of serious fungal infections, including Endocarditis, Meningitis, Septicemia, Urinary tract infections, Pulmonary infections.

Action

Following penetration into fungi, converted to fluorouracil, which interferes with fungal DNA and RNA synthesis. Synergistic action with amphotericin B against some fungi. **Therapeutic Effects:** Fungicidal action against susceptible organisms. **Spectrum:** Active against only a small number of fungi, mainly: *Candida*, *Cryptococcus*.

Adverse Reactions/Side Effects

CNS: SEIZURES, ataxia, confusion, dizziness, drowsiness, fatigue, headache. **CV:** chest pain. **EENT:** hearing loss. **GI:** diarrhea, nausea, vomiting, abdominal pain, dry mouth. **Derm:** photosensitivity, pruritus, rash, urticaria. **Endo:** hypoglycemia. **F and E:** hypokalemia. **GU:** azotemia. **Hemat:** APLASTIC ANEMIA, eosinophilia, leukopenia, pancytopenia, anemia, thrombocytopenia. **Neuro:** peripheral neuropathy. **Resp:** dyspnea. **Misc:** fever.

PHYSICAL THERAPY IMPLICATIONS

Examination and Evaluation

- Be alert for new seizures or increased seizure activity, especially at the onset of drug treatment. Document the number, duration, and severity of seizures, and report these findings to the physician immediately.
- Monitor signs of blood dyscrasias, including aplastic anemia (fatigue, pallor, shortness of breath with exertion), eosinophilia (weakness, myalgia), leukopenia (fever, sore throat, signs of infection), thrombocytopenia (bruising, nose bleeds, bleeding gums), or unusual weakness and fatigue that might be due to other anemias and blood dyscrasias. Notify physician of these signs immediately.
- Monitor signs of peripheral neuropathy (numbness, tingling, muscle weakness). Perform objective tests (nerve conduction, monofilaments) to assess and document any neuropathic changes.
- Assess dizziness, drowsiness, or ataxia that might affect gait, balance, and other functional activities. Report balance problems and functional limitations to the physician, and caution the patient and family/caregivers to guard against falls and trauma.
- Monitor any chest pain or difficult, labored breathing. Attempt to determine if pain is drug induced or caused by cardiovascular and pulmonary dysfunction (e.g., angina that occurs during exercise). Report any problematic cardiorespiratory symptoms.
- Monitor signs of hypoglycemia, including weakness, malaise, irritability, and fatigue. Patients with diabetes mellitus should check blood glucose levels frequently.
- Monitor and report signs of low potassium levels (hypokalemia), such as muscle weakness, aches, and cramps.
- Monitor signs of increased nitrogenous compounds in the blood (azotemia), including confusion, decreased alertness, tachycardia, pallor, fatigue, dry mouth, thirst, and decreased/absent urine production. Notify physician of these signs immediately.

Interventions

- Always wash hands thoroughly and disinfect equipment (whirlpools, electrotherapeutic devices, treatment tables, and so forth) to help prevent the spread of infection. Employ universal precautions or isolation procedures as indicated for specific patients.
- Causes photosensitivity; use care if administering UV treatments. Advise patient to avoid direct sunlight and use sunscreens and protective clothing.

Patient/Client-Related Instruction

- Advise patient to take this drug as directed for the full course of treatment even if feeling better.
- Instruct patient and family/caregivers to report other troublesome side effects such as severe or prolonged headache, fever, hearing loss, skin disorders (rash, hives, itching), or GI problems (nausea, vomiting, diarrhea, abdominal pain, dry mouth).

Pharmacokinetics

Absorption: Well absorbed (80–90%) from the GI tract following oral administration.
Distribution: Widely distributed. Crosses the blood-brain barrier.
Metabolism and Excretion: 80–90% excreted unchanged by the kidneys.
Half-life: 2.5–5 hr (increased in renal impairment).

TIME/ACTION PROFILE (antifungal blood levels)

ROUTE	ONSET	PEAK	DURATION
PO	rapid	1–2 hr	6 hr

Contraindications/Precautions

Contraindicated in: Hypersensitivity; Pregnancy or lactation.
Use Cautiously in: Bone marrow depression (especially following radiation therapy or antineoplastics).
Exercise Extreme Caution in: Renal impairment (blood level monitoring, lower dose, and increased dosage interval recommended if CCr <40 mL/min).

Interactions

Drug-Drug: Additive bone marrow depression with other **bone marrow–depressant drugs**, including **antineoplastics** and **radiation therapy**. **Amphotericin B** may ↑ toxicity of flucytosine but may also ↑ its antifungal activity. **Cytarabine** may ↓ its antifungal activity.

Route/Dosage

PO (Adults): 12.5–37.5 mg/kg q 6 hr.
PO (Children): 12.5–37.5 mg/kg q 6 hr.

Renal Impairment

PO (Adults): *CCr 20–40 mL/min*—12.5 mg/kg q 12 hr; *CCr 10–20 mL/min*—12.5 mg/kg q 24 hr; *CCr <10 mL/min*—12.5 mg/kg q 24–48 hr.

Availability

Capsules: 250 mg, 500 mg.

HIGH ALERT

fludarabine (floo-dar-a-been)

Fludara

Classification
Therapeutic: antineoplastics
Pharmacologic: antimetabolites

Indications

B-cell chronic lymphocytic leukemia unresponsive to standard therapy. **Unlabeled Use:** Non-Hodgkin's lymphoma.

Action

Converted intracellularly to an active phosphorylated metabolite that inhibits DNA synthesis. **Therapeutic Effects:** Death of rapidly replicating cells, particularly malignant ones.

Adverse Reactions/Side Effects

CNS: NEUROTOXICITY, fatigue, agitation, coma, confusion, headache, malaise, weakness. **EENT:** hearing loss, visual disturbances. **Resp:** PULMONARY HYPERSENSITIVITY, cough, pneumonia, dyspnea, sinusitis. **CV:** edema. **GI:** GI BLEEDING, diarrhea, nausea, anorexia, esophagitis, mucositis, stomatitis, vomiting. **GU:** dysuria, hematuria, urinary tract infection. **Derm:** rashes. **Endo:** gonadal suppression. **Hemat:** PANCYTOPENIA, anemia, leukopenia, thrombocytopenia, hemolytic anemia. **MS:** myalgia. **Neuro:** peripheral neuropathy. **Misc:** fever, tumor lysis syndrome.

PHYSICAL THERAPY IMPLICATIONS

Examination and Evaluation

- Monitor signs of CNS toxicity, including confusion, agitation, severe headache, hearing loss, visual disturbances, and decreased consciousness. Notify physician, especially if patient becomes unresponsive or difficult to arouse.
- Assess pulmonary function periodically by measuring lung volumes, breath sounds, and respiratory rate (See Appendices I, J, K). Notify physician or nursing staff immediately if patient experiences signs of pulmonary hypersensitivity (dry cough, dyspnea, tightness in the throat and chest, shortness of breath, cyanosis).
- Monitor signs of GI bleeding, including abdominal pain, vomiting blood, blood in stools, or black, tarry stools. Report these signs to the physician or nursing staff immediately.
- Watch for signs of blood dyscrasias such as leukopenia (fever, sore throat, signs of infection), thrombocytopenia (bleeding gums, bruising, petechiae, hematuria), or unusual weakness and

fatigue that might be due to aplastic anemia or other anemias. Report these signs to the physician or nursing staff immediately.

- Assess peripheral edema using girth measurements, volume displacement, and measurement of pitting edema (See Appendix N). Report increased swelling in feet and ankles or a sudden increase in body weight due to fluid retention.
- Assess numbness, tingling, or weakness that might indicate peripheral neuropathy. Establish baseline electroneuromyographic values using EMG and nerve conduction whenever possible. Periodically reexamine these values to document drug-induced changes in peripheral nerve function.
- Monitor neuromuscular signs of electrolyte imbalances that might indicate tumor lysis syndrome. Signs include severe muscle weakness or paralysis due to increased plasma potassium (hyperkalemia) or muscle hyperexcitability and tetany due to phosphate and calcium imbalances (hyperphosphatemia and hypocalcemia). Notify physician or nursing staff immediately if these signs occur.

Interventions

- For patients who are medically able to begin exercise, implement appropriate resistive exercises and aerobic training to maintain muscle strength and aerobic capacity during cancer chemotherapy or to help restore function after chemotherapy.
- Because of the risk of pulmonary hypersensitivity, assess pulmonary function during exercise, and terminate exercise if patient exhibits untoward symptoms (severe shortness of breath or fatigue) or displays other criteria for exercise termination (See Appendix L).

Patient/Client-Related Instruction

- Because of immunosuppressant effects, advise patient to decrease risk of infections (frequent hand washing, etc.) and avoid contact with persons with contagious diseases.
- Advise patient about the likelihood of GI reactions, including nausea, vomiting, diarrhea, loss of appetite, heartburn, and inflammation in or around the mouth. Instruct patient to report severe or prolonged GI problems or signs of GI bleeding (blood in stools, black, tarry stools).
- Advise patient and family/caregivers that fatigue, weakness, and muscle aches (myalgia) are likely and may be severe. Functional abilities may be limited, and patient may need to use assistive devices during ambulation.
- Advise patient that rash and other skin reactions are likely. Report severe or unexpected skin reactions to the physician.
- Instruct patient and family/caregivers to report other troublesome side effects such as severe or prolonged headache, fever, or problems with urination (urinary tract infection, difficult/painful urination).

Pharmacokinetics

Absorption: Administered IV only, resulting in complete bioavailability.
Distribution: Extensively distributed.
Metabolism and Excretion: Following administration, rapidly converted to an active metabolite, which, when phosphorylated intracellularly, exerts antineoplastic activity; 40% of initial active metabolite excreted unchanged by the kidneys.
Half-life: 20 hr (for initial active metabolite).

TIME/ACTION PROFILE (effects on blood counts)

ROUTE	ONSET	PEAK	DURATION
IV	7 wk*	13–16 days	unknown

*Median time to response.

Contraindications/Precautions

Contraindicated in: Hypersensitivity to fludarabine, mannitol, or sodium hydroxide; Patients taking pentostatin; Pregnancy or lactation; Severe renal impairment (CCr <30 mL/min).
Use Cautiously in: Moderate renal impairment (↓ dose if CCr <70 mL/min); Patients with childbearing potential; Bone marrow depression; Children (safety not established).

Interactions

Drug-Drug: ↑ bone marrow suppression with other **antineoplastics** or **radiation therapy**. Concomitant use with **pentostatin** ↑ risk of potentially fatal pulmonary toxicity (concurrent use not recommended).

Route/Dosage

IV (Adults): 25 mg/m² daily for 5 days; repeat course every 28 days.

Renal Impairment

IV (Adults): *CCr 30–70 mL/min*— decrease dose by 20%.

Availability

Powder for injection: 50 mg/vial. **Solution for injection:** 25 mg/mL in 2-mL vials.

fludrocortisone

(floo-droe-**kor**-ti-sone)

Florinef

Classification

Therapeutic: hormones

Pharmacologic: corticosteroids (mineralocorticoid)

Indications

Sodium loss and hypotension associated with adrenocortical insufficiency (given with hydrocortisone or cortisone). Management of sodium loss due to congenital adrenogenital syndrome (congenital adrenal hyperplasia). **Unlabeled Use:** Idiopathic orthostatic hypotension (with increased sodium intake). Type IV renal tubular acidosis.

Action

Causes sodium reabsorption, hydrogen and potassium excretion, and water retention by its effects on the distal renal tubule. **Therapeutic Effects:** Maintenance of sodium balance and blood pressure in patients with adrenocortical insufficiency.

Adverse Reactions/Side Effects

CNS: dizziness, headache. **CV:** CHF, arrhythmias, edema, hypertension. **GI:** anorexia, nausea. **Endo:** adrenal suppression, weight gain. **F and E:** hypokalemia, hypokalemic alkalosis. **MS:** arthralgia, muscular weakness, tendon contractures. **Neuro:** ascending paralysis. **Misc:** hypersensitivity reactions.

PHYSICAL THERAPY IMPLICATIONS

Examination and Evaluation

- Watch for signs of congestive heart failure, including dyspnea, rales/crackles, peripheral edema, jugular venous distention, and exercise intolerance. Report these signs to the physician immediately.
- Assess heart rate, ECG, and heart sounds, especially during exercise (See Appendices G, H). Report any rhythm disturbances or symptoms of increased arrhythmias, including palpitations, chest discomfort, shortness of breath, fainting, and fatigue/weakness.
- Assess blood pressure (BP) and compare to normal values (See Appendix F). Report a sustained increase in BP (hypertension).
- Monitor and report signs of low potassium levels (hypokalemia) or hypokalemic alkalosis. Signs include headache, lethargy, cardiac arrhythmias, and muscle dysfunction (muscle weakness, aches, cramps). Notify physician immediately if these signs occur.
- Report signs of adrenal suppression, including hypotension, weight loss, weakness, nausea, vomiting, anorexia, lethargy, confusion, and restlessness.
- Watch for weakness in the lower extremities that migrates progressively toward the trunk, arms, and neck (ascending paralysis). Report these symptoms to the physician immediately.
- Be alert for signs of hypersensitivity reactions, including pulmonary symptoms (tightness in the throat and chest, wheezing, cough, dyspnea) or skin reactions (rash, pruritus, urticaria). Notify physician immediately if these reactions occur.
- Assess peripheral edema using girth measurements, volume displacement, and measurement of pitting edema (See Appendix N). Report increased swelling in feet and ankles or a sudden increase in body weight due to fluid retention.
- Assess any joint pain, tendon contractures, or other muscle abnormalities to rule out musculoskeletal pathology; that is, try to determine if pain is drug induced rather than caused by anatomic or biomechanical problems.
- Assess dizziness that might affect gait, balance, and other functional activities (See Appendix C). Report balance problems and functional limitations to the physician, and caution the patient and family/caregivers to guard against falls and trauma.
- Periodically assess body weight and other anthropometric measures (body mass index, body composition). Report a rapid or unexplained weight gain or increased body fat.

Interventions

- Because of an increased risk of cardiac arrhythmias, CHF, and hypertension, use caution during aerobic exercise and endurance conditioning. Terminate exercise if patient exhibits untoward symptoms (chest pain, shortness of breath, unusual fatigue), or displays other criteria for exercise termination (See Appendix L).
- To minimize orthostatic hypotension, patient should move slowly when assuming a more upright position.

Patient/Client-Related Instruction

- Remind patients to take medication as directed to control sodium and water balance even if they are asymptomatic.
- Advise patients on long-term treatment to consult physician before stopping this medication. Stopping the medication suddenly may result in adrenocortical shock (severe hypotension, hypoglycemia, weakness, vomiting). If these signs appear, notify health care professional immediately; may be life threatening.
- Instruct patient or family/caregivers to report other troublesome side effects such as severe or prolonged headache or GI problems (nausea, loss of appetite).

Pharmacokinetics

Absorption: Well absorbed following oral administration.
Distribution: Widely distributed; probably enters breast milk.
Protein Binding: High.
Metabolism and Excretion: Mostly metabolized by the liver.
Half-life: 3.5 hr.

TIME/ACTION PROFILE (mineralocorticoid activity)

ROUTE	ONSET	PEAK	DURATION
PO	unknown	unknown	1–2 days

Contraindications/Precautions

Contraindicated in: Hypersensitivity.
Use Cautiously in: CHF; Addison's disease (patients may have exaggerated response); Pregnancy, lactation, or children (safety not established).

Interactions

Drug-Drug: Use with **thiazide** or **loop diuretics**, **piperacillin**, or **amphotericin B** may result in ↑ risk of hypokalemia. Hypokalemia may ↑ risk of **digoxin** toxicity. May produce prolonged neuromuscular blockade following the use of **nondepolarizing neuromuscular blocking agents. Phenobarbital** or **rifampin** may ↑ metabolism and ↓ effectiveness of fludrocortisone.
Drug-Food: Large amounts of **salt** or **sodium-containing foods** may cause excessive sodium retention and potassium loss.

Route/Dosage

PO (Adults): *Adrenocortical insufficiency*—100 mcg/day (range 100 mcg 3 times weekly—200 mcg daily). Doses as small as 50 mcg daily may be required by some patients. Use with 10–37.5 mg cortisone daily or 10–30 mg hydrocortisone daily. *Adrenogenital syndrome*—100–200 mcg/day. *Idiopathic hypotension*—50–200 mcg/day (unlabeled).
PO (Children): 50–100 mcg/day.

Availability (generic available)

Tablets: 100 mcg (0.1 mg).

flunisolide (floo-nis-oh-lide)

AeroBid, AeroBid-M

Classification
Therapeutic: anti-inflammatories (steroidal)
Pharmacologic: corticosteroids

Indications

Maintenance treatment of asthma as prophylactic therapy. May decrease requirement for or eliminate use of systemic corticosteroids in patients with asthma.

Action

Potent, locally acting anti-inflammatory and immune modifier. **Therapeutic Effects:** Decreased frequency and severity of asthma attacks. Improves asthma symptoms.

Adverse Reactions/Side Effects

CNS: headache, dizziness, irritability, nervousness. **CV:** palpitations. **EENT:** hoarseness, nasal congestion, pharyngitis, dysphonia, oropharyngeal fungal infections, rhinitis, sinusitis. **Resp:** bronchospasm, cough, wheezing. **Derm:** rash. **GI:** diarrhea, nausea, taste disturbances, vomiting, abdominal pain, anorexia, dry mouth. **GU:** menstrual disturbances. **Endo:** adrenal suppression (high-dose, long-term therapy only), decreased growth (children). **Misc:** flu-like syndrome.

PHYSICAL THERAPY IMPLICATIONS

Examination and Evaluation

- Assess pulmonary function periodically by measuring lung volumes, breath sounds, respiratory rate, and other symptoms (wheezing, dyspnea, shortness of breath) (See Appendices I, J, K). Report changes in pulmonary function to help document the effects of drug therapy in treating asthma.
- Observe for paradoxical bronchospasm (cough, wheezing, dyspnea), especially at higher or excessive doses. If condition occurs, advise patient to withhold medication and notify physician immediately.
- Assess muscle strength periodically during long-term use. Although inhalation reduces the risk of systemic musculoskeletal damage, some degree of weakness and bone loss may still occur during prolonged, extensive use.
- Report CNS problems such as headache, dizziness, irritability, and nervousness. Excessive or prolonged CNS symptoms may require a reduction in dose.
- Report signs of adrenal suppression, including hypotension, weight loss, weakness, nausea, vomiting, anorexia, lethargy, confusion, and restlessness.
- Assess growth rate in children receiving chronic therapy; report delayed or stunted growth to the physician.

Interventions

- Implement resistive exercises and weight-bearing activities to minimize muscle wasting and osteoporosis. Use caution to prevent musculoskeletal damage in patients with preexisting muscle and bone loss.

- Design and implement appropriate aerobic exercise and respiratory muscle training programs to maintain optimal cardiovascular and pulmonary function. Work with patient and family/caregivers to find forms of exercise (e.g., swimming) that can help improve respiratory function without triggering asthma attacks.
- Protect skin from breakdown, especially over bony prominences.

Patient/Client-Related Instruction

- Counsel patient on proper use of metered-dose inhaler; observe use of this device whenever possible to ensure proper technique.
- Advise patient not to exceed the recommended dose or frequency of inhalations. Contact physician immediately if bronchospasm is not relieved by medication or is accompanied by severe headache or other symptoms.
- Caution patient not to use this drug to treat acute symptoms. A rapid-acting inhaled beta-adrenergic bronchodilator is typically used for relief of acute asthma attacks.
- Advise patient about the likelihood of upper respiratory tract infection or irritation, including hoarseness, nasal congestion, pharyngitis, sinusitis, and rhinitis. Instruct patient to report severe or prolonged upper respiratory problems to the physician.
- Instruct patient to report any loss of vision that might indicate cataracts or increased intraocular pressure.
- Advise patient that corticosteroids cause immunosuppression and may mask symptoms of infection. Instruct patient to avoid people with known contagious illnesses and to report possible infections immediately.
- Advise patients on long-term treatment to consult physician before stopping this medication. Stopping the medication suddenly may result in adrenocortical shock (severe hypotension, hypoglycemia, weakness, vomiting). If these signs appear, notify physician immediately; may be life threatening.
- Instruct patient and family/caregivers to report other troublesome side effects such as severe or prolonged skin rash, palpitations, flu-like symptoms, menstrual problems, or GI problems (nausea, vomiting, diarrhea, abdominal pain, loss of appetite).

Pharmacokinetics

Absorption: 40%; action is primarily local following inhalation.
Distribution: Crosses placenta; enters breast milk in small amounts.
Metabolism and Excretion: Metabolized by the liver following absorption from lungs; 50% excreted in urine, 50% in feces.
Half-life: 1.8 hr.

TIME/ACTION PROFILE (improvement in symptoms)

ROUTE	ONSET	PEAK	DURATION
inhalation	within 24 hr	1–4 wk*	unknown

*Improvement in pulmonary function; decreased airway responsiveness may take longer.

Contraindications/Precautions

Contraindicated in: Hypersensitivity (product contains chlorofluorocarbon propellants); Acute attack of asthma/status asthmaticus.
Use Cautiously in: Active untreated infections; Diabetes or glaucoma; Underlying immunosuppression (due to disease or concurrent therapy); Systemic corticosteroid therapy (should not be abruptly discontinued when inhalable therapy is started; additional corticosteroids needed in stress or trauma); Pregnancy, lactation, or children <6 yr (safety not established; prolonged or high-dose therapy may lead to complications).

Interactions

Drug-Drug: None known.

Route/Dosage

Inhalation (Adults and Children >15 yr): 2 inhalations twice daily (not to exceed 4 inhalations twice daily).
Inhalation (Children 6–15 yr): 2 inhalations twice daily (not to exceed 2 inhalations twice daily).

Availability

Inhalation aerosol: 250 mcg/metered inhalation in 7-g canisters (delivers 100 metered inhalations) Rx. **Inhalation aerosol-menthol (Aerobid-M):** 250 mcg/metered inhalation in 7-g canisters (delivers 100 metered inhalations) Rx.

fluocinolone
(floo-oh-**sin**-oh-lone)
Derma-Smoothe/FS, ✱Fluoderm, Fluolar, FS Shampoo, Synalar, Synamol

Classification
Therapeutic: anti-inflammatories (steroidal)
Pharmacologic: corticosteroids

Indications

Management of inflammation and pruritus associated with various allergic/immunologic skin problems.

Action
Suppresses normal immune response and inflammation. **Therapeutic Effects:** Suppression of dermatologic inflammation and immune processes.

Adverse Reactions/Side Effects
Derm: allergic contact dermatitis, atrophy, burning, dryness, edema, folliculitis, hypersensitivity reactions, hypertrichosis, hypopigmentation, irritation, maceration, miliaria, perioral dermatitis, secondary infection, striae. **Misc:** adrenal suppression (use of occlusive dressings, long-term therapy).

PHYSICAL THERAPY IMPLICATIONS

Examination and Evaluation
- Assess the area being treated to help document whether drug therapy is successful in resolving skin conditions.
- Monitor any new or increased reactions at the site of application, including inflammation, irritation, infection, burning, swelling, exfoliation, and rash. Report severe or prolonged skin reactions to the physician.
- Report signs of adrenal suppression, including hypotension, weight loss, weakness, nausea, vomiting, anorexia, lethargy, confusion, and restlessness.

Interventions
- Protect skin from breakdown, especially over bony prominences.

Patient/Client-Related Instruction
- Advise patients on long-term treatment to consult physician before stopping this medication. Stopping the medication suddenly may result in adrenocortical shock (severe hypotension, hypoglycemia, weakness, vomiting). If these signs appear, notify physician immediately; may be life threatening.
- Check that the patient and family or caregivers understand topical application procedures and adhere to the recommended dosing schedule.

Pharmacokinetics
Absorption: Minimal. Prolonged use on large surface areas, application of large amounts, or use of occlusive dressings may increase systemic absorption.
Distribution: Remains primarily at site of action.
Metabolism and Excretion: Usually metabolized in skin.
Half-life: Unknown.

TIME/ACTION PROFILE (response depends on condition being treated)

ROUTE	ONSET	PEAK	DURATION
topical	mins–hrs	hrs–days	hrs–days

Contraindications/Precautions
Contraindicated in: Hypersensitivity or known intolerance to corticosteroids or components of vehicles (ointment or cream base, preservative, alcohol); Untreated bacterial or viral infections.
Use Cautiously in: Hepatic dysfunction; Diabetes mellitus, cataracts, glaucoma, or tuberculosis (use of large amounts of high-potency agents may worsen condition); Patients with preexisting skin atrophy; Pregnancy, lactation, or children (chronic high-dose usage may result in adrenal suppression in mother, growth suppression in children; children may be more susceptible to adrenal growth suppression).

Interactions
Drug-Drug: None significant.

Route/Dosage
Topical (Adults): Apply to affected area(s) 2–5 times daily (depends on preparation and condition being treated).
Topical (Children ≥2 yr): Apply to affected area(s) 1–2 times daily (depends on product, preparation, and condition being treated).

Availability
Cream: 0.01% Rx, 0.025% Rx. **Ointment:** 0.025% Rx. **Solution:** 0.01% Rx. **Shampoo:** 0.01% Rx. **Oil:** 0.01% Rx.

fluocinonide
(floo-oh-**sin**-oh-nide)
Fluocin, Licon, 🍁Lidemol, Lidex, Lidex-E, 🍁Lyderm, 🍁Topsyn, Vanos

Classification
Therapeutic: anti-inflammatories (steroidal)
Pharmacologic: corticosteroids

Indications
Management of inflammation and pruritus associated with various allergic/immunologic skin problems.

Action
Suppresses normal immune response and inflammation. **Therapeutic Effects:** Suppression of dermatologic inflammation and immune processes.

Adverse Reactions/Side Effects
Derm: allergic contact dermatitis, atrophy, burning, dryness, edema, folliculitis, hypersensitivity reactions, hypertrichosis, hypopigmentation, irritation, maceration, miliaria, perioral dermatitis, secondary infection, striae. **Misc:** adrenal suppression (use of occlusive dressings, long-term therapy).

PHYSICAL THERAPY IMPLICATIONS

Examination and Evaluation

- Assess the area being treated to help document whether drug therapy is successful in resolving skin conditions.
- Monitor any new or increased reactions at the site of application, including inflammation, irritation, infection, burning, swelling, exfoliation, and rash. Report severe or prolonged skin reactions to the physician.
- Report signs of adrenal suppression, including hypotension, weight loss, weakness, nausea, vomiting, anorexia, lethargy, confusion, and restlessness.

Interventions

- Protect skin from breakdown, especially over bony prominences.

Patient/Client-Related Instruction

- Advise patients on long-term treatment to consult physician before stopping this medication. Stopping the medication suddenly may result in adrenocortical shock (severe hypotension, hypoglycemia, weakness, vomiting). If these signs appear, notify physician immediately; may be life threatening.
- Check that the patient and family or caregivers understand topical application procedures and adhere to the recommended dosing schedule.

Pharmacokinetics

Absorption: Minimal. Prolonged use on large surface areas, or large amounts applied, or use of occlusive dressings may increase systemic absorption.
Distribution: Remains primarily at site of action.
Metabolism and Excretion: Usually metabolized in skin.
Half-life: Unknown.

TIME/ACTION PROFILE (response depends on condition being treated)

ROUTE	ONSET	PEAK	DURATION
topical	mins–hrs	hrs–days	hrs–days

Contraindications/Precautions

Contraindicated in: Hypersensitivity or known intolerance to corticosteroid or components of vehicles (ointment or cream base, preservative, alcohol); Local untreated bacterial or viral infections.
Use Cautiously in: Hepatic dysfunction; Diabetes mellitus, cataracts, glaucoma, or tuberculosis (use of large amounts of high-potency agents may worsen condition); Patients with preexisting skin atrophy; Pregnancy, lactation, or children (chronic high-dose usage may result in adrenal suppression in mother, growth suppression in children; children may be more susceptible to adrenal and growth suppression).

Interactions

Drug-Drug: None significant.

Route/Dosage

Topical (Adults): Apply to affected area(s) 2–4 times daily (depends on product, preparation, and condition being treated).
Topical (Children): Apply to affected area(s) once daily.

Availability (generic available)

Cream: 0.05%, 0.1%. **Gel:** 0.05%. **Ointment:** 0.05%. **Solution:** 0.05%. ***In combination with:*** various other topical preparations. See Appendix B.

HIGH ALERT

fluorouracil (floor-oh-**yoor**-a-sil)

Adrucil, Efudex, Fluoroplex, 5-FU

Classification
Therapeutic: antineoplastics
Pharmacologic: antimetabolites

Indications

IV: Used alone and in combination with other modalities (surgery, radiation therapy, other antineoplastics) in the treatment of Colon cancer, Breast cancer, Rectal cancer, Gastric cancer, Pancreatic carcinoma. **Topical:** Management of multiple actinic (solar) keratoses and superficial basal cell carcinomas.

Action

Inhibits DNA and RNA synthesis by preventing thymidine production (cell-cycle S phase–specific). **Therapeutic Effects:** Death of rapidly replicating cells, particularly malignant ones.

Adverse Reactions/Side Effects

More likely to occur with systemic use than with topical use
CNS: acute cerebellar dysfunction. **GI:** diarrhea, nausea, stomatitis, vomiting. **Derm:** alopecia, maculopapular rash, local inflammatory reactions (topical only), melanosis of nails, nail loss, palmar-plantar erythrodysesthesia, phototoxicity. **Endo:** sterility. **Hemat:** anemia, leukopenia, thrombocytopenia. **Local:** thrombophlebitis. **Misc:** fever.

PHYSICAL THERAPY IMPLICATIONS

Examination and Evaluation

- Monitor signs of acute cerebellar dysfunction, including ataxia, nystagmus, hypotonia, tremor, and dysarthria, Notify physician or nursing staff if these signs occur.
- Be alert for signs of blood dyscrasias such as leukopenia (fever, sore throat, signs of infection),

thrombocytopenia (bleeding gums; bruising; petechiae; blood in stools, urine; vomiting blood), or unusual weakness and fatigue that might be due to anemia. Report these signs to the physician or nursing staff.
- Monitor IV injection site for signs of thrombophlebitis (pain, swelling, inflammation). Report prolonged or excessive injection-site skin reactions to the physician.

Interventions
- For patients who are medically able to begin exercise, implement appropriate resistive exercises and aerobic training to maintain muscle strength and aerobic capacity during cancer chemotherapy or to help restore function after chemotherapy.
- Guard against falls and trauma due to cerebellar dysfunction or severe fatigue and weakness. Implement fall prevention strategies, especially if patient exhibits ataxia, incoordination, or other impairments that affect gait and balance (See Appendix E).
- Causes photosensitivity; use care if administering UV treatments. Advise patient to avoid direct sunlight and use sunscreens and protective clothing.

Patient/Client-Related Instruction
- Instruct patient to decrease risk of infections (frequent hand washing, etc.) and avoid contact with persons with contagious diseases.
- Advise patient that rashes and other skin reactions (hair loss, increased sensitivity to UV light, local inflammation during topical use) are likely. Report severe or unexpected skin reactions to the physician.
- Advise patient about the risk of palmar-plantar erythrodysesthesia (hand-and-foot syndrome), as indicated by pain, redness, and dry, scaly skin on the palms of the hands and soles of the feet. Instruct patient to protect the hands and feet from heat and friction, and to apply lotion to the affected areas. Superficial cold application can also temporarily reduce symptoms.
- Advise patient about the likelihood of GI reactions, including nausea, vomiting, diarrhea, and inflammation in or around the mouth. Instruct patient to report severe or prolonged GI problems.

Pharmacokinetics
Absorption: Minimal absorption (5–10%) after topical application.
Distribution: Widely distributed; concentrates and persists in tumors.
Metabolism and Excretion: Converted to an active metabolite; undergoes hepatic metabolism with small amounts excreted unchanged in urine.
Half-life: 20 hr.

TIME/ACTION PROFILE (IV = effects on blood counts, topical = dermatologic effects)

ROUTE	ONSET	PEAK	DURATION
IV	1–9 days	9–21 days (nadir)	30 days
topical	2–3 days	2–6 wk	1–2 mo

Contraindications/Precautions
Contraindicated in: Hypersensitivity; Pregnancy or lactation.
Use Cautiously in: Infections; Depressed bone marrow reserve; Other chronic debilitating illnesses; Obese patients, patients with edema or ascites (dose should be based on ideal body weight).

Interactions
Drug-Drug: Combination chemotherapy with **irinotecan** may produce unacceptable toxicity (dehydration, neutropenia, sepsis). Additive bone marrow depression with other **bone marrow depressants**, including other **antineoplastics** and **radiation therapy**. May decrease antibody response to **live-virus vaccines** and increase risk of adverse reactions.

Route/Dosage
Doses may vary greatly, depending on tumor, patient condition, and protocol used.

Advanced Colorectal Cancer
IV (Adults): 370 mg/m^2 preceded by leucovorin *or* 425 mg/m^2 preceded by leucovorin daily for 5 days. May be repeated q 4–5 wk.

Other Tumors
IV (Adults): *Initial dose*—12 mg/kg/day for 4 days, then 1 day of rest, then 6 mg/kg every other day for 4–5 doses *or* 7–12 mg/kg/day for 4 days followed by 3-day rest, then 7–10 mg/kg q 3–4 days for 3 doses. *Maintenance*—7–12 mg/kg q 7–10 days *or* 300–500 mg/m^2/day for 4–5 days, repeated monthly (no single daily dose should exceed 800 mg).
Poor-Risk Patients: 3–6 mg/kg/day on days 1–3, 3 mg/kg/day on days 5, 7, 9 (not to exceed 400 mg/dose). Doses of 370–425 mg/m^2/day for 5 days have been used in combination with leucovorin.

Actinic (Solar) Keratoses/Superficial Basal Cell Carcinomas
Topical (Adults): *Actinic/solar keratoses*—1% solution or cream 1–2 times daily to lesions on head, neck, or chest; 2–5% solution or cream may be needed for hands. *Superficial basal cell carcinomas*—5% solution or cream bid for 3–6 wk (up to 12 wk).

Availability

Injection: 50 mg/mL in 10-mL ampules or 10-, 20-, and 100-mL vials. **Cream:** 1%, 5%. **Solution:** 1%, 2%, 5%.

fluoxetine (floo-**ox**-uh-teen)

Prozac, Prozac Weekly, Sarafem

Classification

Therapeutic: antidepressants

Pharmacologic: selective serotonin reuptake inhibitors (SSRIs)

Indications

Major depressive disorder. Obsessive compulsive disorder (OCD). Bulimia nervosa. Panic disorder. Depressive episodes associated with bipolar I disorder (when used with olanzapine). Treatment-resistant depression (when used with olanzapine). **Sarafem:** Premenstrual dysphoric disorder (PMDD). **Unlabeled Use:** Anorexia nervosa, attention-deficit hyperactivity disorder (ADHD), Diabetic neuropathy, Fibromyalgia, Obesity, Raynaud's phenomenon, Social anxiety disorder (social phobia), Posttraumatic stress disorder (PTSD).

Action

Selectively inhibits the reuptake of serotonin in the CNS. **Therapeutic Effects:** Antidepressant action. Decreased behaviors associated with panic disorder, bulimia. Decreased mood alterations associated with PMDD.

Adverse Reactions/Side Effects

CNS: NEUROLEPTIC MALIGNANT SYNDROME, SEIZURES, anxiety, drowsiness, headache, insomnia, nervousness, abnormal dreams, dizziness, fatigue, hypomania, mania, weakness. **EENT:** stuffy nose, visual disturbances. **Resp:** cough. **CV:** chest pain, palpitations. **GI:** diarrhea, abdominal pain, abnormal taste, anorexia, constipation, dry mouth, dyspepsia, nausea, vomiting, weight loss. **GU:** sexual dysfunction, urinary frequency. **Derm:** ↑ sweating, pruritus, erythema nodosum, flushing, rashes. **Endo:** dysmenorrhea. **F and E:** hyponatremia. **MS:** arthralgia, back pain, myalgia. **Neuro:** tremor. **Misc:** SEROTONIN SYNDROME, allergic reactions, fever, flu-like syndrome, hot flashes, sensitivity reaction.

PHYSICAL THERAPY IMPLICATIONS

Examination and Evaluation

- Be alert for new seizures or increased seizure activity, especially at the onset of drug treatment. Document the number, duration, and severity of seizures, and report these findings immediately to the physician.
- Watch for signs of neuroleptic malignant syndrome, including hyperthermia, diaphoresis, generalized muscle rigidity, altered mental status, tachycardia, changes in blood pressure (BP), and incontinence. Symptoms typically occur within 4–14 days after initiation of drug therapy, but can occur at any time during drug use. Report these signs to the physician immediately.
- Monitor and report signs of serotonin syndrome, including hyperthermia, rigidity, myoclonus, and autonomic instability with fluctuating vital signs and extreme agitation that may proceed to delirium and coma. Patients should not take fluoxetine with other drugs that increase serotonin levels (e.g., MAO inhibitors).
- Be alert for increased depression and suicidal thoughts, especially in the initial period of drug therapy and in children and teenagers. Likewise, inform physician or other mental health care professional if patient demonstrates other mood changes such as increased anxiety, nervousness, or abnormal arousal (mania).
- Monitor signs of allergic reactions, including pulmonary symptoms (laryngeal edema, wheezing, dyspnea, cough) or skin reactions (rash, pruritus, urticaria). Notify physician immediately if these reactions occur.
- Assess pain levels periodically to help document drug efficacy when used to treat fibromyalgia, diabetic neuropathy, Raynaud's phenomenon, or other chronic pain syndromes.
- Assess any muscle, joint, or back pain to rule out musculoskeletal pathology; that is, try to determine if pain is drug induced rather than caused by anatomic or biomechanical problems.
- Assess dizziness and drowsiness that might affect gait, balance, and other functional activities (See Appendix C). Report balance problems and functional limitations to the physician, and caution the patient and family/caregivers to guard against falls and trauma.
- Monitor symptoms of chest pain and palpitations, especially during exercise. Report severe or prolonged cardiac symptoms to the physician.
- Monitor signs of low sodium levels (hyponatremia), including headache, confusion, lethargy, irritability, decreased consciousness, and neuromuscular abnormalities (muscle weakness, cramps, tremors). Report severe or prolonged signs to the physician.
- Periodically assess body weight and other anthropometric measures (body mass index, body composition). Report a rapid or unexplained weight loss or decreased body fat.

Interventions

- Guard against falls and trauma (hip fractures, head injury, and so forth), and implement fall-prevention strategies (See Appendix E).

- Help patient explore nonpharmacologic methods (exercise, counseling, support groups, and so forth) to reduce depression and other psychologic disorders.

Patient/Client-Related Instruction

- Advise patient that antidepressant effects may not occur immediately; it may take 2 wk or more before an improvement in mood is observed.
- Advise patient to avoid alcohol and other CNS depressants because of the increased risk of sedation and adverse effects.
- Advise patient that this medication should be tapered at the completion of long-term therapy. Abrupt withdrawal may cause dizziness, sensory disturbances, agitation, anxiety, nausea, and sweating.
- Instruct patient to report severe or prolonged GI problems, including nausea, vomiting, diarrhea, constipation, abdominal pain, abnormal taste, and loss of appetite.
- Instruct patient to report other problematic side effects such as severe or prolonged headache, sleep loss, abnormal dreams, cough, stuffy nose, vision disturbances, urinary frequency, dysmenorrhea, sexual dysfunction, hot flashes, flu-like symptoms (fever, malaise), or skin reactions (rash, itching, flushing, painful reddish nodules, increased sweating).

Pharmacokinetics

Absorption: Well absorbed after oral administration.
Distribution: Crosses the blood-brain barrier.
Protein Binding: 94.5%.
Metabolism and Excretion: Converted by the liver to norfluoxetine, another antidepressant compound; fluoxetine and norfluoxetine are mostly metabolized by the liver; 12% excreted by kidneys as unchanged fluoxetine, 7% as unchanged norfluoxetine.
Half-life: 1–3 days (norfluoxetine 5–7 days).

TIME/ACTION PROFILE (antidepressant effect)

ROUTE	ONSET	PEAK	DURATION
PO	1–4 wk	unknown	2 wk

Contraindications/Precautions

Contraindicated in: Hypersensitivity; Concurrent use or use within 14 days of discontinuing MAO inhibitors (fluoxetine should be discontinued at least 5 wk before MAO therapy is initiated); Concurrent use of pimozide; Concurrent use of thioridazine (fluoxetine should be discontinued at least 5 wk before thioridazine therapy is initiated).
Use Cautiously in: Severe hepatic or renal impairment (lower/less frequent dose may be necessary); History of seizures; Debilitated patients (↑ risk of seizures); Diabetes mellitus; Patients with concurrent chronic illness or multiple drug therapy (dose adjustments may be necessary); Patients with impaired hepatic function (↓ doses/↑ dosing interval may be necessary); May ↑ risk of suicide attempt/ideation, especially during early treatment or dose adjustment; OB: Use during third trimester may result in neonatal serotonin syndrome requiring prolonged hospitalization, respiratory and nutritional support. May cause sedation in infant; Lactation: May cause sedation in infant; discontinue drug or bottle feed; Pedi: Risk of suicide ideation or attempt may be greater in children or adolescents (safe use in children <8 yr not established); Geri: Appears on Beers' list; Geriatric patients are at increased risk for excessive CNS stimulation, sleep disturbances, and agitation.

F

Interactions

Drug-Drug: Discontinue use of **MAO inhibitors** for 14 days before fluoxetine therapy; combined therapy may result in confusion, agitation, seizures, hypertension, and hyperpyrexia (serotonin syndrome). Fluoxetine should be discontinued for at least 5 wk before MAO inhibitor therapy is initiated. Concurrent use with **pimozide** may ↑ risk of QT interval prolongation. ↑ levels of **thioridazine** which may ↑ risk of QT interval prolongation (concurrent use contraindicated; fluoxetine should be discontinued for at least 5 wk before thioridazine is initiated). Inhibits the activity of cytochrome P4502D6 enzyme in the liver and ↑ effects of drugs metabolized by this enzyme system. **Medications that inhibit the P450 enzyme system** (including **ritonavir, saquinavir**, and **efavirenz**) may ↑ risk of developing the serotonin syndrome). For concurrent use with **ritonavir**, ↓ fluoxetine dose by 70%; if initiating fluoxetine, start with 10 mg/day dose. ↓ metabolism and ↑ effects of **alprazolam** (decrease alprazolam dose by 50%). Drugs that affect serotonergic neurotransmitter systems, including **linezolid, tramadol**, and **triptans**, ↑ risk of serotonin syndrome. ↑ CNS depression with **alcohol, antihistamines**, other **antidepressants, opioid analgesics**, or **sedative/hypnotics**. ↑ risk of side effects and adverse reactions with other **antidepressants, risperidone**, or **phenothiazines**. May ↑ effectiveness/risk of toxicity from **carbamazepine, clozapine, digoxin, haloperidol, phenytoin, lithium**, or **warfarin**. May ↓ the effects of **buspirone**. **Cyproheptadine** may ↓ or reverse effects of fluoxetine. May ↑ sensitivity to **adrenergics** and increase the risk of serotonin syndrome. May alter the activity of other **drugs that are highly bound to plasma proteins**. ↑ risk of serotonin syndrome with **5-HT_1 agonists**. ↑ risk of bleeding with **NSAIDS, aspirin, clopidogrel**, or **warfarin**.

Drug-Natural: ↑ risk of serotonin syndrome with **St. John's wort and SAMe.**

Route/Dosage

PO (Adults): *Depression, OCD*—20 mg/day in the morning. After several weeks, may ↑ by 20 mg/day at weekly intervals. Doses greater than 20 mg/day should be given in 2 divided doses, in the morning and at noon (not to exceed 80 mg/day). Patients who have been stabilized on the 20–mg/day dose may be switched over to delayed-release capsules (Prozac Weekly) at dose of 90 mg weekly, initiated 7 days after the last 20-mg dose. *Panic disorder*—10 mg/day initially, may ↑ after 1 wk to 20 mg/day (usual dose is 20 mg, but may be ↑ as needed/tolerated up to 60 mg/day). *Bulimia nervosa*—60 mg/day (may need to titrate up to dosage over several days). *PMDD*—20 mg/day (not to exceed 80 mg/day) *or* 20 mg/day starting 14 days prior to expected onset of menses, continued through first full day of menstruation, repeated with each cycle. *Depressive episodes associated with bipolar I disorder*—20 mg/day with olanzapine 5 mg/day (both given in evening); may ↑ fluoxetine dose up to 50 mg/day and olanzapine dose up to 12.5 mg/day; *Treatment-resistant depression*—20 mg/day with olanzapine 5 mg/day (both given in evening); may ↑ fluoxetine dose up to 50 mg/day and olanzapine dose up to 20 mg/day.

PO (Geriatric Patients): *Depression*—10 mg/day in the morning initially, may be ↑ (not to exceed 60 mg/day).

PO (Children 7–17 yr): *Adolescents and higher weight children*—10 mg/day; may be ↑ after 2 wk to 20 mg/day; additional increases may be made after several more weeks (range 20–60 mg/day); *Lower weight children*—10 mg/day initially; may be ↑ after several more weeks (range 20–30 mg/day).

Availability (generic available)

Tablets: 10 mg, 20 mg. **Capsules:** 10 mg, 20 mg, 40 mg. **Delayed-release capsules (Prozac Weekly):** 90 mg. **Oral solution (mint flavor):** 20 mg/5 mL. ***In combination with:*** olanzapine (Symbyax; See Appendix B).

fluphenazine (floo-fen-a-zeen)

Apo-Fluphenazine, Modecate Concentrate, PMS-Fluphenazine, Prolixin, Prolixin Decanoate

Classification
Therapeutic: antipsychotics
Pharmacologic: phenothiazines

Indications

Acute and chronic psychoses.

Action

Alters the effects of dopamine in the CNS. Has anticholinergic and alpha-adrenergic blocking activity. **Therapeutic Effects:** Diminished signs and symptoms of psychoses.

Adverse Reactions/Side Effects

CNS: NEUROLEPTIC MALIGNANT SYNDROME, extrapyramidal reactions, sedation, tardive dyskinesia. **EENT:** blurred vision, dry eyes. **CV:** hypertension, hypotension, tachycardia. **GI:** anorexia, constipation, drug-induced hepatitis, dry mouth, ileus, nausea, weight gain. **GU:** urinary retention. **Derm:** photosensitivity, pigment changes, rashes. **Endo:** galactorrhea. **Hemat:** AGRANULOCYTOSIS, leukopenia, thrombocytopenia. **Misc:** allergic reactions.

PHYSICAL THERAPY IMPLICATIONS

Examination and Evaluation

- Monitor and report signs of neuroleptic malignant syndrome (hyperthermia, diaphoresis, generalized muscle rigidity, altered mental status, tachycardia, changes in blood pressure [BP], incontinence). Symptoms typically occur within 4–14 days after initiation of drug therapy, but can occur at any time during drug use.
- Monitor signs of agranulocytosis and leukopenia (fever, sore throat, mucosal lesions, signs of infection) or thrombocytopenia (bruising, nose bleeds, bleeding gums). Report these signs to the physician or nursing staff immediately.
- Assess motor function, and be alert for extrapyramidal symptoms. Report these symptoms immediately, especially tardive dyskinesia, because this problem may be irreversible. Common extrapyramidal symptoms include:
  - Tardive dyskinesia (uncontrolled rhythmic movement of mouth, face, and extremities, lip smacking or puckering, puffing of cheeks, uncontrolled chewing, rapid or worm-like movements of tongue).
  - Pseudoparkinsonism (shuffling gait, rigidity, tremor, pill-rolling motion, loss of balance control, difficulty speaking or swallowing, mask-like face).
  - Akathisia (restlessness or desire to keep moving).
  - Other dystonias and dyskinesias (dystonic muscle spasms, twisting motions, twitching, inability to move eyes, weakness of arms or legs).
- Monitor signs of allergic reactions, including pulmonary symptoms (laryngeal edema, wheezing, dyspnea) or skin reactions (rash, pruritus, urticaria). Notify physician or nursing staff immediately if these reactions occur.
- Assess BP and compare to normal values (See Appendix F). Report changes in BP, either

a problematic decrease in BP (hypotension) or a sustained increase in BP (hypertension).

- Assess heart rate, ECG, and heart sounds, especially during exercise (See Appendices G, H). Report an increased heart rate (tachycardia) or symptoms of other arrhythmias, including palpitations, chest discomfort, shortness of breath, fainting, and fatigue/weakness.
- Periodically assess body weight and other anthropometric measures (body mass index, body composition). Report a rapid or unexplained weight gain or increased body fat.

Interventions

- Guard against falls and trauma (hip fractures, head injury, and so forth) caused by drowsiness, blurred vision, or extrapyramidal symptoms; implement fall-prevention strategies (See Appendix E).
- Use caution during aerobic exercise and other forms of therapeutic exercise because of the risk of tachycardia and abnormal BP responses. Assess exercise tolerance frequently (BP, heart rate, fatigue levels), and terminate exercise immediately if any untoward responses occur (See Appendix L).
- To minimize orthostatic hypotension, patient should move slowly when assuming a more upright position.
- Causes photosensitivity; use care if administering UV treatments. Advise patient to avoid direct sunlight and use sunscreens and protective clothing.
- Help patient and family/caregivers explore nonpharmacologic methods (exercise, counseling, support groups) to reduce schizophrenic episodes and behavioral problems.

Patient/Client-Related Instruction

- Advise patient to avoid alcohol and other CNS depressants because of the increased risk of sedation and adverse effects.
- Advise patient about the likelihood of GI reactions (nausea, constipation, dry mouth, loss of appetite). Instruct patient to report severe or prolonged GI problems or signs of drug-induced hepatitis (yellow skin or eyes, abdominal pain, severe nausea and vomiting, fever, sore throat, malaise, weakness, facial edema).
- Instruct patient to report other problematic side effects such as blurred vision, excessive sedation, dry eyes, skin rash, skin discoloration, urinary retention, or nipple discharge.

Pharmacokinetics

Absorption: Well absorbed after PO/IM administration. Decanoate salt in sesame oil has delayed onset and prolonged action because of delayed release from oil vehicle and subsequent delayed release from fatty tissues.
Distribution: Widely distributed. Crosses the blood-brain barrier. Crosses the placenta; enters breast milk.
Protein Binding: ≥90%.
Metabolism and Excretion: Highly metabolized by the liver; undergo enterohepatic recirculation.
Half-life: *Fluphenazine hydrochloride*—33 hr; *fluphenazine decanoate*—6.8–9.6 days.

F

TIME/ACTION PROFILE (antipsychotic activity)

ROUTE	ONSET	PEAK	DURATION
PO hydrochloride	1 hr	unknown	6–8 hr
IM decanoate	24–72 hr	48–96 hr	≥4 wk

Contraindications/Precautions

Contraindicated in: Hypersensitivity; Cross-sensitivity with other phenothiazines may exist; Subcortical brain damage; Severe CNS depression; Coma; Bone marrow depression; Liver disease; Hypersensitivity to sesame oil (decanoate salt); Some products contain alcohol or tartrazine and should be avoided in patients with known intolerance; Concurrent use of drugs that prolong the QT interval; Pedi: Children <6 mo (safety not established).
Use Cautiously in: Cardiovascular disease; Parkinson's disease; Angle-closure glaucoma; Myasthenia gravis; Prostatic hypertrophy; Seizure disorders; OB/Lactation: Enters breast milk, not recommended; Geri: Initial dose reduction may be necessary in geriatric or debilitated patients; ↑ risk of mortality in elderly patients treated for dementia-related psychosis.

Interactions

Drug-Drug: Concurrent use with drugs that prolong the QT interval, including **antiarrhythmics, pimozide, erythromycin, clarithromycin, fluoroquinolones, methadone**, and **tricyclic antidepressants** may ↑ the risk for arrhythmias; concurrent use should be avoided. Additive hypotension with **antihypertensives**. Additive CNS depression with other **CNS depressants**, including **alcohol, antidepressants, antihistamines, opioids, sedative/hypnotics**, or **general anesthetics. Phenobarbital** may ↑ metabolism and ↓ effectiveness of fluphenazine. May ↑ the risk of **lithium** toxicity. **Aluminum-containing antacids** may ↓ oral absorption of fluphenazine. May ↓ antiparkinson activity of **levodopa** and **bromocriptine**. May ↓ the vasopressor response to **epinephrine** and **norepinephrine. Beta blockers, chlorpromazine, chloroquine, delavirdine, fluoxetine, paroxetine, quinidine, quinine, ritonavir**, and **ropinirole** may ↑ the effects of fluphenazine. ↑ risk of anticholinergic effects with other

agents having anticholinergic properties, including **antihistamines, tricyclic antidepressants, disopyramide,** or **quinidine. Metoclopramide** may ↑ the risk of extrapyramidal reactions.

Route/Dosage

Fluphenazine Decanoate

IM (Adults): 12.5–25 mg initially; may be repeated q 3 wk. Dose may be slowly increased as needed (not to exceed 100 mg/dose).

Fluphenazine Hydrochloride

PO (Adults): 0.5–10 mg/day in divided doses q 6–8 hr (maximum dose = 40 mg/day).
PO (Geriatric Patients or Debilitated Patients): 1–2.5 mg/day initially; increase dose every 4–7 days by 1–2.5 mg/day as needed (max dose = 20 mg/day).
IM (Adults): 1.25–2.5 mg q 6–8 hr.

Availability (generic available)

Fluphenazine decanoate injection: 25 mg/mL, 100 mg/mL. **Fluphenazine hydrochloride tablets:** 1 mg, 2.5 mg, 5 mg Rx, 10 mg. **Fluphenazine hydrochloride elixir (orange flavor):** 2.5 mg/5 mL. **Fluphenazine hydrochloride concentrate:** 5 mg/mL. **Fluphenazine hydrochloride injection:** 2.5 mg/mL.

flurandrenolide

(floor-an-**dren**-oh-lide)
Cordran, 🍁Drenison

Classification
Therapeutic: anti-inflammatories (steroidal)
Pharmacologic: corticosteroids

Indications

Management of inflammation and pruritus associated with various allergic/immunologic skin problems.

Action

Suppresses normal immune response and inflammation. **Therapeutic Effects:** Suppression of dermatologic inflammation and immune processes.

Adverse Reactions/Side Effects

Derm: allergic contact dermatitis, atrophy, burning, dryness, edema, folliculitis, hypersensitivity reactions, hypertrichosis, hypopigmentation, irritation, maceration, miliaria, perioral dermatitis, secondary infection, striae. **Misc:** adrenal suppression (use of occlusive dressings, long-term therapy).

PHYSICAL THERAPY IMPLICATIONS

Examination and Evaluation

- Assess the area being treated to help document whether drug therapy is successful in resolving skin conditions.
- Monitor any new or increased reactions at the site of application, including inflammation, irritation, infection, burning, swelling, exfoliation, and rash. Report severe or prolonged skin reactions to the physician.
- Report signs of adrenal suppression, including hypotension, weight loss, weakness, nausea, vomiting, anorexia, lethargy, confusion, and restlessness.

Interventions

- Protect skin from breakdown, especially over bony prominences.

Patient/Client-Related Instruction

- Advise patients on long-term treatment to consult physician before stopping this medication. Stopping the medication suddenly may result in adrenocortical shock (severe hypotension, hypoglycemia, weakness, vomiting). If these signs appear, notify physician immediately; may be life-threatening.
- Check that the patient and family or caregivers understand topical application procedures and adhere to the recommended dosing schedule.

Pharmacokinetics

Absorption: Minimal. Prolonged use on large surface areas or large amounts applied or use of occlusive dressings may increase systemic absorption.
Distribution: Remains primarily at site of action.
Metabolism and Excretion: Usually metabolized in skin.
Half-life: Unknown.

TIME/ACTION PROFILE (response depends on condition being treated)

ROUTE	ONSET	PEAK	DURATION
topical	mins–hrs	hrs–days	hrs–days

Contraindications/Precautions

Contraindicated in: Hypersensitivity or known intolerance to corticosteroids or components of vehicles (ointment or cream base, preservative, alcohol); Untreated bacterial or viral infections.
Use Cautiously in: Hepatic dysfunction; Diabetes mellitus, cataracts, glaucoma, or tuberculosis (use of large amounts of high-potency agents may worsen condition); Patients with preexisting skin atrophy; Pregnancy, lactation, or children (chronic high-dose usage may result in adrenal suppression in mother, growth suppression in children; children may be more susceptible to adrenal and growth suppression).

Interactions

Drug-Drug: None significant.

Route/Dosage

Topical (Adults): Apply to affected area(s) 2–3 times daily (depends on product, preparation, and condition being treated).

Topical (Children): Apply to affected area(s) 1–2 times daily (depends on product, preparation, and condition being treated).

Availability

Cream: 0.025% Rx, 0.05% Rx. **Ointment:** 0.025% Rx, 0.05% Rx. **Lotion:** 0.05% Rx. **Tape:** 4 mcg/cm^2 Rx.

flurazepam (floor-az-e-pam)

Apo-Flurazepam, Dalmane, Novoflupam, Somnol

Classification

Therapeutic: sedative/hypnotics

Pharmacologic: benzodiazepines

Schedule IV

Indications

Short-term management of insomnia (<4 wk).

Action

Depresses the CNS, probably by potentiating gamma-aminobutyric acid (GABA), an inhibitory neurotransmitter. **Therapeutic Effects:** Relief of insomnia.

Adverse Reactions/Side Effects

CNS: abnormal thinking, behavior changes, confusion, daytime drowsiness, decreased concentration, dizziness, hallucinations, headache, lethargy, mental depression, paradoxical excitation, sleep-driving. **EENT:** blurred vision. **GI:** constipation, diarrhea, nausea, vomiting. **Derm:** rashes. **Neuro:** ataxia. **Misc:** physical dependence, psychologic dependence, tolerance.

PHYSICAL THERAPY IMPLICATIONS

Examination and Evaluation

- Monitor daytime drowsiness, short-term memory deficits, and "hangover" symptoms (headache, nausea, malaise, irritability, dysphoria). Repeated or excessive symptoms may require change in dose or medication.
- Assess dizziness or ataxia that might affect gait, balance, and other functional activities (See Appendix C). Report balance problems and functional limitations to the physician, and caution the patient and family/caregivers to guard against falls and trauma.
- Report any behavioral or personality changes such as depression, confusion, decreased concentration, nervousness, excitation, hallucinations, or expression of abnormal thoughts.

Interventions

- Guard against falls and trauma (hip fractures, head injury, and so forth). Implement fall-prevention strategies, especially in older adults or if drowsiness and dizziness carry over into the daytime (See Appendix E).
- Help patient explore nonpharmacologic methods to improve sleep, such as relaxation techniques, regular exercise, avoid caffeine, and so forth.

Patient/Client-Related Instruction

- Instruct patients on prolonged treatment not to discontinue medication without consulting their physician. Long-term use can cause tolerance and physical/psychologic dependence, and increased sleep problems (rebound insomnia) can occur when the drug is suddenly discontinued.
- Advise patient to avoid alcohol and other CNS depressants because of the increased risk of sedation and adverse effects.
- Caution patient and family/caregivers to guard against complex motor behaviors that can occur while asleep, including driving a car.
- Instruct patient to report other bothersome side effects including severe or prolonged headache, blurred vision, skin rash, or GI problems (nausea, vomiting, constipation, diarrhea).

Pharmacokinetics

Absorption: Well absorbed after oral administration.
Distribution: Widely distributed; crosses blood-brain barrier. Probably crosses the placenta and enters breast milk. Accumulation of drug occurs with chronic dosing.
Protein Binding: 97% (one of the active metabolites).
Metabolism and Excretion: Metabolized by the liver; some metabolites have hypnotic activity.
Half-life: 2.3 hr (half-life of active metabolite may be 30–200 hr).

TIME/ACTION PROFILE (hypnotic activity)

ROUTE	ONSET	PEAK	DURATION
PO	15–45 min	0.5–1 hr	7–8 hr

Contraindications/Precautions

Contraindicated in: Impaired respiratory function; Impaired respiratory function; Sleep apnea; Hypersensitivity; Cross-sensitivity with other benzodiazepines may exist; Preexisting CNS depression; Severe uncontrolled pain; Angle-closure glaucoma; OB: Infants may experience withdrawal effects; Lactation: Enters breast milk; discontinue or bottle feed.

Use Cautiously in: Hepatic dysfunction (dosage reduction may be necessary); History of suicide attempt or drug dependence; Geri: Appears on Beers' list and is associated with increased falls risk in geriatric patients; Debilitated patients (initial dose reduction may be necessary); Pedi: Safety not established in children <15 yr.

Interactions

Drug-Drug: Concurrent use with **alcohol, antidepressants, antihistamines,** and **opioids** may result in additive CNS depression. **Cimetidine, hormonal contraceptives, disulfiram, fluoxetine, isoniazid, ketoconazole, metoprolol, propoxyphene, propranolol,** or **valproic acid** may ↓ metabolism of flurazepam, enhancing its actions. May ↓ efficacy of **levodopa. Rifampin** or **barbiturates** may ↑ metabolism and decrease ↓ effectiveness of flurazepam. Sedative effects may be ↓ by **theophylline.**
Drug-Natural: Concomitant use of **kava, valerian, chamomile,** or **hops** can ↑ CNS depression.

Route/Dosage

PO (Adults): 15–30 mg at bedtime.
PO (Geriatric Patients or Debilitated Patients): 15 mg initially, may be increased.

Availability (generic available)

Capsules: 15 mg, 30 mg. **Tablets:** 15 mg, 30 mg.

flurbiprofen (floor-bye-proe-fen)

Ansaid, Apo-Flurbiprofen, Froben, Novo-Flurprofen, Nu-Flurbiprofen

Classification
Therapeutic: antirheumatics, nonsteroidal anti-inflammatory agents
Pharmacologic: propionic acid derivatives

Indications

PO: Inflammatory disorders, including Rheumatoid arthritis, Osteoarthritis. **Unlabeled Use:** Nonopioid analgesic. Antidysmenorrheal.

Action

Inhibits prostaglandin synthesis, resulting in reduced inflammation and pain when administered orally.
Therapeutic Effects: PO: Suppression of pain and inflammation.

Adverse Reactions/Side Effects

CNS: dizziness, drowsiness, headache, insomnia, mental depression, psychic disturbances. **EENT:** blurred vision, corneal opacities, tinnitus. **CV:** changes in blood pressure, edema, palpitations. **GI:** GI BLEEDING, abdominal pain, heartburn, nausea, bloated feeling, constipation, diarrhea, drug-induced hepatitis, stomatitis. **GU:** incontinence. **Derm:** EXFOLIATIVE DERMATITIS, STEVENS-JOHNSON SYNDROME, TOXIC EPIDERMAL NECROLYSIS, increased sweating, rashes. **Hemat: PO:** blood dyscrasias, prolonged bleeding time. **MS:** myalgia. **Misc:** ALLERGIC REACTIONS, INCLUDING ANAPHYLAXIS, chills, fever.

PHYSICAL THERAPY IMPLICATIONS

Examination and Evaluation

- Monitor signs of GI bleeding, including abdominal pain, vomiting blood, blood in stools, or black, tarry stools. Report these signs to the physician immediately.
- Monitor signs of allergic reactions and anaphylaxis, including pulmonary symptoms (laryngeal edema, wheezing, cough, dyspnea) or skin reactions (rash, pruritus, urticaria). Be especially alert for exfoliation, dermatitis, and other severe skin reactions that might indicate serious hypersensitivity reactions (Stevens-Johnson syndrome, toxic epidermal necrolysis). Notify physician immediately if these reactions occur.
- Assess pain and other variables (range of motion, muscle strength) to document whether this drug is successful in helping manage the patient's pain and decreasing impairments.
- Assess blood pressure (BP) periodically and compare to normal values (See Appendix F). NSAIDs can increase BP in certain patients.
- Be alert for signs of prolonged bleeding time such as bleeding gums, nosebleeds, and unusual or excessive bruising. Report these signs to the physician.
- Assess peripheral edema using girth measurements, volume displacement, and measurement of pitting edema (See Appendix N). Report increased swelling in feet and ankles or a sudden increase in body weight due to fluid retention.
- Monitor signs of kidney dysfunction such as painful urination or blood in the urine. Report signs of renal failure immediately, including decreased urine output, increased BP, muscle cramps/twitching, edema/weight gain from fluid retention, yellowish brown skin, and confusion that progresses to seizures and coma.
- Monitor unusual weakness and fatigue that might be due to anemia or other symptoms such as fever, sore throat, mucosal lesions, or signs of infection that might be due to other blood dyscrasias. Notify physician if these signs occur.
- Assess dizziness and drowsiness that might affect gait, balance, and other functional activities (See Appendix C). Report balance problems and functional limitations to the physician, and caution the patient and family/caregivers to guard against falls and trauma.
- Monitor and report confusion, agitation, mental depression, or other psychic disturbances.

Interventions

- Implement appropriate manual therapy techniques, physical agents, and therapeutic exercises to reduce pain and decrease the need for flurbiprofen and other NSAIDs.
- If treating arthritic conditions, recommend orthotic and assistive devices as needed to reduce pain, improve function, and augment the effects of drug therapy.
- Use caution with any physical interventions that could increase bleeding, including wound débridement, chest percussion, joint mobilization, and application of local heat.
- Help patient explore other nonpharmacologic methods to reduce chronic pain, such as relaxation techniques, exercise, counseling, and so forth.

Patient/Client-Related Instruction

- Advise patient that analgesics are usually more effective if given before pain becomes severe; emphasize that adequate pain control will allow better participation in physical therapy.
- Inform patient that NSAIDs may impair bone and cartilage healing. Advise patient to consult physician about NSAID use, especially after fractures, spinal fusion, and other bone surgeries.
- Caution patient about the use of over-the-counter products that contain NSAIDs or acetaminophen while taking prescription doses of flurbiprofen. Use of multiple NSAIDs increases the risk of toxicity and overdose.
- Instruct patient to report excessive or prolonged headache or ringing/buzzing in the ears (tinnitus); these signs may indicate drug toxicity.
- Advise patient about the likelihood of GI reactions, including nausea, vomiting, diarrhea, constipation, heartburn, and inflammation in/around the mouth. Instruct patient to report severe or prolonged GI reactions or signs of drug-induced hepatitis such as anorexia, abdominal pain, severe nausea and vomiting, yellow skin or eyes, skin rashes, flu-like symptoms, and muscle/joint pain.
- Advise patient to reduce alcohol intake because alcohol increases the risk of gastric toxicity.
- Instruct patient and family/caregivers to report other troublesome side effects such as severe or prolonged chills, fever, sleep loss, tremor, heart palpitations, vision disturbances, incontinence, or skin reactions (rash, increased sweating).

Pharmacokinetics

Absorption: Well absorbed after oral administration.
Distribution: Unknown.
Protein Binding: 99%.
Metabolism and Excretion: Mostly metabolized by the liver; 20–25% excreted unchanged by the kidneys.
Half-life: 3–6 hr.

TIME/ACTION PROFILE

ROUTE	ONSET	PEAK	DURATION
PO (anti-inflammatory)	few days–1 wk	1–2 wk	unknown

F

Contraindications/Precautions

Contraindicated in: Hypersensitivity; Cross-sensitivity may exist with other NSAIDs, including aspirin; Active GI bleeding or ulcer disease; Perioperative pain from coronary artery bypass graft (CABG) surgery.
Use Cautiously in: Cardiovascular disease or risk factors for cardiovascular disease (may ↑ risk of serious cardiovascular thrombotic events, myocardial infarction, and stroke, especially with prolonged use); Severe renal or hepatic disease; History of ulcer disease; Diabetes mellitus; Geri: Geriatric patients (↑ risk of GI bleeding); Bleeding disorders; OB: Pregnancy (not recommended for use during second half of pregnancy); OB/Pedi: Lactation or children (safety not established).

Interactions

Drug-Drug: Concurrent use with **aspirin** may ↓ effectiveness. ↑ adverse GI effects with **aspirin**, other **NSAIDs, potassium supplements, corticosteroids,** or **alcohol.** Chronic use with **acetaminophen** may ↑ risk of adverse renal reactions. May ↓ effectiveness of **diuretics** or **antihypertensives.** May ↑ hypoglycemic response to **insulins** or **oral hypoglycemic agents.** ↑ risk of toxicity from **methotrexate. Probenecid** ↑ risk of toxicity from flurbiprofen. ↑ risk of bleeding with **cefotetan, cefoperazone, antiplatelet agents, heparin, thrombolytics, valproic acid,** or **warfarin.** ↑ risk of adverse hematologic reactions with **antineoplastics** or **radiation therapy.** ↑ risk of nephrotoxicity with cyclosporine.
Drug-Natural: ↑ bleeding risk with **arnica, chamomile, clove, dong quai, feverfew, garlic, ginger, ginkgo, *Panax ginseng*,** and others.

Route/Dosage

PO (Adults): *Anti-inflammatory*—200–300 mg daily in 2–4 divided doses (not to exceed 300 mg/day or 100 mg/dose). *Nonopioid analgesic/antidysmenorrheal*—50 mg q 4–6 hr as needed (unlabeled).

Availability (generic available)

Tablets: 50 mg, 100 mg.

flutamide (floo-ta-mide)

Eulexin

Classification

Therapeutic: antineoplastics

Pharmacologic: antiandrogens

Indications

Treatment of prostate carcinoma in conjunction with luteinizing hormone–releasing hormone (LHRH) analogues such as leuprolide.

Action

Antagonizes the effects of androgen (testosterone) at the cellular level. **Therapeutic Effects:** Decreased growth of prostate carcinoma, an androgen-sensitive tumor.

Adverse Reactions/Side Effects

Side effects primarily caused by LHRH antagonist

CNS: anxiety, confusion, drowsiness, mental depression, nervousness. **CV:** edema, hypertension. **GI:** HEPATOTOXICITY, diarrhea, nausea, vomiting. **GU:** erectile dysfunction, loss of libido. **Derm:** photosensitivity, rash. **Endo:** gynecomastia. **Misc:** hot flashes.

PHYSICAL THERAPY IMPLICATIONS

Examination and Evaluation

- Be alert for signs of hepatotoxicity, including anorexia, abdominal pain, severe nausea and vomiting, yellow skin or eyes, fever, sore throat, malaise, weakness, facial edema, lethargy, and unusual bleeding or bruising. Report these signs to the physician immediately.
- Assess blood pressure periodically and compare to normal values (See Appendix F). Report a sustained increase in blood pressure (hypertension) to the physician.
- Assess peripheral edema using girth measurements, volume displacement, and measurement of pitting edema (See Appendix N). Report increased swelling in feet and ankles or a sudden increase in body weight due to fluid retention.
- Be alert for anxiety, confusion, nervousness, drowsiness, or other alterations in mental status. Notify physician if these side effects become problematic (See Appendix D).

Interventions

- For patients who are medically able to begin exercise, implement appropriate resistive exercises and aerobic training to maintain muscle strength and aerobic capacity during cancer chemotherapy or to help restore function after chemotherapy.
- Use caution during aerobic exercise and other forms of therapeutic exercise. Assess exercise tolerance frequently (respiratory symptoms, blood pressure, heart rate, fatigue levels), and terminate exercise immediately if any untoward responses occur (See Appendix L).
- Causes photosensitivity; use care if administering UV treatments. Advise patient to avoid direct sunlight and use sunscreens and protective clothing.

Patient/Client-Related Instruction

- Instruct patient and family/caregivers to report other troublesome side effects such as severe or prolonged skin rash, hot flashes, breast enlargement (gynecomastia), sexual dysfunction (decreased libido, erectile dysfunction), or GI problems (diarrhea, nausea, vomiting).

Pharmacokinetics

Absorption: Well absorbed after oral administration.

Distribution: Unknown.

Metabolism and Excretion: Mostly metabolized by the liver. Some conversion to another antiandrogenic compound (2-hydroxyflutamide).

Half-life: Unknown.

TIME/ACTION PROFILE

ROUTE	ONSET	PEAK	DURATION
PO	unknown	unknown	unknown

Contraindications/Precautions

Contraindicated in: Hypersensitivity; Severe hepatic impairment.

Use Cautiously in: Severe cardiovascular disease.

Interactions

Drug-Drug: Acts synergistically with **LHRH analogues (leuprolide).**

Route/Dosage

PO (Adults): 250 mg q 8 hr; given concurrently with leuprolide.

Availability

Capsules: 125 mg, 250 mg.

fluticasone (floo-tik-a-sone)

Flovent HFA, Flovent Diskus

Classification

Therapeutic: anti-inflammatories (steroidal)

Pharmacologic: corticosteroids

Indications

Maintenance and prophylactic treatment of asthma. May decrease requirement for or avoid use of systemic corticosteroids and delay pulmonary damage that occurs from chronic asthma.

Action

Potent, locally acting anti-inflammatory and immune modifier. **Therapeutic Effects:** Decreases frequency and severity of asthma attacks.

Adverse Reactions/Side Effects

CNS: headache, dizziness. **EENT:** dysphonia, hoarseness, oropharyngeal fungal infections, nasal stuffiness, rhinorrhea, sinusitis. **Resp:** bronchospasm, cough, upper respiratory tract infection, wheezing. **GI:** diarrhea. **Endo:** adrenal suppression (high-dose, long-term therapy only), decreased growth (in children), Cushing's syndrome. **MS:** muscle pain. **Misc:** CHURG-STRAUSS SYNDROME, fever.

PHYSICAL THERAPY IMPLICATIONS

Examination and Evaluation

- Be alert for signs of allergic blood vessel reactions (Churg-Strauss syndrome). Early signs include allergic rhinitis, sinusitis, asthma, or hay fever–like reactions. Symptoms can increase to include fever, skin rash, joint pain, severe pain and numbness (peripheral neuropathy), shortness of breath, coughing up blood, bloody urine, chest pain, arrhythmias, and GI problems (diarrhea, nausea, vomiting, GI bleeding). Notify physician immediately for further evaluation of any signs listed above.
- Assess pulmonary function periodically by measuring lung volumes, breath sounds, respiratory rate, and other symptoms (wheezing, dyspnea, shortness of breath) (See Appendices I, J, K). Report changes in pulmonary function to help document the effects of drug therapy in treating asthma.
- Observe for paradoxical bronchospasm (cough, wheezing, dyspnea), especially at higher or excessive doses. If condition occurs, advise patient to withhold medication and notify physician immediately.
- Assess muscle strength periodically during long-term use. Although inhalation reduces the risk of systemic musculoskeletal damage, some degree of weakness and bone loss may still occur during prolonged, extensive use.
- Assess any muscle pain to rule out musculoskeletal pathology; that is, try to determine if pain is drug induced rather than caused by anatomic or biomechanical problems.
- Report signs of adrenal suppression, including hypotension, weight loss, weakness, nausea, vomiting, anorexia, lethargy, confusion, and restlessness.
- Assess growth rate in children receiving chronic therapy; report delayed or stunted growth to the physician.

Interventions

- Implement resistive exercises and weight-bearing activities to minimize muscle wasting and osteoporosis. Use caution to prevent musculoskeletal damage in patients with preexisting muscle and bone loss.
- Design and implement appropriate aerobic exercise and respiratory muscle–training programs to maintain optimal cardiovascular and pulmonary function. Work with patient and family/caregivers to find forms of exercise (e.g., swimming) that can help improve respiratory function without triggering asthma attacks.
- Protect skin from breakdown, especially over bony prominences.

Patient/Client-Related Instruction

- Counsel patient on proper use of metered-dose inhaler or dry-powder inhaler; observe use of the device whenever possible to ensure proper technique.
- Advise patient not to exceed the recommended dose or frequency of inhalations. Contact physician immediately if bronchospasm is not relieved by medication or is accompanied by severe headache or other symptoms.
- Caution patient not to use this drug to treat acute symptoms. A rapid-acting inhaled beta-adrenergic bronchodilator is typically used for relief of acute asthma attacks.
- Advise patient that corticosteroids cause immunosuppression and may mask symptoms of infection. Instruct patient to avoid people with known contagious illnesses and to report possible infections immediately.
- Advise patient about the likelihood of upper respiratory tract infection or irritation, including pharyngitis, sinusitis, rhinitis, and problems with vocalization (dysphonia). Instruct patient to report severe or prolonged upper respiratory problems to the physician.
- Advise patients on long-term treatment to consult physician before stopping this medication. Stopping the medication suddenly may result in adrenocortical shock (severe hypotension, hypoglycemia, weakness, vomiting). If these signs appear, notify physician immediately; may be life threatening.
- Instruct patient and family/caregivers to report other troublesome side effects such as severe or prolonged fever or diarrhea.

Pharmacokinetics

Absorption: <1% (aerosol), 18% (powder). Action is primarily local after inhalation.

Distribution: 10–25% of inhaled corticosteroids is deposited in the airways if a spacer device is not used. With the use of a spacer, a greater percentage may reach the respiratory tract. Crosses the placenta and enters breast milk in small amounts.
Protein Binding: 91%.
Metabolism and Excretion: Metabolized by the liver after absorption from lungs; <5% excreted in urine; remainder excreted in feces.
Half-life: 7.8 hr.

TIME/ACTION PROFILE (improvement in symptoms)

ROUTE	ONSET	PEAK	DURATION
inhalation	within 24 hr	1–4 wk*	several days after DC

*Improvement in pulmonary function; decreased airway responsiveness may take longer.

Contraindications/Precautions

Contraindicated in: Hypersensitivity (contains propellants); Acute attack of asthma/status asthmaticus.
Use Cautiously in: Active untreated infections; Diabetes or glaucoma; Underlying immunosuppression (due to disease or concurrent therapy); Systemic corticosteroid therapy (should not be abruptly discontinued when inhalable therapy is started; additional corticosteroids needed in stress or trauma); Hepatic dysfunction; Severe milk protein allergy (powder for oral inhalation contains lactose); Pregnancy, lactation, or children <12 yr (for aerosol) or <4 yr (for powder) (safety not established; prolonged or high-dose therapy may lead to complications).

Interactions

Drug-Drug: Ketoconazole ↓ metabolism and ↑ levels of fluticasone. **Ritonavir** significantly ↑ fluticasone serum concentrations and may result in systemic corticosteroid effects (concurrent use is NOT recommended).

Route/Dosage

Aerosol for oral inhalation

Inhalation (Adults and Children ≥12 yr): *Patients whose previous asthma therapy included bronchodilators alone*—88 mcg bid initially, may be increased up to 440 mcg bid; *Patients whose previous therapy included other inhaled corticosteroids*—88–220 mcg bid initially, may be increased up to 440 mcg bid; *Patients whose previous therapy included oral corticosteroids*—440 mcg bid initially, may be increased up to 880 mcg bid.

Powder for oral inhalation

Inhalation (Adults and Children ≥12 yr): *Patients whose previous asthma therapy included bronchodilators alone*—100 mcg bid initially, may be increased up to 500 mcg bid; *Patients whose previous therapy included other inhaled corticosteroids*—100–250 mcg bid initially, may be increased up to 500 mcg bid; *Patients whose previous therapy included oral corticosteroids*—500–1000 mcg bid.
Inhalation (Children 4–11 yr): *Patients whose previous asthma therapy included bronchodilators alone*—50 mcg bid initially, may be increased up to 100 mcg bid; *Patients whose previous therapy included other inhaled corticosteroids*—50 mcg bid initially, may be increased up to 100 mcg bid.

Availability

Inhalation aerosol (Flovent HFA): 44 mcg/metered inhalation in 10.6-g canisters (120 metered inhalations), 110 mcg/metered inhalation in 12-g canisters (120 metered inhalations), 220 mcg/metered inhalation in 12-g canisters (120 metered inhalations).
Powder for inhalation (Flovent Diskus): 50 mcg, 100 mcg, 250 mcg. ***In combination with:*** salmeterol (Advair). See Appendix B.

fluvastatin (floo-va-stat-in)

Lescol, Lescol XL

Classification
Therapeutic: lipid-lowering agents
Pharmacologic: HMG CoA reductase inhibitors

Indications

Adjunctive management of primary hypercholesterolemia and mixed dyslipidemia. Secondary prevention of coronary revascularization in patients with clinically evident coronary heart disease. Slows the progression of coronary atherosclerosis in patients with coronary artery disease.

Action

Inhibits 3-hydroxy-3-methylglutaryl coenzyme A (HMG CoA) reductase, an enzyme which is responsible for catalyzing an early step in the synthesis of cholesterol.
Therapeutic Effects: Lowering of total and LDL cholesterol and triglycerides. Slightly increases HDL cholesterol. Slows the progression of coronary atherosclerosis with resultant decrease in incidence of coronary heart disease–related events.

Adverse Reactions/Side Effects

CNS: headache, dizziness, insomnia, fatigue.
Resp: bronchitis, cough, pharyngitis, rhinitis, sinusitis. **CV:** chest pain, peripheral edema. **GI:** nausea, vomiting, abdominal pain/cramps, constipation, flatulence, dyspepsia, elevated liver enzymes. **Derm:** photosensitivity, rash/pruritus. **MS:** RHABDOMYOLYSIS, arthritis, myopathy, back pain, arthropathy.
Misc: allergic reactions, including anaphylaxis.

PHYSICAL THERAPY IMPLICATIONS

Examination and Evaluation

- Assess any joint pain, muscle pain, tenderness, or weakness, especially if accompanied by fever, malaise, and dark-colored urine. Advise patient that these symptoms may represent drug-induced myopathy, and that myopathy can progress to severe muscle damage (rhabdomyolysis). Report any unexplained musculoskeletal symptoms to the physician immediately, and suspend exercise and gait training until these symptoms can be evaluated.
- Monitor signs of allergic reactions and anaphylaxis, including pulmonary symptoms (tightness in the throat and chest, wheezing, cough, dyspnea) or skin reactions (rash, pruritus, urticaria). Notify physician immediately if these reactions occur.
- Assess dizziness that might affect gait, balance, and other functional activities (See Appendix C). Report balance problems and functional limitations to the physician, and caution the patient and family/caregivers to guard against falls and trauma.
- Assess peripheral edema using girth measurements, volume displacement, and measurement of pitting edema (See Appendix N). Report increased swelling in feet and ankles or a sudden increase in body weight due to fluid retention.
- Monitor any chest pain and attempt to determine if pain is drug induced or caused by cardiovascular dysfunction (e.g., angina that occurs during exercise). Notify physician about suspected cardiac dysfunction.
- Monitor symptoms of bronchitis, including cough, production of sputum, shortness of breath, and wheezing. Report prolonged or severe symptoms to the physician.

Interventions

- In patients with drug-induced myopathy, implement gradual strengthening and other therapeutic exercises to facilitate recovery from muscle pain and weakness. Use caution during early stages to avoid fatigue of affected muscles, and implement assistive devices (walker, cane, crutches) as needed to prevent falls and assist mobility. Increase exercise intensity as tolerated; recovery from myopathy typically takes 4–6 wk, but can be longer in older patients or people with comorbidities.
- Design and implement aerobic exercise and endurance-training programs to improve cardiovascular function and help reduce the risk of coronary heart disease.
- Causes photosensitivity; use care if administering UV treatments. Advise patient to avoid direct sunlight and use sunscreens and protective clothing.

Patient/Client-Related Instruction

- Remind patients to take medication as directed to control hyperlipidemia even though they are asymptomatic.
- Counsel patients about additional interventions to help control lipid disorders and improve cardiovascular health, including dietary modification, regular exercise, moderation of alcohol consumption, and smoking cessation.
- Instruct patient to report prolonged or severe GI reactions, including nausea, constipation, heartburn, abdominal pain, and flatulence.
- Instruct patient and family/caregivers to report other troublesome side effects such as severe or prolonged headache, sleep loss, upper respiratory tract inflammation, or skin problems (rash, itching).

Pharmacokinetics

Absorption: 98% absorbed after oral administration but undergoes extensive first-pass hepatic metabolism resulting in 24% bioavailability.
Distribution: Enters breast milk; remainder of distribution unknown.
Protein Binding: >98%.
Metabolism and Excretion: After extensive hepatic metabolism, 5% is excreted in urine, 90% in feces.
Half-life: 1.2 hr.

TIME/ACTION PROFILE (cholesterol-lowering effect)

ROUTE	ONSET	PEAK	DURATION
PO	1–2 wk	4–6 wk	unknown

Contraindications/Precautions

Contraindicated in: Hypersensitivity; Pregnancy; Lactation; Active liver disease or unexplained persistent elevations in AST & ALT.
Use Cautiously in: History of liver disease; Alcoholism; Renal impairment; Children <18 yr (safety not established).

Interactions

Drug-Drug: Fluvastatin is metabolized by the CYP2C9 metabolic pathway. Concurrent use with **gemfibrozil, erythromycin, cyclosporine, azole antifungal agents,** or **niacin** (nicotinic acid) may ↑ risk of myopathy (concurrent use with gemfibrozil should be avoided, temporarily decrease dose or discontinue if systemic azole antifungals are required). Concurrent ingestion with **cholestyramine** or **colestipol** ↓ absorption of fluvastatin. Blood levels are ↑ by **cimetidine, ranitidine, omeprazole,** and concurrent

ingestion of **alcohol**. Concurrent use with **rifampin** ↓ blood levels. May slightly ↑ serum **digoxin** levels. May ↑ risk of bleeding with **warfarin**.
Drug-Food: Grapefruit juice ↑ blood levels and the risk of rhabdomyolysis.

Route/Dosage

PO (Adults): *Capsules*—20 mg once daily at bedtime. May be increased to 40 mg once daily or 20 mg bid. *Extended-release tablets*—60 mg once daily at bedtime.

Availability

Capsules: 20 mg Rx, 40 mg Rx. **Extended-release tablets:** 80 mg.

fluvoxamine (floo-**vox**-a-meen)

Luvox, Luvox CR

Classification
Therapeutic: antidepressants, antiobsessive agents
Pharmacologic: selective serotonin reuptake inhibitors (SSRIs)

Indications

Obsessive-compulsive disorder (OCD) (immediate and controlled release). Social anxiety disorder (SAD) (controlled release only). **Unlabeled Use:** Depression. Generalized anxiety disorder (GAD). Posttraumatic stress disorder (PSTD).

Action

Inhibits the reuptake of serotonin in the CNS. **Therapeutic Effects:** Decrease in obsessive-compulsive behaviors. Decrease in symptoms of social anxiety disorder.

Adverse Reactions/Side Effects

CNS: NEUROLEPTIC MALIGNANT SYNDROME, sedation, dizziness, drowsiness, headache, insomnia, nervousness, weakness, agitation, anxiety, apathy, emotional lability, manic reactions, mental depression, psychotic reactions, syncope. **EENT:** sinusitis. **Resp:** cough, dyspnea. **CV:** edema, hypertension, palpitations, postural hypotension, tachycardia, vasodilation. **GI:** constipation, diarrhea, dry mouth, dyspepsia, nausea, anorexia, dysphagia, ↑ liver enzymes, flatulence, weight gain (unusual), vomiting. **GU:** ↓ libido/sexual dysfunction. **Derm:** ↑ sweating. **Metab:** weight gain, weight loss. **MS:** hypertonia, myoclonus/twitching. **Neuro:** hypokinesia/hyperkinesia, tremor. **Misc:** SEROTONIN SYNDROME, allergic reactions, chills, flu-like symptoms, tooth disorder/caries, yawning.

PHYSICAL THERAPY IMPLICATIONS

Examination and Evaluation

- Watch for signs of neuroleptic malignant syndrome, including hyperthermia, diaphoresis, generalized muscle rigidity, altered mental status, tachycardia, changes in blood pressure (BP), and incontinence. Symptoms typically occur within 4-14 days after initiation of drug therapy, but can occur at any time during drug use. Report these signs to the physician immediately.
- Monitor and report signs of serotonin syndrome, including hyperthermia, rigidity, myoclonus, and autonomic instability with fluctuating vital signs and extreme agitation that may proceed to delirium and coma. Patients should not take fluvoxamine with other drugs that increase serotonin levels (e.g., MAO inhibitors).
- Be alert for increased depression and suicidal thoughts and ideology, especially when initiating drug treatment, and in children and teenagers. Notify physician or other mental health care professional immediately if patient exhibits worsening depression or expresses thoughts of suicide.
- Monitor other alterations in behavior or mental status, including nervousness, anxiety, agitation, apathy, emotional lability, and manic/psychotic reactions. Notify physician promptly if these symptoms develop.
- Assess BP periodically and compare to normal values (See Appendix F). Report a sustained increase in BP (hypertension) or symptomatic decreases in BP following changes in position (orthostatic hypotension). Document orthostatic hypotension and contact physician when systolic BP falls >20 mm Hg, or diastolic BP falls >10 mm Hg as patient assumes a more upright position.
- Assess heart rate, ECG, and heart sounds, especially during exercise (See Appendices G, H). Report a rapid heart rate (tachycardia) or signs of other arrhythmias, including palpitations, chest discomfort, shortness of breath, fainting, and fatigue/weakness.
- Assess peripheral edema using girth measurements, volume displacement, and measurement of pitting edema (See Appendix N). Report increased swelling in feet and ankles or a sudden increase in body weight due to vasodilation or fluid retention.
- Assess changes in motor activity or muscle function. Report severe or problematic tremor, increased muscle tone, or changes in muscle activity and motor abnormalities (hyperkinesia, hypokinesia).
- Assess dizziness and drowsiness that might affect gait, balance, and other functional activities

(See Appendix C). Report balance problems and functional limitations to the physician, and caution the patient and family/caregivers to guard against falls and trauma.

- Monitor signs of allergic reactions, including pulmonary symptoms (laryngeal edema, wheezing, dyspnea, cough) or skin reactions (rash, pruritus, urticaria). Notify physician if these reactions occur.
- Periodically assess body weight and other anthropometric measures (body mass index, body composition). Report a rapid or unexplained weight gain or weight loss.

Interventions

- Guard against falls and trauma (hip fractures, head injury, and so forth), and implement fall-prevention strategies (See Appendix E).
- Because of the risk of arrhythmias and hypotension, use caution during aerobic exercise and other forms of therapeutic exercise. Assess exercise tolerance frequently (BP, heart rate, fatigue levels), and terminate exercise immediately if any untoward responses occur (See Appendix L).
- To minimize orthostatic hypotension, patient should move slowly when assuming a more upright position.
- Help patient explore nonpharmacologic methods reduce obsessive-compulsive behavior and other psychologic disorders (exercise, counseling, support groups, and so forth).

Patient/Client-Related Instruction

- Advise patient that antidepressant effects may not occur immediately; it may take 2 wk or longer before an improvement in mood is observed.
- Advise patient to avoid alcohol and other CNS depressants because of the increased risk of sedation and adverse effects.
- Instruct patient to report severe or prolonged GI problems, including nausea, vomiting, diarrhea, constipation, indigestion, dry mouth, abdominal pain, and flatulence.
- Instruct patient to report other problematic side effects such as severe or prolonged headache, cough, labored breathing, sinus irritation, increased sweating, sexual dysfunction, or flu-like symptoms (fever, chills, malaise, body aches).

Pharmacokinetics

Absorption: 53% absorbed after oral administration.
Distribution: Excreted in breast milk; enters the CNS. Remainder of distribution not known.
Metabolism and Excretion: Eliminated mostly by the kidneys.
Half-life: 13.6–15.6 hr.

TIME/ACTION PROFILE (improvement on obsessive-compulsive behaviors)

ROUTE	ONSET	PEAK	DURATION
PO	within 2–3 wk	several mos	unknown

Contraindications/Precautions

Contraindicated in: Hypersensitivity to fluvoxamine or other SSRIs; Concurrent use or use within 14 days of discontinuing MAOIs, alosetron, pimozide, thioridazine, or tizanidine.
Use Cautiously in: Impaired hepatic function; May ↑ risk of suicide attempt/ideation, especially during early treatment or dose adjustment; risk may be greater in children or adolescents; OB: Neonates exposed to SSRI in third trimester may develop drug discontinuation syndrome, including respiratory distress, feeding difficulty, and irritability; Lactation: Discontinue drug or bottle feed; Pedi: Safety not established in children <8 yr (for immediate release); Geri: May have ↑ sensitivity; recommend lower initial dose and slower dosage titration.

Interactions

Drug-Drug: Serious, potentially fatal reactions (serotonin syndrome) may occur with **MAO inhibitors. Smoking** may ↓ effectiveness of fluvoxamine. Concurrent use with **tricyclic antidepressants** may ↑ plasma levels of fluvoxamine. Drugs that affect serotonergic neurotransmitter systems, including **linezolid, tramadol**, and **triptans** ↑ risk of serotonin syndrome. ↓ metabolism and may ↑ effects of some **beta blockers (propranolol), alosetron** (avoid concurrent use), some **benzodiazepines** (avoid concurrent **diazepam), carbamazepine, methadone, lithium, theophylline** (↓ dose to 33% of usual dose), **ramelteon** (avoid concurrent use), **warfarin**, and **L-tryptophan**. ↑ risk of bleeding with **NSAIDS, aspirin, clopidogrel**, or **warfarin**. ↑ blood levels and risk of toxicity from **clozapine** (dosage adjustments may be necessary).

Route/Dosage

PO (Adults): *Immediate release (OCD only)*—50 mg daily at bedtime; ↑ by 50 mg q 4–7 days until desired effect is achieved. If daily dose >100 mg, give in two equally divided doses or give a larger dose at bedtime (not to exceed 300 mg/day). *Controlled release (OCD and SAD)*—100 mg at bedtime; ↑ by 50 mg q 7 days until desired effect is achieved, not to exceed 300 mg/day.
PO (Children 8–17 yr): *Immediate release (OCD only)*—25 mg at bedtime, may ↑ by 25 mg/day q 4–7 days (not to exceed 200 mg/day; daily doses >50 mg should be given in divided doses with a larger dose at bedtime).

Hepatic Impairment

PO (Adults): 25 mg daily at bedtime initially, slower titration and longer dosing intervals should be used.

Availability

Tablets: 25 mg, 50 mg, 100 mg. **Controlled-release capsules:** 100 mg, 150 mg.

HIGH ALERT

fondaparinux

(fon-da-**par**-i-nuks)

Arixtra

Classification

Therapeutic: anticoagulants

Pharmacologic: active factor X inhibitors

Indications

Prevention and treatment of deep vein thrombosis (DVT) and pulmonary embolism (PE). **Unlabeled Use:** Systemic anticoagulation for other diagnoses.

Action

Binds selectively to antithrombin III (AT III). This binding potentiates the neutralization (inactivation) of active factor X (Xa). **Therapeutic Effects:** Interruption of the coagulation cascade resulting in inhibition of thrombus formation. Prevention of thrombus formation decreases the risk of pulmonary emboli.

Adverse Reactions/Side Effects

CNS: confusion, dizziness, headache, insomnia. **CV:** edema, hypotension. **GI:** constipation, diarrhea, dyspepsia, increased serum aminotransferases, nausea, vomiting. **GU:** urinary retention. **Derm:** bullous eruption, hematoma, purpura, rash. **Hemat:** bleeding, thrombocytopenia. **F and E:** hypokalemia. **Misc:** fever, increased wound drainage.

PHYSICAL THERAPY IMPLICATIONS

Examination and Evaluation

- Monitor symptoms of DVT (pain, swelling, warmth, redness) to document whether drug therapy is effective in preventing or reducing venous thrombosis. Request or administer objective tests (Doppler ultrasound) if symptoms increase.
- In patients with DVT, watch for signs of PE (shortness of breath, chest pain, cough, bloody sputum). Notify physician immediately if these signs occur.
- Assess signs of bleeding and thrombocytopenia, including bleeding gums, nosebleeds, unusual bruising, black/tarry stools, hematuria, or a sudden fall in hematocrit or blood pressure. Notify physician or nursing staff immediately of these signs.
- Assess blood pressure periodically and compare to normal values (See Appendix F). Report low blood pressure (hypotension), especially if patient experiences dizziness, fatigue, or other symptoms.
- Assess peripheral edema using girth measurements, volume displacement, and measurement of pitting edema (See Appendix N). Report increased swelling in feet and ankles or a sudden increase in body weight due to fluid retention.
- Monitor and report unusual muscle weakness, aches, or cramps that might indicate low potassium levels (hypokalemia).
- Monitor any wounds or suture lines for increased drainage or bleeding. Report prolonged or excessive wound drainage to the physician.
- Assess dizziness that might affect gait, balance, and other functional activities (See Appendix C). Report balance problems and functional limitations to the physician and nursing staff, and caution the patient and family/caregivers to guard against falls and trauma.

Interventions

- Use caution with any physical interventions that could increase bleeding, including wound débridement, chest percussion, joint mobilization, and application of local heat.

Patient/Client-Related Instruction

- Instruct patient to report other bothersome side effects such as severe or prolonged headache, fever, confusion, sleep loss, urinary retention, skin reactions (rash, purplish spots, blood clots), or GI problems (nausea, vomiting, diarrhea, constipation, indigestion).

Pharmacokinetics

Absorption: 100% absorbed following subcutaneous administration.
Distribution: Distributes mainly throughout the intravascular space.
Metabolism and Excretion: Eliminated mainly unchanged in urine.
Half-life: 17–21 hr.

TIME/ACTION PROFILE (anticoagulant effect)

ROUTE	ONSET	PEAK	DURATION
SC	rapid	3 hr	24 hr

Contraindications/Precautions

Contraindicated in: Hypersensitivity; Severe renal impairment (CCr <30 mL/min; increased risk of bleeding); Body weight <50 kg in patients undergoing hip replacement (markedly increased risk of bleeding); Active major bleeding; Bacterial endocarditis; Thrombocytopenia due to fondaparinux antibodies.

Use Cautiously in: Mild-to-moderate renal impairment; Retinopathy (hypertensive or diabetic); Untreated hypertension; Recent history of ulcer disease; History of congenital or acquired bleeding disorder; Geri: Patients >65 yr (increased risk of bleeding); Malignancy; History of heparin-induced thrombocytopenia; OB/Pedi: Pregnancy, lactation, or children (safety not established; use during pregnancy only if clearly needed).

Exercise Extreme Caution in: Severe uncontrolled hypertension; Bleeding disorders; GI bleeding/ulceration/pathology; Hemorrhagic stroke; Recent CNS or ophthalmologic surgery; Active GI bleeding/ulceration; Spinal/epidural anesthesia or spinal puncture (increased risk of spinal/epidural hematoma that may lead to long-term or permanent paralysis).

Interactions

Drug-Drug: Risk of bleeding may be ↑ by concurrent use of **warfarin** or **drugs that affect platelet function**, including **aspirin, NSAIDs, dipyridamole,** some **cephalosporins, valproates, clopidogrel, ticlopidine, abciximab, eptifibatide, tirofiban,** and **dextran**.

Drug-Natural: ↑ risk of bleeding with **arnica, chamomile, clove, dong quai, feverfew, garlic, ginger, gingko,** *Panax ginseng*, and others.

Route/Dosage

Treatment of DVT/PE

SC (Adults): *<50 kg*—5 mg once daily for at least 5 days until therapeutic anticoagulation with warfarin is achieved (INR >2 for 2 consecutive days); warfarin may be started within 72 hr of fondaparinux (has been used for up to 26 days); *50–100 kg*—7.5 mg once daily for at least 5 days until therapeutic anticoagulation with warfarin is achieved (INR >2 for 2 consecutive days); *>100 kg*—10 mg once daily for at least 5 days until therapeutic anticoagulation with warfarin is achieved (INR >2 for 2 consecutive days); warfarin may be started within 72 hr of fondaparinux.

Prevention of DVT/PE

SC (Adults): 2.5 mg once daily, starting 6–8 hr after surgery, continuing for 5–9 days (up to 11 days) following abdominal surgery or knee/hip replacement or continuing for 24 days following hip fracture surgery (up to 32 days).

Availability

Solution for SC injection: 2.5 mg/0.5 mL in prefilled syringes, 5 mg/0.4 mL in prefilled syringes, 7.5 mg/0.6 mL in prefilled syringes, 10 mg/0.8 mL in prefilled syringes.

formoterol (for-mo-te-role)

Foradil, Perforomist

Classification

Therapeutic: bronchodilators

Pharmacologic: adrenergics

F

Indications

Long-term maintenance treatment of asthma. Prevention of bronchospasm in reversible obstructive airways disease, including long-term management of bronchoconstriction associated with COPD, including chronic bronchitis and emphysema. Acute prevention of exercise-induced bronchospasm, when used on an occasional, as needed, basis. Maintenance treatment of emphysema and chronic bronchitis.

Action

Produces accumulation of cyclic adenosine monophosphate (cAMP) at beta-adrenergic receptors, resulting in relaxation of airway smooth muscle. Relatively specific for $beta_2$ (pulmonary) receptors.

Therapeutic Effects: Bronchodilation.

Adverse Reactions/Side Effects

CNS: dizziness, fatigue, headache, insomnia, malaise, nervousness. **Resp:** PARADOXICAL BRONCHOSPASM. **CV:** angina, arrhythmias, hypertension, hypotension, palpitations, tachycardia. **GI:** dry mouth, nausea. **F and E:** hypokalemia. **Metab:** hyperglycemia, metabolic acidosis. **MS:** muscle cramps. **Neuro:** tremor. **Misc:** ALLERGIC REACTIONS, INCLUDING ANAPHYLAXIS.

PHYSICAL THERAPY IMPLICATIONS

Examination and Evaluation

- Monitor signs of paradoxical bronchospasm (wheezing, cough, dyspnea, tightness in chest and throat), especially at higher or excessive doses. If condition occurs, advise patient to withhold medication and notify physician or other health care professional immediately.
- Monitor signs of allergic reactions or anaphylaxis, including pulmonary symptoms (bronchospasm, wheezing, cough, dyspnea) or skin reactions (rash, pruritus, urticaria). Notify physician immediately if these reactions occur.
- Assess pulmonary function at rest and during exercise (See Appendices I, J, K) to document effectiveness of medication in controlling bronchospasm.
- Assess blood pressure periodically and compare to normal values (See Appendix F). Report a sustained increase in blood pressure (BP) (hypertension) or a fall in BP (hypotension) that causes dizziness or fainting.

- Assess heart rate, ECG, and heart sounds, especially during exercise (See Appendices G, H). Report a rapid heart rate (tachycardia) or signs of other arrhythmias, including palpitations, chest discomfort, shortness of breath, fainting, and fatigue/weakness.
- Assess dizziness that might affect gait, balance, and other functional activities (See Appendix C). Report balance problems and functional limitations to the physician, and caution the patient and family/caregivers to guard against falls and trauma.
- Monitor and report signs of CNS toxicity, including nervousness, sleep loss, tremor, or hyperactivity. Sustained or severe CNS signs may indicate overdose or excessive use of this drug.
- Monitor signs of metabolic acidosis, including confusion, lethargy, stupor, shallow rapid breathing, tachycardia, hypotension, nausea, and vomiting. Notify physician immediately if these signs occur.
- Be alert for signs of hyperglycemia, including confusion, drowsiness, flushed/dry skin, fruit-like breath odor, rapid/deep breathing, polyuria, loss of appetite, and unusual thirst. Patients with diabetes mellitus should check blood glucose levels frequently.
- Monitor and report any muscle weakness, aches, or cramps that might indicate low potassium levels (hypokalemia).

Interventions

- When implementing airway clearance techniques or respiratory muscle training, attempt to intervene when the airway is maximally bronchodilated. Peak responses typically occur 1–3 hr after inhalation.
- Use caution during aerobic exercise and endurance conditioning because of the risk of cardiovascular stimulation. Cardiac effects should be minimal at lower doses or occasional inhaled use. Cardiovascular effects such as arrhythmias, angina pectoris, or increased BP may occur at higher doses or during excessive use, and are caused by inadvertent stimulation of beta receptors on the heart.

Patient/Client-Related Instruction

- Advise patient not to exceed the recommended dose or frequency of inhalations. Contact physician immediately if bronchospasm is not relieved by medication or is accompanied by diaphoresis, dizziness, or other symptoms.
- Counsel patient on proper use of inhaler; observe use of this device whenever possible to ensure proper technique.
- Instruct patient and family/caregivers to report severe or prolonged headache, fatigue, or GI problems (nausea, dry mouth).

Pharmacokinetics

Absorption: Following inhalation, majority of inhaled drug is swallowed and absorbed.
Distribution: Unknown.
Metabolism and Excretion: Mostly metabolized by the liver; 10–18% excreted unchanged in urine.
Half-life: 10 hr.

TIME/ACTION PROFILE (bronchodilation)

ROUTE	ONSET	PEAK	DURATION
inhalation	15 min	1–3 hr	12 hr

Contraindications/Precautions

Contraindicated in: Hypersensitivity; Acute attack of asthma (onset of action is delayed).
Use Cautiously in: Cardiovascular disease (including angina and hypertension); Diabetes; Glaucoma; Hyperthyroidism; Pheochromocytoma; Excessive use (may lead to tolerance and paradoxical bronchospasm); OB/Pedi: Pregnancy, lactation, or children <5 yr (may inhibit contractions during labor; use only if potential benefits outweigh risks).

Interactions

Drug-Drug: **Concurrent use with MAO inhibitors, tricyclic antidepressants,** or other **agents that may prolong the QTc interval** may result in serious arrhythmias and should be undertaken with extreme caution. ↑ risk of hypokalemia with **theophylline**, **corticosteroids**, and **potassium-losing diuretics**. **Beta blockers** may ↓ therapeutic effects of formoterol. ↑ adrenergic effects may occur with concurrent use of **adrenergics**.

Route/Dosage

Maintenance Treatment of Asthma

Inhaatioln (Adults and Children ≥5 yr): 1 capsule (12 mcg) every 12 hr using the Aerolizer Inhaler.

Prevention of Exercise-Induced Bronchospasm

Inhalation (Adults and Children ≥12 yr): 1 capsule (12 mcg) at least 15 min before exercise on an occasional as-needed basis.

Maintenance Treatment of Emphysema and Chronic Bronchitis

Inhalation (Adults): 20 mcg/2 mL–unit dose vial twice daily via jet nebulizer.

Availability

Capsule for Aerolizer use: 12 mcg. **Vials for nebulization:** 20 mcg/2 mL. ***In combination with:*** budesonide (Symbicort). See Appendix B.

fosamprenavir

(fos-am-**pren**-a-veer)

Lexiva

Classification

Therapeutic: antiretrovirals

Pharmacologic: protease inhibitors

Indications

With other antiretrovirals in the management of HIV infection.

Action

Inhibits the action of HIV protease and prevents the cleavage of viral polyproteins. **Therapeutic Effects:** Increased CD4 cell counts and decreased viral load with subsequent slowed progression of HIV and its sequelae.

Adverse Reactions/Side Effects

Reflects use with other antiretrovirals

CNS: headache, fatigue, mood disorders. **GI:** diarrhea, nausea, vomiting, abdominal pain, ↑ liver enzymes. **Derm:** rash. **Endo:** glucose intolerance. **Hemat:** neutropenia. **Metab:** fat redistribution, ↑ triglycerides. **Misc:** ALLERGIC REACTIONS, INCLUDING STEVENS-JOHNSON SYNDROME, ANGIOEDEMA, inflammatory response to opportunistic infection.

PHYSICAL THERAPY IMPLICATIONS

Examination and Evaluation

- Monitor rashes or other skin reactions such as hives, itching, raised patches of red or white skin (welts), burning, acne, exfoliation, and abnormal sweating. Notify physician immediately because certain skin responses may indicate serious allergic reactions such as Stevens-Johnson syndrome and angioedema.
- Monitor personality changes and mood disorders, including anxiety, depression, mood swings, severe restlessness, and increased thoughts of suicide. Notify physician if these changes become problematic.
- Watch for signs of neutropenia, including fever, sore throat, and signs of infection. Report these signs to the physician.

Interventions

- Implement resistive exercises and other therapeutic exercises as needed to maintain muscle strength and function and prevent muscle wasting associated with HIV infection and AIDS.
- Design and implement aerobic exercise and endurance-training programs to help prevent heart disease associated with drug-related hyperlipidemia and other problems with lipid and glucose metabolism.

Patient/Client-Related Instruction

- Emphasize the importance of taking fosamprenavir as directed even if the patient is asymptomatic, and that this drug must always be used in combination with other antiretroviral drugs. Do not take more than prescribed amount, and do not stop taking without a consulting health care professional.
- Inform patient that fosamprenavir does not cure HIV or AIDS or prevent associated or opportunistic infections. Fosamprenavir does not reduce the risk of transmission of HIV to others through sexual contact or blood contamination. Caution patient to use a condom, and to avoid sharing needles or donating blood to prevent spreading the AIDS virus to others.
- Advise patient that this drug may cause problems in fat and glucose metabolism (increased triglycerides and glucose intolerance, respectively). Remind patient that periodic blood tests may be needed to monitor plasma lipids.
- Inform patient that redistribution and accumulation of body fat may occur, causing central obesity, thin arms and legs, dorsocervical fat enlargement (buffalo hump), breast enlargement, and other symptoms that resemble Cushing's syndrome (moon face, striations on abdominal skin). Discuss possible effects on body image, and help patient explore coping mechanisms.
- Instruct patient to report other troublesome side effects such as prolonged or severe headache, fatigue, or GI reactions (diarrhea, nausea, vomiting, abdominal pain).

Pharmacokinetics

Absorption: Fosamprenavir is a prodrug. Following oral administration, it is rapidly converted to amprenavir by the gut lining during absorption.
Distribution: Penetration into RBCs is concentration dependent.
Metabolism and Excretion: Mostly metabolized the liver (CYP3A4 enzyme system). Minimal renal excretion.
Half-life: 7.7 hr.

TIME/ACTION PROFILE (blood levels)

ROUTE	ONSET	PEAK	DURATION
PO	rapid	1.5–4 hr	12–24 hr

Contraindications/Precautions

Contraindicated in: Hypersensitivity, sulfonamide/sulfa hypersensitivity; Severe hepatic impairment; Concurrent use of flecainide, propafenone, rifampin, ergot derivatives, St. John's wort, lovastatin, simvastatin, pimozide, delavirdine, midazolam, or triazolam.

Use Cautiously in: Geri: Consider age-related decrease in body mass, cardiac/hepatic/renal impairment, concurrent illness and medications; Mild-to-moderate hepatic impairment; Concurrent use of medications handled by or affecting the CYP3A4 enzyme system (may require serum level monitoring, dose or dosing interval alterations); OB/Pedi: Pregnancy, lactation, children <2 yr (safety not established; breast-feeding not recommended in HIV-infected patients).

Interactions

Drug-Drug: Amprenavir, the active moiety of fosamprenavir is metabolized by **CYP3A4**; it also inhibits and induces this enzyme system. The action of any other medication that is also handled by or affects this system may be altered by concurrent use. Concurrent use of **flecainide, propafenone, rifampin, ergot derivatives (dihydroergotamine, ergotamine, ergonovine, methylergonovine), fluticasone lovastatin, simvastatin, pimozide, delavirdine, midazolam, or triazolam** may result in serious, potentially life-threatening adverse reactions, including arrhythmias, excessive sedation, myopathy, or loss of virologic response and is contraindicated. Blood levels are ↓ by **efavirenz** (additional ritonavir may be required when used together), **nevirapine, lopinavir/ritonavir, saquinavir, carbamazepine, phenobarbital, phenytoin, dexamethasone, histamine H_2 receptor antagonists,** and **proton-pump inhibitors**; monitor for ↓ antiretroviral activity. Levels are ↑ by **indinavir** and **nelfinavir**. May ↓ **methadone** and **paroxetine** levels. ↑ levels and risk of toxicity from **amiodarone, lidocaine, quinidine** (monitor blood levels), **ketoconazole,** and **itraconazole** (dose of itraconazole or ketoconazole should not exceed 200 mg/day when fosamprenavir is used with ritonavir or 400 mg/day when used without), **rifabutin** (monitor for neutropenia, ↓ rifabutin dose by 50% when used with fosamprenavir or by 75% when used with fosamprenavir with ritonavir), **atorvastatin.** and **rosuvastatin** (dose not to exceed 20 mg/day or consider other HMG-CoA reductase inhibitors), **cyclosporine,** or **tacrolimus** (monitor blood levels of immunosuppressants), **calcium channel blockers** (clinical monitoring recommended), some **benzodiazepines (alprazolam, clorazepate, diazepam, flurazepam**; dose reduction of benzodiazepine may be needed), **sildenafil, tadalafil,** and **vardenafil** (use cautiously; ↓ dose of sildenafil to 25 mg q 48 hr, for tadalafil single dose should not exceed 10 mg in any 72 hr period, dose of vardenafil should not exceed 2.5 mg q 24 hr if used without ritonavir or 2.5 mg q 72 hr with ritonavir with monitoring for toxicity), and **tricyclic antidepressants** (blood level monitoring recommended). May alter the effects of **warfarin** (monitor INR) or **hormonal contraceptives** (use alternative method of contraception).

Drug-Natural: Concurrent use of **St. John's wort** is contraindicated; ↓ blood levels and may lead to ↓ virologic response.

Route/Dosage

PO (Adults): *Treatment-naive patients without ritonavir*—1400 mg bid; *Treatment-naive patients with ritonavir*—1400 mg once daily with ritonavir 100 or 200 mg once daily, or 700 mg bid with ritonavir 100 mg bid. *Protease inhibitor–experienced patients*—700 mg bid with ritonavir 100 mg bid. If efavirenz is added to a once daily regimen using both fosamprenavir and ritonavir, an additional 100 mg of ritonavir (total of 300 mg) should be given.

PO (Children 2–5 yr): *Treatment-naive*—30 mg/kg bid, not to exceed 1400 mg bid.

PO (Children ≥6 yr): *Treatment-naive*—30 mg/kg bid, not to exceed 1400 mg bid, or 18 mg/kg bid (not to exceed 700 mg bid) with ritonavir 3 mg/kg bid (not to exceed 100 mg bid); *Protease inhibitor-experienced*—18 mg/kg bid (not to exceed 700 mg bid) with ritonavir 3 mg/kg bid (not to exceed 100 mg bid). When used without ritonavir in children ≥47 kg, may use adult regimen of 1400 mg bid.

Hepatic Impairment

PO (Adults): *Mild hepatic impairment*—700 mg bid without ritonavir (therapy-naive) or 700 mg bid with ritonavir 100 mg once daily (therapy-naive or protease inhibitor experienced); *Moderate hepatic impairment*—700 mg bid without ritonavir (therapy-naive) or 450 mg bid with ritonavir 100 mg once daily (therapy-naive or protease inhibitor–experienced); *Severe hepatic impairment*—350 mg bid without ritonavir (therapy-naive).

Availability

Tablets: 700 mg. **Oral suspension:** 50 mg/mL.

fosaprepitant (injection)

(fos-a-**prep**-i-tant)

Emend

Classification

Therapeutic: antiemetics

Pharmacologic: neurokinin antagonists

Indications
Prevention of nausea and vomiting associated with emetogenic chemotherapy.

Action
Acts as a selective antagonist at substance P/neurokinin$_1$ (NK1) receptors in the brain. **Therapeutic Effects:** Decreased nausea and vomiting associated with chemotherapy.

Adverse Reactions/Side Effects
CNS: dizziness, fatigue, weakness. **GI:** diarrhea. **Misc:** hiccups.

PHYSICAL THERAPY IMPLICATIONS

Examination and Evaluation
- Monitor improvements in GI symptoms (decreased nausea and vomiting, increased appetite) to help document whether drug therapy is successful.
- Assess dizziness, fatigue, or weakness that might affect gait, balance, and other functional activities (See Appendix C). Report balance problems and functional limitations to the physician and nursing staff, and caution the patient and family/caregivers to guard against falls and trauma.

Patient/Client-Related Instruction
- Instruct patient to report bothersome GI side effects such as severe or prolonged diarrhea or hiccups.

Pharmacokinetics
Absorption: Following IV administration, fosaprepitant is rapidly converted to aprepitant, the active component.
Distribution: Crosses the blood-brain barrier; remainder of distribution unknown.
Metabolism and Excretion: Mostly metabolized by the liver (CYP3A4 enzyme system); not renally excreted.
Half-life: *Aprepitant*—9–13 hr.

TIME/ACTION PROFILE (antiemetic effect)

ROUTE	ONSET	PEAK	DURATION
PO	rapid	end of infusion*	24 hr

*Blood level.

Contraindications/Precautions
Contraindicated in: Hypersensitivity; Concurrent use with pimozide (risk of life-threatening adverse cardiovascular reactions); Lactation: May cause unwanted effects in nursing infants.
Use Cautiously in: OB: Use only if clearly needed; Pedi: Safety not established.

Interactions
Drug-Drug: Aprepitant inhibits, induces and is metabolized by the CYP3A4 enzyme system; it also induces the CYP2C9 system. Concurrent use with other medications that are metabolized by CYP3A4 may result in ↑ toxicity from these agents, including **docetaxel, paclitaxel, etoposide, irinotecan, ifosfamide, imatinib, vinorelbine, vinblastine, vincristine, midazolam, triazolam**, and **alprazolam**; concurrent use should be undertaken with caution. Concurrent use with drugs that significantly inhibit the CYP3A4 enzyme system, including **ketoconazole, itraconazole, nefazodone, clarithromycin, ritonavir, nelfinavir**, and **diltiazem**, may ↑ blood levels and effects of aprepitant. Concurrent use with drugs that induce the CYP3A4 enzyme system, including **rifampin, carbamazepine**, and **phenytoin**, may ↓ blood levels and effects of aprepitant. ↑ blood levels and effects of **dexamethasone** (regimen reflects a 50% dose reduction); a similar effect occurs with **methylprednisolone** (IV dose by 25%, PO dose by 50% when used concurrently). May ↓ the effects of **warfarin** (careful monitoring for 2 wk recommended), **oral contraceptives** (use alternate method), **tolbutamide,** and **phenytoin.**

Route/Dosage
IV (Adults): 115 mg 30 min prior to chemotherapy on day 1.

Availability
Lyophilized solid (requires reconstitution prior to injection): 115 mg/10-mL vial.

foscarnet (foss-kar-net)
Foscavir

Classification
Therapeutic: antivirals
Pharmacologic: pyrophosphate analogues

Indications
Treatment of cytomegalovirus (CMV) retinitis in HIV-infected patients (alone or with ganciclovir). Treatment of acyclovir-resistant mucocutaneous herpes simplex virus (HSV) infections in immunocompromised patients.

Action
Prevents viral replication by inhibiting viral DNA-polymerase and reverse transcriptase. **Therapeutic Effects:** Virustatic action against susceptible viruses including CMV.

Adverse Reactions/Side Effects

CNS: SEIZURES, headache, anxiety, confusion, dizziness, fatigue, malaise, mental depression, weakness. EENT: conjunctivitis, eye pain, vision abnormalities. **Resp:** coughing, dyspnea. **CV:** chest pain, ECG abnormalities, edema, palpitations. **GI:** diarrhea, nausea, vomiting, abdominal pain, abnormal taste sensation, anorexia, constipation, dyspepsia. **GU:** renal failure, albuminuria, dysuria, nocturia, polyuria, urinary retention. **Derm:** increased sweating, pruritus, rash, skin ulceration. **F and E:** hypocalcemia, hypokalemia, hypomagnesemia, hyperphosphatemia, hypophosphatemia. **Hemat:** anemia, granulocytopenia, leukopenia. **Local:** pain/inflammation at injection site. **MS:** arthralgia, myalgia, back pain, involuntary muscle contraction. **Neuro:** ataxia, hypoesthesia, neuropathy, paresthesia, tremor. **Misc:** fever, chills, flu-like syndrome, lymphoma, sarcoma.

PHYSICAL THERAPY IMPLICATIONS

Examination and Evaluation

- Be alert for new seizures or increased seizure activity, especially at the onset of drug treatment. Document the number, duration, and severity of seizures, and report these findings immediately to the physician.
- Assess heart rate, ECG, and heart sounds, especially during exercise (See Appendices G, H). Report any rhythm disturbances or symptoms of increased arrhythmias, including palpitations, chest discomfort, shortness of breath, dyspnea, fainting, and fatigue/weakness.
- Assess peripheral edema using girth measurements, volume displacement, and measurement of pitting edema (See Appendix N). Report increased swelling in feet and ankles or a sudden increase in body weight due to fluid retention.
- Monitor signs of leukopenia and granulocytopenia (fever, sore throat, mucosal lesions, signs of infection) or unusual weakness and fatigue that might be due to anemia. Report these signs to the physician.
- Monitor neuromuscular signs of electrolyte imbalances (hypocalcemia, hypokalemia, etc.), including headache, lethargy, weakness, cramping, and muscle hyperexcitability and tetany. Notify physician immediately if these signs occur.
- Monitor signs of renal failure, including decreased urine output, increased blood pressure, muscle cramps/twitching, edema/weight gain from fluid retention, yellowish brown skin, and confusion that progresses to seizures and coma. Report these signs to the physician immediately.
- Assess any joint, muscle, or back pain to rule out musculoskeletal pathology; that is, try to determine if pain is drug induced rather than caused by anatomic or biomechanical problems.
- Monitor signs of peripheral neuropathy and paresthesia (numbness, tingling, muscle weakness). Perform objective tests (nerve conduction, monofilaments) to assess and document any neuropathic changes.
- Be alert for anxiety, confusion, mental depression, or other alterations in mental status. Notify physician promptly if these symptoms develop.
- Be alert for tremor, dizziness, or ataxia that might affect gait, balance, or other functional activities. Report balance problems and functional limitations to the physician, and caution the patient and family/caregivers to guard against falls and trauma.
- Monitor IV injection site for pain, swelling, and irritation. Report prolonged or excessive injection site reactions to the physician.

Interventions

- Because of the risk of arrhythmias, use caution during aerobic exercise and other forms of therapeutic exercise. Assess exercise tolerance frequently (blood pressure, heart rate, fatigue levels), and terminate exercise immediately if any untoward responses occur (See Appendix L).
- Always wash hands thoroughly and disinfect equipment (whirlpools, electrotherapeutic devices, treatment tables, and so forth) to help prevent the spread of infection. Employ universal precautions as indicated for specific patients.

Patient/Client-Related Instruction

- Instruct patient to report any vision disturbances, including blurred vision, decreased visual acuity, and signs of macular abnormalities (blurry or decreased central vision with peripheral vision intact).
- Instruct patient and family/caregivers to report other troublesome side effects, including severe or prolonged headache, flu-like symptoms, skin problems (rash, sweating, itching, ulcerations), or GI problems (diarrhea, nausea, vomiting, constipation, heartburn, abdominal pain, loss of appetite).

Pharmacokinetics

Absorption: IV administration results in complete bioavailability.
Distribution: Variable penetration into CSF. May concentrate in and be slowly released from bone.
Metabolism and Excretion: 80–90% excreted unchanged in urine.
Half-life: 3 hr (in patients with normal renal function); longer half-life of 90 hr may reflect release of drug from bone.

TIME/ACTION PROFILE

ROUTE	ONSET	PEAK	DURATION
IV	rapid	end of infusion	8–24 hr

Contraindications/Precautions

Contraindicated in: Hypersensitivity.
Use Cautiously in: Renal impairment (dose reduction required if CCr ≤1.4–1.6 mL/min/kg; see product information); History of seizures; OB/Pedi: Pregnancy, lactation, or children (safety not established).

Interactions

Drug-Drug: Concurrent use with parenteral **pentamidine** may result in severe, life-threatening hypocalcemia. Risk of nephrotoxicity may be ↑ by concurrent use of other **nephrotoxic agents (amphotericin B, aminoglycosides)**.

Route/Dosage

IV (Adults): *CMV retinitis*—60 mg/kg q 8 hr or 90 mg/kg q 12 hr for 2–3 wk, then 90–120 mg/kg/day as a single dose. Dosage reduction required for any degree of renal impairment; *HSV*—40 mg/kg q 8–12 hr for 2–3 wk or until healing occurs.

Availability (generic available)

Injection: 6000 mg/250 mL, 12,000 mg/500 mL.

fosfomycin (fos-foe-**mye**-sin)

Monurol

Classification
Therapeutic: anti-infectives
Pharmacologic: phosphonic acid derivatives

Indications

Uncomplicated urinary tract infections in women (acute cystitis).

Action

Inactivates an enzyme crucial for bacterial cell wall synthesis. Decreases adherence of bacteria to uroepithelial cells. **Therapeutic Effects:** Bactericidal action against susceptible bacteria. **Spectrum:** Active against *Enterococcus faecalis* and *Escherichia coli*.

Adverse Reactions/Side Effects

CNS: dizziness, headache, weakness. **GI:** PSEUDOMEMBRANOUS COLITIS, diarrhea, dyspepsia, nausea. **GU:** vaginitis.

PHYSICAL THERAPY IMPLICATIONS

Examination and Evaluation

- Be alert for signs of pseudomembranous colitis, including diarrhea, abdominal pain, fever, pus or mucus in stools, or other severe or prolonged GI problems (nausea, cramps, vomiting). Notify physician immediately if these signs occur.
- Assess dizziness and weakness that might affect gait, balance, and other functional activities (See Appendix C). Report balance problems and functional limitations to the physician and nursing staff, and caution the patient and family/caregivers to guard against falls and trauma.

Interventions

- Always wash hands thoroughly and disinfect equipment (whirlpools, electrotherapeutic devices, treatment tables, and so forth) to help prevent the spread of infection. Employ universal precautions or isolation procedures as indicated for specific patients.

Patient/Client-Related Instruction

- Instruct patient to report other bothersome side effects such as severe or prolonged headache, vaginal irritation, or GI problems (nausea, diarrhea, indigestion).

Pharmacokinetics

Absorption: Rapidly absorbed and converted to fosfomycin, its active component, resulting in 37% bioavailability.
Distribution: Distributes to kidneys and bladder wall; crosses the placenta.
Metabolism and Excretion: Excreted unchanged in urine (38%) and feces (18%).
Half-life: 5.7 hr.

TIME/ACTION PROFILE (bactericidal urine levels*)

ROUTE	ONSET	PEAK	DURATION
PO	rapid	2–4 hr	unknown

*Symptoms may take 24–48 hr to subside.

Contraindications/Precautions

Contraindicated in: Hypersensitivity; Pyelonephritis; Lactation: Lactation.
Use Cautiously in: OB/Pedi: Pregnancy or children <12 yr (safety not established).

Interactions

Drug-Drug: Urinary excretion and blood levels are ↓ by **metoclopramide**.

Route/Dosage

PO (Adults and Children ≥18 yr): 3 g single dose.

Availability

Sachet: 3 g.

fosinopril (foe-sin-oh-pril)
Monopril

Classification
Therapeutic: antihypertensives
Pharmacologic: angiotensin-converting enzyme (ACE) inhibitors

Indications
Alone or with other agents in the management of hypertension. Management of heart failure.

Action
ACE inhibitors block the conversion of angiotensin I to the vasoconstrictor angiotensin II. ACE inhibitors also prevent the degradation of bradykinin and other vasodilatory prostaglandins. ACE inhibitors also increase plasma renin levels and reduce aldosterone levels. Net result is systemic vasodilation. **Therapeutic Effects:** Lowering of blood pressure in patients with hypertension. Decreased afterload and symptoms in patients with heart failure.

Adverse Reactions/Side Effects
CNS: dizziness, fatigue, headache, insomnia, weakness. Resp: cough. **CV:** hypotension, chest pain, edema. **GI:** abdominal pain, diarrhea, nausea, vomiting. **GU:** erectile dysfunction, impaired renal function. **Derm:** rashes. **F and E:** hyperkalemia. **MS:** muscle cramps. **Resp:** dyspnea. **Misc:** ANGIOEDEMA.

PHYSICAL THERAPY IMPLICATIONS

Examination and Evaluation
- Monitor signs of angioedema, including rashes, raised patches of red or white skin (welts), burning/itching skin, swelling in the face, and difficulty breathing. Notify physician of these signs immediately.
- Assess blood pressure periodically and compare to normal values (See Appendix F) to help document antihypertensive effects. Report low blood pressure (hypotension), especially if patient experiences dizziness or syncope.
- Assess signs and symptoms of CHF (dyspnea, rales/crackles, jugular venous distention, exercise intolerance) to help document whether drug therapy is effective in reducing these symptoms.
- Assess peripheral edema using girth measurements, volume displacement, and measurement of pitting edema (See Appendix N). Report increased swelling in feet and ankles or a sudden increase in body weight due to fluid retention.
- Watch for signs of impaired renal function, including decreased urine output, cloudy urine, or sudden weight gain due to fluid retention. Report these signs to the physician.
- Monitor symptoms of high plasma potassium levels (hyperkalemia), including bradycardia, fatigue, weakness, numbness, and tingling. Notify physician because severe cases can lead to life-threatening arrhythmias and paralysis.
- Assess dizziness that might affect gait, balance, and other functional activities (See Appendix C). Report balance problems and functional limitations to the physician, and caution the patient and family/caregivers to guard against falls and trauma.

Interventions
- Implement aerobic exercise and cardiac conditioning programs to augment drug therapy and maintain or improve cardiovascular pump function in patients with heart failure and other cardiac conditions.
- Avoid physical therapy interventions that cause systemic vasodilation (large whirlpool, Hubbard tank). Additive effects of this drug and the intervention may cause a dangerous fall in blood pressure.
- To minimize orthostatic hypotension, patient should move slowly when assuming a more upright position.

Patient/Client-Related Instruction
- Remind patients to take medication as directed to control hypertension and other cardiac conditions even if they are asymptomatic.
- Instruct patients with heart failure to weigh themselves every day, and call their physician if they gain 3 lb or more in 1 day or more than 5 lb in 1 week. Sudden weight gain may indicate fluid buildup due to worsening heart failure.
- Counsel patients about additional interventions to help control blood pressure and cardiac dysfunction, including regular exercise, weight loss, sodium restriction, stress reduction, moderation of alcohol consumption, and smoking cessation.
- Instruct patient to notify physician of a prolonged dry cough or difficult, labored breathing; drug therapy may need to be altered to resolve this side effect.
- Instruct patient or family/caregivers to report other troublesome side effects such as severe or prolonged headache, insomnia, erectile dysfunction, skin rash, or GI problems (nausea, vomiting, diarrhea, abdominal pain).

Pharmacokinetics
Absorption: 36% absorbed following oral administration.
Distribution: Crosses the placenta; enters breast milk in small amounts.
Protein Binding: 99.4%.

Metabolism and Excretion: Converted by the liver and GI mucosa to fosinoprilat, the active metabolite: 50% excreted in urine, 50% in feces.
Half-life: 12 hr.
TIME/ACTION PROFILE (effect on blood pressure—single dose*)

ROUTE	ONSET	PEAK	DURATION
PO	within 1 hr	2–6 hr	24 hr

*Full effects may not be noted for several weeks.

Contraindications/Precautions

Contraindicated in: Hypersensitivity; Bilateral renal artery stenosis; History of angioedema with previous use of ACE inhibitors; OB: Can cause injury or death of fetus—if pregnancy occurs, discontinue immediately. Lactation: Appears in breast milk; patient must discontinue fosinopril or provide alternate to breast milk.
Use Cautiously in: Patients with renal impairment, hypovolemia, hyponatremia, and concurrent diuretic therapy; Black patients (monotherapy for hypertension less effective, may require additional therapy; higher risk of angioedema); Surgery/anesthesia (hypotension may be exaggerated); Women of childbearing potential; Pedi: Safety not established in children <6 yr; Geri: Initial dose reduction recommended.
Exercise Extreme Caution in: Family history of angioedema.

Interactions

Drug-Drug: Excessive hypotension may occur with concurrent use of **diuretics**. Additive hypotension with other **antihypertensive agents**. ↑ risk of hyperkalemia with concurrent use of **potassium supplements, potassium-sparing diuretics, potassium-containing salt substitutes,** or **angiotensin II receptor antagonists**. Antihypertensive response may be blunted by **NSAIDs**. Absorption may be decreased by **antacids** (separate administration by 1–2 hr). ↑ levels and may ↑ the risk of **lithium** toxicity.

Route/Dosage

PO (Adults): *Hypertension*—10 mg once daily, may be increased as required up to 80 mg/day. *Heart failure*—10 mg once daily (5 mg once daily in patients who have been vigorously diuresed), may be increased over several weeks up to 40 mg/day.
PO (Children ≥6 yr and >50 kg): *Hypertension*—5–10 mg once daily.

Availability (generic available)

Tablets: 10 mg, 20 mg, 40 mg. ***In combination with:*** hydrochlorothiazide (Monopril-HCTRx). See Appendix B.

fosphenytoin (fos-fen-i-toyn)

Cerebyx

Classification
Therapeutic: anticonvulsants
Pharmacologic: hydantoin derivatives

F

Indications

Short-term (<5 day) parenteral management of generalized, convulsive status epilepticus when use of phenytoin is not feasible. Treatment and prevention of seizures during neurosurgery when use of phenytoin is not feasible.

Action

Limits seizure propagation by altering ion transport. May also decrease synaptic transmission. Fosphenytoin is rapidly converted to phenytoin, which is responsible for its pharmacologic effects. **Therapeutic Effects:** Diminished seizure activity.

Adverse Reactions/Side Effects

CNS: dizziness, drowsiness, nystagmus, agitation, brain edema, headache, stupor, vertigo. **EENT:** amblyopia, deafness, diplopia, tinnitus. **CV:** hypotension (with rapid IV administration), tachycardia. **GI:** dry mouth, nausea, taste perversion, tongue disorder, vomiting. **Derm:** pruritus, rash, STEVENS-JOHNSON SYNDROME. **MS:** back pain. **Neuro:** ataxia, dysarthria, extrapyramidal syndrome, hypesthesia, incoordination, paresthesia, tremor. **Misc:** pelvic pain.

PHYSICAL THERAPY IMPLICATIONS

Examination and Evaluation

- Monitor skin reactions (rash, itching/burning skin, hives, exfoliation, dermatitis). Notify physician immediately about because certain skin reactions may indicate serious hypersensitivity reactions (Stevens-Johnson syndrome).
- Document the number, duration, and severity of seizures to help determine if this drug is effective in reducing seizure activity.
- Assess dizziness and vertigo that might affect gait, balance, and other functional activities (See Appendix C). Report balance problems and functional limitations to the physician and nursing staff, and caution the patient and family/caregivers to guard against falls and trauma.
- Monitor drowsiness, confusion, agitation, stupor, or signs of brain edema (changes in mood and behavior, decreased consciousness, headache, lethargy, seizures, vomiting). Notify physician immediately of these signs.

- Assess gait and motor function and document any signs of incoordination, ataxia, or other motor symptoms that might indicate extrapyramidal syndrome such as involuntary movements of the jaw, limbs, Parkinson-like symptoms, and other dystonias and dyskinesias. Report these signs to the physician.
- Assess signs of tremor, paresthesia (numbness, tingling) or other changes in sensation. Perform objective tests, including electroneuromyography and sensory testing to document any drug-related neuropathic changes.
- Assess blood pressure after IV administration and compare to normal values (See Appendix F). Report low blood pressure (hypotension), especially if patient experiences dizziness or syncope.
- Assess heart rate, ECG, and heart sounds, especially during exercise (See Appendices G, H). Report rapid heart rate (tachycardia) or symptoms of other arrhythmias, including palpitations, chest discomfort, shortness of breath, fainting, and fatigue/weakness.
- Assess any back pain or pelvic pain to rule out musculoskeletal pathology; that is, try to determine if pain is drug induced rather than caused by anatomic or biomechanical problems.

Interventions

- Guard against falls and trauma (hip fractures, head injury, and so forth), especially if drowsiness, dizziness, or motor problems (ataxia, dyskinesias) affect gait and balance. Implement fall prevention strategies, especially if balance is impaired (See Appendix E).
- Because of the risk of tachycardia, use caution during aerobic exercise and other forms of therapeutic exercise. Assess exercise tolerance frequently (blood pressure, heart rate, fatigue levels), and terminate exercise immediately if any untoward responses occur (See Appendix L).
- To minimize orthostatic hypotension, patient should move slowly when assuming a more upright position.

Patient/Client-Related Instruction

- Advise patient to avoid alcohol and other CNS depressants because of the increased risk of sedation and adverse effects.
- Advise patient about the risk of daytime drowsiness and decreased attention and mental focus. Use care if driving or in other activities that require strong concentration and fast responses.
- Instruct patient and family/caregivers to report other troublesome side effects such as severe or prolonged headache, ringing/buzzing in the ears (tinnitus), visual problems (double vision, nystagmus), skin reactions (rash, itching), or GI problems (nausea, vomiting, abnormal taste, dry mouth).

Pharmacokinetics

Absorption: Rapidly converted to phenytoin after IV administration and completely absorbed after IM administration.
Distribution: Distributes into CSF and other body tissues and fluids. Enters breast milk; crosses the placenta, achieving similar maternal/fetal levels. Preferentially distributes into fatty tissue.
Protein Binding: *Fosphenytoin*—95–99%; *phenytoin*—90–95%.
Metabolism and Excretion: Mostly metabolized by the liver; minimal amounts excreted in the urine.
Half-life: *Fosphenytoin*—15 min; *phenytoin*—22 hr (range 7–42 hr).

TIME/ACTION PROFILE (anticonvulsant effect)

ROUTE	ONSET	PEAK	DURATION
IM	unknown	30 min	up to 24 hr
IV	15–45 min	15–60 min	up to 24 hr

Contraindications/Precautions

Contraindicated in: Hypersensitivity; Sinus bradycardia, sinoatrial block, 2nd- or 3rd-degree AV heart block or Adams-Stokes syndrome.
Use Cautiously in: Hepatic or renal disease (↑ risk of adverse reactions; dose reduction recommended for hepatic impairment); OB: Safety not established; may result in fetal hydantoin syndrome if used chronically or hemorrhage in the newborn if used at term; Lactation: Safety not established.

Interactions

Drug-Drug: Disulfiram, acute ingestion of **alcohol, amiodarone, ethosuximide, isoniazid, chloramphenicol, sulfonamides, fluoxetine, gabapentin, H_2 antagonists, benzodiazepines, omeprazole, ketoconazole, fluconazole, estrogens, succinimides, halothane, methylphenidate, phenothiazines, salicylates, ticlopidine, tolbutamide, topiramate, trazodone, felbamate,** and **cimetidine** may ↑ phenytoin blood levels. **Barbiturates, carbamazepine, reserpine,** and chronic ingestion of **alcohol** may ↓ phenytoin blood levels. Phenytoin may ↓ the effects of **amiodarone, benzodiazepines, carbamazepine, chloramphenicol, corticosteroids, disopyramide, warfarin, felbamate, doxycycline, lamotrigine, oral contraceptives, paroxetine, propafenone, rifampin, ritonavir, quinidine, tacrolimus, theophylline, topiramate, tricyclic antidepressants, zonisamide, methadone, cyclosporine,** and **estrogens**. IV phenytoin and **dopamine** may cause additive hypotension. Additive CNS depression with other **CNS depressants,** including **alcohol, antihistamines, antidepressants,**

opioids, and **sedative/hypnotics**. **Antacids** may ↓ absorption of orally administered phenytoin. ↑ systemic clearance of antileukemic drugs **teniposide** and **methotrexate** which has been associated with a worse event free survival, phenytoin use is not recommended in children undergoing chemotherapy for acute lymphocytic leukemia. **Calcium** and **sucralfate** ↓ phenytoin absorption.

Route/Dosage

Note: Doses of fosphenytoin are expressed as phenytoin sodium equivalents (PE).

Status Epilepticus

IV (Adults): 15–20 mg PE/kg.

Nonemergent and Maintenance Dosing

IV, IM (Adults and Children >16 yr): *Loading dose*—10–20 mg PE/kg. *Maintenance dose*—4–6 mg PE/kg/day.
IV, IM (Children 10–16 yr): 6–7 mg PE/kg/day.
IV, IM (Children 7–9 yr): 7–8 mg PE/kg/day.
IV, IM (Children 4–6 yr): 7.5–9 mg PE/kg/day.
IV, IM (Children 0.5–3 yr): 8–10 mg PE kg/day.
IV, IM (Infants): 5 mg PE kg/day.
IV, IM (Neonates): 5–8 mg PE/kg/day.

Availability (generic available)

Injection: 50 mg PE/mL.

frovatriptan (froe-va-**trip**-tan)

Frova

Classification
Therapeutic: vascular headache suppressants
Pharmacologic: 5-HT_1 agonists

Indications

Acute treatment of migraine headache.

Action

Acts as an agonist at specific 5-HT receptor sites in intracranial blood vessels and sensory trigeminal nerves. **Therapeutic Effects:** Cranial vessel vasoconstriction with associated decrease in release of neuropeptides and resultant decrease in migraine headache.

Adverse Reactions/Side Effects

CNS: dizziness, drowsiness, fatigue. **CV:** CORONARY ARTERY VASOSPASM, MI, VENTRICULAR FIBRILLATION, VENTRICULAR TACHYCARDIA, chest pain, myocardial ischemia. **GI:** dry mouth, dyspepsia, nausea. **Derm:** flushing. **MS:** skeletal pain. **Neuro:** paresthesia. **Misc:** pain.

PHYSICAL THERAPY IMPLICATIONS

Examination and Evaluation

- Continually monitor for signs of coronary artery vasospasm and MI, including sudden chest pain, pain radiating into the arm or jaw, shortness of breath, dizziness, sweating, anxiety, and nausea. Seek immediate medical assistance if patient develops these signs.
- Assess heart rate, ECG, and heart sounds, especially during exercise (See Appendices G, H). Report any rhythm disturbances or symptoms of increased arrhythmias, including palpitations, chest discomfort, shortness of breath, dizziness, fainting, and fatigue/weakness.
- Assess the frequency and severity of headaches, and document whether drug therapy is successful in decreasing migraine attacks.
- Assess any skeletal or muscle pain to rule out musculoskeletal pathology; that is, try to determine if pain is drug induced rather than caused by anatomic or biomechanical problems.
- Assess signs of paresthesia (numbness, tingling). Perform objective tests, including electroneuromyography and sensory testing to document any drug-related neuropathic changes.
- Watch for dizziness and drowsiness that affects gait, balance, and other functional activities (See Appendix C). Report balance problems and functional limitations to the physician and nursing staff, and caution the patient and family/caregivers to guard against falls and trauma.

Interventions

- Because of the risk of MI and arrhythmias, use extreme caution during aerobic exercise and other forms of therapeutic exercise. Assess exercise tolerance frequently (blood pressure, heart rate, respiration, fatigue levels), and terminate exercise immediately if any untoward responses occur (See Appendix L).
- Implement appropriate interventions (manual techniques, physical agents, therapeutic exercise) to manage headache pain and reduce the need for drug therapy. Help patient also explore other nonpharmacologic methods to reduce chronic headache pain (relaxation techniques, imagery, and so forth).
- If a headache occurs and drug treatment is needed during a rehabilitation session, allow patient to recover in a quiet, darkened room to allow the drug to achieve maximal effects.

Patient/Client-Related Instruction

- Advise patient and family or caregiver about the signs of MI (see above under Examination and Evaluation), and to seek immediate medical assistance if these signs develop.
- Advise the patient to bring this drug to each therapy session; this drug is most effective when taken at the first signs of a migraine attack.
- Advise patient to adhere to the correct dosing schedule and not to exceed the recommended frequency and number of doses per 30-day period.
- Instruct patient to report other troublesome side effects such as severe or prolonged skin reactions (flushing) or GI problems (nausea, indigestion, dry mouth).

Pharmacokinetics

Absorption: 20–30% following oral administration.
Distribution: Unknown.
Metabolism and Excretion: Mostly metabolized by the liver (P4501A2 enzyme system); some metabolites eliminated in urine, <10% excreted unchanged.
Half-life: 26 hr.

TIME/ACTION PROFILE (blood levels)

ROUTE	ONSET	PEAK	DURATION
PO	unknown	2–4 hr	unknown

Contraindications/Precautions

Contraindicated in: Hypersensitivity; History, symptoms, or findings consistent with ischemic heart disease, coronary artery vasospasm, other significant underlying cardiovascular disease; Cerebrovascular syndromes including strokes of any type, transient ischemic attacks; Uncontrolled hypertension; Hemiplegic or basilar migraine; Peripheral vascular disease, including ischemic bowel disease; Should not be used within 24 hr of any other 5-HT agonist or ergot-type compounds (dihydroergotamine); Children <18 yr.
Use Cautiously in: Elderly patients (may be more susceptible to adverse cardiovascular effects); Pregnancy or lactation (safety not established).
Exercise Extreme Caution in: Cardiovascular risk factors (hypertension, hypercholesterolemia, cigarette smoking, obesity, diabetes, strong family history, menopausal women or men >40 yr); use only if cardiovascular status has been evaluated and determined to be safe and first dose is administered under supervision.

Interactions

Drug-Drug: Blood levels may be ↑ by **hormonal contraceptives** or **propranolol**. Blood levels may be ↓ by **ergotamine**. ↑ risk of serious vasospastic reactions with **dihydroergotamine** (concurrent use contraindicated).

Route/Dosage

PO (Adults): 2.5 mg; if there has been initial relief, a second tablet may be taken after at least 2 hr (daily dose should not exceed 3 tablets and should not be used to treat more than 4 attacks/30-day period).

Availability

Tablets: 2.5 mg.

fulvestrant (ful-**ves**-trant)

Faslodex

Classification
Therapeutic: antineoplastics
Pharmacologic: estrogen receptor antagonists

Indications

Treatment of hormone receptor–positive metastatic breast cancer in postmenopausal women with progressive disease that has not responded to antiestrogen therapy.

Action

Competitively binds to estrogen receptors. Binding results in down-regulation of estrogen receptor protein in cancerous breast tissue. **Therapeutic Effects:** Decreased progression of hormone receptor-positive breast cancer.

Adverse Reactions/Side Effects

CNS: headache, weakness, anxiety, depression, dizziness, insomnia. **EENT:** pharyngitis. **Resp:** dyspnea, increased cough. **CV:** vasodilation (hot flushes), chest pain, edema. **GI:** abdominal pain, constipation, diarrhea, nausea, vomiting, anorexia. **GU:** pelvic pain, urinary tract infection. **Derm:** rash, sweating. **Local:** pain/inflammation at injection site. **Hemat:** anemia. **MS:** back pain, bone pain, arthritis. **Neuro:** paresthesia. **Misc:** fever, flu syndrome.

PHYSICAL THERAPY IMPLICATIONS

Examination and Evaluation

- Monitor signs of anemia, including unusual weakness, fatigue, shortness of breath with exertion, and bruising. Notify physician if these signs occur.
- Assess peripheral edema using girth measurements, volume displacement, and measurement of pitting edema (See Appendix N). Report increased swelling in feet and ankles or a sudden increase in body weight due to fluid retention.
- Monitor any chest pain or difficult, labored breathing. Attempt to differentiate whether symptoms are drug induced or caused by cardiovascular dysfunction (e.g., angina that occurs during exercise).
- Assess any back pain, bone pain, pelvic pain, or other musculoskeletal pain. Suggest additional tests

(radiography, MRI) as needed to rule out fracture.

- Monitor and report depression, anxiety, or other changes in mood and behavior.
- Assess signs of paresthesia (numbness, tingling) or muscle twitching. Perform objective tests, including electroneuromyography and sensory testing to document any drug-related neuropathic changes.
- Monitor IM injection site for pain, swelling, and irritation. Report prolonged or excessive injection-site reactions to the physician.

Interventions

- For patients who are medically able to begin exercise, implement appropriate resistive exercises and aerobic training to maintain muscle strength and aerobic capacity during cancer chemotherapy or to help restore function after chemotherapy.

Patient/Client-Related Instruction

- Instruct patient to report other troublesome side effects such as severe or prolonged headache, sleep loss, cough, throat irritation, hot flashes, flu-like symptoms, urinary tract infection, skin reactions (rash, sweating), or GI problems (nausea, diarrhea, vomiting, constipation, abdominal pain, loss of appetite).

Pharmacokinetics

Absorption: Well absorbed following IM administration.
Distribution: Rapidly and extensively distributed.
Protein Binding: 99%.
Metabolism and Excretion: Mostly metabolized by the liver; negligible renal elimination.
Half-life: 40 days.

TIME/ACTION PROFILE (effect on estrogen receptors)

ROUTE	ONSET	PEAK	DURATION
IM	rapid	7 days	30 days

Contraindications/Precautions

Contraindicated in: Pregnancy or lactation; Children; Hypersensitivity; Bleeding disorders, thrombocytopenia, concurrent anticoagulant therapy.
Use Cautiously in: Moderate-to-severe hepatic impairment.

Interactions

Drug-Drug: None known.

Route/Dosage

IM (Adults): 250 mg once monthly (may be given as a single injection or two injections of 125 mg each).

Availability

Solution for injection: 50 mg/mL in 5-mL prefilled syringes; 50 mg/mL in 2 2.5-mL prefilled syringes.

furosemide (fur-oh-se-mide)

Apo-Furosemide, Lasix, ✱Lasix Special, Novosemide, Nu-Furosemide, PMS-Furosemide

Classification
Therapeutic: diuretics
Pharmacologic: loop diuretics

Indications

Edema due to heart failure, hepatic impairment, or renal disease. Hypertension.

Action

Inhibits the reabsorption of sodium and chloride from the loop of Henle and distal renal tubule. Increases renal excretion of water, sodium, chloride, magnesium, potassium, and calcium. Effectiveness persists in impaired renal function. **Therapeutic Effects:** Diuresis and subsequent mobilization of excess fluid (edema, pleural effusions). Decreased blood pressure.

Adverse Reactions/Side Effects

CNS: blurred vision, dizziness, headache, vertigo.
EENT: hearing loss, tinnitus. **CV:** hypotension.
GI: anorexia, constipation, diarrhea, dry mouth, dyspepsia, nausea, pancreatitis, vomiting. **GU:** excessive urination. **Derm:** photosensitivity, pruritus, rash.
Endo: hyperglycemia, hyperuricemia. **F and E:** dehydration, hypocalcemia, hypochloremia, hypokalemia, hypomagnesemia, hyponatremia, hypovolemia, metabolic alkalosis. **Hemat:** APLASTIC ANEMIA, AGRANULOCYTOSIS, hemolytic anemia, leukopenia, thrombocytopenia.
MS: muscle cramps. **Neuro:** paresthesia. **Misc:** fever, increased BUN, nephrocalcinosis.

PHYSICAL THERAPY IMPLICATIONS

Examination and Evaluation

- Monitor signs of aplastic anemia (fatigue, weakness, shortness of breath, pale skin, dizziness), agranulocytosis (fever, sore throat, mucosal lesions, signs of infection), or other symptoms and bleeding problems that might be due to other blood dyscrasias. Report these signs to the physician immediately.
- Monitor signs of fluid, electrolyte, or acid-base imbalances, including dizziness, drowsiness, blurred vision, confusion, hypotension, or muscle cramps and weakness. Report excessive or prolonged symptoms to the physician.
- Assess dizziness and vertigo that might affect gait, balance, and other functional activities (See Appendix C). Report balance problems and functional limitations

✱ = Canadian drug name; *CAPITALS indicate life-threatening; underlines indicate most frequent.

to the physician, and caution the patient and family/caregivers to guard against falls and trauma.

- Assess blood pressure periodically and compare to normal values (See Appendix F) to help determine antihypertensive effects. Report low blood pressure (hypotension), especially if patient experiences dizziness or syncope.
- When used to treat edema, help determine drug effects by assessing peripheral edema using girth measurements, volume displacement, and measurement of pitting edema (See Appendix N). Also monitor signs of pulmonary edema such as dyspnea and rales/crackles (See Appendix K). Document whether peripheral and pulmonary symptoms are controlled adequately by diuretic therapy.
- Monitor signs of hyperglycemia such as drowsiness, fruity breath, increased urination, and unusual thirst. Patients with diabetes mellitus should check blood glucose levels frequently.

Interventions

- Implement fall-prevention strategies, especially in older adults or if patient exhibits sedation, dizziness, blurred vision, or other impairments that affect gait and balance (See Appendix E).
- Use caution during aerobic exercise, especially in hot environments. Increased sweating will cause fluid and electrolyte loss, and may exaggerate diuretic side effects (dizziness, muscle cramps, and so forth).
- To minimize orthostatic hypotension, patient should move slowly when assuming a more upright position.
- Causes photosensitivity; use care if administering UV treatments.

Patient/Client-Related Instruction

- Remind patients to take medication as directed to control hypertension and other cardiac conditions even if they are asymptomatic.
- Counsel patients about additional interventions to help control blood pressure and cardiac dysfunction, including regular exercise, weight loss, sodium restriction, stress reduction, moderation of alcohol consumption, and smoking cessation.
- Advise patient about the possibility of GI reactions (nausea, vomiting, diarrhea, constipation, loss of appetite). Instruct patient or family and caregivers to report severe or prolonged GI symptoms or signs of pancreatitis (upper abdominal pain after eating, indigestion, weight loss, oily stools).
- Remind patient and family/caregivers that diuretics typically increase urine output. Any unusual problems such as excessive or painful urination or blood in the urine should be reported to the physician.
- Instruct patient to report any hearing loss or ringing/buzzing in the ears (tinnitus).
- Advise patient about photosensitivity, and to use sunscreens, protective clothing, and avoid prolonged sun exposure. Instruct patient to also report any rashes or other skin reactions.

Pharmacokinetics

Absorption: 60–67% absorbed after oral administration (↓ in acute CHF and in renal failure); also absorbed from IM sites.
Distribution: Crosses placenta; enters breast milk.
Protein Binding: 91–99%.
Metabolism and Excretion: Minimally metabolized by liver, some nonhepatic metabolism, some renal excretion as unchanged drug.
Half-life: 30–60 min (↑ in renal impairment).

TIME/ACTION PROFILE (diuretic effect)

ROUTE	ONSET	PEAK	DURATION
PO	30–60 min	1–2 hr	6–8 hr
IM	10–30 min	unknown	4–8 hr
IV	5 min	30 min	2 hr

Contraindications/Precautions

Contraindicated in: Hypersensitivity; Cross-sensitivity with thiazides and sulfonamides may occur; Hepatic coma or anuria; Some liquid products may contain alcohol; avoid in patients with alcohol intolerance.
Use Cautiously in: Severe liver disease (may precipitate hepatic coma; concurrent use with potassium-sparing diuretics may be necessary); Electrolyte depletion; Geri: Geriatric patients may have increased risk of side effects, especially hypotension and electrolyte imbalance, at usual doses; Diabetes mellitus; Increasing azotemia; Pregnancy and lactation; Pedi: Increased risk of renal calculi and patent ductus arteriosus in premature neonates.

Interactions

Drug-Drug: ↑ hypotension with **antihypertensives, nitrates,** or acute ingestion of **alcohol**. ↑ risk of hypokalemia with other **diuretics, amphotericin B, stimulant laxatives,** and **corticosteroids**. Hypokalemia may ↑ risk of **digoxin** toxicity and ↑ risk of arrhythmia in patients taking drugs that prolong the QT interval. ↓ **lithium** excretion, may cause **lithium** toxicity. ↑ risk of ototoxicity with **aminoglycosides**. **NSAIDS** ↓ effects of furosemide. ↓ effects of furosemide when given at same time as **sucralfate, cholestyramine,** or **colestipol**. ↑ risk of **salicylate** toxicity (with use of high-dose **salicylate** therapy).

Route/Dosage

Edema

PO (Adults): 20–80 mg/day as a single dose initially, may repeat in 6–8 hr; may increase dose by 20–40 mg q 6–8 hr until desired response. Maintenance doses may be given once or twice daily (doses up to 2.5 g/day have been used in patients with congestive

heart failure or renal disease). *Hypertension*—40 twice daily initially (when added to regimen, ↓ dose of other antihypertensives by 50%); adjust further dosing based on response; *Hypercalcemia*—120 mg/day in 1–3 doses.
PO (Children >1 month): 2 mg/kg as a single dose; may be increased by 1–2 mg/kg q 6–8 hr (maximum dose = 6 mg/kg).
PO (Neonates): 1–4 mg/kg/dose 1–2 times/day.
IM, IV (Adults): 20–40 mg, may repeat in 1–2 hr and ↑ by 20 mg q 1–2 hr until response is obtained, maintenance dose may be given q 6–12 hr; *Continuous infusion*—Bolus 0.1 mg/kg followed by 0.1 mg/kg/hr, double q 2 hr to a maximum of 0.4 mg/kg/hr.
IM, IV (Children): 1–2 mg/kg/dose q 6–12 hr; *Continuous infusion*—0.05 mg/kg/hr, titrate to clinical effect.
IM, IV (Neonates): 1–2 mg/kg/dose q 12–24 hr.

Hypertension

PO (Adults): 40 bid initially (when added to regimen, ↓ dose of other antihypertensives by 50%); adjust further dosing based on response.

Availability (generic available)

Tablets: 20 mg, 40 mg, 80 mg, 500 mg. **Oral solution (10 mg/mL—orange flavor, 8 mg/mL—pineapple-peach flavor):** 8 mg/mL, 10 mg/mL. **Solution for injection:** 10 mg/mL.

F

gabapentin (ga-ba-pen-tin)

Neurontin

Classification

Therapeutic: analgesic adjuncts, therapeutic, anticonvulsants, mood stabilizers

Indications

Partial seizures (adjunct treatment). Postherpetic neuralgia. **Unlabeled Use:** Chronic pain. Prevention of migraine headache. Bipolar disorder. Anxiety.

Action

Mechanism of action is not known. May affect transport of amino acids across and stabilize neuronal membranes. **Therapeutic Effects:** Decreased incidence of seizures. Decreased postherpetic pain.

Adverse Reactions/Side Effects

CNS: <u>confusion</u>, <u>depression</u>, <u>drowsiness</u>, sedation, anxiety, concentration difficulties (children), dizziness, emotional lability (children), hostility, hyperkinesia (children), malaise, vertigo, weakness. **EENT:** abnormal vision, nystagmus. **CV:** hypertension. **GI:** weight gain, anorexia, flatulence, gingivitis. **MS:** arthralgia. **Neuro:** <u>ataxia</u>, altered reflexes, hyperkinesia, paresthesia. **Misc:** facial edema.

PHYSICAL THERAPY IMPLICATIONS

Examination and Evaluation

- Document the number, duration, and severity of seizures to help determine if this drug is effective in reducing seizure activity.
- Monitor drowsiness, anxiety, confusion, and other changes in mood or behavior (hostility, emotional lability, concentration difficulties). Repeated or excessive symptoms may require change in dose or medication.
- Assess vertigo or dizziness that might affect gait, balance, and other functional activities (See Appendix C). Report balance problems and functional limitations to the physician, and caution the patient and family/caregivers to guard against falls and trauma.
- If treating neuropathic pain or other pain syndromes (migraine, chronic pain, postherpetic neuralgia), use visual analogue scales and other appropriate pain scales to assess the patient's pain and help document the effects of drug therapy.
- If treating anxiety or bipolar disorder, monitor any changes in the patient's mood or behavior. Report manic symptoms (excitement, agitation) or symptoms of depression (sadness, apathy, loss of energy).
- Assess gait and motor function and document any signs of ataxia, increased motor activity (hyperkinesias), or other abnormal motor symptoms. Report these signs to the physician.
- Assess signs of paresthesia (numbness, tingling) or changes in reflex activity. Perform objective tests, including electroneuromyography and sensory testing to document any drug-related neuropathic changes.
- Assess blood pressure periodically and compare to normal values (See Appendix F). Report a sustained increase in blood pressure (hypertension) to the physician.
- Assess any joint pain to rule out musculoskeletal pathology; that is, try to determine if pain is drug induced rather than caused by anatomic or biomechanical problems.
- Periodically assess body weight and other anthropometric measures (body mass index, body composition). Report a substantial or unexplained weight gain or increase in body fat.

Interventions

- Guard against falls and trauma (hip fractures, head injury, and so forth), especially if gait and balance are affected by drowsiness, dizziness, or ataxia. Implement fall prevention strategies, especially if balance is impaired (See Appendix E).
- If treating neuropathic pain or other pain syndromes, implement appropriate interventions (physical agents, manual techniques, therapeutic exercise) to manage pain and reduce the need for drug therapy. Help patient also explore other nonpharmacologic methods to reduce chronic pain such as relaxation techniques, imagery, counseling, and so forth.

Patient/Client-Related Instruction

- Advise patient to avoid alcohol and other CNS depressants because of the increased risk of sedation and adverse effects.
- Advise patients on prolonged antiseizure therapy not to discontinue medication without consulting their physician. Abrupt withdrawal may cause increased seizures.
- Advise patient about the risk of daytime drowsiness and decreased attention and mental focus. Use care if driving or in other activities that require strong concentration or fast responses.

- Encourage patient and family/caregivers to perform rigorous oral hygiene and teeth cleansing to reduce gingival hyperplasia.
- Instruct patient to report other troublesome side effects such as severe or prolonged facial edema, vision problems (double vision, nystagmus), or GI problems (flatulence, loss of appetite).

Pharmacokinetics

Absorption: Well absorbed after oral administration by active transport. At larger doses, transport becomes saturated and absorption decreases (bioavailability ranges from 60% for a 300-mg dose to 35% for a 1600-mg dose).
Distribution: Crosses blood-brain barrier; enters breast milk.
Metabolism and Excretion: Eliminated mostly by renal excretion of unchanged drug.
Half-life: 5–7 hr (normal renal function); up to 132 hr in anuria.

TIME/ACTION PROFILE (blood levels)

ROUTE	ONSET	PEAK	DURATION
PO	rapid	2–4 hr	8 hr

Contraindications/Precautions

Contraindicated in: Hypersensitivity.
Use Cautiously in: All patients (may ↑ risk of suicidal thoughts/behaviors); Renal insufficiency (↓ dose and/or ↑ dosing interval if CCr ≤60 mL/min); Geri: Geriatric patients (because of age-related ↓ in renal function); OB/Pedi: Safety not established for children <3 yr and pregnant women; Lactation: Discontinue drug or bottle feed.

Interactions

Drug-Drug: Antacids may ↓ absorption of gabapentin. ↑ risk of CNS depression with other **CNS depressants**, including **alcohol, antihistamines, opioids**, and **sedative/hypnotics**. **Morphine** ↑ gabapentin levels and may ↑ risk of toxicity, dosage adjustments may be required.
Drug-Natural: Kava, valerian, or **chamomile** can ↑ CNS depression.

Route/Dosage

Epilepsy

PO (Adults and Children >12 yr): 300 mg tidy initially. Titration may be continued until desired (range is 900–1800 mg/day in 3 divided doses; doses should not be more than 12 hr apart). Doses up to 2400–3600 mg/day have been well tolerated.
PO (Children ≥5–12 yr): 10–15 mg/kg/day in 3 divided doses initially titrated upward over 3 days to 25–35 mg/kg/day in 3 divided doses; dosage interval should not exceed 12 hr (doses up to 50 mg/kg/day have been used).
PO (Children 3–4 yrs): 10–15 mg/kg/day in 3 divided doses initially titrated upward over 3 days to 40 mg/kg/day in 3 divided doses; dosage interval should not exceed 12 hr (doses up to 50 mg/kg/day have been used).

Renal Impairment

PO (Adults and Children >12 yr):
CCr 30–60 mL/min—300 mg twice daily;
CCr 15–30 mL/min—300 mg once daily;
CCr <15 mL/min—300 mg once every other day; further adjustments are based on clinical response.

Postherpetic Neuralgia

PO (Adults): 300 mg once daily on first day, 300 mg twice daily on second day, then 300 mg tid on day 3, may then be titrated upward as needed up to 600 mg tid.

Availability (generic available)

Capsules: 100 mg, 300 mg, 400 mg. **Tablets:** 100 mg, 300 mg, 400 mg, 600 mg, 800 mg. **Oral solution (cool strawberry anise flavor):** 250 mg/5 mL.

galsulfase (gal-sul-fase)

Naglazyme

Classification
Therapeutic: replacement enzyme
Pharmacologic: enzymes

Indications

Mucopolysaccharidosis VI (MPS IV).

Action

Replaces a deficient enzyme in MPS IV. Without replacement, glycosaminoglycans accumulate resulting in cell, organ, and tissue dysfunction.
Therapeutic Effects: Improved walking and stair climbing.

Adverse Reactions/Side Effects

CV: malaise. **EENT:** conjunctivitis, corneal opacification, ear pain. **Resp:** dyspnea. **CV:** chest pain, ↑ blood pressure. **Derm:** facial edema. **GI:** gastroenteritis, abdominal pain. **MS:** areflexia. **Misc:** INFUSION REACTIONS, rigors.

PHYSICAL THERAPY IMPLICATIONS

Examination and Evaluation

- Be alert for allergy-like responses (wheezing, laryngeal edema, urticaria, other skin reactions) that occur during and after administration (infusion reactions). Report these responses to the physician or nursing staff immediately.

- Assess ambulation on level surfaces and during stair climbing. Document any changes in functional ability to help document whether drug therapy is effective in maintaining or improving motor function.
- Monitor any changes in muscle tone or deep tendon reflexes. Report increased muscle contractions or decreased reflex activity.
- Assess blood pressure (BP) and compare to normal values (See Appendix F). Report a sustained increase in BP (hypertension) or any chest pain or difficult, labored breathing.
- Monitor and report any vision problems, eye inflammation, or ear pain.

Interventions

- Implement therapeutic exercises (resistive training, coordination exercises, gait training) to complement the effects of drug therapy and help achieve optimal function.

Patient/Client-Related Instruction

- Instruct patient and family/caregivers to report other troublesome side effects such as severe or prolonged malaise, facial swelling, or GI problems (gastroenteritis, abdominal pain).

Pharmacokinetics

Absorption: IV administration results in complete bioavailability.
Distribution: Widely distributed.
Metabolism and Excretion: Unknown.
Half-life: 9 min (after 1 wk of treatment, 26 min (after 24 wk of treatment).

TIME/ACTION PROFILE (improve exercise parameters)

ROUTE	ONSET	PEAK	DURATION
IV	unknown	24 wk	unknown

Contraindications/Precautions

Contraindicated in: None.
Use Cautiously in: Febrile or respiratory illness; Pedi: Children <5 yr (safety not established); OB: Pregnancy or lactation (safety being evaluated).

Interactions

Drug-Drug: None noted.

Route/Dosage

IV (Adults and Children >5 yr): 1 mg/kg once weekly.

Availability

Solution for IV administration (diluted prior to use): 5 mg/5 mL in 5-mL vials.

ganciclovir (gan-sye-kloe-vir)

Cytovene, Vitrasert

Classification
Therapeutic: antivirals
Pharmacologic: guanine nucleoside analogues

Indications

IV: Treatment of cytomegalovirus (CMV) retinitis in immunocompromised patients, including HIV-infected patients (may be used with foscarnet). Prevention of CMV infection in transplant patients at risk. **PO:** Maintenance treatment of stable CMV retinitis in immunocompromised patients after initial IV treatment and prevention of CMV retinitis in patients with advanced HIV infection.

Action

CMV converts ganciclovir to its active form (ganciclovir phosphate) inside the host cell, where it inhibits viral DNA polymerase. **Therapeutic Effects:** Antiviral effect directed preferentially against CMV-infected cells.

Adverse Reactions/Side Effects

CNS: SEIZURES, abnormal dreams, coma, confusion, dizziness, drowsiness, headache, malaise, nervousness. **EENT:** retinal detachment **intravitreal only:** decreased visual acuity, vitreous hemorrhage, hyphema, intraocular pressure spikes, lens opacities, macular abnormalities, optic nerve changes, uveitis. **Resp:** dyspnea. **CV:** arrhythmias, edema, hypertension, hypotension. **GI:** GI BLEEDING, abdominal pain, increased liver enzymes, nausea, vomiting. **GU:** gonadal suppression, hematuria, renal toxicity. **Derm:** alopecia, photosensitivity, pruritus, rash, urticaria. **Endo:** hypoglycemia. **Hemat:** neutropenia, thrombocytopenia, anemia, eosinophilia. **Local:** pain/phlebitis at IV site. **Neuro:** ataxia, tremor. **Misc:** fever.

PHYSICAL THERAPY IMPLICATIONS

Examination and Evaluation

- Be alert for new seizures or increased seizure activity, especially at the onset of drug treatment. Document the number, duration, and severity of seizures, and report these findings to the physician immediately.
- Monitor signs of GI bleeding, including abdominal pain, vomiting blood, blood in stools, or black, tarry stools. Report these signs to the physician immediately.
- Assess heart rate, ECG, and heart sounds, especially during exercise (See Appendices G, H). Report any

rhythm disturbances or symptoms of increased arrhythmias, including palpitations, chest discomfort, shortness of breath, dyspnea, fainting, and fatigue/weakness.

- Assess blood pressure (BP) and compare to normal values (See Appendix F). Report changes in BP, either a problematic decrease in BP (hypotension) or a sustained increase in BP (hypertension).
- Assess peripheral edema using girth measurements, volume displacement, and measurement of pitting edema (see Appendix N). Report increased swelling in feet and ankles or a sudden increase in body weight due to fluid retention.
- Monitor signs of neutropenia (fever, sore throat, signs of infection), eosinophilia (fatigue, weakness, myalgia); thrombocytopenia (bruising, nose bleeds, and bleeding gums), or unusual weakness and fatigue that might be due to anemia. Report these signs to the physician.
- Be alert for nervousness, confusion, excessive drowsiness, lethargy, or other alterations in mental status. Notify physician promptly if these symptoms develop.
- Assess dizziness, tremor, or ataxia that might affect gait, balance, or other functional activities (See Appendices C, E). Report balance problems and functional limitations to the physician, and caution the patient and family/caregivers to guard against falls and trauma.
- Monitor and report signs of hypoglycemia, especially during and after exercise. Common neuromuscular symptoms include anxiety; restlessness; tingling in hands, feet, lips, or tongue; chills; cold sweats; confusion; difficulty in concentration; drowsiness; nightmares or trouble sleeping; excessive hunger; headache; irritability; nervousness; tremor; weakness; unsteady gait.
- Monitor IV injection site for pain, swelling, and irritation. Report prolonged or excessive injection site reactions to the physician.

Interventions

- Because of the risk of arrhythmias and abnormal BP responses, use caution during aerobic exercise and other forms of therapeutic exercise. Assess exercise tolerance frequently (BP, heart rate, fatigue levels), and terminate exercise immediately if any untoward responses occur (See Appendix L).
- Always wash hands thoroughly and disinfect equipment (whirlpools, electrotherapeutic devices, treatment tables, and so forth) to help prevent the spread of infection. Use universal precautions as indicated for specific patients.
- Causes photosensitivity; use care if administering UV treatments.

Patient/Client-Related Instruction

- Instruct patient to report signs of renal toxicity, including blood or pus in urine, decreased urine output, weight gain from fluid retention, and fatigue.
- Instruct patient to report any vision disturbances, including blurred vision, decreased visual acuity, and signs of macular abnormalities (blurry or decreased central vision with peripheral vision intact).
- Advise patient about photosensitivity, and to use sunscreens, protective clothing, and avoid prolonged sun exposure. Advise patient to also report any rashes or other skin reactions.
- Instruct patient and family/caregivers to report other troublesome side effects, including severe or prolonged headache, fever, abnormal dreams, skin problems (rash, hives, itching, hair loss), or GI problems (nausea, vomiting, abdominal pain).

Pharmacokinetics

Absorption: 5–9% absorbed after oral administration. IV administration results in complete bioavailability. Action of intravitreal implant is local.
Distribution: Widely distributed; enters CSF.
Metabolism and Excretion: 90% excreted unchanged by the kidneys.
Half-life: 2.9 hr (increased in renal impairment).

TIME/ACTION PROFILE (antiviral levels)

ROUTE	ONSET	PEAK	DURATION
PO	rapid	1.8–3 hr	3–8 hr
IV	rapid	end of infusion	12–24 hr
Intravitreal	rapid	unknown	5–8 mo

Contraindications/Precautions

Contraindicated in: Hypersensitivity to ganciclovir or acyclovir.
Use Cautiously in: Renal impairment (dose reduction required if CCr <80 mL/min); Geriatric patients (dose reduction recommended); Bone marrow depression or immunosuppression; Pregnancy, lactation, or children (safety not established).

Interactions

Drug-Drug: ↑ risk of bone marrow depression with **antineoplastics, radiation therapy**, or **zidovudine**. Toxicity may be ↑ by **probenecid**. ↑ risk of seizures with **imipenem/cilastatin**. Concurrent use of other **nephrotoxic drugs, cyclosporine**, or **amphotericin B** ↑ risk of nephrotoxicity.

Route/Dosage

IV (Adults): *Induction*—5 mg/kg q 12 hr for 14–21 days. *Maintenance regimen*—5 mg/kg/day or 6 mg/kg for 5 days of each week. If progression occurs,

increase to q 12 hr regimen. *Prevention*—5 mg/kg q 12 hr for 7–14 days, then 5 mg/kg/day or 6 mg/kg for 5 days of each week.
PO (Adults): *Maintenance regimen*—1000 mg tid (with food) or 500 mg 6 times daily; *Prevention of CMV retinitis in advanced HIV infection*—1000 mg tid.
Intravitreal (Adults): 4.5 mg implant.

Availability (generic available)

Capsules: 250 mg, 500 mg. **Powder for injection:** 500 mg/vial. **Intravitreal insert:** 4.5 mg.

gefitinib (je-fit-in-ib)

Iressa

Classification
Therapeutic: antineoplastics
Pharmacologic: enzyme inhibitors

Indications

Patients who are currently benefiting from or have benefited from gefitinib in the past for treatment of non–small cell lung cancer.

Action

Inhibits activation of kinases found in transmembrane cell surface receptors, including epidermal growth factor receptor (EGFR-TK). **Therapeutic Effects:** Death of rapidly replicating cells, particularly malignant ones.

Adverse Reactions/Side Effects

CNS: weakness. **EENT:** aberrant eyelash, conjunctivitis, corneal erosion/ulcer, eye pain, ↓ vision. **CV:** peripheral edema. **Resp:** PULMONARY TOXICITY, dyspnea. **GI:** diarrhea, nausea, vomiting, anorexia, hepatotoxicity, mouth ulceration. **Derm:** acne, dry skin, rash, pruritus. **Metab:** weight loss. **Misc:** ALLERGIC REACTIONS, INCLUDING ANGIOEDEMA.

PHYSICAL THERAPY IMPLICATIONS

Examination and Evaluation

- Monitor signs of allergic reactions and angioedema, including pulmonary symptoms (tightness in the throat and chest, wheezing, cough, dyspnea) or skin reactions (rashes, raised patches of red or white skin, burning/itching skin, swelling in the face). Notify physician or nursing staff immediately if these reactions occur.
- Assess any other breathing problems or signs of pulmonary toxicity such as dry cough, wheezing, chest pain, shortness of breath, and difficult or labored breathing. Monitor pulse oximetry and perform pulmonary function tests (See Appendices I, J, K) to quantify suspected changes in ventilation and respiratory function.
- Assess peripheral edema using girth measurements, volume displacement, and measurement of pitting edema (See Appendix N). Report increased swelling in feet and ankles or a sudden increase in body weight due to fluid retention.
- Monitor any vision disturbances or eye pain and inflammation. Report these signs to the physician.
- Monitor body weight and report any severe or sudden weight loss.

Interventions

- For patients who are medically able to begin exercise, implement appropriate resistive exercises and aerobic training to maintain muscle strength and aerobic capacity during cancer chemotherapy or to help restore function after chemotherapy.
- Use caution during aerobic exercise and endurance conditioning because of potential pulmonary toxicity. Terminate exercise if patient exhibits untoward symptoms (chest pain, shortness of breath, etc.) or displays other criteria for exercise termination (See Appendix L).

Patient/Client-Related Instruction

- Advise patient and family/caregivers that fatigue and weakness are likely and may be severe. Functional abilities may be limited, and patient may need to use assistive devices during ambulation.
- Advise patient about the likelihood of GI reactions such as diarrhea, nausea, vomiting, loss of appetite, and inflammation in/around mouth. Instruct patient to report severe or prolonged GI problems, or signs of hepatotoxicity including anorexia, abdominal pain, severe nausea and vomiting, yellow skin or eyes, fever, sore throat, malaise, weakness, facial edema, lethargy, and unusual bleeding or bruising.
- Advise patient that skin reactions are likely, including rash, acne, pruritus, and dry skin. Report severe or unexpected skin reactions to the physician.

Pharmacokinetics

Absorption: 60% absorbed following oral administration.
Distribution: Extensively distributed.
Metabolism and Excretion: Mostly metabolized by the liver (CYP3A4 enzyme system); excreted in feces, <4% excreted in urine.
Half-life: 48 hr.

G

TIME/ACTION PROFILE

ROUTE	ONSET	PEAK	DURATION
PO	unknown	unknown	unknown

Contraindications/Precautions

Contraindicated in: Hypersensitivity; OB: Pregnancy, lactation, children.

Use Cautiously in: Idiopathic pulmonary fibrosis (↑ risk of pulmonary toxicity); Concurrent use of strong inhibitors of the CYP3A4 enzyme system (may increase risk of toxicity).

Interactions

Drug-Drug: Strong inducers of the CYP3A4 enzyme system, including **rifampin** and **phenytoin,** ↓ blood levels and effects (consider ↑ dose of gefitinib to 500 mg/day). Strong inhibitors of the CYP3A4 enzyme system, including **ketoconazole** and **itraconazole,** ↑ blood levels and effects (use with caution). Absorption and efficacy may be ↓ by **drugs that** ↑ **gastric pH,** including **cimetidine** and **ranitidine**. May ↑ the risk of bleeding with **warfarin**. Concurrent use with **vinorelbine** may ↑ risk/severity of neutropenia.

Route/Dosage

PO (Adults): 250 mg once daily.

Availability

Tablets: 250 mg.

HIGH ALERT

gemcitabine (jem-site-a-been)

Gemzar

Classification

Therapeutic: antineoplastics

Pharmacologic: antimetabolites, nucleoside analogues

Indications

Pancreatic cancer (locally advanced or metastatic). Inoperable locally advanced/metastatic non–small cell lung cancer (with cisplatin). Metastatic breast cancer (with paclitaxel). Advanced ovarian cancer that has relapsed 6 mo after completion of platinum-based therapy (with carboplatin).

Action

Interferes with DNA synthesis (cell-cycle phase–specific). **Therapeutic Effects:** Death of rapidly replicating cells, particularly malignant ones.

Adverse Reactions/Side Effects

Resp: PULMONARY TOXICITY, dyspnea, bronchospasm. **CV:** ARRHYTHMIAS, CEREBROVASCULAR ACCIDENT, MI, edema, hypertension. **GI:** HEPATOTOXICITY, diarrhea, nausea, stomatitis, transient elevation of hepatic transaminases, vomiting. **GU:** HEMOLYTIC UREMIC SYNDROME, hematuria, proteinuria. **Derm:** alopecia, rash. **Hemat:** anemia, leukopenia, thrombocytopenia. **Local:** injection site reactions. **Neuro:** paresthesias. **Misc:** flu-like symptoms, fever, anaphylactoid reactions.

PHYSICAL THERAPY IMPLICATIONS

Examination and Evaluation

- Continually monitor for signs of MI (sudden chest pain, pain radiating into the arm or jaw, shortness of breath, dizziness, sweating, anxiety, nausea) or stroke (sudden severe headache, confusion, nausea, vomiting, paralysis, numbness, speech problems, visual disturbances). Seek immediate medical assistance if patient develops these signs.
- Assess heart rate, ECG, and heart sounds, especially during exercise (See Appendices G, H). Report any rhythm disturbances or symptoms of increased arrhythmias, including palpitations, chest discomfort, shortness of breath, fainting, and fatigue/weakness.
- Assess any breathing problems or signs of pulmonary toxicity, including dyspnea, rales/crackles, decreased breath sounds, pleuritic friction rub, bronchospasm, tachypnea, cough, pleuritic pain, and hemoptysis. Monitor pulse oximetry and perform pulmonary function tests (See Appendices I, J, K) to quantify suspected changes in ventilation and respiratory function.
- Be alert for signs of hepatotoxicity, including anorexia, abdominal pain, severe nausea and vomiting, yellow skin or eyes, fever, sore throat, malaise, weakness, facial edema, lethargy, and unusual bleeding or bruising. Report these signs to the physician immediately.
- Monitor signs of hemolytic uremic syndrome, including fatigue, irritability, abdominal pain, pale skin tones, decreased urine output, small bruises (petechiae), peripheral edema, and weight gain due to fluid retention. Report these signs to the physician immediately.
- Monitor signs of leukopenia (fever, sore throat, signs of infection), thrombocytopenia (bruising, nose bleeds, and bleeding gums), or unusual weakness and fatigue that might be due to anemia. Report these signs to the physician immediately.
- Be alert for signs of hypersensitivity and anaphylactoid reactions, including pulmonary symptoms (tightness in the throat and chest, wheezing, cough, dyspnea) or skin reactions (rash, pruritus, urticaria). Notify physician or nursing staff immediately if these reactions occur.

- Assess signs of paresthesia such as numbness and tingling. Perform objective tests, including electroneuromyography and sensory testing to document any drug-related neuropathic changes.
- Assess blood pressure (BP) and compare to normal values (See Appendix F). Report a sustained increase in BP (hypertension).
- Assess peripheral edema using girth measurements, volume displacement, and measurement of pitting edema (See Appendix N). Report increased swelling in feet and ankles or a sudden increase in body weight due to fluid retention.
- Monitor IV injection site for pain, swelling, and irritation. Report prolonged or excessive injection site reactions to the physician.

Interventions

- For patients who are medically able to begin exercise, implement appropriate resistive exercises and aerobic training to maintain muscle strength and aerobic capacity during cancer chemotherapy or to help restore function after chemotherapy.
- Because of the risk of MI, stroke, and pulmonary toxicity, use extreme caution during aerobic exercise and other forms of therapeutic exercise. Assess exercise tolerance frequently (BP, heart rate, fatigue levels), and terminate exercise immediately if any untoward responses occur (See Appendix L).

Patient/Client-Related Instruction

- Advise patient and family or caregiver about the signs of MI and stroke (see above under Examination and Evaluation), and to seek immediate medical assistance if these signs develop.
- Advise patient and family/caregivers about the risk of infections, to guard against infection (frequent hand washing, etc.), and to avoid crowds and contact with persons with contagious diseases.
- Advise patient about the likelihood of GI reactions such as nausea, vomiting, diarrhea, and irritation of the mouth. Instruct patient to report severe or prolonged GI problems or signs of liver toxicity (see above under Examination and Evaluation).
- Instruct patient and family/caregivers to report other troublesome side effects such as severe or prolonged fever, flu-like symptoms, or skin reactions (rash, hair loss).

Pharmacokinetics

Absorption: IV administration results in complete bioavailability.
Distribution: Unknown.
Metabolism and Excretion: Converted in cells to active diphosphate and triphosphate metabolites; these are excreted primarily by the kidneys.
Half-life: 32–94 min.

TIME/ACTION PROFILE (effect on blood counts)

ROUTE	ONSET	PEAK	DURATION
IV	unknown	unknown	unknown

Contraindications/Precautions

Contraindicated in: Hypersensitivity; OB: Pregnancy or lactation.
Use Cautiously in: History of cardiovascular disease; Impaired hepatic or renal function (increased risk of toxicity); OB: Patients with childbearing potential; Other chronic debilitating illness.

Interactions

Drug-Drug: ↑ bone marrow depression with other **antineoplastics** or **radiation therapy**. May ↓ antibody response to **live-virus vaccines** and ↑ risk of adverse reactions.

Route/Dosage

Other regimens are used.

Pancreatic Cancer

IV (Adults): 1000 mg/m² once weekly for 7 wk, followed by a week of rest. May be followed by cycles of once-weekly administration for 3 wk followed by a week of rest.

Non–Small Cell Lung Cancer (with Cisplatin)

IV (Adults): 1000 mg/m² on days 1, 8, and 15 of each 28-day cycle (cisplatin is also given on day 1) *or* 1250 mg/m² on days 1 and 8 of each 21-day cycle (cisplatin is also given on day 1).

Breast Cancer

IV (Adults): 1250 mg/m² on days 1 and 8 of each 21-day cycle (paclitaxel is also given on day 1).

Ovarian Cancer

IV (Adults): 1000 mg/m² on days 1 and 8 of each 21-day cycle.

Availability

Powder for injection: 200 mg in 10-mL vial, 1 g in 50-mL vial.

gemifloxacin (jem-i-flox-a-sin)

Factive

Classification

Therapeutic: anti-infectives
Pharmacologic: fluoroquinolones

Indications

Treatment of the following bacterial respiratory infections: Acute bacterial exacerbations of chronic bronchitis, Community-acquired pneumonia.

Action

Inhibits bacterial DNS synthesis by inhibiting DNA gyrase enzyme. **Therapeutic Effects:** Death of susceptible bacteria resulting in resolution of infection. **Spectrum:** Active against gram-positive pathogens, including *Streptococcus pneumoniae*. Gram-negative spectrum notable for *Klebsiella pneumoniae, Haemophilus influenzae, H. parainfluenzae, Moraxella catarrhalis*. Additional spectrum includes *Chlamydophylia pneumoniae, Mycoplasma pneumoniae*.

Adverse Reactions/Side Effects

CNS: drowsiness, dizziness, headache, confusion. **CV:** QTc prolongation, ARRHYTHMIAS. **GI:** PSEUDOMEMBRANOUS COLITIS, diarrhea, abdominal pain, nausea, vomiting. **Derm:** photosensitivity, rash. **MS:** tendinitis, tendon rupture.

PHYSICAL THERAPY IMPLICATIONS

Examination and Evaluation

- Monitor symptoms of pseudomembranous colitis (diarrhea, abdominal pain, fever, pus or mucus in stools) or other severe or prolonged GI problems (nausea, cramps, vomiting). Notify physician or nursing staff immediately of these symptoms.
- Assess heart rate, ECG, and heart sounds, especially during exercise (See Appendices G, H). Report any rhythm disturbances or symptoms of increased arrhythmias, including palpitations, chest discomfort, shortness of breath, fainting, and fatigue/weakness.
- Assess any tendon pain. Tendinopathy and rupture can occur, especially in large, weight-bearing tendons (Achilles, patellar tendons). Risk of tendon damage is greater in patients >65-yr-old, transplant recipients (i.e., kidney, heart, lung), patients with preexisting tendon damage, and patients taking corticosteroids concurrently.
- Assess dizziness and drowsiness that might affect gait, balance, and other functional activities (See Appendix C). Report balance problems and functional limitations to the physician and nursing staff, and caution the patient and family/caregivers to guard against falls and trauma.

Interventions

- If tendon symptoms occur, notify the physician and protect the affected area to avoid tendon ruptures. Do not stretch or exercise the affected tendon, and provide crutches, walker, or other assistive devices if lower extremities are involved.
- Because of the arrhythmias, use caution during aerobic exercise and other forms of therapeutic exercise. Assess exercise tolerance frequently (blood pressure, heart rate, fatigue levels), and terminate exercise immediately if any untoward responses occur (See Appendix L).
- Always wash hands thoroughly and disinfect equipment (whirlpools, electrotherapeutic devices, treatment tables, and so forth) to help prevent the spread of infection. Use universal precautions or isolation procedures as indicated for specific patients.
- Causes photosensitivity; use care if administering UV treatments.

Patient/Client-Related Instruction

- Advise patient about photosensitivity, and to use sunscreens, protective clothing, and avoid prolonged sun exposure. Advise patient to also report any rashes or other skin reactions.
- Instruct patient to report other troublesome side effects such as severe or prolonged headache, confusion, or GI problems (nausea, vomiting, diarrhea, abdominal pain).

Pharmacokinetics

Absorption: 71% absorbed following oral administration.
Distribution: Widely distributed; penetrates lung tissue and fluids well.
Metabolism and Excretion: Minimal metabolism; 61% excreted unchanged in feces, 36% excreted unchanged in urine.
Half-life: 7 hr.

TIME/ACTION PROFILE (blood levels)

ROUTE	ONSET	PEAK	DURATION
PO	rapid	0.5–2 hr	24 hr

Contraindications/Precautions

Contraindicated in: Hypersensitivity (cross-sensitivity within class may exist); OB/Lactation/Pedi: Safety not established.

Use Cautiously in: Known or suspected CNS disorder; Renal impairment (decrease dose if CCr ≤40 mL/min); Concurrent use of Class IA antiarrhythmics (disopyramide, quinidine, procainamide), Class III antiarrhythmics (amiodarone, sotalol), some phenothiazines, or tricyclic antidepressants; Congenital long QT syndrome; Concurrent use of corticosteroids (↑ risk of tendinitis/tendon rupture); Kidney, heart, or lung transplant patients (↑ risk of tendinitis/tendon rupture); Geri: ↑ risk of adverse reactions.

Interactions

Drug-Drug: Concurrent use of Class IA and Class III **antiarrhythmics, antipsychotics, tricyclic antidepressants,** or **erythromycin** may ↑ the risk of QTc prolongation and serious, potentially life-threatening arrhythmias (concurrent use should be avoided). Administration with **magnesium and**

aluminum-containing antacids, iron salts, bismuth subsalicylate, sucralfate, didanosine (chewable/buffered tablets or pediatric powder for oral solution), **zinc salts**, and other **metals** ↓ absorption. Concurrent use of **corticosteroids** may ↑ the risk of tendon rupture. May ↑ the risk of nephrotoxicity from **cyclosporine**. Blood levels are ↑ by **probenecid**.

Route/Dosage

Acute bacterial exacerbation of chronic bronchitis (ABECB)

PO (Adults): 320 mg once daily for 5 days.

Community-acquired-pneumonia (CAP)

PO (Adults): 320 mg once daily for 7 days.

Renal Impairment

PO (Adults): *CCr ≤40 mL/min* AECB:160 mg once daily for 5 days; CAP:160 mg once daily for 7 days.

Availability

Tablets: 320 mg.

HIGH ALERT

gemtuzumab ozogamicin

(jem-**tu**-zoo-mab o-zo-ga-**my**-sin)

Mylotarg

Classification

Therapeutic: antineoplastics

Pharmacologic: monoclonal antibodies, antitumor antibiotics

Indications

Treatment of patients with patients with CD33-positive acute myeloid leukemia in first relapse who are ≥60 yr old and who are not considered to be candidates for cytotoxic chemotherapy.

Action

The antibody portion (gemtuzumab) attaches to the CD33 antigen on the surface of acute myeloid leukemic cells. Binding produces a complex that is internalized by the leukemic cells. Once internalized, the antitumor antibiotic portion of the drug (ozogamicin, also know as calicheamicin) is released and binds to DNA resulting in breaks in double-strand DNA and cell death. **Therapeutic Effects:** Death of acute myeloid leukemic cells.

Adverse Reactions/Side Effects

CNS: headache. **Resp:** dyspnea, hypoxia. **CV:** hypotension, hypertension. **GI:** mucositis, nausea, vomiting, hepatotoxicity. **Derm:** rash. **Endo:** hyperglycemia. **F and E:** hypokalemia. **Hemat:** NEUTROPENIA, anemia, bleeding, thrombocytopenia. **Misc:** chills, fever, postinfusion reaction, allergic reactions, infection, tumor lysis syndrome.

PHYSICAL THERAPY IMPLICATIONS

Examination and Evaluation

- Monitor signs of bone marrow suppression, including neutropenia (fever, sore throat, signs of infection), thrombocytopenia (bruising, nose bleeds, and bleeding gums), or unusual weakness and fatigue that might be due to anemia or other blood dyscrasias. Report these signs to the physician or nursing staff immediately.
- Report allergy-like responses (wheezing, tightness in the throat or chest, urticaria, other skin reactions) that occur during and after administration (infusion related events).
- Monitor neuromuscular signs of electrolyte imbalances that might indicate tumor lysis syndrome. Signs include severe muscle weakness or paralysis due to increased plasma potassium (hyperkalemia) or muscle hyperexcitability and tetany due to phosphate and calcium imbalances (hyperphosphatemia and hypocalcemia). Notify physician immediately if these signs occur.
- Assess blood pressure (BP) periodically and compare to normal values (See Appendix F). Report a sustained increase in BP (hypertension) or a decrease in BP (hypotension), especially if symptoms such as dizziness and syncope occur.
- Assess any breathing problems such as difficult or labored breathing. Monitor pulse oximetry and perform pulmonary function tests (See Appendices I, J, K) to quantify suspected changes in ventilation and respiratory function.
- Be alert for signs of hyperglycemia, including confusion, drowsiness, flushed/dry skin, fruit-like breath odor, rapid/deep breathing, polyuria, loss of appetite, and unusual thirst. Patients with diabetes mellitus should check blood glucose levels frequently.

Interventions

- For patients who are medically able to begin exercise, implement appropriate resistive exercises and aerobic training to maintain muscle strength and aerobic capacity during cancer chemotherapy or to help restore function after chemotherapy.
- Because of the risk of abnormal BP responses, blood dyscrasias, and pulmonary problems, use caution during aerobic exercise and endurance conditioning. Terminate exercise if patient exhibits untoward symptoms (chest pain, shortness of breath, etc.), or displays other criteria for exercise termination (See Appendix L).

Patient/Client-Related Instruction

- Advise patient to guard against infection (frequent hand washing, etc.) and to avoid crowds and contact with persons with contagious diseases.
- Advise patient about the likelihood of GI reactions (nausea, vomiting, inflammation of mucous membranes). Instruct patient to report severe or prolonged GI problems, or signs of liver toxicity such as anorexia, abdominal pain, severe nausea and vomiting, yellow skin or eyes, fever, sore throat, malaise, weakness, facial edema, lethargy, and unusual bleeding or bruising.
- Instruct patient or family/caregivers to report other troublesome side effects such as severe or prolonged headache, chills, fever, or skin rash.

Pharmacokinetics

Absorption: IV administration results in complete bioavailability.
Distribution: Binds to CD33 receptor sites, is then internalized by leukemic cells, releasing ozogamicin.
Metabolism and Excretion: Ozogamicin is probably metabolized by the liver.
Half-life: *Total ozogamicin*—45 hr (increased with second dose); *unconjugated ozogamicin*—100 hr.

TIME/ACTION PROFILE

ROUTE	ONSET	PEAK	DURATION
IN	rapid	following infusion	2 wk

Contraindications/Precautions

Contraindicated in: Hypersensitivity; Pregnancy; Lactation.
Use Cautiously in: Patients with hepatic impairment; Children (safety not established).

Interactions

Drug-Drug: None reported to date.

Route/Dosage

IV (Adults ≥60 yr): 9 mg/m^2 as a 2-hr infusion followed by a second dose 14 days later.

Availability

Powder for injection (requires reconstitution): 5 mg/vial.

gentamicin (jen-ta-**mye**-sin)

Cidomycin, Garamycin, G-Mycin, Jenamicin

Classification
Therapeutic: anti-infectives
Pharmacologic: aminoglycosides

Indications

Treatment of serious gram-negative bacterial infections and infections caused by staphylococci when penicillins or other less toxic drugs are contraindicated. In combination with other agents in the management of serious enterococcal infections. Prevention of infective endocarditis. **Topical, Ophth:** Treatment of localized infections due to susceptible organisms.

Action

Inhibits protein synthesis in bacteria at level of 30S ribosome. **Therapeutic Effects:** Bactericidal action. **Spectrum:** Notable for activity against *Pseudomonas aeruginosa, Klebsiella pneumoniae, Escherichia coli, Proteus, Serratia, Acinetobacter, Staphylococcus aureus*. In treatment of enterococcal infections, synergy with a penicillin is required. Not active against Streptococci, Anaerobes.

Adverse Reactions/Side Effects

CNS: ataxia, vertigo. **EENT:** ototoxicity (vestibular and cochlear). **GU:** nephrotoxicity. **MS:** muscle paralysis (high parenteral doses). **Misc:** hypersensitivity reactions.

PHYSICAL THERAPY IMPLICATIONS

Examination and Evaluation

- Monitor signs of hypersensitivity reactions, including pulmonary symptoms (tightness in the throat and chest, wheezing, cough dyspnea) or skin reactions (rash, pruritus, urticaria). Notify physician or nursing staff immediately if these reactions occur.
- Report any muscle weakness or paralysis that occurs following injection of high doses.
- Monitor signs of ataxia and vertigo that might affect gait, balance, and other functional activities. Report balance problems and functional limitations to the physician and nursing staff, and caution the patient and family/caregivers to guard against falls and trauma.
- Monitor signs of ototoxicity, including hearing loss, tinnitus, and balance problems (See Appendix E for fall assessment and prevention). Report these signs to the physician, and caution the patient and family/caregivers to guard against falls and trauma.

Interventions

- Always wash hands thoroughly and disinfect equipment (whirlpools, electrotherapeutic devices, treatment tables, and so forth) to help prevent the spread of infection. Employ universal precautions or isolation procedures as indicated for specific patients.

Patient/Client-Related Instruction

- Advise patient to report signs of nephrotoxicity, including blood or pus in urine, decreased urine output, fatigue, and weight gain from fluid retention.

Pharmacokinetics

Absorption: Well absorbed after IM administration. IV administration results in complete bioavailability. Some absorption follows administration by other routes.

Distribution: Widely distributed throughout extracellular fluid; crosses the placenta; small amounts enter breast milk. Poor penetration into CSF.

Metabolism and Excretion: >90% excreted unchanged by kidneys.

Half-life: Neonates <7 days: 3–11.5 hr; Neonates 7–30 days: 3–6 hr; Infants: 3–5 hr; Children: 1–3 hr; Adolescents: 0.5–2.5 hr; Adults: 2–4 hr (increased in renal impairment).

TIME/ACTION PROFILE (blood levels*)

ROUTE	ONSET	PEAK	DURATION
IM	rapid	30–90 min	8–24 hr
IV	rapid	15–30 min†	8–24 hr

*All parenterally administered aminoglycosides.

†Postdistribution peak occurs 30 min after the end of a 30-min infusion and 15 min after the end of a 1-hr infusion.

Contraindications/Precautions

Contraindicated in: Hypersensitivity to gentamicin or other aminoglycosides; Most parenteral products contain bisulfites and should be avoided in patients with known intolerance; Products containing benzyl alcohol should be avoided in neonates.

Use Cautiously in: Renal impairment (dosage adjustments necessary; blood level monitoring useful in preventing ototoxicity and nephrotoxicity); Hearing impairment; Geriatric patients (difficulty in assessing auditory and vestibular function; age-related renal impairment); Neuromuscular diseases such as myasthenia gravis; Pregnancy and lactation; Neonates (increased risk of neuromuscular blockade; difficulty in assessing auditory and vestibular function; immature renal function) and neonates on extracorporeal oxygenation (ECMO) (require dose adjustments).

Interactions

Drug-Drug: Inactivated by **penicillins** and **cephalosporins** when coadministered to patients with renal insufficiency. Possible respiratory paralysis after **inhalation anesthetics** or **neuromuscular blockers**. Increased incidence of ototoxicity with **loop diuretics**. Increased incidence of nephrotoxicity with other **nephrotoxic drugs**.

Route/Dosage

Many regimens are used; most involve dosing adjusted on the basis of blood level monitoring and assessment of renal function.

IM, IV (Adults): 1–2 mg/kg q 8 hr (up to 6 mg/kg/day in 3 divided doses); *Once-daily dosing (unlabeled)*—4–7 mg/kg q 24 hr.

IM, IV (Children >5 yr): 2–2.5 mg/kg/dose q 8 hr. *Once daily*—5–7.5 mg/kg/dose q 24 hr. *Cystic fibrosis*—2.5–3.3 mg/kg/dose q 6–8 hr. *Hemodialysis*—1.25–1.75 mg/kg/dose postdialysis.

IM, IV (Children 1 mo–5 yr): 2.5 mg/kg/dose q 8 hr. *Once daily*5–7.5 mg/kg/dose q 24 hr. *Cystic fibrosis*—2.5–3.3 mg/kg/dose q 6–8 hr. *Hemodialysis*—1.25–1.75 mg/kg/dose postdialysis.

IM, IV (Neonates full term and/or >1 wk): *Weight < 1200 g*—2.5 mg/kg/dose q 18–24 hr. *Weight 1200–2000 g*—2.5 mg/kg/dose q 8–12 hr. *Weight > 2000 g*—2.5 mg/kg/dose q 8 hr. *ECMO*—2.5 mg/kg/dose q 18 hr, subsequent doses based on serum concentrations. *Once daily*—3.5–5 mg/kg/dose q 24 hr.

IM, IV (Neonates premature and/or ≤1 wk): *Weight < 1000 g*—3.5 mg/kg/dose q 24 hr. *Weight 1000–1200 g*—2.5 mg/kg/dose q 18–24 hr. *Weight > 1200 g*—2.5 mg/kg/dose q 12 hr. *Once daily*—3.5–4 mg/kg/dose q 24 hr.

Intrathecal (Adults): 4–8 mg/day.

Intrathecal (Infants >3 mo and Children): 1–2 mg/day.

Intrathecal (Neonates): 1 mg/day.

Topical (Adults and Children >1 mo): Apply cream or ointment 3–4 times daily.

Renal Impairment

IM, IV (Adults): Initial dose of 2 mg/kg. Subsequent doses/intervals dependent on blood level monitoring and renal function assessment.

Availability

Injection: 10 mg/mL, 40 mg/mL. **Premixed injection:** 40 mg/50 mL, 60 mg/50 mL, 60 mg/100 mL, 70 mg/50 mL, 80 mg/50 mL, 80 mg/100 mL, 90 mg/100 mL, 100 mg/50 mL, 100 mg/100 mL, 120 mg/100 mL.

Topical cream: 0.1%. **Topical ointment:** 0.1%.

glatiramer (gla-tir-a-mer)

Copaxone

Classification

Therapeutic: anti–multiple sclerosis agents

Pharmacologic: immune response modifiers

Indications

Reduction of frequency of relapses in relapsing-remitting multiple sclerosis (MS).

Action

Appears to modify the immune process thought to be responsible for MS. **Therapeutic Effects:** Decreased incidence of relapses in relapsing-remitting MS.

Adverse Reactions/Side Effects

CNS: anxiety, weakness, confusion, migraine, vertigo. **CV:** chest pain, palpitations, edema, syncope, tachycardia, vasodilation. **Derm:** pruritus, rashes, sweating, erythema. **EENT:** rhinitis, nystagmus. **GI:** diarrhea, nausea, anorexia, vomiting. **GU:** urgency. **Local:** injection-site reactions. **MS:** arthralgia, back pain, hypertonia. **Neuro:** tremor. **Resp:** dyspnea. **Misc:** flu-like symptoms, lymphadenopathy, fever, immediate postinjection reaction, infection, pain, weight gain.

PHYSICAL THERAPY IMPLICATIONS

Examination and Evaluation

- Periodically assess balance, coordination, spasticity, and other aspects of neuromuscular function to help document whether this drug is effective in reducing MS exacerbations.
- Assess heart rate, ECG, and heart sounds, especially during exercise (See Appendices G, H). Report an increased heart rate (tachycardia) or symptoms of other arrhythmias, including palpitations, chest pain, shortness of breath, labored breathing, syncope, and fatigue/weakness.
- Assess peripheral edema using girth measurements, volume displacement, and measurement of pitting edema (See Appendix N). Report increased swelling in feet and ankles due to peripheral vasodilation.
- Report allergy-like responses (wheezing, laryngeal edema, urticaria, other skin reactions) that occur immediately after administration (immediate postinjection reaction).
- Assess any back pain, joint pain, tremor, or increased muscle tone to rule out musculoskeletal pathology; that is, try to determine if pain or hypertonicity is drug induced rather than caused by anatomic or biomechanical problems.
- Assess vertigo or weakness that might affect gait, balance, and other functional activities. Report balance problems and functional limitations to the physician and nursing staff, and caution the patient and family/caregivers to guard against falls and trauma.
- Be alert for signs of infection and flu-like symptoms, including fever, sore throat, swollen glands, chills, aches, nausea, vomiting, diarrhea, and localized inflammation. Notify physician or nursing staff of these signs.
- Periodically assess body weight and other anthropometric measures (body mass index, body composition). Report a rapid or unexplained weight gain or increased body fat.
- Assess the subcutaneous injection site for pain, swelling, and irritation. Report prolonged or excessive injection site reactions to the physician.

Interventions

- Design and implement coordination, balance, and other therapeutic exercises to maintain function and complement drug effects in patients with MS.
- Because of the risk of arrhythmias, use caution during aerobic exercise and other forms of therapeutic exercise. Assess exercise tolerance frequently (blood pressure, heart rate, fatigue levels), and terminate exercise immediately if any untoward responses occur (See Appendix L).
- Do not apply massage or physical agents (heat, cold, electrotherapeutic modalities) at or near the subcutaneous application site. These interventions can alter drug absorption from subcutaneous tissues.

Patient/Client-Related Instruction

- Advise patient to guard against infection (frequent hand washing, etc.) and to avoid crowds and contact with persons with contagious diseases.
- Instruct patient to report other troublesome side effects, including severe or prolonged anxiety, confusion, migraine headaches, nasal inflammation/irritation, urinary urgency, skin problems (rash, redness, itching, sweating), or GI problems (diarrhea, nausea, vomiting, loss of appetite).

Pharmacokinetics

Absorption: Some absorption follows subcutaneous administration.
Distribution: Some enters the lymphatic system.
Metabolism and Excretion: Unknown.
Half-life: Unknown.

TIME/ACTION PROFILE

ROUTE	ONSET	PEAK	DURATION
SC	Unknown	unknown	unknown

Contraindications/Precautions

Contraindicated in: Hypersensitivity to glatiramer or mannitol.

Use Cautiously in: Pregnancy, lactation, or children <18 yr (safety not established).

Interactions

Drug-Drug: Unknown.

Route/Dosage

SC (Adults): 20 mg/day.

Availability

Injection: 20 mg/mL in prefilled syringes.

HIGH ALERT

glimepiride (glye-mep-i-ride)

Amaryl

Classification

Therapeutic: antidiabetics

Pharmacologic: sulfonylureas

Indications

PO: Control of blood sugar in type 2 diabetes mellitus when diet therapy fails. Requires some pancreatic function.

Action

Lowers blood sugar by stimulating the release of insulin from the pancreas and increasing the sensitivity to insulin at receptor sites. May also decrease hepatic glucose production. May be used concurrently with metformin when the combination of diet, exercise, and either drug alone fails to produce glycemic control. **Therapeutic Effects:** Lowering of blood sugar in diabetic patients.

Adverse Reactions/Side Effects

CNS: dizziness, drowsiness, headache, weakness. **GI:** constipation, cramps, diarrhea, drug-induced hepatitis, dyspepsia, increased appetite, nausea, vomiting. **Derm:** photosensitivity, rashes. **Endo:** hypoglycemia. **F and E:** hyponatremia.

PHYSICAL THERAPY IMPLICATIONS

Examination and Evaluation

- Be alert for signs of hypoglycemia, especially during and after exercise. Common neuromuscular signs include anxiety; restlessness; tingling in hands, feet, lips, or tongue; chills; cold sweats; confusion; difficulty in concentration; drowsiness; excessive hunger; headache; irritability; nervousness; tremor; weakness; unsteady gait. Report persistent or repeated episodes of hypoglycemia to the physician.
- Assess any dizziness (See Appendix C) or drowsiness that might impair gait, balance, and other complex motor tasks (driving a car). Report balance problems and functional limitations to the physician, and caution the patient and family/caregivers to guard against falls and trauma.
- Monitor signs of low sodium levels (hyponatremia), including headache, confusion, lethargy, irritability, decreased consciousness, and neuromuscular abnormalities (muscle weakness and cramps). Report severe or prolonged signs to the physician.
- Assess blood pressure periodically (See Appendix F). A sudden or sustained increase in blood pressure (hypertension) may indicate problems in diabetes management, and should be reported to the physician.

Interventions

- Implement aerobic exercise and endurance training programs to maintain optimal body weight, improve insulin sensitivity, and reduce the risk of macrovascular disease (heart attack, stroke) and microvascular problems (reduced blood flow to tissues and organs that causes poor wound healing, neuropathy, retinopathy, and nephropathy).
- Provide a source of oral glucose (fruit juice, glucose gels/tablets, etc.) to treat mild hypoglycemia. Call for emergency assistance if symptoms persist or in cases of severe hypoglycemia. Emergency treatment typically consists of IV glucose, glucagon, or epinephrine.
- Causes photosensitivity; use care if administering UV treatments.

Patient/Client-Related Instruction

- Encourage patient to monitor blood glucose before and after exercise and to adjust food intake to maintain normal glycemic levels.
- Emphasize the importance of adhering to nutritional guidelines and the need for periodic assessment of glycemic control (serum glucose and glycosylated hemoglobin levels) throughout the management of diabetes mellitus.
- Advise patient about symptoms of hyperglycemia (confusion, drowsiness; flushed, dry skin; fruit-like breath odor; rapid, deep breathing, polyuria; loss of appetite; unusual thirst). Drug dosages may need to be adjusted to prevent repeated episodes of hyperglycemia.
- Instruct patient to report severe or prolonged GI problems (diarrhea, constipation, cramps) or signs of drug-induced hepatitis (anorexia, abdominal pain, severe nausea and vomiting, yellow skin or eyes, skin rashes, flu-like symptoms, muscle/joint pain).
- Advise patient about photosensitivity, and to use sunscreens, protective clothing, and avoid prolonged sun exposure. Advise patient to also report any rashes or other skin reactions.

Pharmacokinetics

Absorption: Well absorbed following oral administration.
Distribution: Unknown.
Protein Binding: 99.5%.
Metabolism and Excretion: Mostly metabolized by the liver; one metabolite has hypoglycemic activity.
Half-life: 5–9.2 hr.

TIME/ACTION PROFILE (hypoglycemic activity)

ROUTE	ONSET	PEAK	DURATION
PO	unknown	2–3 hr	24 hr

Contraindications/Precautions

Contraindicated in: Hypersensitivity; Hypersensitivity to sulfonamides (cross-sensitivity may occur); Type 1 diabetes; Diabetic coma or ketoacidosis; Severe renal, hepatic, thyroid, or other endocrine disease; Uncontrolled infection, serious burns, or trauma.
Use Cautiously in: Severe cardiovascular or hepatic disease; Geri: Geriatric patients (increased sensitivity; dose reduction may be required); Severe renal disease (increased risk of hypoglycemia); Infection, stress, or changes in diet may alter requirements for control of blood sugar; Impaired thyroid, pituitary, or adrenal function; Malnutrition, high fever, prolonged nausea, or vomiting; OB/Lactation: Pregnancy or lactation (safety not established; insulin recommended during pregnancy).

Interactions

Drug-Drug: Ingestion of **alcohol** may result in disulfiram-like reaction. Effectiveness may be ↓ by concurrent use of **diuretics, corticosteroids, phenothiazines, oral contraceptives, estrogens, thyroid preparations, phenytoin, nicotinic acid, sympathomimetics**, and **isoniazid. Alcohol, androgens (testosterone), chloramphenicol, clofibrate, MAO inhibitors, NSAIDs** (except diclofenac), **salicylates, sulfonamides**, and **warfarin** may ↑ risk of hypoglycemia. Concurrent use with **warfarin** may alter the response to both agents (↑ effects of both initially, then ↓ activity); close monitoring recommended during any changes in dose. **Beta-adrenergic blockers** may mask the signs and symptoms of hypoglycemia.

Route/Dosage

PO (Adults): 1–2 mg once daily initially; may increase q 1–2 wk up to 8 mg/day (usual range 1–4 mg/day).

Availability

Tablets: 1 mg, 2 mg, 4 mg. ***In combination with:*** pioglitazone (Duetact). See Appendix B.

HIGH ALERT

glipizide (glip-i-zide)

Glucotrol, Glucotrol XL

Classification
Therapeutic: antidiabetics
Pharmacologic: sulfonylureas

Indications

PO: Controls blood sugar in type 2 diabetes mellitus when diet therapy fails. Requires some pancreatic function.

Action

Lowers blood sugar by stimulating the release of insulin from the pancreas and increasing the sensitivity to insulin at receptor sites. May also decrease hepatic glucose production. **Therapeutic Effects:** Lowering of blood sugar in diabetic patients.

Adverse Reactions/Side Effects

CNS: dizziness, drowsiness, headache, weakness. **GI:** constipation, cramps, diarrhea, drug-induced hepatitis, dyspepsia, increased appetite, nausea, vomiting. **Derm:** photosensitivity, rashes. **Endo:** hypoglycemia. **F and E:** hyponatremia. **Hemat:** APLASTIC ANEMIA, agranulocytosis, leukopenia, pancytopenia, thrombocytopenia.

PHYSICAL THERAPY IMPLICATIONS

Examination and Evaluation

- Monitor signs of aplastic anemia (fatigue, weakness, shortness of breath with exertion, tachycardia, dizziness, headache), agranulocytosis (fever, sore throat, mucosal lesions, signs of infection, bruising), thrombocytopenia (bruising, nose bleeds, and bleeding gums), or unusual weakness and fatigue that might be due to other blood dyscrasias. Report these signs to the physician immediately.
- Be alert for signs of hypoglycemia, especially during and after exercise. Common neuromuscular signs include anxiety; restlessness; tingling in hands, feet, lips, or tongue; chills; cold sweats; confusion; difficulty in concentration; drowsiness; excessive hunger; headache; irritability; nervousness; tremor; weakness; unsteady gait. Report persistent or repeated episodes of hypoglycemia to the physician.
- Assess any dizziness (See Appendix C) or drowsiness that might impair gait, balance, and other complex motor tasks (driving a car). Report balance problems and functional limitations to the physician, and caution the patient and family/caregivers to guard against falls and trauma.

- Assess blood pressure periodically (See Appendix F). A sudden or sustained increase in blood pressure (hypertension) may indicate problems in diabetes management, and should be reported to the physician.

Interventions

- Implement aerobic exercise and endurance training programs to maintain optimal body weight, improve insulin sensitivity, and reduce the risk of macrovascular disease (heart attack, stroke) and microvascular problems (reduced blood flow to tissues and organs that causes poor wound healing, neuropathy, retinopathy, and nephropathy).
- Provide a source of oral glucose (fruit juice, glucose gels/tablets, etc.) to treat mild hypoglycemia. Call for emergency assistance if symptoms persist or in cases of severe hypoglycemia. Emergency treatment typically consists of IV glucose, glucagon, or epinephrine.
- Causes photosensitivity; use care if administering UV treatments.

Patient/Client-Related Instruction

- Encourage patient to monitor blood glucose before and after exercise, and to adjust food intake to maintain normal glycemic levels.
- Emphasize the importance of adhering to nutritional guidelines and the need for periodic assessment of glycemic control (serum glucose and glycosylated hemoglobin levels) throughout the management of diabetes mellitus.
- Advise patient about symptoms of hyperglycemia (confusion, drowsiness; flushed, dry skin; fruit-like breath odor; rapid, deep breathing, polyuria; loss of appetite; unusual thirst). Drug dosages may need to be adjusted to prevent repeated episodes of hyperglycemia.
- Instruct patient to report severe or prolonged GI problems (diarrhea, constipation, cramps) or signs of drug-induced hepatitis (anorexia, abdominal pain, severe nausea and vomiting, yellow skin or eyes, skin rashes, flu-like symptoms, muscle/joint pain).
- Advise patient about photosensitivity, and to use sunscreens, protective clothing, and avoid prolonged sun exposure. Advise patient to also report any rashes or other skin reactions.

Pharmacokinetics

Absorption: Well absorbed following oral administration.
Distribution: Unknown.
Protein Binding: 99%.
Metabolism and Excretion: Mostly metabolized by the liver.
Half-life: 2.1–2.6 hr.

TIME/ACTION PROFILE (hypoglycemic activity)

ROUTE	ONSET	PEAK	DURATION
PO	15–30 min	1–2 hr	up to 24 hr

Contraindications/Precautions

Contraindicated in: Hypersensitivity; Hypersensitivity to sulfonamides (cross-sensitivity may occur); Insulin-dependent diabetics; Diabetic coma or ketoacidosis; Severe renal, hepatic, thyroid, or other endocrine disease; Uncontrolled infection, serious burns, or trauma.
Use Cautiously in: Severe cardiovascular or hepatic disease; Geri: Increased sensitivity; dosage reduction may be required; Severe renal disease (increased risk of hypoglycemia); Infection, stress, or changes in diet may alter requirements for control of blood sugar; Impaired thyroid, pituitary, or adrenal function; Malnutrition, high fever, prolonged nausea, or vomiting; OB: Pregnancy or lactation (safety not established; insulin recommended during pregnancy).

Interactions

Drug-Drug: Ingestion of **alcohol** may result in disulfiram-like reaction. Effectiveness may be ↓ by concurrent use of **diuretics, corticosteroids, phenothiazines, oral contraceptives, estrogens, thyroid preparations, phenytoin, nicotinic acid, sympathomimetics**, and **isoniazid. Alcohol, androgens (testosterone), chloramphenicol, clofibrate, MAO inhibitors, NSAIDs** (except diclofenac), **salicylates, fluconazole sulfonamides**, and **warfarin** may ↑ risk of hypoglycemia. Concurrent use with **warfarin** may alter the response to both agents (increased effects of both initially, then decreased activity); close monitoring recommended during any changes in dosage. **Beta-adrenergic blockers** may mask the signs and symptoms of hypoglycemia.

Route/Dosage

PO (Adults): 5 mg/day initially, increased as needed (range 2.5–40 mg/day); XL dosage form is given once daily. Doses >15 mg/day may be given as 2 divided doses of regular-release product (not XL).
PO (Geriatric Patients): 2.5 mg/day initially.

Availability (generic available)

Tablets: 5 mg Rx, 10 mg Rx. **Extended-release tablets:** 2.5 mg, 5 mg Rx, 10 mg Rx. ***In combination with:*** metformin (MetaGlip). See Appendix B.

glucagon (gloo-ka-gon)

GlucaGen

Classification

Therapeutic: hormones

Pharmacologic: pancreatics

Indications

Acute management of severe hypoglycemia when administration of glucose is not feasible. Facilitation of radiographic examination of the GI tract. **Unlabeled Use:** Antidote to Beta blockers, Calcium channel blockers.

Action

Stimulates hepatic production of glucose from glycogen stores (glycogenolysis). Relaxes the musculature of the GI tract (stomach, duodenum, small bowel, and colon), temporarily inhibiting movement. Has positive inotropic and chronotropic effects. **Therapeutic Effects:** Increase in blood glucose. Relaxation of GI musculature, facilitating radiographic examination.

Adverse Reactions/Side Effects

CV: hypotension. **GI:** nausea, vomiting. **Misc:** HYPERSENSITIVITY REACTIONS, INCLUDING ANAPHYLAXIS.

PHYSICAL THERAPY IMPLICATIONS

Examination and Evaluation

- Monitor signs of hypersensitivity reactions and anaphylaxis, including pulmonary symptoms (tightness in the throat and chest, wheezing, cough, dyspnea) or skin reactions (rash, pruritus, urticaria). Notify physician or nursing staff immediately if these reactions occur.
- Assess blood pressure periodically and compare to normal values (See Appendix F). Report low blood pressure (hypotension), especially if patient experiences dizziness, fatigue, or syncope.

Interventions

- Because of the risk of recurrent hypoglycemia, use caution during aerobic exercise and other forms of therapeutic exercise. Assess exercise tolerance frequently (blood pressure, heart rate, fatigue levels, dizziness), and terminate exercise immediately if any untoward responses occur (See Appendix L).
- Provide a source of oral glucose (fruit juice, glucose gels/tablets, etc.) to treat mild hypoglycemia. Call for emergency assistance if symptoms persist or in cases of severe hypoglycemia. Emergency treatment typically consists of IV glucose, glucagon, or epinephrine.

Patient/Client-Related Instruction

- Educate patient and family/caregivers about the signs of hypoglycemia (see above in Evaluation and Examination). Emphasize that early recognition and administration of glucose may prevent acute reactions and need for subsequent glucagon administration.
- Instruct patient to report severe or prolonged GI reactions such as nausea and vomiting.

Pharmacokinetics

Absorption: Well absorbed following IM and SC administration.

Distribution: Unknown.

Metabolism and Excretion: Extensively metabolized by the liver, plasma, and kidneys.

Half-life: 8–18 min.

TIME/ACTION PROFILE

ROUTE	ONSET	PEAK	DURATION
IM (hyperglycemic action)	within 10 min	30 min	60–90 12–27 min
IV (hyperglycemic action)	1 min	5– min	9–17 min
SC (hyperglycemic action)	within 10 min	30–45 min	60–90 min
IV (effect on GI musculature)	45 sec (for 0.25–2-mg dose)	unknown	9–17 min (0.25–0.5–mg dose); 22–25 min (2-mg dose)
IM (effect on GI musculature)	8–10 min (1-mg dose); 4–7 min (2-mg dose)	unknown	9–27 min (1-mg dose); 21–32 min (2-mg dose)

Contraindications/Precautions

Contraindicated in: Hypersensitivity; Pheochromocytoma; Some products contain glycerin and phenol—avoid use in patients with hypersensitivities to these ingredients.

Use Cautiously in: History suggestive of insulinoma or pheochromocytoma; Prolonged fasting, starvation, adrenal insufficiency or chronic hypoglycemia (low levels of releasable glucose); When used to inhibit GI motility, use cautiously in geriatric patient with cardiac disease or diabetics; OB: Should be used during pregnancy only if clearly needed; Lactation: Safety not established.

Interactions

Drug-Drug: Large doses may enhance the effect of **warfarin**. Negates the response to **insulin** or **oral hypoglycemic agents**; **phenytoin** inhibits the stimulant effect of glucagon on insulin release. Hyperglycemic effect is intensified and prolonged by **epinephrine**. Patients on concurrent **beta blocker** therapy may have a greater increase in heart rate and blood pressure.

Route/Dosage

Hypoglycemia

IV, IM, SC (Adults and Children ≥20 kg): 1 mg; may be repeated in 15 min if necessary.
IV, IM, SC (Children <20 kg): 0.5 mg or 0.02–0.03 mg/kg; may be repeated in 15 min if necessary.

Radiographic Examination of the GI Tract

IM, IV (Adults): 0.25–2 mg; depending on location and duration of examination (0.5 mg IV or 2 mg IM for relaxation of stomach, for examination of the colon 2 mg IM 10 min before procedure).

Antidote (unlabeled)

IV (Adults): *To beta blockers*—50–150 mcg (0.05–0.15 mg)/kg, followed by 1–5 mg/hr infusion. *To calcium channel blockers*—2 mg; additional doses determined by response.

Availability

Powder for injection: 1-mg (equivalent to 1 unit) vials as an emergency kit for low blood glucose and a diagnostic kit.

HIGH ALERT

glyburide (glye-byoo-ride)

Apo-Glyburide, DiaBeta, ✱Euglucon, Gen-Glybe, Glynase PresTab, Micronase, Novo-Glyburide, Nu-Glyburide

Classification
Therapeutic: antidiabetics
Pharmacologic: sulfonylureas

Indications

PO: Control of blood sugar in type 2 diabetes mellitus when diet therapy fails. Requires some pancreatic function.

Action

Lowers blood sugar by stimulating the release of insulin from the pancreas and increasing the sensitivity to insulin at receptor sites. May also decrease hepatic glucose production. **Therapeutic Effects:** Lowering of blood sugar in diabetic patients.

Adverse Reactions/Side Effects

CNS: dizziness, drowsiness, headache, weakness. **GI:** constipation, cramps, diarrhea, drug-induced hepatitis, dyspepsia, increased appetite, nausea, vomiting. **Derm:** photosensitivity, rashes. **Endo:** hypoglycemia. **F and E:** hyponatremia. **Hemat:** APLASTIC ANEMIA, agranulocytosis, leukopenia, pancytopenia, thrombocytopenia.

PHYSICAL THERAPY IMPLICATIONS

G

Examination and Evaluation

- Monitor signs of aplastic anemia (fatigue, weakness, shortness of breath with exertion, tachycardia, dizziness, headache), agranulocytosis (fever, sore throat, mucosal lesions, signs of infection, bruising), thrombocytopenia (bruising, nose bleeds and bleeding gums), or unusual weakness and fatigue that might be due to other blood dyscrasias. Report these signs to the physician immediately.
- Be alert for signs of hypoglycemia, especially during and after exercise. Common neuromuscular signs include anxiety; restlessness; tingling in hands, feet, lips, or tongue; chills; cold sweats; confusion; difficulty in concentration; drowsiness; excessive hunger; headache; irritability; nervousness; tremor; weakness; unsteady gait. Report persistent or repeated episodes of hypoglycemia to the physician.
- Assess any dizziness (See Appendix C) or drowsiness that might impair gait, balance, and other complex motor tasks (driving a car). Report balance problems and functional limitations to the physician, and caution the patient and family/caregivers to guard against falls and trauma.
- Monitor signs of low sodium levels (hyponatremia), including headache, confusion, lethargy, irritability, decreased consciousness, and neuromuscular abnormalities (muscle weakness and cramps). Report severe or prolonged signs to the physician.
- Assess blood pressure periodically (See Appendix F). A sudden or sustained increase in blood pressure (hypertension) may indicate problems in diabetes management, and should be reported to the physician.

Interventions

- Implement aerobic exercise and endurance training programs to maintain optimal body weight, improve insulin sensitivity, and reduce the risk of macrovascular disease (heart attack, stroke) and microvascular problems (reduced blood flow to tissues and organs that causes poor wound healing, neuropathy, retinopathy, and nephropathy).

- Provide a source of oral glucose (fruit juice, glucose gels/tablets, etc.) to treat mild hypoglycemia. Call for emergency assistance if symptoms persist or in cases of severe hypoglycemia. Emergency treatment typically consists of IV glucose, glucagon, or epinephrine.
- Causes photosensitivity; use care if administering UV treatments.

Patient/Client-Related Instruction

- Encourage patient to monitor blood glucose before and after exercise, and to adjust food intake to maintain normal glycemic levels.
- Emphasize the importance of adhering to nutritional guidelines and the need for periodic assessment of glycemic control (serum glucose and glycosylated hemoglobin levels) throughout the management of diabetes mellitus.
- Advise patient about symptoms of hyperglycemia (confusion, drowsiness; flushed, dry skin; fruit-like breath odor; rapid, deep breathing, polyuria; loss of appetite; unusual thirst). Drug dosages may need to be adjusted to prevent repeated episodes of hyperglycemia.
- Instruct patient to report severe or prolonged GI problems (diarrhea, constipation, cramps) or signs of drug-induced hepatitis (anorexia, abdominal pain, severe nausea and vomiting, yellow skin or eyes, skin rashes, flu-like symptoms, muscle/joint pain).
- Advise patient about photosensitivity, and to use sunscreens, protective clothing, and avoid prolonged sun exposure. Advise patient to also report any rashes or other skin reactions.

Pharmacokinetics

Absorption: Well absorbed following oral administration; micronized forms have better absorption.
Distribution: Reaches high concentrations in bile and crosses the placenta.
Metabolism and Excretion: Mostly metabolized by the liver.
Half-life: 10 hr.

TIME/ACTION PROFILE (hypoglycemic activity)

ROUTE	ONSET	PEAK	DURATION
PO	45–60 min	1.5–3 hr	24 hr

Contraindications/Precautions

Contraindicated in: Hypersensitivity; Hypersensitivity to sulfonamides (cross-sensitivity may occur); Type 1 diabetes; Diabetic coma or ketoacidosis; Severe renal, hepatic, thyroid, or other endocrine disease; Uncontrolled infection, serious burns, or trauma.
Use Cautiously in: Severe cardiovascular or hepatic disease; Geri: Increased sensitivity; dosage reduction may be required; Severe renal disease (increased risk of hypoglycemia); Infection, stress, or changes in diet may alter requirements for control of blood sugar; Impaired thyroid, pituitary, or adrenal function; Malnutrition, high fever, prolonged nausea, or vomiting; OB: Pregnancy or lactation (safety not established; insulin recommended during pregnancy).

Interactions

Drug-Drug: Ingestion of **alcohol** may result in disulfiram-like reaction. Effectiveness may be decreased by concurrent use of **diuretics, corticosteroids, phenothiazines, oral contraceptives, estrogens, thyroid preparations, phenytoin, nicotinic acid, sympathomimetics,** and **isoniazid. Alcohol, androgens (testosterone), chloramphenicol, clofibrate, MAO inhibitors, NSAIDs** (except diclofenac), **salicylates, sulfonamides,** and **warfarin** may ↑ the risk of hypoglycemia. Concurrent use with **warfarin** may alter the response to both agents (↑ effects of both initially, then ↓ activity); close monitoring recommended during any changes in dosage. **Beta-adrenergic blockers** may mask the signs and symptoms of hypoglycemia.

Route/Dosage

PO (Adults): *DiaBeta/Micronase*—2.5–5 mg once daily initially (range 1.25–20 mg/day). *Glynase PresTab* —1.5–3 mg/day initially (range 0.75–12 mg/day; doses >6 mg/day should be given as divided doses). Increments should not exceed 1.5 mg/wk.
PO (Geriatric Patients): *DiaBeta/Micronase*—1.25–2.5 mg/day initially; may be increased by 2.5 mg/day weekly. *Glynase PresTab*—0.75–3 mg/day; may be increased by 1.5 mg/day weekly.

Availability (generic available)

Tablets: 1.25 mg, 2.5 mg, 5 mg. **Micronized tablets:** 1.5 mg, 3 mg, 6 mg. ***In combination with:*** metformin (Glucovance). See Appendix B.

glycopyrrolate

(glye-koe-**pye**-roe-late)
Robinul, Robinul-Forte

Classification
Therapeutic: antispasmodics
Pharmacologic: anticholinergics

Indications

Inhibits salivation and excessive respiratory secretions when given preoperatively. Reverses some of the secretory and vagal actions of cholinesterase inhibitors used to treat nondepolarizing neuromuscular blockade (cholinergic adjunct). Adjunctive management of peptic ulcer disease.

Action

Inhibits the action of acetylcholine at postganglionic sites located in smooth muscle, secretory glands, and the CNS (antimuscarinic activity). Low doses decrease sweating, salivation, and respiratory secretions. Intermediate doses result in increased heart rate. Larger doses decrease GI and GU tract motility. **Therapeutic Effects:** Decreased GI and respiratory secretions.

Adverse Reactions/Side Effects

CNS: confusion, drowsiness. **EENT:** blurred vision, cycloplegia, dry eyes, mydriasis. **CV:** tachycardia, orthostatic hypotension, palpitations. **GI:** dry mouth, constipation. **GU:** urinary hesitancy, retention.

PHYSICAL THERAPY IMPLICATIONS

Examination and Evaluation

- Assess heart rate, ECG, and heart sounds, especially during exercise (See Appendices G, H). Report a rapid heart rate (tachycardia) or signs of other arrhythmias, including palpitations, chest discomfort, shortness of breath, fainting, and fatigue/weakness.
- Assess blood pressure (BP) when patient assumes a more upright position (lying to standing, sitting to standing, lying to sitting). Document orthostatic hypotension and contact physician when systolic BP falls >20 mm Hg or diastolic BP falls >10 mm Hg.
- If used to treat peptic ulcer, monitor any changes in symptoms (i.e., decreased abdominal pain, improved appetite) to help document whether drug therapy is successful.

Interventions

- Because of the risk of arrhythmias and abnormal BP responses, use caution during aerobic exercise and other forms of therapeutic exercise. Assess exercise tolerance frequently (BP, heart rate, fatigue levels), and terminate exercise immediately if any untoward responses occur (See Appendix L).
- To minimize orthostatic hypotension, patient should move slowly when assuming a more upright position.

Patient/Client-Related Instruction

- Instruct patient and family/caregivers to report other troublesome side effects such as severe or prolonged drowsiness, confusion, vision problems, problems with urination, or GI problems (constipation, dry mouth).

Pharmacokinetics

Absorption: Incompletely absorbed (10%) after oral administration. Well absorbed after IM administration.
Distribution: Distribution not fully known. Does not significantly cross the blood-brain barrier or eye. Crosses the placenta.
Metabolism and Excretion: Eliminated primarily unchanged in the feces, via biliary excretion.
Half-life: 1.7 hr (0.6–4.6 hr).

TIME/ACTION PROFILE (anticholinergic effects)

ROUTE	ONSET	PEAK	DURATION
PO	1 hr	unknown	8–12 hr
IM	15–30 min	30–45 min	2–7 hr*
IV	1–10 min	unknown	2–7 hr*

*Antisecretory effect lasts up to 7 hr; vagal blockade lasts 2–3 hr.

Contraindications/Precautions

Contraindicated in: Hypersensitivity; Angle-closure glaucoma; Acute hemorrhage; Tachycardia secondary to cardiac insufficiency or thyrotoxicosis; Pedi: Injection contains benzyl alcohol and should not be given to neonates; Myasthenia gravis; Obstructive uropathy; Paralytic ileus.
Use Cautiously in: Geri: Geriatric patients have increased sensitivity to anticholinergic drugs and are more susceptible to adverse reactions. Pedi: Young children and infants have increased sensitivity to anticholinergic drugs and are more susceptible to adverse reactions; Patients who may have intra-abdominal infections; Prostatic hyperplasia; Chronic renal, hepatic, pulmonary, or cardiac disease; Down's syndrome patients and children with spastic paralysis or brain damage (may be hypersensitive to antimuscarinic effects); Pregnancy and lactation (safety not established).

Interactions

Drug-Drug: Additive anticholinergic effects with other **anticholinergics**, including **antihistamines, phenothiazines, meperidine, amantadine, tricyclic antidepressants, quinidine**, and **disopyramide**. May alter the absorption of other **orally administered drugs** by slowing motility of the GI tract. **Antacids** or **adsorbent antidiarrheal agents** ↓ absorption of anticholinergics. May ↑ GI mucosal lesions in patients taking oral **potassium chloride** tablets. ↑ risk of adverse cardiovascular reactions with **cyclopropane** anesthesia. Concurrent use may ↓ absorption of **ketoconazole** (administer 2 hr after ketoconazole).

Route/Dosage

Control of Secretions During Surgery

IM (Adults): 4.4 mcg/kg 30–60 min preoperative (not to exceed 0.1 mg).

IM (Children >2 yr): 4.4 mcg/kg 30–60 min preoperative.
IM (Children <2 yr): 4.4–8.8 mcg/kg 30–60 min preoperative.

Control of Secretions (chronic)

IM, IV (Children): 4–10 mcg/kg/dose q 3–4 hr.
PO (Children): 40–100 mcg/kg/dose 3–4 times/day.

Cholinergic Adjunct

IV (Adults and Children): 200 mcg for each 1 mg of neostigmine or 5 mg of pyridostigmine given at the same time.

Antiarrhythmic

IV (Adults): 100 mcg, may be repeated q 2–3 min.
IV (Children): 4.4 mcg/kg (up to 100 mcg); may be repeated q 2–3 min.

Peptic Ulcer

PO (Adults): 1–2 mg 2–3 times daily. An additional 2 mg may be given at bedtime; may be decreased to 1 mg bid (not to exceed 8 mg/day).
IM, IV (Adults): 100–200 mcg q 4 hr up to 4 times daily.

Availability (generic available)

Tablets: 1 mg, 2 mg. **Injection:** 200 mcg (0.2 mg)/mL.

gold sodium thiomalate

(gold **soe**-dee-um thye-**oh-ma**-late)
Aurolate

Other Names:
Aurothiomalate

Classification
Therapeutic: antirheumatics, gold compounds
Pharmacologic: disease-modifying antirheumatic drugs (DMARDs)

Indications

Progressive rheumatoid arthritis resistant to conventional therapy.

Action

Inhibits inflammatory process. Modifies immune response (immunomodulating properties).
Therapeutic Effects: Relief of pain and inflammation. Slowing of the disease process in rheumatoid arthritis.

Adverse Reactions/Side Effects

CNS: dizziness, headache, neuropathy, syncope. **EENT:** corneal gold deposition, corneal ulcerations. **Resp:** pneumonitis. **CV:** bradycardia. **GI:** abdominal pain, cramping, diarrhea, metallic taste, stomatitis, anorexia, difficulty swallowing, drug-induced hepatitis, dyspepsia, flatulence, nausea, vomiting. **Derm:** dermatitis, rash, photosensitivity reactions, pruritus. **Hemat:** AGRANULOCYTOSIS, APLASTIC ANEMIA, thrombocytopenia, eosinophilia, leukopenia. **Misc:** ALLERGIC REACTIONS, INCLUDING ANAPHYLAXIS, angioneurotic edema, nitritoid reactions.

PHYSICAL THERAPY IMPLICATIONS

Examination and Evaluation

- Watch for signs of allergic reactions, including anaphylaxis and angioneurotic edema. Signs include pulmonary symptoms such as tightness in the throat and chest, wheezing, cough, and dyspnea, and skin reactions such as rash, pruritus, urticaria, burning/itching skin, and swelling in the face. Notify physician immediately if these reactions occur.
- Monitor and report signs of agranulocytosis (fever, sore throat, mucosal lesions, infection), aplastic anemia (unusual fatigue, shortness of breath with exertion), thrombocytopenia (bruising, nose bleeds, bleeding gums), or other weakness or coagulation problems that might indicate other blood dyscrasias. Periodic blood tests may be needed to monitor WBC and RBC counts.
- Be alert for reactions resembling nitrite poisoning (nitritoid reactions), including flushing of the face, edema of the tongue and lips, vomiting, profuse sweating, and hypotension. Seek immediate medical assistance because these reactions can be severe and life threatening.
- Assess any breathing problems or signs of pneumonitis such as dry cough, wheezing, rales, chest pain, shortness of breath, and difficult or labored breathing. Monitor pulse oximetry and perform pulmonary function tests (See Appendices I, J, K) to quantify suspected changes in ventilation and respiratory function.
- Assess heart rate and ECG, especially during exercise (See Appendix G). Report bradycardia or symptoms of arrhythmias, including chest discomfort, shortness of breath, fainting, and fatigue/weakness.
- Assess dizziness and syncope that might affect gait, balance, and other functional activities (See Appendix C). Report balance problems and functional limitations to the physician, and caution the patient and family/caregivers to guard against falls and trauma.
- Be alert for signs of peripheral neuropathy such as numbness, tingling, and decreased muscle strength. Establish baseline electroneuromyographic values at the beginning of drug treatment whenever possible, and reexamine these values periodically to document drug-induced changes in peripheral nerve function.

- Periodically assess impairments (pain, range of motion), functional ability, and disability to help document whether antirheumatic drug therapy is successful.

Interventions

- Implement appropriate manual therapy techniques, physical agents, therapeutic exercises, and orthotic/assistive devices to reduce pain, improve function, and augment the effects of antirheumatic drug therapy.
- Because of the risk of bradycardia and pneumonitis, use caution during aerobic exercise and other forms of therapeutic exercise. Assess exercise tolerance frequently (blood pressure, heart rate, respiratory function, fatigue levels), and terminate exercise immediately if any untoward responses occur (See Appendix L).
- Help patients with arthritis explore other nonpharmacologic methods to reduce chronic arthritis pain such as relaxation techniques, exercise, counseling, and so forth.
- Causes photosensitivity; use care if administering UV treatments. Advise patient to avoid direct sunlight and use sunscreens and protective clothing.

Patient/Client-Related Instruction

- Advise patient about the likelihood of GI reactions such as nausea, vomiting, diarrhea, abdominal cramps, flatulence, indigestion, loss of appetite, difficulty swallowing, and irritation of the oral mucosa. Instruct patient to report severe or prolonged GI problems, or signs of drug-induced hepatitis such as yellow skin or eyes, abdominal pain, severe nausea and vomiting, fever, sore throat, malaise, weakness, and facial edema.
- Advise patient that rash and other skin reactions (dermatitis, pruritus) are likely. Report severe or unexpected skin reactions to the physician.
- Advise patient to guard against infection (frequent hand washing, etc.) and to avoid crowds and contact with persons with contagious diseases.
- Instruct patient to report other troublesome side effects, including severe or prolonged headache, or eye irritation.

Pharmacokinetics

Absorption: Rapidly absorbed following IM administration.
Distribution: Widely distributed, appears to concentrate in arthritic joints more than in uninvolved joints. Enters breast milk.
Protein Binding: Highly bound to plasma proteins.
Metabolism and Excretion: 60–90% slowly excreted by the kidneys (up to 15 mo); 10–40% excreted in the feces.
Half-life: *Gold*—26 days in blood, 40–128 days in tissue.

TIME/ACTION PROFILE (anti-inflammatory activity)

ROUTE	ONSET	PEAK	DURATION
IM	6–8 wk	unknown	unknown

Contraindications/Precautions

Contraindicated in: Hypersensitivity; Severe hepatic or renal dysfunction; Previous heavy metal toxicity; History of colitis or exfoliative dermatitis; Uncontrolled diabetes; Tuberculosis; CHF; Systemic lupus erythematosus; Recent radiation therapy; Debilitated patients; Pregnancy or lactation.
Use Cautiously in: History of blood dyscrasias; Hypertension; Rashes.

Interactions

Drug-Drug: Bone marrow toxicity may be ↑ with other **myelosuppressive agents (antineoplastic agents, radiation therapy)**. Concurrent use with **penicillamine** ↑ risk of adverse hematologic or renal reactions.

Route/Dosage

IM (Adults): 10 mg initially, then 25 mg 1 wk later, followed by 25–50 mg weekly until improvement or toxicity occurs, up to 1 g total, then 25–50 mg q 2 wk for up to 20 wk, then q 3–4 wk. *History of a previous mild reaction*—Reinstitute with an initial dose of 5 mg, increasing by 5–10 mg weekly or monthly until a dose of 25–50 mg is reached.
IM (Children): 10 mg initially, followed 1 wk later by 1 mg/kg q 2 wk for up to 20 wk, then q 3–4 wk.

Availability (generic available)

Injection: 10 mg/mL, 25 mg/mL, 50 mg/mL.

goserelin (goe-se-rel-lin)

Zoladex

Classification
Therapeutic: antineoplastics, hormones
Pharmacologic: gonadotropin-releasing hormones

Indications

Prostate cancer in patients who cannot tolerate orchiectomy or estrogen therapy (palliative). With flutamide and radiation therapy in the treatment of locally confined stage T2b–T4 (stage B2–C) prostate cancer. Advanced breast cancer in perimenopausal and postmenopausal women (palliative). Endometriosis. Produces thinning of the endometrium before endometrial ablation for dysfunctional uterine bleeding.

Action

Acts as a synthetic form of luteinizing hormone–releasing hormone (LHRH, GnRH). Inhibits the production of gonadotropins by the pituitary gland. Initially, levels of luteinizing hormone (LH), follicle-stimulating hormone (FSH), and testosterone increase. Continued administration leads to decreased production of testosterone and estradiol. **Therapeutic Effects:** Decreased spread of cancer of the prostate or breast. Regression of endometriosis with decreased pain. Thinning of the endometrium.

Adverse Reactions/Side Effects

CNS: headache, anxiety, depression, dizziness, fatigue, insomnia, weakness. **Resp:** dyspnea. **CV:** CEREBROVASCULAR ACCIDENT, MYOCARDIAL INFARCTION, vasodilation, chest pain, hypertension, palpitations. **GI:** anorexia, constipation, diarrhea, nausea, ulcer, vomiting. **GU:** renal insufficiency, urinary obstruction. **Derm:** sweating, rashes. **Endo:** decreased libido, erectile dysfunction, breast swelling, breast tenderness, infertility, ovarian cysts, ovarian hyperstimulation syndrome (with gonadotropins). **F and E:** peripheral edema. **Hemat:** anemia. **Metab:** gout, hyperglycemia, ↑ lipids. **MS:** ↑ bone pain, arthralgia, ↓ bone density. **Misc:** hot flashes, chills, fever, weight gain.

PHYSICAL THERAPY IMPLICATIONS

Examination and Evaluation

- Seek immediate medical assistance if symptoms of MI develop, including sudden chest pain, pain radiating into the arm or jaw, shortness of breath, dizziness, sweating, anxiety, and nausea.
- Seek immediate medical assistance for signs of cerebrovascular accident (stroke), including sudden severe headache, confusion, nausea, vomiting, and increasing neurologic loss (paralysis, numbness, speech problems, visual disturbances).
- Assess blood pressure periodically and compare to normal values (See Appendix F). Report a sustained increase in blood pressure (hypertension) or other cardiopulmonary symptoms (chest pain, palpitations, difficulty breathing).
- Assess any joint or bone pain to rule out musculoskeletal pathology; that is, try to determine if pain is drug induced rather than caused by anatomic or biomechanical problems.
- Assess peripheral edema using girth measurements, volume displacement, and measurement of pitting edema (See Appendix N). Report increased swelling in feet and ankles due to peripheral vasodilation.
- Monitor signs of anemia, including unusual fatigue, shortness of breath with exertion, and bruising, and pale skin. Notify physician immediately if these signs occur.
- Be alert for signs of hyperglycemia, including confusion, drowsiness, flushed/dry skin, fruit-like breath odor, rapid/deep breathing, polyuria, loss of appetite, and unusual thirst. Patients with diabetes mellitus should check blood glucose levels frequently.
- Assess dizziness and weakness that might affect gait, balance, and other functional activities (See Appendix C). Report balance problems and functional limitations to the physician and nursing staff, and caution the patient and family/caregivers to guard against falls and trauma.
- Monitor personality or behavioral changes, including anxiety, depression, sleep loss, or other changes in mood. Notify physician if these changes become problematic.

Interventions

- For patients who are medically able to begin exercise, implement appropriate resistive exercises and aerobic training to maintain muscle strength and aerobic capacity during cancer chemotherapy or to help restore function after chemotherapy.
- Because of the risk of heart attack and stroke, use extreme caution during aerobic exercise and other forms of therapeutic exercise. Assess exercise tolerance frequently (blood pressure, heart rate, respiratory function, fatigue levels), and terminate exercise immediately if any untoward responses occur (See Appendix L).

Patient/Client-Related Instruction

- Advise patient and family or caregiver about the signs of MI and stroke (see above under Examination and Evaluation), and to seek immediate medical assistance if these signs develop.
- Instruct patient to report signs of kidney dysfunction or problems with urination, including cloudy urine, decreased urine output, or inability to empty the bladder completely.
- Advise patient about the likelihood of GI reactions (nausea, vomiting, diarrhea, constipation, loss of appetite). Instruct patient to report severe or prolonged GI reactions, or signs of gastric ulcer (burning pain in the abdomen, indigestion, vomiting blood).
- Advise patient that skin reactions (rash, increased sweating) are likely. Report severe or unexpected skin reactions to the physician.

- Instruct patient or family/caregivers to report other troublesome side effects such as severe or prolonged headache, gout, hot flashes, chills, erectile dysfunction, decreased libido, or breast swelling and tenderness.

Pharmacokinetics

Absorption: Well absorbed from SC implant. Absorption is slower in first 8 days, then is faster and continuous for remainder of 28-day dosing cycle.
Distribution: Unknown.
Metabolism and Excretion: Some metabolism by the liver (<10%), some excretion by kidneys (>90%, only 20% as unchanged drug).
Half-life: 4.2 hr.

TIME/ACTION PROFILE (decrease in serum testosterone levels)

ROUTE	ONSET	PEAK	DURATION
SC	unknown	2–4 wk	length of therapy

Contraindications/Precautions

Contraindicated in: Hypersensitivity; Undiagnosed vaginal bleeding; Pregnancy or lactation.
Use Cautiously in: Lactation or children <18 yr (safety not established).

Interactions

Drug-Drug: None significant.

Route/Dosage

SC (Adults): 3.6 mg q 4 wk or 10.8 mg q 12 wk.
Endometrial thinning—1 or 2 depots given 4 wk apart; if 1 depot used, surgery is performed at 4 wk; if 2 depots used, surgery is performed 2–4 wk after 2nd depot.

Availability

Implant: 3.6 mg, 10.8 mg.

granisetron (gra-nees-e-tron)

Kytril

granisetron (transdermal) (gra-nees-e-tron)

Sancuso

Classification
Therapeutic: antiemetics
Pharmacologic: 5-HT3 antagonists

Indications

Prevention of nausea and vomiting due to: emetogenic chemotherapy, radiation therapy. Prevention and treatment of postoperative nausea and vomiting.

Action

Blocks the effects of serotonin at receptor sites (selective antagonist) located in vagal nerve terminals and in the chemoreceptor trigger zone in the CNS. **Therapeutic Effects:** Decreased incidence and severity of nausea and vomiting following emetogenic chemotherapy, radiation therapy, or surgery.

Adverse Reactions/Side Effects

CNS: headache, agitation, anxiety, CNS stimulation, drowsiness, weakness. **CV:** hypertension. **GI:** constipation, diarrhea, elevated liver enzymes, taste disorder. **Derm:** application-site reactions, photosensitivity. **Misc:** anaphylactoid reactions, fever.

PHYSICAL THERAPY IMPLICATIONS

Examination and Evaluation

- Monitor improvements in GI symptoms (decreased nausea and vomiting, increased appetite) to help document whether drug therapy is successful.
- Monitor signs of allergic and anaphylactoid reactions, including pulmonary symptoms (tightness in the throat and chest, wheezing, cough, dyspnea) or skin reactions (rash, pruritus, urticaria). Notify physician or nursing staff immediately if these reactions occur.
- Assess blood pressure (BP) and compare to normal values (See Appendix F). Report a sustained increase in BP (hypertension).
- Monitor personality changes, including agitation, anxiety, or other signs of CNS excitation. Notify physician if these changes become problematic.
- If applied transdermally, monitor the application site for local irritation or inflammation. Report excessive application-site reactions to the physician.

Patient/Client-Related Instruction

- Instruct patient to report bothersome side effects such as severe or prolonged headache, drowsiness, weakness, fever, or GI problems (diarrhea, constipation, abnormal taste).

Pharmacokinetics

Absorption: 50% absorbed following oral administration.
Distribution: Distributes into erythrocytes; remainder of distribution is unknown.

Metabolism and Excretion: Mostly metabolized by the liver; 12% excreted unchanged in urine.
Half-life: *Patients with cancer*—8–9 hr (range 0.9–31.1 hr); *healthy volunteers* —4.9 hr (range 0.9–15.2 hr); *geriatric patients*—7.7 hr (range 2.6–17.7 hr).

TIME/ACTION PROFILE

ROUTE	ONSET	PEAK	DURATION
PO	rapid	60 min	24 hr
IV	rapid	30 min	up to 24 hr
TD	unknown	48 hr	unknown

Contraindications/Precautions

Contraindicated in: Hypersensitivity; Some products contain benzyl alcohol; avoid use in neonates.
Use Cautiously in: OB/Lactation: Safety not established; Pedi: Children <2 yr (safe use of IV route not established); Pedi: Children <18 yr (safe use of PO route not established).

Interactions

Drug-Drug: ↑ risk of extrapyramidal reactions with other **agents causing extrapyramidal reactions**.

Route/Dosage

Prevention of Nausea and Vomiting Due to Emetogenic Chemotherapy

PO (Adults): 1 mg twice daily; 1st dose given at least 60 min prior to chemotherapy and 2nd dose 12 hr later only on days when chemotherapy is administered; may also be given as 2 mg once daily at least 60 min prior to chemotherapy.
IV (Adults and Children 2–16 yr): 10 mcg/kg within 30 min prior to chemotherapy.
TD (Adults): One 34.3 mg patch (delivers 3.1 mg/24 hr) applied up to 48 hr prior to chemotherapy, leave in place for at least 24 hr following chemotherapy, may be left in place for a total of 7 days.

Prevention of Nausea and Vomiting Associated with Radiation Therapy

PO (Adults): 2 mg taken once daily within 1 hr of radiation therapy.

Prevention and Treatment of Postoperative Nausea and Vomiting

IV (Adults): *Prevention*—1 mg prior to induction of anesthesia or just prior to reversal of anesthesia; *Treatment*—1 mg.

Availability (generic available)

Tablets: 1 mg. **Oral solution (orange flavor):** 2 mg/10 mL in 30-mL bottles. **Solution for injection:** 1 mg/mL. **Transdermal system (patch):** Each patch contains 34.3 mg/52 cm² (delivers 3.1 mg/24 hr).

guaifenesin (gwye-**fen**-e-sin)

Alfen Jr, Altarussin, Benylin-E, Breonesin, Calmylin Expectorant, Diabetic Tussin, Ganidin NR, Guiatuss, Hytuss, Hytuss-2X, Mucinex, Naldecon Senior EX, Organidin NR, Resyl, Robitussin, Scot-tussin Expectorant, Siltussin SA, Siltussin DAS

Classification
Therapeutic: allergy, cold, and cough remedies, expectorant

Indications

Coughs associated with viral upper respiratory tract infections.

Action

Reduces viscosity of tenacious secretions by increasing respiratory tract fluid. **Therapeutic Effects:** Mobilization and subsequent expectoration of mucus.

Adverse Reactions/Side Effects

CNS: dizziness, headache. **GI:** nausea, diarrhea, stomach pain, vomiting. **Derm:** rashes, urticaria.

PHYSICAL THERAPY IMPLICATIONS

Examination and Evaluation

- Assess the quantity and consistency of sputum to help document whether this drug is successful in reducing the viscosity of respiratory secretions.
- Assess dizziness that might affect gait, balance, and other functional activities (See Appendix C). Report balance problems and functional limitations to the physician, and caution the patient and family/caregivers to guard against falls and trauma.

Interventions

- When implementing airway clearance techniques or other pulmonary interventions, attempt to intervene when the drug has produced expectorant effects. Effects typically begin 30 min after oral administration.
- Design and implement breathing exercises to maximize ventilation and help prevent infections caused by pulmonary congestion.

Patient/Client-Related Instruction

- Instruct patient and family/caregivers to report other troublesome side effects such as severe or prolonged headache, skin reactions (rash, welts), or GI problems (diarrhea, nausea, vomiting, stomach pain).

Pharmacokinetics

Absorption: Well absorbed after oral administration.
Distribution: Unknown.
Metabolism and Excretion: Renally excreted as metabolites.
Half-life: Unknown.

TIME/ACTION PROFILE (expectorant action)

ROUTE	ONSET	PEAK	DURATION
PO	30 min	unknown	4–6 hr
PO-ER	unknown	unknown	12 hr

Contraindications/Precautions

Contraindicated in: Hypersensitivity; Some products contain alcohol and should be avoided in patients with known intolerance; Some products contain aspartame and should be avoided in patients with phenylketonuria.
Use Cautiously in: Cough lasting >1 wk or accompanied by fever, rash, or headache; Pregnancy (although safety has not been established, guaifenesin has been used without adverse effects); Patients receiving disulfiram (liquid products may contain alcohol); Diabetic patients (some products may contain sugar); Children (check age limitations on specific dose forms).

Interactions

Drug-Drug: None significant.

Route/Dosage

PO (Adults): 200–400 mg q 4 hr or 600–1200 mg q 12 hr as extended-release product (not to exceed 2400 mg/day).
PO (Children 6–12 yr): 100–200 mg q 4 hr or 600 mg q 12 hr as extended-release product (not to exceed 1200 mg/day).
PO (Children 2–6 yr): 50–100 mg q 4 hr (not to exceed 600 mg/day).

Availability (generic available)

Syrup: 100 mg/5 mL OTC. **Oral solution:** 100 mg/5 mL Rx, OTC, 200 mg/5 mL OTC. **Capsules:** 200 mg OTC. **Tablets:** 100 mg OTC, 200 mg Rx, OTC, 1200 mg. **Extended-release tablets (Mucinex):** 600 mg, 1200 mg. ***In combination with:*** analgesics/antipyretics, antihistamines, decongestants, and cough suppressants Rx, OTC.

guanfacine (gwahn-fa-seen)

Tenex

Classification
Therapeutic: antihypertensives
Pharmacologic: centrally acting antiadrenergics

Indications

Hypertension (with thiazide-type diuretics).

Action

Stimulates CNS $alpha_2$-adrenergic receptors, producing a decrease in sympathetic outflow to heart, kidneys, and blood vessels. Result is decreased blood pressure and peripheral resistance, a slight decrease in heart rate, and no change in cardiac output. **Therapeutic Effects:** Lowering of blood pressure.

Adverse Reactions/Side Effects

CNS: drowsiness, weakness, depression, dizziness, fatigue, headache, insomnia. **EENT:** tinnitus. **Resp:** dyspnea. **CV:** bradycardia, chest pain, palpitations, rebound hypertension. **GI:** constipation, dry mouth, abdominal pain, nausea. **GU:** erectile dysfunction.

PHYSICAL THERAPY IMPLICATIONS

Examination and Evaluation

- Assess blood pressure (BP) periodically and compare to normal values (See Appendix F). Document whether drug therapy is successful in controlling hypertension.
- Assess heart rate, ECG, and heart sounds, especially during exercise (See Appendices G, H). Report an unusually slow heart rate (bradycardia) or signs of other arrhythmias, including palpitations, chest discomfort, shortness of breath, fainting, and fatigue/weakness.
- Assess dizziness and weakness that might affect gait, balance, and other functional activities (See Appendix C). Report balance problems and functional limitations to the physician, and caution the patient and family/caregivers to guard against falls and trauma.
- Be alert for signs of depression or other changes in mood and behavior. Notify physician if these changes become problematic.
- Be alert for a rapid increase in BP if guanfacine is suddenly discontinued (rebound hypertension). Report this increase to the physician immediately.

Interventions

- Because of the risk of arrhythmias and abnormal BP responses, use caution during aerobic exercise and other forms of therapeutic exercise. Assess exercise tolerance frequently (BP, heart rate, fatigue levels), and terminate exercise immediately if any untoward responses occur (See Appendix L).

- Avoid physical therapy interventions that cause systemic vasodilation (large whirlpool, Hubbard tank). Additive effects of this drug and the intervention may cause a dangerous fall in BP.
- To minimize orthostatic hypotension, advise patient to move slowly when assuming a more upright position.

Patient/Client-Related Instruction

- Remind patients to take medication as directed to control hypertension even if they are asymptomatic.
- Counsel patients about additional interventions to help control BP, such as regular exercise, weight loss, sodium restriction, stress reduction, moderation of alcohol consumption, and smoking cessation.
- Instruct patient or family/caregivers to report other bothersome side effects such as severe or prolonged headache, fatigue, drowsiness, sleep loss, ringing/buzzing in the ears (tinnitus), difficult/labored breathing, sexual dysfunction, skin reactions (rash, excessive sweating), or GI problems (constipation, nausea, abdominal pain, dry mouth).

Pharmacokinetics

Absorption: Well absorbed (80%) following oral administration.
Distribution: Appears to be widely distributed.
Metabolism and Excretion: 50% metabolized by the liver, 50% excreted unchanged by the kidneys.
Half-life: 17 hr.

TIME/ACTION PROFILE (antihypertensive effect)

ROUTE	ONSET	PEAK	DURATION
PO (single dose)	unknown	8–12 hr	24 hr
PO (multiple doses)	within 1 wk	1–3 mo	unknown

Contraindications/Precautions

Contraindicated in: Hypersensitivity.
Use Cautiously in: Severe coronary artery disease or recent myocardial infarction; Geriatric patients (↑ sensitivity, ↓ hepatic/cardiac/renal function); Cerebrovascular disease; Severe renal or liver disease; Pregnancy, lactation, or children <12 yr (safety not established).

Interactions

Drug-Drug: ↑ hypotension with other **antihypertensives, nitrates**, and acute ingestion of **alcohol**. ↑ CNS depression may occur with other **CNS depressants**, including **alcohol, antihistamines, opioid analgesics, tricyclic antidepressants**, and **sedative/hypnotics. NSAIDs** may ↓ effectiveness. **Adrenergics** may ↓ effectiveness.

Route/Dosage

PO (Adults): 1 mg daily given at bedtime, may be increased if necessary at 3- to 4-wk intervals up to 2 mg/day; may also be given in 2 divided doses.

Availability (generic available)

Tablets: 1 mg, 2 mg.

halcinonide (hal-sin-oh-nide)

Halog

Classification

Therapeutic: anti-inflammatories (steroidal)
Pharmacologic: corticosteroids

Indications

Management of inflammation and pruritus associated with various allergic and immunologic skin problems.

Action

Suppresses normal immune response and inflammation. **Therapeutic Effects:** Suppression of dermatologic inflammation and immune processes.

Adverse Reactions/Side Effects

Derm: allergic contact dermatitis, atrophy, burning, dryness, edema, folliculitis, hypersensitivity reactions, hypertrichosis, hypopigmentation, irritation, maceration, miliaria, perioral dermatitis, secondary infection, striae. **Misc:** adrenal suppression (use of occlusive dressings, long-term therapy).

PHYSICAL THERAPY IMPLICATIONS

Examination and Evaluation

- Assess the area being treated to help document whether drug therapy is successful in resolving skin conditions.
- Monitor any new or increased reactions at the site of application, including inflammation, irritation, infection, burning, swelling, exfoliation, and rash. Report severe or prolonged skin reactions to the physician.
- Report signs of adrenal suppression, including hypotension, weight loss, weakness, nausea, vomiting, anorexia, lethargy, confusion, and restlessness.

Interventions

- Protect skin from breakdown, especially over bony prominences.

Patient/Client-Related Instruction

- Advise patients on long-term treatment to consult physician before stopping this medication. Stopping the medication suddenly may result in adrenocortical shock (severe hypotension, hypoglycemia, weakness, vomiting). If these signs appear, notify physician immediately; may be life threatening.
- Check that the patient and family or caregivers understand topical application procedures, and adhere to the recommended dosing schedule.

Pharmacokinetics

Absorption: Minimal. Prolonged use on large surface areas or large amounts applied or use of occlusive dressings may increase systemic absorption.
Distribution: Remains primarily at site of action.
Metabolism and Excretion: Usually metabolized in skin.
Half-life: Unknown.

TIME/ACTION PROFILE (response depends on condition being treated)

ROUTE	ONSET	PEAK	DURATION
Topical	mins–hrs	hrs–days	hrs–days

Contraindications/Precautions

Contraindicated in: Hypersensitivity or known intolerance to corticosteroids or components of vehicles (ointment or cream base, preservative, alcohol); Untreated bacterial or viral infections.
Use Cautiously in: Hepatic dysfunction; Diabetes mellitus, cataracts, glaucoma, or tuberculosis (use of large amounts of high-potency agents may worsen condition); Patients with preexisting skin atrophy; Pregnancy, lactation, or children (chronic high-dose usage may result in adrenal suppression in mother and growth suppression in children; children may be more susceptible to adrenal and growth suppression).

Interactions

Drug-Drug: None significant.

Route/Dosage

Topical (Adults): Apply to affected area(s) 1–3 times daily (depends on product, preparation, and condition being treated).
Topical (Children): Apply to affected area(s) once daily.

Availability

Cream: 0.025% Rx, 0.1% Rx. **Ointment:** 0.1% Rx.

halobetasol (hal-oh-bay-ta-sol)

Ultravate

Classification

Therapeutic: anti-inflammatories (steroidal)
Pharmacologic: corticosteroids

Indications

Management of inflammation and pruritus associated with various allergic/immunologic skin problems.

Action
Suppresses normal immune response and inflammation. **Therapeutic Effects:** Suppression of dermatologic inflammation and immune processes.

Adverse Reactions/Side Effects
Derm: allergic contact dermatitis, atrophy, burning, dryness, edema, folliculitis, hypersensitivity reactions, hypertrichosis, hypopigmentation, irritation, maceration, miliaria, perioral dermatitis, secondary infection, striae. **Misc:** adrenal suppression (use of occlusive dressings, long-term therapy).

PHYSICAL THERAPY IMPLICATIONS

Examination and Evaluation
- Assess the area being treated to help document whether drug therapy is successful in resolving skin conditions.
- Monitor any new or increased reactions at the site of application, including inflammation, irritation, infection, burning, swelling, exfoliation, and rash. Report severe or prolonged skin reactions to the physician.
- Report signs of adrenal suppression, including hypotension, weight loss, weakness, nausea, vomiting, anorexia, lethargy, confusion, and restlessness.

Interventions
- Protect skin from breakdown, especially over bony prominences.

Patient/Client-Related Instruction
- Advise patients on long-term treatment to consult physician before stopping this medication. Stopping the medication suddenly may result in adrenocortical shock (severe hypotension, hypoglycemia, weakness, vomiting). If these signs appear, notify physician immediately; may be life threatening.
- Check that the patient and family or caregivers understand topical application procedures and adhere to the recommended dosing schedule.

Pharmacokinetics
Absorption: Minimal. Prolonged use on large surface areas or large amounts applied or use of occlusive dressings may increase systemic absorption.
Distribution: Remains primarily at site of action.
Metabolism and Excretion: Usually metabolized in skin.
Half-life: Unknown.

TIME/ACTION PROFILE (response depends on condition being treated)

ROUTE	ONSET	PEAK	DURATION
Topical	mins–hrs	hrs–days	hrs–days

Contraindications/Precautions
Contraindicated in: Hypersensitivity or known intolerance to corticosteroids or components of vehicles (ointment or cream base, preservative, alcohol); Untreated bacterial or viral infections.
Use Cautiously in: Hepatic dysfunction; Diabetes mellitus, cataracts, glaucoma, or tuberculosis (use of large amounts of high-potency agents may worsen condition); Patients with preexisting skin atrophy; Pregnancy, lactation, or children (chronic high-dose usage may result in adrenal suppression in mother, growth suppression in children; children may be more susceptible to adrenal and growth suppression).

Interactions
Drug-Drug: None significant.

Route/Dosage
Topical (Adults): Apply to affected area(s) 1–2 times daily.

Availability
Cream: 0.05% Rx. **Ointment:** 0.05% Rx.

haloperidol (ha-loe-**per**-i-dole)
Apo-Haloperidol, Haldol, Haldol Decanoate, Haldol LA, Novo-Peridol, Peridol, PMS Haloperidol

Classification
Therapeutic: antipsychotics
Pharmacologic: butyrophenones

Indications
Acute and chronic psychotic disorders, including schizophrenia, manic states, drug-induced psychoses. Schizophrenic patients who require long-term parenteral (IM) antipsychotic therapy. Also useful in managing aggressive or agitated patients. Tourette's syndrome. Severe behavioral problems in children which may be accompanied by unprovoked, combative, explosive hyperexcitability, hyperactivity accompanied by conduct disorders (short-term use when other modalities have failed). Considered second-line treatment after failure with atypical antipsychotic. **Unlabeled Use:** Nausea and vomiting from surgery or chemotherapy.

Action
Alters the effects of dopamine in the CNS. Also has anticholinergic and alpha-adrenergic blocking activity. **Therapeutic Effects:** Diminished signs and symptoms of psychoses. Improved behavior in children with Tourette's syndrome or other behavioral problems.

Adverse Reactions/Side Effects

CNS: SEIZURES, extrapyramidal reactions, confusion, drowsiness, restlessness, tardive dyskinesia. **EENT:** blurred vision, dry eyes. **Resp:** respiratory depression. **CV:** hypotension, tachycardia. **GI:** constipation, dry mouth, anorexia, drug-induced hepatitis, ileus, weight gain. **GU:** urinary retention. **Derm:** diaphoresis, photosensitivity, rashes. **Endo:** galactorrhea, amenorrhea. **Hemat:** anemia, leukopenia. **Metab:** hyperpyrexia. **Misc:** NEUROLEPTIC MALIGNANT SYNDROME, hypersensitivity reactions.

PHYSICAL THERAPY IMPLICATIONS

Examination and Evaluation

- Be alert for new seizures or increased seizure activity, especially at the onset of drug treatment. Document the number, duration, and severity of seizures, and report these findings immediately to the physician.
- Monitor and report signs of neuroleptic malignant syndrome (hyperthermia, diaphoresis, generalized muscle rigidity, altered mental status, tachycardia, changes in blood pressure [BP], incontinence). Symptoms typically occur within 4–14 days after initiation of drug therapy, but can occur at any time during drug use.
- Assess motor function, and be alert for extrapyramidal symptoms. Report these symptoms immediately, especially tardive dyskinesia, because this problem may be irreversible. Common extrapyramidal symptoms include:
  - Tardive dyskinesia (uncontrolled rhythmic movement of mouth, face, and extremities, lip smacking or puckering, puffing of cheeks, uncontrolled chewing, rapid or worm-like movements of tongue).
  - Pseudoparkinsonism (shuffling gait, rigidity, tremor, pill-rolling motion, loss of balance control, difficulty speaking or swallowing, mask-like face).
  - Akathisia (restlessness or desire to keep moving).
  - Other dystonias and dyskinesias (dystonic muscle spasms, twisting motions, twitching, inability to move eyes, weakness of arms or legs).
- Monitor signs of hypersensitivity reactions, including pulmonary symptoms (laryngeal edema, wheezing, dyspnea) or skin reactions (rash, pruritus, urticaria). Notify physician or nursing staff immediately if these reactions occur.
- Assess BP periodically, and compare to normal values (See Appendix F). Report low BP (hypotension), especially if patient experiences dizziness or syncope.
- Assess heart rate, ECG, and heart sounds, especially during exercise (see Appendixes G, H). Report a rapid heart rate (tachycardia) or signs of other arrhythmias, including palpitations, chest discomfort, shortness of breath, fainting, and fatigue/weakness.
- Assess symptoms of respiratory depression (dyspnea, cyanosis). Monitor pulse oximetry and perform pulmonary function tests (See Appendix I) to quantify suspected changes in ventilation and respiratory function. Excessive respiratory depression requires emergency care.
- Watch for report signs of leukopenia (fever, sore throat, mucosal lesions, signs of infection) or unusual weakness and fatigue that might be due to anemia. Report these signs to the physician or nursing staff.
- If used to control nausea and vomiting, monitor the frequency, severity, and duration of GI problems to help document drug effectiveness.
- If used to control behavioral problems in children, document any changes in combative or hyperactive behavior to help determine drug efficacy and appropriate dosing.
- Periodically assess body weight and other anthropometric measures (body mass index, body composition). Report a substantial weight gain or increased body fat.

Interventions

- Guard against falls and trauma (hip fractures, head injury, and so forth) caused by drowsiness, blurred vision, or extrapyramidal symptoms; implement fall prevention strategies (See Appendix E).
- Because of the risk of tachycardia and abnormal BP responses, use caution during aerobic exercise and other forms of therapeutic exercise. Assess exercise tolerance frequently (BP, heart rate, fatigue levels), and terminate exercise immediately if any untoward responses occur (See Appendix L).
- To minimize orthostatic hypotension, patient should move slowly when assuming a more upright position.
- This drug impairs body temperature regulation; use care during exercise and during other activities that increase body temperature (hot whirlpools, saunas, and so forth).
- Help patient and family/caregivers explore non-pharmacologic methods (exercise, counseling, support groups, and so forth) to reduce schizophrenic episodes and behavioral problems.
- Causes photosensitivity; use care if administering UV treatments. Advise patient to avoid direct sunlight and use sunscreens and protective clothing.

Patient/Client-Related Instruction

- Advise patient to avoid alcohol and other CNS depressants because of the increased risk of sedation and adverse effects.
- Advise patient about the likelihood of GI problems such as dry mouth, loss of appetite, and constipation. Instruct patient to report severe of prolonged GI problems, or signs of drug-induced hepatitis, including anorexia, abdominal pain, severe nausea and vomiting, yellow skin or eyes, skin rashes, flu-like symptoms, and muscle/joint pain.
- Instruct patient to report other problematic side effects such as severe or prolonged dry eyes, blurred vision, urinary retention, menstrual irregularities, nipple discharge, fever, or increased sweating.

Pharmacokinetics

Absorption: Well absorbed following PO/IM administration. Decanoate salt is slowly absorbed and has a long duration of action.
Distribution: Concentrates in liver. Crosses placenta; enters breast milk.
Protein Binding: 90%.
Metabolism and Excretion: Mostly metabolized by the liver.
Half-life: 21–24 hr.

TIME/ACTION PROFILE (antipsychotic activity)

ROUTE	ONSET	PEAK	DURATION
PO	2 hr	2–6 hr	8–12 hr
IM	20–30 min	30–45 min	4–8 hr*
IM (decanoate)	3–9 days	unknown	1 mo

*Effect may persist for several days.

Contraindications/Precautions

Contraindicated in: Hypersensitivity; Angle-closure glaucoma; Bone marrow depression; CNS depression; Severe liver or cardiovascular disease (Q-T interval prolonging conditions); Some products contain tartrazine, sesame oil, or benzyl alcohol and should be avoided in patients with known intolerance or hypersensitivity.
Use Cautiously in: Debilitated patients (dose reduction required); Cardiac disease; Diabetes; Respiratory insufficiency; Prostatic hyperplasia; CNS tumors; Intestinal obstruction; Seizures ; OB: Safety not established; Lactation: Discontinue drug or bottle-feed; Geri: Dose reduction required due to increased sensitivity; ↑ risk of mortality in elderly patients treated for dementia-related psychosis.

Interactions

Drug-Drug: ↑ hypotension with **antihypertensives, nitrates**, or acute ingestion of **alcohol**. ↑ anticholinergic effects with **drugs having anticholinergic properties**, including **antihistamines, antidepressants, atropine, phenothiazines, quinidine**, and **disopyramide**. ↑ CNS depression with other **CNS depressants**, including **alcohol, antihistamines, opioid analgesics**, and **sedative/hypnotics**. Concurrent use with **epinephrine** may result in severe hypotension and tachycardia. May ↓ therapeutic effects of **levodopa**. Acute encephalopathic syndrome may occur when used with **lithium**. Dementia may occur with **methyldopa**.
Drug-Natural: Kava, valerian, or **chamomile** can ↑ CNS depression.

Route/Dosage

Haloperidol

PO (Adults): 0.5–5 mg 2–3 times daily. Patients with severe symptoms may require up to 100 mg/day.
PO (Geriatric Patients or Debilitated Patients): 0.5–2 mg twice daily initially; may be gradually increased as needed.
PO (Children 3–12 yr or 15–40 kg): 50 mcg/kg/day in 2–3 divided doses; may increase by 500 mcg (0.5 mg)/day q 5–7 days as needed (up to 75 mcg/kg/day for nonpsychotic disorders or Tourette's syndrome or 150 mcg/kg/day for psychoses).
IM (Adults): 2–5 mg q 1–8 hr (not to exceed 100 mg/day).
IV (Adults): 0.5–5 mg, may be repeated q 30 min (unlabeled).

Haloperidol Decanoate

IM (Adults): 10–15 times the previous daily PO dose but not to exceed 100 mg initially, given monthly (not to exceed 300 mg/mo).

Availability (generic available)

Tablets: 0.5 mg, 1 mg, 2 mg, 5 mg, 10 mg, 20 mg. **Oral concentrate:** 2 mg/mL. **Haloperidol injection:** 5 mg/mL. **Haloperidol decanoate injection:** 50 mg/mL, 100 mg/mL.

HIGH ALERT

heparin (hep-a-rin)

Calcilean, Calciparine, Hepalean, Heparin Leo, Hep-Lock, Hep-Lock U/P

Classification

Therapeutic: anticoagulants
Pharmacologic: antithrombotics

Indications

Prophylaxis and treatment of various thromboembolic disorders, including Venous thromboembolism, pulmonary emboli, atrial fibrillation with embolization, acute and chronic consumptive coagulopathies, peripheral arterial thromboembolism. Used in very low doses (10–100 units) to maintain patency of IV catheters (heparin flush).

Action

Potentiates the inhibitory effect of antithrombin on factor Xa and thrombin. In low doses, prevents the conversion of prothrombin to thrombin by its effects on factor Xa. Higher doses neutralize thrombin, preventing the conversion of fibrinogen to fibrin. **Therapeutic Effects:** Prevention of thrombus formation. Prevention of extension of existing thrombi (full dose).

Adverse Reactions/Side Effects

GI: drug-induced hepatitis. **Derm:** alopecia (long-term use), rashes, urticaria. **Hemat:** BLEEDING, anemia, thrombocytopenia (can occur up to several weeks after discontinuation of therapy). **Local:** pain at injection site. **MS:** osteoporosis (long-term use). **Misc:** fever, hypersensitivity.

PHYSICAL THERAPY IMPLICATIONS

Examination and Evaluation

- Monitor symptoms of deep vein thrombosis (DVT) (pain, swelling, warmth, redness) to determine if drug therapy is effective in preventing or reducing venous thrombosis. Request or administer objective tests (Doppler ultrasound) if symptoms increase.
- In patients with DVT, watch for signs of pulmonary embolism, such as shortness of breath, chest pain, cough, and bloody sputum. Notify physician or nursing staff immediately if these signs occur.
- Assess for signs of bleeding and hemorrhage, including bleeding gums, nosebleeds, unusual bruising, black/tarry stools, hematuria, and fall in hematocrit or blood pressure. Notify physician or nursing staff immediately if heparin causes excessive anticoagulation.
- Monitor signs of allergic reactions and anaphylaxis, including pulmonary symptoms (tightness in the throat and chest, wheezing, cough, dyspnea) or skin reactions (rash, pruritus, urticaria). Notify physician or nursing staff immediately if these reactions occur.
- Be alert for acute arterial or venous thrombosis caused by heparin-induced thrombocytopenia (HIT). In certain patients, heparin initiates an immune reaction where antibodies attack circulating platelets. Although most cases of HIT are minor and asymptomatic, some patients may experience life- or limb-threatening platelet clots, resulting in myocardial infarction, ischemic stroke, acute leg ischemia, or venous thromboembolism. HIT can occur during and up to several weeks after heparin therapy. Any signs of increased clotting should be reported immediately.
- Watch for unusual weakness and fatigue that might be due to anemia. Report these signs to the physician or nursing staff.
- Monitor and report signs of drug-induced hepatitis, including anorexia, abdominal pain, severe nausea and vomiting, yellow skin or eyes, skin rashes, flu-like symptoms, and muscle/joint pain.
- Assess injection site for pain, swelling, and irritation. Report prolonged or excessive injection-site reactions to the physician or nursing staff.

Interventions

- Use caution with any physical interventions that could increase bleeding, including wound débridement, chest percussion, joint mobilization, and application of local heat.
- Recommend or implement other physical methods to decrease DVT and prevent thromboembolism, including graduated compression stockings and intermittent pneumatic compression pumps.
- Implement early mobilization and ambulation to reduce the risk of new or increased DVT. Early ambulation appears to be safe in patients with DVT if the patient is adequately heparinized (INR values in acceptable range), does not have an active pulmonary embolism, or have other risk factors that contraindicate ambulation.
- Institute weight-bearing and resistance exercises during long-term heparin use to maintain or increase bone mineral density and prevent osteoporosis.

Patient/Client-Related Instruction

- Instruct patient immediately to report signs of GI bleeding, including abdominal pain, vomiting blood, blood in stools, or black, tarry stools.

Pharmacokinetics

Absorption: Erratically absorbed following SC or IM administration.

Distribution: Does not cross the placenta or enter breast milk.

Protein Binding: Very high (to low-density lipoproteins, globulins, and fibrinogen).

Metabolism and Excretion: Probably removed by the reticuloendothelial system (lymph nodes, spleen).

Half-life: 1–2 hr (increases with increasing dose); affected by obesity, renal and hepatic function, malignancy, presence of pulmonary embolism, and infections.

TIME/ACTION PROFILE (anticoagulant effect)

ROUTE	ONSET	PEAK	DURATION
Heparin SC	20–60 min	2 hr	8–12 hr
Heparin IV	immediate	5–10 min	2–6 hr

Contraindications/Precautions

Contraindicated in: Hypersensitivity; Uncontrolled bleeding; Severe thrombocytopenia; Open wounds (full dose); Products containing benzyl alcohol should not be used in premature infants.

Use Cautiously in: Severe liver or kidney disease; Retinopathy (hypertensive or diabetic); Untreated hypertension; Ulcer disease; Spinal cord or brain injury; History of congenital or acquired bleeding disorder; Malignancy; OB: May be used during pregnancy, but use with caution during the last trimester and in the immediate postpartum period; Geri: Women >60 yr have increased risk of bleeding.

Exercise Extreme Caution in: Severe uncontrolled hypertension; Bacterial endocarditis, bleeding disorders; GI bleeding/ulceration/pathology; Hemorrhagic stroke; Recent CNS or ophthalmologic surgery; Active GI bleeding/ulceration; History of thrombocytopenia related to heparin.

Interactions

Heparin is frequently used concurrently or sequentially with other agents affecting coagulation. The risk of potentially serious interactions is greatest with full anticoagulation.

Drug-Drug: Risk of bleeding may be ↑ by concurrent use of **drugs that affect platelet function**, including **aspirin, NSAIDs, clopidogrel, dipyridamole, some penicillins, ticlopidine, abciximab, eptifibatide, tirofiban**, and **dextran**. Risk of bleeding may be ↑ by concurrent use of **drugs that cause hypoprothrombinemia**, including **quinidine, cefoperazone, cefotetan**, and **valproic acid**. Concurrent use of **thrombolytics** ↑ risk of bleeding. Heparins affect the prothrombin time used in assessing the response to **warfarin. Digoxin, tetracyclines, nicotine**, and **antihistamines** may ↓ anticoagulant effect of heparin. **Streptokinase** may be followed by relative resistance to heparin.

Drug-Natural: ↑ risk of bleeding with **arnica, anise, chamomile, clove, dong quai, fever few, garlic, ginger**, and ***Panax ginseng***.

Route/Dosage

Therapeutic Anticoagulation

IV (Adults): *Intermittent bolus*—10,000 units, followed by 5000–10,000 units q 4–6 hr. *Continuous infusion*—5000 units (35–70 units/kg), followed by 20,000–40,000 units infused over 24 hr (approx. 1000 units/hr or 15–18 units/kg/hr).

IV (Children >1 yr): *Intermittent bolus*—50–100 units/kg, followed by 50–100 units/kg q 4 hr. *Continuous infusion*—Loading dose 75 units/kg, followed by 20 units/kg/hr, adjust to maintain aPTT of 60–85 sec.

IV (Neonates and Infants <1 yr): *Continuous infusion*—Loading dose 75 units/kg, followed by 28 units/kg/hr, adjust to maintain a PTT of 60–85 sec.

Subcut (Adults): 5000 units IV, followed by initial SC dose of 10,000–20,000 units, then 8000–10,000 units q 8 hr or 15,000–20,000 units q 12 hr.

Prophylaxis of Thromboembolism

SC (Adults): 5000 units q 8–12 hr (may be started 2 hr prior to surgery).

Cardiovascular Surgery

IV (Adults): At least 150 units/kg (300 units/kg if procedure <60 min; 400 units/kg if > 60 min).

IA (Neonates, Infants, and Children): 100–150 units/kg via an artery prior to cardiac catheterization.

Line Flushing

IV (Adults and Children): 10–100 units/mL (10 units/mL for infants <10 kg, 100 units/mL for all others) solution to fill heparin lock set to needle hub; replace after each use.

Total Parenteral Nutrition

IV (Adults and Children): 05–1 units/mL (final solution concentration) to maintain line patency.

Arterial Line Patency

IA (Neonates): 0.5–2 units/mL.

Availability (generic available)

Heparin Sodium

Solution for injection: 10 units/mL, 100 units/mL, 1000 units/mL, 5000 units/mL, 7500 units/mL, 10,000 units/mL, 20,000 units/mL, 40,000 units/mL.
Premixed solution: 1000 units/500 mL, 2000 units/1000 mL, 12,500 units/250 mL, 25,000 units in 250 and 500 mL.

histrelin (his-tre-lin)

Vantas

Classification

Therapeutic: hormones
Pharmacologic: gonadotropin-releasing hormones

Indications

Palliative treatment of advanced prostate cancer.

Action

Continuous administration decreases production of gonadotropins. **Therapeutic Effects:** Suppression of testosterone production. Prevention of disease progression.

Adverse Reactions/Side Effects

CNS: seizures, <u>headache</u>, anxiety, depression, dizziness, insomnia, lethargy, malaise, irritability. **EENT:**

visual disturbances. **Resp:** dyspnea. **CV:** vasodilation, edema, palpitations, tachycardia. **GI:** abdominal discomfort, constipation, nausea, vomiting. **GU:** dysuria, hematuria, polyuria, urinary retention. **Derm:** rash, acne, pruritis, increased sweating. **Endo:** breast discharge, breast pain, genital pruritis, increased breast size. **Hemat:** anemia. **Local:** itching, erythema, and swelling at implantation site. **Metab:** hyperlipidemia, hypercalcemia. **MS:** arthralgia, joint stiffness, muscle cramps, muscle stiffness, myalgia, bone pain. **Neuro:** tremor. **Misc:** ALLERGIC REACTIONS, INCLUDING ANGIOEDEMA, increased appetite, increased pain.

PHYSICAL THERAPY IMPLICATIONS

Examination and Evaluation

- Monitor signs of allergic reactions and angioedema, including pulmonary symptoms (tightness in the throat and chest, wheezing, cough, dyspnea) or skin reactions (rash, raised patches of red or white skin, burning/itching skin, swelling in the face). Notify physician or nursing staff immediately if these reactions occur.
- Be alert for new seizures or increased seizure activity, especially at the onset of drug treatment. Document the number, duration, and severity of seizures, and report these findings to the physician immediately.
- Assess heart rate, ECG, and heart sounds, especially during exercise (see Appendixes G, H). Report increased heart rate (tachycardia) or symptoms of other arrhythmias, including palpitations, chest discomfort, shortness of breath, fainting, and fatigue/weakness.
- Assess peripheral edema using girth measurements, volume displacement, and measurement of pitting edema (see Appendix N). Report increased swelling in feet and ankles due to fluid retention or peripheral vasodilation.
- Assess any joint, bone, or muscle and stiffness to rule out musculoskeletal pathology; that is, try to determine if pain is drug induced (e.g., related to high calcium levels) rather than caused by anatomic or biomechanical problems.
- Report unusual weakness and fatigue that might be due to anemia.
- Monitor personality or behavioral changes such as anxiety, irritability, depression, or difficulty sleeping. Notify physician if these changes become problematic.
- Assess dizziness that might affect gait, balance, and other functional activities (see Appendix C). Report balance problems and functional limitations to the physician and nursing staff, and caution the patient and family/caregivers to guard against falls and trauma.
- Monitor implantation site for pain, itching, and swelling. Report prolonged or excessive implant-site reactions to the physician.

Interventions

- For patients who are medically able to begin exercise, implement appropriate resistive exercises and aerobic training to maintain muscle strength and aerobic capacity during cancer chemotherapy or to help restore function after chemotherapy.
- Because of the risk of arrhythmias, use caution during aerobic exercise and other forms of therapeutic exercise. Assess exercise tolerance frequently (blood pressure, heart rate, fatigue levels), and terminate exercise immediately if any untoward responses occur (see Appendix L).

Patient/Client-Related Instruction

- Instruct patient to report problems with urination, including urinary retention, blood in the urine, increased urination, or difficulty initiating urination.
- Advise patient about the likelihood of GI reactions such as nausea, vomiting, diarrhea, constipation, and abdominal discomfort. Instruct patient to report severe or prolonged GI reactions.
- Advise patient that skin reactions such as rash, itching, acne, and increased sweating are likely. Report severe or unexpected skin reactions to the physician.
- Instruct patient or family/caregivers to report other troublesome side effects such as severe or prolonged headache, vision disturbances, difficulty breathing, or problems with breast tissues (breast pain, tenderness, discharge, increased size).

Pharmacokinetics

Absorption: Highly absorbed (92%) from implant. Peak absorption occurs at 12 hr, and continues over 1-yr period.
Distribution: Unknown.
Protein Binding: 29%.
Metabolism and Excretion: Unknown.
Half-life: 3.92 hours.

TIME/ACTION PROFILE (decrease in LH, FSH, and sex-steroid levels)

ROUTE	ONSET	PEAK	DURATION
SC	unknown	12 hr	52 wk

Contraindications/Precautions

Contraindicated in: Hypersensitivity to any component of the product, GnRH, or GnRH agonist analogues; Women and children.
Use Cautiously in: Patients with metastatic vertebral lesions or urinary tract obstruction (initial transient increase in testosterone may worsen symptoms).

Interactions

Drug-Drug: Unknown.

Route/Dosage

SC

Availability

Injection: 50 mg/implant.

hydralazine (hye-dral-a-zeen)

Apresoline, Novo-Hylazin

Classification

Therapeutic: antihypertensives

Pharmacologic: vasodilators

Indications

Moderate to severe hypertension (with a diuretic). **Unlabeled Use:** CHF unresponsive to conventional therapy with digoxin and diuretics.

Action

Direct-acting peripheral arteriolar vasodilator. **Therapeutic Effects:** Lowering of blood pressure in hypertensive patients and decreased afterload in patients with CHF.

Adverse Reactions/Side Effects

CNS: dizziness, drowsiness, headache. **CV:** tachycardia, angina, arrhythmias, edema, orthostatic hypotension. **GI:** diarrhea, nausea, vomiting. **Derm:** rashes. **F and E:** sodium retention. **MS:** arthralgias, arthritis. **Neuro:** peripheral neuropathy. **Misc:** drug-induced lupus syndrome.

PHYSICAL THERAPY IMPLICATIONS

Examination and Evaluation

- Assess blood pressure periodically and compare to normal values (See Appendix F) to help document antihypertensive effects.
- Assess signs and symptoms of CHF (dyspnea, rales/crackles, peripheral edema, jugular venous distention, exercise intolerance) to help document whether drug therapy is effective in reducing these symptoms.
- Assess heart rate, ECG, and heart sounds, especially during exercise (See Appendices G, H). Report a rapid heart rate (tachycardia) or signs of other arrhythmias, including palpitations, chest discomfort, shortness of breath, fainting, and fatigue/weakness.
- Assess blood pressure (BP) when patient assumes a more upright position (lying to standing, sitting to standing, lying to sitting). Document orthostatic hypotension and contact physician when systolic BP falls >20 mm Hg or diastolic BP falls >10 mm Hg.
- Assess peripheral edema using girth measurements, volume displacement, and measurement of pitting edema (See Appendix N). Report increased swelling in feet and ankles or a sudden increase in body weight due to sodium and fluid retention.
- Assess numbness, tingling, or weakness that might indicate peripheral neuropathy. Establish baseline electroneuromyographic values using EMG and nerve conduction whenever possible. Periodically reexamine these values to document drug-induced changes in peripheral nerve function.
- Assess any joint pain to rule out musculoskeletal pathology; that is, try to determine if pain is drug induced rather than caused by anatomical or biomechanical problems.
- Assess dizziness and drowsiness that might affect gait, balance, and other functional activities (See Appendix C). Report balance problems and functional limitations to the physician, and caution the patient and family/caregivers to guard against falls and trauma.
- Monitor signs of drug-induced lupus syndrome, including increased BP, fever, joint pain, skin rashes, and redness/irritation of the eye (uveitis). Notify physician promptly if these signs appear.

Interventions

- Design and implement aerobic exercise and endurance training programs to reduce hypertension, and improve myocardial pumping ability.
- Because of an increased risk of cardiac arrhythmias (tachycardia, others), use caution during aerobic exercise and endurance conditioning. Terminate exercise if patient exhibits untoward symptoms (chest pain, shortness of breath, unusual fatigue), or displays other criteria for exercise termination (See Appendix L).
- Avoid physical therapy interventions that cause systemic vasodilation (large whirlpool, Hubbard tank). Additive effects of this drug and the intervention may cause a dangerous fall in blood pressure.
- To minimize orthostatic hypotension, patient should move slowly when assuming a more upright position.

Patient/Client-Related Instruction

- Remind patients to take medication as directed to control hypertension and other cardiac conditions even if they are asymptomatic.
- Counsel patients about additional interventions to help control BP and cardiac dysfunction, including regular exercise, weight loss, sodium restriction, stress reduction, moderation of alcohol consumption, and smoking cessation.

- Instruct patient or family/caregivers to report other troublesome side effects such as severe or prolonged headache, skin rash, or GI problems (nausea, vomiting, diarrhea).

Pharmacokinetics

Absorption: Rapidly absorbed following oral administration; well absorbed from IM sites.
Distribution: Widely distributed. Crosses the placenta; enters breast milk in minimal concentrations.
Metabolism and Excretion: Mostly metabolized by the GI mucosa and liver.
Half-life: 2–8 hr.

TIME/ACTION PROFILE (antihypertensive effect)

ROUTE	ONSET	PEAK	DURATION
PO	45 min	2 hr	2–4 hr
IM	10–30 min	1 hr	3–8 hr
IV	5–20 min	15–30 min	2–6 hr

Contraindications/Precautions

Contraindicated in: Hypersensitivity; Some products contain tartrazine and should be avoided in patients with known intolerance.
Use Cautiously in: Cardiovascular or cerebrovascular disease; Severe renal and hepatic disease (dose modification may be necessary); Pregnancy and lactation (has been used safely during pregnancy).

Interactions

Drug-Drug: ↑ hypotension with acute ingestion of **alcohol**, other **antihypertensives**, or **nitrates**. **MAO inhibitors** may exaggerate hypotension. May ↓ pressor response to **epinephrine**. **NSAIDs** may ↓ antihypertensive response. **Beta blockers** ↓ tachycardia from hydralazine (therapy may be combined for this reason). **Metoprolol** and **propranolol** ↑ hydralazine levels. ↑ blood levels of **metoprolol** and **propranolol**.

Route/Dosage

PO (Adults): *Hypertension*—10 mg 4 times daily initially. After 2–4 days may increase to 25 mg 4 times daily for the rest of the 1st week; may then increase to 50 mg 4 times daily (up to 300 mg/day). Once maintenance dose is established, twice-daily dosing may be used. *CHF*—25–37.5 mg 4 times daily; may be increased up to 300 mg/day in 3–4 divided doses.
PO (Children >1 mo): Initial–0.75–1 mg/kg/day in 2–4 divided doses, not to exceed 25 mg/dose; may increase gradually to 5 mg/kg/day in infants and 7.5 mg/kg/day in children (not to exceed 200 mg/day) in 2–4 divided doses.
IM, IV (Adults): *Hypertension*—5–40 mg repeated as needed. *Eclampsia*—5 mg q 15–20 min; if no response after a total of 20 mg, consider an alternative agent.
IM, IV (Children >1 mo): Initial–0.1–0.2 mg/kg/dose (not to exceed 20 mg) q 4–6 hr as needed, up 1.7–3.5 mg/kg/day in 4–6 divided doses.

Availability (generic available)

Tablets: 10 mg, 25 mg, 50 mg, 100 mg. **Injection:** 20 mg/mL. ***In combination with:*** isosorbide dinitrate (BiDil). See Appendix B.

hydrochlorothiazide

(hye-droe-klor-oh-**thye**-a-zide)
Apo-Hydro, Esedrix, HCTZ, Hydro-chlor, Hydro-D, HydroDIURIL, Microzide, Neo-Codema, Novo-Hydrazide, Oretic, ♣Urozide

Classification
Therapeutic: antihypertensives, diuretics
Pharmacologic: thiazides

Indications

Management of mild-to-moderate hypertension. Treatment of edema associated with Congestive heart failure, Renal dysfunction, Cirrhosis, Glucocorticoid therapy, Estrogen therapy.

Action

Increases excretion of sodium and water by inhibiting sodium reabsorption in the distal tubule. Promotes excretion of chloride, potassium, hydrogen, magnesium, phosphate, calcium and bicarbonate. May produce arteriolar dilation. **Therapeutic Effects:** Lowering of blood pressure in hypertensive patients and diuresis with mobilization of edema.

Adverse Reactions/Side Effects

CNS: dizziness, drowsiness, lethargy, weakness. **CV:** hypotension. **GI:** anorexia, cramping, hepatitis, nausea, vomiting. **Derm:** photosensitivity, rashes. **Endo:** hyperglycemia. **F and E:** hypokalemia, dehydration, hypercalcemia, hypochloremic alkalosis, hypomagnesemia, hyponatremia, hypophosphatemia, hypovolemia. **Hemat:** blood dyscrasias. **Metab:** hyperuricemia, hypercholesterolemia. **MS:** muscle cramps. **Misc:** pancreatitis.

PHYSICAL THERAPY IMPLICATIONS

Examination and Evaluation

- Monitor signs of fluid, electrolyte, or acid-base imbalances, including dizziness, drowsiness, blurred vision, confusion, hypotension, or muscle cramps and weakness. Report excessive or prolonged symptoms to the physician.

- Assess dizziness and weakness that might affect gait, balance, and other functional activities (See Appendix C). Report balance problems and functional limitations to the physician, and caution the patient and family/caregivers to guard against falls and trauma.
- Assess blood pressure periodically and compare to normal values (See Appendix F) to help document antihypertensive effects.
- When used to treat edema, help determine drug effects by assessing peripheral edema using girth measurements, volume displacement, and measurement of pitting edema (See Appendix N). Also monitor signs of pulmonary edema such as dyspnea and rales/crackles (See Appendix K). Document whether peripheral and pulmonary symptoms are controlled adequately by diuretic therapy.
- Monitor signs of hyperglycemia (drowsiness, fruity breath, increased urination, unusual thirst). Patients with diabetes mellitus should check blood glucose levels frequently.

Interventions

- Implement fall prevention strategies, especially in older adults or if patient exhibits sedation, dizziness, blurred vision, or other impairments that affect gait and balance (See Appendix E).
- Use caution during aerobic exercise, especially in hot environments. Increased sweating will cause fluid and electrolyte loss, and may exaggerate diuretic side effects (dizziness, muscle cramps, and so forth).
- To minimize orthostatic hypotension, patient should move slowly when assuming a more upright position.
- Causes photosensitivity; use care if administering UV treatments.

Patient/Client-Related Instruction

- Remind patients to take medication as directed to control hypertension and other cardiac conditions even if they are asymptomatic.
- Counsel patients about additional interventions to help control blood pressure and cardiac dysfunction, including regular exercise, weight loss, sodium restriction, stress reduction, moderation of alcohol consumption, and smoking cessation.
- Instruct patient to report signs of thrombocytopenia (bruising, nose bleeds, and bleeding gums), or unusual weakness and fatigue that might be due to anemia or other blood dyscrasias.
- Advise patient about the possibility of GI reactions (cramping, nausea, vomiting, loss of appetite). Instruct patient or family and caregivers to report severe or prolonged GI symptoms, or signs of hepatitis (abdominal pain, severe nausea and vomiting, yellow skin or eyes, fever, sore throat, malaise, weakness, facial edema, lethargy, unusual bleeding or bruising) or pancreatitis (upper abdominal pain after eating, indigestion, weight loss, oily stools).
- Advise patient about photosensitivity, and to use sunscreens, protective clothing, and avoid prolonged sun exposure. Instruct patient to also report any rashes or other skin reactions.
- Advise patient that this drug may cause problems in fat and uric acid metabolism (hypercholesterolemia and hyperuricemia, respectively). Remind patient that periodic blood tests may be needed to monitor plasma lipids and uric acid levels.

Pharmacokinetics

Absorption: Rapidly absorbed after oral administration.
Distribution: Distributed into extracellular space; crosses the placenta and enters breast milk.
Metabolism and Excretion: Excreted mainly unchanged by the kidneys.
Half-life: 6–15 hr.

TIME/ACTION PROFILE (diuretic effect)

ROUTE	ONSET	PEAK	DURATION
PO*	2 hr	3–6 hr	6–12 hr

*Onset of antihypertensive effect is 3–4 days and does not become maximal for 7–14 days of dosing.

Contraindications/Precautions

Contraindicated in: Hypersensitivity (cross-sensitivity with other thiazides or sulfonamides may exist); Some products contain tartrazine and should be avoided in patients with known intolerance; Anuria; Lactation.
Use Cautiously in: Renal or hepatic impairment; Pregnancy (jaundice or thrombocytopenia may be seen in the newborn); Pedi: Avoid use of oral solution in neonates (contains sodium benzoate, a metabolite of benzyl alcohol which causes potentially fatal gasping syndrome).

Interactions

Drug-Drug: Additive hypotension with other **antihypertensives**, acute ingestion of **alcohol**, or **nitrates**. Additive hypokalemia with **corticosteroids, amphotericin B, piperacillin**, or **ticarcillin**. Decreases the excretion of **lithium**. **Cholestyramine** or **colestipol** decreases absorption. Hypokalemia increases risk of **digoxin** toxicity. **NSAIDs** may decrease effectiveness.

Route/Dosage

When used as a diuretic in adults, generally given daily, but may be given every other day or 2–3 days/week.

PO (Adults): 12.5–100 mg/day in 1–2 doses (up to 200 mg/day; not to exceed 50 mg/day for hypertension; doses above 25 mg are associated with greater likelihood of electrolyte abnormalities).
PO (Children >6 mo): 2 mg/kg in 2 divided doses (not to exceed 200 mg/day).
PO (Children <6 mo): Up to 2–4 mg/kg/day in 2 divided doses (not to exceed 37.5 mg/day).

Availability (generic available)

Tablets: 25 mg, 50 mg. **Capsules:** 12.5 mg. **Oral solution:** 10 mg/mL. ***In combination with:*** spironolactone, triamterene, bisoprolol, hydralazine, moexipril, reserpine, timolol. See Appendix B.

HIGH ALERT

hydrocodone
(hye-droe-**koe**-done)
Hycodan, Tussigon (U.S. antitussive formulations contain homatropine)

hydrocodone/acetaminophen
(hye-froe-**koe**-done/a-see-toh-min-oh-fen)
Anexsia, Co-Gesic, Lorcet-HD, Lortab, Norco, Vicodin, Zydone

hydrocodone/aspirin
(hye-froe-**koe**-done/**as**-pi-rin)
Azdone

hydrocodone/ibuprofen
(hye-froe-koe-done/eye-byoo-pro-fen)
Vicoprofen

Classification
Therapeutic: allergy, cold, and cough remedies (antitussive), opioid analgesics
Pharmacologic: opioid agonists/nonopioid analgesic combinations

Schedule III (in combination)
For information on the acetaminophen, aspirin, and ibuprofen components of these formulations, see the acetaminophen, aspirin, and ibuprofen monographs

Indications

Used mainly in combination with nonopioid analgesics (acetaminophen/aspirin/ibuprofen) in the management of moderate-to-severe pain. Antitussive (usually in combination products with decongestants).

Action

Bind to opiate receptors in the CNS. Alter the perception of and response to painful stimuli while producing generalized CNS depression. Suppress the cough reflex via a direct central action. **Therapeutic Effects:** Decrease in severity of moderate pain. Suppression of the cough reflex.

Adverse Reactions/Side Effects

Noted for hydrocodone only; see acetaminophen/aspirin/ibuprofen monographs for specific information on individual components
CNS: confusion, dizziness, sedation, euphoria, hallucinations, headache, unusual dreams. **EENT:** blurred vision, diplopia, miosis. **Resp:** respiratory depression. **CV:** hypotension, bradycardia. **GI:** constipation, dyspepsia, nausea, vomiting. **GU:** urinary retention. **Derm:** sweating. **Misc:** physical dependence, psychologic dependence, tolerance.

PHYSICAL THERAPY IMPLICATIONS

Examination and Evaluation

- Assess symptoms of respiratory depression, including decreased respiratory rate, confusion, bluish color of the skin and mucous membranes (cyanosis), and difficult, labored breathing (dyspnea). Monitor pulse oximetry and perform pulmonary function tests (See Appendix I) to quantify suspected changes in ventilation and respiratory function. Excessive respiratory depression requires emergency care.
- Be alert for excessive sedation or changes in mood and behavior (euphoria, confusion, hallucinations). Notify physician or nurse immediately if patient is unconscious or extremely difficult to arouse.
- Use appropriate pain scales (visual analogue scales, others) to document whether this drug is successful in helping manage the patient's pain.
- Assess blood pressure periodically and compare to normal values (See Appendix F). Report low blood pressure (hypotension), especially if patient experiences dizziness, fainting, or other symptoms.
- Assess heart rate, ECG, and heart sounds, especially during exercise (See Appendices G, H). Report slow heart rate (bradycardia) or symptoms of other arrhythmias, including palpitations, chest discomfort, shortness of breath, fainting, and fatigue/weakness.
- Assess dizziness that might affect gait, balance, and other functional activities (See Appendix C). Report balance problems and functional limitations to the

physician and nursing staff, and caution the patient and family/caregivers to guard against falls and trauma.

- If used as a cough suppressant, assess cough and lung sounds (See Appendix K) and monitor sputum production. Document whether this drug is effective as a cough suppressant.

Interventions

- Implement appropriate manual therapy techniques, physical agents, and therapeutic exercises to reduce pain and help wean patient off opioid analgesics as soon as possible.
- Because of the risk of respiratory depression, bradycardia, and hypotension, use caution during aerobic exercise and other forms of therapeutic exercise. Assess exercise tolerance frequently (blood pressure, heart rate, respiratory rate, fatigue levels), and terminate exercise immediately if any untoward responses occur (See Appendix L).
- Help patient explore other nonpharmacologic methods to reduce chronic pain, such as relaxation techniques, exercise, counseling, and so forth.
- Guard against falls and trauma (hip fractures, head injury). Implement fall prevention strategies (See Appendix E), especially if patient exhibits sedation, dizziness, or blurred vision.
- To minimize orthostatic hypotension, patient should move slowly when assuming a more upright position.

Patient/Client-Related Instruction

- Advise patient that opioid analgesics are usually more effective if given before pain becomes severe; emphasize that adequate pain control will allow better participation in physical therapy.
- Educate patient about the dangers of opioid overdose; encourage patient to adhere to proper dosing schedule.
- Emphasize that the risk of physical addiction (tolerance and dependence) is usually minimal during short-term treatment of pain. Advise patient that addiction is more likely during excessive or inappropriate use of opioid analgesics.
- Advise patient to avoid alcohol and other CNS depressants because of the increased risk of sedation and decreased CNS function.
- Advise patient to increase fluid intake and dietary fiber to avoid constipation. Laxatives may also be helpful in patients susceptible to fecal impaction (e.g., people with spinal cord injury).
- Instruct patient to report other troublesome side effects such as severe or prolonged headache, urinary retention, unusual dreams, excessive sweating, vision disturbances, or GI problems (nausea, vomiting, indigestion).

Pharmacokinetics

Absorption: Well absorbed following oral administration.
Distribution: Unknown.
Metabolism and Excretion: Mostly metabolized by the liver; eliminated in the urine (50–60% as metabolites, 15% as unchanged drug).
Half-life: 2.2 hr.

TIME/ACTION PROFILE (analgesic effect)

ROUTE	ONSET	PEAK	DURATION
PO	10–30 min	30–60 min	4–6 hr

Contraindications/Precautions

Contraindicated in: Hypersensitivity to hydrocodone (cross-sensitivity may exist to other opioids); Hypersensitivity to acetaminophen/aspirin/ibuprofen (for combination products); Aspirin- and ibuprofen-containing products should be avoided in patients with bleeding disorders or thrombocytopenia; Acetaminophen should be avoided in patients with severe hepatic or renal disease; ibuprofen-containing products should be avoided in patients undergoing coronary artery bypass graft surgery; OB/Lactation: Pregnancy or lactation (avoid chronic use); Products containing alcohol, aspartame, saccharin, sugar, or tartrazine (FDC yellow dye #5) should be avoided in patients who have hypersensitivity or intolerance to these compounds.
Use Cautiously in: Head trauma; Increased intracranial pressure; Severe renal, hepatic, or pulmonary disease; Cardiovascular disease (ibuprofen-containing products only); History of peptic ulcer disease (ibuprofen-containing products only); Alcoholism; Geriatric or debilitated patients (initial dosage reduction required; more prone to CNS depression, constipation); Patients with undiagnosed abdominal pain; Prostatic hyperplasia; Pedi: Children (safety not established).

Interactions

Drug-Drug: Use with extreme caution in patients receiving **mao inhibitors** (may produce severe, unpredictable reactions—do not use within 14 days of each other). Additive CNS depression with **alcohol, antihistamines,** and **sedative/hypnotics**. Administration of partial antagonist opioids (**buprenorphine, butorphanol, nalbuphine,** or **pentazocine**) may ↓ analgesia or precipitate opioid withdrawal in physically dependent patients.
Drug-Natural: Concomitant use of **kava, valerian, skullcap, chamomile,** or **hops** can increase CNS depression.

Route/Dosage

PO (Adults): *Analgesic*—2.5–10 mg q 3–6 hr as needed; if using combination products, acetaminophen or aspirin dosage should not exceed 4 g/day and

should not exceed 5 tablets/day of ibuprofen-containing products; *Antitussive*—5 mg q 4–6 hr as needed.
PO (Children): *Analgesic (2–13 yr)*—0.14 mg/kg q 4–6 hr. *Antitussive (6–12 yr)*—2.5 mg q 4–6 hr.

Availability

Hydrocodone

Hydrocodone tablets: 5 mg (Hycodan).
Hydrocodone syrup: 5 mg/mL (Hycodan, Robidone).

Hydrocodone/Acetaminophen (generic available)

Tablets: 2.5 mg hydrocodone/500 mg acetaminophen, 5 mg hydrocodone/400 mg acetaminophen (Zydone), 5 mg hydrocodone/325 mg acetaminophen (Anexsia 5/325, Norco), 5 mg hydrocodone/500 mg acetaminophen (Anexsia 5/500, Co-Gesic, Lorcet, Lortab 5/500, Vicodin), 7.5 mg hydrocodone/325 mg acetaminophen (Anexsia 7.5/325, Norco), 7.5 mg hydrocodone/400 mg acetaminophen (Zydone), 7.5 mg hydrocodone/500 mg acetaminophen, 7.5 mg hydrocodone/650 mg acetaminophen (Anexsia 7.5/650), 7.5 mg hydrocodone/750 mg acetaminophen (Vicodin ES), 10 mg hydrocodone/325 mg acetaminophen(Norco), 10 mg hydrocodone/400 mg acetaminophen (Zydone), 10 mg hydrocodone/500 mg acetaminophen (Lortab 10/500), 10 mg hydrocodone/650 mg acetaminophen, 10 mg hydrocodone/660 mg acetaminophen (Vicodin HP), 10 mg hydrocodone/750 mg acetaminophen (Anexsia 10/750). **Capsules:** 5 mg hydrocodone/500 mg acetaminophen (Lorcet-HD). **Elixir/oral solution:** 2.5 mg hydrocodone plus 167 mg acetaminophen/5 mL.

Hydrocodone/Aspirin

Tablets: 5 mg hydrocodone/500 mg aspirin (Azdone).

Hydrocodone/Ibuprofen

Tablets: 7.5 mg hydrocodone/200 mg ibuprofen.

hydrocortisone

(hye-droe-**kor**-ti-sone)
Cortef, Cortenema, Cortifoam, Solu-Cortef

Classification
Therapeutic: anti-inflammatories (steroidal)
Pharmacologic: corticosteroids

Indications

Management of adrenocortical insufficiency; chronic use in other situations is limited because of mineralocorticoid activity. Used systemically and locally in a wide variety of disorders, including Inflammatory, Allergic, Hematologic, Neoplastic, Autoimmune disorders.

Action

In pharmacologic doses, suppresses inflammation and the normal immune response. Has numerous intense metabolic effects (see Adverse Reactions and Side Effects). Suppresses adrenal function at chronic doses of 20 mg/day. Replaces endogenous cortisol in deficiency states. Also has potent mineralocorticoid (sodium-retaining) activity. **Therapeutic Effects:** Replacement therapy in adrenal insufficiency. Suppression of inflammation and modification of the normal immune response.

Adverse Reactions/Side Effects

Adverse reactions/side effects are much more common with high-dose/long-term therapy

CNS: depression, euphoria, headache, increased intracranial pressure (children only), personality changes, psychoses, restlessness. **EENT:** cataracts, increased intraocular pressure. **CV:** hypertension. **GI:** PEPTI CULCERATION, anorexia, nausea, vomiting. **Derm:** acne, decreased wound healing, ecchymoses, fragility, hirsutism, petechiae. **Endo:** adrenal suppression, hyperglycemia. **F and E:** fluid retention (long-term high doses), hypokalemia, hypokalemic alkalosis. **Hemat:** THROMBOEMBOLISM, thrombophlebitis. **Metab:** weight gain, weight loss. **MS:** muscle wasting, osteoporosis, aseptic necrosis of joints, muscle pain. **Misc:** hypersensitivity reactions, INCLUDING ANAPHYLAXIS, cushingoid appearance (moon face, buffalo hump), increased susceptibility to infection.

PHYSICAL THERAPY IMPLICATIONS

Examination and Evaluation

- Monitor signs of thrombophlebitis (lower extremity swelling, warmth, erythema, tenderness) and thromboembolism (shortness of breath, chest pain, cough, bloody sputum). Notify physician or nursing staff immediately, and request objective tests (Doppler ultrasound, lung scan, others) if thrombosis is suspected.
- Monitor and report signs of peptic ulcer, including heartburn, nausea, vomiting blood, tarry stools, and loss of appetite.
- Monitor signs of hypersensitivity reactions or anaphylaxis, including pulmonary symptoms (tightness in the throat and chest, wheezing, cough, dyspnea) or skin reactions (rash, pruritus, urticaria). Notify physician or nursing staff immediately if these reactions occur.
- Assess any muscle or joint pain. Report persistent or increased musculoskeletal pain to determine

presence of bone or joint pathology (aseptic necrosis, fracture).

- Assess signs of increased intracranial pressure in children, including changes in mood and behavior, decreased consciousness, headache, lethargy, seizures, and vomiting. Notify physician immediately of these signs.
- Assess muscle strength periodically to determine degree of muscle wasting during long- term use.
- Measure blood pressure periodically and compare to normal values (See Appendix F). Report a sustained increase in blood pressure (hypertension) to the physician.
- Assess peripheral edema using girth measurements, volume displacement, and measurement of pitting edema (See Appendix N). Report increased swelling in feet and ankles or a sudden increase in body weight due to fluid retention.
- Monitor personality changes, including depression, euphoria, restlessness, hallucinations, and psychosis. Notify physician if these changes become problematic.
- Be alert for signs of low potassium levels (hypokalemia) and metabolic acidosis, including hyperventilation, cardiac arrhythmias, dizziness, and confusion. Notify physician immediately if these signs occur.
- Report signs of adrenal suppression, including hypotension, weight loss, weakness, nausea, vomiting, anorexia, lethargy, confusion, and restlessness.
- Monitor signs of hyperglycemia (confusion; drowsiness; flushed, dry skin; fruit-like breath odor; rapid, deep breathing; polyuria; loss of appetite; unusual thirst). Insulin dosages may need to be adjusted to prevent repeated episodes of hyperglycemia.
- Periodically assess body weight and other anthropometric measures (body mass index, body composition). Report a rapid or unexplained weight gain or weight loss.

Interventions

- Implement resistive exercises and weight-bearing activities to minimize muscle wasting and osteoporosis. Use caution to prevent musculoskeletal damage in patients with preexisting muscle and bone loss.
- Protect skin from breakdown, especially over bony prominences.

Patient/Client-Related Instruction

- Advise patient that wound healing may be delayed; instruct patient to check skin regularly and report any nonhealing sores.
- Advise patient that corticosteroids cause immunosuppression and may mask symptoms of infection. Instruct patient to avoid people with known contagious illnesses and to report possible infections immediately.
- Advise patients on long-term treatment to consult physician before stopping this medication. Stopping the medication suddenly may result in adrenocortical shock (severe hypotension, hypoglycemia, weakness, vomiting). If these signs appear, notify physician immediately; may be life threatening.
- Instruct patient to report any loss of vision that might indicate cataracts or increased intraocular pressure.
- Advise patient about possible cushingoid appearance, including puffiness in the face (moon face), increased fat in the torso, thin arms and legs, abdominal skin striations, bruising, and deposition of fat at the posterior base of the neck (buffalo hump). Discuss possible effects on body image, and help patient explore coping mechanisms.
- Instruct patient and family/caregivers to report other troublesome side effects such as severe or prolonged headache or skin reactions (acne, hair growth).

Pharmacokinetics

Absorption: Well absorbed following oral administration. Sodium succinate salt is rapidly absorbed following IM administration. Absorption from local sites (intra-articular, intralesional) is slow but complete.

Distribution: Widely distributed, crosses the placenta, and probably enters breast milk.

Metabolism and Excretion: Metabolized mostly by the liver.

Half-life: 1.5–2 hr (plasma), 8–12 hr (tissue); adrenal suppression lasts 1.25–1.5 days.

TIME/ACTION PROFILE (anti-inflammatory activity)

ROUTE	ONSET	PEAK	DURATION
PO	unknown	1–2 hr	1.25–1.5 days
IM	rapid	1 hr	variable
IV	rapid	unknown	unknown

Contraindications/Precautions

Contraindicated in: Active untreated infections (may be used in patients being treated for tuberculous meningitis); Lactation: Avoid chronic use; Known alcohol, bisulfite, or tartrazine hypersensitivity or intolerance (some products contain these and should be avoided in susceptible patients).

Use Cautiously in: Chronic treatment (will lead to adrenal suppression; use lowest possible dose for shortest period of time); Pedi: Chronic use will result in decreased growth; use lowest possible dose for shortest period of time; Hypothyroidism; Cirrhosis; Ulcerative colitis; Stress (surgery, infections); supplemental doses may be needed; Potential infections may mask signs (fever, inflammation); OB: Pregnancy (safety not established).

Interactions

Drug-Drug: Additive hypokalemia with **thiazide, loop diuretics**, or **amphotericin B**. Hypokalemia may increase the risk of **digoxin** toxicity. May ↑ requirement for **insulin** or **oral hypoglycemic agents. Phenytoin, phenobarbital**, and **rifampin** ↑ metabolism; may ↓ effectiveness. **Oral contraceptives** may block metabolism. ↑ risk of adverse GI effects with **NSAIDs** (including **aspirin**). At chronic doses that suppress adrenal function, may ↓ antibody response to and ↑ risk of adverse reactions from **live-virus vaccines**.

Route/Dosage

PO (Adults): 20–240 mg/day in 1–4 divided doses.
PO (Children): *Adrenocortical insufficiency*—0.56 mg/kg (15–20 mg/m²/day) as a single dose or in divided doses. *Other uses*—2–8 mg/kg/day (60–240 mg/m²/day) as a single dose or in divided doses.
Rect (Adults): *Retention enema*—100 mg nightly for 21 days or until remission occurs; *aerosol foam*—90 mg 1–2 times/day for 2–3 wk; then adjusted.
IM, IV (Adults): *Hydrocortisone sodium succinate*—100–500 mg q 2–6 hr (range 100–8000 mg/day).
IM, IV (Children): *Adrenocortical insufficiency: hydrocortisone sodium succinate*—0.186–0.28 mg/kg/day (10–12 mg/m²/day) in 3 divided doses. *Other uses: hydrocortisone sodium succinate*—0.666–4 mg/kg (20–120 mg/m²) q 12–24 hr.

Availability

Tablets: 5 mg, 10 mg, 20 mg. **Enema:** 100 mg. **Rectal aerosol:** 90 mg. **Powder for injection (sodium succinate):** 100 mg, 250 mg, 500 mg, 1 g.

HIGH ALERT

hydromorphone

(hye-droe-**mor**-fone)
Dilaudid, Dilaudid-HP, Hydrostat IR, PMS Hydromorphone

Classification
Therapeutic: allergy, cold, and cough remedies (antitussives), opioid analgesics
Pharmacologic: opioid agonists

Schedule II

Indications

Moderate-to-severe pain (alone and in combination with nonopioid analgesics); extended-release product for opioid-tolerant patients requiring around-the-clock management of persistent pain. Antitussive (lower doses).

Action

Binds to opiate receptors in the CNS. Alters the perception of and response to painful stimuli while producing generalized CNS depression. Suppresses the cough reflex via a direct central action. **Therapeutic Effects:** Decrease in moderate-to-severe pain. Suppression of cough.

Adverse Reactions/Side Effects

CNS: confusion, sedation, dizziness, dysphoria, euphoria, floating feeling, hallucinations, headache, unusual dreams. **EENT:** blurred vision, diplopia, miosis. **Resp:** respiratory depression. **CV:** hypotension, bradycardia. **GI:** constipation, dry mouth, nausea, vomiting. **GU:** urinary retention. **Derm:** flushing, sweating. **Misc:** physical dependence, psychologic dependence, tolerance.

H

PHYSICAL THERAPY IMPLICATIONS

Examination and Evaluation

- Assess symptoms of respiratory depression, including decreased respiratory rate, confusion, bluish color of the skin and mucous membranes (cyanosis), and difficult, labored breathing (dyspnea). Monitor pulse oximetry and perform pulmonary function tests (See Appendix I) to quantify suspected changes in ventilation and respiratory function. Excessive respiratory depression requires emergency care.
- Be alert for excessive sedation or changes in mood and behavior (euphoria, dysphoria, confusion, hallucinations). Notify physician or nurse immediately if patient is unconscious or extremely difficult to arouse.
- Use appropriate pain scales (visual analogue scales, others) to document whether this drug is successful in helping manage the patient's pain.
- Assess blood pressure periodically and compare to normal values (See Appendix F). Report low blood pressure (hypotension), especially if patient experiences dizziness, fainting, or other symptoms.
- Assess heart rate, ECG, and heart sounds, especially during exercise (See Appendices G, H). Report slow heart rate (bradycardia) or symptoms of other arrhythmias, including palpitations, chest discomfort, shortness of breath, fainting, and fatigue/weakness.
- Assess dizziness that might affect gait, balance, and other functional activities (See Appendix C). Report balance problems and functional limitations to the physician and nursing staff, and caution the patient and family/caregivers to guard against falls and trauma.
- If used as a cough suppressant, assess cough and lung sounds (See Appendix K), and monitor sputum

production. Document whether this drug is effective as a cough suppressant.

Interventions

- Implement appropriate manual therapy techniques, physical agents, and therapeutic exercises to reduce pain and help wean patient off opioid analgesics as soon as possible.
- Because of the risk of respiratory depression, bradycardia, and hypotension, use caution during aerobic exercise and other forms of therapeutic exercise. Assess exercise tolerance frequently (blood pressure, heart rate, respiratory rate, fatigue levels), and terminate exercise immediately if any untoward responses occur (See Appendix L).
- Help patient explore other nonpharmacologic methods to reduce chronic pain, such as relaxation techniques, exercise, counseling, and so forth.
- Guard against falls and trauma (hip fractures, head injury). Implement fall-prevention strategies (See Appendix E), especially if patient exhibits sedation, dizziness, or blurred vision.
- To minimize orthostatic hypotension, patient should move slowly when assuming a more upright position.

Patient/Client-Related Instruction

- Advise patient that opioid analgesics are usually more effective if given before pain becomes severe; emphasize that adequate pain control will allow better participation in physical therapy.
- Educate patient about the dangers of opioid overdose; encourage patient to adhere to proper dosing schedule.
- Emphasize that the risk of physical addiction (tolerance and dependence) is usually minimal during short-term treatment of pain. Advise patient that addiction is more likely during excessive or inappropriate use of opioid analgesics.
- Advise patient to avoid alcohol and other CNS depressants because of the increased risk of sedation and decreased CNS function.
- Advise patient to increase fluid intake and dietary fiber to avoid constipation. Laxatives may also be helpful in patients susceptible to fecal impaction (e.g., people with spinal cord injury).
- Instruct patient to report other troublesome side effects such as severe or prolonged headache, urinary retention, unusual dreams, excessive sweating, vision disturbances, or GI problems (nausea, vomiting, dry mouth).

Pharmacokinetics

Absorption: Well absorbed following oral, rectal, SC, and IM administration. Extended-release product results in an initial release of drug, followed by a second sustained phase of absorption.
Distribution: Widely distributed. Crosses the placenta; enters breast milk.
Metabolism and Excretion: Mostly metabolized by the liver.
Half-life: *Oral, immediate release, or injection*—2–4 hr.

TIME/ACTION PROFILE (analgesic effect)

ROUTE	ONSET	PEAK	DURATION
PO	30 min	30–90 min	4–5 hr
SC	15 min	30–90 min	4–5 hr
IM	15 min	30–60 min	4–5 hr
IV	10–15 min	15–30 min	2–3 hr
rectal	15–30 min	30–90 min	4–5 hr

Contraindications/Precautions

Contraindicated in: Hypersensitivity; Some products contain bisulfites and should be avoided in patients with known hypersensitivity; OB/Lactation: Avoid chronic use during pregnancy or lactation.
Use Cautiously in: Head trauma; Increased intracranial pressure; Severe renal, hepatic, or pulmonary disease; Hypothyroidism; Adrenal insufficiency; Alcoholism; Geri: Geriatric or debilitated patients (dose reduction recommended); Undiagnosed abdominal pain; Prostatic hypertrophy.

Interactions

Drug-Drug: Exercise extreme caution with **MAO inhibitors** (may produce severe, unpredictable reactions—reduce initial dose of hydromorphone to 25% of usual dose, discontinue MAO inhibitors 2 wk prior to hydromorphone). ↑ risk of CNS depression with **alcohol, antidepressants, antihistamines,** and **sedative/hypnotics,** including **benzodiazepines** and **phenothiazines**. Administration of partial antagonists (**buprenorphine, butorphanol, nalbuphine,** or **pentazocine**) may precipitate opioid withdrawal in physically dependent patients. **Nalbuphine** or **pentazocine** may ↓ analgesia.
Drug-Natural: Concomitant use of **kava, valerian, chamomile,** or **hops** can ↑ CNS depression.

Route/Dosage

Doses depend on level of pain and tolerance.

Analgesic

PO (Adults ≥50 kg): 4–8 mg q 3–4 hr initially (some patients may respond to doses as small as 2 mg initially).
PO (Adults and Children <50 kg): 0.06 mg/kg q 3–4 hr initially; younger children may require smaller initial doses of 0.03 mg/kg. Maximum dose 5 mg.
IV, IM, SC (Adults ≥50 kg): 1.5 mg q 3–4 hr as needed initially; may be increased.
IV, IM, SC (Adults and Children <50 kg): 0.015 mg/kg mg q 3–4 hr as needed initially; may be increased.

IV (Adults): *Continuous infusion (unlabeled)*—0.2–30 mg/hr depending on previous opioid use. An initial bolus of twice the hourly rate in milligrams may be given with subsequent breakthrough boluses of 50–100% of the hourly rate in milligrams.
Rect (Adults): 3 mg q 6–8 hr initially as needed.

Antitussive

PO (Adults and Children >12 yr): 1 mg q 3–4 hr.
PO (Children 6–12 yr): 0.5 mg q 3–4 hr.

Availability (generic available)

Tablets: 2 mg, 3 mg, 4 mg, 8 mg. **Oral solution:** 5 mg/5 mL. **Injection:** 1 mg/mL, 2 mg/mL, 4 mg/mL, 10 mg/mL. **Suppositories:** 3 mg. ***In combination with:*** guaifenesin and alcohol (Dilaudid Cough Syrup). See Appendix B.

hydroxychloroquine
(hye-drox-ee-**klor**-oh-kwin)
Plaquenil

Classification
Therapeutic: antimalarials, antirheumatics (disease-modifying antirheumatic drugs, DMARDs)

Indications

Suppression/chemoprophylaxis of malaria. Treatment of severe rheumatoid arthritis/systemic lupus erythematosus.

Action

Inhibits protein synthesis in susceptible organisms by inhibiting DNA and RNA polymerase. **Therapeutic Effects:** Death of plasmodia responsible for causing malaria. Also has anti-inflammatory properties.

Adverse Reactions/Side Effects

CNS: SEIZURES, aggressiveness, anxiety, apathy, confusion, fatigue, headache, irritability, personality changes, psychoses. **EENT:** keratopathy, ototoxicity, retinopathy, tinnitus, visual disturbances. **CV:** ECG changes, hypotension. **GI:** abdominal cramps, anorexia, diarrhea, epigastric discomfort, nausea, vomiting, hepatic failure. **Derm:** bleaching of hair, alopecia, hyperpigmentation, photosensitivity, Stevens-Johnson syndrome. **Hemat:** AGRANULOCYTOSIS, APLASTIC ANEMIA, leukopenia, thrombocytopenia. **Neuro:** neuromyopathy, peripheral neuritis.

PHYSICAL THERAPY IMPLICATIONS

Examination and Evaluation

- Be alert for new seizures or increased seizure activity, especially at the onset of drug treatment. Document the number, duration, and severity of seizures, and report these findings to the physician immediately.
- Monitor signs of agranulocytosis and leukopenia (fever, sore throat, mucosal lesions, signs of infection, bruising), thrombocytopenia (bruising, nose bleeds, bleeding gums), or unusual weakness and fatigue that might be due to aplastic anemia. Periodic blood tests may be needed to monitor WBC and RBC counts.
- Monitor rashes or other skin reactions (pruritus, urticaria, exfoliation). Notify physician immediately because certain skin reactions may indicate serious hypersensitivity reactions (Stevens-Johnson syndrome).
- If treating rheumatoid arthritis or lupus erythematosus, periodically assess patient's impairments (pain, range of motion), functional ability, and disability to help document whether antirheumatic drug therapy is successful.
- Be alert for signs of peripheral neuromyopathy and neuritis (numbness, tingling, decreased muscle strength). Establish baseline electroneuromyographic values at the beginning of drug treatment whenever possible, and reexamine these values periodically to document drug-induced changes in peripheral nerve function.
- Assess heart rate, ECG, and heart sounds, especially during exercise (See Appendices G, H). Report any rhythm disturbances or symptoms of increased arrhythmias, including palpitations, chest discomfort, shortness of breath, fainting, and fatigue/weakness.
- Assess blood pressure periodically and compare to normal values (See Appendix F). Report low blood pressure (hypotension), especially if patient experiences dizziness, fatigue, or other symptoms.
- Monitor changes in personality, mood, and behavior, including aggressiveness, anxiety, confusion, irritability, and psychosis. Notify physician if these changes become problematic.
- If treating malaria, monitor any changes in symptoms (decreased fever, chills, sweating) to help document whether antimalarial drug therapy is successful.

Interventions

- Because of the risk of ECG changes and hypotension, use caution during aerobic exercise and other forms of therapeutic exercise. Assess exercise tolerance frequently (blood pressure, heart rate, fatigue levels), and terminate exercise immediately if any untoward responses occur (See Appendix L).
- Implement appropriate manual therapy techniques, physical agents, therapeutic exercises, and

H

orthotic/assistive devices to reduce pain, improve function, and augment the effects of antirheumatic drug therapy.

- Help patient explore other nonpharmacologic methods to reduce chronic pain, such as relaxation techniques, exercise, counseling, and so forth.
- Causes photosensitivity; use care if administering UV treatments. Advise patient to avoid direct sunlight and use sunscreens and protective clothing.

Patient/Client-Related Instruction

- Instruct patient to report visual disturbances (blurred vision, double vision) or hearing problems (ringing in the ears, hearing loss). Visual and auditory problems are more common at higher doses.
- Remind patient to take this drug as directed when treating malaria even if patient is asymptomatic.
- Advise patient about the likelihood of GI reactions such as nausea, vomiting, diarrhea, cramps, and heartburn. Instruct patient to report severe or prolonged GI problems or signs of liver toxicity such as yellow skin or eyes, abdominal pain, severe nausea and vomiting, fever, sore throat, malaise, weakness, and facial edema.
- Instruct patient to report other untoward side effects such as severe or prolonged headache or skin reactions (hyperpigmentation, hair loss).

Pharmacokinetics

Absorption: Highly variable (31–100%) following oral administration.
Distribution: Widely distributed; high concentrations in RBCs; crosses the placenta; excreted into breast milk.
Metabolism and Excretion: Partially metabolized by the liver to active metabolites; partially excreted unchanged by the kidneys.
Half-life: 72–120 hr.

TIME/ACTION PROFILE (blood levels)

ROUTE	ONSET	PEAK	DURATION
PO	Rapid*	1–2 hr	days–weeks

*Onset of antirheumatic action may take 6 wk.

Contraindications/Precautions

Contraindicated in: Hypersensitivity to hydroxychloroquine or chloroquine; Previous visual damage from hydroxychloroquine or chloroquine.
Use Cautiously in: Concurrent use of hepatotoxic drugs; History of liver disease or alcoholism or renal impairment; Severe neurologic disorders; Severe blood disorders; Retinal or visual field changes; G6PD deficiency; Psoriasis; Bone marrow depression; Obesity (determine dose by ideal body weight); Pregnancy or lactation (avoid use unless treating/preventing malaria or treating amebic abscess); Children (long-term use increased sensitivity to effects).

Interactions

Drug-Drug: May ↑ the risk of hepatotoxicity when administered with **hepatotoxic drugs**. May ↑ the risk of hematologic toxicity when administered with **penicillamine**. May ↑ risk of dermatitis when administered with other **agents having dermatologic toxicity**. May decrease serum titers of rabies antibody when given concurrently with **human diploid cell rabies vaccine. Urinary acidifiers** may ↑ renal excretion. May ↑ serum levels of **digoxin**.

Route/Dosage

Antimalarial doses expressed as milligrams of base; antirheumatic and lupus doses expressed as milligrams of hydroxychloroquine sulfate (200 mg hydroxychloroquine sulfate = 155 mg of hydroxychloroquine base).

Malaria

PO (Adults): *Suppression or chemoprophylaxis*—310 mg once weekly; start 1–2 wk prior to entering malarious area; continue for 4 wk after leaving area. *Treatment*—620 mg, then 310 mg at 6 hr, 24 hr, and 48 hr after initial dose.
PO (Children): *Suppression or chemoprophylaxis*—5 mg/kg once weekly; start 1–2 wk prior to entering malarious area; continue for 4 wk after leaving area. *Treatment*—10 mg/kg initially, then 5 mg/kg at 6–8 hr, 24 hr, and 48 hr after initial dose.

Rheumatoid Arthritis

PO (Adults): 400–600 mg once daily initially, maintenance 200–400 mg/day divided 1–2 times/day.
PO (Children): 3–5 mg/kg/day divided 1–2 times/day to a maximum of 400 mg/day; not to exceed 7 mg/kg/day.

Systemic Lupus Erythematosus

PO (Adults): 400 mg once or twice daily, maintenance 200–400 mg/day.
PO (Children): 3–5 mg/kg/day divided 1–2 times/day to a maximum of 400 mg/day; not to exceed 7 mg/kg/day.

Availability

Tablets: 200 mg (155 mg base).

hydroxyurea

(hye-drox-ee-yoo-**ree**-a)
Droxia, Hydrea, Mylocel

Classification
Therapeutic: antineoplastics
Pharmacologic: antimetabolites

Indications

Treatment of head and neck carcinoma. Treatment of ovarian carcinoma. Treatment of resistant chronic myelogenous leukemia. Treatment of melanoma. Reduction of painful crises in sickle cell anemia and decreased need for transfusions in adult patients with a history of recurrent moderate-to-severe crises (at least 3 in the preceding year). **Unlabeled Use:** Used as part of antiretroviral therapy in patients with HIV infection.

Action

Interferes with DNA synthesis (cell-cycle S-phase–specific). May alter characteristics of RBCs. **Therapeutic Effects:** Death of rapidly replicating cells, particularly malignant ones. Decreased frequency of painful crises and decreased need for transfusions in sickle cell anemia.

Adverse Reactions/Side Effects

CNS: drowsiness (large doses). **GI:** anorexia, diarrhea, nausea, vomiting, constipation, hepatitis, stomatitis. **GU:** dysuria, infertility, renal tubular dysfunction. **Derm:** alopecia, exacerbation of postradiation erythema, erythema, pruritus, rashes. **Hemat:** leukopenia, anemia, thrombocytopenia. **Metab:** hyperuricemia. **Misc:** chills, fever, malaise.

PHYSICAL THERAPY IMPLICATIONS

Examination and Evaluation

- Be alert for signs of leukopenia (fever, sore throat, signs of infection), thrombocytopenia (bruising, nose bleeds, bleeding gums), or unusual weakness and fatigue that might be due to anemia or other blood dyscrasias. Report these signs immediately to the physician or nursing staff.
- Assess drowsiness that might affect gait, balance, and other functional activities. Notify physician, nursing staff, and family/caregivers if drowsiness becomes problematic.

Interventions

- For patients who are medically able to begin exercise, implement appropriate resistive exercises and aerobic training to maintain muscle strength and aerobic capacity during cancer chemotherapy or to help restore function after chemotherapy.
- If treating patients with sickle-cell anemia, use caution during aerobic exercise and other forms of therapeutic exercise. Assess exercise tolerance frequently (blood pressure, heart rate, fatigue levels), and terminate exercise immediately if any untoward responses occur (See Appendix L).

Patient/Client-Related Instruction

- Advise patient to guard against infection (frequent hand washing, etc.), and to avoid crowds and contact with persons with contagious diseases.
- Advise patient that rashes and other skin reactions (itching, hair loss, redness, warmth) are likely. Severe or unexpected skin reactions should be reported to the physician.
- Advise patient about the likelihood of GI reactions such as diarrhea, nausea, vomiting, constipation, loss of appetite, and inflammation in/around the mouth. Instruct patient to report severe or prolonged GI problems, or signs of drug-induced hepatitis, including abdominal pain, severe nausea and vomiting, yellow skin or eyes, skin rashes, and muscle/joint pain.
- Advise patient that flu-like symptoms (fever, chills, body aches) are likely, and to report severe or prolonged symptoms.
- Instruct patient to report any urinary problems, including difficult or painful urination.

Pharmacokinetics

Absorption: Well absorbed following oral administration.
Distribution: Crosses the blood-brain barrier; concentrates in RBCs and leukocytes.
Metabolism and Excretion: 50% excreted unchanged by the kidneys; 50% metabolized by the liver and eliminated as respiratory CO.
Half-life: 3–4 hr.

TIME/ACTION PROFILE (effects on blood counts)

ROUTE	ONSET	PEAK	DURATION
PO	7 days	10 days	21 days

Contraindications/Precautions

Contraindicated in: Hypersensitivity; Pregnancy or lactation; Some products contain tartrazine (FDC yellow dye #5) and should be avoided in patients with known hypersensitivity.
Use Cautiously in: Patients with childbearing potential; Renal impairment (close monitoring of hematologic parameters recommended, dosage reduction may be necessary); Hepatic impairment (close monitoring of hematologic parameters recommended); Myeloproliferative disorders (may increase risk of vasculitic ulcerations and gangrene); Active infections; Decreased bone marrow reserve; Other chronic debilitating illness; Geriatric patients (may be more sensitive to effects, lower doses may be required); Obese patients or patients with edema (dose should be determined using ideal body weight).

Interactions

Drug-Drug: Additive bone marrow depression with **agents that depress bone marrow**, including **radiation therapy**. May decrease the antibody response to and increase the risk of adverse reactions to **live-virus vaccines.**

Route/Dosage

Head and Neck Cancer, Ovarian Cancer, Malignant Melanoma

PO (Adults): 60–80 mg/kg (2–3 g/m^2) as a single daily dose q 3 days or 20–30 mg/kg/day as a single dose. Therapy should be initiated 7 days prior to radiation and continued.

Resistant Chronic Myelogenous Leukemia

PO (Adults): 20–30 mg/kg/day in 1–2 divided doses.

Sickle Cell Anemia

PO (Adults and Children): 15 mg/kg/day as a single dose; may increase by 5 mg/kg/day q 12 wk up to 35 mg/kg/day.

Availability (generic available)

Capsules: 200 mg, 250 mg, 300 mg, 400 mg, 500 mg. **Tablets:** 100 mg, 1000 mg.

hydroxyzine (hye-**drox**-i-zeen)

Apo-Hydroxyzine, Atarax, Hyzine-50, Multipax, Novohydroxyzin, Vistaril

Classification

Therapeutic: antianxiety agents, antihistamines, sedative/hypnotics

Indications

Treatment of anxiety. Preoperative sedation. Antiemetic. Antipruritic. May be combined with opioid analgesics.

Action

Acts as a CNS depressant at the subcortical level of the CNS. Has anticholinergic, antihistaminic, and antiemetic properties. Blocks histamine 1 receptors. **Therapeutic Effects:** Sedation. Relief of anxiety. Decreased nausea and vomiting. Decreased allergic symptoms associated with release of histamine, including pruritus.

Adverse Reactions/Side Effects

CNS: drowsiness, agitation, ataxia, dizziness, headache, weakness. **Resp:** wheezing. **GI:** dry mouth, bitter taste, constipation, nausea. **GU:** urinary retention. **Derm:** flushing. **Local:** pain at IM site, abscesses at IM sites. **Misc:** chest tightness.

PHYSICAL THERAPY IMPLICATIONS

Examination and Evaluation

- Monitor any respiratory problems, including wheezing or tightness in the chest and throat. Report severe or prolonged respiratory symptoms to the physician.
- Be alert for increased anxiety or agitation, especially during the initial period of drug therapy. Notify physician about any problematic changes in mood or behavior.
- Assess dizziness, drowsiness, and ataxia that might affect gait, balance, and other functional activities (See Appendix C). Report balance problems and functional limitations to the physician, and caution the patient and family/caregivers to guard against falls and trauma.
- Monitor IM injection site for pain, swelling, and irritation. Report prolonged or excessive injection site reactions to the physician.

Interventions

- Guard against falls and trauma (hip fractures, head injury, and so forth). Implement fall- prevention strategies, especially in older adults or if balance is impaired (See Appendix E).
- Help patient explore nonpharmacologic methods to reduce anxiety, such as relaxation techniques, exercise, counseling, support groups, and so forth.

Patient/Client-Related Instruction

- Advise patient about the risk of daytime drowsiness and decreased attention and mental focus. These problems can be severe in certain people. Use care if driving or in other activities that require quick reactions and strong concentration.
- Advise patient to avoid alcohol and other CNS depressants because of the increased risk of sedation and adverse effects.
- Instruct patient to report other troublesome side effects such as severe or prolonged headache, urinary retention, skin redness/warmth, or GI problems (constipation, nausea, dry mouth, bitter taste).

Pharmacokinetics

Absorption: Well absorbed following PO/IM administration.
Distribution: Unknown.
Metabolism and Excretion: Completely metabolized by the liver; eliminated in the feces via biliary excretion.
Half-life: 3 hr.

TIME/ACTION PROFILE (sedative, antiemetic, antipruritic effects)

ROUTE	ONSET	PEAK	DURATION
PO	15–30 min	2–4 hr	4–6 hr
IM	15–30 min	2–4 hr	4–6 hr

Contraindications/Precautions

Contraindicated in: Hypersensitivity; OB: Potential for congenital defects (oral clefts and hypoplasia of cerebral hemisphere); Lactation: Safety not established.

Use Cautiously in: Severe hepatic dysfunction; OB: Has been used safely during labor; Pedi: Injection contains benzyl alcohol, which can cause potentially fatal gasping syndrome in neonates; Geri: Appears on Beers' list. Geriatric patients are more susceptible to adverse reactions due to anticholinergic effects; dosage reduction recommended.

Interactions

Drug-Drug: Additive CNS depression with other **CNS depressants**, including **alcohol, antidepressants, antihistamines, opioid analgesics**, and **sedative/hypnotics**. Additive anticholinergic effects with other **drugs possessing anticholinergic properties**, including **antihistamines, antidepressants, atropine, haloperidol, phenothiazines, quinidine**, and **disopyramide**. Can antagonize the vasopressor effects of **epinephrine**.

Drug-Natural: Concomitant use of **kava, valerian**, or **chamomile** can ↑ CNS depression. ↑ anticholinergic effects with **angel's trumpet, jimson weed**, and **scopolia**.

Route/Dosage

PO (Adults): *Antianxiety*—25–100 mg 4 times/day, not to exceed 600 mg/day. *Preoperative sedation*—50–100 mg single dose. *Antipruritic*—25 mg 3–4 times daily.

PO (Children): —2 mg/kg/day divided q 6–8 hr.

IM (Adults): *Preoperative sedation*—25–100 mg single dose. *Antiemetic, adjunct to opioid analgesics*—25–100 mg q 4–6 hr as needed.

IM (Children):—0.5–1 mg/kg/dose q 4–6 hr as needed.

Availability (generic available)

Tablets: 10 mg, 25 mg, 50 mg, 100 mg. **Capsules:** 10 mg, 25 mg, 50 mg, 100 mg. **Syrup:** 10 mg/5 mL. **Oral suspension:** 25 mg/5 mL. **Injection:** 25 mg/mL, 50 mg/mL.

hyoscyamine

(hi-oh-**sye**-a-meen)

Anaspaz, A-Spas S/L, Cystospaz, Cystospaz-M, Donnamar, ED-SPAZ, Gastrosed, Levsinex, Levsin, Levbid, L-hyoscyamine, NuLev

Classification

Therapeutic: antispasmodics

Pharmacologic: anticholinergics

Indications

Control of gastric secretion, visceral spasm, hypermotility in spastic colitis, spastic bladder, pylorospasm, and related abdominal cramps. Decreases symptoms of various functional intestinal disorders, including mild dysenteries, diverticulitis, infant colic, biliary and renal colic. Adjunctive therapy in peptic ulcer disease, irritable bowel syndrome, neurogenic bowel disturbances. Decreases pain and hypersecretion associated with pancreatitis. Relief of symptoms of acute rhinitis. Decreases rigidity and tremors associated with parkinsonism and controls related sialorrhea and hyperhidrosis. May also be used to manage anticholinesterase poisoning. Management of cystitis or renal colic. Management of some forms of heart block due to vagal activity. **IM, IV, SC:** Facilitation of diagnostic hypotonic duodenography; may also increase radiologic visibility of the kidneys. Preoperative administration decreases secretions and blocks bradycardia associated with some forms of anesthesia and related surgical agents.

Action

Inhibits the muscarinic effect of acetylcholine in smooth muscle, secretory glands, and the CNS. Small doses ↓ salivary and bronchial secretions and ↓ sweating; intermediate doses dilate the pupil, inhibit accommodation, ↑ heart rate (vagolytic action); large doses ↓ GI and GU motility, further ↑ in dose ↓ gastric acid secretion. **Therapeutic Effects:** ↓ secretions with ↓ GI and GU symptomatology. ↑ heart rate.

Adverse Reactions/Side Effects

CNS: confusion/excitement (especially in geriatric patients), dizziness, flushing, headache, insomnia, lightheadedness (IM, IV, SC), nervousness. **EENT:** blurred vision, cycloplegia, ↑ intraocular pressure, mydriasis, photophobia. **CV:** palpitations, tachycardia. **GI:** dry mouth, altered taste perception, bloated feeling, constipation, nausea, paralytic ileus, vomiting. **GU:** erectile dysfunction, urinary hesitancy/retention. **Derm:** ↓ sweating, urticaria. **Local:** local irritation (IM, IV, SC). **Misc:** ALLERGIC REACTIONS, INCLUDING ANAPHYLAXIS, fever (especially in children), suppression of lactation.

PHYSICAL THERAPY IMPLICATIONS

Examination and Evaluation

- Be alert for signs of allergic reactions and anaphylaxis, including pulmonary symptoms (tightness in the throat and chest, wheezing, cough, dyspnea) or skin reactions (rash, pruritus, urticaria). Notify physician immediately if these reactions occur.
- Assess heart rate, ECG, and heart sounds, especially during exercise (See Appendices G, H). Although intended to treat certain arrhythmias, this drug can unmask or precipitate new arrhythmias (proarrhythmic effect). Report any rhythm disturbances or symptoms of increased arrhythmias, including palpitations, chest pain, shortness of breath, fainting, and fatigue/weakness.

- If used to treat bowel disorders, monitor any improvements such as decreased abdominal pain, decreased diarrhea, and improved appetite to help document whether drug therapy is successful.
- Monitor signs of intestinal paralysis (paralytic ileus), including nausea, lack of bowel sounds or movements, abdominal bloating/distention, and vomiting. Report these signs to the physician immediately.
- Be alert for decreased sweating and altered/increased body temperature (hyperpyrexia). Notify physician of a prolonged or persistent elevation in body temperature.
- Monitor and report excessive confusion, excitement, nervousness, or other alterations in mental status.
- Assess dizziness and light-headedness that might affect gait, balance, and other functional activities (See Appendix C). Report balance problems and functional limitations to the physician, and caution the patient and family/caregivers to guard against falls and trauma.
- Monitor IM injection site for pain and redness. Report prolonged or excessive injection site reactions to the physician.

Interventions

- Because of the risk of arrhythmias and impaired thermoregulation, use caution during aerobic exercise and other forms of therapeutic exercise. Assess exercise tolerance frequently (blood pressure, heart rate, fatigue levels), and terminate exercise immediately if any untoward responses occur (See Appendix L).

Patient/Client-Related Instruction

- Instruct patient and family/caregivers to report other troublesome side effects such as severe or prolonged headache, sleep loss, vision problems, problems with urination, sexual dysfunction, fever, hives, or GI problems (nausea, vomiting, constipation, heartburn, bloating, altered taste, dry mouth).

Pharmacokinetics

Absorption: Well absorbed; food does not affect absorption.
Distribution: Crosses the placenta and blood-brain barrier; enters breast milk.
Metabolism and Excretion: Excreted mostly unchanged by the kidneys.
Half-life: 3.5 hr.

TIME/ACTION PROFILE (GI effects)

ROUTE	ONSET	PEAK	DURATION
PO	20–30 min	unknown	4–6 hr
IM, IV, SC	2–3 min	unknown	4–6 hr

Contraindications/Precautions

Contraindicated in: Hypersensitivity; Angle-closure glaucoma; Synechiae; Tachycardia or unstable cardiovascular status; GI obstructive disease, paralytic ileus, intestinal atony, severe ulcerative colitis; Obstructive uropathy; Myasthenia gravis; Lactation; Products containing benzyl alcohol should not be used in newborn or immature infants; Some products contain alcohol, sulfites, or tartrazine and should be avoided in patients with known intolerance/hypersensitivity; Phenylketonuria (NuLev contains aspartame).
Use Cautiously in: History of cardiovascular disease, including CHF, arrhythmias, hypertension, tachycardia, or coronary artery disease; Renal disease or prostatic hyperplasia; Hepatic disease, early ileus, or reflux esophagitis; Autonomic neuropathy; Hyperthyroidism; Geri: Appears on Beers' list. Geriatric patients have increased sensitivity to anticholinergics; Infants, small children, blondes, Down's syndrome, brain damage, or spastic paralysis (increased sensitivity); Pregnancy (may cause fetal tachycardia; safety not established).

Interactions

Drug-Drug: Concurrent administration with **amantadine** ↑ anticholinergic side effects (may require dose reduction). ↑ effects of **atenolol**; Concurrent use with **phenothiazines** may result in ↓ effect of phenothiazine and ↑ anticholinergic side effects (dose reduction may be necessary); ↑ anticholinergic side effects with **tricyclic antidepressants**.

Route/Dosage

PO, SL (Adults): 0.125–0.25 mg 3–4 times daily or 0.375–0.75 mg as sustained-release form q 12 hr.
PO (Children2–<12 yr): *orally disintegrating tablets (NuLev)*—0.0625–0.125 mg (½–1 tablet) q 4 hr, up to 6 times/day.
PO (Children 34–36 kg): 125–187 mcg q 4 hr as needed.
PO (Children 22.7–33 kg): 94–125 mcg q 4 hr as needed.
PO (Children 13.6–22.6 kg): 63 mcg q 4 hr as needed.
PO (Children 9.1–13.5 kg): 31.3 mcg q 4 hr as needed.
PO (Children 6.8–9 kg): 25 mcg q 4 hr as needed.
PO (Children 4.5–6.7 kg): 18.8 mcg q 4 hr as needed.
PO (Children 3.4–4.4 kg): 15.6 mcg q 4 hr as needed.
PO (Children 2.3–3.3 kg): 12.5 mcg q 4 hr as needed.
IM, IV, SC (Adults): *Gastrointestinal anticholinergic*—0.25–0.5 mg 3–4 times daily as needed; *preoperative prophylaxis of secretions*—0.5 mg or 0.005 mg/kg 30–60 min before anesthesia; *antiarrhythmic*—0.125 mg IV repeated as needed; *cholinergic adjunct (curariform block)*—0.2 mg for each 1 mg of neostigmine.
IM, IV, SC (Children ≥2 yr): *preoperative prophylaxis of secretions*—0.005 mg/kg 30–60 min before anesthesia.

Availability (generic available)

Tablets: 0.125 mg, 0.15 mg. **Sublingual tablets:** 0.125 mg, 0.375 mg. **Orally disintegrating tablets (contains aspartame) (mint):** 0.125 mg. **Extended release tablets:** 0.375 mg. **Timed-release capsules:** 0.375 mg. **Solution (drops) (orange):** 0.125 mg/mL. **Elixir (orange):** 0.125 mg/5 mL. **Injection:** 0.5 mg/mL.

ibandronate (i-ban-dro-nate)

Boniva

Classification

Therapeutic: bone resorption inhibitors

Pharmacologic: bisphosphonates

Indications

Treatment/prevention of postmenopausal osteoporosis.

Action

Inhibits resorption of bone by inhibiting osteoclast activity. **Therapeutic Effects:** Reversal/prevention of progression of osteoporosis with decreased fractures.

Adverse Reactions/Side Effects

GI: diarrhea, dyspepsia, esophagitis, esophageal/gastric ulcer. **MS:** musculoskeletal pain, pain in arms/legs, osteonecrosis (primarily of jaw). **Misc:** injection site reactions.

PHYSICAL THERAPY IMPLICATIONS

Examination and Evaluation

- Assess any muscle or joint pain. Report persistent or increased musculoskeletal pain to determine presence of bone or joint pathology, including fracture. Be especially aware of possible mouth and jaw pain due to osteonecrosis of the jaw.
- Monitor IV injection site for pain, swelling, and irritation. Report prolonged or excessive injection site reactions to the physician.

Interventions

- Institute weight-bearing and resistance exercises as tolerated to maintain or increase bone mineral density. Start with low-impact or aquatic programs in patients with extensive demineralization, and increase exercise intensity slowly to prevent fractures.
- Protect against falls and fractures (See Appendix E). Modify home environment (remove throw rugs, improve lighting, etc.) and provide assistive devices (cane, walker) or other protective devices as needed to improve balance and prevent falls.

Patient/Client-Related Instruction

- Instruct patient on the importance of taking exactly as directed and to remain upright for 60 min following oral dose to facilitate passage to stomach and minimize risk of esophageal irritation.
- Instruct patient to notify physician if pain or difficulty swallowing, retrosternal pain, or new/worsening heartburn occur.
- Instruct patient to report other troublesome GI problems such as severe or prolonged diarrhea or indigestion.
- Advise patient about the benefits of proper diet in sustaining bone mineralization. If necessary, refer patient for nutritional counseling about supplemental calcium and vitamin D.
- Encourage patient to modify behaviors that increase the risk of osteoporosis (stop smoking, reduce alcohol consumption).

Pharmacokinetics

Absorption: 0.6% absorbed following oral administration (significantly decreased by food).
Distribution: Rapidly binds to bone.
Protein Binding: 90.9–99.5%.
Metabolism and Excretion: 50–60% excreted in urine; unabsorbed drug is eliminated in feces.
Half-life: *PO*—10–60 hr; *IV*—4.6–25.5 hr.

TIME/ACTION PROFILE

ROUTE	ONSET	PEAK	DURATION
PO	unknown	0.5–2 hr	up to 1 mo
IV	unknown	3 hr	up to 3 mo

Contraindications/Precautions

Contraindicated in: Hypersensitivity; Uncorrected hypocalcemia; Inability to stand/sit upright for at least 60 min; CCr <30 mL/min.
Use Cautiously in: Geri: Consider age-related ↓ in body mass, renal and hepatic function, concurrent disease states and drug therapy; Concurrent use of NSAIDs or aspirin; Concurrent dental surgery (may ↑ risk of jaw osteonecrosis); OB: Use only if potential benefit outweighs risks to mother and fetus; Lactation: Lactation; Pedi: Children <18 yr (safety not established).

Interactions

Drug-Drug: Calcium-, aluminum-, magnesium-, and **iron**-containing products, including **antacids** ↓ absorption (ibandronate should be taken 60 min before). Concurrent use of **NSAIDs,** including **aspirin,** may ↑ risk of gastric irritation.
Drug-Food: Milk and other foods ↓ absorption.

Route/Dosage

PO (Adults): 2.5 mg once daily or 150 mg once monthly.

IV (Adults): 3 mg 1q 3 mo.

Availability

Tablets: 2.5 mg, 150 mg. **Injection:** 3 mg/3 mL in prefilled single-use syringe.

ibritumomab tiuxetan

(i-bri-**too**-mo-mab tye-**uks**-i-tan)

Zevalin

Classification

Therapeutic: antineoplastics

Pharmacologic: monoclonal antibodies, radioisotopes

Indications

Relapsed or refractory low-grade, follicular, or transformed B-cell non-Hodgkin's lymphoma (including rituximab-resistant).

Action

Ibritumomab tiuxetan is a monoclonal antibody linked to a radioisotope that targets white blood cells, including malignant ones. Used in combination with rituximab as part of a two-step process using indium-111 (step 1) and yttrium-90 (step 2) ibritumomab tiuxetan. **Therapeutic Effects:** Decreased spread of lymphoma.

Adverse Reactions/Side Effects

CNS: anxiety, dizziness. **EENT:** rhinitis. **Resp:** dyspnea, increased cough, bronchospasm. **GI:** abdominal pain, anorexia, diarrhea, nausea, vomiting. **Derm:** ecchymoses, pruritus. **Hemat:** LEUKOPENIA, THROMBOCYTOPENIA, anemia. **MS:** arthralgia. **Misc:** INFECTIONS, INFUSION REACTIONS, ALLERGIC REACTIONS, INCLUDING ANAPHYLAXIS, secondary malignancies.

PHYSICAL THERAPY IMPLICATIONS

Examination and Evaluation

- Be alert for signs of allergic reactions and anaphylaxis. Reactions include pulmonary symptoms (tightness in the throat and chest, wheezing, cough, dyspnea) and skin reactions (rash, pruritus, urticaria, burning skin, swelling in the face). Be especially alert for these signs after drug infusion (infusion reactions). Notify physician or nursing staff immediately if these reactions occur.
- Monitor signs of bone marrow suppression, including leukopenia (fever, sore throat, signs of infection), thrombocytopenia (bruising, nose bleeds, bleeding gums), or unusual weakness and fatigue that might be due to anemia. Notify physician of these signs immediately.
- Be alert for signs of infection, including fever, sore throat, chills, nausea, vomiting, diarrhea, and localized inflammation. Notify physician or nursing staff of these signs immediately.
- Monitor signs of secondary malignancy, including a change in bowel or bladder habits, nonhealing sores, unusual bleeding or discharge, a lump in the breast or other parts of the body, chronic indigestion or difficulty in swallowing, obvious changes in a wart or mole, and persistent coughing or hoarseness. Report these signs to the physician immediately.
- Assess symptoms of bronchospasm (wheezing, coughing, tightness in chest) or other prolonged or severe respiratory problems (difficult or labored breathing). Perform pulmonary function tests to quantify suspected changes in ventilation and respiration (See Appendices I, J, K).
- Assess dizziness that might affect gait, balance, and other functional activities (See Appendix C). Report balance problems and functional limitations to the physician and nursing staff, and caution the patient and family/caregivers to guard against falls and trauma.
- Assess any increased joint pain to rule out musculoskeletal pathology; that is, try to determine if pain is drug induced rather than caused by anatomic or biomechanical problems.

Interventions

- For patients who are medically able to begin exercise, implement appropriate resistive exercises and aerobic training to maintain muscle strength and aerobic capacity during cancer chemotherapy or to help restore function after chemotherapy.

Patient/Client-Related Instruction

- Advise patient to guard against infection (frequent hand washing, etc.), and to avoid crowds and contact with persons with contagious diseases.
- Instruct patient or family/caregivers to report other bothersome side effects such as severe or prolonged anxiety, nasal irritation, or GI problems (nausea, vomiting, abdominal pain, loss of appetite).

Pharmacokinetics

Absorption: IV administration results in complete bioavailability.

Distribution: Distributes to lymphoid tissue in bone marrow, lymph nodes, thymus, spleen, tonsils, and lymphoid nodules in the intestinal tract.
Metabolism and Excretion: Over 7 days, 7.2% of injected radioactivity was excreted in urine.
Half-life: Mean half-life of yttrium-90–ibritumomab tiuxetan activity in blood is 30 hr.

TIME/ACTION PROFILE

ROUTE	B-cell depletion	B-cell recovery	B cells in normal range
IV	4 wk	2 wk	9 mo

Contraindications/Precautions

Contraindicated in: Hypersensitivity to ibritumomab tiuxetan, indium-111, yttrium-90, or murine proteins; OB: Pregnancy or lactation.
Use Cautiously in: Thrombocytopenia (step 2 dose of yttrium-90 ibritumomab tiuxetan should be decreased); Pedi: Children (safety not established).

Interactions

Drug-Drug: May ↓ the antibody response to, and ↑ the risk of adverse reactions from, **live-virus vaccines**. ↑ risk of bleeding with **anticoagulants, antiplatelet agents**, and other **agents that may affect hemostasis**. **Growth factor** should be avoided for 2 wk before and 2 wk following treatment.

Route/Dosage

Step 1

IV (Adults): 5 mCi (1.6 mg total antibody dose) of indium-111 ibritumomab tiuxetan, preceded by rituximab 250 mg/m² within 4 hr.

Step 2

IV (Adults): *7–9 days after step 1*—0.4 mCi/kg of yttrium-90 ibritumomab tiuxetan, preceded by rituximab 250 mg/m² within 4 hr.

Availability

Indium-111 (In-111) Zevalin kit: Contains 1 2-mL vial of 3.2 mg ibritumomab tiuxetan in solution, 1 50-mM sodium acetate vial, 1 formulation buffer vial, and 1 empty reaction vial with 4 identification labels (indium-111 is ordered separately). **Yttrium-90 (Y-90) Zevalin kit:** contains 1 2-mL vial of 3.2 mg ibritumomab tiuxetan in solution, 1 50-mM sodium acetate vial, 1 formulation buffer vial, and 1 empty reaction vial with 4 identification labels (yttrium-90 is shipped directly).

ibuprofen, oral

(eye-byoo-**proe**-fen)

Actiprofen, Advil, Advil Migraine Liqui-Gels, Apo-Ibuprofen, Children's Advil, Children's Motrin, Excedrin IB, Genpril, Haltran, Junior Strength Advil, Menadol, Medipren, Midol Maximum Strength Cramp Formula, Motrin, Motrin Drops, Motrin IB, Motrin Junior Strength, Motrin Migraine Pain, Novo-Profen, Nu-Ibuprofen, Nuprin, PediaCare Children's Fever

Classification
Therapeutic: antipyretics, antirheumatics, nonopioid analgesics, nonsteroidal anti-inflammatory agents
Pharmacologic: nonopioid analgesics

Indications

Mild-to-moderate pain or dysmenorrhea. Inflammatory disorders, including Rheumatoid arthritis (including juvenile), Osteoarthritis. Lowering of fever. **Unlabeled Use:** Slows progression of lung disease in cystic fibrosis patients >5 yrs of age (high doses).

Action

Inhibits prostaglandin synthesis. **Therapeutic Effects:** Decreased pain and inflammation. Reduction of fever.

Adverse Reactions/Side Effects

CNS: headache, dizziness, drowsiness, psychic disturbances. **EENT:** amblyopia, blurred vision, tinnitus. **CV:** arrhythmias, edema. **GI:** GI BLEEDING, HEPATITIS, constipation, dyspepsia, nausea, vomiting, abdominal discomfort. **GU:** cystitis, hematuria, renal failure. **Derm:** EXFOLIATIVE DERMATITIS, STEVENS-JOHNSON SYNDROME, TOXIC EPIDERMAL NECROLYSIS, rashes. **Hemat:** blood dyscrasias, prolonged bleeding time. **Misc:** ALLERGIC REACTIONS, INCLUDING ANAPHYLAXIS.

PHYSICAL THERAPY IMPLICATIONS

Examination and Evaluation

- Monitor signs of GI bleeding, including abdominal pain, vomiting blood, blood in stools, or black, tarry stools. Report these signs to the physician immediately.

- Be alert for signs of drug-induced hepatitis, including anorexia, abdominal pain, severe nausea and vomiting, yellow skin or eyes, skin rashes, flu-like symptoms, and muscle/joint pain. Report these signs to the physician immediately.
- Monitor signs of allergic reactions and anaphylaxis, including pulmonary symptoms (laryngeal edema, wheezing, cough, dyspnea) or skin reactions (rash, pruritus, urticaria). Be especially alert for exfoliation, dermatitis, and other severe skin reactions that might indicate serious hypersensitivity reactions (Stevens-Johnson syndrome, toxic epidermal necrolysis). Notify physician immediately if these reactions occur.
- Assess pain and other variables (range of motion, muscle strength) to document whether this drug is successful in helping manage the patient's pain and decreasing impairments.
- Assess heart rate, ECG, and heart sounds, especially during exercise (See Appendices G, H). Report any rhythm disturbances or symptoms of increased arrhythmias, including palpitations, chest discomfort, shortness of breath, fainting, and fatigue/weakness.
- Assess blood pressure (BP) periodically and compare to normal values (See Appendix F). NSAIDs can increase BP in certain patients.
- Be alert for signs of prolonged bleeding time such as bleeding gums, nosebleeds, and unusual or excessive bruising. Report these signs to the physician.
- Assess peripheral edema using girth measurements, volume displacement, and measurement of pitting edema (See Appendix N). Report increased swelling in feet and ankles or a sudden increase in body weight due to fluid retention.
- Monitor signs of kidney dysfunction such as painful urination or blood in the urine. Report signs of renal failure immediately, including decreased urine output, increased BP, muscle cramps/twitching, edema/weight gain from fluid retention, yellowish brown skin, and confusion that progresses to seizures and coma.
- Monitor unusual weakness and fatigue that might be due to anemia or other symptoms such as fever, sore throat, mucosal lesions, or signs of infection that might be due to other blood dyscrasias. Notify physician if these signs occur.
- Assess dizziness and drowsiness that might affect gait, balance, and other functional activities (See Appendix C). Report balance problems and functional limitations to the physician, and caution the patient and family/caregivers to guard against falls and trauma.
- Monitor and report confusion, agitation, or other psychic disturbances.

Interventions

- Implement appropriate manual therapy techniques, physical agents, and therapeutic exercises to reduce pain and decrease the need for ibuprofen and other NSAIDs.
- Because of the risk of arrhythmias, use caution during aerobic exercise and other forms of therapeutic exercise. Assess exercise tolerance frequently (BP, heart rate, fatigue levels), and terminate exercise immediately if any untoward responses occur (See Appendix L).
- If treating arthritic conditions, recommend orthotic and assistive devices as needed to reduce pain, improve function, and augment the effects of drug therapy.
- Use caution with any physical interventions that could increase bleeding, including wound débridement, chest percussion, joint mobilization, and application of local heat.
- Help patient explore other nonpharmacologic methods to reduce chronic pain, such as relaxation techniques, exercise, counseling, and so forth.

Patient/Client-Related Instruction

- Advise patient that analgesics are usually more effective if given before pain becomes severe; emphasize that adequate pain control will allow better participation in physical therapy.
- Inform patient that NSAIDs may impair bone and cartilage healing. Advise patient to consult physician about NSAID use, especially after fractures, spinal fusion, and other bone surgeries.
- Caution patient about the use of over-the-counter products that contain NSAIDs or acetaminophen while taking prescription doses of ibuprofen. Use of multiple NSAIDs increases the risk of toxicity and overdose.
- Instruct patient to report excessive or prolonged headache or ringing/buzzing in the ears (tinnitus); these signs may indicate drug toxicity.
- Advise patient about the risks of gastric irritation. Instruct patient to notify physician of GI reactions such as severe or prolonged nausea, vomiting, constipation, indigestion, and abdominal pain.
- Advise patient to reduce alcohol intake because alcohol increases the risk of gastric toxicity.

Pharmacokinetics

Absorption: Well absorbed (80%) from the GI tract.
Distribution: Does not enter breast milk in significant amounts.
Protein Binding: 99%.
Metabolism and Excretion: Mostly metabolized by the liver; small amounts (1%) excreted unchanged by the kidneys.
Half-life: Children: 1–2 hr; Adults: 2–4 hr.

TIME/ACTION PROFILE

ROUTE	ONSET	PEAK	DURATION
PO (antipyretic)	0.5–2.5 hr	2–4 hr	6–8 hr
PO (analgesic)	30 min	1–2 hr	4–6 hr
PO (anti-inflammatory)	7 days	1–2 wk	unknown

Contraindications/Precautions

Contraindicated in: Hypersensitivity; Cross-sensitivity may exist with other NSAIDs, including aspirin; Active GI bleeding or ulcer disease; Chewable tablets contain aspartame and should not be used in patients with phenylketonuria; Perioperative pain from coronary artery bypass graft (CABG) surgery.

Use Cautiously in: Cardiovascular disease (may ↑ risk of cardiovascular events); Renal or hepatic disease, dehydration, or patients on nephrotoxic drugs (may ↑ risk of renal toxicity); Aspirin triad patients (asthma, nasal polyps, and aspirin intolerance); can cause fatal anaphylactoid reactions; Geri: ↑ risk of adverse reactions secondary to age-related ↓ in renal and hepatic function, concurrent illnesses, and medications; Chronic alcohol use/abuse; History of ulcer disease (may ↑ risk of GI bleeding); OB: Not recommended for pregnant patients; has been associated with persistent pulmonary hypertension in infants; Lactation: Has been used safely; Pedi: Safety not established for infants <6 mo.

Interactions

Drug-Drug: May limit the cardioprotective effects of low-dose **aspirin**. Concurrent use with **aspirin** may ↓ effectiveness of ibuprofen. Additive adverse GI side effects with **aspirin, oral potassium** and other **NSAIDs, corticosteroids**, or **alcohol**. Chronic use with **acetaminophen** may ↑ risk of adverse renal reactions. May ↓ effectiveness of **diuretics** or **antihypertensives.** May ↑ hypoglycemic effects of **insulin** or **oral hypoglycemic agents**. May slightly ↑ serum **digoxin** levels. May ↑ serum **lithium** levels and risk of toxicity. ↑ risk of toxicity from **methotrexate**. **Probenecid** ↑ risk of toxicity from ibuprofen. ↑ risk of bleeding with **cefotetan, cefoperazone, valproic acid, thrombolytics, warfarin**, and **drugs affecting platelet function**, including **clopidogrel, ticlopidine, abciximab, eptifibatide**, or **tirofiban**. ↑ risk of adverse hematologic reactions with **antineoplastics** or **radiation therapy**. ↑ risk of nephrotoxicity with **cyclosporine**.

Drug-Natural: ↑ bleeding risk with, **arnica, chamomile, feverfew, garlic, ginger, ginkgo, *Panax ginseng***, and others.

Route/Dosage

Analgesia

PO (Adults): *Anti-inflammatory*—400–800 mg 3–4 times daily (not to exceed 3600 mg/day). *Analgesic/antidysmenorrheal/antipyretic* —200–400 mg q 4–6 hr (not to exceed 1200 mg/day).

PO (Children 6 mo–12 yr): *Anti-inflammatory*—30–50 mg/kg/day in 3–4 divided doses (maximum dose 2.4 g/day). *Antipyretic*—5 mg/kg for temperature <102.5°F (39.17°C) or 10 mg/kg for higher temperatures (not to exceed 40 mg/kg/day); may be repeated q 4–6 hr. *Cystic fibrosis (unlabeled)*—20–30 mg/kg/day divided bid.

PO (Infants and Children): *Analgesic*—4–10 mg/kg/dose q 6–8 hr.

Pediatric OTC Dosing

PO (Children 11 yr/72–95 lb): 300 mg q 6–8 hr.
PO (Children 9–10 yr/60–71 lb): 250 mg q 6–8 hr.
PO (Children 6–8 yr/48–59 lb): 200 mg q 6–8 hr.
PO (Children 4–5 yr/36–47 lb): 150 mg q 6–8 hr.
PO (Children 2–3 yr/24–35 lb): 100 mg q 6–8 hr.
PO (Children 12–23 mo/18–23 lb): 75 mg q 6–8 hr.
PO (Infants 6–11 mo/12–17 lb): 50 mg q 6–8 hr.

Availability (generic available)

Tablets: 100 mg OTC, 200 mg OTC, 300 mg, 400 mg, 600 mg, 800 mg. **Capsules (liqui-gels):** 200 mg OTC. **Chewable tablets (fruit, grape, orange, and citrus flavor):** 50 mg OTC, 100 mg OTC. **Liquid (berry flavor):** 100 mg/5 mL OTC. **Oral suspension (fruit, berry, grape flavor):** 100 mg/5 mL OTC, 100 mg/2.5 mL OTC. **Pediatric drops (berry flavor):** 50 mg/1.25 mL OTC. ***In combination with:*** decongestants, OTC, hydrocodone (Vicoprofen), oxycodone (Combunox). See Appendix B.

ibutilide (eye-byoo-ti-lide)

Corvert

Classification

Therapeutic: antiarrhythmics (class III)

Indications

Rapid conversion of recent-onset atrial flutter or fibrillation to normal sinus rhythm, including management of atrial flutter or fibrillation occurring within 1 wk of coronary artery bypass or cardiac valve surgery.

Action

Activates slow inward current of sodium in cardiac tissue, resulting in delayed repolarization, prolonged action potential duration, and increased refractoriness. Mildly slows sinus rate and AV conduction. **Therapeutic Effects:** Conversion to normal sinus rhythm.

Adverse Reactions/Side Effects

CNS: headache. **CV:** arrhythmias. **GI:** nausea.

PHYSICAL THERAPY IMPLICATIONS

Examination and Evaluation

- Assess heart rate, ECG, and heart sounds, especially during exercise (See Appendices G, H). Although intended to treat certain arrhythmias, this drug can unmask or precipitate new arrhythmias (proarrhythmic effect). Report any rhythm disturbances or symptoms of increased arrhythmias, including palpitations, chest pain, shortness of breath, fainting, and fatigue/weakness.

Interventions

- Because of the risk of arrhythmias, use caution during aerobic exercise and other forms of therapeutic exercise. Assess exercise tolerance frequently (blood pressure, heart rate, fatigue levels), and terminate exercise immediately if any untoward responses occur (See Appendix L).

Patient/Client-Related Instruction

- Advise patient and family or caregivers about the signs of arrhythmias (see above under Examination and Evaluation) and to seek immediate medical assistance if these signs develop.
- Instruct patient and family/caregivers to report other side effects such as severe or prolonged headache or nausea.

Pharmacokinetics

Absorption: IV administration results in complete bioavailability.
Distribution: Unknown.
Metabolism and Excretion: Highly metabolized by the liver, 1 metabolite is active; metabolites excreted by kidneys.
Half-life: 6 hr (2–12 hr).

TIME/ACTION PROFILE (antiarrhythmic effect)

ROUTE	ONSET	PEAK	DURATION
IV	within 30–90 min	unknown	up to 24 hr

Contraindications/Precautions

Contraindicated in: Hypersensitivity.
Use Cautiously in: CHF or left ventricular dysfunction (↑ risk of more serious arrhythmias during infusion); Pregnancy, lactation, or children <18 yr (safety not established).

Interactions

Drug-Drug: Amiodarone, disopyramide, procainamide, quinidine, and **sotalol** should not be given concurrently or within 4 hr because of additive effects on refractoriness. Proarrhythmic effects may be ↑ by **phenothiazines, tricyclic** and **tetracyclic antidepressants**, some **antihistamines**, and **histamine H_2 receptor blocking agents**; concurrent use should be avoided.

Route/Dosage

Atrial Fibrillation/Flutter

IV (Adults ≥60 kg): 1 mg infusion; may be repeated 10 min after end of first infusion.
IV (Adults <60 kg): 0.01 mg/kg infusion; may be repeated 10 min after end of first infusion.

Atrial Fibrillation/Flutter After Cardiac Surgery

IV (Adults ≥60 kg): 0.5 mg infusion, may be repeated once.
IV (Adults <60 kg): 0.005 mg/kg infusion, may be repeated once.

Availability

Solution for injection: 0.1 mg/mL in 10-mL vial.

idarubicin (eye-da-roo-bi-sin)

Idamycin

Classification
Therapeutic: antineoplastics
Pharmacologic: anthracyclines

Indications

Acute myelogenous leukemia in adults (with other agents).

Action

Inhibits nucleic acid synthesis. **Therapeutic Effects:** Death of rapidly replicating cells, particularly malignant ones.

Adverse Reactions/Side Effects

CNS: headache, mental status changes. **Resp:** pulmonary toxicity, pulmonary allergic reactions. **CV:** ARRHYTHMIAS, CARDIOTOXICITY, CHF. **GI:** abdominal cramps, diarrhea, mucositis, nausea, vomiting. **Derm:** alopecia, photosensitivity, rashes. **Endo:** gonadal suppression. **Hemat:** BLEEDING, anemia, leukopenia, thrombocytopenia. **Local:** phlebitis at IV site. **Metab:** hyperuricemia. **Neuro:** peripheral neuropathy. **Misc:** fever.

PHYSICAL THERAPY IMPLICATIONS

Examination and Evaluation

- Be alert for signs of cardiotoxicity and heart failure, including dyspnea, rales/crackles, peripheral edema, jugular venous distention, and exercise intolerance. Report these signs to the physician or nursing staff immediately.

- Assess heart rate, ECG, and heart sounds, especially during exercise (See Appendices G, H). Report any rhythm disturbances or symptoms of increased arrhythmias, including palpitations, chest discomfort, shortness of breath, fainting, and fatigue/weakness.
- Watch for signs of bleeding and hemorrhage, including bleeding gums, nosebleeds, unusual bruising, black/tarry stools, hematuria, or a fall in hematocrit or blood pressure. Notify physician or nursing staff immediately if these signs occur.
- Assess for signs of pulmonary toxicity or allergic reactions, including rales/crackles, decreased breath sounds, pleuritic friction rub, fatigue, tachypnea, cough, wheezing, pleuritic pain, fever, hemoptysis, and hypoxia. Notify physician or nursing staff immediately if these signs occur.
- Monitor signs of leukopenia (fever, sore throat, signs of infection), thrombocytopenia (bruising, nose bleeds, bleeding gums), or unusual weakness and fatigue that might be due to anemia. Report these signs to the physician or nursing staff.
- Be alert for signs of peripheral neuropathy (numbness, tingling, decreased muscle strength). Establish baseline electroneuromyographic values using EMG and nerve conduction at the beginning of drug treatment whenever possible, and reexamine these values periodically to document drug-induced changes in peripheral nerve function.
- Assess confusion, agitation, or other alterations in mental status (See Appendix D). Notify physician promptly if these symptoms develop.
- Monitor IV injection site for pain, swelling, and inflammation (phlebitis). Report signs of phlebitis or other prolonged or excessive injection site reactions to the physician.

Interventions

- For patients who are medically able to begin exercise, implement appropriate resistive exercises and aerobic training to maintain muscle strength and aerobic capacity during cancer chemotherapy or to help restore function after chemotherapy.
- Because of the risk of cardiotoxicity and arrhythmias, use caution during aerobic exercise and other forms of therapeutic exercise. Assess exercise tolerance frequently (blood pressure, heart rate, respiratory symptoms, fatigue levels), and terminate exercise immediately if any untoward responses occur (See Appendix L).
- Causes photosensitivity; use care if administering UV treatments. Advise patient to avoid direct sunlight and use sunscreens and protective clothing.

Patient/Client-Related Instruction

- Instruct patient to guard against infection (frequent hand washing, etc.), and to avoid crowds and contact with persons with contagious diseases.
- Advise patient about the likelihood of GI reactions such as diarrhea, nausea, vomiting, abdominal pain, and irritation in or around the mouth. Instruct patient or family and caregivers to report other severe or unexpected GI problems.
- Advise patient that rash, hair loss, and other skin reactions are likely. Report any severe or unexpected skin reactions.
- Advise patient and family/caregivers to report other bothersome side effects such as severe or prolonged headache or fever.

Pharmacokinetics

Absorption: IV administration results in complete bioavailability.
Distribution: Rapidly distributed with extensive tissue binding. High degree of cellular uptake.
Metabolism and Excretion: Extensive hepatic and extrahepatic metabolism. One metabolite is active (idarubicinol). Primarily eliminated via biliary excretion.
Half-life: 22 hr (range 4–46 hr).

TIME/ACTION PROFILE (effects on blood counts)

ROUTE	ONSET	PEAK	DURATION
IV	unknown	10–14 days	21 days

Contraindications/Precautions

Contraindicated in: Pregnancy or lactation.
Use Cautiously in: Children (safety not established); Patients with childbearing potential; Active infection; Decreased bone marrow reserve; Geriatric patients; Other chronic debilitating illnesses; Hepatic impairment (dose reduction may be required; avoid if bilirubin ≥5 mg/dL); Renal impairment; Preexisting cardiac disease; Previous daunorubicin or doxorubicin therapy.

Interactions

Drug-Drug: ↑ myelosuppression with other **antineoplastics** or **radiation therapy**. May ↓ antibody response to and increase risk of adverse reactions from **live-virus vaccines**.

Route/Dosage

IV (Adults): 12 mg/m^2 daily for 3 days in combination with cytarabine.

Availability (generic available)

Powder for injection: 5-mg vials, 10-mg vials.

ifosfamide (eye-fos-fam-ide)

Ifex

Classification

Therapeutic: antineoplastics

Pharmacologic: alkylating agents

Indications

Germ-cell testicular carcinoma (with other agents). Used with mesna, which prevents ifosfamide-induced hemorrhagic cystitis.

Action

Following conversion to active compounds, interferes with DNA replication and RNA transcription, ultimately disrupting protein synthesis (cell-cycle phase–nonspecific). **Therapeutic Effects:** Death of rapidly replicating cells, particularly malignant ones.

Adverse Reactions/Side Effects

CNS: CNS toxicity (somnolence, confusion, hallucinations, coma), cranial nerve dysfunction, disorientation, dizziness. **CV:** cardiotoxicity. **GI:** nausea, vomiting, anorexia, constipation, diarrhea, hepatotoxicity. **GU:** hemorrhagic cystitis, dysuria, sterility, renal toxicity. **Derm:** alopecia. **Hemat:** anemia, leukopenia, thrombocytopenia. **Local:** phlebitis. **Misc:** allergic reactions.

PHYSICAL THERAPY IMPLICATIONS

Examination and Evaluation

- Monitor signs of CNS toxicity, including confusion, disorientation, hallucinations, decreased alertness, or cranial nerve dysfunction. Notify physician or nursing staff immediately because these symptoms can worsen and progress to coma.
- Assess heart rate, ECG, and blood pressure, especially during exercise. Report any abnormal cardiac responses or signs of cardiac toxicity, including arrhythmias, chest discomfort, shortness of breath, fainting, or fatigue/weakness.
- Monitor signs of allergic reactions, including pulmonary symptoms (tightness in the throat and chest, wheezing, cough, dyspnea) or skin reactions (rash, pruritus, urticaria). Notify physician or nursing staff immediately if these reactions occur.
- Watch for signs of leukopenia (fever, sore throat, signs of infection), thrombocytopenia (bruising, nose bleeds and bleeding gums), or unusual weakness and fatigue that might be due to anemia. Report these signs to the physician or nursing staff.
- Monitor and report problems with urination or signs of kidney toxicity, including blood or pus in urine, decreased urine output, weight gain from fluid retention, and fatigue.
- Assess dizziness that might affect gait, balance, and other functional activities (See Appendix C). Report balance problems and functional limitations to the physician and nursing staff, and caution the patient and family/caregivers to guard against falls and trauma.
- Monitor IV injection site for pain, swelling, and inflammation. Report prolonged or excessive injection site reactions to the physician.

Interventions

- For patients who are medically able to begin exercise, implement appropriate resistive exercises and aerobic training to maintain muscle strength and aerobic capacity during cancer chemotherapy or to help restore function after chemotherapy.
- Because of the risk of cardiotoxicity, use caution during aerobic exercise and other forms of therapeutic exercise. Assess exercise tolerance frequently (blood pressure, heart rate, fatigue levels), and terminate exercise immediately if any untoward responses occur (See Appendix L).

Patient/Client-Related Instruction

- Advise patient to guard against infection (frequent hand washing, etc.), and to avoid crowds and contact with persons with contagious diseases.
- Advise patient about the likelihood of GI reactions such as nausea, vomiting, diarrhea, and constipation. Instruct patient or family and caregivers to report severe or prolonged GI problems, and to also report signs of hepatotoxicity, including loss of appetite, abdominal pain, severe nausea and vomiting, yellow skin or eyes, fever, sore throat, malaise, weakness, facial edema, lethargy, and unusual bleeding or bruising.
- Advise patient that hair loss is likely, but to report other severe or unexpected skin reactions to the physician.

Pharmacokinetics

Absorption: Administered IV only; inactive prior to conversion to metabolites.

Distribution: Excreted in breast milk.

Metabolism and Excretion: Metabolized by the liver to active antineoplastic compounds.

Half-life: 15 hr.

TIME/ACTION PROFILE (effects on blood counts)

ROUTE	ONSET	PEAK	DURATION
IV	unknown	7–14 days	21 days

Contraindications/Precautions

Contraindicated in: Hypersensitivity; Pregnancy or lactation.

Use Cautiously in: Patients with childbearing potential; Active infections; ↓ bone marrow reserve; Geriatric patients; Other chronic debilitating illness; Impaired renal function; Children.

Interactions

Drug-Drug: ↑ myelosuppression with other **antineoplastics** or **radiation therapy**. Toxicity may be ↑ by **allopurinol** or **phenobarbital**. May ↓ antibody response to and ↑ risk of adverse reactions from **live-virus vaccines**.

Route/Dosage

Other Regimens are Used

IV (Adults): 1.2 g/m^2/day for 5 days; coadminister with mesna. May repeat cycle q 3 wk.

Availability

Injection: 1- and 3-g vials. ***In combination with:*** In a kit with mesna.

Iloprost (eye-lo-prost)

Ventavis

Classification

Therapeutic: vasodilators

Pharmacologic: prostacyclins

Indications

Management of New York Class III/IV symptoms of pulmonary hypertension, where there is marked limitation of physical activity.

Action

Dilates pulmonary and arterial vasculature. **Therapeutic Effects:** Improved exercise capacity.

Adverse Reactions/Side Effects

CNS: fainting, headache, insomnia. **Resp:** ↑ cough, dyspnea, hemoptysis. **CV:** CHF, vasodilation, chest pain, hypotension, peripheral edema, supraventricular tachycardia. **GI:** nausea, vomiting. **GU:** renal failure. **Derm:** facial flushing. **MS:** back pain, jaw-muscle spasm, muscle cramps.

PHYSICAL THERAPY IMPLICATIONS

Examination and Evaluation

- Assess signs of congestive heart failure, including dyspnea, rales/crackles, peripheral edema, jugular venous distention, and exercise intolerance. Report these signs to the physician immediately.
- Assess heart rate, ECG, and heart sounds, especially during exercise (See Appendices G, H). Report any rhythm disturbances or symptoms of increased arrhythmias, including palpitations, chest pain, shortness of breath, dyspnea, fainting, and fatigue/weakness.
- Assess blood pressure (BP) periodically, and compare to normal values (See Appendix F). Report low BP (hypotension), especially if patient experiences dizziness, fainting, or other symptoms.
- Monitor signs of renal failure, including decreased urine output, increased BP, muscle cramps/twitching, edema/weight gain from fluid retention, yellowish brown skin, and confusion that progresses to seizures and coma. Report these signs to the physician immediately.
- Assess any back pain and muscle cramps or spasms to rule out musculoskeletal pathology; that is, try to determine if pain is drug induced rather than caused by anatomic or biomechanical problems.
- Assess any breathing problems such as increased cough, coughing up blood, or difficult, labored breathing. Report excessive or prolonged respiratory problems to the physician.
- Monitor signs of vasodilation including redness, warmth, flushing, and edema in the face and extremities. Report any problematic vasodilation to the physician.

Interventions

- Because of the risk of arrhythmias and abnormal BP responses, use caution during aerobic exercise and other forms of therapeutic exercise. Assess exercise tolerance frequently (BP, heart rate, fatigue levels), and terminate exercise immediately if any untoward responses occur (See Appendix L).
- Avoid physical therapy interventions that cause systemic vasodilation (large whirlpool, Hubbard tank). Additive effects of this drug and the intervention may cause a dangerous fall in BP.
- To minimize orthostatic hypotension, patient should move slowly when assuming a more upright position.

Patient/Client-Related Instruction

- Instruct patient or family/caregivers to report other troublesome side effects such as severe or prolonged headache, sleep loss, or GI problems (nausea, vomiting).

Pharmacokinetics

Absorption: Unknown.
Distribution: Unknown.
Metabolism and Excretion: Any absorbed iloprost is metabolized.
Half-life: 20–30 min (plasma).

TIME/ACTION PROFILE (improved exercise capacity)

ROUTE	ONSET	PEAK	DURATION
Oral	unknown	unknown	up to 2 hr

Contraindications/Precautions

Contraindicated in: Hypersensitivity; Systolic BP <85 mm Hg; Lactation.

Use Cautiously in: Concurrent use of drugs or coexisting medical conditions which may ↑ risk of syncope; Children (safety not established); Pregnancy (use only if maternal benefit outweighs fetal risk).

Interactions

Drug-Drug: ↑ risk of hypotension with other **vasodilators** or **diuretics**. Risk of bleeding may be ↑ by **anticoagulants**.

Route/Dosage

Inhaln (Adults): 2.5 mcg initially, then 5 mcg/dose 6–9 times daily; not more than q 2 hr.

Availability

Solution for inhalation: 20 mcg/2-mL ampules.

HIGH ALERT

imatinib (i-mat-i-nib)

Gleevec

Classification

Therapeutic: antineoplastics

Pharmacologic: enzyme inhibitors

Indications

Newly diagnosed Philadelphia positive (Ph+) chronic myeloid leukemia (CML). CML in blast crisis, accelerated phase, or in chronic phase after failure of interferon-alpha treatment. Kit (CD117) positive Metastatic/unresectable malignant gastrointestinal stomal tumors (GIST). Pediatric patients with Ph+ CML after failure of bone marrow transplant or resistance to interferon-alpha. Adult patients with relapsed or refractory Ph+ acute lymphoblastic leukemia (ALL). Myelodysplastic/myeloproliferative disease (MDS/MPD). Aggressive systemic mastocytosis (ASM). Hypereosinophilic syndrome and/or Chronic eosinophilic leukemia (HES/CEL). Unresectable, recurrent, or metastatic Dermatofibrosarcoma protuberans (DFSP).

Action

Inhibits kinases which may be produced by malignant cell lines. **Therapeutic Effects:** Inhibits production of malignant cell lines with decreased proliferation of leukemic cells in CML, HES/CEL, and ALL and malignant cells in GIST, MDS/MPD, ASM, and DFSP.

Adverse Reactions/Side Effects

CNS: fatigue, headache, weakness. **Resp:** cough, dyspnea, epistaxis, nasopharyngitis, pneumonia. **GI:** HEPATOTOXICITY, abdominal pain, anorexia, constipation, diarrhea, dyspepsia, nausea, vomiting. **Derm:** petechiae, pruritus, skin rash. **F and E:** edema (including pleural effusion, pericardial infusion, anasarca, superficial edema and fluid retention), hypokalemia. **Hemat:** BLEEDING, NEUTROPENIA, THROMBOCYTOPENIA. **Metab:** weight gain. **MS:** arthralgia, muscle cramps, musculoskeletal pain, myalgia. **Misc:** fever, night sweats.

PHYSICAL THERAPY IMPLICATIONS

Examination and Evaluation

- Be alert for signs of hepatotoxicity, including anorexia, abdominal pain, severe nausea and vomiting, yellow skin or eyes, fever, sore throat, malaise, weakness, facial edema, lethargy, and unusual bleeding or bruising. Report these signs to the physician or nursing staff immediately.
- Monitor signs of neutropenia (fever, sore throat, signs of infection), thrombocytopenia (bruising, nose bleeds, bleeding gums), or any other unusual bleeding. Report these signs immediately to the physician or nursing staff.
- Assess any breathing problems or signs of pneumonia such as cough, fever, chills, and chest pain during inspiration and expiration. Monitor pulse oximetry and perform pulmonary function tests (See Appendices I, J, K) to quantify suspected changes in ventilation and respiratory function.
- Assess peripheral edema using girth measurements, volume displacement, and measurement of pitting edema (See Appendix N). Report increased swelling in feet and ankles or a sudden increase in body weight due to fluid retention.
- Monitor signs of pericardial infusion (chest pain, pressure) or pleural effusion (rales/crackles, decreased breath sounds, pleuritic friction rub, fatigue, dyspnea, tachypnea, cough, wheezing, pleuritic pain, hypoxia). Notify physician of these signs.
- Assess any muscle or joint pain to rule out musculoskeletal pathology; that is, try to determine if pain is drug induced rather than caused by anatomic or biomechanical problems.
- Monitor neuromuscular signs of low potassium levels (hypokalemia), including headache, lethargy, weakness, cramping, and muscle hyperexcitability and tetany. Notify physician immediately if these signs occur.
- Periodically assess body weight, and report a rapid or unexplained weight gain.

Interventions

- For patients who are medically able to begin exercise, implement appropriate resistive exercises and aerobic training to maintain muscle strength and aerobic capacity during cancer chemotherapy or to help restore function after chemotherapy.

- Because of potential pulmonary toxicity and pleural/pericardial edema, use caution during aerobic exercise and endurance conditioning. Terminate exercise if patient exhibits untoward symptoms (chest pain, shortness of breath, etc.), or displays other criteria for exercise termination (See Appendix L).

Patient/Client-Related Instruction

- Advise patient to guard against infection (frequent hand washing, etc.), and to avoid crowds and contact with persons with contagious diseases.
- Advise patient that skin reactions are likely, including rash, pruritus, and bruising. Report severe or unexpected skin reactions to the physician.
- Advise patient about the likelihood of GI reactions (abdominal pain, constipation, diarrhea, nausea, vomiting, loss of appetite, heartburn). Instruct patient to report severe, prolonged GI problems, or signs of liver toxicity as indicated above (See Examination and Evaluation).
- Instruct patient or family/caregivers to report other bothersome side effects such as severe or prolonged headache, fever, nasal irritation, or night sweats.

Pharmacokinetics

Absorption: Well absorbed (98%) following oral administration.
Distribution: Unknown.
Protein Binding: 95%.
Metabolism and Excretion: Mostly metabolized by the CYP3A4 enzyme system to N-dimethyl imatinib, which is as active as imatinib. Excreted mostly in feces as metabolites. 5% excreted unchanged in urine.
Half-life: *Imatinib*—18 hr; *N-dimethyl imatinib*—40 hr.

TIME/ACTION PROFILE (blood levels of imatinib)

ROUTE	ONSET	PEAK	DURATION
PO	unknown	2–4 hr	24 hr

Contraindications/Precautions

Contraindicated in: Hypersensitivity; OB: Potential for fetal harm; Lactation: Potential for serious adverse reactions in nursing infants; breast-feeding should be avoided.
Use Cautiously in: Hepatic impairment (dose reduction recommended if bilirubin >3 times normal or liver transaminases >5 times normal); Cardiac disease (severe congestive heart failure and left ventricular dysfunction may occur); Pedi: Safety not established for children <3 yr; Geri: Increased risk of edema.

Interactions

Drug-Drug: Blood levels and effects are ↑ by concurrent **ketoconazole**. Blood levels and effects may be ↓ by **phenytoin**. ↑ blood levels of **simvastatin**. Imatinib inhibits the following enzyme systems: CYP2C9, CYP2D6, CYP3A4/5, and may be expected to alter the effects of other drugs metabolized by these systems.

Route/Dosage

Chronic myeloid leukemia

PO (Adults): *Chronic phase*—400 mg once daily, may be increased to 600 mg once daily; *accelerated phase or blast crisis*—600 mg once daily; may be increased to 800 mg/day given as 400 mg bid based on response and circumstances.
PO (Children): *Newly diagnosed Ph+ CML*—340 mg/m²/day (not to exceed 600 mg); *CML recurrent after failure of bone marrow transplant or resistance to interferon-alpha*—260 mg/m²/day.

Hepatic Impairment

PO (Adults and Children): Decrease dose by 25% in patients with severe hepatic impairment.

Gastrointestinal Stromal Tumors

PO (Adults): 400 mg/day or 600 mg/day as a single dose.

Ph+ Acute Lymphoblastic Leukemia

PO (Adults): 600 mg/day.

Myelodysplastic/Myeloproliferative diseases

PO (Adults): 400 mg/day.

Aggressive Systemic Mastocytosis

PO (Adults): 400 mg/day. *For patients with eosinophilia*—100 mg/day; increase to 400 mg if well tolerated and response insufficient.

Hypereosinophilic Syndrome and/or Chronic Eosinophilic Leukemia

PO (Adults): 400 mg/day. *For patients with FIP1L1–PDGFRa fusion kinase* 100 mg/day; increase to 400 mg if well tolerated and response insufficient.

Dermatofibrosarcoma Protuberans

PO (Adults): 800 mg/day.

Availability

Tablets: 100 mg, 400 mg.

imiglucerase
(i-mi-**gloo**-ser-ase)
Cerezyme

Classification
Therapeutic: replacement enzymes

Indications
Treatment of symptomatic type 1 Gaucher's disease.

Action
Prevents the accumulation of glucocerebrosides in cells. Replaces glucocerebrosidases that are deficient in type 1 Gaucher's disease. **Therapeutic Effects:** Improvement in symptoms of Gaucher's disease (anemia, thrombocytopenia, bone disease, splenomegaly, and hepatomegaly).

Adverse Reactions/Side Effects
CNS: dizziness, headache. **CV:** mild hypotension. **GI:** abdominal discomfort, nausea. **GU:** decreased urinary frequency. **Derm:** pruritus, rash. **Misc:** antibody production, hypersensitivity reactions, fever.

PHYSICAL THERAPY IMPLICATIONS

Examination and Evaluation
- Monitor signs of hypersensitivity reactions, including pulmonary symptoms (tightness in the throat and chest, wheezing, cough, dyspnea) or skin reactions (rash, pruritus, urticaria). Notify physician or nursing staff immediately if these reactions occur.
- Assess blood pressure periodically and compare to normal values (See Appendix F). Report low blood pressure (hypotension), especially if patient experiences dizziness, fatigue, or syncope.
- Assess dizziness that might affect gait, balance, and other functional activities (See Appendix C). Report balance problems and functional limitations to the physician and nursing staff, and caution the patient and family/caregivers to guard against falls and trauma.

Interventions
- Implement therapeutic exercises (resistive training, coordination exercises, gait training) to complement the effects of drug therapy and help achieve optimal function.

Patient/Client-Related Instruction
- Instruct patient and family/caregivers to report other troublesome side effects such as severe or prolonged headache, fever, urinary retention, skin problems (rash, itching), or GI problems (nausea, abdominal pain).

Pharmacokinetics
Absorption: IV administration results in complete bioavailability.
Distribution: Widely distributed.
Metabolism and Excretion: Excreted mainly by the kidneys.
Half-life: 3.6–10.4 min.

TIME/ACTION PROFILE (improvement in symptoms)

ROUTE	ONSET	PEAK	DURATION
IV	unknown	unknown	unknown

Contraindications/Precautions
Contraindicated in: Hypersensitivity.
Use Cautiously in: Pregnancy or lactation (safety not established).

Interactions
Drug-Drug: None significant.

Route/Dosage
IV (Adults and Children): Range 2.5 units/kg 3 times weekly to 15–60 units/kg q 1–2 wk. Evaluate dosage every 6 mo for possible reduction.

Availability
Injection: 200 units/vial.

imipenem/cilastatin
(im-i-**pen**-em/sye-la-**stat**-in)
Primaxin

Classification
Therapeutic: anti-infectives
Pharmacologic: carbapenems

Indications
Treatment of Lower respiratory tract infections, urinary tract infections, abdominal infections, gynecologic infections, skin and skin structure infections, bone and joint infections, bacteremia, endocarditis, polymicrobic infections.

Action
Imipenem binds to the bacterial cell wall, resulting in cell death. Combination with cilastatin prevents renal inactivation of imipenem, resulting in high urinary concentrations. Imipenem resists the actions of many enzymes that degrades most other penicillins and penicillin-like anti-infectives. **Therapeutic Effects:** Bactericidal action against susceptible bacteria. **Spectrum:** Spectrum is broad. Active against most gram-positive aerobic cocci: *Streptococcus pneumoniae*, Group A beta-hemolytic streptococci, *Enterococcus*, *Staphylococcus aureus*. Active against many gram-negative bacillary organisms: *Escherichia coli*,

Klebsiella, Acinetobacter, Proteus, Serratia, Pseudomonas aeruginosa. Also displays activity against: *Salmonella, Shigella, Neisseria gonorrhoeae,* Numerous anaerobes.

Adverse Reactions/Side Effects

CNS: SEIZURES, dizziness, somnolence. **CV:** hypotension. **GI:** PSEUDOMEMBRANOUS COLITIS, diarrhea, nausea, vomiting. **Derm:** rash, pruritus, sweating, urticaria. **Hemat:** eosinophilia. **Local:** phlebitis at IV site. **Misc:** ALLERGIC REACTION, INCLUDING ANAPHYLAXIS, fever, superinfection.

PHYSICAL THERAPY IMPLICATIONS

Examination and Evaluation

- Watch for seizures; notify physician immediately if patient develops or increases seizure activity.
- Monitor signs of pseudomembranous colitis, including diarrhea, abdominal pain, fever, pus or mucus in stools, and other severe or prolonged GI problems (nausea, vomiting, heartburn). Notify physician or nursing staff immediately of these signs.
- Monitor signs of allergic reactions and anaphylaxis, including pulmonary symptoms (tightness in the throat and chest, wheezing, cough dyspnea) or skin reactions (rash, pruritus, urticaria). Notify physician or nursing staff immediately if these reactions occur.
- Assess blood pressure periodically and compare to normal values (See Appendix F). Report low blood pressure (hypotension), especially if patient experiences dizziness, fatigue, or other symptoms.
- Monitor for signs of eosinophilia (fatigue, weakness, myalgia); report these signs to the physician.
- Assess dizziness or somnolence that might affect gait, balance, and other functional activities (See Appendix C). Report balance problems and functional limitations to the physician and nursing staff, and caution the patient and family/caregivers to guard against falls and trauma.
- Monitor injection site for pain, swelling, and irritation. Report prolonged or excessive injection site reactions to the physician.

Interventions

- Always wash hands thoroughly and disinfect equipment (whirlpools, electrotherapeutic devices, treatment tables, and so forth) to help prevent the spread of infection. Use universal precautions or isolation procedures as indicated for specific patients.

Patient/Client-Related Instruction

- Instruct patient to notify physician immediately of signs of superinfection, including black, furry overgrowth on tongue, vaginal itching or discharge, and loose or foul-smelling stools.
- Instruct patient and family/caregivers to report other troublesome side effects such as severe or prolonged fever, skin problems (rash, hives, itching, sweating), or GI problems (nausea, vomiting, diarrhea).

Pharmacokinetics

Absorption: Well absorbed after IM administration (imipenem 95%, cilastatin 75%). IV administration results in complete bioavailability.
Distribution: Widely distributed. Crosses the placenta; enters breast milk.
Metabolism and Excretion: *Imipenem and cilastatin*—70% excreted unchanged by the kidneys.
Half-life: *Imipenem and cilastatin*—1 hr (prolonged in renal impairment).

TIME/ACTION PROFILE (blood levels)

ROUTE	ONSET	PEAK	DURATION
IM	rapid	1–2 hr	12 hr
IV	rapid	end of infusion	6–8 hr

Contraindications/Precautions

Contraindicated in: Hypersensitivity; Cross-sensitivity may occur with penicillins and cephalosporins.
Use Cautiously in: Previous history of multiple hypersensitivity reactions; Seizure disorders; Geri: Geriatric patients; Renal impairment (dose reduction required if CCr ≤70 mL/min/1.73 m²); OB/Lactation/Pedi: Safety not established.

Interactions

Drug-Drug: Do not admix with **aminoglycosides** (inactivation may occur). **Probenecid** ↓ renal excretion and ↑ blood levels. ↑ risk of seizures with **ganciclovir** or **cyclosporine** (avoid concurrent use of ganciclovir). May ↓ serum **valproate** levels (↑ risk of seizures).

Route/Dosage

IV (Adults): *Mild infections*—250–500 mg q 6 hr. *Moderate infections*—500 mg q 6–8 hr *or* 1 g q 8 hr. *Serious infections*—500 mg q 6 hr to 1 g q 6–8 hr.
IV (Children ≥3 mo [non-CNS infections]): 15–25 mg/kg q 6 hr; higher doses have been used in older children with cystic fibrosis.
IV (Children 4 wk–3 mo): 25 mg/kg q 6 hr.
IV (Children 1–4 wk): 25 mg/kg q 8 hr.
IV (Children <1 wk): 25 mg/kg q 12 hr.
IM (Adults): 500–750 mg q 12 hr.
IM (Children): 10–15 mg/kg q 6 hr.

Renal Impairment

IV (Adults): If dose for normal renal function is 1 g/day: *CCr 41–70 mL/min*—125–250 mg q 6–8 hr,

CCr 21–40 mL/min—125–250 mg q 8–12 hr, *CCr 6–20 mL/min*—125–250 mg q 12 hr; **if dose for normal renal function is 1.5 g/day:** *CCr 41–70 mL/min*—125–250 mg q 6–8 hr, *CCr 21–40 mL/min*—125–250 mg q 8–12 hr, *CCr 6–20 mL/min*—125–250 mg q 12 hr; **if dose for normal renal function is 2 g/day:** *CCr 41–70 mL/min*—125–500 mg q 6–8 hr, *CCr 21–40 mL/min*—125–250 mg q 8–12 hr, *CCr 6–20 mL/min*—125–250 mg q 12 hr; **if dose for normal renal function is 3 g/day:** *CCr 41–70 mL/min*—250–500 mg q 6–8 hr, *CCr 21–40 mL/min*—250–500 mg q 6–8 hr, *CCr 6–20 mL/min*—250–500 mg q 12 hr; **if dose for normal renal function is 4 g/day:** *CCr 41–70 mL/min*—250–750 mg q 6–8 hr, *CCr 21–40 mL/min*—250–500 mg q 6–8 hr, *CCr 6–20 mL/min*—250 –250 mg q 12 hr.

Availability

Powder for IV injection: 250 mg imipenem/250 mg cilastatin, 500 mg imipenem/500 mg cilastatin. **Powder for IM injection:** 500 mg imipenem/500 mg cilastatin, 750 mg imipenem/750 mg cilastatin.

imipramine (im-ip-ra-meen)

Apo-Imipramine, Impril, Norfranil, Novopramine, Tipramine, Tofranil, Tofranil PM

Classification

Therapeutic: antidepressants

Pharmacologic: tricyclic antidepressants

Indications

Various forms of depression. Enuresis in children. **Unlabeled Use:** Adjunct in the management of chronic pain, incontinence (in adults), vascular headache prophylaxis, cluster headache, insomnia.

Action

Potentiates the effect of serotonin and norepinephrine. Has significant anticholinergic properties. **Therapeutic Effects:** Antidepressant action that develops slowly over several weeks.

Adverse Reactions/Side Effects

CNS: drowsiness, fatigue, agitation, confusion, hallucinations, insomnia. **EENT:** blurred vision, dry eyes. **CV:** ARRHYTHMIAS, hypotension, ECG changes. **GI:** constipation, dry mouth, nausea, paralytic ileus, weight gain. **GU:** urinary retention, decreased libido. **Derm:** photosensitivity. **Endo:** gynecomastia. **Hemat:** blood dyscrasias.

PHYSICAL THERAPY IMPLICATIONS

Examination and Evaluation

- Assess heart rate, ECG, and heart sounds, especially during exercise (See Appendices G, H). Report any rhythm disturbances or symptoms of increased arrhythmias, including palpitations, chest discomfort, shortness of breath, fainting, and fatigue/weakness.
- Measure blood pressure periodically and compare to normal values (See Appendix F). Report low blood pressure (hypotension), especially if patient experiences dizziness or syncope.
- Monitor signs of leukopenia (fever, sore throat, signs of infection), thrombocytopenia (bruising, nose bleeds, bleeding gums), or unusual weakness and fatigue that might be due to anemia or other blood dyscrasias. Report these signs to the physician.
- Be alert for increased depression and suicidal thoughts and ideology, especially when initiating drug treatment or in children and teenagers. Notify physician or mental health professional immediately if patient exhibits worsening depression or other changes in mood and behavior.
- Assess confusion, agitation, hallucinations, or other alterations in mental status (See Appendix D). Notify physician promptly if these symptoms develop.
- Be alert for sedation and fatigue, especially in older adults. Report excessive or prolonged symptoms that could affect balance, gait, and functional activities.
- If used to treat chronic pain, assess pain levels periodically to help document drug efficacy.
- Periodically assess body weight and other anthropometric measures (body mass index, body composition). Report a rapid or unexplained weight gain or increased body fat.

Interventions

- Guard against falls and trauma (hip fractures, head injury, and so forth), and implement fall prevention strategies (See Appendix E).
- Because of cardiac arrhythmias and hypotension, use caution during aerobic exercise and endurance conditioning. Assess exercise tolerance frequently (blood pressure, heart rate, fatigue levels), and terminate exercise immediately if any untoward responses occur (See Appendix L).
- To minimize orthostatic hypotension, patient should move slowly when assuming a more upright position.
- Help patient explore nonpharmacologic methods to reduce depression (exercise, counseling, support groups, and so forth).

- If treating neuropathic pain, chronic headache, or other pain syndromes, implement appropriate interventions (physical agents, manual techniques, therapeutic exercise) to manage pain and reduce the need for drug therapy. Help patient also explore other nonpharmacological methods to reduce chronic pain (relaxation techniques, imagery, counseling, and so forth).
- Causes photosensitivity; use care if administering UV treatments. Advise patient to avoid direct sunlight and use sunscreens and protective clothing.

Patient/Client-Related Instruction

- Advise patient that antidepressant effects may not occur immediately; it may take 2 wk or more before an improvement in mood is observed.
- Advise patient to avoid alcohol and other CNS depressants because of the increased risk of sedation and adverse effects.
- Instruct patient to report other troublesome side effects such as severe or prolonged sleep loss, dry eyes, blurred vision, urinary retention, decreased libido, increased breast size in men (gynecomastia), or GI problems (nausea, constipation, dry mouth).

Pharmacokinetics

Absorption: Well absorbed from the GI tract.
Distribution: Widely distributed. Probably crosses the placenta and enters breast milk.
Protein Binding: 89–95%.
Metabolism and Excretion: Extensively metabolized by the liver, mostly on first pass; some conversion to active compounds. Undergoes enterohepatic recirculation and secretion into gastric juices.
Half-life: 8–16 hr.

TIME/ACTION PROFILE (antidepressant effect)

ROUTE	ONSET	PEAK	DURATION
PO, IM	hrs	2–6 wk	wks

Contraindications/Precautions

Contraindicated in: Hypersensitivity; Cross-sensitivity with other antidepressants may occur; Angle-closure glaucoma; Hypersensitivity to tartrazine or sulfites (in some preparations); Recent MI, known history of QTc prolongation, heart failure.
Use Cautiously in: Preexisting cardiovascular disease; Seizures or history of seizure disorder; May ↑ risk of suicide attempt/ideation especially during early treatment or dose adjustment; OB: Drug is present in breast milk; discontinue imipramine or bottle feed; Pedi: Suicide risk may be greater in children or adolescents. Safety not established in children <6 yr; Geri: Geriatric patients (more susceptible to adverse reactions). Geriatric males with prostatic hyperplasia are more susceptible to urinary retention.

Interactions

Drug-Drug: May cause hypotension, tachycardia, and potentially fatal reactions when used with **MAO inhibitors** (avoid concurrent use—discontinue 2 wk prior to imipramine). Concurrent use with **SSRI antidepressants** may result in increased toxicity and should be avoided (**fluoxetine** should be stopped 5 wk before). Concurrent use with **clonidine** may result in hypertensive crisis and should be avoided. Imipramine is metabolized in the liver by the **cytochrome P4502D6 enzyme,** and its action may be affected by drugs that compete for metabolism by this enzyme, including **other antidepressants, phenothiazines, carbamazepine, class 1C antiarrhythmics (propafenone, flecainide)**; when used concurrently, dose reduction of one or the other or both may be necessary. Concurrent use of other drugs that inhibit the activity of the enzyme, including **cimetidine, quinidine, amiodarone**, and **ritonavir**, may result in ↑ effects of imipramine. Concurrent use with **levodopa** may result in delayed/↓ absorption of levodopa or hypertension. Blood levels and effects may be ↓ by **rifamycins.** ↑ CNS depression with other CNS **depressants**, including **alcohol, antihistamines, clonidine, opioids**, and **sedative/hypnotics. Barbiturates** may alter blood levels and effects. **Adrenergic** and **anticholinergic** side effects may be ↑ with other **agents having these properties. Phenothiazines** or **hormonal contraceptives** ↑ levels and may cause toxicity. **Cigarette smoking (nicotine)** may increase metabolism and alter effects.
Drug-Natural: Concomitant use of **kava, valerian,** or **chamomile** can increase CNS depression. ↑ anticholinergic effects with **jimson weed** and **scopolia**.

Route/Dosage

PO (Adults): 25–50 mg 3–4 times daily (not to exceed 300 mg/day); total daily dose may be given at bedtime.
PO (Geriatric Patients): 25 mg at bedtime initially, up to 100 mg/day in divided doses.
PO (Children >12 yr): *Antidepressant*—25–50 mg/day in divided doses (not to exceed 100 mg/day).
PO (Children 6–12 yr): *Antidepressant*—10–30 mg/day in 2 divided doses.
PO (Children ≥6 yr): *Enuresis*—25 mg once daily 1 hr before bedtime; increase if necessary by 25 mg at weekly intervals to 50 mg in children <12 yr, up to 75 mg in children >12 yr.
IM (Adults): Up to 100 mg/day in divided doses (not to exceed 300 mg/day).

I

Availability (generic available)

Tablets: 10 mg, 25 mg, 50 mg, 75 mg. **Capsules:** 75 mg, 100 mg, 125 mg, 150 mg. **Injection:** 12.5 mg/mL.

imiquimod (i-mi-kwi-mod)

Aldara

Classification

Therapeutic: antivirals, immune modifiers
Pharmacologic: immune response modifiers

Indications

External genital or perianal warts/condylomata (condyloma acuminatum). Typical, nonhyperkeratotic, nonhypertrophic actinic keratoses on the face or scalp. Biopsy-confirmed, primary superficial basal cell carcinoma.

Action

May induce the formation of interferons that have antiproliferative and antiviral properties. **Therapeutic Effects:** Regression of external genital or perianal warts/condylomata, actinic keratoses, or basal cell carcinoma lesions.

Adverse Reactions/Side Effects

Local: irritation, pain, pruritus, burning, swelling, fungal infections (women).

PHYSICAL THERAPY IMPLICATIONS

Examination and Evaluation

- Assess skin lesions whenever possible to help determine if drug therapy is successful in controlling infection. Report any local irritation, pain, itching, swelling, or other skin reactions at the application site.

Interventions

- Avoid contact with cutaneous lesions when treating patient.
- Always wash hands thoroughly and disinfect equipment (whirlpools, electrotherapeutic devices, treatment tables, and so forth) to help prevent the spread of infection. Use universal precautions as indicated for specific patients.

Patient/Client-Related Instruction

- Advise patient to apply medication as directed. Imiquimod should not be used more frequently or longer than prescribed.
- For patients with actinic keratosis and basal cell carcinoma, advise patient to use sunscreens, wear protective clothing, and avoid prolonged sun exposure to prevent further skin damage from UV rays.

Pharmacokinetics

Absorption: Minimal absorption.
Distribution: Action is primarily local.
Metabolism and Excretion: <0.9% excreted in urine and feces.
Half-life: Unknown.

TIME/ACTION PROFILE (regression of lesions)

ROUTE	ONSET	PEAK	DURATION
Topical	days–wks	10–16 wk	unknown

Contraindications/Precautions

Contraindicated in: None known.
Use Cautiously in: Previous treatment/surgery in affected area (area should be healed prior to use); Preexisting inflammatory skin lesions (may be exacerbated); Immunocompromised patients (safety not established); Pregnancy, lactation, or children <12 yr (safety not established).

Interactions

Drug-Drug: None known.

Route/Dosage

External Genital Warts

Topical (Adults and children >12 yr): Apply thin layer to warts at bedtime every other day (3 times weekly); leave on for 6–10 hr, then rinse off with mild soap and water. Repeat until lesions are completely cleared or up to 16 wk.

Actinic Keratoses

Topical (Adults): Apply thin layer to clean, dry affected area twice weekly; leave on for 8 hr, then rinse off with mild soap and water. Continue for 16 wk.

Superficial Basal Cell Carcinoma

Topical (Adults): Apply thin layer to clean, dry affected area 5 times per week; leave on for 8 hr, then rinse off with mild soap and water. Continue for 6 wk.

Availability

Cream: 5% in single-use packets in boxes of 12.

HIGH ALERT

inamrinone (in-am-ri-none)

Inocor

Classification

Therapeutic: inotropics
Pharmacologic: bipyridines

Indications

Short-term treatment of CHF unresponsive to digoxin, diuretics, and vasodilators.

Action
Increases myocardial contractility. Decreases preload and afterload by a direct dilating effect on vascular smooth muscle. **Therapeutic Effects:** Increased cardiac output (inotropic effect).

Adverse Reactions/Side Effects
Resp: dyspnea. **CV:** arrhythmias, hypotension. **GI:** diarrhea, hepatotoxicity, nausea, vomiting. **F and E:** hypokalemia. **Hemat:** thrombocytopenia. **Misc:** tachyphylaxis, fever, hypersensitivity reactions.

PHYSICAL THERAPY IMPLICATIONS
Examination and Evaluation
- Assess heart rate, ECG, and heart sounds, especially during exercise (See Appendices G, H). Report any rhythm disturbances or symptoms of increased arrhythmias, including palpitations, chest discomfort, shortness of breath, fainting, and fatigue/weakness.
- Assess signs and symptoms of CHF (dyspnea, rales/crackles, peripheral edema, jugular venous distention, exercise intolerance) to help document whether drug therapy is effective in reducing these symptoms. Be alert for a sudden increase in symptoms that might indicate a rapid decrease in drug effectiveness (tachyphylaxis).
- Monitor signs of hypersensitivity reactions, including pulmonary symptoms (tightness in the throat and chest, wheezing, cough, dyspnea) or skin reactions (rash, pruritus, urticaria). Notify physician or nursing staff immediately if these reactions occur.
- Report any muscle weakness, aches, or cramps that might indicate low potassium levels (hypokalemia).
- Assess blood pressure periodically and compare to normal values (See Appendix F). Report low blood pressure (hypotension), especially if patient experiences dizziness, fatigue, or other symptoms.
- Monitor and report signs of thrombocytopenia, including bruising, nose bleeds, and bleeding gums.

Interventions
- Design and implement aerobic exercise and endurance training programs to improve myocardial pumping ability and reduce symptoms of CHF.
- Use caution during aerobic exercise and endurance conditioning because of an increased risk of cardiac arrhythmias. Terminate exercise if patient exhibits untoward symptoms (chest pain, shortness of breath, etc.) or displays other criteria for exercise termination (See Appendix L).

Patient/Client-Related Instruction
- Remind patients to take medication as directed to control CHF even if they are asymptomatic.
- Instruct patients to weigh themselves every day and to call their physician if they gain 3 lb or more in 1 day or more than 5 lb in 1 week. Sudden weight gain may indicate fluid buildup due to worsening heart failure.
- Counsel patients about additional interventions to help control cardiac dysfunction, including regular exercise, weight loss, sodium restriction, stress reduction, moderation of alcohol consumption, and smoking cessation.
- Advise patient about the likelihood of GI reactions, including nausea, vomiting, and diarrhea. Instruct patient to report severe or prolonged GI problems or signs of liver toxicity (yellow skin or eyes, abdominal pain, severe nausea and vomiting, fever, sore throat, malaise, weakness, facial edema).

Pharmacokinetics
Absorption: IV administration results in complete bioavailability.
Distribution: Unknown.
Metabolism and Excretion: 50% metabolized by the liver; 10–40% excreted unchanged by the kidneys.
Half-life: 3.6–5.8 hr (increased in CHF).

TIME/ACTION PROFILE (inotropic effect)

ROUTE	ONSET	PEAK	DURATION*
IV	2–5 min	10 min	0.5–2 hr

*After infusion is discontinued.

Contraindications/Precautions
Contraindicated in: Hypersensitivity to inamrinone or bisulfites; Idiopathic hypertrophic subaortic stenosis.
Use Cautiously in: Atrial fibrillation or flutter; Recent aggressive diuretic therapy (correct fluid and electrolyte disorders before administering inamrinone); Thrombocytopenia (platelets <100,000/mm^3); Renal impairment (may require dosage adjustment); Geriatric patients (age-related decline in renal function may require dosage adjustment); Pregnancy, lactation, or children (safety not established).

Interactions
Drug-Drug: Inotropic effects may be additive with **digoxin**. Hypotension may be exaggerated by **disopyramide**.

Route/Dosage
IV (Adults): 0.75 mg/kg loading dose; may be repeated in 30 min if necessary, then 5–10 mcg/kg/min infusion (total daily dose should not exceed 10 mg/kg).
IV (Infants): 3–4.5 mg/kg in divided doses followed by an infusion of 10 mcg/kg/min.

IV (Neonates): 3–4.5 mg/kg in divided doses followed by an infusion of 3–5 mcg/kg/min.

Availability

Injection: 5 mg/mL.

indapamide (in-dap-a-mide)

Lozide, Lozol

Classification

Therapeutic: antihypertensives, diuretics
Pharmacologic: thiazide-like diuretics

Indications

Mild-to-moderate hypertension. Edema associated with CHF and other causes.

Action

Increases excretion of sodium and water by inhibiting sodium reabsorption in the distal tubule. Promotes excretion of chloride, potassium, magnesium, and bicarbonate. May produce arteriolar dilation.
Therapeutic Effects: Lowering of blood pressure in hypertensive patients and diuresis with subsequent mobilization of edema.

Adverse Reactions/Side Effects

CNS: dizziness, drowsiness, lethargy. **CV:** arrhythmias, hypotension. **GI:** anorexia, cramping, nausea, vomiting. **Derm:** photosensitivity, rashes. **Endo:** hyperglycemia. **F and E** hypokalemia, dehydration, hypochloremic alkalosis, hyponatremia, hypovolemia. **Metab:** hyperuricemia. **MS:** muscle cramps.

PHYSICAL THERAPY IMPLICATIONS

Examination and Evaluation

- Assess blood pressure periodically and compare to normal values (See Appendix F) to help document antihypertensive effects.
- Assess heart rate, ECG, and heart sounds, especially during exercise (See Appendices G, H). Report any rhythm disturbances or symptoms of increased arrhythmias, including palpitations, chest discomfort, shortness of breath, fainting, and fatigue/weakness.
- Monitor signs of fluid and electrolyte imbalances, including dizziness, drowsiness, blurred vision, confusion, lethargy, hypotension, or muscle cramps and weakness. Report excessive of prolonged symptoms to the physician.
- Assess dizziness and drowsiness that might affect gait, balance, and other functional activities (See Appendix C). Report balance problems and functional limitations to the physician, and caution the patient and family/caregivers to guard against falls and trauma.
- When used to treat edema, help determine drug effects by assessing peripheral edema using girth measurements, volume displacement, and measurement of pitting edema (See Appendix N). Also monitor signs of pulmonary edema such as dyspnea and rales/crackles (See Appendix K). Document whether peripheral and pulmonary symptoms are controlled adequately by diuretic therapy.
- Monitor signs of hyperglycemia such as drowsiness, fruity breath, increased urination, and unusual thirst. Patients with diabetes mellitus should check blood glucose levels frequently.

Interventions

- Implement fall-prevention strategies, especially in older adults of if patient exhibits sedation, dizziness, or other impairments that affect gait and balance (See Appendix E).
- Use caution during aerobic exercise, especially in hot environments. Increased sweating will cause fluid and electrolyte loss, and may exaggerate arrhythmias and diuretic side effects (dizziness, muscle cramps, and so forth).
- To minimize orthostatic hypotension, patient should move slowly when assuming a more upright position.
- Causes photosensitivity; use care if administering UV treatments.

Patient/Client-Related Instruction

- Remind patients to take medication as directed to control hypertension and other cardiac conditions, even if they are asymptomatic.
- Counsel patients about additional interventions to help control blood pressure and cardiac dysfunction, such as regular exercise, weight loss, sodium restriction, stress reduction, moderation of alcohol consumption, and smoking cessation.
- Advise patient about photosensitivity, and to use sunscreens, protective clothing, and avoid prolonged sun exposure. Instruct patient to also report any rashes or other skin reactions.
- Instruct patient to report other troublesome side effects, including severe or prolonged skin rash or GI problems (nausea, vomiting, abdominal cramps, loss of appetite.

Pharmacokinetics

Absorption: Well absorbed from the GI tract after oral administration.
Distribution: Widely distributed.
Metabolism and Excretion: Mostly metabolized by the liver. Small amounts (7%) excreted unchanged by the kidneys.
Half-life: 14–18 hr.

TIME/ACTION PROFILE (antihypertensive effect)

ROUTE	ONSET	PEAK	DURATION
PO (single dose)	unknown	24 hr	unknown
PO (multiple dose)	1–2 wk	8–12 wk	up to 8 wk

Contraindications/Precautions

Contraindicated in: Hypersensitivity; Cross-sensitivity with sulfonamides may occur; Anuria; Lactation.
Use Cautiously in: Renal or severe hepatic impairment; Geriatric patients (increased sensitivity); Pregnancy or children (safety not established).

Interactions

Drug-Drug: Additive hypotension with other **antihypertensives, nitrates**, or acute ingestion of **alcohol**. Additive hypokalemia with **corticosteroids, amphotericin B, piperacillin,** or **ticarcillin**. ↓ the excretion of **lithium**; may cause toxicity. Hypokalemia may ↑ risk of **digoxin** toxicity.
Drug-Natural: Licorice and **stimulant laxative herbs (aloe, senna)** may ↑ risk of potassium depletion.

Route/Dosage

PO (Adults): *Hypertension*—1.25–5 mg daily in the morning; may be increased at 4-wk intervals up to 5 mg/day. *Edema secondary to CHF*—2.5 mg daily in the morning; may be increased after 1 wk to 5 mg/day.

Availability (generic available)

Tablets: 1.25 mg, 2.5 mg.

indinavir (in-din-a-veer)
Crixivan

Classification
Therapeutic: antiretrovirals
Pharmacologic: protease inhibitors

Indications

HIV infection (with other antiretrovirals). **Unlabeled Use:** Prevention of HIV infection after known exposure (with other antiretrovirals).

Action

Inhibits the action of HIV protease and prevents the cleavage of viral polyproteins. **Therapeutic Effects:** Slowing of the progression of HIV infection and its sequelae.

Adverse Reactions/Side Effects

CNS: dizziness, drowsiness, fatigue, headache, insomnia, weakness. **GI:** abdominal pain, acid regurgitation, altered taste, asymptomatic hyperbilirubinemia, diarrhea, nausea, vomiting. **GU:** nephrolithiasis. **Endo:** hyperglycemia. **F and E:** KETOACIDOSIS. **MS:** back pain, flank pain. **Misc:** redistribution of body fat.

PHYSICAL THERAPY IMPLICATIONS

Examination and Evaluation

- Monitor signs of hyperglycemia and ketoacidosis, including confusion, drowsiness, fatigue, weakness, rapid breathing, fruity or pungent breath, excessive thirst, frequent urination, nausea, vomiting, and abdominal pain. Notify physician immediately if these signs occur.
- Assess any back or side pain to rule out musculoskeletal pathology; that is, try to determine if pain is drug induced rather than caused by anatomic or biomechanical problems.
- Assess dizziness and drowsiness that might affect gait, balance, and other functional activities (See Appendix C). Report balance problems and functional limitations to the physician and nursing staff, and caution the patient and family/caregivers to guard against falls and trauma.
- Monitor and report signs of kidney stones (nephrolithiasis), including severe pain in the side and back, pain on urination, bloody urine, and a persistent urge to urinate.

Interventions

- Implement resistive exercises and other therapeutic exercises as tolerated to maintain muscle strength and function and prevent muscle wasting associated with HIV infection and AIDS.
- Because of the risk of ketoacidosis, use caution during aerobic exercise and other forms of therapeutic exercise. Assess exercise tolerance frequently (blood pressure, heart rate, fatigue levels), and terminate exercise immediately if any untoward responses occur (see Appendix L).

Patient/Client-Related Instruction

- Emphasize the importance of taking indinavir as directed even if the patient is asymptomatic, and that this drug must always be used in combination with other antiretroviral drugs. Do not take more than prescribed amount and do not stop taking without consulting health care professional.
- Inform patient that indinavir does not cure HIV or AIDS or prevent associated or opportunistic infections. Indinavir does not reduce the risk of transmission of HIV to others through sexual contact or blood contamination. Caution patient to use a condom, and avoid sharing needles or donating blood to prevent spreading the AIDS virus to others.

- Inform patient that redistribution and accumulation of body fat may occur, causing central obesity, thin arms and legs, dorsocervical fat enlargement (buffalo hump), breast enlargement, and other symptoms that resemble Cushing's syndrome (moon face, striations on abdominal skin). Discuss possible effects on body image, and help patient explore coping mechanisms.
- Instruct patient to report other troublesome side effects such as prolonged or severe headache, sleep loss, or GI problems (diarrhea, nausea, vomiting, heartburn, altered taste, loss of appetite).

Pharmacokinetics

Absorption: Rapidly absorbed after oral administration.
Distribution: Unknown.
Metabolism and Excretion: Mostly metabolized by the liver; <20% excreted unchanged by the kidneys.
Half-life: 1.8 hr.

TIME/ACTION PROFILE (blood levels)

ROUTE	ONSET	PEAK	DURATION
PO	rapid	0.8 hr	8 hr

Contraindications/Precautions

Contraindicated in: Hypersensitivity; Dehydration; Concurrent alprazolam, dihydroergotamine, ergotamine, midazolam, rifampin, triazolam, or St. John's wort.
Use Cautiously in: Hepatic impairment (dose reduction recommended in moderate to severe hepatic insufficiency caused by cirrhosis); Hemophilia (↑ risk of bleeding); Diabetes mellitus; Lactation/Pedi: Safety not established; breast-feeding not recommended in HIV-infected patients.

Interactions

Drug-Drug: Concurrent use with **alprazolam, dihydroergotamine, ergotamine, midazolam, rifampin,** or **triazolam** is contraindicated because of ↑ risk of serious or life-threatening adverse reactions, including arrhythmias, excessive sedation, and vasoconstriction. **Rifampin** and **fluconazole** ↓ blood levels; concurrent use should be avoided. ↑ risk of myopathy with **lovastatin, simvastatin, atorvastatin,** or **rosuvastatin** (consider using **pravastatin** or **fluvastatin** as an alternative). ↑ blood levels of **rifabutin** (↓ dosage of rifabutin by 50%) and **hormonal contraceptives. Rifabutin, nevirapine,** and **efavirenz** ↓ indinavir levels; if concurrent rifabutin or efavirenz therapy is necessary, ↑ indinavir dose to 1000 mg q 8 hr. Blood levels are ↑ by **ketoconazole, itraconazole,** and **delavirdine** (↓ dose of indinavir to 600 mg q 8 hr). Alters absorption of **didanosine.** May ↑ blood levels and effects of **sildenafil, vardenafil** or **tadalafil.**
Drug-Natural: St. John's wort significantly ↓ blood levels and effectiveness of **indinavir** (concurrent use is contraindicated).
Drug-Food: High-fat or **high-protein meals** ↓ absorption.

Route/Dosage

PO (Adults): 800 mg q 8 hr.

Availability

Capsules: 100 mg, 200 mg, 333 mg, 400 mg.

indomethacin

(in-doe-**meth**-a-sin)
✱Apo-Indomethacin, ✱Indameth, ✱Indocid, Indocin, Indocin I.V, ✱Indocin PDA, Indocin SR, Indochron E-R, ✱Novo-Methacin, ✱Nu-Indo

Classification

Therapeutic: antirheumatics, ductus arteriosus patency adjuncts (IV only), nonsteroidal anti-inflammatory agents

Indications

PO: Inflammatory disorders, including Rheumatoid arthritis, gouty arthritis, osteoarthritis , ankylosing spondylitis. Generally reserved for patients who do not respond to less toxic agents. **IV:** Alternative to surgery in the management of patent ductus arteriosus in premature neonates.

Action

Inhibits prostaglandin synthesis. **Therapeutic Effects: PO**—Suppression of pain and inflammation. **IV**—Closure of patent ductus arteriosus (PDA).

Adverse Reactions/Side Effects

CNS: dizziness, drowsiness, headache, psychic disturbances. **EENT:** blurred vision, tinnitus. **CV:** hypertension, edema. **GI: PO**—DRUG-INDUCED HEPATITIS, GI BLEEDING, constipation, dyspepsia, nausea, vomiting, discomfort, necrotizing enterocolitis. **GU:** cystitis, hematuria, renal failure. **Derm:** rashes. **F and E:** hyperkalemia **IV:** dilutional hyponatremia **IV:** hypoglycemia. **Hemat:** thrombocytopenia, blood dyscrasias, prolonged bleeding time. **Local:** phlebitis at IV site. **Misc:** ALLERGIC REACTIONS, INCLUDING ANAPHYLAXIS.

PHYSICAL THERAPY IMPLICATIONS

Examination and Evaluation

- Monitor signs of GI bleeding, including abdominal pain, vomiting blood, blood in stools, or black, tarry stools. Report these signs to the physician immediately.

- Be alert for signs of drug-induced hepatitis, including anorexia, abdominal pain, severe nausea and vomiting, yellow skin or eyes, skin rashes, flu-like symptoms, and muscle/joint pain. Report these signs to the physician immediately.
- Monitor signs of allergic reactions and anaphylaxis, including pulmonary symptoms (laryngeal edema, wheezing, cough, dyspnea) or skin reactions (rash, pruritus, urticaria). Notify physician immediately if these reactions occur.
- Assess pain and other variables (range of motion, muscle strength) to document whether this drug is successful in helping manage the patient's pain and decreasing impairments.
- Assess blood pressure (BP) periodically and compare to normal values (See Appendix F). NSAIDs can increase BP and promote hypertension in certain patients.
- Assess peripheral edema using girth measurements, volume displacement, and measurement of pitting edema (see Appendix N). Report increased swelling in feet and ankles or a sudden increase in body weight due to fluid retention.
- Assess for signs of thrombocytopenia and prolonged bleeding time such as bleeding gums, nosebleeds, and unusual or excessive bruising. Notify physician if these signs occur.
- Report any unusual weakness and fatigue that might be due to anemia.
- Monitor symptoms of high plasma potassium levels (hyperkalemia), including bradycardia, fatigue, weakness, numbness, and tingling. Notify physician because severe cases can lead to life-threatening arrhythmias and paralysis.
- Monitor signs of hypoglycemia, especially during and after exercise. Common neuromuscular symptoms include anxiety; restlessness; tingling in hands, feet, lips, or tongue; chills; cold sweats; confusion; difficulty in concentration; drowsiness; nightmares or trouble sleeping; excessive hunger; headache; irritability; nervousness; tremor; weakness; unsteady gait. Report persistent or repeated episodes of hypoglycemia to the physician.
- Monitor signs of kidney dysfunction such as painful urination or blood in the urine. Report signs of renal failure immediately, including decreased urine output, increased BP, muscle cramps/twitching, edema/weight gain from fluid retention, yellowish brown skin, and confusion that progresses to seizures and coma.
- Assess dizziness and drowsiness that might affect gait, balance, and other functional activities (See Appendix C). Report balance problems and functional limitations to the physician, and caution the patient and family/caregivers to guard against falls and trauma.
- Monitor and report confusion, agitation, or other psychic disturbances.
- Monitor IV injection site for signs of phlebitis including pain, swelling, and inflammation. Report prolonged or excessive injection site reactions to the physician.

Interventions

- Implement appropriate manual therapy techniques, physical agents, and therapeutic exercises to reduce pain and decrease the need for indomethacin and other NSAIDs.
- If treating arthritic conditions, recommend orthotic and assistive devices as needed to reduce pain, improve function, and augment the effects of drug therapy.
- Use caution with any physical interventions that could increase bleeding, including wound débridement, chest percussion, joint mobilization, and application of local heat.
- Help patient explore other nonpharmacologic methods to reduce chronic pain, such as relaxation techniques, exercise, counseling, and so forth.

Patient/Client-Related Instruction

- Advise patient that analgesics are usually more effective if given before pain becomes severe; emphasize that adequate pain control will allow better participation in physical therapy.
- Inform patient that NSAIDs may impair bone and cartilage healing. Advise patient to consult physician about NSAID use, especially after fractures, spinal fusion, and other bone surgeries.
- Caution patient about the use of over-the-counter products that contain NSAIDs or acetaminophen while taking prescription doses of indomethacin. Use of multiple NSAIDs increases the risk of toxicity and overdose.
- Instruct patient to report excessive or prolonged headache or ringing/buzzing in the ears (tinnitus); these signs may indicate drug toxicity.
- Advise patient about the risks of gastric irritation. Instruct patient to notify physician of GI reactions such as severe or prolonged nausea, vomiting, constipation, indigestion, and abdominal pain.
- Advise patient to reduce alcohol intake because alcohol increases the risk of gastric toxicity.
- Instruct patient and family/caregivers to report other troublesome side effects such as severe or prolonged vision disturbances or skin rash.

Pharmacokinetics

Absorption: Well absorbed after oral administration in adults, incomplete oral absorption in neonates.
Distribution: Crosses the blood-brain barrier and the placenta. Enters breast milk.
Protein Binding: 99%.
Metabolism and Excretion: Mostly metabolized by the liver.
Half-life: Neonates <2 weeks: 20 hr; >2 weeks: 11 hr; Adults: 2.6–11 hr.

TIME/ACTION PROFILE

ROUTE	ONSET	PEAK	DURATION
PO (analgesic)	30 min	0.5–2 hr	4–6 hr
PO-ER (analgesic)	30 min	unknown	4–6 hr
PO (anti-inflammatory)	up to 7 days	1–2 wk	4–6 hr
PO-ER (anti-inflammatory)	up to 7 days	1–2 wk	4–6 hr
IV (closure of PDA)	up to 48 hr	unknown	unknown

Contraindications/Precautions

Contraindicated in: Hypersensitivity; Known alcohol intolerance (suspension); Cross-sensitivity may exist with other NSAIDs, including aspirin; Active GI bleeding; Ulcer disease; Proctitis or recent history of rectal bleeding; Necrotizing enterocolitis in neonates; Intraventricular hemorrhage; Thrombocytopenia.
Use Cautiously in: Severe cardiovascular, renal, or hepatic disease; History of ulcer disease; Epilepsy; Hypertension; Geri: Geriatric patients are at increased risk for adverse reactions, including dizziness and GI bleeding ; Pregnancy or lactation (not recommended during 2nd half of pregnancy); Lactation.

Interactions

Drug-Drug: Concurrent use with **aspirin** may ↓ effectiveness. Additive adverse GI effects with **aspirin**, other **NSAIDs**, **corticosteroids**, or **alcohol**. Chronic use of **acetaminophen** ↑ risk of adverse renal reactions. May ↓ effectiveness of **diuretics** or **antihypertensives**. May ↑ hypoglycemia from **insulins** or **oral hypoglycemic agents**. May ↑ risk of toxicity from **lithium** or **zidovudine** (avoid concurrent use with zidovudine). ↑ risk of toxicity from **methotrexate**. **Probenecid** ↑ risk of toxicity from indomethacin. ↑ risk of bleeding with **cefotetan, cefoperazone, valproic acid, thrombolytics, warfarin**, and **drugs affecting platelet function**, including **clopidogrel, ticlopidine, abciximab, eptifibatide**, or **tirofiban**. ↑ risk of adverse hematologic reactions with **antineoplastics** or **radiation therapy**. ↑ risk of nephrotoxicity with **cyclosporine**. Concurrent use with **potassium-sparing diuretics** may result in hyperkalemia. May ↑ levels of **digitalis glycosides, methotrexate, lithium**, and **aminoglycosides** when used IV in neonates.
Drug-Natural: ↑ bleeding risk with **anise, arnica, chamomile, clove, dong quai, feverfew, garlic, ginger, ginkgo, *Panax ginseng***.

Route/Dosage

Anti-inflammatory

PO (Adults): *Antiarthritic*—25–50 mg 2–4 times daily *or* 75-mg extended-release capsule once or bid (not to exceed 200 mg or 150 mg of SR/day). A single bedtime dose of 100 mg may be used. *Antigout*—100 mg initially, followed by 50 mg tisd for relief of pain, then decreased further.
PO (Children >2 yr): 1–2 mg/kg/day in 2–4 divided doses (not to exceed 4 mg/kg/day or 150–200 mg/day).

Closure of Patent Ductus Arteriosus

IV (Neonates): 0.2 mg/kg initially, then 2 subsequent doses at 12- to 24-hr intervals of 0.1 mg/kg if age <48 hr at time of initial dose; 0.2 mg/kg if 2–7 days at initial dose; 0.25 mg/kg if age >7 days at initial dose.

Availability (generic available)

Capsules: 25 mg, 50 mg. **Sustained-release capsules:** 75 mg. **Oral suspension (fruit mint, pineapple coconut mint flavors):** 25 mg/5 mL. **Powder for injection:** 1-mg vials.

infliximab (in-flix-i-mab)

Remicade

Classification
Therapeutic: antirheumatics (disease-modifying antirheumatic drugs, DMARDs), gastrointestinal anti-inflammatories—therapeutic
Pharmacologic: monoclonal antibodies

Indications

Active rheumatoid arthritis (moderate-to-severe, with methotrexate). Active Crohn's disease (moderate-to-severe). Active psoriatic arthritis. Active ankylosing spondylitis. Active ulcerative colitis (moderate-to-severe) with inadequate response to conventional therapy: reducing signs and symptoms, inducing and maintaining clinical remission and mucosal healing, and eliminating corticosteroid use. Plaque psoriasis (chronic severe).

Action

Neutralizes and prevents the activity of tumor necrosis factor-alpha (TNF-alpha), resulting in

anti-inflammatory and antiproliferative activity.
Therapeutic Effects: Decreased pain and swelling, decreased rate of joint destruction and improved physical function in ankylosing spondylitis, rheumatoid or psoriatic arthritis. Reduction and maintenance of closure of fistulae in Crohn's disease. Decreased symptoms, maintaining remission and mucosal healing with decreased corticosteroid use in ulcerative colitis. Decrease in duration, scaling, and erythema of psoriatic lesions.

Adverse Reactions/Side Effects

CNS: fatigue, headache, anxiety, depression, dizziness, insomnia. **EENT:** conjunctivitis. **Resp:** upper respiratory tract infection, bronchitis, cough, dyspnea, laryngitis, pharyngitis, respiratory tract allergic reaction, rhinitis, sinusitis. **CV:** chest pain, hypertension, hypotension, pericardial effusion, tachycardia, CHF. **GI:** abdominal pain, nausea, vomiting, constipation, diarrhea, dyspepsia, flatulence, hepatotoxicity, intestinal obstruction, oral pain, tooth pain, ulcerative stomatitis. **GU:** dysuria, urinary frequency, urinary tract infection. **Derm:** acne, alopecia, dry skin, ecchymosis, eczema, erythema, flushing, hematoma, increased sweating, hot flushes, pruritus, urticaria, rash. **Hemat:** neutropenia. **MS:** arthralgia, arthritis, back pain, involuntary muscle contractions, myalgia. **Neuro:** paresthesia. **Misc:** INFECTIONS (INCLUDING REACTIVATION TUBERCULOSIS, PNEUMONIA AND INVASIVE FUNGAL INFECTIONS), fever, infusion reactions, chills, flu-like syndrome, herpes simplex, herpes zoster, hypersensitivity reactions, ↑ risk of lymphoma, lupus-like syndrome, moniliasis, pain, peripheral edema, vasculitis.

PHYSICAL THERAPY IMPLICATIONS

Examination and Evaluation

- Watch for any signs of infection, especially pulmonary signs associated with pneumonia, invasive fungal infections, or dormant tuberculosis that is reactivated by drug therapy (reactivation tuberculosis). Common pulmonary signs of infection include persistent cough, dyspnea, chest pain, coughing up blood, fatigue, fever, chills, and loss of appetite. Report these signs to the physician immediately.
- Monitor signs of hypersensitivity reactions and anaphylaxis, including pulmonary symptoms (tightness in the throat and chest, wheezing, cough, dyspnea) or skin reactions (rash, pruritus, urticaria). Be especially alert for allergy-like responses that occur during and after administration (infusion reactions). Notify physician immediately if these reactions occur.
- Monitor and report signs of neutropenia such as fever, sore throat, and signs of infection. Periodic blood tests may be needed to monitor WBC and RBC counts.
- Assess any new or increased back, joint, or muscle pain and spasms to rule out musculoskeletal pathology; that is, try to determine if pain is drug induced rather than caused by arthritis or anatomic and biomechanical problems.
- Assess blood pressure (BP) and compare to normal values (See Appendix F). Report changes in BP, either a problematic decrease in BP (hypotension) or a sustained increase in BP (hypertension).
- Assess heart rate, ECG, and heart sounds, especially during exercise (See Appendices G, H). Report a rapid heart rate (tachycardia) or signs of other arrhythmias, including palpitations, chest discomfort, shortness of breath, fainting, and fatigue/weakness.
- Assess signs of congestive heart failure such as dyspnea, rales/crackles, peripheral edema, jugular venous distention, and exercise intolerance. Report these signs to the physician.
- Monitor changes in mood and behavior, including depression, anxiety, and insomnia. Notify physician if these changes become problematic.
- Monitor signs of drug-induced lupus syndrome, including increased BP, fever, joint pain, skin rashes, and redness/irritation of the eye (uveitis). Notify physician promptly if these signs appear.
- If treating arthritic conditions, periodically assess impairments (pain, range of motion), functional ability, and disability to help document whether antirheumatic drug therapy is successful.
- If treating inflammatory bowel diseases, monitor any changes in symptoms such as decreased abdominal pain, decreased diarrhea, and improved appetite to help document whether drug therapy is successful.
- If treating psoriasis, monitor skin responses to help document whether drug therapy is successful in resolving this condition.

Interventions

- If treating arthritic conditions, implement appropriate manual therapy techniques, physical agents, therapeutic exercises, and orthotic/assistive devices to reduce pain, improve function, and augment the effects of antirheumatic drug therapy.
- Because of the risk of CHF, tachycardia, and abnormal BP responses, use caution during aerobic exercise and other forms of therapeutic exercise. Assess exercise tolerance frequently (BP, heart rate, fatigue levels), and terminate exercise immediately if any untoward responses occur (See Appendix L).

I

- Help patients with arthritis explore other nonpharmacologic methods to reduce chronic arthritis pain, such as relaxation techniques, exercise, counseling, and so forth.

Patient/Client-Related Instruction

- Advise patient about the likelihood of GI reactions such as nausea, vomiting, diarrhea, constipation, flatulence, abdominal pain, oral/tooth pain, and irritation of the oral mucosa. Instruct patient to report severe or prolonged GI problems or signs of liver toxicity such as yellow skin or eyes, abdominal pain, severe nausea and vomiting, fever, sore throat, malaise, weakness, and facial edema.
- Advise patient that rash and other skin reactions such as acne, pruritus, urticaria, eczema, flushing, bruising, hair loss, and dry skin are likely. Report severe or unexpected skin reactions to the physician.
- Instruct patient to report any blistering or other skin lesions that might indicate herpes simplex or herpes zoster infections.
- Advise patient to guard against infection (frequent hand washing, etc.), and to avoid crowds and contact with persons with contagious diseases.
- Instruct patient to report problems with urination, including increased urinary frequency, difficult urination, or signs of urinary tract infection (blood in the urine, increased nighttime urination, pain and burning during urination).
- Instruct patient to report other troublesome side effects, including severe or prolonged headache, flu-like syndrome, eye inflammation (conjunctivitis), peripheral edema, or yeast infections in the mouth/throat or vagina.

Pharmacokinetics

Absorption: IV administration results in complete bioavailability.
Distribution: Predominantly distributed within the vascular compartment.
Metabolism and Excretion: Unknown.
Half-life: 9.5 days.

TIME/ACTION PROFILE (symptoms of Crohn's disease)

ROUTE	ONSET	PEAK	DURATION
IV	1–2 wk	unknown	12–48 wk*

*After infusion.

Contraindications/Precautions

Contraindicated in: Hypersensitivity to infliximab, murine (mouse) proteins, or other components in the formulation; OB: Lactation; CHF.
Use Cautiously in: Patients being retreated after 2 yr without treatment (↑ risk of adverse reactions); History of tuberculosis or exposure (latent tuberculosis should be treated prior to infliximab therapy); Geri: Geriatric patients; OB: Pregnancy (use only if clearly needed); Pedi: Children (safety not established).

Interactions

Drug-Drug: None significant.

Route/Dosage

Rheumatoid arthritis

IV (Adults): 3 mg/kg followed by 3 mg/kg 2 and 6 wk after initial dose and then every 8 wk; dose may be adjusted in partial responders up to 10 mg/kg or treatment as often as every 4 wk (used with methotrexate).

Crohn's Disease

IV (Adults): *Moderate-to-severe Crohn's disease*—5 mg/kg as a single infusion. *Fistulizing Crohn's disease*—5 mg/kg repeated 2 and 6 wk after initial infusion; maintenance dose of 5 mg/kg may be given q 8 wk.

Ankylosing spondylitis

IV (Adults): 5 mg/kg given as an infusion repeated 2 and 6 wk later, then q 6 wk.

Psoriatic Arthritis

IV (Adults): 5 mg/kg given as an infusion repeated 2 and 6 wk later, then q 8 wk thereafter (with or without methotrexate).

Ulcerative Colitis

IV (Adults): 5 mg/kg given as an infusion regimen at 0, 2, and 6 wk followed by a maintenance regimen of 5 mg/kg q 8 wk thereafter.

Psoriasis

IV (Adults): 5 mg/kg given as an infusion regimen at 0, 2, and 6 wk followed by a maintenance regimen of 5 mg/kg q 8 wk thereafter.

Availability

Powder for injection: 100 mg/vial.

HIGH ALERT

insulin, regular (injection, concentrated) (in-su-lin)

Humulin R, Insulin-Toronto, Novolin R, Iletin II Regular, Velosulin BR, Humulin R Regular U-500 (Concentrated)

Classification

Therapeutic: antidiabetics, hormones
Pharmacologic: pancreatics

Indications

Control of hyperglycemia in patients with diabetes mellitus. **Concentrated regular insulin U-500:**

Only for use in patients with insulin requirements >200 units/day. **Unlabeled Use:** Treatment of hyperkalemia.

Action

Lowers blood glucose by stimulating glucose uptake in skeletal muscle and fat, inhibiting hepatic glucose production. Other actions of insulin: inhibition of lipolysis and proteolysis, enhanced protein synthesis. **Therapeutic Effects:** Control of hyperglycemia in diabetic patients.

Adverse Reactions/Side Effects

Endo: HYPOGLYCEMIA. **Local:** lipodystrophy, pruritus, erythema, swelling. **Misc:** ALLERGIC REACTIONS, INCLUDING ANAPHYLAXIS.

PHYSICAL THERAPY IMPLICATIONS

Examination and Evaluation

- Monitor signs of hypoglycemia, especially during and after exercise. Common neuromuscular symptoms include anxiety; restlessness; tingling in hands, feet, lips, or tongue; chills; cold sweats; confusion; difficulty in concentration; drowsiness; excessive hunger; headache; irritability; nervousness; tremor; weakness; unsteady gait. Report persistent or repeated episodes of hypoglycemia to the physician.
- Monitor signs of allergic reactions and anaphylaxis, including pulmonary symptoms (tightness in the throat and chest, wheezing, cough, dyspnea) or skin reactions (rash, pruritus, urticaria). Notify physician immediately if these reactions occur.
- Assess blood pressure periodically (see Appendix F). A sudden or sustained increase in blood pressure (hypertension) may indicate problems in diabetes management, and should be reported to the physician.
- Assess body weight periodically. Changes in weight may necessitate changes in insulin dose.
- Assess injection site for redness, swelling, or other reactions. Make sure patient understands the need to rotate injections sites to prevent local damage and lipodystrophy.

Interventions

- Implement aerobic exercise and endurance training programs to maintain optimal body weight, improve insulin sensitivity, and reduce the risk of macrovascular disease (heart attack, stroke) and microvascular problems (reduced blood flow to tissues and organs that causes poor wound healing, neuropathy, retinopathy, and nephropathy).
- Provide a source of oral glucose (fruit juice, glucose gels/tablets, etc.) to treat mild hypoglycemia. Call for emergency assistance if symptoms persist or in cases of severe hypoglycemia. Emergency treatment typically consists of IV glucose, glucagon, or epinephrine.
- Do not apply physical agents (heat, cold, electrotherapeutic modalities) or massage at or near the injection site; these interventions will alter insulin absorption from subcutaneous tissues.

Patient/Client-Related Instruction

- Encourage patient to monitor blood glucose before and after exercise and to adjust insulin dose accordingly based on exercise duration and intensity.
- Emphasize the importance of adhering to nutritional guidelines and the need for periodic assessment of glycemic control (serum glucose and glycosylated hemoglobin levels) throughout the management of diabetes mellitus.
- Advise patient about symptoms of hyperglycemia (confusion, drowsiness; flushed, dry skin; fruit-like breath odor; rapid, deep breathing, polyuria; loss of appetite; unusual thirst). Insulin dosages may need to be adjusted to prevent repeated episodes of hyperglycemia.

Pharmacokinetics

Absorption: Rapidly absorbed from subcutaneous administration sites. U-100 regular insulin is absorbed slightly more quickly than U-500.
Distribution: Identical to endogenous insulin.
Metabolism and Excretion: Metabolized by liver, spleen, kidney, and muscle.
Half-life: 30–60 min.

TIME/ACTION PROFILE (hypoglycemic effect)

ROUTE	ONSET	PEAK	DURATION
regular insulin IV	10–30 min	15–30 min	30–60 min
regular insulin subcutaneous	30–60 min	2–4 hr	5–7 hr

Contraindications/Precautions

Contraindicated in: Hypoglycemia; Allergy or hypersensitivity to a particular type of insulin, preservatives, or other additives.
Use Cautiously in: Stress or infection, may temporarily increase insulin requirements; Renal/hepatic impairment, may ↓ insulin requirements; OB: Pregnancy may temporarily ↑ insulin requirements.

Interactions

Drug-Drug: Beta blockers, clonidine, and **reserpine** may mask some of the signs and symptoms of hypoglycemia. **Corticosteroids, thyroid supplements, estrogens, isoniazid, niacin,**

phenothiazines, and **rifampin** may ↑ insulin requirements. **Alcohol, ACE inhibitors, MAO inhibitors, octreotide, oral hypoglycemic agents,** and **salicylates,** may ↓ insulin requirements. **Drug-Natural: Glucosamine** may worsen blood glucose control. **Fenugreek, chromium,** and **coenzyme Q10** may produce additive hypoglycemic effects.

Route/Dosage

Dose depends on blood glucose, response, and many other factors.

Ketoacidosis—Regular (100 units/mL) Insulin Only

IV (Adults): 0.1 unit/kg/hr as a continuous infusion.
IV (Children): Loading dose—0.1 unit/kg, then maintenance continuous infusion 0.05–0.2 unit/kg/hr, titrate to optimal rate of decrease of serum glucose of 80–100 mg/dL/hr.

Maintenance Therapy

Subcut (Adults and Children): 0.5–1 unit/kg/day in divided doses. *Adolescents during rapid growth*—0.8–1.2 unit/kg/day in divided doses.

Treatment of Hyperkalemia

SC, IV (Adults and Children): dextrose 0.5–1 g/kg combined with insulin 1 unit for q 4–5 g dextrose given.

Availability

Insulin injection (regular insulin): 100 units/mL OTC, 100 units/mL in PenFill cartridges. **Regular (concentrated) insulin injection:** 500 units/mL. ***In combination with:*** NPH insulins (Humulin 70/30, Novolin 70/30).

interferon alfacon-1

(in-ter-**feer**-on **al**-fa-kon-won)
Infergen

Classification
Therapeutic: immune modifiers
Pharmacologic: interferons

Indications

Treatment of chronic hepatitis C infection (HCV).

Action

Antiproliferative, antiviral, and immunomodulatory effects. **Therapeutic Effects:** Improvement in liver function studies, liver histology, and decreased hepatitis C viral RNA concentration.

Adverse Reactions/Side Effects

CNS: anxiety, depression, dizziness, insomnia, nervousness, malaise, suicidal ideation. **EENT:** loss of visual acuity or visual field, tinnitus. **GI:** abdominal pain, anorexia, diarrhea, dyspepsia, vomiting, constipation, dry mouth, flatulence. **Derm:** alopecia, pruritus, rash. **Endo:** hypothyroidism. **Hemat:** ANEMIA, LEUKOPENIA, THROMBOCYTOPENIA. **Local:** injection site reactions. **MS:** body pain. **Neuro:** paresthesia. **Misc:** ALLERGIC REACTIONS, INCLUDING ANAPHYLAXIS, flu-like symptoms (headache, fatigue, fever).

PHYSICAL THERAPY IMPLICATIONS

Examination and Evaluation

- Monitor signs of leukopenia (fever, sore throat, signs of infection), thrombocytopenia (bruising, nose bleeds, bleeding gums), or unusual weakness and fatigue that might be due to anemias or other blood dyscrasias. Report these signs to the physician immediately.
- Monitor signs of allergic reactions and anaphylaxis, including pulmonary symptoms (tightness in the throat and chest, wheezing, cough, dyspnea), or skin reactions (rash, pruritus, urticaria, dermatitis). Notify physician or nursing staff immediately if these reactions occur.
- Monitor personality changes, including anxiety, nervousness, depression, and increased thoughts of suicide. Notify physician if these changes become problematic.
- Assess any joint pain or muscle pain to rule out musculoskeletal pathology; that is, try to determine if pain is drug induced rather than caused by anatomic or biomechanical problems.
- Monitor signs of paresthesia (numbness, tingling). Perform objective tests (nerve conduction, monofilaments) to document any neuropathic changes.
- Monitor and report any signs of hypothyroidism, including bradycardia, lethargy, cold intolerance, weight gain, and muscle weakness.
- Assess dizziness that might affect gait, balance, and other functional activities (See Appendix C). Report balance problems and functional limitations to the physician and nursing staff, and caution the patient and family/caregivers to guard against falls and trauma.
- Assess injection site for pain, swelling, and irritation. Report prolonged or excessive injection site reactions to the physician.

Interventions

- Implement resistive exercises and other therapeutic exercises as tolerated to maintain muscle strength and function in patients with chronic hepatitis.

Patient/Client-Related Instruction

- Advise patient about the likelihood of GI reactions, including nausea, vomiting, diarrhea, constipation, flatulence, dry mouth, and loss of appetite. Instruct patient to report severe or prolonged GI problems.
- Instruct patient to report other troublesome side effects such as prolonged or severe vision disturbances, ringing/buzzing in the ears (tinnitus), flu-like symptoms, or skin problems (rash, itching, hair loss)

Pharmacokinetics

Absorption: Well absorbed following SC administration.
Distribution: Unknown.
Metabolism and Excretion: Unknown.
Half-life: Up to 7 hr.

TIME/ACTION PROFILE

ROUTE	ONSET	PEAK	DURATION
SC	unknown	unknown	unknown

Contraindications/Precautions

Contraindicated in: Hypersensitivity to alfa interferons or *Escherichia coli*–derived products.
Use Cautiously in: History of severe psychiatric illness, depression, or suicide attempt; Underlying myelosuppression; Endocrine disorders; Autoimmune disorders; Pregnancy, lactation, or patients <18 yr (safety not established).

Interactions

Drug-Drug: Concurrent use of **antineoplastics** or **agents known to cause myelosuppression** ↑ the risk of myelosuppression. May alter the effects of other **drugs sharing common liver metabolic pathways.**
Drug-Natural: Avoid concomitant use with immunomodulating products, such as **astragalus, echinacea,** and **melatonin**.

Route/Dosage

SC (Adults): 9 mcg 3 times weekly for 24 wk; may be increased to 15 mcg 3 times weekly if patient has tolerated the lower dose, but has not responded or has relapsed. Dose reduction to 7.5 mcg may be considered in patients who do not tolerate the initial dose.

Availability

Solution for injection: 9 mcg/0.3 mL, 15 mcg/0.5 mL.

interferon beta-1a
(in-ter-feer-on bay-ta won-aye)
Avonex, Rebif

Classification
Therapeutic: anti–multiple sclerosis agents, immune modifiers
Pharmacologic: interferons

Indications

Relapsing forms of multiple sclerosis.

Action

Antiviral and immunoregulatory properties produced by interacting with specific receptor sites on cell surfaces may explain beneficial effects. Produced by recombinant DNA technology. **Therapeutic Effects:** Reduce incidence of relapse (neurologic dysfunction) and slow physical disability.

Adverse Reactions/Side Effects

CNS: SEIZURES, depression, dizziness, fatigue, headache, drowsiness, incoordination, rigors, suicidal ideation. **EENT:** sinusitis, vision abnormalities. **Resp:** upper respiratory tract infection. **CV:** chest pain, heart failure. **GI:** abdominal pain, nausea, autoimmune hepatitis, dry mouth, elevated liver function studies. **GU:** urinary tract infection, urinary incontinence, polyuria. **Derm:** alopecia, rash. **Endo:** hyperthyroidism, hypothyroidism, spontaneous abortion. **Hemat:** neutropenia, anemia, thrombocytopenia. **Local:** injection-site reactions, injection site necrosis. **MS:** myalgia, arthralgia, back pain, muscle spasm. **Misc:** allergic reactions, including anaphylaxis, chills, fever, flu-like symptoms, pain.

PHYSICAL THERAPY IMPLICATIONS

Examination and Evaluation

- Be alert for new seizures or increased seizure activity, especially at the onset of drug treatment. Document the number, duration, and severity of seizures, and report these findings to the physician immediately.
- Monitor signs of allergic reactions and anaphylaxis, including pulmonary symptoms (tightness in the throat and chest, wheezing, cough, dyspnea), or skin reactions (rash, pruritus, urticaria, dermatitis). Notify physician or nursing staff immediately if these reactions occur.
- Periodically assess balance, coordination, spasticity, and other aspects of neuromuscular function to

help document this drug's effectiveness in reducing MS exacerbations.

- Monitor personality changes, including depression and increased thoughts of suicide. Notify physician if these changes become problematic.
- Monitor any chest pain or signs of heart failure, including dyspnea, rales/crackles, peripheral edema, jugular venous distention, and exercise intolerance. Report these signs to the physician.
- Assess any joint, back, or muscle pain and spasm to rule out musculoskeletal pathology; that is, try to determine if pain is drug induced rather than caused by anatomic or biomechanical problems.
- Monitor and report any increase or decrease in metabolism that might indicate thyroid disorders. Signs of hyperthyroidism include tachycardia, nervousness, heat intolerance, weight loss, and muscle wasting. Hypothyroidism is typically indicated by bradycardia, lethargy, cold intolerance, weight gain, and muscle weakness.
- Assess dizziness that might affect gait, balance, and other functional activities (See Appendix C). Report balance problems and functional limitations to the physician and nursing staff, and caution the patient and family/caregivers to guard against falls and trauma.
- Assess injection site for pain, swelling, and irritation. Report prolonged or excessive injection site reactions to the physician.

Interventions

- Design and implement coordination, balance, and other therapeutic exercises to maintain function and complement drug effects in patients with MS.

Patient/Client-Related Instruction

- Instruct patient to report severe or prolonged nausea or signs of drug-induced hepatitis such as yellow skin or eyes, abdominal pain, severe nausea and vomiting, fever, sore throat, malaise, weakness, and facial edema.
- Instruct patient to report other troublesome side effects such as prolonged or severe headache, vision disturbances, sinus inflammation, flu-like symptoms, or skin problems (rash, hair loss).

Pharmacokinetics

Absorption: 50% absorbed following SC administration.
Distribution: Unknown.
Metabolism and Excretion: Unknown.
Half-life: 69 hr (SC), 10 hr (IM).

TIME/ACTION PROFILE (serum concentrations)

ROUTE	ONSET	PEAK	DURATION
IM	unknown	3–15 hr	unknown
SC	unknown	16 hr	unknown

Contraindications/Precautions

Contraindicated in: Hypersensitivity to natural or recombinant interferon beta or human albumin.
Use Cautiously in: Patients with a history of suicide attempt or depression; History of seizures; Cardiovascular disease; Liver disease; History of alcohol abuse; Patients with childbearing potential; OB/Lactation/Pedi: Safety not established.

Interactions

Drug-Drug: ↑ myelosuppression may occur with other myelosuppressives, including **antineoplastics**. Concurrent use of **hepatotoxic agents** may ↑ the risk of hepatotoxicity (↑ liver enzymes).
Drug-Natural: Avoid concomitant use with immunomodulating natural products such as **astragalus, echinacea,** and **melatonin**.

Route/Dosage

Avonex

IM (Adults): 30 mcg once weekly.

Rebif

SC (Adults): *Target dose of 22 mcg 3 times/wk*—Start with 4.4 mcg 3 times/wk for 2 wk, then increase to 11 mcg 3 times/wk for 2 wk, then increase to maintenance dose of 22 mcg 3 times/wk; *Target dose of 44 mcg 3 times/wk*—Start with 8.8 mcg 3 times/wk for 2 wk, then increase to 22 mcg 3 times/wk for 2 wk, then increase to maintenance dose of 44 mcg 3 times/wk.

Availability

Avonex

Powder for injection: 30 mcg/vial Rx. **Prefilled syringes:** 30 mcg/0.5 mL Rx.

Rebif

Prefilled syringes: 22 mcg/0.5 mL Rx, 44 mcg/0.5 mL Rx, titration pack of 6 syringes prefilled with 8.8 mcg/0.2 mL and 6 syringes prefilled with 22 mcg/0.5 mL Rx.

interferon beta-1b

(in-ter-**feer**-on **bay**-ta won-bee)
Betaseron

Classification
Therapeutic: anti–multiple sclerosis agents, immune modifiers
Pharmacologic: interferons

Indications

Relapsing forms of multiple sclerosis (MS). MS patients who have experienced a first clinical episode and have MRI features consistent with the disease.

Action

Antiviral and immunoregulatory properties produced by interacting with specific receptor sites on cell surfaces may explain beneficial effects. Produced by recombinant DNA technology. **Therapeutic Effects:** Reduce incidence of relapse (neurologic dysfunction) and slowing of physical disability.

Adverse Reactions/Side Effects

CNS: depression, headache, incoordination, insomnia, suicidal ideation. **Resp:** dyspnea. **CV:** edema, chest pain, hypertension. **GI:** abdominal pain, constipation, nausea, vomiting, autoimmune hepatitis, elevated liver function studies. **GU:** urgency, erectile dysfunction. **Derm:** rash. **Endo:** menstrual disorders, hyperthyroidism, hypothyroidism, menorrhagia, spontaneous abortion. **Hemat:** neutropenia, anemia, thrombocytopenia. **Local:** injection-site reactions, injection site necrosis. **MS:** myalgia, muscle spasm. **Misc:** allergic reactions, including anaphylaxis, chills, fever, flu-like symptoms, pain.

PHYSICAL THERAPY IMPLICATIONS

- Monitor signs of allergic reactions and anaphylaxis, including pulmonary symptoms (tightness in the throat and chest, wheezing, cough, dyspnea), or skin reactions (rash, pruritus, urticaria, dermatitis). Notify physician or nursing staff immediately if these reactions occur.
- Monitor signs of neutropenia (fever, sore throat, signs of infection), thrombocytopenia (bruising, nose bleeds, bleeding gums), or unusual weakness and fatigue that might be due to anemia. Report these signs to the physician immediately.
- Periodically assess balance, coordination, spasticity, and other aspects of neuromuscular function to help document this drug's effectiveness in reducing MS exacerbations.
- Monitor personality changes, including depression and increased thoughts of suicide. Notify physician if these changes become problematic.
- Assess blood pressure (BP) and compare to normal values (See Appendix F). Report a sustained increase in BP (hypertension).
- Assess peripheral edema using girth measurements, volume displacement, and measurement of pitting edema (See Appendix N). Report increased swelling in feet and ankles or a sudden increase in body weight due to fluid retention.
- Monitor any chest pain or difficult/labored breathing. Report prolonged or severe cardiopulmonary problems to the physician, especially if these problems are exacerbated by exercise.
- Assess any muscle pain or spasms to rule out musculoskeletal pathology; that is, try to determine if pain is drug induced rather than caused by anatomic or biomechanical problems.
- Monitor and report any increase or decrease in metabolism that might indicate thyroid disorders. Signs of hyperthyroidism include tachycardia, nervousness, heat intolerance, weight loss, and muscle wasting. Hypothyroidism is typically indicated by bradycardia, lethargy, cold intolerance, weight gain, and muscle weakness.
- Assess dizziness that might affect gait, balance, and other functional activities (See Appendix C). Report balance problems and functional limitations to the physician and nursing staff, and caution the patient and family/caregivers to guard against falls and trauma.
- Assess injection site for pain, swelling, and irritation. Report prolonged or excessive injection site reactions to the physician.

I

Interventions

- Design and implement coordination, balance, and other therapeutic exercises to maintain function and complement drug effects in patients with MS.

Patient/Client-related Instruction

- Advise patient about the likelihood of GI reactions such as nausea, vomiting, and constipation. Instruct patient to report severe or prolonged GI problems or signs of hepatitis (yellow skin or eyes, abdominal pain, severe nausea and vomiting, fever, sore throat, malaise, weakness, facial edema).
- Instruct patient to report other troublesome side effects such as prolonged or severe headache, sleep loss, urinary urgency, menstrual disorders, erectile dysfunction, flu-like symptoms, or skin rash.

Pharmacokinetics

Absorption: 50% absorbed following SC administration.
Distribution: Unknown.
Metabolism and Excretion: Unknown.
Half-life: 8 min–4.3 hr.

TIME/ACTION PROFILE (serum concentrations)

ROUTE	ONSET	PEAK	DURATION
SC	rapid	1–8 hr	unknown

Contraindications/Precautions

Contraindicated in: Hypersensitivity to natural or recombinant interferon beta or human albumin.
Use Cautiously in: Patients with a history of suicide attempt or depression; Patients with childbearing potential; OB/Lactation/Pedi: Safety not established.

Interactions

Drug-Drug: Not known.

Route/Dosage

Subcut (Adults): Initiate with 0.0625 mg every other day and then increase over 6 wk to 0.25 mg every other day.

Availability

Powder for injection: 0.3 mg/vial.

interferon gamma-1b

(in-ter-**feer**-on **gam**-ma won-bee)
Actimmune

Classification
Therapeutic: immune modifiers
Pharmacologic: interferons

Indications

Diminished severity and frequency of infectious complications of chronic granulomatous disease. Slow disease progression in severe, malignant osteopetrosis.

Action

A protein produced by recombinant DNA technology that is capable of activating phagocytes, enhancing their ability to kill pathogens, including *Staphylococcus aureus*, *Toxoplasma gondii*, *Leishmania donovani*, *Listeria monocytogenes*, *Mycobacterium avium intracellulare*. Interferon gamma has antiproliferative effects superior to interferons alpha and beta. **Therapeutic Effects:** Decreased incidence and severity of infection in patients with chronic granulomatous disease. Slowed disease progression of severe, malignant osteopetrosis.

Adverse Reactions/Side Effects

CNS: headache, decreased mental status, dizziness. **GI:** nausea, vomiting, abdominal pain. **Derm:** rash. **Hemat:** neutropenia, thrombocytopenia. **Local:** edema or tenderness at injection site. **MS:** arthralgia, myalgia, back pain. **Neuro:** gait disturbances. **Misc:** chills, fever.

PHYSICAL THERAPY IMPLICATIONS

- Monitor signs of neutropenia (fever, sore throat, signs of infection) or thrombocytopenia (bruising, nose bleeds, bleeding gums). Report these signs to the physician immediately.
- Assess any gait abnormalities that might be drug induced. Attempt to rule out neuromuscular causes of gait problems, and report any unexplained gait disturbances to the physician.
- Monitor personality changes or decreased mental status. Notify physician if these changes become problematic.
- Assess any joint, muscle, or back pain to rule out musculoskeletal pathology; that is, try to determine if pain is drug-induced rather than caused by anatomic problems or problems related directly to the underlying condition (osteopetrosis or joint infections).
- Assess dizziness that might affect gait, balance, and other functional activities (See Appendix C). Report balance problems and functional limitations to the physician and nursing staff, and caution the patient and family/caregivers to guard against falls and trauma.
- Assess injection site for pain, swelling, and irritation. Report prolonged or excessive injection site reactions to the physician.

Interventions

- Use caution during therapeutic exercises to avoid fracture in patients with osteopetrosis. Implement appropriate resistive exercises as tolerated to maintain muscle strength and promote normal bone mineralization.

Patient/Client-Related Instruction

- Instruct patient to report other troublesome side effects such as prolonged or severe headache, chills, fever, skin rash, or GI problems (nausea, vomiting, abdominal pain).

Pharmacokinetics

Absorption: Well absorbed after SC administration.
Distribution: Unknown.
Metabolism and Excretion: Unknown.
Half-life: 5.9 hr.

TIME/ACTION PROFILE (blood levels)

ROUTE	ONSET	PEAK	DURATION
SC	unknown	4 hr	unknown

Contraindications/Precautions

Contraindicated in: Hypersensitivity to interferon gamma, *Escherichia coli*–derived products, mannitol, or polysorbate.
Use Cautiously in: Cardiovascular disease; Bone marrow depression; Pregnancy, lactation, or children <1 yr (safety not established).

Interactions

Drug-Drug: May have additive bone marrow–depressing effects with **antineoplastics** or **radiation therapy**.

Route/Dosage

Body Surface Area >0.5 m²

SC (Children): 50 mcg/m² (1 million units/m²) 3 times weekly.

Body Surface Area ≤0.5 m²

SC (Children >1 yr): 1.5 mcg/kg 3 times weekly.

Availability

Injection: 100 mcg (3 million units)/vial.

INTERFERONS, ALPHA
(in-ter-feer-onz, al-fa)

peginterferon alpha-2a
Pegasys

interferon alpha-2b (recombinant)
Intron A

peginterferon alpha-2b (pegylated)
Pegintron

interferon alpha-n3 (human)
Alferon N

Classification
Therapeutic: immune modifiers
Pharmacologic: interferons

Indications
Peginterferon alpha-2a: Treatment of: Chronic hepatitis C (alone or with ribavirin), Chronic hepatitis B. **Interferon alpha-2b:** Treatment of: Hairy cell leukemia, Malignant melanoma, AIDS-related Kaposi's sarcoma, Condylomata acuminata (intralesional), Chronic hepatitis B, Chronic hepatitis C (with oral ribavirin) which has relapsed following previous treatment with interferon alone, Follicular non-Hodgkin's lymphoma. **Peginterferon alpha-2b:** Chronic hepatitis C (alone or with ribavirin). **Interferon alpha-n3:** Treatment of condylomata acuminata (intralesional).

Action
Interferons are proteins capable of modifying the immune response and have antiproliferative action against tumor cells. Interferon alpha-2b is produced by recombinant DNA techniques, peginterferon is a "pegylated" formulation of interferon alpha-2b formulated to have a longer duration of action; interferon alpha-n3 is from pooled human leukocytes. Interferons also have antiviral activity. **Therapeutic Effects:** Antineoplastic, antiviral, and antiproliferative activities. Decreased progression of hepatic damage (for patients with hepatitis).

Adverse Reactions/Side Effects
All are more prominent with SC, IV, or IM administration

CNS: NEUROPSYCHIATRIC DISORDERS, confusion, depression, dizziness, fatigue, headache, insomnia, irritability, anxiety. **EENT:** blurred vision, nose bleeds, rhinitis. **CV:** ISCHEMIC DISORDERS, arrhythmias, chest pain, edema. **GI:** COLITIS, PANCREATITIS, anorexia, abdominal pain, diarrhea, dry mouth, nausea, taste disorder, vomiting, weight loss, drug-induced hepatitis, flatulence. **Derm:** alopecia, dry skin, pruritus, rash, sweating. **Endo:** thyroid disorders. **Hemat:** LEUKOPENIA, THROMBOCYTOPENIA, anemia, hemolytic anemia (with ribavirin). **MS:** arthralgia, myalgia, leg cramps. **Neuro:** paresthesia. **Resp:** cough, dyspnea. **Local:** injection site reactions. **Misc:** AUTOIMMUNE DISORDERS, INFECTIOUS DISORDERS, allergic reactions, including anaphylaxis, chills, fever, flu-like syndrome.

PHYSICAL THERAPY IMPLICATIONS

Examination and Evaluation
- Continually monitor for signs of ischemic disorders, including MI (sudden chest pain, pain radiating into the arm or jaw, shortness of breath, dizziness, sweating, anxiety, nausea), stroke (sudden severe headache, confusion, nausea, vomiting, paralysis, numbness, speech problems, visual disturbances), or peripheral ischemia (extreme coldness in the hands and feet, cyanosis, muscle cramping). Seek immediate medical assistance if patient develops these signs.
- Be alert for signs of colitis (diarrhea, abdominal pain, cramps, nausea, fecal incontinence) and pancreatitis (upper abdominal pain especially after eating, indigestion, weight loss, oily stools). Notify physician immediately of these signs.
- Monitor signs of leukopenia (fever, sore throat, signs of infection), thrombocytopenia (bruising, nose bleeds, bleeding gums), or unusual weakness and fatigue that might be due to anemias or other blood dyscrasias. Report these signs to the physician immediately.
- Be alert for signs of autoimmune reactions and infectious disorders, including muscle and joint pain, weakness, fever, dyspnea, skin reactions (rash, itching), and other unexplained symptoms. Notify physician of these signs immediately.
- Monitor signs of neuropsychiatric disorders such as confusion, anxiety, irritability, delirium, and hallucinations. Notify physician promptly if these signs occur.
- Monitor signs of hypersensitivity reactions and anaphylaxis, including pulmonary symptoms (tightness in the throat and chest, wheezing, cough, dyspnea), or skin reactions (rash, pruritus, urticaria, dermatitis). Notify physician or nursing staff immediately if these reactions occur.
- Assess heart rate, ECG, and heart sounds, especially during exercise (See Appendices G, H). Report any rhythm disturbances or symptoms of

increased arrhythmias, including palpitations, chest discomfort, shortness of breath, fainting, and fatigue/weakness.

- Assess peripheral edema using girth measurements, volume displacement, and measurement of pitting edema (See Appendix N). Report increased swelling in feet and ankles or a sudden increase in body weight due to fluid retention.
- Assess any joint pain, muscle pain, or leg cramps to rule out musculoskeletal pathology; that is, try to determine if pain is drug induced rather than caused by anatomic or biomechanical problems.
- Monitor signs of paresthesia (numbness, tingling). Perform objective tests (nerve conduction, monofilaments) to document any neuropathic changes.
- Monitor and report any increase or decrease in metabolism that might indicate thyroid disorders. Signs of hyperthyroidism include tachycardia, nervousness, heat intolerance, weight loss, and muscle wasting. Hypothyroidism is typically indicated by bradycardia, lethargy, cold intolerance, weight gain, and muscle weakness.
- Assess dizziness that might affect gait, balance, and other functional activities (See Appendix C). Report balance problems and functional limitations to the physician and nursing staff, and caution the patient and family/caregivers to guard against falls and trauma.
- Assess injection site for pain, swelling, and irritation. Report prolonged or excessive injection site reactions to the physician.

Interventions

- Implement resistive exercises and other therapeutic exercises as tolerated to maintain muscle strength and function and prevent muscle wasting associated with cancer, chronic hepatitis, and HIV infections.
- Because of the risk of ischemic disorders and arrhythmias, use extreme caution during aerobic exercise and other forms of therapeutic exercise. Assess exercise tolerance frequently (blood pressure, heart rate, fatigue levels), and terminate exercise immediately if any untoward responses occur (See Appendix L).

Patient/Client-Related Instruction

- Advise patient about the likelihood of GI reactions (nausea, vomiting, diarrhea, flatulence, loss of appetite). Instruct patient to report severe or prolonged GI problems, or signs of drug-induced hepatitis (yellow skin or eyes, abdominal pain, severe nausea and vomiting, fever, sore throat, malaise, weakness, facial edema).
- Instruct patient to report other troublesome side effects such as prolonged or severe headache, sleep loss, blurred vision, nose bleeds, flu-like symptoms, or skin problems (rash, itching, hair loss, increased sweating)

Pharmacokinetics

Absorption: Not absorbed orally. Well absorbed (>80%) following IM and SC administration. Minimal systemic absorption follows intralesional administration.

Distribution: Unknown.

Metabolism and Excretion: Filtered by the kidneys and subsequently degraded in the renal tubule; *peginterferon alpha-2b*—30% renally excreted.

Half-life: *Peginterferon alpha-2a*—50–160 hr; *interferon alpha-2b*—2–3 hr; *peginterferon alpha-2b*—40 hr.

TIME/ACTION PROFILE (clinical effects)

ROUTE	ONSET	PEAK	DURATION
interferon alpha-2b IM, SC	1–3 mo	unknown	unknown (CR)
interferon alpha-2b IM, SC	unknown	3–5 days	3–5 days (BC)
interferon alpha-2b IM, SC	2 wk	unknown	unknown (LFT)
interferons alpha-2b IM, SC and alpha-n3 SC	unknown	4–8 wk	unknown (IL)
peginterferon alpha-2b SC	unknown	6 mos or more	unknown

BC = effects on platelet counts; CR = clinical response; RL= regression of lesions; LFT = effects on liver function in patients with hepatitis.

Contraindications/Precautions

Contraindicated in: Hypersensitivity to alpha interferons or human serum albumin; Autoimmune hepatitis; Hepatic decompensation (Child-Pugh classes B and C) before or during therapy; Pedi: Products containing benzyl alcohol should not be used in neonates.

Use Cautiously in: Severe cardiovascular, pulmonary, renal, or hepatic disease; Active infections; Underlying CNS pathology or psychiatric history; Decreased bone marrow reserve or underlying immunosuppression; Current history of chickenpox, herpes zoster, or herpes labialis (may reactivate or disseminate disease); Previous or concurrent radiation therapy; Autoimmune disorders (may ↑ risk of exacerbation); Geri: ↑ risk of adverse reactions; OB/Pedi: Childbearing potential, pregnancy, lactation and children <3 yr (safety not established).

Exercise Extreme Caution in: History of depression/suicide attempt.

Interactions

Drug-Drug: Additive myelosuppression with other **antineoplastic agents** or **radiation therapy**. ↑ CNS depression may occur with **CNS depressants**, including **alcohol**, **antihistamines**, **sedative/hypnotics**, and **opioids**. May ↓ metabolism and ↑ blood levels and toxicity of **theophylline** and **methadone**. ↑ risk of adverse reactions with **zidovudine**. **Ribavirin** ↑ risk of hemolytic anemia, especially if CCr <50 mL/min (avoid if possible). May ↓ effects of **immunosuppressant agents**.

Route/Dosage

Peginterferon alpha-2a

SC (Adults): *Chronic hepatitis C*180 mcg once weekly for 48 wk for genotypes 1, 4 (24 wk for genotypes 2, 3). *Patients with chronic hepatitis C coinfected with HIV*—180 mcg once weekly for 48 wk.

Interferon alpha-2b

IV (Adults): *Malignant melanoma (induction)*—20 million units/m² for 5 days of each week for 4 wk initially, followed by SC maintenance dosing.

IM, SC (Adults): *Hairy cell leukemia*—2 million units/m² IM or SC 3 times weekly for up to 6 mo. *Malignant melanoma (maintenance)*—10 million units/m² SC 3 times weekly for 48 wk, following initial IV dosing. *AIDS-related Kaposi's sarcoma*—30 million units/m² IM or SC 3 times weekly until disease progression or maximum response has been achieved after 16 wk. *Chronic hepatitis C*—3 million units IM or SC 3 times weekly. If normalization of ALT occurs after 16 wk of therapy, continue treatment for total of 18–24 mo. If normalization of ALT does not occur after 16 wk of therapy, may consider discontinuing treatment. *Chronic hepatitis B*—5 million units/day IM or SC *or* 10 million units IM or SC 3 times weekly for 16 wk. *Follicular non Hodgkin's lymphoma*—5 million units SC 3 times weekly for up to 18 mo (to be used following completion of anthracycline-containing chemotherapy).

SC (Children> 3 yr): *Chronic hepatitis B*—3 million units/m² 3 times weekly for the first week of therapy, then increase to 6 million units/m² 3 times weekly (not to exceed 10 million units/dose) for 16–24 wk.

IL (Adults): *Condylomata acuminata*—1 million units/lesion 3 times weekly for 3 wk; treat only 5 lesions per course. An additional course of treatment may be initiated at 12–16 wk.

Peginterferon alpha-2b

Monotherapy

SC (Adults): *137–160 kg*—150 mcg once weekly for 1 yr. *107–136 kg*—120 mcg once weekly for 1 yr. *89–106 kg*—96 mcg once weekly for 1 yr. *73–88 kg*—80 mcg once weekly for 1 year. *57–72 kg*—64 mcg once weekly for 1 yr. *46–56 kg*—50 mcg once weekly for 1 yr. *37–45 kg*—40 mcg once weekly for 1 yr.

In Combination with Ribavirin (Rebetol)

SC (Adults): *>85 kg*—150 mcg once weekly. *76–85 kg*—120 mcg once weekly. *61–75 kg*—96 mcg once weekly. *51–60 kg*—80 mcg once weekly. *40–50 kg*—64 mcg once weekly. *<40 kg*—50 mcg once weekly.

Interferon alpha-n3

IL (Adults): 250,000 units/lesion twice weekly for up to 8 wk; for large lesions, divide dose and inject at several sites.

Availability

Peginterferon alpha-2a

Solution for injection: 180 mcg/mL in single-use vials. **Prefilled syringes:** 180 mcg/0.5 mL.

Interferon alpha-2b

Powder for injection: 10-million unit single-use vial, 18-million unit single-use vial, 50-million unit single-use vial. **Solution for injection:** 10-million unit single-use vial, 18-million unit single-use vial, 18-million unit multidose pen, 25-million unit multidose vial, 30-million unit multidose pen, 60-million unit multidose pen. ***In combination with:*** oral ribavirin (Rebetol) as a combination package (Rebetron). See Appendix B (in various dosage packages).

Peginterferon alpha-2b

Powder for injection (Redipen system or vials): 50 mcg/0.5 mL, 80 mcg/0.5 mL, 120 mcg/0.5 mL, 150 mcg/0.5 mL.

Interferon Alpha-n3

Solution for injection: 5-million units/mL.

ipilimumab (i-pil-li-moo-mab)

Yervoy

Classification

Therapeutic: antineoplastics

Pharmacologic: monoclonal antibodies

Indications

Treatment of unresectable/metastatic melanoma.

Action

Binds to cytotoxic T-lymphocyte–associated antigen 4 (CTLA-4). CTLA-4 is a negative regulator of T-cell activation; binding results in augmented T-cell activation and proliferation. **Therapeutic Effects:** ↓ spread of melanoma.

Adverse Reactions/Side Effects

CNS: fatigue. **EENT:** immune-mediated ocular disease. **GI:** IMMUNE-MEDIATED COLITIS, IMMUNE-MEDIATED HEPATITIS, colitis, diarrhea. **Derm:** IMMUNE-MEDIATED DERMATITIS, INCLUDING TOXIC EPIDERMAL NECROLYSIS, pruritus, rash. **Endo:** IMMUNE-MEDIATED ENDROCRINOPATHIES, INCLUDING HYPOPITUITARISM, HYPOTHYROIDISM, HYPERTHYROIDISM, ADRENAL INSUFFICIENCY, CUSHING'S SYNDROME, AND HYPOGONADISM. **Neuro:** IMMUNE-MEDIATED NEUROPATHY.

PHYSICAL THERAPY IMPLICATIONS

Examination and Evaluation

- Watch for the following immune-mediated responses, and report these responses to the physician or nursing staff immediately.
  - Colitis (diarrhea, abdominal pain, cramps, nausea, fecal incontinence).
  - Hepatitis (anorexia, abdominal pain, severe nausea and vomiting, yellow skin or eyes, skin rashes, flu-like symptoms, muscle/joint pain).
  - Skin reactions (severe rash, dermatitis, exfoliation, epidermal necrolysis).
  - Thyroid dysfunction, including hyperthyroidism (tachycardia, nervousness, heat intolerance, weight loss, muscle wasting), or hypothyroidism (bradycardia, lethargy, cold intolerance, weight gain, muscle weakness).
  - Neuropathy (numbness, tingling, pain, weakness).
  - Adrenal dysfunction, including adrenal insufficiency (hypotension, weight loss, weakness, nausea, vomiting, anorexia, lethargy, confusion, restlessness) or Cushing's syndrome (puffiness in the face, increased abdominal fat, thin arms and legs, abdominal skin striations, changes in skin pigmentation, bruising, deposition of fat behind the base of the neck).
  - Hypopituitarism (fatigue, weight loss, decreased libido, hot flashes in women, cold intolerance, anemia, alopecia, stunted growth in children).
  - Ocular disease (blurred vision, loss of vision, other vision problems).

Interventions

- For patients who are medically able to begin exercise, implement appropriate resistive exercises and aerobic training to maintain muscle strength and aerobic capacity during cancer chemotherapy or to help restore function after chemotherapy.
- Because of numerous immune-mediated problems, use caution during aerobic exercise and endurance conditioning because of potential pulmonary toxicity. Terminate exercise if patient exhibits untoward symptoms (chest pain, shortness of breath, unusual fatigue) or displays other criteria for exercise termination (See Appendix L).

Patient/Client-Related Instruction

- Instruct patient or family/caregivers to report other bothersome side effects such as severe or prolonged skin reactions (rash, itching) or GI problems (diarrhea, abdominal pain).

Pharmacokinetics

Absorption: IV administration results in complete bioavailability.
Distribution: Crosses the placenta
Metabolism and Excretion: Unknown
Half-life: 14.7 days

TIME/ACTION PROFILE

ROUTE	ONSET	PEAK	DURATION
IV	unknown	unknown	unknown

Contraindications/Precautions

Contraindicated in: Lactation: Avoid breast-feeding.
Use Cautiously in: OB: Use only if potential maternal benefit justifies potential risk to the fetus; may cause fetal harm; Pedi: safe and effective use in children has not been established.

Interactions

Drug-Drug: None noted.

Route/Dosage

IV (Adults): 3 mg/kg every 3 wk for a total of 4 doses.

Availability

Solution for IV infusion (requires further dilution): 50 mg/10-mL vial; 200 mg/40-mL vial.

ipratropium (ip-ra-**troe**-pee-um)

Atrovent HFA

Classification
Therapeutic: allergy, cold, and cough remedies, bronchodilators
Pharmacologic: anticholinergics

Indications

Inhalation: Maintenance therapy of reversible airway obstruction due to COPD, including chronic bronchitis and emphysema. **Intranasal:** Rhinorrhea associated with allergic and nonallergic perennial rhinitis (0.03% solution) or the common cold (0.06% solution). **Unlabeled Use: Inhalation:** Adjunctive management of bronchospasm caused by asthma.

Action

Inhalation: Inhibits cholinergic receptors in bronchial smooth muscle, resulting in decreased concentrations of cyclic guanosine monophosphate (cGMP). Decreased levels of cGMP produce local bronchodilation. **Intranasal:** Local application inhibits secretions from glands lining the nasal mucosa.
Therapeutic Effects: Inhalation—Bronchodilation without systemic anticholinergic effects. **Intranasal:** Decreased rhinorrhea.

Adverse Reactions/Side Effects

CNS: dizziness, headache, nervousness. **EENT:** blurred vision, sore throat, **nasal only:** epistaxis, nasal dryness/irritation. **Resp:** bronchospasm, cough. **CV:** hypotension, palpitations. **GI:** GI irritation, nausea. **Derm:** rash. **Misc:** allergic reactions.

PHYSICAL THERAPY IMPLICATIONS

Examination and Evaluation

- Assess pulmonary function at rest and during exercise (See Appendices I, J, K) to document effectiveness of medication in controlling bronchospasm in asthma and COPD.
- Monitor signs of paradoxical bronchospasm (wheezing, cough, dyspnea, tightness in chest and throat), especially at higher or excessive doses. If condition occurs, advise patient to withhold medication and notify physician immediately.
- Be alert for signs of allergic reactions, including pulmonary symptoms (tightness in the throat and chest, wheezing, cough, dyspnea) or skin reactions (rash, pruritus, urticaria). Notify physician or nursing staff immediately if these reactions occur.
- Assess blood pressure periodically and compare to normal values (See Appendix F). Report low blood pressure (hypotension), especially if patient experiences dizziness or syncope.
- Assess dizziness that might affect gait, balance, and other functional activities (See Appendix C). Report balance problems and functional limitations to the physician, and caution the patient and family/caregivers to guard against falls and trauma.

Interventions

- Design and implement appropriate aerobic exercise and respiratory muscle training programs to maintain optimal cardiovascular and pulmonary function. Work with patient and family/caregivers to find forms of exercise (e.g., swimming) that can help improve respiratory function without triggering bronchoconstrictive attacks.
- When implementing airway clearance techniques or respiratory muscle training, attempt to intervene when the airway is maximally bronchodilated. Peak responses typically occur 1–2 hr after inhalation.

Patient/Client-Related Instruction

- Advise patient to not exceed the recommended dose or frequency of inhalations. Contact physician immediately if bronchospasm is not relieved by medication or is accompanied by diaphoresis, dizziness, or other symptoms.
- Counsel patient on proper use of inhaler or nebulizer; observe use of these devices whenever possible to ensure proper technique.
- Instruct patient and family/caregivers to report troublesome side effects such as severe or prolonged headache, nervousness, blurred vision, sore throat, nose bleeds, skin rash, or GI problems (nausea, GI irritation).

Pharmacokinetics

Absorption: Minimal systemic absorption (2% for inhalation solution; 20% for inhalation aerosol; <20% following nasal use).
Distribution: 15% of dose reaches lower airways after inhalation.
Metabolism and Excretion: Small amounts absorbed are metabolized by the liver.
Half-life: 2 hr.

TIME/ACTION PROFILE (bronchodilation)

ROUTE	ONSET	PEAK	DURATION
Inhalation	1–3 min	1–2 hr	4–6 hr
Intranasal	15 min	unknown	6–12 hr

Contraindications/Precautions

Contraindicated in: Hypersensitivity to ipratropium, atropine, belladonna alkaloids, or bromide; Avoid use during acute bronchospasm; **Note: Atrovent HFA has replaced the discontinued Atrovent CFC (chlorofluorocarbon). Soy and CFC-allergic patients can now safely use the Atrovent HFA formulation. However, Combivent (ipratropium/albuterol combination) MDI does contain soya lecithin and is contraindicated in patients with a history of hypersensitivity to soy and peanut.**
Use Cautiously in: Patients with bladder neck obstruction, prostatic hyperplasia, glaucoma, or urinary retention; Geri: May be more sensitive to effects.

Interactions

Drug-Drug: ↑ anticholinergic properties with other **drugs having anticholinergic properties (antihistamines, phenothiazines, disopyramide).**

Route/Dosage

Inhalation (Adults and Children >12 yr): *Metered-dose inhaler (nonacute)*—2 inhalations 4 qid (not to exceed 12 inhalations/24 hr or more frequently than q 4 hr). *Acute exacerbations*—4–8 puffs using a spacer device as needed. *Via nebulization (nonacute)*—2504 times daily given q 6 hr. *Acute exacerbations*—500 mcg q 30 min for 3 doses then q 2–4 hr as needed.

Inhalation (Children 5–12 yr): *Metered-dose inhaler (nonacute)*—1–2 inhalations q 6 hr as needed (not to exceed 12 inhalations/24 hr). *Acute exacerbations*—4–8 puffs as needed. *Via nebulization (nonacute)*—250–500 mcg qid daily given q 6 hr. *Acute exacerbations*—250 mcg q 20 min for 3 doses then q 2–4 hr as needed.
Inhalation (Infants): *Nebulization*—125–250 mcg tid.
Inhalation (Neonates): *Nebulization*—25 mcg/kg/dose tid.
Intranasal (Adults and Children >6 yr): *0.03 % solution*—2 sprays in each nostril 2–3 times daily (21 mcg/spray).
Inhalation (Adults and Children >5 yr): *0.06% solution*—2 sprays in each nostril 3–4 times daily (42 mcg/spray).

Availability (generic available)

Aerosol inhaler (HFA) (chlorofluorocarbon-free): 17 mcg/spray in 12.9-g canister (200 inhalations). **Inhalation solution:** 0.0125%, 0.02% in single-dose vials containing 500 mcg, 0.025%. **Nasal spray:** 0.03% solution—21 mcg/spray in 30-mL bottle (345 sprays/bottle), 0.06% solution—42 mcg/spray in 15-mL bottle (165 sprays). ***In combination with:*** albuterol (Combivent, DuoNeb). See Appendix B.

irbesartan (ir-be-sar-tan)

Avapro

Classification
Therapeutic: antihypertensives
Pharmacologic: angiotensin II receptor antagonists

Indications

Alone or with other agents in the management of hypertension. Treatment of diabetic nephropathy in patients with type 2 diabetes and hypertension.

Action

Blocks the vasoconstrictor and aldosterone-secreting effects of angiotensin II at various receptor sites, including vascular smooth muscle and the adrenal glands. **Therapeutic Effects:** Lowering of blood pressure in patients with hypertension. Decreased progression of diabetic nephropathy.

Adverse Reactions/Side Effects

CNS: anxiety, dizziness, fatigue, headache. **CV:** chest pain, edema, hypotension, tachycardia. **Derm:** rashes. **GI:** abdominal pain, diarrhea, dyspepsia, nausea, vomiting. **GU:** impaired renal function. **F and E:** hyperkalemia. **MS:** pain. **Misc:** ANGIOEDEMA.

PHYSICAL THERAPY IMPLICATIONS

Examination and Evaluation

- Watch for signs of angioedema, including rashes, raised patches of red or white skin (welts), burning/itching skin, swelling in the face, and difficulty breathing. Notify physician immediately of these signs.
- Assess blood pressure periodically and compare to normal values (See Appendix F) to help document antihypertensive effects. Report low blood pressure (hypotension), especially if patient experiences dizziness or syncope.
- Assess heart rate, ECG, and heart sounds, especially during exercise (See Appendices G, H). Report a rapid heart rate (tachycardia) or signs of other arrhythmias, including palpitations, chest discomfort, shortness of breath, fainting, and fatigue/weakness.
- Assess peripheral edema using girth measurements, volume displacement, and measurement of pitting edema (See Appendix N). Report increased swelling in feet and ankles or a sudden increase in body weight due to vasodilation or fluid retention.
- If treating diabetic neuropathy, establish baseline electroneuromyographic values at the beginning of drug treatment whenever possible. Periodically reexamine these values to monitor peripheral nerve function and document whether drug therapy delays the progression of neuropathic disease.
- Assess any muscle or joint pain to rule out musculoskeletal pathology; that is, try to determine if pain is drug induced rather than caused by anatomic or biomechanical problems.
- Monitor signs of high plasma potassium levels (hyperkalemia), including bradycardia, fatigue, weakness, numbness, and tingling. Notify physician because severe cases can lead to life-threatening arrhythmias and paralysis.
- Watch for signs of impaired renal function, including decreased urine output, cloudy urine, or sudden weight gain due to fluid retention. Report these signs to the physician.
- Assess dizziness that might affect gait, balance, and other functional activities (See Appendix C). Report balance problems and functional limitations to the physician, and caution the patient and family/caregivers to guard against falls and trauma.

Interventions

- Because of an increased risk of cardiac arrhythmias (tachycardia), use caution during aerobic exercise and endurance conditioning. Terminate exercise if patient exhibits untoward symptoms (chest pain, shortness of breath, etc.) or displays other criteria for exercise termination (See Appendix L).

- Avoid physical therapy interventions that cause systemic vasodilation (large whirlpool, Hubbard tank). Additive effects of this drug and the intervention may cause a dangerous fall in blood pressure.
- To minimize orthostatic hypotension, patient should move slowly when assuming a more upright position.

Patient/Client-Related Instruction

- Remind patients to take medication as directed to control hypertension and diabetic neuropathy even if they are asymptomatic.
- Counsel patients about additional interventions to help control blood pressure and diabetes mellitus, including regular exercise, weight loss, sodium restriction, stress reduction, moderation of alcohol consumption, and smoking cessation.
- Instruct patient or family/caregivers to report other troublesome side effects such as severe or prolonged headache, anxiety, chest pain, skin rash, or GI problems (nausea, vomiting, diarrhea, indigestion, abdominal pain).

Pharmacokinetics

Absorption: 60–80% absorbed following oral administration.
Distribution: Crosses the placenta.
Protein Binding: 90%.
Metabolism and Excretion: Some hepatic metabolism; 20% excreted in urine, 80% in feces.
Half-life: 11–15 hr.

TIME/ACTION PROFILE (antihypertensive effect with chronic dosing)

ROUTE	ONSET	PEAK	DURATION
PO	within 2 hr	2 wk	24 hr

Contraindications/Precautions

Contraindicated in: Hypersensitivity; Bilateral renal artery stenosis; OB: Can cause injury or death of fetus; Lactation: Appears in breast milk; patient must discontinue irbesartan or provide alternate to breast milk.
Use Cautiously in: Volume- or salt-depleted patients or patients receiving high doses of diuretics (correct deficits before initiating therapy or initiate at lower doses); Black patients (may not be as effective); Impaired renal function due to primary renal disease or heart failure (may worsen renal function); Women of childbearing potential—if pregnancy occurs, discontinue immediately; Pedi: Safety not established in children <18 yr.

Interactions

Drug-Drug: Antihypertensive effect may be blunted by **NSAIDs**. Additive hypotension with other **antihypertensives**. Excessive hypotension may occur with concurrent use of **diuretics**. ↑ risk of hyperkalemia with concurrent use of **sulfamethoxazole/trimethoprim (high dose) potassium supplements, potassium-containing salt substitutes, angiotensin-converting enzyme inhibitors,** or **potassium-sparing diuretics**. May ↑ the levels/effects of **amiodarone, fluoxetine, glimepiride, glipizide, phenytoin, rosiglitazone,** and **warfarin**.

I

Route/Dosage

PO (Adults): *Hypertension*—150 mg once daily; may be increased to 300 mg once daily. Initiate therapy at 75 mg once daily in patients who are receiving diuretics or are volume depleted. *Nephropathy in patients with type 2 diabetes*—300 mg once daily.

Availability

Tablets: 75 mg Rx, 150 mg Rx, 300 mg Rx. ***In combination with:*** hydrochlorothiazide (Avalide). See Appendix B.

irinotecan (eye-ri-noe-tee-kan)
Camptosar

Classification
Therapeutic: antineoplastics
Pharmacologic: enzyme inhibitors

Indications

Metastatic colorectal cancer (with 5-fluorouracil and leucovorin).

Action

Interferes with DNA synthesis by inhibiting the enzyme topoisomerase. **Therapeutic Effects:** Death of rapidly replicating cells, particularly malignant ones.

Adverse Reactions/Side Effects

CNS: dizziness, headache, insomnia, weakness. **EENT:** rhinitis. **Resp:** coughing, dyspnea. **CV:** edema, vasodilation. **GI:** DIARRHEA, ELEVATED LIVER ENZYMES, abdominal pain/cramping, anorexia, constipation, dyspepsia, flatulence, nausea, stomatitis, vomiting, abdominal enlargement, colonic ulceration. **Derm:** alopecia, rash, sweating. **F and E:** dehydration. **Hemat:** anemia, leukopenia, neutropenia, thrombocytopenia. **Local:** injection-site reactions. **Metab:** weight loss. **MS:** back pain. **Misc:** chills, fever.

PHYSICAL THERAPY IMPLICATIONS

Examination and Evaluation

- Be alert for severe diarrhea or signs of hepatotoxicity, including severe nausea and vomiting, yellow skin or eyes, fever, sore throat, malaise, weakness, facial edema, lethargy, and unusual bleeding or bruising. Report these signs to the physician or nursing staff immediately.
- Watch for signs of leukopenia (fever, sore throat, signs of infection), thrombocytopenia (bruising, nose bleeds, bleeding gums), or unusual weakness and fatigue that might be due to anemia or other blood dyscrasias. Report these signs to the physician or nursing staff immediately.
- Monitor respiratory side effects, including cough, nasal irritation, or difficult, labored breathing. Report severe or troublesome respiratory problems to the physician or nursing staff.
- Assess peripheral edema using girth measurements, volume displacement, and measurement of pitting edema (See Appendix N). Report increased swelling in feet and ankles caused by peripheral vasodilation.
- Assess dizziness that might affect gait, balance, and other functional activities (See Appendix C). Report balance problems and functional limitations to the physician and nursing staff, and caution the patient and family/caregivers to guard against falls and trauma.
- Assess any back pain to rule out musculoskeletal pathology; that is, try to determine if pain is drug induced rather than caused by anatomic or biomechanical problems.
- Periodically assess body weight and other anthropometric measures (body mass index, body composition). Report a rapid or substantial weight loss.
- Monitor IV injection site for pain, swelling, and inflammation. Report prolonged or excessive injection site reactions to the physician.

Interventions

- For patients who are medically able to begin exercise, implement appropriate resistive exercises and aerobic training to maintain muscle strength and aerobic capacity during cancer chemotherapy or to help restore function after chemotherapy.
- Make sure patient maintains adequate fluid intake to avoid dehydration, especially during exercise.

Patient/Client-Related Instruction

- Advise patient to guard against infection (frequent hand washing, etc.), and toavoid crowds and contact with persons with contagious diseases.
- Advise patient and family/caregivers that fatigue and weakness are likely and may be severe. Functional abilities may be limited, and patient may need to use assistive devices during ambulation.
- Advise patient that hair loss and other skin reactions (rashes, hives, itching) are likely. Instruct patient to report severe or unexpected skin problems.
- Instruct patient and family to report severe or prolonged GI reactions such as nausea, constipation, indigestion, flatulence, abdominal pain, loss of appetite, and irritation in or around the mouth.
- Instruct patient and family/caregivers to report other bothersome side effects such as severe or prolonged headache, insomnia, or flu-like symptoms (chills, fever).

Pharmacokinetics

Absorption: IV administration results in complete bioavailability.
Distribution: Unknown.
Protein Binding: *Irinotecan*—30–68%; *SN-38 (active metabolite)*—95%.
Metabolism and Excretion: Converted by the liver to SN-38, its active metabolite, which is also metabolized by the liver. Small amounts excreted by kidneys.
Half-life: 6 hr.

TIME/ACTION PROFILE (hematologic effects)

ROUTE	ONSET	PEAK	DURATION
IV	unknown	21–29 days	27–34 days

Contraindications/Precautions

Contraindicated in: Hypersensitivity; OB/Lactation: Pregnancy or lactation.
Use Cautiously in: Previous pelvic or abdominal irradiation or age ≥65 yr (increased risk of myelosuppression); Presence of infection, underlying bone marrow depression, or concurrent chronic illness; History of prior pelvic/abdominal irradiation and serum bilirubin >1–2 mg/dL (initial dosage reduction recommended); Geri: ↑ sensitivity to adverse effects (myelosuppression); initiate at lower dose; Previous severe myelosuppression or diarrhea (reinstitute at lower dose following resolution); Patients with genetically reduced UGT1A1 activity (↑ risk of neutropenia); OB: Patients with childbearing potential; Pedi: Safety not established.

Interactions

Drug-Drug: Combination with **fluorouracil** may result in serious toxicity (dehydration, neutropenia, sepsis). ↑ bone marrow depression may occur with other **antineoplastics** or **radiation therapy**. **Laxatives** should be avoided (diarrhea may be ↑). **Diuretics** ↑ risk of dehydration (may discontinue during therapy). **Dexamethasone** used as an antiemetic ↑ risk of hyperglycemia and lymphocytopenia.

Prochlorperazine given on the same day as irinotecan ↑ risk of akathisia.
Drug-Natural: St. John's wort ↑ increases levels and risk of toxicity.

Route/Dosage

Other regimens are used; careful modification required for all levels of toxicity/tolerance.

Single Agent

IV (Adults): *Weekly dosage schedule*—125 mg/m^2 once weekly for 4 wk, followed by a 2-wk rest period. Cycle may be repeated using doses which depend on patient tolerance and degree of toxicity encountered. *Once every 3-wk schedule*—350 mg/m^2 once every 3 wk.
IV (Geriatric Patients >70 yr): Initiate at 300 mg/m^2 every 3 wk.

Hepatic Impairment

IV (Adults): *Bilirubin 1–2 mg/dL and history of prior pelvic/abdominal irradiation—Weekly dosage schedule*—Initiate therapy at lower dose (100 mg/m^2); once weekly for 4 wk, followed by a 2-wk rest period. Cycle may be repeated with dose adjusted as tolerated. *Once every 3-wk schedule*—300 mg/m^2 once every 3 wk, dose adjusted as tolerated as low as 200 mg/m^2 and further adjusted in 50-mg increments.

As Part of Combination Therapy with Leucovorin and 5-Fluorouracil

IV (Adults): *Regimen 1 (Bolus regimen)*—125 mg/m^2 once weekly for 4 wk, followed by a 2-wk rest period. Cycle may be repeated using doses that depend on patient tolerance and degree of toxicity encountered; *Regimen 2 (Infusional regimen)*—180 mg/m^2 every 2 wk for 3 doses, followed by a 3-wk rest period. Cycle may be repeated using doses that depend on patient tolerance and degree of toxicity encountered.

Availability (generic available)

Solution for injection: 20 mg/mL in 2-mL and 5-mL vials.

isocarboxazid

(eye-soe-kar-**box**-a-zid)
Marplan

Classification
Therapeutic: antidepressants
Pharmacologic: monamine oxidase (MAO) inhibitors

Indications

Treatment of depression (usually reserved for patients who do not tolerate or respond to other modes of therapy [e.g., tricyclic antidepressants, SSRIs, SSNRIs, or electroconvulsive therapy]).

Action

Inhibits the enzyme monoamine oxidase, resulting in an accumulation of various neurotransmitters (dopamine, epinephrine, norepinephrine, and serotonin) in the body. **Therapeutic Effects:** Improved mood in depressed patients.

Adverse Reactions/Side Effects

CNS: SEIZURES, dizziness, headache, akathisia, anxiety, ataxia, drowsiness, euphoria, insomnia, restlessness, weakness. **EENT:** blurred vision. **CV:** HYPERTENSIVE CRISIS, orthostatic hypotension. **GI:** nausea, black tongue, constipation, diarrhea, dry mouth. **GU:** dysuria, sexual dysfunction, urinary incontinence, urinary retention. **Derm:** photosensitivity.

PHYSICAL THERAPY IMPLICATIONS

Examination and Evaluation

- Be alert for new seizures or increased seizure activity, especially at the onset of drug treatment. Document the number, duration, and severity of seizures, and report these findings to the physician immediately.
- Measure blood pressure (BP) periodically and compare to normal values (See Appendix F). Immediately report a large, rapid increase in BP (hypertensive crisis). Signs and symptoms of hypertensive crisis include chest pain, tachycardia or bradycardia, severe headache, nausea, vomiting, neck stiffness, sweating, and enlarged pupils. The risk of hypertensive crisis is increased when this drug is taken with other antidepressants, excessive caffeine, other drugs that increase BP, or foods that contain tyramine (e.g., fermented wines, cheeses).
- Assess BP when patient assumes a more upright position (lying to standing, sitting to standing, lying to sitting). Document orthostatic hypotension and contact physician when systolic BP falls >20 mm Hg, or diastolic BP falls >10 mm Hg.
- Be alert for increased depression and suicidal thoughts and ideology, especially when initiating drug treatment or in children and teenagers. Notify physician or mental health professional immediately if patient exhibits worsening depression or other changes in mood and behavior such as anxiety, euphoria, or severe restlessness.

- Assess dizziness, drowsiness, and ataxia that might affect gait, balance, and other functional activities (See Appendix C). Report balance problems and functional limitations to the physician and nursing staff, and caution the patient and family/caregivers to guard against falls and trauma.

Interventions

- Guard against falls and trauma (hip fractures, head injury, and so forth), and implement fall-prevention strategies in patients with dizziness, ataxia, or other conditions that affect balance (See Appendix E).
- To minimize orthostatic hypotension, patient should move slowly when assuming a more upright position.
- Help patient explore nonpharmacologic methods to reduce depression (exercise, counseling, support groups, and so forth).
- Causes photosensitivity; use care if administering UV treatments. Advise patient to avoid direct sunlight and use sunscreens and protective clothing.

Patient/Client-Related Instruction

- Advise patient that antidepressant effects may not occur immediately; it may take 2 wk or longer before an improvement in mood is observed.
- Advise patient to avoid alcohol and other CNS depressants because of the increased risk of sedation and adverse effects.
- Instruct patient to report other troublesome side effects such as severe or prolonged headache, blurred vision, problems with urination, sexual dysfunction, or GI problems (nausea, constipation, diarrhea, black tongue, dry mouth).

Pharmacokinetics

Absorption: Unknown.
Distribution: Unknown.
Metabolism and Excretion: Unknown.
Half-life: Unknown.

TIME/ACTION PROFILE (antidepressant effect)

ROUTE	ONSET	PEAK	DURATION
PO	Unknown	3–6 wk	unknown

Contraindications/Precautions

Contraindicated in: Hypersensitivity; Liver disease; Severe renal disease; Cerebrovascular disease; Cardiovascular disease; Uncontrolled hypertension; Pheochromocytoma; History of severe or frequent headaches; Patients undergoing elective surgery requiring general anesthesia (should be discontinued at least 10 days before surgery); Excessive consumption of caffeine; Concurrent use of meperidine, SSRI antidepressants, SSNRI antidepressants, tricyclic antidepressants, tetracyclic antidepressants, nefazodone, trazodone, procarbazine, selegiline, linezolid, carbamazepine, cyclobenzaprine, bupropion, buspirone, sympathomimetics, other MAO inhibitors, dextromethorphan, narcotics, alcohol, general anesthetics, diuretics, tryptophan, or antihistamines; Concurrent use of foods containing high concentrations of tyramine; Lactation; Children <16 yr (safety and effectiveness not established).

Use Cautiously in: Patients who may be suicidal or have a history of drug dependency; Pedi: May ↑ risk of suicide attempt/ideation especially during first 1–2 mo of treatment or with dose adjustments (approved for use in children ≥16 yr); Hyperthyroidism; Schizophrenia; Bipolar disorder; Seizure disorders; Diabetes (↑ risk of hypoglycemia); Geri: Geriatric patients (↑ risk of adverse reactions); Pregnancy (safety not established).

Interactions

Drug-Drug: Serious, potentially fatal adverse reactions may occur with concurrent use of other **antidepressants** (**SSRIs, SSNRIs, bupropion, tricyclics, tetracyclics, nefazodone, trazodone**), **carbamazepine, cyclobenzaprine, sibutramine, procarbazine**, or **selegiline**. Avoid using within 2 wk of each other (wait 5 wk from end of **fluoxetine** therapy). Hypertensive crisis may occur with **amphetamines, methyldopa, levodopa, dopamine, epinephrine, norepinephrine, reserpine, methylphenidate**, or **vasoconstrictors**. Hypertension or hypotension, coma, seizures, respiratory depression, and death may occur with **meperidine** (avoid using within 2–3 wk of MAO inhibitor therapy). Concurrent use with **dextromethorphan** may produce psychosis or bizarre behavior. Hypertension may occur with concurrent use of **buspirone**; avoid using within 10 days of each other. Additive hypotension may occur with **antihypertensives, spinal anesthesia, opioids,** or **barbiturates**. Additive hypoglycemia may occur with **insulins** or **oral hypoglycemic agents**. Risk of seizures may be ↑ with **tramadol**.

Drug-Natural: Serious, potentially fatal adverse effects (serotonin syndrome) may occur with concomitant use of **St. John's wort** and **SAMe**. Hypertensive crises may occur with large amounts of **caffeine**-containing herbs (**cola nut, guarana**, or **malt**). Insomnia, headache, tremor, hypomania may occur with **ginseng**. Hypertensive crises, disorientation, and memory impairment may occur with **tryptophan** or supplements containing **tyrosine** or **phenylalanine**.

Drug-Food: Hypertensive crisis may occur with ingestion of foods containing high concentrations of **tyramine** (See Appendix L). Consumption of foods or beverages with high **caffeine** content increases the risk of hypertension and arrhythmias.

Route/Dosage

PO (Adults): 10 mg twice daily; may be increased every 2–4 days by 10 mg, up to 40 mg/day by the end of the first week, then may increase by up to 20 mg every week, up to 60 mg/day in 2–4 divided doses. After optimal response is obtained, dose should be slowly decreased to lowest effective amount (40 mg/day or less).

Availability

Tablets: 10 mg Rx.

isoniazid (eye-soe-nye-a-zid)

INH, ✱Isotamine, Nydrazid, ✱PMS Isoniazid, Laniazid

Classification

Therapeutic: antituberculars

Indications

First-line therapy of active tuberculosis, in combination with other agents. Prevention of tuberculosis in patients exposed to active disease (alone).

Action

Inhibits mycobacterial cell wall synthesis and interferes with metabolism. **Therapeutic Effects:** Bacteriostatic or bactericidal action against susceptible mycobacteria.

Adverse Reactions/Side Effects

CNS: psychosis, seizures. **EENT:** visual disturbances. **GI:** DRUG-INDUCED HEPATITIS, nausea, vomiting. **Derm:** rashes. **Endo:** gynecomastia. **Hemat:** blood dyscrasias. **Neuro:** peripheral neuropathy. **Misc:** fever.

PHYSICAL THERAPY IMPLICATIONS

Examination and Evaluation

- Be alert for signs of drug-induced hepatitis, including anorexia, abdominal pain, severe nausea and vomiting, yellow skin or eyes, fever, sore throat, malaise, weakness, facial edema, lethargy, and unusual bleeding or bruising. Report these signs to the physician or nursing staff immediately.
- Watch for seizures; notify physician immediately if patient develops or increases seizure activity.
- Be alert for signs of peripheral neuropathy (numbness, tingling, decreased muscle strength). Establish baseline electroneuromyographic values at the beginning of drug treatment whenever possible, and reexamine these values periodically to document drug-induced changes in peripheral nerve function.
- Monitor psychosis or other alterations in mental status. Notify the physician promptly if these symptoms develop (See Appendix D)
- Monitor signs of blood dyscrasias such as leukopenia (fever, sore throat, signs of infection), thrombocytopenia (bruising, nose bleeds and bleeding gums), or unusual weakness and fatigue that might be due to anemia. Report these signs to the physician.

Interventions

- Always wash hands thoroughly and disinfect equipment (whirlpools, electrotherapeutic devices, treatment tables, and so forth) to help prevent the spread of infection. Employ universal precautions or isolation procedures as indicated for specific patients.

Patient/Client-Related Instruction

- Instruct patient and family/caregivers to report other troublesome side effects such as severe or prolonged fever, skin rash, vision problems, breast enlargement in men, or GI problems (nausea, vomiting).

Pharmacokinetics

Absorption: Well absorbed following PO/IM administration.
Distribution: Widely distributed; readily crosses the blood-brain barrier. Crosses the placenta; enters breast milk in concentrations equal to plasma.
Metabolism and Excretion: 50% metabolized by the liver at rates that vary widely among individuals; 50% excreted unchanged by the kidneys.
Half-life: 1–4 hr.

TIME/ACTION PROFILE (blood levels)

ROUTE	ONSET	PEAK	DURATION
PO	rapid	1–2 hr	up to 24 hr
IM	rapid	1–2 hr	up to 24 hr

Contraindications/Precautions

Contraindicated in: Hypersensitivity; Acute liver disease; Previous hepatitis from isoniazid.
Use Cautiously in: History of liver damage or chronic alcohol ingestion; Black and Hispanic women, women in the postpartum period, or patients >50 yr (increased risk of drug-induced hepatitis); Severe renal impairment (dosage reduction may be necessary); Malnourished patients, patients with diabetes, or chronic alcoholics (increased risk of neuropathy); Pregnancy and lactation (although safety is not established, isoniazid has been used with ethambutol to treat tuberculosis in pregnant women without harm to the fetus).

Interactions

Drug-Drug: Additive CNS toxicity with other **antituberculars. BCG vaccine** may not be effective during isoniazid therapy. Isoniazid inhibits the metabolism of **phenytoin. Aluminum-containing antacids** may ↓ absorption. Psychotic reactions and coordination difficulties may result with **disulfiram**. Concurrent administration of **pyridoxine** may prevent neuropathy. ↑ risk of hepatotoxicity with other **hepatotoxic agents,** including **alcohol** and **rifampin**. Isoniazid may ↓ blood levels and effectiveness of **ketoconazole**. Concurrent use with **carbamazepine** ↑ carbamazepine blood levels and risk of hepatotoxicity.
Drug-Food: Severe reactions may occur with ingestion of foods containing high concentrations of **tyramine**.

Route/Dosage

PO, IM (Adults): 300 mg/day (5 mg/kg) *or* 15 mg/kg (up to 900 mg) 2–3 times weekly.
PO, IM (Children): 10–20 mg/kg/day (up to 300 mg/day) *or* 20–40 mg/kg (up to 900 mg) 2–3 times weekly.

Availability (generic available)

Tablets: 50 mg, 100 mg, 300 mg. **Syrup (orange, raspberry flavor):** 50 mg/5 mL. **Injection:** 100 mg/mL. ***In combination with:*** rifampin (Rifamate) or with rifampin and pyrazinamide (Rifater).

HIGH ALERT

isoproterenol

(eye-soe-proe-**ter**-e-nole)
Isuprel, Medihaler-Iso

Classification
Therapeutic: antiarrhythmics, bronchodilators
Pharmacologic: adrenergics

Indications

Management of bronchospasm during anesthesia. Treatment of asthma or COPD. Management of bradycardia (IV only).

Action

Results in the accumulation of cyclic adenosine monophosphate (cAMP) at beta-adrenergic receptors. Produces bronchodilation. Inhibits the release of mediators of immediate hypersensitivity reactions from mast cells. Has additional significant beta (cardiac)–adrenergic action, which results in positive inotropic and chronotropic effects.
Therapeutic Effects: Bronchodilation. Increased heart rate.

Adverse Reactions/Side Effects

CNS: nervousness, restlessness, tremor, headache, insomnia. **CV:** ARRHYTHMIAS, angina, hypertension, tachycardia. **GI:** nausea, vomiting, xerostomia. **Endo:** hyperglycemia. **Misc:** pink/red discoloration of saliva.

PHYSICAL THERAPY IMPLICATIONS

Examination and Evaluation

- Assess heart rate, ECG, and heart sounds, especially during exercise (See Appendices G, H). Immediately report any rhythm disturbances or symptoms of increased arrhythmias, including palpitations, chest discomfort, shortness of breath, fainting, and fatigue/weakness.
- Assess pulmonary function at rest and during exercise (See Appendices I, J, K) to document effectiveness of medication in controlling bronchospasm.
- Assess blood pressure (BP) periodically and compare to normal values (See Appendix F). Report a sustained increase in BP (hypertension) to the physician.
- Monitor and report signs of CNS toxicity, including nervousness, restlessness, or tremor. Sustained or severe CNS signs may indicate overdose or excessive use of this drug.
- Be alert for signs of hyperglycemia, including confusion, drowsiness, flushed/dry skin, fruit-like breath odor, rapid/deep breathing, polyuria, loss of appetite, and unusual thirst. Patients with diabetes mellitus should check blood glucose levels frequently.

Interventions

- When implementing airway clearance techniques or respiratory muscle training, attempt to intervene when the airway is maximally bronchodilated. Drug effect is usually rapid (within 5 min) after inhalation, so chest physical therapy interventions can begin soon after drug administration.
- Because of the risk of cardiovascular stimulation, use extreme caution during aerobic exercise and endurance conditioning. Cardiovascular effects such as arrhythmias, angina pectoris, or increased BP occur more commonly with isoproterenol compared to other bronchodilators because isoproterenol stimulates beta-1 receptors of the heart as well as beta-2 receptors on the lungs.

Patient/Client-Related Instruction

- Advise patient not to exceed the recommended dose or frequency of inhalations. Contact physician immediately if bronchospasm is not relieved by medication or is accompanied by diaphoresis, dizziness, or other symptoms.

- Counsel patient on proper use of inhaler; observe use of this device whenever possible to ensure proper technique.
- Instruct patient and family/caregivers to report severe or prolonged headache, sleep loss, or GI problems (nausea, vomiting, dry mouth).

Pharmacokinetics

Absorption: Well absorbed following IM or SC administration; IV administration results in complete bioavailability.
Distribution: Unknown.
Metabolism and Excretion: Metabolism occurs in the lung, liver, and other tissues; 50% excreted unchanged by the kidneys after IV administration.
Half-life: 2.5–5 min.

TIME/ACTION PROFILE (bronchodilation)

ROUTE	ONSET	PEAK	DURATION
Inhalation	2–5 min	unknown	0.5–2 hr
IV	immediate	unknown	<1 hr

Contraindications/Precautions

Contraindicated in: Hypersensitivity to adrenergic amines or bisulfites.
Use Cautiously in: Cardiovascular disease (including hypertension and coronary artery disease); Hyperthyroidism; Diabetes; Glaucoma; Geri: Geriatric patients are more susceptible to adverse reactions, may require dosage reduction; Pregnancy (near term) and lactation; Pedi: Safety not established in children, pediatric use has been associated with serious adverse reactions.

Interactions

Drug-Drug: Concurrent use with other **adrenergic agents** (sympathomimetics) will have additive adrenergic side effects. Use with **MAO inhibitors** may lead to hypertensive crisis. May ↑ **theophylline** elimination. **Beta blockers** may negate therapeutic effect.

Route/Dosage

IV (Adults): *Heart block, Adams-Stokes attacks, and cardiac arrest*—0.02–0.06 mg may be followed by additional doses of 0.01–0.02 mg *or* 5 mcg/min infusion; *bronchospasm during anesthesia*—0.01–0.02 mg, repeated as needed).
IV (Neonates, Infants, and Children): 0.05–2 mcg/kg/min via continuous infusion.
IM (Adults): *Heart block, Adams-Stokes attacks, and cardiac arrest*—0.2 mg; subsequent range 0.02–1 mg.
SC (Adults): *Heart block, Adams-Stokes attacks, and cardiac arrest*—0.2 mg; subsequent range 0.15 mg–0.2 mg.
Intracardiac (Adults): *Heart block, Adams-Stokes attacks, and cardiac arrest*—0.02 mg.

Availability (generic available)

Injection: 20 mcg (0.02 mg)/mL, 200 mcg (0.2 mg)/mL.

Isosorbide

isosorbide dinitrate

(eye-soe-**sor**-bide dye-**nye**-trate)
Apo-ISDN, Cedocard-SR, Coronex, Dilatrate-SR, Isordil, Novosorbide, PMS-Isosorbide

isosorbide mononitrate

(eye-soe-**sor**-bide mon-oh-**nye**-trate)
Apo-ISMN, Imdur ISMO, Monoket

Classification
Therapeutic: antianginals
Pharmacologic: nitrates

I

Indications

Acute treatment of anginal attacks (sublingual only). Prophylactic management of angina pectoris. Treatment of chronic CHF (unlabeled).

Action

Produce vasodilation (venous greater than arterial). Decrease left ventricular end-diastolic pressure and left ventricular end-diastolic volume (preload). Net effect is reduced myocardial oxygen consumption. Increase coronary blood flow by dilating coronary arteries and improving collateral flow to ischemic regions.
Therapeutic Effects: Relief and prevention of anginal attacks.

Adverse Reactions/Side Effects

CNS: dizziness, headache. **CV:** hypotension, tachycardia, paradoxic bradycardia, syncope. **GI:** nausea, vomiting. **Misc:** flushing, tolerance.

PHYSICAL THERAPY IMPLICATIONS

Examination and Evaluation

- Assess episodes of angina pectoris at rest and during exercise. Document whether drug therapy is helpful in reducing the frequency and severity of anginal attacks.
- Assess heart rate, ECG, and heart sounds, especially during exercise (See Appendices G, H). Report any rhythm disturbances (tachycardia, bradycardia, others) or symptoms of increased arrhythmias,

including palpitations, chest discomfort, shortness of breath, fainting, and fatigue/weakness.

- Assess dizziness and syncope that might affect gait, balance, and other functional activities (See Appendix C). Report balance problems and functional limitations to the physician, and caution the patient and family/caregivers to guard against falls and trauma.
- If used to treat CHF, assess signs and symptoms (dyspnea, rales/crackles, peripheral edema, jugular venous distention, exercise intolerance) to help document whether drug therapy is effective in reducing these symptoms.
- Report signs of drug tolerance during long-term use, as indicated by increased episodes of angina or CHF symptoms. This problem may be resolved by instituting nitrate-free periods; that is, the physician may recommend removing the nitroglycerin patch for several hours each day.

Interventions

- Design and implement aerobic exercise and endurance training programs to improve coronary perfusion, reduce angina, and improve myocardial pumping ability.
- Because of an increased risk of angina and arrhythmias, or in conditions such as CHF, use caution during aerobic exercise and endurance conditioning. Terminate exercise if patient exhibits untoward symptoms (chest pain, shortness of breath, etc.) or displays other criteria for exercise termination (See Appendix L).
- Avoid physical therapy interventions that cause systemic vasodilation (large whirlpool, Hubbard tank). Additive effects of this drug and these interventions may cause a dangerous fall in blood pressure.
- To minimize orthostatic hypotension, patient should move slowly when assuming a more upright position.
- If used to treat acute angina, make sure patient brings isosorbide sublingual tablets to all physical therapy appointments, and that this drug is readily available during exercise and other interventions.

Patient/Client-Related Instruction

- During acute angina attacks, advise patient to sit or lie down and use medication at first sign of angina. Relief usually occurs within 5 min. Dose may be repeated if pain is not relieved in 5–10 min. Call health care professional or go to nearest emergency room if angina pain is not relieved by 3 tablets in 15 min.
- Remind patients to take medication as directed to control angina or CHF even if they are asymptomatic. Patients with CHF should weigh themselves every day, and call their physician if they gain 3 lb or more in 1 day or more than 5 lb in 1 week.
- Counsel patients about additional interventions to help control angina and cardiac dysfunction such as regular exercise, weight loss, sodium restriction, stress reduction, moderation of alcohol consumption, and smoking cessation.
- Advise patient to protect sublingual tablets from light, heat, and moisture, and to make sure the prescription is renewed periodically to maintain drug potency.
- Inform patient that headache is a common side effect that should decrease with continuing therapy. Notify health care professional if headache is persistent or severe.
- Instruct patient or family/caregivers to report severe or prolonged GI problems (nausea, vomiting).

Pharmacokinetics

Absorption: Isosorbide dinitrate undergoes extensive first-pass metabolism by the liver, resulting in 25% bioavailability; isosorbide mononitrate has 100% bioavailability (does not undergo first-pass metabolism).
Distribution: Unknown.
Metabolism and Excretion: Isosorbide dinitrate is metabolized by the liver to 2 active metabolites (5-mononitrate and 2-mononitrate). Isosorbide mononitrate is primarily metabolized by the liver to inactive metabolites; primarily excreted in urine as metabolites.
Half-life: *Isosorbide dinitrate*—1 hr; *isosorbide mononitrate*—5 hr.

TIME/ACTION PROFILE (cardiovascular effects)

ROUTE	ONSET	PEAK	DURATION
ISDN-SL	2–10 min	unknown	1–2 hr
ISDN-PO	45–60 min	unknown	4 hr
ISDN-PO-ER	30 min	unknown	up to 12 hr
ISMN-PO	30–60 min	unknown	7 hr
ISMN-ER	unknown	unknown	12 hr

Contraindications/Precautions

Contraindicated in: Hypersensitivity; Concurrent use of sildenafil, vardenafil, or tadalafil.
Use Cautiously in: Volume-depleted patients; Right ventricular infarction; Hypertrophic cardiomyopathy; Geri: Older patients may be more sensitive to hypotension (start with lower doses); OB: Pregnancy (may compromise maternal/fetal circulation) or lactation; Pedi: Children (safety not established).

Interactions

Drug-Drug: Concurrent use of **sildenafil, tadalafil,** or **vardenafil** may result in significant and potentially fatal hypotension (do not use these drugs within 24 hr of isosorbide dinitrate or mononitrate). Additive hypotension with **antihypertensives**, acute ingestion of **alcohol**, **beta blockers**, **calcium channel blockers**, and **phenothiazines**.

Route/Dosage

Isosorbide Dinitrate

SL (Adults): *Acute attack of angina pectoris*—2.5–5 mg may be repeated q 5–10 min for 3 doses in 15–30 min. *Prophylaxis of angina pectoris*—2.5–5 mg given 15 mm prior to activities known to provoke angina.

PO (Adults): *Prophylaxis of angina pectoris*—5–20 mg 2–3 times daily; usual maintenance dose is 10–40 mg q 6 hr (immediate-release) or 40–80 mg q 8–12 hr (sustained-release).

Isosorbide Mononitrate

PO (Adults): *ISMO, Monoket*—5–20 mg twice daily with the 2 doses given 7 hr apart. *Imdur*—30–60 mg once daily; may increase to 120 mg once daily (maximum dose = 240 mg/day).

Availability (generic available)

Isosorbide Dinitrate

Sublingual tablets: 2.5 mg, 5 mg. **Tablets:** 5 mg, 10 mg, 20 mg, 30 mg, 40 mg. **Extended-release tablets:** 20 mg, 40 mg. **Sustained-release capsules:** 40 mg. ***In combination with:*** hydralazine (BiDil). See Appendix B.

Isosorbide Mononitrate (generic available)

Tablets (ISMO, Monoket): 10 mg, 20 mg. **Extended-release tablets (Imdur):** 30 mg, 60 mg, 120 mg.

isotretinoin

(eye-soe-**tret**-i-noyn)

Amnesteem

Classification

Therapeutic: antiacne agents

Pharmacologic: retinoids

Indications

Management of severe nodular acne resistant to more conventional therapy, including topical therapy and systemic antibiotics. Not to be used under any circumstances in pregnant patients.

Action

A metabolite of vitamin A (retinol); reduces sebaceous gland size and differentiation. **Therapeutic Effects:** Diminution and resolution of severe acne. May also prevent abnormal keratinization.

Adverse Reactions/Side Effects

CNS: SUICIDE ATTEMPT, behavior changes, depression, PSEUDOTUMOR CEREBRI, psychosis, suicidal ideation. **EENT:** conjunctivitis, epistaxis, blurred vision, contact lens intolerance, corneal opacities, decreased night vision, dry eyes. **CV:** edema. **GI:** cheilitis, dry mouth, nausea, vomiting, abdominal pain, anorexia, hepatitis, pancreatitis, increased appetite. **Derm:** pruritus, palmar desquamation, photosensitivity, skin infections, thinning of hair. **Hemat:** anemia. **Metab:** decreased high-density lipoproteins, hypercholesterolemia, hypertriglyceridemia, hyperglycemia, hyperuricemia. **MS:** arthralgia, back pain, muscle/bone pain (↑ in adolescents), hyperostosis. **Misc:** SEVERE BIRTH DEFECTS, increased thirst.

PHYSICAL THERAPY IMPLICATIONS

Evaluation and Examination

- Be alert for signs of intracranial swelling caused by pseudotumor cerebri. Signs include headache, dizziness, ringing in the ears, nausea, vomiting, pain in the neck/back/shoulders, and vision disturbances (blurred vision, double vision, flashes of light, brief periods of blindness). Notify physician of these signs immediately.
- Be alert for signs of depression and changes in behavior that suggest suicidal thoughts. Notify physician promptly if these signs develop (See Appendix D).
- Monitor signs of anemia, including unusual fatigue, pallor, shortness of breath with exertion, and bruising. Notify physician immediately if these signs occur.
- Assess any muscle, joint, or bone pain to rule out musculoskeletal pathology; that is, try to determine if pain is drug induced rather than caused by anatomic or biomechanical problems.
- Assess peripheral edema using girth measurements, volume displacement, and measurement of pitting edema (See Appendix N). Report increased swelling in feet and ankles or a sudden increase in body weight due to fluid retention.

Interventions

- Causes photosensitivity; use care if administering UV treatments. Advise patient to avoid direct sunlight and use sunscreens and protective clothing.

Patient/Client-Related Instruction

- Remind patient about the risk of birth defects, and that pregnancy must be avoided when using this medication. Instruct patient to consult physician about adequate forms of contraception, and remind patient that adherence to contraceptive strategies is essential.

- Advise patient about the likelihood of vision problems, including eye inflammation, blurred vision, and decreased night vision. Instruct patient to report severe or unexpected vision disturbances.
- Advise patient about the likelihood of GI reactions such as nausea, vomiting, abdominal pain, and a change in appetite. Instruct patient to report severe or prolonged GI problems, signs of liver toxicity (yellow skin or eyes, abdominal pain, severe nausea and vomiting, fever, sore throat, malaise, weakness, facial edema), or signs of pancreatitis (upper abdominal pain after eating, indigestion, weight loss, oily stools).
- Advise patient that acne may worsen initially during treatment and that other skin reactions may occur, including itching, infections, skin loss from palms, and thinning hair). Report severe or unexpected skin reactions to the physician.

Pharmacokinetics

Absorption: Rapidly absorbed following (23–25%) oral administration; absorption increases when taken with a high-fat meal.
Distribution: Appears to be widely distributed; crosses the placenta.
Protein Binding: 99.9%.
Metabolism and Excretion: Metabolized by the liver and excreted in the urine and feces.
Half-life: 10–20 hr.

TIME/ACTION PROFILE (diminution of acne)

ROUTE	ONSET	PEAK	DURATION
PO	unknown	up to 8 wk	unknown

Contraindications/Precautions

Contraindicated in: Hypersensitivity to retinoids, glycerin, soybean oil, or parabens; Pregnant patients; Women of childbearing age who may become or who intend to become pregnant; Lactation; Patients planning to donate blood.
Use Cautiously in: Preexisting hypertriglyceridemia; Diabetes mellitus; History of alcohol abuse, psychosis, depression, or suicide attempt; Obese patients; Inflammatory bowel disease.

Interactions

Drug-Drug: Additive toxicity with **vitamin A** and **drugs having anticholinergic properties.** ↑ risk of pseudotumor cerebri with **tetracycline** or **minocycline**. Concurrent use with **alcohol** ↑ hypertriglyceridemia. Drying effects ↑ by concurrent use of **benzoyl peroxide, sulfur, tretinoin,** and **other topical agents**.
Drug-Natural: If **hormonal contraceptives** are being used, **St. John's wort** should be avoided; may ↓ effectiveness.
Drug-Food: Excessive ingestion of **foods high in vitamin A** may result in additive toxicity.

Route/Dosage

PO (Adults): 0.5–1 mg/kg/day (up to 2 mg/kg/day) in 2 divided doses for 15–20 wk. Once discontinued, if relapse occurs, therapy may be reinstituted after an 8-wk rest period.

Availability (generic available)

Capsules: 10 mg, 20 mg, 40 mg.

isradipine (is-rad-i-peen)

DynaCirc, DynaCirc CR

Classification
Therapeutic: antianginals, antihypertensives
Pharmacologic: calcium channel blockers

Indications

Management of hypertension, angina pectoris, and vasospastic (Prinzmetal's) angina.

Action

Inhibits the transport of calcium into myocardial and vascular smooth muscle cells, resulting in inhibition of excitation-contraction coupling and subsequent contraction. **Therapeutic Effects:** Systemic vasodilation resulting in decreased blood pressure. Coronary vasodilation resulting in decreased frequency and severity of attacks of angina.

Adverse Reactions/Side Effects

CNS: abnormal dreams, anxiety, confusion, dizziness, drowsiness, headache, nervousness, psychiatric disturbances, weakness. **EENT:** blurred vision, disturbed equilibrium, epistaxis, tinnitus. **Resp:** cough, dyspnea. **CV:** ARRHYTHMIAS, CHF, peripheral edema, bradycardia, chest pain, hypotension, palpitations, syncope, tachycardia. **GI:** abnormal liver function studies, anorexia, constipation, diarrhea, dry mouth, dysgeusia, dyspepsia, nausea, vomiting. **GU:** dysuria, nocturia, polyuria, sexual dysfunction, urinary frequency. **Derm:** dermatitis, erythema multiforme, flushing, increased sweating, photosensitivity, pruritus/urticaria, rash. **Endo:** gynecomastia, hyperglycemia. **Hemat:** anemia, leukopenia, thrombocytopenia. **Metab:** weight gain. **MS:** joint stiffness, muscle cramps. **Neuro:** paresthesia, tremor. **Misc:** STEVENS-JOHNSON SYNDROME, gingival hyperplasia.

PHYSICAL THERAPY IMPLICATIONS

Examination and Evaluation

- Assess heart rate, ECG, and heart sounds, especially during exercise (See Appendices G, H). Report any

rhythm disturbances or symptoms of increased arrhythmias, including palpitations, chest pain, shortness of breath, fainting, and fatigue/weakness.

- Monitor rashes or other skin reactions (hives, abnormal sweating, itching/burning, exfoliation). Notify physician immediately because certain skin reactions may indicate serious hypersensitivity reactions (Stevens-Johnson syndrome).
- Assess routinely for signs of CHF and pulmonary edema (dyspnea, cough, shortness of breath, rales/crackles, jugular venous distention). Report these signs to the physician.
- Assess blood pressure periodically and compare to normal values (See Appendix F) to help document antihypertensive effects.
- Assess episodes of angina pectoris at rest and during exercise. Document whether drug therapy is helpful in reducing the frequency and severity of anginal attacks.
- Assess peripheral edema using girth measurements, volume displacement, and measurement of pitting edema (See Appendix N). Report increased swelling in feet and ankles due to peripheral vasodilation.
- Assess signs of paresthesia (numbness, tingling) or muscle twitching. Perform objective tests, including electroneuromyography and sensory testing to document any drug-related neuropathic changes.
- Watch for signs of hyperglycemia, including confusion, drowsiness, flushed/dry skin, fruit-like breath odor, rapid/deep breathing, polyuria, loss of appetite, and unusual thirst. Insulin dosages may need to be adjusted to prevent repeated episodes of hyperglycemia.
- Monitor and report signs of leukopenia (fever, sore throat, signs of infection), thrombocytopenia (bruising, nose bleeds, and bleeding gums), or unusual weakness and fatigue that might be due to anemia.
- Assess any joint stiffness or muscle cramping to rule out musculoskeletal pathology; that is, try to determine if pain is drug induced rather than caused by anatomic or biomechanical problems.
- Assess dizziness and weakness that might affect gait, balance, and other functional activities (See Appendix C). Report balance problems and functional limitations to the physician, and caution the patient and family/caregivers to guard against falls and trauma.
- Monitor mood and personality changes, including anxiety, nervousness, confusion, or other psychiatric disturbances. Notify physician if these changes become problematic.

Interventions

- Design and implement aerobic exercise and endurance training programs to normalize blood pressure, improve coronary perfusion, reduce angina, and improve myocardial pumping ability.
- Because of the risk of cardiac arrhythmias and CHF, use caution during aerobic exercise and other forms of therapeutic exercise. Assess exercise tolerance frequently (blood pressure, heart rate, fatigue levels), and terminate exercise immediately if any untoward responses occur (See Appendix L).
- Guard against falls and trauma (hip fractures, head injury). Implement fall prevention strategies, especially if patient exhibits dizziness or disturbed equilibrium (See Appendix E).
- To minimize orthostatic hypotension, patient should move slowly when assuming a more upright position.
- Causes photosensitivity; use care if administering UV treatments.

Patient/Client-Related Instruction

- Remind patients to take medication as directed to control hypertension and other cardiac conditions even if they are asymptomatic.
- Counsel patients about additional interventions to help control blood pressure and cardiac dysfunction, including regular exercise, weight loss, sodium restriction, stress reduction, moderation of alcohol consumption, and smoking cessation.
- Advise patient about photosensitivity and to use sunscreens, protective clothing, and avoid prolonged sun exposure. Advise patient to also report any rashes or other skin reactions.
- Instruct patient or family/caregivers to report other troublesome side effects such as severe or prolonged headache, tinnitus, nightmares, tremor, weight gain, problems with urination, sexual dysfunction, breast enlargement in men (gynecomastia), or GI problems (nausea, vomiting, constipation, diarrhea, indigestion, loss of appetite).

Pharmacokinetics

Absorption: Well absorbed following oral administration but extensively metabolized, resulting in decreased bioavailability.
Distribution: Unknown.
Protein Binding: 95%.
Metabolism and Excretion: Completely metabolized by the liver.
Half-life: 8 hr.

TIME/ACTION PROFILE (cardiovascular effects†)

ROUTE	ONSET	PEAK	DURATION
PO	<2 hr	2–3 hr	12 hr
PO-CR	2 hr	8–10 hr	24 hr

†For single doses, maximal antihypertensive effect during chronic dosing may take 2–4 wk.

Contraindications/Precautions

Contraindicated in: Hypersensitivity; Sick sinus syndrome; 2nd- or 3rd-degree AV block (unless an artificial pacemaker is in place); Blood pressure <90 mm Hg.

Use Cautiously in: Severe hepatic impairment (dose reduction recommended); Geri: Geriatric patients (dose reduction recommended for most agents; increased risk of hypotension); Severe renal impairment; History of serious ventricular arrhythmias or CHF; OB/Lactation/Pedi: Pregnancy, lactation, or children (safety not established).

Interactions

Drug-Drug: Additive hypotension may occur when used concurrently with **fentanyl**, other **antihypertensives**, **nitrates**, acute ingestion of **alcohol**, or **quinidine**. Antihypertensive effects may be ↓ by concurrent use of **NSAIDs**. Concurrent use with **beta blockers**, **digoxin**, **disopyramide**, or **phenytoin** may result in bradycardia, conduction defects, or CHF.

Drug-Food: Grapefruit and Grapefruit juice ↑ serum levels and effect.

Route/Dosage

PO (Adults): 2.5 mg twice daily; may be ↑ q 2–4 wk by 5 mg/day (not to exceed 20 mg/day) *or* 5 mg once daily as CR tablets; may be ↑ q 2–4 wk by 5 mg/day (not to exceed 20 mg/day).

Availability

Capsules: 2.5 mg, 5 mg. **Controlled-release tablets:** 5 mg, 10 mg.

itraconazole (it-tra-**kon**-a-zole)

Sporanox

Classification

Therapeutic: antifungals (systemic)

Indications

Histoplasmosis. Blastomycosis. Aspergillosis. Dermatophyte infection of fingernails or toenails in nonimmunocompromised patients (oral capsules only). Oropharyngeal esophageal candidiasis.

Action

Inhibits enzymes necessary for integrity of the fungal cell membrane. **Therapeutic Effects:** Fungistatic effects against susceptible organisms. **Spectrum:** Active against *Histoplasma capsulatum*, *Blastomyces dermatitidis*, *Cryptococcus neoformans*, *Aspergillus fumigatus*, *Trichophyton* spp., *Candida*, and other fungi that cause nail infections (tinea unguium).

Adverse Reactions/Side Effects

CNS: dizziness, drowsiness, fatigue, headache, malaise. **EENT:** tinnitus. **CV:** CHF, edema, hypertension. **GI:** HEPATOTOXICITY, nausea, abdominal pain, anorexia, diarrhea, flatulence, vomiting. **GU:** albuminuria, decreased libido, erectile dysfunction. **Derm:** TOXIC EPIDERMAL NECROLYSIS, photosensitivity, pruritus, rash. **Endo:** adrenal insufficiency. **F and E:** hypokalemia. **MS:** rhabdomyolysis. **Misc:** allergic reactions including anaphylaxis, fever.

PHYSICAL THERAPY IMPLICATIONS

Examination and Evaluation

- Be alert for signs of hepatotoxicity, including anorexia, abdominal pain, severe nausea and vomiting, yellow skin or eyes, fever, sore throat, malaise, weakness, facial edema, lethargy, and unusual bleeding or bruising. Notify physician of these signs immediately.
- Monitor rashes or other severe skin reactions such as exfoliation, hives, itching, raised patches of red or white skin (welts), burning, acne, and abnormal sweating. Notify physician immediately because certain skin responses may indicate serious hypersensitivity reactions.
- Monitor other signs of allergic reactions and anaphylaxis, including pulmonary symptoms such as tightness in the throat and chest, wheezing, cough, and dyspnea. Notify physician immediately if these reactions occur.
- Assess signs of congestive heart failure (dyspnea, rales/crackles, peripheral edema, jugular venous distention, exercise intolerance). Report these signs to the physician.
- Assess blood pressure (BP) and compare to normal values (See Appendix F). Report a sustained increase in BP (hypertension).
- Assess peripheral edema using girth measurements, volume displacement, and measurement of pitting edema (See Appendix N). Report increased swelling in feet and ankles or a sudden increase in body weight due to fluid retention.
- Assess any muscle pain, tenderness, or weakness, especially if accompanied by fever, malaise, and dark-colored urine. Advise patient that these symptoms may represent drug-induced myopathy, and that myopathy can progress to severe muscle damage (rhabdomyolysis). Report any unexplained musculoskeletal symptoms to the physician immediately.

- Monitor any muscle weakness, aches, or cramps that might indicate low potassium levels (hypokalemia). Notify physician immediately if these signs occur.
- Report signs of adrenal insufficiency, including hypotension, weight loss, weakness, nausea, vomiting, anorexia, lethargy, confusion, and restlessness.
- Assess dizziness or drowsiness that might affect gait, balance, and other functional activities (See Appendix C). Report balance problems and functional limitations to the physician and nursing staff, and caution the patient and family/caregivers to guard against falls and trauma.

Interventions

- Always wash hands thoroughly and disinfect equipment (whirlpools, electrotherapeutic devices, treatment tables, and so forth) to help prevent the spread of infection. Employ universal precautions or isolation procedures as indicated for specific patients.

Patient/Client-Related Instruction

- Advise patient to take this drug as directed for the full course of treatment even if feeling better.
- Instruct patient to report other troublesome side effects such as prolonged or severe headache, fever, ringing/buzzing in the ears (tinnitus), decreased libido, erectile dysfunction, skin problems (rash, itching), or GI reactions (diarrhea, nausea, vomiting, flatulence, abdominal pain).

Pharmacokinetics

Absorption: Oral absorption is enhanced by food.
Distribution: Tissue concentrations are higher than plasma concentrations. Does not enter CSF; enters breast milk.
Protein Binding: *Itraconazole*—99.8%; *hydroxyitraconazole*—99.5%.
Metabolism and Excretion: Mostly metabolized by the liver and excreted in feces. Hydroxyitraconazole, the major metabolite, has antifungal activity.
Half-life: 21 hr.

TIME/ACTION PROFILE (blood levels)

ROUTE	ONSET	PEAK	DURATION
PO	rapid	4 hr	12–24 hr
IV	unknown	end of infusion	12–24 hr

Contraindications/Precautions

Contraindicated in: Hypersensitivity. Cross-sensitivity with other azole antifungals (**miconazole, ketoconazole**) may occur; OB: Lactation; Concurrent **quinidine, dofetilide, pimozide**, oral **midazolam, triazolam, ergot alkaloids (dihydroergotamine, ergonovine, ergotamine, methylergonovine)**, **simvastatin**, or **lovastatin**; Severe renal impairment (CCr <30 mL/min); CHF or other evidence of ventricular dysfunction.
Use Cautiously in: Patients with hepatic impairment (dosage reduction may be required); Patients with achlorhydria or hypochlorhydria (absorption will be decreased); OB/Pedi: Pregnancy or children (safety not established).

Interactions

Drug-Drug: Itraconazole is a potent inhibitor of the P4503A hepatic enzyme, which can ↑ blood levels and effects of other drugs which are metabolized by this system. ↑ risk of potentially fatal arrhythmias with **quinidine, dofetilide**, or **pimozide** (concurrent use is contraindicated and may result in QTc prolongation, torsades de pointes, ventricular arrhythmias, and sudden death). ↑ risk of excessive sedation with **midazolam** or **triazolam**, ↑ risk of adverse CNS reactions with **pimozide**, and ↑ risk of myopathy with **simvastatin** or **lovastatin** (concurrent use contraindicated). Concurrent use with **ergot alkaloids (dihydroergotamine, ergonovine, ergotamine, methylergonovine)** ↑ risk of vasoconstriction and is contraindicated. May also ↑ blood levels and the risk of toxicity from **warfarin, ritonavir, indinavir, saquinavir, vinca alkaloids, busulfan, cilostazol, diazepam, eletriptan, felodipine, isradipine, nicardipine, nifedipine, nimodipine, cyclosporine, vardenafil, tacrolimus, sildenafil, methylprednisolone, digoxin**, and **quinidine**. May also ↓ metabolism and ↑ effects of **budesonide, dexamethasone**, and **methylprednisolone**. Absorption ↓ by **antacids, histamine H_2 blockers, sucralfate, gastric acid–pump inhibitors**, or other **agents that increase gastric pH**, including the buffer in **didanosine** (take 2 hr after itraconazole). **Phenytoin, phenobarbital, isoniazid, rifampin, rifabutin**, and **carbamazepine** ↑ metabolism and ↓ blood levels of itraconazole (↑ dosage may be necessary). Itraconazole ↓ metabolism and may ↑ effects of **phenytoin** and **oral hypoglycemic agents**. If hypokalemia occurs, the risk of **digoxin** toxicity is ↑. Blood levels of itraconazole may be ↑ by **clarithromycin, erythromycin, ritonavir, and indinavir**.
Drug-Food: Food increases absorption.

Route/Dosage

Aspergillosis

PO (Adults): 200 mg once or twice daily for a minimum of 3 mo.

Blastomycosis, Histoplasmosis

PO (Adults): 200 mg once daily; may be increased by 100 mg/day up to 200 mg twice daily.

Onychomycosis

PO (Adults): *Toenail fungus with or without fingernail fungus*—200 mg/day for 12 consecutive wk. *Fingernail fungu*—200 mg twice daily for 1 wk, then 3 wk without therapy, then 200 mg twice daily an additional 1 wk–6 mo.

Candidiasis

PO (Adults): *Oropharyngeal candidiasis*—200 mg (20 mL) daily for 1–2 wk. *Oropharyngeal candidiasis unresponsive to fluconazole*—100 mg (10 mL) twice daily for at least 2–4 wk. *Esophageal candidiasis*—100 mg (10 mL) once daily for at least 3 wk.

Availability

Capsules: 100 mg. **Oral solution (cherry caramel):** 10 mg/mL.

ixabepilone (ix-a-bep-i-lone)

Ixempra

Classification

Therapeutic: antineoplastics

Pharmacologic: epothilone B analog

Indications

Combination use with capecitabine for the treatment of metastatic or locally advanced breast cancer currently resistant to a taxane and anthracycline or resistant to a taxane and cannot tolerate further anthracycline. May also be used as monotherapy for breast cancers that are not responding to anthracyclines, taxane, or capecitabine.

Action

Binds to β-tubulin subunits on microtubules; this action blocks cells in mitosis, leading to cell death. Also has antiangiogenic activity. **Therapeutic Effects:** Decreased spread of breast cancer.

Adverse Reactions/Side Effects

CNS: fatigue, weakness, dizziness, headache, insomnia. **EENT:** ↑ lacrimation. **CV:** chest pain, edema, myocardial ischemia, ventricular dysfunction. **Resp:** dyspnea. **GI:** abdominal pain, anorexia, constipation, diarrhea, mucositis, nausea, stomatitis, vomiting, altered taste. **Derm:** alopecia, hyperpigmentation, nail disorder, palmar-plantar erythrodysesthesia (combination therapy with capecitabine), exfoliation, pruritus, rash, hot flushes. **Hemat:** MYELOSUPPRESSION. **MS:** arthralgia, musculoskeletal pain, myalgia. **Neuro:** peripheral neuropathy. **Misc:** hypersensitivity reactions.

PHYSICAL THERAPY IMPLICATIONS

Examination and Evaluation

- Monitor signs of bone marrow suppression (myelosuppression) as indicated by blood dyscrasias such as neutropenia (fever, sore throat, signs of infection), thrombocytopenia (bruising, nose bleeds, bleeding gums), or anemia (unusual weakness and fatigue, shortness of breath on exertion, pallor, cyanosis). Report these signs to the physician immediately.
- Monitor signs of hypersensitivity reactions, including pulmonary symptoms (tightness in the throat and chest, wheezing, cough, dyspnea) or skin reactions (rash, pruritus, urticaria). Notify physician or nursing staff immediately if these reactions occur.
- Monitor any chest pain or other signs of cardiac dysfunction (palpitations, fatigue upon exertion, altered heart rate). Notify physician if cardiac symptoms increase during exercise or limit functional ability.
- Assess peripheral edema using girth measurements, volume displacement, and measurement of pitting edema (See Appendix N). Report increased swelling in feet and ankles or a sudden increase in body weight due to fluid retention.
- Assess any joint or muscle pain to rule out musculoskeletal pathology; that is, try to determine if pain is drug-induced rather than caused by anatomical or biomechanical problems.
- Be alert for signs of peripheral neuropathy (numbness, tingling, decreased muscle strength). Establish baseline electroneuromyographic values using EMG and nerve conduction at the beginning of drug treatment whenever possible, and reexamine these values periodically to document drug-induced changes in peripheral nerve function.
- Assess dizziness and weakness that might affect gait, balance, and other functional activities (See Appendix C). Report balance problems and functional limitations to the physician and nursing staff, and caution the patient and family/caregivers to guard against falls and trauma.

Interventions

- For patients who are medically able to begin exercise, implement appropriate resistive exercises and aerobic training to maintain muscle strength and aerobic capacity during cancer chemotherapy or to help restore function after chemotherapy.
- Because of the risk of ventricular dysfunction, use caution during aerobic exercise and other forms of therapeutic exercise. Assess exercise tolerance frequently (blood pressure, heart rate, fatigue levels), and terminate exercise immediately if any untoward responses occur (See Appendix L).

Patient/Client-Related Instruction

- Advise patient and family/caregivers about the risk of infections, and to guard against infection (frequent hand washing, etc.), and to avoid crowds and contact with persons with contagious diseases.

- Advise patient and family/caregivers that fatigue and weakness are likely and may be severe. Functional abilities may be limited, and patient may need to use assistive devices during ambulation.
- Advise patient and family/caregivers about the likelihood of GI reactions such as nausea, vomiting, diarrhea, constipation, abdominal pain, irritation of the oral mucosa, and abnormal taste. Instruct patient to report severe or prolonged GI problems.
- Advise patient that skin rashes and other skin reactions are likely, including rash, itching, exfoliation, and changes in pigmentation. Palmar-plantar erythrodysesthesia (hand-and-foot syndrome) may also occur as indicated by pain, redness, and dry, scaly skin on the palms of the hands and soles of the feet. Instruct patient to protect the hands and feet from heat and friction and to apply lotion to the affected areas. Superficial cold application can also temporarily reduce symptoms.
- Instruct patient to report other troublesome side effects such as severe or prolonged headache, sleep loss, excessive nasal/eye discharge, or hot flashes.

Pharmacokinetics

Absorption: IV administration results in complete bioavailability.
Distribution: Unknown.
Metabolism and Excretion: Extensively metabolized by the liver, primarily by the CYP3A4 enzyme system Metabolites are not active and are excreted mainly by the kidneys.
Half-life: 52 hr.

TIME/ACTION PROFILE (blood levels)

ROUTE	ONSET	PEAK	DURATION
IV	unknown	end of infusion	unknown

Contraindications/Precautions

Contraindicated in: Previous hypersensitivity to any medications containing Cremophor EL or similar derivatives (polyoxyethylated castor oil); Neutrophils <1500 cells/m^3 or platelets <100,000 cells/m^3; Severe hepatic impairment; Use with capecitabine is contraindicated for hepatic impairment (AST or ALT >2.5 × upper limits of normal or bilirubin >1 × upper limit of normal) due to ↑ risk of toxicity and death associated with neutropenia; OB: Pregnancy or lactation.
Use Cautiously in: Toxicity; dose adjustments may be required for neuropathy/arthralgia/myalgia/fatigue, neutropenia, thrombocytopenia, moderate hepatic impairment or palmar-plantar erythrodysesthesia; Diluent contains dehydrated alcohol; consider possible CNS effects; Diabetes or history of neuropathy (↑ risk of severe neuropathy); History of cardiac disease (may ↑ risk of myocardial ischemia or ventricular dysfunction); OB: Patients with child-bearing potential.

Interactions

Drug-Drug: Strong CYP3A4 inhibitors, including **ketoconazole, itraconazole, voriconazole, clarithromycin, telithromycin, atazanavir, delavirdine, ritonavir, saquinavir,** or **nefazodone,** ↑ blood levels and the risk of serious toxicities; concurrent use should be avoided if possible. If concurrent use is required, dose reduction of ixabepilone is recommended. Inducers of the **CYP3A4 enzyme system,** including **dexamethasone, phenytoin, carbamazepine, phenobarbital, rifampin, rifampicin,** or **rifabutin,** may ↓ levels and effectiveness; avoid if possible.
Drug-Natural: St. John's wort may ↓ blood levels and should be avoided.
Drug-Food: Grapefruit juice may ↑ blood levels and toxicity; avoid concurrent use.

Route/Dosage

IV (Adults): 40 mg/m^2 every 3 wk; not to exceed dose greater than that calculated for 2.2 m^2 (88 mg/dose).

Hepatic Impairment

IV (Adults): *Moderate impairment*—20 mg/m^2 every 3 wk; not to exceed 30 mg/m^2.

Availability

Powder for injection (requires specific diluent for initial reconstitution): 15-mg vial (contains 16 mg ixabepilone to allow for withdrawal losses) with 8 mL of diluent in a separate vial as a kit; 45-mg vial (contains 47 mg ixabepilone to allow for withdrawal losses) with 23.5 mL of diluent in a separate vial.

kanamycin (kan-a-**mye**-sin)

Kantrex

Classification

Therapeutic: anti-infectives

Pharmacologic: aminoglycosides

Indications

IM, IV: Treatment of serious infections when other less toxic drugs are contraindicated.

Action

Inhibits protein synthesis in bacteria at level of 30S ribosome. **Therapeutic Effects:** Bactericidal action. **Spectrum:** Notable for activity against *Klebsiella pneumoniae, Escherichia coli, Proteus, Serratia marcescens, Enterobacter aerogenes, Acinetobacter, Staphylococcus aureus.*

Adverse Reactions/Side Effects

EENT: ototoxicity (vestibular and cochlear). **GU:** nephrotoxicity. **MS:** muscle paralysis (high parenteral doses). **Misc:** hypersensitivity reactions.

PHYSICAL THERAPY IMPLICATIONS

Examination and Evaluation

- Monitor signs of hypersensitivity reactions, including pulmonary symptoms (tightness in the throat and chest, wheezing, cough dyspnea) or skin reactions (rash, pruritus, urticaria). Notify physician or nursing staff immediately if these reactions occur.
- Report any muscle weakness or paralysis that occurs following injection of high doses.
- Monitor signs of ototoxicity, including hearing loss, tinnitus, and balance problems (See Appendix E for Fall Assessment and Prevention). Report these signs, and caution the patient and family/caregivers to guard against falls and trauma.

Interventions

- Always wash hands thoroughly and disinfect equipment (whirlpools, electrotherapeutic devices, treatment tables, and so forth) to help prevent the spread of infection. Use universal precautions or isolation procedures as indicated for specific patients.

Patient/Client-Related Instruction

- Advise patient to report signs of nephrotoxicity, including blood or pus in urine, decreased urine output, fatigue, and weight gain from fluid retention.

Pharmacokinetics

Absorption: Well absorbed after IM administration. IV administration results in complete bioavailability.
Distribution: Widely distributed throughout extracellular fluid; crosses the placenta; small amounts enter breast milk. Some penetration into CSF when meninges are inflamed.
Metabolism and Excretion: Excretion is >90% renal.
Half-life: 2–4 hr (increased in renal impairment).

TIME/ACTION PROFILE (blood levels*)

ROUTE	ONSET	PEAK	DURATION
IM	rapid	30–90 min	N/A
IV	rapid	15–30 min†	N/A

*All parenterally administered aminoglycosides.
†Postdistribution peak occurs 30 min after the end of a 30-min infusion and 15 min after the end of a 1-hr infusion.

Contraindications/Precautions

Contraindicated in: Hypersensitivity to kanamycin or other aminoglycosides; Pregnancy.
Use Cautiously in: Renal impairment (dosage adjustments necessary; blood level monitoring useful in preventing ototoxicity and nephrotoxicity); Hearing impairment; Geriatric patients and premature infants (difficulty in assessing auditory and vestibular function; age-related renal impairment); Neonates (increased risk of neuromuscular blockade; difficulty in assessing auditory and vestibular function; immature renal function); Neuromuscular diseases such as myasthenia gravis; Lactation (safety not established).

Interactions

Drug-Drug: Inactivated by **penicillins** and **cephalosporins** when coadministered to patients with renal insufficiency. Possible respiratory paralysis after **inhalation anesthetics** or **neuromuscular blockers.** ↑ incidence of ototoxicity with **loop diuretics.** ↑ incidence of nephrotoxicity with other **nephrotoxic drugs.**

Route/Dosage

All parenteral doses should be adjusted on the basis of serum levels and renal function. Dose should be based on ideal body weight.
IM, IV (Adults and Children and Infants): 5 mg/kg q 8 hr, or 7.5 mg/kg q 12 hr (not to exceed 15 mg/kg/day).
Intraperitoneal: (Adults): 500 mg.
Inhalation (Adults): 250 mg 2–4 times daily.

Renal Impairment

IM, IV (Adults): 7.5 mg/kg; further dosing and intervals determined by blood level monitoring and assessment of renal function.

Availability (generic available)

Injection: 37.5 mg/mL, 250 mg/mL, 333.3 mg/mL.

ketamine (ket-a-meen)

Ketalar

Classification

Therapeutic: general anesthetics

Indications

Anesthesia for short-term diagnostic and surgical procedures. As induction before the use of other anesthetics. As a supplement to other anesthetics. **Unlabeled Use:** Provides sedation and analgesia.

Action

Blocks afferent impulses of pain perception. Suppresses spinal cord activity. Affects CNS transmitter systems. **Therapeutic Effects:** Anesthesia with profound analgesia, minimal respiratory depression, and minimal skeletal muscle relaxation.

Adverse Reactions/Side Effects

CNS: emergence reactions, elevated intracranial pressure. **EENT:** diplopia, increased intraocular pressure, nystagmus. **Resp:** laryngospasm, respiratory depression and apnea (rapid IV administration of large doses). **CV:** hypertension, tachycardia, arrhythmias, bradycardia, hypotension. **GI:** excessive salivation, nausea, vomiting. **Derm:** erythema, rash. **Local:** pain at injection site. **MS:** increased skeletal muscle tone.

PHYSICAL THERAPY IMPLICATIONS*

**Implications refer primarily to any residual effects that occur typically within 24 hr after anesthesia.*

Examination and Evaluation

- Assess respiration and notify physician immediately if patient exhibits any interruption in respiratory rate (apnea) or signs of respiratory depression, including decreased respiratory rate, confusion, bluish color of the skin and mucous membranes (cyanosis), and difficult, labored breathing (dyspnea). Monitor pulse oximetry and perform pulmonary function tests (See Appendix I) to quantify suspected changes in ventilation and respiratory function. Apnea or excessive respiratory depression requires emergency care.
- Monitor signs of laryngeal spasm, including tightness in the throat and chest, wheezing, cough, and severe shortness of breath. Notify physician or nursing staff immediately if these reactions occur.
- Assess signs of increased intracranial pressure, including decreased consciousness, headache, lethargy, seizures, and vomiting (See Appendix D). Notify physician or nursing staff immediately of these signs.
- Be alert for signs of emergence reactions, including nightmares, hallucinations, and other changes in mood and behavior. Report these signs to the physician or nursing staff.
- Assess blood pressure (BP) and compare to normal values (See Appendix F). Report changes in BP, either a problematic decrease in BP (hypotension) or a sustained increase in BP (hypertension).
- Assess heart rate, ECG, and heart sounds, especially during exercise (See Appendices G, H). Report abnormal heart rhythms or symptoms of arrhythmias, including palpitations, chest discomfort, shortness of breath, fainting, and fatigue/weakness.
- Be alert for residual muscle rigidity and increased skeletal muscle tone. Report a sustained increase in muscle tone.
- Monitor injection site for pain, swelling, and irritation. Report prolonged or excessive injection site reactions to the physician.

Interventions

- Implement breathing activities and other therapeutic exercises to encourage ventilation and help overcome any residual effects of the anesthetic.
- Because of the risk of respiratory depression, arrhythmias, and abnormal BP responses, use caution during aerobic exercise and other forms of therapeutic exercise. Assess exercise tolerance frequently (BP, heart rate, respiratory rate, fatigue levels), and terminate exercise immediately if any untoward responses occur (See Appendix L).
- Because of the risk of intracranial hypertension, avoid activities that might increase intracranial pressure such as elevating the feet above the head (Trendelenburg's position) or holding breath and straining during a bowel movement (Valsalva's maneuver).
- To minimize orthostatic hypotension, patient should move slowly when assuming a more upright position.

Patient/Client-Related Instruction

- Advise patient to avoid alcohol or other CNS depressants for 24 hr after anesthesia.
- Instruct patient to report other troublesome side effects such as severe or prolonged vision disturbances, skin reactions (rash, warmth, redness), or GI problems (nausea, vomiting, excessive salivation).

Pharmacokinetics

Absorption: Rapidly absorbed after IM administration.
Distribution: Rapidly distributed. Enters the CNS; crosses the placenta.
Metabolism and Excretion: Mostly metabolized by the liver. Some conversion to another active compound.
Half-life: 2.5 hr.

TIME/ACTION PROFILE (anesthesia)

ROUTE	ONSET	PEAK	DURATION
IV	30 sec	unknown	5–10 min
IM	3–4 min	unknown	12–25 min

Contraindications/Precautions

Contraindicated in: Hypersensitivity; Psychiatric disturbances; Hypertension; Elevated intracranial pressure; Pregnancy or lactation.
Use Cautiously in: Cardiovascular disease; Procedures involving larynx, pharynx, or bronchial tree (muscle relaxants required); Gastroesophageal reflux; Hepatic dysfunction; History of alcohol abuse; Cerebral trauma; Intracerebral mass or hemorrhage; Hyperthyroidism; History of psychiatric problems; Increased cerebrospinal fluid (CSF) pressure; Increased intraocular pressure; Severe eye trauma.

Interactions

Drug-Drug: Use with **barbiturates, hydroxyzine,** and **opioid analgesics** may result in prolonged recovery time. Use with **halothane** may result in ↓ BP, cardiac output, and heart rate. Use with **tubocurarine** or **nondepolarizing neuromuscular blocking agents** may result in prolonged respiratory depression. Concurrent use with **thyroid hormone** ↑ the risk of tachycardia and hypertension. Concurrent administration with **diazepam** may ↓ the incidence of emergence reaction. Concurrent administration with **atropine** may ↑ the incidence of unpleasant dreams.

Route/Dosage

General Anesthesia

IV (Adults): *Induction*—1–2 mg/kg (range 1–4.5 mg/kg)–2 mg/kg produces 5–10 min of surgical anesthesia or 1–2 mg/kg as a single injection or infused at 0.5 mg/min. May be used with concurrent diazepam. *Maintenance*—Increments of ½ to the full induction dose may be repeated as needed. If given with concurrent diazepam, an infusion of 0.1–0.5 mg/min may be used, augmented by 2–5 mg doses of diazepam.
IV (Children): 0.5–2 mg/kg, use smaller doses (0.5–1 mg/kg) for minor procedures.
IM (Adults): 3–8 mg/kg (10 mg/kg produces 12–25 min of surgical anesthesia).
IM (Children): 3–7 mg/kg.
PO (Children): 6–10 mg/kg for 1 dose (mix in cola or other beverage) 30 min prior to procedure.

Sedation/Analgesia (Unlabeled)

IV (Adults): 200–750 mcg (0.2–0.75 mg)/kg over 2–3 min initially, followed by 5–20 mcg (0.005–0.02 mg)/kg/min as an infusion.
IV (Children): 5–20 mcg/kg/min.
IM (Adults): 2–4 mg/kg initially, then 5–20 mcg (0.005–0.02 mg)/kg/min as an IV infusion.

Availability (generic available)

Injection: 10 mg/mL, 50 mg/mL, 100 mg/mL.

K

ketoconazole (systemic)

(kee-toe-**koe**-na-zole)
Nizoral

ketoconazole (topical)

(kee-toe-**kon**-a-zole)
Extina, Nizoral, Nizoral A-D, Xolegel

Classification
Therapeutic: antifungals (systemic)
Pharmacologic: imidazole

Indications

Systemic: treatment of Candidiasis (disseminated and mucocutaneous), Chromomycosis, Coccidioidomycosis, Histoplasmosis, Paracoccidioidomycosis.
Unlabeled Use: Treatment of advanced prostate cancer. Treatment of Cushing's syndrome.
Topical: treatment of a variety of cutaneous fungal infections, including cutaneous candidiasis, tinea pedis (athlete's foot), tinea cruris (jock itch), tinea corporis (ringworm), dandruff (as a shampoo), seborrheic dermatitis, and tinea versicolor.

Action

Disrupts fungal cell membrane. Interferes with fungal metabolism. Also inhibits the production of adrenal steroids. **Therapeutic Effects:** Fungistatic or fungicidal action against susceptible organisms, depending on organism and site of infection. **Spectrum:** Active against many pathogenic fungi, including *Blastomyces*, *Candida*, *Coccidioides*, *Cryptococcus*, *Histoplasma*, Many dermatophytes.

Adverse Reactions/Side Effects

CNS: dizziness, drowsiness. **EENT:** photophobia.
GI: DRUG-INDUCED HEPATITIS, nausea, vomiting,

abdominal pain, constipation, diarrhea, flatulence. **GU:** azoospermia, ↓ male libido, menstrual irregularities, oligospermia. **Derm:** rashes, ↑ hair loss (shampoo). **Endo:** gynecomastia. **Local:** burning, itching, local hypersensitivity reactions, redness, stinging.

PHYSICAL THERAPY IMPLICATIONS

Examination and Evaluation

- Be alert for signs of drug-induced hepatitis, including anorexia, abdominal pain, severe nausea and vomiting, yellow skin or eyes, fever, sore throat, malaise, weakness, facial edema, lethargy, and unusual bleeding or bruising. Notify physician immediately of these signs.
- Monitor rashes or other severe skin reactions such as exfoliation, hives, itching, raised patches of red or white skin (welts), burning, acne, and abnormal sweating. Notify physician immediately because certain skin responses may indicate serious hypersensitivity reactions.
- Assess dizziness or drowsiness that might affect gait, balance, and other functional activities (See Appendix C). Report balance problems and functional limitations to the physician and nursing staff, and caution the patient and family/caregivers to guard against falls and trauma.
- For cutaneous infections, assess healing of skin lesions to help document drug effectiveness.

Interventions

- Avoid contact with cutaneous lesions when treating patient.
- Always wash hands thoroughly and disinfect equipment (whirlpools, electrotherapeutic devices, treatment tables, and so forth) to help prevent the spread of infection. Use universal precautions or isolation procedures as indicated for specific patients.

Patient/Client-Related Instruction

- Advise patient to take or apply this drug as directed for the full course of treatment even if feeling better.
- Advise patient to report any increased local sensitivity to topical application of this drug (pain, burning, itching, swelling) or extensive hair loss when used as a shampoo.
- Instruct patients with cutaneous infections about proper hygiene; e.g., thoroughly wash and dry the affected area, wear clean socks and ventilated shoes for tinea pedis, and so forth.
- Inform patient that early relief of cutaneous symptoms may be seen in 2–3 days. Full therapeutic response may take 2 wk for candidiasis, tinea cruris, tinea corporis, and tinea versicolor, and 4–6 wk for tinea pedis.
- Advise patient to seek medical help if infections persist or recur after the full treatment. Recurrent fungal infections may be a sign of systemic illness.
- Instruct patient on systemic doses to report other troublesome side effects such as prolonged or severe headache, increased visual sensitivity to light (photophobia), fever, ringing/buzzing in the ears (tinnitus), decreased libido, breast enlargement in men, menstrual irregularities, skin problems (rash, itching), or GI reactions (diarrhea, nausea, vomiting, constipation, flatulence, abdominal pain).

Pharmacokinetics

Absorption: Absorption from the GI tract is pH dependent; increasing pH decreases absorption.
Distribution: Widely distributed. CNS penetration is unpredictable and minimal. Crosses the placenta; enters breast milk.
Protein Binding: 99%.
Metabolism and Excretion: Partially metabolized by the liver. Excreted in feces via biliary excretion.
Half-life: 8 hr.

TIME/ACTION PROFILE (blood levels)

ROUTE	ONSET	PEAK	DURATION
PO	rapid	1–4 hr	24 hr
topical	unknown	unknown	Unknown

Contraindications/Precautions

Systemic use contraindicated in: Hypersensitivity; Pregnancy or lactation; Concurrent triazolam.
Use Cautiously in: *Systemic*—History of liver disease; Achlorhydria or hypochlorhydria; Alcoholism.
Topical— Nail and scalp infections (may require additional systemic therapy); OB/Lactation: Safety not established.

Interactions

Drug-Drug: Ketoconazole inhibits the hepatic P4503A4 enzyme system, which results in ↓ metabolism and possibly ↑ effects and/or toxicity from **cyclosporine, tacrolimus, corticosteroids** (dosage reduction may be necessary), **calcium channel blockers, sulfonylurea, oral hypoglycemic agents, quinidine, buspirone, clarithromycin, troleandomycin, erythromycin, cyclophosphamide, phenytoin, warfarin** (↑ risk of bleeding), **tamoxifen, tricyclic antidepressants, carbamazepine, nisoldipine, zolpidem, vinca alkaloids, ifosfamide**, some **benzodiazepines** (effect may persist for several days; use of triazolam is contraindicated), **alfentanil, fentanyl, sufentanil, donepezil, atorvastatin, lovastatin, simvastatin, amprenavir, indinavir** (dosage ↓ of indinavir recommended), **nelfinavir, ritonavir, saquinavir, quinidine, sildenafil** and **vardenafil** (dosage adjustments may be necessary). May alter the effectiveness of **hormonal contraceptives** (alternative method of contraception recommended). Drugs that ↑ gastric pH, including **antacids**, **histamine H_2 antagonists**, **didanosine** (chewable tablets, because of buffer), and **gastric acid–pump inhibitors** ↓ absorption (wait 2 hr before administration of ketoconazole). **Sucralfate** and **isoniazid** also ↓ bioavailability. ↑ hepatotoxicity with other **hepatotoxic agents**, including **alcohol**. Disulfiram-like reaction may occur with **alcohol**. **Rifampin** or **isoniazid** may ↓ levels and effectiveness. May ↓ absorption and effectiveness of **theophylline**.

Route/Dosage

PO (Adults): *Antifungal*—200–400 mg/day, single dose. *Prostate cancer*—400 mg tid (unlabeled).
PO (Children >2 yr): 3.3–6.6 mg/kg/day, single dose.
Topical (Adults and Children ≥12 yr): Apply cream once daily for cutaneous candidiasis, tinea corporis, tinea cruris, tinea pedia, and tinea versicolor. Apply cream twice daily for seborrheic dermatitis. Patients with cutaneous candidiasis, tinea cruris, tinea corporis, and tinea versicolor should be treated for 2 wk. Patients with tinea pedis should be treated for 6 wk. Patients with seborrheic dermatitis should be treated for 4 wk (2 wk with gel). For dandruff, use shampoo twice weekly (wait 3–4 days between treatments) for 4 wk, then intermittently.

Availability (generic available)

Tablets: 200 mg. **Oral suspension:** 100 mg/5 mL. **Cream:** 2%. **Shampoo:** 1% OTC. **Foam:** 2%. **Gel:** 2%.

ketoprofen (kee-toe-**proe**-fen)

Actron, ✤Apo-Keto, ✤Apo-Keto-E, Orudis, ✤Orudis-E, Orudis KT, ✤Orudis-SR, Oruvail, ✤Rhodis

Classification

Therapeutic: antipyretics, antirheumatics, nonopioid analgesics, nonsteroidal anti-inflammatory agents
Pharmacologic: nonopioid analgesics

Indications

Inflammatory disorders, including Rheumatoid arthritis, Osteoarthritis. Mild-to-moderate pain, including dysmenorrhea and fever.

Action

Inhibits prostaglandin synthesis. **Therapeutic Effects:** Suppression of pain and inflammation. Reduction of fever.

Adverse Reactions/Side Effects

CNS: drowsiness, headache, dizziness. **EENT:** blurred vision, tinnitus. **CV:** edema. **GI:** DRUG-INDUCED HEPATITIS, GI BLEEDING, constipation, diarrhea, dyspepsia, nausea, vomiting, anorexia, discomfort, flatulence. **GU:** cystitis, hematuria, renal failure. **Derm:** EXFOLIATIVE DERMATITIS, STEVENS-JOHNSON SYNDROME, TOXIC EPIDERMAL NECROLYSIS, photosensitivity, rashes. **Endo:** gynecomastia. **Hemat:** blood dyscrasias, prolonged bleeding time. **MS:** myalgia. **Misc:** ALLERGIC REACTIONS, INCLUDING ANAPHYLAXIS, fever.

PHYSICAL THERAPY IMPLICATIONS

K

Examination and Evaluation

- Monitor signs of GI bleeding, including abdominal pain, vomiting blood, blood in stools, or black, tarry stools. Report these signs to the physician immediately.
- Be alert for signs of drug-induced hepatitis, including anorexia, abdominal pain, severe nausea and vomiting, yellow skin or eyes, skin rashes, flu-like symptoms, and muscle/joint pain. Report these signs to the physician immediately.
- Monitor signs of allergic reactions and anaphylaxis, including pulmonary symptoms (laryngeal edema, wheezing, cough, dyspnea) or skin reactions (rash, pruritus, urticaria). Be especially alert for exfoliation, dermatitis, and other severe skin reactions that might indicate serious hypersensitivity reactions (Stevens-Johnson syndrome, toxic epidermal necrolysis). Notify physician immediately if these reactions occur.
- Assess pain and other variables (range of motion, muscle strength) to document whether if this drug is successful in helping manage the patient's pain and decreasing impairments.
- Assess blood pressure (BP) periodically and compare to normal values (See Appendix F). NSAIDs can increase BP in certain patients.
- Be alert for signs of prolonged bleeding time such as bleeding gums, nosebleeds, and unusual or excessive bruising. Report these signs to the physician.
- Assess peripheral edema using girth measurements, volume displacement, and measurement of pitting edema (See Appendix N). Report increased swelling in feet and ankles or a sudden increase in body weight due to fluid retention.
- Monitor signs of kidney dysfunction such as painful urination or blood in the urine. Report signs of renal failure immediately, including decreased urine output, increased BP, muscle cramps/twitching, edema/weight gain from fluid retention, yellowish brown skin, and confusion that progresses to seizures and coma.

- Monitor unusual weakness and fatigue that might be due to anemia or other symptoms such as fever, sore throat, mucosal lesions, or signs of infection that might be due to other blood dyscrasias. Notify physician if these signs occur.
- Assess dizziness and drowsiness that might affect gait, balance, and other functional activities (See Appendix C). Report balance problems and functional limitations to the physician, and caution the patient and family/caregivers to guard against falls and trauma.

Interventions

- Implement appropriate manual therapy techniques, physical agents, and therapeutic exercises to reduce pain and decrease the need for ketoprofen and other NSAIDs.
- If treating arthritic conditions, recommend orthotic and assistive devices as needed to reduce pain, improve function, and augment the effects of drug therapy.
- Use caution with any physical interventions that could increase bleeding, including wound débridement, chest percussion, joint mobilization, and application of local heat.
- Help patient explore other nonpharmacologic methods to reduce chronic pain, such as relaxation techniques, exercise, counseling, and so forth.
- Causes photosensitivity; use care if administering UV treatments. Advise patient to avoid direct sunlight and use sunscreens and protective clothing.

Patient/Client-Related Instruction

- Advise patient that analgesics are usually more effective if given before pain becomes severe; emphasize that adequate pain control will allow better participation in physical therapy.
- Inform patient that NSAIDs may impair bone and cartilage healing. Advise patient to consult physician about NSAID use, especially after fractures, spinal fusion, and other bone surgeries.
- Caution patient about the use of over-the-counter products that contain NSAIDs or acetaminophen while taking prescription doses of ketoprofen. Use of multiple NSAIDs increases the risk of toxicity and overdose.
- Instruct patient to report excessive or prolonged headache or ringing/buzzing in the ears (tinnitus); these signs may indicate drug toxicity.
- Advise patient about the risks of gastric irritation. Instruct patient to notify physician of GI reactions such as severe or prolonged nausea, vomiting, constipation, diarrhea, indigestion, and flatulence.
- Advise patient to reduce alcohol intake because alcohol increases the risk of gastric toxicity.
- Instruct patient and family/caregivers to report other troublesome side effects such as severe or prolonged fever, vision disturbances, skin rash, or breast enlargement in men (gynecomastia).

Pharmacokinetics

Absorption: Well absorbed from the GI tract.
Distribution: Unknown.
Protein Binding: 99%.
Metabolism and Excretion: Mostly (60%) metabolized by the liver; some renal excretion.
Half-life: 2–4 hr.

TIME/ACTION PROFILE

ROUTE	ONSET	PEAK	DURATION
PO (analgesic)	within 60 min	1 hr	4–6 hr
PO (anti-inflammatory)	few days–1 wk	unknown	up to 24 hr (SR products)

Contraindications/Precautions

Contraindicated in: Hypersensitivity; Cross-sensitivity may exist with other NSAIDs, including aspirin; Active GI bleeding; Ulcer disease; Some products contain tartrazine and should be avoided in patients with known intolerance; Perioperative pain from coronary artery bypass graft (CABG) surgery.
Use Cautiously in: Cardiovascular disease or risk factors for cardiovascular disease (may ↑ risk of serious cardiovascular thrombotic events, myocardial infarction, and stroke, especially with prolonged use); Severe renal or hepatic disease; History of ulcer disease; Renal impairment (dosage reduction suggested); Geri: Extended-release product should not be used in geriatric patients, patients of small stature, or patients with renal impairment; Geriatric patients (increased risk of GI bleeding); Chronic alcohol use/abuse; OB/Pedi: Pregnancy, lactation, or children (safety not established; avoid use during 2nd half of pregnancy).

Interactions

Drug-Drug: Aspirin alters distribution, metabolism, and excretion of ketoprofen (concurrent use not recommended). ↑ adverse GI effects with other **NSAIDs, corticosteroids**, or **alcohol**. Chronic use with **acetaminophen** may ↑ risk of adverse renal reactions. May ↓ effectiveness of **diuretics** or **antihypertensives**. May ↑ hypoglycemic effects of **insulin** or sulfonylurea **oral hypoglycemic agents**. May ↑ serum **lithium** levels and increase the risk of toxicity. ↑ risk of toxicity from **methotrexate**. **Probenecid** ↑ risk of toxicity from ketoprofen (concurrent use not recommended). ↑ risk of bleeding with **cefotetan, cefoperazone, valproic acid, thrombolytic agents, clopidogrel, ticlopidine, eptifibatide, tirofiban**, or **anticoagulants**. ↑ risk of adverse hematologic reactions with **antineoplastics** or **radiation therapy**. ↑ risk of nephrotoxicity with **cyclosporine**.
Drug-Natural: ↑ bleeding risk with **arnica, chamomile, clove, dong quai, feverfew, garlic, ginger, ginkgo**, and ***Panax ginseng***.

Route/Dosage

PO (Adults): *Anti-inflammatory*—150–300 mg/day in 3–4 divided doses or 150–200 mg once daily as extended-release product. *Analgesic*—25–50 mg q 6–8 hr. *OTC analgesic/antipyretic*—12.5 mg q 4–6 hr; if relief is not obtained 1 hr after first dose, an additional dose may be given. An initial dose of 25 mg may be used (not to exceed 25 mg/4–6 hr or 75 mg/24 hr).

Availability (generic available)

Tablets: 12.5 mg OTC. **Capsules:** 25 mg, 50 mg, 75 mg. **Extended-release capsules:** 100 mg, 150 mg, 200 mg.

ketorolac (kee-toe-role-ak)

🍁 Toradol

Classification

Therapeutic: nonsteroidal anti-inflammatory agents, nonopioid analgesics
Pharmacologic: pyrrolizine carboxylic acid

Indications

Short-term management of pain (not to exceed 5 days total for all routes combined).

Action

Inhibits prostaglandin synthesis, producing peripherally mediated analgesia. Also has antipyretic and anti-inflammatory properties. **Therapeutic Effects:** Decreased pain.

Adverse Reactions/Side Effects

CNS: drowsiness, abnormal thinking, dizziness, euphoria, headache. **Resp:** asthma, dyspnea. **CV:** edema, pallor, vasodilation. **GI:** GI BLEEDING, abnormal taste, diarrhea, dry mouth, dyspepsia, GI pain, nausea. **GU:** oliguria, renal toxicity, urinary frequency. **Derm:** EXFOLIATIVE DERMATITIS, STEVENS-JOHNSON SYNDROME, TOXIC EPIDERMAL NECROLYSIS, pruritus, purpura, sweating, urticaria. **Hemat:** prolonged bleeding time. **Local:** injection site pain. **Neuro:** paresthesia. **Misc:** allergic reactions, including, anaphylaxis.

PHYSICAL THERAPY IMPLICATIONS

Examination and Evaluation

- Monitor signs of GI bleeding, including abdominal pain, vomiting blood, blood in stools, or black, tarry stools. Report these signs to the physician immediately.
- Monitor signs of allergic reactions and anaphylaxis, including pulmonary symptoms (laryngeal edema, wheezing, cough, dyspnea) or skin reactions (rash, pruritus, urticaria). Be especially alert for exfoliation, dermatitis, and other severe skin reactions that might indicate serious hypersensitivity reactions (Stevens-Johnson syndrome, toxic epidermal necrolysis). Notify physician immediately if these reactions occur.
- Assess pain and other variables (range of motion, muscle strength) to document whether this drug is successful in helping manage the patient's pain and decreasing impairments.
- Assess signs of paresthesia, including numbness and tingling. Perform objective tests, including electroneuromyography and sensory testing to document any drug-related neuropathic changes.
- Assess blood pressure (BP) periodically and compare to normal values (See Appendix F). NSAIDs can increase BP in certain patients.
- Be alert for signs of prolonged bleeding time such as bleeding gums, nosebleeds, and unusual or excessive bruising. Report these signs to the physician.
- Assess peripheral edema using girth measurements, volume displacement, and measurement of pitting edema (See Appendix N). Report increased swelling in feet and ankles or a sudden increase in body weight due to fluid retention.
- Assess symptoms of bronchospasm and asthma, including wheezing, coughing, dyspnea, and tightness in chest. Perform pulmonary function tests to quantify suspected changes in ventilation and respiration (See Appendices I, J, K).
- Monitor signs of kidney toxicity, including blood or pus in urine, increased urinary frequency, decreased urine output, weight gain from fluid retention, and fatigue. Report these signs to the physician.
- Assess dizziness and drowsiness that might affect gait, balance, and other functional activities (See Appendix C). Report balance problems and functional limitations to the physician, and caution the patient and family/caregivers to guard against falls and trauma.
- Monitor and report euphoria, abnormal thinking, or other psychic disturbances.
- Monitor injection site for pain, swelling, and irritation. Report prolonged or excessive injection site reactions to the physician.

Interventions

- Implement appropriate manual therapy techniques, physical agents, and therapeutic exercises to reduce pain and decrease the need for ketorolac and other NSAIDs.
- If treating arthritic conditions, recommend orthotic and assistive devices as needed to reduce pain, improve function, and augment the effects of drug therapy.
- Use caution with any physical interventions that could increase bleeding, including wound débridement,

chest percussion, joint mobilization, and application of local heat.

- Help patient explore other nonpharmacologic methods to reduce chronic pain, such as relaxation techniques, exercise, counseling, and so forth.

Patient/Client-related Instruction

- Advise patient that analgesics are usually more effective if given before pain becomes severe; emphasize that adequate pain control will allow better participation in physical therapy.
- Inform patient that NSAIDs may impair bone and cartilage healing. Advise patient to consult physician about NSAID use, especially after fractures, spinal fusion, and other bone surgeries.
- Caution patient about the use of over-the-counter products that contain NSAIDs or acetaminophen while taking prescription doses of ketorolac. Use of multiple NSAIDs increases the risk of toxicity and overdose.
- Instruct patient to report excessive or prolonged headache or ringing/buzzing in the ears (tinnitus); these signs may indicate drug toxicity.
- Advise patient about the risks of gastric irritation. Instruct patient to notify physician of GI reactions such as severe or prolonged nausea, diarrhea, indigestion, abnormal taste, and abdominal pain.
- Advise patient to reduce alcohol intake because alcohol increases the risk of gastric toxicity.
- Instruct patient and family/caregivers to report other troublesome side effects such as severe or prolonged headache or skin reactions (rash, hives, itching, bruising).

Pharmacokinetics

Absorption: Rapidly and completely absorbed following all routes of administration.
Distribution: Enters breast milk in low concentrations.
Metabolism and Excretion: <50% metabolized by the liver. Ketorolac and its metabolites are excreted primarily by the kidneys (92%); 6% excreted in feces.
Half-life: 4.5 hr (range 3.8–6.3 hr; increased in geriatric patients and patients with impaired renal function).

TIME/ACTION PROFILE (analgesic effects)

ROUTE	ONSET	PEAK	DURATION
PO	unknown	2–3 hr	4–6 hr or longer
IM, IV	10 min	1–2 hr	6 hr or longer

Contraindications/Precautions

Contraindicated in: Hypersensitivity; Cross-sensitivity with other NSAIDs may exist; OB: Labor, delivery or lactation; Preoperative or perioperative use; Known alcohol intolerance (injection only); Perioperative pain from coronary artery bypass graft (CABG) surgery.

Use Cautiously in: Cardiovascular disease or risk factors for cardiovascular disease (may ↑ risk of serious cardiovascular thrombotic events, myocardial infarction, and stroke, especially with prolonged use); History of GI bleeding; Renal impairment (dosage reduction may be required); Geri: Appears on Beers' list. Geriatric patients have increased risk of GI bleeding; OB/Pedi: Pregnancy and children (use not recommended during 2nd half of pregnancy).

Interactions

Drug-Drug: Concurrent use with **aspirin** may ↓ effectiveness. ↑ adverse GI effects with **aspirin**, other **NSAIDs**, **potassium supplements, corticosteroids**, or **alcohol**. Chronic use with **acetaminophen** may ↑ risk of adverse renal reactions. May ↓ effectiveness of **diuretics** or **antihypertensives**. May ↑ serum **lithium** levels and ↑ risk of toxicity. ↑ risk of toxicity from **methotrexate**. ↑ risk of bleeding with **cefotetan, cefoperazone, valproic acid, clopidogrel, ticlopidine, tirofiban, eptifibatide, thrombolytic agents**, or **anticoagulants**. ↑ risk of adverse hematologic reactions with **antineoplastics** or **radiation therapy**. May ↑ risk of nephrotoxicity from **cyclosporine. Probenecid** ↑ ketorolac blood levels and the risk of adverse reactions (concurrent use should be avoided).

Drug-Natural: ↑ bleeding risk with **arnica, chamomile, clove, dong quai, feverfew, garlic, ginger, ginkgo, *Panax ginseng***.

Route/Dosage

Oral therapy is indicated only as a continuation of parenteral therapy; parenteral therapy should not exceed 20 doses/5 days. Total duration of therapy by all routes should not exceed 5 days.

PO (Adults <65 yr): 20 mg initially, followed by 10 mg q 4–6 hr as needed (not to exceed 40 mg/day).

PO (Adults ≥65 yr, <50 kg, or with renal impairment): 10 mg q 4–6 hr as needed (not to exceed 40 mg/day).

IM (Adults <65 yr): *Single dose*—60 mg. *Multiple dosing*—30 mg q 6 hr (not to exceed 120 mg/day).

IM (Adults ≥65 yr; <50 kg, or with renal impairment): *Single dose*—30 mg. *Multiple dosing*—15 mg q 6 hr (not to exceed 60 mg/day).

IV (Adults <65 yr): *Single dose*—30 mg. *Multiple dosing*—30 mg q 6 hr (not to exceed 120 mg/day).

IV (Adults ≥65 yr; <50 kg, or with renal impairment): *Single dose*—15 mg. *Multiple dosing*—15 mg q 6 hr (not to exceed 60 mg/day).

Availability (generic available)

Tablets: 10 mg. **Injection:** 15 mg/mL in 1-mL preloaded syringes, 30 mg/mL in 1- and 2-mL preloaded syringes.

HIGH ALERT

labetalol (la-bet-a-lole)

Trandate

Classification

Therapeutic: antianginals, antihypertensives

Pharmacologic: beta blockers

Indications

Management of hypertension.

Action

Blocks stimulation of $beta_1$ (myocardial)– and $beta_2$ (pulmonary, vascular, and uterine)–adrenergic receptor sites. Also has $alpha_1$-adrenergic blocking activity, which may result in more orthostatic hypotension. **Therapeutic Effects:** Decreased blood pressure.

Adverse Reactions/Side Effects

CNS: fatigue, weakness, anxiety, depression, dizziness, drowsiness, insomnia, memory loss, mental status changes, nightmares. **EENT:** blurred vision, dry eyes, nasal stuffiness. **Resp:** bronchospasm, wheezing. **CV:** ARRHYTHMIAS, BRADYCARDIA, CHF, PULMONARY EDEMA, orthostatic hypotension. **GI:** constipation, diarrhea, nausea. **GU:** erectile dysfunction, decreased libido. **Derm:** itching, rashes. **Endo:** hyperglycemia, hypoglycemia. **MS:** arthralgia, back pain, muscle cramps. **Neuro:** paresthesia. **Misc:** drug-induced lupus syndrome.

PHYSICAL THERAPY IMPLICATIONS

Examination and Evaluation

- Assess heart rate, ECG, and heart sounds, especially during exercise (See Appendices G, H). Report any rhythm disturbances or symptoms of increased arrhythmias, including palpitations, chest discomfort, shortness of breath, fainting, and fatigue/weakness.
- Assess routinely for signs of CHF and pulmonary edema, including dyspnea, rales/crackles, weight gain, peripheral edema, and jugular venous distention. Report these signs to the physician immediately.
- Assess blood pressure (BP) periodically and compare to normal values (See Appendix F) to help document antihypertensive effects. Be alert for a fall in BP when patient assumes a more upright position (lying to standing, sitting to standing, lying to sitting). Document orthostatic hypotension and contact physician when systolic BP falls >20 mm Hg, or diastolic BP falls >10 mm Hg.
- Assess symptoms of bronchospasm (wheezing, coughing, tightness in chest). Perform pulmonary function tests to quantify suspected changes in ventilation and respiration (See Appendices I, J, K). Repeated or prolonged bronchoconstriction may require a change in dose or medication (e.g., switch to a more cardioselective beta blocker).
- Watch for signs of hypoglycemia (weakness, malaise, irritability, fatigue) or hyperglycemia (drowsiness, fruity breath, increased urination, unusual thirst). Patients with diabetes mellitus should check blood glucose levels frequently. Medication may mask some signs of hypoglycemia, but dizziness and sweating may still occur.
- Monitor excessive fatigue or weakness. Beta blockers often cause some degree of fatigue and weakness, but any sudden or severe change in muscle strength or energy levels should be reported.
- Assess any back or joint pain to rule out musculoskeletal pathology; that is, try to determine if pain is drug induced rather than caused by anatomic or biomechanical problems.
- Assess signs of paresthesia (numbness, tingling) or muscle cramping. Perform objective tests, including electroneuromyography and sensory testing to document any drug-related neuropathic changes.
- Monitor mood and personality changes, including depression, anxiety, memory loss, or other changes in behavior. Notify physician if these changes become problematic.
- Assess dizziness and drowsiness that might affect gait, balance, and other functional activities (see Appendix C). Report balance problems and functional limitations to the physician, and caution the patient and family/caregivers to guard against falls and trauma.
- Monitor signs of drug-induced lupus syndrome, including increased BP, fever, joint pain, skin rashes, and redness/irritation of the eye (uveitis). Notify physician promptly if these signs appear.

Interventions

- Because of an increased risk of cardiac arrhythmias and CHF, use caution during aerobic exercise and endurance conditioning. Terminate exercise if patient exhibits untoward symptoms (chest pain, shortness of breath, unusual fatigue), or displays other criteria for exercise termination (See Appendix L).
- Establish aerobic exercise workloads that account for the effects of beta blockers on heart rate. Some

L

heart rate guidelines may not be appropriate because beta blockers typically decrease maximal HR by 20–30 bpm. Use other guidelines such as rating of perceived exertion (RPE, modified Borg scale) to determine exercise workloads.
- To minimize orthostatic hypotension, patient should move slowly when assuming a more upright position.

Patient/Client-Related Instruction

- Remind patients to take medication as directed to control hypertension even if they are asymptomatic.
- Counsel patients about additional interventions to help control BP, including regular exercise, weight loss, sodium restriction, stress reduction, moderation of alcohol consumption, and smoking cessation.
- Instruct patient to report other troublesome side effects such as severe or prolonged insomnia, nightmares, blurred vision, dry eyes, stuffy nose, skin rash/itching, sexual problems (decreased libido, erectile dysfunction), or GI problems (nausea, constipation, diarrhea).

Pharmacokinetics

Absorption: Well absorbed but rapidly undergoes extensive first-pass hepatic metabolism, resulting in 25% bioavailability.
Distribution: Some CNS penetration; crosses the placenta.
Metabolism and Excretion: Undergoes extensive hepatic metabolism.
Half-life: 3–8 hr.

TIME/ACTION PROFILE (cardiovascular effects)

ROUTE	ONSET	PEAK	DURATION
PO	20 min–2 hr	1–4 hr	8–12 hr
IV	2–5 min	5 min	16–18 hr

Contraindications/Precautions

Contraindicated in: Uncompensated CHF; Pulmonary edema; Cardiogenic shock; Bradycardia or heart block.
Use Cautiously in: Renal impairment; Hepatic impairment; Geriatric patients (increased sensitivity to beta blockers; initial dosage reduction recommended); Pulmonary disease (including asthma); Diabetes mellitus (may mask signs of hypoglycemia); Thyrotoxicosis (may mask symptoms); Patients with a history of severe allergic reactions (intensity of reactions may be increased); Pregnancy, lactation, or children (safety not established; may cause fetal/neonatal bradycardia, hypotension, hypoglycemia, or respiratory depression).

Interactions

Drug-Drug: General anesthesia, IV, and **verapamil** may cause additive myocardial depression. Additive bradycardia may occur with **digoxin**. Additive hypotension may occur with other **antihypertensives**, acute ingestion of **alcohol**, or **nitrates**. Concurrent **thyroid** administration may ↓ effectiveness. May alter the effectiveness of **insulin** or **oral hypoglycemic agents** (dose adjustments may be necessary). May ↓ the effectiveness of **adrenergic bronchodilators** and **theophylline**. May ↓ beneficial beta cardiovascular effects of **dopamine** or **dobutamine**. Use cautiously within 14 days of **MAO inhibitor** therapy (may result in hypertension). Effects may be ↑ by **propranolol** or **cimetidine**. Concurrent **NSAIDs** may ↓ antihypertensive action.

Route/Dosage

PO (Adults): 100 mg bid initially, may be increased by 100 mg tid q 2–3 days as needed (usual range 400–800 mg/day in 2–3 divided doses; doses up to 1.2–2.4 g/day have been used).
IV (Adults): 20 mg (0.25 mg/kg) initially, additional doses of 40–80 mg may be given q 10 min as needed (not to exceed 300 mg total dose) *or* 2 mg/min infusion (range 50–300 mg total dose required).

Availability (generic available)

Tablets: 100 mg, 200 mg, 300 mg. **Injection:** 5 mg/mL.

lacosamide (la-**kose**-a-mide)
Vimpat

Classification
Therapeutic: anticonvulsants

Indications

Adjunctive therapy of partial-onset seizures.

Action

Mechanism is not known, but may involve enhancement of slow inactivation of sodium channels with resultant membrane stabilization; also binds to collapsin response mediator protein-2 (CRMP-2) which is involved in neural differentiation and growth. **Therapeutic Effects:** Decreased incidence and severity of partial-onset seizures.

Adverse Reactions/Side Effects

CNS: dizziness, headache, syncope, vertigo. **EENT:** diplopia. **CV:** PR interval prolongation. **GI:** nausea, vomiting. **Neuro:** ataxia. **Misc:** multiorgan hypersensitivity reactions (Drug Reaction with eosinophilia and systemic symptoms—DRESS).

PHYSICAL THERAPY IMPLICATIONS

Examination and Evaluation

- Be alert for hypersensitivity responses that might indicate DRESS. These responses include fever, skin reactions (rash that progresses to exfoliative dermatitis), blood dyscrasias (eosinophilia, neutrophilia, neutropenia, thrombopenia, anemia), and involvement of one or more internal organs leading to hepatitis, pneumonitis, nephritis, myocarditis, pericarditis, myositis, pancreatitis, or thyroiditis. Notify physician of these reactions immediately.
- Document the number, duration, and severity of seizures to help determine if this drug is effective in reducing seizure activity.
- Assess dizziness, syncope, and vertigo that might affect gait, balance, and other functional activities (See Appendix C). Report balance problems and functional limitations to the physician, and caution the patient and family/caregivers to guard against falls and trauma.
- Assess any ataxia or gait disturbances to rule out neuromuscular pathology; that is, try to determine if neurologic signs are drug-induced rather than caused by neurologic pathology.
- Assess heart rate, ECG, and heart sounds, especially during exercise (See Appendixes G, H). Report any rhythm disturbances (prolonged PR interval) or symptoms of increased arrhythmias, including palpitations, chest discomfort, shortness of breath, fainting, and fatigue/weakness.

Interventions

- Guard against falls and trauma (hip fractures, head injury, and so forth), especially if dizziness or ataxia affect gait and balance. Implement fall prevention strategies, especially if balance is impaired (See Appendix E).
- Because of the risk of cardiac arrhythmias (prolonged PR interval), use caution during aerobic exercise and other forms of therapeutic exercise. Assess exercise tolerance frequently (blood pressure, heart rate, fatigue levels), and terminate exercise immediately if any untoward responses occur (See Appendix L).

Patient/Client-Related Instruction

- Advise patient to avoid alcohol and other CNS depressants because of the increased risk of sedation and adverse effects.
- Advise patients on prolonged antiseizure therapy not to discontinue medication without consulting their physician. Abrupt withdrawal may cause increased seizures.
- Instruct patient and family/caregivers to report other troublesome side effects such as severe or prolonged vision problems or GI reactions problems (nausea, vomiting).

Pharmacokinetics

Absorption: 100% absorbed following oral administration; IV administration results in complete bioavailability.
Distribution: Unknown.
Metabolism and Excretion: Partially metabolized by the liver; 40% excreted in urine as unchanged drug, 30% as a metabolite.
Half-life: 13 hr.

TIME/ACTION PROFILE (blood levels)

ROUTE	ONSET	PEAK	DURATION
PO	unknown	1–4 hr	12 hr
IV	unknown	end of infusion	12 hr

Contraindications/Precautions

Contraindicated in: Hypersensitivity; Severe hepatic impairment; Lactation: Avoid use during breast-feeding.
Use Cautiously in: CCr <30 mL/min (use lower daily dose); Mild-to-moderate hepatic impairment; titrate dose carefully, use lower daily dose; Known cardiac conduction problems or severe cardiac disease (MI or CHF); History of suicidal ideation or suicide attempt; Geri: Titrate dose carefully in elderly patients; OB: Use during pregnancy only if potential benefit justifies risk to the fetus; Pedi: Safety and effectiveness have not been established in children <17 yr.

Interactions

Drug-Drug: Use cautiously with other **drugs that affect cardiac conduction.**

Route/Dosage

PO, IV (Adults): 50 mg bid; may be increased weekly by 100 mg/day in 2 divided doses up to a maintenance dose of 200–400 mg/day given in 2 divided doses
Severe renal impairment (CCR ≤30 mL/min) or mild-to-moderate hepatic impairment—daily dose should not exceed 300 mg.

Availability

Tablets: 50 mg, 150 mg, 200 mg. **Solution for IV injection:** 200 mg/20 mL single-use vials, 200 mg.

lamivudine (la-miv-yoo-deen)

Epivir, Epivir HBV, 3TC

Classification

Therapeutic: antiretrovirals, antivirals

Pharmacologic: nucleoside reverse transcriptase inhibitors

Indications

HIV infection (with other antiretrovirals). Chronic hepatitis B infection. **Unlabeled Use:** Part of HIV-post-exposure prophylaxis with zidovudine and indinavir.

Action

After intracellular conversion to its active form (lamivudine-5-triphosphate), inhibits viral DNA synthesis by inhibiting the enzyme reverse transcriptase. **Therapeutic Effects:** Slows the progression of HIV infection and decreases the occurrence of its sequelae. Increases CD4 cell counts and decreases viral load. Protection from liver damage caused by chronic hepatitis B infection; decreases viral load.

Adverse Reactions/Side Effects

Noted for combination of lamivudine plus zidovudine

CNS: SEIZURES, fatigue, headache, insomnia, malaise, depression, dizziness. **Resp:** cough. **GI:** HEPATOMEGALY WITH STEATOSIS, PANCREATITIS (↑ IN PEDIATRIC PATIENTS), anorexia, diarrhea, nausea, vomiting, abdominal discomfort, abnormal liver function studies, dyspepsia. **Derm:** alopecia, erythema multiforme, rashes, urticaria. **Endo:** hyperglycemia. **F and E:** lactic acidosis. **Hemat:** anemia, neutropenia, pure red cell aplasia. **MS:** musculoskeletal pain, arthralgia, muscle weakness, myalgia, rhabdomyolysis. **Neuro:** neuropathy. **Misc:** HYPERSENSITIVITY REACTIONS, INCLUDING ANAPHYLAXIS AND STEVENS-JOHNSON SYNDROME.

PHYSICAL THERAPY IMPLICATIONS

Examination and Evaluation

- Be alert for new seizures or increased seizure activity, especially at the onset of drug treatment. Document the number, duration, and severity of seizures, and report these findings immediately to the physician.
- Be alert for signs of enlarged, fatty liver (hepatomegaly with steatosis) that can progress to liver dysfunction and liver failure. Signs of liver disease include anorexia, abdominal pain, abdominal swelling (ascites), severe nausea and vomiting, yellow skin or eyes, fever, sore throat, malaise, weakness, facial edema, lethargy, and unusual bleeding or bruising. Notify physician of these signs immediately.
- Monitor signs of pancreatitis, including upper abdominal pain (especially after eating), indigestion, weight loss, and oily stools. Report these signs to the physician immediately.
- Monitor signs of hypersensitivity reactions and anaphylaxis, including pulmonary symptoms (tightness in the throat and chest, wheezing, cough, dyspnea) or skin reactions that could indicate Stevens-Johnson syndrome (rash, pruritus, urticaria, dermatitis, exfoliation). Notify physician or nursing staff immediately if these reactions occur.
- Monitor signs of lactic acidosis, including confusion, lethargy, stupor, shallow rapid breathing, tachycardia, hypotension, nausea, and vomiting. Notify physician immediately if these signs occur.
- Assess any musculoskeletal pain, muscle tenderness, or weakness, especially if accompanied by fever, malaise, and dark-colored urine. These symptoms may represent drug-induced myopathy, and that myopathy can progress to severe muscle damage (rhabdomyolysis). Report any unexplained musculoskeletal symptoms to the physician immediately.
- Be alert for signs of peripheral neuropathy (numbness, tingling, decreased muscle strength). Establish baseline electroneuromyographic values using EMG and nerve conduction at the beginning of drug treatment whenever possible, and reexamine these values periodically to assess drug-induced changes in peripheral nerve function.
- Monitor signs of neutropenia (fever, sore throat, mucosal lesions, signs of infection, bruising, bleeding), or unusual weakness and fatigue that might be due to anemia and other blood dyscrasias. Report these signs to the physician.
- Assess dizziness that might affect gait, balance, and other functional activities (See Appendix C). Report balance problems and functional limitations to the physician and nursing staff, and caution the patient and family/caregivers to guard against falls and trauma.
- Monitor signs of hyperglycemia (confusion; drowsiness; flushed, dry skin; fruit-like breath odor; rapid, deep breathing, polyuria; loss of appetite; unusual thirst). Insulin dosages may need to be adjusted to prevent repeated episodes of hyperglycemia.

Interventions

- Implement resistive exercises and other therapeutic exercises as tolerated to maintain muscle strength and function and prevent muscle wasting associated with HIV infection and AIDS.

- Because of the risk of lactic acidosis and myopathy, use caution during aerobic exercise and other forms of therapeutic exercise. Assess exercise tolerance frequently (blood pressure, heart rate, fatigue levels), and terminate exercise immediately if any untoward responses occur (See Appendix L).

Patient/Client-Related Instruction

- Emphasize the importance of taking lamivudine as directed even if the patient is asymptomatic, and that this drug must always be used in combination with other antiretroviral drugs. Do not take more than prescribed amount, and do not stop taking without consulting health care professional.
- Inform patient that lamivudine does not cure HIV or AIDS or prevent associated or opportunistic infections. Lamivudine does not reduce the risk of transmission of HIV to others through sexual contact or blood contamination. Caution patient to use a condom, and avoid sharing needles or donating blood to prevent spreading the AIDS virus to others.
- Instruct patient to report other troublesome side effects such as prolonged or severe headache, sleep loss, depression, cough, skin problems (rash, hives, redness, hair loss), or GI problems (diarrhea, nausea, vomiting, abdominal pain, loss of appetite).

Pharmacokinetics

Absorption: Well absorbed after oral administration (86% in adults, 66% in infants and children).
Distribution: Distributes into the extravascular space. Some penetration into CSF; remainder of distribution unknown.
Metabolism and Excretion: Mostly excreted unchanged in urine; <5% metabolized by the liver.
Half-life: *Adults*—3.7 hr; *children*—2 hr.

TIME/ACTION PROFILE (blood levels)

ROUTE	ONSET	PEAK	DURATION
PO	unknown	0.9 hr*	12 hr

*On an empty stomach; peak levels occur at 3.2 hr if lamivudine is taken with food. Food does not affect total amount of drug absorbed.

Contraindications/Precautions

Contraindicated in: Hypersensitivity; Lactation: Lactation.
Use Cautiously in: Impaired renal function (↑ dosing interval/↓ dose recommended if CCr <50 mL/min); Women, prolonged exposure, obesity, history of liver disease (↑ risk of lactic acidosis and severe hepatomegaly with steatosis); Coinfection with hepatitis B (hepatitis may recur after discontinuation of lamivudine); Geri: Dosage reduction may be necessary; OB/Pedi: Pregnancy or children <3 mo (safety not established).
Exercise Extreme Caution in: Pedi: Pediatric patients with a history of pancreatitis (use only if no alternative).

Interactions

Drug-Drug: Trimethoprim/sulfamethoxazole ↑ lamivudine blood levels (dose alteration may be necessary in renal impairment). ↑ risk of pancreatitis with concurrent use of other **drugs causing pancreatitis**. ↑ risk of neuropathy with concurrent use of other **drugs causing neuropathy**. Combination therapy with **tenofovir** and **abacavir** may lead to virologic nonresponse and should not be used.

Route/Dosage

HIV infection

PO (Adults and Children >16 yr and ≥50 kg): 150 mg bid or 300 mg once daily.
PO (Adults <50 kg): 2 mg/kg twice daily.
PO (Children 3 mo–16 yr): *Oral solution*–4 mg/bid.

Renal Impairment

PO (Adults): *CCr 30–49 mL/min*—150 mg once daily; *CCr 15–29 mL/min*—150 mg first dose, then 100 mg once daily; *CCr 5–14 mL/min*—150 mg first dose, then 50 mg once daily; *CCr <5 mL/min*—50 mg first dose, then 25 mg once daily.

Chronic Hepatitis B

PO (Adults): 100 mg once daily.

Renal Impairment

PO (Adults): *CCr 30–49 mL/min*—100 mg first dose, then 50 mg once daily; *CCr 15–29 mL/min*—100 mg first dose, then 25 mg once daily; *CCr 5–14 mL/min*—35 mg first dose, then 15 mg once daily; *CCr <5 mL/min*—35 mg first dose, then 10 mg once daily.
PO (Children 2–17 yr): 3 mg/kg once daily (up to 100 mg/day).

Availability

Epivir

Tablets: 150 mg, 300 mg. **Oral solution (strawberry-banana flavor):** 10 mg/mL in 240-mL bottles.

Epivir HBV

Tablets: 100 mg. **Oral solution (strawberry-banana flavor):** 5 mg/mL in 240-mL bottles. ***In combination with:*** zidovudine (Combivir); zidovudine and abacavir (Trizivir). See Appendix B.

lamotrigine (la-moe-tri-jeen)

Lamictal

Classification

Therapeutic: anticonvulsants

Pharmacologic: phenyltriazine derivative

Indications

Adjunct treatment of partial seizures in adults with epilepsy. Lennox-Gastaut syndrome. Primary generalized tonic-clonic seizures in adults and children ≥2 yr. Conversion to monotherapy in adults with partial seizures receiving a single enzyme-inducing antiepileptic drug. Maintenance treatment of bipolar disorder.

Action

Stabilizes neuronal membranes by inhibiting sodium transport. **Therapeutic Effects:** Decreased incidence of seizures. Delayed time to recurrence of mood episodes.

Adverse Reactions/Side Effects

CNS: <u>ataxia</u>, <u>dizziness</u>, <u>headache</u>, behavior changes, depression, drowsiness, insomnia, tremor. **EENT:** blurred vision, double vision, rhinitis. **GI:** <u>nausea</u>, <u>vomiting</u>. **GU:** vaginitis. **Derm:** <u>photosensitivity</u>, <u>rash (higher incidence in children, patients taking valproic acid (VPA), high initial doses, or rapid dose increases)</u>. **MS:** arthralgia. **Misc:** allergic or hypersensitivity reactions including Stevens-Johnson syndrome.

PHYSICAL THERAPY IMPLICATIONS

Examination and Evaluation

- Monitor signs of allergic and hypersensitivity reactions, including pulmonary symptoms (tightness in the throat and chest, wheezing, cough, dyspnea) or skin reactions (rash, pruritus, urticaria). Be especially alert for severe skin reactions (exfoliation, dermatitis) that might indicate Stevens-Johnson syndrome. Notify physician immediately if these reactions occur.
- Document the number, duration, and severity of seizures to help determine if this drug is effective in reducing seizure activity.
- If treating bipolar disorder, monitor any changes in the patient's mood or behavior. Report manic symptoms (excitement, agitation) or symptoms of depression (sadness, apathy, loss of energy).
- Assess dizziness, ataxia, or tremor that might affect gait, balance, and other functional activities (See Appendix C). Report balance problems and functional limitations to the physician, and caution the patient and family/caregivers to guard against falls and trauma.
- Monitor daytime drowsiness, depression, or other changes in behavior. Repeated or excessive symptoms may require change in dose or medication.
- Assess any joint pain to rule out musculoskeletal pathology; that is, try to determine if pain is drug-induced rather than caused by anatomic or biomechanical problems.

Interventions

- Guard against falls and trauma (hip fractures, head injury, and so forth), especially if dizziness or ataxia affect gait and balance. Implement fall-prevention strategies, especially if balance is impaired (See Appendix E).
- Causes photosensitivity; use care if administering UV treatments. Advise patient to avoid direct sunlight and use sunscreens and protective clothing.

Patient/Client-Related Instruction

- Advise patient to avoid alcohol and other CNS depressants because of the increased risk of sedation and adverse effects.
- Advise patients on prolonged antiseizure therapy not to discontinue medication without consulting their physician. Abrupt withdrawal may cause increased seizures.
- Advise patient about the risk of daytime drowsiness and decreased attention and mental focus. Use care if driving or in other activities that require strong concentration and fast responses.
- Advise patient about the likelihood of skin rash, especially in children, patients taking other antiseizure drugs, or when initiating or changing doses of lamotrigine. Instruct patient to report severe or prolonged skin reactions.
- Instruct patient and family/caregivers to report other troublesome side effects such as severe or prolonged headache, sleep loss, vision problems, nasal irritation, vaginal inflammation, or GI reactions (nausea, vomiting).

Pharmacokinetics

Absorption: 98% absorbed following oral administration.

Distribution: Enters breast milk. Highly bound to melanin-containing tissues (eyes, pigmented skin).

Metabolism and Excretion: Mostly metabolized by the liver to inactive metabolites; 10% excreted unchanged by the kidneys.

Half-life: Children taking enzyme-inducing antiepileptic drugs (AEDs): 7–10 hr; Children taking enzyme inducers and VPA: 15–27 hr; Children taking VPA: 44–94 hr; Adults: 25.4 hr (during chronic therapy of lamotrigine alone).

TIME/ACTION PROFILE (blood levels)

ROUTE	ONSET	PEAK	DURATION
PO	unknown	1.4–4.8 hr	unknown

Contraindications/Precautions

Contraindicated in: Hypersensitivity; Lactation: Lactation.

Use Cautiously in: All patients (may ↑ risk of suicidal thoughts/behaviors); Patients with renal dysfunction, impaired cardiac function, and hepatic dysfunction (lower maintenance doses may be required); Prior history of rash with lamotrigine; OB: Exposure during first trimester (may ↑ risk of cleft lip/palate).

Interactions

Drug-Drug: Concurrent use with **carbamazepine** may result in ↓ levels of lamotrigine and ↑ levels of an active metabolite of carbamazepine. Lamotrigine levels are ↓ by concurrent use of **phenobarbital**, **phenytoin**, or **primidone**. Concurrent use with **VPA** results in a twofold ↑ in lamotrigine levels, ↑ incidence of rash, and a ↓ in VPA level (lamotrigine dose should be ↓ by at least 50%). **Oral contraceptives** may ↓ serum levels of lamotrigine (dose adjustments may be necessary when starting and stopping oral contraceptives).

Route/Dosage

Epilepsy

In combination with Other Antiepileptic Agents

PO (Adults and Children >12 yr): *Patients taking carbamazepine, phenobarbital, phenytoin, or primidone*—50 mg daily as a single dose for first 2 wk, then 50 mg twice daily for next 2 wk; then ↑ by 100 mg/day on a weekly basis to maintenance dose of 150–250 mg bid (not to exceed 500 mg/day). *Patients taking carbamazepine, phenobarbital, phenytoin, or primidone with VPA*—25 mg every other day for first 2 wk, then 25 mg once daily for next 2 wk; then ↑ by 25–50 mg/day q 1–2 wk to maintenance dose of 50–200 mg bid (not to exceed 400 mg/day).

PO (Children 2–12 yr): *Patients taking carbamazepine, phenobarbital, phenytoin, or primidone*—0.6 mg/kg/day in 2 divided doses (rounded down to nearest whole tablet) for first 2 wk, then 1.2 mg/kg in 2 divided doses (rounded down to nearest whole tablet) for next 2 wk; then ↑ by 1.2 mg/kg/day (rounded down to nearest whole tablet) q 1–2 wk to maintenance dose of 5–15 mg/kg day (not to exceed 400 mg/day in 2 divided doses). *Patients taking VPA*—0.15 mg/kg/day in 1–2 divided doses (rounded down to nearest whole tablet) for first 2 wk; (if initial calculated dose is 2.5–5 mg/day, then initial dose should be 5 mg every other day for 2 wk; if patient weighs between 6.7–14 kg, use 2 mg every other day for 2 wk). Then 0.3 mg/kg in 1–2 divided doses (rounded down to nearest whole tablet) for next 2 wk; then ↑ by 0.3 mg/kg/day (rounded down to nearest whole tablet) q 1–2 wk to maintenance dose of 1–5 mg/kg day (not to exceed 200 mg/day in 1–2 divided doses). *Patients taking antiepileptic drugs other than carbamazepine, phenobarbital, phenytoin, primidone, or valproate*—0.3 mg/kg/day in 2 divided doses (rounded down to nearest whole tablet) for first 2 wk, then 0.6 mg/kg in 2 divided doses (rounded down to nearest whole tablet) for next 2 wk; then ↑ by 0.6 mg/kg/day (rounded down to nearest whole tablet) q 1–2 wk to maintenance dose of 5–15 mg/kg day (not to exceed 300 mg/day in 2 divided doses).

Conversion to Monotherapy

PO (Adults ≥16 yr): 50 mg/day for 2 wk, then 50 mg twice daily for 2 wk, then ↑ by 100 mg/day q 1–2 wk to maintenance dose of 300–500 mg/day in 2 divided doses; when target level is reached, ↓ other antiepileptics by 20% weekly over 4 wk.

Bipolar disorder

Escalation regimen

PO (Adults): *Patients not taking carbamazepine, valproate, or other enzyme-inducing drugs*—25 mg/day for 2 wk; then 50 mg/day for 2 wk; then 100 mg/day for 1 wk; then 200 mg/day. *Patients taking valproate*—25 mg every other day for 2 wk; then 25 mg/day for 2 wk; then 50 mg/day for 1 wk; then 100 mg/day. *Patients taking carbamazepine (or other enzyme inducers), but not taking valproate*—50 mg/day for 2 wk; then 100 mg/day (in divided doses) for 2 wk; then 200 mg/day (in divided doses) for 1 wk; then 300 mg/day (in divided doses) for 1 wk; then up to 400 mg/day (in divided doses).

Dosage adjustment following discontinuation of other psychotropics

PO (Adults): *Following discontinuation of other psychotropics*—maintain previous dose; *following discontinuation of valproate*—100 mg/day, then ↑ to 150 mg/day for 1 wk, then 200 mg/day; *following discontinuation of carbamazepine or other enzyme-inducers*—400 mg/day for 1 wk, then 300 mg/day for 1 wk, then 200 mg/day.

Availability (generic available)

Tablets: 25 mg, 100 mg, 150 mg, 200 mg. **Chewable dispersible tablets:** 2 mg, 5 mg, 25 mg.

lanreotide (lan-ree-oh-tide)

Somatuline Depot

Classification

Therapeutic: hormones

Pharmacologic: somatostatin analogue

Indications

Long-term management of acromegaly which cannot be treated by or has not responded to surgery and/or radiation therapy.

Action

Acts as an analogue of somatostatin, inhibiting growth hormone (GH) and insulin-like growth factor-1 (IGF-1) in patients with acromegaly. **Therapeutic Effects:** Decreased levels of GH and IGF-1 in acromegalic patients resulting in decreased manifestations of acromegaly.

Adverse Reactions/Side Effects

CV: bradycardia, hypertension. **GI:** abdominal pain, diarrhea, gallstones. **Endo:** hyperglycemia, hypoglycemia. **Hemat:** anemia. **Local:** injection-site reactions.

PHYSICAL THERAPY IMPLICATIONS

Examination and Evaluation

- Assess blood pressure (BP) and compare to normal values (See Appendix F). Report a sustained increase in BP (hypertension).
- Assess heart rate, ECG, and heart sounds, especially during exercise (See Appendices G, H). Report slow heart rate (bradycardia) or symptoms of other arrhythmias, including palpitations, chest discomfort, shortness of breath, fainting, and fatigue/weakness.
- Monitor signs of hypoglycemia (weakness, malaise, irritability, fatigue) or hyperglycemia (drowsiness, fruity breath, increased urination, unusual thirst). Patients with diabetes mellitus should check blood glucose levels frequently.
- Monitor signs of anemia, including unusual fatigue, pallor, shortness of breath with exertion, and bruising. Notify physician immediately if these signs occur.
- Monitor injection site for pain, swelling, and irritation. Report prolonged or excessive injection site reactions to the physician.

Interventions

- Because of the risk of arrhythmias and anemia, use caution during aerobic exercise and other forms of therapeutic exercise. Assess exercise tolerance frequently (BP, heart rate, respiratory rate, fatigue levels), and terminate exercise immediately if any untoward responses occur (See Appendix L).

Patient/Client-Related Instruction

- Instruct patient to report other troublesome GI side effects such as diarrhea, or abdominal pain that might indicate gallstones (e.g., sudden intense pain in the abdomen or right side, jaundice, chills, fever).

Pharmacokinetics

Absorption: Following SC administration, lanreotide precipitates in body tissues acting as a depot formulation from which drug is slowly released (75% bioavailability).

Distribution: Unknown.

Metabolism and Excretion: Minimal renal/fecal excretion, some biliary excretion.

Half-life: 23–30 days.

TIME/ACTION PROFILE

ROUTE	ONSET	PEAK	DURATION
SC	unknown	first 24 hr	1 mo

Contraindications/Precautions

Contraindicated in: OB: Lactation.

Use Cautiously in: Diabetic patients; Underlying heart disease, especially bradycardia; OB: Use only if maternal benefit outweighs risk to fetus; Pedi: Safe use in children has not been established.

Interactions

Drug-Drug: ↑ risk of bradycardia with other **drugs that may cause ↓ heart rate,** including **beta blockers**. May ↓ absorption of **cyclosporine** (dose adjustment may be necessary). May alter the effects of **antidiabetic agents** (monitor blood sugar). May ↓ activity or CYP450 enzyme system; use cautiously with drugs metabolized by that system, including **quinidine**.

Route/Dosage

SC (Adults): 90 mg every 4 wk for 3 mo; further adjustments are made on the basis of GH and IGF-1 levels as follows: *GH >1 to ≤2.5 ng/mL, IGF-1 normal with good symptom control*—maintain dose at 90 mg q 4 wk; *GH >2.5 ng/mL, IGF-1 elevated and/or uncontrolled symptoms*—increase to 120 mg q 4 wk; *GH ≤1 mg/mL, IGF-1 symptoms currently controlled*—decrease dose to 60 mg q 4 wk.

Hepatic/Renal Impairment

SC (Adults): *Moderate-to-severe hepatic or renal impairment*—60 mg q 4 wk; further adjustments are made on the basis of GH and IGF-1 levels.

Availability

Semisolid in prefilled syringes: 60 mg, 90 mg, 120 mg.

lansoprazole (lan-soe-pra-zole)

Prevacid

Classification

Therapeutic: antiulcer agents

Pharmacologic: proton-pump inhibitors

Indications

Erosive esophagitis. Duodenal ulcers (with or without anti-infectives for *Helicobacter pylori*). Active benign gastric ulcer. Short-term treatment of symptomatic GERD. Healing and risk reduction of NSAID-associated gastric ulcer. Pathologic hypersecretory conditions, including Zollinger-Ellison syndrome.

Action

Binds to an enzyme in the presence of acidic gastric pH, preventing the final transport of hydrogen ions into the gastric lumen. **Therapeutic Effects:** Diminished accumulation of acid in the gastric lumen, with lessened acid reflux. Healing of duodenal ulcers and esophagitis.

Adverse Reactions/Side Effects

CNS: dizziness, headache. **GI:** diarrhea, abdominal pain, nausea. **Derm:** rash.

PHYSICAL THERAPY IMPLICATIONS

Examination and Evaluation

- Monitor improvements in GI symptoms (gastritis, heartburn, and so forth) to help determine if drug therapy is successful.
- Assess dizziness that might affect gait, balance, and other functional activities (See Appendix C). Report balance problems and functional limitations to the physician, and caution the patient and family/caregivers to guard against falls and trauma.

Interventions

- In cases of NSAID-induced gastritis, implement appropriate manual therapy techniques, physical agents, and therapeutic exercises to reduce pain and decrease the need for aspirin and other NSAIDs.

Patient/Client-Related Instruction

- Advise patient to avoid alcohol and foods that may cause an increase in GI irritation.
- Instruct patient to report bothersome or prolonged side effects, including headache, skin rash, or GI effects (nausea, diarrhea, abdominal pain).

Pharmacokinetics

Absorption: 80% absorbed after oral administration.
Distribution: Unknown.
Protein Binding: 97%.
Metabolism and Excretion: Extensively metabolized by the liver to inactive compounds. Converted intracellularly to at least two other antisecretory compounds.
Half-life: Children: 1.2–1.5 hr; Adults: 1.3–1.7 hr (↑ in geriatric patients and patients with impaired hepatic function).

TIME/ACTION PROFILE (acid suppression)

ROUTE	ONSET	PEAK	DURATION
PO	rapid	1.7 hr	>24 hr

Contraindications/Precautions

Contraindicated in: Hypersensitivity.
Use Cautiously in: Geri: Maintenance dose should not exceed 30 mg/day unless additional acid suppression is required; SoluTabs contain aspartame; use caution when used in phenylketonurics; Severe hepatic impairment (not to exceed 30 mg/day in these patients); OB/Lactation/Pedi: Pregnancy, lactation, or children <1 yr (safety not established).

Interactions

Drug-Drug: Sucralfate ↓ absorption of lansoprazole (take 30 min before sucralfate). May ↓ absorption of drugs requiring acid pH, including **ketoconazole, itraconazole, atazanavir, ampicillin esters, iron salts,** and **digoxin.** May ↑ risk of bleeding with warfarin (monitor INR/PT).

Route/Dosage

PO (Adults and children ≥12 yr): *Short-term treatment of duodenal ulcer*—15 mg once daily for 4 wk; *H. pylori eradication to reduce the risk of duodenal ulcer recurrence*—30 mg bid with clarithromycin 500 mg bid and amoxicillin 1000 mg bid for 10–14 days (triple therapy) or 30 mg tid daily with 1000 mg amoxicillin tid for 14 days (dual therapy); *maintenance of healed duodenal ulcers*—15 mg once daily; *short-term treatment of gastric ulcers/healing of NSAID-associated gastric ulcer*—30 mg once daily for up to 8 wk; *risk reduction of NSAID-associated gastric ulcer*—15 mg once daily for up to 12 wk; *short-term treatment of symptomatic GERD*—15 mg once daily for up to 8 wk; *short-term treatment of erosive esophagitis*—30 mg once daily for up to 8 wk (8 additional weeks may be necessary); *maintenance of healing of erosive esophagitis*—15 mg once daily; *pathologic hypersecretory conditions*—60 mg once daily initially, up to 90 mg bid (daily dose >120 mg should be given in divided doses).
PO (Children 1–11 yr and >30 kg): *GERD*—30 mg once to bid.
PO (Children 1–11 yr and 10–30 kg): *GERD*—15 mg once or bid.

PO (Children 1–11 yr and <10 kg): *GERD*—7.5 mg once daily.
PO (Children 3 mo–14 yr): *Alternative weight-based dosing*—0.5–1.6 mg/kg once daily.

Availability

Delayed-release capsules: 15 mg, 30 mg. **Delayed-release orally disintegrated tablets (SoluTabs):** 15 mg, 30 mg. **Delayed-release oral suspension packets:** 15 mg, 30 mg. ***In combination with:*** amoxicillin and clarithromycin as part of a compliance package (Prevpac). Naproxen as part of a combination package (Prevacid NapraPac). See Appendix B.

lapatinib (la-pat-i-nib)

Tykerb

Classification
Therapeutic: antineoplastics
Pharmacologic: enzyme inhibitors

Indications

Advanced metastatic breast cancer with tumor overexpression of the human epidermal receptor type 2 (HER2) and past therapy with an anthracycline, a taxane, and trastuzumab; used in combination with capecitabine (Xeloda).

Action

Acts as an inhibitor of intracellular tyrosine kinase affecting epidermal growth factor (EGFR, ErbB1) and HER2 (ErbB2). Inhibits the growth of ErbB-driven tumors. Effect is additive with capecitabine. **Therapeutic Effects:** Decreased/slowed spread of metastatic breast cancer.

Adverse Reactions/Side Effects

CNS: fatigue, insomnia. **Resp:** dyspnea, interstitial lung disease, pneumonitis. **CV:** ↓ left ventricular ejection fraction. **GI:** HEPATOTOXICITY, diarrhea, nausea, vomiting, dyspepsia, ↑ liver enzymes, stomatitis. **Derm:** palmar-plantar erythrodysesthesia, rash, dry skin. **Hemat:** neutropenia. **MS:** back pain, extremity pain.

PHYSICAL THERAPY IMPLICATIONS

Examination and Evaluation

- Be alert for signs of hepatotoxicity, including anorexia, abdominal pain, severe nausea and vomiting, yellow skin or eyes, fever, sore throat, malaise, weakness, facial edema, lethargy, and unusual bleeding or bruising. Report these signs to the physician or nursing staff immediately.
- Assess any breathing problems and signs of pneumonitis or interstitial lung disease. Signs include dry cough, wheezing, chest pain, shortness of breath, and difficult or labored breathing. Monitor pulse oximetry and perform pulmonary function tests (See Appendices I, J, K) to quantify suspected changes in ventilation and respiratory function.
- Be alert for palmer-planter erythrodysesthesia, as indicated by pain, redness, and dry, scaly skin on the palms of the hands and soles of the feet. Report these signs to the physician or nursing staff. Instruct patient also to protect the hands and feet from heat and friction, and to apply lotion to the affected areas. Superficial cold application can also temporarily reduce symptoms.
- Monitor signs of neutropenia, including fever, sore throat, and other signs of infection. Report these signs to the physician or nursing staff.
- Assess any back or extremity pain to rule out musculoskeletal pathology; that is, try to determine if pain is drug induced rather than caused by anatomic or biomechanical problems.

Interventions

- For patients who are medically able to begin exercise, implement appropriate resistive exercises and aerobic training to maintain muscle strength and aerobic capacity during cancer chemotherapy or to help restore function after chemotherapy.
- Because of potential cardiac problems (decreased left ventricular function) and pulmonary toxicity, use caution during aerobic exercise and endurance conditioning. Terminate exercise if patient exhibits untoward symptoms (chest pain, shortness of breath, unusual fatigue) or displays other criteria for exercise termination (See Appendix L).

Patient/Client-Related Instruction

- Advise patient to guard against infection (frequent hand washing, etc.), and to avoid crowds and contact with persons with contagious diseases.
- Advise patient about the likelihood of GI reactions such as nausea, vomiting, diarrhea, and indigestion. Instruct patient to report severe or prolonged GI problems.
- Instruct patient to report other bothersome side effects such as severe or prolonged fatigue, sleep loss, or skin reactions (rash, dry skin).

Pharmacokinetics

Absorption: Incompletely and variably absorbed following oral administration; blood levels are increased by food.
Distribution: Unknown.
Protein Binding: >99%.

Metabolism and Excretion: Extensively metabolized by, mostly by CYP3A4 and CYP3A5 enzyme systems; <2% excreted by kidneys.
Half-life: 24 hr.

TIME/ACTION PROFILE (blood levels)

ROUTE	ONSET	PEAK	DURATION
PO	unknown	4 hr	24 hr

Contraindications/Precautions

Contraindicated in: Decreased left ventricular ejection fraction (Grade 2 or greater); OB/Lactation: Pregnancy or lactation.
Use Cautiously in: Concurrent use of CYP3A4 inhibitors, including ketoconazole, itraconazole, clarithromycin, atazanavir, indinavir, nefazodone, nelfinavir, ritonavir, saquinavir, telithromycin, and voriconazole, should be avoided (if necessary, dose reduction of lapatinib is required); Concurrent use of CYP3A4 inducers, including dexamethasone, phenytoin, carbamazepine, rifampin, rifabutin, rifapentine and Phenobarbital, may decrease levels and effectiveness and should be avoided (if necessary, dose of lapatinib may be titrated upward to 4500 mg/day as tolerated); Severe hepatic impairment (dose reduction recommended for Child-Pugh Class C); Known QTc prolongation or coexisting risk factors of QTc prolongation, including hypokalemia, hypomagnesemia, concurrent antiarrhythmics, or medications that are known to prolong QTc; Geri: May be more sensitive to effects; Pedi: Safety not established.

Interactions

Drug-Drug: Lapatinib inhibits CYP3A4, CYP28, and P-glycoprotein; concurrent use of drugs which are substrates for these enzyme should be undertaken with caution. Concurrent use of **CYP3A4 inhibitors,** including **ketoconazole, itraconazole, clarithromycin, atazanavir, indinavir, nefazodone, nelfinavir, ritonavir, saquinavir, telithromycin,** and **voriconazole,** may ↑ blood levels and the risk of toxicity. Concurrent use should be avoided, but if necessary, dosage of lapatinib should be decreased. Concurrent use of **CYP3A4 inducers,** including **dexamethasone, phenytoin, carbamazepine, rifampin, rifabutin, rifapentine,** and **Phenobarbital,** may ↓ blood levels and effectiveness and should be avoided. If necessary, dosage of lapatinib may be titrated upward to 4500 mg/day as tolerated.
Drug-Food: Concurrent **grapefruit** may ↑ blood levels and the risk of toxicity and should be avoided.

Route/Dosage

PO (Adults): 1250 mg (5 tablets) once daily for 21 days.

Hepatic Impairment

PO (Adults): *Severe hepatic impairment*—750 mg/day.

Availability

Tablets: 250 mg.

laronidase (la-ron-i-dase)

Aldurazyme

Classification

Therapeutic: replacement enzymes
Pharmacologic: enzymes

L

Indications

Mucopolysaccharidosis I (MPS I; specifically Hurler and Hurler-Scheie form or Scheie form) with moderate to severe symptoms.

Action

Replaces the naturally occurring enzyme α-L-iduronidase which is deficient in MPS I. Without replacement, the glucosaminoglycans dermatan and heparan accumulate in tissues. **Therapeutic Effects:** Decreased cellular, tissue, and organ damage due to MPS accumulation resulting in improved pulmonary function and walking capacity.

Adverse Reactions/Side Effects

Resp: respiratory tract infections. **Derm:** rash. **Local:** injection site reactions. **Misc:** ALLERGIC REACTIONS, INCLUDING ANAPHYLAXIS, infusion-related reactions.

PHYSICAL THERAPY IMPLICATIONS

Examination and Evaluation

- Monitor signs of allergic reactions and anaphylaxis, including pulmonary symptoms (tightness in the throat and chest, wheezing, cough, dyspnea) or skin reactions (rash, pruritus, urticaria). Be especially alert for allergy-like responses that occur during and after administration (infusion-related reactions). Notify physician immediately if these reactions occur.
- Assess ambulation on level surfaces and during stair climbing. Document any changes in functional ability to help determine if drug therapy is effective in maintaining or improving motor function.
- Assess for signs of respiratory tract infections such as fever, cough, sputum production, shortness of breath, difficulty breathing, and fatigue. Notify physician if these signs occur.

- Monitor IV infusion site for pain, swelling, and irritation. Report prolonged or excessive infusion-site reactions to the physician.

Interventions

- Implement therapeutic exercises (resistive training, coordination exercises, gait training) to complement the effects of drug therapy and help achieve optimal function.

Pharmacokinetics

Absorption: IV administration results in complete bioavailability.
Distribution: Unknown.
Metabolism and Excretion: Unknown.
Half-life: 1.5–3.6 hr.

TIME/ACTION PROFILE

ROUTE	ONSET	PEAK	DURATION
IV	unknown	unknown	1 wk

Contraindications/Precautions

Contraindicated in: None known.
Use Cautiously in: Pregnancy (use only if clearly needed); Lactation (safety not established).

Interactions

Drug-Drug: None known.

Route/Dosage

IV (Adults and Children): 0.58 mg/kg once weekly, pretreat with antipyretics and/or antihistamines.

Availability

Solution for injection: 2.9 mg/5 mL-vial.

leflunomide (le-flu-noe-mide)

Arava

Classification

Therapeutic: antirheumatics (disease-modifying antirheumatic drugs, DMARDs)
Pharmacologic: immune response modifiers

Indications

Rheumatoid arthritis (disease-modifying agent).

Action

Inhibits an enzyme required for pyrimidine synthesis; has antiproliferative and anti-inflammatory effects. **Therapeutic Effects:** Decreased pain and inflammation, slowed structural progression, and improved physical function.

Adverse Reactions/Side Effects

CNS: headache, dizziness, weakness. **Resp:** bronchitis, increased cough, pharyngitis, pneumonia, respiratory infection, rhinitis, sinusitis. **CV:** chest pain, hypertension. **GI:** diarrhea, nausea, abdominal pain, abnormal liver enzymes, hepatotoxicity (rare), anorexia, dyspepsia, gastroenteritis, mouth ulcers, vomiting. **GU:** urinary tract infection. **Derm:** alopecia, rash, dry skin, eczema, pruritus. **F and E:** hypokalemia. **Metab:** weight loss. **MS:** arthralgia, back pain, joint disorder, leg cramps, synovitis, tenosynovitis. **Neuro:** paresthesia. **Misc:** allergic reactions, flu syndrome, infections, including sepsis, pain.

PHYSICAL THERAPY IMPLICATIONS

Examination and Evaluation

- Assess pulmonary function periodically by measuring lung volumes, breath sounds, and respiratory rate (See Appendices I, J, K). Notify physician immediately if patient experiences signs of pneumonia (cough, fever, chills, chest pain during inspiration and expiration) or other respiratory problems (bronchitis, rhinitis, sinusitis, pharyngitis).
- Periodically assess impairments (pain, range of motion), functional ability, and disability to help determine if antirheumatic drug therapy is successful.
- Assess any new or increased back pain, joint pain, or other musculoskeletal problems to rule out musculoskeletal pathology; that is, try to determine if pain is drug induced rather than caused by arthritis or anatomic and biomechanical problems.
- Assess signs of paresthesia (numbness, tingling) or muscle twitching. Perform objective tests, including electroneuromyography and sensory testing to document any drug-related neuropathic changes.
- Monitor any other muscle weakness, aches, or cramps that might indicate low potassium levels (hypokalemia).
- Monitor signs of allergic reactions, including pulmonary symptoms (tightness in the throat and chest, wheezing, cough, dyspnea) or skin reactions (rash, pruritus, urticaria). Notify physician immediately if these reactions occur.
- Assess dizziness or weakness that might affect gait, balance, and other functional activities (See Appendix C). Report balance problems and functional limitations to the physician, and caution the patient and family/caregivers to guard against falls and trauma.
- Assess blood pressure (BP) periodically and compare to normal values (See Appendix F). Report a sustained increase in BP (hypertension) or recurrent episodes of chest pain.

Interventions

- Implement appropriate manual therapy techniques, physical agents, therapeutic exercises, and orthotic/assistive devices to reduce pain, improve function, and augment the effects of anti-rheumatic drug therapy.

- Help patients with arthritis explore other nonpharmacologic methods to reduce chronic arthritis pain, such as relaxation techniques, exercise, counseling, and so forth.

Patient/Client-Related Instruction

- Advise patient about the likelihood of GI reactions (nausea, vomiting, diarrhea, mouth sores, heartburn). Instruct patient to report severe or prolonged GI problems, or signs of hepatic toxicity (abdominal pain, severe nausea and vomiting, yellow skin or eyes, fever, sore throat, malaise, weakness, facial edema, lethargy, unusual bleeding or bruising).
- Advise patient that rash and other skin reactions (pruritus, eczema, hair loss, dry skin) are likely. Report severe or unexpected skin reactions to the physician.
- Advise patient to guard against infection (frequent hand washing, etc.), and to avoid crowds and contact with persons with contagious diseases.
- Instruct patient to report other troublesome side effects including severe or prolonged headache, flu-like symptoms, or signs of infection including urinary tract infection (blood in the urine, increased nighttime urination, pain and burning during urination).

Pharmacokinetics

Absorption: Tablets are 80% absorbed following oral administration; rapidly converted to the M1 metabolite, which is responsible for pharmacologic activity.
Distribution: Crosses the placenta.
Protein Binding: 99%.
Metabolism and Excretion: Extensively metabolized with metabolites excreted in urine (43%) and feces (48%). Also undergoes biliary recycling.
Half-life: 14–18 days.

TIME/ACTION PROFILE (antirheumatic effect)

ROUTE	ONSET	PEAK	DURATION
PO	1 mo	3–6 mo	wks–mos*

*Due to persistence of active metabolite.

Contraindications/Precautions

Contraindicated in: Hypersensitivity; OB: Women who are or may become pregnant; Compromised immune function, including bone marrow dysplasia or severe uncontrolled infection; Concurrent vaccination with live vaccines; Pedi: Children <18 yr; OB: Lactation.
Use Cautiously in: Renal insufficiency; OB: Women with childbearing potential; OB: Men attempting to father a child.
Exercise Extreme Caution in: Significant hepatic impairment, including positive serology for hepatitis B or C; or concurrent use of other hepatotoxic agents (↑ risk of hepatotoxicity).

Interactions

Drug-Drug: Cholestyramine and **activated charcoal** cause a rapid and significant ↓ in blood levels of active metabolite. Concurrent use of **methotrexate** and other **hepatotoxic drugs** ↑ risk of hepatotoxicity. Concurrent administration of **rifampin** ↑ blood levels of the active metabolite. May ↑ risk of bleeding with **warfarin**.

Route/Dosage

PO (Adults): *Loading dose*—100 mg daily for 3 days; *maintenance dosing*—20 mg/day (if intolerance occurs, dose may be decreased to 10 mg/day).

Availability

Tablets: 10 mg, 20 mg, 100 mg.

L

lenalidomide (len-a-lid-o-mide)

Revlimid

Classification
Therapeutic: antianemics
Pharmacologic: immune response modifiers

Indications

Transfusion-dependent anemia due to specific myelodysplastic syndromes associated with deletion 5q cytogenetic abnormality.

Action

Lenalidomide is a structural analogue of thalidomide. Inhibits secretion of proinflammatory cytokines and increases secretion of anti-inflammatory cytokines.
Therapeutic Effects: Decreased anemia in certain myelodysplastic syndromes with a decreased requirement for transfusions.

Adverse Reactions/Side Effects

CNS: dizziness, fatigue, headache, insomnia, depression. **Resp:** cough, pharyngitis. **CV:** PULMONARY EMBOLISM, edema, chest pain, deep vein thrombosis, palpitations. **GI:** abdominal pain, constipation, diarrhea, nausea, vomiting, abnormal taste, anorexia, dry mouth. **Derm:** STEVENS-JOHNSON SYNDROME, pruritus, rash, dry skin, sweating. **Endo:** hypothyroidism. **F and E**

hypokalemia, hypomagnesemia. **Hemat:** NEUTROPENIA, THROMBOCYTOPENIA. **MS:** arthralgia, myalgia. **Misc:** fever, chills.

PHYSICAL THERAPY IMPLICATIONS

Examination and Evaluation

- Monitor signs of deep vein thrombosis (lower extremity swelling, warmth, erythema, tenderness) and pulmonary embolism (shortness of breath, chest pain, cough, bloody sputum). Notify physician or nursing staff immediately, and request objective tests (Doppler ultrasound, lung scan, others) if thrombosis is suspected.
- Monitor rashes or other skin reactions (hives, acne, abnormal sweating, exfoliation). Notify physician immediately because certain skin reactions may indicate serious hypersensitivity reactions (Stevens-Johnson syndrome).
- Be alert for signs of neutropenia (fever, sore throat, signs of infection) or thrombocytopenia (bruising, nose bleeds, bleeding gums). Report these signs to the physician or nursing staff immediately.
- Assess peripheral edema using girth measurements, volume displacement, and measurement of pitting edema (See Appendix N). Report increased swelling in feet and ankles or a sudden increase in body weight due to fluid retention.
- Monitor and report signs of decreased metabolism that might indicate hypothyroidism. Signs include bradycardia, lethargy, cold intolerance, weight gain, and muscle weakness.
- Report signs of electrolyte imbalances, including low potassium levels (headache, lethargy, weakness, cramping, muscle hyperexcitability, tetany) or low magnesium levels (irritability, insomnia, muscle tremors, confusion).
- Assess any joint or muscle pain to rule out musculoskeletal pathology; that is, try to determine if pain is drug induced rather than caused by anatomic or biomechanical problems.
- Assess dizziness that might affect gait, balance, and other functional activities (See Appendix C). Report balance problems and functional limitations to the physician and nursing staff, and caution the patient and family/caregivers to guard against falls and trauma.

Interventions

- For patients who are medically able to begin exercise, implement appropriate resistive exercises and aerobic training to maintain or restore muscle strength and aerobic capacity.
- Because of the risk of pulmonary thrombosis, use caution during aerobic exercise and other forms of therapeutic exercise. Assess exercise tolerance frequently (blood pressure, heart rate, fatigue levels), and terminate exercise immediately if any untoward responses occur (See Appendix L).

Patient/Client-Related Instruction

- Advise patient to guard against infection (frequent hand washing, etc.), and to avoid crowds and contact with persons with contagious diseases.
- Inform patient about the likelihood of GI problems such as nausea, vomiting, diarrhea, constipation, abnormal taste, abdominal pain, and loss of appetite. Instruct patient to report severe or unusual GI reactions.
- Instruct patient or family/caregivers to report other bothersome side effects such as severe or prolonged headache, sleep loss, depression, cough, pharyngitis, chest pain, palpitations, fever, chills, or skin reactions (rash, itching, sweating, dry skin).

Pharmacokinetics

Absorption: Well absorbed following oral administration. Levels are higher in multiple myeloma patients.
Distribution: Crosses the placenta.
Metabolism and Excretion: 66% excreted unchanged in urine; some renal excretion involves active secretion.
Half-life: 3 hr.

TIME/ACTION PROFILE (decreased need for transfusions)

ROUTE	ONSET	PEAK	DURATION
PO	within 3 mo	unknown	unknown

Contraindications/Precautions

Contraindicated in: Hypersensitivity; OB: Pregnancy (contraception must be used in males and females); Lactation: Lactation.
Use Cautiously in: OB: Patients with childbearing potential; Renal impairment (may ↑ risk of adverse reactions); Geri: Consider age-related ↓ in renal function; Pedi: Safety not established.

Interactions

Drug-Drug: Risk of neutropenia and thrombocytopenia may ↑ with **antineoplastics, immunosuppressants**, and **radiation therapy**.

Route/Dosage

PO (Adults): 10 mg once daily; dose alteration is required for hematologic toxicity.

Availability

Capsules: 5 mg, 10 mg.

lepirudin (rDNA)
(le-peer-yoo-din)
Refludan

Classification
Therapeutic: anticoagulants
Pharmacologic: thrombin inhibitors

Indications
Management of thromboembolic disease and prevention of its complications in patients who have experienced heparin-induced thrombocytopenia.

Action
Acts as an anticoagulant by inhibiting the action of thrombin. Produced by recombinant DNA technology. **Therapeutic Effects:** Anticoagulation with prevention of thromboembolic complications.

Adverse Reactions/Side Effects
Hemat: BLEEDING. **Misc:** ALLERGIC REACTIONS, INCLUDING ANAPHYLAXIS.

PHYSICAL THERAPY IMPLICATIONS

Examination and Evaluation
- Assess signs of bleeding and hemorrhage (bleeding gums, nosebleed, unusual bruising, black, tarry stools, hematuria, fall in hematocrit or blood pressure). Notify physician or nursing staff immediately of these signs.
- Monitor signs of allergic reactions and anaphylaxis, including pulmonary symptoms (tightness in the throat and chest, wheezing, cough, dyspnea) or skin reactions (rash, pruritus, urticaria). Notify physician or nursing staff immediately if these reactions occur.

Interventions
- Use caution with any physical interventions that could increase bleeding, including wound débridement, chest percussion, joint mobilization, and application of local heat.

Patient/Client-Related Instruction
- Instruct patient immediately to report signs of GI bleeding, including abdominal pain, vomiting blood, blood in stools, or black, tarry stools.

Pharmacokinetics
Absorption: IV administration results in complete bioavailability.
Distribution: Distributes mainly to extracellular fluids.
Metabolism and Excretion: Metabolized by release of amino acids caused by breakdown of drug; 48% excreted unchanged in urine.
Half-life: 1.3 hr.

TIME/ACTION PROFILE (anticoagulant effect)

ROUTE	ONSET	PEAK	DURATION
IV	within 30–90 min	unknown	up to 24 hr

Contraindications/Precautions
Contraindicated in: Hypersensitivity.
Use Cautiously in: Recent puncture of large vessels/organ biopsy; Vessel/organ anomaly; Recent CVA, stroke, intracerebral surgery or other neuroaxial procedure; Severe uncontrolled hypertension; Severe renal impairment (CCr <15 mL/min); Bacterial endocarditis ; Hemorrhagic diatheses; Recent major surgery; Recent major bleeding; Severe liver impairment; Moderate renal impairment (reduced bolus and maintenance infusion rate recommended if CCr 15 <50 mL/min); Pregnancy, lactation or children (safety not established).

Interactions
Drug-Drug: ↑ risk of bleeding with **thrombolytic agents, NSAIDs, valproic acid, cefotetan, cefoperazone**, platelet aggregation inhibitors, including **aspirin, dipyridamole, clopidogrel, ticlopidine, tirofiban**, and **eptifibatide**.

Route/Dosage
IV (Adults): 0.4 mg/kg (not to exceed 44 mg) as a bolus over 15–20 sec, followed by 0.15 mg/kg/hr (not to exceed 16.5 mg/hr) initially; further adjustments made on the basis of laboratory assessment (aPTT) but should not exceed infusion rate of 0.21 mg/kg/hr without checking for coagulation abnormalities.

Renal Impairment
IV (Adults): 0.2 mg/kg as a bolus over 15–20 sec, then if *CCr 45–60 mL/min*—0.075 mg/kg/hr; if *CCr 30–44 mL/min*—0.045 mg/kg/hr; if *CCr 15–29 mL/min*—0.0225 mg/kg/hr.

Availability
Powder for injection: 50 mg/vial.

letrozole (let-roe-zole)
Femara

Classification
Therapeutic: antineoplastics
Pharmacologic: aromatase inhibitors

Indications
First-line treatment of postmenopausal women with hormone receptor–positive or hormone receptor

unknown metastatic or advanced breast cancer. Advanced breast cancer in postmenopausal patients with disease progression despite antiestrogen therapy. Extended adjuvant treatment of postmenopausal early breast cancer already treated with 5 yr of tamoxifen.

Action

Inhibits the enzyme aromatase, which is partially responsible for conversion of precursors to estrogen. **Therapeutic Effects:** Lowers levels of circulating estrogen, which may halt progression of estrogen-sensitive breast cancer. Decreased risk of recurrence/metastatic disease.

Adverse Reactions/Side Effects

CNS: anxiety, depression, dizziness, drowsiness, fatigue, headache, vertigo, weakness. **Resp:** coughing, dyspnea, pleural effusion. **CV:** chest pain, edema, hypertension, cerebrovascular events, thromboembolic events. **GI:** nausea, abdominal pain, anorexia, constipation, diarrhea, dyspepsia, vomiting. **Derm:** alopecia, hot flashes, increased sweating, pruritus, rash. **F and E:** hypercalcemia. **Metab:** hypercholesterolemia, weight gain. **MS:** musculoskeletal pain, arthralgia, fractures.

PHYSICAL THERAPY IMPLICATIONS

Examination and Evaluation

- Monitor signs of stroke (sudden severe headache, confusion, nausea, vomiting, paralysis, numbness, speech problems, visual disturbances) or pulmonary embolism (sudden shortness of breath, chest pain, cough, bloody sputum). Notify physician of these signs immediately.
- Monitor signs of pleural effusion, including cough, shortness of breath, chest pain, or labored breathing. Report these signs to the physician immediately.
- Assess any joint, muscle, or other musculoskeletal pain. Suggest additional tests (radiography, MRI) as needed to rule out fracture.
- Assess blood pressure periodically and compare to normal values (See Appendix F). Report a sustained increase in blood pressure (hypertension) to the physician.
- Assess peripheral edema using girth measurements, volume displacement, and measurement of pitting edema (See Appendix N). Report increased swelling in feet and ankles or a sudden increase in body weight due to fluid retention.
- Monitor signs of high calcium levels (hypercalcemia), including muscle pain, weakness, joint pain, confusion, and lethargy. Notify physician because severe cases can lead to life-threatening arrhythmias and paralysis.
- Monitor personality changes, including anxiety and depression. Notify physician if these changes become problematic.
- Assess dizziness, weakness, or vertigo that might affect gait, balance, and other functional activities (See Appendix C). Report balance problems and functional limitations to the physician and nursing staff, and caution the patient and family/caregivers to guard against falls and trauma.
- Periodically assess body weight and other anthropometric measures (body mass index, body composition). Report a rapid or unexplained weight gain. Blood tests may also be necessary to monitor high cholesterol levels.

Interventions

- For patients who are medically able to begin exercise, implement appropriate resistive exercises and aerobic training to maintain muscle strength and aerobic capacity during cancer chemotherapy or to help restore function after chemotherapy.
- Because of potential cardiopulmonary problems, use caution during aerobic exercise and other forms of therapeutic exercise. Assess exercise tolerance frequently (respiratory symptoms, blood pressure, heart rate, fatigue levels), and terminate exercise immediately if any untoward responses occur (See Appendix L).

Patient/Client-Related Instruction

- Advise patient and family or caregiver about the signs of stroke and pulmonary embolism (see above under Examination and Evaluation) and to seek immediate medical assistance if these signs develop.
- Advise patient and family/caregivers that fatigue and weakness are likely and may be severe. Functional abilities may be limited, and patient may need to use assistive devices during ambulation.
- Advise patient about the likelihood of GI reactions such as diarrhea, nausea, vomiting, constipation, abdominal pain, indigestion, and loss of appetite. Instruct patient or family and caregivers to report severe or unexpected GI reactions.
- Advise patient that rashes and other skin reactions (hair loss, itching, increased sweating) are likely. Report other severe or unexpected skin reactions to the physician.
- Instruct patient to report other troublesome side effects such as severe or prolonged headaches or hot flashes.

Pharmacokinetics

Absorption: Rapidly and completely absorbed.
Distribution: Unknown.
Metabolism and Excretion: Mostly metabolized by the liver.
Half-life: 2 days.

TIME/ACTION PROFILE (effect on lowering of serum estradiol levels)

ROUTE	ONSET	PEAK	DURATION
PO	unknown	2–3 days	unknown

Contraindications/Precautions

Contraindicated in: Hypersensitivity; Premenopausal women; OB: Pregnancy.
Use Cautiously in: Severe hepatic impairment; OB/Pedi: Lactation or children (safety not established).

Interactions

Drug-Drug: None significant.

Route/Dosage

PO (Adults): 2.5 mg daily.

Availability

Tablets: 2.5 mg.

leuprolide (loo-proe-lide)

Eligard, Lupron, Lupron Depot, Lupron Depot-PED, Lupron Depot-3 Month, Lupron Depot-4 Month

Classification
Therapeutic: antineoplastics
Pharmacologic: hormones, gonadotropin-releasing hormones

Indications

Injection, depot, or implant: Advanced prostate cancer in patients who are unable to tolerate orchiectomy or estrogen therapy (may be used in combination with flutamide or bicalutamide): Management of central precocious puberty (CPP). **3.75-mg depot only:** Endometriosis: Uterine fibroids (with iron therapy).

Action

A synthetic analogue of luteinizing hormone–releasing hormone (LHRH). Initially causes a transient increase in testosterone; however, with continuous administration, testosterone levels are decreased. Reduces gonadotropins, testosterone, and estradiol. **Therapeutic Effects:** Decreased testosterone levels and resultant decrease in spread of prostate cancer. Reduction of pain/lesions in endometriosis. Decreased growth of fibroids. Delayed puberty.

Adverse Reactions/Side Effects

CNS: dizziness, headache, syncope; **depot**—drowsiness, personality disorder. **SC**—anxiety, lethargy, memory disorder, mood swings. **EENT:** blurred vision; **SC**—hearing disorder. **Resp:** hemoptysis; **depot**—epistaxis, throat nodules; **SC**—cough, pleural rub, pulmonary fibrosis, pulmonary infiltrate. **CV:** MI, PULMONARY EMBOLI, angina, arrhythmias; **depot**—vasodilation; **SC**—transient ischemic attack/stroke. **GI:** anorexia, diarrhea, dysphagia, nausea, vomiting; **depot**—gingivitis; **SC**—GI BLEEDING, hepatic dysfunction, peptic ulcer, rectal polyps, taste disorders. **GU:** decreased testicular size, dysuria, incontinence, testicular pain; **depot**—cervix disorder; **SC**—bladder spasm, penile swelling, prostate pain, urinary obstruction. **Derm: depot**—hair growth, rash; **SC**—dry skin, hair loss, pigmentation, skin cancer, skin lesions. **Endo:** breast swelling, breast tenderness, diabetes. **F and E:** hypercalcemia, lower extremity edema. **Local:** burning, itching, swelling at injection site. **Metab: depot**—hyperuricemia, increased bone density. **MS:** fibromyalgia, transient increase in bone pain (prostate cancer only); **SC**—ankylosing spondylitis, joint pain, pelvic fibrosis, temporal bone pain. **Neuro: SC**—peripheral neuropathy. **Misc:** hot flashes, chills, decreased libido, fever; **depot**—body odor, epistaxis.

PHYSICAL THERAPY IMPLICATIONS

Examination and Evaluation

- See immediate medical assistance if symptoms of MI develop, including sudden chest pain, pain radiating into the arm or jaw, shortness of breath, dizziness, sweating, anxiety, and nausea.
- Assess pulmonary function periodically by measuring lung volumes, breath sounds, and respiratory rate (See Appendices I, J, K). Notify physician immediately if patient experiences signs of pulmonary fibrosis (dry cough, dyspnea, shortness of breath, cyanosis) or pulmonary embolism (sudden shortness of breath, chest pain, cough, bloody sputum).
- Watch for signs of GI bleeding, including abdominal pain, vomiting blood, blood in stools, or black, tarry stools. Report these signs to the physician immediately.
- Monitor and report signs of TIA or stroke, including sudden severe headache, confusion, nausea, vomiting, and increasing neurologic loss (paralysis, numbness, speech problems, visual disturbances).
- Assess heart rate, ECG, and heart sounds, especially during exercise (See Appendices G, H). Report any rhythm disturbances or symptoms of increased arrhythmias, including palpitations, chest discomfort, shortness of breath, fainting, and fatigue/weakness.
- Assess dizziness that might affect gait, balance, and other functional activities (See Appendix C). Report increased dizziness, syncope, and similar problems

that might affect function and increase the risk of falls.

- Assess any muscle, joint, or back pain to rule out musculoskeletal pathology; that is, try to determine if pain is drug induced rather than caused by anatomic or biomechanical problems.
- Establish baseline electroneuromyographic values at the beginning of drug treatment whenever possible. Periodically reexamine these values to document drug-induced changes in peripheral nerve function.
- Monitor neuromuscular signs of high calcium levels (hypercalcemia), including muscle pain, weakness, joint pain, confusion, and lethargy. Notify physician immediately if these signs occur.
- Assess peripheral edema using girth measurements, volume displacement, and measurement of pitting edema (See Appendix N). Report increased swelling in feet and ankles or a sudden increase in body weight due to fluid retention.
- Monitor personality or behavioral changes, including anxiety, memory loss, mood swings, or other changes in mood. Notify physician if these changes become problematic.
- Monitor injection site for pain, burning, itching, or swelling. Report prolonged or excessive injection site reactions to the physician.

Interventions

- For patients who are medically able to begin exercise, implement appropriate resistive exercises and aerobic training to maintain muscle strength and aerobic capacity during cancer chemotherapy, or to help restore function after chemotherapy.
- Because of the risk of cardiac and pulmonary dysfunction, use caution during aerobic exercise and other forms of therapeutic exercise. Assess exercise tolerance frequently (blood pressure, heart rate, respiratory function, fatigue levels), and terminate exercise immediately if any untoward responses occur (see Appendix L).

Patient/Client-Related Instruction

- Advise patient and family or caregiver about the signs of MI, pulmonary embolism, and GI bleeding (see above under Examination and Evaluation), and to seek immediate medical assistance if these signs develop.
- Advise patient about the likelihood of GI reactions such as nausea, vomiting, diarrhea, and indigestion. Instruct patient to report severe or prolonged GI problems, and also to report signs of hepatic dysfunction, including severe nausea and vomiting, yellow skin or eyes, skin rashes, flu-like symptoms, and muscle/joint pain.
- Advise patient that rash other skin reactions are likely, including hair loss, abnormal hair growth, dry skin, and changes in pigmentation. Report severe/unexpected skin reactions or any suspicious skin lesions to the physician.
- Instruct patient or family/caregivers to report other troublesome side effects such as severe or prolonged headache, drowsiness, blurred vision, hearing problems, hot flashes, chills, nose bleeds, body odor, or breast swelling and tenderness.

Pharmacokinetics

Absorption: Rapidly and almost completely absorbed following subcut administration. More slowly absorbed following IM administration of depot form.
Distribution: Unknown.
Metabolism and Excretion: Unknown.
Half-life: 3 hr.

TIME/ACTION PROFILE (effect on hormone levels)

ROUTE	ONSET*	PEAK†	DURATION‡
SC	within 1st week	2–4 wk	4–12 wk
IM	within 1st week	2–4 wk	4–12 wk
IM-depot	within 1st week	2–4 wk	4–12 wk

*Initial transient increase in testosterone and estradiol levels.
†Maximum decline in testosterone and estradiol levels.
‡Restoration of normal pituitary-gonadal function; in amenorrheic patients, normal menses usually returns 60–90 days after treatment is discontinued.

Contraindications/Precautions

Contraindicated in: Intolerance to synthetic analogues of LHRH (GnRH); OB/Lactation: Pregnancy or lactation (depot form).
Use Cautiously in: Hypersensitivity to benzyl alcohol (results in induration and erythema at SC site).

Interactions

Drug-Drug: ↑ antineoplastic effects with **antiandrogens (megestrol, flutamide)**.

Route/Dosage

Prostate Cancer

SC (Adults): 1 mg/day *or* 7.5 mg once monthly, 22.5 mg q 3 mo, 30 mg q 4 mo or 45 mg q 6 mo as long-acting/depot injection.
IM (Adults): 7.5 mg once monthly, 22.5 mg q 3 mo or 30 mg q 4 mo.

Endometriosis/Fibroids

IM (Adults): 3.75 mg once monthly, or 11.25 q 3 mo, or 30 mg q 4 mo.

Central Precocious Puberty (CPP)

SCb (Children): 50 mcg/kg/day, may be increased by 10 mcg/kg/day as required.
IM (Children >37.5 kg): 15 mg q 4 wk.
IM (Children 25–37.5 kg): 11.25 mg q 4 wk.
IM (Children ≤25 kg): 7.5 mg q 4 wk.

Availability (generic available)

Solution for injection (Lupron and others): 5 mg/mL in 2.8-mL vial. **Lyophilized microspheres for depot injection (Lupron Depot):** 3.75-mg single-use vial, 7.5-mg single-use vial. **Lyophilized microspheres for pediatric depot injection (Lupron Depot-Ped):** 7.5 mg, 11.25 mg, 15-mg single-use kits. **Lyophilized microspheres for 3-mo depot injection (Lupron Depot-3 month):** 22.5-mg single-use kits. **Lyophilized microspheres for 4-mo depot injection (Lupron Depot-4 month:** 30 mg. **Polymeric matrix injectable formulation for SC use (Eligard):** 7.5 mg, 22.5 mg, 30 mg, 45 mg.

levalbuterol

(leev-al-**byoo**-ter-ole)
Xopenex, Xopenex HFA

Classification
Therapeutic: bronchodilators
Pharmacologic: adrenergics

Indications

Bronchospasm due to reversible airway disease (short-term control agent).

Action

R-enantiomer of racemic albuterol. Binds to $beta_2$-adrenergic receptors in airway smooth muscle leading to activation of adenyl cyclase and increased levels of cyclic-3′,5′-adenosine monophosphate (cAMP). Increases in cAMP activate kinases, which inhibit the phosphorylation of myosin and decrease intracellular calcium. Decreased intracellular calcium relaxes bronchial smooth muscle. **Therapeutic Effects:** Relaxation of airway smooth muscle with subsequent bronchodilation. Relatively selective for $beta_2$ (pulmonary) receptors.

Adverse Reactions/Side Effects

CNS: anxiety, dizziness, headache, nervousness. **Resp:** increased cough, paradoxical bronchospasm, turbinate edema. **CV:** tachycardia. **GI:** dyspepsia, vomiting. **Endo:** hyperglycemia. **F and E:** hypokalemia. **Neuro:** tremor.

PHYSICAL THERAPY IMPLICATIONS

Examination and Evaluation

- Monitor signs of paradoxical bronchospasm (wheezing, cough, dyspnea, tightness in chest and throat), especially at higher or excessive doses. If condition occurs, advise patient to withhold medication and notify physician or other health care professional immediately.
- Assess pulmonary function at rest and during exercise (See Appendices I, J, K) to document effectiveness of medication in controlling bronchospasm.
- Assess heart rate, ECG, and heart sounds, especially during exercise (See Appendices G, H). Report tachycardia or symptoms of other arrhythmias, including palpitations, chest pain, shortness of breath, fainting, and fatigue/weakness.
- Monitor and report signs of CNS toxicity, including anxiety, nervousness, and tremor. Sustained or severe CNS signs may indicate overdose or excessive use of this drug.
- Assess dizziness that might affect gait, balance, and other functional activities (See Appendix C). Report balance problems and functional limitations to the physician, and caution the patient and family/caregivers to guard against falls and trauma.
- Monitor signs of hyperglycemia, including drowsiness, fruity breath, increased urination, and unusual thirst. Patients with diabetes mellitus should check blood glucose levels frequently.
- Monitor and report any muscle weakness, aches, or cramps that might indicate low potassium levels (<u>hypokalemia</u>).

Interventions

- When implementing airway clearance techniques or respiratory muscle training, attempt to intervene when the airway is maximally bronchodilated. Responses usually begin 15 min after inhalation and peak approximately 90 min after inhalation.
- Because of the risk of cardiovascular stimulation, use caution during aerobic exercise and endurance conditioning. Cardiac effects should be minimal at lower doses or occasional inhaled use. Cardiovascular effects such as arrhythmias, angina pectoris, or increased blood pressure (BP) may occur at higher doses or during excessive use and are caused by inadvertent stimulation of beta receptors on the heart.

Patient/Client-Related Instruction

- Advise patient to not exceed the recommended dose or frequency of inhalations. Contact physician immediately if bronchospasm is not relieved by medication or is accompanied by diaphoresis, dizziness, or other symptoms.
- Counsel patient on proper use of inhaler; observe use of this device whenever possible to ensure proper technique.
- Instruct patient and family/caregivers to report severe or prolonged headache, cough, nasal

congestion/swelling (turbinate edema), or GI problems (indigestion, vomiting).

Pharmacokinetics

Absorption: Some absorption occurs following inhalation.
Distribution: Unknown.
Metabolism and Excretion: Metabolized in the liver to an inactive sulfate and 3–6% excreted unchanged in the urine.
Half-life: 3.3–4 hr.

TIME/ACTION PROFILE (bronchodilation)

ROUTE	ONSET	PEAK	DURATION
Inhalation	10–17 min	90 min	5–6 hr

Contraindications/Precautions

Contraindicated in: Hypersensitivity to levalbuterol or albuterol.
Use Cautiously in: Cardiovascular disorders (including coronary insufficiency, hypertension, and arrhythmias); History of seizures; Hypokalemia; Hyperthyroidism; Diabetes mellitus; Unusual sensitivity to adrenergic amines; OB/Lactation/Pedi: Pregnancy, lactation, or children <6 yr (for nebulized solution) or <4 yr (for metered-dose inhaler) (safety not established).
Exercise Extreme Caution in: Concurrent use or use within 2 wk of **tricyclic antidepressants** or **MAO inhibitors** (may ↑ risk of adverse cardiovascular reactions).

Interactions

Drug-Drug: Concurrent use or use within 2 wk of **tricyclic antidepressants** or **mao inhibitors** may ↑ risk of adverse cardiovascular reactions (use with extreme caution). **Beta blockers** block the beneficial pulmonary effects of adrenergic bronchodilators (choose cardioselective beta blockers if necessary and with caution). May ↑ risk of hypokalemia from **potassium-losing diuretics**. May ↓ serum **digoxin** levels. May ↑ risk of arrhythmias with **hydrocarbon inhalation anesthetics** or **cocaine**.
Drug-Natural: Use with caffeine-containing herbs (**guarana, tea, coffee**) ↑ stimulant effect.

Route/Dosage

Inhalation (Adults and Children ≥4 yr): 2 inhalations q 4–6 hr; some patients may respond to 1 inhalation q 4 hr.
Inhalation (Adults and Children >12 yr): 0.63 mg via nebulization tid (q 6–8 hr); may be increased to 1.25 mg tid (q 6–8 hr).
Inhalation (Children 6–11 yr): 0.31 mg tid (not exceed 0.63 mg tid).
Inhalation (Children 2–11 yr): 0.16–1.25 mg single doses have been used safely.

Availability (generic available)

Metered-dose inhaler: 45 mcg/actuation in 8.5-g (80 actuations) and 15-g (200-metered actuations) canisters.
Inhalation solution: 0.31 mg/3 mL in green foil pouch containing 12 vials, 0.63 mg/3 mL in yellow foil pouch containing 12 vials, 1.25 mg/3 mL in red foil pouch containing 12 vials, 1.25 mg/0.5 mL in unit-dose vials.

levetiracetam

(le-ve-teer-**aye**-se-tam)
Keppra

Classification
Therapeutic: anticonvulsants
Pharmacologic: pyrrolidines

Indications

Partial-onset seizures (adjunct). Primary generalized tonic-clonic seizures in patients 6 years of age and older. Myoclonic seizures in adults with myoclonic epilepsy (adjunct).

Action

Appears to inhibit burst firing without affecting normal neuronal excitability and may selectively prevent hypersynchronization of epileptiform burst firing and propagation of seizure activity. **Therapeutic Effects:** Decreased incidence and severity of seizures.

Adverse Reactions/Side Effects

CNS: dizziness, fatigue/somnolence, weakness, behavioral abnormalities. **Neuro:** coordination difficulties (adults only).

PHYSICAL THERAPY IMPLICATIONS

Examination and Evaluation

- Document the number, duration, and severity of seizures to help determine if this drug is effective in reducing seizure activity.
- Assess dizziness or weakness that might affect gait, balance, and other functional activities (See Appendix C). Report balance problems and functional limitations to the physician, and caution the patient and family/caregivers to guard against falls and trauma.
- Monitor daytime drowsiness, somnolence, or other changes in behavior. Repeated or excessive symptoms may require change in dose or medication.
- Assess any incoordination to rule out neuromusculoskeletal pathology; that is, try to determine if incoordination is drug induced rather than caused by neurologic or musculoskeletal problems.

Interventions
- Guard against falls and trauma (hip fractures, head injury, and so forth), especially if dizziness or incoordination affect gait and balance. Implement fall-prevention strategies, especially if balance is impaired (See Appendix E).

Patient/Client-Related Instruction
- Advise patient to avoid alcohol and other CNS depressants because of the increased risk of sedation and adverse effects.
- Advise patients on prolonged antiseizure therapy not to discontinue medication without consulting their physician. Abrupt withdrawal may cause increased seizures.
- Advise patient about the risk of daytime drowsiness and decreased attention and mental focus. Use care if driving or in other activities that require strong concentration and fast responses.

Pharmacokinetics
Absorption: Rapidly and completely absorbed following oral administration.
Distribution: Unknown.
Metabolism and Excretion: 66% excreted unchanged by the kidneys; some metabolism by the liver (metabolites inactive).
Half-life: 7.1 hr (increased in renal impairment).

TIME/ACTION PROFILE (blood levels)

ROUTE	ONSET	PEAK	DURATION
PO	rapid	1–1.5 hr*	12 hr

*1 hr in the fasting state, 1.5 hr when taken with food.

Contraindications/Precautions
Contraindicated in: Hypersensitivity; OB: Lactation.
Use Cautiously in: Geri: Renal elimination decreased; dose reduction may be necessary; Renal impairment (dose reduction recommended if CCr ≤80 mL/min); Pedi: Children <4 yr (safety not established); OB: Use only during pregnancy if potential benefit justifies potential risk to fetus.

Interactions
Drug-Drug: None noted.

Route/Dosage
PO, IV (Adults): 500 mg twice daily initially; may be increased by 1000 mg/day at 2-wk intervals up to 3000 mg/day.
PO (Children 6–16 yr): 10 mg/kg twice daily; may be increased at 2-wk intervals by 20 mg/kg increments up to 60 mg/kg/day.

Renal Impairment
PO (Adults): *CCr 50–80 mL/min*—500–1000 mg q 12 hr initially; *CCr 30–50 mL/min*—250–750 mg q 12 hr initially; *CCr <30 mL/min*—250–500 mg q 12 hr initially.
PO (Children and adolescents 4–15 yr): 20 mg/kg/day in 2 divided doses initially; may be increased by 20 mg/kg/day every 2 wk up to 60 mg/kg/day in 2 divided doses as tolerated.

Availability
Tablets: 250 mg, 500 mg, 750 mg, 100 mg. **Oral solution (grape-flavored):** 100 mg/mL in 480-mL bottles. **Injection:** 100 mg/mL in 5-mL vials.

L

levocetirizine
(lee-vo-se-**teer**-i-zeen)
Xyzal

Classification
Therapeutic: antihistamines
Pharmacologic: piperazines

Indications
Management of seasonal/perennial allergic rhinitis. Management of chronic idiopathic urticaria.

Action
Antagonizes the effects of histamine at H_1 receptor sites; does not bind to or inactivate histamine.
Therapeutic Effects: Decreased symptoms of histamine excess (rhinitis, itching).

Adverse Reactions/Side Effects
CNS: drowsiness, fatigue, weakness. **GI:** dry mouth.

PHYSICAL THERAPY IMPLICATIONS

Examination and Evaluation
- Monitor symptoms of seasonal allergies (sneezing, rhinitis, itching eyes, cough) or chronic idiopathic urticaria (rash, hives, itching) to help document benefits of this drug in treating these disorders.

Interventions
- Guard against falls and trauma (hip fractures, head injury, and so forth). Implement fall-prevention strategies (See Appendix E), especially in older adults or patients with excessive drowsiness, weakness, or fatigue.

Patient/Client-Related Instruction
- Advise patient about the risk of daytime drowsiness and decreased attention and mental focus. Although

the risk of drowsiness is considerably lower with this drug compared to traditional antihistamines, patients should use care if driving or in other activities that require quick reactions and strong concentration.

- Advise patient to avoid alcohol and other CNS depressants because of the increased risk of sedation and adverse effects.
- Instruct patient to report other troublesome side effects including dry mouth or upper respiratory tract irritation.

Pharmacokinetics

Absorption: Well absorbed following oral administration.
Distribution: Unknown.
Metabolism and Excretion: Excreted mostly unchanged by the kidneys (85%).
Half-life: 8 hr.

TIME/ACTION PROFILE

ROUTE	ONSET	PEAK	DURATION
PO	rapid	0.9 hr	24 hr

Contraindications/Precautions

Contraindicated in: Hypersensitivity to levocetirizine or cetirizine; Severe renal impairment (CCr <10 mL/min); Pedi: Pediatric patients with impaired renal function; Lactation: Lactation.
Use Cautiously in: Geri: Consider age-related ↓ in renal function and concurrent disease states; OB: Use in pregnancy only if clearly needed; Pedi: Children <6 yr (safety not established).

Interactions

Drug-Drug: ↑ blood levels of **ritonavir**. ↑ CNS depression may occur with **alcohol**, **opioid analgesics**, or **sedative hypnotics**.

Route/Dosage

PO (Adults and Children ≥12 yr): 5 mg once daily in the evening; some patients may respond to 2.5 mg once daily.
PO (Children 6–11 yr): 2.5 mg once daily in the evening.

Renal Impairment

PO (Adults and Children ≥12 yr): *CCr 50–80 mL/min*—2.5 mg once daily; *CCr 30–50 mL/min*—2.5 mg every other day; *CCr 10–30 mL/min*—2.5 mg twice weekly (q 3–4 days).

Availability

Tablets: 5 mg. **Oral solution:** 2.5 mg/5 mL.

levodopa (lee-voe-doe-pa)

Dopar, Larodopa, L-dopa

carbidopa/levodopa (kar-bi-doe-pa/lee-voe-doe-pa)

Parcopa, Sinemet, Sinemet CR

Classification
Therapeutic: antiparkinson agents
Pharmacologic: dopamine agonists

Indications

Parkinson's disease. Not useful for drug-induced extrapyramidal reactions.

Action

Levodopa is converted to dopamine in the CNS, where it serves as a neurotransmitter. Carbidopa, a decarboxylase inhibitor, prevents peripheral destruction of levodopa. **Therapeutic Effects:** Relief of tremor and rigidity in Parkinson's syndrome.

Adverse Reactions/Side Effects

CNS: involuntary movements, anxiety, dizziness, hallucinations, memory loss, psychiatric problems. **EENT:** blurred vision, mydriasis. **GI:** nausea, vomiting, anorexia, dry mouth, hepatotoxicity. **Derm:** melanoma. **Hemat:** hemolytic anemia, leukopenia. **Misc:** darkening of urine or sweat.

PHYSICAL THERAPY IMPLICATIONS

Examination and Evaluation

- Assess patient's gait and motor function to help determine antiparkinson effects, especially when starting drug therapy, or during dosing changes or addition of other antiparkinson drugs. Motor function should be assessed at different times of the day, such as when drugs are reaching peak therapeutic levels (i.e., 30–60 min after oral dose), as well as when drug effects are minimal (just before the next dose).
- Document increased side effects such as involuntary movements (dyskinesias) or fluctuations in response (on-off phenomenon, end-of-dose akinesia). Notify physician because increased side effects might require dose adjustment or a change in medication regimen.
- Monitor anxiety, hallucinations, memory deficits, and other psychologic problems. Repeated or excessive symptoms may require change in dose or medication.
- Assess dizziness and drowsiness that might affect gait, balance, and other functional activities

(See Appendix C). Report balance problems and functional limitations to the physician, and caution the patient and family/caregivers to guard against falls and trauma.

- Monitor signs of blood dyscrasias, including leukopenia (fever, sore throat, signs of infection) and hemolytic anemia (unusual weakness and fatigue, dizziness, jaundice, pallor, abdominal pain). Report these signs to the physician.
- Assess any skin changes because levodopa can activate malignant melanoma.

Interventions

- Implement therapeutic exercises (coordination exercises, gait training, cardiovascular conditioning) to complement the effects of drug therapy and help achieve optimal function.
- Guard against falls and trauma (hip fractures, head injury, and so forth). Implement fall- prevention strategies (See Appendix E), especially if patient exhibits Parkinson's symptoms (postural instability, rigidity) combined with drug side effects (dizziness, blurred vision, dyskinesias).

Patient/Client-Related Instruction

- Inform patient that beneficial drug effects may occur within 2–3 wk, but may also take up to 6 mo to reach full therapeutic effect. Therapeutic effects may also begin to diminish after several years of continuous use.
- Advise patient to avoid large amounts of protein in a single meal (i.e., space out daily protein intake over several meals). Levodopa is typically administered with food to reduce stomach irritation, but dietary protein can impair levodopa absorption.
- Advise patient about the likelihood of GI reactions, including nausea, vomiting, dry mouth, and loss of appetite. Instruct patient to report severe or prolonged GI problems or signs of liver toxicity such as yellow skin or eyes, anorexia, abdominal pain, severe nausea and vomiting, fever, sore throat, malaise, weakness, facial edema, lethargy, and unusual bleeding or bruising.

Pharmacokinetics

Absorption: Well absorbed following oral administration.
Distribution: Widely distributed. *Levodopa*—enters the CNS in small concentrations. *Carbidopa*—does not cross the blood-brain barrier but does cross the placenta. Both enter breast milk.
Metabolism and Excretion: *Levodopa*—mostly metabolized by the GI tract and liver. *Carbidopa*—30% excreted unchanged by the kidneys.
Half-life: *Levodopa*—1 hr; *carbidopa*—1–2 hr.

TIME/ACTION PROFILE (antiparkinson effects)

ROUTE	ONSET	PEAK	DURATION
carbidopa	unknown	unknown	5–24 hr
levodopa	10–15 min	unknown	5–24 hr or more
carbidopa/ levodopa sustained release	unknown	2 hr	12 hr

Contraindications/Precautions

Contraindicated in: Hypersensitivity; Angle-closure glaucoma; MAO inhibitor therapy; Malignant melanoma; Undiagnosed skin lesions; OB: Lactation; Some products contain tartrazine, phenylalanine, or aspartame and should be avoided in patients with known hypersensitivity.
Use Cautiously in: History of cardiac, psychiatric, or ulcer disease; OB/Pedi: Pregnancy or children <18 yr (safety not established).

Interactions

Drug-Drug: Use with **MAO inhibitors** may result in hypertensive reactions. ↑ risk of arrhythmias with **inhalation hydrocarbon anesthetics** (especially **halothane**; if possible, discontinue 6–8 hr before anesthesia). **Phenothiazines, haloperidol, papaverine, phenytoin**, and **reserpine** may ↓ effect of levodopa. Large doses of **pyridoxine** may ↓ beneficial effects of levodopa. Concurrent use with **methyldopa** may alter the effectiveness of levodopa and ↑ risk of CNS side effects. ↑ hypotension may result with concurrent **antihypertensives. Anticholinergics** may ↓ absorption of levodopa. ↑ risk of adverse reactions with **selegiline** or **cocaine**.
Drug-Natural: Kava may ↓ levodopa effectiveness.
Drug-Food: Ingestion of foods containing large amounts of **pyridoxine** may ↓ effect of levodopa.

Route/Dosage

Levodopa

PO (Adults): 250 mg 2–4 times daily; may increase by 100–750 mg q 3–7 days until desired effect is achieved (not to exceed 8 g/day).

Carbidopa/Levodopa

Tablets contain 10/100, 25/100, 25/250 mg
PO (Adults): *Patients not currently receiving levodopa*—10 mg carbidopa/100 mg levodopa 3–4 times daily or 25 mg carbidopa/100 mg levodopa 3 times daily; may be increased every 1–2 days until desired effect is achieved. *Conversion from levodopa alone (<1.5 g/day)*—25 mg carbidopa/100 mg levodopa

3–4 times daily; may be increased every 1–2 days until desired effect is achieved. *Conversion from levodopa alone (>1.5 g/day)*—25 mg carbidopa/250 mg levodopa 3–4 times daily; may be increased every 1–2 days until desired effect is achieved.

Carbidopa/Levodopa Extended Release

Extended-release (ER) tablets contain 25/100 or 50/200 of carbidopa and levodopa, respectively.

PO (Adults): *Patients not currently receiving levodopa*—50 mg carbidopa/200 mg levodopa bid (minimum of 6 hr apart) initially. *Conversion from levodopa alone*—initiate therapy at 25% of the daily dose of levodopa; for moderate disease, start with 50 mg carbidopa/200 mg levodopa bid. *Conversion from standard carbidopa/levodopa*—initiate therapy with at least 10% more levodopa content/day (may need up to 30% more) given at 4- to 8-hr intervals while awake. Allow 3 days between dosage changes; some patients may require larger doses and shorter dosing intervals.

Availability

Levodopa (generic available)

Tablets: 100 mg, 250 mg, 500 mg. **Capsules:** 100 mg, 250 mg, 500 mg.

Carbidopa/Levodopa (generic available)

Tablets: 10 mg carbidopa/100 mg levodopa, 25 mg carbidopa/100 mg levodopa, 25 mg carbidopa/250 mg levodopa. **Orally disintegrating tablets (mint):** 10 mg carbidopa/100 mg levodopa, 25 mg carbidopa/100 mg levodopa, 25 mg carbidopa/250 mg levodopa. **Extended-release tablets:** 25 mg carbidopa/100 mg levodopa, 50 mg carbidopa/200 mg levodopa. ***In combination with:*** entacapone (Stalevo Rx). See Appendix B.

levofloxacin (le-voe-**flox**-a-sin)

Levaquin

Classification

Therapeutic: anti-infectives

Pharmacologic: fluoroquinolones

Indications

PO, IV: Treatment of the following bacterial infections: Urinary tract infections, including cystitis, pyelonephritis, and prostatitis; Respiratory tract infections, including acute sinusitis, acute exacerbations of chronic bronchitis, community-acquired pneumonia, and nosocomial pneumonia; Uncomplicated and complicated skin and skin structure infections. Postexposure treatment of inhalational anthrax.

Action

Inhibits bacterial DNA synthesis by inhibiting DNA gyrase enzyme. **Therapeutic Effects:** Death of susceptible bacteria. **Spectrum:** Active against gram-positive pathogens, including *Staphylococcus aureus, S. epidermidis, S. saprophyticus, Streptococcus pyogenes, S. pneumoniae, Enterococcus faecalis, Bacillus anthracis.* Gram-negative spectrum notable for activity against: *Escherichia coli, Klebsiella pneumoniae, Enterobacter cloacae, Proteus mirabilis, Pseudomonas aeruginosa, Serratia marcescens, Haemophilus influenzae, Moraxella catarrhalis.* Additional spectrum includes *Chlamydophylia pneumoniae, Legionella pneumoniae, Mycoplasma pneumoniae.*

Adverse Reactions/Side Effects

CNS: SEIZURES, dizziness, drowsiness, headache, insomnia, agitation, confusion. **CV:** QTc prolongation, ARRHYTHMIAS. **GI:** HEPATOTOXICITY, PSEUDOMEMBRANOUS COLITIS, abdominal pain, diarrhea, nausea, vomiting. **GU:** vaginitis. **Derm:** photosensitivity, rash. **Endo:** hyperglycemia, hypoglycemia. **Local:** phlebitis at IV site. **Neuro:** peripheral neuropathy. **MS:** arthralgia, tendinitis, tendon rupture. **Misc:** HYPERSENSITIVITY REACTIONS, INCLUDING ANAPHYLAXIS.

PHYSICAL THERAPY IMPLICATIONS

Examination and Evaluation

- Watch for seizures; notify physician immediately if patient develops or increases seizure activity.
- Monitor signs of hypersensitivity reactions and anaphylaxis, including pulmonary symptoms (tightness in the throat and chest, wheezing, cough, dyspnea) or skin reactions (rash, angioedema, pruritus, urticaria). Notify physician or nursing staff immediately if these reactions occur.
- Assess heart rate, ECG, and heart sounds, especially during exercise (See Appendices G, H). Report any rhythm disturbances or symptoms of increased arrhythmias, including palpitations, chest discomfort, shortness of breath, fainting, and fatigue/weakness.
- Monitor signs of pseudomembranous colitis, including diarrhea, abdominal pain, fever, pus or mucus in stools, and other severe or prolonged GI problems (nausea, vomiting, heartburn). Notify physician or nursing staff immediately of these signs.
- Be alert for signs of hepatotoxicity, including anorexia, abdominal pain, severe nausea and vomiting, yellow skin or eyes, fever, sore throat, malaise, weakness, facial edema, lethargy, and unusual bleeding or bruising. Report these signs to the physician.
- Assess any tendon pain or joint pain. Tendinopathy and rupture can occur, especially in large, weight-bearing tendons (Achilles, patellar tendons). Risk of tendon damage is greater in patients >65 yr old, transplant recipients (i.e., kidney, heart, lung), patients with preexisting tendon

damage, and patients taking corticosteroids concurrently.

- Monitor signs of peripheral neuropathy (numbness, tingling). Perform objective tests (nerve conduction, monofilaments) to document any neuropathic changes.
- Assess dizziness and drowsiness that might affect gait, balance, and other functional activities (See Appendix C). Report balance problems and functional limitations to the physician and nursing staff, and caution the patient and family/caregivers to guard against falls and trauma.
- Be alert for confusion, agitation, or other alterations in mental status. Notify the physician promptly if these symptoms develop.
- Monitor signs of hypoglycemia (weakness, malaise, irritability, fatigue) or hyperglycemia (drowsiness, fruity breath, increased urination, unusual thirst). Patients with diabetes mellitus should check blood glucose levels frequently.
- Monitor IV injection site for pain, swelling, and irritation. Report prolonged or excessive injection site reactions to the physician.

Interventions

- If tendon symptoms occur, notify the physician and protect the affected area to avoid tendon ruptures. Do not stretch or exercise the affected tendon, and provide crutches, walker, or other assistive devices if lower extremities are involved.
- Because of the risk of arrhythmias, use caution during aerobic exercise and other forms of therapeutic exercise. Assess exercise tolerance frequently (blood pressure, heart rate, fatigue levels), and terminate exercise immediately if any untoward responses occur (See Appendix L).
- Always wash hands thoroughly and disinfect equipment (whirlpools, electrotherapeutic devices, treatment tables, and so forth) to help prevent the spread of infection. Employ universal precautions or isolation procedures as indicated for specific patients.
- Causes photosensitivity; use care if administering UV treatments.

Patient/Client-Related Instruction

- Advise patient about photosensitivity and to use sunscreens, protective clothing, and avoid prolonged sun exposure. Advise patient also to report any rashes or other skin reactions.
- Instruct patient to report other troublesome side effects such as severe or prolonged headache, sleep loss, vaginal irritation, or GI problems (nausea, vomiting, diarrhea, abdominal pain).

Pharmacokinetics

Absorption: Well absorbed (99%) after oral administration; IV administration results in complete bioavailability.

Distribution: Widely distributed. High tissue and urinary levels are achieved. Appears to cross the placenta.

Metabolism and Excretion: 87% excreted unchanged in urine, small amounts metabolized.

Half-life: 8 hr.

TIME/ACTION PROFILE (blood levels)

ROUTE	ONSET	PEAK	DURATION
PO	rapid	1–2 hr	24 hr
IV	rapid	end of infusion	24 hr

Contraindications/Precautions

Contraindicated in: Hypersensitivity (cross-sensitivity within class may exist); Pedi: Children <18 yr (except for inhalational anthrax [postexposure]); OB: Pregnancy.

Use Cautiously in: Known or suspected CNS disorder; Renal impairment (dose reduction recommended if CCr ≤50 mL/min); Cirrhosis; Concurrent use of corticosteroids (↑ risk of tendinitis/tendon rupture); Kidney, heart, or lung transplant patients (↑ risk of tendinitis/tendon rupture); Geri: Geriatric patients, dialysis patients (↑ risk of adverse reactions); Lactation: Safety not established.

Interactions

Drug-Drug: ↑ serum **theophylline** levels and may lead to toxicity. Administration with **antacids, iron salts, bismuth subsalicylate, sucralfate,** and **zinc salts** ↓ absorption. May ↑ the effects of **warfarin**. Serum levels may be ↓ by **antineoplastic agents**. **Cimetidine** may interfere with elimination. **Probenecid** ↓ renal elimination. May ↑ the risk of nephrotoxicity from **cyclosporine**. Concurrent therapy with **corticosteroids** may ↑ the risk of tendon rupture.

Drug-Food: Absorption is impaired by concurrent enteral feeding (because of metal cations).

Route/Dosage

PO, IV (Adults): *Most infections*—250–750 mg q 24 hr; *Inhalational anthrax (postexposure)*—500 mg daily for 60 days.

PO, IV (Adults and Children >50 kg): *Inhalational anthrax (postexposure)*—500 mg daily for 60 days.

PO, IV (Children <50 kg): *Inhalational anthrax (postexposure)*—8 mg/kg (max: 250 mg/dose) q 12 hr for 60 days.

Renal Impairment

PO, IV (Adults): Most infections: *CCr 20–49 mL/min*—500 mg initially then 250 mg q 24 hr; *CCr 10–19 mL/min*—500 mg initially then 250 mg q 48 hr. **Urinary tract infections:** *CCr 10–19 mL/min*—250 mg q 48 hr.

Availability

Tablets: 250 mg, 500 mg, 750 mg. **Oral solution:** 25 mg/mL in 480-mL bottles. **Solution for injection:** 25 mg/mL in 20-mL and 30-mL vials. **Premixed solution for injection:** 250 mg/50 mL D5W, 500 mg/100 mL D5W, 750 mg/150 mL D5W.

levoleucovorin calcium

(lee-vo-loo-koe-**vor**-in **kal**-see-um)

Fusilev

Classification

Therapeutic: antidotes (for methotrexate), vitamins

Pharmacologic: folic acid analogues

Indications

Used as "rescue" following high-dose methotrexate treatment of osteosarcoma. Decreases toxicity which may follow impaired methotrexate elimination or unintended toxicity of other folic acid antagonists.

Action

The reduced form of folic acid that serves as a cofactor in the synthesis of DNA and RNA; does not require dihydrofolate reductase for activity. **Therapeutic Effects:** Reversal of toxic effects of folic acid antagonists, including methotrexate, that inhibit dihydrofolate reductase.

Adverse Reactions/Side Effects

(all patients also received methotrexate)

CNS: confusion. **Resp:** dyspnea. **GI:** nausea, stomatitis, vomiting, altered taste, diarrhea, dyspepsia. **Derm:** dermatitis. **GU:** abnormal renal function. **Neuro:** neuropathy. **Misc:** allergic reactions.

PHYSICAL THERAPY IMPLICATIONS

Examination and Evaluation

- Monitor signs of allergic reactions, including pulmonary symptoms (tightness in the throat and chest, wheezing, cough, dyspnea) or skin reactions (rash, pruritus, urticaria). Notify physician or nursing staff immediately if these reactions occur.
- Watch for signs of kidney dysfunction, including hematuria, increased frequency, cloudy urine, and decreased urine output. Report these signs to the physician.
- Monitor signs of peripheral neuropathy (numbness, tingling). Perform objective tests (nerve conduction, monofilaments) to document any neuropathic changes.

Interventions

- For patients who are medically able to begin exercise, implement appropriate resistive exercises and aerobic training to maintain muscle strength and aerobic capacity during cancer chemotherapy or to help restore function after chemotherapy or toxicity from other drugs.

Patient/Client-Related Instruction

- Instruct patient and family/caregivers to report any bothersome side effects such as severe or prolonged confusion, dermatitis, or GI problems (indigestion, nausea, vomiting, diarrhea, altered taste, inflammation in/around the mouth).

Pharmacokinetics

Absorption: IV administration results on complete bioavailability.

Distribution: Transported actively and passively across cell membranes; enters CSF.

Metabolism and Excretion: Extensively converted to tetrahydrofolic derivatives.

Half-life: *Total tetrahydrofolic acid*—5.1 hr.

TIME/ACTION PROFILE

ROUTE	ONSET	PEAK	DURATION
IV	unknown	end of infusion	3–6 hr

Contraindications/Precautions

Contraindicated in: Hypersensitivity to folic acid or folinic acid.

Use Cautiously in: Concurrent use of anticonvulsants; may increase risk of seizures; OB: Use in pregnancy only if clearly needed, use cautiously during lactation; Pedi: Has been used safely in pediatric patients.

Interactions

Drug-Drug: ↑ risk of toxicity from **fluorouracil**. May ↓ effectiveness of **phenobarbital, phenytoin**, or **primidone** leading to ↑ risk of seizures. May ↓ effectiveness of **trimethoprim-sulfamethoxazole** when used to treat *Pneumocystis carnii* pneumonia in HIV-infected patients.

Route/Dosage

Levoleucovorin rescue following high-dose methotrexate—based on a methotrexate dose of 12 g/m^2 IV over 4 hr and concurrent with hydration and maintenance of urine pH ≥7.

IV (Adults): *Normal methotrexate elimination*—7.5 mg (5 mg/m^2) every 6 hr for 10 doses starting 24 hr after the start of the methotrexate infusion; *Delayed* *late methotrexate elimination*—7.5 mg (5 mg/m^2) every 6 hr starting 24 hr after the start of the methotrexate infusion; continue until methotrexate level $<5 \times 10^{-8}$ (0.05 micromolar); *delayed early methotrexate elimination and/or evidence of acute renal injury*—75 mg (5 mg/m^2) every 3 hr starting 24 hr after the start of the methotrexate infusion; continue until methotrexate level is <1 micromolar, then 7.5 mg every 3 hr (until 0.05 micromolar).

Levoleucovorin rescue following inadvertent overdosage of methotrexate

IV (Adults): 7.5 mg (approximately 5 mg/m^2) every 6 hr until serum methotrexate level is less than 10^{-8} M. Determine creatinine and methotrexate levels at 24 hr intervals. If 24 hour serum creatinine has increased 50% over baseline or 24 hr methotrexate level is greater than 5×10^{-6} M or 48 hr level is greater than 9×10^{-7} M, ↑ dose to 50 mg/m^2 IV every 3 hr until methotrexate level is less than 10^{-8} M. Maintain hydration and urinary alkalinization (pH ≥7). Initiate as soon as possible and within 24 hr of methotrexate when there is delayed excretion; as time interval increases, effectiveness ↓.

Availability

Lyophilized powder for injection (requires reconstitution): 50 mg vial (contains mannitol).

HIGH ALERT

levorphanol (lee-vor-fan-ole)

Levo-Dromoran, Levorphan

Classification

Therapeutic: opioid analgesics
Pharmacologic: opioid agonists

Schedule II

Indications

Moderate-to-severe pain.

Action

Binds to opiate receptors in the CNS, altering perception of and response to pain. Produces generalized CNS depression. **Therapeutic Effects:** Decreased pain.

Adverse Reactions/Side Effects

CNS: confusion, sedation, dysphoria, euphoria, dizziness, floating feeling, hallucinations, headache, unusual dreams. **EENT:** blurred vision, diplopia, miosis. **Resp:** respiratory depression. **CV:** hypotension, bradycardia. **GI:** constipation, dry mouth, nausea, vomiting. **GU:** urinary retention. **Derm:** flushing, sweating, pruritus. **Misc:** physical dependence, psychological dependence, tolerance.

PHYSICAL THERAPY IMPLICATIONS

Examination and Evaluation

- Assess symptoms of respiratory depression, including decreased respiratory rate, confusion, bluish color of the skin and mucous membranes (cyanosis), and difficult, labored breathing (dyspnea). Monitor pulse oximetry and perform pulmonary function tests (See Appendix I) to quantify suspected changes in ventilation and respiratory function. Excessive respiratory depression requires emergency care.
- Be alert for excessive sedation or changes in mood and behavior (euphoria, dysphoria, confusion, hallucinations). Notify physician or nurse immediately if patient is unconscious or extremely difficult to arouse.
- Use appropriate pain scales (visual analogue scales, others) to document whether this drug is successful in helping manage the patient's pain.
- Assess blood pressure periodically and compare to normal values (See Appendix F). Report low blood pressure (hypotension), especially if patient experiences dizziness, fainting, or other symptoms.
- Assess heart rate, ECG, and heart sounds, especially during exercise (See Appendices G, H). Report slow heart rate (bradycardia) or symptoms of other arrhythmias, including palpitations, chest discomfort, shortness of breath, fainting, and fatigue/weakness.
- Assess dizziness that might affect gait, balance, and other functional activities (See Appendix C). Report balance problems and functional limitations to the physician and nursing staff, and caution the patient and family/caregivers to guard against falls and trauma.

Interventions

- Implement appropriate manual therapy techniques, physical agents, and therapeutic exercises to reduce pain and help wean patient off opioid analgesics as soon as possible.
- Because of the risk of respiratory depression, bradycardia, and hypotension, use caution during aerobic exercise and other forms of therapeutic exercise. Assess exercise tolerance frequently (blood pressure, heart rate, respiratory rate, fatigue levels), and terminate exercise immediately if any untoward responses occur (See Appendix L).
- Help patient explore other nonpharmacologic methods to reduce chronic pain, such as relaxation techniques, exercise, counseling, and so forth.

- Guard against falls and trauma (hip fractures, head injury). Implement fall-prevention strategies (See Appendix E), especially if patient exhibits sedation, dizziness, or blurred vision.
- To minimize orthostatic hypotension, patient should move slowly when assuming a more upright position.

Patient/Client-Related Instruction

- Advise patient that opioid analgesics are usually more effective if given before pain becomes severe; emphasize that adequate pain control will allow better participation in physical therapy.
- Educate patient about the dangers of opioid overdose; encourage patient to adhere to proper dosing schedule.
- Emphasize that the risk of physical addiction (tolerance and dependence) is usually minimal during short-term treatment of pain. Advise patient that addiction is more likely during excessive or inappropriate use of opioid analgesics.
- Advise patient to avoid alcohol and other CNS depressants because of the increased risk of sedation and decreased CNS function.
- Advise patient to increase fluid intake and dietary fiber to avoid constipation. Laxatives may also be helpful in patients susceptible to fecal impaction (e.g., people with spinal cord injury).
- Instruct patient to report other troublesome side effects such as severe or prolonged headache, urinary retention, unusual dreams, vision disturbances, skin reactions (itching, flushing, excessive sweating), or GI problems (nausea, vomiting, dry mouth).

Pharmacokinetics

Absorption: Well absorbed following oral and SC administration.
Distribution: Extensive.
Metabolism and Excretion: Mostly metabolized by the liver.
Half-life: 12–16 hr; may be as long as 30 hr with chronic dosing.

TIME/ACTION PROFILE (analgesic effect)

ROUTE	ONSET	PEAK	DURATION
PO	10–60 min	90–120 min	4–5 hr
SC	unknown	60–90 min	4–5 hr
IV	unknown	within 20 min	4–5 hr

Contraindications/Precautions

Contraindicated in: Hypersensitivity; Avoid chronic use during pregnancy or lactation.
Use Cautiously in: Head trauma; Increased intracranial pressure; Severe renal, hepatic, or pulmonary disease; Hypothyroidism; Adrenal insufficiency; Alcoholism; Undiagnosed abdominal pain; Prostatic hyperplasia; Geriatric or debilitated patients (dosage reduction suggested).

Interactions

Drug-Drug: Use with extreme caution in patients receiving **MAO inhibitors** (may result in unpredictable, severe reactions—decrease initial dose of levorphanol to 25% of usual dose). Additive CNS depression with **alcohol, antihistamines/antidepressants**, and **sedative/hypnotics**. Administration of **partial-antagonist opioid analgesics** may precipitate withdrawal in physically dependent patients. **Nalbuphine** or **pentazocine** may ↓ analgesia.
Drug-Natural: Concomitant use of **kava, valerian, skullcap, chamomile**, or **hops** can ↑ CNS depression.

Route/Dosage

Larger doses may be required during chronic use.
PO (Adults ≥50 kg): *Initial dosing in opioid-naive patients*—4 mg q 6–8 hr.
PO (Adults and Children <50 kg): *Initial dosing in opioid-naive patients*—0.04 mg/kg q 6–8 hr (unlabeled for use in children).
SC, IV (Adults ≥50 kg): *Initial dosing in opioid-naive patients*—2 mg q 6–8 hr. *Preoperative use*—1–2 mg SCt 90 min prior to procedure.
Subcut, IV (Adults and Children <50 kg): *Initial dosing in opioid-naive patients*—0.02 mg/kg mg q 6–8 hr (unlabeled for use in children).

Availability (generic available)

Tablets: 2 mg. **Solution for injection:** 2 mg/mL.

levothyroxine

(lee-voe-thye-**rox**-een)
Eltroxin, Levo-T, Levothroid, Levoxyl, Novothyrox, PMS-Levothyroxine Sodium, Synthroid, T_4, Tirosint, Unithroid

Classification
Therapeutic: hormones
Pharmacologic: thyroid preparations

Indications

Thyroid supplementation in hypothyroidism. Treatment or suppression of euthyroid goiters. Adjunctive treatment for thyrotropin-dependent thyroid cancer.

Action

Replacement of or supplementation to endogenous thyroid hormones. Principal effect is increasing metabolic rate of body tissues: Promote gluconeogenesis, Increase utilization and mobilization of glycogen stores, Stimulate protein synthesis,

Promote cell growth and differentiation, Aid in the development of the brain and CNS. **Therapeutic Effects:** Replacement in hypothyroidism to restore normal hormonal balance. Suppression of thyroid cancer.

Adverse Reactions/Side Effects

Usually only seen when excessive doses cause iatrogenic hyperthyroidism

CNS: insomnia, irritability, headache. **CV:** arrhythmias, tachycardia, angina pectoris. **GI:** abdominal cramps, diarrhea, vomiting. **Derm:** hyperhidrosis. **Endo:** hyperthyroidism, menstrual irregularities. **Metab:** weight loss, heat intolerance. **MS:** accelerated bone maturation in children.

PHYSICAL THERAPY IMPLICATIONS

Examination and Evaluation

- Monitor and report signs of excessive or inadequate dosing. Excessive doses mimic hyperthyroidism, as indicated by nervousness, weight loss, muscle wasting, tachycardia, and heat intolerance. Inadequate doses mimic hypothyroidism, as indicated by lethargy, weight gain, bradycardia, and cold intolerance.
- Assess heart rate, ECG, and heart sounds, especially during exercise (See Appendices G, H). Report any rhythm disturbances or symptoms of increased arrhythmias, including palpitations, chest discomfort, shortness of breath, fainting, and fatigue/weakness.
- Assess episodes of angina pectoris at rest and during exercise. Attempt to determine if pain is drug related or caused by cardiovascular dysfunction (e.g., angina that occurs during exercise).
- Assess height in children periodically; inform physician of delayed growth that might indicate premature skeletal maturation and closure of epiphyseal plates.
- Monitor and report signs of CNS toxicity, including irritability and sleep loss. Sustained or severe CNS signs are typically consistent with hyperthyroidism and may require an adjustment in drug dose.

Interventions

- Because of the risk of arrhythmias and angina, use caution during aerobic exercise and endurance conditioning. Assess heart rate and exercise tolerance frequently, and terminate exercise immediately if any untoward responses occur (See Appendix L).

Patient/Client-Related Instruction

- Caution patient about the risk of increased sweating (hyperhidrosis), and advise patient about proper skin care (thoroughly cleanse and dry the affected areas; apply astringent powders if necessary).
- Instruct patient to report other troublesome side effects including severe or prolonged headache, menstrual irregularities, or GI problems (nausea, vomiting, abdominal cramps).

Pharmacokinetics

Absorption: Levothyroxine is variably (40–80%) absorbed from the GI tract.
Distribution: Distributed into most body tissues. Thyroid hormones do not readily cross the placenta; minimal amounts enter breast milk.
Protein Binding: > 99%.
Metabolism and Excretion: Metabolized by the liver and other tissues to active T_3. Thyroid hormone undergoes enterohepatic recirculation and is excreted in the feces via the bile.
Half-life: 6–7 days.

TIME/ACTION PROFILE

ROUTE	ONSET	PEAK	DURATION
levothyroxine PO	unknown	1–3 wk	1–3 wk
levothyroxine IV	6–8 hr	24 hr	unknown

Contraindications/Precautions

Contraindicated in: Hypersensitivity; Recent MI; Hyperthyroidism.
Use Cautiously in: Cardiovascular disease (initiate therapy with lower doses); Severe renal insufficiency; Uncorrected adrenocortical disorders; Pedi: Monitor neonates and infants for cardiac overload, arrhythmias, and aspiration during first 2 wk of therapy; Geri: Extremely sensitive to thyroid hormones; initial dose should be reduced.

Interactions

Drug-Drug: Bile acid sequestrants and **orlistat** ↓ absorption of orally administered thyroid preparations. Alters the effectiveness of **warfarin** (INR will increase with thyroid hormone supplementation). May ↑ requirement for **insulin** or **oral hypoglycemic agents** in diabetics. Concurrent **estrogen** therapy may ↑ thyroid replacement requirements. ↑ cardiovascular effects with **adrenergics** (sympathomimetics).
Drug-Food: Foods or supplements containing high amounts of calcium, iron, magnesium, or zinc may bind levothyroxine and prevent complete absorption.

Route/Dosage

PO (Adults): *Hypothyroidism*—50 mcg as a single dose initially; may be increased q 2–3 wk by 25 mcg/day; usual maintenance dose is 75–125 mcg/day (1.5 mcg/kg/day).

PO (Geriatric Patients and Patients with Increased Sensitivity to Thyroid Hormones): 12.5–25 mcg as a single dose initially; may be increased q 6–8 wk; usual maintenance dose is 75 mcg/day.
PO (Children >12 yr): 2–3 mcg/kg/day (≥150 mcg/day).
PO (Children 6–12 yr): 4–5 mcg/kg/day (100–125 mcg/day).
PO (Children 1–5 yr): 5–6 mcg/kg/day (75–100 mcg/day).
PO (Children 6–12 mo): 6–8 mcg/kg/day (50–75 mcg/day).
PO (Infants 3–6 mo): 8–10 mcg/kg/day (25–50 mcg/day).
PO (Infants 0–3 mo or Infants at Risk for Cardiac Failure): 10–15 mcg/kg/day or 25 mcg/day; may be increased after 4–6 wks to 50 mcg.
IM, IV (Adults): *Hypothyroidism*—50–100 mcg/day as a single dose. *Myxedema coma/stupor*—200–500 mcg IV; additional 100–300 mcg may be given on 2nd day, followed by daily administration of smaller doses.
IM, IV (Children): *Hypothyroidism*—approximately 50–75% of the oral dose.

Availability (generic available)

Tablets: 25 mcg, 50 mcg, 75 mcg, 88 mcg, 100 mcg, 112 mcg, 125 mcg, 137 mcg, 150 mcg, 175 mcg, 200 mcg, 300 mcg. **Soft Gel capsules:** 12.5 mcg, 25 mcg, 50 mcg, 75 mcg, 125 mcg, 150 mcg. **Powder for injection:** 200 mcg/vial, 500 mcg/vial.

HIGH ALERT

LIDOCAINE

lidocaine (parenteral)
(lye-doe-kane)
LidoPen, Xylocaine, Xylocard

lidocaine (local anesthetic)
Xylocaine

lidocaine (mucosal)
Anestacon, Xylocaine Viscous

lidocaine patch
Lidoderm

lidocaine (topical)
L-M-X 4, L-M-X 5, Solarcaine Aloe Extra Burn Relief, Xylocaine, Zilactin-L

Classification
Therapeutic: anesthetics (topical/local); antiarrhythmics (class IB)
Pharmacologic: aminoethylamides

Indications

IV: Ventricular arrhythmias. **IM:** Self-injected or when IV unavailable (during transport to hospital facilities). **Local:** Infiltration/mucosal/topical anesthetic. **Patch:** Pain due to postherpetic neuralgia.

Action

IV, IM: Suppresses automaticity and spontaneous depolarization of the ventricles during diastole by altering the flux of sodium ions across cell membranes with little or no effect on heart rate. **Local:** Produces local anesthesia by inhibiting transport of ions across neuronal membranes, thereby preventing initiation and conduction of normal nerve impulses. **Therapeutic Effects:** Control of ventricular arrhythmias. Local anesthesia.

Adverse Reactions/Side Effects

Applies mainly to systemic use
CNS: SEIZURES, confusion, drowsiness, blurred vision, dizziness, nervousness, slurred speech, tremor. **EENT: mucosal use**—decreased or absent gag reflex. **CV:** CARDIAC ARREST, arrhythmias, bradycardia, heart block, hypotension. **GI:** nausea, vomiting. **Resp:** bronchospasm. **Local:** stinging, burning, contact dermatitis, erythema. **Misc:** ALLERGIC REACTIONS, INCLUDING ANAPHYLAXIS.

PHYSICAL THERAPY IMPLICATIONS

Examination and Evaluation

- Be alert for new seizures or increased seizure activity, especially during IV or IM administration. Document the number, duration, and severity of seizures, and report these findings immediately to the physician.
- Monitor cardiac symptoms at rest and during exercise. Seek immediate medical assistance if symptoms of cardiac arrest develop, including sudden chest pain, pain radiating into the arm or jaw, shortness of breath, dizziness, sweating, anxiety, and nausea.
- Monitor signs of allergic reactions and anaphylaxis, including pulmonary symptoms (laryngeal edema, bronchospasm, wheezing, cough, dyspnea) or skin reactions (rash, pruritus, urticaria). Notify physician or nursing staff immediately if these reactions occur.
- Assess heart rate, ECG, and heart sounds, especially during exercise (See Appendices G, H). Although intended to treat certain arrhythmias, this drug can unmask or precipitate new arrhythmias (proarrhythmic effect). Report any rhythm disturbances or symptoms of increased arrhythmias, including palpitations, chest pain, shortness of breath, fainting, and fatigue/weakness.

- Be alert for other signs of toxicity during continuous systemic administration or prolonged use of lidocaine patches. Signs of toxicity include confusion, nervousness, tremor, blurred or double vision, nausea, vomiting, slurred speech, ringing in ears, tremors, twitching, difficulty breathing, severe dizziness or fainting, and unusually slow heart rate. Report these signs to physician or nursing staff immediately.
- When used for regional pain control or neuropathic pain, use appropriate pain scales and sensory testing to document level of local anesthesia and analgesic effects.
- Assess dizziness and drowsiness that might affect gait, balance, and other functional activities (See Appendix C). Report balance problems and functional limitations to the physician and nursing staff, and caution the patient and family/caregivers to guard against falls and trauma.
- Monitor skin reactions during local or topical use. Report severe or prolonged reactions such as stinging, burning, or irritation.

Interventions

- Because of the risk of arrhythmias and cardiac arrest, use extreme caution during aerobic exercise and other forms of therapeutic exercise. Assess exercise tolerance frequently (blood pressure, heart rate, fatigue levels), and terminate exercise immediately if any untoward responses occur (See Appendix L).
- When administered via a patch, be aware of patch location and do not apply thermal agents or massage on or near the patch.

Patient/Client-Related Instruction

- Advise patient and family or caregivers about the signs of cardiac arrest (see above under Examination and Evaluation) and to seek immediate medical assistance if these signs develop.
- Instruct patient and family/caregivers to report other severe or prolonged side effects such as bronchospasm or GI reactions (nausea, vomiting).

Pharmacokinetics

Absorption: Well absorbed after administration into the deltoid muscle; some absorption follows local use.
Distribution: Widely distributed. Concentrates in adipose tissue. Crosses the blood-brain barrier and placenta; enters breast milk.
Metabolism and Excretion: Mostly metabolized by the liver; <10% excreted in urine as unchanged drug.
Half-life: Biphasic—initial phase, 7–30 min; terminal phase, 90–120 min; increased in CHF and liver impairment.

TIME/ACTION PROFILE (IV, IM = antiarrhythmic effects; local = anesthetic effects)

ROUTE	ONSET	PEAK	DURATION
IV	immediate	immediate	10–20 min (up to several hours after continuous infusion)
IM	5–15 min	20–30 min	60–90 min
local	rapid	unknown	1–3 hr

Contraindications/Precautions

Applies mainly to systemic use
Contraindicated in: Hypersensitivity; cross-sensitivity may occur; Third-degree heart block.
Use Cautiously in: Liver disease, CHF, patients weighing <50 kg, and geriatric patients (reduce bolus and/or maintenance dose); Respiratory depression; Shock; Heart block; Pregnancy or lactation (safety not established); Children (safety not established for transdermal patch).

Interactions

Applies mainly to systemic use
Drug-Drug: ↑ cardiac depression and toxicity with **phenytoin, amiodarone, quinidine, procainamide,** or **propranolol. Cimetidine, azole antifungals, clarithromycin, erythromycin, fluoxetine, nefazodone, paroxetine, protease inhibitors, ritonavir, verapamil,** and **beta blockers** may ↓ metabolism and ↑ risk of toxicity. Lidocaine may ↑ levels of **calcium channel blockers,** certain **benzodiazepines, cyclosporine, fluoxetine, lovastatin, simvastatin, mirtazapine, paroxetine, ritonavir, tacrolimus, theophylline, tricyclic antidepressants,** and **venlafaxine.** Effects of lidocaine may be ↓ by **carbamazepine, phenobarbital, phenytoin,** and **rifampin.**

Route/Dosage

Ventricular Tachycardia (with a Pulse) or Pulseless Ventricular Tachycardia/Ventricular Fibrillation

IV (Adults): 1–1.5 mg/kg bolus; may repeat doses of 0.5–0.75 mg/kg q 5–10 min up to a total dose of 3 mg/kg; may then start continuous infusion of 1–4 mg/min.
Endotracheal:(Adults): Give 2–2.5 times the IV loading dose down the endotracheal tube, followed by a 10 mL saline flush.
IV (Children): 1 mg/kg bolus (not to exceed 100 mg), followed by 20–50 mcg/kg/min continuous infusion (range 20–50 mcg/kg/min); may administer second

bolus of 0.5–1 mg/kg if delay between bolus and continuous infusion.
Endotracheal (Children): Give 2–3 mg/kg down the endotracheal tube followed by a 5-mL saline flush.
IM (Adults and Children ≥50 kg): 300 mg (4.5 mg/kg); may be repeated in 60–90 min.

Local

Infiltration (Adults and Children): Infiltrate affected area as needed (increased amount and frequency of use increases likelihood of systemic absorption and adverse reactions).
Topical (Adults): Apply to affected area 2–3 times daily.
Mucosal (Adults): *For anesthetizing oral surfaces*—20 mg as 2 sprays/quadrant (not to exceed 30 mg/quadrant) may be used. 15 mL of the viscous solution may be used q 3 hr for oral or pharyngeal pain. *For anesthetizing the female urethra*—3–5 mL of the jelly or 20 mg as 2% solution may be used. *For anesthetizing the male urethra*—5–10 mL of the jelly or 5–15 mL of 2% solution may be used before catheterization or 30 mL of jelly before cystoscopy or similar procedures. Topical solutions may be used to anesthetize mucous membranes of the larynx, trachea, or esophagus.
Patch: (Adults): Up to 3 patches may be applied once for up to 12 hr in any 24-hr period; consider smaller areas of application in geriatric or debilitated patients.

Availability (generic available)

Autoinjector for IM injection: 300 mg/3 mL. **Direct IV injection:** 10 mg/mL (1%), 20 mg/mL (2%). **For IV admixture:** 100 mg/mL (10%). **Premixed solution for IV infusion:** 4 mg/mL (0.4%), 8 mg/mL (0.8%). **Injection for local infiltration/nerve block:** 0.5%, 1%, 2%, 4%. ***In combination with:*** epinephrine for local infiltration. **Cream:** 4% OTC. **Gel:** 0.5% OTC, 2.5% OTC. **Jelly:** 2%. **Liquid:** 5%. **Ointment:** 5%. **Transdermal system:** 5% patch Cost: $189.98/box of 30 patches. **Solution:** 4%. **Spray:** 10%. **Viscous solution:** 2%. ***In combination with:*** prilocaine (as EMLA cream, Oraquix); with tetracaine (Synera); with bupivacaine (Duocaine); with epinephrine (LidoSite).

lindane (lin-dane)

G-Well, ✱Hexit, ✱PMS Lindane, Scabene

Other Names:
Gamma-benzene hexachloride, ✱GBH

Classification
Therapeutic: pediculicides, scabicides

Indications

Second-line treatment of parasitic arthropod infestation (scabies and head, body, and crab lice) for use only in patients who are intolerant to or do not respond to less toxic agents.

Action

Causes seizures and death in parasitic arthropods.
Therapeutic Effects: Cure of infestation by parasitic arthropods.

Adverse Reactions/Side Effects

All adverse reactions except dermatologic are signs of systemic absorption and toxicity
CNS: SEIZURES, headache. **CV:** tachycardia. **GI:** nausea, vomiting. **Derm:** contact dermatitis (repeated application), local irritation.

PHYSICAL THERAPY IMPLICATIONS

Examination and Evaluation

- Monitor signs of systemic absorption and toxicity. Signs include headache, seizures, fast heart rate (tachycardia), and GI reactions (nausea, vomiting). Report these signs to the physician immediately.
- Monitor the administration site(s) for local irritation or inflammation. Report severe or prolonged skin reactions to the physician.

Patient/Client-Related Instruction

- Check that the patient and family or caregivers understand topical application procedures and adhere to the recommended dosing schedule.
- Instruct patient about proper hygiene, e.g., thoroughly wash and dry the affected areas, do not share combs or hair brushes, avoid sexual contact with carriers of lice or crabs, and so forth.

Pharmacokinetics

Absorption: Significant systemic absorption (9–13%) greater with topical application to damaged skin.
Distribution: Stored in fat.
Metabolism and Excretion: Metabolized by the liver.
Half-life: 17–22 hr (infants and children).

TIME/ACTION PROFILE (antiparasitic action)

ROUTE	ONSET	PEAK	DURATION
topical	rapid	6 hr	190 min

Contraindications/Precautions

Contraindicated in: Hypersensitivity; Areas of skin rash, abrasion, or inflammation (absorption is increased); History of seizures; Lactation; Premature neonates(increased risk of CNS toxicity).
Use Cautiously in: Pregnancy (do not exceed recommended dose; do not use >2 courses of therapy); Children ≤2 yr, geriatric patients, patients with skin

conditions (increased risk of systemic absorption and CNS side effects).

Interactions

Drug-Drug: Concurrent use of **medications that lower seizure threshold** (may ↑ risk of seizures). Simultaneous topical use of **skin, scalp,** or **hair** products may increase systemic absorption.

Route/Dosage

Scabies

Topical (Adults and Children >1 mo): 1% lotion applied to all skin surfaces from neck to toes; wash off 6 hr after application in infants, after 6–8 hr in children or after 8–12 hr in adults; may require a 2nd treatment 1 wk later.

Head Lice or Crab Lice

Topical (Adults and Children): 15–30 mL of shampoo applied and lathered for 4 min; may require a 2nd treatment 1 wk later.

Availability (generic available)

Lotion: 1%. **Shampoo:** 1%.

linezolid (li-nez-oh-lid)

Zyvox

Classification

Therapeutic: anti-infectives

Pharmacologic: oxazolidinones

Indications

Treatment of Infections caused by vancomycin-resistant *Enterococcus faecium*, Nosocomial pneumonia caused by *Staphylococcus aureus* (methicillin-susceptible and methicillin-resistant strains), Complicated skin/skin structure infections caused by *S. aureus* (methicillin-susceptible and methicillin-resistant strains), *Streptococcus pyogenes* or *S. agalactiae* (including diabetic foot infections), Uncomplicated skin/skin structure infections caused by *S. aureus* (methicillin-susceptible and methicillin-resistant strains), *S. pyogenes*, Community-acquired pneumonia caused by *Streptococcus pneumoniae* (including multidrug-resistant strains) or *S. aureus* (methicillin-susceptible strains only).

Action

Inhibits bacterial protein synthesis at the level of the 23S ribosome of the 50S subunit. **Therapeutic Effects:** Bactericidal action against streptococci; bacteriostatic action against enterococci and staphylococci.

Adverse Reactions/Side Effects

CV: headache, insomnia. **GI:** PSEUDOMEMBRANOUS COLITIS, diarrhea, increased liver function tests, nausea, taste alteration, vomiting. **F and E:** lactic acidosis. **Hemat:** thrombocytopenia. **Neuro:** optic neuropathy, peripheral neuropathy.

PHYSICAL THERAPY IMPLICATIONS

Examination and Evaluation

- Monitor signs of pseudomembranous colitis, including diarrhea, abdominal pain, fever, pus or mucus in stools, and other severe or prolonged GI problems (nausea, vomiting, heartburn). Notify physician or nursing staff immediately of these signs.
- Monitor signs of lactic acidosis, including confusion, lethargy, stupor, shallow rapid breathing, tachycardia, hypotension, nausea, and vomiting. Notify physician or nursing staff immediately if these signs occur.
- Assess heart rate, ECG, and heart sounds, especially during exercise (See Appendices G, H). Report any rhythm disturbances or symptoms of increased arrhythmias, including palpitations, chest discomfort, shortness of breath, fainting, and fatigue/weakness.
- Assess blood pressure periodically and compare to normal values (See Appendix F). Report low blood pressure (hypotension), especially if patient experiences dizziness, fatigue, or other symptoms.
- Be alert for signs of peripheral neuropathy (numbness, tingling, decreased muscle strength). Establish baseline electroneuromyographic values at the beginning of drug treatment whenever possible, and reexamine these values periodically to document drug-induced changes in peripheral nerve function.
- Report signs of thrombocytopenia, including bruising, nose bleeds, and bleeding gums.
- Monitor injection site for pain, swelling, and irritation. Report prolonged or excessive injection site reactions to the physician or nursing staff.

Interventions

- Always wash hands thoroughly and disinfect equipment (whirlpools, electrotherapeutic devices, treatment tables, and so forth) to help prevent the spread of infection. Use universal precautions or isolation procedures as indicated for specific patients.
- Because of the risk of lactic acidosis, use caution during aerobic exercise and other forms of therapeutic exercise. Assess exercise tolerance frequently (blood pressure, heart rate, fatigue levels), and terminate exercise immediately if any untoward responses occur (See Appendix L).

L

Patient/Client-Related Instruction

- Advise patient to report any vision disturbances (blurred vision, double vision) that might indicate optic neuropathy.
- Advise patient about the likelihood of GI reactions (nausea, vomiting, diarrhea, taste abnormalities). Instruct patient to report severe or prolonged GI problems.
- Instruct patient and family/caregivers to report other troublesome side effects such as severe or prolonged headache or insomnia.

Pharmacokinetics

Absorption: Rapidly and extensively (100%) absorbed following oral administration.
Distribution: Readily distributes to well-perfused tissues.
Metabolism and Excretion: 65% metabolized, mostly by the liver; 30% excreted unchanged by the kidneys.
Half-life: 6.4 hr.

TIME/ACTION PROFILE

ROUTE	ONSET	PEAK	DURATION
PO	rapid	1–2 hr	12 hr
IV	rapid	end of infusion	12 hr

Contraindications/Precautions

Contraindicated in: Hypersensitivity; Phenylketonuria (suspension contains aspartame); Uncontrolled HTN, pheochromocytoma, thyrotoxicosis, or concurrent use of sympathomimetic agents, vasopressors, or dopaminergic agents (↑ risk of hypertensive response); Concurrent or recent (<2 wk) use of monoamine oxidase (MAO) inhibitors (↑ risk of hypertensive response); Carcinoid syndrome or concurrent use of SSRIs, TCAs, triptans, meperidine, or buspirone (↑ risk of serotonin syndrome).
Use Cautiously in: Thrombocytopenia, concurrent use of antiplatelet agents or bleeding diathesis (platelet counts should be monitored more frequently); OB: Safety not established.

Interactions

Drug-Drug: ↑ risk of hypertensive response with **MAO inhibitors, sympathomimetics** (e.g., **pseudoephedrine**), **vasopressors** (e.g., **epinephrine, norepinephrine**), and **dopaminergic agents** (e.g., **dopamine, dobutamine**); concurrent or recent use should be avoided. ↑ risk of serotonin syndrome with **SSRIs, TCAs, 5-HT$_1$ agonists, meperidine**, or **buspirone**; concurrent use should be avoided.
Drug-Food: Because of MAO inhibitory properties, consumption of large amounts of foods or beverages containing tyramine should be avoided (↑ risk of pressor response. See Appendix L).

Route/Dosage

Vancomycin-resistant *Enterococcus faecium* infections

PO, IV (Adults): 600 mg every 12 hr for 14–28 days.
PO, IV (Children birth–11 yr): (in the first week of life, preterm neonates may initially receive 10 mg/kg every 12 hr).

Pneumonia, complicated skin/skin structure infections

PO, IV (Adults): 600 mg every 12 hr for 10–14 days.
PO, IV (Children birth–11 yr): 10 mg/kg every 8 hr for 10–14 days (in the first week of life, preterm neonates may initially receive 10 mg/kg every 12 hr).

Uncomplicated skin/skin structure infections

PO (Adults): 400 mg q 12 hr for 10–14 days.
PO, IV (Children 5–11 yr): 10 mg/kg every 12 hr for 10–14 days.
PO, IV (Children < 5 yr): 10 mg/kg every 8 hr for 10–14 days (in the first week of life, preterm neonates may initially receive 10 mg/kg every 12 hr).

Availability (generic available)

Oral suspension: (orange): 20 mg/mL. **Tablets:** 400 mg, 600 mg. **Premixed infusion:** 200 mg/100 mL, 400 mg/200 mL, 600 mg/300 mL.

liothyronine
(lye-oh-**thye**-roe-neen)
Cytomel, L-triiodothyronine, T_3, Triostat

Classification
Therapeutic: hormones
Pharmacologic: thyroid preparations

Indications

Thyroid supplementation in hypothyroidism. Treatment or suppression of euthyroid goiters. Diagnostic agent for suppression tests to differentiate mild hyperthyroidism from thyroid gland autonomy. Treatment of myxedema coma (IV formulation).

Action

Replacement of or supplementation to endogenous thyroid hormones. Principal effect is increasing metabolic rate of body tissues: Promote gluconeogenesis, Increase utilization and mobilization of glycogen stores, Stimulate protein synthesis, Promote cell growth and differentiation, Aid in the development of the brain and CNS. **Therapeutic Effects:** Replacement in hypothyroidism to restore normal hormonal balance.

Adverse Reactions/Side Effects

Usually only seen when excessive doses cause iatrogenic hyperthyroidism

CNS: insomnia, irritability, headache. **CV:** arrhythmias, tachycardia, angina pectoris. **GI:** abdominal cramps, diarrhea, vomiting. **Derm:** hyperhidrosis. **Endo:** hyperthyroidism, menstrual irregularities. **Metab:** weight loss, heat intolerance. **MS:** accelerated bone maturation in children.

PHYSICAL THERAPY IMPLICATIONS

Examination and Evaluation

- Monitor and report signs of excessive or inadequate dosing. Excessive doses mimic hyperthyroidism, as indicated by nervousness, weight loss, muscle wasting, tachycardia, and heat intolerance. Inadequate doses mimic hypothyroidism, as indicated by lethargy, weight gain, bradycardia, and cold intolerance.
- Assess heart rate, ECG, and heart sounds, especially during exercise (See Appendices G, H). Report any rhythm disturbances or symptoms of increased arrhythmias, including palpitations, chest discomfort, shortness of breath, fainting, and fatigue/weakness.
- Assess episodes of angina pectoris at rest and during exercise. Attempt to determine if pain is drug related, or caused by cardiovascular dysfunction (e.g., angina that occurs during exercise).
- Assess height in children periodically; inform physician of delayed growth that might indicate premature skeletal maturation and closure of epiphyseal plates.
- Monitor and report signs of CNS toxicity, including irritability and sleep loss. Sustained or severe CNS signs are typically consistent with hyperthyroidism and may require an adjustment in drug dose.

Interventions

- Because of the risk of arrhythmias and angina, use caution during aerobic exercise and endurance conditioning. Assess heart rate and exercise tolerance frequently, and terminate exercise immediately if any untoward responses occur (See Appendix L).

Patient/Client-Related Instruction

- Caution patient about the risk of increased sweating (hyperhidrosis) and advise patient about proper skin care (thoroughly cleanse and dry the affected areas; apply astringent powders if necessary).
- Instruct patient to report other troublesome side effects, including severe or prolonged headache, menstrual irregularities, or GI problems (nausea, vomiting, abdominal cramps).

Pharmacokinetics

Absorption: Liothyronine is well absorbed.
Distribution: Distributed into most body tissues. Thyroid hormones do not readily cross the placenta; minimal amounts enter breast milk.
Metabolism and Excretion: Metabolized by the liver and other tissues. Thyroid hormone undergoes enterohepatic recirculation and is excreted in the feces via the bile.
Half-life: 1–2 days.

TIME/ACTION PROFILE

ROUTE	ONSET	PEAK	DURATION
liothyronine PO	unknown	24–72 hr	72 hr
liothyronine IV	unknown	unknown	unknown

Contraindications/Precautions

Contraindicated in: Hypersensitivity; Recent MI; Hyperthyroidism.
Use Cautiously in: Cardiovascular disease (initiate therapy with lower doses); Severe renal insufficiency; Uncorrected adrenocortical disorders; Geri: Geriatric patients are extremely sensitive to thyroid hormones; initial dosage should be reduced.

Interactions

Drug-Drug: Bile acid sequestrants ↓ absorption of orally administered thyroid preparations. Alters the effectiveness of **warfarin** (INR will increase with thyroid hormone supplementation). May ↑ requirement for **insulin** or **oral hypoglycemic agents** in diabetics. Concurrent **estrogen** therapy may ↑ thyroid replacement requirements. ↑ cardiovascular effects with **adrenergics** (sympathomimetics).

Route/Dosage

PO (Adults): *Mild hypothyroidism*—25 mcg once daily; may increase by 12.5–25 mcg/day q 1- to 2-wk intervals; usual maintenance dose is 25–50 mcg/day. *Myxedema*—2.5–5 mcg once daily initially; increase by 5–10 mcg/day q 1–2 wk up to 25 mcg/day, then increase by 12.5–25 mcg/day; usual maintenance dose is 25–50 mcg/day. *Simple goiter*—5 mcg once daily initially; increase by 5–10 mcg/day q 1–2 wk up to 25 mcg/day, then increase by 12.5–25 mcg/day q wk until desired effect is obtained; usual maintenance dose is 50–100 mcg/day. *T_3 suppression test*—75–100 mcg daily for 7 days. Radioactive ^{131}I is administered before and after 7-day course.
PO (Geriatric Patients or Patients with Cardiovascular Disease): 5 mcg /day initially; increase by no more than 5 mcg/day q 2 wk.

IV (Adults): *Myxedema coma*—25–50 mcg initially (if cardiovascular disease is present, initial dose should be 10–20 mcg). Additional doses may be given, to a total of at least 65 mcg/day (not to exceed 100 mcg/day). Doses should be at least 4 hr but not more than 12 hr apart.

Availability

Tablets: 5 mcg, 25 mcg, 50 mcg. **Injection:** 10 mcg/mL in 1-mL vials.

liotrix (lye-oh-trix)

T_3/T_4, Thyrolar

Classification

Therapeutic: hormones
Pharmacologic: thyroid preparations

Indications

Thyroid supplementation in hypothyroidism. Treatment or suppression of euthyroid goiters and thyroid cancer. Diagnostic agent for suppression tests to differentiate mild hyperthyroidism from thyroid gland autonomy.

Action

Replacement of or supplementation to endogenous thyroid hormones. Principal effect is increasing metabolic rate of body tissues: Promote gluconeogenesis, Increase utilization and mobilization of glycogen stores, Stimulate protein synthesis, Promote cell growth and differentiation, Aid in the development of the brain and CNS. Contain T_3 (triiodothyronine) and T_4 (thyroxine) activity. **Therapeutic Effects:** Replacement in deficiency states with restoration of normal hormonal balance.

Adverse Reactions/Side Effects

Usually only seen when excessive doses cause iatrogenic hyperthyroidism

CNS: insomnia, irritability, headache. **CV:** arrhythmias, tachycardia, angina pectoris. **GI:** abdominal cramps, diarrhea, vomiting. **Derm:** hyperhidrosis. **Endo:** hyperthyroidism, menstrual irregularities. **Metab:** weight loss, heat intolerance. **MS:** accelerated bone maturation in children.

PHYSICAL THERAPY IMPLICATIONS

Examination and Evaluation

- Monitor and report signs of excessive or inadequate dosing. Excessive doses mimic hyperthyroidism, as indicated by nervousness, weight loss, muscle wasting, tachycardia, and heat intolerance. Inadequate doses mimic hypothyroidism, as indicated by lethargy, weight gain, bradycardia, and cold intolerance.
- Assess heart rate, ECG, and heart sounds, especially during exercise (See Appendices G, H). Report any rhythm disturbances or symptoms of increased arrhythmias, including palpitations, chest discomfort, shortness of breath, fainting, and fatigue/weakness.
- Assess episodes of angina pectoris at rest and during exercise. Attempt to determine if pain is drug related or caused by cardiovascular dysfunction (e.g., angina that occurs during exercise).
- Assess height in children periodically; inform physician of delayed growth that might indicate premature skeletal maturation and closure of epiphyseal plates.
- Monitor and report signs of CNS toxicity, including irritability and sleep loss. Sustained or severe CNS signs are typically consistent with hyperthyroidism and may require an adjustment in drug dose.

Interventions

- Because of the risk of arrhythmias and angina, use caution during aerobic exercise and endurance conditioning. Assess heart rate and exercise tolerance frequently, and terminate exercise immediately if any untoward responses occur (See Appendix L).

Patient/Client-Related Instruction

- Caution patient about the risk of increased sweating (hyperhidrosis), and advise patient about proper skin care (thoroughly cleanse and dry the affected areas; apply astringent powders if necessary).
- Instruct patient to report other troublesome side effects, including severe or prolonged headache, menstrual irregularities, or GI problems (nausea, vomiting, abdominal cramps).

Pharmacokinetics

Absorption: Levothyroxine is variably (50–80%) absorbed from the GI tract. Liothyronine is well absorbed.

Distribution: Distributed into most body tissues. Thyroid hormones do not readily cross the placenta; minimal amounts enter breast milk.

Metabolism and Excretion: Metabolized by the liver and other tissues. Thyroid hormone undergoes enterohepatic recirculation and is excreted in the feces via the bile.

Half-life: *T_3 (liothyronine)*—1–2 days; *T_4 (thyroxine)*—6–7 days.

TIME/ACTION PROFILE

ROUTE	ONSET	PEAK	DURATION
levothyroxine PO	unknown	1–3 wk	1–3 wk
liothyronine PO	unknown	24–72 hr	72 hr

Contraindications/Precautions

Contraindicated in: Hypersensitivity; Recent MI; Hyperthyroidism.
Use Cautiously in: Cardiovascular disease (initiate therapy with lower doses); Severe renal insufficiency; Uncorrected adrenocortical disorders; Geri: Geriatric patients are extremely sensitive to thyroid hormones; initial dosage should be reduced.

Interactions

Drug-Drug: Bile acid sequestrants ↓ absorption of orally administered thyroid preparations. Alters the effectiveness of **warfarin** (INR will increase with thyroid hormone supplementation). May ↑ requirement for **insulin** or **oral hypoglycemic agents** in diabetics. Concurrent **estrogen** therapy may ↑ thyroid replacement requirements. ↑ cardiovascular effects with **adrenergics** (sympathomimetics).

Route/Dosage

Liotrix

Contains T_4 and T_3 in a ratio of 4:1
PO (Adults): *Hypothyroidism*—Start with 50 mcg levothyroxine/12.5 mcg liothyronine; increase by 50 mcg levothyroxine/12.5 mcg liothyronine q 2–4 wk until desired effect is obtained; usual maintenance dose is 50–100 mcg levothyroxine/12.5–25 mcg liothyronine daily. *Myxedema/hypothyroidism with cardiovascular disease*—12.5 mcg levothyroxine/3.1 mcg liothyronine/day; increase by 12.5 mcg levothyroxine/3.1 mcg liothyronine q 2–4 wk until desired effect is obtained.
PO (Geriatric Patients): 12.5–25 mcg levothyroxine/3.1–6.2 mcg liothyronine/day; increase by 12.5–25 mcg levothyroxine/3.1–6.2 mcg liothyronine q 6–8 wk until desired effect is obtained.

Availability

Tablets: 12.5 mcg levothyroxine/3.1 mcg liothyronine, 25 mcg levothyroxine/6.25 mcg liothyronine, 50 mcg levothyroxine/12.5 mcg liothyronine, 100 mcg levothyroxine/25 mcg liothyronine, 150 mcg levothyroxine/37.5 mcg liothyronine.

liraglutide (lir-a-gloo-tide)

Victoza

Classification
Therapeutic: antidiabetics
Pharmacologic: glucagon-like peptide-1 (GLP-1) receptor agonists

Indications

Adjunct treatment to diet and exercise in the management of adults with type 2 diabetes mellitus; not recommended as first line therapy, a substitute for insulin, use in patients with type 1 diabetes or ketoacidosis.

Action

Acts as an acylated human Glucagon-Like Peptide-1 (GLP-1, an incretin) receptor agonist; ↑ intracellular cyclic AMP (cAMP) leading to insulin release when glucose is elevated, which then subsides as blood glucose ↓ toward euglycemia. Also ↓ glucagon secretion and delays gastric emptying. **Therapeutic Effects:** Improved glycemic control.

Adverse Reactions/Side Effects

CNS: headache. **GI:** diarrhea, nausea, vomiting, constipation, pancreatitis. **Local:** injection-site reactions.

PHYSICAL THERAPY IMPLICATIONS

Examination and Evaluation

- Monitor signs of pancreatitis, including upper abdominal pain (especially after eating), indigestion, weight loss, and oily stools. Report these signs to the physician immediately.
- Be alert for signs of hypoglycemia, especially during and after exercise. Common neuromuscular signs include anxiety; restlessness; tingling in hands, feet, lips, or tongue; chills; cold sweats; confusion; difficulty in concentration; drowsiness; excessive hunger; headache; irritability; nervousness; tremor; weakness; unsteady gait. Report persistent or repeated episodes of hypoglycemia to the physician.
- Assess blood pressure periodically (See Appendix F). A sudden or sustained increase in blood pressure (hypertension) may indicate problems in diabetes management, and should be reported to the physician.
- Assess injection site for redness, swelling, or other reactions. Make sure patient understands the need to rotate injections sites to prevent local damage and lipodystrophy.

Interventions

- Implement aerobic exercise and endurance training programs to maintain optimal body weight, improve insulin sensitivity, and reduce the risk of macrovascular disease (heart attack, stroke) and microvascular problems (reduced blood flow to tissues and organs that causes poor wound healing, neuropathy, retinopathy, and nephropathy).

Patient/Client-Related Instruction

- Encourage patient to monitor blood glucose before and after exercise and to adjust food intake to maintain normal glycemic levels.

- Emphasize the importance of adhering to nutritional guidelines and the need for periodic assessment of glycemic control (serum glucose and glycosylated hemoglobin levels) throughout the management of diabetes mellitus.
- Advise patient about symptoms of hyperglycemia, including confusion, drowsiness, flushed, dry skin, fruit-like breath odor, rapid/deep breathing, polyuria, loss of appetite, and unusual thirst. Drug dosages may need to be adjusted to prevent repeated episodes of hyperglycemia.
- Instruct patient to report other troublesome side effects such as severe or prolonged headache or GI problems (nausea, vomiting, diarrhea, constipation).

Pharmacokinetics

Absorption: 55% absorbed following subcutaneous injection.
Distribution: unknown
Protein Binding: >98%.
Metabolism and Excretion: Endogenously metabolized.
Half-life: 13 hr.

TIME/ACTION PROFILE (decrease in HbA_{1c})

ROUTE	ONSET	PEAK	DURATION
SC	within 4 wk	8 wk	unknown

Contraindications/Precautions

Contraindicated in: Personal or family history of Medullary Thyroid Carcinoma (MTC)/Multiple Endocrine Neoplasia syndrome type 2 (MEN 2)
Lactation: Avoid use; Pedi: Not recommended.
Use Cautiously in: History of pancreatitis; Hepatic/renal impairment; OB: Use only if potential benefit justifies potential risk to fetus.

Interactions

Drug-Drug: Concurrent use with **agents that ↑ insulin secretion**, including **sulfonylureas**, may ↑ the risk of serious hypoglycemia, use cautiously and consider dose reduction of agent ↑ insulin secretion; May alter absorption of concomitantly administered **oral medications** due to delayed gastric emptying.

Route/Dosage

SC (Adults): 0.6 mg once daily initially, may be ↑ at weekly intervals up to 1.8 mg/day.

Availability

Solution for subcutaneous injection: prefilled, multidose pen that delivers doses of 0.6 mg, 1.2 mg, or 1.8 mg.

lisdexamfetamine
(lis-deks-am-**fet**-a-meen)
Vyvanse

Classification
Therapeutic: central nervous system stimulants
Pharmacologic: sympathomimetics

Schedule II

Indications

Management of attention deficit hyperactivity disorder (ADHD) (in adults and children).

Action

Blocks reuptake and increases release of norepinephrine and dopamine resulting in increased levels in extraneuronal space. **Therapeutic Effects:** Improved attention span in ADHD.

Adverse Reactions/Side Effects

CNS: behavioral disturbances, dizziness, hallucinations, insomnia, irritability, mania, psychomotor hyperactivity, thought disorder, tics. **EENT:** blurred vision, poor accommodation. **GI:** abdominal pain, ↓ appetite, dry mouth, nausea, vomiting. **Derm:** rash. **Metab:** ↓ weight. **Misc:** long-term growth suppression.

PHYSICAL THERAPY IMPLICATIONS

Examination and Evaluation

- Monitor attentiveness and behavior in patients with ADHD. Report any changes in attention and hyperactivity, and document whether this drug appears to be producing the desired effects.
- Be alert for signs of excessive CNS stimulation, including increased activity, hallucinations, mania, irritability, tics, disordered thoughts, or behavioral disturbances. Report these signs to the physician.
- Assess dizziness that might affect gait, balance, and other functional activities (See Appendix C). Report balance problems and functional limitations to the physician, and caution the patient and family/caregivers to guard against falls and trauma.
- Assess growth rate in children receiving chronic therapy; report delayed or stunted growth to the physician.
- Periodically assess body weight and other anthropometric measures (body mass index, body composition). Report a rapid or unexplained weight loss or decreased body fat.

Patient/Client-Related Instruction

- Instruct patient and family/caregivers to report other troublesome side effects, including severe or prolonged sleep loss, vision disturbances, skin rash, or GI problems (nausea, vomiting, decreased appetite, abdominal pain, dry mouth).

Pharmacokinetics

Absorption: Rapidly absorbed and converted to dextroamphetamine, the active drug.
Distribution: Unknown.
Metabolism and Excretion: 42% excreted in urine as amphetamine.
Half-life: <1 hr for lisdexamfetamine.

TIME/ACTION PROFILE

ROUTE	ONSET	PEAK	DURATION
PO	rapid	1 hr	24 hr

Contraindications/Precautions

Contraindicated in: Hypersensitivity to lisdexamfetamine or other sympathomimetic amines; Advanced arteriosclerosis; Symptomatic cardiovascular disease, including known structural cardiac abnormalities (may increase the risk of sudden death); Moderate-to-severe hypertension; Glaucoma; Agitation; OB: Lactation; History of substance abuse; During or within 14 days of monoamine oxidase inhibitor therapy.
Use Cautiously in: History of preexisting psychosis, bipolar disorder, aggression, tics, Tourette's syndrome or seizures (may exacerbate condition); OB: Use in pregnancy only if maternal benefit outweighs fetal risk.

Interactions

Drug-Drug: Serious adverse reactions, including hyperpyrexia and hypertension, may occur with **monamine oxidase inhibitors**; avoid use within 14 days. Concurrent use of other **sympathomimetic amines** may result in additive effects and ↑ risk of adverse reactions. **Urinary acidifying agents,** including **ammonium chloride** and **sodium acid phosphate,** ↑ excretion and ↓ blood levels and may result in ↓ effectiveness. May ↓ effectiveness of **adrenergic blockers.** ↑ risk of adverse cardiovascular reactions with **tricyclic antidepressants.** May ↓ sedating effects of **antihistamines.** May ↓ effectiveness of **antihypertensives.** Effects may be ↓ by **haloperidol, lithium,** or **chlorpromazine.** May ↓ absorption of **phenobarbital** or **phenytoin.**

Route/Dosage

PO (Adults and Children 6–12 yr): 30 mg daily; may ↑ by 10–20 mg/day at weekly intervals, up to 70 mg/day.

Availability

Capsules: 20 mg, 30 mg, 40 mg, 50 mg, 60 mg, 70 mg.

lisinopril (lyse-in-oh-pril)

Prinivil, Zestril

Classification
Therapeutic: antihypertensives
Pharmacologic: angiotensin-converting enzyme (ACE) inhibitors

Indications

Alone or with other agents in the management of hypertension. Management of heart failure. Reduction of risk of death or development of heart failure after myocardial infarction.

Action

ACE inhibitors block the conversion of angiotensin I to the vasoconstrictor angiotensin II. ACE inhibitors also prevent the degradation of bradykinin and other vasodilatory prostaglandins. ACE inhibitors also increase plasma renin levels and reduce aldosterone levels. Net result is systemic vasodilation. **Therapeutic Effects:** Lowering of blood pressure in hypertensive patients. Increased survival and decreased symptoms in patients with heart failure. Increased survival after myocardial infarction.

Adverse Reactions/Side Effects

CNS: dizziness, fatigue, headache, weakness. **Resp:** cough. **CV:** hypotension, chest pain. **GI:** abdominal pain, diarrhea, nausea, vomiting. **GU:** erectile dysfunction, impaired renal function. **Derm:** rashes. **F and E:** hyperkalemia. **Misc:** ANGIOEDEMA.

PHYSICAL THERAPY IMPLICATIONS

Examination and Evaluation

- Watch for signs of angioedema, including rashes, raised patches of red or white skin (welts), burning/itching skin, swelling in the face, and difficulty breathing. Notify physician immediately of these signs.
- Assess blood pressure periodically and compare to normal values (See Appendix F) to help document antihypertensive effects. Report low blood pressure (hypotension), especially if patient experiences dizziness or syncope.
- Assess signs and symptoms of CHF (dyspnea, rales/crackles, peripheral edema, jugular venous distention, exercise intolerance) to help document whether drug therapy is effective in reducing these symptoms.
- Watch for signs of impaired renal function, including decreased urine output, cloudy urine, or sudden weight gain due to fluid retention. Report these signs to the physician.

- Assess dizziness that might affect gait, balance, and other functional activities (See Appendix C). Report balance problems and functional limitations to the physician, and caution the patient and family/caregivers to guard against falls and trauma.
- Monitor symptoms of high plasma potassium levels (hyperkalemia), including bradycardia, fatigue, weakness, numbness, and tingling. Notify physician because severe cases can lead to life-threatening arrhythmias and paralysis.

Interventions

- Implement aerobic exercise and cardiac conditioning programs to augment drug therapy and maintain or improve cardiovascular pump function.
- Use caution during aerobic exercise and endurance conditioning in patients with heart failure or recovering from MI. Terminate exercise if patient exhibits untoward symptoms (chest pain, shortness of breath, unusual fatigue) or displays other criteria for exercise termination (See Appendix L).
- Avoid physical therapy interventions that cause systemic vasodilation (large whirlpool, Hubbard tank). Additive effects of this drug and the intervention may cause a dangerous fall in blood pressure.
- To minimize orthostatic hypotension, patient should move slowly when assuming a more upright position.

Patient/Client-Related Instruction

- Remind patients to take medication as directed to control hypertension and other cardiac conditions even if they are asymptomatic.
- Instruct patients with heart failure to weigh themselves every day, and call their physician if they gain 3 lb or more in 1 day or more than 5 lb in 1 week. Sudden weight gain may indicate fluid buildup due to worsening heart failure.
- Counsel patients about additional interventions to help control blood pressure and cardiac dysfunction, including regular exercise, weight loss, sodium restriction, stress reduction, moderation of alcohol consumption, and smoking cessation.
- Instruct patient to notify physician of a prolonged dry cough; drug therapy may need to be altered to resolve this side effect.
- Instruct patient to report other troublesome side effects such as severe or prolonged headache, erectile dysfunction, or GI problems (nausea, vomiting, diarrhea, abdominal pain).

Pharmacokinetics

Absorption: 25% absorbed following oral administration (much interindividual variability).
Distribution: Crosses the placenta; may enter breast milk.
Metabolism and Excretion: 100% eliminated by the kidneys.
Half-life: 12 hr (increased in renal impairment).

TIME/ACTION PROFILE (effect on blood pressure—single dose*)

ROUTE	ONSET	PEAK	DURATION
PO	1 hr	6 hr	24 hr

*Full effects may not be noted for several weeks.

Contraindications/Precautions

Contraindicated in: Hypersensitivity; History of angioedema with previous use of ACE inhibitors; OB: Can cause injury or death of fetus—if pregnancy occurs, discontinue immediately. Lactation: Appears in breast milk; discontinue lisinopril or breast-feeding.
Use Cautiously in: Patients with renal impairment, hypovolemia, hyponatremia, and concurrent diuretic therapy (initial dosage reduction recommended); Black patients (monotherapy of hypertension less effective, may require additional therapy; higher risk of angioedema); Surgery/anesthesia (hypotension may be exaggerated); Women of childbearing potential; Pedi: Safety not established children <6 yr; Geri: Initial dosage reduction recommended.
Exercise Extreme Caution in: Family history of angioedema.

Interactions

Drug-Drug: Excessive hypotension may occur with concurrent use of **diuretics**. Additive hypotension with other **antihypertensive agents**. Increased risk of hyperkalemia with concurrent use of **potassium supplements, potassium-sparing diuretics, potassium-containing salt substitutes**, or **angiotensin II receptor antagonists**. Antihypertensive response may be blunted by **NSAIDs**. Increases levels and may increase the risk of **lithium** toxicity.

Route/Dosage

Hypertension

PO (Adults): 10 mg once daily, can be increased up to 20–40 mg/day (initiate therapy at 5 mg/day in patients receiving diuretics).
PO (Children ≥6 yr): 0.07 mg/kg once daily (up to 5 mg/day); may be titrated every 1–2 wk up to 0.6 mg/kg/day (or 40 mg/day).

Renal Impairment

PO (Adults): *CCr 10–30 mL/min*—Initiate therapy at 5 mg daily; may be slowly titrated up to 40 mg/day. *CCr <10 mL/min*—Initiate therapy at 2.5 mg once daily; may be slowly titrated up to 40 mg/day.

Renal Impairment

(Children ≥6 yr): *CCr <30 mL/min*—Contraindicated.

Heart Failure

PO (Adults): 5 mg once daily, may be titrated every 2 wk up to 40 mg/day; initiate therapy at 2.5 mg once daily in patients with hyponatremia (serum sodium <130 mEq/L).

Renal Impairment

(Adults): *CCr ≤30 mL/min*—Initiate therapy at 2.5 mg once daily.

Acute Myocardial Infarction

PO (Adults): 5 mg once daily for 2 days, then 10 mg daily.

Renal Impairment

PO (Adults): Initiate with caution in patients with serum creatinine >2 mg/dL.

Availability (generic available)

Tablets: 2.5 mg, 5 mg, 10 mg, 20 mg, 30mg, 40 mg. ***In combination with:*** hydrochlorothiazide (Prinzide), (Zestoretic).

lithium (lith-ee-um)

✱Carbolith, Duralith, Eskalith, Lithizine, Lithobid

Classification

Therapeutic: mood stabilizers

Indications

Manic episodes of manic depressive illness (treatment, maintenance, prophylaxis).

Action

Alters cation transport in nerve and muscle. May also influence reuptake of neurotransmitters. **Therapeutic Effects:** Prevents/decreases incidence of acute manic episodes.

Adverse Reactions/Side Effects

CNS: SEIZURES, fatigue, headache, impaired memory, ataxia, sedation, confusion, dizziness, drowsiness, psychomotor retardation, restlessness, stupor. **EENT:** aphasia, blurred vision, dysarthria, tinnitus. **CV:** ARRHYTHMIAS, ECG changes, edema, hypotension. **GI:** abdominal pain, anorexia, bloating, diarrhea, nausea, dry mouth, metallic taste. **GU:** polyuria, glycosuria, nephrogenic diabetes insipidus, renal toxicity. **Derm:** acneiform eruption, folliculitis, alopecia, diminished sensation, pruritus. **Endo:** hypothyroidism, goiter, hyperglycemia, hyperthyroidism. **F and E:** hyponatremia. **Hemat:** leukocytosis. **Metab:** weight gain. **MS:** muscle weakness, hyperirritability, rigidity. **Neuro:** tremors.

PHYSICAL THERAPY IMPLICATIONS

Note: Many symptoms listed below may indicate lithium toxicity. Mild toxicity is associated with metallic taste, fine tremor, nausea, and weakness. Moderate levels include vomiting, diarrhea, increased tremor, dizziness, incoordination, and blurred vision. Severe lithium toxicity is associated with confusion, hallucinations, nystagmus, dysarthria, and fasciculations. Be alert for these symptoms, and notify the physician about any increase in the signs of lithium toxicity.

Examination and Evaluation

- Be alert for new seizures or increased seizure activity, especially at the onset of drug treatment or following an increase in dose. Document the number, duration, and severity of seizures, and report these findings immediately to the physician.
- Assess heart rate, ECG, and heart sounds, especially during exercise (See Appendices G, H). Report arrhythmias or symptoms of rhythm disturbances, including palpitations, chest discomfort, shortness of breath, fainting, and fatigue/weakness.
- Assess blood pressure (BP) periodically and compare to normal values (See Appendix F). Report low BP (hypotension), especially if patient experiences dizziness, fatigue, or other symptoms.
- Assess peripheral edema using girth measurements, volume displacement, and measurement of pitting edema (See Appendix N). Report increased swelling in feet and ankles or a sudden increase in body weight due to fluid retention.
- Monitor personality and behavioral changes such as restlessness, confusion, impaired memory, mental slowness, and stupor. Notify physician if these changes become problematic.
- Assess any muscle weakness, rigidity, or other changes in muscle tone and excitability. Try to determine if symptoms are drug induced rather than caused by neurologic or musculoskeletal pathology.
- Monitor and report any increase or decrease in metabolism that might indicate thyroid disorders. Signs of hyperthyroidism include tachycardia, nervousness, heat intolerance, weight loss, muscle wasting, and goiter. Hypothyroidism is typically indicated by bradycardia, lethargy, cold intolerance, weight gain, and muscle weakness.
- Watch for signs of hyperglycemia such as drowsiness, fruity breath, increased urination, and unusual thirst. Patients with diabetes mellitus should check blood glucose levels frequently.
- Monitor signs of low sodium levels (hyponatremia), including headache, confusion, lethargy, irritability, decreased consciousness, and neuromuscular abnormalities (muscle weakness and cramps). Report severe or prolonged signs to the physician.

- Be alert for signs of increased white blood cell counts (leukocytosis), including fever, weakness, weight loss, loss of appetite, dizziness, fainting, dyspnea, bleeding/bruising, or pain or tingling in the arms, legs, or abdomen. Report these signs to the physician immediately.
- Assess dizziness, drowsiness, tremors, and ataxia that might affect gait, balance, and other functional activities (See Appendix C). Report balance problems and functional limitations to the physician, and caution the patient and family/caregivers to guard against falls and trauma.
- Periodically assess body weight and other anthropometric measures (body mass index, body composition). Report a substantial weight gain or increased body fat.

Interventions

- Guard against falls and trauma (hip fractures, head injury, and so forth) caused by drowsiness, dizziness, blurred vision, or ataxia; implement fall-prevention strategies (See Appendix E).
- Because of the risk of arrhythmias and abnormal BP responses, use caution during aerobic exercise and other forms of therapeutic exercise Assess exercise tolerance frequently (BP, heart rate, fatigue levels), and terminate exercise immediately if any untoward responses occur (See Appendix L).
- Help patient explore non-pharmacological methods to reduce bipolar episodes and mood disorders (exercise, counseling, support groups, and so forth).

Patient/Client-Related Instruction

- Advise patient that increased urination is likely, but to report signs of kidney toxicity such as blood or pus in urine, decreased urine output, weight gain from fluid retention, and unusual fatigue.
- Advise patient that skin reactions such as itching, hair loss, acne, follicular irritation are likely. Report severe or unexpected skin reactions to the physician.
- Instruct patient to report severe or prolonged GI problems, including nausea, diarrhea, abdominal pain, bloating, dry mouth, or appetite loss.
- Instruct patient to report other problematic side effects such as severe or prolonged headache, fatigue, blurred vision, or speech and hearing disturbances.

Pharmacokinetics

Absorption: Completely absorbed after oral administration.
Distribution: Widely distributed into many tissues and fluids; CSF levels are 50% of plasma levels. Crosses the placenta; enters breast milk.
Metabolism and Excretion: Excreted almost entirely unchanged by the kidneys.
Half-life: 20–27 hr.

TIME/ACTION PROFILE (antimanic effects)

ROUTE	ONSET	PEAK	DURATION
PO, PO-ER	5–7 days	10–21 days	days

Contraindications/Precautions

Contraindicated in: Hypersensitivity; Severe cardiovascular or renal disease; Dehydrated or debilitated patients; Should be used only where therapy, including blood levels, may be closely monitored; Some products contain alcohol or tartrazine and should be avoided in patients with known hypersensitivity or intolerance.
Use Cautiously in: Any degree of cardiac, renal, or thyroid disease; Diabetes mellitus; **Pregnancy/Lactation:** Safety not established; Geri: Initial dosage reduction recommended.

Interactions

Drug-Drug: May prolong the action of **neuromuscular blocking agents**. ↑ risk of neurologic toxicity with **haloperidol** or **molindone**. **Diuretics, methyldopa, probenecid, fluoxetine,** and **NSAIDs** may ↑ risk of toxicity. Blood levels may be ↑ by **ACE inhibitors**. Lithium may ↓ effects of **chlorpromazine**. **Chlorpromazine** may mask early signs of lithium toxicity. Hypothyroid effects may be additive with **potassium iodide** or **antithyroid agents**. **Aminophylline, phenothiazines,** and **drugs containing large amounts of sodium** ↑ renal elimination and ↓ effectiveness. **Psyllium** can ↓ **lithium** levels.
Drug-Natural: Caffeine-containing herbs (**cola nut, guarana, mate, tea, coffee**) may ↓ **lithium** serum levels and efficacy.
Drug-Food: Large changes in **sodium** intake may alter the renal elimination of lithium. ↑ sodium intake will ↑ renal excretion.

Route/Dosage

Precise dosing is based on serum lithium levels. 300 mg lithium carbonate contains 8–12 mEq lithium.
PO (Adults and children ≥12 yr): *Tablets/capsules*—300–600 mg tid initially; usual maintenance dose is 300 mg tid or qid. *Slow-release capsules*—200–300 mg tid initially; increased up to 1800 mg/day in divided doses. Usual maintenance dose is 300–400 mg tid. *Extended-release tablets*—450–900 mg bid *or* 300–600 mg tid initially; usual maintenance dose is 450 mg bid *or* 300 mg tid.
PO (Children <12 yr): 15–20 mg (0.4–0.5 mEq)/kg/day in 2–3 divided doses; dosage may be adjusted weekly.

Availability (generic available)

Capsules: 150 mg, 300 mg, 600 mg. **Tablets:** 300 mg. **Controlled-release tablets:** 300 mg, 450 mg. **Slow-release tablets:** 300 mg. **Syrup:** 300 mg (8 mEq lithium)/5 mL.

lomustine (loe-mus-teen)

CCNU, CeeNu

Classification

Therapeutic: antineoplastics

Pharmacologic: alkylating agents

Indications

Used alone or with other agents for primary and metastatic brain tumors, Hodgkin's disease.

Action

Inhibits DNA and RNA synthesis by alkylation (cell-cycle phase–nonspecific). **Therapeutic Effects:** Death of rapidly replicating cells, particularly malignant ones.

Adverse Reactions/Side Effects

CNS: ataxia, disorientation, dysarthria, lethargy. **Resp:** fibrosis, pulmonary infiltrates. **GI:** nausea, vomiting, anorexia, hepatotoxicity, stomatitis. **GU:** azotemia, renal failure. **Derm:** alopecia. **Endo:** infertility. **Hemat:** leukopenia, thrombocytopenia, anemia. **Metab:** hyperuricemia. **Misc:** secondary malignancy (long-term use).

PHYSICAL THERAPY IMPLICATIONS

Examination and Evaluation

- Assess pulmonary function periodically by measuring lung volumes, breath sounds, and respiratory rate (See Appendices I, J, K). Notify physician or nursing staff immediately if patient experiences signs of pulmonary fibrosis or pulmonary infiltrates (dry cough, dyspnea, chest pain, shortness of breath, cyanosis).
- Watch for signs of leukopenia (fever, sore throat, signs of infection), thrombocytopenia (bruising, nose bleeds, bleeding gums), or unusual weakness and fatigue that might be due to anemia. Report these signs to the physician or nursing staff.
- Monitor and report signs of CNS toxicity including ataxia, disorientation, garbled speech, or lethargy.
- Monitor signs of renal failure, including decreased urine output, increased blood pressure, muscle cramps/twitching, edema/weight gain from fluid retention, yellowish brown skin, and confusion that progresses to seizures and coma. Report these signs to the physician or nursing staff immediately.
- Watch for signs of a secondary malignancy, including a change in bowel or bladder habits, nonhealing sores, unusual bleeding or discharge, a lump in the breast or other parts of the body, chronic indigestion or difficulty in swallowing, obvious changes in a wart or mole, and persistent coughing or hoarseness. Report these signs to the physician immediately.

Interventions

- For patients who are medically able to begin exercise, implement appropriate resistive exercises and aerobic training to maintain muscle strength and aerobic capacity during cancer chemotherapy or to help restore function after chemotherapy.
- Because of the risk of pulmonary fibrosis, use caution during aerobic exercise and other forms of therapeutic exercise. Assess exercise tolerance frequently (blood pressure, heart rate, fatigue levels), and terminate exercise immediately if any untoward responses occur (See Appendix L).

Patient/Client-related Instruction

- Advise patient to guard against infection (frequent hand washing, etc.), and to avoid crowds and contact with persons with contagious diseases.
- Advise patient about the likelihood of GI reactions such as nausea, vomiting, loss of appetite, and irritation in or around the mouth. Instruct patient to report severe or prolonged GI problems, and to also report signs of liver toxicity, including abdominal pain, severe nausea and vomiting, yellow skin or eyes, fever, sore throat, malaise, weakness, facial edema, lethargy, and unusual bleeding or bruising.
- Advise patient that hair loss and other skin reactions (rash, itching) are likely. Report severe or unexpected skin reactions to the physician.

Pharmacokinetics

Absorption: Rapidly absorbed following oral administration.

Distribution: Widely distributed. Active metabolites enter the CSF well. Enters breast milk.

Metabolism and Excretion: Mostly metabolized by the liver. Some metabolites are active antineoplastic agents. Metabolites are excreted by the kidneys.

Half-life: 1–2 days (active metabolites).

TIME/ACTION PROFILE (effects on blood counts)

ROUTE	ONSET	PEAK	DURATION
PO	unknown	4–7 wk	1–2 wk

Contraindications/Precautions

Contraindicated in: Hypersensitivity; Pregnancy or lactation.

Use Cautiously in: Patients with childbearing potential; Active infections; Decreased bone marrow reserve (dosage reduction required); Geriatric patients or patients with other chronic debilitating illnesses; Impaired liver function.

Interactions

Drug-Drug: ↑ bone marrow depression with other **antineoplastics** or **radiation therapy.** May ↓ antibody response to **live-virus vaccines** and ↑ risk of adverse reactions.

Route/Dosage

PO (Adults and Children): 100–130 mg/m² as a single dose every 6 wk (adjustments required for concurrent therapy or decreased blood counts).

Availability

Capsules: 10 mg, 40 mg, 100 mg.

lopinavir/ritonavir

(loe-**pin**-a-veer/ri-**toe**-na-veer)

Kaletra

Classification

Therapeutic: antiretrovirals

Pharmacologic: protease inhibitors, metabolic inhibitors

Indications

HIV infection (with other antiretrovirals).

Action

Lopinavir: Inhibits HIV viral protease. **Ritonavir:** Although ritonavir has antiretroviral activity of its own (inhibits the action of HIV protease and prevents the cleavage of viral polyproteins), it is combined with lopinavir to inhibit the metabolism of lopinavir, thus increasing its plasma levels. **Therapeutic Effects:** Increased CD4 cell counts and decreased viral load with subsequent slowed progression of HIV infection and its sequelae.

Adverse Reactions/Side Effects

CNS: headache, insomnia, weakness. **GI:** diarrhea (↑ in children), abdominal pain, nausea, pancreatitis, taste aversion (in children), vomiting (↑ in children). **Derm:** rash.

PHYSICAL THERAPY IMPLICATIONS

Examination and Evaluation

- Monitor fatigue and weakness. Some degree of weakness is expected, but excessive or unusual weakness should be reported.

Interventions

- Implement resistive exercises and other therapeutic exercises as needed to maintain muscle strength and function, and prevent muscle wasting associated with HIV infection and AIDS.

Patient/Client-Related Instruction

- Emphasize the importance of taking lopinavir as directed even if the patient is asymptomatic and that this drug must always be used in combination with other antiretroviral drugs. Do not take more than prescribed amount, and do not stop taking without consulting health care professional.
- Inform patient that lopinavir does not cure HIV or AIDS or prevent associated or opportunistic infections. Lopinavir does not reduce the risk of transmission of HIV to others through sexual contact or blood contamination. Caution patient to use a condom, and to avoid sharing needles or donating blood to prevent spreading the AIDS virus to others.
- Advise patient about the likelihood of GI reactions (nausea, diarrhea, vomiting, taste changes). Instruct patient to report severe or prolonged GI problems or signs of pancreatitis such as upper abdominal pain (especially after eating), indigestion, weight loss, and oily stools.
- Instruct patient to report other troublesome side effects such as prolonged or severe headache, skin rash, or sleep loss.

Pharmacokinetics

Absorption: Well absorbed following oral administration; food enhances absorption.

Distribution: *Ritonavir*—poor CNS penetration.

Protein Binding: *Lopinavir*—98–99% bound to plasma proteins.

Metabolism and Excretion: *Lopinavir*—completely metabolized in the liver by cytochrome P450P3A (CYP450P3A); ritonavir is a potent inhibitor of this enzyme. Ritonavir—highly metabolized by the liver (by CYP450P3A and CYP2D6 enzymes); one metabolite has antiretroviral activity; 3.5% excreted unchanged in urine.

Half-life: *Lopinavir*—5–6 hr; Ritonavir—3–5 hr.

TIME/ACTION PROFILE (blood levels)

ROUTE	ONSET	PEAK	DURATION
lopinavir PO	rapid	4 hr	12 hr
ritonavir PO	rapid	4 hr*	12 hr

*Nonfasting.

Contraindications/Precautions

Contraindicated in: Hypersensitivity; Concurrent use of dihydroergotamine, ergotamine, ergonovine, flecainide, methylergonovine, midazolam, pimozide, propafenone, amiodarone, and triazolam, which are highly dependent on CYP3A or CYP2D6 for metabolism and for which ↑ blood levels may result in serious and/or life-threatening events; Concurrent use with simvastatin, lovastatin, St. John's wort (hypericum perforatum) is not recommended; Hypersensitivity or intolerance to alcohol or castor oil (present in capsules and liquid).

Use Cautiously in: Known alcohol intolerance (oral solution contains alcohol); Concurrent use with atorvastatin (may increase risk of rhabdomyolysis);

Concurrent use of antiarrhythmics, including lidocaine and quinidine (therapeutic blood level monitoring recommended); Concurrent use of anticonvulsants, including carbamazepine, Phenobarbital, or phenytoin (may decrease effectiveness of lopinavir); Concurrent use of dihydropyridine calcium channel blockers, including felodipine, nifedipine, and nicardipine (clinical monitoring recommended due to increased levels of calcium channel blocker); Impaired hepatic function, history of hepatitis (for ritonavir content); OB: Pregnancy or lactation (safety not established; breast-feeding not recommended in HIV-infected patients).

Exercise Extreme Caution in: Concurrent use with sildenafil, vardenafil, or tadalafil should be undertaken with extreme caution and may result in hypotension, syncope, visual changes, and prolonged erection.

Interactions

Drug-Drug: Concurrent use of **flecainide, amiodarone, propafenone, dihydroergotamine, ergonovine, ergotamine, methylergonovine, pimozide, midazolam,** and **triazolamis** contraindicated because of the risk of potentially serious, life-threatening drug interactions. Concurrent use with **sildenafil, vardenafil,** or **tadalafil** should be undertaken with extreme caution and may result in hypotension, syncope, visual changes, and prolonged erection (dose reduction of sildenafil to 25 mg every 48 hr with monitoring recommended). Concurrent use with **rifampin** ↓ effectiveness of antiretroviral therapy and should not be undertaken. Should not be used concurrently with **simvastatin** or **lovastatin** due to ↑ risk of rhabdomyolysis; similar risk exists for **atorvastatin** (use lowest possible dose with careful monitoring). Concurrent use with **efavirenz** or **nevirapine** ↓ lopinavir/ritonavir levels and effectiveness; dose increase may be necessary. **Delavirdine** ↑ lopinavir levels. ↑ levels of **lidocaine** and **quinidine** (blood level monitoring recommended). Concurrent use of anticonvulsants, including **carbamazepine, phenobarbital,** or **phenytoin,** may ↓ effectiveness of lopinavir. ↑ levels of dihydropyridine calcium channel blockers, including **felodipine, nifedipine,** and **nicardipine** (clinical monitoring recommended). May alter levels and effectiveness of **warfarin.** ↑ levels of **clarithromycin** (dose reduction recommended for patients with CCr ≤60 mL/min. ↑ blood levels of **itraconazole** and **ketoconazole** (high antifungal doses not recommended). ↑ levels of **rifabutin** (dose reduction recommended). ↓ blood levels of **atovaquone** (may require dosage increase). **Dexamethasone** ↓ blood levels and may ↓ effectiveness of lopinavir. Oral solution contains alcohol and may produce intolerance when administered with **disulfiram** or **metronidazole.** May ↑ levels and risk of toxicity with immunosuppressants, including **cyclosporine** or **tacrolimus** (blood level monitoring recommended). May ↓ levels and effects of **methadone** (dose of **methadone** may need to be ↑). May ↓ levels and contraceptive efficacy of some estrogen-based **hormonal contraceptives,** including **ethinyl estradiol** (alternative or additional methods of contraception recommended). ↑ levels of **fluticasone** by inhalation; avoid concurrent use.

Drug-Natural: Concurrent use with **St. John's wort** may ↓ levels and beneficial effect of lopinavir/ritonavir.

Route/Dosage

PO (Adults and Children >40 kg): 400/100 mg (3 capsules or 5 mL oral solution) bid *or* may be given as a single daily dose of 800/200 mg (6 capsules or 10 mL oral solution); single dose approved for adults only.

PO (Children 15–40 kg): 10 mg/kg lopinavir content bid.

PO (Children 7–15 kg): 12 mg/kg lopinavir content bid.

With concurrent efavirenz or nevirapine

PO (Adults and Children >40 kg): 533/133 mg (4 capsules or 6.5 mL oral solution) bid.

PO (Children 15–50 kg): 11 mg/kg lopinavir content bid.

PO (Children 7–15 kg): 13 mg/kg lopinavir content bid.

Availability

Capsules: 133.3 mg lopinavir/33 mg ritonavir. **Oral solution (cotton candy or vanilla):** 80 mg lopinavir/20 mg ritonavir per milliliter (contains 42.4% alcohol) in 60-mL bottles.

loratadine (lor-at-a-deen)

Alavert, ✱Claritin, Claritin 24–Hour Allergy, Claritin Hives Relief, Children's Loratidine, Claritin Reditabs, Clear-Atadine, Dimetapp Children's ND Non-Drowsy Allergy, Non-Drowsy Allergy Relief for Kids, Tavist ND

Classification

Therapeutic: antihistamines

Pharmacologic: piperidines

Indications

Relief of symptoms of seasonal allergies. Management of chronic idiopathic urticaria. Management of hives.

Action
Blocks peripheral effects of histamine released during allergic reactions. **Therapeutic Effects:** Decreased symptoms of allergic reactions (nasal stuffiness; red, swollen eyes; itching).

Adverse Reactions/Side Effects
CNS: confusion, drowsiness (rare), paradoxical excitation. **EENT:** blurred vision. **GI:** dry mouth, GI upset. **Derm:** photosensitivity, rash. **Metab:** weight gain.

PHYSICAL THERAPY IMPLICATIONS
Examination and Evaluation
- Monitor symptoms of seasonal allergies (sneezing, rhinitis, itching eyes, cough) or chronic idiopathic urticaria (rash, hives, itching) to help document benefits of this drug in treating these disorders.
- Monitor signs of increased excitation, including restlessness, agitation, and hyperactivity. Severe or problematic excitation may require a change in dose or drug.
- Periodically assess body weight and other anthropometric measures (body mass index, body composition). Report a rapid or unexplained weight gain or increased body fat.

Interventions
- Guard against falls and trauma (hip fractures, head injury, and so forth). Implement fall- prevention strategies, especially in older adults or if balance is impaired (See Appendix E).
- Causes photosensitivity; use care if administering UV treatments. Advise patient to avoid direct sunlight and use sunscreens and protective clothing. Also report any rashes and other skin reactions.

Patient/Client-Related Instruction
- Advise patient about the risk of daytime drowsiness, confusion, and decreased attention and mental focus. Although the risk of drowsiness is considerably lower with this drug compared to traditional antihistamines, patients should use care if driving or in other activities that require quick reactions and strong concentration.
- Advise patient to avoid alcohol and other CNS depressants because of the increased risk of sedation and adverse effects.
- Instruct patient to report other troublesome side effects including severe or prolonged dry mouth, skin rash, or GI upset.

Pharmacokinetics
Absorption: Rapidly absorbed after oral administration (80%).
Distribution: Unknown.
Protein Binding: *Loratadine*—97%; *descarboethoxyloratadine*—73–77%.
Metabolism and Excretion: Rapidly and extensively metabolized during first pass through the liver. Much is converted to descarboethoxyloratadine, an active metabolite.
Half-life: *Loratadine*—7.8–11 hr; *descarboethoxyloratadine*—20 hr.

TIME/ACTION PROFILE (antihistaminic effects)

ROUTE	ONSET	PEAK	DURATION
PO	1–3 hr	8–12 hr	>24 hr

Contraindications/Precautions
Contraindicated in: Hypersensitivity; OB: Lactation.
Use Cautiously in: Patients with hepatic impairment or CCr <30 mL/min (↓ dose to 10 mg every other day); Patients receiving drugs known to affect hepatic metabolism of drugs; Geri: ↑ risk of adverse reactions; OB/Pedi: Pregnancy or children <2 yr (safety not established).

Interactions
Drug-Drug: The following interactions may occur, but are less likely to occur with loratadine that with more sedating antihistamines. **MAO inhibitors** may intensify and prolong effects of antihistamines. ↑ CNS depression may occur with other **CNS depressants**, including **alcohol, antidepressants, opioid analgesics,** and **sedative/hypnotics**.
Drug-Natural: Kava, valerian, or **chamomile** can ↑ CNS depression.

Route/Dosage
PO (Adults and Children ≥6 yr): 10 mg once daily.
PO (Children ≥2–5 yr): 5 mg once daily.

Renal Impairment
PO (Adults): *CCr <30 mL/min*—10 mg every other day.

Hepatic Impairment
PO (Adults): 10 mg every other day.

Availability (generic available)
Rapidly disintegrating tablets (mint): 5 mg, 10 mg OTC. **Tablets:** 10 mg OTC, 10 mg. **Capsules:** 10 mg OTC. **Chewable tablets:** 5 mg OTC (grape flavored). **Syrup (grape, fruit):** 5 mg/5 ml OTC. ***In combination with:*** pseudoephedrine (Claritin-D) OTC. See Appendix B.

lorazepam (lor-az-e-pam)
Apo-Lorazepam, Ativan, Novo-Lorazem, Nu-Loraz

Classification
Therapeutic: analgesic adjuncts, antianxiety agents, sedative/hypnotics
Pharmacologic: benzodiazepines

Schedule IV

Indications
Anxiety disorder (oral). Preoperative sedation (injection). Decreases preoperative anxiety and provides amnesia. **Unlabeled Use: IV:** Antiemetic prior to chemotherapy. Insomnia, panic disorder, as an adjunct with acute mania or acute psychosis.

Action
Depresses the CNS, probably by potentiating gamma-aminobutyric acid (GABA), an inhibitory neurotransmitter. **Therapeutic Effects:** Sedation. Decreased anxiety. Decreased seizures.

Adverse Reactions/Side Effects
CNS: dizziness, drowsiness, lethargy, hangover, headache, ataxia, slurred speech, forgetfulness, confusion, mental depression, rhythmic myoclonic jerking in preterm infants, paradoxical excitation. **EENT:** blurred vision. **Resp:** respiratory depression. **CV: rapid IV use only:** APNEA, CARDIA CARREST, bradycardia, hypotension. **GI:** constipation, diarrhea, nausea, vomiting, weight gain (unusual). **Derm:** rashes. **Misc:** physical dependence, psychologic dependence, tolerance.

PHYSICAL THERAPY IMPLICATIONS

Examination and Evaluation
- Assess respiration after rapid IV administration. Notify physician immediately if patient exhibits any interruption in respiratory rate (apnea) or signs of respiratory depression such as rapid labored breathing, cyanosis, confusion, irritability, sleepiness, headache, and oxygen desaturation. Monitor pulse oximetry and perform pulmonary function tests (See Appendices I, J, K) to quantify suspected changes in ventilation and respiratory function.
- Continually monitor for signs of cardiac arrest, especially after rapid IV administration. Signs include sudden chest pain, pain radiating into the arm or jaw, shortness of breath, dizziness, sweating, anxiety, nausea, and loss of consciousness. Seek immediate medical assistance if patient develops these signs.
- Assess blood pressure periodically and compare to normal values (See Appendix F). Report low blood pressure (hypotension), especially if patient experiences dizziness or syncope.
- Assess heart rate, ECG, and heart sounds, especially during exercise (See Appendices G, H). Report an unusually slow heart rate (bradycardia) or signs of other arrhythmias, including palpitations, chest discomfort, shortness of breath, fainting, and fatigue/weakness.
- Monitor daytime drowsiness and "hangover" symptoms (headache, nausea, irritability, lethargy, dysphoria). Repeated or excessive symptoms may require change in dose or medication.
- Report any behavioral or personality changes such as confusion, forgetfulness, slurred speech, decreased mental acuity, or excessive excitation.
- Assess dizziness, drowsiness, and ataxia that might affect gait, balance, and other functional activities (See Appendix C). Report balance problems and functional limitations to the physician, and caution the patient and family/caregivers to guard against falls and trauma.

Interventions
- Guard against falls and trauma (hip fractures, head injury, and so forth). Implement fall prevention strategies, especially in older adults or if drowsiness and dizziness carry over into the daytime (See Appendix E).
- Because of the risk of cardiac arrest and respiratory depression, use extreme caution during aerobic exercise and other forms of therapeutic exercise. Assess exercise tolerance frequently (blood pressure, heart rate, fatigue levels), and terminate exercise immediately if any untoward responses occur (See Appendix L).
- Help patient explore nonpharmacologic methods to reduce anxiety or insomnia, such as relaxation techniques, exercise, counseling, support groups, and so forth.

Patient/Client-Related Instruction
- Instruct patients on prolonged treatment not to discontinue medication without consulting their physician. Prolonged use can cause tolerance and dependence, and abrupt withdrawal can cause insomnia, unusual irritability or nervousness, and seizures.
- Advise patient to avoid alcohol and other CNS depressants because of the increased risk of sedation and adverse effects.
- Instruct patient to report other bothersome side effects such as severe or prolonged headache, blurred vision, skin rash, or GI problems (nausea, vomiting, diarrhea, constipation).

Pharmacokinetics
Absorption: Well absorbed following oral administration. Rapidly and completely absorbed following IM administration. Sublingual absorption is more rapid than oral and is similar to IM.
Distribution: Widely distributed. Crosses the blood-brain barrier. Crosses the placenta; enters breast milk.
Metabolism and Excretion: Highly metabolized by the liver.

Half-life: Full-term neonates: 18–73 hr; Older children: 6–17 hr; Adults: 10–16 hr.

TIME/ACTION PROFILE (sedation)

ROUTE	ONSET	PEAK	DURATION
PO	15–60 min	1–6 hr	8–12 hr
IM	30–60 min	1–2 hr†	8–12 hr
IV	15–30 min	15–20 min	8–12 hr

†Amnestic response

Contraindications/Precautions

Contraindicated in: Hypersensitivity; Cross-sensitivity with other benzodiazepines may exist; Comatose patients or those with preexisting CNS depression; Uncontrolled severe pain; Angle-closure glaucoma; Severe hypotension; Sleep apnea; OB: Use in pregnancy and lactation may cause CNS depression, flaccidity, feeding difficulties, hypothermia, seizures, and respiratory problems in the neonate; Lactation: Recommend to discontinue drug or bottle-feed.

Use Cautiously in: Severe hepatic/renal/pulmonary impairment; Myasthenia gravis; Depression; Psychosis; History of suicide attempt or drug abuse; COPD; Sleep apnea; Pedi: Use cautiously in children under 12 yr. In ↑ doses, benzyl alcohol in injection may cause potentially fatal gasping syndrome in neonates; Geri: Lower doses recommended for geriatric or debilitated patients; Hypnotic use should be short term; **OVERDOSE:** Administer Flumazenil (do not use with patients with seizure disorder. May induce seizures.

Interactions

Drug-Drug: Additive CNS depression with other **CNS depressants,** including **alcohol, antihistamines, antidepressants, opioid analgesics, clozapine,** and other **sedative/hypnotics,** including other benzodiazepines. May ↓ the efficacy of **levodopa. Smoking** may ↑ metabolism and ↓ effectiveness. **Valproate** can ↑ serum concentrations and ↓ clearance (↓ dose by 50%). **Probenecid** may ↓ metabolism of lorazepam, enhancing its actions (↓ dose by 50%). **Oral contraceptives** may ↑ clearance and ↓ concentration of lorazepam.

Drug-Natural: Concomitant use of **kava, valerian** or, **chamomile** can ↑ CNS depression.

Route/Dosage

PO (Adults): *Anxiety*—1–3 mg bid–tid (up to 10 mg/day). *Insomnia*—2–4 mg at bedtime.

PO (Geriatric Patients or Debilitated Patients): *Anxiety*—0.5–2 mg/day in divided doses initially. *Insomnia*—0.25–1 mg initially; increased as needed.

PO (Children): *Anxiety/sedation*—0.02–0.1 mg/kg/dose (not to exceed 2 mg) q 4–8 hr. *Preoperative sedation*—0.02–0.09 mg/kg/dose.

PO (Infants): *Anxiety/sedation*—0.02–0.1 mg/kg/dose (not to exceed 2 mg) q 4–8 hr. *Preoperative sedation*—0.02–0.09 mg/kg/dose.

SL (Adults and adolescents >18 yr): *Anxiety*—2–3 mg/day in divided doses, not to exceed 6 mg/day; *Preoperative sedation*—0.05 mg/kg, up to 4 mg total given 1–2 hr before surgery.

SL (Geriatric Patients and debilitated patients): 0.5 mg/da;, dose may be adjusted as necessary.

IM (Adults): *Preoperative sedation*—50 mcg (0.05 mg)/kg 2 hr before surgery (not to exceed 4 mg).

IM (Children): *Preoperative sedation*—0.02–0.09 mg/kg/dose.

IM (Infants): *Preoperative sedation*—0.02–0.09 mg/kg/dose.

IV (Adults): *Preoperative sedation*—44 mcg (0.044 mg)/kg (not to exceed 2 mg) 15–20 min before surgery. *Operative amnestic effect*—up to 50 mcg/kg (not to exceed 4 mg). *Antiemetic*—2 mg 30 min prior to chemotherapy; may be repeated q 4 hr as needed (unlabeled). *Anticonvulsant*—50 mcg (0.05 mg)/kg, up to 4 mg; may be repeated after 10–15 min (not to exceed 8 mg/12 hr; unlabeled).

IV (Children): *Preoperative sedation*—0.02–0.09 mg/kg/dose; may use smaller doses (0.01–0.03 mg/kg) and repeat q 20 min. *Antiemetic*—Single dose: 0.04–0.08 mg/kg/dose prior to chemotherapy (not to exceed 4 mg). Multiple doses: 0.02–0.05 mg/kg/dose q 6 hr prn (not to exceed 2 mg). *Anxiety/sedation*—0.02–0.1 mg/kg (not to exceed 2 mg) q 4–8 hr. *Status epilepticus*—0.1 mg/kg over 2–5 min (not to exceed 4 mg); may repeat with 0.05 mg/kg if needed.

IV (Infants): *Preoperative sedation*—0.02–0.09 mg/kg/dose; may use smaller doses (0.01–0.03 mg/kg) and repeat q 20 min. *Anxiety/sedation*—0.02–0.1 mg/kg/dose (not to exceed 2 mg) q 4–8 hr. *Status epilepticus*—0.1 mg/kg over 2–5 min (not to exceed 4 mg); may repeat with 0.05 mg/kg if needed.

IV (Neonates): *Status epilepticus*—0.05 mg/kg over 2–5 min; may repeat in 10–15 min.

Availability (generic available)

Tablets: 0.5 mg, 1 mg, 2 mg. **Concentrated oral solution:** 0.5 mg/5 mL, 2 mg/mL. **Sublingual tablets:** 0.5 mg, 1 mg, 2 mg. **Injection:** 2 mg/mL, 4 mg/mL.

losartan (loe-**sar**-tan)

Cozaar

Classification

Therapeutic: antihypertensives

Pharmacologic: angiotensin II receptor antagonists

Indications

Alone or with other agents in the management of hypertension. Treatment of diabetic nephropathy in patients with type 2 diabetes. Prevention of stroke in patients with hypertension and left ventricular hypertrophy.

Action

Blocks the vasoconstrictor and aldosterone-secreting effects of angiotensin II at various receptor sites, including vascular smooth muscle and the adrenal glands. **Therapeutic Effects:** Lowering of blood pressure in hypertensive patients. Decreased progression of diabetic nephropathy. Decreased incidence of stroke in patients with hypertension and left ventricular hypertrophy (effect may be less in black patients).

Adverse Reactions/Side Effects

CNS: dizziness, fatigue, headache, insomnia, weakness. **CV:** chest pain, edema, hypotension. **EENT:** nasal congestion. **Endo:** hypoglycemia, weight gain. **GI:** diarrhea, abdominal pain, dyspepsia, nausea. **GU:** impaired renal function. **F and E:** hyperkalemia. **MS:** back pain, myalgia. **Misc:** ANGIOEDEMA, fever.

PHYSICAL THERAPY IMPLICATIONS

Examination and Evaluation

- Monitor signs of angioedema, including rashes, raised patches of red or white skin (welts), burning/itching skin, swelling in the face, and difficulty breathing. Notify physician immediately of these signs.
- Assess blood pressure periodically and compare to normal values (See Appendix F) to help document antihypertensive effects. Report low blood pressure (hypotension), especially if patient experiences dizziness or syncope.
- Assess peripheral edema using girth measurements, volume displacement, and measurement of pitting edema (See Appendix N). Report increased swelling in feet and ankles or a sudden increase in body weight due to fluid retention.
- If treating diabetic neuropathy, establish baseline electroneuromyographic values at the beginning of drug treatment whenever possible. Periodically reexamine these values to monitor peripheral nerve function and document whether drug therapy delays the progression of neuropathic disease.
- Assess any muscle pain or back pain to rule out musculoskeletal pathology; that is, try to determine if pain is drug-induced rather than caused by anatomical or biomechanical problems.
- Monitor symptoms of high plasma potassium levels (hyperkalemia), including bradycardia, fatigue, weakness, numbness, and tingling. Notify physician because severe cases can lead to life-threatening arrhythmias and paralysis.
- Monitor signs of hypoglycemia, especially during and after exercise. Common neuromuscular symptoms include anxiety; restlessness; tingling in hands, feet, lips, or tongue; chills; cold sweats; confusion; difficulty in concentration; drowsiness; nightmares or trouble sleeping; excessive hunger; headache; irritability; nervousness; tremor; weakness; unsteady gait. Patients with diabetes mellitus should check blood glucose levels frequently.
- Watch for and report signs of impaired renal function, including decreased urine output, cloudy urine, or sudden weight gain due to fluid retention.
- Assess dizziness that might affect gait, balance, and other functional activities (See Appendix C). Report balance problems and functional limitations to the physician, and caution the patient and family/caregivers to guard against falls and trauma.
- Assess body weight periodically and report any substantial weight gains.

Interventions

- Avoid physical therapy interventions that cause systemic vasodilation (large whirlpool, Hubbard tank). Additive effects of this drug and the intervention may cause a dangerous fall in blood pressure.
- To minimize orthostatic hypotension, patient should move slowly when assuming a more upright position.
- Provide a source of oral glucose (fruit juice, glucose gels/tablets, etc.) to treat mild hypoglycemia. Call for emergency assistance if symptoms persist or in cases of severe hypoglycemia. Patients with diabetes mellitus should check blood glucose levels frequently.

Patient/Client-Related Instruction

- Remind patients to take medication as directed to control hypertension and diabetic neuropathy even if they are asymptomatic.
- Counsel patients about additional interventions to help control blood pressure and diabetes mellitus such as regular exercise, weight loss, sodium restriction, stress reduction, moderation of alcohol consumption, and smoking cessation.
- Instruct patient or family/caregivers to report other troublesome side effects such as severe or prolonged headache, insomnia, chest pain, nasal congestion, fever, or GI problems (nausea, diarrhea, abdominal pain, indigestion).

Pharmacokinetics

Absorption: Well absorbed but undergoes extensive first-pass hepatic metabolism, resulting in 33% bioavailability.
Distribution: Crosses the placenta.
Protein Binding: 99%.
Metabolism and Excretion: Undergoes extensive first-pass hepatic metabolism; 14% is converted to an

active metabolite. 4% excreted unchanged in urine; 6% excreted in urine as active metabolite; some biliary elimination also occurs.
Half-life: 2 hr (6–9 hr for metabolite).

TIME/ACTION PROFILE (antihypertensive effect*)

ROUTE	ONSET	PEAK	DURATION
PO	6 hr	3–6 wks	24 hr

*Onset of antihypertensive effect with chronic dosing.

Contraindications/Precautions
Contraindicated in: Hypersensitivity; Bilateral renal artery stenosis; OB: Potential for injury or death of fetus. If pregnancy occurs, discontinue immediately; Lactation: Discontinue drug or use formula.
Use Cautiously in: Volume- or salt-depleted patients or patients receiving high doses of diuretics (correct deficits before initiating therapy or initiate at lower doses); Black patients (reduction in stroke risk may not apply to this patient population); Impaired renal function due to primary renal disease or heart failure (may worsen renal function); Hepatic impairment (lower initial doses recommended); Women of childbearing potential; Pedi: Safety not established for children <6 yr.

Interactions
Drug-Drug: Additive hypotension with other **antihypertensives**. Excessive hypotension may occur with concurrent use of **diuretics**. ↑ risk of hyperkalemia with concurrent use of **potassium supplements, potassium-containing salt substitutes, angiotensin-converting enzyme inhibitors**, or **potassium-sparing diuretics. NSAIDs** and **rifampin** may ↓ antihypertensive effects. May ↑ the effects of **amiodarone, fluoxetine, glimepiride, glipizide, phenytoin, rosiglitazone, sertraline,** and **warfarin**.

Route/Dosage
PO (Adults): *Hypertension*—50 mg once daily initially (range 25–100 mg/day as a single daily dose or 2 divided doses) (initiate therapy at 25 mg once daily in patients who are receiving diuretics or are volume depleted). *Prevention of stroke in patients with hypertension and left ventricular hypertrophy*—50 mg once daily initially; hydrochlorothiazide 12.5 mg once daily should be added and/or dose of losartan increased to 100 mg once daily followed by an increase in hydrochlorothiazide to 25 mg once daily based on blood pressure response; *Nephropathy in patients with type 2 diabetes*—50 mg once daily, may increase to 100 mg once daily depending on blood pressure response.

Hepatic Impairment
PO (Adults): *Patients with hypertension*—25 mg once daily initially; may be increased as tolerated.
PO (Children ≥6 yr): *Hypertension*—0.7 mg/kg once daily (up to 50 mg/day); may be titrated up to 1.4 mg/kg/day (or 100 mg/day).

Renal Impairment
(Children ≥6 yr): *CCr < 30 mL/min*—Contraindicated.

Availability
Tablets: 25 mg, 50 mg, 100 mg. ***In combination with:*** hydrochlorothiazide (HyzaarRx). See Appendix B.

lovastatin (loe-va-sta-tin)
Mevacor

Classification
Therapeutic: lipid-lowering agents
Pharmacologic: HMG CoA reductase inhibitors (statin)

Indications
Adjunctive management of primary hypercholesterolemia and mixed dyslipidemias. Primary prevention of coronary heart disease (myocardial infarction, unstable angina, and coronary revascularization) in asymptomatic patients with increased total and low-density lipoprotein (LDL) cholesterol and decreased high-density lipoprotein (HDL) cholesterol. Slows the progression of coronary atherosclerosis in patients with coronary artery disease.

Action
Inhibits 3-hydroxy-3-methylglutaryl coenzyme A (HMG CoA) reductase, an enzyme which is responsible for catalyzing an early step in the synthesis of cholesterol.
Therapeutic Effects: Lowering of total and LDL cholesterol and triglycerides. Slightly increases HDL cholesterol. Slows the progression of coronary atherosclerosis with resultant decrease in coronary heart disease-related events.

Adverse Reactions/Side Effects
CNS: dizziness, headache, insomnia, weakness. **EENT:** blurred vision. **GI:** abdominal cramps, constipation, diarrhea, flatus, heartburn, altered taste, drug-induced hepatitis, dyspepsia, elevated liver enzymes, nausea, pancreatitis. **GU:** erectile dysfunction. **Derm:** rashes, pruritus. **MS:** RHABDOMYOLYSIS, arthralgia, myalgia, myositis. **Misc:** hypersensitivity reactions.

PHYSICAL THERAPY IMPLICATIONS
Examination and Evaluation
- Assess any joint pain, or muscle pain, tenderness, or weakness, especially if accompanied by fever, malaise, and dark-colored urine. Advise patient that these symptoms may represent drug-induced myopathy, and that myopathy can progress to severe muscle damage (rhabdomyolysis). Report any unexplained musculoskeletal symptoms to the

physician immediately and suspend exercise and gait training until these symptoms can be evaluated.

- Monitor signs of hypersensitivity reactions, including pulmonary symptoms (tightness in the throat and chest, wheezing, cough, dyspnea) or skin reactions (rash, pruritus, urticaria). Notify physician immediately if these reactions occur.

Interventions

- In patients with drug-induced myopathy, implement gradual strengthening and other therapeutic exercises to facilitate recovery from muscle pain and weakness. Use caution during early stages to avoid fatigue of affected muscles, and implement assistive devices (walker, cane, crutches) as needed to prevent falls and assist mobility. Increase exercise intensity as tolerated; recovery from myopathy typically takes 4–6 wk, but can be longer in older patients or people with comorbidities.
- Design and implement aerobic exercise and endurance training programs to improve cardiovascular function and help reduce the risk of coronary heart disease.

Patient/Client-Related Instruction

- Remind patients to take medication as directed to control hyperlipidemia even though they are asymptomatic.
- Counsel patients about additional interventions to help control lipid disorders and improve cardiovascular health, including dietary modification, regular exercise, moderation of alcohol consumption, and smoking cessation.
- Instruct patient to report signs of drug-induced hepatitis (anorexia, abdominal pain, severe nausea and vomiting, yellow skin or eyes, skin rashes, flu-like symptoms) or pancreatitis (upper abdominal pain after eating, indigestion, weight loss, oily stools)
- Instruct patient to report other prolonged or severe GI reactions, including nausea, constipation, diarrhea, heartburn, altered taste, or flatulence.
- Advise patient to consult physician if erectile dysfunction or other sexual problems occur.
- Instruct patient and family/caregivers to report other troublesome side effects such as severe or prolonged headache, sleep loss, blurred vision, or skin reactions (rash, itching).

Pharmacokinetics

Absorption: Poorly and variably absorbed after oral administration.
Distribution: Crosses the blood-brain barrier and placenta.
Metabolism and Excretion: Extensively metabolized by the liver, most during first pass; excreted in bile and feces. 10% excreted unchanged by the kidneys.
Half-life: 3 hr.

TIME/ACTION PROFILE (cholesterol-lowering effect)

ROUTE	ONSET	PEAK	DURATION
PO, PO-ER	2 wk	4–6 wk	6 wk*

*After discontinuation.

Contraindications/Precautions

Contraindicated in: Hypersensitivity; Active liver disease or unexplained persistent elevations in AST & ALT; OB: Pregnancy or lactation.
Use Cautiously in: History of liver disease; Alcoholism; Renal impairment; Concurrent use of gemfibrozil, azole antifungals, protease inhibitors, niacin, cyclosporine, amiodarone, or verapamil (higher risk of myopathy/rhabdomyolysis); Pedi: Children <10 yr (safety not established); Women of childbearing age.

Interactions

Drug-Drug: Cholesterol-lowering effect may be ↑ with **cholestyramine** and **colestipol**, but bioavailability may be ↓. Risk of myopathy is ↑ by concurrent **amiodarone, cyclosporine, gemfibrozil, clofibrate, diltiazem, clarithromycin, telithromycin, erythromycin, danazol** (do not exceed 20 mg lovastatin/day), **nefazodone, amprenavir, nelfinavir, ritonavir, saquinavir**, large doses of **niacin, azole, antifungal agents,** and **verapamil** (combined use with clofibrate or gemfibrozil not recommended; use ↓ doses with cyclosporine, amiodarone, verapamil, niacin). May increase effects of **warfarin**. Levels may be significantly ↑ by **azole antifungals** (temporarily discontinue lovastatin). **Isradipine** may ↓ the effectiveness.
Drug-Natural: St. John's wort may ↓ levels and effectiveness.
Drug-Food: Grapefruit juice ↑ blood levels and the risk of rhabdomyolysis. Food enhances blood levels of lovastatin.

Route/Dosage

PO (Adults): 20 mg once daily with evening meal. Increase at 4-wk intervals to a maximum of 80 mg/day in single or divided doses (initiate at 10 mg/day in patients receiving niacin, cyclosporine, or other immunosuppressants and do not exceed 20 mg/day; should not exceed 40 mg/day if receiving verapamil or amiodarone or 20 mg /day if receiving danazol).

Renal Impairment

PO (Adults): *CCr <30 mL/min*—dosage should not exceed 20 mg/day unless carefully titrated.
PO (Children/Adolescents 10–17 yr): *Familial heterozygous hypercholesterolemia*—10–40 mg/day; adjusted at 4- wk intervals.

Availability

Tablets: 10 mg, 20 mg, 40 mg. **Extended-release tablets:** 10 mg, 20 mg, 40 mg, 60 mg. ***In combination with:*** Niacin (Advicor). See Appendix B.

loxapine (lox-a-peen)

Loxapac, Loxitane, Loxitane C, Loxitane IM

Classification

Therapeutic: antipsychotics

Pharmacologic: tricyclic dibenzoxazepine

Indications

Schizophrenia. Considered second-line treatment after failure of atypical antipsychotic. **Unlabeled Use:** Other psychotic disorders. Bipolar disorder.

Action

Appears to block dopamine and serotonin at postsynaptic receptor sites in the CNS. **Therapeutic Effects:** Diminution of psychotic behavior.

Adverse Reactions/Side Effects

CNS: NEUROLEPTIC MALIGNANT SYNDROME, confusion, dizziness, drowsiness, extrapyramidal reactions, headache, insomnia, syncope, tardive dyskinesia, weakness. **EENT:** blurred vision, lens opacities, nasal congestion. **CV:** orthostatic hypotension, tachycardia. **GI:** constipation, drug-induced hepatitis, dry mouth, ileus, nausea, vomiting. **GU:** urinary retention. **Derm:** dermatitis, edema, facial photosensitivity, pigment changes, rashes, seborrhea. **Endo:** galactorrhea. **Hemat:** AGRANULOCYTOSIS. **Neuro:** ataxia. **Misc:** allergic reactions.

PHYSICAL THERAPY IMPLICATIONS

Examination and Evaluation

- Monitor and report signs of neuroleptic malignant syndrome, including hyperthermia, diaphoresis, generalized muscle rigidity, altered mental status, tachycardia, changes in blood pressure (BP), and incontinence. Symptoms typically occur within 4–14 days after initiation of drug therapy, but can occur at any time during drug use.
- Watch for signs of agranulocytosis, including fever, sore throat, mucosal lesions, and other signs of infection. Report these signs to the physician immediately.
- Assess motor function, and be alert for extrapyramidal symptoms. Report these symptoms immediately, especially tardive dyskinesia, because this problem may be irreversible. Common extrapyramidal symptoms include:
  - Tardive dyskinesia (uncontrolled rhythmic movement of mouth, face, and extremities, lip smacking or puckering, puffing of cheeks, uncontrolled chewing, rapid or worm-like movements of tongue).
  - Pseudoparkinsonism (shuffling gait, rigidity, tremor, pill-rolling motion, loss of balance control, difficulty speaking or swallowing, mask-like face).
  - Akathisia (restlessness or desire to keep moving).
  - Other dystonias and dyskinesias (dystonic muscle spasms, twisting motions, twitching, inability to move eyes, weakness of arms or legs).
- Assess heart rate, ECG, and heart sounds, especially during exercise (See Appendices G, H). Report a rapid heart rate (tachycardia) or signs of other arrhythmias, including palpitations, chest discomfort, shortness of breath, fainting, and fatigue/weakness.
- Assess BP when patient assumes a more upright position (lying to standing, sitting to standing, lying to sitting). Document orthostatic hypotension and contact physician when systolic BP falls >20 mm Hg or diastolic BP falls >10 mm Hg.
- Monitor signs of allergic reactions, including pulmonary symptoms (tightness in the throat and chest, wheezing, cough, dyspnea) or skin reactions (rash, pruritus, urticaria). Notify physician immediately if these reactions occur.
- Assess dizziness, drowsiness, and ataxia that might affect gait, balance, and other functional activities (See Appendix C). Report balance problems and functional limitations to the physician and nursing staff, and caution the patient and family/caregivers to guard against falls and trauma.

Interventions

- Guard against falls and trauma (hip fractures, head injury, and so forth) caused by drowsiness, ataxia, blurred vision, or extrapyramidal symptoms; implement fall- prevention strategies (See Appendix E).
- Because of the risk of tachycardia and abnormal BP responses, use caution during aerobic exercise and other forms of therapeutic exercise. Assess exercise tolerance frequently (BP, heart rate, fatigue levels), and terminate exercise immediately if any untoward responses occur (See Appendix L).
- To minimize orthostatic hypotension, patient should move slowly when assuming a more upright position.
- Causes photosensitivity; use care if administering UV treatments. Advise patient to avoid direct sunlight and use sunscreens and protective clothing.
- Help patient and family/caregivers explore nonpharmacologic methods such as exercise, counseling, and support groups to reduce schizophrenic episodes and behavioral problems.

Patient/Client-Related Instruction

- Advise patient to avoid alcohol and other CNS depressants because of the increased risk of sedation and adverse effects.
- Advise patient about the likelihood of GI problems such as nausea, vomiting, constipation, and dry mouth. Instruct patient to report severe or prolonged GI reactions, and to also report signs of drug-induced hepatitis, including anorexia, abdominal pain, severe nausea and vomiting, yellow skin or eyes, skin rashes, flu-like symptoms, and muscle/joint pain.
- Instruct patient to report other problematic side effects such as severe or prolonged headache, sleep loss, dry eyes, nasal congestion, visual disturbances, nipple discharge, urinary retention, or skin reactions (rash, skin discoloration, dermatitis, oily discharge).

Pharmacokinetics

Absorption: Well absorbed after IM administration; bioavailability with oral administration is approximately 30%.
Distribution: Unknown.
Metabolism and Excretion: Extensively metabolized by the liver; some conversion to active antipsychotic compounds.
Half-life: *PO*—3–4 hr; *IM*—12 hr.

TIME/ACTION PROFILE (antipsychotic effect)

ROUTE	ONSET	PEAK	DURATION
PO, IM	30 min	1.5–3 hr	12 hr

Contraindications/Precautions

Contraindicated in: Hypersensitivity or intolerance to loxapine or amoxapine; Coma; CNS depression; OB: Safety not established; weigh potential benefit against possible risks to fetus; Lactation: Discontinue loxapine or bottle-feed.
Use Cautiously in: Glaucoma; Intestinal obstruction; History of seizures; Alcoholism; Cardiovascular disease; Impaired liver function; Geriatric men or men with prostatic hyperplasia (more prone to urinary retention); Geri: More susceptible to adverse reactions; ↑ risk of mortality in elderly patients treated for dementia-related psychosis; Pedi: Children <16 yr (safety not established).

Interactions

Drug-Drug: ↓ the antihypertensive effects of **guanadrel**. Blocks the alpha-adrenergic effects of **epinephrine** (may result in hypotension and tachycardia). Additive CNS depression with other **CNS depressants**, including **alcohol, antihistamines, opioid analgesics**, and **sedative/hypnotics**. **Antacids** or **adsorbent antidiarrheals** may ↓ absorption. Use with **antidepressants** or **MAO inhibitors** may result in prolonged CNS depression and ↑ anticholinergic effects.
Drug-Natural: Concomitant use of **kava, valerian, skullcap, chamomile**, or **hops** can ↑ CNS depression.

Route/Dosage

PO (Adults): 10 mg bid, may be increased gradually over the first 7–10 days as needed and tolerated. Usual maintenance dose is 60–100 mg/day.
IM (Adults): 12.5–50 mg q 4–6 hr as needed and tolerated; some patients respond to twice daily dosing.

Availability

Capsules: 5 mg, 10 mg, 25 mg, 50 mg. **Tablets:** 5 mg, 10 mg, 25 mg, 50 mg. **Oral concentrate:** 25 mg/mL. **Injection:** 50 mg/mL.

L

lurasidone (loo-ras-i-done)

Latuda

Classification
Therapeutic: antipsychotics
Pharmacologic: benzoisothiazole

Indications

Treatment of schizophrenia.

Action

Effect may mediated via effects on central dopamine type 2 (D_2) and serotonin type 2 ($5HT_{2A}$) receptor antagonism. **Therapeutic Effects:** ↓ schizophrenic behavior.

Adverse Reactions/Side Effects

CNS: NEUROLEPTIC MALIGNANT SYNDROME, SEIZURES, akathisia, drowsiness, parkinsonism, agitation, anxiety, cognitive/motor impairment, dizziness, dystonia, tardive dyskinesia. **EENT:** blurred vision. **CV:** bradycardia, orthostatic hypotension, syncope, tachycardia. **GI:** nausea, esophageal dysmotility. **Derm:** pruritus, rash. **Endo:** hyperglycemia, hyperprolactinemia. **Hemat:** AGRANULOCYTOSIS, anemia, leukopenia. **Metab:** dyslipidemia, weight gain

PHYSICAL THERAPY IMPLICATIONS

Examination and Evaluation

- Be alert for new seizures or increased seizure activity, especially at the onset of drug treatment. Document the number, duration, and severity of seizures, and report these findings immediately to the physician.
- Monitor and report signs of neuroleptic malignant syndrome, including hyperthermia, diaphoresis,

generalized muscle rigidity, altered mental status, tachycardia, changes in blood pressure (BP), and incontinence. Symptoms typically occur within 4–14 days after initiation of drug therapy, but can occur at any time during drug use.

- Watch for signs of agranulocytosis and leukopenia (fever, sore throat, mucosal lesions, other signs of infection) or unusual weakness and fatigue that might be due to anemia. Report these signs to the physician immediately.
- Assess motor function, and be alert for extrapyramidal symptoms. Report these symptoms immediately, especially tardive dyskinesia, because this problem may be irreversible. Common extrapyramidal symptoms include:
  - Tardive dyskinesia (uncontrolled rhythmic movement of mouth, face, and extremities, lip smacking or puckering, puffing of cheeks, uncontrolled chewing, rapid or worm-like movements of tongue).
  - Pseudoparkinsonism (shuffling gait, rigidity, tremor, pill-rolling motion, loss of balance control, difficulty speaking or swallowing, mask-like face).
  - Akathisia (restlessness or desire to keep moving).
  - Other dystonias and dyskinesias (dystonic muscle spasms, twisting motions, twitching, inability to move eyes, weakness of arms or legs).
- Assess heart rate, ECG, and heart sounds, especially during exercise (See Appendices G, H). Report any rhythm disturbances or symptoms of increased arrhythmias, including palpitations, chest discomfort, shortness of breath, fainting, and fatigue/weakness.
- Assess BP when patient assumes a more upright position (lying to standing, sitting to standing, lying to sitting). Document orthostatic hypotension and contact physician when systolic BP falls >20 mm Hg or diastolic BP falls >10 mm Hg.
- Monitor behavioral changes such as anxiety, agitation, and cognitive/motor impairment. Notify physician if these changes become problematic.
- Assess dizziness, drowsiness, and syncope that might affect gait, balance, and other functional activities (See Appendix C). Report balance problems and functional limitations to the physician, and caution the patient and family/caregivers to guard against falls and trauma.
- Watch for signs of hyperglycemia, including drowsiness, fruity breath, increased urination, and unusual thirst. Patients with diabetes mellitus should check blood glucose levels frequently.
- Periodically assess body weight and other anthropometric measures (body mass index, body composition). Report a rapid or substantial weight gain or increased body fat.

Interventions

- Guard against falls and trauma (hip fractures, head injury, and so forth) caused by drowsiness, dizziness, blurred vision, or extrapyramidal symptoms; implement fall prevention strategies (See Appendix E).
- Because of the risk of arrhythmias and blood dyscrasias, use caution during aerobic exercise and other forms of therapeutic exercise Assess exercise tolerance frequently (BP, heart rate, fatigue levels), and terminate exercise immediately if any untoward responses occur (See Appendix L).
- To minimize orthostatic hypotension, patient should move slowly when assuming a more upright position.
- Help patient and family/caregivers explore nonpharmacologic methods (exercise, counseling, support groups) to reduce schizophrenic episodes and behavioral problems.

Patient/Client-Related Instruction

- Advise patient to avoid alcohol and other CNS depressants because of the increased risk of sedation and adverse effects.
- Advise patient that this drug may cause problems in fat and glucose metabolism (hyperlipidemia and hyperglycemia, respectively). Remind patient that periodic blood tests may be needed to monitor plasma lipids and blood glucose.
- Instruct patient to report other problematic side effects such as severe or prolonged blurred vision, skin reactions (rash, itching), or GI problems (nausea, indigestion, gastroesophageal reflux)

Pharmacokinetics

Absorption: 9–19% absorbed following oral administration.
Distribution: Unknown
Protein Binding: >99%
Metabolism and Excretion: Mostly metabolized by the CYP3A4 enzyme system. Two metabolites are pharmacologically active; 80% eliminated in feces, 8% in urine primarily as metabolites
Half-life: 18 hr

TIME/ACTION PROFILE

ROUTE	ONSET	PEAK	DURATION
PO	unknown	1–3 hr*	24 hr

*Blood level.

Contraindications/Precautions

Contraindicated in: Hypersensitivity.
Use Cautiously in: Renal/hepatic impairment (dose adjustment recommended for CCr of 10 mL/min–<50 mL/min or Child-Pugh Classes B and C); History of suicide attempt; Diabetes mellitus; Overheating/dehydration

(may ↑ risk of serious adverse reactions); History of leukopenia or previous drug-induced leukopenia/neutropenia; Geri: ↑ risk of seizures; elderly patients with dementia-related psychoses (↑ risk of cerebrovascular adverse reactions); use cautiously in elderly females (↑ risk of tardive dyskinesia); OB: Use in pregnancy only if potential benefit justifies potential risk to fetus; Lactation: breast-feeding should only be considered if potential benefit justifies risk to child; Pedi: Safe and effective use in children has not been established.

Interactions

Drug-Drug: Strong inhibitors of the CYP3A4 enzyme system, including **ketoconazole**; ↑ blood levels and risk of adverse reactions; concurrent use should be avoided; **Moderate inhibitors of the CYP3A4 enzyme system**, including **diltiazem**, ↑ blood levels; if used concurrently, dose of lurasidone should not exceed 40 mg/day; **Strong inducers of the CYP3A4 enzyme system**, including **rifampin**, ↓ blood levels and effectiveness; concurrent use should be avoided; ↑ sedation may occur with other **CNS depressants**, including **alcohol, sedative/hypnotics, opioids**, some **antidepressants**, and **antihistamines.**

Route/Dosage

PO (Adults): 40 mg once daily; not to exceed 80 mg once daily. *Concurrent use of moderate CYP3A4 inhibitors*—dose should not exceed 40 mg once daily.

Renal Impairment

PO (Adults): *CCr of 10 mL/min–<50 mL/min*—dose should not exceed 40 mg once daily.

Hepatic Impairment

PO (Adults): *Child-Pugh Classes B and C*—dose should not exceed 40 mg once daily.

Availability

Tablets: 40 mg, 80 mg.

HIGH ALERT

lymphocyte immune globulin

(lim-foe-site im-**myoon** **glob**-yoo-lin)

ATG, antilymphocyte globulin, Atgam, LIG

Classification

Therapeutic: immunosuppressants

Pharmacologic: immune globulins

Indications

Management of allograft rejection in renal transplant patients. Treatment of aplastic anemia in patients who are not candidates for bone marrow transplantation.

Action

Decreases the circulating number of T lymphocytes, which are involved in both cell-mediated and humoral immunity. **Therapeutic Effects:** Resolution of rejection of renal allografts. Remission of aplastic anemia.

Adverse Reactions/Side Effects

CNS: headache. **Resp:** dyspnea. **CV:** chest pain, hypotension. **GI:** diarrhea, nausea, stomatitis, vomiting. **Derm:** dermatologic reactions, erythema, itching. **Hemat:** leukopenia, thrombocytopenia, anemia, hemolysis. **Local:** pain/phlebitis at IV site. **MS:** arthralgia. **Misc:** ALLERGIC REACTIONS, INCLUDING ANAPHYLAXIS, chills, fever, serum sickness–like reactions, clotted AV fistula, night sweats.

PHYSICAL THERAPY IMPLICATIONS

Examination and Evaluation

- Be alert for signs of allergic reactions and anaphylaxis, including pulmonary symptoms (tightness in the throat and chest, wheezing, cough, dyspnea) or skin reactions (rash, pruritus, urticaria). Notify physician or nursing staff immediately if these reactions occur.
- Monitor signs of serum sickness–like reactions, including muscle aches, joint pains, fever, and skin rash. Notify physician or nursing staff immediately if these reactions occur.
- Monitor signs of leukopenia (fever, sore throat, signs of infection), thrombocytopenia (bruising, nose bleeds, and bleeding gums), or unusual weakness and fatigue that might be due to anemia or other blood dyscrasias. Report these signs to the physician or nursing staff.
- Assess blood pressure periodically and compare to normal values (See Appendix F). Report low blood pressure (hypotension), especially if patient experiences dizziness, fatigue, or other symptoms.
- Assess any joint pain to rule out musculoskeletal pathology; that is, try to determine if pain is drug-induced rather than caused by arthritis or anatomic and biomechanical problems.
- Monitor IV injection site for pain, swelling, and irritation. Report prolonged or excessive injection site reactions to the physician.

Patient/Client-Related Instruction

- Because of immunosuppressant effects, advise patient to guard against infection (frequent hand washing, etc.), and to avoid crowds and contact with persons with contagious diseases.

- Instruct patient to report other untoward side effects such as severe or prolonged headache, chest pain, difficulty breathing, chills, fever, night sweats, skin reactions (rash, redness, warmth, itching), or GI problems (diarrhea, nausea, vomiting, inflammation in/around the mouth).

Pharmacokinetics

Absorption: IV administration results in complete bioavailability.

Distribution: Unknown.

Metabolism and Excretion: Unknown.

Half-life: 5.7 days.

TIME/ACTION PROFILE (decreased circulating T lymphocytes)

ROUTE	ONSET	PEAK	DURATION
IV	rapid	unknown	unknown

Contraindications/Precautions

Contraindicated in: History of hypersensitivity during previous courses of therapy or systemic reaction to skin testing; Hypersensitivity to thimerosal; Hypersensitivity to equine gamma globulin preparations.

Use Cautiously in: Pregnancy or lactation (safety not established).

Interactions

Drug-Drug: Concurrent use of **corticosteroids** and **immunosuppressants** may mask some adverse reactions.

Route/Dosage

Skin Test

Intradermal (Adults): 0.1 mL of 1:1000 dilution (5 mcg of horse serum).

Renal Allograft Recipients

IV (Adults): 10–30 mg/kg/day for 14 days, then every other day for 14 days.

IV (Children): 5–25 mg/kg/day for 14 days, then every other day for 14 days.

Aplastic Anemia

IV (Adults): 10–20 mg/kg/day for 8–14 days, then every other day for 21 doses total.

Availability

Injection: 50 mg/mL.

magnesium salicylate
(mag-**neez**-ee-um sal-**is**-il-ate)
🍁 Doan's Backache Pills, Doan's Regular Strength Tablets, Magan, Mobidin

Classification
Therapeutic: antipyretics, nonopioid analgesics
Pharmacologic: salicylates

Indications

Inflammatory disorders, including Rheumatoid arthritis, Osteoarthritis. Mild-to-moderate pain. Fever.

Action

Produce analgesia and reduce inflammation and fever by inhibiting the production of prostaglandins.
Therapeutic Effects: Analgesia. Reduction of inflammation. Reduction of fever.

Adverse Reactions/Side Effects

EENT: tinnitus. **GI:** GI BLEEDING, dyspepsia, epigastric distress, nausea, abdominal pain, anorexia, hepatotoxicity, vomiting. **Misc:** ALLERGIC REACTIONS, INCLUDING ANAPHYLAXIS AND LARYNGEAL EDEMA.

PHYSICAL THERAPY IMPLICATIONS

Examination and Evaluation

- Monitor signs of GI bleeding, including abdominal pain, vomiting blood, blood in stools, or black, tarry stools. Report these signs to the physician immediately.
- Monitor signs of allergic reactions and anaphylaxis, including pulmonary symptoms (laryngeal edema, wheezing, cough, dyspnea) or skin reactions (rash, pruritus, urticaria). Notify physician immediately if these reactions occur. Allergic reactions are more common in people with asthma, nasal polyps, or aspirin-induced allergies.
- Be alert for signs of liver toxicity, including abdominal pain, severe nausea and vomiting, yellow skin or eyes, loss of appetite, skin rashes, flu-like symptoms, and muscle/joint pain. Report these signs to the physician immediately.
- Assess pain and other variables (range of motion, muscle strength) to document whether this drug is successful in helping manage the patient's pain and decrease impairments.

Interventions

- Implement appropriate manual therapy techniques, physical agents, and therapeutic exercises to reduce pain and decrease the need for salicylates and other NSAIDs.
- Help patient explore other nonpharmacologic methods to reduce chronic pain, such as relaxation techniques, exercise, counseling, and so forth.

Patient/Client-Related Instruction

- Advise patient that analgesics are usually more effective if given before pain becomes severe; emphasize that adequate pain control will allow better participation in physical therapy.
- Caution patient about the use of over-the-counter products that contain aspirin, other NSAIDs, or acetaminophen while taking high doses of salicylates. Use of multiple NSAIDs increases the risk of toxicity and overdose.
- Advise patient about the risks of gastric irritation. Instruct patient to notify physician of GI effects such as severe or prolonged nausea, heartburn, indigestion, abdominal pain, vomiting, and loss of appetite.
- Advise patient to reduce alcohol intake because alcohol increases the risk of gastric toxicity.
- Inform patient that salicylates and other NSAIDs may impair bone and cartilage healing. Advise patient to consult physician about salicylate use, especially after fractures, spinal fusion, and other bone surgeries.
- Instruct patient to report excessive or prolonged headache or ringing/buzzing in the ears (tinnitus); these signs may indicate salicylate toxicity.

Pharmacokinetics

Absorption: Well absorbed after oral administration.
Distribution: Rapidly and widely distributed; crosses the placenta and enter breast milk.
Metabolism and Excretion: Extensively metabolized by the liver; inactive metabolites excreted by the kidneys. Amount excreted unchanged by the kidneys depends on urine pH; as pH increases, amount excreted unchanged increases from 2–3% up to 80%.
Half-life: 2–3 hr for low doses; up to 15–30 hr with larger doses because of saturation of liver metabolism.

TIME/ACTION PROFILE

ROUTE	ONSET	PEAK	DURATION
PO	5–30 min	1–3 hr	3–6 hr

Contraindications/Precautions

Contraindicated in: Hypersensitivity to aspirin or other salicylates; Cross-sensitivity with other NSAIDs may exist (less with nonaspirin salicylates); Children or adolescents with viral infections (may increase the risk of Reye's syndrome).
Use Cautiously in: History of GI bleeding or ulcer disease; Chronic alcohol use/abuse; Severe renal disease

(magnesium toxicity may occur); Severe hepatic disease; Geriatric patients (↑ risk of adverse reactions especially GI bleeding; more sensitive to toxic levels); OB: Salicylates may have adverse effects on fetus and mother and in general should be avoided during pregnancy, especially during the 3rd trimester; Lactation: Safety not established.

Interactions

Drug-Drug: May ↑ activity of **penicillins, phenytoin, methotrexate, valproic acid, oral hypoglycemic agents**, and **sulfonamides**. May ↓ beneficial effects of **probenecid** or **sulfinpyrazone**. **Urinary acidification** ↑ reabsorption and may ↑ serum salicylate levels. **Alkalinization of the urine** or the ingestion of large amounts of **antacids** ↑ excretion and ↓ serum salicylate levels. May blunt the therapeutic response to **diuretics** or other **antihypertensives**. ↑ risk of GI irritation with **NSAIDs**.

Drug-Food: Foods capable of acidifying the urine may ↑ serum salicylate levels.

Route/Dosage

PO (Adults): 304 mg q 4 hr or 467 mg q 6 hr.

Availability

Tablets: 304 mg OTC, 467 mg OTC, 545 mg, 600 mg, 650 mg.

malathion (ma-la-thye-on)

Ovide

Classification

Therapeutic: pediculocides

Pharmacologic: acetylcholinesterase inhibitor

Indications

Treatment of head lice and their eggs (*Pediculus humanus capitus*).

Action

Acts as a cholinesterase inhibitor, causing death of lice and their eggs. **Therapeutic Effects:** Eradication of head lice and their eggs.

Adverse Reactions/Side Effects

EENT: ocular irritation (with accidental eye exposure). **Derm:** scalp irritation.

PHYSICAL THERAPY IMPLICATIONS

Examination and Evaluation

- Monitor the scalp for local irritation or inflammation. Report severe or prolonged scalp reactions to the physician.

Interventions

- Avoid touching the affected area. Use care to wash hands thoroughly, change pillowcases, and disinfect equipment (whirlpools, electrotherapeutic devices, treatment tables, and so forth) to help prevent the spread of head lice.

Patient/Client-Related Instruction

- Check that the patient and family or caregivers understand topical application procedures and adhere to the recommended dosing schedule.
- Caution patient and family/caregivers about avoiding accidental contact with the eyes. If this occurs, eyes should be flushed thoroughly with water. Health care professional should be contacted if eye irritation persists.
- Instruct patient about proper hygiene; e.g., do not share combs or hair brushes, thoroughly wash hats or clothing that may be infested, and so forth.

Pharmacokinetics

Absorption: Minimal absorption (<10%) with topical application.

Distribution: Binds to hair shaft, which may protect against reinfestation.

Metabolism and Excretion: Metabolized to malaoxon and excreted.

Half-life: 8 hr.

TIME/ACTION PROFILE (pediculicidal effect)

ROUTE	ONSET[†]	PEAK	DURATION
Topical	6 hr	12 hr	persists after application*

*Due to binding to hair shaft.

Contraindications/Precautions

Contraindicated in: Hypersensitivity; Known alcohol intolerance.

Use Cautiously in: Pregnancy (use only if needed); lactation (use cautiously, safety not established); children <2 yr (safety not established).

Interactions

Drug-Drug: These interactions would only occur if large amounts of malathion were absorbed. Additive toxicity may occur with **carbamate** or **organophosphate-type insecticides/pesticides**. May cause additive respiratory depression with parenteral **aminoglycosides**. ↑ risk of systemic toxicity with **ester-type local anesthetics**, **antimyasthenics**, or **cholinesterase inhibitors** (including ophthalmics). May alter the response to **edrophonium** in patients with myasthenic weakness.

Route/Dosage

Topical (Adults and Children ≥2 yr): Apply lotion to dry hair and rub until scalp is moistened; follow 8–12 hr later with nonmedicated shampoo; additional application may be required after 7–9 days.

Availability

Lotion: 0.5% in 59-mL bottles (contains 78% isopropyl alcohol, terpineol, dipentene, and pine needle oil).

maraviroc (ma-rav-i-rok)
Selzentry

Classification
Therapeutic: antiretrovirals
Pharmacologic: chemokine receptor antagonist

Indications
HIV infection (with other antiretrovirals), specifically in patients with only CCR5-tropic HIV-1 detectable, with evidence of viral replication and HIV-1 strains displaying multiple resistance to other antiretrovirals. Use should be determined by treatment history and tropism testing.

Action
Blocks a specific receptor on CD-4 and T-cell surfaces which prevents CCR5-tropic HIV-1 from entering. **Therapeutic Effects:** Decreased invasion of CD-4 and T-cells by CCR5-tropic HIV-1 virus resulting in viral replication.

Adverse Reactions/Side Effects
CNS: dizziness. **Resp:** cough, upper respiratory tract infection. **GI:** abdominal pain, appetite disorder, HEPATOTOXICITY. **Derm:** RASH. **MS:** musculoskeletal pain. **Misc:** ALLERGIC REACTIONS, fever, immune reconstitution syndrome, ↑ risk of infection.

PHYSICAL THERAPY IMPLICATIONS

Examination and Evaluation
- Be alert for signs of liver toxicity, including anorexia, abdominal pain, severe nausea and vomiting, yellow skin or eyes, fever, sore throat, malaise, weakness, facial edema, lethargy, and unusual bleeding or bruising. Report these signs to the physician or nursing staff immediately.
- Monitor signs of allergic reactions, including pulmonary symptoms (tightness in the throat and chest, wheezing, dyspnea) or skin reactions (rash, pruritus, urticaria). Notify physician or nursing staff immediately if these reactions occur.
- Be alert for signs of an unusually aggressive immune reaction to opportunistic infection (immune reconstitution syndrome). Signs include fever, pain, warmth and redness and swelling at the site of infection. Notify physician of these signs immediately.
- Assess for signs of upper respiratory tract infection, including cough, fever, difficulty breathing, shortness of breath, increased sputum production, and malaise/fatigue. Report these signs to the physician or nursing staff.
- Assess any musculoskeletal pain, muscle tenderness, or weakness, especially if accompanied by fever, malaise, and dark-colored urine. These symptoms may represent drug-induced myopathy, and advise the patient that myopathy can progress to severe muscle damage (rhabdomyolysis). Report any unexplained musculoskeletal symptoms to the physician immediately.
- Assess dizziness that might affect gait, balance, and other functional activities (See Appendix C). Report balance problems and functional limitations to the physician and nursing staff, and caution the patient and family/caregivers to guard against falls and trauma.

Interventions
- Implement resistive exercises and other therapeutic exercises as tolerated to maintain muscle strength and function and prevent muscle wasting associated with HIV infection and AIDS.

Patient/Client-Related Instruction
- Emphasize the importance of taking maraviroc as directed even if the patient is asymptomatic, and that this drug must always be used in combination with other antiretroviral drugs. Do not take more than prescribed amount, and do not stop taking without consulting health care professional.
- Inform patient that maraviroc does not cure HIV or AIDS or prevent associated or opportunistic infections. Maraviroc does not reduce the risk of transmission of HIV to others through sexual contact or blood contamination. Caution patient to use a condom, and to avoid sharing needles or donating blood to prevent spreading the AIDS virus to others.
- Advise patient to guard against infection (frequent hand washing, etc.), and to avoid crowds and contact with persons with contagious diseases.
- Instruct patient to report other troublesome GI side effects such as prolonged or severe abdominal pain or loss of appetite.

Pharmacokinetics
Absorption: 2–33% absorbed following oral administration.
Distribution: Unknown.
Metabolism and Excretion: Mostly metabolized by the liver (CYP3A enzyme system); 8% renal excretion as unchanged drug.
Half-life: 14–18 hr.

TIME/ACTION PROFILE (blood levels)

ROUTE	ONSET	PEAK	DURATION
PO	unknown	0.5–4 hr	1–2 hr

M

Contraindications/Precautions

Contraindicated in: Dual/mixed or CXCR4-tropic HIV-1; OB: Lactation (breast-feeding not recommended for HIV-infected patients).

Use Cautiously in: Preexisting liver disease, including Hepatitis B or C (may ↑ risk of hepatotoxicity); Cardiovascular disease or risk factors (↑ risk of cardiovascular events); Hepatic impairment; Renal impairment (if CCr <50 mL/min and using a CYP3A inhibitor use only if necessary); Treatment-naive adults (safety/efficacy not established); Geri: Consider age-related ↓ in renal/hepatic function, concurrent drug therapy, and concomitant disease; OB: Use only if clearly needed; Pedi: Safe use in children <16 yr not established.

Interactions

Drug-Drug: Levels are ↑ by **CYP3A inhibitors,** including **protease inhibitors** (excluding tipranavir/ritonavir), **delavirdine, ketoconazole, lopinavir/ritonavir, saquinavir,** and **atazanavir.** Levels are ↓ by **CYP3A inducers,** including **efavirenz** and **rifampin.**

Route/Dosage

PO (Adults): *Concurrent CYP3A inhibitors (except tipranavir/ritonavir) or delavirdine*—150 mg bid; *Concurrent NRTIs, tipranavir/ritonavir, nevirapine, and other drugs that are not strong inhibitors/inducers of CYP3A*—300 mg bid; *Concurrent CYP3A inducers including efavirenz*—600 mg bid.

Availability

Tablets: 150 mg, 300 mg.

mecasermin (me-**kaz**-er-men)

Increlex

Classification

Therapeutic: hormones

Pharmacologic: growth hormones

Indications

Long-term treatment of growth failure in children due to primary insulin-like growth factor-1 (IGF) deficiency or growth hormone gene deletion with antibodies to growth hormone.

Action

Under normal conditions, growth hormone attaches to receptors resulting in increased production of IGF-1. IGF-1 stimulates uptake of glucose, fatty acids, and amino acids which support tissue growth. These processes signal and support statural growth. **Therapeutic Effects:** Replacement of IGF-1 in deficiency states resulting in achievement of optimal potential statural growth.

Adverse Reactions/Side Effects

CNS: SEIZURES, dizziness, headache, intracranial hypertension. **Resp:** tonsillar hypertrophy, snoring. **GI:** vomiting. **Endo:** HYPOGLYCEMIA. **Local:** bruising, lipohypertrophy. **MS:** arthralgia, extremity pain. **Misc:** thymus hypertrophy.

PHYSICAL THERAPY IMPLICATIONS

Examination and Evaluation

- Be alert for new seizures or increased seizure activity, especially at the onset of drug treatment. Document the number, duration, and severity of seizures, and report these findings to the physician immediately.
- Monitor signs of hypoglycemia, especially during and after exercise. Common neuromuscular symptoms include anxiety; restlessness; tingling in hands, feet, lips, or tongue; chills; cold sweats; confusion; difficulty in concentration; drowsiness; nightmares or trouble sleeping; excessive hunger; headache; irritability; nervousness; tremor; weakness; and unsteady gait. Report repeated or severe episodes of hypoglycemia to the physician.
- Periodically assess height and weight in children to help document the effects of drug therapy.
- Be alert for signs of intracranial hypertension, including headache, dizziness, ringing in the ears, nausea, vomiting, pain in the neck/back/shoulders, and vision disturbances (blurred vision, double vision, flashes of light, brief periods of blindness). Notify physician of these signs immediately.
- Assess any joint pain or extremity pain to rule out musculoskeletal pathology; that is, try to determine if pain is drug induced rather than caused by anatomic or biomechanical problems.
- Monitor subcutaneous injection site for bruising or increased fat accumulation (lipohypertrophy). Report prolonged or excessive injection site reactions to the physician.

Interventions

- Design and implement therapeutic exercise programs to capitalize on growth hormone effects and increase muscle strength and function in children.
- Do not apply physical agents (heat, cold, electrotherapeutic modalities) or massage over the injection site; these interventions can alter drug absorption from subcutaneous tissues.
- Provide a source of oral glucose (fruit juice, glucose gels/tablets, etc.) to treat mild hypoglycemia. Call for emergency assistance if symptoms persist or in cases of severe hypoglycemia. Emergency treatment typically consists of IV glucose, glucagon, or epinephrine.

Patient/Client-Related Instruction

- Instruct patient to report other bothersome side effects such as severe or prolonged headache, dizziness, vomiting, or problems related to tonsillar hypertrophy (snoring, difficulty breathing).

Pharmacokinetics
Absorption: Well absorbed following SC administration.
Distribution: Bound to various binding proteins.
Metabolism and Excretion: Some metabolism in liver and kidney.
Half-life: 5.8 hr.

TIME/ACTION PROFILE (blood levels)

ROUTE	ONSET	PEAK	DURATION
SC	rapid	3 hr	12 hr

Contraindications/Precautions
Contraindicated in: Hypersensitivity; Contains benzyl alcohol, avoid in neonates; Closed epiphyses; Active/suspected neoplasia.
Use Cautiously in: Adults or children <2 yr (safety not established); Pregnancy/lactation (safety not established).

Interactions
Drug-Drug: None noted.

Route/Dosage
Subcut (Children): 0.04–0.08 mg/kg twice daily; may be increased weekly by 0.04 mg/kg/dose up to 0.12 mg/kg twice daily.

Availability
Solution for injection: 10 mg/mL in 4-mL vials.

mechlorethamine
(me-klor-**eth**-a-meen)
Mustargen

OTHER NAMES:
Nitrogen mustard

Classification
Therapeutic: antineoplastics
Pharmacologic: alkylating agents

Indications
Part of combination therapy of Hodgkin's disease and malignant lymphomas. Used palliatively in Bronchogenic carcinoma, Leukemias. Administered into cavities (pleural, peritoneal) to prevent reaccumulation of malignant effusions.

Action
Interferes with DNA and RNA synthesis by cross-linking strands (cell-cycle phase–nonspecific). **Therapeutic Effects:** Death of rapidly replicating cells, particularly malignant ones.

Adverse Reactions/Side Effects
CNS: SEIZURES, drowsiness, headache, vertigo, weakness. **GI:** nausea, vomiting, anorexia, diarrhea. **GU:** infertility. **Derm:** rashes, alopecia. **Hemat:** LEUKOPENIA, THROMBOCYTOPENIA, anemia. **Local:** tissue necrosis, phlebitis at IV site. **Metab:** hyperuricemia. **Misc:** reactivation of herpes zoster.

PHYSICAL THERAPY IMPLICATIONS

Examination and Evaluation
- Be alert for new seizures or increased seizure activity. Document the number, duration, and severity of seizures, and report these findings to the physician or nursing staff immediately.
- Monitor signs of leukopenia (fever, sore throat, signs of infection), thrombocytopenia (bruising, nose bleeds, bleeding gums), or unusual weakness and fatigue that might be due to anemia. Report these signs to the physician or nursing staff immediately.
- Assess balance and risk of falls, especially if patient exhibits vertigo or excessive weakness or drowsiness (See Appendix E). Report balance problems and functional limitations to the physician and nursing staff, and caution the patient and family/caregivers to guard against falls and trauma.
- Monitor IV injection site for pain, phlebitis, and local tissue necrosis. Report injection site reactions to the physician or nursing staff.

Interventions
- For patients who are medically able to begin exercise, implement appropriate resistive exercises and aerobic training to maintain muscle strength and aerobic capacity during cancer chemotherapy or to help restore function after chemotherapy.

Patient/Client-Related Instruction
- Advise patient to guard against infection (frequent hand washing, etc.), and to avoid crowds and contact with persons with contagious diseases.
- Instruct patient to report other bothersome side effects such as severe or prolonged headache, skin reactions (rash, hair loss, reactivation of herpes zoster lesions), or GI problems (nausea, vomiting, diarrhea, loss of appetite).

Pharmacokinetics
Absorption: Administered IV and intracavitary only. Some absorption occurs after intracavitary instillation.
Distribution: Unknown.
Metabolism and Excretion: Rapidly degraded in body tissues and fluids.

M

Half-life: Unknown.

TIME/ACTION PROFILE (effects on blood counts)

ROUTE	ONSET	PEAK	DURATION
WBCs	24 hr	7–14 days	10–21 days
platelets	unknown	9–16 days	20 days

Contraindications/Precautions

Contraindicated in: Hypersensitivity; Pregnancy; Lactation.

Use Cautiously in: Infections; Decreased bone marrow reserve; Previous radiotherapy or chemotherapy (dose reduction required); Obesity or severe edema (dose should be based on ideal dry body weight); Geri: Geriatric patients or patients with chronic debilitating illnesses; Patients with childbearing potential.

Interactions

Drug-Drug: ↑ myelosuppression with other **antineoplastics** or **radiation therapy**. May ↓ antibody response to **live-virus vaccines** and ↑ risk of adverse reactions.

Route/Dosage

IV (Adults and Children): 0.4 mg/kg as single dose or divided over 2–4 days (not to exceed 0.2–0.3 mg/kg in patients who have received previous chemotherapy or radiation therapy); *as part of MOPP regimen for Hodgkin's lymphoma in adults*—6 mg/m^2 on days 1 and 8 of 28-day cycle; doses in subsequent cycles are determined by blood counts.

Intracavitary: (Adults): 0.4 mg/kg.

Intrapericardial: (Adults): 0.2 mg/kg.

Availability

Injection: 10-mg vials.

meclizine (mek-li-zeen)

Antivert, Antrizine, Bonamine, Bonine, Dramamine Less Drowsy Formula, Meni-D, Vergon

Classification

Therapeutic: antiemetics, antihistamines

Pharmacologic: piperazines

Indications

Management/prevention of Motion sickness, Vertigo.

Action

Has central anticholinergic, CNS depressant, and antihistaminic properties. Decreases excitability of the middle ear labyrinth and depresses conduction in middle ear vestibular-cerebellar pathways. **Therapeutic Effects:** Decreased motion sickness. Decreased vertigo from vestibular pathology.

Adverse Reactions/Side Effects

CNS: drowsiness, fatigue. **EENT:** blurred vision. **GI:** dry mouth.

PHYSICAL THERAPY IMPLICATIONS

Examination and Evaluation

- Monitor any improvements in symptoms (nausea, vomiting, dizziness, vertigo) to help document the effects of this drug.

Interventions

- Guard against falls and trauma (hip fractures, head injury, and so forth). Implement fall prevention strategies, especially in older adults or if balance is impaired (See Appendix E).
- In patients with chronic vertigo, implement therapeutic exercise and vestibular training activities to help reduce symptoms.

Patient/Client-Related Instruction

- Advise patient about the risk of daytime drowsiness and decreased attention and mental focus. These problems can be severe in certain people. Use care if driving or in other activities that require quick reactions and strong concentration.
- Advise patient to avoid alcohol and other CNS depressants because of the increased risk of sedation and adverse effects.
- Instruct patient to report other troublesome side effects including severe or prolonged fatigue, dry mouth, or blurred vision.

Pharmacokinetics

Absorption: Absorbed after oral administration.

Distribution: Unknown.

Metabolism and Excretion: Unknown.

Half-life: 6 hr.

TIME/ACTION PROFILE (antihistaminic effects)

ROUTE	ONSET	PEAK	DURATION
PO	1 hr	unknown	8–24 hr

Contraindications/Precautions

Contraindicated in: Hypersensitivity; Pregnancy.

Use Cautiously in: Prostatic hyperplasia; Angle-closure glaucoma; Geriatric (increased sensitivity; increased risk of adverse reactions); Children or lactation (safety not established).

Interactions

Drug-Drug: Additive CNS depression with other **CNS depressants**, including **alcohol**, other **antihistamines**, **opioid analgesics**, and **sedative/hypnotics**. Additive anticholinergic effects with other **drugs possessing anticholinergic properties**, including some **antihistamines**, **antidepressants**, **atropine**, **haloperidol**, **phenothiazines**, **quinidine**, and **disopyramide**.

Route/Dosage

PO (Adults): *Motion sickness*—25–50 mg 1 hr before exposure; may repeat in 24 hr; *vertigo*—25–100 mg/day in divided doses.

Availability

Tablets: 12.5 mg, 25 mg Rx, OTC, 50 mg. **Chewable tablets:** 25 mg Rx, OTC. **Capsules:** 15 mg OTC, 25 mg, 30 mg OTC.

meclofenamate

(me-kloe-**fen**-am-ate)

Meclomen

Classification

Therapeutic: antirheumatics, nonopioid analgesics

Pharmacologic: fenamate

Indications

Management of mild-to-moderate pain, including rheumatoid arthritis, osteoarthritis, dysmenorrhea. Management of excessive menstrual flow.

Action

Inhibits prostaglandin synthesis. **Therapeutic Effects:** Suppression of pain and inflammation.

Adverse Reactions/Side Effects

CNS: dizziness, headache, drowsiness. **EENT:** tinnitus, visual disturbances. **CV:** edema. **GI:** GI BLEEDING, DRUG-INDUCED HEPATITIS, diarrhea, dyspepsia, nausea, vomiting, anorexia, constipation, discomfort, flatulence, stomatitis. **GU:** renal failure. **Derm:** hives, itching. **Hemat:** blood dyscrasias. **Misc:** ALLERGIC REACTIONS, INCLUDING ANAPHYLAXIS AND STEVENS-JOHNSON SYNDROME, drug-induced systemic lupus erythematosus–like syndrome.

PHYSICAL THERAPY IMPLICATIONS

Examination and Evaluation

- Monitor signs of GI bleeding, including abdominal pain, vomiting blood, blood in stools, or black, tarry stools. Report these signs to the physician immediately.
- Be alert for signs of drug-induced hepatitis, including anorexia, abdominal pain, severe nausea and vomiting, yellow skin or eyes, skin rashes, flu-like symptoms, and muscle/joint pain. Report these signs to the physician immediately.
- Monitor signs of allergic reactions and anaphylaxis, including pulmonary symptoms (laryngeal edema, wheezing, cough, dyspnea) or skin reactions (rash, pruritus, urticaria). Be especially alert for exfoliation, dermatitis, and other severe skin reactions that might indicate serious hypersensitivity reactions (Stevens-Johnson syndrome, toxic epidermal necrolysis). Notify physician immediately if these reactions occur.
- Assess pain and other variables (range of motion, muscle strength) to document whether this drug is successful in helping manage the patient's pain and decreasing impairments.
- Assess blood pressure (BP) periodically and compare to normal values (See Appendix F). NSAIDs can increase BP in certain patients.
- Be alert for signs of prolonged bleeding time such as bleeding gums, nosebleeds, and unusual or excessive bruising. Report these signs to the physician.
- Monitor unusual weakness and fatigue that might be due to anemia or other symptoms such as fever, sore throat, mucosal lesions, or signs of infection that might be due to other blood dyscrasias. Notify physician if these signs occur.
- Assess peripheral edema using girth measurements, volume displacement, and measurement of pitting edema (See Appendix N). Report increased swelling in feet and ankles or a sudden increase in body weight due to fluid retention.
- Monitor signs of drug-induced lupus syndrome, including increased BP, fever, joint pain, skin rashes, and redness/irritation of the eye (uveitis). Notify physician promptly if these signs appear.
- Monitor signs of kidney dysfunction such as painful urination or blood in the urine. Report signs of renal failure immediately, including decreased urine output, increased BP, muscle cramps/twitching, edema/weight gain from fluid retention, yellowish brown skin, and confusion that progresses to seizures and coma.
- Assess dizziness and drowsiness that might affect gait, balance, and other functional activities (See Appendix C). Report balance problems and functional limitations to the physician, and caution the patient and family/caregivers to guard against falls and trauma.

Interventions

- Implement appropriate manual therapy techniques, physical agents, and therapeutic exercises to reduce pain and decrease the need for meclofenamate and other NSAIDs.
- If treating arthritic conditions, recommend orthotic and assistive devices as needed to reduce pain, improve function, and augment the effects of drug therapy.
- Use caution with any physical interventions that could increase bleeding, including wound

débridement, chest percussion, joint mobilization, and application of local heat.
- Help patient explore other nonpharmacologic methods to reduce chronic pain, such as relaxation techniques, exercise, counseling, and so forth.

Patient/Client-Related Instruction

- Advise patient that analgesics are usually more effective if given before pain becomes severe; emphasize that adequate pain control will allow better participation in physical therapy.
- Inform patient that NSAIDs may impair bone and cartilage healing. Advise patient to consult physician about NSAID use, especially after fractures, spinal fusion, and other bone surgeries.
- Caution patient about the use of over-the-counter products that contain NSAIDs or acetaminophen while taking prescription doses of meclofenamate. Use of multiple NSAIDs increases the risk of toxicity and overdose.
- Instruct patient to report excessive or prolonged headache or ringing/buzzing in the ears (tinnitus); these signs may indicate drug toxicity.
- Advise patient about the risks of gastric irritation. Instruct patient to notify physician of GI reactions such as severe or prolonged nausea, vomiting, constipation, diarrhea, indigestion, flatulence, inflammation in/around the mouth, and loss of appetite.
- Advise patient to reduce alcohol intake because alcohol increases the risk of gastric toxicity.
- Instruct patient and family/caregivers to report other troublesome side effects such as severe or prolonged vision disturbances or skin reactions (hives, itching).

Pharmacokinetics

Absorption: Well absorbed from the GI tract.
Distribution: Unknown.
Protein Binding: >99%.
Metabolism and Excretion: Metabolized by the liver; some active metabolites.
Half-life: 40 min–2 hr.

TIME/ACTION PROFILE

ROUTE	ONSET	PEAK	DURATION
PO (analgesic)	within 1 hr	unknown	4–6 hr
PO (anti-inflammatory)	days	2–3 wk	days

Contraindications/Precautions

Contraindicated in: Hypersensitivity; Cross-sensitivity may occur with other NSAIDs, including aspirin; Active GI bleeding or ulcer disease.
Use Cautiously in: Severe cardiovascular, renal, or hepatic disease; History of ulcer disease; Pregnancy, lactation, or children <14 yr (safety not established; avoid use during 2nd half of pregnancy).

Interactions

Drug-Drug: Concurrent use with **aspirin** may ↓ meclofenamate blood levels and may ↓ effectiveness. May ↑ risk of bleeding with **thrombolytic agents, cefoperazone, cefotetan, valproic acid, clopidogrel, ticlopidine, eptifibatide**, and **tirofiban**. Additive adverse GI side effects with **aspirin, alcohol, corticosteroids, potassium supplements**, and other **NSAIDs**. **Probenecid** ↑ blood levels and may ↑ toxicity. Chronic use with **acetaminophen** or **gold compounds** may increase the risk of adverse renal reactions. May ↓ the effectiveness of **antihypertensives** or **diuretics**. May ↑ hypoglycemia from **oral hypoglycemic agents** or **insulins**. ↑ risk of hematologic adverse reactions with **antineoplastics** or **radiation therapy**. May ↑ blood levels and toxicity from **lithium** or **methotrexate**. ↑ risk of nephrotoxicity with **cyclosporine**.
Drug-Natural: ↑ bleeding risk with **anise, arnica, chamomile, clove, feverfew, garlic, ginger, ginkgo, *Panax ginseng***, and others.

Route/Dosage

PO (Adults): *Anti-inflammatory*—200–400 mg/day in 3–4 divided doses. *Analgesic*—50–100 mg q 4–6 hr (not to exceed 400 mg/day). *Dysmenorrhea/excessive menstrual flow*—100 mg 3 times daily for up to 6 days or until cessation of menses.

Availability (generic available)

Capsules: 50 mg, 100 mg.

medroxyprogesterone

(me-**drox**-ee-proe-**jess**-te-rone)
Alti-MPA, Amen, Curretab, Cycrin, Depo-Provera, Depo-Sub Q Provera 104, Gen-Medroxy, Novo-Medrone, Provera, Provera Pak, Ratio-MPA

Classification

Therapeutic: antineoplastics, contraceptive hormones
Pharmacologic: hormones, progestins

Indications

To decrease endometrial hyperplasia in postmenopausal women receiving concurrent estrogen (0.625 mg/day conjugated estrogens). Treatment of secondary amenorrhea and abnormal uterine bleeding caused by hormonal imbalance. **IM:** Treatment of advanced unresponsive endometrial or renal carcinoma; Management of endometriosis-associated pain (Depo-Sub Q Provera 104 only). **Unlabeled Use:** Obesity-hypoventilation (pickwickian) syndrome, sleep apnea, hypersomnolence.

Action

A synthetic form of progesterone—actions include secretory changes in the endometrium, increases in basal body temperature, histologic changes in vaginal epithelium, relaxation of uterine smooth muscle, mammary alveolar tissue growth, pituitary inhibition, and withdrawal bleeding in the presence of estrogen. **Therapeutic Effects:** Decreased endometrial hyperplasia in postmenopausal women receiving concurrent estrogen (combination with estrogen decreases vasomotor symptoms and prevents osteoporosis). Restoration of hormonal balance with control of uterine bleeding. Management of endometrial or renal cancer. Prevention of pregnancy.

Adverse Reactions/Side Effects

CNS: depression. **EENT:** retinal thrombosis. **CV:** PULMONARY EMBOLISM, thromboembolism, thrombophlebitis. **GI:** drug-induced hepatitis, gingival bleeding. **GU:** cervical erosions. **Derm:** chloasma, melasma, rashes. **Endo:** amenorrhea, breakthrough bleeding, breast tenderness, changes in menstrual flow, galactorrhea, hyperglycemia, spotting. **F and E:** edema. **Metab:** bone loss. **Misc:** ALLERGIC REACTIONS, INCLUDING ANAPHYLAXIS AND ANGIOEDEMA, weight gain, weight loss.

PHYSICAL THERAPY IMPLICATIONS

Examination and Evaluation

- Monitor signs of thrombophlebitis (localized pain, swelling, warmth, erythema, tenderness) and pulmonary embolism (shortness of breath, chest pain, cough, bloody sputum). Notify physician immediately, and request objective tests (Doppler ultrasound, lung scan, others) if thromboembolism is suspected.
- Monitor signs of allergic reactions including anaphylaxis and angioedema. Signs include pulmonary symptoms (tightness in the chest and throat, wheezing, cough, dyspnea) or skin reactions (rash, pruritus, urticaria, swelling in the face). Notify physician immediately if these reactions occur.
- Assess peripheral edema using girth measurements, volume displacement, and measurement of pitting edema (See Appendix N). Report increased swelling in feet and ankles or a sudden increase in body weight due to fluid retention.
- Report signs of drug-induced hepatitis, including anorexia, abdominal pain, severe nausea and vomiting, yellow skin or eyes, skin rashes, flu-like symptoms, and muscle/joint pain.
- Monitor and report depression or other changes in mood and behavior.
- Periodically assess body weight and other anthropometric measures (body mass index, body composition). Report a rapid or sustained weight loss or gain, or a substantial change in lean body mass.

Interventions

- Because of the risk of thromboembolism, use caution during aerobic exercise and other forms of therapeutic exercise. Assess exercise tolerance frequently (blood pressure, heart rate, fatigue levels), and terminate exercise immediately if any untoward responses occur (See Appendix L).
- Institute weight-bearing and resistance exercises as tolerated to maintain bone mineral density and minimize bone loss.

Patient/Client-Related Instruction

- Caution patient and family/caregivers about risks of thromboembolism, and review warning signs of a pulmonary embolism (sudden shortness of breath, dyspnea, bloody sputum, cough).
- Caution patient that cigarette smoking may increase the risk of infarction and thromboembolic disease, especially for women older than 35.
- Advise women about possible changes in menstrual function. Instruct patient to notify the physician about any abnormal bleeding.
- Instruct patient to report other troublesome side effects such as visual problems, bleeding gums, or skin disorders (rash, discoloration).

Pharmacokinetics

Absorption: 0.6–10% absorbed after oral administration.
Distribution: Enters breast milk.
Metabolism and Excretion: Metabolized by the liver.
Half-life: *1st phase*—52 min; *2nd phase*—230 min; *biological*—14.5 hr.

TIME/ACTION PROFILE (IM = antineoplastic effects)

ROUTE	ONSET	PEAK	DURATION
PO	unknown	unknown	unknown
IM	wks–mos	Mo	unknown*
SC	unknown	1 wk	3 mo

*Contraceptive effect lasts 3 mo.

Contraindications/Precautions

Contraindicated in: Hypersensitivity; Hypersensitivity to parabens (IM suspension only); Pregnancy; Missed abortion; Thromboembolic disease; Cerebrovascular disease; Severe liver disease; Breast or genital cancer; Porphyria.
Use Cautiously in: History of liver disease; Renal disease; Cardiovascular disease; Seizure disorders; Mental depression; Lactation: Lactation (when used as a contraceptive, wait until 6 wk after delivery if breastfeeding).

Interactions

Drug-Drug: May ↓ effectiveness of **bromocriptine** when used concurrently for galactorrhea/amenorrhea. Contraceptive effectiveness may be ↓ by **carbamazepine**, **phenobarbital**, **phenytoin**, **rifampin**, or **rifabutin**. **Aminoglutethimide** may ↓ oral absorption.

Route/Dosage

Postmenopausal Women Receiving Concurrent Estrogen

PO (Adults): 2.5–5 mg daily concurrently with 0.625 mg conjugated estrogens (monophasic regimen) *or* 5 mg daily on days 15–28 of the cycle with 0.625 mg conjugated estrogens taken daily throughout cycle (biphasic regimen).

Secondary Amenorrhea

PO (Adults): 5–10 mg/day for 5–10 days; start at any time in cycle.

Dysfunctional Uterine Bleeding/Induction of Menses

PO (Adults): 5–10 mg/day for 5–10 days, starting on day 16 or day 21 of menstrual cycle.

Renal or Endometrial Carcinoma

IM (Adults): 400–1000 mg, may be repeated weekly; if improvement occurs, attempt to decrease dosage to 400 mg monthly.

Endometriosis-associated pain

SC (Adults): 104 mg every 12–14 wk (3 mo), beginning on day 5 of normal menses (not recommended for more than 2 years).

Availability (generic available)

Tablets: 2.5 mg, 5 mg, 10 mg, 100 mg. **Suspension for depot injection:** 50 mg/mL, 100 mg/mL, 150 mg/mL, 400 mg/mL. **Suspension for subcutaneous injection (Depo-Sub Q Provera 104):** 104 mg/0.65 mL in single-use syringes. ***In combination with:*** conjugated estrogens as Prempro (single combination tablet of 0.626 mg conjugated estrogens plus 2.5 or 5 mg medroxyprogesterone) or Premphase (0.625 mg conjugated estrogens tablet for 14 days followed by combination tablet of 0.625 mg conjugated estrogens plus 5 mg medroxyprogesterone for days 15–28) in convenience packages.
See Appendix B.

megestrol (me-jes-trole)

Megace

Classification

Therapeutic: antineoplastics, hormones
Pharmacologic: progestins

Indications

Palliative treatment of endometrial and breast carcinoma, either alone or with surgery or radiation (tablets only). Treatment of anorexia, weight loss, and cachexia associated with AIDS (oral suspension only).

Action

Antineoplastic effect may result from inhibition of pituitary function. **Therapeutic Effects:** Regression of tumor. Increased appetite and weight gain in patients with AIDS.

Adverse Reactions/Side Effects

CV: THROMBOEMBOLISM, edema. **GI:** GI irritation. **Derm:** alopecia. **Endo:** asymptomatic adrenal suppression (chronic therapy). **Hemat:** thrombophlebitis. **MS:** carpal tunnel syndrome.

PHYSICAL THERAPY IMPLICATIONS

Examination and Evaluation

- Monitor signs of thrombophlebitis (localized pain, swelling, warmth, erythema, tenderness) and pulmonary embolism (shortness of breath, chest pain, cough, bloody sputum). Notify physician immediately, and request objective tests (Doppler ultrasound, lung scan, others) if thromboembolism is suspected.
- Assess peripheral edema using girth measurements, volume displacement, and measurement of pitting edema (See Appendix N). Report increased swelling in feet and ankles or a sudden increase in body weight due to fluid retention.
- Assess signs of carpal tunnel syndrome, and implement physical therapy interventions (physical agents, exercise, splinting, and so forth) to decrease symptoms. Periodically reevaluate condition with sensory and motor tests to help document treatment effects.

Interventions

- Because of the risk of thromboembolism, use caution during aerobic exercise and other forms of therapeutic exercise. Assess exercise tolerance frequently (blood pressure, heart rate, fatigue levels), and terminate exercise immediately if any untoward responses occur (See Appendix L).
- If treating weight loss and debilitation in people with AIDS, implement strengthening and conditioning exercises as tolerated.

Patient/Client-Related Instruction

- Caution patient and family/caregivers about risks of thromboembolism, and review warning signs of a pulmonary embolism (sudden shortness of breath, dyspnea, bloody sputum, cough).
- Caution patient that cigarette smoking may increase the risk of infarction and thromboembolic disease, especially for women older than 35.

- Instruct patient to report other troublesome side effects such as GI irritation or hair loss.

Pharmacokinetics

Absorption: Well absorbed from the GI tract.
Distribution: Unknown.
Protein Binding: ≥90%.
Metabolism and Excretion: Completely metabolized by the liver.
Half-life: 38 hr (range 13–104 hr).

TIME/ACTION PROFILE (antineoplastic activity)

ROUTE	ONSET	PEAK	DURATION
PO	wks–mos	2 mo	unknown

Contraindications/Precautions

Contraindicated in: Hypersensitivity; OB: Pregnancy, missed abortion, or lactation; Undiagnosed vaginal bleeding; Severe liver disease; Suspension contains alcohol and should be avoided in patients with known intolerance.
Use Cautiously in: Diabetes; Mental depression; Renal disease; History of thrombophlebitis; Cardiovascular disease; Seizure disorders.

Interactions

Drug-Drug: None significant.

Route/Dosage

PO (Adults): *Breast carcinoma*—160 mg/day single dose or divided doses; *endometrial/ovarian carcinoma*—40–320 mg/day in divided doses; *anorexia associated with AIDS*—800 mg day; may decrease to 400 mg/day after 1 mo (range 400–800 mg/day).

Availability (generic available)

Tablets: 20 mg, 40 mg. **Oral suspension (lemon-lime flavor):** 40 mg/mL in 10-mL, 20-mL, 240-mL, and 480-mL bottles, 125 mg/mL in 150-mL bottles (Megace ES).

meloxicam (me-lox-i-kam)

Mobic

Classification
Therapeutic: nonsteroidal anti-inflammatory agents
Pharmacologic: nonopioid analgesics

Indications

Relief of signs and symptoms of osteoarthritis and rheumatoid arthritis (including juvenile rheumatoid arthritis).

Action

Inhibits prostaglandin synthesis, probably by inhibiting the enzyme cyclooxygenase. **Therapeutic Effects:** Decreased pain and inflammation associated with osteoarthritis. Also decreases fever.

Adverse Reactions/Side Effects

CV: edema. **GI:** GI BLEEDING, abnormal liver function tests, diarrhea, dyspepsia, nausea. **Derm:** EXFOLIATIVE DERMATITIS, STEVENS-JOHNSON SYNDROME, TOXIC EPIDERMAL NECROLYSIS, pruritus. **Hemat:** anemia, leukopenia, thrombocytopenia.

PHYSICAL THERAPY IMPLICATIONS

Examination and Evaluation

- Watch for signs of GI bleeding, including abdominal pain, vomiting blood, blood in stools, or black, tarry stools. Report these signs to the physician immediately.
- Monitor rashes or other skin reactions (itching, hives, acne, abnormal sweating, exfoliation). Notify physician immediately because certain skin reactions may indicate serious hypersensitivity reactions such as Stevens-Johnson syndrome or toxic epidermal necrolysis.
- Assess pain and other variables (range of motion, muscle strength) to document whether this drug is successful in helping manage the patient's pain and decreasing impairments.
- Monitor signs of leukopenia (fever, sore throat, signs of infection), thrombocytopenia (bruising, nose bleeds, bleeding gums), or unusual weakness and fatigue that might be due to anemia. Report these signs to the physician.
- Assess blood pressure (BP) periodically and compare to normal values (See Appendix F). NSAIDs can increase BP and promote hypertension in certain patients.
- Assess peripheral edema using girth measurements, volume displacement, and measurement of pitting edema (See Appendix N). Report increased swelling in feet and ankles or a sudden increase in body weight due to fluid retention.

Interventions

- Implement appropriate manual therapy techniques, physical agents, and therapeutic exercises to reduce pain and decrease the need for meloxicam and other NSAIDs.
- If treating arthritic conditions, recommend orthotic and assistive devices as needed to reduce pain, improve function, and augment the effects of drug therapy.
- Help patient explore other nonpharmacologic methods to reduce chronic pain, such as relaxation techniques, exercise, counseling, and so forth.

Patient/Client-Related Instruction

- Advise patient that analgesics are usually more effective if given before pain becomes severe;

M

emphasize that adequate pain control will allow better participation in physical therapy.

- Inform patient that NSAIDs may impair bone and cartilage healing. Advise patient to consult physician about NSAID use, especially after fractures, spinal fusion, and other bone surgeries.
- Caution patient about the use of over-the-counter products that contain NSAIDs or acetaminophen while taking prescription doses of meloxicam. Use of multiple NSAIDs increases the risk of toxicity and overdose.
- Advise patient about the risks of gastric irritation. Instruct patient to notify physician of GI reactions such as severe or prolonged nausea, diarrhea, and indigestion.
- Advise patient to reduce alcohol intake because alcohol increases the risk of gastric toxicity.

Pharmacokinetics

Absorption: Well absorbed following oral administration.
Distribution: Unknown.
Protein Binding: 99.4%.
Metabolism and Excretion: Mostly metabolized to inactive metabolites by the liver via the P450 enzyme system; metabolites are excreted in urine and feces.
Half-life: 20.1 hr.

TIME/ACTION PROFILE

ROUTE	ONSET	PEAK*	DURATION
PO	unknown	5–6 hr	24 hr

*Blood levels.

Contraindications/Precautions

Contraindicated in: Hypersensitivity; Cross-sensitivity may occur with other NSAIDs, including aspirin; Severe renal impairment (CCr ≤15 mL/min); Concurrent use of aspirin (increased risk of adverse reactions); Perioperative pain from coronary artery bypass graft (CABG) surgery.
Use Cautiously in: Cardiovascular disease or risk factors for cardiovascular disease (may ↑ risk of serious cardiovascular thrombotic events, myocardial infarction, and stroke, especially with prolonged use); Dehydration (correct deficits before initiating therapy); Geri: Impaired renal function, heart failure, liver dysfunction, geriatric patients (≥65 yr), concurrent ACE inhibitor, or diuretic therapy (↑ risk of reversible renal dysfunction); Coagulation disorders or concurrent anticoagulant therapy (may ↑ risk of bleeding); Geri: Geriatric patients (↑ risk of GI bleeding); OB/Pedi: Pregnancy, lactation, or children <2 yr (safety not established; avoid use late in pregnancy).

Interactions

Drug-Drug: May ↓ antihypertensive effects of **ACE inhibitors**. May ↓ diuretic effects of **furosemide** or **thiazide diuretics**. Concurrent use with **aspirin** ↑ meloxicam blood levels and may ↑ risk of adverse reactions. Concurrent use with **cholestyramine** ↓ blood levels. ↑ plasma **lithium** levels (close monitoring recommended when meloxicam is introduced or withdrawn). May ↑ risk of bleeding with **anticoagulants**, including **warfarin**.

Route/Dosage

PO (Adults): 7.5 mg once daily; some patients may require 15 mg/day.
PO (Children 2–17 yr and >12 kg): 0.125 mg/kg once daily up to 7.5 mg/day.

Availability (generic available)

Tablets: 7.5 mg, 15 mg. **Oral suspension (raspberry flavor):** 7.5 mg/5 mL in 100-mL bottles.

melphalan (mel-fa-lan)

Alkeran, L-PAM

OTHER NAMES:
phenylalanine mustard

Classification
Therapeutic: antineoplastics
Pharmacologic: alkylating agents

Indications

Alone or with other therapies for Multiple myeloma, Ovarian cancer. **Unlabeled Use:** Breast cancer. Prostate cancer. Testicular carcinoma. Chronic myelogenous leukemia. Osteogenic sarcoma.

Action

Inhibits DNA and RNA synthesis by alkylation (cell-cycle phase–nonspecific). **Therapeutic Effects:** Death of rapidly replicating cells, particularly malignant ones. Also has immunosuppressive properties.

Adverse Reactions/Side Effects

Resp: bronchopulmonary dysplasia, pulmonary fibrosis. **GI:** diarrhea, hepatitis, nausea, stomatitis, vomiting. **GU:** infertility. **Derm:** alopecia, pruritus, rashes. **Endo:** menstrual irregularities. **Hemat:** leukopenia, thrombocytopenia, anemia. **Metab:** hyperuricemia. **Misc:** ALLERGIC REACTIONS, INCLUDING ANAPHYLAXIS (MORE COMMON AFTER IV USE).

PHYSICAL THERAPY IMPLICATIONS

Examination and Evaluation

- Monitor signs of allergic reactions or anaphylaxis, including pulmonary symptoms (tightness in the throat and chest, wheezing, cough, dyspnea) or skin reactions (rash, pruritus, urticaria). Notify physician or nursing staff immediately if these reactions occur.
- Assess pulmonary function periodically by measuring lung volumes, breath sounds, and respiratory

rate (See Appendices I, J, K). Notify physician immediately if patient experiences signs of pulmonary fibrosis or bronchopulmonary dysplasia (dry cough, dyspnea, chest pain, shortness of breath, abnormal breath sounds, cyanosis).

- Watch for signs of leukopenia (fever, sore throat, signs of infection), thrombocytopenia (bruising, nose bleeds, bleeding gums), or unusual weakness and fatigue that might be due to anemia. Report these signs to the physician or nursing staff.

Interventions

- For patients who are medically able to begin exercise, implement appropriate resistive exercises and aerobic training to maintain muscle strength and aerobic capacity during cancer chemotherapy or to help restore function after chemotherapy.
- Because of the risk of pulmonary fibrosis, use caution during aerobic exercise and other forms of therapeutic exercise. Assess exercise tolerance frequently (blood pressure, heart rate, fatigue levels), and terminate exercise immediately if any untoward responses occur (See Appendix L).

Patient/Client-Related Instruction

- Advise patient to guard against infection (frequent hand washing, etc.), and to avoid crowds and contact with persons with contagious diseases.
- Advise patient about the likelihood of GI reactions such as nausea, vomiting, diarrhea, loss of appetite, and irritation in or around the mouth. Instruct patient to report severe or prolonged GI reactions, and to also report signs of drug-induced hepatitis, including abdominal pain, severe nausea and vomiting, yellow skin or eyes, fever, sore throat, malaise, weakness, facial edema, lethargy, and unusual bleeding or bruising.
- Advise patient that hair loss and other skin reactions (rash, pruritus) are likely. Report severe or unexpected skin reactions to the physician.
- Advise women about possible changes in menstrual function. Instruct patient to notify health care professional about any severe or prolonged menstrual irregularities.

Pharmacokinetics

Absorption: Incompletely and variably absorbed following oral administration.
Distribution: Rapidly distributed throughout total body water.
Protein Binding: ≤30%.
Metabolism and Excretion: Rapidly metabolized in the bloodstream. Small amounts (10%) excreted unchanged by the kidneys.
Half-life: 1.5 hr.

TIME/ACTION PROFILE (effects on blood counts)

ROUTE	ONSET	PEAK	DURATION
PO	5 days	2–3 wk	5–6 wk

Contraindications/Precautions

Contraindicated in: Hypersensitivity to melphalan or chlorambucil; Pregnancy or lactation.
Use Cautiously in: Patients with childbearing potential; Active infections; Decreased bone marrow reserve; Geri: Geriatric patients or patients with other chronic debilitating illnesses; Impaired renal function (dose reduction recommended if BUN ≥30 mg/dL); Pedi: Children (safety not established).

Interactions

Drug-Drug: ↑ bone marrow depression with other **antineoplastics** or **radiation therapy**. May ↓ antibody response to **live-virus vaccines** and ↑ risk of adverse reactions. May ↑ the risk of pulmonary toxicity with **carmustine**. Concurrent IV use with **cyclosporine** may ↑ risk of renal failure. Risk of enterocolitis may be ↑ with concurrent **nalidixic acid**.

Route/Dosage

Multiple Myeloma

PO (Adults): 150 mcg (0.15 mg)/kg/day for 7 days, followed by 3-wk rest, then 50 mcg (0.05 mg)/kg/day maintenance dose *or* 100–150 mcg/kg/day or 250 mg (0.25 mg)/kg/day for 4 days followed by 2- to 4-wk rest, then 2–4 mg/day maintenance dose *or* 7 mg/m^2 *or* 250 mcg (0.25 mg)/kg daily for 5 days q 5–6 wk.
IV (Adults): 16 mg/m^2 q 2 wk for 4 doses, then q 4 wk.

Ovarian Carcinoma

PO (Adults): 200 mcg (0.2 mg)/kg/day for 5 days q 4–5 wk.

Availability

Tablets: 2 mg. **Powder for injection:** 50 mg.

memantine (me-man-teen)

Namenda

Classification
Therapeutic: anti-Alzheimer's agents
Pharmacologic: N-methyl-D-aspartate antagonist

Indications

Moderate-to-severe Alzheimer's dementia.

Action

Binds to CNS N-methyl-D-aspartate (NMDA) receptor sites, preventing binding of glutamate, an excitatory neurotransmitter. **Therapeutic Effects:** Decreased symptoms of dementia. Does not slow progression. Cognitive enhancement. Does not cure disease.

Adverse Reactions/Side Effects

CNS: dizziness, fatigue, headache, sedation. **CV:** hypertension. **Derm:** rash. **GI:** weight gain. **GU:** urinary frequency. **Hemat:** anemia.

PHYSICAL THERAPY IMPLICATIONS

Examination and Evaluation

- Assess blood pressure (BP) and compare to normal values (See Appendix F). Report a sustained increase in BP (hypertension).
- Monitor signs of anemia, including unusual fatigue, shortness of breath with exertion, pallor, and bruising. Notify physician if these signs occur.
- Assess dizziness and drowsiness that might affect gait, balance, and other functional activities (See Appendix C). Report balance problems and functional limitations to the physician and nursing staff, and caution the patient and family/caregivers to guard against falls and trauma.
- Periodically assess body weight and other anthropometric measures (body mass index, body composition). Report a substantial weight gain or increased body fat.

Interventions

- Guard against falls and trauma (hip fractures, head injury, and so forth) caused by drowsiness, dizziness, or other drugs; implement fall prevention strategies (See Appendix E).
- Help patient and family/caregivers explore nonpharmacologic methods to reduce combative episodes and mood disorders (exercise, structured activities, validation therapies, and so forth).

Patient/Client-Related Instruction

- Instruct patient and family/caregivers to report other bothersome side effects such as severe or prolonged headache, skin rash, or urinary frequency.

Pharmacokinetics

Absorption: Well absorbed after oral administration.
Distribution: Unknown.
Metabolism and Excretion: 57–82% excreted unchanged in urine by active tubular secretion moderated by pH- dependent tubular reabsorption. Remainder metabolized; metabolites are not pharmacologically active.
Half-life: 60–80 hr.

TIME/ACTION PROFILE (blood levels)

ROUTE	ONSET	PEAK	DURATION
PO	unknown	3–7 hr	12 hr

Contraindications/Precautions

Contraindicated in: Severe renal impairment.
Use Cautiously in: Moderate renal impairment (consider ↓ dose); Concurrent use of other NMDA antagonists (amantadine, rimantadine, ketamine, dextromethorphan); Concurrent use of drugs or diets that cause alkaline urine; Conditions that ↑ urine pH including severe urinary tract infections or renal tubular acidosis (lead to ↓ excretion and ↑ levels); OB/Lactation/Pedi: Safety not established. Discontinue drug or bottle-feed.

Interactions

Drug-Drug: Medications that ↑ urine pH lead to ↓ excretion and ↑ blood levels (**carbonic anhydrase inhibitors, sodium bicarbonate**).

Route/Dosage

PO (Adults): 5 mg once daily initially, increased at weekly intervals to 10 mg/day (5 mg bid), then 15 mg/day (5 mg once daily, 10 mg once daily as separate doses), then to target dose of 20 mg/day (as 10 mg bid).

Availability

Tablets: 5 mg, 10 mg, titration package containing 28 5-mg tablets and 21 10-mg tablets. **Oral solution, sugar-free, alcohol-free (peppermint):** 2 mg/mL in 360-mL bottles.

HIGH ALERT

meperidine (me-per-i-deen)

Demerol

OTHER NAMES:
Pethidine

Classification
Therapeutic: opioid analgesics
Pharmacologic: opioid agonists

Schedule II

Indications

Moderate or severe pain (alone or with nonopioid agents). Anesthesia adjunct, analgesic during labor, preoperative sedation. **Unlabeled Use:** Rigors.

Action

Binds to opiate receptors in the CNS. Alters the perception of and response to painful stimuli, while producing generalized CNS depression. **Therapeutic Effects:** Decrease in severity of pain.

Adverse Reactions/Side Effects

CNS: SEIZURES, confusion, sedation, dysphoria, euphoria, floating feeling, hallucinations, headache, unusual dreams. **EENT:** blurred vision, diplopia, miosis. **Resp:** respiratory depression. **CV:** hypotension, bradycardia. **GI:** constipation, nausea, vomiting. **GU:** urinary retention. **Derm:** flushing, sweating.

Misc: physical dependence, psychologic dependence, tolerance.

PHYSICAL THERAPY IMPLICATIONS

Examination and Evaluation

- Be alert for new seizures or increased seizure activity, especially at the onset of drug treatment. Document the number, duration, and severity of seizures, and report these findings immediately to the physician.
- Assess symptoms of respiratory depression, including decreased respiratory rate, confusion, bluish color of the skin and mucous membranes (cyanosis), and difficult, labored breathing (dyspnea). Monitor pulse oximetry and perform pulmonary function tests (See Appendix I) to quantify suspected changes in ventilation and respiratory function. Excessive respiratory depression requires emergency care.
- Be alert for excessive sedation or changes in mood and behavior (euphoria, dysphoria, confusion, hallucinations). Notify physician or nurse immediately if patient is unconscious or extremely difficult to arouse.
- Use appropriate pain scales (visual analogue scales, others) to document whether this drug is successful in helping manage the patient's pain.
- Assess blood pressure periodically and compare to normal values (See Appendix F). Report low blood pressure (hypotension), especially if patient experiences dizziness, fainting, or other symptoms.
- Assess heart rate, ECG, and heart sounds, especially during exercise (See Appendices G, H). Report slow heart rate (bradycardia) or symptoms of other arrhythmias, including palpitations, chest discomfort, shortness of breath, fainting, and fatigue/weakness.

Interventions

- Implement appropriate manual therapy techniques, physical agents, and therapeutic exercises to reduce pain and help wean patient off opioid analgesics as soon as possible.
- Because of the risk of respiratory depression, bradycardia, and hypotension, use caution during aerobic exercise and other forms of therapeutic exercise. Assess exercise tolerance frequently (blood pressure, heart rate, respiratory rate, fatigue levels), and terminate exercise immediately if any untoward responses occur (See Appendix L).
- Help patient explore other nonpharmacologic methods to reduce chronic pain, such as relaxation techniques, exercise, counseling, and so forth.
- Guard against falls and trauma (hip fractures, head injury). Implement fall prevention strategies (See Appendix E), especially if patient exhibits sedation, dizziness, or blurred vision.
- To minimize orthostatic hypotension, patient should move slowly when assuming a more upright position.

Patient/Client-Related Instruction

- Advise patient that opioid analgesics are usually more effective if given before pain becomes severe; emphasize that adequate pain control will allow better participation in physical therapy.
- Educate patient about the dangers of opioid overdose; encourage patient to adhere to proper dosing schedule.
- Emphasize that the risk of physical addiction (tolerance and dependence) is usually minimal during short-term treatment of pain. Advise patient that addiction is more likely during excessive or inappropriate use of opioid analgesics.
- Advise patient to avoid alcohol and other CNS depressants because of the increased risk of sedation and decreased CNS function.
- Advise patient to increase fluid intake and dietary fiber to avoid constipation. Laxatives may also be helpful in patients susceptible to fecal impaction (e.g., people with spinal cord injury).
- Instruct patient to report other troublesome side effects such as severe or prolonged headache, urinary retention, unusual dreams, excessive sweating, vision disturbances, or GI problems (nausea, vomiting).

Pharmacokinetics

Absorption: 50% from the GI tract; well absorbed from IM sites. Oral doses are about half as effective as parenteral doses.
Distribution: Widely distributed. Crosses the placenta; enters breast milk.
Protein Binding: Neonates: 52%; Infants 3–18 months: 85%; Adults: 60–80%.
Metabolism and Excretion: Mostly metabolized by the liver; some converted to normeperidine, which may accumulate and cause seizures. 5% excreted unchanged by the kidneys.
Half-life: Neonates: 12–39 hr; Infants 3–18 months: 2.3 hr; Children 5–8 yr: 3 hr; Adults: 2.5–4 hr (prolonged in impaired renal or hepatic function [7–11 hr]).

TIME/ACTION PROFILE (analgesia)

ROUTE	ONSET	PEAK	DURATION
PO	15 min	60 min	2–4 hr
IM	10–15 min	30–50 min	2–4 hr
SC	10–15 min	40–60 min	2–4 hr
IV	immediate	5–7 min	2–3 hr

Contraindications/Precautions

Contraindicated in: Hypersensitivity; Hypersensitivity to bisulfites (some injectable products); Pregnancy or lactation (chronic use); Recent (14–21 days) MAO inhibitor therapy.

Use Cautiously in: Head trauma; Increased intracranial pressure; Severe renal, hepatic, or pulmonary disease; Hypothyroidism; Adrenal insufficiency; Alcoholism; Geri: Appears on Beers' list. Geriatric patients (morphine recommended); Debilitated patients (dose reduction suggested); Undiagnosed abdominal pain or prostatic hyperplasia; Labor (respiratory depression may occur in the newborn); Patients with renal impairment, or extensive burns; High dose or prolonged therapy (>600 mg/day or >2 days; increased risk of CNS stimulation and seizures due to accumulation of normeperidine); Sickle cell anemia (may require reduced initial doses); Pedi: Neonates (syrup contains benzyl alcohol); Pedi: Children (increased risk of seizures due to accumulation of normeperidine).

Interactions

Drug-Drug: **Do not use in patients receiving MAO inhibitors or procarbazine** (may cause fatal reaction—contraindicated within 14–21 days of MAO inhibitor therapy). ↑ CNS depression with **alcohol, antihistamines**, and **sedative/hypnotics**. Administration of **agonist/antagonist opioid analgesics** may precipitate opioid withdrawal in physically dependent patients. **Nalbuphine** or **pentazocine** may ↓ analgesia. **Protease inhibitor antiretrovirals** may ↑ effects and adverse reactions (concurrent use should be avoided). **Phenytoin** ↑ metabolism and may ↓ effects. **Chlorpromazine** and **thioridazine** may ↑ the risk of adverse reactions (concurrent use should be avoided). May aggravate side effects of **isoniazid**. **Acyclovir** may increase plasma concentrations of meperidine and normeperidine.

Drug-Natural: Concomitant use of **kava, valerian,** or **chamomile** can ↓ CNS depression. **St. John's wort** may increase serious side effects, concurrent use is not recommended.

Route/Dosage

PO, IM, SC, IV (Adults): *Analgesia*—50–150 mg q 3–4 hr. *Analgesia during labor*—50–100 mg IM or SC when contractions become regular; may repeat q 1–3 hr. *Preoperative sedation*—50–100 mg IM or SC 30–90 min before anesthesia.

PO, IM, SC, IV (Children): *Analgesia*—1–1.5 mg/kg q 3–4 hr (should not exceed 100 mg/dose). *Preoperative sedation*—1–2 mg/kg 30–90 min before anesthesia (not to exceed adult dose).

IV (Adults): 15–35 mg/hr as a continuous infusion; *PCA*—10 mg initially; with a range 0f 1–5 mg/ incremental dose, recommended lockout interval is 6–10 min (minimum 5 min).

IV (Children): *Continuous infusion*—0.5–1 mg/kg loading dose followed by 0.3 mg/kg/hr, titrate to effect up to 0.5–0.7 mg/kg/hr.

Availability (generic available)

Tablets: 50 mg, 100 mg. **Syrup (banana flavor):** 50 mg/5 mL. **Injection:** 10 mg/mL, 25 mg/mL, 50 mg/mL, 75 mg/mL, 100 mg/mL. ***In combination with:*** promethazine (Mepergan) and atropine. See Appendix B.

meprobamate

(me-proe-**bam**-ate)

Apo-Meprobamate, Equanil, Miltown

Classification

Therapeutic: antianxiety agents, sedative/hypnotics

Pharmacologic: carbamates

Schedule IV

Indications

Anxiety disorders (provides sedation).

Action

Produces CNS depression by acting at multiple sites in the CNS. **Therapeutic Effects:** Sedation.

Adverse Reactions/Side Effects

CNS: drowsiness. **EENT:** blurred vision. **CV:** hypotension. **GI:** anorexia, diarrhea, nausea, vomiting. **Derm:** pruritus, rashes, urticaria. **Neuro:** ataxia. **Misc:** hypersensitivity reactions, physical dependence, psychological dependence, tolerance.

PHYSICAL THERAPY IMPLICATIONS

Examination and Evaluation

- Monitor daytime drowsiness and "hangover" symptoms (headache, nausea, irritability, dysphoria). Repeated or excessive symptoms may require change in dose or medication.
- Assess balance and risk of falls (See Appendix E), especially in older adults, or in patients exhibiting sedation, dizziness, blurred vision, or ataxia.
- Monitor signs of hypersensitivity reactions, including pulmonary symptoms (tightness in the throat and chest, wheezing, cough, dyspnea) or skin reactions (rash, pruritus, urticaria). Notify physician immediately if these reactions occur.
- Assess blood pressure periodically and compare to normal values (See Appendix F). Report low blood pressure (hypotension), especially if patient experiences dizziness, fatigue, or other symptoms.

Interventions

- Guard against falls and trauma (hip fractures, head injury, and so forth). Implement fall prevention strategies, especially in older adults or if drowsiness and dizziness carry over into the daytime (See Appendix E).

- Help patient explore nonpharmacologic methods to reduce anxiety, such as relaxation techniques, exercise, counseling, support groups, and so forth.
- To minimize orthostatic hypotension, patient should move slowly when assuming a more upright position.

Patient/Client-Related Instruction

- Instruct patients on prolonged treatment not to discontinue medication without consulting their physician. Abrupt withdrawal may cause insomnia, unusual irritability or nervousness, and seizures.
- Advise patient about the risk of daytime drowsiness and decreased attention and mental focus. These problems can be severe in certain people. Use care if driving or in other activities that require quick reactions and strong concentration.
- Advise patient to avoid alcohol and other CNS depressants because of the increased risk of sedation and adverse effects.
- Instruct patient to report other bothersome side effects such as severe or prolonged skin reactions (rash, hives, itching), blurred vision, or GI problems (nausea, vomiting, diarrhea, loss of appetite).

Pharmacokinetics

Absorption: Well absorbed after oral administration.
Distribution: Widely distributed. Crosses the placenta; enters breast milk in high concentrations.
Metabolism and Excretion: Metabolized by the liver.
Half-life: 6–16 hr.

TIME/ACTION PROFILE (sedation)

ROUTE	ONSET	PEAK	DURATION
PO	<1 hr	1–3 hr	6–12 hr
PO-ER	unknown	unknown	12 hr

Contraindications/Precautions

Contraindicated in: Hypersensitivity; Comatose patients or those with preexisting CNS depression; Uncontrolled severe pain; Pregnancy and lactation.
Use Cautiously in: Hepatic dysfunction or severe renal impairment; History of suicide attempt or drug abuse; Geri: Appears on Beers' list and is associated with falls. Dosage reduction suggested.

Interactions

Drug-Drug: Additive CNS depression with other **CNS depressants**, including **alcohol, antihistamines, opioid analgesics**, and other **sedative/hypnotics**.
Drug-Natural: Concomitant use of **kava, valerian, skullcap, chamomile**, or **hops** can increase CNS depression.

Route/Dosage

PO (Adults): 400 mg 3–4 times daily or 600 mg bid.
Extended-release capsules—400–800 mg bid daily (not to exceed 2400 mg/day).
PO (Children 6–12 yr): 100–200 mg 2–3 bid–tid.
Extended-release capsules—200 mg bid.

Availability (generic available)

Tablets: 200 mg, 400 mg, 600 mg. ***In combination with:*** aspirin (Equagesic). See Appendix B.

HIGH ALERT

mercaptopurine

(mer-kap-toe-**pyoor**-een)

Purinethol

Classification

Therapeutic: antineoplastics

Pharmacologic: antimetabolites

Indications

Leukemias (with other agents), including Acute lymphocytic leukemia, Acute myelogenous leukemia.
Unlabeled Use: Treatment of Some lymphomas, Polycythemia vera, Crohn's disease, Psoriatic arthritis.

Action

Disrupts DNA and RNA synthesis (cell-cycle S phase–specific). **Therapeutic Effects:** Death of rapidly proliferating cells, especially malignant ones. Also has immunosuppressant properties.

Adverse Reactions/Side Effects

CNS: weakness. **GI:** HEPATOTOXICITY, anorexia, diarrhea, nausea, vomiting. **Derm:** alopecia, hyperpigmentation. **Endo:** gonadal suppression, oligospermia. **Hemat:** anemia, leukopenia, thrombocytopenia. **Metab:** hyperuricemia. **Misc:** fever.

PHYSICAL THERAPY IMPLICATIONS

Examination and Evaluation

- Be alert for signs of hepatotoxicity, including anorexia, abdominal pain, severe nausea and vomiting, yellow skin or eyes, fever, sore throat, malaise, weakness, facial edema, lethargy, and unusual bleeding or bruising. Report these signs to the physician or nursing staff immediately.
- Instruct patient to report signs of leukopenia (fever, sore throat, signs of infection), thrombocytopenia (bruising, nose bleeds, bleeding gums), or unusual weakness and fatigue that might be due to anemia. Report these signs to the physician or nursing staff.

Interventions

- For patients who are medically able to begin exercise, implement appropriate resistive exercises and aerobic training to maintain muscle strength and aerobic capacity during cancer chemotherapy or to help restore function after chemotherapy.

Patient/Client-Related Instruction

- Because of immunosuppressant effects, advise patient to decrease risk of infections (frequent hand washing, etc.) and avoid contact with persons with contagious diseases.
- Advise patient and family/caregivers that fatigue and weakness are likely and may be severe. Functional abilities may be limited, and patient may need to use assistive devices during ambulation.
- Advise patient that hair loss, changes in skin color, and other skin reactions are likely. Report severe or unexpected skin reactions to the physician.
- Instruct patient to report other troublesome side effects such as severe or prolonged fever or GI problems (nausea, vomiting, diarrhea, loss of appetite).

Pharmacokinetics

Absorption: Variably and incompletely (5–50%) absorbed after oral administration.
Distribution: Widely distributed throughout total body water.
Metabolism and Excretion: Metabolized by liver. Some metabolism by the GI mucosa. Nearly 50% is excreted unchanged by the kidneys.
Half-life: Three phases—45 min, 2.5 hr, 10 hr.

TIME/ACTION PROFILE (effects on blood counts)

ROUTE	ONSET	PEAK	DURATION
PO	7–10 days	14 days	21 days

Contraindications/Precautions

Contraindicated in: Hypersensitivity; Pregnancy or lactation; Severe liver disease.
Use Cautiously in: Infections; ↓ bone marrow reserve; **Geri:** ↑ risk of adverse reactions; Other chronic debilitating illnesses; **OB:** Patients with childbearing potential.

Interactions

Drug-Drug: Allopurinol ↓ metabolism and ↑ risk of toxicity from mercaptopurine (↓ dose of mercaptopurine to 25–33% of the usual dose). A similar effect may occur with **olsalazine, sulfasalazine,** and **mesalamine**. May ↑ risk of bleeding with **warfarin**. ↑ risk of hepatotoxicity with other **hepatotoxic agents**. ↑ bone marrow depression with **trimethoprim/sulfamethoxazole**, other **antineoplastics**, or **radiation therapy**. May alter the effect of **warfarin**. ↓ antibody response to **live-virus vaccines** and ↑ risk of adverse reactions.
Drug-Natural: Concomitant use with **echinacea** and **melatonin** may interfere with immunosuppression.

Route/Dosage

PO (Adults): *Initial dose*—2.5 mg/kg (80–100 mg/m²)/day as a single dose or divided doses; after 4 wk, if necessary, dose may be slowly increased to 5 mg/kg/day (dose should be rounded to the nearest 25 mg); *maintenance dose*—1.5–2.5 mg/kg (50–100 mg/m²)/day.
PO (Children): 2.5 mg/kg/day (75 mg/m²) single dose or divided doses (dose should be rounded to the nearest 25 mg).

Availability (generic available)

Tablets: 50 mg.

meropenem (mer-oh-**pen**-em)

Merrem

Classification

Therapeutic: anti-infectives
Pharmacologic: carbapenems

Indications

Treatment of Intra-abdominal infections, Bacterial meningitis. Skin and skin structure infections. **Unlabeled Use:** Febrile neutropenia. Hospital-acquired pneumonia and sepsis.

Action

Binds to bacterial cell wall, resulting in cell death. Meropenem resists the actions of many enzymes that degrade most other penicillins and penicillin-like anti-infectives. **Therapeutic Effects:** Bactericidal action against susceptible bacteria. **Spectrum:** Active against the following gram-positive organisms: *Staphylococcus aureus, Streptococcus pneumoniae,* Viridans group streptococci, *Enterococcus faecalis*. Also active against the following gram-negative pathogens: *Escherichia coli, Haemophilus influenzae, Klebsiella pneumoniae, Neisseria meningitidis, Pseudomonas aeruginosa, Proteus mirabilis*. Active against the following anaerobes: *Bacteroides fragilis, B. fragilis* group, *Peptostreptococcus* species.

Adverse Reactions/Side Effects

CNS: SEIZURES, dizziness, headache. **Resp:** APNEA.
GI: PSEUDOMEMBRANOUS COLITIS, constipation, diarrhea, glossitis (increased in children), nausea, thrush (increased in children), vomiting. **Derm:** moniliasis (children only), pruritus, rash. **Local:** inflammation at injection site, phlebitis. **Misc:** ALLERGIC REACTIONS, INCLUDING ANAPHYLAXIS.

PHYSICAL THERAPY IMPLICATIONS

Examination and Evaluation

- Watch for seizures; notify physician immediately if patient develops or increases seizure activity.
- Assess respiration, and notify physician immediately if patient exhibits any interruption in respiratory rate (apnea) or other signs of respiratory failure (rapid labored breathing, cyanosis, confusion, irritability, sleepiness, headache, oxygen desaturation).
- Monitor signs of pseudomembranous colitis, including diarrhea, abdominal pain, fever, pus or mucous in stool, and other severe or prolonged GI problems (nausea, vomiting, heartburn). Notify physician or nursing staff immediately of these signs.
- Monitor signs of allergic reactions and anaphylaxis, including pulmonary symptoms (tightness in the throat and chest, wheezing, cough dyspnea) or skin reactions (rash, pruritus, urticaria). Notify physician or nursing staff immediately if these reactions occur.
- Assess dizziness that might affect gait, balance, and other functional activities (See Appendix C). Report balance problems and functional limitations to the physician and nursing staff, and caution the patient and family/caregivers to guard against falls and trauma.
- Monitor injection site for pain, swelling, and irritation. Report prolonged or excessive injection site reactions to the physician.

Interventions

- Always wash hands thoroughly and disinfect equipment (whirlpools, electrotherapeutic devices, treatment tables, and so forth) to help prevent the spread of infection. Employ universal precautions or isolation procedures as indicated for specific patients.

Patient/Client-Related Instruction

- Instruct children and family/caregiver to report signs of thrush and moniliasis, including painful, creamy white lesions on the tongue and inside the mouth.
- Instruct patient and family/caregivers to report other troublesome side effects such as severe or prolonged headache, skin problems (rash, itching), or GI problems (nausea, vomiting, diarrhea, constipation).

Pharmacokinetics

Absorption: IV administration results in complete bioavailability.
Distribution: Widely distributed into body tissues and fluids; enters CSF when meninges are inflamed.
Metabolism and Excretion: 65–83% excreted unchanged by the kidneys.
Half-life: Premature neonates: 3 hr; Term neonates: 2 hr; Infants 3 mo–2 yr: 1.4 hr; Children >2 yr and Adults: 1 hr (increased in renal impairment).

TIME/ACTION PROFILE (blood levels)

ROUTE	ONSET	PEAK	DURATION
IV	rapid	end of infusion	8 hr

Contraindications/Precautions

Contraindicated in: Hypersensitivity to meropenem or imipenem; Serious hypersensitivity to other beta-lactams (penicillins or cephalosporins; cross-sensitivity may occur).
Use Cautiously in: Renal impairment (↑ risk of thrombocytopenia and seizures; dose reduction recommended if CCr <50 mL/min); History of seizures, brain lesions, or meningitis; OB/Lactation/Pedi: Pregnancy, lactation, or children <3 mo (safety not established).

Interactions

Drug-Drug: Probenecid ↓ renal excretion and ↑ blood levels (coadministration not recommended). May ↓ serum **valproate** levels (↑ risk of seizures).

Route/Dosage

IV (Adults): 0.5–1 g q 8 hr. *Meningitis*—2 g q 8 hr.
IV (Children ≥3 mo–12 yr): *Intra-abdominal infections*—20 mg/kg q 8 hr; *meningitis*—40 mg/kg q 8 hr (maximum 2 g q 8 hr).
IV (Neonates <7 days): 20 mg/kg/dose q 12 hr. *Neonates >7 days, 1200–2000 g*—20 mg/kg/dose q 12 hr. *Neonates >7 days, >2000 g*—20 mg/kg/dose q 8 hr.

Renal Impairment

IV (Adults): *CCr 26–50 mL/min*—1 g q 12 hr; *CCr 10–25 mL/min*—500 mg q 12 hr; *CCr <10 mL/min*—500 mg q 24 hr.

Availability

Powder for injection: 500 mg, 1 g.

mesalamine (me-sal-a-meen)

Asacol, Canasa, Lialda, Pentasa, Rowasa, ✱Salofalk

Classification
Therapeutic: gastrointestinal anti-inflammatories—therapeutic
Pharmacologic: salicylates

Indications

Inflammatory bowel diseases, including Ulcerative colitis, Proctitis, Proctosigmoiditis.

Action

Locally acting anti-inflammatory action in the colon, where activity is probably due to inhibition of prostaglandin synthesis. **Therapeutic Effects:** Reduction in the symptoms of inflammatory bowel disease.

Adverse Reactions/Side Effects

CNS: headache, dizziness, malaise, weakness. **EENT:** pharyngitis, rhinitis. **CV:** pericarditis. **GI:** diarrhea, eructation (PO), flatulence, nausea, vomiting. **GU:** interstitial nephritis, pancreatitis, renal failure. **Derm:** hair loss, rash. **Local:** anal irritation (enema, suppository). **MS:** back pain. **Misc:** ANAPHYLAXIS, acute intolerance syndrome, fever.

PHYSICAL THERAPY IMPLICATIONS

Examination and Evaluation

- Monitor signs of allergic reactions and anaphylaxis, including pulmonary symptoms (tightness in the throat and chest, wheezing, cough, dyspnea) or skin reactions (rash, pruritus, urticaria). Notify physician immediately if these reactions occur.
- Be alert for signs of pericarditis, including sharp chest pain, shortness of breath when reclining, dry cough, abdominal or leg edema, low-grade fever, weakness, fatigue, and malaise. Report these signs to the physician.
- Monitor signs of kidney inflammation and kidney failure, including decreased urine output, increased blood pressure, muscle cramps/twitching, edema/weight gain from fluid retention, yellowish brown skin, and confusion that progresses to seizures and coma. Report these signs to the physician immediately.
- Monitor improvements in GI symptoms (decreased abdominal pain, cramps, diarrhea, and so forth) to help document whether drug therapy is successful.
- Assess any back pain to rule out musculoskeletal pathology; that is, try to determine if pain is drug induced rather than caused by anatomic or biomechanical problems.
- Assess dizziness that might affect gait, balance, and other functional activities (See Appendix C). Report balance problems and functional limitations to the physician, and caution the patient and family/caregivers to guard against falls and trauma.

Patient/Client-Related Instruction

- Advise patient to avoid alcohol and foods that may cause an increase in GI irritation.
- Advise patient about the likelihood of GI problems such as nausea, diarrhea, vomiting, belching, flatulence, and anal irritation. Instruct patient to report severe or prolonged GI reactions, or signs of pancreatitis such as upper abdominal pain (especially after eating), indigestion, weight loss, and oily stools.
- Instruct patient to report other bothersome side effects such as severe or prolonged headache, fever, nasal/pharyngeal irritation, or skin problems (rash, hair loss).

Pharmacokinetics

Absorption: 28% absorbed following oral administration; 10–30% absorbed from the colon, depending on retention time, following rectal administration.
Distribution: Unknown.
Metabolism and Excretion: Some metabolism occurs, site unknown; mostly eliminated unchanged in the feces.
Half-life: 12 hr PO (range 2–15 hr); 0.5–1.5 hr rectal.

TIME/ACTION PROFILE (clinical improvement)

ROUTE	ONSET	PEAK	Duration
PO	unknown	unknown	6–8 hr
extended release	2 hr	9–12 hr	24 hr
rectal	3–21 days	unknown	24 hr

Contraindications/Precautions

Contraindicated in: Hypersensitivity reactions to sulfonamides, salicylates, mesalamine, or sulfasalazine; Cross-sensitivity with furosemide, sulfonylurea hypoglycemic agents, or carbonic anhydrase inhibitors may exist; G6PD deficiency; Hypersensitivity to bisulfites (mesalamine enema only); Urinary tract or intestinal obstruction; Porphyria.
Use Cautiously in: Severe hepatic or renal impairment; OB: Pregnancy or lactation (safety not established).

Interactions

Drug-Drug: May ↓ metabolism and ↑ effects/toxicity of **mercaptopurine** or **thioguanine**.

Route/Dosage

PO (Adults): 800 mg tid for 6 wk as delayed-release tablets *or* 1 g qid as controlled-release capsules *or* 2–4 1.2-g tablets once daily with a meal for a total daily dose of 2.4 or 4.8 g of Lialda.
Rect (Adults): 4-g enema (60 mL) at bedtime, retained for 8 hr for 3–6 wk *or* 1 g at bedtime.

Availability (generic available)

Delayed-release tablets: 250 mg, 400 mg, 500 mg, 1.2 g (Lialda). **Controlled-release capsules:** 250 mg, 500 mg. **Suppositories:** 1 g. **Rectal suspension:** 4 g/60 mL.

metaproterenol

(met-a-proe-**ter**-e-nole)
Alupent

Classification
Therapeutic: bronchodilators
Pharmacologic: adrenergics

Indications

Treatment/prevention of bronchospasm due to reversible airway disease (a short-term control agent).

Action

Results in the accumulation of cyclic adenosine monophosphate (cAMP) at $beta_2$-adrenergic receptors. Produces bronchodilation. Inhibits the release of mediators of immediate hypersensitivity reactions from mast cells. Relatively selective for $beta_2$ (pulmonary)–adrenergic receptor sites, with less effect on $beta_1$ (cardiac)–adrenergic receptors. **Therapeutic Effects:** Bronchodilation.

Adverse Reactions/Side Effects

CNS: nervousness, restlessness, tremor, headache, insomnia. **Resp:** PARADOXICAL BRONCHOSPASM (EXCESSIVE USE OF INHALERS). **CV:** angina, arrhythmias, hypertension, tachycardia. **GI:** nausea, vomiting. **Endo:** hyperglycemia.

PHYSICAL THERAPY IMPLICATIONS

Examination and Evaluation

- Watch for signs of paradoxical bronchospasm, including wheezing, cough, dyspnea, shortness of breath, and tightness in chest and throat. These signs are more common at higher doses or during excessive use of the inhaler. If condition occurs, advise patient to withhold medication and notify physician or other health care professional immediately.
- Assess pulmonary function at rest and during exercise (See Appendices I, J, K) to document effectiveness of medication in controlling bronchospasm.
- Assess heart rate, ECG, and heart sounds, especially during exercise (See Appendices G, H). Report any rhythm disturbances or symptoms of increased arrhythmias, including palpitations, chest pain, shortness of breath, fainting, and fatigue/weakness.
- Assess blood pressure (BP) periodically and compare to normal values (See Appendix F). Report a sustained increase in BP (hypertension).
- Monitor and report signs of CNS toxicity, including nervousness, restlessness, or tremor. Sustained or severe CNS signs may indicate overdose or excessive use of this drug.
- Be alert for signs of hyperglycemia, including confusion, drowsiness, flushed/dry skin, fruit-like breath odor, rapid/deep breathing, polyuria, loss of appetite, and unusual thirst. Patients with diabetes mellitus should check blood glucose levels frequently.

Interventions

- When implementing airway clearance techniques or respiratory muscle training, attempt to intervene when the airway is maximally bronchodilated. Peak responses typically occur about 1 hr after inhalation or oral administration.
- Because of the risk of cardiovascular stimulation, use caution during aerobic exercise and endurance conditioning. Cardiac effects should be minimal at lower doses or occasional inhaled use. Cardiovascular effects such as arrhythmias, angina pectoris, or increased BP may occur at higher doses or during excessive use, and are caused by inadvertent stimulation of beta receptors on the heart.

Patient/Client-Related Instruction

- Advise patient to not exceed the recommended dose or frequency of inhalations. Contact physician immediately if bronchospasm is not relieved by medication or is accompanied by diaphoresis, dizziness, or other symptoms.
- Counsel patient on proper use of inhaler; observe use of this device whenever possible to ensure proper technique.
- Instruct patient and family/caregivers to report severe or prolonged headache, sleep loss, or GI problems (nausea, vomiting).

Pharmacokinetics

Absorption: Small amounts may be systemically absorbed following inhalation, but rapidly undergo extensive metabolism.
Distribution: Unknown.
Metabolism and Excretion: Extensively metabolized by the liver and other tissues.
Half-life: Unknown.

TIME/ACTION PROFILE (bronchodilation)

ROUTE	ONSET	PEAK	DURATION
oral	30 min	1 hr	1–5 hr
inhalation-aerosol	within 1 min	1 hr	1–5 hr
inhalation-IPPB	5–30 min	unknown	2–6 hr

Contraindications/Precautions

Contraindicated in: Hypersensitivity to adrenergic amines; Selected products may contain bisulfites, alcohol (in some oral liquid preparations), or fluorocarbons (in some inhalers) and should be avoided in patients with known hypersensitivity or intolerance.
Use Cautiously in: Cardiac disease; Hypertension; Hyperthyroidism; Diabetes; Glaucoma; Elderly patients (more susceptible to adverse reactions; may require dosage reduction); Excessive use may lead to tolerance and paradoxical bronchospasm (inhaler); Pregnancy (near term) and lactation.

Interactions

Drug-Drug: Concurrent use with other **adrenergics (sympathomimetic)** will have additive adrenergic

side effects. Use with **MAO inhibitors** may lead to hypertensive crisis. **Beta blockers** may negate therapeutic effect.
Drug-Natural: Use with caffeine-containing herbs **(cola nut, guarana, mate, tea, coffee)** increases stimulant effect.

Route/Dosage

PO (Adults and Children >9 yr): 20 mg tid–qid.
PO (Children 6–9 yr): 10 mg tid–qid.
PO (Children 2–6 yr): 1.3–2.6 mg/kg/day divided q 6–8 hr.
PO (Children <2 yr): 0.4 mg/kg/dose tid–qid; may give q 8–12 hr in infants.
Inhaln (Adults and Children >12 yr): *Metered-dose inhaler*—2–3 inhalations q 3–4 hr (not to exceed 12 inhalations/day). *IPPB*—0.2–0.3 mL of 5% solution or 2.5 mL of 0.4–0.6% solution for nebulization tid–qid (not to exceed q 4 hr use).
Inhaln (Children >1 mo): 0.5–1 mg/kg (0.01–0.02 mL/kg) of 5% solution via nebulization q 4–6 hr; minimum dose 0.1 mL (5 mg) maximum dose 0.3 mL (15 mg).

Availability (generic available)

Oral syrup: 10 mg/5 mL Rx. **Tablet:** 10 mg Rx, 20 mg Rx. **Inhalation aerosol:** 650 mcg/spray (100 inhalations/5 mL), 750 mcg/spray (100 inhalations/5 mL). **Inhalation solution:** 0.4%, 0.6%, 5%.

metaxalone (me-tax-a-lone)

Skelaxin

Classification

Therapeutic: skeletal muscle relaxants (centrally acting)

Indications

Muscle spasm associated with acute painful musculoskeletal conditions (with rest and physical therapy).

Action

Skeletal muscle relaxation, probably as a result of CNS depression. **Therapeutic Effects:** Skeletal muscle relaxation.

Adverse Reactions/Side Effects

CNS: drowsiness, dizziness, confusion, headache, irritability, nervousness. **GI:** nausea, anorexia, dry mouth, GI upset, vomiting. **GU:** urinary retention.

PHYSICAL THERAPY IMPLICATIONS

Examination and Evaluation

- Assess patient's pain, stiffness, and ROM to help document antispasm effects.
- Assess dizziness that might affect gait, balance, and other functional activities (See Appendix C). Report balance problems and functional limitations to the physician, and caution the patient and family/caregivers to guard against falls and trauma.
- Be alert for confusion, irritability nervousness, or other alterations in mental status (see Appendix D). Notify physician promptly if these symptoms become problematic.

Interventions

- Implement appropriate manual therapy techniques, physical agents, and therapeutic exercises to reduce pain and wean patient off muscle relaxants as soon as possible.
- Help patient explore other nonpharmacologic methods to reduce chronic pain, such as relaxation techniques, exercise, counseling, and so forth.
- Implement fall-prevention strategies, especially if balance is impaired (See Appendix E).

Patient/Client-Related Instruction

- Inform patient that long-term use can cause tolerance and dependence; encourage adherence to physical therapy so that drug therapy can be discontinued as soon as possible.
- Inform patient that this drug may cause severe drowsiness, dizziness, and reduced psychomotor skills. Patients should avoid driving or other activities that require concentration and fast reactions.
- Advise patient to avoid alcohol and other CNS depressants because of the increased risk of sedation and adverse effects.
- Warn patient about anticholinergic effects such as dry mouth, constipation, urinary retention, sedation, and weakness; anticholinergic effects are often more severe in older adults.
- Instruct patient and family/caregivers to report other GI problems such as prolonged or severe nausea, vomiting, indigestion, or loss of appetite.

Pharmacokinetics

Absorption: Well absorbed following oral administration.
Distribution: Unknown.
Metabolism and Excretion: Mostly metabolized by the liver; metabolites excreted in urine.
Half-life: 2–3 hr.

TIME/ACTION PROFILE

ROUTE	ONSET	PEAK	DURATION
PO	1 hr	2 hr	4–6 hr

Contraindications/Precautions

Contraindicated in: Hypersensitivity; Significant hepatic/renal impairment; History of drug-induced hemolytic anemia or other anemia.
Use Cautiously in: History of seizures; Geri: Appears on Beers' list. Poorly tolerated due to anticholinergic effects; Pregnancy, lactation, or children ≤12 yr (safety

not established; use only in pregnancy/lactation if possible benefits outweigh potential risks).

Interactions

Drug-Drug: ↑ CNS depression with other **CNS depressants**, including **alcohol, antihistamines, opioid analgesics**, and **sedative/hypnotics**.
Drug-Natural: Concomitant use of **kava, valerian,** or **chamomile** can ↑ CNS depression.

Route/Dosage

PO (Adults): 800 mg 3–4 times daily.

Availability

Tablets: 800 mg.

metformin (met-for-min)

Fortamet, Glumetza, Glucophage, Glucophage XR, Novo-Metformin, Riomet

Classification
Therapeutic: antidiabetics
Pharmacologic: biguanides

Indications

Management of type 2 diabetes mellitus; may be used with diet, insulin, or sulfonylurea oral hypoglycemics.

Action

Decreases hepatic glucose production. Decreases intestinal glucose absorption. Increases sensitivity to insulin. **Therapeutic Effects:** Maintenance of blood glucose.

Adverse Reactions/Side Effects

GI: abdominal bloating, diarrhea, nausea, vomiting, unpleasant metallic taste. **Endo:** hypoglycemia. **F and E:** LACTIC ACIDOSIS. **Misc:** ↓ vitamins B_1 and B_2 levels.

PHYSICAL THERAPY IMPLICATIONS

Examination and Evaluation

- Monitor signs of lactic acidosis, especially during exercise. Signs include confusion, lethargy, stupor, shallow rapid breathing, tachycardia, hypotension, nausea, and vomiting. Notify physician immediately if these signs occur.
- Be alert for signs of hypoglycemia, especially during and after exercise. Common neuromuscular signs include anxiety; restlessness; tingling in hands, feet, lips, or tongue; chills; cold sweats; confusion; difficulty in concentration; drowsiness; excessive hunger; headache; irritability; nervousness; tremor; weakness; unsteady gait. Report persistent or repeated episodes of hypoglycemia to the physician.
- Report signs of vitamin B deficiencies, including neurologic disorders (agitation, confusion, paresthesias), skin lesions (cracked, dry lips, dermatitis), and cardiovascular problems (palpitations, tachycardia). Blood tests can confirm low vitamin B levels, and vitamin or dietary supplements may be needed to resolve this problem.
- Assess blood pressure periodically (See Appendix F). A sudden or sustained increase in blood pressure (hypertension) may indicate problems in diabetes management, and should be reported to the physician.

Interventions

- Implement aerobic exercise and endurance training programs to maintain optimal body weight, improve insulin sensitivity, and reduce the risk of macrovascular disease (heart attack, stroke) and microvascular problems (reduced blood flow to tissues and organs that causes poor wound healing, neuropathy, retinopathy, and nephropathy).
- Use caution during aerobic exercise and endurance conditioning because of an increased risk of lactic acidosis. Terminate exercise if patient exhibits untoward symptoms (chest pain, shortness of breath, etc.), or displays other criteria for exercise termination (See Appendix L).
- Provide a source of oral glucose (fruit juice, glucose gels/tablets, etc.) to treat mild hypoglycemia. Call for emergency assistance if symptoms persist or in cases of severe hypoglycemia. Emergency treatment typically consists of IV glucose, glucagon, or epinephrine.

Patient/Client-Related Instruction

- Encourage patient to monitor blood glucose before and after exercise and to adjust food intake to maintain normal glycemic levels.
- Emphasize the importance of adhering to nutritional guidelines and the need for periodic assessment of glycemic control (serum glucose and glycosylated hemoglobin levels) throughout the management of diabetes mellitus.
- Advise patient about symptoms of hyperglycemia (confusion, drowsiness; flushed, dry skin; fruit-like breath odor; rapid, deep breathing, polyuria; loss of appetite; unusual thirst). Drug dosages may need to be adjusted to prevent repeated episodes of hyperglycemia.
- Instruct patient to report troublesome GI problems, including severe or prolonged diarrhea, nausea, vomiting, or abdominal pain and bloating.

Pharmacokinetics

Absorption: 50–60% absorbed after oral administration.

Distribution: Enters breast milk in concentrations similar to plasma.
Metabolism and Excretion: Eliminated almost entirely unchanged by the kidneys.
Half-life: 17.6 hr.

TIME/ACTION PROFILE (blood levels)

ROUTE	ONSET	PEAK	DURATION
PO	unknown	unknown	12 hr
XR	unknown	4–8 hr	24 hr

Contraindications/Precautions

Contraindicated in: Hypersensitivity; Metabolic acidosis; Dehydration, sepsis, hypoxemia, hepatic impairment, excessive alcohol use (acute or chronic); Renal dysfunction (serum creatinine >1.5 mg/dL in men or >1.4 mg/dL in women); Radiographic studies requiring IV iodinated contrast media (withhold metformin); CHF.
Use Cautiously in: Concurrent renal disease; Geri: Geriatric/debilitated patients (↓ doses may be required; avoid in patients >80 yr unless renal function is normal); Chronic alcohol use/abuse; Serious medical conditions (MI, stroke); Patients undergoing stress (infection, surgical procedures); Hypoxia; Pituitary deficiency or hyperthyroidism; OB/Lactation/Pedi: Pregnancy, lactation, or children <10 yr (safety not established; extended release for use in patients >17 yr only).

Interactions

Drug-Drug: Acute or chronic **alcohol** ingestion or **iodinated contrast media** ↑ risk of lactic acidosis. **Amiloride, digoxin, morphine, procainamide, quinidine, ranitidine, triamterene, trimethoprim, calcium channel blockers**, and **vancomycin** may compete for elimination pathways with metformin. Altered responses may occur. **Cimetidine** and **furosemide** may ↑ effects of metformin. **Nifedipine** ↑ absorption and effects.
Drug-Natural: Glucosamine may worsen blood glucose control. **Chromium**, and **coenzyme Q10** may produce ↑ hypoglycemic effects.

Route/Dosage

PO (Adults and children >17 yr): 500 mg bid; may increase by 500 mg at weekly intervals up to 2000 mg/day. If doses >2000 mg/day are required, give in 3 divided doses (not to exceed 2500 mg/day) or 850 mg once daily; may increase by 850 mg at 2-wk intervals (in divided doses) up to 2550 mg/day in divided doses (up to 850 mg tid); *Extended-release tablets*—500–1000 mg once daily with evening meal, may increase by 500 mg at weekly intervals up to 2500 mg once daily. If 2000 mg once daily is inadequate, 1000 mg bid may be used.
PO (Children >10 yr): 500 mg bid, may be increased by 500 mg/day at 1-wk intervals, up to 2000 mg/day in 2 divided doses.

Availability (generic available)

Tablets: 500 mg, 850 mg, 1000 mg. **Extended-release tablets (Fortamet, Glucophage XR, Glumetza):** 500 mg, 750 mg, 1000 mg. **Oral solution (Cherry flavor):** 500 mg/5mL in 120- and 480-mL bottles. ***In combination with:*** glyburide (Glucovance) glipizide (Metaglip), pioglitazone (ACTOplus), repaglinide (PrandiMet), rosiglitazone (Avandamet), and sitagliptin (Janumet). See Appendix B.

HIGH ALERT

methadone (meth-a-done)

Methadose

Classification
Therapeutic: opioid analgesics
Pharmacologic: opioid agonists

Schedule II

Indications

Severe pain. Suppresses withdrawal symptoms in opioid detoxification.

Action

Binds to opiate receptors in the CNS. Alters the perception of and response to painful stimuli, while producing generalized CNS depression. **Therapeutic Effects:** Decrease in severity of pain. Suppression of withdrawal symptoms during detoxification and maintenance from heroin and other opioids.

Adverse Reactions/Side Effects

CNS: confusion, sedation, dizziness, dysphoria, euphoria, floating feeling, hallucinations, headache, unusual dreams. **EENT:** blurred vision, diplopia, miosis. **Resp:** respiratory depression. **CV:** hypotension, bradycardia, QT prolongation, torsades de pointes. **GI:** constipation, nausea, vomiting. **GU:** urinary retention. **Derm:** flushing, sweating. **Misc:** physical dependence, psychologic dependence, tolerance.

PHYSICAL THERAPY IMPLICATIONS

Examination and Evaluation

- Assess symptoms of respiratory depression, including decreased respiratory rate, confusion, bluish color of the skin and mucous membranes (cyanosis), and difficult, labored breathing (dyspnea). Monitor pulse oximetry and perform pulmonary function tests (See Appendix I) to quantify suspected changes in ventilation and respiratory function. Excessive respiratory depression requires emergency care.
- Be alert for excessive sedation or changes in mood and behavior (euphoria, dysphoria, confusion, hallucinations). Notify physician or nurse immediately

if patient is unconscious or extremely difficult to arouse.

- Use appropriate pain scales (visual analog scales, others) to document whether this drug is successful in helping manage the patient's pain.
- Assess blood pressure periodically and compare to normal values (See Appendix F). Report low blood pressure (hypotension), especially if patient experiences dizziness, fainting, or other symptoms.
- Assess heart rate, ECG, and heart sounds, especially during exercise (See Appendices G, H). Report slow heart rate (bradycardia), ECG changes, or symptoms of other arrhythmias including palpitations, chest discomfort, shortness of breath, fainting, and fatigue/weakness.
- Assess dizziness that might affect gait, balance, and other functional activities (See Appendix C). Report balance problems and functional limitations to the physician and nursing staff, and caution the patient and family/caregivers to guard against falls and trauma.

Interventions

- Implement appropriate manual therapy techniques, physical agents, and therapeutic exercises to reduce pain and help wean patient off opioid analgesics as soon as possible.
- Because of the risk of respiratory depression, arrhythmias, and hypotension, use caution during aerobic exercise and other forms of therapeutic exercise. Assess exercise tolerance frequently (blood pressure, heart rate, respiratory rate, fatigue levels), and terminate exercise immediately if any untoward responses occur (See Appendix L).
- Help patient explore other nonpharmacologic methods to reduce chronic pain, such as relaxation techniques, exercise, counseling, and so forth.
- Guard against falls and trauma (hip fractures, head injury). Implement fall-prevention strategies (See Appendix E), especially if patient exhibits sedation, dizziness, or blurred vision.
- To minimize orthostatic hypotension, patient should move slowly when assuming a more upright position.

Patient/Client-Related Instruction

- Advise patient that opioid analgesics are usually more effective if given before pain becomes severe; emphasize that adequate pain control will allow better participation in physical therapy.
- Educate patient about the dangers of opioid overdose; encourage patient to adhere to proper dosing schedule.
- Emphasize that the risk of physical addiction (tolerance and dependence) is usually minimal during short-term treatment of pain. Advise patient that addiction is more likely during excessive or inappropriate use of opioid analgesics.
- Advise patient to avoid alcohol and other CNS depressants because of the increased risk of sedation and decreased CNS function.
- Advise patient to increase fluid intake and dietary fiber to avoid constipation. Laxatives may also be helpful in patients susceptible to fecal impaction (e.g., people with spinal cord injury).
- Instruct patient to report other troublesome side effects such as severe or prolonged headache, urinary retention, unusual dreams, excessive sweating, vision disturbances, or GI problems (nausea, vomiting).

Pharmacokinetics

Absorption: Well absorbed from all sites (50% absorbed following oral administration).
Distribution: Widely distributed. Crosses the placenta; enters breast milk.
Protein Binding: High.
Metabolism and Excretion: Mostly metabolized by the liver; some metabolites are active and may accumulate with chronic administration.
Half-life: 15–25 hr; increases with chronic use.

TIME/ACTION PROFILE (analgesic effect)

ROUTE	ONSET	PEAK	DURATION
PO	30–60 min	90–120 min	4–12 hr
IM, SC	10–20 min	60–120 min	4–6 hr

Contraindications/Precautions

Contraindicated in: Hypersensitivity; Known alcohol intolerance (some oral solutions); Concurrent MAO inhibitor therapy.
Use Cautiously in: Cardiac hypertrophy, concomitant diuretic use, hypokalemia, hypomagnesemia, history of cardiac conduction abnormalities, concurrent medications affecting cardiac conduction, or other risk factor of arrhythmias; Head trauma; Increased intracranial pressure; Severe renal, hepatic, or pulmonary disease; Hypothyroidism; Adrenal insufficiency; Alcoholism; Undiagnosed abdominal pain; Prostatic hyperplasia or ureteral stricture; OB: Use with addiction control: weigh risk against potential for illicit drug use. Counsel mother about potential harm to fetus; Lactation: Appears in breast milk. Weigh risks against potential for illicit drug use. Counsel mother about potential harm to infant and to wean breast-feeding slowly to prevent abstinence syndrome; Geri: Dose reduction suggested.

Interactions

Drug-Drug: Use with extreme caution in patients receiving **MAO inhibitors** (may result in severe,

M

unpredictable reactions—reduce initial dose of methadone to 25% of usual dose). Use with extreme caution with any drug known potentially to prolong QT interval, including **classes I and III antiarrhythmics**, some **neuroleptics** and **tricyclic antidepressants**, and **calcium channel blockers**. Concurrent use of **laxatives, diuretics**, and **mineralocorticoids** may ↑ risk of hypomagnesemia or hypokalemia and ↑ risk of arrhythmias. ↑ CNS depression with **alcohol, antihistamines**, and **sedative/hypnotics**. Administration of **agonist/antagonist opioids** may precipitate opioid withdrawal in physically dependent patients. **Nalbuphine** or **pentazocine** may ↓ analgesia. **Interferons (alpha)** may ↓ metabolism and ↑ effects. **Nevirapine, efavirenz, ritonavir, ritonavir/lopinavir, phenobarbital, carbamazepine, phenytoin**, and **rifampin** may ↑ metabolism and decrease analgesia; withdrawal may occur. **Fluvoxamine** may increase CNS depression; with **fluvoxamine**, opioid withdrawal may occur. May ↑ blood levels and effects of **zidovudine** and **desipramine**. May ↓ level and effects of **didanosine** and **stavudine**.
Drug-Natural: St. John's Wort ↑ metabolism and ↓ blood levels; concurrent use may result in withdrawal. **Kava, valerian,** or **chamomile** can ↑ CNS depression.

Route/Dosage

Larger doses may be required for analgesia during chronic therapy; interval may be ↓/dose ↑ if pain recurs.
PO (Adults and Children ≥50 kg): *Analgesic*—20 mg q 6–8 hr. *Opioid detoxification*—15–40 mg once daily or amount needed to prevent withdrawal. Dose may be ↓ q 1–2 days; maintenance dose is determined on an individual basis.
PO (Adults and Children <50 kg): *Analgesic*—0.2 mg/kg q 6–8 hr.
IM, SC (Adults and Children ≥50 kg): *Analgesic*—10 mg q 6–8 hr. *Opioid detoxification*—15–40 mg once daily or amount needed to prevent withdrawal. Dose may be ↓ q 1–2 days; maintenance dose is determined on an individual basis.
IM, SC (Adults and Children <50 kg): 0.1 mg/kg mg q 6–8 hr.

Availability (generic available)

Tablets: 5 mg, 10 mg. **Dispersible tablets (diskettes):** 40 mg (available only to licensed detoxification/maintenance programs). **Oral solution (contains alcohol) (citrus):** 5 mg/5 mL, 10 mg/5 mL. **Oral concentrate (cherry and unflavored):** 10 mg/mL.

methazolamide
(meth-a-**zole**-a-mide)
GlaucTabs, Neptazane

Classification
Therapeutic: diuretics
Pharmacologic: carbonic anhydrase inhibitors

Indications

Lowering of intraocular pressure in the treatment of glaucoma.

Action

Inhibition of carbonic anhydrase in the eye results in decreased secretion of aqueous humor. Inhibit renal carbonic anhydrase, resulting in self-limiting urinary excretion of sodium, potassium, bicarbonate, and water. **Therapeutic Effects:** Lowering of intraocular pressure.

Adverse Reactions/Side Effects

CNS: depression, tiredness, weakness, drowsiness. **EENT:** transient nearsightedness. **GI:** anorexia, metallic taste, nausea, vomiting. **GU:** crystalluria, renal calculi. **Derm:** rashes. **Endo:** hyperglycemia. **F and E:** hyperchloremic acidosis, hypokalemia. **Hemat:** APLASTIC ANEMIA, HEMOLYTIC ANEMIA, LEUKOPENIA. **Metab:** weight loss, hyperuricemia. **Neuro:** paresthesias. **Misc:** allergic reactions.

PHYSICAL THERAPY IMPLICATIONS

Examination and Evaluation

- Monitor signs of leukopenia (fever, sore throat, signs of infection) or various anemias (unusual fatigue, shortness of breath, dizziness, headache, coldness in your hands and feet, pale skin, chest pain, bruising). Report these signs to the physician immediately.
- Monitor signs of fluid, electrolyte, or acid-base imbalances, including dizziness, drowsiness, blurred vision, confusion, hypotension, or muscle cramps and weakness. Report excessive or prolonged symptoms to the physician.
- Monitor signs of allergic reactions, including pulmonary symptoms (tightness in the throat and chest, wheezing, cough, dyspnea) or skin reactions (rash, pruritus, urticaria). Notify physician or nursing staff immediately if these reactions occur.
- Be alert for signs of hyperglycemia, including confusion, drowsiness, flushed/dry skin, fruit-like breath odor, rapid/deep breathing, polyuria, loss of appetite, and unusual thirst. Patients with diabetes mellitus should check blood glucose levels frequently.

- Assess signs of paresthesia such as numbness, tingling, and muscle weakness. Perform objective tests, including electroneuromyography and sensory testing to document any drug-related neuropathic changes.
- Monitor and report depression or other changes in mood and behavior.

Interventions

- Implement fall-prevention strategies, especially in older adults or if patient exhibits weakness, tiredness, drowsiness, nearsightedness, or other impairments that affect gait and balance (See Appendix E).

Patient/Client-Related Instruction

- Instruct patient to report any problems with urination or signs of renal calculi (kidney stones) such as severe pain in the side and back, pain on urination, bloody urine, and a persistent urge to urinate.
- Instruct patient to report other bothersome side effects such as severe or prolonged skin rash or GI problems (nausea, vomiting, metallic taste).

Pharmacokinetics

Absorption: Well absorbed after oral administration.
Distribution: Crosses the placenta.
Metabolism and Excretion: 15–30% excreted unchanged in urine.
Half-life: 14 hr.

TIME/ACTION PROFILE (lowering of intraocular pressure)

ROUTE	ONSET	PEAK	DURATION
PO	2–4 hr	6–8 hr	10–18 hr

Contraindications/Precautions

Contraindicated in: Hypersensitivity or cross-sensitivity with sulfonamides may occur; Avoid during first trimester of pregnancy; Concurrent use of oral and ophthalmic carbonic anhydrase inhibitors (dorzolamide) is not recommended.
Use Cautiously in: Chronic respiratory disease; Electrolyte abnormalities; Renal or hepatic disease; Diabetes mellitus; Second or third trimester of pregnancy or lactation (safety not established).

Interactions

Drug-Drug: Excretion of **barbiturates, aspirin,** and **lithium** is ↑ and may lead to ↓ effectiveness. Excretion of **amphetamines, quinidine, procainamide, cyclosporine,** and possibly **tricyclic antidepressants** is ↓ and may lead to toxicity.

Route/Dosage

PO (Adults): 50–100 mg 2–3 times daily.

Availability (generic available)

Tablets: 25 mg Rx, 50 mg Rx.

methocarbamol

(meth-oh-**kar**-ba-mole)
Carbacot, Robaxin

Classification
Therapeutic: skeletal muscle relaxants (centrally acting)

Indications

Adjunctive treatment of muscle spasm associated with acute painful musculoskeletal conditions (with rest and physical therapy).

Action

Skeletal muscle relaxation, probably as a result of CNS depression. **Therapeutic Effects:** Skeletal muscle relaxation.

Adverse Reactions/Side Effects

CNS: SEIZURES (IV, IM ONLY), dizziness, drowsiness, lightheadedness. **EENT:** blurred vision, nasal congestion. **CV: IV:** bradycardia, hypotension. **GI:** anorexia, GI upset, nausea. **GU:** brown, black, or green urine. **Derm:** flushing (IV only), pruritus, rashes, urticaria. **Local:** pain at IM site, phlebitis at IV site. **Misc:** ALLERGIC REACTIONS, INCLUDING ANAPHYLAXIS (IM, IV USE ONLY), fever.

PHYSICAL THERAPY IMPLICATIONS

Examination and Evaluation

- Be alert for new seizures or increased seizure activity, especially during IV or IM administration. Document the number, duration, and severity of seizures, and report these findings immediately to the physician.
- Monitor signs of allergic reactions and anaphylaxis, including skin reactions such as rash, itching, burning, welts, and swelling in the face, and pulmonary symptoms such as tightness in the throat and chest, wheezing, cough, and dyspnea. Seek immediate medical assistance if these reactions occur.
- Assess patient's pain, stiffness, and ROM to help document antispasm effects.
- Assess heart rate, ECG, and heart sounds, especially during exercise (See Appendices G, H). Report slow heart rate (bradycardia) or symptoms of other arrhythmias, including palpitations, chest discomfort, shortness of breath, fainting, and fatigue/weakness.

M

- Assess blood pressure periodically and compare to normal values (See Appendix F). Report low blood pressure (hypotension), especially if patient experiences dizziness, light-headedness, or other symptoms.
- Assess dizziness that might affect gait, balance, and other functional activities (See Appendix C). Report balance problems and functional limitations to the physician, and caution the patient and family/caregivers to guard against falls and trauma.

Interventions

- Implement appropriate manual therapy techniques, physical agents, and therapeutic exercises to reduce pain and wean patient off muscle relaxants as soon as possible.
- Help patient explore other nonpharmacologic methods to reduce chronic pain, such as relaxation techniques, exercise, counseling, and so forth.
- Implement fall-prevention strategies, especially if balance is impaired (See Appendix E).

Patient/Client-Related Instruction

- Inform patient that long-term use can cause tolerance and physical/psychologic dependence; encourage adherence to physical therapy so that drug therapy can be discontinued as soon as possible.
- Inform patient that this drug may cause severe drowsiness, dizziness, and reduced psychomotor skills. Patients should avoid driving or other activities that require concentration and fast reactions.
- Advise patient to avoid alcohol and other CNS depressants because of the increased risk of sedation and adverse effects.
- Warn patient about anticholinergic effects such as dry mouth, constipation, urinary retention, sedation, and weakness; anticholinergic effects are often more severe in older adults.
- Instruct patient and family/caregivers to report other troublesome side effects such as severe or prolonged fever, skin reactions (rash, itching, hives), or GI problems (nausea, indigestion, loss of appetite).

Pharmacokinetics

Absorption: Rapidly absorbed from the GI tract.
Distribution: Widely distributed. Crosses the placenta; enters breast milk in small amounts.
Metabolism and Excretion: Metabolized by the liver.
Half-life: 1–2 hr.

TIME/ACTION PROFILE (skeletal muscle relaxation)

ROUTE	ONSET	PEAK	DURATION
PO	30 min	2 hr	unknown
IM	rapid	unknown	unknown
IV	immediate	end of infusion	unknown

Contraindications/Precautions

Contraindicated in: Hypersensitivity; Hypersensitivity to polyethylene glycol (parenteral only); Renal impairment (parenteral form).
Use Cautiously in: Pregnancy, lactation, and children (safety not established); Geri: Appears on Beers' list. Poorly tolerated due to anticholinergic effects; Seizure disorders (parenteral form).

Interactions

Drug-Drug: Additive CNS depression with other **CNS depressants**, including **alcohol, antihistamines, opioid analgesics,** and **sedative/hypnotics**.
Drug-Natural: Concomitant use of **kava, valerian, chamomile,** or **hops** can ↑ CNS depression.

Route/Dosage

PO (Adults): 1.5 g qid initially (up to 8 g/day) for 2–3 days, then 4–4.5 g/day in 3–6 divided doses; may be followed by maintenance dosing of 750 mg q 4 hr or 1 g qid or 1.5 g tid.
IM, IV (Adults): 1–3 g/day for not more than 3 days; course may be repeated after a 48-hr rest.

Availability (generic available)

Tablets: 500 mg, 750 mg. **Injection:** 100 mg/mL in 10-mL ampules, 100 mg/mL in 10-mL vials. ***In combination with:*** aspirin (Robaxisal). See Appendix B.

methohexital (meth-o-**hex**-i-tal)

Brevital, Brietal

Classification
Therapeutic: general anesthetics
Pharmacologic: barbiturates

Schedule IV

Indications

Induction of general anesthesia. Sole anesthesia in short (<15 min), minimally painful procedures. Supplement to other anesthetic agents. To produce unconsciousness during balanced anesthesia.

Action

Produces anesthesia by depressing the CNS, probably by potentiating gamma-aminobutyric acid (GABA), an inhibitory neurotransmitter. **Therapeutic Effects:** Unconsciousness and general anesthesia.

Adverse Reactions/Side Effects

CNS: SEIZURES, anxiety, emergence delirium, headache, restlessness. **EENT:** rhinitis. **Resp:** APNEA, LARYNGOSPASM, bronchospasm, coughing, dyspnea, respiratory depression. **CV:** CARDIORESPIRATORY ARREST, hypotension. **GI:** abdominal pain, hiccups, nausea, salivation, vomiting. **Derm:** erythema, pruritus, urticaria. **Local:** pain at IM site, phlebitis at IV site. **MS:** muscle twitching. **Misc:** shivering, allergic reactions.

PHYSICAL THERAPY IMPLICATIONS*

**Implications refer primarily to any residual effects that occur typically within 24 hr after anesthesia.*

Examination and Evaluation

- Assess respiration and notify physician or nursing staff immediately if patient exhibits any interruption in respiratory rate (apnea) or signs of cardiorespiratory arrest. Signs include decreased or absent respiration, confusion, bluish color of the skin and mucous membranes (cyanosis), and difficult/labored breathing (dyspnea). Monitor pulse oximetry and perform pulmonary function tests (See Appendix I) to quantify suspected changes in ventilation and respiratory function. Apnea or cardiorespiratory arrest requires emergency care.
- Be alert for seizures, and document the number, duration, and severity of seizures. Report these findings immediately to the physician or nursing staff.
- Monitor signs of laryngeal spasm and bronchospasm, including tightness in the throat and chest, wheezing, cough, and severe shortness of breath. Notify physician or nursing staff immediately if these reactions occur.
- Be alert for signs of emergence reactions, including delirium, nightmares, hallucinations, anxiety, and other changes in mood and behavior. Report these signs to the physician or nursing staff.
- Assess blood pressure periodically and compare to normal values (See Appendix F). Report low blood pressure (hypotension), especially if patient experiences dizziness, fatigue, or other symptoms.
- Be alert for residual muscle twitching and increased skeletal muscle tone. Report a sustained increase in muscle excitability.
- Monitor injection site for pain, swelling, and inflammation consistent with phlebitis. Report prolonged or excessive injection site reactions to the physician.

Interventions

- Implement breathing activities and other therapeutic exercises to encourage ventilation and help overcome any residual effects of the anesthetic.
- Because of the risk of cardiorespiratory arrest, use extreme caution during aerobic exercise and other forms of therapeutic exercise until the residual anesthetic effects have diminished. Assess exercise tolerance frequently (blood pressure, heart rate, respiratory rate, fatigue levels), and terminate exercise immediately if any untoward responses occur (See Appendix L).
- To minimize orthostatic hypotension, patient should move slowly when assuming a more upright position.

Patient/Client-Related Instruction

- Advise patient to avoid alcohol or other CNS depressants for 24 hr after anesthesia.
- Instruct patient to report other troublesome side effects such as severe or prolonged headache, nasal irritation, shivering, skin reactions (hives, itching, warmth, redness), or GI problems (nausea, vomiting, hiccups, abdominal pain, excessive salivation).

Pharmacokinetics

Absorption: IV administration results in complete bioavailability.
Distribution: Accumulates and may be slowly rereleased from lipoid tissues; rapidly crosses the blood-brain barrier. Crosses the placenta.
Metabolism and Excretion: Mostly metabolized by the liver; some metabolism in kidneys and brain.
Half-life: 1.5–5 hr (increased in geriatric patients).

TIME/ACTION PROFILE (anesthesia)

ROUTE	ONSET	PEAK	DURATION
IV	within 60 sec	unknown	5–7 min
IM*	2–10 min	unknown	unknown

*In pediatric patients.

Contraindications/Precautions

Contraindicated in: Hypersensitivity; Intra-arterial injection; Porphyria; Lactation: Lactation.
Use Cautiously in: Addison's disease; Severe anemia; Severe CV or hepatic disease; Myxedema; Shock or hypotension; Pulmonary disease; Debilitated patients; Geri: Appears on Beers' list. Geriatric patients are at increased risk for side effects (dosage reduction recommended); OB: Safety not established.

Interactions

Drug-Drug: Additive CNS depression with **alcohol, antihistamines, opioid analgesics,** and **sedative/hypnotics.**
Drug-Natural: See **sedative** drug-drug interactions. **St. John's wort** may affect methohexital levels and effectiveness; avoid use. Concomitant use of **kava, valerian, skullcap, chamomile,** or **hops** can increase CNS depression.

Route/Dosage

All doses must be individualized.
IV (Adults): *Induction*—1–1.5 mg/kg. *Maintenance*—20–40 mg q 4–7 min as intermittent doses *or* 3 mL of a 0.2% solution/min.
IM (Children >1 mo): *Induction*—6.6–10 mg/kg of a 5% solution.

Rect (Children >1 mo): *Induction*—25 mg/kg using a 1% solution.

Availability (generic available)

Powder for injection: 500 mg, 2.5 g, 5 g.

HIGH ALERT

methotrexate

(meth-oh-**trex**-ate)

Folex, Folex PFS, Rheumatrex, Trexall

OTHER NAMES:

Amethopterin

Classification

Therapeutic: antineoplastics, antirheumatics (disease-modifying antirheumatic drugs, DMARDs), immunosuppressants

Pharmacologic: antimetabolites

Indications

Alone or with other treatment modalities in the treatment of: Trophoblastic neoplasms (choriocarcinoma, chorioadenoma destruens, hydatidiform mole), Leukemias, Breast carcinoma, Head carcinoma, Neck carcinoma, Lung carcinoma. Treatment of severe psoriasis and rheumatoid arthritis unresponsive to conventional therapy. Treatment of mycosis fungoides (cutaneous T-cell lymphoma).

Action

Interferes with folic acid metabolism. Result is inhibition of DNA synthesis and cell reproduction (cell-cycle S-phase–specific). Also has immunosuppressive activity. **Therapeutic Effects:** Death of rapidly replicating cells, particularly malignant ones, and immunosuppression.

Adverse Reactions/Side Effects

CNS: arachnoiditis (IT use only), dizziness, drowsiness, headaches, malaise. **EENT:** blurred vision, dysarthria, transient blindness. **Resp:** PULMONARY FIBROSIS, intestinal pneumonitis. **GI:** anorexia, hepatotoxicity, nausea, stomatitis, vomiting. **GU:** infertility. **Derm:** alopecia, painful plaque erosions (during psoriasis treatment), photosensitivity, pruritus, rashes, skin ulceration, urticaria. **Hemat:** APLASTIC ANEMIA, anemia, leukopenia, thrombocytopenia. **Metab:** hyperuricemia. **MS:** osteonecrosis, stress fracture. **Misc:** nephropathy, chills, fever, soft tissue necrosis.

PHYSICAL THERAPY IMPLICATIONS

NOTE: Higher doses used to treat cancer will cause more numerous and severe reactions. Use of methotrexate to treat arthritis is at a much lower dose and frequency—often just once a week.

Examination and Evaluation

- Assess pulmonary function periodically by measuring lung volumes, breath sounds, and respiratory rate (See Appendices I, J, K). Notify physician immediately if patient experiences signs of pulmonary fibrosis or pneumonitis such as dry cough, dyspnea, shortness of breath, cyanosis, and fever.
- Monitor any unusual weakness and fatigue that might be due to aplastic anemia. Report signs of anemia or other blood dyscrasias such as leukopenia (fever, sore throat, signs of infection), or thrombocytopenia (bleeding gums; bruising; petechiae; blood in stools, urine, or emesis).
- Report signs of arachnoiditis, especially following IT administration. Signs include tingling, numbness, or weakness in the legs; strange sensations such as insects crawling on skin or water trickling down the legs; muscle cramps, spasms, or twitching; and bowel, bladder, or sexual dysfunction.
- Assess any musculoskeletal pain that might indicate osteonecrosis, stress fracture, or soft tissue necrosis. Report signs of musculoskeletal lesions and suggest the need for additional diagnostic testing (radiographs, MRI).
- If treating rheumatoid arthritis, periodically assess patient's impairments (pain, range of motion), functional ability, and disability to help document whether antirheumatic drug therapy is successful.
- If treating psoriasis or cutaneous fungal infections, assess healing of skin lesions to help document drug effectiveness.
- Assess dizziness (See Appendix C) that might affect gait, balance, and other functional activities. Report balance problems and functional limitations to the physician, and caution the patient and family/caregivers to guard against falls and trauma.

Interventions

- If treating rheumatoid arthritis, implement appropriate manual therapy techniques, physical agents, therapeutic exercises, and orthotic/assistive devices to reduce pain, improve function, and augment the effects of antirheumatic drug therapy.
- Help patients with arthritis explore other nonpharmacologic methods to reduce chronic arthritis pain, such as relaxation techniques, exercise, counseling, and so forth.
- For patients with cancer who are medically able to begin exercise, implement appropriate resistive exercises and aerobic training to maintain muscle strength and aerobic capacity during cancer chemotherapy or to help restore function after chemotherapy.
- Because of the risk of pulmonary fibrosis, assess pulmonary function during exercise, and terminate exercise if patient exhibits untoward symptoms (severe shortness of breath or fatigue) or

displays other criteria for exercise termination (See Appendix L).

- Causes photosensitivity; use care if administering UV treatments. Advise patient to avoid direct sunlight and use sunscreens and protective clothing.

Patient/Client-Related Instruction

- Instruct patient to report signs of nephrotoxicity, including hematuria, increased frequency, cloudy urine, and decreased urine output.
- Advise patient about the likelihood of GI reactions such as nausea, vomiting, diarrhea, and loss of appetite. Instruct patient to report severe or prolonged GI problems or signs of hepatic toxicity such as abdominal pain, severe nausea and vomiting, yellow skin or eyes, fever, sore throat, malaise, weakness, facial edema, lethargy, and unusual bleeding or bruising.
- Advise patient that hair loss and other skin reactions such as rash, pruritus, urticaria, and skin ulcerations are likely. Report severe or unexpected skin reactions to the physician.
- Because of immunosuppressant effects, advise patient to guard against infection (frequent hand washing, etc.), and to avoid crowds and contact with persons with contagious diseases.
- Instruct patient or family/caregivers to report other troublesome side effects, including severe or prolonged headache, drowsiness, vision problems, or difficulty speaking.

Pharmacokinetics

Absorption: Small doses are well absorbed from the GI tract. Larger doses incompletely absorbed.
Distribution: Actively transported across cell membranes, widely distributed. Does not reach therapeutic concentrations in the CSF. Crosses placenta; enters breast milk in low concentrations. Absorption in children is variable (23–95%) and dose dependent.
Metabolism and Excretion: Excreted mostly unchanged by the kidneys.
Half-life: *Low dose*—3–10 hr; *high dose*—8–15 hr (increased in renal impairment).

TIME/ACTION PROFILE (effects on blood counts)

ROUTE	ONSET	PEAK	DURATION
PO, IM, IV	4–7 days	7–14 days	21 days

Contraindications/Precautions

Contraindicated in: Hypersensitivity; Pregnancy or lactation; Products containing benzyl alcohol should not be used in neonates.
Use Cautiously in: Renal impairment (CCr must be ≥60 mL/min prior to therapy); Patients with childbearing potential; Active infections; Decreased bone marrow reserve; Geri: Geriatric patients or patients with other chronic debilitating illnesses.

Interactions

Drug-Drug: The following drugs may ↑ hematologic toxicity of methotrexate: high-dose **salicylates, NSAIDs, oral hypoglycemic agents (sulfonylureas), phenytoin, tetracyclines, probenecid, trimethoprim/sulfamethoxazole, pyrimethamine,** and **chloramphenicol.** ↑ hepatotoxicity with other **hepatotoxic drugs,** including **azathioprine, sulfasalazine,** and **retinoids.** ↑ nephrotoxicity with other **nephrotoxic drugs.** ↑ bone marrow depression with other **antineoplastics** or **radiation therapy. Radiation therapy** ↑ risk of soft tissue necrosis and osteonecrosis. May ↓ antibody response to **live-virus vaccines** and ↑ risk of adverse reactions. ↑ risk of neurologic reactions with **acyclovir** (IT methotrexate only). **Asparaginase** may ↓ effects of methotrexate.
Drug-Natural: Concomitant use with **echinacea** and **melatonin** may interfere with immunosuppression. **Caffeine** may ↓ efficacy of methotrexate; similar effect may occur with **guarana.**

Route/Dosage

Trophoblastic Neoplasms

PO, IM (Adults): 15–30 mg/day for 5 days; repeat after 1 or more weeks for 3–5 courses.

Breast Cancer

IV (Adults): 40 mg/m^2 on days 1 and 8 (with other agents; many regimens are used).

Leukemia

PO (Adults): *Induction*—3.3 mg/m^2/day, usually with prednisone.
PO, IM (Adults): *Maintenance*—20–30 mg/m^2 twice weekly.
IV (Adults): 2.5 mg/kg q 2 wk.
IT (Adults): 12 mg/m^2 or 15 mg.
IT (Children ≥3 yr): 12 mg.
IT (Children 2 yr): 10 mg.
IT (Children 1 yr): 8 mg.
IT (Children <1 yr): 6 mg.

Osteosarcoma

IV (Adults): 12 g/m^2 as a 4-hr infusion followed by leucovorin rescue, usually as part of a combination chemotherapeutic regimen (or increase dose until peak serum methotrexate level is 1×10^{-3} M/L but not to exceed 15 g/m^2; 12 courses are given starting 4 wk after surgery and repeated at scheduled intervals.

Psoriasis

Therapy may be preceded by a 5- to 10-mg test dose

PO (Adults): 2.5–5 mg q 12 hr for 3 doses *or* q 8 hr for 4 doses once weekly (not to exceed 30 mg/wk).
PO, IM, IV (Adults): 10–25 mg/weekly (not to exceed 30 mg/wk).

Arthritis

Therapy may be preceded by a 5- to 10-mg test dose in adults.
PO (Adults): 7.5 mg weekly (2.5 mg q 12 hr for 3 doses or single dose, not to exceed 20 mg/wk); when response is obtained, dosage should be decreased.
PO (Children): 10 mg/m^2 once weekly initially, may be increased up to 20–30 mg/m^2, however, response may be better if doses >20 mg/m^2 are given IM or SC.

Mycosis Fungoides

PO, IM, SC (Adults): 5–50 mg once weekly, if response is poor, dose may be changed to 15–37.5 mg twice weekly.
IM (Adults): 50 mg once weekly or 25 mg twice weekly.

Availability (generic available)

Tablets: 2.5 mg, 5 mg, 7.5 mg, 10 mg, 15 mg. **Injection:** 2.5 mg/mL, 25 mg/mL, 20 mg, 50 mg, 100 mg, 250 mg, 1 g. **Preservative-free injection:** 25 mg/mL.

methoxypolyethylene glycol–epoetin beta

(meth-**oks**-ee-**pol**-ee-**eth**-il-een **glye**-kol–e-**poe**-e-tin **bay**-ta)

Mircera

Classification

Therapeutic: antianemics

Pharmacologic: hormones

Indications

Anemia due to chronic renal failure.

Action

Stimulates erythropoiesis (production of red blood cells). **Therapeutic Effects:** Maintains and may elevate RBCs, decreasing the need for transfusions.

Adverse Reactions/Side Effects

CNS: SEIZURES, headaches. **CV:** CARDIOVASCULAR AND THROMBOTIC EVENTS, hypertension, hypotension. **GI:** diarrhea, constipation, vomiting. **Hemat:** PURE RED APLASIA. **Misc:** ALLERGIC REACTIONS, INCLUDING ANAPHYLAXIS, fistula complications.

PHYSICAL THERAPY IMPLICATIONS

Examination and Evaluation

- Monitor continually and seek immediate medical assistance if patient develops any of the following signs or syndromes:
  - Myocardial infarction, as indicated by sudden chest pain, pain radiating into the arm or jaw, shortness of breath, dizziness, sweating, anxiety, and nausea.
  - Stroke, as indicated by severe headache, confusion, nausea, vomiting, paralysis, numbness, speech problems, and visual disturbances.
  - Seizures, as indicated by various symptoms depending on the type of seizure such as decreased consciousness, changes in muscle tone, muscle twitches/jerking, convulsions, automatisms (lip smacking, chewing), and strange auditory, visual, and other sensations.
  - Lack of red blood cells and their precursors (red cell aplasia), as indicated by unusual fatigue, shortness of breath with exertion, pallor, and bruising.
  - Hypersensitivity reactions and anaphylaxis, including pulmonary symptoms (tightness in the throat and chest, wheezing, cough, dyspnea) or skin reactions (rash, pruritis, urticaria).
- Assess blood pressure (BP) and compare to normal values (See Appendix F). Report changes in BP, either a problematic decrease in BP (hypotension) or a sustained increase in BP (hypertension).

Interventions

- Because of the risk of thrombosis, use caution during aerobic exercise and other forms of therapeutic exercise. Assess exercise tolerance frequently (BP, heart rate, fatigue levels), and terminate exercise immediately if any untoward responses occur (See Appendix L).
- If administered via subcutaneous injection, do not apply massage or physical agents (heat, cold, electrotherapeutic modalities) at or near the application site. These interventions can alter drug absorption from subcutaneous tissues.

Patient/Client-Related Instruction

- Caution patient and family/caregivers about risks of coronary thrombosis, stroke, seizures, anemia, and hypersensitivity reactions. Review warning signs of these problems (see above under Evaluation and Examination), and instruct patient and family/caregivers to report any suspicious symptoms to the physician.
- Instruct patient to report other troublesome side effects such as severe or prolonged headache or GI problems (vomiting, diarrhea, constipation).

Pharmacokinetics

Absorption: Well absorbed (62%) following subcutaneous administration; IV administration results in complete bioavailability.
Distribution: Unknown.
Metabolism and Excretion: Unknown.
Half-life: 134 hr.

TIME/ACTION PROFILE (effect on hemoglobin)

ROUTE	ONSET	PEAK	DURATION
IV, SC	7–15 days	unknown	2–4 wk

Contraindications/Precautions

Contraindicated in: Hypersensitivity; Uncontrolled hypertension; Treatment of anemia due to cancer chemotherapy.

Use Cautiously in: Patients with hypertension or cardiovascular disease (monitor closely); Dialysis patients (IV route recommended to decrease immunogenicity); Predialysis patients (may require lower doses); Geri: Use lower doses, consider age related decrease in metabolic function, concurrent disease states and medications; OB/Lactation: Use during pregnancy only if maternal benefit outweighs fetal risk; Pedi: Safe use not established.

Interactions

Drug-Drug: None noted.

Route/Dosage

SC (Adults): 0.6 mcg/kg once every 2 wk; dosing based on hemoglobin values. Once every 2-wks dose is determined, may be given monthly at twice the every 2-wks dose.

Availability

Vials of solution for injection: 50 mcg/mL, 100 mcg/mL, 200 mcg/mL, 300 mcg/mL, 400 mcg/mL, 600 mcg/mL, 1000 mcg/mL. **Prefilled syringes of solution:** 50 mcg/0.3 mL, 75 mcg/0.3 mL, 100 mcg/0.3 mL, 150 mcg/0.3 mL, 200 mcg/0.3 mL, 250 mcg/0.3 mL, 400 mcg/0.6 mL, 600 mcg/0.6 mL, 800 mcg/0.6 mL.

methyl aminolevulinate

(meth-il a-meen-oh-lev-yoo-lin-late)

Metvix

Classification

Therapeutic: antineoplastics

Pharmacologic: photodynamic agents

Indications

Thin and moderately thick nonhyperkeratotic, nonpigmented actinic keratoses of the face/scalp in immunocompetent patients (with débridement and specific wavelength red light therapy).

Action

Converted to photoactive porphyrins which when exposed to specific wavelength red light result in a photodynamic cytotoxic reaction. **Therapeutic Effects:** Resolution of precancerous lesions.

Adverse Reactions/Side Effects

Derm: burning, contact sensitization, erythema, irritation, itching, pain in area of application, edema at site.

PHYSICAL THERAPY IMPLICATIONS

Examination and Evaluation

- Assess the area being treated to help document whether drug therapy is successful in resolving skin lesions.
- Watch for any new or increased reactions at the site of application, including irritation, burning, itching, and swelling. Report severe or prolonged skin reactions to the physician.

Patient/Client-Related Instruction

- Make sure patient understands how this drug works; that is, red light exposure activates the cytotoxic effects and decreases cell growth in precancerous skin lesions.
- Instruct patient to prevent new lesions by limiting sun exposure, using sunscreens, and wearing protective clothing.

Pharmacokinetics

Absorption: Unknown.
Distribution: Unknown.
Metabolism and Excretion: Unknown.
Half-life: Unknown.

TIME/ACTION PROFILE (lesion resolution)

ROUTE	ONSET	PEAK	DURATION
topical	within days	unknown	3 mo

Contraindications/Precautions

Contraindicated in: Cutaneous photosensitivity or allergy to porphyrins, peanuts or almonds; Lactation/Pedi: Lactation or children.

Use Cautiously in: Bleeding disorders; OB: Use only if clearly needed.

Interactions

Drug-Drug: Concurrent use with other **photosensitizing agents** may result in an exaggerated reaction.

Route/Dosage

Topical (Adults): Following local débridement, apply a 1-mm layer of cream to lesion and surrounding 5 mm of skin (not to exceed 1 g/treatment), cover with occlusive, nonabsorbent dressing for 3 hr. Dressing is then removed, excess cream rinsed off, and skin exposed to red light treatment. Treatment is repeated 7 days later.

Availability

16.8% Cream: 2-g tubes.

methyldopa (meth-il-doe-pa)

Aldomet, Apo-Methyldopa, Dopamet, Novamedopa, Nu-Medopa

Classification

Therapeutic: antihypertensives
Pharmacologic: centrally acting antiadrenergics

Indications

Management of moderate-to-severe hypertension (with other agents).

Action

Stimulates CNS alpha-adrenergic receptors, producing a decrease in sympathetic outflow to heart, kidneys, and blood vessels. Result is ↓ blood pressure and peripheral resistance, a slight ↓ in heart rate, and no change in cardiac output. **Therapeutic Effects:** Lowering of blood pressure.

Adverse Reactions/Side Effects

CNS: sedation, ↓ mental acuity, depression. **EENT:** nasal stuffiness. **CV:** MYOCARDITIS, bradycardia, edema, orthostatic hypotension. **GI:** DRUG-INDUCED HEPATITIS, diarrhea, dry mouth. **GU:** erectile dysfunction. **Hemat:** eosinophilia, hemolytic anemia. **Misc:** fever.

PHYSICAL THERAPY IMPLICATIONS

Examination and Evaluation

- Watch for signs of myocarditis, including chest pain, arrhythmias, fatigue, shortness of breath, peripheral/pulmonary edema, and difficult or labored breathing. Report these signs to the physician immediately.
- Be alert for signs of drug-induced hepatitis, including anorexia, abdominal pain, severe nausea and vomiting, yellow skin or eyes, skin rashes, flu-like symptoms, and muscle/joint pain. Report these signs to the physician immediately.
- Assess blood pressure (BP) periodically and compare to normal values (See Appendix F). Document whether drug therapy is successful in controlling hypertension. Also measure BP when patient assumes a more upright position (lying to standing, sitting to standing, lying to sitting). Document orthostatic hypotension and contact physician when systolic BP falls >20 mm Hg or diastolic BP falls >10 mm Hg.
- Assess heart rate, ECG, and heart sounds, especially during exercise (See Appendices G, H). Report an unusually slow heart rate (bradycardia) or signs of other arrhythmias, including palpitations, chest discomfort, shortness of breath, fainting, and fatigue/weakness.
- Assess peripheral edema using girth measurements, volume displacement, and measurement of pitting edema (See Appendix N). Report increased swelling in feet and ankles or a sudden increase in body weight due to fluid retention.
- Monitor signs of eosinophilia (fatigue, weakness, myalgia) and hemolytic anemia (unusual fatigue, shortness of breath, dizziness, headache, coldness in your hands and feet, pale skin, chest pain). Report these signs to the physician.
- Be alert for signs of depression, decreased mental alertness, or other changes in mood and behavior. Notify physician if these changes become problematic.

Interventions

- Because of the risk of arrhythmias and abnormal BP responses, use caution during aerobic exercise and other forms of therapeutic exercise. Assess exercise tolerance frequently (BP, heart rate, fatigue levels), and terminate exercise immediately if any untoward responses occur (See Appendix L).
- Avoid physical therapy interventions that cause systemic vasodilation (large whirlpool, Hubbard tank). Additive effects of this drug and the intervention may cause a dangerous fall in BP.
- To minimize orthostatic hypotension, advise patient to move slowly when assuming a more upright position.

Patient/Client-Related Instruction

- Remind patients to take medication as directed to control hypertension even if they are asymptomatic.
- Counsel patients about additional interventions to help control BP, such as regular exercise, weight loss, sodium restriction, stress reduction, moderation of alcohol consumption, and smoking cessation.
- Instruct patient or family/caregivers to report other bothersome side effects such as severe or prolonged sedation, nasal congestion, fever, sexual dysfunction, or GI problems (diarrhea, dry mouth).

Pharmacokinetics

Absorption: 50% absorbed from the GI tract. Parenteral form, methyldopate hydrochloride, is slowly converted to methyldopa.
Distribution: Crosses the blood-brain barrier. Crosses the placenta; small amounts enter breast milk.
Metabolism and Excretion: Partially metabolized by the liver, partially excreted unchanged by the kidneys.
Half-life: 1.7 hr.

TIME/ACTION PROFILE (antihypertensive effect)

ROUTE	ONSET	PEAK	DURATION
PO	4–6 hr	12–24 hr	24–48 hr
IV	4–6 hr	unknown	10–16 hr

Contraindications/Precautions

Contraindicated in: Hypersensitivity; Active liver disease; Oral suspension contains alcohol and

bisulfites and should be avoided in patients with known intolerance.
Use Cautiously in: Previous history of liver disease; Geri: ↑ risk of adverse reactions; consider age-related impairment of hepatic, renal, and cardiovascular function as well as other chronic illnesses. Appears on Beers' list. May cause bradycardia and exacerbate depression in geriatric patients; OB: Has been used safely; Lactation: Lactation.

Interactions

Drug-Drug: Additive hypotension with other **antihypertensives**, acute ingestion of **alcohol, anesthesia**, and **nitrates**. **Amphetamines, barbiturates, tricyclic antidepressants, NSAIDs**, and **phenothiazines** may ↓ antihypertensive effect of methyldopa. ↑ effects and risk of psychoses with **haloperidol**. Excess sympathetic stimulation may occur with concurrent use of **MAO inhibitors** or other **adrenergics**. May ↑ effects of **tolbutamide**. May ↑ **lithium** toxicity. Additive hypotension and CNS toxicity with **levodopa**. Additive CNS depression may occur with **alcohol, antihistamines, sedative/hypnotics**, some **antidepressants**, and **opioid analgesics**. Concurrent use with **nonselective beta blockers** may rarely cause paradoxical hypertension.

Route/Dosage

PO (Adults): 250–500 mg bid–tid daily (not to exceed 500 mg/day if used with other agents); may be increased q 2 days as needed; usual maintenance dose is 500 mg–2 g/day (not to exceed 3 g/day).
PO (Children): 10 mg/kg/day (300 mg/m²/day); may be increased q 2 days up to 65 mg/kg/day in divided doses (not to exceed 3 g/day).
IV (Adults): 250–500 mg q 6 hr (up to 1 g q 6 hr).
IV (Children): 5–10 mg/kg q 6 hr; up to 65 mg/kg/day in divided doses (not to exceed 3 g/day).

Availability (generic available)

Tablets: 125 mg, 250 mg, 500 mg. **Oral suspension (orange-pineapple flavor, contains bisulfites):** 250 mg/5 mL. **Injection:** 250 mg/5 mL in 5- and 10-mL vials. ***In combination with:*** hydrochlorothiazide (Aldoril) or chlorothiazide (Aldoclor). See Appendix B.

methylergonovine

(meth-il-er-goe-**noe**-veen)
Methergine

Classification
Therapeutic:
Pharmacologic: ergot alkaloids

Indications

Prevention and treatment of postpartum or postabortion hemorrhage caused by uterine atony or subinvolution.

Action

Directly stimulates uterine and vascular smooth muscle. **Therapeutic Effects:** Uterine contraction.

Adverse Reactions/Side Effects

CNS: dizziness, headache. **EENT:** tinnitus. **Resp:** dyspnea. **CV:** HYPERTENSION, arrhythmias, chest pain, palpitations. **GI:** nausea, vomiting. **GU:** cramps. **Derm:** diaphoresis. **Misc:** allergic reactions.

PHYSICAL THERAPY IMPLICATIONS

Examination and Evaluation

- Assess blood pressure (BP) and compare to normal values (See Appendix F). Report increased BP (hypertension) to the physician immediately.
- Assess heart rate, ECG, and heart sounds, especially during exercise (See Appendices G, H). Report any rhythm disturbances or symptoms of increased arrhythmias, including palpitations, chest pain, shortness of breath, difficulty breathing, fainting, and fatigue/weakness.
- Assess dizziness that affects gait, balance, and other functional activities (See Appendix C). Report balance problems and functional limitations to the physician, and caution the patient and family/caregivers to guard against falls and trauma.
- Assess any abdominal or pelvic pain and cramping. Notify physician if pain/cramping does not subside or continues to worsen.

Interventions

- Because of the risk of hypertension and arrhythmias, use caution during aerobic exercise and other forms of therapeutic exercise. Assess exercise tolerance frequently (BP, heart rate, respiration, fatigue levels), and terminate exercise immediately if any untoward responses occur (see Appendix L).

Patient/Client-Related Instruction

- Instruct patient to report other troublesome side effects such as severe or prolonged headache, ringing/buzzing in the ears, sweating, or GI problems (nausea, vomiting).

Pharmacokinetics

Absorption: Well absorbed following oral or IM administration.
Distribution: Unknown. Enters breast milk in small quantities.
Metabolism and Excretion: Probably metabolized by the liver.

Half-life: 30–120 min.

TIME/ACTION PROFILE (effects on uterine contractions)

ROUTE	ONSET	PEAK	DURATION
PO	5–15 min	unknown	3 hr
IM	2–5 min	unknown	3 hr
IV	immediate	unknown	45 min–3 hr

Contraindications/Precautions

Contraindicated in: Hypersensitivity; Should not be used to induce labor.
Use Cautiously in: Hypertensive or eclamptic patients (more susceptible to hypertensive and arrhythmogenic side effects); Severe hepatic or renal disease; Sepsis.
Exercise Extreme Caution in: 3rd stage of labor.

Interactions

Drug-Drug: Excessive vasoconstriction may result when used with heavy cigarette smoking (**nicotine**) or other **vasopressors** such as **dopamine**.

Route/Dosage

PO (Adults): 200–400 mcg (0.4–0.6 mg) q 6–12 hr for 2–7 days.
IM, IV (Adults): 200 mcg (0.2 mg) q 2–4 hr for up to 5 doses.

Availability

Tablets: 200 mcg (0.2 mg). **Injection:** 200 mcg (0.2 mg)/mL in 1-mL ampules.

methylphenidate

(meth-il-**fen**-i-date)

Concerta, Metadate CD, Metadate ER, Methylin, Methylin ER, PMS-Methylphenidate, Riphenidate, Ritalin, Ritalin LA, Ritalin-SR

Classification
Therapeutic: central nervous system stimulants
Pharmacologic: amphetamine derivatives

Schedule II

Indications

Treatment of ADHD (adjunct). Symptomatic treatment of narcolepsy. **Unlabeled Use:** Management of some forms of refractory depression.

Action

Produces CNS and respiratory stimulation with weak sympathomimetic activity. **Therapeutic Effects:** Increased attention span in ADHD. Increased motor activity, mental alertness, and diminished fatigue in narcoleptic patients.

Adverse Reactions/Side Effects

CNS: hyperactivity, insomnia, restlessness, tremor, dizziness, headache, irritability. **EENT:** blurred vision. **CV:** hypertension, palpitations, tachycardia, hypotension. **GI:** anorexia, constipation, cramps, diarrhea, dry mouth, metallic taste, nausea, vomiting. **Derm:** rashes. **Neuro:** akathisia, dyskinesia. **Misc:** fever, hypersensitivity reactions, physical dependence, psychological dependence, suppression of weight gain (children), tolerance.

PHYSICAL THERAPY IMPLICATIONS

Examination and Evaluation

- Be alert for signs of excessive CNS stimulation, including hyperactivity, restlessness, tremor, or irritability. Report these signs to the physician.
- Monitor attentiveness and behavior in patients with ADHD. Report any changes in attention and hyperactivity, and document whether this drug appears to be producing the desired effects.
- Monitor alertness in patients with narcolepsy; document the frequency and duration of sleeping episodes to help document the effects of drug therapy
- Assess heart rate, ECG, and heart sounds, especially during exercise (See Appendices G, H). Report fast heart rate (tachycardia) or symptoms of other arrhythmias, including palpitations, chest discomfort, shortness of breath, fainting, and fatigue/weakness.
- Assess blood pressure (BP) and compare to normal values (See Appendix F). Report changes in BP, either a problematic decrease in BP (hypotension) or a sustained increase in BP (hypertension).
- Be alert for abnormal muscle tone and movements (dyskinesias), extreme restlessness (akathisia), or other signs of motor dysfunction. Report problematic movement disorders to the physician.
- Monitor signs of hypersensitivity reactions, including pulmonary symptoms (tightness in the throat and chest, wheezing, cough, dyspnea) or skin reactions (rash, pruritus, urticaria). Notify physician if these reactions occur.
- Assess body weight in children receiving chronic therapy; report decreased body weight or an inability to gain weight.

Interventions

- Because of the risk of arrhythmias and abnormal BP responses, use caution during aerobic exercise and other forms of therapeutic exercise. Assess exercise tolerance frequently (BP, heart rate, fatigue levels), and terminate exercise immediately if any untoward responses occur (See Appendix L).

Patient/Client-Related Instruction

- Advise patient or family/caregivers about the potential risk of tolerance and physical/psychologic dependence. Emphasize that addiction is more likely during prolonged, excessive, or inappropriate use of this drug.

- Instruct patient and family/caregivers to report other troublesome side effects including severe or prolonged headache, fever, blurred vision, sleep loss, skin rash, or GI problems (loss of appetite, nausea, vomiting, constipation, diarrhea, abdominal cramps, metallic taste, dry mouth).

Pharmacokinetics

Absorption: Slow and incomplete after oral administration; absorption of sustained or extended-release tablet (SR) is delayed and provides continuous release. *Metadate CD, Concerta, Ritalin LA*—provides initial rapid release followed by a second continuous release (biphasic release).
Distribution: Unknown.
Metabolism and Excretion: Mostly metabolized (80%) by the liver.
Half-life: 2–4 hr.

TIME/ACTION PROFILE (CNS stimulation)

ROUTE	ONSET	PEAK	DURATION
PO	unknown	1–3 hr	4–6 hr
PO-ER	unknown	4–7 hr	3–12 hr*

*Depends on formulation.

Contraindications/Precautions

Contraindicated in: Hypersensitivity; Hyperexcitable states; Hyperthyroidism; Patients with psychotic personalities or suicidal or homicidal tendencies; Tourette's syndrome; Glaucoma; Motor tics; Concurrent use or use within 14 days of MAO inhibitors.
Use Cautiously in: History of cardiovascular disease; Hypertension; Diabetes mellitus; Geriatric or debilitated patients; Continual use (may result in psychologic or physical dependence); Pedi: Growth suppression may occur in children with long-term use; Seizure disorders (may lower seizure threshold); Concerta product should be used cautiously in patients with esophageal motility disorders or severe GI narrowing (may ↑ the risk of obstruction); Pregnancy or lactation (safety not established).

Interactions

Drug-Drug: ↑ sympathomimetic effects with other **adrenergics**, including **vasoconstrictors**, and **decongestants**. Use with **MAO inhibitors** or **vasopressors** may result in hypertensive crisis (concurrent use or use within 14 days of MAO inhibitors is contraindicated). Metabolism of **warfarin, phenytoin, phenobarbital, primidone, selective serotonin reuptake inhibitors,** and **tricyclic antidepressants** may be ↓ and effects ↑. Avoid concurrent use with **pimozide** (may mask cause of tics). Concurrent use with **clonidine** may result in serious ECG abnormalities (a 40% dose reduction of methylphenidate is necessary).
Drug-Natural: Use with caffeine-containing herbs **(guarana, tea, coffee)** ↑ stimulant effect. **St. John's wort** may ↑ serious side effects (concurrent use is NOT recommended).
Drug-Food: Excessive use of **caffeine**-containing foods or beverages **(coffee, cola, tea)** may cause ↑ CNS stimulation.

Route/Dosage

PO (Adults): *ADHD*—5–20 mg bid–tid daily as prompt-release tablets. When maintenance dose is determined, may change to extended-release formulation. *Narcolepsy*—10 mg bid–tid times/day; maximum dose 60 mg/day.
PO (Children >6 yr): *Prompt-release tablets*—0.3 mg/kg/dose or 2.5–5 mg before breakfast and lunch; increase by 0.1 mg/kg/dose or by 5–10 mg/day at weekly intervals (not to exceed 60 mg/day or 2 mg/kg/day). When maintenance dose is determined, may change to extended-release formulation. *Ritalin SR, Metadate ER*— may be used in place of the prompt-release tablets when the 8-hr dosage corresponds to the titrated 8-hr dosage of the prompt-release tablets; *Ritalin LA*—can be used in place of bid regimen given once daily at same total dose or in place of SR product at same dose; *Concerta (patients who have not taken methylphenidate previously)*—18 mg once daily in the morning initially, may be titrated as needed up to 54 mg/day. *Concerta (patients are currently taking other forms of methylphenidate)*—18 mg once daily in the morning if previous dose was 5 mg bid–tid times daily or 20 mg daily as SR product, 36 mg once daily in the morning if previous dose was 10 mg 2–3 times daily or 40 mg daily as SR product, 54 mg once daily in the morning if previous dose was 15 mg bid–tid times daily or 60 mg once daily as SR product. *Metadate CD*—20 mg once daily. Dosage may be adjusted in weekly 20-mg increments to a maximum of 60 mg/day taken once daily in the morning.

Availability (generic available)

Immediate-release tablets: 5 mg, 10 mg, 20 mg. **Extended-release tablets (Metadate ER, Methylin ER):** 10 mg, 20 mg. **Extended-release tablets (Concerta):** 18 mg, 27 mg, 36 mg, 54 mg. **Sustained-release tablets (Ritalin SR):** 20 mg. **Extended-release capsules (Metadate CD):** 10 mg, 20 mg, 30 mg. **Extended-release capsules (Ritalin LA):** 10 mg, 20 mg, 30 mg, 40 mg. **Chewable tablets (Methylin) (grape flavor):** 2.5 mg, 5 mg, 10 mg. **Oral solution (Methylin) (grape flavor):** 5 mg/5 mL, 10 mg/5 mL.

M

methylprednisolone

(meth-il-pred-**nis**-oh-lone)

A-Methapred, depMedalone, Depoject, Depo-Medrol, Depopred, Depo-Predate, Duralone, Medralone, Medrol, Meprolone, Rep-Pred, Solu-Medrol

Classification

Therapeutic: anti-inflammatories (steroidal), immunosuppressants

Pharmacologic: corticosteroids

Indications

Used systemically and locally in a variety of chronic diseases, including inflammatory, allergic, hematologic, neoplastic, autoimmune disorders, immunosuppressant. May be suitable for alternate-day dosing in the management of chronic illness. Replacement therapy in adrenal insufficiency. **Unlabeled Use:** Adjunctive therapy of hypercalcemia. Management of acute spinal cord injury. Adjunctive management of nausea and vomiting from chemotherapy.

Action

Suppresses inflammation and the normal immune response. Has numerous intense metabolic effects (see Adverse Reactions and Side Effects). Suppresses adrenal function at chronic doses of 4 mg/day. Has negligible mineralocorticoid activity. **Therapeutic Effects:** Suppression of inflammation and modification of the normal immune response. Replacement therapy in adrenal insufficiency.

Adverse Reactions/Side Effects

Adverse reactions/side effects are much more common with high-dose/long-term therapy

CNS: depression, euphoria, headache, increased intracranial pressure (children only), personality changes, psychoses, restlessness. **EENT:** cataracts, increased intraocular pressure. **CV:** hypertension. **GI:** PEPTIC ULCERATION, anorexia, nausea, vomiting. **Derm:** acne, decreased wound healing, ecchymoses, fragility, hirsutism, petechiae. **Endo:** adrenal suppression, hyperglycemia. **F and E:** fluid retention (long-term high doses), hypokalemia, hypokalemic alkalosis. **Hemat:** THROMBOEMBOLISM, thrombophlebitis. **Metab:** weight gain, weight loss. **MS:** muscle wasting, osteoporosis, aseptic necrosis of joints, muscle pain. **Misc:** cushingoid appearance (moon face, buffalo hump), increased susceptibility to infection.

PHYSICAL THERAPY IMPLICATIONS

Examination and Evaluation

- Monitor signs of thrombophlebitis (lower extremity swelling, warmth, erythema, tenderness) and thromboembolism (shortness of breath, chest pain, cough, bloody sputum). Notify physician immediately, and request objective tests (Doppler ultrasound, lung scan, others) if thrombosis is suspected. Avoid exercise to the affected extremity and ambulation activities while awaiting further tests and evaluation.
- Monitor and report signs of peptic ulcer, including heartburn, nausea, vomiting blood, tarry stools, and loss of appetite.
- Assess signs of increased intracranial pressure in children, including changes in mood and behavior, decreased consciousness, headache, lethargy, seizures, and vomiting. Notify physician of these signs immediately.
- Assess any muscle or joint pain. Report persistent or increased musculoskeletal pain to determine presence of bone or joint pathology (aseptic necrosis, fracture).
- Assess muscle strength periodically to determine degree of muscle wasting during long-term use.
- Measure blood pressure periodically and compare to normal values (See Appendix F). Report a sustained increase in blood pressure (hypertension) to the physician.
- Assess peripheral edema using girth measurements, volume displacement, and measurement of pitting edema (See Appendix N). Report increased swelling in feet and ankles or a sudden increase in body weight due to fluid retention.
- Monitor personality changes, including depression, euphoria, restlessness, hallucinations, and psychosis. Notify physician if these changes become problematic.
- Be alert for signs of low potassium levels (hypokalemia) and metabolic acidosis, including hyperventilation, cardiac arrhythmias, dizziness, and confusion. Notify physician immediately if these signs occur.
- Report signs of adrenal suppression, including hypotension, weight loss, weakness, nausea, vomiting, anorexia, lethargy, confusion, and restlessness.
- Monitor signs of hyperglycemia (confusion; drowsiness; flushed, dry skin; fruit-like breath odor; rapid, deep breathing; polyuria; loss of appetite; unusual thirst). Insulin dosages may need to be adjusted to prevent repeated episodes of hyperglycemia.
- Periodically assess body weight and other anthropometric measures (body mass index, body composition). Report a rapid or unexplained weight gain or weight loss.
- If used to treat acute spinal cord injury, assess motor and sensory function to help determine the extent of recovery and return of neurologic function.

Interventions

- Implement resistive exercises and weight bearing activities to minimize muscle wasting and

osteoporosis. Use caution to prevent musculoskeletal damage in patients with preexisting muscle and bone loss.
- Protect skin from breakdown, especially over bony prominences.

Patient/Client-Related Instruction
- Advise patient that wound healing may be delayed; instruct patient to check skin regularly and report any nonhealing sores.
- Advise patient that corticosteroids cause immunosuppression and may mask symptoms of infection. Instruct patient to avoid people with known contagious illnesses and to report possible infections immediately.
- Advise patients on long-term treatment to consult physician before stopping this medication. Stopping the medication suddenly may result in adrenocortical shock (severe hypotension, hypoglycemia, weakness, vomiting). If these signs appear, notify physician immediately; may be life threatening.
- Instruct patient to report any loss of vision that might indicate cataracts or increased intraocular pressure.
- Advise patient about possible cushingoid appearance, including puffiness in the face (moon face), increased fat in the torso, thin arms and legs, abdominal skin striations, bruising, and deposition of fat at the posterior base of the neck (buffalo hump). Discuss possible effects on body image, and help patient explore coping mechanisms.
- Instruct patient and family/caregivers to report other troublesome side effects such as severe or prolonged headache, GI reactions (nausea, vomiting, loss of appetite), or skin reactions (acne, hair growth).

Pharmacokinetics
Absorption: Well absorbed after oral administration. Succinate salt is rapidly absorbed after IM administration. Acetate salt is slowly but completely absorbed after IM administration. Absorption from local sites (intra-articular, intralesional) is slow but complete.
Distribution: Widely distributed, crosses the placenta, and probably enters breast milk.
Metabolism and Excretion: Metabolized mostly by the liver.
Half-life: >3.5 hr (plasma), 18–36 hr (tissue); adrenal suppression lasts 1.25–1.5 days.

TIME/ACTION PROFILE (anti-inflammatory activity)

ROUTE	ONSET	PEAK	DURATION
PO	unknown	1–2 hr	1.25–1.5 days
IM (acetate)	6–48 hr	4–8 days	1–4 wk
IM, IV (succinate)	rapid	unknown	unknown

Contraindications/Precautions
Contraindicated in: Active untreated infections (may be used in patients being treated for tuberculous meningitis); Lactation (avoid chronic use); Known alcohol, bisulfite, or tartrazine hypersensitivity or intolerance (some products contain these and should be avoided in susceptible patients); Administration of live-virus vaccines.
Use Cautiously in: Chronic treatment (will lead to adrenal suppression; use lowest possible dose for shortest period of time); Children (chronic use will result in decreased growth; use lowest possible dose for shortest period of time); Stress (surgery, infections); supplemental doses may be needed; Potential infections may mask signs (fever, inflammation); Pregnancy (safety not established); Neonates (avoid use of benzyl alcohol containing injectable preparations; use preservative-free formulations).

M

Interactions
Drug-Drug: Additive hypokalemia with **thiazide** and **loop diuretics, amphotericin B, piperacillin,** or **ticarcillin**. Hypokalemia may ↑ the risk of **digitalis glycoside** toxicity. May ↑ requirement for **insulins** or **oral hypoglycemic agents. Phenytoin, phenobarbital,** and **rifampin** stimulate metabolism; may ↓ effectiveness. **Oral contraceptives** may block metabolism. ↑ risk of adverse GI effects with **NSAIDs** (including **aspirin**). At chronic doses that suppress adrenal function, may ↓ the antibody response to and ↑ the risk of adverse reactions from **live-virus vaccines**. May ↑ serum concentrations of **cyclosporine** and **tacrolimus**. May ↑ the risk of tendon rupture from **fluoroquinolones**.

Route/Dosage
PO (Adults): *Multiple sclerosis*—160 mg/day for 7 days, then 64 mg every other day for 1 mo. *Other uses*—2–60 mg/day as a single dose or in 2–4 divided doses. *Asthma exacerbations*—120–180 mg/day in divided doses tid–qid 48 hr, then 60–80 mg/day divided bid.
PO (Children): *Anti-inflammatory/Immunosuppressive*—0.5–1.7 mg/kg/day or 5–25 mg/m^2/day in divided doses q 6–12 hr. *Asthma exacerbations*—1 mg/kg q 6 hr for 48 hr, then 1–2 mg/kg/day (maximum: 60 mg/day) divided bid.
Rect (Adults): 40 mg 3–7 times weekly for at least 2 wk.
IM, IV (Adults): *Most uses: methylprednisolone sodium succinate*—40–250 mg q 4–6 hr. *High-dose "pulse" therapy: methylprednisolone sodium succinate*—30 mg/kg IV q 4–6 hr for up to 72 hr. *Multiple sclerosis: methylprednisolone sodium succinate*—160 mg/day for 7 days, then 64 mg every

other day for 1 mo. *Adjunctive therapy of* Pneumocystis carinii *pneumonia in AIDS patients: methylprednisolone sodium succinate*—30 mg bid for 5 days, then 30 mg once daily for 5 days, 15 mg once daily for 10 days. *Acute spinal cord injury: methylprednisolone sodium succinate*—30 mg/kg over 15 min initially, followed 45 min later with 5.4 mg/kg/hr for 23 hr (unlabeled).
IM, IV (Children): *Anti-inflammatory/ Immunosuppressive*— 0.5–1.7 mg/kg/day or 5–25 mg/m²/day in divided doses q 6–12 hr. *Acute spinal cord injury: methylprednisolone sodium succinate*—30 mg/kg over 15 min initially, then 45 min later initiate continuous infusion of 5.4 mg/kg/hr for 23 hr (unlabeled). *Status asthmaticus*—2 mg/kg/dose, then 0.5–1 mg/kg/dose q 6 hr. *Lupus nephritis*—30 mg/kg IV every other day for 6 doses.
IM (Adults): *Methylprednisolone acetate*—40–120 mg daily, weekly, or every 2 wk.

Availability (generic available)

Tablets: 2 mg, 4 mg, 8 mg, 16 mg, 24 mg, 32 mg. **Solution for injection:** 40 mg, 125 mg, 500 mg, 1 g, 2 g. **Suspension for injection:** 20 mg/mL, 40 mg/mL, 80 mg/mL. **Enema:** 40 mg.

metoclopramide

(met-oh-**kloe**-pra-mide)
Apo-Metoclop, Clopra, Emex, Maxeran, Octamide, Octamide-PFS, Reclomide, Reglan

Classification

Therapeutic: antiemetics
Pharmacologic: dopamine receptor antagonists

Indications

Prevention of chemotherapy-induced emesis. Treatment of postsurgical and diabetic gastric stasis. Facilitation of small bowel intubation in radiographic procedures. Management of esophageal reflux. Treatment and prevention of postoperative nausea and vomiting when nasogastric suctioning is undesirable. **Unlabeled Use:** Treatment of hiccups. Adjunct management of migraine headaches.

Action

Blocks dopamine receptors in chemoreceptor trigger zone of the CNS. Stimulates motility of the upper GI tract and accelerates gastric emptying. **Therapeutic Effects:** Decreased nausea and vomiting. Decreased symptoms of gastric stasis. Easier passage of nasogastric tube into small bowel.

Adverse Reactions/Side Effects

CNS: <u>drowsiness</u>, <u>extrapyramidal reactions</u>, <u>restlessness</u>, NEUROLEPTIC MALIGNANT SYNDROME, anxiety, depression, irritability, tardive dyskinesia. **CV:** arrhythmias (supraventricular tachycardia, bradycardia), hypertension, hypotension. **GI:** constipation, diarrhea, dry mouth, nausea. **Endo:** gynecomastia. **Hemat:** methemoglobinemia, neutropenia, leukopenia, agranulocytosis.

PHYSICAL THERAPY IMPLICATIONS

Examination and Evaluation

- Monitor signs of neuroleptic malignant syndrome, including hyperthermia, diaphoresis, generalized muscle rigidity, altered mental status, tachycardia, changes in blood pressure (BP), and incontinence. Symptoms typically occur within 4–14 days after initiation of drug therapy, but can occur at any time during drug use. Report these signs to the physician or nursing staff immediately.
- Assess motor function, and be alert for extrapyramidal symptoms. Report these symptoms immediately, especially tardive dyskinesia, because this problem may be irreversible. Common extrapyramidal symptoms include:
    - Tardive dyskinesia (uncontrolled rhythmic movement of mouth, face, and extremities, lip smacking or puckering, puffing of cheeks, uncontrolled chewing, rapid or worm-like movements of tongue).
    - Pseudoparkinsonism (shuffling gait, rigidity, tremor, pill-rolling motion, loss of balance control, difficulty speaking or swallowing, mask-like face).
    - Akathisia (restlessness or desire to keep moving).
    - Other dystonias and dyskinesias (dystonic muscle spasms, twisting motions, twitching, inability to move eyes, weakness of arms or legs).
- Monitor the frequency, severity, and duration of GI problems (nausea, vomiting, heartburn, hiccups) to help document drug effectiveness.
- Assess heart rate, ECG, and heart sounds, especially during exercise (See Appendices G, H). Report any disturbances in cardiac rhythm or symptoms of arrhythmias, including palpitations, chest discomfort, shortness of breath, fainting, and fatigue/weakness.
- Assess BP and compare to normal values (See Appendix F). Report changes in BP, either a problematic decrease in BP (hypotension) or a sustained increase in BP (hypertension).
- Monitor signs of agranulocytosis, neutropenia, and leukopenia (fever, sore throat, signs of infection) or methemoglobinemia (bluish coloring of the skin, lips fingernails; headache; shortness of breath; lack of energy). Report these signs to the physician or nursing staff.

- If used to treat migraines, assess the frequency and severity of headaches and document whether drug therapy is successful in decreasing migraine attacks.

Interventions

- Guard against falls and trauma (hip fractures, head injury, and so forth) caused by drowsiness, blurred vision, or extrapyramidal symptoms; implement fall prevention strategies (See Appendix E).
- Because of the risk of ECG changes and abnormal BP responses, use caution during aerobic exercise and other forms of therapeutic exercise. Assess exercise tolerance frequently (BP, heart rate, fatigue levels), and terminate exercise immediately if any untoward responses occur (See Appendix L).

Patient/Client-Related Instruction

- Instruct patient to report other problematic side effects such as severe or prolonged GI problems (nausea, diarrhea, constipation, dry mouth) or increased breast size in men (gynecomastia).

Pharmacokinetics

Absorption: Well absorbed from the GI tract, from rectal mucosa, and from IM sites.
Distribution: Widely distributed into body tissues and fluids. Crosses blood-brain barrier and placenta. Enters breast milk in concentrations greater than plasma.
Metabolism and Excretion: Partially metabolized by the liver; 25% eliminated unchanged in the urine.
Half-life: 2.5–6 hr.

TIME/ACTION PROFILE (effects on peristalsis)

ROUTE	ONSET	PEAK	DURATION
PO	30–60 min	unknown	1–2 hr
IM	10–15 min	unknown	1–2 hr
IV	1–3 min	immediate	1–2 hr

Contraindications/Precautions

Contraindicated in: Hypersensitivity; Possible GI obstruction or hemorrhage; History of seizure disorders; Pheochromocytoma; Parkinson's disease.
Use Cautiously in: History of depression; Diabetes (may alter response to insulin); Renal impairment (reduce dose in CCr <50 mL/min); OB/Lactation: Safety not established; Pedi: some syrup products contain benzoate, a metabolite of benzyl alcohol, which can cause potentially fatal gasping syndrome in neonates. Prolonged clearance in neonates can result in high serum concentrations and increase the risk for methemoglobinemia. Side effects are more common in children, especially extrapyramidal reactions; Geri: More susceptible to oversedation and extrapyramidal reactions.

Interactions

Drug-Drug: Additive CNS depression with other **CNS depressants**, including **alcohol, antidepressants, antihistamines, opioid analgesics,** and **sedative/hypnotics**. May ↑ absorption and risk of toxicity from **cyclosporine**. May affect the GI absorption of other **orally administered drugs** as a result of effect on GI motility. May exaggerate hypotension during **general anesthesia**. ↑ risk of extrapyramidal reactions with agents such as **haloperidol** or **phenothiazines**. **Opioids** and **anticholinergics** may antagonize the GI effects of metoclopramide. Use cautiously with **MAO inhibitors** (causes release of catecholamines). May ↑ neuromuscular blockade from **succinylcholine**. May ↓ effectiveness of **levodopa**. May ↑ **tacrolimus** serum levels.

M

Route/Dosage

Prevention of Chemotherapy-Induced Vomiting

PO, IV (Adults and Children): 1–2 mg/kg 30 min before chemotherapy. Additional doses of 1–2 mg/kg may be given q 2–4 hr; pretreatment with diphenhydramine will ↓ the risk of extrapyramidal reactions to this dosage.

Facilitation of Small Bowel Intubation

IV (Adults and Children >14 yr): 10 mg over 1–2 min.
IV (Children 6–14 yr): 2.5–5 mg (dose should not exceed 0.5 mg/kg) over 1–2 min.
IV (Children <6 yr): 0.1 mg/kg over 1–2 min.

Diabetic Gastroparesis

PO, IV (Adults): 10 mg 30 min before meals and at bedtime for 2–8 wk.

Gastroesophageal Reflux

PO, IM, IV (Adults): 10–15 mg 30 min before meals and at bedtime (not to exceed 0.5 mg/kg/day). A single dose of 20 mg may be given preventively. Some patients may respond to doses as small as 5 mg.
PO, IM, IV (Neonates, Infants, and Children): 0.4–0.8 mg/kg/day in 4 divided doses.

Postoperative Nausea/Vomiting

IM, IV (Adults and Children >14 yr): 10 mg at the end of surgical procedure; repeat in 6–8 hr if needed.
IM, IV (Children <14 yr): 0.1–0.2 mg/kg/dose; repeat in 6–8 hr if needed.

Treatment of Hiccups

PO, IM (Adults): 10–20 mg qid PO; may be preceded by a single 10-mg dose IM (unlabeled).

Availability (generic available)

Tablets: 5 mg, 10 mg. **Concentrated solution:** 10 mg/mL. **Syrup (apricot-peach flavor):** 5 mg/5 mL. **Injection:** 5 mg/mL.

metolazone (me-tole-a-zone)

Zaroxolyn

Classification

Therapeutic: antihypertensives, diuretics
Pharmacologic: thiazide-like diuretics

Indications

Mild-to-moderate hypertension. Edema associated with CHF or the nephrotic syndrome.

Action

Increases excretion of sodium and water by inhibiting sodium reabsorption in the distal tubule. Promotes excretion of chloride, potassium, magnesium, and bicarbonate. May produce arteriolar dilation. **Therapeutic Effects:** Lowering of blood pressure in hypertensive patients. Diuresis with subsequent mobilization of edema. Effect may continue in renal impairment.

Adverse Reactions/Side Effects

CNS: drowsiness, lethargy. **CV:** chest pain, hypotension, palpitations. **GI:** anorexia, bloating, cramping, drug-induced hepatitis, nausea, vomiting. **Derm:** photosensitivity, rashes. **Endo:** hyperglycemia. **F and E:** hypokalemia, dehydration, hypercalcemia, hypochloremic alkalosis, hypomagnesemia, hyponatremia, hypophosphatemia, hypovolemia. **Hemat:** blood dyscrasias. **Metab:** hyperuricemia. **MS:** muscle cramps. **Misc:** chills, pancreatitis.

PHYSICAL THERAPY IMPLICATIONS

Examination and Evaluation

- Monitor signs of fluid, electrolyte, or acid-base imbalances, including dizziness, drowsiness, blurred vision, confusion, hypotension, or muscle cramps and weakness. Report excessive or prolonged symptoms to the physician.
- Assess dizziness and weakness that might affect gait, balance, and other functional activities (See Appendix C). Report balance problems and functional limitations to the physician, and caution the patient and family/caregivers to guard against falls and trauma.
- Assess blood pressure periodically and compare to normal values (See Appendix F) to help document antihypertensive effects. Report low blood pressure (hypotension) or other cardiac symptoms such as chest pain or palpitations.
- When used to treat edema, help determine drug effects by assessing peripheral edema using girth measurements, volume displacement, and measurement of pitting edema (See Appendix N). Also monitor signs of pulmonary edema such as dyspnea and rales/crackles (See Appendix K). Document whether peripheral and pulmonary symptoms are controlled adequately by diuretic therapy.
- Monitor signs of hyperglycemia (drowsiness, fruity breath, increased urination, unusual thirst). Patients with diabetes mellitus should check blood glucose levels frequently.

Interventions

- Implement fall-prevention strategies, especially in older adults or if patient exhibits sedation, dizziness, blurred vision, or other impairments that affect gait and balance (See Appendix E).
- Use caution during aerobic exercise, especially in hot environments. Increased sweating will cause fluid and electrolyte loss, and may exaggerate diuretic side effects (dizziness, muscle cramps, and so forth).
- To minimize orthostatic hypotension, patient should move slowly when assuming a more upright position.
- Causes photosensitivity; use care if administering UV treatments.

Patient/Client-Related Instruction

- Remind patients to take medication as directed to control hypertension and other cardiac conditions even if they are asymptomatic.
- Counsel patients about additional interventions to help control blood pressure and cardiac dysfunction, including regular exercise, weight loss, sodium restriction, stress reduction, moderation of alcohol consumption, and smoking cessation.
- Instruct patient to report signs of thrombocytopenia (bruising, nose bleeds, and bleeding gums) or unusual weakness and fatigue that might be due to anemia or other blood dyscrasias.
- Advise patient about the possibility of GI reactions (cramping, bloating, nausea, vomiting, loss of appetite). Instruct patient or family and caregivers to report severe or prolonged GI symptoms or signs of hepatitis (abdominal pain, severe nausea and vomiting, yellow skin or eyes, fever, sore throat, malaise, weakness, facial edema, lethargy, unusual bleeding or bruising) or pancreatitis (upper abdominal pain after eating, indigestion, weight loss, oily stools).
- Advise patient about photosensitivity and to use sunscreens, protective clothing, and avoid prolonged sun exposure. Instruct patient also to report any rashes or other skin reactions.
- Advise patient that this drug may cause problems in fat and uric acid metabolism (hypercholesterolemia and hyperuricemia, respectively). Remind patient

that periodic blood tests may be needed to monitor plasma lipids and uric acid levels.

Pharmacokinetics

Absorption: Absorption is variable.
Distribution: Unknown.
Metabolism and Excretion: Excreted mainly unchanged by the kidneys.
Half-life: 8 hr.

TIME/ACTION PROFILE (diuretic effect*)

ROUTE	ONSET	PEAK	DURATION
PO	1 hr	2 hr	12–24 hr

*Full antihypertensive effect may take days–weeks.

Contraindications/Precautions

Contraindicated in: Hypersensitivity; Cross-sensitivity with other sulfonamides may exist; Anuria; OB: Lactation.
Use Cautiously in: Severe hepatic impairment; Geri: ↑ sensitivity; OB/Pedi: Pregnancy or children (safety not established; children may be more susceptible to diuretic and hypokalemic effects).

Interactions

Drug-Drug: ↑ risk of hypotension with **nitrates**, acute ingestion of **alcohol**, or other **antihypertensives**. ↑ risk of hypokalemia with **corticosteroids**, **amphotericin B**, **piperacillin**, or **ticarcillin**. May ↑ the risk of **digoxin** toxicity. ↓ the excretion of **lithium**; may cause toxicity. May ↓ the effectiveness of **methenamine**. **Stimulant laxatives** (including **aloe, senna**) may ↑ risk of potassium depletion.
Drug-Food: Food may ↑ extent of absorption.

Route/Dosage

PO (Adults): *Hypertension*—2.5–5 mg/day; *edema*—5–20 mg/day.

Availability (generic available)

Tablets: 2.5 mg, 5 mg, 10 mg.

HIGH ALERT

metoprolol (me-toe-proe-lole)

Beloc, Beloc-ZOK, Betaloc Durules, Betaloc-ZOK, ✱Lopresor, ✱Lopresor SR, Lopressor, Metoprol, Novo-metoprol, Seloken-ZOK, Toprol-XL

Classification
Therapeutic: antianginals, antihypertensives
Pharmacologic: beta blockers

Indications

Hypertension. Angina pectoris. Prevention of MI and decreased mortality in patients with recent MI. Management of stable, symptomatic (class II or III) heart failure due to ischemic, hypertensive, or cardiomyopathic origin (may be used with ACE inhibitors, diuretics, and/or digoxin; Toprol-XL 25 mg only). **Unlabeled Use:** Ventricular arrhythmias/tachycardia. Migraine prophylaxis. Tremors. Aggressive behavior. Drug-induced akathisia. Anxiety.

Action

Blocks stimulation of $beta_1$ (myocardial)–adrenergic receptors. Does not usually affect $beta_2$ (pulmonary, vascular, uterine)–adrenergic receptor sites. **Therapeutic Effects:** Decreased blood pressure and heart rate. Decreased frequency of attacks of angina pectoris. Decreased rate of cardiovascular mortality and hospitalization in patients with heart failure.

Adverse Reactions/Side Effects

CNS: <u>fatigue</u>, <u>weakness</u>, anxiety, depression, dizziness, drowsiness, insomnia, memory loss, mental status changes, nervousness, nightmares. **EENT:** blurred vision, stuffy nose. **Resp:** bronchospasm, wheezing. **CV:** BRADYCARDIA, CHF, PULMONARY EDEMA, hypotension, peripheral vasoconstriction. **GI:** constipation, diarrhea, drug-induced hepatitis, dry mouth, flatulence, gastric pain, heartburn, increased liver function studies, nausea, vomiting. **GU:** <u>erectile dysfunction</u>, decreased libido, urinary frequency. **Derm:** rashes. **Endo:** hyperglycemia, hypoglycemia. **MS:** arthralgia, back pain, joint pain. **Misc:** drug-induced lupus syndrome.

PHYSICAL THERAPY IMPLICATIONS

Examination and Evaluation

- Assess heart rate, ECG, and heart sounds, especially during exercise (See Appendices G, H). Although intended to treat certain arrhythmias, this drug can unmask or precipitate new arrhythmias (proarrhythmic effect). Report an unusually slow heart rate (bradycardia) or signs of other arrhythmias, including palpitations, chest pain, shortness of breath, fainting, and fatigue/weakness.
- Watch for signs of CHF and pulmonary edema, including dyspnea, rales/crackles, weight gain, peripheral edema, and jugular venous distention. Report any new or increased signs of heart failure, but also determine if drug therapy is effective in reducing these symptoms in patients with preexisting heart failure.
- Assess blood pressure periodically and compare to normal values (See Appendix F) to help document antihypertensive effects. Report low blood pressure (hypotension), especially if patient experiences dizziness or syncope.
- If used to prevent migraine headaches, monitor the incidence and severity of migraine attacks to document

✱ = Canadian drug name; *CAPITALS indicate life-threatening; <u>underlines</u> indicate most frequent.

whether this drug is successful in helping manage the patient's pain.

- Assess exercise tolerance and episodes of angina pectoris. Document improvements in these variables, but also report any decline in exercise tolerance or increased frequency/severity of anginal attacks.
- Assess symptoms of bronchospasm (wheezing, coughing, tightness in chest). Perform pulmonary function tests to quantify suspected changes in ventilation and respiration (See Appendices I, J, K). Repeated or prolonged bronchoconstriction may require a change in dose or medication.
- Monitor signs of peripheral vasoconstriction, such as extreme coldness in the hands and feet, cyanosis, and muscle cramping. Notify physician of severe or prolonged signs of vasoconstriction.
- Assess dizziness and drowsiness that might affect gait, balance, and other functional activities (See Appendix C). Report balance problems and functional limitations to the physician, and caution the patient and family/caregivers to guard against falls and trauma.
- Monitor excessive fatigue or weakness. Beta blockers often cause some degree of fatigue and weakness, but any sudden or severe change in muscle strength or energy levels should be reported.
- Watch for signs of hypoglycemia (weakness, malaise, irritability, fatigue) or hyperglycemia (drowsiness, fruity breath, increased urination, unusual thirst). Medication may mask some signs of hypoglycemia, but dizziness and sweating may still occur. Patients with diabetes mellitus should check blood glucose levels frequently.
- Assess any back pain or joint pain to rule out musculoskeletal pathology; that is, try to determine if pain is drug-induced rather than caused by anatomic or biomechanical problems.
- Monitor mood and personality changes, including depression, anxiety, nervousness, memory loss, or other changes in behavior. Notify physician if these changes become problematic.
- Monitor signs of drug-induced lupus syndrome, including increased BP, fever, joint pain, skin rashes, and redness/irritation of the eye (uveitis). Notify physician promptly if these signs appear.

Interventions

- Design and implement aerobic exercise and endurance training programs to improve coronary perfusion, reduce angina, and improve myocardial pumping ability.
- Because of an increased risk of cardiac arrhythmias (bradycardia, others), use caution during aerobic exercise and endurance conditioning. Likewise, monitor patients closely during treatment of other cardiac problems (angina, CHF, recent MI). Terminate exercise if patient exhibits untoward symptoms (chest pain, shortness of breath, unusual fatigue), or displays other criteria for exercise termination (See Appendix L).
- Establish aerobic exercise workloads that account for the effects of beta blockers on heart rate. Some heart rate guidelines may not be appropriate because beta blockers typically decrease maximal HR by 20–30 bpm. Use other guidelines such as rating of perceived exertion (RPE, modified Borg scale) to determine exercise workloads.
- To minimize orthostatic hypotension, patient should move slowly when assuming a more upright position.

Patient/Client-Related Instruction

- Remind patients to take medication as directed to control hypertension and other cardiac conditions even if they are asymptomatic.
- Instruct patients with heart failure to weigh themselves every day, and call their physician if they gain 3 lb or more in 1 day or more than 5 lb in 1 week. Sudden weight gain may indicate fluid buildup due to worsening heart failure.
- Counsel patients about additional interventions to help control blood pressure and cardiac dysfunction, including regular exercise, weight loss, sodium restriction, stress reduction, moderation of alcohol consumption, and smoking cessation.
- Instruct patient to report severe or prolonged GI problems (constipation, diarrhea, flatulence, heartburn, dry mouth) or signs of drug-induced hepatitis (anorexia, abdominal pain, severe nausea and vomiting, yellow skin or eyes, skin rashes, flu-like symptoms, muscle/joint pain).
- Instruct patient or family/caregivers to report other troublesome side effects such as severe or prolonged insomnia, nightmares, blurred vision, stuffy nose, increased urination, skin rash, or sexual problems (decreased libido, erectile dysfunction).

Pharmacokinetics

Absorption: Well absorbed after oral administration.
Distribution: Crosses the blood-brain barrier, crosses the placenta; small amounts enter breast milk.
Metabolism and Excretion: Mostly metabolized by the liver.
Half-life: 3–7 hr.

TIME/ACTION PROFILE (cardiovascular effects)

ROUTE	ONSET	PEAK	DURATION
PO*	15 min	Unknown	6–12 hr
PO–ER	unknown	6–12 hr	24 hr
IV	immediate	20 min	5–8 hr

*Maximal effects on blood pressure (chronic therapy) may not occur for 1 wk. Hypotensive effects may persist for up to 4 wk after discontinuation.

Contraindications/Precautions

Contraindicated in: Uncompensated CHF; Pulmonary edema; Cardiogenic shock; Bradycardia or heart block.

Use Cautiously in: Renal impairment; Hepatic impairment; Geri: Geriatric patients (↑ sensitivity to beta blockers; initial dose reduction recommended); Pulmonary disease (including asthma; beta$_1$ selectivity may be lost at higher doses); Diabetes mellitus (may mask signs of hypoglycemia); Thyrotoxicosis (may mask symptoms); Patients with a history of severe allergic reactions (intensity of reactions may be increased); OB: Pregnancy, lactation, or children (safety not established; all agents cross the placenta and may cause fetal/neonatal bradycardia, hypotension, hypoglycemia, or respiratory depression).

Interactions

Drug-Drug: General anesthesia, **IV phenytoin**, and **verapamil** may cause ↑ myocardial depression. ↑ bradycardia may occur with **digoxin**. ↑ hypotension may occur with other **antihypertensives**, acute ingestion of **alcohol**, or **nitrates**. Concurrent use with **amphetamines, cocaine, ephedrine, epinephrine, norepinephrine, phenylephrine**, or **pseudoephedrine** may result in unopposed alpha-adrenergic stimulation (excessive hypertension, bradycardia). Concurrent administration of **thyroid** administration may ↓ effectiveness. May alter the effectiveness of **insulins** or **oral hypoglycemic agents** (dosage adjustments may be necessary). May ↓ the effectiveness of **theophylline**. May ↓ the beneficial beta$_1$ cardiovascular effects of **dopamine** or **dobutamine**. Use cautiously within 14 days of **MAO inhibitor** therapy (may result in hypertension).

Route/Dosage

PO (Adults): *Antihypertensive/antianginal*—25–100 mg/day as a single dose initially or 2 divided doses; may be increased q 7 days as needed up to 450 mg/day (for angina, give in divided doses). Extended-release products are given once daily. *MI*—25–50 mg (starting 15 min after last IV dose) q 6 hr for 48 hr, then 100 mg twice daily for a minimum of 3 mo. *Heart failure*—12.5–25 mg once daily, can be doubled every 2 wk up to 200 mg/day. *Migraine prevention*—50–100 mg 2–4 times daily (unlabeled).

IV (Adults): *MI*—5 mg q 2 min for 3 doses, followed by oral dosing.

Availability (generic available)

Tablets (tartrate): 25 mg, 50 mg, 100 mg. **Extended-release tablets (succinate; Toprol-XL):** 25 mg, 50 mg, 100 mg, 200 mg. **Injection:** 1 mg/mL. ***In combination with:*** hydrochlorothiazide (Lopressor HCT). See Appendix B.

metronidazole

(me-troe-**nye**-da-zole)

Apo-Metronidazole, Flagyl, Flagyl ER, Metric 21, MetroCream, MetroGel, MetroGel-Vaginal, MetroLotion, Metro IV, Metryl, 🍁Nidagel, Noritate, 🍁Novonidazol, Protostat, 🍁Trikacide

Classification

Therapeutic: anti-infectives, antiprotozoals, antiulcer agents

Pharmacologic: Nitroimidazole derivatives

Indications

PO, IV: Treatment of the following anaerobic infections: Intra-abdominal infections (may be used with a cephalosporin), Gynecologic infections, Skin and skin structure infections, Lower respiratory tract infections, Bone and joint infections, CNS infections, Septicemia, Endocarditis. **IV:** Perioperative prophylactic agent in colorectal surgery. **PO:** Amebicide in the management of amebic dysentery, amebic liver abscess, and trichomoniasis: Treatment of peptic ulcer disease caused by *Helicobacter pylori*. **Topical:** Treatment of acne rosacea. **Vaginal:** Management of bacterial vaginosis. **Unlabeled Use:** Treatment of giardiasis. Treatment of anti-infective–associated pseudomembranous colitis.

Action

Disrupts DNA and protein synthesis in susceptible organisms. **Therapeutic Effects:** Bactericidal, trichomonacidal, or amebicidal action. **Spectrum:** Most notable for activity against anaerobic bacteria, including *Bacteroides*, *Clostridium*. In addition, is active against *Trichomonas vaginalis*, *Entamoeba histolytica*, *Giardia lamblia*, *H. pylori*, *C. difficile*.

Adverse Reactions/Side Effects

CNS: SEIZURES, dizziness, headache. **EENT:** tearing (topical only). **GI:** abdominal pain, anorexia, nausea, diarrhea, dry mouth, furry tongue, glossitis, unpleasant taste, vomiting. **Derm:** rashes, urticaria; **topical only—** burning, mild dryness, skin irritation, transient redness. **Hemat:** leukopenia. **Local:** phlebitis at IV site. **Neuro:** peripheral neuropathy. **Misc:** superinfection, disulfiram-type reaction with alcohol.

PHYSICAL THERAPY IMPLICATIONS

Examination and Evaluation

- Watch for seizures; notify physician immediately if patient develops or increases seizure activity.
- Monitor signs of peripheral neuropathy (numbness, tingling). Perform objective tests (nerve

conduction, monofilaments) to document any neuropathic changes.

- Monitor signs of disulfiram-like reaction (i.e., toxicity occurring when this drug is taken with alcohol). Signs include throbbing headache, difficulty breathing, nausea, vomiting, sweating, thirst, chest pain, palpitations, tachycardia, hypotension, syncope, agitation, confusion, weakness, vertigo, and blurred vision. Report these signs to the physician immediately.
- Assess dizziness that might affect gait, balance, and other functional activities (see Appendix C). Report balance problems and functional limitations to the physician and nursing staff, and caution the patient and family/caregivers to guard against falls and trauma.
- Be alert for confusion, agitation, headache, or other alterations in mental status. Notify the physician promptly if these symptoms develop.
- Monitor IV injection site for pain, swelling, and irritation. Report prolonged or excessive injection site reactions to the physician.

Interventions

- Always wash hands thoroughly and disinfect equipment (whirlpools, electrotherapeutic devices, treatment tables, and so forth) to help prevent the spread of infection. Employ universal precautions or isolation procedures as indicated for specific patients.

Patient/Client-Related Instruction

- Instruct patient to report signs of leukopenia, including fever, sore throat, and signs of infection.
- Instruct patient to notify physician immediately of signs of superinfection, including black, furry overgrowth on tongue, vaginal itching or discharge, and loose or foul-smelling stools.
- Advise patient about the likelihood of GI reactions, including nausea, vomiting, diarrhea, loss of appetite, and abdominal pain. Instruct patient to report severe or prolonged GI problems.
- Advise patient about the likelihood of skin reactions, including rash, hives, and local irritation during topical application. Report severe or unexpected skin reactions to the physician.

Pharmacokinetics

Absorption: 80% absorbed after oral administration. Minimal absorption after topical or vaginal application.

Distribution: Widely distributed into most tissues and fluids, including CSF. Crosses the placenta and enters fetal circulation rapidly; enters breast milk in concentrations equal to plasma levels.

Metabolism and Excretion: Partially metabolized by the liver (30–60%), partially excreted unchanged in the urine, 6–15% eliminated in the feces.

Half-life: Neonates: 25–75 hr; Children and adults: 6–12 hr.

TIME/ACTION PROFILE (PO, IV = blood levels; topical = improvement in rosacea)

ROUTE	ONSET	PEAK	DURATION
PO	rapid	1–3 hr	8 hr
PO-ER	rapid	unknown	up to 24 hr
IV	rapid	end of infusion	6–8 hr
topical	3 wk	9 wk	12 hr
vaginal	unknown	6–12 hr	12 hr

Contraindications/Precautions

Contraindicated in: Hypersensitivity; Hypersensitivity to parabens (topical only); 1st trimester of pregnancy.

Use Cautiously in: History of blood dyscrasias; History of seizures or neurologic problems; Severe hepatic impairment (dose reduction suggested); Pregnancy (although safety not established, has been used to treat trichomoniasis in 2nd- and 3rd-trimester pregnancy—but not as single-dose regimen); Lactation (if needed, use single dose and interrupt nursing for 24 hr thereafter); Patients receiving corticosteroids or predisposed to edema (injection contains 28 mEq sodium/g metronidazole).

Interactions

Drug-Drug: Cimetidine may ↓ the metabolism of metronidazole. **Phenobarbital** and **rifampin** ↑ metabolism and may ↓ effectiveness. Metronidazole ↑ the effects of **phenytoin, lithium,** and **warfarin**. Disulfiram-like reaction may occur with **alcohol** ingestion. May cause acute psychosis and confusion with **disulfiram**. ↑ risk of leukopenia with **fluorouracil** or **azathioprine**.

Route/Dosage

PO (Adults): *Anaerobic infections*—7.5 mg/kg q 6 hr (not to exceed 4 g/day). *Trichomoniasis*—250 mg q 8 hr for 7 days *or* single 2-g dose *or* 1 g bid for 1 day. *Amebiasis*—500–750 mg q 8 hr for 5–10 days. *H. pylori*—250 mg qid *or* 500 mg bid for 1–2 wk (with other agents). *Bacterial vaginoses*—750 mg once daily as ER tablets for 7 days. *Antibiotic-associated pseudomembranous colitis*—250–500 mg tid–qid times/day for 10–14 days.

PO (Infants and Children): *Anaerobic infections*—30 mg/kg/day divided q 6 hr, maximum dose: 4 g/day. *Trichomoniasis*—15–30 mg/kg/day divided q 8 hr for 7–10 days. *Amebiasis*—35–50 mg/kg/day divided q 8 hr for 5–10 days (not to exceed 750 mg/dose). *Antibiotic-associated pseudomembranous colitis*—30 mg/kg/day divided q 6 hr for 7–10 days. *H. pylori*—15–20 mg/kg/day divided bid for 4 wk.

IV, PO (Neonates 0–4 weeks, <1200 g): 7.5 mg/kg q 48 hr. *Postnatal age <7 days, 1200–2000 g*—7.5 mg/kg/day q 24 hr. *Postnatal age <7 days, >2000 g*—15 mg/kg/day divided q 12 hr. *Postnatal*

age >7 days, 1200–2000 g—15 mg/kg/day divided q 12 hr. *Postnatal age >7 days, >2000 g*—30 mg/kg/day divided q 12 hr.
IV (Adults): *Anaerobic infections*—Initial dose 15 mg/kg, then 7.5 mg/kg q 6–8 hr *or* 500 mg q 6–8 hr (not to exceed 4 g/day). *Perioperative prophylaxis*—Initial dose 15 mg/kg 1 hr before surgery, then 7.5 mg/kg 6 and 12 hr later. *Amebiasis*—500–750 mg q 8 hr for 5–10 days.
IV (Children): *Anaerobic infections*—30 mg/kg/day divided q 6 hr, maximum dose 4 g/day.
Topical (Adults): *Acne rosacea*—apply thin film to affected area bid.
Vaginal (Adults): *Bacterial vaginosis*—1 applicator full (5 g) bid for 5 days.

Availability (generic available)

Tablets: 250 mg, 500 mg. **Extended-release (ER) tablets:** 750 mg. **Capsules:** 375 mg, 500 mg. **Premixed injection:** 500 mg/100 mL RTU (ready-to-use). **Topical gel:** 0.75% in 45-g and 60-g tubes. **Topical cream:** 0.75% in 45-g tubes, 1% in 60-g tubes. **Topical lotion:** 0.75% in 59-mL bottle. **Vaginal gel:** 0.75% (37.5 mg/5 g applicator full) in 70-g tubes. ***In combination with:*** bismuth subsalicylate tablets and tetracycline capsules (Helidac) as part of a compliance package; bismuth subcitrate potassium and tetracycline (Pylera). See Appendix B.

mexiletine (mex-il-e-teen)

Mexitil

Classification
Therapeutic: antiarrhythmics (class IB)

Indications

Prophylaxis/treatment of serious ventricular arrhythmias, including ventricular tachycardia (VT) and premature ventricular contractions (PVCs). **Unlabeled Use:** Management of chronic neuropathic pain.

Action

Decreases the duration of the action potential and effective refractory period in cardiac conduction tissue by altering transport of sodium across myocardial cell membranes. Has little or no effect on heart rate. **Therapeutic Effects:** Control of ventricular arrhythmias.

Adverse Reactions/Side Effects

CNS: dizziness, nervousness, confusion, fatigue, headache, sleep disorder. **EENT:** blurred vision, tinnitus. **Resp:** dyspnea. **CV:** ARRHYTHMIAS, chest pain, edema, palpitations. **GI:** HEPATIC NECROSIS, heartburn, nausea, vomiting. **Derm:** rashes. **Hemat:** blood dyscrasias. **Neuro:** tremor, coordination difficulties, paresthesia.

PHYSICAL THERAPY IMPLICATIONS

Examination and Evaluation

- Assess heart rate, ECG, and heart sounds, especially during exercise (See Appendices G, H). Although intended to treat certain arrhythmias, this drug can unmask or precipitate new arrhythmias (proarrhythmic effect). Report any rhythm disturbances or symptoms of increased arrhythmias, including palpitations, chest pain, shortness of breath, fainting, and fatigue/weakness.
- Be alert for signs of liver dysfunction and hepatic necrosis, including anorexia, abdominal pain, severe nausea and vomiting, yellow skin or eyes, fever, sore throat, malaise, weakness, facial edema, lethargy, and unusual bleeding or bruising. Report these signs to the physician immediately.
- Monitor signs of blood dyscrasias including agranulocytosis (fever, sore throat, mucosal lesions, other signs of infection), thrombocytopenia (bruising, nose bleeds, bleeding gums), or anemia (unusual fatigue, shortness of breath, dizziness, headache, coldness in your hands and feet, pale skin, chest pain). Report these signs to the physician.
- Assess peripheral edema using girth measurements, volume displacement, and measurement of pitting edema (See Appendix N). Report increased swelling in feet and ankles or a sudden increase in body weight due to fluid retention.
- Assess signs of parasthesia (numbness, tingling) or tremor. Perform objective tests including electroneuromyography and sensory testing to document any drug-related neuropathic changes.
- If treating neuropathic pain, use visual analogue scales and other appropriate pain scales to assess the patient's pain and help document the effects of drug therapy.
- Monitor nervousness, confusion, or other changes in mood and behavior. Notify physician if these changes become problematic.
- Assess dizziness or incoordination that might affect gait, balance, and other functional activities (See Appendix C). Report balance problems and functional limitations to the physician, and caution the patient and family/caregivers to guard against falls and trauma.

Interventions

- Because of the risk of serious cardiac arrhythmias, use extreme caution during aerobic exercise and other forms of therapeutic exercise.

M

Assess exercise tolerance frequently (blood pressure, heart rate, fatigue levels), and terminate exercise immediately if any untoward responses occur (See Appendix L).

- If treating chronic neuropathic pain, implement appropriate interventions (physical agents, manual techniques, therapeutic exercise) to manage pain and reduce the need for drug therapy. Help patient also explore other non-pharmacological methods to reduce chronic pain such as relaxation techniques, imagery, counseling, and so forth.

Patient/Client-Related Instruction

- Advise patient and family/caregivers about the signs of cardiac arrhythmias (see above under Examination and Evaluation) and to seek immediate medical assistance if these signs develop.
- Instruct patient and family/caregivers to report other side effects such as severe or prolonged headache, sleep disorders, vision problems, difficult/labored breathing, ringing/buzzing in the ears (tinnitus), tremor, fatigue, skin rash, or GI problems (nausea, vomiting, heartburn).

Pharmacokinetics

Absorption: Well absorbed from the GI tract.
Distribution: Enters breast milk in concentrations similar to plasma.
Metabolism and Excretion: Mostly metabolized by the liver; 10% excreted unchanged by the kidneys.
Half-life: 10–12 hr.

TIME/ACTION PROFILE (antiarrhythmic effects*)

ROUTE	ONSET	PEAK	DURATION
PO	30 min–2 hr	2–3 hr	8–12 hr

*Provided a loading dose has been given.

Contraindications/Precautions

Contraindicated in: Hypersensitivity; Cardiogenic shock; 2nd- or 3rd-degree heart block (if a pacemaker has not been inserted); Lactation.
Use Cautiously in: Sinus node or intraventricular conduction abnormalities; Hypotension; CHF; Severe hepatic impairment (dosage reduction suggested); Pregnancy or children (safety not established).

Interactions

Drug-Drug: Opioid analgesics, atropine, and **antacids** may slow absorption. **Metoclopramide** may speed absorption. **Phenytoin, rifampin, cigarette smoking**, or **phenobarbital** may ↑ metabolism and ↓ effectiveness. **Cimetidine** may ↑ or ↓ mexiletine levels. May ↑ blood levels and risk of toxicity from **theophylline**. Additive cardiac effects may occur with other **antiarrhythmics. Drugs that drastically alter urine pH** may alter blood levels (alkalinization ↑ reabsorption and blood levels; acidification ↑ excretion and ↓ blood levels).
Drug-Food: Foods that drastically alter urine pH may alter blood levels. Alkalinization ↑ reabsorption and ↑ blood levels. Acidification ↑ excretion and may ↓ effectiveness (See Appendix L).

Route/Dosage

PO (Adults): 400-mg loading dose initially, then 200 mg 8 hr later, then 200–400 mg q 8 hr; dosage alterations of 50–100 mg may be made q 2–3 days. If controlled on ≤300 mg q 8 hr, can give same daily dose at 12-hr intervals (not to exceed 1200 mg/day). Some patients may require q 6 hr dosing.

Availability

Capsules: 100 mg, 150 mg, 200 mg, 250 mg.

micafungin (mye-ka-fun-jin)

Mycamine

Classification
Therapeutic: antifungals
Pharmacologic: echinocandins

Indications

Esophageal candidiasis. Candidemia/acute disseminated candidiasis/Candidal peritonitis and abscesses. Prophylaxis of *Candida* infections during hematopoietic stem cell transplantation.

Action

Inhibits synthesis of glucan required for the formation of fungal cell wall. **Therapeutic Effects:** Death of susceptible fungi. **Spectrum:** Active against the following *Candida* spp.: *C. albicans*, *C. glabrata*, *C. krusei*, *C. parapsilosis*, *C. tropicalis*.

Adverse Reactions/Side Effects

GI: worsening hepatic function/hepatitis. **GU:** renal impairment. **Hemat:** hemolysis/hemolytic anemia. **Local:** injection-site reactions. **Misc:** ALLERGIC REACTIONS, INCLUDING ANAPHYLAXIS (RARE).

PHYSICAL THERAPY IMPLICATIONS

Examination and Evaluation

- Monitor signs of allergic reactions and anaphylaxis, including pulmonary symptoms (tightness in the throat and chest, wheezing, cough, dyspnea) or skin reactions (rash, pruritus, urticaria). Notify physician or nursing staff immediately if these reactions occur.
- Be alert for signs of liver dysfunction and hepatitis, including anorexia, abdominal pain, severe nausea and vomiting, yellow skin or eyes, fever, sore throat, malaise, weakness, facial edema, lethargy, and unusual bleeding or bruising. Report these signs to the physician immediately.

- Monitor and report signs of hemolytic anemia, including unusual weakness and fatigue, dizziness, jaundice, and abdominal pain.
- Monitor IV injection site for pain, swelling, and irritation. Report prolonged or excessive injection-site reactions to the physician.

Interventions

- Always wash hands thoroughly and disinfect equipment (whirlpools, electrotherapeutic devices, treatment tables, and so forth) to help prevent the spread of infection. Use universal precautions or isolation procedures as indicated for specific patients.

Patient/Client-Related Instruction

- Instruct patient to report signs of renal impairment, including decreased urine output, cloudy urine, and sudden weight gain due to fluid retention.

Pharmacokinetics

Absorption: IV administration results in complete bioavailability.
Distribution: Unknown.
Protein Binding: >99 %.
Metabolism and Excretion: Mostly metabolized; 71% fecal elimination.
Half-life: 15 hr.

TIME/ACTION PROFILE

ROUTE	ONSET	PEAK	DURATION
IV	rapid	end of infusion	24 hr

Contraindications/Precautions

Contraindicated in: Hypersensitivity.
Use Cautiously in: Severe hepatic impairment; OB/Lactation/Pedi: Lactation or children (safety not established), pregnancy (use only if clearly needed).

Interactions

Drug-Drug: ↑ blood levels and risk of toxicity with **sirolimus** and **nifedipine** (dose adjustments may be necessary).

Route/Dosage

IV (Adults): *Esophageal candidiasis*—150 mg/day for 15 days (range 10–30 days); *Candidemia/acute disseminated candidiasis/*Candida *peritonitis and abscesses*—100 mg/day for 15 days (range 10–47 days); *Prevention of* Candida *infections in stem cell transplantation*—50 mg/day.

Availability

Lyophilized powder for injection: 50 mg/vial, 100 mg/vial.

miconazole (topical)

(mye-**kon**-a-zole)
Fungoid, Lotrimin AF, Micatin, ✱ Micozole, Monistat-Derm, Zeasorb-AF

miconazole (vaginal)

(mye-**kon**-a-zole)
Monistat-1, Monistat-3, Monistat-7, Vagistat-3

Classification
Therapeutic: antifungals (topical, vaginal)
Pharmacologic: imidazoles

M

Indications

Treatment of a variety of cutaneous fungal infections, including tinea pedis (athlete's foot), tinea cruris (jock itch), tinea corporis (ringworm). Treatment of vulvovaginal candidiasis.

Action

Affects the synthesis of the fungal cell wall, allowing leakage of cellular contents. **Therapeutic Effects:** Decrease in symptoms of fungal infection.

Adverse Reactions/Side Effects

Local: burning, itching, local hypersensitivity reactions, redness, stinging.

PHYSICAL THERAPY IMPLICATIONS

Examination and Evaluation

- Monitor symptoms and healing of skin lesions to help document drug effectiveness.

Interventions

- Avoid contact with cutaneous lesions when treating patient.
- Always wash hands thoroughly and disinfect equipment (whirlpools, electrotherapeutic devices, treatment tables, and so forth) to help prevent the spread of infection.

Patient/Client-Related Instruction

- Advise patient to report any increased local sensitivity to this drug (pain, burning, itching, swelling).
- Instruct patient about proper hygiene; e.g., thoroughly wash and dry the affected area, wear clean socks and ventilated shoes for tinea pedis, and so forth.
- Advise patient to apply the drug as directed for the full course of treatment, even if feeling better.
- Inform patient that early relief of cutaneous symptoms may be seen in 2–3 days. Full therapeutic

response may take 2 wk for tinea cruris and tinea corporis and 3–4 wk for tinea pedis.

- Vaginal infections: therapeutic response is usually seen after 1 wk. Therapy should be continued during menstrual period.
- Advise patient to seek medical help if infections persist or recur after the full treatment. Recurrent fungal infections may be a sign of systemic illness.

Pharmacokinetics

Absorption: Absorption through intact skin is minimal.
Distribution: Distribution after topical administration is primarily local.
Metabolism and Excretion: Systemic metabolism and excretion not known following local application.
Half-life: Not applicable.

TIME/ACTION PROFILE

ROUTE	ONSET	PEAK	DURATION
topical	unknown	unknown	unknown
intravaginal	unknown	unknown	unknown

Contraindications/Precautions

Contraindicated in: Hypersensitivity to active ingredients, additives, preservatives, or bases; Some products contain alcohol or bisulfites and should be avoided in patients with known intolerance.
Use Cautiously in: Nail and scalp infections (may require additional systemic therapy); OB/Lactation: Safety not established.

Interactions

Drug-Drug: Not known.

Route/Dosage

Topical (Adults and Children >2 yr): Apply twice daily. Treat patients with tinea cruris for 2 wk and patients with tinea pedis or tinea corporis for 4 wk.
Vaginal (Adults and Children ≥12 yr): *Vaginal suppositories*—1 100-mg suppository at bedtime for 7 days, *or* 1 200-mg suppository at bedtime for 3 days, *or* 1 1200-mg suppository as a single dose. *Vaginal cream*—1 applicatorful of 2% cream at bedtime for 7 days *or* 1 applicatorful of 4% cream at bedtime for 3 days. *Combination packs*—contain a cream or suppositories as well as an external vaginal cream (may be used bid daily for up to 7 days, as needed, for symptomatic management of itching).

Availability (generic available)

Cream: 2% Rx, OTC. **Lotion powder:** 2% OTC. **Ointment:** 2% OTC. **Powder:** 2% OTC. **Solution:** 2% OTC. **Spray liquid:** 2% OTC. **Spray powder:** 2% OTC. **Tincture:** 2% OTC. ***In combination with:*** zinc oxide (Vusion) Rx Appendix B.
Vaginal cream: 2% OTC, 4% OTC. **Vaginal suppositories:** 100 mg OTC, 200 mg Rx, OTC. ***In combination with:*** combination package of 3 200-mg suppositories and 2% external cream OTC; 1 1200-mg suppository and 2% external cream OTC; 4% vaginal cream and 2% external cream OTC; 7 100-mg suppositories and 2% external cream OTC; 2% vaginal cream and 2% external cream OTC.

HIGH ALERT

midazolam (me-daz-oh-lam)

Versed

Classification
Therapeutic: antianxiety agents, sedative/hypnotics
Pharmacologic: benzodiazepines

Schedule IV

Indications

PO: Preprocedural sedation and anxiolysis in pediatric patients. **IM, IV:** Preoperative sedation/anxiolysis/amnesia. **IV:** Provides sedation/anxiolysis/amnesia during therapeutic, diagnostic, or radiographic procedures (conscious sedation): Aids in the induction of anesthesia and as part of balanced anesthesia. As a continuous infusion, provides sedation of mechanically ventilated patients during anesthesia or in a critical care setting, status epilepticus.

Action

Acts at many levels of the CNS to produce generalized CNS depression. Effects may be mediated by gamma-aminobutyric acid (GABA), an inhibitory neurotransmitter. **Therapeutic Effects:** Short-term sedation. Postoperative amnesia.

Adverse Reactions/Side Effects

CNS: agitation, drowsiness, excess sedation, headache. **EENT:** blurred vision. **Resp:** APNEA, LARYNGOSPASM, RESPIRATORY DEPRESSION, bronchospasm, coughing. **CV:** CARDIAC ARREST, arrhythmias. **GI:** hiccups, nausea, vomiting. **Derm:** rashes. **Local:** phlebitis at IV site, pain at IM site.

PHYSICAL THERAPY IMPLICATIONS*

**Implications refer primarily to any residual effects that occur typically within 24 hr after anesthesia.*

Examination and Evaluation

- Continually monitor for signs of cardiac arrest such as sudden chest pain, pain radiating into the arm or jaw, shortness of breath, dizziness, sweating, anxiety, nausea, and loss of consciousness. Seek immediate medical assistance if patient develops these signs.
- Assess respiration and notify physician or nursing staff immediately if patient exhibits any interruption

in respiratory rate (apnea) or signs of respiratory depression. Signs include decreased or absent respiration, confusion, bluish color of the skin and mucous membranes (cyanosis), and difficult, labored breathing (dyspnea). Monitor pulse oximetry and perform pulmonary function tests (See Appendix I) to quantify suspected changes in ventilation and respiratory function. Apnea or severe respiratory depression requires emergency care.

- Monitor signs of laryngeal spasm and bronchospasm, including tightness in the throat and chest, wheezing, cough, and severe shortness of breath. Notify physician or nursing staff immediately if these reactions occur.
- Assess heart rate, ECG, and heart sounds, especially during exercise (See Appendices G, H). Report any rhythm disturbances or symptoms of increased arrhythmias, including palpitations, chest discomfort, shortness of breath, fainting, and fatigue/weakness.
- Report excessive or prolonged sedation, agitation, or blurred vision; that is, CNS symptoms that persist more than 12 hr after the drug has been discontinued.
- If used to stop a severe, prolonged seizure (status epilepticus), watch for seizures after midazolam is discontinued. Report a return of seizure activity to the physician or nursing staff immediately.
- If used during mechanical ventilation, observe whether the patient is adequately sedated and the chest wall is relaxed and compliant with ventilation. Notify physician or nursing staff if the patient is agitated or appears to be resisting mechanical ventilation.
- Monitor injection site for pain, swelling, and inflammation consistent with phlebitis. Report prolonged or excessive injection site reactions to the physician.

Interventions

- Implement breathing activities and other therapeutic exercises to encourage ventilation and help overcome any residual effects of the anesthetic.
- Because of the risk of cardiorespiratory arrest, use extreme caution during aerobic exercise and other forms of therapeutic exercise until the residual anesthetic effects have diminished. Assess exercise tolerance frequently (blood pressure, heart rate, respiratory rate, fatigue levels), and terminate exercise immediately if any untoward responses occur (See Appendix L).

Patient/Client-Related Instruction

- Advise patient to avoid alcohol or other CNS depressants for 24 hr after anesthesia.
- Instruct patient to report other troublesome side effects such as severe or prolonged headache, skin rash, or GI problems (nausea, vomiting, hiccups).

Pharmacokinetics

Absorption: Rapidly absorbed following oral and nasal administration; undergoes substantial intestinal and first-pass hepatic metabolism. Well absorbed following IM administration; IV administration results in complete bioavailability.
Distribution: Crosses the blood-brain barrier and placenta.
Protein Binding: 97%.
Metabolism and Excretion: Almost exclusively metabolized by the liver, resulting in conversion to hydroxymidazolam, an active metabolite, and 2 other inactive metabolites (metabolized by cytochrome P4503A4 enzyme system); metabolites are excreted in urine.
Half-life: Preterm neonates: 2.6–17.7 hr; Neonates: 4–12 hr; Children: 3–7 hr; Adults: 2–6 hr (increased in renal impairment, CHF, or cirrhosis).

TIME/ACTION PROFILE (sedation)

ROUTE	ONSET	PEAK	DURATION
IN	5 min	10 min	30–60 min
IM	15 min	30–60 min	2–6 hr
IV	1.5–5 min	Rapid	2–6 hr

Contraindications/Precautions

Contraindicated in: Hypersensitivity; Cross-sensitivity with other benzodiazepines may occur; Shock; Comatose patients or those with preexisting CNS depression; Uncontrolled severe pain; Products containing benzyl alcohol should not be used in neonates; Pregnancy; Acute angle-closure glaucoma.
Use Cautiously in: Pulmonary disease; CHF; Renal impairment; Severe hepatic impairment; Obese pediatric patients (calculate dose on the basis of ideal body weight); Geriatric or debilitated patients (especially patients >70 yr) more susceptible to cardiorespiratory depressant effects; dosage reduction required; Lactation (safety not established).

Interactions

Drug-Drug: ↑ CNS depression with **alcohol, antihistamines, opioid analgesics**, and other **sedative/hypnotics** (↓ midazolam dose by 30–50% if used concurrently). ↑ risk of hypotension with **antihypertensives, opioid analgesics**, acute ingestion of **alcohol**, or **nitrates**. Midazolam is metabolized by the cytochrome P4503A4 enzyme system; drugs that induce or inhibit this system may be expected to alter the effects of midazolam. **Carbamazepine, phenytoin, rifampin, rifabutin**, and **phenobarbital** ↓ levels of midazolam. The following agents ↓ midazolam

metabolism and may ↑ its effects: **erythromycin, cimetidine, ranitidine, diltiazem, verapamil, fluconazole, itraconazole,** and **ketoconazole**.
Drug-Natural: Concomitant use of **kava, valerian,** or **chamomile** can ↑ CNS depression. Long-term use of **St. John's wort** may significantly ↓ serum concentrations of oral midazolam.
Drug-Food: Grapefruit juice ↓ metabolism and may ↑ effects of midazolam.

Route/Dosage

Dose must be individualized, taking caution to reduce dose in geriatric patients and in those who are already sedated.

Preoperative Sedation/Anxiolysis/Amnesia

PO (Children 6 mo–16 yr): 0.25–0.5 mg/kg, may require up to 1 mg/kg (dose should not exceed 20 mg); *patients with cardiac/respiratory compromise or concurrent CNS depressants*—0.25 mg/kg.
IM (Adults Otherwise Healthy and <60 yr): 0.07–0.08 mg/kg 1 hr before surgery (usual dose 5 mg).
IM (Adults ≥60 yr; Debilitated or Chronically Ill): 0.02–0.03 mg/kg 1 hr before surgery (usual dose 1–3 mg).
IM (Children): 0.1–0.15 mg/kg up to 0.5 mg/kg 30–60 min prior to procedure; not to exceed 10 mg/dose.

Conscious Sedation for Short Procedures

IV (Adults and Children Otherwise Healthy >12 yr and <60 yr): 1–1.5 mg initially; dose may be increased further as needed. Total doses >3.5 mg are rarely needed (reduce dose by 30% if other CNS depressants are used). Maintenance doses of 25% of the dose required for initial sedation may be given as necessary.
IV (Children 6–12 yr): 0.025–0.05 mg/kg initially, then titrate dose carefully; may need up to 0.4 mg/kg total, maximum dose 10 mg.
IV (Children 6 mo–5 yr): 0.05 mg/kg initially, then titrate dose carefully; may need up to 0.6 mg/kg total, maximum dose 6 mg.
IV (Geriatric Patients ≥60 yr; Debilitated or Chronically Ill): 1–2.5 mg initially; dosage may be increased further as needed. Total doses >5 mg are rarely needed (reduce dose by 50% if other CNS depressants are used). Maintenance doses of 25% of the dose required for initial sedation may be given as necessary.
Intranasal (Children): 0.2–0.3 mg/kg, may repeat in 5–15 min.

Status Epilepticus

IV (Children >2 mo): 0.15 mg/kg load followed by a continuous infusion of 1 mcg/kg/min. Titrate dose upward q 5 min until seizure controlled, range: 1–18 mcg/kg/min.

Induction of Anesthesia (Adjunct)

May give additional dose of 25% of initial dose if needed
IV (Adults Otherwise Healthy and <55 yr): 300–350 mcg/kg initially (up to 600 mcg/kg total). If patient is premedicated, initial dose should be further reduced.
IV (Geriatric Patients >55 yr): 150–300 mcg/kg as initial dose. If patient is premedicated, initial dose should be further reduced.
IV (Adults—Debilitated): 150–250 mcg/kg initial dose. If patient is premedicated, initial dose should be further reduced.

Sedation in Critical Care Settings

IV (Adults): 0.01–0.05 mg/kg (0.5–4 mg in most adults) initially if a loading dose is required; may repeat q 10–15 min until desired effect is obtained; may be followed by infusion at 0.02–0.1 mg/kg/hr (1–7 mg/hr in most adults).
IV (Children): *Intubated patients only*—0.05–0.2 mg/kg initially as a loading dose; follow with infusion at 0.06–0.12 mg/kg/min (1–2 mcg/kg/min), titrate to effect, range: 0.4–6 mcg/kg/min.
IV (Neonates >32 wk): *Intubated patients only*—0.06 mg/kg/hr (1 mcg/kg/min).
IV (Neonates <32 wk): *Intubated patients only*—0.03 mg/kg/hr (0.5 mcg/kg/min).

Availability (generic available)

Injection: 1 mg/mL, 5 mg/mL. **Syrup (cherry flavor):** 2 mg/mL.

midodrine (mye-doe-dreen)

ProAmatine

Classification
Therapeutic: vasopressors
Pharmacologic: alpha-1 agonists

Indications

Symptomatic management of refractory orthostatic hypotension in patients whose lives are impaired.
Unlabeled Use: Urinary incontinence.

Action

Activation of alpha$_1$-adrenergic receptors in arteries and veins. **Therapeutic Effects:** ↑ in vascular tone and blood pressure.

Adverse Reactions/Side Effects

CNS: anxiety, confusion, head pressure/fullness, headache, nervousness. **CV:** supine hypertension, bradycardia. **GU:** urinary urge/retention/frequency, dysuria. **Derm:** facial flushing, piloerection, pruritus, rash. **Neuro:** paresthesia. **Misc:** chills, pain.

PHYSICAL THERAPY IMPLICATIONS

Examination and Evaluation

- Assess blood pressure (BP) when the patient assumes a more upright position (lying to standing, sitting to standing, lying to sitting). Document whether drug therapy is successful in reducing the incidence and severity of orthostatic hypotension; that is, reduced episodes where systolic BP falls >20 mm Hg, or diastolic BP falls >10 mm Hg.

- Assess BP when patient is lying down. Compare to normal values (See Appendix F), and report a sustained increase in BP (hypertension) to the physician.
- Assess heart rate, ECG, and heart sounds, especially during exercise (See Appendices G, H). Report a slow heart rate (bradycardia) or symptoms of other arrhythmias, including angina, palpitations, shortness of breath, fainting, and fatigue/weakness.
- Monitor and report signs of CNS toxicity, including nervousness, anxiety, confusion, or feelings of pressure or fullness in the head. Sustained or severe CNS signs may indicate overdose or excessive use of this drug.
- Assess signs of paresthesia, including numbness, tingling, and muscle weakness. Perform objective tests, including electroneuromyography and sensory testing to document any drug-related neuropathic changes.
- If used to treat urinary incontinence, monitor the frequency of incontinent episodes to help determine if drug therapy is successful in reducing these episodes.

Interventions

- Because of the risk of cardiovascular stimulation, use caution during aerobic exercise and endurance conditioning. Assess exercise tolerance frequently (BP, heart rate, fatigue levels), and terminate exercise immediately if any untoward responses occur (See Appendix L).

Patient/Client-Related Instruction

- Instruct patient and family/caregivers to report other troublesome side effects such as severe or prolonged headache, chills, pain, skin reactions (rash, itching flushing, goose bumps), or urinary problems (urgency, increased frequency, urinary retention, difficulty initiating urination).

Pharmacokinetics

Absorption: 93% absorbed following oral administration; rapidly converted to desglymidodrine, the active metabolite.
Distribution: Desglymidodrine crosses the blood-brain barrier poorly.
Metabolism and Excretion: Desglymidodrine is 80% excreted by the kidneys.
Half-life: *Midodrine*—25 min; *desglymidodrine*—3–4 hr.

TIME/ACTION PROFILE (blood levels of active metabolite)

ROUTE	ONSET	PEAK	DURATION
PO	rapid	1–2 hr	2–3 hr

Contraindications/Precautions

Contraindicated in: Urinary retention; Severe organic heart disease; Acute renal disease; Persistent/excessive supine hypertension; Pheochromocytoma; Thyrotoxicosis.
Use Cautiously in: History of hypertension; Renal impairment (↓ initial dose); Hepatic impairment; Diabetes mellitus, visual problems, concurrent fludrocortisone (↑ risk of visual disturbances); **OB, Pedi:** Pregnancy, lactation or children (safety not established).

Interactions

Drug-Drug: ↑ risk of bradycardia with **digoxin, beta blockers**, and **antipsychotics**. Concurrent use with other **alpha-adrenergic agonists**, including **phenylephrine, ephedrine, pseudoephedrine**, and **dihydroergotamine**, may result in ↑ pressor effect. Effects may be ↓ by **alpha-adrenergic blockers**, including **prazosin, terazosin**, and **doxazosin**. ↑ Effects of **fludrocortisone** (↓ initial dose of fludrocortisone or ↓ salt intake prior to midodrine).

Route/Dosage

PO (Adults): *Orthostatic hypotension*—10 mg tid; *urinary incontinence*—2.5–5 mg bid–tid.

Renal Impairment

PO (Adults): 2.5 mg tid.

Availability (generic available)

Tablets: 2.5 mg, 5 mg, 10 mg.

mifepristone (mi-fe-pris-tone)

Mifeprex

Classification
Therapeutic: abortifacients
Pharmacologic: antiprogestational agents

Indications

Medical termination of intrauterine pregnancy up to day 49 of pregnancy.

Action

Antagonizes endometrial and myometrial effects of progesterone. Sensitizes the myometrium to contraction-inducing activity of prostaglandins.
Therapeutic Effects: Termination of pregnancy.

Adverse Reactions/Side Effects

CNS: dizziness, fainting, headache, weakness. **GI:** abdominal pain, diarrhea, nausea, vomiting. **GU:** uterine bleeding, uterine cramping, ruptured ectopic pregnancy, pelvic pain.

PHYSICAL THERAPY IMPLICATIONS

Examination and Evaluation

- Assess dizziness, fainting, and weakness that might affect gait, balance, and other functional activities (See Appendix C). Report persistent balance problems and functional limitations to the physician, and caution the patient and family/caregivers to guard against falls and trauma.

Patient/Client-Related Instruction

- Instruct patient to notify health care professional immediately if she develops weakness, nausea, vomiting, diarrhea, with or without abdominal pain or fever more than 24 hr after taking mifepristone; may indicate life-threatening sepsis.
- Inform patient that vaginal bleeding and uterine cramping will probably occur. Bleeding or spotting occurs for an average of 9–16 days, but may continue for more than 30 days. Instruct patient to report any severe or unusual cramping, bleeding, or pelvic pain that extends beyond the expected time periods.

Pharmacokinetics

Absorption: Rapidly absorbed following oral administration (69% bioavailability).
Distribution: Unknown.
Protein Binding: 98%.
Metabolism and Excretion: Mostly metabolized by the liver (cytochrome CYP4503A4 [CY P4503A4] enzyme system).
Half-life: 18 hr.

TIME/ACTION PROFILE (termination of pregnancy)

ROUTE	ONSET	PEAK	DURATION
PO	unknown	within 2 days	unknown

Contraindications/Precautions

Contraindicated in: Presence of an intrauterine device (IUD); Confirmed or suspected ectopic pregnancy; Undiagnosed adnexal mass; Chronic adrenal failure; Concurrent long-term corticosteroid therapy; Bleeding disorders or concurrent anticoagulant therapy; Inherited porphyrias.
Use Cautiously in: Chronic medical conditions such as cardiovascular, hypertensive, hepatic, renal, or respiratory disease (safety and efficacy not established); Women >35 yrs old or who smoke ≥10 cigarettes/day.

Interactions

Drug-Drug: Blood levels and therapeutic effectiveness may be ↑ by **ketoconazole, itraconazole**, and **erythromycin**. Blood levels and effects may be ↓ by **rifampin, dexamethasone, phenytoin, phenobarbital**, and **carbamazepine**. Mifepristone may ↓ metabolism and ↑ effects of other **drugs metabolized by the CYP4503A4 enzyme system**, including **some agents used during general anesthesia**.
Drug-Natural: Blood levels and effects may be ↓ by **St. John's wort**.
Drug-Food: Blood levels and effects may be ↑ by **grapefruit juice**.

Route/Dosage

PO (Adults): *Day 1*—600 mg (given as 3 200-mg tablets) as a single dose, followed on *day 3* by 400 mcg misoprostol (Cytotec), unless abortion has occurred and has been confirmed by clinical or ultrasonographic examination (see misoprostol monograph).

Availability

Tablets: 200 mg.

miglitol (mi-gli-tole)

Glyset

Classification
Therapeutic: antidiabetics
Pharmacologic: alpha-glucosidase inhibitors

Indications

Management of non–insulin-dependent diabetes mellitus (type 2) in conjunction with dietary therapy; may be used concurrently with sulfonylurea oral hypoglycemic agents.

Action

Lowers blood glucose by inhibiting the enzyme alpha-glucosidase in the GI tract, resulting in delayed glucose absorption. **Therapeutic Effects:** Lowering of blood glucose in diabetic patients, especially postprandial hyperglycemia.

Adverse Reactions/Side Effects

GI: abdominal pain, diarrhea, flatulence. **Hemat:** low serum iron.

PHYSICAL THERAPY IMPLICATIONS

Examination and Evaluation

- Be alert for signs of hypoglycemia, especially during and after exercise. Common neuromuscular signs include anxiety; restlessness; tingling in hands, feet, lips, or tongue; chills; cold sweats; confusion; difficulty in concentration; drowsiness; excessive hunger; headache; irritability; nervousness; tremor; weakness; unsteady gait. Report persistent or repeated episodes of hypoglycemia to the physician.

- Assess blood pressure periodically (See Appendix F). A sudden or sustained increase in blood pressure (hypertension) may indicate problems in diabetes management, and should be reported to the physician.
- Monitor signs of low iron levels and subsequent anemia, including fatigue, weakness, shortness of breath, chest pain, and pale skin. Report these signs to the physician for further evaluation.

Interventions

- Implement aerobic exercise and endurance training programs to maintain optimal body weight, improve insulin sensitivity, and reduce the risk of macrovascular disease (heart attack, stroke) and microvascular problems (reduced blood flow to tissues and organs that causes poor wound healing, neuropathy, retinopathy, and nephropathy).

Patient/Client-Related Instruction

- Encourage patient to monitor blood glucose before and after exercise, and to adjust food intake to maintain normal glycemic levels.
- Emphasize the importance of adhering to nutritional guidelines, and the need for periodic assessment of glycemic control (serum glucose and glycosylated hemoglobin levels) throughout the management of diabetes mellitus.
- Advise patient about symptoms of hyperglycemia (confusion, drowsiness; flushed, dry skin; fruit-like breath odor; rapid, deep breathing, polyuria; loss of appetite; unusual thirst). Drug dosages may need to be adjusted to prevent repeated episodes of hyperglycemia.
- Instruct patient to report troublesome GI problems, including severe or prolonged diarrhea, flatulence, and abdominal pain.

Pharmacokinetics

Absorption: Completely absorbed at lower doses (25 mg); 50–70% absorbed at higher doses (100 mg).
Distribution: Distributes primarily into extracellular fluid; small amounts enter breast milk.
Metabolism and Excretion: Not metabolized; action is primarily local in the GI tract; amounts that are absorbed are excreted mostly unchanged in urine.
Half-life: 2 hr.

TIME/ACTION PROFILE (effect on glucose absorption)

ROUTE	ONSET	PEAK	DURATION
PO	rapid	within 1 hr	unknown

Contraindications/Precautions

Contraindicated in: Hypersensitivity; Diabetic ketoacidosis; Inflammatory bowel disease or other chronic intestinal conditions resulting in impaired absorption or predisposition to obstruction; Lactation.
Use Cautiously in: Patients with fever, infection, trauma, or stress (may cause hyperglycemia requiring alternate therapy); Renal impairment (use not recommended if creatinine >2 mg/dL); Pregnancy or children (safety not established).

Interactions

Drug-Drug: May ↓ absorption of **ranitidine** and **propranolol**. Effects may be ↓ by **intestinal adsorbents** (such as **charcoal**) and **digestive enzyme products**; concurrent use should be avoided.
Drug-Food: Concurrent **carbohydrates** may ↑ diarrhea.

Route/Dosage

PO (Adults): 25 mg tid; may begin with 25 mg once daily; may be increased up to 100 mg tid.

Availability

Tablets: 25 mg, 50 mg, 100 mg.

M

miglustat (mi-gloo-stat)

Zavesca

Classification
Therapeutic: none assigned
Pharmacologic: enzyme inhibitors (D-glucose analogue)

Indications

Mild-to-moderate type 1 Gaucher's disease when enzyme replacement therapy is not an option.

Action

Competitively and reversibly inhibits glucosylceramide synthase, which is the initial step in the production of glycosphingolipids. The glycosphingolipid glucosylceramide accumulates in tissues in Gaucher's disease.
Therapeutic Effects: Decreased production/accumulation of glycosphingolipid glucosylceramide with decreased tissue damage.

Adverse Reactions/Side Effects

CNS: headache. **GI:** abdominal pain, diarrhea, flatulence, nausea, weight loss, anorexia, dyspepsia. **GU:** ↓ male fertility. **Hemat:** thrombocytopenia. **Metab:** weight loss. **Neuro:** paresthesia, peripheral neuropathy, tremor.

PHYSICAL THERAPY IMPLICATIONS

Examination and Evaluation

- Be alert for signs of paresthesias and peripheral neuropathy, as indicated by numbness, tingling, and decreased muscle strength. Establish baseline electroneuromyographic values using EMG and nerve conduction at the beginning of drug treatment whenever possible, and reexamine these values periodically to document drug-induced changes in peripheral nerve function.

- Monitor signs of thrombocytopenia such as bruising, nose bleeds, and bleeding gums. Report these signs to the physician.
- Periodically assess body weight and other anthropometric measures (body mass index, body composition). Report a rapid or unexplained weight loss or decreased body fat.

Interventions

- Implement therapeutic exercises (resistive exercises, gait training) to complement the effects of drug therapy and help maintain bone density.

Patient/Client-Related Instruction

- Instruct patient to report other troublesome side effects, including prolonged or severe headache, tremor, or GI problems such as nausea, diarrhea, indigestion, loss of appetite, abdominal pain, and flatulence.

Pharmacokinetics

Absorption: Well absorbed following oral administration.
Distribution: Distributes into extravascular tissues.
Metabolism and Excretion: Not metabolized; excreted mostly unchanged in urine.
Half-life: 6–7 hr.

TIME/ACTION PROFILE (blood levels)

ROUTE	ONSET	PEAK	DURATION
PO	unknown	2–2.5 hr	8 hr

Contraindications/Precautions

Contraindicated in: Hypersensitivity; OB/Lactation: Pregnancy or lactation; Severe renal impairment (<30 mL/min).
Use Cautiously in: Mild-to-moderate renal impairment (dose alteration recommended if CCr <70 mL/min); Geri: Consider age related decrease in body mass, cardiac, renal and hepatic function, other chronic illnesses and concurrent drug therapies; Pedi: Children <18 yr (safety not established).

Interactions

Drug-Drug: ↑ clearance of imiglucerase (should not be used concurrently).

Route/Dosage

PO (Adults): 100 mg tid at regular intervals.

Renal Impairment

PO (Adults): *CCr 50–70 mL/min*—100 mg bid; *CCr 30–50 mL/min*—100 mg once daily.

Availability

Capsules: 100 mg.

milnacipran (mil-na-sip-ran)

Savella

Classification

Therapeutic: antifibromyalgia agents
Pharmacologic: selective norepinephrine reuptake inhibitors

Indications

Management of fibromyalgia.

Action

Inhibits neuronal reuptake of norepinephrine and serotonin. **Therapeutic Effects:** Decreased pain associated with fibromyalgia.

Adverse Reactions/Side Effects

CNS: dizziness, headache, insomnia. **CV:** hypertension, tachycardia. **GI:** constipation, dry mouth, liver function abnormalities, nausea, vomiting. **Derm:** hot flushes, hyperhydrosis.

PHYSICAL THERAPY IMPLICATIONS

Examination and Evaluation

- Assess pain using visual analogue scales and other appropriate pain scales. Document any changes in pain to help determine the effects of drug therapy in treating fibromyalgia.
- Assess dizziness that might affect gait, balance, and other functional activities (See Appendix C). Report balance problems and functional limitations to the physician, and caution the patient and family/caregivers to guard against falls and trauma.
- Assess blood pressure (BP) and compare to normal values (See Appendix F). Report a sustained increase in BP (hypertension).
- Assess heart rate, ECG, and heart sounds, especially during exercise (See Appendices G, H). Report a rapid heart rate (tachycardia) or symptoms of other arrhythmias, including palpitations, chest discomfort, shortness of breath, fainting, and fatigue/weakness.

Interventions

- Implement appropriate interventions (physical agents, manual techniques, therapeutic exercise) to help manage pain and reduce the need for drug therapy.
- Because of the risk of hypertension and tachycardia, use caution during aerobic exercise and other forms of therapeutic exercise. Assess exercise tolerance frequently (BP, heart rate, fatigue levels), and terminate exercise immediately if any untoward responses occur (See Appendix L).

- Help patient explore other nonpharmacologic methods to reduce chronic pain such as relaxation techniques, imagery, counseling, and so forth.

Patient/Client-Related Instruction

- Instruct patient to report other troublesome side effects such as severe or prolonged headache, sleep loss, excessive sweating, hot flashes, or GI problems (nauseas, vomiting, constipation, dry mouth).

Pharmacokinetics

Absorption: 85–90% absorbed following oral administration.
Distribution: Unknown.
Metabolism and Excretion: Mostly excreted urine as unchanged drug (55%) and inactive metabolites.
Half-life: *D*-isomer 8–10 hr; *L*-isomer 4–6 hr.

TIME/ACTION PROFILE (decrease in pain)

ROUTE	ONSET	PEAK	DURATION
PO	1 wk	unknown	unknown

Contraindications/Precautions

Contraindicated in: Uncontrolled narrow-angle glaucoma; Concurrent use of or in close temporal proximity to MAO inhibitors; End-stage renal disease; Significant history of alcohol use/abuse; Chronic liver disease.
Use Cautiously in: History of suicide risk or attempt; History of seizures; Moderate-to-severe renal impairment; for CCr <30 mL/min reduced dose is required; Severe hepatic impairment; Obstructive uropathy (↑ risk of adverse genitourinary effects); Geri: Consider age-related decrease in renal function, chronic disease state, and concurrent drug therapy; OB: Use only if clearly required during pregnancy, weighing benefit to mother versus potential harm to fetus; Lactation: Potential for serious adverse reactions in infant; discontinue drug or discontinue breast-feeding; Pedi: Increased risk of suicidal thinking and behavior (suicidality) in adolescents and young adults up to 24 yr with Major Depressive Disorder (MDD) and other psychiatric disorders.

Interactions

Drug-Drug: Concurrent use with **MAO inhibitors** may result in serious, potentially fatal reactions; wait at least 14 days following discontinuation of MAO inhibitor before initiation of milnacipran. Wait at least 5 days after discontinuing milnacipran before initiation of MAO inhibitor. Concurrent use with **MAO inhibitors** may result in serious, potentially fatal reactions. Concurrent use of **serotonergic drugs** (including **triptans**, **lithium**, and **tramadol**) may ↑ the risk of serotonin syndrome; also ↑ risk of coronary vasoconstriction and hypertension. Concurrent use of **NSAIDs**, **aspirin**, or other **drugs that affect coagulation** may ↑ the risk of bleeding. May ↓ antihypertensive effectiveness of **clonidine**. ↑ risk of hypertension and arrhythmias with **epinephrine** or **norepinephrine**. ↑ risk of euphoria and hypotension when switching from **clomipramine**. Concurrent use with **digoxin** may result in adverse hemodynamics, including hypotension and tachycardia; avoid concurrent use with IV digoxin.

Route/Dosage

PO (Adults): *Day 1*—12.5 mg; *Days 2–3* —12.5 mg bid; *Day 4–7* —25 mg bid; *After Day 7*—50 mg bid. Some patients may require up to 100 mg bid depending on response.

Renal Impairment

PO (Adults): *CCr 5–29 mL/min*—maintenance dose is 25 mg twice daily; some patients may be require up to 50 mg bid depending on response.

Availability

Tablets (contain tartrazine): 12.5 mg, 25 mg, 50 mg, 100 mg.

M

HIGH ALERT

milrinone (mil-ri-none)

Primacor

Classification

Therapeutic: inotropics
Pharmacologic: phosphodiesterase-3 inhibitors

Indications

Short-term treatment of CHF unresponsive to conventional therapy with digoxin, diuretics, and vasodilators.

Action

Increases myocardial contractility. Decreases preload and afterload by a direct dilating effect on vascular smooth muscle. **Therapeutic Effects:** Increased cardiac output (inotropic effect).

Adverse Reactions/Side Effects

CNS: headache, tremor. **CV:** VENTRICULAR ARRHYTHMIAS, angina pectoris, hypotension, supraventricular arrhythmias. **CV:** skin rash. **GI:** liver function abnormalities. **F and E:** hypokalemia. **Hemat:** thrombocytopenia.

PHYSICAL THERAPY IMPLICATIONS

Examination and Evaluation

- Assess heart rate, ECG, and heart sounds, especially during exercise (See Appendices G, H). Report any rhythm disturbances or symptoms of increased arrhythmias, including palpitations, chest discomfort, shortness of breath, fainting, and fatigue/weakness.
- Assess signs and symptoms of CHF (dyspnea, rales/crackles, peripheral edema, jugular venous distention, exercise intolerance) to help document whether drug therapy is effective in reducing these symptoms.
- Assess blood pressure periodically and compare to normal values (See Appendix F). Report low blood pressure (hypotension), especially if patient experiences dizziness, fatigue, or other symptoms.
- Report any muscle weakness, aches, or cramps that might indicate low potassium levels (hypokalemia).
- Monitor and report signs of thrombocytopenia (bruising, nose bleeds, bleeding gums).

Interventions

- Design and implement aerobic exercise and endurance training programs to improve myocardial pumping ability and reduce symptoms of CHF.
- Use caution during aerobic exercise and endurance conditioning because of an increased risk of cardiac arrhythmias. Terminate exercise if patient exhibits untoward symptoms (chest pain, shortness of breath, etc.), or displays other criteria for exercise termination (See Appendix L).

Patient/Client-Related Instruction

- Remind patients to take medication as directed to control CHF even if they are asymptomatic.
- Instruct patients to weigh themselves every day, and call their physician if they gain 3 lb or more in 1 day or more than 5 lb in 1 week. Sudden weight gain may indicate fluid buildup due to worsening heart failure.
- Counsel patients about additional interventions to help control cardiac dysfunction, including regular exercise, weight loss, sodium restriction, stress reduction, moderation of alcohol consumption, and smoking cessation.
- Instruct patient to report signs of liver dysfunction, including yellow skin or eyes, abdominal pain, severe nausea and vomiting, fever, sore throat, malaise, weakness, and facial edema.
- Instruct patient or family/caregivers to report other troublesome side effects such as severe or prolonged headache, tremor, or skin rash.

Pharmacokinetics

Absorption: IV administration results in complete bioavailability.
Distribution: Unknown.
Metabolism and Excretion: 80–90% excreted unchanged by the kidneys.
Half-life: 2.3 hr (increased in renal impairment).

TIME/ACTION PROFILE (hemodynamic effects)

ROUTE	ONSET	PEAK	DURATION
IV	5–15 min	unknown	3–6 hr

Contraindications/Precautions

Contraindicated in: Hypersensitivity; Severe aortic or pulmonic valvular heart disease; Hypertrophic subaortic stenosis (may increase outflow tract obstruction).
Use Cautiously in: History of arrhythmias, electrolyte abnormalities, abnormal digoxin levels, or insertion of vascular catheters (↑ risk of ventricular arrhythmias); Renal impairment (reduced infusion rate recommended if CCr is <50 mL/min); OB/Lactation/Pedi: Safety not established.

Interactions

Drug-Drug: None significant.

Route/Dosage

IV (Adults): *Loading dose*—50 mcg/kg followed by *infusion* at 0.50 mcg/kg/min (range 0.375–0.75 mcg/kg/min).

Availability (generic available)

Injection: 1 mg/mL in 10-, 20-, and 50-mL vials. **Premixed infusion:** 20 mg/100 mL, 40 mg/200 mL.

minocycline (min-oh-sye-kleen)

Apo-Minocycline, Arestin, DOM-Minocycline, Dynacin, Enca, Gen-Minocycline, Minocin, Novo-Minocycline, PMS-Minocycline, Ratio-Minocycline, Riva-Minocycline, Solodyn

Classification
Therapeutic: anti-infectives
Pharmacologic: tetracyclines

Indications

Treatment of various infections caused by unusual organisms, including *Mycoplasma*, *Chlamydia*, *Rickettsia*. Treatment of gonorrhea and syphilis in penicillin-allergic patients. Prevention of exacerbations of chronic bronchitis. Treatment of acne. Inflammatory lesions of nonnodular acne vulgaris (Solodyn).

Action

Inhibit bacterial protein synthesis at the level of the 30S bacterial ribosome. **Therapeutic Effects:** Bacteriostatic action against susceptible bacteria.

Spectrum: Include activity against some gram-positive pathogens: *Bacillus anthracis*, *Clostridium perfringens*, *C. tetani*, *Listeria monocytogenes*, *Nocardia*, *Propionibacterium acnes*, *Actinomyces israelii*. Active against some gram-negative pathogens: *Haemophilus influenzae*, *Legionella pneumophila*, *Yersinia enterocolitica*, *Y. pestis*, *Neisseria gonorrhoeae*, *N. meningitidis*. Also active against several other pathogens, including *Mycoplasma*, *Treponema pallidum*, *Chlamydia*, *Rickettsia*.

Adverse Reactions/Side Effects

CNS: benign intracranial hypertension (increased risk in children), dizziness. **EENT:** vestibular reactions. **GI:** diarrhea, nausea, vomiting, esophagitis, hepatotoxicity, pancreatitis. **Derm:** photosensitivity, rash, pigmentation of skin and mucous membranes. **Hemat:** blood dyscrasias. **MS:** lupus-like syndrome. **Misc:** hypersensitivity reactions, superinfection.

PHYSICAL THERAPY IMPLICATIONS

Examination and Evaluation

- Monitor signs of hypersensitivity reactions or anaphylaxis, including pulmonary symptoms (tightness in the throat and chest, wheezing, cough dyspnea) or skin reactions (rash, angioedema, pruritus, urticaria). Notify physician or nursing staff immediately if these reactions occur.
- Monitor signs of leukopenia (fever, sore throat, signs of infection), thrombocytopenia (bruising, nose bleeds, and bleeding gums), or unusual weakness and fatigue that might be due to anemia or other blood dyscrasias. Report these signs to physician or nursing staff.
- Monitor and report signs of benign intracranial hypertension, especially in children. Signs include dizziness, headache, tinnitus, nausea, and disturbed vision (e.g., blurry or double vision).
- Assess dizziness or vestibular reactions that might affect gait, balance, and other functional activities (See Appendix C). Report balance problems and functional limitations to the physician and nursing staff, and caution the patient and family/caregivers to guard against falls and trauma.
- Monitor signs of drug-induced lupus-like syndrome, including increased blood pressure (BP), fever, joint pain, skin rashes, and redness/irritation of the eye (uveitis). Notify physician promptly if these signs appear.

Interventions

- Always wash hands thoroughly and disinfect equipment (whirlpools, electrotherapeutic devices, treatment tables, and so forth) to help prevent the spread of infection. Employ universal precautions or isolation procedures as indicated for specific patients.
- Because of the risk of intracranial hypertension, avoid activities that might increase intracranial pressure such as elevating the feet above the head (Trendelenburg's position) or holding breath and straining during a bowel movement (Valsalva's maneuver).
- Causes photosensitivity; use care if administering UV treatments.

Patient/Client-Related Instruction

- Instruct patient to notify physician immediately of signs of superinfection, including black, furry overgrowth on tongue, vaginal itching or discharge, and loose or foul-smelling stools.
- Advise patient about the likelihood of GI reactions (nausea, vomiting, diarrhea, heartburn). Instruct patient to report severe or prolonged GI problems, signs of liver toxicity (yellow skin or eyes, abdominal pain, severe nausea and vomiting, fever, sore throat, malaise, weakness, facial edema), or pancreatitis (upper abdominal pain after eating, indigestion, weight loss, oily stools).
- Advise patient about photosensitivity and to use sunscreens, protective clothing, and avoid prolonged sun exposure. Advise patient to also report any rashes, pigmentation problems, or other skin reactions.

Pharmacokinetics

Absorption: Well absorbed from the GI tract.
Distribution: Widely distributed, some CSF and good bone penetration; crosses the placenta and enters breast milk.
Metabolism and Excretion: 5–20% excreted unchanged by the urine; some metabolism by the liver with enterohepatic circulation and excretion in bile and feces.
Half-life: 11–26 hr.

TIME/ACTION PROFILE (blood levels)

ROUTE	ONSET	PEAK	DURATION
PO	rapid	2–3 hr	6–12 hr
PO extended-release	unknown	3.5–4 hr	24 hr

Contraindications/Precautions

Contraindicated in: Hypersensitivity; Some products contain alcohol or bisulfites and should be avoided in patients with known hypersensitivity or intolerance; Pedi: Children <8 yr (permanent staining of teeth); OB: Risk of permanent staining of teeth in infant if used during last half of pregnancy; Lactation.

M

Use Cautiously in: Cachectic or debilitated patients; Renal disease; Hepatic impairment; Nephrogenic diabetes insipidus.

Interactions

Drug-Drug: May enhance the effect of **warfarin**. May ↓ the effectiveness of **estrogen-containing oral contraceptives. Antacids, calcium, iron supplements,** and **magnesium salts** form insoluble compounds (chelates) and ↓ absorption of tetracyclines. **Sucralfate** may bind to tetracycline and prevent its absorption from the GI tract. **Cholestyramine** or **colestipol** ↓ oral absorption of tetracyclines. **Adsorbent antidiarrheals** may ↓ absorption.
Drug-Food: Calcium in foods or **dairy products** ↓ absorption by forming insoluble compounds (chelates).

Route/Dosage

PO (Adults): 100–200 mg initially, then 100 mg q 12 hr or 50 mg q 6 hr.
PO (Children ≥8 yr): 4 mg/kg initially, then 2 mg/kg q 12 hr.
PO (Adults and Children ≥12 yr and 91–136 kg): *(Extended-release)*—135 mg once daily for 12 wk.
PO (Adults and Children ≥12 yr and 60–90 kg): *(Extended-release)*—90 mg once daily for 12 wk.
PO (Adults and Children ≥12 yr and 45–59 kg): *(Extended-release)*—45 mg once daily for 12 wk.

Availability (generic available)

Capsules: 50 mg, 100 mg. **Tablets:** 50 mg, 100 mg. **Oral suspension (custard flavor):** 50 mg/5 mL. **Extended-release tablets:** 45 mg, 90 mg, 135 mg.

minoxidil (systemic)

(mi-**nox**-i-dil)
Loniten

Classification
Therapeutic: antihypertensives
Pharmacologic: vasodilators

Indications

Severe symptomatic hypertension or hypertension associated with end-organ damage that has failed to respond to combinations of more conventional therapy.

Action

Directly relaxes vascular smooth muscle, probably by inhibiting the enzyme phosphodiesterase. Results in vasodilation, which is more pronounced in arterioles than veins. **Therapeutic Effects:** Lowering of blood pressure.

Adverse Reactions/Side Effects

CNS: headache. **Resp:** PULMONARY EDEMA. **CV:** CHF, ECG changes (alteration in T waves), tachycardia, angina, pericardial effusion. **GI:** nausea. **Derm:** hypertrichosis, pigment changes, rashes. **Endo:** gynecomastia, menstrual irregularities. **F and E:** sodium and water retention. **Misc:** intermittent claudication.

PHYSICAL THERAPY IMPLICATIONS

Examination and Evaluation

- Watch for signs of CHF and pulmonary edema, including dyspnea, cough, shortness of breath, rales/crackles, exercise intolerance, and jugular venous distention. Report these signs to the physician immediately.
- Assess blood pressure periodically and compare to normal values (See Appendix F) to help document antihypertensive effects.
- Assess heart rate, ECG, and heart sounds, especially during exercise (See Appendces G, H). Report a rapid heart rate (tachycardia) or signs of other arrhythmias, including palpitations, chest discomfort, shortness of breath, fainting, and fatigue/weakness.
- Monitor signs of intermittent claudication, including pain, cramping, and fatigue in the lower extremities that occurs when walking. Report severe symptoms or signs of claudication that fail to subside when at rest.
- Assess peripheral edema using girth measurements, volume displacement, and measurement of pitting edema (See Appendix N). Report increased swelling in feet and ankles or a sudden increase in body weight due to sodium and water retention.

Interventions

- Design and implement aerobic exercise and endurance training programs to reduce hypertension and improve myocardial pumping ability.
- Because of an increased risk of cardiac arrhythmias (tachycardia, others), use caution during aerobic exercise and endurance conditioning. Terminate exercise if patient exhibits untoward symptoms (chest pain, shortness of breath, unusual fatigue) or displays other criteria for exercise termination (See Appendix L).
- Avoid physical therapy interventions that cause systemic vasodilation (large whirlpool, Hubbard tank). Additive effects of this drug and the intervention may cause a dangerous fall in blood pressure.
- To minimize orthostatic hypotension, patient should move slowly when assuming a more upright position.

Patient/Client-Related Instruction

- Remind patients to take medication as directed to control hypertension even if they are asymptomatic.
- Counsel patients about additional interventions to help control blood pressure, including regular

exercise, weight loss, sodium restriction, stress reduction, moderation of alcohol consumption, and smoking cessation.

- Instruct patient or family/caregivers to report other troublesome side effects such as severe or prolonged headache, nausea, excessive hair growth, breast enlargement in men, menstrual irregularities in women, or skin reactions (rash, changes in pigmentation).

Pharmacokinetics

Absorption: Well absorbed following oral administration.
Distribution: Widely distributed; enters breast milk.
Metabolism and Excretion: 90% metabolized by the liver.
Half-life: 4.2 hr.

TIME/ACTION PROFILE (antihypertensive effect)

ROUTE	ONSET	PEAK	DURATION
PO	30 min	2–3 hr	2–5 days

Contraindications/Precautions

Contraindicated in: Hypersensitivity; Pheochromocytoma.
Use Cautiously in: Recent MI; Severe renal impairment (can be used in moderate renal impairment); Geriatric patients (may be more sensitive to effects; consider age-related decline in body mass, hepatic/renal/cardiovascular function); Pregnancy or lactation (safety not established).

Interactions

Drug-Drug: Additive hypotensive effects with other **antihypertensives**, acute ingestion of **alcohol** or **nitrates. NSAIDs** may ↓ the antihypertensive effectiveness of minoxidil.

Route/Dosage

PO (Adults and Children >12 yr): *Hypertension*—5 mg once daily or in 2 divided doses; may double at 3-day intervals; usual range 10–40 mg/day (for rapid control with careful monitoring, doses may be adjusted q 6 hr; up to 100 mg/day have been used).
PO (Children <12 yr): *Hypertension*—0.2 mg/kg/day (5 mg maximum) as a single dose or 2 divided doses; may be gradually increased at 3-day intervals in increments of 50–100% until response is obtained; usual range 0.25–1 mg/kg/day (for rapid control, doses may be adjusted q 6 hr; not to exceed 50 mg/day).

Availability (generic available)

Tablets: 2.5 mg, 10 mg.

mirtazapine (meer-taz-a-peen)

Remeron, Remeron Soltabs

Classification
Therapeutic: antidepressants
Pharmacologic: tetracyclic antidepressants

Indications

Major Depressive Disorder. **Unlabeled Use:** Panic Disorder. Generalized Anxiety Disorder (GAD). Posttraumatic Stress Disorder (PTSD).

Action

Potentiates the effects of norepinephrine and serotonin. **Therapeutic Effects:** Antidepressant action, which may develop only after several weeks.

Adverse Reactions/Side Effects

CNS: drowsiness, abnormal dreams, abnormal thinking, agitation, anxiety, apathy, confusion, dizziness, malaise, weakness. **EENT:** sinusitis. **Resp:** dyspnea, increased cough. **CV:** edema, hypotension, vasodilation. **GI:** constipation, dry mouth, increased appetite, abdominal pain, anorexia, elevated liver enzymes, nausea, vomiting. **GU:** urinary frequency. **Derm:** pruritus, rash. **F and E:** increased thirst. **Hemat:** AGRANULOCYTOSIS. **Metab:** weight gain, hypercholesterolemia, increased triglycerides. **MS:** arthralgia, back pain, myalgia. **Neuro:** hyperkinesia, hypesthesia, twitching. **Misc:** flu-like syndrome.

PHYSICAL THERAPY IMPLICATIONS

Examination and Evaluation

- Watch for signs of agranulocytosis, including fever, sore throat, mucosal lesions, signs of infection, and bruising. Report these signs to the physician immediately.
- Be alert for increased depression and suicidal thoughts and ideology, especially when initiating drug treatment, and in children and teenagers. Notify physician or other mental health care professional immediately if patient exhibits worsening depression or other changes in mood and behavior.
- Monitor any confusion, anxiety, agitation, apathy, or other alterations in mental status. Notify physician promptly if these symptoms develop (See Appendix D).
- Assess changes in motor activity or muscle function. Report severe or problematic twitching, increased muscle tone, or changes in muscle activity and motor abnormalities (hyperkinesia, hypokinesia).
- Assess dizziness and drowsiness that might affect gait, balance, and other functional activities (See

Appendix C). Report balance problems and functional limitations to the physician, and caution the patient and family/caregivers to guard against falls and trauma.

- Assess blood pressure periodically and compare to normal values (See Appendix F). Report low blood pressure (hypotension), especially if patient experiences dizziness and syncope.
- Assess any back, joint, or muscle pain to rule out musculoskeletal pathology; that is, try to determine if pain is drug induced rather than caused by anatomic or biomechanical problems.
- Assess peripheral edema using girth measurements, volume displacement, and measurement of pitting edema (See Appendix N). Report increased swelling in feet and ankles or a sudden increase in body weight due to fluid retention.
- Periodically assess body weight and other anthropometric measures (body mass index, body composition). Report a rapid or unexplained weight gain or increased body fat.

Interventions

- Guard against falls and trauma (hip fractures, head injury, and so forth), and implement fall-prevention strategies (See Appendix E).
- To minimize orthostatic hypotension, patient should move slowly when assuming a more upright position.
- Help patient explore nonpharmacologic methods reduce depression and other psychologic disorders (exercise, counseling, support groups, and so forth).

Patient/Client-Related Instruction

- Advise patient that antidepressant effects may not occur immediately; it may take 2 wk or more before an improvement in mood is observed.
- Advise patient to avoid alcohol and other CNS depressants because of the increased risk of sedation and adverse effects.
- Advise patient that this drug may cause problems in fat metabolism (increased plasma cholesterol and triglycerides). Remind patient that periodic blood tests may be needed to monitor plasma lipids.
- Instruct patient to report severe or prolonged GI problems, including constipation, vomiting, abdominal pain, dry mouth, or a change in appetite.
- Instruct patient to report other problematic side effects such as severe or prolonged cough, labored breathing, increased thirst, increased urge to urinate, upper respiratory tract irritation, skin reactions (rash, itching), or flu-like symptoms (fever, malaise, body aches).

Pharmacokinetics

Absorption: Well absorbed but rapidly metabolized, resulting in 50% bioavailability.
Distribution: Unknown.
Protein Binding: 85%.
Metabolism and Excretion: Extensively metabolized by the liver (P4502D6, 1A2, and 3A enzymes involved); metabolites excreted in urine (75%) and feces (15%).
Half-life: 20–40 hr.

TIME/ACTION PROFILE (antidepressant effect)

ROUTE	ONSET	PEAK	DURATION
PO	1–2 wk	6 wk or more	unknown

Contraindications/Precautions

Contraindicated in: Hypersensitivity; Concurrent MAO inhibitor therapy.
Use Cautiously in: History of seizures; History of suicide attempt; May ↑ risk of suicide attempt/ideation, especially during early treatment or dose adjustment; History of mania/hypomania; Patients with hepatic or renal impairment; OB: Safety not established; Lactation: Discontinue drug or bottle-feed; Pedi: Safety not established. Suicide risk may be greater in children or adolescents; Geri: ↑ sensitivity to CNS effects and oversedation. Begin at lower doses and titrate carefully.

Interactions

Drug-Drug: May cause hypertension, seizures, and death when used with **MAO inhibitors**; do not use within 14 days of MAO inhibitor therapy. ↑ CNS depression with other **CNS depressants**, including **alcohol** and **benzodiazepines**. **Drugs affecting P450 enzymes, CYP2D6, CYP1A2,** and **CYP3A4** may alter the effects of mirtazapine.
Drug-Natural: Concomitant use of **kava, valerian, skullcap, chamomile, or hops** can ↑ CNS depression. ↑ risk of serotonergic side effects including serotonin syndrome with **St. John's wort** and **SAMe.**

Route/Dosage

PO (Adults): 15 mg/day as a single bedtime dose initially; may be increased q 1–2 wk up to 45 mg/day.

Availability (generic available)

Tablets: 15 mg, 30 mg, 45 mg. **Orally disintegrating tablets (orange flavor):** 15 mg, 30 mg, 45 mg.

misoprostol (mye-soe-prost-ole)
Cytotec

Classification
Therapeutic: antiulcer agents, cytoprotective agents
Pharmacologic: prostaglandins

Indications

Prevention of gastric mucosal injury from NSAIDs, including aspirin, in high-risk patients (geriatric patients, debilitated patients, or those with a history of ulcers). With mifepristone for termination of pregnancy. **Unlabeled Use:** Treatment of duodenal ulcers.

Action

Acts as a prostaglandin analogue, decreasing gastric acid secretion (antisecretory effect) and increasing the production of protective mucus (cytoprotective effect). Causes uterine contractions. **Therapeutic Effects:** Prevention of gastric ulceration from NSAIDs. With mifepristone terminates pregnancy of less than 49 days.

Adverse Reactions/Side Effects

CNS: headache. **GI:** abdominal pain, diarrhea, constipation, dyspepsia, flatulence, nausea, vomiting. **GU:** miscarriage, menstrual disorders.

PHYSICAL THERAPY IMPLICATIONS

Examination and Evaluation

- Monitor improvements in GI symptoms (gastritis, heartburn, and so forth) to help document whether drug therapy is successful in preventing gastric damage or duodenal ulcers.

Interventions

- In cases of NSAID-induced gastritis, implement appropriate manual therapy techniques, physical agents, and therapeutic exercises to reduce musculoskeletal pain and decrease the need for aspirin and other NSAIDs.

Patient/Client-Related Instruction

- Advise patient to avoid alcohol and foods that may cause an increase in GI irritation.
- Inform patient that misoprostol will cause spontaneous abortion. Women of childbearing age must be informed of this effect through verbal and written information and must use contraception throughout drug treatment. If pregnancy is suspected, the woman should stop taking misoprostol and notify her health care professional immediately.
- If used with mifepristone to terminate pregnancy, inform patient that vaginal bleeding and uterine cramping will probably occur. Bleeding or spotting occurs for an average of 9–16 days, but may continue for more than 30 days. Instruct patient to report any severe or unusual cramping, bleeding, or pelvic pain that extends beyond the expected time periods.
- Instruct patient to report bothersome side effects, including severe or prolonged headache, menstrual irregularities, or GI problems (nausea, diarrhea, vomiting, constipation, heartburn, flatulence, abdominal pain).

Pharmacokinetics

Absorption: Well absorbed following oral administration and rapidly converted to its active form (misoprostol acid).
Distribution: Unknown.
Protein Binding: 85%.
Metabolism and Excretion: Undergoes some metabolism and is then excreted by the kidneys.
Half-life: 20–40 min.

TIME/ACTION PROFILE (effect on gastric acid secretion)

ROUTE	ONSET	PEAK	DURATION
PO	30 min	unknown	3–6 hr

Contraindications/Precautions

Contraindicated in: Hypersensitivity to prostaglandins; Pregnancy or lactation (when used to prevent NSAID-induced gastric injury).
Use Cautiously in: Patients with childbearing potential; Children <18 yr (safety not established).
Exercise Extreme Caution in: When used for cervical ripening (unlabeled use), may cause uterine rupture; risk factors are late trimester pregnancy, previous cesarian section or uterine surgery, or ≥5 previous pregnancies.

Interactions

Drug-Drug: ↑ risk of diarrhea with **magnesium-containing antacids**.

Route/Dosage

PO (Adults): *Antiulcer*—200 mcg qid with or after meals and at bedtime, *or* 400 mcg bid, with the last dose at bedtime. If intolerance occurs, dosage may be decreased to 100 mcg qid. *Termination of Pregnancy*—400 mcg single dose 2 days after mifepristone if abortion has not occurred.

Availability (generic available)

Tablets: 100 mcg (0.1 mg), 200 mcg (0.2 mg).
In combination with: 50 mg diclofenac/200 mcg misoprostol and 75 mg diclofenac/200 mcg misoprostol (Arthrotec). See Appendix B.

mitomycin (mye-toe-mye-sin)

MitoExtra, Mutamycin

Classification
Therapeutic: antineoplastics
Pharmacologic: antitumor antibiotics

Indications

Used with other agents in the management of disseminated adenocarcinoma of the stomach or pancreas.

Unlabeled Use: Palliative treatment of Carcinoma of the colon or breast, Head and neck tumors, Advanced biliary, lung, and cervical squamous cell carcinomas.

Action

Primarily inhibits DNA synthesis by causing cross-linking; also inhibits RNA and protein synthesis (cell-cycle phase–nonspecific but is most active in S and G phases). **Therapeutic Effects:** Death of rapidly replicating cells, particularly malignant ones.

Adverse Reactions/Side Effects

Resp: PULMONARY TOXICITY. **CV:** edema. **GI:** nausea, vomiting, anorexia, stomatitis. **GU:** infertility, renal failure. **Derm:** alopecia, desquamation. **Hemat:** leukopenia, thrombocytopenia, anemia. **Local:** phlebitis at IV site. **Misc:** HEMOLYTIC UREMIC SYNDROME, fever, prolonged malaise.

PHYSICAL THERAPY IMPLICATIONS

Examination and Evaluation

- Assess pulmonary function periodically by measuring lung volumes, breath sounds, and respiratory rate (See appendixes I, J, K). Report immediately any signs of pulmonary toxicity, including rales/crackles, dyspnea, shortness of breath, decreased breath sounds, pleuritic friction rub, tachypnea, cough, wheezing, pleuritic pain, fever, fatigue, hemoptysis, and hypoxia.
- Monitor signs of renal failure and hemolytic uremic syndrome, including decreased urine output, increased blood pressure, muscle cramps/twitching, edema/weight gain from fluid retention, pale or yellowish brown skin, small bruises (petechiae), and confusion that progresses to seizures and coma. Report these signs to the physician or nursing staff immediately.
- Watch for signs of leukopenia (fever, sore throat, signs of infection), thrombocytopenia (bruising, nose bleeds, bleeding gums), or unusual weakness and fatigue that might be due to anemia. Report these signs to the physician or nursing staff.
- Assess peripheral edema using girth measurements, volume displacement, and measurement of pitting edema (see Appendix N). Report increased swelling in feet and ankles or a sudden increase in body weight due to fluid retention.
- Assess IV injection site for pain, swelling, and inflammation (phlebitis). Report signs of phlebitis or other prolonged or excessive injection site reactions to the physician.

Interventions

- For patients who are medically able to begin exercise, implement appropriate resistive exercises and aerobic training to maintain muscle strength and aerobic capacity during cancer chemotherapy or to help restore function after chemotherapy.
- Because of the risk of pulmonary toxicity, use caution during aerobic exercise and other forms of therapeutic exercise. Assess exercise tolerance frequently (respiratory symptoms, blood pressure, heart rate, fatigue levels), and terminate exercise immediately if any untoward responses occur (See Appendix L).

Patient/Client-Related Instruction

- Instruct patient to guard against infection (frequent hand washing, etc.), and to avoid crowds and contact with persons with contagious diseases.
- Advise patient about the likelihood of GI reactions, including nausea, vomiting, loss of appetite, and irritation in or around the mouth. Instruct patient or family and caregivers to report other severe or unexpected GI problems.
- Advise patient that hair loss and other skin reactions are likely. Report any severe or unexpected skin reactions.

Pharmacokinetics

Absorption: IV administration results in complete bioavailability.
Distribution: Widely distributed, concentrates in tumor tissue. Does not enter CSF.
Metabolism and Excretion: Mostly metabolized by the liver. Small amounts (<10%) excreted unchanged by the kidneys and in bile.
Half-life: 50 min.

TIME/ACTION PROFILE (effects on blood counts)

ROUTE	ONSET	PEAK	DURATION
IV	3–8 wk	4–8 wk	up to 3 mo

Contraindications/Precautions

Contraindicated in: Hypersensitivity; Pregnancy or lactation.
Use Cautiously in: Patients with childbearing potential; Active infections; Decreased bone marrow reserve; Geri: Geriatric patients or patients with other chronic debilitating illnesses; Impaired liver function; History of pulmonary problems.

Interactions

Drug-Drug: Additive bone marrow depression with other **antineoplastics** or **radiation therapy**. May ↓ antibody response to **live-virus vaccines** and ↑ risk of adverse reactions. Concurrent or sequential use with **vinca alkaloids** may result in respiratory toxicity.

Route/Dosage

IV (Adults): 20 mg/m^2 every 6–8 wk.

Availability

Injection: 5-mg, 20-mg, and 40-mg vials.

mitotane (mye-toe-tane)

p'-DDD, Lysodren

Classification

Therapeutic: antineoplastics

Pharmacologic: adrenocortical suppressants

Indications

Inoperable carcinoma of the adrenal cortex.
Unlabeled Use: Cushing's syndrome due to pituitary disorders.

Action

Suppresses adrenal function. Has a direct cytotoxic effect on adrenal tumors. Structurally related to DDT (an insecticide). **Therapeutic Effects:** Regression of adrenal cortical tumors.

Adverse Reactions/Side Effects

CNS: lethargy, somnolence, brain damage, dizziness, fatigue, functional impairment (high-dose, long-term therapy), headache, irritability, mental depression, tremors, vertigo, weakness. **EENT:** blurred vision, decreased hearing, diplopia, lens opacities, optic neuritis, toxic retinopathy. **Resp:** shortness of breath, wheezing. **CV:** hypertension, hypotension. **GI:** anorexia, diarrhea, nausea, vomiting, increased salivation. **GU:** albuminuria, hematuria, hemorrhagic cystitis. **Derm:** maculopapular rash, flushing. **Endo:** adrenal suppression, gynecomastia. **Metab:** hypercholesterolemia, hypouricemia. **MS:** aching, arthralgia, myalgia. **Misc:** fever.

PHYSICAL THERAPY IMPLICATIONS

Examination and Evaluation

- Monitor signs of CNS toxicity, including irritability, headache, dizziness, decreased mental acuity, lethargy, tremors, vertigo, and functional impairments. Notify physician because toxicity can lead to permanent brain damage.
- Assess blood pressure (BP) periodically, and compare to normal values (See Appendix F). Report a sustained increase in BP (hypertension) or low blood pressure (hypotension) that causes dizziness and syncope.
- Assess any muscle pain, joint pain, or body aches to rule out musculoskeletal pathology; that is, try to determine if pain is drug induced rather than caused by anatomic or biomechanical problems.
- Monitor any breathing problems such as wheezing or shortness of breath. Report severe or prolonged respiratory impairments.

Interventions

- For patients who are medically able to begin exercise, implement appropriate resistive exercises and aerobic training to maintain muscle strength and aerobic capacity during cancer chemotherapy or to help restore function after chemotherapy.
- Because of cardiovascular and pulmonary impairments (changes in BP, respiratory problems), use caution during aerobic exercise and endurance conditioning. Terminate exercise if patient exhibits untoward symptoms (chest pain, shortness of breath, etc.) or displays other criteria for exercise termination (See Appendix L).

Patient/Client-Related Instruction

- Advise patient and family/caregivers that fatigue and weakness are likely and may be severe. Functional abilities may be limited, and patient may need to use assistive devices during ambulation.
- Instruct patient to report any hearing loss or vision problems (blurred vision, double vision).
- Advise patient about the likelihood of GI reactions such as diarrhea, nausea, vomiting, and loss of appetite. Instruct patient to report severe or prolonged GI problems.
- Instruct patient to report signs of kidney dysfunction, including blood in the urine and painful or difficult urination.
- Instruct patient or family/caregivers to report other bothersome side effects such as severe or prolonged fever, skin warmth/flushing, or breast enlargement in men.

Pharmacokinetics

Absorption: 30–40% absorbed following oral administration.
Distribution: Widely distributed to all body tissues; accumulates in fatty tissue.
Metabolism and Excretion: Slowly released from fatty tissue. Mostly metabolized by the liver; 10% excreted by the kidneys; 15% excreted in bile.
Half-life: 18–159 days.

TIME/ACTION PROFILE (clinical effects*)

ROUTE	ONSET	PEAK	DURATION
PO	2–4 wk	6 wk	unknown

*Onset = inhibition of adrenocortical function; peak = tumor response.

Contraindications/Precautions

Contraindicated in: Hypersensitivity.
Use Cautiously in: Obesity (↑ risk of adverse reactions); Pregnancy, lactation, or children (especially 1st trimester of pregnancy; safety not established).

Exercise Extreme Caution in: Shock or severe trauma; discontinue temporarily and administer exogenous steroids.

Interactions

Drug-Drug: Stimulates hepatic drug-metabolizing enzymes, which may decrease the effectiveness of **drugs that are highly metabolized (warfarin, phenytoin)**. Additive CNS depression with other **CNS depressants**, including **alcohol, antihistamines, antidepressants, opioid analgesics**, or **sedative/hypnotics**. **Spironolactone** may block the effects of mitotane in Cushing's disease.

Route/Dosage

Adrenocortical Carcinoma

PO (Adults): 2–6 g/day in 3–4 divided doses; may be increased as tolerated (range 2–16 g/day).

Cushing's Syndrome

PO (Adults): 3–6 g/day in 3–4 divided doses initially, decreased to maintenance dose of 500 mg twice weekly to 2 g/day (unlabeled use).

Availability

Tablets: 500 mg.

mitoxantrone

(mye-toe-**zan**-trone)

Novantrone

Classification

Therapeutic: antineoplastics, immune modifiers

Pharmacologic: antitumor antibiotics

Indications

Acute nonlymphocytic leukemia (ANLL) in adults (with other antineoplastics). Initial chemotherapy for patients with pain associated with advanced hormone-refractory prostate cancer. Secondary (chronic) progressive, progressive relapsing, or worsening relapsing-remitting multiple sclerosis (MS). **Unlabeled Use:** Breast cancer, liver cancer, and non-Hodgkin's lymphoma.

Action

Inhibits DNA synthesis (cell-cycle phase–nonspecific). **Therapeutic Effects:** Death of rapidly replicating cells, particularly malignant ones. Decreased pain in patients with advanced prostate cancer. Decreased disability and slowed progression of MS.

Adverse Reactions/Side Effects

CNS: SEIZURES, headache. **EENT:** blue-green sclera, conjunctivitis. **Resp:** cough, dyspnea. **CV:** CARDIOTOXICITY, arrhythmias, ECG changes. **GI:** abdominal pain, diarrhea, hepatic toxicity, nausea, stomatitis, vomiting. **GU:** blue-green urine, gonadal suppression, renal failure. **Derm:** alopecia, rashes. **Hemat:** anemia, leukopenia, secondary leukemia, thrombocytopenia. **Metab:** hyperuricemia. **Misc:** fever, hypersensitivity reactions.

PHYSICAL THERAPY IMPLICATIONS

Examination and Evaluation

- Be alert for new seizures or increased seizure activity. Document the number, duration, and severity of seizures, and report these findings to the physician immediately.
- Assess heart rate, ECG, and blood pressure, especially during exercise (See Appendices F, G, H). Report immediately any arrhythmias or other signs of cardiac toxicity, including chest discomfort, shortness of breath, dyspnea, rales/crackles, peripheral edema, jugular venous distention, fainting, or severe fatigue and weakness.
- Monitor signs of hypersensitivity reactions, including pulmonary symptoms (tightness in the throat and chest, wheezing, cough, dyspnea) or skin reactions (rash, pruritus, urticaria). Notify physician or nursing staff immediately if these reactions occur.
- Monitor signs of renal failure, including decreased urine output, increased blood pressure, muscle cramps/twitching, edema/weight gain from fluid retention, yellowish brown skin, and confusion that progresses to seizures and coma. Report these signs to the physician or nursing staff immediately.
- Watch for signs of leukopenia (fever, sore throat, signs of infection), thrombocytopenia (bruising, nose bleeds, bleeding gums), or unusual weakness and fatigue that might be due to anemia or other blood dyscrasias. Report these signs to the physician or nursing staff.

Interventions

- For patients who are medically able to begin exercise, implement appropriate resistive exercises and aerobic training to maintain muscle strength and aerobic capacity during cancer chemotherapy or to help restore function after chemotherapy.
- Because of the risk of cardiotoxicity, use caution during aerobic exercise and other forms of therapeutic exercise. Assess exercise tolerance frequently (blood pressure, heart rate, fatigue levels), and terminate exercise immediately if any untoward responses occur (See Appendix L).

Patient/Client-Related Instruction

- Instruct patient to guard against infection (frequent hand washing, etc.), and to avoid crowds and contact with persons with contagious diseases.
- Advise patient about the likelihood of GI reactions such as diarrhea, nausea, vomiting, abdominal pain, and irritation in or around the mouth.

Instruct patient or family and caregivers to report severe or prolonged GI reactions, and also to report signs of hepatotoxicity, including loss of appetite, abdominal pain, severe nausea and vomiting, yellow skin or eyes, fever, sore throat, malaise, weakness, facial edema, lethargy, and unusual bleeding or bruising.

- Advise patient that hair loss and skin rashes are likely but to report other severe or unexpected skin reactions to the physician.
- Instruct patient or family/caregivers to report other bothersome side effects such as severe or prolonged headache, eye inflammation, fever, or cough.

Pharmacokinetics

Absorption: IV administration results in complete bioavailability.
Distribution: Widely distributed; limited penetration of CSF.
Metabolism and Excretion: Mostly eliminated by hepatobiliary clearance; <10% excreted unchanged by the kidneys.
Half-life: 5.8 days.

TIME/ACTION PROFILE (effects on blood counts)

ROUTE	ONSET	PEAK	DURATION
IV	unknown	10 days	21 days

Contraindications/Precautions

Contraindicated in: Hypersensitivity; OB: Pregnancy or lactation.
Use Cautiously in: Previous cardiac disease; OB: Patients with childbearing potential; Active infections; Depressed bone marrow reserve; Previous mediastinal radiation; Geri: Geriatric patients or patients with other chronic debilitating illness; Pedi: Safety not established; Impaired hepatobiliary function or decreased blood counts (dose reduction required).

Interactions

Drug-Drug: ↑ bone marrow depression with other **antineoplastics** or **radiation therapy**. Risk of cardiomyopathy ↑ by previous **anthracycline antineoplastics (daunorubicin, doxorubicin, idarubicin)** or **mediastinal radiation**. May ↓ antibody response to **live-virus vaccines** and ↑ risk of adverse reactions.

Route/Dosage

Acute Nonlymphatic Leukemia

IV (Adults): *Induction*—12 mg/m²/day for 3 days (usually given with cytosine arabinoside 100 mg/m²/day for 7 days); if incomplete remission occurs, a 2nd induction may be given. *Consolidation*—12 mg/m²/day for 2 days (usually given with cytosine arabinoside 100 mg/m²/day for 5 days), given 6 wk after induction with another course 4 wk later.

Advanced Prostate Cancer

IV (Adults): 12–14 mg/m² single dose as a short infusion (with corticosteroids).

Multiple Sclerosis

IV (Adults): 12 mg/m² q 3 mo.

Availability (generic available)

Injection: 2 mg/mL in 10-, 12.5-, and 15-mL vials.

modafinil (mo-daf-i-nil)

Provigil

Classification

Therapeutic: central nervous system stimulants

M

Indications

To improve wakefulness in patients with excessive daytime drowsiness due to narcolepsy, obstructive sleep apnea, or shift work sleep disorder.

Action

Produces CNS stimulation. **Therapeutic Effects:** Decreased daytime drowsiness in patients with narcolepsy and obstructive sleep apnea. Decreased drowsiness during work in patients with shift work sleep disorder.

Adverse Reactions/Side Effects

CNS: headache, amnesia, anxiety, cataplexy, confusion, depression, dizziness, insomnia, nervousness. **EENT:** rhinitis, abnormal vision, amblyopia, epistaxis, pharyngitis. **Resp:** dyspnea, lung disorder. **CV:** arrhythmias, chest pain, hypertension, hypotension, syncope, vasodilation. **GI:** nausea, abnormal liver function, anorexia, diarrhea, gingivitis, mouth ulcers, thirst, vomiting. **GU:** abnormal ejaculation, albuminuria, urinary retention. **Derm:** dry skin, herpes simplex. **Endo:** hyperglycemia. **Hemat:** eosinophilia. **MS:** joint disorder, neck pain. **Neuro:** ataxia, dyskinesia, hypertonia, paresthesia, tremor. **Misc:** infection.

PHYSICAL THERAPY IMPLICATIONS

Examination and Evaluation

- Monitor alertness in patients with narcolepsy; document the frequency and duration of sleeping episodes to help determine the effects of drug therapy.
- Be alert for signs of adverse changes in mood and behavior, including anxiety, confusion, nervousness, depression, or memory loss. Report these signs to the physician.
- Assess heart rate, ECG, and heart sounds, especially during exercise (See Appendices G, H). Report any

rhythm disturbances or symptoms of arrhythmias, including palpitations, chest discomfort, shortness of breath, fainting, and fatigue/weakness.

- Assess blood pressure (BP) and compare to normal values (See Appendix F). Report changes in BP, either a problematic decrease in BP (hypotension) or a sustained increase in BP (hypertension).
- Monitor any breathing problems, and report difficult/labored breathing, reduced pulse oximetry values, or other signs of lung dysfunction.
- Monitor for signs of eosinophilia such as fatigue, weakness, and myalgia. Report these signs to the physician.
- Be alert for signs of hyperglycemia, including confusion, drowsiness, flushed/dry skin, fruit-like breath odor, rapid/deep breathing, polyuria, loss of appetite, and unusual thirst. Patients with diabetes mellitus should check blood glucose levels frequently.
- Be alert for tremor, ataxia, abnormal muscle tone and movements (dyskinesias, hypertonia), extreme restlessness (akathisia), sudden loss of muscle tone (cataplexy), or other signs of motor dysfunction. Report problematic movement disorders to the physician.
- Assess signs of parasthesia such as numbness, tingling, and muscle weakness. Perform objective tests, including electroneuromyography and sensory testing to document any drug-related neuropathic changes.
- Assess any joint pain or neck pain to rule out musculoskeletal pathology; that is, try to determine if pain is drug-induced rather than caused by anatomic or biomechanical problems.
- Assess dizziness or syncope that might affect gait, balance, and other functional activities (See Appendix C). Report balance problems and functional limitations to the physician, and caution the patient and family/caregivers to guard against falls and trauma.

Interventions

- Because of the risk of arrhythmias and abnormal BP responses, use caution during aerobic exercise and other forms of therapeutic exercise. Assess exercise tolerance frequently (BP, heart rate, fatigue levels), and terminate exercise immediately if any untoward responses occur (See Appendix L).

Patient/Client-Related Instruction

- Instruct patient and family/caregivers to report other troublesome side effects, including severe or prolonged headache, sleep loss, vision disturbances, nasal/pharyngeal irritation, nosebleeds, infection, skin problems (dry skin, herpes eruptions), urinary retention, or GI problems (nausea, vomiting, diarrhea, mouth ulcers, inflamed gums).

Pharmacokinetics

Absorption: Rapidly absorbed; bioavailability unknown.
Distribution: Well distributed; moderately (60%) bound to plasma proteins.
Metabolism and Excretion: Highly (90%) metabolized by the liver; <10% eliminated unchanged.
Half-life: 15 hr.

TIME/ACTION PROFILE (blood levels)

ROUTE	ONSET	PEAK	DURATION
PO	Rapid	2–4 hr	24 hr

Contraindications/Precautions

Contraindicated in: Hypersensitivity; History of left ventricular hypertrophy or ischemic ECG changes, chest pain, arrhythmia, or other significant manifestations of mitral valve prolapse in association with CNS stimulant use.
Use Cautiously in: History of MI or unstable angina; Severe hepatic impairment with or without cirrhosis (dosage reduction recommended); Concurrent use of MAO inhibitors; Geriatric patients (lower doses may be necessary); Pregnancy, lactation, or children <16 yr (safety not established).

Interactions

Drug-Drug: May ↓ the metabolism and increase the effects of **diazepam, phenytoin, propranolol**, or **tricyclic antidepressants** (dosage adjustments may be necessary). May ↑ metabolism and ↓ effects of **hormonal contraceptives, cyclosporine**, and **theophylline** (dosage adjustments or additional methods of contraception may be necessary).
Drug-Natural: Use with **caffeine-containing herbs (cola nut, guarana, mate, tea, coffee)** may increase stimulant effect.

Route/Dosage

PO (Adults): 200 mg/day as a single dose.

Hepatic Impairment

PO (Adults): *Severe hepatic impairment*—100 mg/day as a single dose.

Availability

Tablets: 100 mg, 200 mg.

moexipril (moe-eks-i-pril)

Univasc

Classification

Therapeutic: antihypertensives
Pharmacologic: angiotensin-converting enzyme (ACE) inhibitors

Indications

Alone or with other agents in the management of hypertension.

Action

ACE inhibitors block the conversion of angiotensin I to the vasoconstrictor angiotensin II. ACE inhibitors also prevent the degradation of bradykinin and other vasodilatory prostaglandins. ACE inhibitors also increase plasma renin levels and reduce aldosterone levels. Net result is systemic vasodilation. **Therapeutic Effects:** Lowering of blood pressure in hypertensive patients.

Adverse Reactions/Side Effects

CNS: dizziness, fatigue, headache. **Resp:** cough. **CV:** hypotension, chest pain, edema. **GI:** diarrhea, dyspepsia. **GU:** impaired renal function. **Derm:** flushing, rashes. **F and E:** hyperkalemia. **MS:** myalgia. **Misc:** ANGIOEDEMA, flu-like symptoms.

PHYSICAL THERAPY IMPLICATIONS

Examination and Evaluation

- Monitor signs of angioedema, including rashes, raised patches of red or white skin (welts), burning/itching skin, swelling in the face, and difficulty breathing. Notify physician immediately of these signs.
- Assess blood pressure periodically and compare to normal values (See Appendix F) to help document antihypertensive effects. Report low blood pressure (hypotension), especially if patient experiences dizziness or syncope.
- Monitor symptoms of high plasma potassium levels (hyperkalemia), including bradycardia, fatigue, weakness, numbness, and tingling. Notify physician because severe cases can lead to life-threatening arrhythmias and paralysis.
- Watch for signs of impaired renal function, including decreased urine output, cloudy urine, or sudden weight gain due to fluid retention. Report these signs to the physician.
- Assess peripheral edema using girth measurements, volume displacement, and measurement of pitting edema (See Appendix N). Report increased swelling in feet and ankles or a sudden increase in body weight due to fluid retention or peripheral vasodilation.
- Assess dizziness that might affect gait, balance, and other functional activities (See Appendix C). Report balance problems and functional limitations to the physician, and caution the patient and family/caregivers to guard against falls and trauma.

Interventions

- Avoid physical therapy interventions that cause systemic vasodilation (large whirlpool, Hubbard tank). Additive effects of this drug and the intervention may cause a dangerous fall in blood pressure.
- To minimize orthostatic hypotension, patient should move slowly when assuming a more upright position.

Patient/Client-Related Instruction

- Remind patients to take medication as directed to control hypertension even if they are asymptomatic.
- Counsel patients about additional interventions to help control blood pressure, including regular exercise, weight loss, sodium restriction, stress reduction, moderation of alcohol consumption, and smoking cessation.
- Instruct patient to notify physician of a prolonged dry cough; drug therapy may need to be altered to resolve this side effect.
- Instruct patient or family/caregivers to report other troublesome side effects such as severe or prolonged headache, chest pain, flu-like symptoms, skin reactions (rash, flushing), or GI problems (diarrhea, indigestion).

M

Pharmacokinetics

Absorption: 13% bioavailability as moexiprilat following oral administration (decreased by food).
Distribution: Crosses the placenta.
Protein Binding: Moexipril: 90%; Moexiprilat: 50–70%.
Metabolism and Excretion: Converted by liver and GI mucosa to moexiprilat, the active metabolite; 13% excreted in urine, 53% excreted in feces.
Half-life: *Moexipril:* 1 hr; *Moexiprilat:* 2–9 hr (increased in renal impairment).

TIME/ACTION PROFILE (antihypertensive effect with chronic dosing)

ROUTE	ONSET	PEAK	DURATION
PO	within 1 hr	4 wk	up to 24 hr

Contraindications/Precautions

Contraindicated in: Hypersensitivity; History of angioedema with previous use of ACE inhibitors; OB: Can cause injury or death of fetus—if pregnancy occurs, discontinue immediately.
Use Cautiously in: Patients with renal impairment, hypovolemia, hyponatremia, and concurrent diuretic therapy; Geri: In patients over 65 yr—initial dosage reduction recommended; Black patients (monotherapy for hypertension less effective, may require additional therapy; higher risk of angioedema); Surgery/anesthesia (hypotension may be exaggerated); Women of childbearing potential; Lactation/Pedi: Safety not established.
Exercise Extreme Caution in: Family history of angioedema.

Interactions

Drug-Drug: Excessive hypotension may occur with concurrent use of **diuretics**. Additive hypotension with other **antihypertensive agents**. ↑ risk of hyperkalemia with concurrent use of **potassium supplements, potassium-sharing diuretics, potassium-containing salt substitutes**, or **angiotensin II receptor antagonists**. Antihypertensive response may be blunted by **NSAIDs**. ↑ levels and may ↑ the risk of **lithium** toxicity.
Drug-Food: Food significantly reduces absorption. Administer moexipril 1 hr before meals.

Route/Dosage

PO (Adults): 7.5 mg once daily, may be increased up to 30 mg/day in 1–2 divided doses (initiate therapy with 3.75 mg/day in patients receiving diuretics).

Renal Impairment

PO (Adults): *CCr ≤40 mL/min*—Initiate therapy at 3.75 mg once daily; may be titrated upward carefully to 15 mg/day.

Availability (generic available)

Tablets: 7.5 mg, 15 mg. ***In combination with:*** hydrochlorothiazide (Uniretic). See Appendix B.

molindone (moe-lin-done)

Moban

Classification

Therapeutic: antipsychotics
Pharmacologic: dihydroindolones

Indications

Schizophrenia. Second-line treatment after failure with atypical antipsychotics. **Unlabeled Use:** Other psychotic disorders. Bipolar Disorder.

Action

Blocks the effects of dopamine in the reticular-activating and limbic systems in the brain. **Therapeutic Effects:** Diminished psychoses associated with schizophrenic behavior.

Adverse Reactions/Side Effects

CNS: NEUROLEPTIC MALIGNANT SYNDROME, extrapyramidal reactions, sedation, depression, dizziness, euphoria, headache, insomnia, tardive dyskinesia. **EENT:** blurred vision, dry eyes, nasal congestion. **CV:** hypotension, tachycardia. **GI:** constipation, dry mouth, anorexia, drug-induced hepatitis, nausea. **Derm:** photosensitivity, rashes. **Endo:** galactorrhea, increased libido, irregular menses. **Misc:** allergic reactions.

PHYSICAL THERAPY IMPLICATIONS

Examination and Evaluation

- Monitor and report signs of neuroleptic malignant syndrome, including hyperthermia, diaphoresis, generalized muscle rigidity, altered mental status, tachycardia, changes in blood pressure (BP), and incontinence. Symptoms typically occur within 4–14 days after initiation of drug therapy, but can occur at any time during drug use.
- Assess motor function, and be alert for extrapyramidal symptoms. Report these symptoms immediately, especially tardive dyskinesia, because this problem may be irreversible. Common extrapyramidal symptoms include:
  - Tardive dyskinesia (uncontrolled rhythmic movement of mouth, face, and extremities, lip smacking or puckering, puffing of cheeks, uncontrolled chewing, rapid or worm-like movements of tongue).
  - Pseudoparkinsonism (shuffling gait, rigidity, tremor, pill-rolling motion, loss of balance control, difficulty speaking or swallowing, mask-like face).
  - Akathisia (restlessness or desire to keep moving).
  - Other dystonias and dyskinesias (dystonic muscle spasms, twisting motions, twitching, inability to move eyes, weakness of arms or legs).
- Be alert for depression, euphoria, or other changes in mood and behavior. Notify physician if these changes become problematic.
- Monitor signs of allergic reactions, including pulmonary symptoms (laryngeal edema, wheezing, dyspnea) or skin reactions (rash, pruritus, urticaria). Notify physician immediately if these reactions occur.
- Assess heart rate, ECG, and heart sounds, especially during exercise (See Appendices G, H). Report a rapid heart rate (tachycardia) or signs of other arrhythmias, including palpitations, chest discomfort, shortness of breath, fainting, and fatigue/weakness.
- Assess BP periodically and compare to normal values (See Appendix F). Report low BP (hypotension), especially if patient experiences dizziness or syncope.
- Assess dizziness and drowsiness that might affect gait, balance, and other functional activities (See Appendix C). Report balance problems and functional limitations to the physician, and caution the patient and family/caregivers to guard against falls and trauma.

Interventions

- Guard against falls and trauma (hip fractures, head injury, and so forth) caused by drowsiness, blurred vision, or extrapyramidal symptoms; implement fall prevention strategies (See Appendix E).

- Because of the risk of tachycardia and abnormal BP responses, use caution during aerobic exercise and other forms of therapeutic exercise. Assess exercise tolerance frequently (BP, heart rate, fatigue levels), and terminate exercise immediately if any untoward responses occur (See Appendix L).
- To minimize orthostatic hypotension, patient should move slowly when assuming a more upright position.
- Causes photosensitivity; use care if administering UV treatments. Advise patient to avoid direct sunlight and use sunscreens and protective clothing.
- Help patient and family/caregivers explore nonpharmacologic methods such as exercise, counseling, and support groups to reduce schizophrenic episodes and behavioral problems.

Patient/Client-Related Instruction

- Advise patient to avoid alcohol and other CNS depressants because of the increased risk of sedation and adverse effects.
- Advise patient about the likelihood of GI problems such as constipation, dry mouth, or loss of appetite. Instruct patient to report severe or prolonged GI problems, and also to report signs of drug-induced hepatitis, including anorexia, abdominal pain, severe nausea and vomiting, yellow skin or eyes, skin rashes, flu-like symptoms, and muscle/joint pain.
- Instruct patient to report other problematic side effects such as severe or prolonged headache, blurred vision, sleep loss, dry eyes, nasal congestion, skin rash, increased libido, nipple discharge, or menstrual disturbances.

Pharmacokinetics

Absorption: Rapidly absorbed following oral administration.
Distribution: Appears to be widely distributed; probably enters the CNS and enters breast milk.
Metabolism and Excretion: Mainly (>90%) metabolized by the liver. Small (<3%) amounts excreted unchanged by the kidneys.
Half-life: 1.5 hr.

TIME/ACTION PROFILE (peak = blood levels; duration = antipsychotic effects)

ROUTE	ONSET	PEAK	DURATION
PO	unknown	1.5 hr	24–36 hr

Contraindications/Precautions

Contraindicated in: Hypersensitivity to molindone; Cross-sensitivity with other antipsychotics may exist; Severe nervous system depression; Lactation: Discontinue drug or bottle-feed.

Use Cautiously in: Diabetes mellitus; Respiratory disease; Prostatic hyperplasia; CNS tumors; Epilepsy; Intestinal obstruction; OB/Pedi: Safety not established; Geri: Lower initial doses recommended; ↑ risk of mortality in elderly patients treated for dementia-related psychosis.

Interactions

Drug-Drug: Additive CNS depression with other **CNS depressants**, including **alcohol, antihistamines, antidepressants, MAO inhibitors, opioid analgesics**, and **sedative/hypnotics**. Additive anticholinergic properties with **agents having anticholinergic effects**, including **phenothiazines, haloperidol, antihistamines, MAO inhibitors**, or **disopyramide**. Encephalopathy may occur with **lithium**. Molindone may mask early signs of **lithium** toxicity. May negate the beneficial effects of **levodopa**.
Drug-Natural: Concomitant use of **kava, valerian, skullcap, chamomile**, or **hops** can increase CNS depression.

Route/Dosage

PO (Adults): 50–75 mg/day in 3–4 divided doses initially; may be increased to 100 mg/day after 3–4 days. Usual maintenance dose is 5–25 mg tid–qid times daily. (Divided doses up to 225 mg/day have been used in severe psychoses.).
PO (Adults—elderly or debilitated): initiate therapy at lower doses.

Availability

Tablets: 5 mg, 10 mg, 25 mg, 50 mg, 100 mg.

mometasone (topical)

(moe-**met**-a-sone)

✱ Elocom, Elocon

Classification
Therapeutic: anti-inflammatories (steroidal)
Pharmacologic: corticosteroids

Indications

Management of inflammation and pruritus associated with various allergic/immunologic skin problems.

Action

Suppresses normal immune response and inflammation. **Therapeutic Effects:** Suppression of dermatologic inflammation and immune processes.

Adverse Reactions/Side Effects

Derm: allergic contact dermatitis, atrophy, burning, dryness, edema, folliculitis, hypersensitivity reactions, hypertrichosis, hypopigmentation, irritation, maceration, miliaria, perioral dermatitis, secondary infection, striae. **Misc:** adrenal suppression (use of occlusive dressings, long-term therapy).

PHYSICAL THERAPY IMPLICATIONS

Examination and Evaluation

- Assess the area being treated to help document whether drug therapy is successful in resolving skin conditions.
- Monitor any new or increased reactions at the site of application, including inflammation, irritation, infection, burning, swelling, exfoliation, and rash. Report severe or prolonged skin reactions to the physician.
- Report signs of adrenal suppression, including hypotension, weight loss, weakness, nausea, vomiting, anorexia, lethargy, confusion, and restlessness.

Interventions

- Protect skin from breakdown, especially over bony prominences.

Patient/Client-Related Instruction

- Advise patients on long-term treatment to consult physician before stopping this medication. Stopping the medication suddenly may result in adrenocortical shock (severe hypotension, hypoglycemia, weakness, vomiting). If these signs appear, notify physician immediately; may be life threatening.
- Check that the patient and family or caregivers understand topical application procedures and adhere to the recommended dosing schedule.

Pharmacokinetics

Absorption: Minimal. Prolonged use on large surface areas or large amounts applied or use of occlusive dressings may increase systemic absorption.
Distribution: Remains primarily at site of action.
Metabolism and Excretion: Usually metabolized in skin.
Half-life: Unknown.

TIME/ACTION PROFILE (response depends on condition being treated)

ROUTE	ONSET	PEAK	DURATION
topical	mins–hrs	hrs–days	hrs–days

Contraindications/Precautions

Contraindicated in: Hypersensitivity or known intolerance to corticosteroids or components of vehicles (ointment or cream base, preservative, alcohol); Untreated bacterial or viral infections.
Use Cautiously in: Hepatic dysfunction; Diabetes mellitus, cataracts, glaucoma, or tuberculosis (use of large amounts of high-potency agents may worsen condition); Patients with preexisting skin atrophy; OB/Lactation/Pedi: Chronic high-dose use may result in adrenal suppression in mother, growth suppression in children; children may be more susceptible to adrenal and growth suppression.

Interactions

Drug-Drug: None significant.

Route/Dosage

Topical (Adults): Apply to affected area(s) once daily.

Availability (generic available)

Cream: 0.1%. **Ointment:** 0.1%. **Lotion:** 0.1%.

montelukast (mon-te-loo-kast)

Singulair

Classification

Therapeutic: allergy, cold, and cough remedies, bronchodilators
Pharmacologic: leukotriene antagonists

Indications

Prevention and chronic treatment of asthma. Management of seasonal allergic rhinitis. Prevention of exercise-induced bronchoconstriction in patients 15 yr and older.

Action

Antagonizes the effects of leukotrienes, which mediate the following: Airway edema, Smooth muscle constriction, Altered cellular activity. Result is decreased inflammatory process, which is part of asthma and allergic rhinitis. **Therapeutic Effects:** Decreased frequency and severity of acute asthma attacks. Decreased severity of allergic rhinitis. Decreased attacks of exercise-induced bronchoconstriction.

Adverse Reactions/Side Effects

CNS: anxiety, depression, fatigue, headache, suicidal thoughts/behaviors, weakness. **EENT:** otitis (children), sinusitis (children). **Resp:** cough, rhinorrhea. **GI:** abdominal pain, diarrhea (children), dyspepsia, nausea (children), increased liver enzymes. **Neuro:** tremor. **Derm:** rash. **Misc:** EOSINOPHILIC CONDITIONS (INCLUDING CHURG-STRAUSS SYNDROME), fever.

PHYSICAL THERAPY IMPLICATIONS

Examination and Evaluation

- Be alert for signs of eosinophilic conditions and allergic blood vessel reactions, including Churg-Strauss syndrome. Early signs include allergic rhinitis, sinusitis, asthma, or hay fever-like reactions. Symptoms can increase to include fever, skin rash, joint pain, severe pain and numbness (peripheral neuropathy), shortness of breath, coughing up blood, bloody urine, chest pain, arrhythmias, and GI problems (diarrhea, nausea, vomiting, GI bleeding). Notify physician immediately for further evaluation of any signs listed above.

- Assess pulmonary function at rest and during exercise (See Appendices I, J, K) to determine effectiveness of medication in controlling bronchoconstriction.
- Monitor and report any changes in mood or behavior, including anxiety, depression, and suicidal thoughts.
- Monitor any muscle weakness or tremor. Report any neuromuscular problems that affect gait or other functional activities.

Interventions

- When implementing airway clearance techniques or respiratory muscle training, attempt to intervene when the airway is maximally bronchodilated. Peak responses typically occur 2–4 hr after oral administration.

Patient/Client-Related Instruction

- Advise patient not to exceed the recommended dose or frequency of administration. Contact physician if bronchospasm is not adequately controlled by the current medication regimen or if respiratory symptoms continue to worsen.
- Instruct patient and family/caregivers to report other troublesome side effects, including severe or prolonged headache, fever, cough, ear pain, sinus inflammation, nasal discharge, skin rash, or GI problems (nausea, diarrhea, indigestion, abdominal pain).

Pharmacokinetics

Absorption: Rapidly absorbed (63–73%) following oral administration.
Distribution: Unknown.
Protein Binding: 99%.
Metabolism and Excretion: Mostly metabolized by the liver (by P4503A4 and 2C9 enzyme systems); metabolites eliminated in feces via bile; negligible renal excretion.
Half-life: 2.7–5.5 hr.

TIME/ACTION PROFILE (improved symptoms of asthma)

ROUTE	ONSET	PEAK*	DURATION
PO (swallow)	within 24 hr	3–4 hr	24 hr
PO (chew)	within 24 hr	2–2.5 hr	24 hr

*Blood levels.

Contraindications/Precautions

Contraindicated in: Hypersensitivity.
Use Cautiously in: Acute attacks of asthma; Phenylketonuria (chewable tablets contain aspartame); Hepatic impairment (may need lower doses); Reduction of corticosteroid therapy (may increase the risk of eosinophilic conditions); OB/Pedi/Lactation: Pregnancy, lactation, or children <1 yr (safety not established).

Interactions

Drug-Drug: Drugs which induce the CYP450 enzyme system (**phenobarbital** and **rifampin**) may decrease the effects of montelukast.

Route/Dosage

Asthma and Allergic Rhinitis

PO (Adults and Children ≥14 yr): 10 mg once daily.
PO (Children 6–14 yr): 5 mg once daily (as chewable tablet).
PO (Children 2–5 yr): 4 mg once daily (as chewable tablet or granules).
PO (Children 6–23 mo): 4 mg once daily (as oral granules).

Exercise-Induced Bronchoconstriction (EIB)

PO (Adults and Children ≥15 yr): 10 mg at least 2 hr before exercise. Do not take within 24 hr of another dose; if taking daily doses, do not take dose for EIB.

Availability

Tablets: 10 mg. **Chewable tablets (cherry flavor):** 4 mg, 5 mg. **Oral granules:** 4 mg/packet in 30-packet cartons.

M

HIGH ALERT

morphine (mor-feen)

Astramorph, Astramorph PF, Avinza, Duramorph, DepoDur, ✱Epimorph, Infumorph, Kadian, ✱M-Eslon, ✱Morphine H.P, ✱Morphitec, ✱M.O.S, ✱M.O.S.-S.R, MS, MS Contin, ✱MS • IR, MSIR, MSO_4, OMS Concentrate, Oramorph SR, RMS, Roxanol, Roxanol Rescudose, Roxanol-T, ✱Statex

Classification

Therapeutic: opioid analgesics
Pharmacologic: opioid agonists

Schedule II

Indications

Severe pain. Pulmonary edema. Pain associated with MI.

Action

Binds to opiate receptors in the CNS. Alters the perception of and response to painful stimuli while producing generalized CNS depression. **Therapeutic Effects:** Decrease in severity of pain.

Adverse Reactions/Side Effects

CNS: confusion, sedation, dizziness, dysphoria, euphoria, floating feeling, hallucinations, headache, unusual dreams. **EENT:** blurred vision, diplopia, miosis. **Resp:** RESPIRATORY DEPRESSION. **CV:** hypotension, bradycardia. **GI:** constipation, nausea, vomiting. **GU:** urinary retention. **Derm:** flushing, itching, sweating. **Misc:** physical dependence, psychologic dependence, tolerance.

PHYSICAL THERAPY IMPLICATIONS

Examination and Evaluation

- Assess symptoms of respiratory depression, including decreased respiratory rate, confusion, bluish color of the skin and mucous membranes (cyanosis), and difficult, labored breathing (dyspnea). Monitor pulse oximetry and perform pulmonary function tests (See Appendix I) to quantify suspected changes in ventilation and respiratory function. Excessive respiratory depression requires emergency care.
- Be alert for excessive sedation or changes in mood and behavior (euphoria, dysphoria, confusion, hallucinations). Notify physician or nurse immediately if patient is unconscious or extremely difficult to arouse.
- Use appropriate pain scales (visual analogue scales, others) to document whether this drug is successful in helping manage the patient's pain.
- Assess blood pressure periodically and compare to normal values (See Appendix F). Report low blood pressure (hypotension), especially if patient experiences dizziness, fainting, or other symptoms.
- Assess heart rate, ECG, and heart sounds, especially during exercise (See Appendices G, H). Report slow heart rate (bradycardia) or symptoms of other arrhythmias, including palpitations, chest discomfort, shortness of breath, fainting, and fatigue/weakness.
- If treating pulmonary edema, monitor symptoms such as shortness of breath, chest pain, and labored breathing to help determine if drug therapy is beneficial in resolving the anxiety and apprehension associated with pulmonary edema. Document any changes in respiratory symptoms.
- Assess dizziness that might affect gait, balance, and other functional activities (See Appendix C). Report balance problems and functional limitations to the physician and nursing staff, and caution the patient and family/caregivers to guard against falls and trauma.

Interventions

- Implement appropriate manual therapy techniques, physical agents, and therapeutic exercises to reduce pain and help wean patient off opioid analgesics as soon as possible.
- Because of the risk of respiratory depression, bradycardia, and hypotension, use caution during aerobic exercise and other forms of therapeutic exercise. Assess exercise tolerance frequently (blood pressure, heart rate, respiratory rate, fatigue levels), and terminate exercise immediately if any untoward responses occur (See Appendix L).
- Help patient explore other nonpharmacologic methods to reduce chronic pain, such as relaxation techniques, exercise, counseling, and so forth.
- Guard against falls and trauma (hip fractures, head injury). Implement fall-prevention strategies (See Appendix E), especially if patient exhibits sedation, dizziness, or blurred vision.
- To minimize orthostatic hypotension, patient should move slowly when assuming a more upright position.

Patient/Client-Related Instruction

- Advise patient that opioid analgesics are usually more effective if given before pain becomes severe; emphasize that adequate pain control will allow better participation in physical therapy.
- Educate patient about the dangers of opioid overdose; encourage patient to adhere to proper dosing schedule.
- Emphasize that the risk of physical addiction (tolerance and dependence) is usually minimal during short-term treatment of pain. Advise patient that addiction is more likely during excessive or inappropriate use of opioid analgesics.
- Advise patient to avoid alcohol and other CNS depressants because of the increased risk of sedation and decreased CNS function.
- Advise patient to increase fluid intake and dietary fiber to avoid constipation. Laxatives may also be helpful in patients susceptible to fecal impaction (e.g., people with spinal cord injury).
- Instruct patient to report other troublesome side effects such as severe or prolonged headache, urinary retention, unusual dreams, vision disturbances, skin reactions (itching, flushing, excessive sweating), or GI problems (nausea, vomiting).

Pharmacokinetics

Absorption: Variably absorbed (about 30%) following oral administration. More reliably absorbed from rectal, SC, and IM sites. Following epidural administration, systemic absorption and absorption into the intrathecal space via the meninges occurs.
Distribution: Widely distributed. Crosses the placenta; enters breast milk in small amounts.

Protein Binding: Premature infants: <20%; Adults: 35%.
Metabolism and Excretion: Mostly metabolized by the liver. Active metabolites excreted renally.
Half-life: Premature neonates: 10–20 hr; Neonates: 7.6 hr; Infants 1–3 mo: 6.2 hr; Children 6 mo–2.5 yr: 2.9 hr; Children 3–6 yr: 1–2 hr; Children 6–19 yr with sickle cell disease: 1.3 hr; Adults: 2–4 hr.

TIME/ACTION PROFILE (analgesia)

ROUTE	ONSET	PEAK	DURATION
PO	unknown	60 min	4–5 hr
PO-ER, SR	unknown	3–4 hr	8–24 hr
IM	10–30 min	30–60 min	4–5 hr
SC	20 min	50–90 min	4–5 hr
Rect	unknown	20–60 min	3–7 hr
IV	rapid	20 min	4–5 hr
Epidural	6–30 min	1 hr	up to 24 hr (48 hr for liposomal injection)
IT	rapid (min)	unknown	up to 24 hr

Contraindications/Precautions

Contraindicated in: Hypersensitivity; Some products contain tartrazine, bisulfites, or alcohol and should be avoided in patients with known hypersensitivity.
Use Cautiously in: Head trauma; ↑ intracranial pressure; Severe renal, hepatic, or pulmonary disease; Hypothyroidism; Adrenal insufficiency; History of substance abuse; Geri: Geriatric or debilitated patients (dose reduction suggested); Undiagnosed abdominal pain; Prostatic hyperplasia; Patients undergoing procedures that rapidly ↓ pain (cordotomy, radiation); long-acting agents should be discontinued 24 hr before and replaced with short-acting agents; OB: Pregnancy or lactation (avoid chronic use; has been used during labor but may cause respiratory depression in the newborn); Pedi: Children <18 yr (epidural liposomal injection only—not recommended); Neonates and infants <3 mo (more susceptible to respiratory depression); Neonates (oral solution contains sodium benzoate which can cause potentially fatal gasping syndrome).

Interactions

Drug-Drug: Use with **extreme caution** in patients receiving **MAO inhibitors** within 14 days prior (may result in unpredictable, severe reactions—↓ initial dose of morphine to 25% of usual dose). ↑ CNS depression with **alcohol, sedative/hypnotics, clomipramine, barbiturates, tricyclic antidepressants,** and **antihistamines**. Administration of **partial-antagonist opioid analgesics** may precipitate opioid withdrawal in physically dependent patients. **Buprenorphine, nalbuphine, butorphanol,** or **pentazocine** may ↓ analgesia. May ↑ the anticoagulant effect of **warfarin**. **Cimetidine** ↓ metabolism and may ↑ effects. Epidural test dose of lidocaine/epinephrine may alter release of liposomal injection.
Drug-Natural: Concomitant use of **kava, valerian,** or **chamomile** can ↑ CNS depression.

Route/Dosage

Larger doses may be required during chronic therapy.
PO, Rectal (Adults ≥50 kg): *Usual starting dose for moderate- to-severe pain in opioid-naive patients*—30 mg q 3–4 hr initially *or* once 24-hr opioid requirement is determined, convert to controlled, extended, *or* sustained-release morphine by administering total daily oral morphine dose every 24 hr (as *Kadian* or *Avinza*), 50% of the total daily oral morphine dose every 12 hr (as *Oramorph SR, Kadian, MS Contin*), or 33% of the total daily oral morphine dose every 8 hr (as *MS Contin*). See equianalgesic chart, Appendix J. *Avinza* dose should not exceed 1600 mg/day because of fumaric acid in formulation.
PO, Rectal (Adults and Children <50 kg): *Usual starting dose for moderate-to-severe pain in opioid-naive patients*—0.3 mg/kg q 3–4 hr initially.
PO (Children >1 mo): *Prompt-release tablets and solution*—0.2–0.5 mg/kg/dose q 4–6 hr as needed. *Controlled- release tablet*—0.3–0.6 mg/kg/dose q 12 hr.
IM, IV, SC (Adults ≥50 kg): *Usual starting dose for moderate-to-severe pain in opioid-naive patients*—4–10 mg q 3–4 hr. *MI*—8–15 mg; for very severe pain, additional smaller doses may be given every 3–4 hr.
IM, IV, SC (Adults and Children <50 kg): *Usual starting dose for moderate-to-severe pain in opioid-naive patients*—0.05–0.2 mg/kg q 3–4 hr; maximum 15 mg/dose.
IM, IV, SC (Neonates): 0.05 mg/kg q 4–8 hr; maximum dose 0.1 mg/kg. Use preservative-free formulation.
IV, SC (Adults): *Continuous infusion*—0.8–10 mg/hr; may be preceded by a bolus of 15 mg (infusion rates vary greatly; up to 400 mg/hr have been used).
IV, SC (Children >1 mo): *Continuous infusion, postoperative pain*—0.01–0.04 mg/kg/hr. *Continuous infusion, sickle cell or cancer pain*—0.02–2.6 mg/kg/hr.
IV (Neonates): *Continuous infusion*—0.01–0.03 mg/kg/hr.
Epidural (Adults): *Intermittent injection*—5 mg/day (initially); if relief is not obtained at 60 min, 1- to 2-mg increments may be made (total dose not to exceed 10 mg/day). *Continuous infusion*—2–4 mg/24 hr; may increase by 1–2 mg/day (up to 30 mg/day); *single-dose extended-release liposomal*

M

injection—lower extremity orthopedic surgery: 15 mg, lower abdominal/pelvic surgery: 10–15 mg, cesarean section: 10 mg. Use preservative-free formulation.
Epidural (Children >1 mo): 0.03–0.05 mg/kg, maximum dose 0.1 mg/kg or 5 mg/24 hr. Use preservative-free formulation.
Intrathecal (Adults): 0.2–1 mg. Use preservative-free formulation.

Availability (generic available)

Soluble tablets: 10 mg, 15 mg, 30 mg. **Tablets:** 15 mg, 30 mg. **Extended (controlled, sustained)-release tablets:** 15 mg, 30 mg, 60 mg, 100 mg, 200 mg. **Sustained-release capsules (Kadian):** 10 mg, 20 mg, 30 mg, 50 mg, 60 mg, 80 mg, 200 mg. **Extended-release capsules (Avinza):** 30 mg, 60 mg, 90 mg, 120 mg. **Oral solution (Roxanol-T—20 mg/mL fruit and mint flavor; also unflavored):** 10 mg/5 mL, 20 mg/5 mL, 100 mg/5 mL, 2 mg/mL, 4 mg/mL, 20 mg/mL (concentrate). **Rectal suppositories:** 5 mg, 10 mg, 20 mg, 30 mg. **Solution for IM, SC, IV injection:** 1 mg/mL, 2 mg/mL, 4 mg/mL, 5 mg/mL, 8 mg/mL, 10 mg/mL, 15 mg/mL, 25 mg/mL, 50 mg/mL. **Solution for epidural, IV injection (preservative-free):** 0.5 mg/mL, 1 mg/mL. **Solution for epidural or IT use (continuous microinfusion device; preservative-free):** 10 mg/mL in 20-mL vial, 25 mg/mL in 20-mL vial. **Extended-release liposome injection for epidural use:** 10 mg/mL in 1-, 2.5-, and 2-mL vials. **Solution for IV injection (PCA device):** 1 mg/mL, 2 mg/mL, 3 mg/mL, 5 mg/mL.

moxifloxacin (mox-i-flox-a-sin)

Avelox

Classification
Therapeutic: anti-infectives
Pharmacologic: fluoroquinolones

Indications

Treatment of the following bacterial infections: Respiratory tract infections, including acute sinusitis, acute exacerbations of chronic bronchitis, and community-acquired pneumonia (CAP), Uncomplicated and complicated skin and skin structure infections.

Action

Inhibits bacterial DNA synthesis by inhibiting DNA gyrase enzyme. **Therapeutic Effects:** Death of susceptible bacteria. **Spectrum:** Active against gram-positive pathogens, including *Staphylococcus aureus*, *Streptococcus pyogenes*, *S. pneumoniae* (including multi-drug-resistant strains). Gram-negative spectrum notable for activity against *Escherichia coli*, *Klebsiella pneumoniae*, *Haemophilus influenzae*, *H. parainfluenzae*, *Moraxella catarrhalis*. Additional spectrum includes *Chlamydophylia pneumoniae*, *Mycoplasma pneumoniae*.

Adverse Reactions/Side Effects

CNS: agitation, anxiety, dizziness, headache, insomnia. **CV:** QTc prolongation, ARRHYTHMIAS. **GI:** PSEUDOMEMBRANOUS COLITIS, abdominal pain, abnormal liver function tests, diarrhea, dyspepsia, nausea, vomiting. **Derm:** photosensitivity. **MS:** tendinitis, tendon rupture. **Misc:** HYPERSENSITIVITY REACTIONS, INCLUDING ANAPHYLAXIS.

PHYSICAL THERAPY IMPLICATIONS

Examination and Evaluation

- Watch for seizures; notify physician immediately if patient develops or increases seizure activity.
- Monitor signs of hypersensitivity reactions and anaphylaxis, including pulmonary symptoms (tightness in the throat and chest, wheezing, cough, dyspnea) or skin reactions (rash, angioedema, pruritus, urticaria). Notify physician or nursing staff immediately if these reactions occur.
- Assess heart rate, ECG, and heart sounds, especially during exercise (See Appendices G, H). Report any rhythm disturbances or symptoms of increased arrhythmias, including palpitations, chest discomfort, shortness of breath, fainting, and fatigue/weakness.
- Monitor signs of pseudomembranous colitis, including diarrhea, abdominal pain, fever, pus or mucus in stools, and other severe or prolonged GI problems (nausea, vomiting, heartburn). Notify physician or nursing staff immediately of these signs.
- Be alert for signs of hepatotoxicity, including anorexia, abdominal pain, severe nausea and vomiting, yellow skin or eyes, fever, sore throat, malaise, weakness, facial edema, lethargy, and unusual bleeding or bruising. Report these signs to the physician.
- Assess any tendon pain. Tendinopathy and rupture can occur, especially in large, weight-bearing tendons (Achilles, patellar tendons). Risk of tendon damage is greater in patients >65 yrs old, transplant recipients (i.e., kidney, heart, lung), patients with preexisting tendon damage, and patients taking corticosteroids concurrently.
- Monitor signs of peripheral neuropathy (numbness, tingling). Perform objective tests (nerve conduction, monofilaments) to document any neuropathic changes.
- Assess dizziness that might affect gait, balance, and other functional activities (See Appendix C). Report balance problems and functional limitations to the physician and nursing staff, and caution the patient and family/caregivers to guard against falls and trauma.

- Be alert for anxiety, agitation, or other alterations in mental status. Notify physician promptly if these symptoms develop.

Interventions

- If tendon symptoms occur, notify the physician and protect the affected area to avoid tendon ruptures. Do not stretch or exercise the affected tendon, and provide crutches, walker, or other assistive devices if lower extremities are involved.
- Because of the risk of arrhythmias, use caution during aerobic exercise and other forms of therapeutic exercise. Assess exercise tolerance frequently (blood pressure, heart rate, fatigue levels), and terminate exercise immediately if any untoward responses occur (See Appendix L).
- Always wash hands thoroughly and disinfect equipment (whirlpools, electrotherapeutic devices, treatment tables, and so forth) to help prevent the spread of infection. Employ universal precautions or isolation procedures as indicated for specific patients.
- Causes photosensitivity; use care if administering UV treatments.

Patient/Client-Related Instruction

- Advise patient about photosensitivity, and to use sunscreens, protective clothing, and avoid prolonged sun exposure. Advise patient to also report any rashes or other skin reactions.
- Instruct patient to report other troublesome side effects such as severe or prolonged headache, sleep loss, or GI problems (nausea, vomiting, diarrhea, abdominal pain, indigestion).

Pharmacokinetics

Absorption: Well absorbed (90%) following oral administration.
Distribution: Widely distributed; tissue concentrations may exceed plasma concentrations.
Metabolism and Excretion: Mostly metabolized by the liver; 20% excreted unchanged in urine, 25% excreted unchanged in feces.
Half-life: 12 hr.

TIME/ACTION PROFILE (blood levels)

ROUTE	ONSET	PEAK	DURATION
PO	within 1 hr	1–3 hr	24 hr

Contraindications/Precautions

Contraindicated in: Hypersensitivity (cross-sensitivity within class may exist); Concurrent use of amiodarone, disopyramide, erythromycin, pentamidine, phenothiazines, procainamide, quinidine, some antipsychotics, sotalol, or tricyclic antidepressants.

Use Cautiously in: Known or suspected CNS disorder; Concurrent use of Class IA antiarrhythmics (disopyramide, quinidine, procainamide) or Class III antiarrhythmics (amiodarone, sotalol), erythromycin, some phenothiazines, and tricyclic antidepressants (increased risk of QTc prolongation and resultant arrhythmias); Congenital long QT syndrome; Concurrent use of corticosteroids (↑ risk of tendinitis/tendon rupture); Kidney, heart, or lung transplant patients (↑ risk of tendinitis/tendon rupture); Geri: ↑ risk of adverse reactions; OB/Lactation/Pedi: Pregnancy, lactation, or children <18 yr (safety not established).

Interactions

Drug-Drug: Concurrent use of **amiodarone, disopyramide, erythromycin, pentamidine,** phenothiazines, **procainamide, quinidine,** some **antipsychotics, sotalol,** or tricyclic **antidepressants** ↑ risk of potentially dangerous arrhythmias in susceptible individuals. May ↑ risk of bleeding with **warfarin. Iron** supplements and aluminum-, calcium-, or magnesium-containing **antacids, bismuth subsalicylate, sucralfate,** multivitamins with **zinc,** or **didanosine** (chewable/buffered tablets of pediatric suspension) ↓ absorption (take at least 2 hr before or 4 hr). Serum levels of fluoroquinolones may be ↓ by **antineoplastics. Cimetidine** may interfere with elimination of fluoroquinolones. May ↑ risk of nephrotoxicity from **cyclosporine.** Concurrent **corticosteroid** therapy may ↑ risk of tendon rupture.

Route/Dosage

PO (Adults): *Most infections*—400 mg once daily (for 5–21 days, depending on infection).

Availability

Tablets: 400 mg.

mupirocin (myoo-peer-oh-sin)

Bactroban, Bactroban Nasal

Classification

Therapeutic: anti-infectives
Pharmacologic: monoxycarbolic acids

Indications

Topical: Treatment of Impetigo, Secondarily infected traumatic skin lesions (up to 10 cm in length or 100 cm^2 area) caused by *Staphylococcus aureus* and *Streptococcus pyogenes*. **Intranasal:** Eradicates nasal colonization with methicillin-resistant *S. aureus*.

Action

Inhibits bacterial protein synthesis. **Therapeutic Effects:** Inhibition of bacterial growth and reproduction.

Spectrum: Greatest activity against gram-positive organisms, including: *S. aureus*, Beta-hemolytic streptococci. Resolution of impetigo. Eradication of *S. aureus* carrier state.

Adverse Reactions/Side Effects

CNS: nasal only: headache. **EENT: nasal only:** cough, itching, pharyngitis, rhinitis, upper respiratory tract congestion. **GI:** nausea **nasal only:** altered taste. **Derm: topical only:** burning, itching, pain, stinging.

PHYSICAL THERAPY IMPLICATIONS

Examination and Evaluation

- Monitor any upper respiratory tract irritation, inflammation, cough, or congestion following nasal administration. Notify physician of severe or prolonged symptoms.
- If applied topically to skin lesions, monitor any new or increased skin reactions, including localized pain, burning, itching, or stinging. Report severe or prolonged skin reactions to the physician.

Interventions

- Always wash hands thoroughly and disinfect equipment (whirlpools, electrotherapeutic devices, treatment tables, and so forth) to help prevent the spread of infection. Use universal precautions or isolation procedures as indicated for specific patients.

Patient/Client-Related Instruction

- Instruct patient with skin lesions to avoid itching or scratching the affected area. Patients should avoid contact with other individuals (e.g., other athletes) during the active phase of the infection.
- Check that the patient and family or caregivers understand topical application procedures, adhere to the recommended dosing schedule, and wash hands thoroughly after applying the drug topically.

Pharmacokinetics

Absorption: Minimal systemic absorption.
Distribution: Remains in the stratum corneum after topical use for prolonged periods of time (72 hr).
Metabolism and Excretion: Metabolized in the skin, removed by desquamation.
Half-life: 17–36 min.

TIME/ACTION PROFILE (anti-infective effect)

ROUTE	ONSET	PEAK	DURATION
nasal	unknown	unknown	12 hr
topical*	unknown	3–5 days	72 hr

*Resolution of lesions.

Contraindications/Precautions

Contraindicated in: Hypersensitivity to mupirocin or polyethylene glycol.
Use Cautiously in: Pregnancy or lactation (safety not established); Impaired renal function; Burn patients.

Interactions

Drug-Drug: Nasal mupirocin should not be used concurrently with other **nasal products**.

Route/Dosage

Topical (Adults and Children ≥2 mo): Ointment: Apply 3–5 times daily for 5–14 days.
Topical (Adults and Children ≥3 mo): Cream: Apply small amount 3 times/day for 10 days.
Intranasal (Adults and Children ≥1 yr): Apply small amount nasal ointment to each nostril 2–4 times/day for 5–14 days.

Availability (generic available)

Ointment: 2% in 0.9-, 15-, 22-, and 30-g tubes, 2% in 15- and 30-g tubes OTC. **Cream:** 2% in 15- and 30-g tubes. **Nasal ointment:** 2% in 1-g single-use tubes.

muromonab-CD3

(myoo-**roe**-moe-nab-CD3)
Orthoclone OKT3

Classification
Therapeutic: immunosuppressants
Pharmacologic: monoclonal antibodies

Indications

Acute renal allograft rejection reactions in transplant patients that have occurred despite conventional antirejection therapy. Acute corticosteroid-resistant hepatic or cardiac allograft rejection reactions.

Action

A purified immunoglobulin antibody that acts as an immunosuppressant by interfering with normal T-cell function. **Therapeutic Effects:** Reversal of graft rejection in transplant patients.

Adverse Reactions/Side Effects

CNS: tremor, aseptic meningitis, dizziness. **Resp:** PULMONARY EDEMA, dyspnea, shortness of breath, wheezing. **CV:** chest pain. **GI:** diarrhea, nausea, vomiting. **Misc:** CYTOKINE RELEASE SYNDROME, INFECTIONS, chills, fever, hypersensitivity reactions, increased risk of lymphoma.

PHYSICAL THERAPY IMPLICATIONS

Examination and Evaluation

- Assess any breathing problems or signs of pulmonary edema, including cough, wheezing, shortness of breath, chest pain, and labored breathing. Monitor pulse oximetry and perform pulmonary function tests (See Appendices I, J, K) and immediately report any adverse changes in ventilation and respiratory function.
- Watch for signs of increased cytokine release from T cells that are affected by this drug (cytokine release syndrome). Signs include hypotension, high fever,

chills, shivering, and malaise. Report these signs to the physician or nursing staff immediately.

- Monitor signs of aseptic meningitis, including severe headache, high fever, neck stiffness, nausea, vomiting, confusion, drowsiness, sensitivity to light, loss of appetite, skin rash, and seizures. Notify physician or nurse immediately if patient exhibits these signs.
- Be alert for signs of other infections, including fever, sore throat, mucosal lesions, chills, nausea, vomiting, diarrhea, and localized inflammation. Notify physician or nursing staff of these signs immediately.
- Monitor signs of lymphoma, including swollen lymph glands, unexplained weight loss, fatigue, weakness, fever, night sweats, dyspnea, cough, and abdominal pain/bloating. Report these signs to the physician immediately.
- Be alert for signs of hypersensitivity reactions, including pulmonary symptoms (tightness in the throat and chest, wheezing, cough, dyspnea) or skin reactions (rash, pruritus, urticaria). Notify physician or nursing staff immediately if these reactions occur.
- Assess dizziness that might affect gait, balance, and other functional activities (See Appendix C). Report balance problems and functional limitations to the physician and nursing staff, and caution the patient and family/caregivers to guard against falls and trauma.

Interventions

- Implement appropriate strengthening, aerobic, and other therapeutic exercises to improve function and promote recovery following organ transplants.
- Because of the risk of pulmonary edema, use caution during aerobic exercise and other forms of therapeutic exercise. Assess exercise tolerance frequently (blood pressure, heart rate, fatigue levels), and terminate exercise immediately if any untoward responses occur (See Appendix L).

Patient/Client-Related Instruction

- Because of immunosuppressant effects, advise patient to guard against infection (frequent hand washing, etc.), and to avoid crowds and contact with persons with contagious diseases.
- Instruct patient to report other bothersome side effects such as severe or prolonged tremor, chest pain, or GI problems (nausea, vomiting, diarrhea).

Pharmacokinetics

Absorption: Administered IV only, resulting in complete bioavailability.
Distribution: Unknown.
Metabolism and Excretion: Eliminated by binding to T lymphocytes.
Half-life: 18 hr.

TIME/ACTION PROFILE (noted as levels of circulating CD3-positive T cells)

ROUTE	ONSET	PEAK	DURATION
IV	mins	2–7 days	1 wk

Contraindications/Precautions

Contraindicated in: Hypersensitivity to muromonab-CD3, murine (mouse) proteins, or polysorbate; Previous muromonab therapy; Fluid overload; Fever >37.8°C or 100°F; Chickenpox or recent exposure to chickenpox; Herpes zoster.
Use Cautiously in: Active infections; Depressed bone marrow reserve; Chronic debilitating illnesses; CHF; Pregnancy, lactation, or children <2 yr (safety not established).

Interactions

Drug-Drug: Additive immunosuppression with other **immunosuppressives**. Concurrent **prednisone** and **azathioprine** dosages should be reduced during muromonab therapy (↑ risk of infection and lymphoproliferative disorders). **Cyclosporine** should be reduced or discontinued during muromonab-CD3 therapy (↑ risk of infection and lymphoproliferative disorders). ↑ risk of adverse CNS reactions with **indomethacin**. May ↓ antibody response to and ↑ risk of adverse reactions from **live-virus vaccines**.
Drug-Natural: Concomitant use with **astragalus, echinacea**, and **melatonin** may interfere with immunosuppression.

Route/Dosage

IV (Adults): 5 mg/day for 10–14 days (pretreatment with corticosteroids, acetaminophen, and/or antihistamines recommended).
IV (Children): 0.1 mg (100 mcg)/kg/day for 10–14 days.

Availability

Solution for injection: 1 mg/mL in 5-mL ampules.

M

mycophenolate mofetil
(mye-koe-**fen**-oh-late **moe**-fe-til)
CellCept

mycophenolic acid
(mye-koe-fe-**nol**-ik **as**-id)
Myfortic

Classification
Therapeutic: immunosuppressants

Indications

Mycophenolate mofetil: Prevention of rejection in allogenic renal, hepatic, and cardiac transplantations (used concurrently with cyclosporine and corticosteroids).
Mycophenolic acid: Prevention of rejection in allogenic renal transplantation (used concurrently with cyclosporine and corticosteroids).

Action

Inhibits the enzyme inosine monophosphate dehydrogenase, which is involved in purine synthesis. This inhibition results in suppression of T- and B-lymphocyte proliferation. **Therapeutic Effects:** Prevention of heart, kidney, or liver transplant rejection.

Adverse Reactions/Side Effects

CNS: PROGRESSIVE MULTIFOCAL LEUKOENCEPHALOPATHY, anxiety, dizziness, headache, insomnia, paresthesia, tremor. **CV:** edema, hypertension, hypotension, tachycardia. **Derm:** rashes. **Endo:** hypercholesterolemia, hyperglycemia, hyperkalemia, hypocalcemia, hypokalemia, hypomagnesemia. **GI:** GI BLEEDING, anorexia, constipation, diarrhea, nausea, vomiting, abdominal pain. **GU:** renal dysfunction. **Hemat:** leukocytosis, leukopenia, thrombocytopenia, anemia. **Resp:** cough, dyspnea. **Misc:** fever, infection, increased risk of malignancy.

PHYSICAL THERAPY IMPLICATIONS

Examination and Evaluation

- Be alert for signs of progressive multifocal leukoencephalopathy. Signs include memory lapses, decreased cognition, vision loss, speech problems, incoordination, ataxia, and muscle weakness that can progress to paralysis, seizures, and coma. Report these signs to the physician or nursing staff immediately.
- Monitor signs of GI bleeding, including abdominal pain, vomiting blood, blood in stools, or black, tarry stools. Report these signs to the physician or nursing staff immediately.
- Assess blood pressure (BP) periodically and compare to normal values (See Appendix F). Report a sustained increase in BP (hypertension) or a fall in BP (hypotension) that causes dizziness or fainting.
- Assess heart rate, ECG, and heart sounds, especially during exercise (See Appendices G, H). Report a rapid heart rate (tachycardia) or signs of other arrhythmias, including palpitations, chest discomfort, shortness of breath, fainting, and fatigue/weakness.
- Assess peripheral edema using girth measurements, volume displacement, and measurement of pitting edema (See Appendix N). Report increased swelling in feet and ankles or a sudden increase in body weight due to fluid retention.
- Assess any breathing problems, and report persistent or severe cough or difficult, labored breathing.
- Monitor signs of leukopenia (fever, sore throat, mucosal lesions, signs of infection, bruising), thrombocytopenia (bruising, nose bleeds, bleeding gums), or unusual weakness and fatigue that might be due to anemia. Periodic blood tests may be needed to monitor WBC and RBC counts.
- Be alert for signs of increased white blood cell counts (leukocytosis), including fever, weakness, weight loss, loss of appetite, dizziness, fainting, dyspnea, bleeding/bruising, or pain or tingling in the arms, legs, or abdomen. Report these signs to the physician or nursing staff immediately.
- Be alert for signs of hyperglycemia, including confusion, drowsiness, flushed/dry skin, fruit-like breath odor, rapid/deep breathing, polyuria, loss of appetite, and unusual thirst. Patients with diabetes mellitus should check blood glucose levels frequently.
- Watch for signs of renal dysfunction, including decreased urine output, cloudy urine, and sudden weight gain due to fluid retention. Report these signs to the physician.
- Monitor signs of malignancy, including a change in bowel or bladder habits, nonhealing sores, unusual bleeding or discharge, a lump in the breast or other parts of the body, chronic indigestion or difficulty in swallowing, obvious changes in a wart or mole, and persistent coughing or hoarseness. Report these signs to the physician immediately.
- Be alert for signs of paresthesia (numbness, tingling) or hyperesthesia (increased sensitivity to touch, pain). Establish baseline electroneuromyographic values at the beginning of drug treatment whenever possible, and reexamine these values periodically to document drug-induced changes in peripheral nerve function.
- Monitor neuromuscular signs of electrolyte imbalances (hypocalcemia, hypokalemia, hyperkalemia, hypomagnesemia), including headache, lethargy, irritability, insomnia, confusion, weakness, cramping, tremors, and changes in muscle excitability. Notify physician immediately if these signs occur.
- Assess dizziness that might affect gait, balance, and other functional activities (See Appendix C). Report balance problems and functional limitations to the physician and nursing staff, and caution the patient and family/caregivers to guard against falls and trauma.

Interventions

- Implement appropriate strengthening, aerobic, and other therapeutic exercises to improve function and promote recovery following organ transplants.

- Because of the risk of arrhythmias and abnormal BP responses, use caution during aerobic exercise and other forms of therapeutic exercise. Assess exercise tolerance frequently (BP, heart rate, fatigue levels), and terminate exercise immediately if any untoward responses occur (See Appendix L).

Patient/Client-Related Instruction

- Because of immunosuppressant effects, advise patient to guard against infection (frequent hand washing, etc.), and to avoid crowds and contact with persons with contagious diseases.
- Advise patient that this drug may cause problems in fat metabolism (hyperlipidemia). Remind patient that periodic blood tests may be needed to monitor plasma lipids.
- Instruct patient to report other bothersome side effects such as severe or prolonged headache, sleep loss, infections, skin rash, or GI problems (nausea, vomiting, diarrhea, constipation, loss of appetite, abdominal pain).

Pharmacokinetics

Absorption: Following oral and IV administration, mycophenolate mofetil is rapidly hydrolyzed to mycophenolic acid (MPA), the active metabolite. Absorption of enteric-coated mycophenolic acid (Myfortic) is delayed compared to mycophenolate mofetil (CellCept).
Distribution: Cross the placenta and enter breast milk.
Protein Binding: *MPA*—97%.
Metabolism and Excretion: MPA is extensively metabolized; <1% excreted unchanged in urine. Some enterohepatic recirculation of MPA occurs.
Half-life: *MPA*—8–18 hr.

TIME/ACTION PROFILE (blood levels of MPA)

ROUTE	ONSET	PEAK	DURATION
mycophenolate mofetil—PO	rapid	0.25–1.25 hr	N/A
mycophenolic acid	rapid	1.5–2.75 hr	N/A

Contraindications/Precautions

Contraindicated in: Hypersensitivity; Hypersensitivity to polysorbate 80 (for IV mycophenolate mofetil); OB/Lactation: ↑ risk of congenital anomalies or spontaneous abortion.
Use Cautiously in: Active serious pathology of the GI tract (including history of ulcer disease or GI bleeding); Phenylketonuria (oral suspension contains aspartame); Severe chronic renal impairment (dose not to exceed 1 g bid [CellCept] if CCr <25 mL/min/1.73 m^2); careful monitoring recommended; Delayed graft function following transplantation (observe for increased toxicity); Geri: Increased risk of adverse reactions related to immunosuppression; OB: Patients with childbearing potential; Pedi: Mycophenolate mofetil approved in children ≥3 mo for renal transplant; mycophenolic acid approved in children ≥5 yr for renal transplant; safety not established for other age groups.

Interactions

Drug-Drug: Combined use with **azathioprine** is not recommended (effects unknown). **Acyclovir** and **ganciclovir** compete with MPA for renal excretion and, in patients with renal dysfunction, may ↑ each other's toxicity. **Magnesium** and **aluminum hydroxide** antacids ↓ the absorption of MPA (avoid simultaneous administration). **Cholestyramine** and **colestipol** ↓ the absorption of MPA (avoid concurrent use). May interfere with the action of **oral contraceptives** (additional contraceptive method should be used). May ↓ the antibody response to and ↑ risk of adverse reactions from **live-virus vaccines**, although influenza vaccine may be useful.
Drug-Food: When administered with food, peak blood levels of MPA are significantly ↓ (should be administered on an empty stomach).

Route/Dosage

Mycophenolate mofetil (CellCept)

Renal Transplantation

PO, IV (Adults): 1 g bid; IV should be started ≤24 hr after transplantation and switched to PO as soon as possible (IV not recommended for ≥14 days).
PO (Children 3 mo–18 yr): 600 mg/m^2 bid (not to exceed 2 g/day).

Hepatic Transplantation

PO, IV (Adults): 1 g bid IV, or 1.5 g bid PO. IV should be started ≤24 hr after transplantation and switched to PO as soon as possible (IV not recommended for ≥14 days).

Cardiac Transplantation

PO, IV (Adults): 1.5 g bid; IV should be started ≤24 hr after transplantation and switched to PO as soon as possible (IV not recommended for ≥14 days).

Renal Impairment

PO, IV (Adults): *CCr <25 mL/min*—daily dose should not exceed 2 g.

M

Mycophenolic acid (Myfortic)

Mycophenolate mofetil and MPA acid should not be used interchangeably without the advice of a health care professional.

Renal Transplantation

PO (Adults): 720 mg bid.

PO (Children 5–16 yr and ≥1.19 m²): 400 mg/m² bid (not to exceed 720 mg bid).

Availability

Mycophenolate mofetil (Cellcept)

Capsules: 250 mg. **Tablets:** 500 mg. **Oral suspension (fruit flavor):** 200 mg/mL in 225-mL bottles. **Powder for injection:** 500 mg vial.

Mycophenolic acid (Myfortic)

Delayed-release tablets (Myfortic): 180 mg, 360 mg.

nabilone (nab-il-own)

Cesamet

Classification

Therapeutic: antiemetics

Pharmacologic: cannabinoids

Schedule II

Indications

Treatment of nausea and vomiting due to chemotherapy that has not responded to other conventional antiemetics.

Action

Antiemetic action may be due to interaction with cannabinoid receptor system in the brain. **Therapeutic Effects:** Decreased nausea and vomiting due to emetogenic chemotherapy.

Adverse Reactions/Side Effects

CNS: concentration difficulty, drowsiness, euphoria, sleep disturbance, vertigo, altered mental state, anxiety, depression, detachment, disorientation, headache, panic, paranoia, psychotomimetic reactions. **CV:** hypotension, tachycardia. **GI:** dry mouth, increased appetite, nausea. **Neuro:** ataxia, physical dependence, psychologic dependence.

PHYSICAL THERAPY IMPLICATIONS

Examination and Evaluation

- Monitor improvements in GI symptoms (decreased nausea and vomiting, increased appetite) to help document whether drug therapy is successful.
- Assess vertigo or ataxia that might affect gait, balance, and other functional activities. Report balance problems and functional limitations to the physician and nursing staff, and caution the patient and family/caregivers to guard against falls and trauma.
- Monitor changes in mood and behavior such as anxiety, euphoria, depression, disorientation, paranoia, memory lapses, impaired concentration, paranoia, panic, psychosis-like reactions, or other changes in mental state. Notify physician if these changes become problematic.
- Assess heart rate, ECG, and heart sounds, especially during exercise (See Appendices G, H). Report fast heart rate (tachycardia) and symptoms of other arrhythmias, including palpitations, chest discomfort, shortness of breath, fainting, and fatigue/weakness.
- Assess blood pressure (BP) periodically and compare to normal values (See Appendix F). Report low BP (hypotension), especially if patient experiences dizziness, fatigue, or other symptoms.

Interventions

- Guard against falls and trauma (hip fractures, head injury, and so forth) caused by vertigo or ataxia; implement fall-prevention strategies (See Appendix E).
- Because of the risk of arrhythmias and abnormal BP responses, use caution during aerobic exercise and other forms of therapeutic exercise. Assess exercise tolerance frequently (BP, heart rate, fatigue levels), and terminate exercise immediately if any untoward responses occur (See Appendix L).

Patient/Client-Related Instruction

- Advise patient about the risk of daytime drowsiness and decreased attention and mental focus. Avoid driving, and use caution in other activities that require strong concentration.
- Educate patient about the risk of physical and psychologic dependence during excessive or prolonged use; encourage patient to adhere to proper dosing schedule.
- Instruct patient to report bothersome side effects such as severe or prolonged headache, nausea, increased appetite, or dry mouth.

Pharmacokinetics

Absorption: Completely absorbed following oral administration.

Distribution: Unknown.

Protein Binding: Highly protein bound.

Metabolism and Excretion: Highly metabolized with extensive first pass hepatic metabolism; metabolites excreted in feces (67%) and urine (22%).

Half-life: 2 hr.

TIME/ACTION PROFILE

ROUTE	ONSET	PEAK	DURATION
PO	unknown	1–3 hr	8–12 hr*

*Psychoactive effects may persist for 72 hr.

Contraindications/Precautions

Contraindicated in: Hypersensitivity; OB: Lactation.

Use Cautiously in: History of substance abuse or mental illness/psychiatric disorder; Geri: Increased risk of hypotension, tachycardia, and psychoactive effects in patients >65 yr; OB: Use in pregnancy only if maternal benefit outweighs fetal risk; Pedi: Safe use in children <18 yr not established; increased risk of psychoactive reactions.

Interactions

Drug-Drug: ↑ risk of CNS depression with other **CNS depressants,** including **alcohol, antihistamines,**

barbiturates, benzodiazepines, buspirone, lithium, muscle relaxants, opioids, sedative/hypnotics, or **other CNS depressants**. ↑ risk of hypertension, tachycardia, and cardiotoxicity with **amphetamines, cocaine,** and **other sympathomimetic agents**. ↑ risk of tachycardia or drowsiness with **atropine, scopolamine, antihistamines,** or **other anticholinergics**. ↑ risk of tachycardia, hypertension, and drowsiness with **tricyclic antidepressants**. May displace, be displaced by, or otherwise interfere with other **highly protein-bound drugs**. May cause reversible hypomanic reaction with **disulfiram** or **fluoxetine**. May ↓ clearance and ↑ effects of **barbiturates**. May ↑ clearance and ↓ effects of **theophylline**. Cross-tolerance and potentiation of effects may occur with **opioids. Naltrexone** may enhance effects. **Alcohol** may ↑ mood effects.

Route/Dosage

PO (Adults): 1 or 2 mg bid; initial dose should be given 1–3 hr prior to chemotherapy. May be given as 1 or 2 mg the night before. Not to exceed 6 mg/day (2 mg tid). May be used during entire course of each cycle of chemotherapy and for 48 hr after the last dose if needed.

Availability

Capsules: 1 mg.

nabumetone (na-byoo-me-tone)

Relafen

Classification

Therapeutic: antirheumatics, nonsteroidal anti-inflammatory agents

Pharmacologic: enolic acid derviatives

Indications

Symptomatic management of rheumatoid arthritis and osteoarthritis.

Action

Inhibits prostaglandin synthesis. **Therapeutic Effects:** Suppression of pain and inflammation.

Adverse Reactions/Side Effects

CNS: agitation, anxiety, confusion, depression, dizziness, drowsiness, fatigue, headache, insomnia, malaise, weakness. **EENT:** abnormal vision, tinnitus. **Resp:** dyspnea, hypersensitivity pneumonitis. **CV:** edema, fluid retention, vasculitis. **GI:** GI BLEEDING, abdominal pain, diarrhea, abnormal liver function tests, anorexia, constipation, dry mouth, dyspepsia, flatulence, gastritis, gastroenteritis, increased appetite, nausea, stomatitis, vomiting. **GU:** albuminuria, azotemia, interstitial nephritis. **Derm:** EXFOLIATIVE DERMATITIS, STEVENS-JOHNSON SYNDROME, TOXIC EPIDERMAL NECROLYSIS, increased sweating, photosensitivity, pruritus, rash. **Hemat:** prolonged bleeding time. **Metab:** weight gain. **Neuro:** paresthesia, tremor. **Misc:** ALLERGIC REACTIONS, INCLUDING ANAPHYLAXIS, ANGIONEUROTIC EDEMA.

PHYSICAL THERAPY IMPLICATIONS

Examination and Evaluation

- Monitor signs of GI bleeding, including abdominal pain, vomiting blood, blood in stools, or black, tarry stools. Report these signs to the physician immediately.
- Monitor signs of allergic reactions and anaphylaxis or angioneurotic edema, including pulmonary symptoms (laryngeal edema, wheezing, cough, dyspnea) or skin reactions (rash, pruritus, urticaria, swelling in the face). Be especially alert for exfoliation, dermatitis, and other severe skin reactions that might indicate serious hypersensitivity reactions (Stevens-Johnson syndrome, toxic epidermal necrolysis). Notify physician immediately if these reactions occur.
- Assess pain and other variables (range of motion, muscle strength) to document whether this drug is successful in helping manage the patient's pain and decreasing impairments.
- Assess blood pressure (BP) periodically and compare to normal values (See Appendix F). NSAIDs can increase BP in certain patients.
- Be alert for signs of difficult, labored breathing (dyspnea) or other signs of pneumonitis such as cough, shortness of breath, fever, and abnormal breath sounds (rales; See Appendix K). Report these signs to the physician.
- Be alert for signs of prolonged bleeding time such as bleeding gums, nosebleeds, and unusual or excessive bruising. Report these signs to the physician.
- Assess peripheral edema using girth measurements, volume displacement, and measurement of pitting edema (See Appendix N). Report increased swelling in feet and ankles or a sudden increase in body weight due to fluid retention.
- Monitor signs of interstitial nephritis (blood in urine, decreased urine output, weight gain from fluid retention) or signs of increased nitrogenous compounds in the blood (azotemia) such as confusion, decreased alertness, tachycardia, pallor, fatigue, dry mouth, thirst, and decreased/absent urine production. Notify physician of these signs.
- Assess any tremors or signs of paresthesia (numbness, tingling). Perform objective tests including electroneuromyography and sensory testing to document any drug-related neuropathic changes.
- Be alert for signs of vasculitis, including fatigue, weakness, muscle pain, joint pain, fever, loss of

appetite, and weight loss. Report these signs to the physician.

- Assess dizziness and drowsiness that might affect gait, balance, and other functional activities (See Appendix C). Report balance problems and functional limitations to the physician, and caution the patient and family/caregivers to guard against falls and trauma.
- Monitor and report confusion, agitation, anxiety, depression, or other psychic disturbances.

Interventions

- Implement appropriate manual therapy techniques, physical agents, and therapeutic exercises to reduce pain and decrease the need for nabumetone and other NSAIDs.
- If treating arthritic conditions, recommend orthotic and assistive devices as needed to reduce pain, improve function, and augment the effects of drug therapy.
- Use caution with any physical interventions that could increase bleeding, including wound débridement, chest percussion, joint mobilization, and application of local heat.
- Help patient explore other nonpharmacologic methods to reduce chronic pain, such as relaxation techniques, exercise, counseling, and so forth.
- Causes photosensitivity; use care if administering UV treatments. Advise patient to avoid direct sunlight and use sunscreens and protective clothing, and to report any untoward skin reactions (rash, itching, excessive sweating).

Patient/Client-Related Instruction

- Advise patient that analgesics are usually more effective if given before pain becomes severe; emphasize that adequate pain control will allow better participation in physical therapy.
- Inform patient that NSAIDs may impair bone and cartilage healing. Advise patient to consult physician about NSAID use, especially after fractures, spinal fusion, and other bone surgeries.
- Caution patient about the use of over-the-counter products that contain NSAIDs or acetaminophen while taking prescription doses of nabumetone. Use of multiple NSAIDs increases the risk of toxicity and overdose.
- Instruct patient to report excessive or prolonged headache or ringing/buzzing in the ears (tinnitus); these signs may indicate drug toxicity.
- Advise patient about the risks of gastric irritation. Instruct patient to notify physician of GI reactions such as severe or prolonged nausea, vomiting, diarrhea, constipation, indigestion, heartburn, flatulence, and abdominal pain.
- Advise patient to reduce alcohol intake because alcohol increases the risk of gastric toxicity.
- Instruct patient and family/caregivers to report other troublesome side effects such as severe or prolonged sleep loss or vision disturbances.

Pharmacokinetics

Absorption: Nabumetone (a prodrug) is 80% absorbed after oral administration; 35% is rapidly converted to 6-methoxy-2-naphthylacetic acid (6-MNA), which is the active drug.
Distribution: Unknown.
Protein Binding: >99%.
Metabolism and Excretion: 6-MNA is metabolized by the liver to inactive compounds.
Half-life: 24 hr (increased in severe renal impairment).

TIME/ACTION PROFILE (analgesia/anti-inflammatory effects)

ROUTE	ONSET	PEAK	DURATION
PO	1–2 days	few days–2 wk	12–24 hr

Contraindications/Precautions

Contraindicated in: Hypersensitivity; Use with other NSAIDs, including aspirin; cross-sensitivity may occur; Active GI bleeding or ulcer disease; Perioperative pain from coronary artery bypass graft (CABG) surgery.
Use Cautiously in: Severe renal, or hepatic disease; History of ulcer disease; OB/Lactation/Pedi: Safety not established; avoid using during 2nd half of pregnancy.

Interactions

Drug-Drug: ↑ adverse GI effects with **aspirin**, other **NSAIDs, potassium supplements, corticosteroids,** or **alcohol**. Chronic use with **acetaminophen** may ↑ risk of adverse renal reactions. May ↓ effectiveness of **diuretics** or **antihypertensives**. May ↑ hypoglycemic effects of **insulins** or **oral hypoglycemic agents**. ↑ risk of toxicity from **methotrexate**. ↑ risk of bleeding with **cefotetan, cefoperazone, valproic acid, anticoagulants, ticlopidine, clopidogrel, eptifibatide, tirofiban,** or **thrombolytic agents**. ↑ risk of adverse hematologic reactions with **antineoplastics** or **radiation therapy**. Concurrent use with **cyclosporine** may ↑ risk of renal toxicity.

Route/Dosage

PO (Adults): 1000 mg/day as a single dose or divided dose bid; may be increased up to 2000 mg/day; use lowest effective dose during chronic therapy.

Availability (generic available)

Tablets: 500 mg, 750 mg.

nadolol (nay-doe-lole)
Corgard, ✱Syn-Nadolol

Classification
Therapeutic: antianginals, antihypertensives
Pharmacologic: beta blockers

Indications
Management of hypertension. Management of angina pectoris. **Unlabeled Use:** Arrhythmias. Migraine prophylaxis. Tremors (essential, lithium-induced, parkinsonian). Aggressive behavior. Antipsychotic-associated akathisia. Situational anxiety. Esophageal varices. Reduction of intraocular pressure.

Action
Blocks stimulation of $beta_1$ (myocardial) and $beta_2$ (pulmonary, vascular, and uterine) receptor sites. **Therapeutic Effects:** Decreased heart rate and blood pressure.

Adverse Reactions/Side Effects
CNS: fatigue, weakness, anxiety, depression, dizziness, drowsiness, insomnia, memory loss, mental status changes, nightmares. **EENT:** blurred vision, dry eyes, nasal stuffiness. **Resp:** bronchospasm, wheezing. **CV:** ARRHYTHMIAS, BRADYCARDIA, CHF, PULMONARY EDEMA, orthostatic hypotension, peripheral vasoconstriction. **GI:** constipation, diarrhea, nausea. **GU:** erectile dysfunction, decreased libido. **Derm:** itching, rashes. **Endo:** hyperglycemia, hypoglycemia. **MS:** arthralgia, back pain, muscle cramps. **Neuro:** paresthesia. **Misc:** drug-induced lupus syndrome.

PHYSICAL THERAPY IMPLICATIONS

Examination and Evaluation
- Assess heart rate, ECG, and heart sounds, especially during exercise (See Appendices G, H). Although intended to treat certain arrhythmias, this drug can unmask or precipitate new arrhythmias (proarrhythmic effect). Report an unusually slow heart rate (bradycardia) or signs of other arrhythmias, including palpitations, chest pain, shortness of breath, fainting, and fatigue/weakness.
- Watch for signs of CHF and pulmonary edema, including dyspnea, rales/crackles, weight gain, peripheral edema, and jugular venous distention. Report any new or increased signs of heart failure, but also determine if drug therapy is effective in reducing these symptoms in patients with preexisting heart failure.
- Assess blood pressure (BP) periodically and compare to normal values (See Appendix F) to help document antihypertensive effects. Also assess BP when patient assumes a more upright position (lying to standing, sitting to standing, lying to sitting). Document orthostatic hypotension and contact physician when systolic BP falls >20 mm Hg, or diastolic BP falls >10 mm Hg.
- Assess exercise tolerance and episodes of angina pectoris. Document improvements in these variables, but also report any decline in exercise tolerance or increased frequency/severity of anginal attacks.
- Assess symptoms of bronchospasm (wheezing, coughing, tightness in chest). Perform pulmonary function tests to quantify suspected changes in ventilation and respiration (See Appendices I, J, K). Repeated or prolonged bronchoconstriction may require a change in dose or medication.
- Monitor signs of peripheral vasoconstriction, such as extreme coldness in the hands and feet, cyanosis, and muscle cramping. Notify physician of severe or prolonged signs of vasoconstriction.
- Assess dizziness and drowsiness that might affect gait, balance, and other functional activities (See Appendix C). Report balance problems and functional limitations to the physician, and caution the patient and family/caregivers to guard against falls and trauma.
- Monitor excessive fatigue or weakness. Beta blockers often cause some degree of fatigue and weakness, but any sudden or severe change in muscle strength or energy levels should be reported.
- Watch for signs of hypoglycemia (weakness, malaise, irritability, fatigue) or hyperglycemia (drowsiness, fruity breath, increased urination, unusual thirst). Medication may mask some signs of hypoglycemia, but dizziness and sweating may still occur. Patients with diabetes mellitus should check blood glucose levels frequently.
- Assess any back pain or joint pain to rule out musculoskeletal pathology; that is, try to determine if pain is drug-induced rather than caused by anatomic or biomechanical problems.
- Assess signs of paresthesia (numbness, tingling) or muscle twitching. Perform objective tests including electroneuromyography and sensory testing to document any drug-related neuropathic changes.
- If used to treat aggressive behavior, anxiety, or extreme restlessness (akathisia), document whether drug therapy is successful in decreasing these behaviors. Also notify physician of any worsening in mood or behavior, including increased depression, anxiety, nervousness, or memory loss.
- If used to prevent migraine headaches, monitor the incidence and severity of attacks to document

whether this drug is successful in helping manage the patient's pain.

- Monitor signs of drug-induced lupus syndrome, including increased BP, fever, joint pain, skin rashes, and redness/irritation of the eye (uveitis). Notify physician promptly if these signs appear.

Interventions

- Design and implement aerobic exercise and endurance training programs to improve coronary perfusion, reduce angina, and improve myocardial pumping ability.
- Because of an increased risk of cardiac arrhythmias (bradycardia, others), use caution during aerobic exercise and endurance conditioning. Likewise, monitor patients closely during treatment of other cardiac problems (angina, CHF, recent MI). Terminate exercise if patient exhibits untoward symptoms (chest pain, shortness of breath, unusual fatigue) or displays other criteria for exercise termination (See Appendix L).
- Establish aerobic exercise workloads that account for the effects of beta blockers on heart rate. Some heart rate guidelines may not be appropriate because beta blockers typically decrease maximal HR by 20–30 bpm. Use other guidelines such as rating of perceived exertion (RPE, modified Borg scale) to determine exercise workloads.
- To minimize orthostatic hypotension, patient should move slowly when assuming a more upright position.

Patient/Client-Related Instruction

- Remind patients to take medication as directed to control hypertension even if they are asymptomatic.
- Counsel patients about additional interventions to help control BP, including regular exercise, weight loss, sodium restriction, stress reduction, moderation of alcohol consumption, and smoking cessation.
- Instruct patient or family/caregivers to report other troublesome side effects such as severe or prolonged insomnia, nightmares, skin rash/itching, blurred vision, dry eyes, stuffy nose, sexual problems (decreased libido, erectile dysfunction), or GI problems (nausea, constipation, diarrhea).

Pharmacokinetics

Absorption: 30% absorbed after oral administration.
Distribution: Minimal penetration of the CNS. Crosses the placenta and enters breast milk.
Metabolism and Excretion: 70% excreted unchanged by the kidneys.
Half-life: 10–24 hr (increased in renal impairment).

TIME/ACTION PROFILE (anithypertensive effects)

ROUTE	ONSET	PEAK	DURATION
PO*	up to 5 days	6–9 days	24 hr

*With chronic dosing.

Contraindications/Precautions

Contraindicated in: Uncompensated CHF; Pulmonary edema; Cardiogenic shock; Bradycardia or heart block.
Use Cautiously in: Renal impairment (CCr <50 mL/min); Hepatic impairment; Geriatric patients (increased sensitivity to beta blockers; initial dosage reduction recommended); Pulmonary disease (including asthma); Diabetes mellitus (may mask signs of hypoglycemia); Thyrotoxicosis (may mask symptoms); Patients with a history of severe allergic reactions (intensity of reactions may be increased); Pregnancy, lactation, or children (safety not established; crosses the placenta and may cause fetal/neonatal bradycardia, hypotension, hypoglycemia, or respiratory depression).

N

Interactions

Drug-Drug: General anesthesia, IV phenytoin, diltiazem, and **verapamil** may cause additive myocardial depression. Additive bradycardia may occur with **digoxin**. Additive hypotension may occur with other **antihypertensives**, acute ingestion of **alcohol**, or **nitrates**. Concurrent use with **amphetamines, cocaine, ephedrine, epinephrine, norepinephrine, phenylephrine**, or **pseudoephedrine** may result in unopposed alpha-adrenergic stimulation (excessive hypertension, bradycardia). Concurrent use with **clonidine** ↑ hypotension and bradycardia. Concurrent **thyroid** administration may ↓ effectiveness. May alter the effectiveness of **insulins** or **oral hypoglycemic agents** (dosage adjustments may be necessary). May ↓ the effectiveness of **theophylline**. May ↓ the beneficial beta cardiovascular effects of **dopamine** or **dobutamine**. Use cautiously within 14 days of **MAO inhibitor therapy** (may result in hypertension). Concurrent **NSAIDs** may ↓ antihypertensive action.

Route/Dosage

PO (Adults): *Antianginal*—40 mg once daily initially; may increase by 40–80 mg/day q 3–7 days as needed (up to 240 mg/day). *Antihypertensive*—40 mg once daily initially; may increase by 40–80 mg/day q 7 days as needed (up to 320 mg/day).

Renal Impairment

PO (Adults): *CCr 31–50 mL/min*—increase dosing interval to 24–36 hr; *CCr 10–30 mL/min*—increase dosing interval to 24–48 hr; *CCr <10 mL/min*—increase dosing interval to 40–60 hr.

Availability (generic available)

Tablets: 20 mg, 40 mg, 80 mg, 120 mg, 160 mg. ***In combination with:*** bendroflumethiazide (Corzide). See Appendix B.

nafarelin (na-fare-e-lin)

Synarel

Classification

Therapeutic: hormones

Pharmacologic: gonadotropin-releasing hormones

Indications

Management of endometriosis. Management of central precocious puberty (gonadotropin-dependent) in children.

Action

Acts as a synthetic analogue of gonadotropin-releasing hormone (GnRH). Initially increases pituitary production of luteinizing hormone (LH) and follicle-stimulating hormone (FSH), which cause ovarian steroid production. Chronic administration leads to decreased production of gonadotropins. Endometriotic lesions are sensitive to ovarian hormones. **Therapeutic Effects:** Reduction in lesions and associated pain in endometriosis. Arrest and regression of puberty in children with central precocious puberty.

Adverse Reactions/Side Effects

CNS: emotional instability, headaches, depression, insomnia. **EENT:** nasal irritation. **CV:** edema. **GU:** vaginal dryness. **Derm:** acne, hirsutism, seborrhea. **Endo:** cessation of menses, impaired fertility, reduced breast size. **MS:** decreased bone density, myalgia. **Misc:** decreased libido, hot flashes, hypersensitivity reactions, weight gain.

PHYSICAL THERAPY IMPLICATIONS

Examination and Evaluation

- Monitor signs of hypersensitivity reactions, including pulmonary symptoms (tightness in the throat and chest, wheezing, cough, dyspnea) or skin reactions (rash, pruritus, urticaria). Notify physician immediately if these reactions occur.
- Assess peripheral edema using girth measurements, volume displacement, and measurement of pitting edema (See Appendix N). Report increased swelling in feet and ankles due to peripheral vasodilation.
- Monitor personality or behavioral changes, including emotional instability, depression, sleep loss, or other changes in mood. Notify physician if these changes become problematic.
- Assess any muscle pain to rule out musculoskeletal pathology; that is, try to determine if pain is drug induced rather than caused by anatomic or biomechanical problems.
- Periodically assess body weight and other anthropometric measures (body mass index, body composition). Report a rapid or unexplained weight gain or increased body fat.

Interventions

- Institute weight-bearing and resistance exercises as tolerated to maintain bone mineral density and prevent demineralization.

Patient/Client-Related Instruction

- Instruct patient or family/caregivers to report other troublesome side effects such as severe or prolonged headache, nasal irritation, hot flashes, menstrual irregularities, vaginal dryness, hot flashes, reduced breast size, decreased libido, or skin reactions (acne, oily skin increased hair growth).

Pharmacokinetics

Absorption: Well absorbed following intranasal administration.
Distribution: Unknown.
Metabolism and Excretion: 20–40% excreted in feces; 3% excreted unchanged by the kidneys.
Half-life: 3 hr.

TIME/ACTION PROFILE (decreased ovarian steroid production)

ROUTE	ONSET	PEAK	DURATION
Intranasal	within 4 wk	3–4 wk	3–6 mo*

*Relief of symptoms of endometriosis following discontinuation.

Contraindications/Precautions

Contraindicated in: Hypersensitivity to GnRH, its analogues, or sorbitol; Pregnancy or lactation.
Use Cautiously in: Rhinitis.

Interactions

Drug-Drug: Concurrent **topical nasal decongestants** may reduce absorption of nafarelin (administer decongestant at least 2 hr after nafarelin).

Route/Dosage

Intranasal (Adults): *Endometriosis*—1 spray (200 mcg) in 1 nostril in the morning and 1 spray in the other nostril in the evening (400 mcg/day). May be increased to 1 spray in each nostril in the morning and evening (800 mcg/day).
Intranasal (Children): *Central precocious puberty*—2 sprays in each nostril in the morning and in the evening (1600 mcg/day); may be increased up to

1800 mcg/day (3 sprays in alternating nostrils 3 times daily).

Availability

Nasal spray: 2 mg/mL in 10-mL bottle (200 mcg/spray).

nafcillin (naf-sil-in)

Nallpen, Unipen

Classification

Therapeutic: anti-infectives

Pharmacologic: penicillinase-resistant penicillins

Indications

Treatment of the following infections due to penicillinase-producing staphylococci: Respiratory tract infections; Sinusitis; Skin and skin structure infections; Bone and joint infections; Urinary tract infections; Endocarditis; Bacteremia; Meningitis.

Action

Bind to bacterial cell wall, leading to cell death. Not inactivated by penicillinase enzymes. **Therapeutic Effects:** Bactericidal action. **Spectrum:** Active against most gram-positive aerobic cocci. Spectrum is notable for activity against Penicillinase-producing strains of *Staphylococcus aureus*, *S. epidermidis*. Not active against methicillin-resistant bacteria.

Adverse Reactions/Side Effects

CNS: SEIZURES. **GI:** PSEUDOMEMBRANOUS COLITIS, diarrhea, epigastric distress, nausea, vomiting. **GU:** interstitial nephritis. **Derm:** rash, urticaria. **Hemat:** eosinophilia, leukopenia. **Local:** pain at IM site, phlebitis at IV site. **Misc:** ALLERGIC REACTIONS, INCLUDING ANAPHYLAXIS AND SERUM SICKNESS, superinfection.

PHYSICAL THERAPY IMPLICATIONS

Examination and Evaluation

- Watch for seizures; notify physician immediately if patient develops or increases seizure activity.
- Monitor signs of pseudomembranous colitis, including diarrhea, abdominal pain, fever, pus or mucus in stools, and other severe or prolonged GI problems (nausea, vomiting, heartburn). Notify physician or nursing staff immediately of these signs.
- Monitor signs of allergic reactions and anaphylaxis, including pulmonary symptoms (tightness in the throat and chest, wheezing, cough dyspnea) or skin reactions (rash, pruritus, urticaria). Notify physician or nursing staff immediately if these reactions occur.
- Assess muscle aches and joint pain (arthralgia) that may be caused by serum sickness. Notify physician if these symptoms seem to be drug-related rather than caused by musculoskeletal injury or if muscle and joint pain are accompanied by allergy-like reactions (fever, rashes, etc.)
- Monitor signs of eosinophilia (fatigue, weakness, myalgia) or leukopenia (fever, sore throat, signs of infection); report these signs to the physician.
- Monitor injection site for pain, swelling, and irritation. Report prolonged or excessive injection-site reactions to the physician or nursing staff.

Interventions

- Always wash hands thoroughly and disinfect equipment (whirlpools, electrotherapeutic devices, treatment tables, and so forth) to help prevent the spread of infection. Use universal precautions or isolation procedures as indicated for specific patients.

N

Patient/Client-Related Instruction

- Instruct patient to notify physician immediately if signs of the following occur:
    - Superinfection (black, furry overgrowth on tongue; vaginal itching or discharge; loose or foul-smelling stools).
    - Interstitial nephritis (blood in urine, decreased urine output, weight gain from fluid retention).
- Instruct patient and family/caregivers to report other troublesome side effects such as severe or prolonged skin problems (rash, itching) or GI problems (nausea, vomiting, diarrhea, heartburn).

Pharmacokinetics

Absorption: Completely absorbed following IV administration; well absorbed from IM sites.

Distribution: Widely distributed; penetration into CSF is minimal but sufficient in the presence of inflamed meninges; cross the placenta and enter breast milk.

Metabolism and Excretion: Partially metabolized by the liver (60%), partially excreted unchanged by the kidneys.

Half-life: Neonates: 1–5 hr; Children 1 mo–14 yr: 0.75–1.9 hr; Adults: 0.5–1.5 hr (increased in renal impairment).

TIME/ACTION PROFILE

ROUTE	ONSET	PEAK	DURATION
Nafcillin IM	30 min	60–120 min	4–6 hr
Nafcillin IV	rapid	end of infusion	4–6 hr

Contraindications/Precautions

Contraindicated in: Previous hypersensitivity to penicillins (cross-sensitivity exists with cephalosporins and other beta-lactam antibiotics).

Use Cautiously in: Severe renal or hepatic impairment.

Interactions

Drug-Drug: Nafcillin may ↓ effectiveness of oral contraceptive agents. **Probenecid** ↓ renal excretion and ↑ blood levels of nafcillin (therapy may be combined for this purpose). Concurrent use with **methotrexate** ↓ methotrexate elimination and ↑ risk of serious toxicity.

Route/Dosage

IM (Adults): 500 mg q 4–6 hr.
IM, IV (Children and Infants): 50–200 mg/kg/day divided q 4–6 hr, maximum: 12 g/day.
IM, IV (Neonates 0–4 wk, <1200 g): 50 mg/kg/day divided q 12 hr.
IV (Adults): 500–2000 mg q 4–6 hr.
IM, IV (Neonates 1.2–2 kg): 50 mg/kg/day divided q 12 hr for the first 7 days of life, then 75 mg/kg/day divided q 8 hr.
IM, IV (Neonates >2 kg): 75 mg/kg/day divided q 8 hr for the first 7 days of life, then 100 mg/kg/day divided q 6 hr.

Availability (generic available)

Powder for injection: 1-, 2-, and 10-g vials.

naftifine (naf-ti-feen)

Naftin

Classification
Therapeutic: antifungals (topical)
Pharmacologic: allylamines

Indications

Treatment of a variety of cutaneous fungal infections, including tinea pedis (athlete's foot), tinea cruris (jock itch), and tinea corporis (ringworm).

Action

Affects the synthesis of the fungal cell wall.
Therapeutic Effects: Decrease in symptoms of fungal infection.

Adverse Reactions/Side Effects

Local: burning, dryness, itching, local hypersensitivity reactions, redness, stinging.

PHYSICAL THERAPY IMPLICATIONS

Examination and Evaluation

- Assess healing of skin lesions to help document drug effectiveness.

Interventions

- Avoid contact with cutaneous lesions when treating patient.
- Always wash hands thoroughly and disinfect equipment (whirlpools, electrotherapeutic devices, treatment tables, and so forth) to help prevent the spread of infection.

Patient/Client-Related Instruction

- Advise patient to report any increased local sensitivity to this drug (pain, burning, itching, swelling).
- Instruct patient about proper hygiene; e.g., thoroughly wash and dry the affected area, wear clean socks and ventilated shoes for tinea pedis, and so forth.
- Advise patient to apply the drug as directed for the full course of treatment even if feeling better.
- Inform patient that early relief of cutaneous symptoms may be seen in 2–3 days. Full therapeutic response may take up to 4 wk.
- Advise patient to seek medical help if infections persist or recur after the full treatment. Recurrent fungal infections may be a sign of systemic illness.

Pharmacokinetics

Absorption: Absorption through intact skin is minimal.
Distribution: Distribution after topical administration is primarily local.
Metabolism and Excretion: Systemic metabolism and excretion not known following local application.
Half-life: Not applicable.

TIME/ACTION PROFILE

ROUTE	ONSET	PEAK	DURATION
Topical	unknown	unknown	unknown

Contraindications/Precautions

Contraindicated in: Hypersensitivity to active ingredients, additives, preservatives, or bases; Contains alcohol and should be avoided in patients with known intolerance.
Use Cautiously in: Nail and scalp infections (may require additional systemic therapy); OB/Lactation: Safety not established.

Interactions

Drug-Drug: Not known.

Route/Dosage

Topical (Adults): Apply cream once daily for up to 4 wk. Apply gel bid for up to 4 wk.

Availability

Cream: 1%. **Gel:** 1%.

HIGH ALERT

nalbuphine (nal-byoo-feen)

Nubain

Classification

Therapeutic: opioid analgesics
Pharmacologic: opioid agonists/analgesics

Indications

Moderate-to-severe pain. Also provides Analgesia during labor, Sedation before surgery, Supplement to balanced anesthesia.

Action

Binds to opiate receptors in the CNS. Alters the perception of and response to painful stimuli while producing generalized CNS depression. In addition, has partial antagonist properties, which may result in opioid withdrawal in physically dependent patients. **Therapeutic Effects:** Decreased pain.

Adverse Reactions/Side Effects

CNS: dizziness, headache, sedation, confusion, dysphoria, euphoria, floating feeling, hallucinations, unusual dreams. **EENT:** blurred vision, diplopia, miosis (high doses). **Resp:** respiratory depression. **CV:** hypertension, orthostatic hypotension, palpitations. **GI:** dry mouth, nausea, vomiting, constipation, ileus. **GU:** urinary urgency. **Derm:** clammy feeling, sweating. **Misc:** physical dependence, psychologic dependence, tolerance.

PHYSICAL THERAPY IMPLICATIONS

Examination and Evaluation

- Assess symptoms of respiratory depression, including decreased respiratory rate, confusion, bluish color of the skin and mucous membranes (cyanosis), and difficult, labored breathing (dyspnea). Monitor pulse oximetry and perform pulmonary function tests (See Appendix I) to quantify suspected changes in ventilation and respiratory function. Excessive respiratory depression requires emergency care.
- Be alert for excessive sedation or changes in mood and behavior (euphoria, dysphoria, confusion, hallucinations). Notify physician or nurse immediately if patient is unconscious or extremely difficult to arouse.
- Use appropriate pain scales (visual analogue scales, others) to document whether this drug is successful in helping manage the patient's pain.
- Assess blood pressure (BP) and compare to normal values (See Appendix F). Report a sustained increase in BP (hypertension) or a fall in BP when patient assumes a more upright position (lying to standing, sitting to standing, lying to sitting). Document orthostatic hypotension and contact physician when systolic BP falls >20 mm Hg, or diastolic BP falls >10 mm Hg.
- Assess dizziness that might affect gait, balance, and other functional activities (See Appendix C). Report balance problems and functional limitations to the physician and nursing staff, and caution the patient and family/caregivers to guard against falls and trauma.

Interventions

- Implement appropriate manual therapy techniques, physical agents, and therapeutic exercises to reduce pain and help wean patient off opioid analgesics as soon as possible.
- Because of the risk of abnormal BP responses, use caution during aerobic exercise and other forms of therapeutic exercise. Assess exercise tolerance frequently (BP, heart rate, fatigue levels), and terminate exercise immediately if any untoward responses occur (See Appendix L).
- Help patient explore other nonpharmacologic methods to reduce chronic pain, such as relaxation techniques, exercise, counseling, and so forth.
- Guard against falls and trauma (hip fractures, head injury). Implement fall-prevention strategies (See Appendix E), especially if patient exhibits sedation, dizziness, or blurred vision.
- To minimize orthostatic hypotension, patient should move slowly when assuming a more upright position.

Patient/Client-Related Instruction

- Advise patient that opioid analgesics are usually more effective if given before pain becomes severe; emphasize that adequate pain control will allow better participation in physical therapy.
- Educate patient about the dangers of opioid overdose; encourage patient to adhere to proper dosing schedule.
- Emphasize that the risk of physical addiction (tolerance and dependence) is usually minimal during short-term treatment of pain. Advise patient that addiction is more likely during excessive or inappropriate use of opioid analgesics.
- Advise patient to avoid alcohol and other CNS depressants because of the increased risk of sedation and decreased CNS function.
- Advise patient to increase fluid intake and dietary fiber to avoid constipation. Laxatives may also be helpful in patients susceptible to fecal impaction (e.g., people with spinal cord injury).
- Instruct patient to report other troublesome side effects such as severe or prolonged headache, unusual dreams, heart palpitations, excessive

N

sweating, vision disturbances, increased urge to urinate, or GI problems (nausea, vomiting, dry mouth).

Pharmacokinetics

Absorption: Well absorbed after IM and SC administration.
Distribution: Probably crosses the placenta and enters breast milk.
Metabolism and Excretion: Mostly metabolized by the liver and eliminated in the feces via biliary excretion. Minimal amounts excreted unchanged by the kidneys.
Half-life: 5 hr.

TIME/ACTION PROFILE (analgesia)

ROUTE	ONSET	PEAK	DURATION
IM	<15 min	60 min	3–6 hr
SC	<15 min	unknown	3–6 hr
IV	2–3 min	30 min	3–6 hr

Contraindications/Precautions

Contraindicated in: Hypersensitivity to nalbuphine or bisulfites; Patients who are physically dependent on opioids and have not been detoxified (may precipitate withdrawal).
Use Cautiously in: Head trauma; Increased intracranial pressure; Severe renal, hepatic, or pulmonary disease; Hypothyroidism; Adrenal insufficiency; Alcoholism; Geriatric or debilitated patients (dose reduction suggested); Undiagnosed abdominal pain; Prostatic hyperplasia; Patients who have recently received opioid agonists; OB: Pregnancy (has been used during labor but may cause respiratory depression in the newborn); Lactation or children (safety not established).

Interactions

Drug-Drug: Use with extreme caution in patients receiving **MAO inhibitors** (may result in unpredictable, severe reactions—reduce initial dose of nalbuphine to 25% of usual dose). Additive CNS depression with **alcohol, antihistamines**, and **sedative/hypnotics**. May precipitate withdrawal in patients who are physically dependent on **opioid agonists**. Avoid concurrent use with other **opioid analgesic agonists** (may diminish analgesic effect).
Drug-Natural: Concomitant use of **kava, valerian, skullcap, chamomile**, or **hops** can ↑ CNS depression.

Route/Dosage

Analgesia

IM, SC, IV (Adults): Usual dose is 10 mg q 3–6 hr (single dose not to exceed 20 mg; total daily dose not to exceed 160 mg).

Supplement to Balanced Anesthesia

IV (Adults): *Initial*—0.3–3 mg/kg over 10–15 min. *Maintenance*—0.25–0.5 mg/kg as needed.

Availability (generic available)

Injection: 10 mg/mL in 1- and 10-mL vials, 20 mg/mL in 1- and 10-mL vials and 1-mL preloaded syringes.

naloxone (nal-**ox**-one)

Narcan

Classification

Therapeutic: antidotes (for opioids)
Pharmacologic: opioid antagonists

Indications

Reversal of CNS depression and respiratory depression because of suspected opioid overdose. **Unlabeled Use:** Opioid-induced pruritus (low dose IV infusion). Management of refractory circulatory shock.

Action

Competitively blocks the effects of opioids, including CNS and respiratory depression, without producing any agonist (opioid-like) effects. **Therapeutic Effects:** Reversal of signs of opioid excess.

Adverse Reactions/Side Effects

CV: hypertension, hypotension, ventricular fibrillation, ventricular tachycardia. **GI:** nausea, vomiting.

PHYSICAL THERAPY IMPLICATIONS

Examination and Evaluation

- Report any remaining signs of opioid-induced CNS depression such as euphoria, dysphoria, confusion, and hallucinations.
- Be alert for any residual symptoms of respiratory depression, including decreased respiratory rate, confusion, bluish color of the skin and mucous membranes, and difficult/labored breathing. Monitor pulse oximetry and perform pulmonary function tests (See Appendix I) to document whether ventilation and respiratory function have returned to normal levels.
- Assess blood pressure (BP) and compare to normal values (See Appendix F). Report changes in BP, either a problematic decrease in BP (hypotension) or a sustained increase in BP (hypertension).
- Assess heart rate, ECG, and heart sounds, especially during exercise (See Appendices G, H). Report any rhythm disturbances or symptoms of arrhythmias, including palpitations, chest discomfort, shortness of breath, fainting, and fatigue/weakness.
- If used to treat opioid-induced itching (pruritus), monitor symptoms to help document whether drug therapy is successful in reducing itching.

Interventions

- Implement appropriate manual therapy techniques, physical agents, and therapeutic exercises to reduce pain and help wean patient off opioid analgesics as soon as possible.
- Because of the risk of arrhythmias and abnormal BP responses, use caution during aerobic exercise and other forms of therapeutic exercise. Assess exercise tolerance frequently (BP, heart rate, respiratory rate, fatigue levels), and terminate exercise immediately if any untoward responses occur (See Appendix L).

Patient/Client-Related Instruction

- Educate patient about the dangers of opioid overdose; encourage patient to adhere to proper dosing schedule.
- Instruct patient to report other troublesome side effects such as severe or prolonged GI problems (nausea, vomiting).

Pharmacokinetics

Absorption: Well absorbed after IM or SC administration.
Distribution: Rapidly distributed to tissues. Crosses the placenta.
Metabolism and Excretion: Metabolized by the liver.
Half-life: 60–90 min (up to 3 hr in neonates).

TIME/ACTION PROFILE (reversal of opioid effects)

ROUTE	ONSET	PEAK	DURATION
IV	1–2 min	unknown	45 min
IM, SC	2–5 min	unknown	>45 min

Contraindications/Precautions

Contraindicated in: Hypersensitivity.
Use Cautiously in: Cardiovascular disease; Patients physically dependent on opioids (may precipitate severe withdrawal); Pregnancy (may cause withdrawal in mother and fetus if mother is opioid dependent); Lactation (safety not established); Neonates of opioid-dependent mothers.

Interactions

Drug-Drug: Can precipitate withdrawal in patients physically dependent on **opioid analgesics**. Larger doses may be required to reverse the effects of **buprenorphine, butorphanol, nalbuphine, pentazocine**, or **propoxyphene**. Antagonizes postoperative **opioid analgesics**.

Route/Dosage

Postoperative Opioid-Induced Respiratory Depression

IV (Adults): 0.02–0.2 mg q 2–3 min until response obtained; repeat q 1–2 hr if needed.
IV (Children): 0.01 mg/kg; may repeat q 2–3 min until response obtained. Additional doses may be given q 1–2 hr if needed.
IM, IV, SC (Neonates): 0.01 mg/kg; may repeat q 2–3 min until response obtained. Additional doses may be given q 1–2 hr if needed.

Opioid-Induced Respiratory Depression during Chronic (>1 wk) Opioid Use

IV, IM, SC (Adults >40 kg): 20–40 mcg (0.02–0.04 mg) given as small, frequent (q min) boluses or as an infusion titrated to improve respiratory function without reversing analgesia.
IV, IM, SC (Adults and Children <40 kg): 0.005–0.02 mg/dose given as small, frequent (q min) boluses or as an infusion titrated to improve respiratory function without reversing analgesia.

Overdose of Opioids

IV, IM, SC (Adults): *Patients not suspected of being opioid dependent*—0.4 mg (10 mcg/kg); may repeat q 2–3 min (IV route is preferred). Some patients may require up to 2 mg. *Patients suspected to be opioid dependent*—Initial dose should be decreased to 0.1–0.2 mg q 2–3 min. May also be given by IV infusion at rate adjusted to patient's response.
IV, IM, SC (Children >5 yr or >20 kg): 2 mg/dose; may repeat q 2–3 min.
IV, IM, SC (Infants up to 5 yr or 20 kg): 0.1 mg/kg; may repeat q 2–3 min.

Opioid-Induced Pruritus

IV (Children): 2 mcg/kg/hr continuous infusion; may increase by 0.5 mcg/kg/hr every few hours if pruritus continues.

Availability (generic available)

Injection: 0.4 mg/mL in 1-mL prefilled syringes and 10-mL vials, 1 mg/mL in 2-mL prefilled syringes.
In combination with: pentazocine (Talwin NX). See Appendix B.

N

naltrexone (nal-trex-one)

ReVia, Vivitrol

Classification
Therapeutic: alcohol abuse therapy adjuncts
Pharmacologic: opioid antagonists

Indications

Provides opioid antagonism in the management of opioid dependence (oral only). Management of alcohol dependence.

Action

Competitively blocks the effects of opioids, including CNS and respiratory depression, without producing any agonist (opioid-like) effects. Mechanism in managing alcohol dependence may involve the endogenous opioid system. **Therapeutic Effects:** Blocks the effects of opioids in previously dependent patients. Reduced alcohol-dependent behavior.

Adverse Reactions/Side Effects

CV: anxiety, fatigue, headache, insomnia, nervousness, depression, dizziness, increased energy, sedation, suicidal ideation. **EENT:** hoarseness, runny/stuffy nose, sinus problems, sneezing. **Resp:** EOSINOPHILIC PNEUMONIA (INJECTION), cough. **CV:** palpitations. **GI:** HEPATOTOXICITY, abdominal cramps/pain, nausea, constipation, ↓ appetite, diarrhea, vomiting. **GU:** delayed ejaculation, erectile dysfunction. **Hemat:** eosinophilia, thrombocytopenia. **Derm:** skin rash. **Local:** injection site reactions. **MS:** muscle/joint pain. **Misc:** chills, ↑ thirst.

PHYSICAL THERAPY IMPLICATIONS

Examination and Evaluation

- Monitor any breathing difficulties. Notify physician immediately if patient experiences signs of eosinophilic pneumonia, such as cough, fever, chills, night sweats, and chest pain during inspiration and expiration.
- Be alert for signs of hepatotoxicity, including anorexia, abdominal pain, severe nausea and vomiting, yellow skin or eyes, fever, sore throat, malaise, weakness, facial edema, lethargy, and unusual bleeding or bruising. Notify physician immediately if these signs occur.
- Monitor changes in mood and behavior such as anxiety, nervousness, depression, sedation, suicidal thoughts, or other changes in mental state. Notify physician if these changes become problematic.
- Monitor signs of eosinophilia (fatigue, weakness, myalgia) or thrombocytopenia (bruising, nose bleeds, and bleeding gums). Report these signs to the physician.
- Assess any muscle or joint pain to rule out musculoskeletal pathology; that is, try to determine if pain is drug induced rather than caused by anatomic or biomechanical problems.
- Assess dizziness that might affect gait, balance, and other functional activities (See Appendix C). Report balance problems and functional limitations to the physician, and caution the patient and family/caregivers to guard against falls and trauma.
- Monitor IM injection site for pain, swelling, and irritation. Report prolonged or excessive injection site reactions to the physician.

Patient/Client-Related Instruction

- Instruct patient to report bothersome side effects such as severe or prolonged headache, cough, nasal problems, palpitations, erectile dysfunction, skin rash, chills, or GI problems (nausea, vomiting, diarrhea, constipation, abdominal cramps, decreased appetite, increased thirst).

Pharmacokinetics

Absorption: Well absorbed orally, but undergoes extensive first-pass hepatic metabolism resulting in 5–40% bioavailability. Well absorbed following IM administration.

Distribution: Enters breast milk.

Metabolism and Excretion: Extensively metabolized by the liver. Major metabolite (6-beta-naltrexol) has opioid antagonist activity. Metabolites are excreted in urine.

Half-life: Oral: *Naltrexone*—4 hr; *6-beta-naltrexol*—13 hr; IM: *Naltrexone*—5–10 days; *6-beta-naltrexol*—5–10 days.

TIME/ACTION PROFILE (opioid blockade)

ROUTE	ONSET	PEAK	DURATION
50 mg PO	5 min–1 hr*	unknown	24 hr*
100 mg PO	5 min–1 hr*	unknown	48 hr*
150 mg PO	5 min–1 hr*	unknown	72 hr*
IM	unknown	unknown	4 wk
IM-extended release	unknown	2 hr, 2–3 days	>1 mo

*Determined by blockade of effects of 25 mg heroin IV.

Contraindications/Precautions

Contraindicated in: Hypersensitivity; Concurrent use of opioid analgesics or physiologic opioid dependence; Acute opioid withdrawal; Positive urine screen for opioids; Failure of a naloxone challenge test; Acute hepatitis/liver failure.

Use Cautiously in: History of hepatic impairment/damage; Moderate-to-severe renal impairment; History of depression or suicidal behavior/attempt; OB: Pregnancy (use only if maternal benefit outweighs fetal risk); Lactation/Pedi: Lactation or children <18 yr (safety not established).

Interactions

Drug-Drug: Concurrent use with **thioridazine** may ↑ CNS depression. May prevent therapeutic effects of **opioid analgesics, antidiarrheals,** and **antitussives.**

Route/Dosage

Opioid dependence

PO (Adults): Following a negative naloxone challenge and 7–10 days of opioid abstinence (longer for methadone), initial dose is 25 mg. If opioid withdrawal does not occur within 1 hr, additional 25 may be given. Maintenance dose is 50 mg daily as a single dose, *or* 50 mg once daily on weekdays and 100 mg on Saturday, *or* 100 mg every other day, *or* 150 mg every third day, *or* 100 mg on Monday and Wednesday and 150 mg on Friday.

Alcohol dependence

PO (Adults): 50 mg daily as a single dose, *or* 50 mg once daily on weekdays and 100 mg on Saturday, *or* 100 mg every other day, *or* 150 mg every third day, *or* 100 mg on Monday and Wednesday and 150 mg on Friday.
IM (Adults): 380 mg every 4 wk or once monthly.

Availability

Tablets: 50 mg. **Microspheres for injection (requires diluent):** 380 mg/vial.

nandrolone decanoate

(nan-dro-lone dek-a-**noe**-ate)
Deca-Durabolin, Hybolin Decanoate, Kabolin

Classification
Therapeutic: antianemics, hormones
Pharmacologic: anabolic steroids

Schedule III

Indications

Treatment of anemia associated with renal insufficiency.

Action

Stimulates erythropoietin production and may have a direct stimulant action on bone marrow. **Therapeutic Effects:** Increased hemoglobin and RBC volume.

Adverse Reactions/Side Effects

CNS: insomnia. **CV:** edema. **GI:** abdominal fullness, diarrhea, hepatic dysfunction. **GU:** changes in libido, erectile dysfunction, prostatic hyperplasia. **Derm:** acne. **Endo:** virilism in women and prepubertal men. **F and E:** hypercalcemia. **MS:** muscle cramps. **Misc:** chills.

PHYSICAL THERAPY IMPLICATIONS

Examination and Evaluation

- Watch for signs of hepatic dysfunction, including anorexia, abdominal pain, severe nausea and vomiting, yellow skin or eyes, fever, sore throat, malaise, weakness, facial edema, lethargy, and unusual bleeding or bruising. Report these signs to the physician.
- Measure blood pressure periodically and compare to normal values (See Appendix F). Report a sustained increase in blood pressure (hypertension) to the physician.
- Assess peripheral edema using girth measurements, volume displacement, and measurement of pitting edema (See Appendix N). Report increased swelling in feet and ankles or a sudden increase in body weight due to fluid retention.
- Report signs of high calcium levels, including muscle pain, cramps, weakness, joint pain, confusion, and lethargy.
- Periodically assess body weight and other anthropometric measures (body mass index, body composition). A rapid or unexplained weight gain or increase in muscle mass may indicate androgen abuse.
- Monitor personality changes, including irritability and increased aggression. Aggressive behaviors ("roid rage") may indicate inappropriate or excessive androgen use.
- Monitor IM injection site for pain, swelling, and irritation. Report prolonged or excessive injection site reactions to the physician.

Interventions

- Design and implement aerobic exercise programs as tolerated to capitalize on increased RBC production and help improve cardiovascular fitness and oxygen delivery to tissues.
- Do not apply physical agents (heat, cold, electrotherapeutic modalities) or massage over the injection site; these interventions can alter drug absorption from subcutaneous tissues.

Patient/Client-Related Instruction

- Advise patient against use of nandrolone and other androgens to artificially increase muscle mass and enhance athletic performance. Androgen abuse is not safe and can cause liver damage, cardiovascular disease, and other serious side effects.
- Advise men about the risk of sexual side effect, including erectile dysfunction and changes in libido. Notify physician if these side effects become persistent or troublesome.
- Instruct men to report signs of prostate enlargement, including difficulty urinating and increased urge to urinate.
- Advise women that masculine side effects are likely, including deepening of voice, unusual hair growth, clitoral enlargement, and menstrual irregularities.
- Instruct patient to report other troublesome side effects such as severe or prolonged sleep loss, chills, acne, or GI problems (diarrhea, abdominal pain/fullness).

Pharmacokinetics

Absorption: Well absorbed following IM administration.

N

Distribution: Unknown.
Metabolism and Excretion: Unknown.
Half-life: Unknown.

TIME/ACTION PROFILE (blood levels)

ROUTE	ONSET	PEAK	DURATION
IM	unknown	3–6 days	unknown

Contraindications/Precautions

Contraindicated in: Hypersensitivity; Pregnancy or lactation; Some products contain sesame oil and should be avoided in patients with known hypersensitivity; Advanced breast cancer with associated hypercalcemia; Breast cancer in males; Severe hepatic impairment; Hypercalcemia; Nephrosis or nephrotic phase of nephritis; Prostate cancer.
Use Cautiously in: Cardiac or hepatic impairment; Coronary artery disease or history of MI; Diabetes mellitus; Benign prostatic hyperplasia; Children; Geriatric patients.

Interactions

Drug-Drug: ↑ risk of hepatotoxicity with other **hepatotoxic agents**. ↑ risk of bleeding with **warfarin, NSAIDs**, and **salicylates**.

Route/Dosage

IM (Adults and Children ≥14 yr): *Women*—50–100 mg q wk; *men*—100–200 mg q wk.
IM (Children 2–13 yr): 25–50 mg q 3–4 wk.

Availability (generic available)

Injection: 100 mg/mL in 2-mL vial, 200 mg/mL in 1-mL vial.

naproxen (na-prox-en)

Aleve, Anaprox, Anaprox DS, ✱Apo-Napro-Na, Apo-Napro-Na DS, ✱Apo-Naproxen, EC-Naprosyn, Naprelan, Napron X, Naprosyn, ✱Naprosyn-E, ✱Naprosyn-SR, ✱Naxen, ✱Novo-Naprox, ✱Novo-Naprox Sodium DS, ✱Nu-Naprox, ✱Synflex, ✱Synflex DS

Classification
Therapeutic: nonopioid analgesics, nonsteroidal anti-inflammatory agents, antipyretics
Pharmacologic: propionic acid derivatives

Indications

Mild-to-moderate pain. Dysmenorrhea. Fever. Inflammatory disorders, including Rheumatoid arthritis (adults and children), Osteoarthritis.

Action

Inhibits prostaglandin synthesis. **Therapeutic Effects:** Decreased pain. Reduction of fever. Suppression of inflammation.

Adverse Reactions/Side Effects

CNS: dizziness, drowsiness, headache. **EENT:** tinnitus, visual disturbances. **Resp:** dyspnea. **CV:** edema, palpitations, tachycardia. **GI:** DRUG-INDUCED HEPATITIS, GI BLEEDING, constipation, dyspepsia, nausea, anorexia, diarrhea, discomfort, flatulence, vomiting. **GU:** cystitis, hematuria, renal failure. **Derm:** photosensitivity, rashes, sweating, pseudoporphyria (12% incidence in children with juvenile rheumatoid arthritis—discontinue therapy if this occurs). **Hemat:** blood dyscrasias, prolonged bleeding time. **Misc:** ALLERGIC REACTIONS, INCLUDING ANAPHYLAXIS AND STEVENS-JOHNSON SYNDROME.

PHYSICAL THERAPY IMPLICATIONS

Examination and Evaluation

- Monitor signs of GI bleeding, including abdominal pain, vomiting blood, blood in stools, or black, tarry stools. Report these signs to the physician immediately.
- Be alert for signs of drug-induced hepatitis, including anorexia, abdominal pain, severe nausea and vomiting, yellow skin or eyes, skin rashes, flu-like symptoms, and muscle/joint pain. Report these signs to the physician immediately.
- Monitor signs of allergic reactions and anaphylaxis, including pulmonary symptoms (laryngeal edema, wheezing, cough, dyspnea) or skin reactions (rash, pruritus, urticaria). Be especially alert for exfoliation, dermatitis, and other severe skin reactions that might indicate serious hypersensitivity reactions such as Stevens-Johnson syndrome. Notify physician immediately if these reactions occur.
- Assess pain and other variables (range of motion, muscle strength) to document whether this drug is successful in helping manage the patient's pain and decreasing impairments.
- Assess heart rate, ECG, and heart sounds, especially during exercise (See Appendices G, H). Report rapid heart rate (tachycardia) or symptoms of other arrhythmias such as palpitations, chest discomfort, shortness of breath, fainting, and fatigue/weakness.
- Assess blood pressure (BP) periodically and compare to normal values (See Appendix F). NSAIDs can increase BP in certain patients.
- Be alert for signs of prolonged bleeding time such as bleeding gums, nosebleeds, and unusual or excessive bruising. Report these signs to the physician.
- Assess peripheral edema using girth measurements, volume displacement, and measurement of pitting edema (See Appendix N). Report increased swelling

in feet and ankles or a sudden increase in body weight due to fluid retention.

- Monitor signs of kidney dysfunction such as painful urination or blood in the urine. Report signs of renal failure immediately, including decreased urine output, increased BP, muscle cramps/twitching, edema/weight gain from fluid retention, yellowish brown skin, and confusion that progresses to seizures and coma.
- Monitor unusual weakness and fatigue that might be due to anemia, or other symptoms such as fever, sore throat, mucosal lesions, or signs of infection that might be due to other blood dyscrasias. Notify physician if these signs occur.
- Assess dizziness and drowsiness that might affect gait, balance, and other functional activities (See Appendix C). Report balance problems and functional limitations to the physician, and caution the patient and family/caregivers to guard against falls and trauma.

Interventions

- Implement appropriate manual therapy techniques, physical agents, and therapeutic exercises to reduce pain and decrease the need for naproxen and other NSAIDs.
- Because of the risk of arrhythmias, use caution during aerobic exercise and other forms of therapeutic exercise. Assess exercise tolerance frequently (BP, heart rate, fatigue levels), and terminate exercise immediately if any untoward responses occur (See Appendix L).
- If treating arthritic conditions, recommend orthotic and assistive devices as needed to reduce pain, improve function, and augment the effects of drug therapy.
- Use caution with any physical interventions that could increase bleeding, including wound débridement, chest percussion, joint mobilization, and application of local heat.
- Help patient explore other nonpharmacologic methods to reduce chronic pain, such as relaxation techniques, exercise, counseling, and so forth.
- Causes photosensitivity; use care if administering UV treatments. Advise patient to avoid direct sunlight and use sunscreens and protective clothing, and to report any untoward skin reactions (rash, excessive sweating).

Patient/Client-Related Instruction

- Advise patient that analgesics are usually more effective if given before pain becomes severe; emphasize that adequate pain control will allow better participation in physical therapy.
- Inform patient that NSAIDs may impair bone and cartilage healing. Advise patient to consult physician about NSAID use, especially after fractures, spinal fusion, and other bone surgeries.
- Caution patient about the use of over-the-counter products that contain NSAIDs or acetaminophen while taking prescription doses of naproxen. Use of multiple NSAIDs increases the risk of toxicity and overdose.
- Instruct patient to report excessive or prolonged headache or ringing/buzzing in the ears (tinnitus); these signs may indicate drug toxicity.
- Advise patient about the risks of gastric irritation. Instruct patient to notify physician of GI reactions such as severe or prolonged nausea, vomiting, constipation, diarrhea, indigestion, flatulence, loss of appetite, and abdominal pain.
- Advise patient to reduce alcohol intake because alcohol increases the risk of gastric toxicity.
- Instruct patient and family/caregivers to report other troublesome side effects such as severe or prolonged vision disturbances or difficult, labored breathing.

Pharmacokinetics

Absorption: Completely absorbed from the GI tract. Sodium salt (Anaprox) is more rapidly absorbed.
Distribution: Crosses the placenta; enters breast milk in low concentrations.
Protein Binding: >99%.
Metabolism and Excretion: Mostly metabolized by the liver.
Half-life: Children <8 yr: 8–17 hr; Children 8–14 yr: 8–10 hr; Adults: 10–20 hr.

TIME/ACTION PROFILE

ROUTE	ONSET	PEAK	DURATION
PO (analgesic)	1 hr	unknown	8–12 hr
PO (anti-inflammatory)	14 days	2–4 wk	unknown

Contraindications/Precautions

Contraindicated in: Hypersensitivity; Cross-sensitivity may occur with other NSAIDs, including aspirin; Active GI bleeding; Ulcer disease; Lactation: Passes into breast milk and should not be used by nursing mothers.
Use Cautiously in: Severe cardiovascular, renal, or hepatic disease; History of ulcer disease or any other history of gastrointestinal bleeding (may ↑ risk of GI bleeding); Underlying cardiovascular disease (may ↑ risk of MI or stroke); Chronic alcohol use/abuse; Geri: Increased risk of adverse reactions; OB: Avoid using during 3rd trimester of pregnancy; may cause

N

premature closure of the ductus arteriosus; Pedi: Children <2 yr (safety not established).

Interactions

Drug-Drug: Concurrent use with **aspirin** ↓ naproxen blood levels and may ↓ effectiveness. ↑ risk of bleeding with **anticoagulants, thrombolytic agents, eptifibatide, tirofiban, cefotetan, cefoperazone, valproic acid, clopidogrel**, and **ticlopidine**. Additive adverse GI side effects with **aspirin**, **corticosteroids**, and other **NSAIDs**. **Probenecid** ↑ blood levels and may ↑ toxicity. ↑ risk of photosensitivity with other **photosensitizing agents**. May ↑ risk of toxicity from **methotrexate, antineoplastics**, or **radiation therapy**. May ↑ serum levels and risk of toxicity from **lithium**. ↑ risk of adverse renal effects with **cyclosporine** or chronic use of **acetaminophen**. May ↓ response to **ACE inhibitors, angiotensin II antagonists**, or **furosemide**. May ↑ risk of hypoglycemia with **insulin** or **oral hypoglycemic agents. Oral potassium supplements** may ↑ GI adverse effects.
Drug-Natural: ↑ anticoagulant effect and bleeding risk with **anise, arnica, chamomile, clove, dong quai, feverfew, garlic, ginger, ginkgo, *Panax ginseng*, licorice**, and others.

Route/Dosage

275 mg naproxen sodium is equivalent to 250 mg naproxen.

Anti-inflammatory/Analgesic/ Antidysmenorrheal

PO (Adults): *Naproxen*—250–500 mg bid (up to 1.5 g/day). *Delayed-release naproxen*—375–500 mg bid. *Naproxen sodium*—275–550 mg bid (up to 1.65 g/day).
PO (Children >2 yr): *Analgesia:* 5–7 mg/kg/dose every 8–12 hr. *Inflammatory disease:* 10–15 mg/kg/day divided q 12 hr, maximum: 1000 mg/day.

Antigout

PO (Adults): *Naproxen*—750 mg naproxen initially, then 250 mg q 8 hr. *Naproxen sodium*—825 mg initially, then 275 mg q 8 hr.

OTC Use (naproxen sodium)

PO (Adults): 200 mg q 8–12 hr or 400 mg followed by 200 mg q 12 hr (not to exceed 600 mg/24 hr).
PO (Geriatric Patients >65 yr): Not to exceed 200 mg q 12 hr.

Availability

Naproxen (generic available)

Tablets (Naprosyn [Apo-Naproxen, Naxen, Novo-Naprox, Nu-Naprox]): 125 mg, 250 mg, 375 mg, 500 mg. **Controlled-release tablets (Naprelan):** 375 mg, 500 mg. **Delayed-release tablets (EC-Naprosyn, Naprosyn-E):** 250 mg, 375 mg, 500 mg. **Extended-release tablets (Naprosyn-SR):** 750 mg. **Oral suspension (Naprosyn):** 125 mg/5 Ll. **Suppositories (Naprosyn, Naxen):** 500 mg.

Naproxen Sodium

Tablets (Aleve, Anaprox, Anaprox DS, Apo-Napro-Na, Novo-Naprox Sodium, Novo-Naprox Sodium DS, Synaflex, Synaflex DS): 220 mg OTC, 275 mg, 550 mg. ***In combination with:*** lansoprazole in a combination package (Prevacid NapraPac), pseudoephedrine (Aleve Cold and Sinus Tablets, Aleve Sinus and Headache Tablets), sumatriptan (Treximet). See Appendix B.

naratriptan (nar-a-trip-tan)

Amerge

Classification

Therapeutic: vascular headache suppressants
Pharmacologic: 5-HT1 agonists

Indications

Acute treatment of migraine headache.

Action

Acts as an agonist at specific 5-HT_1 receptor sites in intracranial blood vessels and sensory trigeminal nerves. **Therapeutic Effects:** Cranial vessel vasoconstriction with resultant decrease in migraine headache.

Adverse Reactions/Side Effects

CNS: dizziness, drowsiness, malaise/fatigue. **CV:** CORONARY ARTERY VASOSPASM, MI, VENTRICULAR FIBRILLATION, VENTRICULAR TACHYCARDIA, myocardial ischemia. **GI:** nausea. **Neuro:** paresthesia. **Misc:** pain/pressure sensation in throat/neck.

PHYSICAL THERAPY IMPLICATIONS

Examination and Evaluation

- Continually monitor for signs of coronary artery vasospasm and MI, including sudden chest pain, pain radiating into the arm or jaw, shortness of breath, dizziness, sweating, anxiety, and nausea. Seek immediate medical assistance if patient develops these signs.
- Assess heart rate, ECG, and heart sounds, especially during exercise (See Appendices G, H). Report any rhythm disturbances or symptoms of increased arrhythmias, including palpitations, chest discomfort, shortness of breath, dizziness, fainting, and fatigue/weakness.
- Assess the frequency and severity of headaches, and document whether drug therapy is successful in decreasing the intensity of migraine attacks.

- Watch for dizziness that affects gait, balance, and other functional activities (See Appendix C). Report balance problems and functional limitations to the physician, and caution the patient and family/caregivers to guard against falls and trauma.
- Assess any neck or throat pain and pressure to rule out musculoskeletal pathology; that is, try to determine if pain is drug induced rather than caused by anatomic or biomechanical problems.
- Assess signs of paresthesia (numbness, tingling). Perform objective tests, including electroneuromyography and sensory testing to document any drug-related neuropathic changes.

Interventions

- Because of the risk of MI and ventricular arrhythmias, use extreme caution during aerobic exercise and other forms of therapeutic exercise. Assess exercise tolerance frequently (blood pressure, heart rate, respiration, fatigue levels), and terminate exercise immediately if any untoward responses occur (See Appendix L).
- Implement appropriate interventions (manual techniques, physical agents, therapeutic exercise) to manage headache pain and reduce the need for drug therapy. Help patient also explore other non-pharmacologic methods to reduce chronic headache pain, such as relaxation techniques, imagery, and so forth.
- If a headache occurs and drug treatment is needed during a rehabilitation session, allow patient to recover in a quiet, darkened room to allow the drug to achieve maximal effects.

Patient/Client-Related Instruction

- Advise patient and family or caregiver about the signs of MI (see above under Examination and Evaluation), and to seek immediate medical assistance if these signs develop.
- Advise the patient to bring this drug to each therapy session; this drug is most effective when taken at the first signs of a migraine attack.
- Advise patient to adhere to the correct dosing schedule, and to not exceed the recommended frequency and number of doses per 24-hr period.
- Instruct patient to report other troublesome side effects such as severe or prolonged drowsiness, malaise, fatigue, or nausea.

Pharmacokinetics

Absorption: Well absorbed (70%) following oral administration.
Distribution: Unknown.
Metabolism and Excretion: 60% excreted unchanged in urine; 30% metabolized by the liver.
Half-life: 6 hr (increased in renal impairment).

TIME/ACTION PROFILE (decreased migraine pain)

ROUTE	ONSET	PEAK	DURATION
PO	30–60 min	2–3 hr*	up to 24 hr

*3–4 hr during migraine attack.

Contraindications/Precautions

Contraindicated in: Hypersensitivity; Geriatric patients; Ischemic cardiovascular, cerebrovascular, or peripheral vascular syndromes; History of significant cardiovascular disease; Uncontrolled hypertension; Severe renal impairment (CCr <15 mL/min); Severe hepatic impairment; Should not be used within 24 hr of other 5-HT_1 agonists or ergot-type compounds (dihydroergotamine).
Use Cautiously in: Mild-to-moderate renal or hepatic impairment (dose should not exceed 2.5 mg/24 hr; initial dose should be decreased); Pregnancy, lactation, or children (safety not established).
Exercise Extreme Caution in: Cardiovascular risk factors (hypertension, hypercholesterolemia, cigarette smoking, obesity, diabetes, strong family history, menopausal women or men >40 yr); use only if cardiovascular status has been evaluated and determined to be safe and 1st dose is administered under supervision.

Interactions

Drug-Drug: Concurrent use with **SSRI antidepressants** may result in weakness, hyperreflexia, and incoordination. **Cigarette smoking** increases the metabolism of naratriptan. Blood levels and effects are increased by **hormonal contraceptives**. Avoid concurrent use (within 24 hr of each other) with **ergot-containing drugs (dihydroergotamine);** may result in prolonged vasospastic reactions. Avoid concurrent (within 2 wk) use with **MAO inhibitors**; produces increased systemic exposure and risk of adverse reactions to naratriptan. Serotonin syndrome may occur with **sibutramine**.
Drug-Natural: ↑ risk of serotonergic side effects, including serotonin syndrome with **St. John's wort** and **SAMe**.

Route/Dosage

PO (Adults): 1 or 2.5 mg; dose may be repeated in 4 hr if response is inadequate (not to exceed 5 mg/24 hr or treatment of more than 4 headaches/mo).

Availability

Tablets: 1 mg, 2.5 mg.

N

natalizumab (na-tal-iz-yoo-mab)

Tysabri

Classification

Therapeutic: anti–multiple sclerosis agents
Pharmacologic: monoclonal antibodies

Indications

To reduce the frequency of exacerbations of relapsing multiple sclerosis (MS).

Action

Binds to integrin receptors on nonneutrophil leukocytes which may alter adhesion and migration characteristics involved in the crossing of activated inflammatory cells into the CNS. **Therapeutic Effects:** Fewer exacerbations of relapsing multiple sclerosis.

Adverse Reactions/Side Effects

CNS: depression, fatigue. **GI:** cholelithiasis. **Misc:** allergic reactions, including anaphylaxis, infections, PROGRESSIVE MULTIFOCAL LEUKOENCEPHALOPATHY (PML), infusion-related reactions.

PHYSICAL THERAPY IMPLICATIONS

Examination and Evaluation

- Be alert for signs of PML. Signs include memory lapses, decreased cognition, vision loss, speech problems, incoordination, ataxia, and muscle weakness that can progress to paralysis, seizures, and coma. Report these signs to the physician or nursing staff immediately.
- Monitor signs of allergic reactions and anaphylaxis, including pulmonary symptoms (tightness in the throat and chest, wheezing, cough, dyspnea) or skin reactions (rash, pruritus, urticaria, dermatitis). Be especially alert for responses that occur during and after administration (infusion related reactions). Notify physician or nursing staff immediately if these reactions occur.
- Periodically assess balance, coordination, spasticity, and other aspects of neuromuscular function to help document this drug's effectiveness in reducing MS exacerbations.
- Monitor personality changes, including depression and increased thoughts of suicide. Notify physician if these changes become problematic.
- Report signs of gallstones (cholelithiasis), including sudden intense pain in the abdomen or right side, jaundice, chills, and fever.

Interventions

- Design and implement coordination, balance, and other therapeutic exercises to maintain function, and complement drug effects in patients with MS.

Patient/Client-Related Instruction

- Advise patient to guard against infection (frequent hand washing, etc.), and to avoid crowds and contact with persons with contagious diseases.
- Instruct patient to report other troublesome side effects such as prolonged or severe fatigue or signs of infection.

Pharmacokinetics

Absorption: IV administration results in complete bioavailability.
Distribution: Unknown.
Metabolism and Excretion: Unknown.
Half-life: 7–15 days.

TIME/ACTION PROFILE

ROUTE	ONSET	PEAK	DURATION
IV	unknown	unknown	unknown

Contraindications/Precautions

Contraindicated in: Hypersensitivity; Concurrent use of immunosuppressants; History of PML; Children <18 yr.
Use Cautiously in: History of depression or suicide attempt; Pregnancy (use only if clearly needed).

Interactions

Drug-Drug: ↑ risk of infections with **immunosuppressants** (avoid concurrent use).

Route/Dosage

NOTE: Because of the risk of PML, natalizumab is available only under a special restricted distribution program, the TOUCH Prescribing Program. Prescribers, pharmacies, and patients must be enrolled in the program to obtain the drug.
IV (Adults): 300 mg q 4 wk.

Availability

Concentrate for IV infusion: 300 mg/15-mL vial.

nateglinide (na-teg-li-nide)

Starlix

Classification

Therapeutic: antidiabetics
Pharmacologic: meglitinides

Indications

To improve glycemic control in patients with type 2 diabetes (with diet and exercise); may also be used with metformin or a thiazolidinedione (pioglitazone, rosiglitazone).

Action

Stimulates the release of insulin from pancreatic beta cells by closing potassium channels, which results in the opening of calcium channels in beta cells. This is followed by release of insulin. Requires functioning pancreatic beta cells. **Therapeutic Effects:** Lowering of blood glucose.

Adverse Reactions/Side Effects

CNS: dizziness. **Resp:** bronchitis, coughing, upper respiratory infection. **GI:** diarrhea. **Endo:** HYPOGLYCEMIA. **MS:** arthropathy, back pain. **Misc:** flu symptoms.

PHYSICAL THERAPY IMPLICATIONS

Examination and Evaluation

- Be alert for signs of hypoglycemia, especially during and after exercise. Common neuromuscular signs include anxiety; restlessness; tingling in hands, feet, lips, or tongue; chills; cold sweats; confusion; difficulty in concentration; drowsiness; excessive hunger; headache; irritability; nervousness; tremor; weakness; unsteady gait. Report episodes of severe hypoglycemia to the physician immediately.
- Monitor symptoms of upper respiratory tract infection and bronchitis, including cough, production of mucous, wheezing, chest discomfort, shortness of breath, fatigue, chills, and fever. Report severe or prolonged symptoms to the physician.
- Assess dizziness that might affect gait, balance, and other functional activities (See Appendix C). Report balance problems to the physician, and caution the patient and family/caregivers to guard against falls and trauma.
- Assess any back or joint pain to rule out musculoskeletal pathology; that is, try to determine if pain is drug induced rather than caused by anatomic or biomechanical problems.
- Assess blood pressure periodically (See Appendix F). A sudden or sustained increase in blood pressure (hypertension) may indicate problems in diabetes management, and should be reported to the physician.

Interventions

- Implement aerobic exercise and endurance training programs to maintain optimal body weight, improve insulin sensitivity, and reduce the risk of macrovascular disease (heart attack, stroke) and microvascular problems (reduced blood flow to tissues and organs that causes poor wound healing, neuropathy, retinopathy, and nephropathy).
- Provide a source of oral glucose (fruit juice, glucose gels/tablets, etc.) to treat mild hypoglycemia. Call for emergency assistance if symptoms persist or in cases of severe hypoglycemia. Emergency treatment typically consists of IV glucose, glucagon, or epinephrine.

Patient/Client-Related Instruction

- Encourage patient to monitor blood glucose before and after exercise and to adjust food intake to maintain normal glycemic levels.
- Emphasize the importance of adhering to nutritional guidelines, and the need for periodic assessment of glycemic control (serum glucose and glycosylated hemoglobin levels) throughout the management of diabetes mellitus.
- Advise patient about symptoms of hyperglycemia (confusion, drowsiness; flushed, dry skin; fruit-like breath odor; rapid, deep breathing, polyuria; loss of appetite; unusual thirst). Drug dosages may need to be adjusted to prevent repeated episodes of hyperglycemia.
- Instruct patient to report other troublesome side effects such as severe or prolonged diarrhea or flu-like symptoms.

Pharmacokinetics

Absorption: Well absorbed (73%) following oral administration; absorption is rapid.
Distribution: Unknown.
Protein Binding: 98%.
Metabolism and Excretion: Mostly metabolized by the liver (cytochrome P2C9 and P3A4 [CYP2C9 and CYP3A4] enzyme systems); 16% excreted unchanged in urine.
Half-life: 1.5 hr.

TIME/ACTION PROFILE (effect on blood glucose)

ROUTE	ONSET	PEAK	DURATION
PO	within 20 min	1 hr	4 hr

Contraindications/Precautions

Contraindicated in: Hypersensitivity; OB: Pregnancy or lactation (insulin recommended to control diabetes during pregnancy); Diabetic ketoacidosis; Type 1 diabetes.
Use Cautiously in: Geri: Elderly patients, malnourished patients, patients with pituitary or adrenal insufficiency (increased susceptibility to hypoglycemia); Strenuous physical exercise, insufficient caloric intake (increased risk of hypoglycemia); Autonomic neuropathy (hypoglycemia may be masked); Moderate-to-severe liver impairment; Fever, infection, trauma, or surgery (may lead to transient loss of glycemic control; insulin may be required); Pedi: Children (safety not established).

Interactions

Drug-Drug: Concurrent use with **beta blockers** may mask hypoglycemia. **Alcohol**, combination with other **antidiabetics, NSAIDs, MAO inhibitors,** or **nonselective beta blockers** may ↑ the risk of hypoglycemia.

Hypoglycemic effects may be ↓ by **thiazide diuretics, corticosteroids, thyroid supplements**, or **sympathomimetic (adrenergic) agents**.
Drug-Food: Blood levels and effects are significantly ↓ when administered prior to a **liquid meal**.

Route/Dosage

PO (Adults): 120 mg tid before meals; patients who are approaching glycemic control may be started at 60 mg tid.

Availability

Tablets: 60 mg, 120 mg.

nebivolol (ne-biv-oh-lol)

Bystolic

Classification
Therapeutic: antihypertensives
Pharmacologic: beta blockers (selective)

Indications

Hypertension (alone and with other antihypertensives).

Action

Blocks stimulation of beta-adrenergic receptor sites; selective for beta$_1$ (myocardial) receptors in most patients. In some patients (poor metabolizers, higher blood levels may result in some beta$_2$ [pulmonary, vascular, uterine] adrenergic) blockade.
Therapeutic Effects: Lowering of blood pressure.

Adverse Reactions/Side Effects

CNS: dizziness, fatigue, headache.

PHYSICAL THERAPY IMPLICATIONS

Examination and Evaluation

- Assess blood pressure periodically and compare to normal values (See Appendix F) to help document antihypertensive effects.
- Assess dizziness that might affect gait, balance, and other functional activities (See Appendix C). Report balance problems and functional limitations to the physician, and caution the patient and family/caregivers to guard against falls and trauma.
- Monitor excessive fatigue or weakness. Beta blockers often cause some degree of fatigue and weakness, but any sudden or severe change in muscle strength or energy levels should be reported.

Interventions

- Establish aerobic exercise workloads that account for the effects of beta blockers on heart rate. Some heart rate guidelines may not be appropriate because beta blockers typically decrease maximal HR by 20–30 bpm. Use other guidelines such as rating of perceived exertion (RPE, modified Borg scale) to determine exercise workloads.
- To minimize orthostatic hypotension, patient should move slowly when assuming a more upright position.

Patient/Client-Related Instruction

- Remind patients to take medication as directed to control hypertension even if they are asymptomatic.
- Counsel patients about additional interventions to help control blood pressure such as regular exercise, weight loss, sodium restriction, stress reduction, moderation of alcohol consumption, and smoking cessation.

Pharmacokinetics

Absorption: Well absorbed following oral administration.
Distribution: Unknown.
Protein Binding: 98%.
Metabolism and Excretion: Mostly metabolized by the liver, including the CYP2D6 enzyme system; some have antihypertensive action; minimal excretion of unchanged drug.
Half-life: *Extensive metabolizers*—12 hr; *poor metabolizers*—19 hr.

TIME/ACTION PROFILE (blood levels)

ROUTE	ONSET	PEAK	DURATION
PO	unknown	1.5–4 hr	24 hr

Contraindications/Precautions

Contraindicated in: Hypersensitivity; Severe bradycardia, heart block greater than 1st degree, cardiogenic shock, decompensated heart failure or sick sinus syndrome (without pacemaker); Severe hepatic impairment (Child-Pugh >B); Bronchospastic disease; OB: Lactation.
Use Cautiously in: Coronary artery disease (rapid cessation should be avoided); Compensated congestive heart failure; Major surgery (anesthesia may augment myocardial depression); Diabetes mellitus (may mask signs of hypoglycemia); Thyrotoxicosis (may mask symptoms); Moderate hepatic impairment (↓ metabolism); Severe renal impairment (↓ initial dose if CCr <30 mL/min); History of severe allergic reactions (↑ intensity of reactions); Pheochromocytoma (alpha blockers required prior to beta blockers); Geri: Consider increased sensitivity, concurrent chronic diseases, medications, and presence of age-related decrease in clearance; OB: Use in pregnancy only if maternal benefit outweighs fetal risk; Pedi: Safe use in children <18 yr not established.

Interactions

Drug-Drug: Drugs that affect the CYP2D6 enzyme system are expected to alter levels and possibly effects of nebivolol; dose alterations may be required. **Fluoxetine**, a known inhibitor of CYP2D6, ↑ levels and effects; similar effects may be expected from **quinidine, propafenone,** and **paroxetine**. Blood levels are also ↑ by **cimetine. Anesthetic agents,** including **ether, trichloroethylene**, and **cyclopropane** as well as **other myocardial depressants** or **inhibitors of AV conduction** such as **diltiazem** and **verapamil,** may ↑ risk of myocardial depression and bradycardia. Avoid concurrent use with **beta blockers**. Concurrent use with **reserpine** or **guanethidine** may excessively reduce sympathetic activity. If used concurrently with **clonidine**, nebivolol should be tapered and discontinued several days prior to gradual withdrawal of clonidine.

Route/Dosage

PO (Adults): 5 mg once daily initially; may increase at 2-wk intervals up to 40 mg/day.

Hepatic/Renal Impairment

PO (Adults): 2.5 mg once daily initially; titrate upward cautiously.

Availability

Tablets: 2.5 mg, 5 mg, 10 mg.

nefazodone (ne-faz-oh-done)

Classification
Therapeutic: antidepressants

Indications

Major depression. **Unlabeled Use:** Panic disorder, posttraumatic stress disorder (PTSD).

Action

Inhibits the reuptake of serotonin and norepinephrine by neurons. Antagonizes $alpha_1$-adrenergic receptors. **Therapeutic Effects:** Antidepressant action, which may develop only after several weeks.

Adverse Reactions/Side Effects

CNS: dizziness, insomnia, somnolence, agitation, confusion, weakness. **EENT:** abnormal vision, blurred vision, eye pain, tinnitus. **Resp:** dyspnea. **CV:** bradycardia, hypotension. **GI:** HEPATIC FAILURE, HEPATOTOXICITY, constipation, dry mouth, nausea, gastroenteritis. **GU:** erectile dysfunction. **Derm:** rashes. **Hemat:** decreased hematocrit.

PHYSICAL THERAPY IMPLICATIONS

Examination and Evaluation

- Be alert for signs of hepatotoxicity and liver failure, including anorexia, abdominal pain, severe nausea and vomiting, yellow skin or eyes, fever, sore throat, malaise, weakness, facial edema, lethargy, and unusual bleeding or bruising. Report these signs to the physician immediately.
- Be alert for increased depression and suicidal thoughts and ideology, especially when initiating drug treatment or in children and teenagers. Notify physician or other mental health care professional immediately if patient exhibits worsening depression or other changes in mood and behavior.
- Assess blood pressure periodically and compare to normal values (See Appendix F). Report low blood pressure (hypotension), especially if patient experiences dizziness or syncope.
- Assess heart rate, ECG, and heart sounds, especially during exercise (See Appendixes G, H). Report an unusually slow heart rate (bradycardia) or signs of other arrhythmias, including palpitations, chest discomfort, shortness of breath, fainting, and fatigue/weakness.
- Assess dizziness and drowsiness that might affect gait, balance, and other functional activities (See Appendix C). Report balance problems and functional limitations to the physician, and caution the patient and family/caregivers to guard against falls and trauma.
- Be alert for agitation, confusion, or other alterations in mental status. Notify physician promptly if these symptoms develop (See Appendix D).

Interventions

- Guard against falls and trauma (hip fractures, head injury, and so forth), and implement fall prevention strategies (See Appendix E).
- Because of the risk of bradycardia and other arrhythmias, use caution during aerobic exercise and other forms of therapeutic exercise. Assess exercise tolerance frequently (blood pressure, heart rate, fatigue levels), and terminate exercise immediately if any untoward responses occur (See Appendix L).
- To minimize orthostatic hypotension, patient should move slowly when assuming a more upright position.
- Help patient explore nonpharmacologic methods reduce depression and other psychologic disorders (exercise, counseling, support groups, and so forth).

Patient/Client-Related Instruction

- Advise patient that antidepressant effects may not occur immediately; it may take 2 wk or more before an improvement in mood is observed.
- Advise patient to avoid alcohol and other CNS depressants because of the increased risk of sedation and adverse effects.

N

- Instruct patient to report other problematic side effects such as severe or prolonged insomnia, vision disturbances, ringing/buzzing in the ears (tinnitus), erectile dysfunction, skin rashes, GI problems (nausea, constipation, dry mouth), or signs of GI infection (diarrhea, vomiting, abdominal cramps, fever).

Pharmacokinetics

Absorption: Well absorbed but undergoes extensive and variable first-pass hepatic metabolism (bioavailability about 20%).
Distribution: Widely distributed; enters the CNS.
Protein Binding: ≥99%.
Metabolism and Excretion: Extensively metabolized. One metabolite (hydroxynefazodone) has antidepressant activity.
Half-life: *Nefazodone*—2–4 hr; *hydroxynefazodone*—1.5–4 hr.

TIME/ACTION PROFILE (antidepressant action)

ROUTE	ONSET	PEAK	DURATION
PO	days–wks	several wk	unknown

Contraindications/Precautions

Contraindicated in: Hypersensitivity; Concurrent MAO inhibitor therapy; Active liver disease or baseline elevated serum transaminases.
Use Cautiously in: May ↑ risk of suicide attempt/ideation, especially during dose early treatment or dose adjustment; History of suicide attempt or drug abuse; Underlying cardiovascular or cerebrovascular disease; History of mania; OB: Safety no established; Lactation: Discontinue drug or bottle-feed; Pedi: Safety not established in children; suicide risk may be greater in children and adolescents; Geri: Initiate therapy at lower doses.

Interactions

Drug-Drug: Serious, potentially fatal reactions may occur during concurrent use with **MAO inhibitors** (do not use concurrently or within 2 wk of MAO inhibitors; discontinue nefazodone at least 14 days before starting MAO inhibitor therapy). ↑ CNS depression with other CNS depressants, including **alcohol, antihistamines, opioid analgesics,** and **sedative/hypnotics**. May ↑ blood levels and effects of **alprazolam** or **triazolam**. May increase serum **digoxin** levels. Additive hypotension may occur with **antihypertensives, nitrates,** or acute ingestion of **alcohol**. May ↑ risk of myopathy with **HMG CoA reductase inhibitors**. Decreased **antidepressant** action with concomitant use of **carabazepine**. May reduce clearance of **haloperidol,** so **haloperidol** dose may need to be decreased.
Drug-Natural: ↑ risk of seritonergic side effects, including serotonin syndrome with **St. John's wort** and **SAMe**. **Kava, valerian,** or **chamomile** can ↑ CNS depression.

Route/Dosage

PO (Adults): 100 mg bid initially; may be ↑ weekly up to 600 mg/day in 2 divided doses.
PO (Geriatric Patients): 50 mg bid initially; may be ↑ weekly as tolerated.

Availability (generic available)

Tablets: 50 mg, 100 mg, 150 mg, 200 mg, 250 mg.

nelarabine (ne-lar-a-been)

Arranon

Classification

Therapeutic: antineoplastics
Pharmacologic: antimetabolites

Indications

T-cell acute lymphoblastic leukemia or T-cell lymphoblastic lymphoma unresponsive to at least 2 other previous chemotherapy regimens.

Action

Converted intracellularly to arabinosylguanine (ara-G) and then to arabinosylguanine triphosphate (ara-GTP). In leukemic cells, it is incorporated into DNA, leading to inhibition of DNA synthesis and cell death. **Therapeutic Effects:** Decreased proliferation of leukemic cells.

Adverse Reactions/Side Effects

Hemat: anemia, leukopenia, neutropenia, thrombocytopenia. **Neuro:** SEVERE NEUROLOGIC EVENTS.

PHYSICAL THERAPY IMPLICATIONS

Examination and Evaluation

- Be alert for signs of CNS neurotoxicity, including confusion, agitation, severe headache, hearing loss, visual disturbances, decreased consciousness, and seizures. Notify physician immediately, especially if patient becomes unresponsive or difficult to arouse.
- Monitor signs of leukopenia and neutropenia (fever, sore throat, signs of infection), thrombocytopenia (bruising, nose bleeds, bleeding gums), or anemia (unusual weakness, fatigue, shortness of breath, pallor). Report these signs to the physician.

Interventions

- For patients who are medically able to begin exercise, implement appropriate resistive exercises and aerobic training to maintain muscle strength and aerobic capacity during cancer chemotherapy or to help restore function after chemotherapy.

Patient/Client-Related Instruction

- Advise patient to decrease risk of infections (frequent hand washing, etc.) and to avoid contact with persons with contagious diseases.

Pharmacokinetics

Absorption: IV administration results in complete bioavailability. Intracellular conversion is required for activation of prodrug.
Distribution: Extensively distributed.
Metabolism and Excretion: Mostly metabolized intracellularly. Partially eliminated by the kidneys as nelarabine and ara-G.
Half-life: Unknown.

TIME/ACTION PROFILE

ROUTE	ONSET	PEAK	DURATION
IV	unknown	end of infusion	unknown

Contraindications/Precautions

Contraindicated in: Hypersensitivity; CCr <50 mL/min; OB: Pregnancy, lactation.
Use Cautiously in: OB: Patients with childbearing potential; Geri: Risk of neurologic events may be ↑; Severe hepatic impairment (bilirubin >3.0 mg/dL).

Interactions

Drug-Drug: Decreases antibody response to and ↑ risk of adverse reactions from **live-virus vaccines**.

Route/Dosage

IV (Adults): 1500 mg/m^2 on days 1, 3, and 5 of every 21-day cycle.
IV (Children): 650 mg/m^2/day for first 5 days of every 21-day cycle.

Availability

Solution for IV injection: 5 mg/mL in 50-mL vials (250 mg/vial).

nelfinavir (nel-fin-a-veer)

Viracept

Classification
Therapeutic: antiretrovirals
Pharmacologic: protease inhibitors

Indications

HIV infection (with other antiretrovirals).

Action

Inhibits HIV protease and prevents cleavage of viral polyproteins. **Therapeutic Effects:** Increased CD4 cell count and decreased viral load. Slowed progression of HIV infection with less sequela.

Adverse Reactions/Side Effects

CNS: SEIZURES, anxiety, depression, dizziness, drowsiness, emotional lability, headache, hyperkinesia, malaise, migraine headache, sleep disorders, suicidal ideation, weakness. **EENT:** acute iritis, pharyngitis, rhinitis, sinusitis. **Resp:** dyspnea. **GI:** diarrhea, anorexia, dyspepsia, elevated liver function studies, epigastric pain, flatulence, GI bleeding, hepatitis, nausea, oral ulcerations, pancreatitis, vomiting. **GU:** nephrolithiasis, sexual dysfunction. **Derm:** pruritus, rash, sweating, urticaria. **Endo:** fat redistribution, hyperglycemia. **F and E:** dehydration. **Hemat:** anemia, leukopenia, thrombocytopenia. **Metab:** hyperlipidemia, hyperuricemia. **MS:** arthralgia, arthritis, back pain, myalgia, myopathy. **Neuro:** myasthenia, paresthesia. **Misc:** allergic reactions, fever.

PHYSICAL THERAPY IMPLICATIONS

Examination and Evaluation

- Be alert for new seizures or increased seizure activity, especially at the onset of drug treatment. Document the number, duration, and severity of seizures, and report these findings immediately to the physician.
- Be alert for signs of peripheral neuropathy (numbness, tingling) and myopathy (muscle pain, weakness). Establish baseline electroneuromyographic values using EMG and nerve conduction at the beginning of drug treatment whenever possible, and reexamine these values periodically to document drug-induced changes in nerve and muscle function.
- Assess any back pain or joint pain to rule out musculoskeletal pathology; that is, try to determine if pain is drug induced rather than caused by anatomic or biomechanical problems.
- Monitor signs of allergic reactions, including pulmonary symptoms (tightness in the throat and chest, wheezing, dyspnea) or skin reactions (rash, pruritus, urticaria). Notify physician or nursing staff immediately if these reactions occur.
- Be alert for signs of hyperglycemia, including confusion, drowsiness, flushed/dry skin, fruit-like breath odor, rapid/deep breathing, polyuria, loss of appetite, and unusual thirst. Patients with diabetes mellitus should check blood glucose levels frequently.
- Monitor signs of leukopenia (fever, sore throat, signs of infection), thrombocytopenia (bruising, nose bleeds, and bleeding gums), or unusual weakness and fatigue that might be due to anemia. Report these signs to the physician.
- Monitor and report signs of kidney stones (nephrolithiasis), including severe pain in the side and back, pain on urination, bloody urine, and a persistent urge to urinate.
- Assess dizziness and drowsiness that might affect gait, balance, and other functional activities

N

(See Appendix C). Report balance problems and functional limitations to the physician and nursing staff, and caution the patient and family/caregivers to guard against falls and trauma.
- Monitor personality changes, including anxiety, depression, mood swings, severe restlessness, and increased thoughts of suicide. Notify physician if these changes become problematic.

Interventions
- Implement resistive exercises and other therapeutic exercises as needed to maintain muscle strength and function and prevent muscle wasting associated with HIV infection and AIDS.
- Design and implement aerobic exercise and endurance training programs to help prevent heart disease associated with drug-related hyperlipidemia and other problems with lipid and glucose metabolism.
- Make sure that fluid intake is adequate during and after exercise; this drug increases the risk of dehydration.

Patient/Client-Related Instruction
- Emphasize the importance of taking nelfinavir as directed even if the patient is asymptomatic, and that this drug must always be used in combination with other antiretroviral drugs. Do not take more than prescribed amount, and do not stop taking nelinavir without consulting a health care professional.
- Inform patient that nelfinavir does not cure HIV or AIDS or prevent associated or opportunistic infections. Nelfinavir does not reduce the risk of transmission of HIV to others through sexual contact or blood contamination. Caution patient to use a condom, and to avoid sharing needles or donating blood to prevent spreading the AIDS virus to others.
- Advise patient that this drug may cause problems in fat metabolism (hyperlipidemia). Remind patient that periodic blood tests may be needed to monitor plasma lipids.
- Inform patient that redistribution and accumulation of body fat may occur, causing central obesity, thin arms and legs, dorsocervical fat enlargement (buffalo hump), breast enlargement, and other symptoms that resemble Cushing's syndrome (moon face, striations on abdominal skin). Discuss possible effects on body image, and help patient explore coping mechanisms.
- Instruct patient to immediately report signs of GI bleeding, including abdominal pain, vomiting blood, blood in stools, or black, tarry stools.
- Advise patient about the likelihood of other GI reactions, including diarrhea, nausea, vomiting, flatulence, heartburn, oral ulcerations, and loss of appetite. Instruct patient to report severe or prolonged GI problems, signs of liver toxicity (yellow skin or eyes, abdominal pain, severe nausea and vomiting, fever, sore throat, malaise, weakness, facial edema), or pancreatitis (upper abdominal pain especially after eating, indigestion, weight loss, oily stools).
- Instruct patient to report other troublesome side effects such as prolonged or severe headache, migraines, sleep loss, vision problems, sexual dysfunction, or upper respiratory tract irritation (rhinitis, sinusitis, pharyngitis).

Pharmacokinetics
Absorption: Well absorbed after oral administration.
Distribution: Unknown.
Protein Binding: >98%.
Metabolism and Excretion: Mostly metabolized (CYP3A4 enzyme system) and excreted in feces as metabolites (78%) or unchanged drug (22%); minimal renal excretion.
Half-life: 3.5–5 hr.

TIME/ACTION PROFILE (plasma levels)

ROUTE	ONSET	PEAK	DURATION
PO	rapid	2–4 hr	8 hr

Contraindications/Precautions
Contraindicated in: Hypersensitivity; Concurrent amiodarone, ergot derivatives, midazolam, quinidine, rifampin, pimozide, simvastatin, lovastatin, St. John's wort, or triazolam; Lactation: Breast-feeding should be avoided by HIV-infected patients.
Use Cautiously in: Hemophiliacs (↑ risk of bleeding); Diabetes mellitus (may exacerbate condition); Hepatic impairment.

Interactions
Drug-Drug: Concurrent **amiodarone**, **dihydroergotamine**, **ergotamine**, **methylergonovine**, **ergonovine**, **midazolam**, **simvastatin**, **lovastatin**, **pimozide**, **quinidine**, or **triazolam** should be avoided; nelfinavir inhibits the action of the CYP3A4 enzyme system and concurrent use may result in excess sedation, vasoconstriction, rhabdomyolysis or serious cardiac arrhythmias. Since nelfinavir is also metabolized by the CYP3A4 enzyme system, potent inducers of the enzyme such as **rifampin** may ↓ blood levels of nelfinavir and promote resistance to its effects; concurrent use should be avoided. ↓ metabolism may ↑ effects of **rifabutin** (dose of rifabutin should be ↓ by 50%), **carbamazepine**, **phenobarbital**, or **phenytoin** (concurrent use with rifampin should be avoided). Plasma levels and effectiveness may be ↑ by **ketoconazole**, **indinavir**, **delavirdine**, or **ritonavir**. May ↓ levels of **methadone**; dose of methadone may need to be ↑. ↑ plasma levels of **indinavir**, **saquinavir**, **cyclosporine**, **tacrolimus**, **sirolimus**, and **azithromycin**. ↑ levels and effects of **sildenafil** (sildenafil dose should not exceed 25 mg in 48 hr).

↑ levels and risk of toxicity from **atorvastatin** (use lowest dose of these agents or consider fluvastatin or pravastatin). Blood levels may be ↓ by **nevirapine**. Should not be given at the same time as **didanosine**. May ↓ plasma levels and effectiveness of **hormonal contraceptives** or **delavirdine**. May ↑ concentrations of phosphodiesterase type 5 inhibitors (PDE5) causing hypotension, visual changes, priapism; ↓ starting doses not to exceed 25 mg within 48 hr for **sildenafil**, 2.5 mg every 72 hr for **vardenafil** and 10 mg every 72 hr for **tadalafil**.
Drug-Natural: St. John's wort induces metabolism of nelfinavir, ↓ blood levels, and may promote resistance to its effects.
Drug-Food: Food ↑ absorption.

Route/Dosage

PO (Adults and Children >13 yr): 750 mg tid *or* 1250 mg bid.
PO (Children 2–13 yr): 20–30 mg/kg tid (not to exceed 750 mg tid).

Availability

Tablets: 250 mg, 625 mg. **Oral powder:** 50 mg nelfinavir/1 g powder (1 g powder/level scoopful).

neomycin (nee-oh-mye-sin)

Neo-Fradin

Classification
Therapeutic: anti-infectives
Pharmacologic: aminoglycosides

Indications

Preparation of the GI tract for surgery. Treatment of diarrhea caused by *Escherichia coli*. To decrease the number of ammonia-producing bacteria in the gut as part of the management of hepatic encephalopathy.

Action

Inhibits protein synthesis in bacteria at level of 30S ribosome. **Therapeutic Effects:** Bactericidal action. **Spectrum:** Notable for activity against *Klebsiella pneumoniae, E. coli, Proteus, Serratia, Acinetobacter, Staphylococcus aureus*.

Adverse Reactions/Side Effects

GI: diarrhea, nausea, vomiting. **Misc:** hypersensitivity reactions.

PHYSICAL THERAPY IMPLICATIONS

Examination and Evaluation

- Monitor signs of hypersensitivity reactions, including pulmonary symptoms (tightness in the throat and chest, wheezing, cough dyspnea) or skin reactions (rash, pruritus, urticaria). Notify physician or nursing staff immediately if these reactions occur.

Interventions

- Always wash hands thoroughly and disinfect equipment (whirlpools, electrotherapeutic devices, treatment tables, and so forth) to help prevent the spread of infection. Use universal precautions or isolation procedures as indicated for specific patients.

Patient/Client-Related Instruction

- Advise patient about the likelihood of GI reactions, including diarrhea, nausea, and vomiting. Instruct patient to report severe or prolonged GI problems.

Pharmacokinetics

Absorption: Minimal systemic absorption, but may accumulate in patients with renal failure.
Distribution: Widely distributed throughout extracellular fluid; crosses the placenta; small amounts enter breast milk. Poor penetration into CSF.
Metabolism and Excretion: Excretion is >90% renal.
Half-life: 2–4 hr (increased in renal impairment).

TIME/ACTION PROFILE (blood levels)

ROUTE	ONSET	PEAK	DURATION
PO	rapid	1–4 hr	N/A

Contraindications/Precautions

Contraindicated in: Hypersensitivity to neomycin or other aminoglycosides; Intestinal obstruction.
Use Cautiously in: Renal impairment (lower doses are recommended); Hearing impairment; Geriatric patients; Neuromuscular diseases such as myasthenia gravis; Pregnancy, lactation, infants, and neonates (safety not established).

Interactions

Interactions are listed for systemically absorbed drug

Drug-Drug: May enhance possible respiratory paralysis after **inhalation anesthetics** or **neuromuscular blockers**. ↑ incidence of ototoxicity with **loop diuretics**. ↑ incidence of nephrotoxicity with other **nephrotoxic drugs**. May ↑ the anticoagulant effects of **warfarin**. May ↓ the absorption of **digoxin** and **methotrexate**.

Route/Dosage

Preoperative Intestinal Antisepsis

PO (Adults): 1 g q hr for 4 doses, then 1 g q 4 hr for 5 doses *or* 1 g at 1 PM, 2 PM, and 11 PM on day before surgery.

N

PO (Children): 15 mg/kg q 4 hr for 2 days *or* 25 mg/kg at 1 PM, 2 PM, and 11 PM on day before surgery.

Hepatic Encephalopathy

PO (Adults): 1–3 g q 6 hr for 5–6 days; may be followed by 4 g/day chronically.

PO (Children): 12.5–25 mg/kg q 6 hr for 5–6 days (max dose 12 g/day).

Availability (generic available)

Oral solution: 125 mg/5 mL. **Tablets:** 500 mg. ***In combination with:*** other topical antibiotics or anti-inflammatory agents for skin, ear, and eye infections. See Appendix B.

HIGH ALERT

nesiritide (ne-sir-i-tide)

Natrecor

Classification

Therapeutic: none assigned

Pharmacologic: vasodilators (human B-type natriuretic peptide)

Indications

Acutely decompensated CHF in hospitalized patients who have dyspnea at rest or with minimal activity; has been used with digoxin, diuretics, and angiotensin-converting enzyme (ACE) inhibitors. Should not be used for intermittent outpatient infusion, scheduled repetitive use, as a diuretic or to improve renal function.

Action

Binds to guanyl cyclase receptors in vascular smooth muscle and endothelial cells, producing increased intracellular guanosine 3′5′-cyclic monophosphate (cGMP) and smooth muscle cell relaxation. cGMP acts as a "second messenger" to dilate veins and arteries. **Therapeutic Effects:** Dose-dependent reduction in pulmonary capillary wedge pressure (PCWP) and systemic arterial pressure in patients with heart failure with resultant decrease in dyspnea.

Adverse Reactions/Side Effects

CNS: anxiety, confusion, dizziness, headache, insomnia, drowsiness. **EENT:** amblyopia. **Resp:** APNEA, cough, hemoptysis. **CV:** hypotension, arrhythmias, bradycardia. **GI:** abdominal pain, nausea, vomiting. **GU:** ↑ creatinine, renal failure. **Derm:** itching, rash, sweating. **Hemat:** anemia. **Local:** injection site reactions. **MS:** back pain, leg cramps. **Neuro:** paresthesia, tremor. **Misc:** fever.

PHYSICAL THERAPY IMPLICATIONS

Examination and Evaluation

- Assess respiration, and notify physician or nursing staff immediately if patient exhibits any interruption in respiratory rate (apnea) or other severe respiratory symptoms (coughing up blood).
- Assess signs and symptoms of CHF (dyspnea, rales/crackles, peripheral edema, jugular venous distention, exercise intolerance) to help document whether drug therapy is effective in reducing these symptoms.
- Assess heart rate, ECG, and heart sounds, especially during exercise (See Appendices G, H). Report a slow heart rate (bradycardia) or symptoms of other arrhythmias, including palpitations, chest pain, shortness of breath, fainting, and fatigue/weakness.
- Assess blood pressure periodically and compare to normal values (See Appendix F). Report low blood pressure (hypotension), especially if patient experiences dizziness, fatigue, or other symptoms.
- Monitor signs of anemia, including unusual fatigue, shortness of breath with exertion, and bruising. Notify physician or nursing staff immediately if these signs occur.
- Monitor signs of renal failure, including decreased urine output, increased blood pressure, muscle cramps/twitching, edema/weight gain from fluid retention, yellowish brown skin, and confusion that progresses to seizures and coma. Report these signs to the physician or nursing staff immediately.
- Assess signs of parasthesia (numbness, tingling). Perform objective tests, including electroneuromyography and sensory testing to document any drug-related neuropathic changes.
- Assess any back pain or leg cramps to rule out musculoskeletal pathology; that is, try to determine if pain is drug induced rather than caused by anatomic or biomechanical problems.
- Assess dizziness and drowsiness that might affect gait, balance, and other functional activities (See Appendix C). Report balance problems and functional limitations to the physician and nursing staff, and caution the patient and family/caregivers to guard against falls and trauma.
- Monitor personality or behavioral changes, including anxiety, confusion, or other changes in mood. Notify physician if these changes become problematic.
- Monitor IV injection site for pain, swelling, and irritation. Report prolonged or excessive injection site reactions to the physician or nursing staff.

Interventions

- Design and implement aerobic exercise and endurance training programs as tolerated to help improve myocardial pumping ability.
- Because of an increased risk of bradycardia and other arrhythmias, use caution during aerobic exercise and endurance conditioning. Terminate exercise if patient exhibits untoward symptoms (chest pain, shortness of breath, unusual fatigue) or displays other criteria for exercise termination (See Appendix L).

- Avoid physical therapy interventions that cause systemic vasodilation (large whirlpool, Hubbard tank). Additive effects of this drug and the intervention may cause a dangerous fall in blood pressure.
- To minimize orthostatic hypotension, patient should move slowly when assuming a more upright position.

Patient/Client-Related Instruction

- Counsel patients about additional interventions to help cardiac dysfunction, including regular exercise, weight loss, sodium restriction, stress reduction, moderation of alcohol consumption, and smoking cessation.
- Instruct patient or family/caregivers to report other troublesome side effects such as severe or prolonged headache, double vision, tremor, fever, skin problems (rash, itching, sweating), or GI problems (nausea, vomiting, abdominal pain).

Pharmacokinetics

Absorption: IV administration results in complete bioavailability.
Distribution: Unknown.
Metabolism and Excretion: Cleared from circulation by binding to cell surface clearance receptors resulting in cellular internalization and proteolysis, proteolytic breakdown by endopeptidases, and renal filtration.
Half-life: 18 min.

TIME/ACTION PROFILE (effects on cardiovascular parameters)

ROUTE	ONSET	PEAK	DURATION
IV	15 min	1 hr	60 min*

*Longer with higher than recommended doses.

Contraindications/Precautions

Contraindicated in: Hypersensitivity; Cardiogenic shock; Systolic blood pressure (BP) <90 mm Hg; Low cardiac filling pressure, significant valvular stenosis, restrictive/subtractive cardiomyopathy, constrictive pericarditis/cardiac tamponade, or other conditions in which cardiac output is dependent on venous return.
Use Cautiously in: Heart failure where renal function is dependent on activity of the renin/angiotensin/aldosterone system (may cause azotemia); BP <90 mm Hg (increased risk of hypotension); Geri: Geriatric patients (some may be more sensitive to effects); Cardiogenic shock (should not be used as primary therapy); OB: Pregnancy, lactation; Pedi: Children (safety not established).

Interactions

Drug-Drug: None reported.

Route/Dosage

IV (Adults): 2 mcg/kg bolus followed by 0.01 mcg/kg/min as a continuous infusion. May increase by 0.005 mcg/kg/min every 3 hr up to a maximum infusion rate of 0.03 mcg/kg/min (based on response).

Availability

Lyophilized powder for injection (requires reconstitution): 1.5 mg/vial.

HIGH ALERT

NEUROMUSCULAR BLOCKING AGENTS (nondepolarizing)

atracurium (a-tra-kyoor-ee-um)
Tracrium

cisatracurium (sis-a-tra-**kyoor**-ee-um)
Nimbex

doxacurium (dox-a-kyoor-ee-um)
Nuromax

gallamine (gal-a-meen)
Flaxedil

metocurine (me-toe-kyoor-een)
Metubine

mivacurium (miv-a-kyoor-ee-um)
Mivacron

pancuronium (pan-kyoor-**oh**-nee-um)
Pavulon

pipecuronium (pip-e-**kyoor**-oh-nee-um)
Arduan

rocuronium (roe-kyoor-**own**-ee-um)
Zemuron

tubocurarine (too-boh-kyoor-ar-een)
Tubarine

vecuronium (ve-kyoor-**oh**-nee-um)
Norcuron

Classification
Therapeutic: neuromuscular blocking agents—nondepolarizing

N

Indications

Induction of skeletal muscle paralysis and facilitation of intubation after induction of anesthesia in surgical procedures. Facilitation of compliance during mechanical ventilation. **Metocurine, tubocurarine:** Adjunct to electroconvulsive therapy. **Tubocurarine:** Diagnostic agent for myasthenia gravis.

Action

Prevent neuromuscular transmission by blocking the effect of acetylcholine at the myoneural junction. Have no analgesic or anxiolytic properties. **Therapeutic Effects:** Skeletal muscle paralysis.

Adverse Reactions/Side Effects

Resp: bronchospasm. **CV: tubocurarine:** arrhythmias; **atracurium, metocurine, tubocurarine:** hypotension (↑ with tubocurarine); **pancuronium, gallamine:** hypertension (↑ with gallamine); **atracurium, pancuronium, gallamine:** tachycardia (↑ with gallamine). **GI: pancuronium:** excessive salivation. **Derm:** rash; **atracurium:** skin flushing. **Misc:** *ALLERGIC REACTIONS, INCLUDING ANAPHYLAXIS*.

PHYSICAL THERAPY IMPLICATIONS

Examination and Evaluation

- Monitor signs of allergic reactions and anaphylaxis, including pulmonary symptoms (tightness in the throat and chest, wheezing, cough, dyspnea) or skin reactions (rash, pruritus, urticaria). Notify physician or nursing staff immediately if these reactions occur.
- Be alert for residual skeletal muscle weakness that persists after the patient recovers from surgery. Report any strength deficits that might affect gait, balance, and other functional activities.
- Assess blood pressure (BP) and compare to normal values (See Appendix F). Report changes in BP, either a problematic decrease in BP (hypotension) or a sustained increase in BP (hypertension).
- Assess symptoms of bronchospasm (wheezing, coughing, tightness in chest) or decreased respiratory muscle function. Perform pulmonary function tests to quantify suspected changes in ventilation and respiration (See Appendix I).
- Assess heart rate, ECG, and heart sounds, especially during exercise (See Appendices G, H). Report any rhythm disturbances or symptoms of increased arrhythmias, including palpitations, chest discomfort, shortness of breath, fainting, and fatigue/weakness.
- If used during mechanical ventilation, observe whether the chest wall is relaxed and compliant with ventilation. Notify physician or nursing staff if the patient is agitated or appears to be resisting mechanical ventilation.

Patient/Client-Related Instruction

- Instruct patient to report other troublesome side effects such as excessive salivation or skin problems (rash, flushing).

Pharmacokinetics

Absorption: Following IV administration, absorption is essentially complete. *Tubocurarine*—Although well absorbed following IM administration, effect is delayed as compared with IV administration.

Distribution: *Atracurium, gallamine*—Distribute into extracellular space; cross the placenta. *Metocurine*—Extensively distributed; crosses the placenta. *Mivacurium*—Tissue distribution is limited. *Pancuronium*—Rapidly distributes into extracellular fluid; small amounts cross the placenta. *Tubocurarine*—Extensively distributed and subsequently redistributed to various tissue compartments; saturation of compartments occurs, explaining prolonged duration of action following repeated doses. *Vecuronium*—Rapidly distributed in extracellular fluid; minimal penetration of the CNS.

Metabolism and Excretion: *Atracurium, mivacurium*—Metabolized in plasma. *Cisatracurium*—Undergoes pH-dependent breakdown, which is responsible for 80% of metabolism; remainder eliminated by liver and kidneys. *Doxacurium*—Excreted primarily unchanged in urine and bile. *Gallamine*—Excreted almost entirely unchanged by the kidneys. *Metocurine*—50% excreted unchanged in urine. *Pancuronium*—Excreted mostly unchanged by the kidneys; small amounts are eliminated in bile. *Pipecuronium*—>75% excreted by the kidneys, mostly as unmetabolized drug. *Rocuronium*—Mostly metabolized by the liver. *Tubocurarine*—30–75% excreted unchanged by the kidneys; 11% excreted in bile; small amounts are metabolized by the liver. *Vecuronium*—Some metabolism by the liver (20%), with conversion to at least 1 active metabolite; 35% excreted unchanged by the kidneys.

Half-life: *Atracurium*—Infants: 20 min; Children: 17 min; Adults: 16 min; *cisatracurium*—22–31 min; *doxacurium*—1.5 hr (increased to 3.7 hr in renal dysfunction and 1.9 hr in liver dysfunction); *gallamine*—2.5 hr; *metocurine*—3.6 hr; *mivacurium*—Trans-trans isomer: 2.3 min; cis-trans isomer 2.1 min; *pancuronium*—2 hr; *pipecuronium*—1.7 hr (prolonged in renal impairment); *rocuronium*—Infants 3–12 mo: 0.8–1.8 hr; Children 1–3 yr: 0.4–1.8 hr; Children 3–8 yr: 0.5–1.1 hr; Adults: 1.4–2.4 hr (increased to 4.3 hr in hepatic impairment and 2.4 hr in renal impairment); *tubocurarine*—2 hr; *vecuronium*—Infants: 65 min; Children: 41 min; Adults: 65–75 min (↓ near term in pregnant patients; ↑ in patients with hepatic impairment).

TIME/ACTION PROFILE (neuromuscular blockade)

ROUTE	ONSET	PEAK	DURATION
atracurium IV	1–4 min	3–5 min	20–35 min
cisatracurium IV	2–3 min	3–5 min	28–50 min
doxacurium IV	5–11 min	unknown	12–54 min
gallamine IV	1–2 min	3–5 min	15–30 min
metocurine IV	within min	6 min	25–90 min*
mivacurium IV (adults)	1–3 min	3.3 min	26 min
mivacurium IV (children)	rapid	1.9 min	19 min
pancuronium IV	30–45 sec	2–3 min	40–60 min
pipecuronium IV	2.5–3 min	5 min	1–2 hr
rocuronium IV	1 min	0.5–1 min (peds) 1–3.7 min (adults)	26–40 min (peds) 31 min†
tubocurarine IV	1 min	2–5 min	2–90 min
tubocurarine IM	15–25 min	unknown	unknown
vecuronium IV	1–3 min	3–5 min	30–40 min

*Total recovery of function may take several hours.

†Following 0.6 mg/kg dose in adult patients.

Contraindications/Precautions

Contraindicated in: Hypersensitivity; Hypersensitivity to bromides (pancuronium, vecuronium only); Hypersensitivity to iodides/iodine (gallamine, metocurine only); Products containing benzyl alcohol should be avoided in neonates.

Use Cautiously in: Patients with underlying cardiovascular disease (↑ risk of arrhythmias; less with atracurium or vecuronium); Dehydration or electrolyte abnormalities (should be corrected); Situations in which histamine release would be problematic (worse with atracurium, mivacurium, and doxacurium; less with cisatracurium and vecuronium); Fractures or muscle spasm; Geriatric patients or patients with impaired renal function (slower onset to complete paralysis with cisatracurium; ↓ elimination of gallamine, metocurine, pancuronium, tubocurarine); Hyperthermia (↑ duration/intensity of paralysis); Patients with significant hepatic impairment (↓ metabolism of vecuronium, altered response to others); Shock (prolonged paralysis from gallamine, metocurine, tubocurarine); Extensive burns (may be more resistant to effects of cisatracurium); Low plasma pseudocholinesterase levels (may be seen in association with anemia, dehydration, cholinesterase inhibitors/insecticides, severe liver disease, pregnancy, or hereditary predisposition); Obese patients; Pregnancy, lactation, or children (safety not established for some agents; most agents have been used safely in pregnant women undergoing cesarean section; selected agents have been used safely in children).

Exercise Extreme Caution in: Patients with neuromuscular diseases such as myasthenia gravis (small test dose may be used to assess response).

Interactions

Drug-Drug: Intensity and duration of paralysis may be prolonged by pretreatment with **succinylcholine, general anesthesia** (inhalation), **aminoglycosides, vancomycin, tetracyclines, polymyxin B, colistin, clindamycin, lidocaine**, and other **local anesthetics, lithium, quinidine, procainamide, beta-adrenergic blocking agents, potassium-losing diuretics**, or **magnesium**. Effects of cisatracurium may be enhanced by concurrent **enflurane** or **isoflurane** (dosage requirements may be decreased by 30–40%; smaller boluses and lower infusion rates may be necessary). Higher infusion rates may be required and duration of action may be shortened in patients receiving long-term **carbamazepine** or **phenytoin**.

Route/Dosage

Atracurium

IV (Adults and Children >2 yr): 0.4–0.5 mg/kg initially (0.25–0.35 mg/kg if administered after steady-state anesthesia with enflurane or isoflurane or 0.3–0.4 mg/kg following succinylcholine) then may repeat 0.08–0.1 mg/kg 20–45 min after initial dose as needed, or by continuous infusion at 0.4–0.8 mg/kg/hr.

IV (Neonates, Infants, and Children up to 2 yr): 0.3–0.4 mg/kg initially followed by maintenance doses of 0.3–0.4 mg/kg as needed or 0.6–1.2 mg/kg/hr via continuous infusion.

Cisatracurium

IV (Adults and Children >12 yr): *Initial intubating dose*—0.15–0.2 mg/kg, additional maintenance doses of 0.03 mg/kg may be used 40–65 min later; *continuous infusion*—1–3 mcg/kg/min.

IV (Children 2–12 yr): *Initial intubating dose*—0.1 mg/kg followed by a maintenance dose of 0.03 mg/kg as needed; *continuous infusion*—1–4 mcg/kg/min.

Doxacurium

IV (Adults and Children >12 yr): 25–50 mcg/kg (may need up to 80 mcg/kg for prolonged effect; 25 mcg/kg for succinylcholine-assisted intubation) initially, followed 60–100 min later by 5–10 mcg/kg, repeated as required or 6–12 mcg/kg/hr via continuous infusion.

IV (Children 2–12 yr): 30–50 mcg/kg initially; maintenance doses of 5–10 mcg/kg may be required more frequently than in adults or 6–12 mcg/kg/hr via continuous infusion.

Gallamine

IV (Adults and Children): 1 mg/kg (not to exceed 100 mg/dose), then 0.5–1 mg/kg may be given 30–40 min later if needed during prolonged procedures; dose cautiously in patients <5 kg.

Metocurine

IV (Adults): 150–400 mcg/kg initially; may give additional doses of 0.5–1 mg q 30–90 min. *Adjunct to electroconvulsive therapy*—2–3 mg (range 1.75–5.5 mg).

Mivacurium

IV (Adults): 150–200 mcg/kg initially, then 100 mcg/kg as bolus doses every 15 min or as a continuous infusion at 9–10 mcg/kg/min. If infusion is begun at the same time as initial dose, start with rate of 4 mcg/kg/min. Infusion rates may range from 1–20 mcg/kg/min.

IV (Children 2–12 yr): 200 mcg/kg initially; may be repeated as needed or continued as an infusion at 10–14 mcg/kg/min (range 5–31 mcg/kg/min).

Pancuronium

IV (Adults and Children >12 yr): 0.15 mg/kg initially; repeat doses may be given q 30–60 min to maintain paralysis. *Continuous infusion*—0.02–0.04 mg/kg/hr.

IV (Children 1–12 yr): 0.15 mg/kg initially; repeat doses may be given q 30–60 min to maintain paralysis. *Continuous infusion*—0.03–0.1 mg/kg/hr.

IV (Neonates and Infants up to 1 yr): 0.1 mg/kg initially; repeat doses may be given q 30–60 min to maintain paralysis. *Continuous infusion*—0.02–0.04 mg/kg/hr.

Pipecuronium

IV (Adults): 70–85 mcg/kg (if given following recovery from succinylcholine during intubation, decrease dose to 50 mcg/kg; 70–85 mcg/kg if longer paralysis desired). Additional doses of 10–15 mcg/kg may be required as maintenance (dosage reduction recommended if using concurrent inhalation anesthetics). Dose should be determined on the basis of ideal body weight in obese patients and may require adjustments in patients with renal impairment.

IV (Children 1–14 yr): 57 mcg/kg initial dose.

IV (Infants 3 mo–1 yr): 40 mcg/kg initial dose.

Rocuronium

IV (Adults and Children >12 yr): *Rapid sequence tracheal intubation*—0.6–1.2 mg/kg; *maintenance dosing*—0.1–0.2 mg/kg; *continuous infusion*—10–12 mcg/kg/min (range 4–16 mcg/kg/min).

IV (Children): *Intubation dose*—0.6 mg)/kg; *maintenance dose*— 0.075–0.125 mg/kg; *continuous infusion*—10–12 mcg/kg/min (range 4–16 mcg/kg/min).

IV (Infants): 0.5 mg/kg/dose q 20–30 min as needed.

Tubocurarine

Preferred route is IV, but IM may be used in infants or other patients without venous access.

IM, IV (Adults): 6–9 mg initially, followed by 3–4.5 mg after 3–5 min if needed. Additional doses of 3 mg (0.165 mg/kg) may be given as needed. *Provision of relaxation to allow mechanical ventilation*—1 mg IV (16.5 mcg/kg); subsequent doses may be given as necessary; *adjunct to electroconvulsive therapy*—165 mcg/kg IV (initial doses should be 3 mg less than calculated dose); *diagnosis of myasthenia gravis*—4–33 mcg/kg IV. Profound myasthenic symptoms may occur.

IV (Infants and Children): 500 mcg/kg.

IV (Neonates–4 wk): 250–500 mcg/kg initially, then additional increments of $\frac{1}{5}$–$\frac{1}{6}$ of initial dose may be given.

Vecuronium

IV (Adults and Children >10 yr): *Intubation*—80–100 mcg/kg for intubation (60–85 mcg/kg if given after steady-state anesthesia achieved or 40–60 mcg/kg after succinylcholine-assisted intubation and anesthesia; wait for disappearance of succinylcholine effects; or 50–60 mcg/kg during balanced anesthesia). Up to 150–280 mcg/kg have been used in some patients; *maintenance*—10–15 mcg/kg 25–40 min after initial dose, then q 12–15 min as needed or as a continuous infusion at 1.5–2 mcg/kg/min.

IV (Children >1 yr): 100 mcg/kg q 1 hr as needed or as a continuous infusion of 1.5–2.5 mcg/kg/min.

IV (Infants >7 wk–1 yr): 100 mcg/kg q 1 hr as needed or as a continuous infusion of 1–1.5 mcg/kg/min.

IV (Neonates): 100 mcg/kg initially then 30–150 mcg/kg/dose q 1–2 hr as needed.

Availability

Atracurium (generic available)

Injection: 10 mg/mL in 5-mL ampules and 10-mL vials.

Cisatracurium

Solution for injection: 2 mg/mL in 5-mL single-use vials or 10-mL multiple-dose vials (with benzyl alcohol), 10 mg/mL in 20 mL vials Rx.

Doxacurium

Injection: 1 mg/mL in 5-mL vials.

Gallamine

Injection: 20 mg/mL in 10-mL vials.

Metocurine (generic available)

Injection: 2 mg/mL in 20-mL vials.

Mivacurium
Injection: 0.5 mg/mL premixed infusion in 50 mL D5W, 2 mg/mL in 5- and 10-mL vials.

Pancuronium
Injection: 1 mg/mL in 10-mL vials, 2 mg/mL in 2- and 5-mL ampules.

Pipecuronium
Powder for injection: 10 mg/vial.

Rocuronium
Injection: 10 mg/mL in 5-mL vials.

Tubocurarine (generic available)
Injection: 3 mg (20 units)/min 10- and 20-mL vials and 5-mL syringes.

Vecuronium (generic available)
Powder for injection: 10 mg and 20 mg vials.

nevirapine (ne-veer-a-peen)

Viramune

Classification
Therapeutic: antiretrovirals
Pharmacologic: nonnucleoside reverse transcriptase inhibitors

Indications

Management of HIV infection in combination with a nucleoside analogue.

Action

Binds to the enzyme reverse transcriptase, which results in disruption of DNA synthesis. **Therapeutic Effects:** Slowed progression of HIV infection and decreased occurrence of sequelae.

Adverse Reactions/Side Effects

Reflects combination therapy

CNS: headache. **GI:** HEPATOTOXICITY, elevated liver enzyme levels, nausea, abdominal pain, diarrhea, hepatitis, ulcerative stomatitis. **Derm:** RASH (MAY PROGRESS TO TOXIC EPIDERMAL NECROLYSIS). **Hemat:** granulocytopenia (increased in children). **MS:** myalgia. **Neuro:** paresthesia, peripheral neuropathy. **Misc:** STEVENS-JOHNSON SYNDROME, fever.

PHYSICAL THERAPY IMPLICATIONS

Examination and Evaluation

- Monitor skin rash and other skin reactions (dermatitis, exfoliation). Report skin problems immediately because they may represent serious hypersensitivity reactions (Stevens-Johnson Syndrome).
- Be alert for signs of hepatotoxicity, including anorexia, abdominal pain, severe nausea and vomiting, yellow skin or eyes, fever, sore throat, malaise, weakness, facial edema, lethargy, and unusual bleeding or bruising. Report these signs to the physician immediately.
- Be alert for signs of paresthesia and peripheral neuropathy (numbness, tingling, decreased muscle strength). Establish baseline electroneuromyographic values using EMG and nerve conduction at the beginning of drug treatment whenever possible, and reexamine these values periodically to document drug-induced changes in peripheral nerve function.
- Assess any muscle pain to rule out musculoskeletal pathology; that is, try to determine if pain is drug induced rather than caused by anatomic or biomechanical problems.

Interventions

- Implement resistive exercises and other therapeutic exercises as tolerated to maintain muscle strength and function and prevent muscle wasting associated with HIV infection and AIDS.

Patient/Client-Related Instruction

- Emphasize the importance of taking nevirapine as directed even if the patient is asymptomatic, and that this drug must always be used in combination with other antiretroviral drugs. Do not take more than prescribed amount, and do not stop taking without consulting a health care professional.
- Inform patient that nevirapine does not cure HIV or AIDS or prevent associated or opportunistic infections. Nevirapine does not reduce the risk of transmission of HIV to others through sexual contact or blood contamination. Caution patient to use a condom, and to avoid sharing needles or donating blood to prevent spreading the AIDS virus to others.
- Instruct children and family/caregivers to report symptoms of granulocytopenia, including fever, sore throat, mucosal lesions, signs of infection, and bruising.
- Instruct patient to report other troublesome side effects such as prolonged or severe headache, fever, or GI reactions (nausea, diarrhea, abdominal pain, and inflammation/ulceration in/around the mouth).

Pharmacokinetics

Absorption: >90% absorbed after oral administration.
Distribution: Crosses placenta and enters breast milk; CSF levels are 45% of those in plasma.
Metabolism and Excretion: Mostly metabolized by the liver (CYP3A4 enzyme system); minor amounts excreted unchanged in urine.

Half-life: 25–30 hr (during multiple dosing).

TIME/ACTION PROFILE (blood levels)

ROUTE	ONSET	PEAK	DURATION
PO	rapid	4 hr	12 hr

Contraindications/Precautions

Contraindicated in: Hypersensitivity; Concurrent ketoconazole, rifampin, or St. John's wort; Moderate-to-severe hepatic impairment (Child-Pugh Class B or C); Women with CD4+ cell counts >250 cells/mm^3 (↑ risk of liver toxicity).
Use Cautiously in: Women (↑ risk of liver toxicity); Hepatic or renal impairment; Concurrent clarithromycin, fluconazole, methadone, or rifabutin (careful monitoring required; alternative therapy should be considered); OB/Lactation/Pedi: Safety not established; breast-feeding not recommended in HIV-infected patients.

Interactions

Drug-Drug: Nevirapine induces the hepatic CYP3A4 enzyme system and can affect the behavior of drugs metabolized by this system. Significantly ↓ **ketoconazole** levels (concurrent use contraindicated). May induce **methadone** withdrawal within 2 wk of starting therapy in patients physically dependent on methadone. May ↓ levels and effectiveness **hormonal contraceptives** (concurrent use of hormonal contraceptives should be avoided). **Rifampin** significantly ↓ levels and effectiveness of nevirapine (concurrent use contraindicated). ↓ levels and effectiveness of **clarithromycin** (consider other agents). Also may ↓ levels and effectiveness of the following: **lopinavir, saquinavir, nelfinavir, indinavir, efavirenz, amiodarone, disopyramide, lidocaine, itraconazole, carbamazepine, clonazepam, ethosuximide, diltiazem, nifedipine, verapamil, cyclosporine, tacrolimus, sirolimus, cyclophosphamide, ergotamine fentanyl, rifabutin** (use together only with careful monitoring). **Fluconazole** ↑ nevirapine levels and risk of toxicity. May ↑ risk of bleeding with **warfarin**. Use of **prednisone** during first 2 wk of therapy may ↑ risk of rash. Initiating other **drugs that often cause rash**, including **trimethoprim/sulfamethoxazole** and **abacavir** simultaneously with nevirapine may ↑ risk of rash.
Drug-Natural: St. John's wort may ↓ efficacy.

Route/Dosage

PO (Adults): 200 mg daily for the first 2 wk, then 200 mg bid (in combination with a nucleoside analogue antiretroviral).
PO (Children ≥15 days): 150 mg/m^2 once daily for first 2 wk, then 150 mg/m^2 bid.

Availability

Tablets: 200 mg. **Oral suspension:** 50 mg/5 mL.

niacin (nye-a-sin)

Edur-Acin, Nia-Bid, Niac, Niacels, Niacor, Niaspan, Nicobid, Nico-400, Nicolar, Nicotinex, Novo-Niacin, Slo-Niacin

Other Names:
Nicotinic acid, Vitamin B

niacinamide (nye-a-sin-a-mide)

Nicotinamide

Classification
Therapeutic: lipid-lowering agents, vitamins
Pharmacologic: water-soluble vitamins

Indications

Treatment and prevention of niacin deficiency (pellagra). Adjunctive therapy in certain hyperlipidemias (niacin only).

Action

Required as coenzymes (for lipid metabolism, glycogenolysis, and tissue respiration). Large doses decrease lipoprotein and triglyceride synthesis by inhibiting the release of free fatty acids from adipose tissue and decreasing hepatic lipoprotein synthesis (niacin only). Cause peripheral vasodilation in large doses (niacin only). **Therapeutic Effects:** Decreased blood lipids (niacin only). Supplementation in deficiency states.

Adverse Reactions/Side Effects

Adverse reactions and side effects refer to IV administration or doses used to treat hyperlipidemias
CNS: nervousness, panic. **EENT:** blurred vision, loss of central vision, proptosis, toxic amblyopia. **CV:** orthostatic hypotension. **GI:** HEPATOTOXICITY (ER ORAL FORM ONLY), GI upset, bloating, diarrhea, dry mouth, flatulence, heartburn, hunger pains, nausea, peptic ulceration. **Derm:** flushing of the face and neck, pruritus, burning, dry skin, hyperpigmentation, increased sebaceous gland activity, rashes, stinging or tingling of skin. **Metab:** glycosuria, hyperglycemia, hyperuricemia.

PHYSICAL THERAPY IMPLICATIONS

Examination and Evaluation

- Be alert for signs of hepatotoxicity, including anorexia, abdominal pain, severe nausea and vomiting, yellow skin or eyes, fever, sore throat, malaise, weakness, facial edema, lethargy, and unusual bleeding or bruising. Report these signs to the physician immediately.
- Assess any muscle pain, tenderness, or weakness, especially if niacin is used with other lipid-lowering drugs (statins, fibric acids). Advise patient that these

symptoms may represent drug-induced myopathy, and that myopathy can progress to severe muscle damage (rhabdomyolysis). Report any unexplained musculoskeletal symptoms to the physician immediately, and suspend exercise and gait training until these symptoms can be evaluated.
- Assess blood pressure (BP) when patient assumes a more upright position (lying to standing, sitting to standing, lying to sitting). Document orthostatic hypotension and contact physician when systolic BP falls >20 mm Hg, or diastolic BP falls >10 mm Hg.
- Report signs of CNS toxicity including nervousness, panic attacks, or vision disturbances.
- Monitor any rash or other skin reactions (burning/itching skin, dryness, increased pigmentation). Report severe or unexpected skin reactions to the physician.

Interventions

- In patients with drug-induced myopathy, implement gradual strengthening and other therapeutic exercises to facilitate recovery from muscle pain and weakness. Use caution during early stages to avoid fatigue of affected muscles, and implement assistive devices (walker, cane, crutches) as needed to prevent falls and assist mobility. Increase exercise intensity as tolerated; recovery from myopathy typically takes 4–6 wk, but can be longer in older patients or people with comorbidities.
- Design and implement aerobic exercise and endurance training programs to improve cardiovascular function and help reduce the risk of coronary heart disease.
- To minimize orthostatic hypotension, patient should move slowly when assuming a more upright position.

Patient/Client-Related Instruction

- Remind patients to take medication as directed to control hyperlipidemia even though they are asymptomatic.
- Counsel patients about additional interventions to help control lipid disorders and improve cardiovascular health, such as dietary modification, regular exercise, moderation of alcohol consumption, and smoking cessation.
- Advise patient that cutaneous flushing and a sensation of warmth may occur within the first 2 hr after taking the drug. These sensations often occur in the face, neck, and ears, and may also include itching, tingling, and headache. These effects are usually transient and subside with continued therapy.
- Advise patient about symptoms of hyperglycemia (confusion, drowsiness; flushed, dry skin; fruit-like breath odor; rapid, deep breathing, polyuria; loss of appetite; unusual thirst). Insulin dosages may need to be adjusted to prevent repeated episodes of hyperglycemia.
- Instruct patient to report prolonged or severe GI reactions including diarrhea, heartburn, flatulence, dry mouth, and abdominal bloating.

Pharmacokinetics

Absorption: Well absorbed following oral administration.
Distribution: Widely distributed following conversion to niacinamide. Enters breast milk.
Metabolism and Excretion: Amounts required for metabolic processes are converted to niacinamide. Large doses of niacin are excreted unchanged in the urine.
Half-life: 45 min.

TIME/ACTION PROFILE (effects on blood lipids)

ROUTE	ONSET	PEAK	DURATION
PO (cholesterol)	several days	unknown	unknown
PO (triglycerides)	several hrs	unknown	unknown

Contraindications/Precautions

Contraindicated in: Hypersensitivity to niacin; Some products may contain tartrazine and should be avoided in patients with known hypersensitivity; Alcohol intolerance (Nicotinex only).
Use Cautiously in: Liver disease; Arterial bleeding; History of peptic ulcer disease; Gout; Glaucoma; Diabetes mellitus.

Interactions

Drug-Drug: ↑ risk of myopathy with concurrent use of **HMG CoA reductase inhibitors.** Additive hypotension with ganglionic blocking agents (**guanadrel**). Large doses may ↓ uricosuric effects of **probenecid** or **sulfinpyrazone.**

Route/Dosage

PO (Adults and Children): *Dietary supplement*—10–20 mg/day. *Dietary deficiency*—Up to 500 mg/day in divided doses. *Hyperlipidemias (Niacin only)*—100–500 mg/day initially; increase slowly up to 1–2 g tid (up to 8 g/day).
PO (Children 7–10 yr): *Prevention of deficiency*—13 mg/day.
PO (Children 4–6 yr): *Prevention of deficiency*—12 mg/day.
PO (Children birth–3 yr): *Prevention of deficiency*—5–9 mg/day.

Availability

Niacin (generic available)

Tablets: 25 mg OTC, 50 mg OTC, 100 mg OTC, 125 mg OTC, 250 mg OTC, 400 mg OTC, 500 mg Rx, OTC.

Extended-release tablets: 125 mg Rx, OTC, 250 mg Rx, OTC, 400 mg OTC, 500 mg Rx, OTC, 750 mg Rx, OTC, 1000 mg OTC. **Extended-release capsules:** 125 mg Rx, OTC, 250 mg Rx, OTC, 300 mg Rx, OTC, 400 mg Rx, OTC, 500 mg Rx, OTC. **Elixir:** 50 mg/5 mL in pints and gallons OTC. ***In combination with:*** lovastatin (Advicor); simvastatin (Simcor). See Appendix B.

Niacinamide (generic available)

Tablets: 50 mg OTC, 100 mg OTC, 125 mg OTC, 250 mg OTC, 500 mg Rx, OTC.

nicardipine (nye-kar-di-peen)

Cardene, Cardene SR, Cardene IV

Classification

Therapeutic: antianginals, antihypertensives

Pharmacologic: calcium channel blockers

Indications

Management of Hypertension, Angina pectoris, Vasospastic (Prinzmetal's) angina. **Unlabeled Use:** Management of CHF.

Action

Inhibits the transport of calcium into myocardial and vascular smooth muscle cells, resulting in inhibition of excitation-contraction coupling and subsequent contraction. **Therapeutic Effects:** Systemic vasodilation resulting in decreased blood pressure. Coronary vasodilation resulting in decreased frequency and severity of attacks of angina.

Adverse Reactions/Side Effects

CNS: abnormal dreams, anxiety, confusion, dizziness, drowsiness, headache, jitteriness, nervousness, psychiatric disturbances, weakness. **EENT:** blurred vision, disturbed equilibrium, epistaxis, tinnitus. **Resp:** cough, dyspnea, shortness of breath. **CV:** ARRHYTHMIAS, CHF, peripheral edema, bradycardia, chest pain, hypotension, palpitations, syncope, tachycardia. **GI:** abnormal results in liver function studies, anorexia, constipation, diarrhea, dry mouth, dysgeusia, dyspepsia, nausea, vomiting. **GU:** dysuria, nocturia, polyuria, sexual dysfunction, urinary frequency. **Derm:** dermatitis, erythema multiforme, flushing, increased sweating, photosensitivity, pruritus/urticaria, rash. **Endo:** gynecomastia, hyperglycemia. **Hemat:** anemia, leukopenia, thrombocytopenia. **Metab:** weight gain. **MS:** joint stiffness, muscle cramps. **Neuro:** paresthesia, tremor. **Misc:** STEVENS-JOHNSON SYNDROME, gingival hyperplasia.

PHYSICAL THERAPY IMPLICATIONS

Examination and Evaluation

- Assess heart rate, ECG, and heart sounds, especially during exercise (See Appendices G, H). Report any rhythm disturbances or symptoms of increased arrhythmias, including palpitations, chest pain, shortness of breath, fainting, and fatigue/weakness.
- Monitor rashes or other skin reactions (hives, abnormal sweating, itching/burning, exfoliation). Notify physician immediately because certain skin reactions may indicate serious hypersensitivity reactions (Stevens-Johnson syndrome).
- Assess routinely for signs of CHF and pulmonary edema (dyspnea, cough, shortness of breath, rales/crackles, jugular venous distention). Report the appearance of these signs in patients who do not have CHF, or any improvement in symptoms if this drug is used to help manage CHF.
- Assess blood pressure periodically and compare to normal values (See Appendix F) to help document antihypertensive effects.
- Assess episodes of angina pectoris at rest and during exercise. Document whether drug therapy is helpful in reducing the frequency and severity of anginal attacks.
- Assess peripheral edema using girth measurements, volume displacement, and measurement of pitting edema (See Appendix N). Report increased swelling in feet and ankles due to peripheral vasodilation.
- Watch for signs of hyperglycemia, including confusion, drowsiness, flushed/dry skin, fruit-like breath odor, rapid/deep breathing, polyuria, loss of appetite, and unusual thirst. Insulin dosages may need to be adjusted to prevent repeated episodes of hyperglycemia.
- Monitor and report signs of leukopenia (fever, sore throat, signs of infection), thrombocytopenia (bruising, nose bleeds, and bleeding gums), or unusual weakness and fatigue that might be due to anemia.
- Assess signs of paresthesia (numbness, tingling) or muscle twitching. Perform objective tests, including electroneuromyography and sensory testing to document any drug-related neuropathic changes.
- Assess any joint stiffness or muscle cramping to rule out musculoskeletal pathology; that is, try to determine if pain is drug induced rather than caused by anatomic or biomechanical problems.
- Assess dizziness and weakness that might affect gait, balance, and other functional activities (See Appendix C). Report balance problems and functional limitations to the physician, and caution the patient and family/caregivers to guard against falls and trauma.
- Monitor mood and personality changes, including anxiety, nervousness, confusion, or other psychiatric disturbances. Notify physician if these changes become problematic.

Interventions

- Design and implement aerobic exercise and endurance training programs to normalize blood pressure, improve coronary perfusion, reduce angina, and improve myocardial pumping ability.
- Because of the risk of cardiac arrhythmias and CHF, use caution during aerobic exercise and other forms of therapeutic exercise. Assess exercise tolerance frequently (blood pressure, heart rate, fatigue levels), and terminate exercise immediately if any untoward responses occur (See Appendix L).
- Guard against falls and trauma (hip fractures, head injury). Implement fall prevention strategies, especially if patient exhibits dizziness or disturbed equilibrium (See Appendix E).
- To minimize orthostatic hypotension, patient should move slowly when assuming a more upright position.
- Causes photosensitivity; use care if administering UV treatments.

Patient/Client-Related Instruction

- Remind patients to take medication as directed to control hypertension and other cardiac conditions even if they are asymptomatic.
- Counsel patients about additional interventions to help control blood pressure and cardiac dysfunction, including regular exercise, weight loss, sodium restriction, stress reduction, moderation of alcohol consumption, and smoking cessation.
- Advise patient about photosensitivity, and to use sunscreens, protective clothing, and avoid prolonged sun exposure. Advise patient to also report any rashes or other skin reactions.
- Instruct patient or family/caregivers to report other troublesome side effects such as severe or prolonged headache, tinnitus, nightmares, tremor, weight gain, problems with urination, sexual dysfunction, breast enlargement in men (gynecomastia), or GI problems (nausea, vomiting, constipation, diarrhea, indigestion, loss of appetite).

Pharmacokinetics

Absorption: Well absorbed following oral administration but extensively metabolized, resulting in decreased bioavailability.
Distribution: Unknown.
Metabolism and Excretion: Mostly metabolized by the liver; ≤10% excreted unchanged by kidneys.
Half-life: 2–4 hr.

TIME/ACTION PROFILE (cardiovascular effects)

ROUTE	ONSET	PEAK	DURATION
PO	20 min	0.5–2 hr	8 hr
PO-ER	unknown	unknown	12 hr
IV	within min	45 min	50 hr*

*Following discontinuation.

Contraindications/Precautions

Contraindicated in: Hypersensitivity; Sick sinus syndrome; 2nd- or 3rd-degree AV block (unless an artificial pacemaker is in place); BP <90 mm Hg; Advanced aortic stenosis.
Use Cautiously in: Severe hepatic impairment (dose reduction recommended); Geri: Geriatric patients (dose reduction/slower IV infusion rates recommended for most agents; increased risk of hypotension); Severe renal impairment (dose reduction may be necessary); History of serious ventricular arrhythmias or CHF; OB/Lactation/Pedi: Pregnancy, lactation, or children (safety not established).

Interactions

Drug-Drug: Additive hypotension may occur when used concurrently with **fentanyl**, other **antihypertensives, nitrates**, acute ingestion of **alcohol**, or **quinidine**. Antihypertensive effects may be ↓ by concurrent use of **NSAIDs**. Concurrent use with **beta blockers, digoxin, disopyramide**, or **phenytoin** may result in bradycardia, conduction defects, or CHF. **Cimetidine** and **propranolol** may ↓ metabolism and increase the risk of toxicity. May ↓ the metabolism of and ↑ risk of toxicity from **cyclosporine, prazosin, quinidine**, or **carbamazepine**.
Drug-Food: Grapefruit and Grapefruit juice ↑ serum levels and effect.

Route/Dosage

PO (Adults): 20 mg 3 times daily, may increase q 3 days (range 20–40 mg tid); or 30 mg bid as sustained-release form (up to 60 mg bid).
IV (Adults): *To replace PO use*—0.5–2.2 mg/hr continuous infusion. *For acute hypertensive episodes*—5 mg/hr titrated as needed (up to 15 mg/hr).

Availability (generic available)

Capsules: 20 mg, 30 mg. **Sustained-release capsules:** 30 mg, 45 mg, 60 mg. **Injection:** 2.5 mg/mL in 10-mL amps.

nifedipine (nye-**fed**-i-peen)

🍁 Adalat, Adalat CC, Adalat PA, 🍁 Adalat XL, Afeditab CR, Apo-Nifed, Nifedical XL, Novo-Nifedin, Nu-Nifed, Procardia, Procardia XL

Classification
Therapeutic: antianginals, antihypertensives
Pharmacologic: calcium channel blockers

Indications

Management of Hypertension (extended-release only), Angina pectoris, Vasospastic (Prinzmetal's) angina.

Unlabeled Use: Prevention of migraine headache. Management of CHF or cardiomyopathy.

Action

Inhibits calcium transport into myocardial and vascular smooth muscle cells, resulting in inhibition of excitation-contraction coupling and subsequent contraction. **Therapeutic Effects:** Systemic vasodilation, resulting in decreased blood pressure. Coronary vasodilation, resulting in decreased frequency and severity of attacks of angina.

Adverse Reactions/Side Effects

CNS: headache, abnormal dreams, anxiety, confusion, dizziness, drowsiness, jitteriness, nervousness, psychiatric disturbances, weakness. **EENT:** blurred vision, disturbed equilibrium, epistaxis, tinnitus. **Resp:** cough, dyspnea, shortness of breath. **CV:** ARRHYTHMIAS, CHF, peripheral edema, bradycardia, chest pain, hypotension, palpitations, syncope, tachycardia. **GI:** abnormal liver function studies, anorexia, constipation, diarrhea, dry mouth, dysgeusia, dyspepsia, nausea, vomiting. **GU:** dysuria, nocturia, polyuria, sexual dysfunction, urinary frequency. **Derm:** flushing, dermatitis, erythema multiforme, increased sweating, photosensitivity, pruritus/urticaria, rash. **Endo:** gynecomastia, hyperglycemia. **Hemat:** anemia, leukopenia, thrombocytopenia. **Metab:** weight gain. **MS:** joint stiffness, muscle cramps. **Neuro:** paresthesia, tremor. **Misc:** STEVENS-JOHNSON SYNDROME, gingival hyperplasia.

PHYSICAL THERAPY IMPLICATIONS

Examination and Evaluation

- Assess heart rate, ECG, and heart sounds, especially during exercise (See Appendices G, H). Report any rhythm disturbances or symptoms of increased arrhythmias, including palpitations, chest pain, shortness of breath, fainting, and fatigue/weakness.
- Monitor rashes or other skin reactions (hives, abnormal sweating, itching/burning, exfoliation). Notify physician immediately because certain skin reactions may indicate serious hypersensitivity reactions (Stevens-Johnson syndrome).
- Assess routinely for signs of CHF and pulmonary edema (dyspnea, cough, shortness of breath, rales/crackles, jugular venous distention). Report these signs to the physician.
- Assess blood pressure periodically and compare to normal values (See Appendix F) to help document antihypertensive effects.
- Assess episodes of angina pectoris at rest and during exercise. Document whether drug therapy is helpful in reducing the frequency and severity of anginal attacks.
- If used to prevent migraine headaches, monitor the incidence and severity of attacks to document whether nifedipine is successful in helping manage the patient's pain.
- Assess peripheral edema using girth measurements, volume displacement, and measurement of pitting edema (See Appendix N). Report increased swelling in feet and ankles or a sudden increase in body weight due to peripheral vasodilation.
- Watch for signs of hyperglycemia, including confusion, drowsiness, flushed/dry skin, fruit-like breath odor, rapid/deep breathing, polyuria, loss of appetite, and unusual thirst. Insulin dosages may need to be adjusted to prevent repeated episodes of hyperglycemia.
- Monitor and report signs of leukopenia (fever, sore throat, signs of infection), thrombocytopenia (bruising, nose bleeds, and bleeding gums), or unusual weakness and fatigue that might be due to anemia.
- Assess signs of paresthesia (numbness, tingling) or muscle twitching. Perform objective tests, including electroneuromyography and sensory testing to document any drug-related neuropathic changes.
- Assess any joint pain or muscle cramping to rule out musculoskeletal pathology; that is, try to determine if pain is drug induced rather than caused by anatomic or biomechanical problems.
- Assess dizziness and weakness that might affect gait, balance, and other functional activities (See Appendix C). Report balance problems and functional limitations to the physician, and caution the patient and family/caregivers to guard against falls and trauma.
- Monitor mood and personality changes, including anxiety, nervousness, confusion, memory loss, or other changes in behavior. Notify physician if these changes become problematic.

Interventions

- Design and implement aerobic exercise and endurance training programs to normalize blood pressure, improve coronary perfusion, reduce angina, and improve myocardial pumping ability.
- Because of the risk of cardiac arrhythmias and CHF, use caution during aerobic exercise and other forms of therapeutic exercise. Assess exercise tolerance frequently (blood pressure, heart rate, fatigue levels), and terminate exercise immediately if any untoward responses occur (See Appendix L).
- Guard against falls and trauma (hip fractures, head injury). Implement fall-prevention strategies, especially if patient exhibits dizziness or disturbed equilibrium (See Appendix E).
- To minimize orthostatic hypotension, patient should move slowly when assuming a more upright position.
- Causes photosensitivity; use care if administering UV treatments.

Patient/Client-Related Instruction

- Remind patients to take medication as directed to control hypertension and other cardiac conditions even if they are asymptomatic.
- Counsel patients about additional interventions to help control blood pressure and cardiac dysfunction, including regular exercise, weight loss, sodium restriction, stress reduction, moderation of alcohol consumption, and smoking cessation.
- Advise patient about photosensitivity, and to use sunscreens, protective clothing, and avoid prolonged sun exposure. Advise patient to also report any rashes or other skin reactions.
- Instruct patient or family/caregivers to report other troublesome side effects such as severe or prolonged headache, nightmares, tremor, problems with urination, sexual dysfunction, breast enlargement in men (gynecomastia), or GI problems (nausea, vomiting, constipation, diarrhea, loss of appetite).

Pharmacokinetics

Absorption: Well absorbed after oral administration, but large amounts are rapidly metabolized (primarily by CYP3A4 enzyme system), resulting in decreased bioavailability (45–70%); bioavailability is increased (80%) with long-acting (CC, PA, XL) forms.
Distribution: Unknown.
Protein Binding: 92–98%.
Metabolism and Excretion: Mostly metabolized by the liver.
Half-life: 2–5 hr.

TIME/ACTION PROFILE

ROUTE	ONSET	PEAK	DURATION
PO	20 min	unknown	6–8 hr
PO–PA	unknown	4 hr	12 hr
PO–CC, PA, XL	unknown	6 hr	24 hr

Contraindications/Precautions

Contraindicated in: Hypersensitivity; Sick sinus syndrome; 2nd- or 3rd-degree AV block (unless an artificial pacemaker is in place); Blood pressure <90 mm Hg; Coadministration with grapefruit juice.
Use Cautiously in: Severe hepatic impairment (↓ dose recommended); History of porphyria; Geri: Short-acting forms appear on Beers' list due to increased risk of hypotension and constipation in geriatric patients (↓ dose recommended). Is also associated with increased incidence of falls; Severe renal impairment (↓ dose may be necessary); History of serious ventricular arrhythmias or CHF; OB/Lactation/Pedi: Pregnancy, lactation, or children (safety not established).

Interactions

Drug-Drug: Additive hypotension may occur when used concurrently with **fentanyl**, other **antihypertensives, nitrates**, acute ingestion of **alcohol**, or **quinidine**. Antihypertensive effects may be ↓ by concurrent use of **NSAIDs**. May ↑ serum levels and risk of toxicity from **digoxin**. Concurrent use with **beta blockers, digoxin, disopyramide**, or **phenytoin** may result in bradycardia, conduction defects, or CHF. **Cimetidine** and **propranolol** may ↓ metabolism and ↑ risk of toxicity. May ↓ metabolism of and ↑ risk of toxicity from **cyclosporine, prazosin, quinidine**, or **carbamazepine**.
Drug-Food: Grapefruit and **Grapefruit juice** ↑ serum levels and effect.

Route/Dosage

PO (Adults): 10–30 mg 3 times daily (not to exceed 180 mg/day), *or* 10–20 mg twice daily as PA form, *or* 30–90 mg once daily as sustained-release (CC, XL) form (not to exceed 90–120 mg/day).

Availability (generic available)

Capsules: 5 mg, 10 mg, 20 mg. **Tablets:** 10 mg. **Extended-release tablets, (Adalat CC, Afeditab CR, Nifedical XL, Procardia XL):** 10 mg, 20 mg, 30 mg, 60 mg, 90 mg.

N

nilotinib (ni-lo-ti-nib)

Tasigna

Classification
Therapeutic: antineoplastics
Pharmacologic: enzyme inhibitors

Indications

Chronic or accelerated phase Philadelphia chromosome–positive chronic myelogenous leukemia which has not responded to other treatment, including imatinib.

Action

Inhibits kinases which may be produced by malignant cell lines. **Therapeutic Effects:** Inhibits production of malignant cells lines with decreased proliferation of leukemic cells.

Adverse Reactions/Side Effects

CNS: fatigue, headache, dizziness. **EENT:** vertigo. **CV:** ARRHYTHMIAS, hypertension, palpitations, QT prolongation. **GI:** constipation, diarrhea, nausea, vomiting, abdominal discomfort, anorexia, dyspepsia, flatulence, hepatotoxicity. **Derm:** pruritus, rash, alopecia, flushing. **F and E:** hyperkalemia, hypocalcemia, hypokalemia, hyponatremia, hypophosphatemia. **Hemat:** MYELOSUPRESSION. **Metab:** ↑ lipase, hyperglycemia. **MS:** musculoskeletal pain. **Neuro:** paresthesia. **Misc:** fever, night sweats.

PHYSICAL THERAPY IMPLICATIONS

Examination and Evaluation

- Monitor signs of myelosuppression, including fatigue, dizziness, fever, chills, sore throat, shortness of breath, chest pain, pallor, and unusual bruising or bleeding. Report these signs to the physician or nursing staff immediately.
- Assess heart rate, ECG, and heart sounds, especially during exercise (See Appendices G, H). Report any rhythm disturbances or symptoms of increased arrhythmias, including palpitations, chest discomfort, shortness of breath, fainting, and fatigue/weakness.
- Assess blood pressure (BP) and compare to normal values (See Appendix F). Report a sustained increase in BP (hypertension).
- Be alert for vertigo that might affect gait, balance, and other functional activities. Report balance problems and functional limitations to the physician and nursing staff, and caution the patient and family/caregivers to guard against falls and trauma.
- Assess any muscle or joint pain to rule out musculoskeletal pathology; that is, try to determine if pain is drug induced rather than caused by anatomic or biomechanical problems.
- Assess signs of paresthesia (numbness, tingling) or muscle twitching. Perform objective tests, including electroneuromyography and sensory testing to document any drug-related neuropathic changes.
- Monitor neuromuscular signs of electrolyte imbalances (hypocalcemia, hyperkalemia, hypokalemia, others), including headache, lethargy, weakness, cramping, and muscle hyperexcitability and tetany. Notify physician or nursing staff if these signs occur.
- Monitor signs of hyperglycemia, including confusion, drowsiness, skin flushing, dry skin, fruit-like breath odor, rapid breathing, polyuria, loss of appetite, and unusual thirst. Insulin dosages may need to be adjusted to prevent repeated episodes of hyperglycemia.

Interventions

- For patients who are medically able to begin exercise, implement appropriate resistive exercises and aerobic training to maintain muscle strength and aerobic capacity during cancer chemotherapy or to help restore function after chemotherapy.
- Because of the risk of serious arrhythmias, use caution during aerobic exercise and endurance conditioning. Terminate exercise if patient exhibits untoward symptoms (chest pain, shortness of breath, unusual fatigue) or displays other criteria for exercise termination (See Appendix L).

Patient/Client-Related Instruction

- Advise patient to guard against infection (frequent hand washing, etc.), and to avoid crowds and contact with persons with contagious diseases.
- Advise patient about the likelihood of GI reactions such as nausea, vomiting, constipation, diarrhea, abdominal discomfort, loss of appetite, indigestion, and flatulence. Instruct patient to report severe or prolonged GI problems or signs of liver toxicity including yellow skin or eyes, abdominal pain, severe nausea and vomiting, fever, sore throat, malaise, weakness, and facial edema.
- Instruct patient to report other bothersome side effects such as severe or prolonged fever, night sweats, or skin reactions (rash, itching, flushing, hair loss).

Pharmacokinetics

Absorption: Well absorbed following oral administration. Blood levels are significantly increased by food.
Distribution: Unknown.
Metabolism and Excretion: Mostly metabolized by the liver; metabolites are not active.
Half-life: 17 hr.

TIME/ACTION PROFILE (blood levels)

ROUTE	ONSET	PEAK	DURATION
PO	unknown	3 hr	12 hr

Contraindications/Precautions

Contraindicated in: Hypokalemia or hypomagnesemia; Long QT syndrome; Concurrent use of medications known to prolong QT interval; Concurrent use of strong inhibitors of the CYP3A4 enzyme system (increased risk of toxicity); Concurrent use of strong inducers of the CYP3A4 enzyme system (may ↓ effectiveness); Concurrent grapefruit juice (may ↑ risk of toxicity); Galactose intolerance, severe lactase deficiency or glucose-galactose malabsorption (capsules contain lactose); OB: Pregnancy or lactation.
Use Cautiously in: Concurrent use of other drugs that prolong QT interval; Electrolyte abnormalities; correct prior to administration to ↓ risk of arrhythmias; Hepatic impairment (↓ dose required for Grade 3 elevated bilirubin, transaminases, or lipase); OB: Women with childbearing potential (effective contraception required); Pedi: Safe use in children has not been established.

Interactions

Drug-Drug: Strong **inhibitors of the CYP3A4 enzyme system**, including **ketoconazole, itraconazole, voriconazole, clarithromycin, telithromycin, atazanavir, indinavir, nelfinavir, indinavir, ritonavir, saquinavir**, and **nefazodone**, may result in ↑ blood levels and toxicity and should be avoided; if concurrent use in necessary, dose reduction by 50% (400 mg once daily) may be required. Strong **inducers of the CYP3A4 enzyme system**, including **carbamazepine, dexamethasone, phenobarbital, phenytoin, rifabutin, rifampin**, and **rifapentine**,

may ↓ blood levels and effectiveness and should be avoided if possible; if required, dose ↑ may be necessary. Nilotinib inhibits the following enzyme systems: **CYP3A4**, **CYP2C8**, **CYP2C9**, and **CYP2D6**; concurrent use of drugs metabolized by these systems may result in toxicity of these agents. Nilotinib induces the following enzyme systems: **CYP2D6**, **CYP2C8**, **CYP2C9**; concurrent use of drugs metabolized by these systems may result ↓ therapeutic effectiveness of these agents. Concurrent use of other **drugs that prolong QT interval**; may ↑ risk of serious arrhythmias.
Drug-Natural: St. John's wort may ↓ levels and effectiveness; avoid concurrent use.
Drug-Food: Grapefruit juice may ↑ blood levels and should be avoided.

Route/Dosage

PO (Adults): 400 mg twice daily; adjustment may be required for toxicity and/or drug interactions.

Availability

Capsules: 200 mg.

nilutamide (nye-**loot**-a-mide)

✱ Anandron, Nilandron

Classification
Therapeutic: antineoplastics
Pharmacologic: antiandrogens

Indications

Management of metastatic prostate cancer (with surgical castration).

Action

Blocks the effects of androgen (testosterone) at the cellular level. **Therapeutic Effects:** Decreased spread of prostate cancer.

Adverse Reactions/Side Effects

CNS: dizziness. **EENT:** impaired adaptation to darkness, abnormal vision. **Resp:** interstitial pneumonitis. **CV:** hypertension. **GI:** HEPATOTOXICITY, constipation, hepatitis, increased liver enzymes, nausea. **Derm:** hot flashes, hair loss, sweating.

PHYSICAL THERAPY IMPLICATIONS

Examination and Evaluation

- Be alert for signs of hepatotoxicity, including anorexia, abdominal pain, severe nausea and vomiting, yellow skin or eyes, fever, sore throat, malaise, weakness, facial edema, lethargy, and unusual bleeding or bruising. Report these signs to the physician immediately.
- Monitor signs of interstitial pneumonitis, including dyspnea, dry cough, shortness of breath, fever, and rales. Report these signs to the physician.
- Assess blood pressure periodically and compare to normal values (See Appendix F). Report a sustained increase in blood pressure (hypertension) to the physician.
- Assess dizziness that might affect gait, balance, and other functional activities (See Appendix C). Report balance problems and functional limitations to the physician and nursing staff, and caution the patient and family/caregivers to guard against falls and trauma.

Interventions

- For patients who are medically able to begin exercise, implement appropriate resistive exercises and aerobic training to maintain muscle strength and aerobic capacity during cancer chemotherapy, or to help restore function after chemotherapy.
- Because of possible pulmonary or blood pressure problems, use caution during aerobic exercise and other forms of therapeutic exercise. Assess exercise tolerance frequently (respiratory symptoms, blood pressure, heart rate, fatigue levels), and terminate exercise immediately if any untoward responses occur (See Appendix L).

Patient/Client-Related Instruction

- Advise patient about the likelihood of vision problems, including the impaired ability to adapt to darkness. Patients should use caution when entering a dark room, and implement better lighting conditions whenever possible.
- Instruct patient and family/caregivers to report other troublesome side effects such as severe or prolonged hot flashes, skin reactions (hair loss, increased sweating), or GI problems (nausea, constipation).

Pharmacokinetics

Absorption: Rapidly and completely absorbed following oral administration.
Distribution: Unknown.
Metabolism and Excretion: Extensively metabolized by the liver; 2 metabolites have antiandrogenic activity; <2% excreted unchanged in urine.
Half-life: 41–49 hr.

TIME/ACTION PROFILE (antiandrogenic effects)

ROUTE	ONSET	PEAK	DURATION
PO	rapid	unknown	24 hr

Contraindications/Precautions

Contraindicated in: Hypersensitivity; Severe hepatic impairment; Severe respiratory insufficiency.

Use Cautiously in: History of liver disease or alcoholism; History of respiratory problems; Pregnancy, lactation, or children (safety not established).

Interactions

Drug-Drug: May ↑ the effects of **warfarin, phenytoin,** and **theophylline**. May cause **alcohol** intolerance.

Route/Dosage

PO (Adults): 300 mg once daily for 30 days; then 150 mg once daily.

Availability

Tablets: 150 mg, 100 mg.

nimodipine (nye-moe-di-peen)

Nimotop

Classification

Therapeutic: subarachnoid hemorrhage therapy agents

Pharmacologic: calcium channel blockers

Indications

Management of subarachnoid hemorrhage.

Action

Inhibits the transport of calcium into vascular smooth muscle cells, resulting in inhibition of excitation-contraction coupling and subsequent contraction. Potent peripheral vasodilator. **Therapeutic Effects:** Prevention of vascular spasm after subarachnoid hemorrhage, resulting in decreased neurologic impairment.

Adverse Reactions/Side Effects

CNS: abnormal dreams, anxiety, confusion, dizziness, drowsiness, headache, nervousness, psychiatric disturbances, weakness. **EENT:** blurred vision, disturbed equilibrium, epistaxis, tinnitus. **Resp:** cough, dyspnea. **CV:** ARRHYTHMIAS, CHF, bradycardia, chest pain, hypotension, palpitations, peripheral edema, syncope, tachycardia. **GI:** abnormal liver function studies, anorexia, constipation, diarrhea, dry mouth, dysgeusia, dyspepsia, nausea, vomiting. **GU:** dysuria, nocturia, polyuria, sexual dysfunction, urinary frequency. **Derm:** dermatitis, erythema multiforme, flushing, increased sweating, photosensitivity, pruritus/urticaria, rash. **Endo:** gynecomastia, hyperglycemia. **Hemat:** anemia, leukopenia, thrombocytopenia. **Metab:** weight gain. **MS:** joint stiffness, muscle cramps. **Neuro:** paresthesia, tremor. **Misc:** STEVENS-JOHNSON SYNDROME, gingival hyperplasia.

PHYSICAL THERAPY IMPLICATIONS

Examination and Evaluation

- Assess heart rate, ECG, and heart sounds, especially during exercise (See Appendices G, H). Report any rhythm disturbances or symptoms of increased arrhythmias, including palpitations, chest pain, shortness of breath, fainting, and fatigue/weakness.
- Monitor rashes or other skin reactions (hives, abnormal sweating, itching/burning, exfoliation). Notify physician immediately because certain skin reactions may indicate serious hypersensitivity reactions (Stevens-Johnson syndrome).
- Assess routinely for signs of CHF and pulmonary edema (dyspnea, cough, shortness of breath, rales/crackles, jugular venous distention). Report these signs to the physician.
- Assess patient's neurologic status (level of consciousness, sensory and motor function) periodically following administration to help determine benefits in treating subarachnoid hemorrhage. Notify physician of any sudden decline in alertness, cognition, or motor function.
- Assess peripheral edema using girth measurements, volume displacement, and measurement of pitting edema (See Appendix N). Report increased swelling in feet and ankles due to peripheral vasodilation.
- Watch for signs of hyperglycemia, including confusion, drowsiness, flushed/dry skin, fruit-like breath odor, rapid/deep breathing, polyuria, loss of appetite, and unusual thirst. Insulin dosages may need to be adjusted to prevent repeated episodes of hyperglycemia.
- Monitor and report signs of leukopenia (fever, sore throat, signs of infection), thrombocytopenia (bruising, nose bleeds, and bleeding gums), or unusual weakness and fatigue that might be due to anemia.
- Assess signs of paresthesia (numbness, tingling) or muscle twitching. Perform objective tests, including electroneuromyography and sensory testing to document any drug-related neuropathic changes.
- Assess any joint stiffness or muscle cramping to rule out musculoskeletal pathology; that is, try to determine if pain is drug induced rather than caused by anatomic or biomechanical problems.
- Assess dizziness and weakness that might affect gait, balance, and other functional activities (See Appendix C). Report balance problems and functional limitations to the physician, and caution the patient and family/caregivers to guard against falls and trauma.
- Monitor mood and personality changes, including anxiety, nervousness, confusion, or other psychiatric disturbances. Notify physician if these changes become problematic.

Interventions

- Because of the risk of cardiac arrhythmias and CHF, use caution during aerobic exercise and other forms of therapeutic exercise. Assess exercise tolerance frequently (blood pressure, heart rate, fatigue levels), and terminate exercise immediately if any untoward responses occur (See Appendix L).

- Guard against falls and trauma (hip fractures, head injury). Implement fall-prevention strategies, especially if patient exhibits dizziness or disturbed equilibrium (See Appendix E).
- To minimize orthostatic hypotension, patient should move slowly when assuming a more upright position.
- Causes photosensitivity; use care if administering UV treatments.

Patient/Client-Related Instruction

- Advise patient about photosensitivity and to use sunscreens, protective clothing, and avoid prolonged sun exposure. Advise patient to also report any rashes or other skin reactions.
- Instruct patient or family/caregivers to report other troublesome side effects such as severe or prolonged headache, tinnitus, nightmares, tremor, weight gain, problems with urination, sexual dysfunction, breast enlargement in men (gynecomastia), or GI problems (nausea, vomiting, constipation, diarrhea, indigestion, loss of appetite).

Pharmacokinetics

Absorption: Well absorbed following oral administration but extensively metabolized, resulting in decreased bioavailability.
Distribution: Crosses the blood-brain barrier; remainder of distribution unknown.
Protein Binding: >95%.
Metabolism and Excretion: Mostly metabolized by the liver; ≤10% excreted unchanged by kidneys.
Half-life: 1–2 hr.

TIME/ACTION PROFILE (vasodilation)

ROUTE	ONSET	PEAK	DURATION
PO	unknown	1 hr	4 hr

Contraindications/Precautions

Contraindicated in: Hypersensitivity; Sick sinus syndrome; 2nd- or 3rd-degree AV block (unless an artificial pacemaker is in place); BP <90 mm Hg.
Use Cautiously in: Severe hepatic impairment (dose reduction recommended); Geri: Dose reduction recommended; ↑ risk of hypotension; Severe renal impairment; History of serious ventricular arrhythmias or CHF; OB/Lactation/Pedi: Safety not established.

Interactions

Drug-Drug: Additive hypotension may occur when used concurrently with **fentanyl**, other **antihypertensives, nitrates**, acute ingestion of **alcohol**, or **quinidine**. Concurrent use with **beta blockers, digoxin, disopyramide**, or **phenytoin** may result in bradycardia, conduction defects, or CHF.
Drug-Natural: Grapefruit and **Grapefruit juice** ↑ serum levels and effect.

Route/Dosage

PO (Adults): 60 mg q 4 hr for 21 days; therapy should be started within 96 hr of subarachnoid hemorrhage.

Hepatic Impairment

PO (Adults): 30 mg q 4 hr for 21 days; therapy should be started within 96 hr of subarachnoid hemorrhage.

Availability (generic available)

Capsules: 30 mg.

nisoldipine (nye-sole-di-peen)

Sular

Classification
Therapeutic: antihypertensives
Pharmacologic: calcium channel blockers

Indications

Management of hypertension.

Action

Inhibits the transport of calcium into vascular smooth muscle cells, resulting in inhibition of vasoconstriction and dilation of arterioles. **Therapeutic Effects:** Systemic vasodilation, resulting in decreased blood pressure.

Adverse Reactions/Side Effects

CNS: headache, dizziness. **EENT:** pharyngitis, sinusitis. **CV:** peripheral edema, chest pain, hypotension, palpitations. **GI:** nausea. **Derm:** rash.
Endo: gynecomastia.

PHYSICAL THERAPY IMPLICATIONS

Examination and Evaluation

- Assess blood pressure periodically and compare to normal values (See Appendix F) to help document antihypertensive effects. Report an excessive fall in blood pressure (hypotension), especially if patient experiences dizziness, fatigue, palpitations, or other symptoms.
- Assess peripheral edema using girth measurements, volume displacement, and measurement of pitting edema (See Appendix N). Report increased swelling in feet and ankles due to peripheral vasodilation.
- Assess dizziness that might affect gait, balance, and other functional activities (See Appendix C). Report balance problems and functional limitations to the physician and nursing staff, and caution the patient

and family/caregivers to guard against falls and trauma.

Interventions

- Because of potential cardiovascular problem (hypotension, palpitations), use caution during aerobic exercise and other therapeutic exercise. Terminate exercise if patient exhibits untoward symptoms (chest pain, shortness of breath, unusual fatigue), or displays other criteria for exercise termination (See Appendix L).
- Avoid physical therapy interventions that cause systemic vasodilation (large whirlpool, Hubbard tank). Additive effects of this drug and the intervention may cause a dangerous fall in blood pressure.
- To minimize orthostatic hypotension, patient should move slowly when assuming a more upright position.

Patient/Client-Related Instruction

- Counsel patients about additional interventions to help control blood pressure, including regular exercise, weight loss, sodium restriction, stress reduction, moderation of alcohol consumption, and smoking cessation.
- Instruct patient or family/caregivers to report other troublesome side effects such as severe or prolonged headache, skin rash, nausea, nasal/sinus irritation, and breast enlargement in men (gynecomastia).

Pharmacokinetics

Absorption: Well absorbed (87%) following oral administration but rapidly and extensively metabolized in the gut wall, resulting in 5% bioavailability.
Distribution: Unknown.
Metabolism and Excretion: Highly metabolized CYP3A4 enzyme system.
Half-life: 7–12 hr.

TIME/ACTION PROFILE (antihypertensive effects)

ROUTE	ONSET	PEAK	DURATION
PO	unknown	6–12 hr	24 hr

Contraindications/Precautions

Contraindicated in: Hypersensitivity; Cross-sensitivity with calcium channel blockers may occur; Concurrent phenytoin use.
Use Cautiously in: CHF/left ventricular dysfunction; Hepatic impairment (dose reduction may be necessary); Geri: Dose ↓ may be necessary); Coronary artery disease (may precipitate angina); OB/Lactation/Pedi: Safety not established.

Interactions

Drug-Drug: Additive hypotension may occur with other **antihypertensives**, acute ingestion of **alcohol**, or **nitrates**. Antihypertensive effects may be ↓ by concurrent use of **NSAIDs**. **Phenytoin** or **other CYP3A4 inducers** ↓ blood levels and effectiveness (avoid concurrent use).
Drug-Food: Grapefruit and **Grapefruit juice** ↑ serum levels and effect. Blood levels are ↑ by concurrent ingestion of a **high-fat meal** and should be avoided.

Route/Dosage

PO (Adults): *Extended-release tablets*—20 mg/day as a single dose initially; may be ↑ by 10 mg/day q 7 days, up to 60 mg/day (usual range 20–40 mg/day); *Geomatric extended-release tablets*—17 mg/day as a single dose initially; may be ↑ by 8.5 mg/day q 7 days, up to 34 mg/day (usual range 8.5–34 mg/day).

Hepatic Impairment

PO (Adults): *Geomatric extended-release tablets*—Initial dose should not exceed 8.5 mg/day.

Availability (generic available)

Extended-release tablets: 20 mg, 30 mg, 40 mg.
Geomatrix extended-release tablets: 8.5 mg, 17 mg, 25.5 mg, 34 mg.

nitazoxanide (nit-a-zox-a-nide)

Alinia

Classification
Therapeutic: antiprotozoals
Pharmacologic: benzamides

Indications

Treatment of diarrhea due to *Cryptosporidium parvum* and *Giardia lamblia*. Not effective for *C. Parvum* diarrhea in HIV-infected patients.

Action

Interferes with electron transfer reaction necessary for anaerobic energy metabolism of offending organisms.
Therapeutic Effects: Antiprotozoal action resulting in decreased diarrhea.

Adverse Reactions/Side Effects

CNS: dizziness. **EENT:** yellow eye discoloration. **GI:** abdominal pain, diarrhea, vomiting. **GU:** discolored urine. **Derm:** pruritus, sweating. **Misc:** fever.

PHYSICAL THERAPY IMPLICATIONS

Examination and Evaluation

- Assess dizziness that might affect gait, balance, and other functional activities (See Appendix C). Report balance problems and functional limitations to the physician and nursing staff, and caution the patient and family/caregivers to guard against falls and trauma.

Interventions

- Make sure patient remains adequately hydrated to offset fluid loss from diarrhea.

Patient/Client-Related Instruction

- Instruct patient and family/caregivers to report other troublesome side effects such as severe or prolonged fever, skin reactions (itching, increased swearing), or GI problems (diarrhea, vomiting, abdominal pain).

Pharmacokinetics

Absorption: Following oral administration, nitazoxanide is rapidly converted to tizoxanide, which is the active metabolite; tizoxanide is further metabolized.
Distribution: Unknown.
Protein Binding: >99%.
Metabolism and Excretion: *Tizoxanide*—excreted in urine, bile and feces; inactive metabolites excreted in urine, bile, and feces.
Half-life: Unknown.

TIME/ACTION PROFILE (blood levels)

ROUTE	ONSET	PEAK	DURATION
PO	unknown*	1–4 hr	12 hr

*Onset of antidiarrheal activity is 24–48 hr.

Contraindications/Precautions

Contraindicated in: Hypersensitivity.
Use Cautiously in: Hepatic and/or renal impairment; Diabetics (contains 1.48 g sucrose/5 mL); **Pedi, OB:** Children <1 pregnancy or lactation (safety not established).

Interactions

Drug-Drug: May interact with other **highly protein-bound drugs** by competing for binding sites.

Route/Dosage

PO (Adults and children ≥12 yr): 500 mg every 12 hr for 3 days.
PO (Children 4–11 yr): 200 mg (10 mL) every 12 hr for 3 days.
PO (Children 1–4 yr): 100 mg (5 mL) every 12 hr for 3 days.

Availability

Tablets: 500 mg. **Oral suspension (strawberry):** 100 mg/5 mL in 60-mL bottle.

nitrofurantoin

(nye-troe-fyoor-**an**-toyn)
✱ Apo-Nitrofurantoin, Furadantin, Macrobid, Macrodantin

Classification
Therapeutic: anti-infectives

Indications

Prevention and treatment of urinary tract infections caused by susceptible organisms; not effective in systemic bacterial infections.

Action

Interferes with bacterial enzymes. **Therapeutic Effects:** Bactericidal or bacteriostatic action against susceptible organisms. **Spectrum:** Many gram-negative and some gram-positive organisms, specifically *Citrobacter*, *Corynebacterium*, *Enterobacter*, *Escherichia coli*, *Klebsiella*, *Neisseria*, *Salmonella*, *Shigella*, *Staphylococcus aureus*, *S.*, *Enterococcus*.

Adverse Reactions/Side Effects

CNS: dizziness, drowsiness, headache. **EENT:** nystagmus. **Resp:** pneumonitis. **CV:** chest pain. **GI:** PSEUDOMEMBRANOUS COLITIS, anorexia, nausea, vomiting, abdominal pain, diarrhea, drug-induced hepatitis. **GU:** rust/brown discoloration of urine. **Derm:** photosensitivity. **Hemat:** blood dyscrasias, hemolytic anemia. **Neuro:** peripheral neuropathy. **Misc:** hypersensitivity reactions.

N

PHYSICAL THERAPY IMPLICATIONS

Examination and Evaluation

- Monitor signs of pseudomembranous colitis, including diarrhea, abdominal pain, fever, pus or mucus in stools, and other severe or prolonged GI problems (nausea, vomiting, heartburn). Notify physician of these signs immediately.
- Assess any breathing problems or signs of pneumonitis such as cough, shortness of breath, fever, rales, chest pain, and difficult, labored breathing. Monitor pulse oximetry and perform pulmonary function tests (See Appendices I, J, K) to quantify suspected changes in ventilation and respiratory function.
- Monitor signs of hypersensitivity reactions, including pulmonary symptoms (tightness in the throat and chest, wheezing, cough, dyspnea) or skin reactions (rash, pruritus, urticaria). Notify physician immediately if these reactions occur.
- Be alert for signs of peripheral neuropathy (numbness, tingling, decreased muscle strength). Establish baseline electroneuromyographic values at the beginning of drug treatment whenever possible, and reexamine these values periodically to document drug-induced changes in peripheral nerve function.
- Assess dizziness or drowsiness that might affect gait, balance, and other functional activities (See Appendix C). Report balance problems and functional limitations to the physician, and caution the patient

and family/caregivers to guard against falls and trauma.

- Monitor signs of blood dyscrasias including hemolytic anemia (unusual weakness and fatigue, dizziness, jaundice, abdominal pain), leukopenia (fever, sore throat, signs of infection), and thrombocytopenia (bruising, nose bleeds, bleeding gums). Report these signs to the physician.

Interventions

- Always wash hands thoroughly and disinfect equipment (whirlpools, electrotherapeutic devices, treatment tables, and so forth) to help prevent the spread of infection. Employ universal precautions or isolation procedures as indicated for specific patients.
- Causes photosensitivity; use care if administering UV treatments.

Patient/Client-Related Instruction

- Advise patient about the likelihood of GI reactions, including nausea, vomiting, diarrhea, loss of appetite. Instruct patient to report severe or prolonged GI problems or signs of drug-induced hepatitis (yellow skin or eyes, abdominal pain, severe nausea and vomiting, fever, sore throat, malaise, weakness, facial edema).
- Advise patient about photosensitivity and to use sunscreens, protective clothing, and avoid prolonged sun exposure. Advise patient to also report any rashes or other skin reactions.
- Instruct patient and family/caregivers to report other troublesome side effects such as severe or prolonged headache, abnormal eye movements (nystagmus), or discolored urine.

Pharmacokinetics

Absorption: Readily absorbed after oral administration. Absorption is slower but more complete with macrocrystals (Macrodantin).
Distribution: Crosses placenta; enters breast milk.
Protein Binding: 40%.
Metabolism and Excretion: Partially metabolized by the liver; 30–50% excreted unchanged by the kidneys.
Half-life: 20 min (increased in renal impairment).

TIME/ACTION PROFILE (urine levels)

ROUTE	ONSET	PEAK	DURATION
PO	unknown	30 min	6–12 hr

Contraindications/Precautions

Contraindicated in: Hypersensitivity; Hypersensitivity to parabens (suspension); Oliguria, anuria, or significant renal impairment (CCr <60 mL/min); G6PD deficiency; OB/Pedi: Infants <1 mo and pregnancy near term (↑ risk of hemolytic anemia in newborn).
Use Cautiously in: Patients with diabetes or debilitated patients (neuropathy may be more common); Lactation/OB: Safety not established but has been used safely in pregnant women. May cause hemolysis in G6PD-deficient infants who are breastfed; Geri: Appears on Beers' list; at ↑ risk for renal, hepatic, and pulmonary reactions.

Interactions

Drug-Drug: Probenecid and **sulfinpyrazone** prevent high urinary concentrations; may ↓ effectiveness. **Antacids** may ↓ absorption. ↑ risk of neurotoxicity with **neurotoxic drugs**. ↑ risk of hepatotoxicity with **hepatotoxic drugs**. ↑ risk of pneumonitis with **drugs having pulmonary toxicity**.

Route/Dosage

PO (Adults): *Treatment of active infection*—50–100 mg q 6–8 hr *or* 100 mg q 12 hr as extended-release product. *Chronic suppression*—50–100 mg single evening dose.
PO (Children >1 mo): *Treatment of active infection*—5–7 mg/kg/day divided q 6 hr; maximum dose: 400 mg/day. *Chronic suppression*—1–2 mg/kg/day as a single dose at bedtime; maximum dose 100 mg/day(unlabeled).

Availability (generic available)

Tablets: 50 mg, 100 mg. **Oral suspension:** 25 mg/5 mL. **Capsules:** 25 mg, 50 mg, 100 mg. **Extended-release capsules:** 100 mg.

nitroglycerin
(nye-troe-**glis**-er-in)

extended-release capsules
Nitro-Time, Nitrogard SR

intravenous
Nitro-Bid IV, Tridil

translingual spray
Nitrolingual, Nitromist

ointment
Nitro-Bid

sublingual
Nitrostat, NitroQuick

transdermal system
Minitran, Nitrek, Nitro-Dur

Classification
Therapeutic: antianginals
Pharmacologic: nitrates

Indications

Acute (**translingual and SL**) and long-term prophylactic (**oral, transdermal**) management of angina pectoris. **PO:** Adjunct treatment of CHF. **IV:** Adjunct treatment of acute MI. Production of controlled hypotension during surgical procedures. Treatment of CHF associated with acute MI.

Action

Increases coronary blood flow by dilating coronary arteries and improving collateral flow to ischemic regions. Produces vasodilation (venous greater than arterial). Decreases left ventricular end-diastolic pressure and left ventricular end-diastolic volume (preload). Reduces myocardial oxygen consumption. **Therapeutic Effects:** Relief or prevention of anginal attacks. Increased cardiac output. Reduction of blood pressure.

Adverse Reactions/Side Effects

CNS: dizziness, headache, apprehension, restlessness, weakness. **EENT:** blurred vision. **CV:** hypotension, tachycardia, syncope. **GI:** abdominal pain, nausea, vomiting. **Derm:** contact dermatitis (transdermal or ointment). **Misc:** alcohol intoxication (large IV doses only), cross-tolerance, flushing, tolerance.

PHYSICAL THERAPY IMPLICATIONS

Examination and Evaluation

- Assess episodes of angina pectoris at rest and during exercise. Document whether drug therapy is helpful in reducing the frequency and severity of angina attacks.
- Assess signs and symptoms of CHF (dyspnea, rales/crackles, peripheral edema, jugular venous distention, exercise intolerance) to help document whether drug therapy is effective in reducing these symptoms.
- Assess dizziness and syncope that might affect gait, balance, and other functional activities (See Appendix C). Report balance problems and functional limitations to the physician and nursing staff, and caution the patient and family/caregivers to guard against falls and trauma.
- Assess blood pressure periodically and compare to normal values (See Appendix F). Report low blood pressure (hypotension), especially if patient experiences dizziness, fainting, or other symptoms.
- Assess heart rate, ECG, and heart sounds, especially during exercise (See Appendices G, H). Report fast heart rate (tachycardia) or symptoms of other arrhythmias, including palpitations, chest discomfort, shortness of breath, fainting, and fatigue/weakness.
- If administered by a patch or ointment, monitor application site for redness and irritation. Report prolonged or excessive skin reactions to the physician or nursing staff.
- Report signs of drug tolerance during long-term use, as indicated by increased episodes of angina or CHF symptoms. This problem may be resolved by instituting nitrate-free periods; that is, the physician may recommend removing the nitroglycerin patch for several hours each day.

Interventions

- Design and implement aerobic exercise and endurance training programs to improve coronary perfusion, reduce angina, and improve myocardial pumping ability.
- Because of an increased risk of angina, arrhythmias, or in conditions such as CHF or recent MI, use caution during aerobic exercise and endurance conditioning. Terminate exercise if patient exhibits untoward symptoms (chest pain, shortness of breath, etc.) or displays other criteria for exercise termination (See Appendix L).
- Avoid physical therapy interventions that cause systemic vasodilation (large whirlpool, Hubbard tank). Additive effects of this drug and these interventions may cause a dangerous fall in blood pressure.
- To minimize orthostatic hypotension, patient should move slowly when assuming a more upright position.
- Make sure patient brings nitroglycerin tablets or translingual sprays to all physical therapy appointments, and that this drug is readily available during exercise and other interventions. If taken sublingually during physical therapy, have the patient lie down or sit with legs elevated and avoid exercise, ambulation, or application of local heat for the duration of drug effects (usually 30–60 min).

Patient/Client-Related Instruction

- Advise patient to sit or lie down and use medication at first sign of an angina attack. Relief usually occurs within 5 min. Dose may be repeated if pain is not relieved in 5–10 min. Call health care professional or go to nearest emergency room if angina pain is not relieved by 3 tablets in 15 min.
- Remind patients to take medication as directed to control angina or CHF even if they are asymptomatic. Patients with CHF should weigh themselves every day and call their physician if they gain 3 lb or more in 1 day or more than 5 lb in 1 wk.
- Counsel patients about additional interventions to help control angina and cardiac dysfunction, including regular exercise, weight loss, sodium restriction, stress reduction, moderation of alcohol consumption, and smoking cessation.
- Advise patient to protect sublingual tablets from light, heat, and moisture and to make sure the prescription is renewed periodically to maintain drug potency.

- Inform patient that headache is a common side effect that should decrease with continuing therapy. Notify health care professional if headache is persistent or severe.
- Instruct patient or family/caregivers to report other troublesome side effects such as severe or prolonged restlessness, apprehension, weakness, blurred vision, or GI problems (nausea, vomiting, abdominal pain).

Pharmacokinetics

Absorption: Well absorbed after oral, buccal, and sublingual administration. Also absorbed through skin. Orally administered nitroglycerin is rapidly metabolized, leading to decreased bioavailability.
Distribution: Unknown.
Metabolism and Excretion: Undergoes rapid and almost complete metabolism by the liver; also metabolized by enzymes in bloodstream.
Half-life: 1–4 min.

TIME/ACTION PROFILE (cardiovascular effects)

ROUTE	ONSET	PEAK	DURATION
SL	1–3 min	unknown	30–60 min
PO-ER	40–60 min	unknown	8–12 hr
TD-ointment	20–60 min	unknown	4–8 hr
TD-patch	40–60 min	unknown	8–24 hr
IV	immediate	unknown	several mins

Contraindications/Precautions

Contraindicated in: Hypersensitivity; Severe anemia; Pericardial tamponade; Constrictive pericarditis; Alcohol intolerance (large IV doses only); Concurrent use of PDE5 inhibitor (sildenafil, tadalafil, vardenafil).
Use Cautiously in: Head trauma or cerebral hemorrhage; Glaucoma; Hypertrophic cardiomyopathy; Severe liver impairment; Malabsorption or hypermotility (PO); Hypovolemia (IV); Normal or decreased pulmonary capillary wedge pressure (IV); Cardioversion (remove transdermal patch before procedure); OB: May compromise maternal/fetal circulation; Pedi/Lactation: Safety not established.

Interactions

Drug-Drug: Concurrent use of nitrates in any form with **sildenafil**, **tadalafil**, and **vardenafil** ↑ risk of serious and potentially fatal hypotension; concurrent use is contraindicated. Additive hypotension with **antihypertensives**, acute ingestion of **alcohol**, **beta blockers**, **calcium channel blockers**, **haloperidol**, or **phenothiazines**. Agents having anticholinergic properties (**tricyclic antidepressants**, **antihistamines**, **phenothiazines**) may ↓ absorption of lingual, or sublingual nitroglycerin.

Route/Dosage

SL (Adults): 0.3–0.6 mg; may repeat q 5 min for 2 additional doses for acute attack.
Translingual Spray: (Adults): 1–2 sprays; may be repeated q 5 min for 2 additional doses for acute attack. Both may also be used prophylactically 5–10 min before activities that may precipitate an acute attack.
PO (Adults): 2.5–9 mg q 8–12 hr.
IV (Adults): 5 mcg/min; increase by 5 mcg/min q 3–5 min to 20 mcg/min; if no response, increase by 10–20 mcg/min q 3–5 min (dosing determined by hemodynamic parameters; max 200 mcg/min).
Transdermal (Adults): *Ointment*—1–2 in. q 6–8 hr. *Transdermal patch*—0.2–0.4 mg/hr initially; may titrate up to 0.4–0.8 mg/hr. Patch should be worn 12–14 hr/day and then taken off for 10–12 hr/day.

Availability (generic available)

Extended-release capsules: 2.5 mg, 6.5 mg, 9 mg. **Sublingual tablets:** 0.3 mg, 0.4 mg, 0.6 mg. **Translingual spray (Nitrolingual):** 400 mcg/spray in 14.5-g canister (200 doses), NitroMist 400 mcg/spray in 8.5 g canister (230 doses). **Transdermal systems:** 0.1 mg/hr, 0.2 mg/hr, 0.3 mg/hr, 0.4 mg/hr, 0.6 mg/hr, 0.8 mg/hr. **Transdermal ointment:** 2%. **Injection:** 5 mg/mL. **Premixed solution:** 25 mg/250 mL, 50 mg/250 mL, 50 mg/500 mL, 100 mg/250 mL, 200 mg/500 mL.

nitroprusside

(nye-troe-**prus**-ide)
Nitropress

Classification
Therapeutic: antihypertensives
Pharmacologic: vasodilators

Indications

Hypertensive crises. Controlled hypotension during anesthesia. Cardiac pump failure or cardiogenic shock (alone or with dopamine).

Action

Produces peripheral vasodilation by a direct action on venous and arteriolar smooth muscle. **Therapeutic Effects:** Rapid lowering of blood pressure. ↓ cardiac preload and afterload.

Adverse Reactions/Side Effects

CNS: dizziness, headache, restlessness. **EENT:** blurred vision, tinnitus. **CV:** dyspnea, hypotension, palpitations. **GI:** abdominal pain, nausea, vomiting. **F and E:** acidosis. **Local:** phlebitis at IV site. **Misc:** CYANIDE TOXICITY, thiocyanate toxicity.

PHYSICAL THERAPY IMPLICATIONS

Examination and Evaluation

- Watch for signs of cyanide or thiocyanate toxicity, including weakness, malaise, confusion, combativeness, giddiness, vertigo, shortness of breath, apnea, seizures, and coma. Report these signs to the physician or nursing staff immediately.
- Assess blood pressure (BP), and determine if BP is maintained in the normal range (See Appendix F). Be alert for any residual hypotension following surgery.
- Monitor any cardiac palpitations or difficult, labored breathing. Report prolonged or severe cardiac or pulmonary symptoms.
- Monitor signs of acidosis, including headache, lethargy, confusion, and rapid breathing. Notify physician or nursing staff immediately if these signs occur.
- Assess dizziness that might affect gait, balance, and other functional activities (See Appendix C). Report balance problems and functional limitations to the physician and nursing staff, and caution the patient and family/caregivers to guard against falls and trauma.
- Assess IV site during and after IV administration, and report signs of phlebitis (local pain, swelling, inflammation).

Interventions

- Avoid physical therapy interventions that cause systemic vasodilation (large whirlpool, Hubbard tank) until drug effects have been completely resolved. Additive effects of this drug and the intervention may cause a dangerous fall in blood pressure.
- To minimize orthostatic hypotension, patient should move slowly when assuming a more upright position.

Patient/Client-Related Instruction

- Counsel patients about additional interventions to help with the long-term control of BP and cardiac dysfunction, including regular exercise, weight loss, sodium restriction, stress reduction, moderation of alcohol consumption, and smoking cessation.
- Instruct patient or family/caregivers to report residual side effects such as severe or prolonged headache, restlessness, blurred vision, ringing/buzzing in the ears (tinnitus), or GI problems (nausea, vomiting, abdominal pain).

Pharmacokinetics

Absorption: IV administration results in complete bioavailability.
Distribution: Unknown.
Metabolism and Excretion: Rapidly metabolized in RBCs and tissues to cyanide and subsequently by the liver to thiocyanate.
Half-life: 2 min.

TIME/ACTION PROFILE (hypotensive effect)

ROUTE	ONSET	PEAK	DURATION
IV	immediate	rapid	1–10 min

Contraindications/Precautions

Contraindicated in: Hypersensitivity; Decreased cerebral perfusion.
Use Cautiously in: Renal disease (↑ risk of thiocyanate accumulation); Hepatic disease (↑ risk of cyanide accumulation); Geriatric patients (↑ sensitivity); Hypothyroidism; Hyponatremia; Vitamin B deficiency; Pregnancy or lactation (safety not established).

Interactions

Drug-Drug: ↑ hypotensive effect with **ganglionic blocking agents, general anesthetics**, and other **antihypertensives. Estrogens** and **sympathomimetics** may ↓ the response to nitroprusside.

Route/Dosage

IV (Adults and Children): 0.3 mcg/kg/min initially; may be increased as needed up to 10 mcg/kg/min (usual dose is 3 mcg/kg/min; not to exceed 10 min of therapy at 10 mcg/kg/min infusion rate).

Availability (generic available)

Injection: 25 mg/mL in 2-mL vials.

N

nizatidine (ni-za-ti-deen)

Axid, Axid AR

Classification
Therapeutic: antiulcer agents
Pharmacologic: histamine H_2 antagonists

Indications

Duodenal ulcers and benign gastric ulcers. Maintenance therapy for duodenal ulcers after healing of active ulcer(s). Gastroesophageal reflux disease (GERD). Treatment/prevention of heartburn, acid indigestion, and sour stomach (OTC use).

Action

Inhibits the action of histamine at the H_2 receptor site located primarily in gastric parietal cells, resulting in inhibition of gastric acid secretion. **Therapeutic Effects:** Healing and prevention of ulcers. Decreased symptoms of gastroesophageal reflux. Decreased secretion of gastric acid.

Adverse Reactions/Side Effects

CNS: confusion, dizziness, drowsiness, hallucinations, headache. **CV:** ARRHYTHMIAS. **GI:** constipation, diarrhea, drug-induced hepatitis (nizatidine), nausea. **GU:** decreased sperm count, erectile dysfunction. **Endo:** gynecomastia. **Hemat:** AGRANULOCYTOSIS, APLASTIC ANEMIA, anemia, neutropenia, thrombocytopenia. **Misc:** hypersensitivity reactions.

PHYSICAL THERAPY IMPLICATIONS

Examination and Evaluation

- Assess heart rate, ECG, and heart sounds, especially during exercise (See Appendices G, H). Report any rhythm disturbances or symptoms of increased arrhythmias, including palpitations, chest discomfort, shortness of breath, fainting, and fatigue/weakness.
- Report signs of agranulocytosis and neutropenia (fever, sore throat, mucosal lesions, signs of infection, bruising), aplastic anemia (unusual fatigue, weakness), or thrombocytopenia (bruising, bleeding gums, nose bleeds).
- Monitor signs of hypersensitivity reactions, including pulmonary symptoms (tightness in the throat or chest, wheezing, cough, dyspnea) or skin reactions (rash, pruritus, urticaria). Notify physician if these reactions occur.
- Assess dizziness and drowsiness that might affect gait, balance, and other functional activities (See Appendix C). Report balance problems and functional limitations to the physician, and caution the patient and family/caregivers to guard against falls and trauma.
- Monitor other CNS symptoms such as confusion, hallucinations, and headache. Excessive or prolonged CNS symptoms may require a reduction in dose.

Interventions

- Use caution during aerobic exercise and endurance conditioning because of an increased risk of cardiac arrhythmias. Terminate exercise if patient exhibits untoward symptoms (chest pain, shortness of breath, etc.), or displays other criteria for exercise termination (See Appendix L).

Patient/Client-Related Instruction

- Advise patient to avoid alcohol and foods that may cause an increase in GI irritation.
- Instruct patient to report troublesome GI effects (constipation, diarrhea, nausea) or signs of drug-induced hepatitis (anorexia, abdominal pain, severe nausea and vomiting, yellow skin or eyes, skin rashes, flu-like symptoms, muscle/joint pain).
- Advise men to consult their physician if they experience erectile dysfunction or breast enlargement (gynecomastia).

Pharmacokinetics

Absorption: 70–95% absorbed after oral administration.
Distribution: Enters breast milk and cerebrospinal fluid.
Metabolism and Excretion: 60% excreted unchanged by the kidneys; some hepatic metabolism; at least 1 metabolite has histamine-blocking activity.
Half-life: 1.6 hr.

TIME/ACTION PROFILE

ROUTE	ONSET	PEAK	DURATION
PO	unknown	unknown	8–12 hr

Contraindications/Precautions

Contraindicated in: Hypersensitivity; Some oral liquids contain alcohol and should be avoided in patients with known intolerance.
Use Cautiously in: Geriatric patients (more susceptible to adverse CNS reactions; dosage reduction recommended); Renal impairment (more susceptible to adverse CNS reactions; ↑ dosage interval recommended if CCr ≤50 mL/min); Pregnancy or lactation.

Interactions

Drug-Drug: ↓ absorption of **ketoconazole. Antacids** and **sucralfate** ↓ absorption.

Route/Dosage

PO (Adults): *Short-term treatment of active ulcers*—300 mg once daily at bedtime. *Duodenal ulcer prophylaxis*—150 mg once daily at bedtime. *GERD*—150 mg bid. *OTC use*—75 mg 30–60 min before foods/beverages expected to cause symptoms.

Renal Impairment

PO (Adults): *Short-term treatment of active ulcers—CCr 20–50 mL/min—* 150 mg once daily; *CCr <20 mL/min*—150 mg every other day; *Duodenal ulcer prophylaxis—CCr 20–50 mL/min—* 150 mg every other day; *CCr <20 mL/min*—150 mg q 3 days.

Availability

Tablets: 75 mg OTC. **Capsules:** 150 mg Rx, 300 mg Rx.

HIGH ALERT

norepinephrine

(nor-ep-i-**nef**-rin)
Levophed

Classification
Therapeutic: vasopressors
Pharmacologic: adrenergics

Indications

Produces vasoconstriction and myocardial stimulation, which may be required after adequate fluid replacement in the treatment of severe hypotension and shock.

Action

Stimulates alpha-adrenergic receptors located mainly in blood vessels, causing constriction of both capacitance and resistance vessels. Also has minor beta-adrenergic activity (myocardial stimulation). **Therapeutic Effects:** Increased blood pressure. Increased cardiac output.

Adverse Reactions/Side Effects

CNS: anxiety, dizziness, headache, insomnia, restlessness, tremor, weakness. **Resp:** dyspnea. **CV:** arrhythmias, bradycardia, chest pain, hypertension. **GU:** decreased urine output, renal failure. **Endo:** hyperglycemia. **F and E:** metabolic acidosis. **Local:** phlebitis at IV site. **Misc:** fever.

PHYSICAL THERAPY IMPLICATIONS

Examination and Evaluation

- Assess blood pressure periodically and compare to normal values (See Appendix F). Report a sustained increase in blood pressure (hypertension) to the physician.
- Assess heart rate, ECG, and heart sounds, especially during exercise (See Appendices G, H). Report a slow heart rate or symptoms of other arrhythmias, including chest pain, palpitations, shortness of breath, fainting, and fatigue/weakness.
- Monitor signs of renal failure, including decreased urine output, increased blood pressure, muscle cramps/twitching, edema/weight gain from fluid retention, yellowish brown skin, and confusion that progresses to seizures and coma. Report these signs to the physician immediately.
- Monitor signs of metabolic acidosis, including headache, lethargy, stupor, seizures, vision disturbances, increased respiration, cardiac arrhythmias, weakness, and GI symptoms (nausea, vomiting, abdominal pain). Notify physician or nursing staff immediately if these signs occur.
- Be alert for signs of hyperglycemia, including confusion, drowsiness, flushed/dry skin, fruit-like breath odor, rapid/deep breathing, polyuria, loss of appetite, and unusual thirst. Patients with diabetes mellitus should check blood glucose levels frequently.
- Monitor and report signs of CNS toxicity, including anxiety, restlessness, insomnia, or tremor. Sustained or severe CNS signs may indicate overdose or excessive use of this drug.
- Assess dizziness that might affect gait, balance, and other functional activities (See Appendix C). Report balance problems and functional limitations to the physician and nursing staff, and caution the patient and family/caregivers to guard against falls and trauma.
- Assess IV site during and after IV administration, and report signs of phlebitis (local pain, swelling, inflammation).

Interventions

- Because of the risk of arrhythmias, angina pectoris, and increased BP, use caution during aerobic exercise and other forms of therapeutic exercise. Assess exercise tolerance frequently (blood pressure, heart rate, fatigue levels), and terminate exercise immediately if any untoward responses occur (See Appendix L).

Patient/Client-Related Instruction

- Instruct patient and family/caregivers to report severe or prolonged fever or difficult, labored breathing.

Pharmacokinetics

Absorption: IV administration results in complete bioavailability.
Distribution: Concentrates in sympathetic nervous tissue. Does not cross the blood-brain barrier but readily crosses the placenta.
Metabolism and Excretion: Taken up and metabolized rapidly by sympathetic nerve endings.
Half-life: Unknown.

TIME/ACTION PROFILE (effects on blood pressure)

ROUTE	ONSET	PEAK	DURATION
IV	immediate	rapid	1–2 min

Contraindications/Precautions

Contraindicated in: Vascular, mesenteric, or peripheral thrombosis; Pregnancy (reduces uterine blood flow); Hypoxia; Hypercarbia; Hypotension secondary to hypovolemia (without appropriate volume replacement); Hypersensitivity to bisulfites.
Use Cautiously in: Hypertension; Concurrent use of MAO inhibitors, tricyclic antidepressants, or cyclopropane or halothane anesthetics; Hyperthyroidism; Cardiovascular disease; Lactation (safety not established).

Interactions

Drug-Drug: Use with **cyclopropane** or **halothane anesthesia, cardiac glycosides, doxapram,** or local use of **cocaine** may result in ↑ myocardial irritability. Use with **MAO inhibitors, methyldopa, doxapram,**

or **tricyclic antidepressants** may result in severe hypertension. **Alpha-adrenergic blockers** can prevent pressor response. **Beta blockers** may exaggerate hypertension or block cardiac stimulation. Concurrent use with **ergot alkaloids (ergotamine, ergonovine, methylergonovine**, or **oxytocin** may result in enhanced vasoconstriction and hypertension).

Route/Dosage

IV (Adults): 0.5–1 mcg/min initially, followed by maintenance infusion of 2–12 mcg/min titrated by blood pressure response (average rate 2–4 mcg/min, up to 30 mcg/min for refractory shock have been used).

IV (Children): 0.1 mcg/kg/min initially; may be followed by infusion titrated to blood pressure response, up to 1 mcg/kg/min.

Availability

Injection: 1 mg/mL in 4-mL ampules.

norfloxacin (nor-**flox**-a-sin)

Noroxin

Classification

Therapeutic: anti-infectives

Pharmacologic: fluoroquinolones

Indications

Treatment of the following bacterial infections: Urinary tract and gynecologic infections, including cystitis, gonorrhea, and prostatitis.

Action

Inhibits bacterial DNA synthesis by inhibiting DNA gyrase enzyme. **Therapeutic Effects:** Death of susceptible bacteria. **Spectrum:** Active against gram-positive pathogens, including *Staphylococcus aureus*, *S. epidermidis*, *Streptococcus agalactiae*, *Enterococcus faecalis*. Gram-negative spectrum notable for activity against *Escherichia coli*, *Klebsiella pneumoniae*, *Enterobacter aerogenes*, *Proteus mirabilis*, *Proteus vulgaris*.

Adverse Reactions/Side Effects

CNS: SEIZURES, dizziness, drowsiness, headache, insomnia, agitation, confusion. **CV:** ARRHYTHMIAS, QTc prolongation. **GI:** HEPATOTOXICITY, PSEUDOMEMBRANOUS COLITIS, abdominal pain, diarrhea, nausea. **GU:** vaginitis. **Derm:** photosensitivity, rash. **Endo:** hyperglycemia, hypoglycemia. **MS:** tendinitis, tendon rupture. **Neuro:** peripheral neuropathy. **Misc:** HYPERSENSITIVITY REACTIONS, INCLUDING ANAPHYLAXIS.

PHYSICAL THERAPY IMPLICATIONS

Examination and Evaluation

- Watch for seizures; notify physician immediately if patient develops or increases seizure activity.
- Monitor signs of hypersensitivity reactions and anaphylaxis, including pulmonary symptoms (tightness in the throat and chest, wheezing, cough, dyspnea) or skin reactions (rash, angioedema, pruritus, urticaria). Notify physician or nursing staff immediately if these reactions occur.
- Assess heart rate, ECG, and heart sounds, especially during exercise (See Appendices G, H). Report any rhythm disturbances or symptoms of increased arrhythmias, including palpitations, chest discomfort, shortness of breath, fainting, and fatigue/weakness.
- Monitor signs of pseudomembranous colitis, including diarrhea, abdominal pain, fever, pus or mucus in stools, and other severe or prolonged GI problems (nausea, vomiting, heartburn). Notify physician or nursing staff immediately of these signs.
- Be alert for signs of hepatotoxicity, including anorexia, abdominal pain, severe nausea and vomiting, yellow skin or eyes, fever, sore throat, malaise, weakness, facial edema, lethargy, and unusual bleeding or bruising. Report these signs to the physician.
- Assess any tendon pain or joint pain. Tendinopathy and rupture can occur, especially in large, weight-bearing tendons (Achilles, patellar tendons). Risk of tendon damage is greater in patients >65 yrs old, transplant recipients (i.e., kidney, heart, lung), patients with pre-existing tendon damage, and patients taking corticosteroids concurrently.
- Monitor signs of peripheral neuropathy (numbness, tingling). Perform objective tests (nerve conduction, monofilaments) to document any neuropathic changes.
- Assess dizziness and drowsiness that might affect gait, balance, and other functional activities (See Appendix C). Report balance problems and functional limitations to the physician and nursing staff, and caution the patient and family/caregivers to guard against falls and trauma.
- Be alert for confusion, agitation, or other alterations in mental status. Notify the physician promptly if these symptoms develop.
- Monitor signs of hypoglycemia (weakness, malaise, irritability, fatigue) or hyperglycemia (drowsiness, fruity breath, increased urination, unusual thirst). Patients with diabetes mellitus should check blood glucose levels frequently.

Interventions

- If tendon symptoms occur, notify the physician and protect the affected area to avoid tendon ruptures. Do not stretch or exercise the affected tendon, and provide crutches, walker, or other assistive devices if lower extremities are involved.
- Because of the risk of arrhythmias, use caution during aerobic exercise and other forms of therapeutic

exercise. Assess exercise tolerance frequently (blood pressure, heart rate, fatigue levels), and terminate exercise immediately if any untoward responses occur (See Appendix L).

- Always wash hands thoroughly and disinfect equipment (whirlpools, electrotherapeutic devices, treatment tables, and so forth) to help prevent the spread of infection. Employ universal precautions or isolation procedures as indicated for specific patients.
- Causes photosensitivity; use care if administering UV treatments.

Patient/Client-Related Instruction

- Advise patient about photosensitivity and to use sunscreens, protective clothing, and avoid prolonged sun exposure. Advise patient to also report any rashes or other skin reactions.
- Instruct patient to report other troublesome side effects such as severe or prolonged headache, sleep loss, vaginal irritation, or GI problems (nausea, diarrhea, abdominal pain).

Pharmacokinetics

Absorption: Well absorbed (30–40%) following oral administration.
Distribution: Widely distributed. High concentrations are achieved in the urine and tissues of the urinary tract. Appears to cross the placenta.
Metabolism and Excretion: 10% metabolized by the liver, 30% excreted unchanged by the kidneys, 30% excreted unchanged in feces.
Half-life: 6.5 hr.

TIME/ACTION PROFILE (blood levels)

ROUTE	ONSET	PEAK	DURATION
PO	rapid	2–3 hr	12 hr

Contraindications/Precautions

Contraindicated in: Hypersensitivity (cross-sensitivity within class may exist); Pedi: Children; OB: Pregnancy.
Use Cautiously in: Known or suspected CNS disorder; Renal impairment (dosage reduction recommended if CCr ≤30 mL/min); Cirrhosis; Underlying conduction abnormalities (may rarely cause QTc prolongation); Concurrent use of corticosteroids (↑ risk of tendinitis/tendon rupture); Kidney, heart, or lung transplant patients (↑ risk of tendinitis/tendon rupture); Geri: Geriatric patients, dialysis patients (↑ risk of adverse reactions); Lactation: Safety not established.

Interactions

Drug-Drug: Concurrent use of **amiodarone, disopyramide, procainamide, quinidine, dofetilide,** or **sotalol** ↑ risk of potentially dangerous arrhythmias in susceptible individuals. ↑ serum **theophylline** levels and may lead to toxicity. Administration with **antacids, iron salts, bismuth subsalicylate, sucralfate,** and **zinc salts** ↓ absorption. May ↑ effects of **warfarin**. Serum levels may be ↓ by **antineoplastic agents. Cimetidine** may interfere with elimination. **Probenecid** ↓ renal elimination. May ↑ risk of nephrotoxicity from **cyclosporine**. Concurrent **corticosteroid** therapy may ↑ risk of tendon rupture. May ↑ effects of some **oral antidiabetic agents.**
Drug-Food: Absorption is impaired by **concurrent enteral feeding** (because of metal cations). Absorption of norfloxacin is ↓ by **food** and/or **dairy products** (take 1 hr before or 2 hr after).

Route/Dosage

PO (Adults): *Urinary tract infections*—400 mg q 12 hr (for 3–21 days, depending on severity of infection). *Gonorrhea*—800 mg single dose. *Prostatitis*—400 mg q 12 hr (for 28 days).

Renal Impairment

PO (Adults): *CCr ≤30 mL/min*—400 mg once daily.

Availability

Tablets: 400 mg.

nortriptyline (nor-trip-ti-leen)

Aventyl, Pamelor

Classification
Therapeutic: antidepressants
Pharmacologic: tricyclic antidepressants

Indications

Various forms of depression. **Unlabeled Use:** Management of chronic neurogenic pain.

Action

Potentiates the effect of serotonin and norepinephrine. Has significant anticholinergic properties. **Therapeutic Effects:** Antidepressant action that develops slowly over several weeks.

Adverse Reactions/Side Effects

CNS: drowsiness, fatigue, lethargy, agitation, confusion, extrapyramidal reactions, hallucinations, headache, insomnia. **EENT:** blurred vision, dry eyes, dry mouth. **CV:** ARRHYTHMIAS, hypotension, ECG changes. **GI:** constipation, nausea, paralytic ileus, unpleasant taste, weight gain. **GU:** urinary retention. **Derm:** photosensitivity. **Endo:** gynecomastia. **Hemat:** blood dyscrasias.

PHYSICAL THERAPY IMPLICATIONS

Examination and Evaluation

- Assess heart rate, ECG, and heart sounds, especially during exercise (See Appendices G, H). Report any rhythm disturbances or symptoms of increased arrhythmias, including palpitations, chest discomfort, shortness of breath, fainting, and fatigue/weakness.
- Be alert for increased depression and suicidal thoughts and ideology, especially when initiating drug treatment or in children and teenagers. Notify physician or mental health professional immediately if patient exhibits worsening depression or other changes in mood and behavior.
- Assess blood pressure (BP) periodically and compare to normal values (See Appendix F). Report low BP (hypotension), especially if patient experiences dizziness or syncope.
- Watch for signs of leukopenia (fever, sore throat, signs of infection), thrombocytopenia (bruising, nose bleeds, bleeding gums), or unusual weakness and fatigue that might be due to anemia or other blood dyscrasias. Report these signs to the physician.
- Be alert for sedation, confusion, agitation, lethargy, hallucinations, or other alterations in mental status. Notify physician if these symptoms become problematic.
- Assess motor function, and be alert for extrapyramidal reactions including Parkinson-like symptoms, dyskinesias, dystonias, or other motor abnormalities. Report any motor problems that might affect gait, balance, and other functional activities.
- If used to treat chronic pain, assess pain levels periodically to help document drug efficacy.
- Periodically assess body weight and other anthropometric measures (body mass index, body composition). Report a rapid or unexplained weight gain or increased body fat.

Interventions

- Guard against falls and trauma (hip fractures, head injury, and so forth), and implement fall-prevention strategies (See Appendix E).
- Because of cardiac arrhythmias and abnormal BP responses, use caution during aerobic exercise and endurance conditioning. Assess exercise tolerance frequently (BP, heart rate, fatigue levels), and terminate exercise immediately if any untoward responses occur (See Appendix L).
- To minimize orthostatic hypotension, patient should move slowly when assuming a more upright position.
- Help patient explore nonpharmacologic methods to reduce depression (exercise, counseling, support groups, and so forth).
- If treating neuropathic pain or other pain syndromes, implement appropriate interventions (physical agents, manual techniques, therapeutic exercise) to manage pain and reduce the need for drug therapy. Help patient also explore other nonpharmacological methods to reduce chronic pain (relaxation techniques, imagery, counseling, and so forth).
- Causes photosensitivity; use care if administering UV treatments. Advise patient to avoid direct sunlight and use sunscreens and protective clothing.

Patient/Client-Related Instruction

- Advise patient that antidepressant effects may not occur immediately; it may take 2 wk or more before an improvement in mood is observed.
- Advise patient to avoid alcohol and other CNS depressants because of the increased risk of sedation and adverse effects.
- Instruct patient to report other troublesome side effects such as severe or prolonged headache, sleep loss, dry eyes, blurred vision, urinary retention, increased breast growth in men (gynecomastia), or GI problems (nausea, constipation, dry mouth, unpleasant taste).

Pharmacokinetics

Absorption: Well absorbed after oral administration.
Distribution: Widely distributed. Enters breast milk in small amounts; probably crosses the placenta.
Protein Binding: 92%.
Metabolism and Excretion: Extensively metabolized by the liver, much of it on its first pass. Some is converted to active compounds. Undergoes enterohepatic recirculation and secretion into gastric juices.
Half-life: 18–28 hr.

TIME/ACTION PROFILE (antidepressant effect)

ROUTE	ONSET	PEAK	DURATION
PO	2–3 wk	6 wk	unknown

Contraindications/Precautions

Contraindicated in: Hypersensitivity; Angle-closure glaucoma; Alcohol intolerance (solution only).
Use Cautiously in: Preexisting cardiovascular disease; History of seizures; Asthma; May ↑ risk of suicide attempt/ideation, especially during early treatment or dose adjustment; risk may be greater in children and adolescents; OB: Use only if clearly needed and maternal benefits outweigh risk to fetus; Lactation: May result in sedation in infant; discontinue drug or bottle-feed; Pedi: Safety not established; Geri: More susceptible to adverse reactions; dose reduction recommended). Preexisting cardiovascular disease. Geriatric men with prostatic hyperplasia may be more susceptible to urinary retention.

Interactions

Drug-Drug: May cause hypertension, hyperpyrexia, seizures, and death when used with **MAO inhibitors**

(avoid concurrent use—discontinue 2 wk before starting nortriptyline). May prevent the therapeutic response to most **antihypertensives**. Hypertensive crisis may occur with **clonidine**. ↑ CNS depression with other **CNS depressants**, including **alcohol, antihistamines, opioids**, and **sedative/hypnotics**. Adrenergic effects may be ↑ with other **adrenergic agents**, including **vasoconstrictors** and **decongestants**. ↑ anticholinergic effects with other **drugs possessing anticholinergic properties**, including **antihistamines, antidepressants, atropine, haloperidol, phenothiazines, quinidine**, and **disopyramide**. **Cimetidine, fluoxetine**, or **hormonal contraceptives** ↑ blood levels and risk of toxicity. ↑ risk of agranulocytosis with **antithyroid agents**.
Drug-Natural: Concomitant use of **kava, valerian**, or **chamomile** can ↑ CNS depression. **St. John's wort** may ↓ serum concentrations and efficacy. ↑ anticholinergic effects with **jimson weed** and **scopolia**.

Route/Dosage

PO (Adults): 25 mg tid–qid, up to 150 mg/day.
PO (Geriatric Patients or adolescents): 30–50 mg/day in divided doses or as a single dose.

Availability (generic available)

Capsules: 10 mg, 25 mg, 50 mg, 75 mg.
Oral solution: 10 mg/5 mL.

nystatin (topical) (nye-**stat**-in)

Mycostatin, ✱Nyaderm, Nystop

nystatin (oral/local) (nye-**stat**-in)

Mycostatin, ✱Nadostine, Nilstat, Nystex, ✱PMS-Nystatin

nystatin (vaginal) (nye-**stat**-in)

Mycostatin

Classification
Therapeutic: antifungals
Pharmacologic: polyenes

Indications

Cream, powder: Treatment of a variety of cutaneous fungal infections, including cutaneous candidiasis, tinea pedis (athlete's foot), tinea cruris (jock itch), tinea corporis (ringworm), and tinea versicolor.
Lozenges, oral suspension: Local treatment of oropharyngeal candidiasis. Treatment of intestinal candidiasis.
Vaginal tablets: Treatment of vulvovaginal candidiasis.

Action

Affects the permeability of the fungal cell wall, allowing leakage of cellular contents. **Therapeutic Effects:** Decreased symptoms of fungal infection.

Adverse Reactions/Side Effects

Local: burning, itching, local hypersensitivity reactions, redness, stinging. **GI:** diarrhea, nausea, stomach pain (large doses), vomiting. **Derm:** contact dermatitis, Stevens-Johnson syndrome. **GU:** irritation, sensitization.

PHYSICAL THERAPY IMPLICATIONS

Examination and Evaluation

- Monitor symptoms and healing of skin lesions to help document drug effectiveness.
- Notify physician immediately of severe rashes or dermatitis because certain conditions may indicate serious hypersensitivity reactions (e.g., Stevens-Johnson syndrome).

Interventions

- Avoid contact with cutaneous lesions when treating patient.
- Always wash hands thoroughly and disinfect equipment (whirlpools, electrotherapeutic devices, treatment tables, and so forth) to help prevent the spread of infection.

Patient/Client-Related Instruction

- Advise patient to report any increased local sensitivity to this drug (pain, burning, itching, swelling).
- Instruct patient about proper hygiene; e.g., thoroughly wash and dry the affected area, wear clean socks and ventilated shoes for tinea pedis, and so forth.
- Advise patient to apply the drug as directed for the full course of treatment, even if feeling better.
- Inform patient that early relief of cutaneous symptoms may be seen in 2–3 days. Full therapeutic response may take 2 wk for cutaneous candidiasis, tinea cruris, tinea versicolor, and tinea corporis, and 6 wk for tinea pedis.
- Vaginal infections: therapeutic response is usually seen after 1 wk. Therapy should be continued during menstrual period.
- Instruct patient to notify physician of severe or prolonged GI effects (nausea, vomiting, diarrhea) during oral administration.
- Advise patient to seek medical help if infections persist or recur after the full treatment. Recurrent fungal infections may be a sign of systemic illness.

Pharmacokinetics

Absorption: Absorption through intact skin is minimal.
Distribution: Distribution after topical administration is primarily local.

N

Metabolism and Excretion: Systemic metabolism and excretion is negligible with local application.
Half-life: Not applicable.

TIME/ACTION PROFILE (resolution of symptoms/lesions)

ROUTE	ONSET	PEAK	DURATION
topical	unknown	unknown	unknown
topical/oral	rapid	unknown	2 hr*
intravaginal	unknown	unknown	unknown

*Maintenance of saliva levels required to inhibit growth of *Candida* species after oral dissolution of 2 lozenges.

Contraindications/Precautions

Contraindicated in: Hypersensitivity to active ingredients, additives, preservatives, or bases; Some products contain alcohol or bisulfites and should be avoided in patients with known intolerance.
Use Cautiously in: Nail and scalp infections (may require additional systemic therapy); Denture wearers (dentures require soaking in nystatin suspension); Pedi: Children <5 yr (lozenges, pastilles, troches). OB/Lactation: Safety not established.

Interactions

Drug-Drug: None significant.

Route/Dosage

Topical (Adults and Children): Apply cream, ointment, or powder bid–tid until healing is complete.
PO (Adults and Children): 400,000–600,000 units qid as oral suspension or 200,000–400,000 units 4–5 times daily as pastilles (lozenges).
PO (Infants): 200,000 units qid or 100,000 units to each side of the mouth qid.
PO (Neonates, Premature, and Low Birth Weight): 100,000 units qid or 50,000 units to each side of the mouth qid.
Vag (Adults): *Vaginal tablets*—100,000 units (1 tablet) daily for 2 wk.

Availability (generic available)

Cream: 100,000 units/g. **Ointment:** 100,000 units/g. **Powder:** 100,000 units/g. ***In combination with:*** triamcinolone Rx. See Appendix B.
Oral suspension: 100,000 units/mL in 5-, 60-, and 480-mL containers. **Oral pastilles (lozenges, troches):** 200,000 units/troche. **Powder for oral suspension:** $\frac{1}{8}$ tsp = 500,000 units in 50-, 150-, and 500-million, 1-, 2-, and 5-billion-unit containers. **Oral tablets:** 500,000 units.
Vaginal tablets: 100,000 units.

ofatumumab

(oh-fa-**too**-moo-mab)

Azerra

Classification

Therapeutic: antineoplastics

Pharmacologic: monoclonal antibodies

Indications

Chronic lymphocytic leukemia (CLL) refractory to fludarabine and alemtuzumab.

Action

A monoclonal antibody that specifically binds to CD20 molecule found on the surface of B lymphocytes, resulting in B-cell lysis. **Therapeutic Effects:** ↓ numbers of leukemic cells in CLL

Adverse Reactions/Side Effects

CNS: weakness. **CV:** peripheral edema. **GI:** INTESTINAL OBSTRUCTION, REACTIVATION OF HEPATITIS B. **Derm:** sweating. **Hemat:** anemia, neutropenia, thrombocytopenia. **MS:** back pain, muscle spasm. **Neuro:** PROGRESSIVE MULTIFOCAL LEUKOENCEPHALOPATHY (PML). **Misc:** INFECTIONS, INFUSION REACTIONS, chills, fever.

PHYSICAL THERAPY IMPLICATIONS

Examination and Evaluation

- Be alert for signs of progressive multifocal leukoencephalopathy. Signs include memory lapses, decreased cognition, vision loss, speech problems, incoordination, ataxia, and muscle weakness that can progress to paralysis, seizures, and coma. Report these signs to the physician or nursing staff immediately.
- Report allergy-like responses such as wheezing, laryngeal edema, urticaria, and other skin reactions that occur during and after administration (infusion related events).
- Watch for signs of reactivation of hepatitis B, including anorexia, abdominal pain, severe nausea and vomiting, yellow skin or eyes, skin rashes, flu-like symptoms, and muscle/joint pain. Report these signs to the physician or nursing staff immediately.
- Monitor signs of severe constipation and intestinal obstruction, including lack of bowel movements, abdominal pain, and abdominal distension. Report these signs to the physician or nursing staff immediately.
- Be alert for signs of infection, including fever, sore throat, chills, nausea, vomiting, diarrhea, and localized inflammation. Notify physician or nursing staff of these signs immediately.
- Monitor and report signs of bone marrow suppression, including neutropenia (fever, sore throat, signs of infection), thrombocytopenia (bruising, nose bleeds, bleeding gums), or unusual weakness and fatigue that might be due to anemia or other blood dyscrasias.
- Assess peripheral edema using girth measurements, volume displacement, and measurement of pitting edema (See Appendix N). Report increased swelling in feet and ankles or a sudden increase in body weight due to fluid retention.
- Assess any back pain or muscle spasms to rule out musculoskeletal pathology; that is, try to determine if pain is drug induced rather than caused by anatomic or biomechanical problems.

Interventions

- For patients who are medically able to begin exercise, implement appropriate resistive exercises and aerobic training to maintain muscle strength and aerobic capacity during cancer chemotherapy or to help restore function after chemotherapy.

Patient/Client-Related Instruction

- Advise patient to guard against infection (frequent hand washing, etc.), and to avoid crowds and contact with persons with contagious diseases.
- Instruct patient or family/caregivers to report other side effects such as severe or prolonged weakness, chills, fever, or excessive sweating.

Pharmacokinetics

Absorption: IV administration results in complete bioavailability.
Distribution: Unknown.
Metabolism and Excretion: Unknown.
Half-life: 14 days (range: 2.3–61.5 days).

TIME/ACTION PROFILE

ROUTE	ONSET	PEAK	DURATION
IV	end of infusion	unknown	7 days

Contraindications/Precautions

Contraindicated in: None noted.
Use Cautiously in: History of hepatitis B infection (may reactivate); OB: Use during pregnancy only if potential benefit to mother justifies potential risk to fetus; Lactation: Use cautiously during lactation; Pedi: Safe and effectiveness in children has not been established.

Interactions

Drug-Drug: May ↓ antibody response to and ↑ risk of adverse reactions from **live-virus vaccines.**

Route/Dosage

IV (Adults): 300 mg initial initially, followed 1 wk later by 2000 mg weekly for 7 doses, followed 4 wk later by 2000 mg q 4 wk for 4 doses (total regimen is 12 doses).

Availability

Solution for IV administration (requires further dilution): 100 mg/5 mL vial.

ofloxacin (oh-flox-a-sin)

Floxin

Classification

Therapeutic: anti-infectives
Pharmacologic: fluoroquinolones

Indications

PO: Treatment of the following bacterial infections: Urinary tract and gynecologic infections, including cystitis, gonorrhea, nongonococcal urethritis and cervicitis, acute pelvic inflammatory disease, and prostatitis; Respiratory tract infections, including acute exacerbations of chronic bronchitis and community-acquired pneumonia; Uncomplicated skin and skin structure infections.

Action

Inhibits bacterial DNA synthesis by inhibiting DNA gyrase enzyme. **Therapeutic Effects:** Death of susceptible bacteria. **Spectrum:** Active against gram-positive pathogens, including *Staphylococcus aureus*, *S. epidermidis*, *Streptococcus pyogenes*, *S. pneumoniae*. Gram-negative spectrum notable for activity against *Escherichia coli*, *Klebsiella pneumoniae*, *Enterobacter aerogenes*, *Proteus mirabilis*, *Haemophilus influenzae*, *Neisseria gonorrhoeae*, *Moraxella catarrhalis*. Additional spectrum includes *Chlamydophylia pneumoniae*, *Legionella pneumoniae*, *Mycoplasma pneumoniae*.

Adverse Reactions/Side Effects

CNS: SEIZURES, dizziness, drowsiness, headache, insomnia, agitation, confusion. **GI:** PSEUDOMEMBRANOUS COLITIS, abdominal pain, diarrhea, nausea, vomiting. **GU:** vaginitis. **Derm:** photosensitivity, rash. **Endo:** hyperglycemia, hypoglycemia. **MS:** tendinitis, tendon rupture. **Neuro:** peripheral neuropathy. **Misc:** HYPERSENSITIVITY REACTIONS, INCLUDING ANAPHYLAXIS.

PHYSICAL THERAPY IMPLICATIONS

Examination and Evaluation

- Watch for seizures; notify physician immediately if patient develops or increases seizure activity.
- Monitor signs of hypersensitivity reactions and anaphylaxis, including pulmonary symptoms (tightness in the throat and chest, wheezing, cough, dyspnea) or skin reactions (rash, angioedema, pruritus, urticaria). Notify physician or nursing staff immediately if these reactions occur.
- Monitor signs of pseudomembranous colitis, including diarrhea, abdominal pain, fever, pus or mucus in stools, and other severe or prolonged GI problems (nausea, vomiting, heartburn). Notify physician or nursing staff immediately of these signs.
- Assess any tendon pain or joint pain. Tendinopathy and rupture can occur, especially in large, weight-bearing tendons (Achilles, patellar tendons). Risk of tendon damage is greater in patients >65 yr old, transplant recipients (i.e., kidney, heart, lung), patients with preexisting tendon damage, and patients taking corticosteroids concurrently.
- Monitor signs of peripheral neuropathy (numbness, tingling). Perform objective tests (nerve conduction, monofilaments) to document any neuropathic changes.
- Assess dizziness and drowsiness that might affect gait, balance, and other functional activities (See Appendix C). Report balance problems and functional limitations to the physician and nursing staff, and caution the patient and family/caregivers to guard against falls and trauma.
- Be alert for confusion, agitation, or other alterations in mental status. Notify the physician promptly if these symptoms develop.
- Monitor signs of hypoglycemia (weakness, malaise, irritability, fatigue) or hyperglycemia (drowsiness, fruity breath, increased urination, unusual thirst). Patients with diabetes mellitus should check blood glucose levels frequently.

Interventions

- If tendon symptoms occur, notify the physician and protect the affected area to avoid tendon ruptures. Do not stretch or exercise the affected tendon, and provide crutches, walker, or other assistive devices if lower extremities are involved.
- Always wash hands thoroughly and disinfect equipment (whirlpools, electrotherapeutic devices, treatment tables, and so forth) to help prevent the spread of infection. Use universal precautions or isolation procedures as indicated for specific patients.
- Causes photosensitivity; use care if administering UV treatments.

Patient/Client-Related Instruction

- Advise patient about photosensitivity and to use sunscreens, protective clothing, and avoid prolonged sun exposure. Advise patient to also report any rashes or other skin reactions.
- Instruct patient to report other troublesome side effects such as severe or prolonged headache, sleep loss, vaginal irritation, or GI problems (nausea, diarrhea, abdominal pain).

Pharmacokinetics

Absorption: Well absorbed (98%) following oral administration.

Distribution: Widely distributed. High tissue and urinary levels are achieved. Appears to cross the placenta; enters breast milk.

Metabolism and Excretion: 70–80% excreted unchanged by the kidneys.

Half-life: 5–7 hr.

TIME/ACTION PROFILE (blood levels)

ROUTE	ONSET	PEAK	DURATION
PO	rapid	1–2 hr	12 hr

Contraindications/Precautions

Contraindicated in: Hypersensitivity (cross-sensitivity within class may exist); Pedi: Children <18 yr; OB: Pregnancy.

Use Cautiously in: Known or suspected CNS disorder; Renal impairment (dose reduction recommended if CCr ≤50 mL/min); Cirrhosis; Concurrent use of corticosteroids (↑ risk of tendinitis/tendon rupture); Kidney, heart, or lung transplant patients (↑ risk of tendinitis/tendon rupture); Geri: ↑ risk of adverse reactions; Lactation: Safety not established.

Interactions

Drug-Drug: ↑ serum **theophylline** levels and may lead to toxicity. Administration with **antacids, iron salts, bismuth subsalicylate, sucralfate**, and **zinc salts** ↓ absorption. May ↑ the effects of **warfarin**. Serum levels may be ↓ by **antineoplastic agents**. **Cimetidine** may interfere with elimination. **Probenecid** ↓ renal elimination. May ↑ risk of nephrotoxicity from **cyclosporine**. Concurrent **corticosteroid** therapy may ↑ risk of tendon rupture.

Drug-Food: Absorption is impaired by **concurrent enteral feeding** (because of metal cations). Absorption of ofloxacin is ↓ by **foods** and/or **dairy products**.

Route/Dosage

PO (Adults): *Most infections*—400 mg q 12 hr (for 3–10 days depending infection). *Urethritis/cervicitis*—300 mg q 12 hr (for 7 days). *Prostatitis*—300 mg q 12 hr (for 6 wk). *Urinary tract infections*—200 mg q 12 hr. *Gonorrhea*—400 mg single dose.

Renal Impairment

PO (Adults): *CCr 20–50 mL/min*—100% of the usual dose q 24 hr; *CCr <20 mL/min*—50% of the usual dose q 24 hr.

Otic (Adults and Children ≥6 mo): *Otitis externa 6 mo–13 yr*—5 drops instilled into affected ear once daily for 7 days; *Otitis externa ≥13 yr*—10 drops instilled into affected ear once daily for 7 days. *Acute otitis media in pediatric patients 1–12 yr old with tympanostomy tubes*—5 drops instilled into the affected ear bid for 10 days. *Chronic suppurative otitis media with perforated tympanic membranes in patients ≥12 yr*—10 drops instilled into the affected ear bid for 14 days.

Availability (generic available)

Tablets: 200 mg Rx, 300 mg Rx, 400 mg Rx. **Otic solution:** 0.3% in 5- and 10-mL dropper bottles and 0.25-mL single-dispensing containers.

olanzapine (oh-lan-za-peen)

Zyprexa, Zyprexa Zydis

Classification

Therapeutic: antipsychotics, mood stabilizers

Pharmacologic: thienobenzodiazepines

O

Indications

Psychotic disorders: Acute manic episodes associated with bipolar disorder (may be used with lithium or valproate), long-term maintenance therapy of bipolar disorder, long-term treatment/maintenance of schizophrenia, agitation due to schizophrenia or mania (IM). **Unlabeled Use:** Management of anorexia nervosa. Treatment of nausea and vomiting related to highly emetogenic chemotherapy.

Action

Antagonizes dopamine and serotonin type 2 in the CNS. Also has anticholinergic, antihistaminic, and anti–alpha$_1$-adrenergic effects. **Therapeutic Effects:** Decreased manifestations of psychoses.

Adverse Reactions/Side Effects

CNS: NEUROLEPTIC MALIGNANT SYNDROME, SEIZURES, agitation, dizziness, headache, restlessness, sedation, weakness, dystonia, insomnia, mood changes, personality disorder, speech impairment, tardive dyskinesia. **EENT:** amblyopia, rhinitis, increased salivation, pharyngitis. **Resp:** cough, dyspnea. **CV:** orthostatic hypotension, tachycardia, chest pain. **GI:** constipation, dry mouth, abdominal pain, increased appetite, weight loss or gain, nausea, increased thirst. **GU:** decreased libido, urinary incontinence. **Derm:** photosensitivity. **Endo:** hyperglycemia, goiter. **Metab:** dyslipidemia. **MS:** hypertonia, joint pain. **Neuro:** tremor. **Misc:** fever, flu-like syndrome.

PHYSICAL THERAPY IMPLICATIONS

Examination and Evaluation

- Monitor and report signs of neuroleptic malignant syndrome, including hyperthermia, diaphoresis, generalized muscle rigidity, altered mental status, tachycardia, changes in blood pressure (BP), and incontinence. Symptoms typically occur within 4–14 days after initiation of drug therapy, but can occur at any time during drug use.
- Be alert for new seizures or increased seizure activity, especially at the onset of drug treatment. Document the number, duration, and severity of seizures, and report these findings to the physician immediately.
- Assess motor function, and be alert for extrapyramidal symptoms. Report these symptoms immediately, especially tardive dyskinesia, because this problem may be irreversible. Common extrapyramidal symptoms include:
  - Tardive dyskinesia (uncontrolled rhythmic movement of mouth, face, and extremities, lip smacking or puckering, puffing of cheeks, uncontrolled chewing, rapid or worm-like movements of tongue).
  - Pseudoparkinsonism (shuffling gait, rigidity, tremor, pill-rolling motion, loss of balance control, difficulty speaking or swallowing, mask-like face).
  - Akathisia (restlessness or desire to keep moving).
  - Other dystonias and dyskinesias (dystonic muscle spasms, twisting motions, twitching, inability to move eyes, weakness of arms or legs).
- Assess heart rate, ECG, and heart sounds, especially during exercise (See Appendices G, H). Report a rapid heart rate (tachycardia) or signs of other arrhythmias, including palpitations, chest pain, shortness of breath, fainting, and fatigue/weakness.
- Assess BP when patient assumes a more upright position (lying to standing, sitting to standing, lying to sitting). Document orthostatic hypotension and contact physician when systolic BP falls >20 mm Hg or diastolic BP falls >10 mm Hg.
- Report any troublesome respiratory problems, including severe or prolonged cough, nasopharyngeal irritation, or difficult/labored breathing.
- Be alert for signs of hyperglycemia, including confusion, drowsiness, flushed/dry skin, fruit-like breath odor, rapid/deep breathing, polyuria, loss of appetite, and unusual thirst. Patients with diabetes mellitus should check blood glucose levels frequently.
- Monitor changes in behavior, including agitation, restlessness, and other changes in mood and personality. Notify physician if these changes become problematic.
- Assess dizziness and weakness that might affect gait, balance, and other functional activities (See Appendix C). Report balance problems and functional limitations to the physician, and caution the patient and family/caregivers to guard against falls and trauma.
- Assess any joint pain and increased muscle tone to rule out neuromusculoskeletal pathology; that is, try to determine if pain is drug induced rather than caused by anatomic or biomechanical problems.
- Periodically assess body weight and other anthropometric measures (body mass index, body composition). Report a substantial weight gain or weight loss.

Interventions

- Guard against falls and trauma (hip fractures, head injury, and so forth) caused by drowsiness, dizziness, blurred vision, or extrapyramidal symptoms; implement fall-prevention strategies (See Appendix E).
- Because of the risk of arrhythmias and abnormal BP responses, use caution during aerobic exercise and other forms of therapeutic exercise Assess exercise tolerance frequently (BP, heart rate, fatigue levels), and terminate exercise immediately if any untoward responses occur (See Appendix L).
- To minimize orthostatic hypotension, patient should move slowly when assuming a more upright position.
- Causes photosensitivity; use care if administering UV treatments. Advise patient to avoid direct sunlight and use sunscreens and protective clothing.
- Help patient and family/caregivers explore nonpharmacologic methods (exercise, counseling, support groups) to reduce schizophrenic episodes and behavioral problems.

Patient/Client-Related Instruction

- Advise patient to avoid alcohol and other CNS depressants because of the increased risk of sedation and adverse effects.
- Advise patient that this drug may cause problems in fat and glucose metabolism (dyslipidemia and hyperglycemia, respectively). Remind patient that periodic blood tests may be needed to monitor plasma lipids and blood glucose.
- Instruct patient to report other problematic side effects such as severe or prolonged headache, vision disturbances, speech impairments, fever, flu-like symptoms, goiter, urinary incontinence, decreased libido, or GI problems (nausea, constipation, abdominal pain, dry mouth).

Pharmacokinetics

Absorption: Well absorbed but rapidly metabolized by first-pass effect, resulting in 60% bioavailability.

Conventional tablets and orally disintegrating tablets (Zydis) are bioequivalent. IM administration results in significantly higher blood levels (5 times that of oral).
Distribution: Extensively distributed.
Protein Binding: 93%.
Metabolism and Excretion: Highly metabolized (mostly by the hepatic P450CYP1A2 system); 7% excreted unchanged in urine.
Half-life: 21–54 hr.

TIME/ACTION PROFILE (antipsychotic effects)

ROUTE	ONSET	PEAK*	DURATION
PO	unknown	6 hr	unknown
IM	rapid	15–45 min	2–4 hr

*Blood levels.

Contraindications/Precautions

Contraindicated in: Hypersensitivity; Lactation: Discontinue drug or bottle feed; **Orally disintegrating tablets only:** Phenylketonuria (orally disintegrating tablets contain aspartame).
Use Cautiously in: Patients with hepatic impairment; Patients at risk for aspiration; Cardiovascular or cerebrovascular disease; History of seizures; History of attempted suicide; Diabetes or risk factors for diabetes (may worsen glucose control); Prostatic hyperplasia; Angle-closure glaucoma; History of paralytic ileus; Dysphagia and aspiration have been associated with antipsychotic drug use; use with caution in patients at risk for aspiration; OB/Pedi: Safety not established; Geri: Geriatric patients (may require ↓ doses; ↑ risk of mortality in elderly patients treated for dementia-related psychosis).

Interactions

Drug-Drug: Effects may be ↓ by concurrent **carbamazepine, omeprazole,** or **rifampin.** ↑ hypotension may occur with **antihypertensives.** ↑ CNS depression may occur with concurrent use of **alcohol** or other **CNS depressants.** May antagonize the effects of **levodopa** or other **dopamine agonists. Nicotine** can ↓ olanzapine levels.

Route/Dosage

PO (Adults—Most Patients): *Schizophrenia*—5–10 mg/day initially; may increase at weekly intervals by 5 mg/day (not to exceed 20 mg/day). *Bipolar mania*—10–15 mg/day initially; may increase every 24 hr by 5 mg/day (not to exceed 20 mg/day).
PO (Adults—Debilitated or Nonsmoking Female Patients ≥65 yr): Initiate therapy at 5 mg/day.
IM (Adults): *Acute agitation*—5–10 mg, may repeat in 2 hr, then 4 hr later.

Availability

Tablets: 2.5 mg, 5 mg, 7.5 mg, 10 mg, 15 mg, 20 mg. **Orally disintegrating tablets (Zydis):** 5 mg, 10 mg, 15 mg, 20 mg. **Powder for injection:** 10 mg/vial. ***In combination with:*** fluoxetine (Symbyax). See Appendix B.

olmesartan medoxomil

(ole-me-**sar**-tan me-**dox**-oh-mil)
Benicar

Classification
Therapeutic: antihypertensives
Pharmacologic: angiotensin II receptor antagonists

Indications

Hypertension (alone or with other agents).

Action

Blocks vasoconstrictor and aldosterone-secreting effects of angiotensin II at various receptor sites, including vascular smooth muscle and the adrenal glands. **Therapeutic Effects:** Lowering of blood pressure.

Adverse Reactions/Side Effects

CNS: dizziness. **CV:** hypotension. **F and E:** hyperkalemia. **GU:** impaired renal function.
Misc: ANGIOEDEMA.

PHYSICAL THERAPY IMPLICATIONS

Examination and Evaluation

- Be alert for signs of angioedema, including rashes, raised patches of red or white skin (welts), burning/itching skin, swelling in the face, and difficulty breathing. Notify physician immediately if these signs occur.
- Assess blood pressure periodically and compare to normal values (See Appendix F) to help determine antihypertensive effects. Report an excessive fall in blood pressure (hypotension), especially if patient experiences dizziness, fatigue, palpitations, or other symptoms.
- Assess dizziness that might affect gait, balance, and other functional activities (See Appendix C). Report balance problems and functional limitations to the physician, and caution the patient and family/caregivers to guard against falls and trauma.
- Assess any unusual weakness and fatigue that might be due to high potassium levels (hyperkalemia) or other electrolyte imbalances.

O

Interventions

- Avoid physical therapy interventions that cause systemic vasodilation (large whirlpool, Hubbard tank). Additive effects of this drug and the intervention may cause a dangerous fall in blood pressure.
- To minimize orthostatic hypotension, patient should move slowly when assuming a more upright position.

Patient/Client-related Instruction

- Remind patients to take medication as directed to control hypertension even if they are asymptomatic.
- Counsel patients about additional interventions to help control blood pressure, including regular exercise, weight loss, sodium restriction, stress reduction, moderation of alcohol consumption, and smoking cessation.
- Instruct patient to report signs of impaired renal function, including decreased urine output, cloudy urine, or sudden weight gain due to fluid retention.

Pharmacokinetics

Absorption: Olmesartan medoxomil is a prodrug that is converted to olmesartan (the active component); 26% bioavailability of olmesartan.
Distribution: Crosses the placenta.
Protein Binding: 99%.
Metabolism and Excretion: No further metabolism following conversion of prodrug to active drug; 35–50% excreted unchanged in urine; remainder eliminated in feces via bile.
Half-life: 13 hr.

TIME/ACTION PROFILE (antihypertensive effect with chronic dosing)

ROUTE	ONSET	PEAK	DURATION
PO	within 1 wk	2 wk	24 hr

Contraindications/Precautions

Contraindicated in: Hypersensitivity; Bilateral renal artery stenosis; OB: Can cause injury or death of fetus—if pregnancy occurs, discontinue immediately; Lactation: Discontinue olmesartan or provide formula.
Use Cautiously in: Volume- or salt-depleted patients or patients receiving high doses of diuretics (correct deficits before initiating therapy or initiate at lower doses); Black patients (may not be as effective); Impaired renal function due to primary renal disease or CHF (may worsen renal function); Patients with childbearing potential; Pedi: Safety not established for children <18 yr.

Interactions

Drug-Drug: Additive hypotension with other **antihypertensives**. Excessive hypotension may occur with concurrent use of **diuretics**. Antihypertensive effect may be blunted by **NSAIDs**. ↑ risk of hyperkalemia with concurrent use of **potassium supplements, potassium-containing salt substitutes, angiotensin-converting enzyme inhibitors,** or **potassium-sparing diuretics.**

Route/Dosage

PO (Adults): 20 mg once daily; may be increased up to 40 mg daily (initiate therapy at a lower dose in patients receiving diuretics or who are volume depleted).

Availability

Tablets: 5 mg, 20 mg, 40 mg. ***In combination with:*** hydrochlorothiazide (Benicar HCT), amlodipine (Azor). See Appendix B.

olopatadine (nasal spray)

(oh-loe-**pat**-ah-deen)

Patanase

Classification

Therapeutic: allergy, cold, and cough remedies
Pharmacologic: antihistamines

Indications

Relief of symptoms of allergic rhinitis.

Action

Antagonizes the effects of histamine at histamine$_1$ receptor sites; does not bind to or inactivate histamine.
Therapeutic Effects: Decreased symptoms of histamine excess, including rhinorrhea, sneezing, and nasal itching.

Adverse Reactions/Side Effects

CNS: drowsiness, headache. **EENT:** epistaxis, nasal perforation, nasal ulcerations, pharyngolaryngeal pain, postnasal drip. **GI:** bitter taste. **Resp:** cough.

PHYSICAL THERAPY IMPLICATIONS

Examination and Evaluation

- Report signs of nasal or pharyngeal problems such as nosebleeds, nasal pain, ulceration, or increased postnasal drip.

Patient/Client-Related Instruction

- Advise patient not to exceed the recommended dose or frequency of intranasal applications.
- Advise patient to avoid alcohol and other CNS depressants because of the increased risk of sedation and adverse effects.
- Instruct patient and family/caregivers to report other troublesome side effects such as severe or prolonged headache, drowsiness, cough, or bitter taste.

Pharmacokinetics

Absorption: 57% absorbed from nasal mucosa.
Distribution: Unknown.

Metabolism and Excretion: Minimal metabolism; 70% eliminated in urine mostly as unchanged drug; 17% fecal elimination.
Half-life: 8–12 hr.

TIME/ACTION PROFILE

ROUTE	ONSET	PEAK	DURATION
nasal	rapid	unknown	12 hr

Contraindications/Precautions

Contraindicated in: None noted.
Use Cautiously in: Nasal pathology other than allergic rhinitis; Geri: Dose cautiously in elderly patients; consider age-related decrease in organ function and concurrent medications; Lactation/OB: Use in pregnancy or lactation only when maternal benefit outweighs fetal risk; Pedi: Safe use in children <12 yr not established.

Interactions

Drug-Drug: ↑ CNS depression may occur with **alcohol**; avoid concurrent use.

Route/Dosage

Intranasal (Adults and Children ≥12 yr): 2 sprays in each nostril bid.

Availability

Nasal spray: 665 mcg/100 μL (0.6%) spray in 30.5-g bottle (provides 240 metered sprays).

olsalazine (ole-sal-a-zeen)

Dipentum

Classification
Therapeutic: gastrointestinal anti-inflammatories—therapeutic
Pharmacologic: salicylic acid derivatives

Indications

Ulcerative colitis (when patients cannot tolerate sulfasalazine).

Action

Locally acting anti-inflammatory action in the colon, where activity is probably due to inhibition of prostaglandin synthesis. **Therapeutic Effects:** Reduction in the symptoms of inflammatory bowel disease.

Adverse Reactions/Side Effects

CNS: ataxia, confusion, dizziness, drowsiness, headache, mental depression, psychosis, restlessness. **GI:** diarrhea, abdominal pain, anorexia, exacerbation of colitis, drug-induced hepatitis, nausea, vomiting. **Derm:** itching, rash. **Hemat:** blood dyscrasias.

PHYSICAL THERAPY IMPLICATIONS

Examination and Evaluation

- Monitor any changes in symptoms (decreased abdominal pain, decreased diarrhea, improved appetite) to help document whether drug therapy is successful.
- Monitor and report signs of blood dyscrasias such as agranulocytosis (fever, sore throat, mucosal lesions, signs of infection), thrombocytopenia (bruising, nose bleeds, bleeding gums), or anemias (unusual weakness, fatigue, pallor, shortness of breath upon exertion).
- Assess dizziness, drowsiness, or ataxia that might affect gait, balance, and other functional activities (See Appendix C). Report balance problems and functional limitations to the physician and nursing staff, and caution the patient and family/caregivers to guard against falls and trauma.
- Monitor changes in mood and behavior, including depression, confusion, restlessness, and psychosis. Notify physician if these changes become problematic.

Patient/Client-Related Instruction

- Advise patient to guard against infection (frequent hand washing, etc.), and to avoid crowds and contact with persons with contagious diseases.
- Advise patient about the likelihood of GI reactions (nausea, vomiting, diarrhea, loss of appetite). Instruct patient to report severe or prolonged GI problems, increased symptoms of colitis, or signs of drug-induced hepatitis (yellow skin or eyes, abdominal pain, severe nausea and vomiting, fever, sore throat, malaise, weakness, facial edema).
- Instruct patient to report other untoward side effects such as severe or prolonged headache or skin reactions (rash, itching).

Pharmacokinetics

Absorption: Acts locally in colon, where 98–99% is converted to mesalamine (5-aminosalicylic acid).
Distribution: Action is primarily local and remains in the colon.
Metabolism and Excretion: 2% absorbed into systemic circulation is rapidly metabolized; mostly eliminated as mesalamine in the feces.
Half-life: 0.9 hr.

TIME/ACTION PROFILE (levels)

ROUTE	ONSET	PEAK	DURATION
PO	unknown	1 hr; 4–8 hr	12 hr

O

Contraindications/Precautions

Contraindicated in: Hypersensitivity reactions to salicylates; Cross-sensitivity with furosemide, sulfonylurea hypoglycemic agents, or carbonic anhydrase inhibitors may exist; G6PD deficiency; Urinary tract or intestinal obstruction; Pedi: Children <2 yr (safe use not established); Porphyria.
Use Cautiously in: Severe hepatic or renal impairment; OB: Pregnancy; Geri: Geriatric patients (consider ↓ body mass, hepatic/renal/cardiac function, intercurrent illness, and drug therapies; Renal impairment (↑ risk of renal tubular damage); Lactation: Lactation (safety not established).

Interactions

Drug-Drug: ↑ risk of bleeding after neuraxial anesthesia with **low molecular weight heparins** and **heparinoids**; discontinue olsalazine before initiation of therapy or monitor closely if discontinuation not possible. May ↓ metabolism, and ↑ effects/toxicity of **mercaptopurine** or **thioguanine** with and ↑ risk of myelosuppression (use lowest possible dose and monitor closely). ↑ risk of developing Reye's syndrome; avoid olsalazine during 6 wk after **varicella vaccine**.

Route/Dosage

PO (Adults): 500 mg bid.

Availability

Capsules: 250 mg.

PHYSICAL THERAPY IMPLICATIONS

Examination and Evaluation

- Be alert for signs of allergic reactions and anaphylaxis, including pulmonary symptoms (tightness in the throat and chest, wheezing, cough, dyspnea) or skin reactions (rash, pruritus, urticaria). Notify physician immediately if these reactions occur.
- Monitor signs of malignancy, including a change in bowel or bladder habits, nonhealing sores, unusual bleeding or discharge, a lump in the breast or other parts of the body, chronic indigestion or difficulty in swallowing, obvious changes in a wart or mole, and persistent coughing or hoarseness. Report these signs to the physician immediately.
- Assess pulmonary function periodically by measuring lung volumes, breath sounds, respiratory rate, and other symptoms (wheezing, dyspnea, shortness of breath) (See Appendices I, J, K). Report changes in pulmonary function to help document the effects of drug therapy in treating asthma.
- Monitor subcutaneous injection sites for pain, swelling, and irritation. Report prolonged or excessive injection site reactions to the physician.

Interventions

- Design and implement appropriate aerobic exercise and respiratory muscle training programs to maintain optimal cardiovascular and pulmonary function. Work with patient and family/caregivers to find forms of exercise (e.g., swimming) that can help improve respiratory function without triggering asthma attacks.

Patient/Client-Related Instruction

- Advise patients to consult physician before stopping this medication or other asthma medications. Stopping these medications suddenly may result in increased bronchoconstriction.

Pharmacokinetics

Absorption: 62% absorbed slowly from SC sites.
Distribution: Enters breast milk.
Metabolism and Excretion: Degraded similarly to IgG via binding degradation, reticuloendothelial system, and the liver.
Half-life: 26 days.

TIME/ACTION PROFILE (effects on IgE levels)

ROUTE	ONSET	PEAK	DURATION
SC	within 1 hr	unknown	up to 1 yr

omalizumab

(oh-ma-liz-yoo-mab)
Xolair

Classification
Therapeutic: antiasthmatics
Pharmacologic: monoclonal antibodies

Indications

Moderate-to-severe asthma not controlled by inhaled corticosteroids.

Action

Inhibits binding of IgE to receptors on mast cells and eosinophils, preventing the release of mediators of the allergic response. Also decreases amount of IgE receptors on basophils. **Therapeutic Effects:** ↓ incidence of exacerbations of asthma.

Adverse Reactions/Side Effects

Local: <u>injection site reactions</u>. **Misc:** ALLERGIC REACTIONS, INCLUDING ANAPHYLAXIS, ↑ risk of malignancy.

Contraindications/Precautions

Contraindicated in: Hypersensitivity; Acute bronchospasm.
Use Cautiously in: Chronic use of inhaled corticosteroids; Pregnancy, lactation, or children <12 yr

(safety not established; use in pregnancy only if clearly needed).

Interactions

Drug-Drug: None noted.

Route/Dosage

SC (Adults and Children >12 yr): 150–375 mg every 2–4 wk (determined by pretreatment serum IgE level and body weight).

Availability

Sterile powder for SC injection (requires reconstitution): 150 mg/vial.

omeprazole (o-mep-ra-zole)

✱ Losec, Prilosec, Prilosec OTC, Zegerid

Classification

Therapeutic: antiulcer agents

Pharmacologic: proton-pump inhibitors

Indications

GERD/maintenance of healing in erosive esophagitis. Duodenal ulcers (with or without anti-infectives for *Helicobacter pylori*). Short-term treatment of active benign gastric ulcer. Pathologic hypersecretory conditions, including Zollinger-Ellison syndrome. Reduction of risk of GI bleeding in critically ill patients. **OTC:** Heartburn occurring ≥ twice/wk.

Action

Binds to an enzyme on gastric parietal cells in the presence of acidic gastric pH, preventing the final transport of hydrogen ions into the gastric lumen. **Therapeutic Effects:** Diminished accumulation of acid in the gastric lumen with lessened gastroesophageal reflux. Healing of duodenal ulcers.

Adverse Reactions/Side Effects

CNS: dizziness, drowsiness, fatigue, headache, weakness. **CV:** chest pain. **GI:** abdominal pain, acid regurgitation, constipation, diarrhea, flatulence, nausea, vomiting. **Derm:** itching, rash. **Misc:** allergic reactions.

PHYSICAL THERAPY IMPLICATIONS

Examination and Evaluation

- Monitor improvements in GI symptoms (gastritis, heartburn, and so forth) to help determine if drug therapy is successful.
- Assess dizziness that might affect gait, balance, and other functional activities (See Appendix C). Report balance problems and functional limitations to the physician, and caution the patient and family/caregivers to guard against falls and trauma.
- Monitor other CNS side effects (drowsiness, fatigue, weakness, headache), and report severe or prolonged effects.
- Monitor any chest pain and attempt to determine if pain is drug induced or caused by cardiovascular dysfunction (e.g., angina that occurs during exercise).

Interventions

- In cases of NSAID-induced gastritis, implement appropriate manual therapy techniques, physical agents, and therapeutic exercises to reduce pain and decrease the need for aspirin and other NSAIDs.

Patient/Client-Related Instruction

- Advise patient to avoid alcohol and foods that may cause an increase in GI irritation.
- Instruct patient to report bothersome or prolonged side effects, including skin problems (itching, rash) or GI effects (nausea, diarrhea, vomiting, constipation, heartburn, flatulence, abdominal pain).

Pharmacokinetics

Absorption: Rapidly absorbed following oral administration; immediate release formulation contains bicarbonate to prevent acid degradation.
Distribution: Good distribution into gastric parietal cells.
Protein Binding: 95%.
Metabolism and Excretion: Extensively metabolized by the liver.
Half-life: 0.5–1 hr (increased in liver disease to 3 hr).

TIME/ACTION PROFILE (antisecretory effects)

ROUTE	ONSET	PEAK	DURATION
PO—delayed release	within 1 hr	within 2 hr	72–96 hr
PO—immediate release	rapid	30 min	24 hr

Contraindications/Precautions

Contraindicated in: Hypersensitivity; Metabolic alkalosis and hypocalcemia (Zegerid only).
Use Cautiously in: Liver disease (dose reduction may be necessary); Geri: Increased risk of hip fractures in patients using high-doses for >1 yr; Bartter's syndrome, hypokalemia, and respiratory alkalosis (Zegerid only); OB/Lactation/Pedi: Pregnancy, lactation, or children <1 yr (safety not established).

Interactions

Drug-Drug: Omeprazole is metabolized by the CYP450 enzyme system and may compete with other agents metabolized by this system. ↓ metabolism and may ↑ effects of Rx **antifungal agents, atazanavir,**

diazepam, digoxin, flurazepam, triazolam, cyclosporine, disulfiram, phenytoin, tacrolimus, and **warfarin**. May ↓ absorption of drugs requiring acid pH, including **ketoconazole, itraconazole, atazanavir, ampicillin, iron salts**, and **digoxin**. Has been used safely with **antacids**. May ↑ risk of bleeding with **warfarin** (monitor INR/PT).

Route/Dosage

PO (Adults): *GERD/erosive esophagitis*—20 mg once daily. *Duodenal ulcers associated with* H. pylori—40 mg daily in the morning with clarithromycin for 2 wk, then 20 mg once daily for 2 wk *or* 20 mg bid with clarithromycin 500 mg bid and amoxicillin 1000 mg bid for 10 days (if ulcer is present at beginning of therapy, continue omeprazole 20 mg daily for 18 more days); has also been used with clarithromycin and metronidazole. *Gastric ulcer*—40 mg once daily for 4–6 wk. *Reduction of the risk of GI bleeding in critically ill patients*—40 mg initially, then another 40 mg 6–8 hr later, followed by 40 mg once daily for up to 14 days. *Gastric hypersecretory conditions*—60 mg once daily initially; may be increased up to 120 mg tid (doses >80 mg/day should be given in divided doses); *OTC*—20 mg once daily for up to 14 days.

PO (Children 1–16 yr and 5–9 kg): *GERD/erosive esophagitis*—5 mg once daily.

PO (Children 1–16 yr and 10–19 kg): *GERD/erosive esophagitis*—10 mg once daily.

PO (Children 1–16 yr and ≥20 kg): *GERD/erosive esophagitis*—20 mg once daily.

Availability (generic available)

Delayed-release capsules: 10 mg, 20 mg Rx, OTC, 40 mg. **Delayed-release powder for oral suspension (peach-mint):** 2.5-mg packet, 10-mg packet.

ondansetron (on-dan-se-tron)

Zofran

Classification

Therapeutic: antiemetics

Pharmacologic: 5-HT_3 antagonists

Indications

Prevention of nausea and vomiting associated with chemotherapy or radiation therapy. **IM, IV:** Prevention and treatment of postoperative nausea and vomiting.

Action

Blocks the effects of serotonin at 5-HT_3 receptor sites (selective antagonist) located in vagal nerve terminals and the chemoreceptor trigger zone in the CNS. **Therapeutic Effects:** Decreased incidence and severity of nausea and vomiting following chemotherapy or surgery.

Adverse Reactions/Side Effects

CNS: headache, dizziness, drowsiness, fatigue, weakness. **GI:** constipation, diarrhea, abdominal pain, dry mouth, increased liver enzymes. **Neuro:** extrapyramidal reactions.

PHYSICAL THERAPY IMPLICATIONS

Examination and Evaluation

- Monitor improvements in GI symptoms (decreased nausea and vomiting, increased appetite) to help document whether drug therapy is successful.
- Assess motor function, and report any extrapyramidal reactions. Common extrapyramidal symptoms include:
  - Tardive dyskinesia (uncontrolled rhythmic movement of mouth, face, and extremities, lip smacking or puckering, puffing of cheeks, uncontrolled chewing, rapid or worm-like movements of tongue).
  - Pseudoparkinsonism (shuffling gait, rigidity, tremor, pill-rolling motion, loss of balance control, difficulty speaking or swallowing, mask-like face).
  - Akathisia (restlessness or desire to keep moving).
  - Other dystonias and dyskinesias (dystonic muscle spasms, twisting motions, twitching, inability to move eyes, weakness of arms or legs).
- Assess dizziness and drowsiness that might affect gait, balance, and other functional activities (see Appendix C). Report balance problems and functional limitations to the physician and nursing staff, and caution the patient and family/caregivers to guard against falls and trauma.

Patient/Client-Related Instruction

- Instruct patient to report bothersome side effects such as severe or prolonged headache, weakness, fatigue, or GI problems (diarrhea, constipation, abdominal pain, dry mouth).

Pharmacokinetics

Absorption: IV administration results in complete bioavailability; 50% absorbed following oral administration.

Distribution: Unknown.

Metabolism and Excretion: Extensively metabolized by the liver; 5% excreted unchanged by the kidneys.

Half-life: 3.5–5.5 hr.

TIME/ACTION PROFILE (antiemetic effect)

ROUTE	ONSET	PEAK	DURATION
PO, IV	rapid	15–30 min	4–8 hr
IM	rapid	40 min	unknown

Contraindications/Precautions

Contraindicated in: Hypersensitivity; Orally disintegrating tablets contain aspartame and should not be used in patients with phenylketonuria.

Use Cautiously in: Liver impairment (daily dose not to exceed 8 mg); Abdominal surgery (may mask ileus); OB/Pedi: Pregnancy, lactation, or children ≤3 yr (safety not established).

Interactions

Drug-Drug: May be affected by **drugs altering the activity of liver enzymes.**

Route/Dosage

PO (Adults and Children ≥12 yr): *Prevention of chemotherapy-induced nausea/vomiting*—8 mg 30 min prior to chemotherapy and repeated 8 hr later; 8 mg q 12 hr may be given for 1–2 days following chemotherapy. *Prevention of radiation-induced nausea/vomiting*—8 mg 1–2 hr prior to radiation; may be repeated q 8 hr, depending on type, location, and extent of radiation. *Prevention of postoperative nausea/vomiting*—16 mg 1 hr before induction of anesthesia.

PO (Children 4–11 yr): *Prevention of chemotherapy-induced nausea/vomiting*—4 mg 30 min prior to chemotherapy and repeated 4 and 8 hr later; 4 mg q 8 hr may be given for 1–2 days following chemotherapy.

IV (Adults): *Prevention of chemotherapy-induced nausea/vomiting*—0.15 mg/kg 15–30 min prior to chemotherapy, repeated 4 and 8 hr later, or 32-mg single dose 30 min prior to chemotherapy (lower doses have been used).

IM, IV (Adults): *Prevention of postoperative nausea/vomiting*—4 mg before induction of anesthesia or postoperatively.

IV (Children 4–18 yr): *Prevention of chemotherapy-induced nausea/vomiting*—0.15 mg/kg 15–30 min prior to chemotherapy, repeated 4 and 8 hr later.

IV (Children 2–12 yr and ≤40 kg): *Prevention of postoperative nausea/vomiting*—0.15 mg/kg.

IV (Children >40 kg): *Prevention of postoperative nausea/vomiting*—4 mg.

Hepatic Impairment

PO, IM, IV (Adults): Not to exceed 8 mg/day.

Availability (generic available)

Orally disintegrating tablets (contain aspartame) (strawberry flavor): 4 mg, 8 mg. **Tablets:** 4 mg, 8 mg, 24 mg. **Oral solution (strawberry flavor):** 4 mg/5 mL. **Solution for injection:** 2 mg/mL in 2- and 20-mL vials. **Premixed injection:** 32 mg/50 mL D5W.

oprelvekin (oh-prel-ve-kin)

Neumega

Classification

Therapeutic: colony-stimulating factors

Pharmacologic: interleukins, thrombopoietic growth factors

Indications

Prevention of severe thrombocytopenia and reduction of the need for platelet transfusions following myelosuppressive chemotherapy in patients with nonmyeloid malignancies at risk for thrombocytopenia.

Action

Stimulates production of megakaryocytes and platelets. **Therapeutic Effects:** Increased platelet count.

O

Adverse Reactions/Side Effects

These effects occurred in patients who had recently received myelosuppressive chemotherapy

CNS: dizziness, headache, insomnia, nervousness, weakness. **EENT:** conjunctival hemorrhage, blurred vision, changes in visual acuity, blindness, papilledema, pharyngitis, rhinitis. **Resp:** cough, dyspnea, pleural effusions. **CV:** atrial fibrillation, edema, palpitations, syncope, tachycardia, vasodilation, ventricular arrhythmias. **GI:** anorexia, constipation, diarrhea, dyspepsia, mucositis, nausea, oral moniliasis, vomiting, abdominal pain. **Derm:** alopecia, ecchymoses, rash. **F and E:** sodium and water retention. **Local:** injection site reactions. **MS:** bone pain, myalgia. **Misc:** chills, fever, infection, pain.

PHYSICAL THERAPY IMPLICATIONS

Examination and Evaluation

- Assess heart rate, ECG, and heart sounds, especially during exercise (See Appendices G, H). Report any rhythm disturbances or symptoms of increased arrhythmias, including palpitations, chest discomfort, shortness of breath, fainting, and fatigue/weakness.
- Monitor respiratory function at rest and during exercise. Notify physician if patient experiences signs of pleural effusion, including cough, shortness of breath, chest pain, or labored breathing.
- Assess dizziness that might affect gait, balance, and other functional activities (See Appendix C). Report balance problems and functional limitations to the physician and nursing staff, and caution the patient

and family/caregivers to guard against falls and trauma.

- Assess peripheral edema using girth measurements, volume displacement, and measurement of pitting edema (See Appendix N). Report increased swelling in feet and ankles or a sudden increase in body weight due to fluid retention.
- Assess any muscle or bone pain to rule out musculoskeletal pathology; that is, try to determine if pain is drug induced rather than caused by anatomic or biomechanical problems.
- Monitor subcutaneous injection site for pain, swelling, and irritation. Report prolonged or excessive injection site reactions to the physician.

Interventions

- Because of the risk of arrhythmias and pleural effusion, use caution during aerobic exercise and other forms of therapeutic exercise. Assess exercise tolerance frequently (blood pressure, heart rate, fatigue levels), and terminate exercise immediately if any untoward responses occur (See Appendix L).
- Do not apply massage or physical agents (heat, cold, electrotherapeutic modalities) at or near the subcutaneous application site. These interventions can alter drug absorption from subcutaneous tissues.

Patient/Client-Related Instruction

- Advise patient to report any vision disturbances or eye pain and redness.
- Advise patient and family/caregivers about the likelihood of GI problems such as nausea, vomiting, constipation, diarrhea, abdominal pain, indigestion, loss of appetite, and ulcers/infection in and around the mouth. Instruct patient to report severe or prolonged GI problems.
- Instruct patient to report other troublesome side effects such as severe or prolonged headache, nervousness, nasal/pharyngeal irritation, signs of infection, chills, fever, or skin reaction (rash, bruising, hair loss).

Pharmacokinetics

Absorption: >80% absorbed following SC administration.
Distribution: Unknown.
Metabolism and Excretion: Appears to be mostly metabolized, with metabolites eliminated by kidneys.
Half-life: 6.9 hr.

TIME/ACTION PROFILE (increase in platelet count)

ROUTE	ONSET	PEAK	DURATION
SC	5–9 days	unknown	7–14 days*

*Counts continue to rise for 7 days following discontinuation and then return to baseline by 14 days.

Contraindications/Precautions

Contraindicated in: Hypersensitivity; Lactation.
Use Cautiously in: Any condition in which sodium and water retention would pose problems (CHF, renal disease); Preexisting pericardial effusion or ascites (may be exacerbated); History of atrial arrhythmias (especially if receiving cardiac medications or previous doxorubicin therapy); Preexisting papilledema or tumors of the CNS; OB/Pedi: Pregnancy or children (safety not established).

Interactions

Drug-Drug: None significant.

Route/Dosage

Subcut (Adults): 50 mcg/kg once daily for 10–21 days.

Availability

Powder for injection: 5-mg vial.

orlistat (or-li-stat)

Xenical

Classification

Therapeutic: weight-control agents
Pharmacologic: lipase inhibitors

Indications

Obesity management (weight loss and maintenance) when used in conjunction with a reduced-calorie diet in patients with an initial BMI ≥ 30 kg/m^2 or ≥ 27 kg/m^2 in the presence of additional risk factors (diabetes, hypertension, hyperlipidemia). Reduces the risk of weight regain after prior loss. May delay onset of type 2 diabetes in prediabetic patients.

Action

Decreases the absorption of dietary fat by reversibly inhibiting enzymes (lipases), which are necessary for the breakdown and subsequent absorption of fat. **Therapeutic Effects:** Weight loss and maintenance in obese patients. Delayed onset of type 2 diabetes.

Adverse Reactions/Side Effects

With initial use; incidence decreases with prolonged use

GI: fecal urgency, flatus with discharge, increased defecation, oily evacuation, oily spotting, fecal incontinence.

PHYSICAL THERAPY IMPLICATIONS

Examination and Evaluation

- Periodically assess body weight and other anthropometric measures (body mass index, body composition). Document whether drug therapy is helping reduce body weight and decrease percentage of body fat.

Interventions

- Design and implement aerobic exercise and endurance training programs to help decrease obesity and maintain weight loss.

Patient/Client-Related Instruction

- Counsel patients about additional interventions to help control obesity and improve cardiovascular health, including dietary modification, regular exercise, moderation of alcohol consumption, and smoking cessation.
- Advise patient about the likelihood of GI problems, including increased bowel movements, flatulence, and possible incontinence. Instruct patient to report severe or prolonged GI problems.

Pharmacokinetics

Absorption: Minimal systemic absorption.
Distribution: Action is local, within the GI tract.
Protein Binding: Minimally absorbed drug is >99% bound to plasma proteins.
Metabolism and Excretion: Major route is fecal elimination of unabsorbed drug.
Half-life: 1–2 hr.

TIME/ACTION PROFILE (effects on fecal fat)

ROUTE	ONSET	PEAK	DURATION
PO	24–48 hr	unknown	48–72 hr*

*Following discontinuation.

Contraindications/Precautions

Contraindicated in: Hypersensitivity; Chronic malabsorption syndrome or cholestasis; OB: Pregnancy or lactation.
Use Cautiously in: Pedi: Children <16 yr (safety not established).

Interactions

Drug-Drug: Reduces the absorption of some **fat-soluble vitamins** and **beta-carotene**.

Route/Dosage

PO (Adults and adolescents ≥16 yr): 60–120 mg tid with each meal containing fat.

Availability

Capsules: 120 mg, 60 mg OTC.

orphenadrine (or-fen-a-dreen)

Antiflex, Banflex, Disipal, Flexoject, Flexon, Mio-Rel, Myolin, Myotrol, Norflex, Orfro, Orphenate

Classification
Therapeutic: skeletal muscle relaxants (centrally acting)
Pharmacologic: diphenhydramine analogues

Indications

Adjunct to rest and physical therapy in the treatment of muscle spasm associated with acute painful musculoskeletal conditions. Adjunct therapy of Parkinson's disease (Canadian labeling only).

Action

Skeletal muscle relaxation, probably due to CNS depression. **Therapeutic Effects:** Skeletal muscle relaxation, with decreased discomfort.

Adverse Reactions/Side Effects

CNS: CNS excitation, confusion, dizziness, drowsiness. **EENT:** blurred vision, dry eyes. **CV:** orthostatic hypotension, tachycardia. **GI:** constipation, dry mouth. **GU:** urinary retention.

PHYSICAL THERAPY IMPLICATIONS

Examination and Evaluation

- Assess patient's pain, stiffness, and ROM to help document antispasm effects.
- Assess blood pressure (BP) when patient assumes a more upright position (lying to standing, sitting to standing, lying to sitting). Document orthostatic hypotension and contact physician when systolic BP falls >20 mm Hg, or diastolic BP falls >10 mm Hg.
- Assess heart rate, ECG, and heart sounds, especially during exercise (See Appendices G, H). Report rapid heart rate (tachycardia) or symptoms of other arrhythmias, including palpitations, chest discomfort, shortness of breath, fainting, and fatigue/weakness.
- Assess dizziness that might affect gait, balance, and other functional activities (See Appendix C). Report balance problems and functional limitations to the physician, and caution the patient and family/caregivers to guard against falls and trauma.

O

- Be alert for confusion, irritability nervousness, or other signs of CNS excitation (See Appendix D). Notify physician promptly if these symptoms become problematic.

Interventions

- Implement appropriate manual therapy techniques, physical agents, and therapeutic exercises to reduce pain and wean patient off muscle relaxants as soon as possible.
- Help patient explore other nonpharmacologic methods to reduce chronic pain, such as relaxation techniques, exercise, counseling, and so forth.
- Implement fall prevention strategies, especially if balance is impaired (See Appendix E).
- To minimize orthostatic hypotension, patient should move slowly when assuming a more upright position.

Patient/Client-Related Instruction

- Inform patient that long-term use can cause tolerance and dependence; encourage adherence to physical therapy so that drug therapy can be discontinued as soon as possible.
- Inform patient that this drug may cause severe drowsiness, dizziness, and reduced psychomotor skills. Patients should avoid driving or other activities that require concentration and fast reactions.
- Advise patient to avoid alcohol and other CNS depressants because of the increased risk of sedation and adverse effects.
- Warn patient about anticholinergic effects such as dry mouth, constipation, urinary retention, sedation, and weakness; anticholinergic effects are often more severe in older adults.
- Instruct patient to report vision disturbances, including blurred vision or excessively dry eyes.

Pharmacokinetics

Absorption: Readily absorbed after oral and IM administration; IV administration results in complete bioavailability.
Distribution: Unknown.
Metabolism and Excretion: Mostly metabolized by the liver.
Half-life: 14 hr.

TIME/ACTION PROFILE (skeletal muscle effects)

ROUTE	ONSET	PEAK	DURATION
PO-ER	within 1 hr	6–8 hr	12 hr
IM	5 min	30 min	12 hr
IV	immediate	unknown	12 hr

Contraindications/Precautions

Contraindicated in: Hypersensitivity; Bladder neck obstruction, prostatic hyperplasia, glaucoma, myasthenia gravis, peptic ulcer disease, GI obstruction.
Use Cautiously in: Underlying cardiovascular disease; Impaired renal function; Geri: Appears on Beers' list. Geriatric patients are more susceptible to sedation and anticholinergic effects; OB/Pedi: Pregnancy, lactation, or children (safety not established).

Interactions

Drug-Drug: Concurrent use of other **anticholinergics** ↑ risk of anticholinergic side effects. ↑ risk of CNS depression with other **CNS depressants,** including **alcohol, antihistamines, antidepressants, sedative/hypnotics,** or **opioid analgesics.**
Drug-Natural: Kava, valerian, chamomile, or **hops** can ↑ CNS depression.

Route/Dosage

Skeletal muscle relaxation

PO (Adults): 100 mg bid.
IV, IM (Adults): 60 mg q 12 hr.

Adjunctive therapy of Parkinson's disease

PO (Adults): 50 mg tid (lower doses if used with other agents).

Availability (generic available)

Tablets: 50 mg OTC. **Extended-release tablets:** 100 mg. **Injection:** 30 mg/mL.

oseltamivir (oh-sel-tam-i-vir)

Tamiflu

Classification
Therapeutic: antivirals
Pharmacologic: neuramidase inhibitors

Indications

Treatment of uncomplicated acute illness due to influenza infection in adults and children ≥1 yr who have had symptoms for ≤2 days. Prevention of influenza in patients ≥1 yr.

Action

Inhibits the enzyme neuramidase, which may alter virus particle aggregation and release. **Therapeutic Effects:** Reduced duration or prevention of flu-related symptoms.

Adverse Reactions/Side Effects

CNS: SEIZURES, abnormal behavior, agitation, confusion, delirium, hallucinations, insomnia, nightmares, vertigo. **Resp:** bronchitis. **GI:** nausea, vomiting.

PHYSICAL THERAPY IMPLICATIONS

Examination and Evaluation

- Be alert for new seizures or increased seizure activity, especially at the onset of drug treatment. Document the number, duration, and severity of

seizures, and report these findings immediately to the physician.

- Be alert for agitation, confusion, delirium, hallucinations, or other abnormal behaviors. Notify physician or nursing staff promptly if these symptoms develop.
- Be alert for vertigo that might affect gait, balance, or other functional activities. Report balance problems and functional limitations to the physician and nursing staff, and caution the patient and family/caregivers to guard against falls and trauma.
- Assess any breathing problems, and report signs of prolonged or severe bronchitis (cough, mucous production, shortness of breath, wheezing, chest discomfort, fatigue, fever, chills).

Interventions

- Always wash hands thoroughly and disinfect equipment (whirlpools, electrotherapeutic devices, treatment tables, and so forth) to help prevent the spread of infection. Use universal precautions as indicated for specific patients.

Patient/Client-Related Instruction

- Instruct patient and family/caregivers to report other troublesome side effects, including severe or prolonged insomnia, nightmares, or GI problems (nausea, vomiting).

Pharmacokinetics

Absorption: Rapidly absorbed from the GI tract and converted by the liver to the active form, oseltamivir carboxylate. 75% reaches systemic circulation as the active drug.
Distribution: Unknown.
Metabolism and Excretion: Rapidly metabolized by the liver to oseltamivir carboxylate, the active drug. Oseltamivir is >99% excreted unchanged in urine.
Half-life: *Oseltamivir carboxylate*—6–10 hr.

TIME/ACTION PROFILE (blood levels)

ROUTE	ONSET	PEAK	DURATION
PO	unknown	unknown	12 hr

Contraindications/Precautions

Contraindicated in: Hypersensitivity; Pedi: Children <1 yr.
Use Cautiously in: Pedi: Children ≥1 yr (may be at ↑ risk for neuropsychiatric events); OB/Lactation: Safety not established; use only if potential benefits outweigh possible risks.

Interactions

Drug-Drug: None significant.

Route/Dosage

Treatment of Influenza

PO (Adults and Children >40 kg): 75 mg bid for 5 days.
PO (Children 23–40 kg): 60 mg bid.
PO (Children 15–23 kg): 45 mg bid.
PO (Children ≤15 kg and ≥1 yr): 30 mg bid.

Renal Impairment

PO (Adults): *CCr < 30 mL/min*—75 mg once daily for 5 days.

Influenza Prevention

PO (Adults and Children ≥13 yrs): 75 mg once daily for at least 10 days.
PO (Children >40 kg): 75 mg once daily for 10 days.
PO (Children 23–40 kg): 60 mg once daily for 10 days.
PO (Children 15–23 kg): 45 mg once daily for 10 days.
PO (Children ≤15 kg and ≥1 yr): 30 mg once daily.

Renal Impairment

PO (Adults and Children ≥13 yr):
CCr 10–30 mL/min—75 mg every other day *or* 30 mg every day.

Availability

Capsules: 30 mg, 45 mg, 75 mg. **Oral suspension (tutti-frutti flavor):** 12 mg/mL in 25-mL bottle.

oxacillin (ox-a-**sil**-in)

Bactocill

Classification

Therapeutic: anti-infectives
Pharmacologic: penicillinase-resistant penicillins

Indications

Treatment of the following infections due to penicillinase-producing staphylococci: Respiratory tract infections; Sinusitis; Skin and skin structure infections; Bone and joint infections; Urinary tract infections; Endocarditis; Bacteremia; Meningitis.

Action

Bind to bacterial cell wall, leading to cell death. Not inactivated by penicillinase enzymes. **Therapeutic Effects:** Bactericidal action. **Spectrum:** Active against most gram-positive aerobic cocci. Spectrum is notable for activity against Penicillinase-producing strains of *Staphylococcus aureus*, *S. epidermidis*. Not active against methicillin-resistant bacteria.

O

Adverse Reactions/Side Effects

CNS: SEIZURES. **GI:** diarrhea, epigastric distress, nausea, vomiting, pseudomembranous colitis. **GU:** interstitial nephritis. **Derm:** rash, urticaria. **Hemat:** eosinophilia, leukopenia. **Local:** pain at IM site, phlebitis at IV site. **Misc:** ALLERGIC REACTIONS, INCLUDING ANAPHYLAXIS AND SERUM SICKNESS, superinfection.

PHYSICAL THERAPY IMPLICATIONS

Examination and Evaluation

- Watch for seizures; notify physician immediately if patient develops or increases seizure activity.
- Monitor signs of allergic reactions and anaphylaxis, including pulmonary symptoms (tightness in the throat and chest, wheezing, cough dyspnea) or skin reactions (rash, pruritus, urticaria). Notify physician or nursing staff immediately if these reactions occur.
- Assess muscle aches and joint pain (arthralgia) that may be caused by serum sickness. Notify physician if these symptoms seem to be drug-related rather than caused by musculoskeletal injury or if muscle and joint pain are accompanied by allergy-like reactions (fever, rashes, etc.)
- Monitor signs of eosinophilia (fatigue, weakness, myalgia) or leukopenia (fever, sore throat, signs of infection); report these signs to the physician.
- Monitor injection site for pain, swelling, and irritation. Report prolonged or excessive injection site reactions to the physician.

Interventions

- Always wash hands thoroughly and disinfect equipment (whirlpools, electrotherapeutic devices, treatment tables, and so forth) to help prevent the spread of infection. Use universal precautions or isolation procedures as indicated for specific patients.

Patient/Client-Related Instruction

- Instruct patient to notify physician immediately if signs of the following occur:
  - Pseudomembranous colitis (diarrhea, abdominal pain, fever, pus or mucus in stools) or other severe or prolonged GI problems (nausea, vomiting, heartburn).
  - Superinfection (black, furry overgrowth on tongue; vaginal itching or discharge; loose or foul-smelling stools).
  - Interstitial nephritis (blood in urine, decreased urine output, weight gain from fluid retention).
- Instruct patient and family/caregivers to report other troublesome side effects such as severe or prolonged skin problems (rash, itching) or GI problems (nausea, vomiting, diarrhea, heartburn).

Pharmacokinetics

Absorption: Completely absorbed following IV administration; well absorbed from IM sites.
Distribution: Widely distributed; penetration into CSF is minimal but sufficient in the presence of inflamed meninges; cross the placenta and enter breast milk.
Metabolism and Excretion: Partially metabolized by the liver (9%), partially excreted unchanged by the kidneys.
Half-life: Neonates: 1.6 hr; Children up to 2 yr: 0.9–1.8 hr; Adults: 0.3–0.8 hr (increased in severe hepatic impairment).

TIME/ACTION PROFILE

ROUTE	ONSET	PEAK	DURATION
oxacillin IM	rapid	30 min	4–6 hr
oxacillin IV	rapid	end of infusion	4–6 hr

Contraindications/Precautions

Contraindicated in: Previous hypersensitivity to penicillins (cross-sensitivity exists with cephalosporins and other beta-lactam antibiotics).
Use Cautiously in: Severe renal or hepatic impairment.

Interactions

Drug-Drug: Oxacillin may ↓ effectiveness of oral contraceptive agents. **Probenecid** ↓ renal excretion and ↑ blood levels of oxacillin (therapy may be combined for this purpose). Concurrent use with **methotrexate** ↓ methotrexate elimination and ↑ risk of serious toxicity.

Route/Dosage

IM, IV (Adults and Children ≥40 kg): 250–2000 mg q 4–6 hr (up to 12 g/day).
IM, IV (Children <40 kg): 100–200 mg/kg/day divided q 4–6 hr, maximum: 12 g/day.
IM, IV (Neonates <1200 g): —50 mg/kg/day divided q 12 hr.
IM, IV (Neonates ≥2 kg): —75 mg/kg/day divided q 8 hr for the first 7 days of life, then 100 mg/kg/day divided q 6 hr.
IM, IV (Neonates 1.2–2 kg): —50 mg/kg/day divided q 12 hr for the first 7 days of life, then 75 mg/kg/day divided q 8 hr.

Availability (generic available)

Powder for injection: 250-mg, 500-mg, 2-g, 4-g, and 10-g vials.

oxaliplatin (ox-al-i-**pla**-tin)

Eloxatin

Classification

Therapeutic: antineoplastics

Pharmacologic: platinum coordination complexes

Indications

Used in combination with 5-fluorouracil and leucovorin in the treatment of advanced or metastatic colon or rectal cancer. **Unlabeled Use:** Treatment of ovarian cancer that has progressed despite treatment with other agents.

Action

Inhibits DNA replication and transcription by incorporating platinum into normal cross-linking (cell-cycle–nonspecific). **Therapeutic Effects:** Death of rapidly replicating cells, particularly malignant ones.

Adverse Reactions/Side Effects

Adverse reactions are noted for the combination of oxaliplatin, 5-FU, and leucovorin

CNS: fatigue. **CV:** chest pain, edema, thromboembolism. **Resp:** PULMONARY FIBROSIS, coughing, dyspnea. **GI:** diarrhea, nausea, vomiting, abdominal pain, anorexia, gastroesophageal reflux, stomatitis. **F and E:** dehydration, hypokalemia. **Hemat:** leukopenia, NEUTROPENIA, THROMBOCYTOPENIA, anemia. **Local:** injection site reactions. **MS:** back pain. **Neuro:** neurotoxicity. **Misc:** ANAPHYLAXIS/ANAPHYLACTOID REACTIONS, fever.

PHYSICAL THERAPY IMPLICATIONS

Examination and Evaluation

- Monitor signs of allergic reactions including anaphylaxis. Reactions include pulmonary symptoms (tightness in the throat and chest, wheezing, cough, dyspnea) and skin reactions (rash, pruritus, urticaria, burning skin). Notify physician or nursing staff immediately if these reactions occur.
- Assess any breathing problems or signs of pulmonary fibrosis such as dry cough, wheezing, chest pain, shortness of breath, and difficult or labored breathing. Monitor pulse oximetry and perform pulmonary function tests (See Appendices I, J, K) to quantify suspected changes in ventilation and respiratory function.
- Monitor signs of leukopenia/neutropenia (fever, sore throat, signs of infection), thrombocytopenia (bruising, nose bleeds, bleeding gums), or unusual weakness and fatigue that might be due to anemia or other blood dyscrasias. Notify physician of these signs immediately.
- Monitor signs of venous thrombosis (lower extremity swelling, warmth, erythema, tenderness) and thromboembolism (shortness of breath, chest pain, cough, bloody sputum). Notify physician immediately, and request objective tests (Doppler ultrasound, lung scan, others) if thrombosis is suspected.
- Assess peripheral edema using girth measurements, volume displacement, and measurement of pitting edema (See Appendix N). Report increased swelling in feet and ankles or a sudden increase in body weight due to fluid retention.
- Monitor signs of neurotoxicity, including peripheral neuropathy (numbness, tingling, weakness). Establish baseline electroneuromyographic values at the beginning of drug treatment whenever possible. Periodically reexamine these values to document drug-induced changes in peripheral nerve function.
- Monitor and report any muscle weakness, aches, or cramps that might indicate low potassium levels (hypokalemia).
- Assess any back pain to rule out musculoskeletal pathology; that is, try to determine if pain is drug-induced rather than caused by anatomic or biomechanical problems.
- Monitor IV injection site for pain, swelling, and irritation. Report prolonged or excessive injection site reactions to the physician.

Interventions

- For patients who are medically able to begin exercise, implement appropriate resistive exercises and aerobic training to maintain muscle strength and aerobic capacity during cancer chemotherapy or to help restore function after chemotherapy.
- Make sure patient maintains adequate fluid intake to avoid dehydration, especially during exercise.

Patient/Client-Related Instruction

- Advise patient to guard against infection (frequent hand washing, etc.), and to avoid crowds and contact with persons with contagious diseases.
- Make sure patient and family or caregivers understand the need to immediately report allergic responses or signs of blood dyscrasias as listed above (see Examination and Evaluation).
- Advise patient about the likelihood of GI reactions, including nausea, vomiting, diarrhea, constipation, abdominal pain, heartburn, and irritation of the oral mucosa. Instruct patient to report severe or prolonged GI problems.
- Advise patient and family/caregivers that fatigue and weakness are likely and may be severe. Functional abilities may be limited, and patient may need to use assistive devices during ambulation.

O

Pharmacokinetics

Absorption: IV administration results in complete bioavailability.
Distribution: Extensive tissue distribution.
Protein Binding: >90% (platinum).
Metabolism and Excretion: Undergoes rapid and extensive nonenzymatic biotransformation; excreted mostly by the kidneys.
Half-life: 391 hours.

TIME/ACTION PROFILE

ROUTE	ONSET	PEAK	DURATION
IV	unknown	unknown	unknown

Contraindications/Precautions

Contraindicated in: Hypersensitivity; Hypersensitivity to other platinum compounds; Pregnancy or lactation.
Use Cautiously in: Renal impairment; Geri: Geriatric patients (increased risk of adverse reactions); Pedi: Children (safety not established).

Interactions

Drug-Drug: Concurrent use of **nephrotoxic agents** may ↑ toxicity.

Route/Dosage

IV (Adults): *Day 1*—85 mg/m^2 with leucovorin 200 mg/m^2 at the same time over 2 hr, followed by 5-FU 400 mg/m^2 bolus over 2–4 min, then 5-FU 600 mg/m^2 as a 22 hr infusion. *Day 2*—leucovorin 200 mg/m^2 over 2 hr, followed by 5-FU 400 mg/m^2 bolus over 2–4 min, then 5-FU 600 mg/m^2 as a 22-hr infusion. Cycle is repeated every 2 wk. Dosage reduction/alteration may be required for neurotoxicity or other serious adverse effects.

Availability

Solution for injection: 5 mg/mL in 10-mL vials (50 mg), 5 mg/mL in 20-mL vials (100 mg).

oxaprozin (ox-a-**proe**-zin)

Daypro

Classification
Therapeutic: antirheumatics, nonsteroidal anti-inflammatory agents
Pharmacologic: propionic acid derivatives

Indications

Rheumatoid arthritis and osteoarthritis.

Action

Inhibits prostaglandin synthesis. **Therapeutic Effects:** Suppression of pain and inflammation.

Adverse Reactions/Side Effects

CNS: agitation, anxiety, confusion, depression, dizziness, drowsiness, fatigue, headache, insomnia, malaise, weakness. **EENT:** abnormal vision, tinnitus. **Resp:** dyspnea, hypersensitivity pneumonitis. **CV:** edema, vasculitis. **GI:** GI BLEEDING, abdominal pain, diarrhea, dyspepsia, abnormal liver function tests, anorexia, cholestatic jaundice, constipation, dry mouth, duodenal ulcer, flatulence, gastritis, increased appetite, nausea, stomatitis, vomiting. **GU:** albuminuria, azotemia, interstitial nephritis. **Derm:** EXFOLIATIVE DERMATITIS, STEVENS-JOHNSON SYNDROME, TOXIC EPIDERMAL NECROLYSIS, increased sweating, photosensitivity, pruritus, rash. **Hemat:** prolonged bleeding time. **Metab:** weight gain. **Neuro:** paresthesia, tremor. **Misc:** ALLERGIC REACTIONS, INCLUDING ANAPHYLAXIS, ANGIONEUROTIC EDEMA.

PHYSICAL THERAPY IMPLICATIONS

Examination and Evaluation

- Monitor signs of GI bleeding, including abdominal pain, vomiting blood, blood in stools, or black, tarry stools. Report these signs to the physician immediately.
- Monitor signs of allergic reactions and anaphylaxis or angioneurotic edema, including pulmonary symptoms (laryngeal edema, wheezing, cough, dyspnea) or skin reactions (rash, pruritus, urticaria, swelling in the face). Be especially alert for exfoliation, dermatitis, and other severe skin reactions that might indicate serious hypersensitivity reactions (Stevens-Johnson syndrome, toxic epidermal necrolysis). Notify physician immediately if these reactions occur.
- Assess pain and other variables (range of motion, muscle strength) to document whether this drug is successful in helping manage the patient's pain and decreasing impairments.
- Assess blood pressure (BP) periodically and compare to normal values (See Appendix F). NSAIDs can increase BP in certain patients.
- Be alert for signs of difficult, labored breathing (dyspnea) or other signs of pneumonitis such as cough, shortness of breath, fever, and abnormal breath sounds (rales; See Appendix K). Report these signs to the physician.
- Be alert for signs of prolonged bleeding time such as bleeding gums, nosebleeds, and unusual or excessive bruising. Report these signs to the physician.
- Assess peripheral edema using girth measurements, volume displacement, and measurement of pitting edema (See Appendix N). Report increased swelling in feet and ankles or a sudden increase in body weight due to fluid retention.

- Monitor signs of interstitial nephritis (blood in urine, decreased urine output, weight gain from fluid retention), or signs of increased nitrogenous compounds in the blood (azotemia) such as confusion, decreased alertness, tachycardia, pallor, fatigue, dry mouth, thirst, and decreased/absent urine production. Notify physician of these signs.
- Assess any tremors or signs of paresthesia (numbness, tingling). Perform objective tests including electroneuromyography and sensory testing to document any drug-related neuropathic changes.
- Be alert for signs of vasculitis, including fatigue, weakness, muscle pain, joint pain, fever, loss of appetite, and weight loss. Report these signs to the physician.
- Assess dizziness and drowsiness that might affect gait, balance, and other functional activities (See Appendix C). Report balance problems and functional limitations to the physician, and caution the patient and family/caregivers to guard against falls and trauma.
- Monitor and report confusion, agitation, anxiety, depression, or other psychic disturbances.

Interventions

- Implement appropriate manual therapy techniques, physical agents, and therapeutic exercises to reduce pain and decrease the need for oxaprozin and other NSAIDs.
- If treating arthritic conditions, recommend orthotic and assistive devices as needed to reduce pain, improve function, and augment the effects of drug therapy.
- Use caution with any physical interventions that could increase bleeding, including wound débridement, chest percussion, joint mobilization, and application of local heat.
- Help patient explore other nonpharmacologic methods to reduce chronic pain, such as relaxation techniques, exercise, counseling, and so forth.
- Causes photosensitivity; use care if administering UV treatments. Advise patient to avoid direct sunlight and use sunscreens and protective clothing, and to report any untoward skin reactions (rash, itching, excessive sweating).

Patient/Client-Related Instruction

- Advise patient that analgesics are usually more effective if given before pain becomes severe; emphasize that adequate pain control will allow better participation in physical therapy.
- Inform patient that NSAIDs may impair bone and cartilage healing. Advise patient to consult physician about NSAID use, especially after fractures, spinal fusion, and other bone surgeries.
- Caution patient about the use of over-the-counter products that contain NSAIDs or acetaminophen while taking prescription doses of oxaprozin. Use of multiple NSAIDs increases the risk of toxicity and overdose.
- Instruct patient to report excessive or prolonged headache or ringing/buzzing in the ears (tinnitus); these signs may indicate drug toxicity.
- Advise patient about the risks of gastric irritation. Instruct patient to notify physician of GI reactions such as severe or prolonged nausea, vomiting, diarrhea, constipation, indigestion, heartburn, flatulence, inflammation in/around the mouth, and abdominal pain.
- Advise patient to reduce alcohol intake because alcohol increases the risk of gastric toxicity.
- Instruct patient and family/caregivers to report other troublesome side effects such as severe or prolonged sleep loss or vision disturbances.

Pharmacokinetics

Absorption: Well absorbed following oral administration (80%); 35% is rapidly converted to an active metabolite.
Distribution: Unknown.
Protein Binding: 99.9%.
Metabolism and Excretion: The active metabolite is metabolized by the liver to inactive compounds.
Half-life: 42–50 hr.

TIME/ACTION PROFILE (antirheumatic action)

ROUTE	ONSET	PEAK	DURATION
PO	within 7 days	unknown	unknown

Contraindications/Precautions

Contraindicated in: Hypersensitivity; Cross-sensitivity may exist with other NSAIDs, including aspirin; Active GI bleeding or ulcer disease; Perioperative pain from coronary artery bypass graft (CABG) surgery.
Use Cautiously in: Cardiovascular disease or risk factors for cardiovascular disease (may ↑ risk of serious cardiovascular thrombotic events, myocardial infarction, and stroke, especially with prolonged use); Severe hepatic disease; Renal impairment (lower initial dose may be necessary); History of ulcer disease; Geri: Appears on Beers' list. Geriatric patients are at ↑ risk of GI bleeding. May require dose adjustments due to age-related decrease in renal function); Pedi: Pregnancy, lactation, or children (safety not established; not recommended for use during the second half of pregnancy).

Interactions

Drug-Drug: ↑ adverse GI effects and toxicity with **aspirin**, other **NSAIDs, potassium supplements,**

O

corticosteroids, or **alcohol**. Chronic use with **acetaminophen** may ↑ risk of adverse renal reactions. May ↓ effectiveness of **diuretics** or **antihypertensive** therapy. May ↑ hypoglycemic effects of **insulin** or **oral hypoglycemic agents**. ↑ risk of toxicity from **methotrexate**. ↑ risk of bleeding with **cefotetan, cefoperazone, thrombolytic agents, anticoagulants, ticlopidine, clopidogrel, eptifibatide**, or **tirofiban**. ↑ risk of adverse hematologic reactions with **antineoplastics** or **radiation therapy**.
Drug-Natural: ↑ anticoagulant effect and bleeding risk with **arnica, chamomile, clove, feverfew, garlic, ginger, ginkgo,** ***Panax ginseng***, and others.

Route/Dosage

PO (Adults): 1200 mg once daily; onset may be more rapid with an initial 1800-mg dose. Patients with low body weight, mild disease, or renal impairment may be started at 600 mg/day (not to exceed 1800 mg/day or 26 mg/kg/day). Daily doses >1200 mg should be given in 2–3 divided doses. Consideration should be given to ↓ dose to lowest effective amount.

Availability (generic available)

Tablets: 600 mg.

oxazepam (ox-az-e-pam)

Apo-Oxazepam, Novoxapam, Serax

Classification

Therapeutic: antianxiety agents, sedative/hypnotics
Pharmacologic: benzodiazepines

Schedule IV

Indications

Management of anxiety, anxiety associated with depression. Symptomatic treatment of alcohol withdrawal.

Action

Depresses the CNS, probably by potentiating gamma-aminobutyric acid (GABA), an inhibitory neurotransmitter. **Therapeutic Effects:** Decreased anxiety. Diminished symptoms of alcohol withdrawal.

Adverse Reactions/Side Effects

CNS: dizziness, drowsiness, confusion, hangover, headache, impaired memory, mental depression, paradoxical excitation, slurred speech. **EENT:** blurred vision. **Resp:** respiratory depression. **CV:** tachycardia. **GI:** constipation, diarrhea, drug-induced hepatitis, nausea, vomiting, weight gain (unusual). **GU:** urinary problems. **Derm:** rashes. **Hemat:** leukopenia. **Misc:** physical dependence, psychologic dependence, tolerance.

PHYSICAL THERAPY IMPLICATIONS

Examination and Evaluation

- Be alert for signs of respiratory depression, including dyspnea, shortness of breath, and cyanosis. Monitor pulse oximetry and perform pulmonary function tests (See Appendices I, J, K) to document suspected changes in ventilation and respiratory function.
- Assess heart rate, ECG, and heart sounds, especially during exercise (See Appendices G, H). Report a rapid heart rate (tachycardia) or signs of other arrhythmias, including palpitations, chest discomfort, shortness of breath, fainting, and fatigue/weakness.
- Watch for signs of leukopenia including fever, sore throat, and other signs of infection. Report these signs to the physician.
- Monitor daytime drowsiness and "hangover" symptoms (headache, nausea, irritability, lethargy, dysphoria). Repeated or excessive symptoms may require change in dose or medication.
- Report any behavioral or personality changes such as confusion, forgetfulness, slurred speech, decreased mental acuity, or excessive excitation.
- Assess dizziness and drowsiness that might affect gait, balance, and other functional activities (See Appendix C). Report balance problems and functional limitations to the physician, and caution the patient and family/caregivers to guard against falls and trauma.

Interventions

- Guard against falls and trauma (hip fractures, head injury, and so forth). Implement fall prevention strategies, especially in older adults or if drowsiness and dizziness carry over into the daytime (See Appendix E).
- Because of the risk of arrhythmias and respiratory depression, use caution during aerobic exercise and other forms of therapeutic exercise. Assess exercise tolerance frequently (blood pressure, heart rate, fatigue levels), and terminate exercise immediately if any untoward responses occur (See Appendix L).
- Help patient explore nonpharmacologic methods to decrease anxiety and depression (relaxation techniques, regular exercise, support groups, and so forth).

Patient/Client-Related Instruction

- Instruct patients on prolonged treatment not to discontinue medication without consulting a health care professional. Long-term use can cause tolerance and physical/psychologic dependence, and abrupt withdrawal can cause insomnia, unusual irritability or nervousness, and seizures.

- Advise patient to avoid alcohol and other CNS depressants because of the increased risk of sedation and adverse effects.
- Advise patient about the likelihood of GI problems such as nausea, vomiting, constipation, and diarrhea. Instruct patient to report severe or prolonged GI reactions, and also to report signs of drug-induced hepatitis, including anorexia, abdominal pain, severe nausea and vomiting, yellow skin or eyes, skin rash, flu-like symptoms, and muscle/joint pain.
- Instruct patient to report other bothersome side effects, including severe or prolonged headache, blurred vision, skin rash, or problems with urination.

Pharmacokinetics

Absorption: Well absorbed following oral administration. Absorption is slower than with other benzodiazepines.
Distribution: Widely distributed. Crosses the blood-brain barrier. May cross the placenta and enter breast milk. Recommend to discontinue drug or bottle-feed.
Metabolism and Excretion: Metabolized by the liver to inactive compounds.
Protein Binding: 97%.
Half-life: 5–15 hr.

TIME/ACTION PROFILE (sedation)

ROUTE	ONSET	PEAK	DURATION
PO	45–90 min	unknown	6–12 hr

Contraindications/Precautions

Contraindicated in: Hypersensitivity; Cross-sensitivity with other benzodiazepines may exist; Comatose patients or those with preexisting CNS depression; Uncontrolled severe pain; Angle-closure glaucoma; Pregnancy and lactation; Some products contain tartrazine and should be avoided in patients with known intolerance.
Use Cautiously in: Hepatic dysfunction (may be preferred over some benzodiazepines due to short half-life); History of suicide attempt or drug abuse; Debilitated patients (initial dosage reduction recommended); Severe chronic obstructive pulmonary disease; Myasthenia gravis; Geri: Elderly patients have increased sensitivity to benzodiazepines. Appears on Beers' list and is associated with increased risk of falls (↓ dose required).

Interactions

Drug-Drug: Additive CNS depression with other **CNS depressants**, including **alcohol, antihistamines, antidepressants, opioid analgesics**, and other **sedative/hypnotics** (including other **benzodiazepines**). May ↓ the therapeutic effectiveness of **levodopa**. **Hormonal contraceptives** or **phenytoin** may ↓ effectiveness. **Theophylline** may ↓ sedative effects of oxazepam.
Drug-Natural: Concomitant use of **kava, valerian, skullcap, chamomile,** or **hops** can ↑ CNS depression.

Route/Dosage

PO (Adults): *Antianxiety agent*—10–30 mg tid–qid. *Sedative/hypnotic/management of alcohol withdrawal*—15–30 mg tid–qid.
PO (Geriatric Patients): 5 mg 1–2 times daily initially or 10 mg tid; may be increased as needed.

Availability (generic available)

Capsules: 10 mg, 15 mg, 30 mg. **Tablets:** 10 mg, 15 mg, 30 mg.

O

oxcarbazepine

(ox-kar-**baz**-e-peen)
Trileptal

Classification
Therapeutic: anticonvulsants
Pharmacologic: carbamazepine analogues

Indications

Monotherapy or adjunctive therapy of partial seizures in adults and children 4 yr and older with epilepsy. Adjunctive therapy in patients 2–16 yr with epilepsy. **Unlabeled Use:** Management of trigeminal neuralgia.

Action

Blocks sodium channels in neural membranes, stabilizing hyperexcitable states, inhibiting repetitive neuronal firing, and decreasing propagation of synaptic impulses. **Therapeutic Effects:** Decreased incidence of seizures.

Adverse Reactions/Side Effects

CNS: dizziness/vertigo, drowsiness/fatigue, headache, cognitive symptoms. **EENT:** abnormal vision, diplopia, nystagmus. **GI:** abdominal pain, dyspepsia, nausea, vomiting, thirst. **Derm:** acne, rash, urticaria. **F and E:** hyponatremia. **Neuro:** ataxia, gait disturbances, tremor. **Misc:** allergic reactions, hypersensitivity reactions, including Stevens-Johnson syndrome and multiorgan reactions, lymphadenopathy.

PHYSICAL THERAPY IMPLICATIONS

Examination and Evaluation

- Monitor signs of allergic and hypersensitivity reactions, including pulmonary symptoms (tightness in the throat and chest, wheezing, cough, dyspnea) or skin reactions (rash, pruritus, urticaria). Be especially alert for severe skin reactions (exfoliation, dermatitis) that might indicate Stevens-Johnson syndrome. Notify physician immediately if these reactions occur.

- Document the number, duration, and severity of seizures to help determine if this drug is effective in reducing seizure activity.
- Assess vertigo or dizziness that might affect gait, balance, and other functional activities (See Appendix C). Report balance problems and functional limitations to the physician, and caution the patient and family/caregivers to guard against falls and trauma.
- Assess any gait disturbances, tremor, or ataxia. Attempt to determine if these problems are drug induced rather than caused by neuromuscular pathology.
- Monitor daytime drowsiness, agitation, confusion, or other cognitive impairments. Repeated or excessive symptoms may require change in dose or medication.
- Monitor signs of low sodium levels (hyponatremia), including headache, confusion, lethargy, irritability, decreased consciousness, and neuromuscular abnormalities (muscle weakness and cramps). Report severe or prolonged signs to the physician.
- If used to treat trigeminal neuralgia or other types of neurogenic pain, assess pain using visual analogue scales or other appropriate pain scales to document whether this drug is successful in helping manage the patient's pain.

Interventions

- Guard against falls and trauma (hip fractures, head injury, and so forth), especially if dizziness, vertigo, or ataxia affect gait and balance. Implement fall-prevention strategies, especially if balance is impaired (See Appendix E).

Patient/Client-Related Instruction

- Advise patient to avoid alcohol and other CNS depressants because of the increased risk of sedation and adverse effects.
- Advise patients on prolonged antiseizure therapy not to discontinue medication without consulting their physician. Abrupt withdrawal may cause increased seizures.
- Advise patient about the risk of daytime drowsiness and decreased attention and mental focus. Use care if driving or in other activities that require strong concentration and fast responses.
- Instruct patient and family/caregivers to report other troublesome side effects such as severe or prolonged headache, visual problems (double vision, nystagmus), swollen/tender lymph nodes, skin problems (rash, acne, itching), or GI problems (nausea, vomiting, indigestion, abdominal pain).

Pharmacokinetics

Absorption: Rapidly absorbed after oral administration and rapidly converted to the active 10-hydroxy metabolite (MHD).
Distribution: Enters breast milk in significant amounts.
Metabolism and Excretion: Extensively converted to MHD, which is then primarily excreted by the kidneys.
Half-life: *Oxcarbazepine*—2 hr; *MHD*—9 hr.

TIME/ACTION PROFILE (blood levels)

ROUTE	ONSET	PEAK	DURATION
PO 12 hr	PO	rapid	4.5 hr*

*Steady-state levels of MHD are reached after 2–3 days during bid dosing.

Contraindications/Precautions

Contraindicated in: Hypersensitivity; cross-sensitivity with carbamazepine may occur; OB: Lactation.
Use Cautiously in: Renal impairment (dose reduction recommended if CCR <30 mL/min); OB: Pregnancy (use only if potential benefit justifies the potential risk to the fetus); Pedi: Children <4 yr (safety not established).

Interactions

Drug-Drug: Oxcarbazepine may inhibit the CYP2C19 enzyme system and would be expected to alter the effects of other drugs that are metabolized by this system. Oxcarbazepine and MHD induce the P4503A4/5 enzyme systems and would be expected to alter the effects of other drugs that are metabolized by this system. This may result in decreased levels and effectiveness of **hormonal contraceptives, felodipine, isradipine, nicardipine, nifedipine,** and **nimodipine.** In addition, oxcarbazepine itself is metabolized by cytochrome P450 system and other **drugs that alter the activity of this system.** ↑ CNS depression may occur with other CNS depressants, including **alcohol, antihistamines, antidepressants, sedative/hypnotics,** and **opioids. Carbamazepine, phenobarbital, phenytoin, valproic acid,** and **verapamil** ↓ levels. May ↑ serum levels and effects of **phenytoin** (dosage reduction of phenytoin may be required).

Route/Dosage

(Tablets and oral suspension can be interchanged at equal doses).
PO (Adults): *Adjunctive therapy*—300 mg bid, may be increased by up to 600 mg/day at weekly intervals up to 1200 mg/day (up to 2400 mg/day may be needed); *conversion to monotherapy*—300 mg bid; may be increased by 600 mg/day at weekly intervals,

whereas other antiepileptic drugs are tapered over 3–6 wk; dose of oxcarbazepine should be increased up to 2400 mg/day over a period of 2–4 wk; *initiation of monotherapy*—300 mg bid, increase by 300 mg/day every third day, up to 1200 mg/day. Maximum maintenance dose should be achieved over 2–4 wk.
PO (Children 2–16 yr): *Adjunctive therapy*—4–5 mg/kg bid (up to 600 mg/day), increased over 2 wk to achieve 900 mg/day in patients 20–29 kg, 1200 mg/day in patients 29.1–39 kg and 1800 mg/day in patients >39 kg (range 6–51 mg/kg/day). In patients <20 kg, initial dose of 16–20 mg/kg/day may be used not to exceed 60 mg/kg/day. *conversion to monotherapy*—8–10 mg/kg/day given bid; may be increased by 10 mg/kg/day at weekly intervals, whereas other antiepileptic drugs are tapered over 3–6 wk; dose of oxcarbazepine should be increased up to 600–900 mg/day in patient ≤20 kg, 900–1200 mg/day in patients 25–30 kg, 900–1500 mg/day in patients 35–40 kg. 1200–1500 mg/day in patients 45 kg, 1200–1800 mg/day in patients 50–55 kg, 1200–2100 mg/day in patients 60–65 kg, and 1500–2100 mg/day in patients 70 kg. Maximum maintenance dose should be achieved over 2–4 wk.

Renal Impairment

PO (Adults): *CCr <30 mL/min*—Initiate therapy at 300 mg/day and increase slowly to achieve desired response.

Availability (generic available)

Tablets: 150 mg, 300 mg, 600 mg. **Oral suspension:** 60 mg/mL in 250-mL bottle.

oxiconazole (ox-i-**kon**-a-zole)

Oxistat

Classification
Therapeutic: antifungals (topical)
Pharmacologic: imidazoles

Indications

Treatment of a variety of cutaneous fungal infections, including tinea pedis (athlete's foot), tinea cruris (jock itch), tinea corporis (ringworm), and tinea versicolor (cream only).

Action

Affects the synthesis of the fungal cell wall. **Therapeutic Effects:** Decrease in symptoms of fungal infection.

Adverse Reactions/Side Effects

Local: burning, itching, local hypersensitivity reactions, redness, stinging.

PHYSICAL THERAPY IMPLICATIONS

Examination and Evaluation

- Assess healing of skin lesions to help document drug effectiveness.

Interventions

- Avoid contact with cutaneous lesions when treating patient.
- Always wash hands thoroughly and disinfect equipment (whirlpools, electrotherapeutic devices, treatment tables, and so forth) to help prevent the spread of infection.

Patient/Client-Related Instruction

- Advise patient to report any increased local sensitivity to this drug (pain, burning, itching, swelling).
- Instruct patient about proper hygiene; e.g., thoroughly wash and dry the affected area, wear clean socks and ventilated shoes for tinea pedis, and so forth.
- Advise patient to apply the drug as directed for the full course of treatment even if feeling better.
- Inform patient that early relief of cutaneous symptoms may be seen in 2–3 days. Full therapeutic response may take 2 wk for tinea cruris, tinea corporis, and tinea versicolor and 4 wk for tinea pedis.
- Advise patient to seek medical help if infections persist or recur after the full treatment. Recurrent fungal infections may be a sign of systemic illness.

Pharmacokinetics

Absorption: Absorption through intact skin is minimal.
Distribution: Distribution after topical administration is primarily local.
Metabolism and Excretion: Systemic metabolism and excretion not known following local application.
Half-life: Not applicable.

TIME/ACTION PROFILE

ROUTE	ONSET	PEAK	DURATION
topical	unknown	unknown	unknown

Contraindications/Precautions

Contraindicated in: Hypersensitivity to active ingredients, additives, preservatives, or bases.
Use Cautiously in: Nail and scalp infections (may require additional systemic therapy); OB/Lactation: Safety not established.

Interactions

Drug-Drug: Not known.

O

Route/Dosage

Topical (Adults and Children): Apply cream or lotion once or twice daily in patients with tinea pedis, tinea corporis, or tinea cruris. Apply cream once daily in patients with tinea versicolor. Patients with tinea corporis, tinea cruris, or tinea versicolor should be treated for 2 wk. Patients with tinea pedis should be treated for 4 wk.

Availability

Cream: 1%. **Lotion:** 1%.

OXYBUTYNIN (ox-i-byoo-ti-nin)

oxybutynin (oral)

Ditropan, Ditropan XL

oxybutynin (transdermal)

Oxytrol

Classification

Therapeutic: urinary tract antispasmodics
Pharmacologic: anticholinergics

Indications

Urinary symptoms that may be associated with neurogenic bladder, including Frequent urination, Urgency, Nocturia, Urge incontinence. Overactive bladder with symptoms of urge incontinence, urgency, and frequency.

Action

Inhibits the action of acetylcholine at postganglionic receptors. Has direct spasmolytic action on smooth muscle, including smooth muscle lining the GU tract, without affecting vascular smooth muscle. **Therapeutic Effects:** Increased bladder capacity. Delayed desire to void. Decreased urge incontinence, urinary urgency, and frequency and decreased number of urinary accidents associated with overactive bladder.

Adverse Reactions/Side Effects

CNS: dizziness, drowsiness, agitation, confusion, hallucinations, headache. **EENT:** blurred vision. **CV:** tachycardia. **GI:** constipation, dry mouth, nausea, abdominal pain, diarrhea. **GU:** urinary retention. **Derm:** decreased sweating, *transdermal only:* application site reactions. **Metab:** hyperthermia.

PHYSICAL THERAPY IMPLICATIONS

Examination and Evaluation

- Monitor signs of urine retention (difficult urination, painful or distended abdomen). Excessive urinary retention may require dose adjustment by physician.
- Assess heart rate, ECG, and heart sounds, especially during exercise (See Appendices G, H). Report a rapid heart rate (tachycardia) or signs of other arrhythmias, including palpitations, chest discomfort, shortness of breath, fainting, and fatigue/weakness.
- Be alert for decreased sweating and increased body temperature (hyperthermia), especially during exercise. Notify physician of a prolonged or persistent elevation in body temperature.
- Monitor changes in mood and behavior, including confusion, agitation, and hallucinations. Notify physician if these changes become problematic.
- Assess dizziness that might affect gait, balance, and other functional activities (See Appendix C). Report balance problems and functional limitations to the physician, and caution the patient and family/caregivers to guard against falls and trauma.
- Monitor transdermal application site for pain, swelling, and irritation. Report prolonged or excessive reactions to the physician.

Interventions

- When appropriate, implement pelvic floor muscle strengthening activities and other therapeutic exercises to help maintain bladder control.
- Because of the risk of arrhythmias and impaired thermoregulation, use caution during aerobic exercise and other forms of therapeutic exercise. Assess exercise tolerance frequently (blood pressure, heart rate, fatigue levels), and terminate exercise immediately if any untoward responses occur (See Appendix L).

Patient/Client-Related Instruction

- Advise patient to increase fluid intake and dietary fiber to avoid constipation. Laxatives may also be helpful in patients susceptible to fecal impaction.
- Instruct patient and family/caregivers to report other troublesome side effects such as severe or prolonged headache, blurred vision, or GI problems (nausea, diarrhea, constipation, dry mouth, abdominal pain).

Pharmacokinetics

Absorption: Rapidly absorbed following oral administration, but undergoes extensive first-pass metabolism; XL tablets provide extended release. Transdermal absorption occurs by passive diffusion through intact skin and bypasses the first-pass effect.
Distribution: Widely distributed.
Metabolism and Excretion: Extensively metabolized by the liver (CYP3A4 enzyme system); one metabolite is pharmacologically active; metabolites are renally excreted with negligible (<0.1%) excretion of unchanged drug.
Half-life: 7–8 hr.

TIME/ACTION PROFILE (urinary spasmolytic effect)

ROUTE	ONSET	PEAK	DURATION
PO	30–60 min	3–6 hr	6–10 hr (up to 24 hr with XL tablet)
transdermal	within 24 hr	36 hr	3–4 days

Contraindications/Precautions

Contraindicated in: Hypersensitivity; Uncontrolled angle-closure glaucoma; Intestinal obstruction or atony; Urinary retention.
Use Cautiously in: Hepatic/renal impairment; Bladder outflow obstruction; Ulcerative colitis; Benign prostatic hyperplasia; Cardiovascular disease; Reflux esophagitis or gastrointestinal obstructive disorders; Patients with dementia receiving acetylcholinesterase inhibitors; Myasthenia gravis; OB/Lactation: Safety not established; Geri: Appears on Beers' list. Poorly tolerated due to anticholinergic effects; Pedi: Children <5 yr (safety not established).

Interactions

Drug-Drug: ↑ anticholinergic effects with other **agents having anticholinergic properties**, including **amantadine, antidepressants, phenothiazines, disopyramide**, and **haloperidol**. Additive CNS depression with other **CNS depressants**, including **alcohol, antihistamines, antidepressants, opioids**, and **sedative/hypnotics**. **Ketoconazole, itraconazole, erythromycin**, and **clarithromycin** may ↑ effects.

Route/Dosage

PO (Adults): *Immediate-release tablets*—5 mg bid–tid times daily (not to exceed 5 mg qid) (may start with 2.5 mg bid–tid in elderly). *Extended-release tablets*—5–10 mg once daily; may ↑, as needed (in 5-mg increments), up to maximum dose of 30 mg/day.
PO (Children >5 yr): *Immediate-release tablets*—5 mg bid–tid (not to exceed 15 mg/day). *Extended-release tablets (children ≥6 yr)*—5 mg once daily; may ↑, as needed (in 5-mg increments), up to maximum dose of 20 mg/day.
Transdermal (Adults): 1 3.9-mg system applied twice weekly (q 3–4 days).

Availability (generic available)

Tablets: 5 mg. **Extended-release tablets:** 5 mg, 10 mg, 15 mg. **Syrup:** 5 mg/5 mL. **Transdermal system:** 3.9 mg/day system.

HIGH ALERT

oxycodone (ox-i-koe-done)

OxyContin, OxyFAST, OxyIR, Percolone, Roxicodone, ✱Supeudol

Classification

Therapeutic: opioid analgesics
Pharmacologic: opioid agonists, opioid agonists/nonopioid analgesic combinations

Schedule II

Indications

Moderate-to-severe pain.

Action

Binds to opiate receptors in the CNS. Alters the perception of and response to painful stimuli, while producing generalized CNS depression. **Therapeutic Effects:** Decreased pain.

O

Adverse Reactions/Side Effects

CNS: confusion, sedation, dizziness, dysphoria, euphoria, floating feeling, hallucinations, headache, unusual dreams. **EENT:** blurred vision, diplopia, miosis. **Resp:** RESPIRATORY DEPRESSION. **CV:** orthostatic hypotension. **GI:** constipation, dry mouth, nausea, vomiting. **GU:** urinary retention. **Derm:** flushing, sweating. **Misc:** physical dependence, psychologic dependence, tolerance.

PHYSICAL THERAPY IMPLICATIONS

Examination and Evaluation

- Assess symptoms of respiratory depression, including decreased respiratory rate, confusion, bluish color of the skin and mucous membranes (cyanosis), and difficult, labored breathing (dyspnea). Monitor pulse oximetry and perform pulmonary function tests (See Appendix I) to quantify suspected changes in ventilation and respiratory function. Excessive respiratory depression requires emergency care.
- Be alert for excessive sedation or changes in mood and behavior (euphoria, dysphoria, confusion, hallucinations). Notify physician or nurse immediately if patient is unconscious or extremely difficult to arouse.
- Use appropriate pain scales (visual analogue scales, others) to document whether this drug is successful in helping manage the patient's pain.
- Assess blood pressure (BP) when patient assumes a more upright position (lying to standing, sitting to standing, lying to sitting). Document orthostatic

hypotension and contact physician when systolic BP falls >20 mm Hg, or diastolic BP falls >10 mm Hg.
- Assess dizziness that might affect gait, balance, and other functional activities (See Appendix C). Report balance problems and functional limitations to the physician and nursing staff, and caution the patient and family/caregivers to guard against falls and trauma.

Interventions
- Implement appropriate manual therapy techniques, physical agents, and therapeutic exercises to reduce pain and help wean patient off opioid analgesics as soon as possible.
- Because of the risk of respiratory depression and orthostatic hypotension, use caution during aerobic exercise and other forms of therapeutic exercise. Assess exercise tolerance frequently (BP, heart rate, respiratory rate, fatigue levels), and terminate exercise immediately if any untoward responses occur (See Appendix L).
- Help patient explore other nonpharmacologic methods to reduce chronic pain, such as relaxation techniques, exercise, counseling, and so forth.
- Guard against falls and trauma (hip fractures, head injury). Implement fall-prevention strategies (See Appendix E), especially if patient exhibits sedation, dizziness, or blurred vision.
- To minimize orthostatic hypotension, patient should move slowly when assuming a more upright position.

Patient/Client-Related Instruction
- Advise patient that opioid analgesics are usually more effective if given before pain becomes severe; emphasize that adequate pain control will allow better participation in physical therapy.
- Educate patient about the dangers of opioid overdose; encourage patient to adhere to proper dosing schedule.
- Emphasize that the risk of physical addiction (tolerance and dependence) is usually minimal during short-term treatment of pain. Advise patient that addiction is more likely during excessive or inappropriate use of opioid analgesics.
- Advise patient to avoid alcohol and other CNS depressants because of the increased risk of sedation and decreased CNS function.
- Advise patient to increase fluid intake and dietary fiber to avoid constipation. Laxatives may also be helpful in patients susceptible to fecal impaction (e.g., people with spinal cord injury).
- Instruct patient to report other troublesome side effects such as severe or prolonged headache, urinary retention, unusual dreams, excessive sweating, vision disturbances, or GI problems (nausea, vomiting, dry mouth).

Pharmacokinetics
Absorption: Well absorbed from the GI tract.
Distribution: Widely distributed. Crosses the placenta; enters breast milk.
Metabolism and Excretion: Mostly metabolized by the liver.
Half-life: 2–3 hr.

TIME/ACTION PROFILE (analgesic effects)

ROUTE	ONSET	PEAK	DURATION
PO	10–15 min	60–90 min	3–6 hr
PO-CR*	10–15 min	3 hr	12 hr

*Controlled release.

Contraindications/Precautions
Contraindicated in: Hypersensitivity; Some products contain alcohol or bisulfites and should be avoided in patients with known intolerance or hypersensitivity.
Use Cautiously in: Head trauma; Increased intracranial pressure; Severe renal, hepatic, or pulmonary disease; Hypothyroidism; Adrenal insufficiency; Alcoholism; Geri: Elderly or debilitated patients (initial dose reduction recommended); Undiagnosed abdominal pain; Prostatic hyperplasia; **OB:** Pregnancy or lactation (avoid chronic use; weight maternal benefit against fetal risks).

Interactions
Drug-Drug: Use with caution in patients receiving **MAO inhibitors** (may result in unpredictable reactions—decrease initial dose of oxycodone to 25% of usual dose). Additive CNS depression with **alcohol**, **antihistamines**, and **sedative/hypnotics**. Administration of **partial-antagonist opioid analgesics** may precipitate withdrawal in physically dependent patients. **Nalbuphine, buprenorphine,** or **pentazocine** may ↓ analgesia.

Route/Dosage
Larger doses may be required during chronic therapy.
PO (Adults ≥50 kg): 5–10 mg q 3–4 hr initially, as needed. CR tablets (OxyContin) may be given q 12 hr.
PO (Adults <50 kg or Children): 0.2 mg/kg q 3–4 hr initially, as needed.

Rect (Adults): 10–40 mg tid–qid times daily initially, as needed.

Availability (generic available)

Tablets (Percolone, Roxicodone): 5 mg, 15 mg, 30 mg. **Immediate-release capsules (OxyIR):** 5 mg. **CR tablets (OxyContin):** 10 mg, 20 mg, 40 mg, 80 mg. **Oral solution (Roxicodone) (burgundy cherry):** 5 mg/5 mL in 500-mL bottle. **Concentrated oral solution (Roxicodone Intensol, OxyFAST):** 20 mg/mL in 30-mL bottle with dropper. **Suppositories:** 10 mg, 20 mg. ***In combination with:*** ibuprofen (Combunox), aspirin (Endodan, Percodan), acetaminophen (Endocet, Magnacet, Oxycet, Percocet, Roxicet, Tylox). See Appendix B.

oxymorphone (ox-i-mor-fone)

Opana, Opana ER

Classification

Therapeutic: opioid analgesics
Pharmacologic: opioid agonists

Schedule II

Indications

Management of moderate-to-severe pain. Extended-release tablets should only be used in patients who require continuous 24-hr management of chronic pain. Supplement in balanced anesthesia.

Action

Binds to opiate receptors in the CNS. Alters the perception of and response to painful stimuli, while producing generalized CNS depression. **Therapeutic Effects:** Decrease in pain.

Adverse Reactions/Side Effects

CNS: confusion, sedation, dizziness, dysphoria, euphoria, floating feeling, hallucinations, headache, unusual dreams. **EENT:** blurred vision, diplopia, miosis. **Resp:** RESPIRATORY DEPRESSION. **CV:** orthostatic hypotension. **GI:** constipation, dry mouth, nausea, vomiting. **GU:** urinary retention. **Derm:** flushing, sweating. **Misc:** physical dependence, psychologic dependence, tolerance.

PHYSICAL THERAPY IMPLICATIONS

Examination and Evaluation

- Assess symptoms of respiratory depression, including decreased respiratory rate, confusion, bluish color of the skin and mucous membranes (cyanosis), and difficult, labored breathing (dyspnea). Monitor pulse oximetry and perform pulmonary function tests (See Appendix I) to quantify suspected changes in ventilation and respiratory function. Excessive respiratory depression requires emergency care.
- Be alert for excessive sedation or changes in mood and behavior (euphoria, dysphoria, confusion, hallucinations). Notify physician or nurse immediately if patient is unconscious or extremely difficult to arouse.
- Use appropriate pain scales (visual analogue scales, others) to document whether this drug is successful in helping manage the patient's pain.
- Assess blood pressure (BP) when patient assumes a more upright position (lying to standing, sitting to standing, lying to sitting). Document orthostatic hypotension and contact physician when systolic BP falls >20 mm Hg, or diastolic BP falls >10 mm Hg.
- Assess dizziness that might affect gait, balance, and other functional activities (See Appendix C). Report balance problems and functional limitations to the physician and nursing staff, and caution the patient and family/caregivers to guard against falls and trauma.

Interventions

- Implement appropriate manual therapy techniques, physical agents, and therapeutic exercises to reduce pain and help wean patient off opioid analgesics as soon as possible.
- Because of the risk of respiratory depression and orthostatic hypotension, use caution during aerobic exercise and other forms of therapeutic exercise. Assess exercise tolerance frequently (BP, heart rate, respiratory rate, fatigue levels), and terminate exercise immediately if any untoward responses occur (See Appendix L).
- Help patient explore other nonpharmacologic methods to reduce chronic pain, such as relaxation techniques, exercise, counseling, and so forth.
- Guard against falls and trauma (hip fractures, head injury). Implement fall-prevention strategies (See Appendix E), especially if patient exhibits sedation, dizziness, or blurred vision.

O

- To minimize orthostatic hypotension, patient should move slowly when assuming a more upright position.

Patient/Client-Related Instruction

- Advise patient that opioid analgesics are usually more effective if given before pain becomes severe; emphasize that adequate pain control will allow better participation in physical therapy.
- Educate patient about the dangers of opioid overdose; encourage patient to adhere to proper dosing schedule.
- Emphasize that the risk of physical addiction (tolerance and dependence) is usually minimal during short-term treatment of pain. Advise patient that addiction is more likely during excessive or inappropriate use of opioid analgesics.
- Advise patient to avoid alcohol and other CNS depressants because of the increased risk of sedation and decreased CNS function.
- Advise patient to increase fluid intake and dietary fiber to avoid constipation. Laxatives may also be helpful in patients susceptible to fecal impaction (e.g., people with spinal cord injury).
- Instruct patient to report other troublesome side effects such as severe or prolonged headache, urinary retention, unusual dreams, excessive sweating, vision disturbances, or GI problems (nausea, vomiting, dry mouth).

Pharmacokinetics

Absorption: 10% absorbed following oral administration. Food and alcohol significantly ↑ absorption (38%). Well absorbed following IM, SC, or rectal administration.
Distribution: Widely distributed; crosses placenta, enters breast milk.
Metabolism and Excretion: Mostly metabolized by the liver; at least 2 metabolites are pharmacologically active, <1% excreted unchanged in urine.
Half-life: 2.6–4 hr.

TIME/ACTION PROFILE (analgesic effects)

ROUTE	ONSET	PEAK	DURATION
PO	unknown	unknown	4–6 hr
PO-ER	unknown	unknown	12 hr
IM	10–15 min	30–90 min	3–6 hr
IV	5–10 min	15–30 min	3–6 hr
SC	10–20 min	unknown	3–4 hr

Contraindications/Precautions

Contraindicated in: Hypersensitivity; Concurrent alcohol; Moderate/severe hepatic impairment; Respiratory depression (unless monitoring and resuscitative equipment are readily available); Known/suspected paralytic ileus.
Use Cautiously in: Acute alcoholism or delirium tremens or other toxic psychoses; Mild hepatic impairment; Head injury/increased intracranial pressure (may obscure neurologic signs and further increase pressure); Volume depletion or drugs that may cause hypotension, including diuretics and phenothiazines (↑ risk of severe hypotension); Geri: Blood levels are ↑; dose accordingly; Circulatory shock (may ↑ risk of severe hypotension); Adrenocortical insufficiency; Hypothyroidism; Prostatic hypertrophy or ureteral stricture; Severe pulmonary or renal impairment; Biliary tract disease or pancreatitis; OB: Use only in pregnancy if maternal benefit outweighs fetal risk; may enter breast milk and ↑ the risk of sedation/respiratory depression in infant.
Exercise Extreme Caution in: Conditions association with hypoxia, hypercapnea, ↓ respiratory reserve (including asthma, COPD, cor pulmonale, morbid obesity, sleep apnea, myxedema, kyphoscoliosis, CNS depression, and coma).

Interactions

Drug-Drug: Use with caution in patients receiving **MAO inhibitors** (may result in unpredictable reactions—↓ initial dose of oxymorphone to 25% of usual dose). ↑ risk of CNS depression, hypotension, and respiratory depression with **alcohol**, other **opioids**, or **CNS depressants,** including **sedatives, hypnotics, general anesthetics, phenothiazines, tranquilizers, skeletal muscle relaxants,** or **sedating antihistamines**; may initiate therapy with $\frac{1}{2}$ to $\frac{1}{2}$ usual starting dose. **Drugs that may cause volume depletion or hypotension,** including **diuretics** and **phenothiazines,** may ↑ risk of severe hypotension. Administration of **partial-antagonist opioid analgesics** may precipitate withdrawal in physically dependent patients. **Nalbuphine, buprenorphine**, or **pentazocine** ↓ analgesia.
Drug-Natural: Concomitant use of **kava, valerian,** or **chamomile** can ↑ CNS depression.

Route/Dosage

Larger doses may be required during chronic therapy.
PO (Adults): *Opioid-naive patients* 10–20 mg q 4–6 hr; some patients may require initial dose of 5 mg, not to exceed 20 mg. Once optimal analgesia is obtained, chronic pain patients may be converted to an equivalent 24-hr dose given as extended-release tablets q 12 hr.
Subcut, IM (Adults): 1–1.5 mg q 3–6 hr as needed. *Analgesia during labor*—0.5–1 mg.

IV (Adults): 0.5 mg q 3–6 hr as needed; increase as needed.

Availability

Tablets (Opana): 5 mg, 10 mg. **Extended-release tablets (Opana ER):** 5 mg, 7.5 mg, 10 mg, 15 mg, 20 mg, 30 mg, 40 mg. **Injection:** 1 mg/mL in 1-mL ampules, 1.5 mg/mL in 1-ml ampules and 10-mL vials.

oxytocin (ox-i-toe-sin)

Pitocin, Syntocinon

Classification

Therapeutic: hormones

Pharmacologic: oxytocics

Indications

IV: Induction of labor at term. Facilitation of uterine contractions at term. Facilitation of threatened abortion. Postpartum control of bleeding after expulsion of the placenta. **Intranasal:** Used to promote milk letdown in lactating women. **Unlabeled Use:** Evaluation of fetal competence (fetal stress test).

Action

Stimulates uterine smooth muscle, producing uterine contractions similar to those in spontaneous labor. Stimulates mammary gland smooth muscle, facilitating lactation. Has vasopressor and antidiuretic effects. **Therapeutic Effects:** Induction of labor (IV). Milk letdown (intranasal).

Adverse Reactions/Side Effects

Maternal adverse reactions are noted for IV use only

CNS: maternal: COMA, SEIZURES **fetal:** INTRACRANIAL HEMORRHAGE. **Resp: fetal:** ASPHYXIA, hypoxia. **CV: maternal:** hypotension; **fetal:** arrhythmias. **F and E: maternal:** hypochloremia, hyponatremia, water intoxication. **Misc: maternal:** increased uterine motility, painful contractions, abruptio placentae, decreased uterine blood flow, hypersensitivity.

PHYSICAL THERAPY IMPLICATIONS

Examination and Evaluation

- If administered IV during childbirth, be alert for maternal seizures or decreased consciousness that progresses to coma. Report seizures or coma-like responses to the physician or nursing staff immediately.
- Monitor any signs of fetal distress or asphyxia, such as decreased fetal heart rate, arrhythmias, meconium discharge, or decreased or absent fetal movements. Report these signs to the physician or nursing staff immediately.
- Assess maternal blood pressure periodically and compare to normal values (See Appendix F). Report low blood pressure (hypotension), especially if patient experiences dizziness, fatigue, or other symptoms.
- Monitor signs of maternal fluid and electrolyte imbalances, such as low sodium levels (hyponatremia), low chloride levels (hypochloremia), or a relative increase in body fluid (water intoxication). Signs include headache, confusion, lethargy, irritability, decreased consciousness, and neuromuscular abnormalities (muscle weakness and cramps). Report these signs to the physician or nursing staff.

Interventions

- During childbirth, implement physical agents, relaxation techniques, and manual therapies (massage, others) as needed to help reduce pain during uterine contractions.

Patient/Client-Related Instruction

- If used intranasally to facilitate breast-feeding, make sure patient uses proper administration technique and does not exceed the recommended dose or frequency of intranasal applications.

Pharmacokinetics

Absorption: Well absorbed from the nasal mucosa.
Distribution: Widely distributed in extracellular fluid. Small amounts reach fetal circulation.
Metabolism and Excretion: Rapidly metabolized by liver and kidneys.
Half-life: 3–9 min.

TIME/ACTION PROFILE (IV = uterine contractions; intranasal = milk letdown)

ROUTE	ONSET	PEAK	DURATION
IV	immediate	unknown	1 hr
IM	3–5 min	unknown	30–60 min
intranasal	few mins	unknown	20 min

Contraindications/Precautions

Contraindicated in: Hypersensitivity; Anticipated nonvaginal delivery; Pregnancy (intranasal).
Use Cautiously in: 1st and 2nd stages of labor.

Interactions

Drug-Drug: Severe hypertension may occur if oxytocin follows administration of **vasopressors**. Concurrent use with **cyclopropane** anesthesia may result in excessive hypotension.

Route/Dosage

Induction/Stimulation of Labor

IV (Adults): 0.5–2 milliunits/min; increase by 1–2 milliunits/min q 15–60 min until pattern established (usually 5–6 milliunits/min; maximum 20 milliunits/min), then decrease dose.

Postpartum Hemorrhage

IV (Adults): 10 units infused at 20–40 milliunits/min.
IM (Adults): 10 units after delivery of placenta.

Incomplete/Inevitable Abortion

IV (Adults): 10 units at a rate of 20–40 milliunits/min.

Promotion of Milk Letdown

Intranasal (Adults): 1 spray in 1 or both nostrils 2–3 min before breast-feeding or pumping breasts.

Fetal Stress Test

IV (Adults): 0.5 milliunits/min; may be doubled q 20 min until 3 moderate contractions occur in one 10-min period (usually 5–6 milliunits/min) to a maximum of 20 milliunits/min with maternal/fetal monitoring.

Availability (generic available)

Solution for injection: 10 units/mL in 0.5- and 1-mL ampules, 1-mL prefilled syringes, 1-mL and 10-mL vials.
Nasal spray: 40 units/mL in 2- and 5-mL containers.

paclitaxel (pak-li-tax-el)
Onxol, Taxol

paclitaxel protein-bound particles (albumin-bound)
Abraxane

Classification
Therapeutic: antineoplastics
Pharmacologic: taxoids

Indications
Paclitaxel: Advanced ovarian cancer (with cisplatin). Non–small-cell lung cancer when potentially curative surgery and/or radiation therapy is not an option. Metastatic breast cancer unresponsive to other therapy. Node-positive breast cancer when administered sequentially to standard combination chemotherapy that includes doxorubicin. Treatment of AIDS-related Kaposi's sarcoma. **Paclitaxel (albumin-bound):** Metastatic breast cancer after treatment failure or relapse where therapy included an anthracycline.

Action
Interferes with the normal cellular microtubule function that is required for interphase and mitosis. **Therapeutic Effects:** Death of rapidly replicating cells, particularly malignant ones.

Adverse Reactions/Side Effects
CV: ECG changes, hypotension, bradycardia. **GI:** abnormal liver function tests, diarrhea, mucositis, nausea, vomiting. **Derm:** alopecia. **Hemat:** anemia, neutropenia, thrombocytopenia. **MS:** arthralgia, myalgia. **Neuro:** peripheral neuropathy. **Resp:** cough, dyspnea. **Local:** injection site reactions. **Misc:** HYPERSENSITIVITY REACTIONS, INCLUDING ANAPHYLAXIS AND STEVENS-JOHNSON SYNDROME, TOXIC EPIDERMAL NECROLYSIS.

PHYSICAL THERAPY IMPLICATIONS

Examination and Evaluation
- Monitor signs of hypersensitivity reactions and anaphylaxis, including pulmonary symptoms (tightness in the throat and chest, wheezing, cough, dyspnea) or skin reactions (rash, pruritus, urticaria). Notify physician or nursing staff immediately, especially regarding skin problems because certain skin reactions may indicate serious hypersensitivity reactions (Stevens-Johnson syndrome, toxic epidermal necrosis).
- Assess heart rate, ECG, and heart sounds, especially during exercise (See Appendices G, H). Report an unusually slow heart rate (bradycardia) or signs of other arrhythmias, including palpitations, chest discomfort, shortness of breath, fainting, and fatigue/weakness.
- Assess blood pressure periodically and compare to normal values (See Appendix F). Report low blood pressure (hypotension), especially if patient experiences dizziness or syncope.
- Monitor respiratory side effects, including cough and difficult or labored breathing. Report severe or troublesome respiratory problems.
- Instruct patient to report signs of leukopenia (fever, sore throat, signs of infection), thrombocytopenia (bruising, nose bleeds, bleeding gums), or unusual weakness and fatigue that might be due to anemia. Report these signs to the physician or nursing staff.
- Be alert for signs of peripheral neuropathy (numbness, tingling, decreased muscle strength). Establish baseline electroneuromyographic values using EMG and nerve conduction at the beginning of drug treatment whenever possible, and reexamine these values periodically to document drug-induced changes in peripheral nerve function.
- Assess any muscle or joint pain to rule out musculoskeletal pathology; that is, try to determine if pain is drug induced rather than caused by anatomical or biomechanical problems.
- Monitor IV injection site for pain, swelling, and inflammation. Report prolonged or excessive injection site reactions to the physician.

Interventions
- For patients who are medically able to begin exercise, implement appropriate resistive exercises and aerobic training to maintain muscle strength and aerobic capacity during cancer chemotherapy or to help restore function after chemotherapy.
- Because of the risk of arrhythmias and abnormal blood pressure responses, use caution during aerobic exercise and other forms of therapeutic exercise. Assess exercise tolerance frequently (blood pressure, heart rate, fatigue levels), and terminate exercise immediately if any untoward responses occur (See Appendix L).

Patient/Client-Related Instruction
- Advise patient to guard against infection (frequent hand washing, etc.), and to avoid crowds and contact with persons with contagious diseases.
- Advise patient about the likelihood of GI reactions, including diarrhea, nausea, vomiting, and irritation in or around the mouth. Instruct patient or family and caregivers to report severe or prolonged GI reactions, and to also report signs of hepatotoxicity, including severe nausea and vomiting, yellow skin or eyes, fever, sore throat, malaise, weakness, facial edema, lethargy, and unusual bleeding or bruising.

P

- Advise patient that hair loss and other skin reactions are likely. Instruct patient to report severe or unexpected skin problems.

Pharmacokinetics

Absorption: IV administration results in complete bioavailability.
Distribution: Cross the placenta.
Protein Binding: 89–98%.
Metabolism and Excretion: Highly metabolized by the liver, <10% excreted unchanged in urine.
Half-life: *Paclitaxel*—13–52 hr; *Paclitaxel protein-bound particles (albumin-bound)*—27 hr.

TIME/ACTION PROFILE (effect on WBCs)

ROUTE	ONSET	PEAK	DURATION
IV	unknown	11 days	3 weeks

Contraindications/Precautions

Contraindicated in: Hypersensitivity to paclitaxel or to castor oil (non–protein-bound vehicle contains polyoxyethylated castor oil); Known alcohol intolerance; OB: Pregnancy or lactation; ANC $\leq 1500/mm^3$ in patients with ovarian, lung, or breast cancer; ANC $\leq 1000/mm^3$ in patients with AIDS-related Kaposi's sarcoma.
Use Cautiously in: Severe hepatic impairment; Geri: ↑ risk of neuropathy, myelosuppression, and cardiovascular events; OB: Childbearing potential; Active infection; Decreased bone marrow reserve; Pedi: Children (safety and effectiveness not established).

Interactions

Drug-Drug: Ketoconazole, verapamil, quinidine, cyclosporine, diazepam, dexamethasone, teniposide, etoposide, or **vincristine** may ↓ metabolism and ↑ risk of serious toxicity; concurrent use should be undertaken with caution. ↑ risk of myelosuppression with other **antineoplastics** or **radiation therapy**. Myelosuppression ↑ when given after **cisplatin**. May ↑ levels and toxicity of **doxorubicin**. May ↓ antibody response to and ↑ risk of adverse reactions from **live-virus vaccines**.

Route/Dosage

Many other regimens are used.

Paclitaxel

Ovarian Cancer

IV (Adults): *Previously untreated patients*—175 mg/m² over 3 hr q 3 wk, or 135 mg/m² over 24 hr q 3 wk, followed by cisplatin; *Previously treated patients*—135 mg/m² or 175 mg/m² over 3 hr q 3 wk.

Breast Cancer

IV (Adults): *Adjuvant treatment of node-positive breast cancer*—175 mg/m² over 3 hr q 3 wk for 4 courses administered sequentially to doxorubicin-containing combination chemotherapy; *Failure of initial therapy for metastatic disease or relapse within 6 mo of adjuvant therapy*—175 mg/m² over 3 hr q 3 wk.

Non–Small-Cell Lung Cancer

IV (Adults): 135 mg/m² over 24 hr q 3 wk, followed by cisplatin.

AIDS-Related Kaposi's Sarcoma

IV (Adults): 135 mg/m² over 3 hr q 3 wk or 100 mg/m² over 3 hr q 2 wk (dose reduction/adjustment may be necessary in patients with advanced HIV infection).

Paclitaxel Protein-Bound Particles (albumin-bound)

IV (Adults): 260 mg/m² over 30 min q 3 wk.

Availability

Paclitaxel (generic available)
Solution for injection: 6 mg/mL in 5-mL, 16.7-mL, 25-mL, and 50-mL vials.
Paclitaxel Protein-Bound Particles (albumin-bound)
Powder for injection: 100 mg/vial.

palifermin (pa-lif-er-min)

Kepivance

Classification
Therapeutic: cytoprotective agents
Pharmacologic: keratinocyte growth factors (rDNA)

Indications

To decrease incidence/duration of severe oral mucositis associated with myelotoxic therapy requiring stem cell support for hematologic malignancies.

Action

Enhances proliferation of epithelial cells. **Therapeutic Effects:** Decreased incidence/duration of mucositis.

Adverse Reactions/Side Effects

Derm: skin toxicity. **GI:** oral toxicity. **Metab:** ↑ amylase, ↑ lipase. **MS:** arthralgia. **Neuro:** dysesthesia.

PHYSICAL THERAPY IMPLICATIONS

Examination and Evaluation

- Monitor any skin reactions, including rash, itching, irritation, and exfoliation. Report any suspicious or toxic skin reactions to the physician or nursing staff.
- Assess any joint pain to rule out musculoskeletal pathology; that is, try to determine if pain is

drug induced rather than caused by anatomic or biomechanical problems.

- Monitor and report any changes in taste or other unusual sensations such as burning, tingling, or painful responses to touch (dysesthesia).

Patient/Client-Related Instruction

- Instruct patient to report any increase in oral lesions.

Pharmacokinetics

Absorption: IV administration results in complete bioavailability.

Distribution: Distributes into extravascular space.

Metabolism and Excretion: Unknown.

Half-life: 4.5 hr.

TIME/ACTION PROFILE (levels)

ROUTE	ONSET	PEAK	DURATION
IV	unknown	end of dose	unknown

Contraindications/Precautions

Contraindicated in: Hypersensitivity to palifermin or other *Escherichia coli*–derived proteins.

Use Cautiously in: OB: Pregnancy (use only if maternal benefit outweighs fetal risk); Pedi: Children, lactation (safety not established).

Interactions

Drug-Drug: Binds to and inactivates **heparin** (flush tubing between use). Administration within 24 hr after **myelotoxic therapy (chemotherapy/radiation)** ↑ severity and duration of mucositis.

Route/Dosage

IV (Adults): 60 mcg/kg/day for 3 days before and 3 days after myelotoxic therapy.

Availability

Powder for injection: 6.25 mg/vial.

paliperidone (pal-i-per-i-done)

Invega

Classification

Therapeutic: antipsychotics

Pharmacologic: benzisoxazoles

Indications

Schizophrenia.

Action

May act by antagonizing dopamine and serotonin in the CNS. Paliperidone is the active metabolite of risperidone. **Therapeutic Effects:** Decreased manifestations of schizophrenia.

Adverse Reactions/Side Effects

CNS: NEUROLEPTIC MALIGNANT SYNDROME, drowsiness, headache, anxiety, confusion, dizziness, extrapyramidal disorders (dose related), fatigue, parkinsonism (dose related), syncope, tardive dyskinesia, weakness. **EENT:** blurred vision. **Resp:** dyspnea, cough. **CV:** palpitations, tachycardia (dose related), bradycardia, orthostatic hypotension, ↑ QTc interval. **GI:** abdominal pain, dry mouth, dyspepsia, nausea, swollen tongue. **Endo:** hyperglycemia. **MS:** back pain, dystonia (dose related). **Neuro:** akathisia, dyskinesia, tremor (dose related). **Misc:** fever.

PHYSICAL THERAPY IMPLICATIONS

Examination and Evaluation

- Monitor and report signs of neuroleptic malignant syndrome (hyperthermia, diaphoresis, generalized muscle rigidity, altered mental status, tachycardia, changes in blood pressure (BP), incontinence). Symptoms typically occur within 4–14 days after initiation of drug therapy, but can occur at any time during drug use.
- Assess motor function, and be alert for extrapyramidal symptoms. Report these symptoms immediately, especially tardive dyskinesia, because this problem may be irreversible. Common extrapyramidal symptoms include:
  - Tardive dyskinesia (uncontrolled rhythmic movement of mouth, face, and extremities, lip smacking or puckering, puffing of cheeks, uncontrolled chewing, rapid or worm-like movements of tongue).
  - Pseudoparkinsonism (shuffling gait, rigidity, tremor, pill-rolling motion, loss of balance control, difficulty speaking or swallowing, mask-like face).
  - Akathisia (restlessness or desire to keep moving).
  - Other dystonias and dyskinesias (dystonic muscle spasms, twisting motions, twitching, inability to move eyes, weakness of arms or legs).
- Monitor personality changes such as anxiety and confusion. Notify physician if these changes become problematic.
- Assess dizziness, drowsiness, and syncope that might affect gait, balance, and other functional activities (See Appendix C). Report balance problems and functional limitations to the physician, and caution the patient and family/caregivers to guard against falls and trauma.
- Assess heart rate, ECG, and heart sounds, especially during exercise (See Appendices G, H). Report any rhythm disturbances or symptoms of increased arrhythmias, including palpitations, chest discomfort, shortness of breath, fainting, and fatigue/weakness.

- Assess any back pain to rule out musculoskeletal pathology; that is, try to determine if pain is drug induced rather than caused by anatomic or biomechanical problems.
- Assess BP when patient assumes a more upright position (lying to standing, sitting to standing, lying to sitting). Document orthostatic hypotension and contact physician when systolic BP falls >20 mm Hg, or diastolic BP falls >10 mm Hg.
- Report any troublesome respiratory problems, including severe or prolonged cough or difficult/labored breathing.
- Monitor signs of hyperglycemia, including drowsiness, fruity breath, increased urination, and unusual thirst. Patients with diabetes mellitus should check blood glucose levels frequently.

Interventions

- Guard against falls and trauma (hip fractures, head injury, and so forth) caused by drowsiness, dizziness, blurred vision, or extrapyramidal symptoms; implement fall-prevention strategies (See Appendix E).
- Use caution during aerobic exercise and other forms of therapeutic exercise because of the risk of arrhythmias. Assess exercise tolerance frequently (blood pressure, heart rate, fatigue levels), and terminate exercise immediately if any untoward responses occur (See Appendix L).
- To minimize orthostatic hypotension, patient should move slowly when assuming a more upright position.
- Help patient and family/caregivers explore nonpharmacologicl methods (exercise, counseling, support groups) to reduce schizophrenic episodes and behavioral problems.

Patient/Client-Related Instruction

- Advise patient to avoid alcohol and other CNS depressants because of the increased risk of sedation and adverse effects.
- Instruct patient to report other problematic side effects such as severe or prolonged headache, blurred vision, or GI problems (nausea, abdominal pain, dry mouth, indigestion).

Pharmacokinetics

Absorption: 28% absorbed following oral administration; food increases absorption.
Distribution: Unknown.
Metabolism and Excretion: 59% excreted unchanged in urine; 32% excreted in urine as metabolites.
Half-life: 23 hr.

TIME/ACTION PROFILE (blood levels)

ROUTE	ONSET	PEAK	DURATION
PO	unknown	24 hr	24 hr

Contraindications/Precautions

Contraindicated in: Hypersensitivity to paliperidone or risperidone; Concurrent use of drugs known to cause QTc prolongation (including quinidine, procainamide, sotalol, amiodarone, chlorpromazine, thioridazine, moxifloxacin); History of congenital QTc prolongation or other cardiac arrhythmias; Bradycardia, hypokalemia, hypomagnesemia (increased risk of QTc prolongation); Preexisting severe GI narrowing (due to nature of tablet formulation); Lactation: Discontinue drug or bottle-feed.
Use Cautiously in: Patients with Parkinson's Disease or Dementia with Lewy Bodies (↑ sensitivity to effects of antipsychotics); History of suicide attempt; Patients at risk for aspiration pneumonia; History of seizures; Conditions which may ↑ body temperature (strenuous exercise, exposure to extreme heat, concurrent anticholinergics or risk of dehydration); ↓ GI transit time (may ↑ blood levels); May mask symptoms of some drug overdoses, intestinal obstruction, Reye's syndrome, or brain tumor (due to antiemetic effect); Diabetes mellitus; Severe hepatic impairment; Renal impairment (dose reduction recommended if CCr <80 mL/min); OB: Safety not established; use only if maternal benefit outweighs fetal risk; Pedi: Safety not established; Geri: ↑ risk of mortality in elderly patients treated for dementia-related psychosis; consider age-related ↓ in renal function.

Interactions

Drug-Drug: ↑ risk of CNS depression with other **CNS depressants**, including **alcohol, antihistamines, sedative/hypnotics**, or **opioid analgesics**. May antagonize the effects of **levodopa** or other **dopamine agonists**. ↑ risk of orthostatic hypotension with **antihypertensives, nitrates**, or other **agents that lower blood pressure**. **Carbamazepine** may ↓ levels/effects.

Route/Dosage

PO (Adults): 6 mg/day; may be titrated as needed (range 3–12 mg/day).

Renal Impairment

PO (Adults): *CCr 50–80 mL/min*—dose should not exceed 6 mg/day; *CCr 10–<50 mL/min*—dose should not exceed 3 mg/day.

Availability

Extended-release tablets: 1.5 mg, 3 mg, 6 mg, 9 mg.

palivizumab (pal-i-vi-zoo-mab)
Synagis

Classification
Therapeutic: antivirals
Pharmacologic: monoclonal antibodies

Indications
Prevention of serious respiratory tract disease due to respiratory syncytial virus (RSV) in children at high risk (infants with bronchopulmonary dysplasia, history of prematurity, or hemodynamically significant congenital heart disease).

Action
Neutralizes and inhibits fusion of RSV virus; subsequently inhibits viral replication. **Therapeutic Effects:** Prevents serious sequelae of RSV disease in susceptible children.

Adverse Reactions/Side Effects
GI: diarrhea, vomiting. **Local:** erythema, induration. **Misc:** HYPERSENSITIVITY REACTIONS, INCLUDING ANAPHYLACTOID REACTIONS AND ANAPHYLAXIS.

PHYSICAL THERAPY IMPLICATIONS

Examination and Evaluation
- Monitor signs of hypersensitivity reactions and anaphylaxis, including pulmonary symptoms (tightness in the throat and chest, wheezing, cough, dyspnea) or skin reactions (rash, pruritus, urticaria). Notify physician or nursing staff immediately if these reactions occur.
- Monitor intramuscular injection site for pain, redness, warmth, and hardening of local tissues. Report prolonged or excessive injection site reactions to the physician.

Interventions
- Always wash hands thoroughly and disinfect equipment (whirlpools, electrotherapeutic devices, treatment tables, and so forth) to help prevent the spread of infection. Employ universal precautions as indicated for specific patients.

Patient/Client-Related Instruction
- Instruct family/caregivers to report other troublesome side effects, including severe or prolonged GI problems (vomiting, diarrhea).

Pharmacokinetics
Absorption: Well absorbed after IM administration.
Distribution: Unknown.
Metabolism and Excretion: Unknown.
Half-life: 20 days.

TIME/ACTION PROFILE (antibody levels)

ROUTE	ONSET	PEAK	DURATION
IM	rapid	unknown	30 days

Contraindications/Precautions
Contraindicated in: Hypersensitivity.
Use Cautiously in: History of thrombocytopenia or bleeding disorders.

Interactions
Drug-Drug: None known.

Route/Dosage
IM (Children): 15 mg/kg/mo during RSV season (first dose should be administered prior to the RSV season; RSV season is November through April in most Northern Hemisphere countries).

Availability
Lyophilized powder for reconstitution and injection: 100 mg/vial. **Solution for injection:** 50 mg/0.5-mL vial, 100 mg/1-mL vial.

palonosetron
(pal-oh-**noe**-se-tron)
Aloxi

Classification
Therapeutic: antiemetics
Pharmacologic: 5-HT_3 antagonists

Indications
Prevention of acute and delayed nausea and vomiting caused by initial or repeat courses of moderate or highly emetogenic chemotherapy (intravenous). Prevention of acute nausea and vomiting caused by initial or repeat courses of moderately emetogenic chemotherapy (oral). Prevention of postoperative nausea and vomiting (PONV) for up to 24 hr after surgery (intravenous).

Action
Blocks the effects of serotonin at receptor sites (selective antagonist) located in vagal nerve terminals and in the chemoreceptor trigger zones in the CNS. **Therapeutic Effects:** Decreased incidence and severity of nausea and vomiting following emetogenic chemotherapy or surgery.

Adverse Reactions/Side Effects
CNS: dizziness, headache. **GI:** constipation, diarrhea.

PHYSICAL THERAPY IMPLICATIONS

Examination and Evaluation
- Monitor improvements in GI symptoms (decreased nausea and vomiting, increased appetite) to help document whether drug therapy is successful.
- Assess dizziness that might affect gait, balance, and other functional activities (See Appendix C). Report balance problems and functional limitations to the physician and nursing staff, and caution the patient and family/caregivers to guard against falls and trauma.

Patient/Client-Related Instruction

- Instruct patient to report bothersome side effects such as severe or prolonged headache or GI problems (diarrhea, constipation).

Pharmacokinetics

Absorption: IV administration results in complete bioavailability; oral bioavailability = 97%.
Distribution: Unknown.
Metabolism and Excretion: 50% metabolized; 40% excreted unchanged in urine.
Half-life: 40 hr.

TIME/ACTION PROFILE

ROUTE	ONSET	PEAK	DURATION
IV	within 30 min	unknown	7 days
PO	within 1 hr	unknown	7 days

Contraindications/Precautions

Contraindicated in: Hypersensitivity; cross-sensitivity with other 5-HT_3 antagonists may occur; Lactation: Lactation.
Use Cautiously in: OB/Pedi: Safety not established.

Interactions

Drug-Drug: None significant.

Route/Dosage

IV (Adults): *Prevention of chemotherapy-induced nausea/vomiting*—0.25 mg 30 min before start of chemotherapy; *Prevention of PONV*—0.075 mg given immediately before induction of anesthesia.
PO (Adults): 0.5 mg 1 hr before start of chemotherapy.

Availability

Solution for IV injection: 0.075 mg/1.5 mL, 0.25 mg/5 mL. **Capsules:** 0.5 mg.

pamidronate (pa-mid-roe-nate)

Aredia

Classification
Therapeutic: bone resorption inhibitors
Pharmacologic: bisphosphonates, hypocalcemics

Indications

Moderate-to-severe hypercalcemia associated with malignancy. Osteolytic bone lesions associated with multiple myeloma or breast cancer. Moderate-to-severe Paget's disease.

Action

Inhibits resorption of bone. **Therapeutic Effects:** Decreased serum calcium. Decreased skeletal destruction in multiple myeloma or breast cancer. Decreased skeletal complications in Paget's disease.

Adverse Reactions/Side Effects

CNS: fatigue. **EENT:** conjunctivitis, blurred vision, eye pain/inflammation, rhinitis. **Resp:** rales. **CV:** arrhythmias, hypertension, syncope, tachycardia. **GI:** nausea, abdominal pain, anorexia, constipation, vomiting. **F and E:** hypocalcemia, hypokalemia, hypomagnesemia, hypophosphatemia, fluid overload. **GU:** nephrotoxicity. **Hemat:** leukopenia, anemia. **Local:** phlebitis at injection site. **Metab:** hypothyroidism. **MS:** muscle stiffness, musculoskeletal pain, osteonecrosis (primarily of jaw). **Misc:** fever, generalized pain.

PHYSICAL THERAPY IMPLICATIONS

Examination and Evaluation

- Assess any muscle pain/stiffness or bone pain. Report persistent or increased musculoskeletal pain to determine presence of bone or joint pathology, including fracture. Be especially aware of possible mouth and jaw pain due to osteonecrosis of the jaw. Bone pain may persist or increase in patients with Paget's disease, but usually subsides days to months after therapy is discontinued.
- Assess heart rate, ECG, and heart sounds, especially during exercise (See Appendices G, H). Report a rapid heart rate (tachycardia) or signs of other arrhythmias, including palpitations, chest discomfort, shortness of breath, fainting, and fatigue/weakness.
- Assess blood pressure periodically and compare to normal values (See Appendix F). Report a sustained increase in blood pressure (hypertension).
- Monitor any breathing problems, and report rales or other abnormal breath sounds.
- Watch for signs of leukopenia (fever, sore throat, other signs of infection) or unusual weakness and fatigue that might be due to anemia. Report these signs to the physician.
- Monitor neuromuscular signs of electrolyte imbalances (hypocalcemia, hypokalemia, etc.), including headache, lethargy, weakness, cramping, and muscle hyperexcitability and tetany. Notify physician immediately if these signs occur.
- Watch for signs of hypercalcemic relapse, including bone pain, anorexia, nausea, vomiting, thirst, and lethargy. Report these signs to the physician.
- Be alert for signs of nephrotoxicity, including hematuria, increased urinary frequency, cloudy urine, and decreased urine output. Report these signs to the physician.
- Report signs of hypothyroidism, including lethargy, weight gain, bradycardia, and cold intolerance.
- Assess IV site after IV administration, and report signs of phlebitis and venous thrombosis (local pain, swelling, inflammation).

Interventions

- Protect against falls and fractures (See Appendix E). Modify home environment (remove throw rugs, improve lighting, etc.) and provide assistive devices (cane, walker) or other protective devices as needed to improve balance and prevent falls.
- Because of the risk of cardiac arrhythmias (tachycardia, other), use caution during aerobic exercise and endurance conditioning. Terminate exercise if patient exhibits untoward symptoms (chest pain, shortness of breath, unusual fatigue) or displays other criteria for exercise termination (See Appendix L).

Patient/Client-Related Instruction

- Instruct patient to report troublesome side effects such as severe or prolonged vision disturbances, eye pain/inflammation, fever, or GI problems (nausea, vomiting, constipation, abdominal pain, loss of appetite).

Pharmacokinetics

Absorption: IV administration results in complete bioavailability.
Distribution: Rapidly absorbed by bone. Reaches high concentrations in bone, liver, spleen, teeth, and tracheal cartilage. Approximately 50% of a dose is retained by bone and then slowly released.
Metabolism and Excretion: 50% is excreted unchanged in the urine.
Half-life: Elimination half-life from plasma is biphasic—1st phase 1.6 hr, 2nd phase 27.2 hr. Elimination half-life from bone is 300 days.

TIME/ACTION PROFILE (effect on serum calcium)

ROUTE	ONSET	PEAK	DURATION
IV	24 hr	7 days	unknown

Contraindications/Precautions

Contraindicated in: Hypersensitivity to pamidronate, other bisphosphonates, or mannitol; OB: Pregnancy.
Use Cautiously in: Underlying cardiovascular disease, especially CHF (initiate saline hydration cautiously); Concurrent dental surgery (may ↑ risk of jaw osteonecrosis); Renal impairment (dose reduction recommended); Lactation/Pedi: Safety not established.

Interactions

Drug-Drug: Hypokalemia and hypomagnesemia may ↑ risk of **digoxin** toxicity. **Calcium** and **vitamin D** will antagonize the beneficial effects of pamidronate.

Route/Dosage

Single doses should not exceed 90 mg.

Hypercalcemia of Malignancy

IV (Adults): *Moderate hypercalcemia*—30–90 mg; may be repeated after 7 days.

Osteolytic Lesions from Multiple Myeloma

IV (Adults): 90 mg monthly.

Osteolytic Lesions from Metastatic Breast Cancer

IV (Adults): 90 mg q 3–4 wk.

Paget's Disease

IV (Adults): 90–180 mg/treatment; may be given as 30 mg daily for 3 days up to 30 mg/wk for 6 wk. Single doses of 60–90 mg may also be effective.

Availability (generic available)

Injection: 30 mg/vial, 90 mg/vial.

panitumumab

(pan-i-**too**-mu-mab)
Vectibix

Classification
Therapeutic: antineoplastics
Pharmacologic: monoclonal antibodies

P

Indications

Treatment of metastatic colorectal cancer that expresses EGFR (epidermal growth factor receptor) and has failed conventional treatments (to be used as monotherapy).

Action

Binds to EGFR resulting in inactivation of kinases that regulate proliferation and transformation. **Therapeutic Effects:** Decreased progression of colorectal cancer.

Adverse Reactions/Side Effects

CNS: fatigue. **EENT:** OCULAR TOXICITY, eyelash growth. **Resp:** PULMONARY FIBROSIS, cough. **GI:** abdominal pain, constipation, diarrhea, nausea, vomiting, stomatitis. **Derm:** DERMATOLOGIC TOXICITY, paronychia, photosensitivity. **F and E:** edema, hypocalcemia, hypomagnesemia. **Misc:** INFUSION REACTIONS.

PHYSICAL THERAPY IMPLICATIONS

Examination and Evaluation

- Assess any breathing problems or signs of pulmonary fibrosis such as dry cough, wheezing, chest pain, shortness of breath, and difficult or labored breathing. Monitor pulse oximetry and perform pulmonary function tests (See Appendices I, J, K) to quantify suspected changes in ventilation and respiratory function.
- Identify signs of skin toxicity such as rash, itching, scaling, redness, warmth, and rapid skin loss. Report these signs to the physician or nursing staff immediately.
- Report allergy-like responses (wheezing, laryngeal edema, urticaria, other skin reactions) that occur

♣ = Canadian drug name; *CAPITALS indicate life-threatening; underlines indicate most frequent.

during and after administration (infusion related reactions).

- Monitor any vision disturbances, eye pain, or inflammation that might indicate ocular toxicity. Report vision problems to the physician or nursing staff immediately.
- Assess peripheral edema using girth measurements, volume displacement, and measurement of pitting edema (See Appendix N). Report increased swelling in feet and ankles or a sudden increase in body weight due to fluid retention.
- Monitor neuromuscular signs of electrolyte imbalances such as low calcium levels (headache, lethargy, weakness, cramping, muscle hyperexcitability and tetany) and low magnesium levels (irritability, insomnia, muscle tremors, confusion). Notify physician or nursing staff of these signs.

Interventions

- For patients who are medically able to begin exercise, implement appropriate resistive exercises and aerobic training to maintain muscle strength and aerobic capacity during cancer chemotherapy or to help restore function after chemotherapy.
- Use caution during aerobic exercise and endurance conditioning because of potential pulmonary toxicity. Terminate exercise if patient exhibits untoward symptoms (chest pain, shortness of breath, unusual fatigue) or displays other criteria for exercise termination (See Appendix L).
- Causes photosensitivity; use care if administering UV treatments. Advise patient to avoid direct sunlight and use sunscreens and protective clothing.

Patient/Client-Related Instruction

- Advise patient about the likelihood of GI reactions, including abdominal pain, constipation, diarrhea, nausea, vomiting, and inflammation in/around mouth. Instruct patient to report severe or prolonged GI problems.
- Instruct patient or family/caregivers to report other bothersome side effects such as severe or prolonged cough, fatigue, or infections in the fingernails or toenails.

Pharmacokinetics

Absorption: IV administration results in complete bioavailability.
Distribution: Monoclonal antibodies cross the placenta and enter breast milk.
Metabolism and Excretion: Unknown.
Half-life: 7.5 days.

TIME/ACTION PROFILE

ROUTE	ONSET	PEAK	DURATION
IV	unknown	end of infusion	unknown

Contraindications/Precautions

Contraindicated in: Concurrent leucovorin; OB/Lactation: Pregnancy or lactation.
Use Cautiously in: Pedi: Safety not established.

Interactions

Drug-Drug: None noted.

Route/Dosage

IV (Adults): 6 mg/kg as a 60-min infusion every 14 days; decreased infusion rates and dose modifications are recommended for infusion reactions and other serious toxicities.

Availability

Solution for IV administration (requires dilution): 20 mg/mL in 5-mL vials (100 mg/vial).

pantoprazole (pan-toe-pra-zole)

Pantoloc, Protonix, Protonix IV

Classification
Therapeutic: antiulcer agents
Pharmacologic: proton-pump inhibitors

Indications

Erosive esophagitis associated with gastroesophageal reflux disease (GERD). Decrease relapse rates of daytime and nighttime heartburn symptoms on patients with GERD. Pathologic gastric hypersecretory conditions. **Unlabeled Use:** Adjunctive treatment of duodenal ulcers associated with *Helicobacter pylori*.

Action

Binds to an enzyme in the presence of acidic gastric pH, preventing the final transport of hydrogen ions into the gastric lumen. **Therapeutic Effects:** Diminished accumulation of acid in the gastric lumen, with lessened acid reflux. Healing of duodenal ulcers and esophagitis. Decreased acid secretion in hypersecretory conditions.

Adverse Reactions/Side Effects

CNS: headache. **GI:** abdominal pain, diarrhea, eructation, flatulence. **Endo:** hyperglycemia.

PHYSICAL THERAPY IMPLICATIONS

Examination and Evaluation

- Monitor improvements in GI symptoms (gastritis, heartburn, and so forth) to help determine if drug therapy is successful.
- Monitor signs of hyperglycemia (drowsiness, fruity breath, increased urination, unusual thirst). Patients with diabetes mellitus should check blood glucose levels frequently.

Interventions

- In cases of NSAID-induced gastritis, implement appropriate manual therapy techniques, physical agents, and therapeutic exercises to reduce pain and decrease the need for aspirin and other NSAIDs.

Patient/Client-Related Instruction

- Advise patient to avoid alcohol and foods that may cause an increase in GI irritation.
- Instruct patient to report bothersome or prolonged side effects, including headache or GI effects (diarrhea, flatulence, belching, abdominal pain).

Pharmacokinetics

Absorption: Tablet is enteric coated; absorption occurs only after tablet leaves the stomach.
Distribution: Unknown.
Protein Binding: 98%.
Metabolism and Excretion: Mostly metabolized by the liver via the cytochrome P450 (CYP) system; inactive metabolites are excreted in urine (71%) and feces (18%).
Half-life: 1 hr.

TIME/ACTION PROFILE (effect on acid secretion)

ROUTE	ONSET*	PEAK	DURATION*
PO	2.5 hr	unknown	1 wk
IV	15–30 min	2 hr	unknown

*Onset = 51% inhibition; duration = return to normal following discontinuation.

Contraindications/Precautions

Contraindicated in: Hypersensitivity; OB: Should be used during pregnancy only if clearly needed. Lactation: Discontinue breast-feeding due to potential for serious adverse reactions in infants.
Use Cautiously in: Pedi: Safety not established.

Interactions

Drug-Drug: May ↓ absorption of drugs requiring acid pH, including **ketoconazole, itraconazole, atazanavir, ampicillin esters, iron salts**, and **digoxin**. May ↑ risk of bleeding with **warfarin** (monitor INR/PT).

Route/Dosage

PO (Adults): *GERD*—40 mg once daily; *Gastric hypersecretory conditions*—40 mg bid, up to 120 mg bid.
PO (Children): 0.5–1 mg/kg/day.
IV (Adults): *GERD*—40 mg once daily for 7–10 days. *Gastric hypersecretory conditions*—80 mg q 12 hr (up to 240 mg/day).

Availability (generic available)

Delayed-release tablets: 20 mg, 40 mg. **Powder for injection:** 40 mg/vial.

paricalcitol (par-i-kal-si-tole)

Zemplar

Classification
Therapeutic: vitamins
Pharmacologic: fat-soluble vitamins

Indications

Prevention and treatment of secondary hyperparathyroidism in patients with Stage 3 or 4 (PO) or Stage 5 (IV) chronic kidney disease.

Action

Paricalcitol is a synthetic analogue of calcitriol (the active form of vitamin D_3. Promotes the absorption of calcium and decreases parathyroid hormone concentrations. **Therapeutic Effects:** Improved calcium and phosphorus homeostasis in patients with chronic kidney disease.

Adverse Reactions/Side Effects

Seen primarily as manifestations of toxicity (hypercalcemia)
CNS: dizziness, headache, somnolence, weakness.
EENT: conjunctivitis, photophobia, rhinorrhea.
CV: arrhythmias, edema, hypertension, palpitations.
GI: anorexia, constipation, diarrhea, dry mouth, liver function test elevation, metallic taste, nausea, PANCREATITIS, polydipsia, vomiting, weight loss. **GU:** albuminuria, azotemia, decreased libido. **Derm:** pruritus, rash. **Endo:** gout. **F and E:** hypercalcemia. **Metab:** hyperthermia. **MS:** bone pain, metastatic calcification, muscle pain.

PHYSICAL THERAPY IMPLICATIONS

**Note: Many drug implications listed below are related directly to vitamin D toxicity and subsequent hypercalcemia.*

Examination and Evaluation

- Be alert for signs of pancreatitis, including upper abdominal pain (especially after eating), indigestion, weight loss, oily stools. Report these signs to the physician or nursing staff immediately.
- Assess heart rate, ECG, and heart sounds, especially during exercise (See Appendices G, H). Report any rhythm disturbances or symptoms of increased arrhythmias, including palpitations, chest discomfort, shortness of breath, fainting, and fatigue/weakness.
- Assess blood pressure (BP) and compare to normal values (See Appendix F). Report a sustained increase in BP (hypertension).
- Assess peripheral edema using girth measurements, volume displacement, and measurement of pitting edema (See Appendix N). Report increased swelling

in feet and ankles or a sudden increase in body weight due to fluid retention.

- Assess any muscle or bone pain to rule out musculoskeletal pathology; that is, try to determine if pain is drug induced rather than caused by anatomic or biomechanical problems. Request additional tests for suspicious bone pain that may indicate metastatic calcification.
- Monitor signs of electrolyte imbalances such as high calcium levels (hypercalcemia). Neuromuscular signs include muscle pain and weakness, joint pain, confusion, and lethargy. Notify physician because severe cases can lead to life-threatening arrhythmias and paralysis.
- Assess dizziness that might affect gait, balance, and other functional activities (See Appendix C). Report balance problems and functional limitations to the physician, and caution the patient and family/caregivers to guard against falls and trauma.

Interventions

- Because of the risk of arrhythmias, use caution during aerobic exercise and other forms of therapeutic exercise. Assess exercise tolerance frequently (BP, heart rate, fatigue levels), and terminate exercise immediately if any untoward responses occur (See Appendix L).
- Protect against falls and fractures (See Appendix E). Modify home environment (remove throw rugs, improve lighting, etc.) and provide assistive devices (cane, walker) or other protective devices as needed to improve balance and prevent falls.

Patient/Client-Related Instruction

- Advise patient about the likelihood of GI problems, including nausea, vomiting, diarrhea, constipation, dry mouth, increased thirst, metallic taste, and loss of appetite. Instruct patient to report severe or unexpected GI problems.
- Instruct patient to report other troublesome side effects such as severe or prolonged headache, weakness, vision disturbances, nasal discharge, decreased libido, or skin problems (rash, itching).

Pharmacokinetics

Absorption: IV administration results in complete bioavailability; well absorbed following oral administration.
Distribution: Crosses the placenta.
Protein Binding: 99.9%.
Metabolism and Excretion: Primarily metabolized by the liver and excreted via hepatobiliary elimination.
Half-life: 14–20 hr.

TIME/ACTION PROFILE

ROUTE	ONSET	PEAK	DURATION
PO	unknown	2–4 wk	unknown
IV	unknown	2–4 wk	unknown

Contraindications/Precautions

Contraindicated in: Hypersensitivity; Hypercalcemia; Vitamin D toxicity; OB: Lactation.
Use Cautiously in: Patients receiving digoxin; OB: Pregnancy (safety not established).

Interactions

Drug-Drug: Cholestyramine, colestipol, or **mineral oil** ↓ absorption of vitamin D analogues. Use with **thiazide diuretics** may result in hypercalcemia. **Corticosteroids** ↓ effectiveness of vitamin D analogues. Use with **digoxin** ↑ risk of arrhythmias. Concurrent use of **magnesium-containing drugs** may lead to hypermagnesemia. **Calcium-containing drugs** may ↑ risk of hypercalcemia. Concurrent use of other **Vitamin D supplements** (↑ risk of hypercalcemia). **Agents that induce liver enzymes (phenobarbital, rifampin)** and **agents that inhibit liver enzymes (atazanavir, clarithromycin, erythromycin, indinavir, itraconazole, ketoconazole, nefazodone, nelfinavir, ritonavir, saquinavir, verapamil, voriconazole)** may alter requirements for paricalcitol (monitoring of calcium and phosphorus recommended).
Drug-Food: Ingestion of **foods high in calcium content** (See Appendix L) may lead to hypercalcemia.

Route/Dosage

PO (Adults): *Baseline intact PTH concentration ≤500 pg/mL*—Initiate with 1 mcg/day or 2 mcg 3 times weekly; *Baseline intact PTH concentration >500 pg/mL*—Initiate with 2 mcg/day or 4 mcg 3 times weekly; doses can be adjusted at 2- to 4-wk intervals based on intact PTH concentrations.
IV (Adults and Children ≥5 yr): 0.04–0.1 mcg/kg 3 times weekly during dialysis; dose can be adjusted by 2–4 mcg at 2- to 4-wk intervals based on intact PTH concentrations (doses up to 0.24 mcg/kg have been used).

Availability

Capsules: 1 mcg, 2 mcg, 4 mcg. **Injection:** 2 mcg/mL in 1-mL vials, 5 mcg/mL in 1- and 2-mL vials.

paromomycin

(par-oh-**moe**-mye-sin)
Humatin

Classification
Therapeutic: amebicide
Pharmacologic: aminoglycosides

Indications
Treatment of acute and chronic intestinal amebiasis. Management of hepatic coma as adjunctive therapy (i.e., used to control intestinal bacteria that can produce ammonia and worsen encephalopathy related to liver failure).

Action
Inhibits protein synthesis in bacteria at level of 30S ribosome. **Therapeutic Effects:** Resolution of amebic infections. **Spectrum:** Notable for activity against *Entamoeba histolytica*, *Dientamoeba fragilis*, *Diphyllobothrium latum*, *Taenia saginata*, *Cryptosporidium*, *Giardia lamblia*.

Adverse Reactions/Side Effects
GI: abdominal cramps, diarrhea, nausea, vomiting. **Misc:** hypersensitivity reactions.

PHYSICAL THERAPY IMPLICATIONS

Examination and Evaluation
- Monitor signs of hypersensitivity reactions, including pulmonary symptoms (tightness in the throat and chest, wheezing, cough, dyspnea) or skin reactions (rash, pruritus, urticaria). Notify physician or nursing staff immediately if these reactions occur.

Interventions
- Make sure patient remains adequately hydrated to offset fluid loss from diarrhea.

Patient/Client-Related Instruction
- Instruct patient and family/caregivers to report severe or prolonged GI problems including diarrhea, nausea, vomiting, and abdominal cramps.

Pharmacokinetics
Absorption: Minimal to no systemic absorption.
Distribution: Unknown.
Metabolism and Excretion: 100% excreted in feces.
Half-life: Unknown.

TIME/ACTION PROFILE

ROUTE	ONSET	PEAK	DURATION
PO	unknown	unknown	unknown

Contraindications/Precautions
Contraindicated in: Hypersensitivity to paromomycin or other aminoglycosides; Intestinal obstruction.
Use Cautiously in: Renal impairment; Ulcerative bowel lesions; Pregnancy, lactation, infants, and neonates (safety not established).

Interactions
Interactions are listed for systemically absorbed drug
Drug-Drug: May enhance possible respiratory paralysis after **inhalation anesthetics** or **neuromuscular blockers.** ↑ incidence of ototoxicity with **loop diuretics.** May ↑ the anticoagulant effects of **warfarin.** May ↓ the absorption of **digoxin** and **methotrexate.**

Route/Dosage

Intestinal Amebiasis
PO (Adults and Children): 8.33–11.67 mg/kg tid with meals for 5–10 days.

Hepatic Coma
PO (Adults): 4 g/day in 2–4 divided doses for 5–6 days.

Availability
Capsules: 250 mg.

paroxetine hydrochloride
(par-**ox**-e-teen)
Paxil, Paxil CR

paroxetine mesylate
Pexeva

Classification
Therapeutic: antianxiety agents, antidepressants
Pharmacologic: selective serotonin reuptake inhibitors (SSRIs)

P

Indications
Paxil, Paxil CR, Pexeva: Major depressive disorder, panic disorder. **Paxil, Pexeva:** Obsessive compulsive disorder (OCD), generalized anxiety disorder (GAD). **Paxil, Paxil CR:** Social anxiety disorder. **Paxil:** Posttraumatic stress disorder (PTSD). **Paxil CR:** Premenstrual dysphoric disorder (PMDD).

Action
Inhibits neuronal reuptake of serotonin in the CNS, thus potentiating the activity of serotonin; has little effect on norepinephrine or dopamine. **Therapeutic Effects:** Antidepressant action. Decreased frequency of panic attacks, OCD, or anxiety. Improvement in manifestations of posttraumatic stress disorder. Decreased dysphoria prior to menses.

Adverse Reactions/Side Effects
CNS: anxiety, dizziness, drowsiness, headache, insomnia, weakness, agitation, amnesia, confusion, emotional lability, hangover, impaired concentration, malaise, mental depression, suicidal behavior, syncope. **EENT:** blurred vision, rhinitis. **Resp:** cough, pharyngitis, respiratory disorders, yawning. **CV:** chest pain, edema, hypertension, palpitations, orthostatic hypotension, tachycardia, vasodilation. **GI:** constipation, diarrhea, dry mouth, nausea, abdominal pain, decreased appetite, dyspepsia, flatulence, increased

appetite, taste disturbances, vomiting. **GU:** ejaculatory disturbance, decreased libido, genital disorders, urinary disorders, urinary frequency. **Derm:** sweating, photosensitivity, pruritus, rash. **Metab:** weight gain, weight loss. **MS:** back pain, myalgia, myopathy. **Neuro:** paresthesia, tremor. **Misc:** chills, fever.

PHYSICAL THERAPY IMPLICATIONS

Examination and Evaluation

- Be alert for increased depression and suicidal thoughts and ideology, especially when initiating drug treatment, and in children and teenagers. Notify physician or other mental health care professional immediately if patient exhibits worsening depression.
- Inform physician if patient demonstrates other mood changes such as increased anxiety, agitation, impaired memory, impaired concentration, emotional lability, or confusion (See Appendix D).
- Assess blood pressure (BP) periodically and compare to normal values (See Appendix F). Report a sustained increase in BP (hypertension). Also, assess BP when patient assumes a more upright position (lying to standing, sitting to standing, lying to sitting). Document orthostatic hypotension and contact physician when systolic BP falls >20 mm Hg or diastolic BP falls >10 mm Hg.
- Assess heart rate, ECG, and heart sounds, especially during exercise (See Appendices G, H). Report a rapid heart rate (tachycardia) or signs of other arrhythmias, including palpitations, chest discomfort, shortness of breath, fainting, and fatigue/weakness.
- Assess peripheral edema using girth measurements, volume displacement, and measurement of pitting edema (See Appendix N). Report increased swelling in feet and ankles or a sudden increase in body weight due to fluid retention.
- Assess any breathing problems, and report signs of respiratory disorders such as shortness of breath, cough, pharyngitis, and labored or difficult breathing.
- Assess any muscle pain or back pain to rule out musculoskeletal pathology; that is, try to determine if pain is drug induced rather than caused by anatomic or biomechanical problems.
- Assess parethesias (numbness, tingling) or tremor. Perform objective tests, including electroneuromyography, and sensory testing to document any drug-related neuropathic changes.
- Assess dizziness, drowsiness, and syncope that might affect gait, balance, and other functional activities (See Appendix C). Report balance problems and functional limitations to the physician, and caution the patient and family/caregivers to guard against falls and trauma.
- Periodically assess body weight and other anthropometric measures (body mass index, body composition). Report a rapid or unexplained weight gain or weight loss.

Interventions

- Guard against falls and trauma (hip fractures, head injury, and so forth) and implement fall-prevention strategies (See Appendix E).
- Because of the risk of cardiac arrhythmias and changes in BP, use caution during aerobic exercise and endurance conditioning. Assess exercise tolerance frequently (BP, heart rate, fatigue levels), and terminate exercise immediately if any untoward responses occur (see Appendix L).
- To minimize orthostatic hypotension, patient should move slowly when assuming a more upright position.
- Causes photosensitivity; use care if administering UV treatments. Advise patient to avoid direct sunlight and use sunscreens and protective clothing.
- Help patient explore nonpharmacologic methods (exercise, counseling, support groups, and so forth) to reduce depression and other psychologic disorders.

Patient/Client-Related Instruction

- Advise patient that antidepressant effects may not occur immediately; it may take 2 wk or more before an improvement in mood is observed.
- Advise patient to avoid alcohol and other CNS depressants because of the increased risk of sedation and adverse effects.
- Advise patient that this medication should be tapered at the completion of long-term therapy. Abrupt withdrawal may cause dizziness, sensory disturbances, agitation, anxiety, nausea, and sweating.
- Instruct patient to report other problematic side effects such as severe of prolonged headache, blurred vision, urinary frequency, sexual dysfunction, flu-like symptoms (fever, malaise), skin reactions (rash, itching, increased sweating), or GI problems (nausea, vomiting, diarrhea, constipation, indigestion, abdominal pain, flatulence, dry mouth, taste disturbances, changes in appetite).

Pharmacokinetics

Absorption: Completely absorbed following oral administration. Controlled-release tablets are enteric coated and control medication release over 4–5 hr.
Distribution: Widely distributed throughout body fluids and tissues, including the CNS; cross the placenta and enter breast milk.
Protein Binding: 95%.
Metabolism and Excretion: Highly metabolized by the liver (partly by P4502D6 enzyme system); 2% excreted unchanged in urine.
Half-life: 21 hr.

TIME/ACTION PROFILE (antidepressant action)

ROUTE	ONSET	PEAK	DURATION
PO	1–4 wk	unknown	unknown

Contraindications/Precautions

Contraindicated in: Hypersensitivity; Concurrent MAO inhibitor, thioridazine, or pimozide therapy.
Use Cautiously in: Risk of suicide (may ↑ risk of suicide attempt/ideation, especially during early treatment or dose adjustment); History of seizures; History of bipolar disorder; OB: Use during the 1st trimester may be associated with an increased risk of cardiac malformations—consider fetal risk/maternal benefit; use during 3rd trimester may result in neonatal serotonin syndrome requiring prolonged hospitalization, respiratory and nutritional support; Lactation: Safety not established; discontinue drug or bottle-feed; Pedi: May ↑ risk of suicide attempt/ideation, especially during early treatment or dose adjustment may be greater in children and adolescents (safety in children/adolescents not established); Geri: Severe renal hepatic impairment; geriatric or debilitated patients (daily dose should not exceed 40 mg); history of mania/risk of suicide.

Interactions

Drug-Drug: Serious, potentially fatal reactions (hyperthermia, rigidity, myoclonus, autonomic instability, with fluctuating vital signs and extreme agitation, which may proceed to delirium and coma) may occur with concurrent **MAO inhibitor** therapy. MAO inhibitors should be stopped at least 14 days prior to paroxetine therapy. Paroxetine should be stopped at least 14 days prior to MAO inhibitor therapy. May ↓ metabolism and ↑ effects of certain **drugs that are metabolized by the liver**, including other **antidepressants, phenothiazines, class IC antiarrhythmics, risperidone, atomoxetine, theophylline, procyclidine**, and **quinidine**. Concurrent use should be undertaken with caution. Concurrent use with **pimozide** or **thioridazine** may ↑ risk of QT interval prolongation and torsades de pointes. Concurrent use is contraindicated. **Cimetidine** ↑ blood levels. **Phenobarbital** and **phenytoin** may ↓ effectiveness. Concurrent use with **alcohol** is not recommended. May ↓ the effectiveness of **digoxin**. May ↑ risk of bleeding with **warfarin, aspirin**, or **NSAIDS**. Concurrent use with **5-HT$_1$ agonists (frovatriptan, naratriptan, rizatriptan, sumatriptan, zolmitriptan), linezolid, lithium**, or **tramadol** may result in increased serotonin levels and lead to serotonin syndrome.
Drug-Natural: ↑ risk of serotonergic side effects, including serotonin syndrome with **St. John's wort, SAMe**, and **tryptophan**.

Route/Dosage

Depression

PO (Adults): 20 mg as a single dose in the morning; may be ↑ by 10 mg/day at weekly intervals (not to exceed 50 mg/day). *Controlled-release tablets*—25 mg once daily initially. May ↑ at weekly intervals by 12.5 mg (not to exceed 62.5 mg/day).
PO (Geriatric Patients or Debilitated Patients): 10 mg/day initially; may be slowly ↑ (not to exceed 40 mg/day). *Controlled-release tablets*—12.5 mg once daily initially; may be slowly ↑ (not to exceed 50 mg/day).

Obsessive-Compulsive Disorder

PO (Adults): 20 mg/day initially; ↑ by 10 mg/day at weekly intervals up to 40 mg (not to exceed 60 mg/day).

Panic Disorder

PO (Adults): 10 mg/day initially; ↑ by 10 mg/day at weekly intervals up to 40 mg (not to exceed 60 mg/day). *Controlled-release tablets*—12.5 mg/day initially; ↑ by 12.5 mg/day at weekly intervals (not to exceed 75 mg/day).

Social Anxiety Disorder

PO (Adults): 20 mg/day. *Controlled-release tablets*—12.5 mg/day initially; may ↑ by 12.5 mg/day weekly intervals (not to exceed 37.5 mg/day).

Generalized anxiety disorder

PO (Adults): 20 mg once daily initially; ↑ by 10 mg/day at weekly intervals (not to exceed 50 mg/day).

Posttraumatic Stress Disorder

PO (Adults): 20 mg/day initially; may be ↑ by 10 mg/day at weekly intervals (not to exceed 50 mg/day).

Premenstrual Dysphoric Disorder

PO (Adults): *Controlled-release tablets*—12.5 mg once daily throughout menstrual cycle or during luteal phase of menstrual cycle only; may be ↑ to 25 mg/day after one week.

Hepatic Impairment

PO (Adults): *Severe hepatic impairment*—10 mg/day initially; may be slowly ↑ (not to exceed 40 mg/day). *Controlled-release tablets*—12.5 mg once daily initially; may be slowly ↑ (not to exceed 50 mg/day).

Renal Impairment

PO (Adults): *Severe renal impairment*—10 mg/day initially; may be slowly ↑ (not to exceed 40 mg/day). *Controlled-release tablets*—12.5 mg once daily initially; may be slowly ↑ increased (not to exceed 50 mg/day).

Availability (generic available)

Paroxetine hydrochloride tablets: 10 mg, 20 mg, 30 mg, 40 mg. **Paroxetine hydrochloride controlled-release tablets:** 12.5 mg, 25 mg, 37.5 mg. **Paroxetine hydrochloride oral suspension**

P

(orange flavor): 10 mg/5 mL. **Paroxetine mesylate tablets:** 10 mg, 20 mg, 30 mg, 40 mg.

pazopanib (pa-zoe-puh-nib)
Votrient

Classification
Therapeutic: antineoplastics
Pharmacologic: kinase inhibitors

Indications
Treatment of advanced renal cell carcinoma.

Action
Acts as a tyrosine kinase inhibitor of several vascular endothelial growth factor (VEGF) receptors, platelet-derived growth factor receptor, fibroblast growth factor receptor, cytokine receptor, interleukin-2 receptor inducible T-cell kinase, leukocyte-specific protein tyrosine kinase, and transmembrane glycoprotein receptor tyrosine kinase. Overall effect is decreased angiogenesis in tumors. **Therapeutic Effects:** Decreased growth and spread of renal cell carcinoma.

Adverse Reactions/Side Effects
CNS: fatigue, weakness. **CV:** PROLONGED QT INTERVAL PROLONGATION, hypertension, chest pain. **GI:** GI PERFORATION/FISTULA, HEPATOTOXICITY, abdominal pain, anorexia, diarrhea, nausea, vomiting altered taste, dyspepsia. **GU:** proteinuria. **Derm:** alopecia, facial edema, palmar-plantar erythrodysesthesia (hand-foot syndrome), rash, skin depigmentation. **Endo:** hypothyroidism. **Hemat:** BLEEDING, arterial thrombosis. **Metab:** ↑ lipase, weight loss. **Misc:** hair color changes (depigmentation)

PHYSICAL THERAPY IMPLICATIONS

Examination and Evaluation
- Assess heart rate, ECG, and heart sounds, especially during exercise (See Appendices G, H). Report any rhythm disturbances or symptoms of increased arrhythmias, including palpitations, chest discomfort, shortness of breath, fainting, and fatigue/weakness.
- Watch for signs of bleeding, including bleeding gums, nosebleeds, unusual bruising, black/tarry stools, hematuria, and a fall in hematocrit or blood pressure (BP). Notify physician or nursing staff immediately if these signs occur.
- Be alert for signs of hepatotoxicity, including anorexia, abdominal pain, severe nausea and vomiting, yellow skin or eyes, fever, sore throat, malaise, weakness, facial edema, lethargy, and unusual bleeding or bruising. Report these signs to the physician or nursing staff immediately.
- Watch for signs of GI perforation or fistula, including severe abdominal pain, nausea, vomiting, chills, and fever. Report these signs to the physician or nursing staff immediately.
- Monitor signs of arterial thrombosis, including extreme coldness in the hands and feet, cyanosis, and muscle cramping. Notify physician immediately, and request objective tests (Doppler ultrasound, others) if thrombosis is suspected.
- Assess BP and compare to normal values (See Appendix F). Report a sustained increase in BP (hypertension).
- Be alert for palmer-planter erythrodysesthesia, as indicated by pain, redness, and dry, scaly skin on the palms of the hands and soles of the feet. Report these signs immediately to the physician. Instruct patient to also protect the hands and feet from heat and friction, and to apply lotion to the affected areas. Superficial cold application can also temporarily reduce symptoms.
- Monitor signs of hypothyroidism, including bradycardia, lethargy, cold intolerance, weight gain, and muscle weakness. Report these signs to the physician or nursing staff.
- Periodically assess body weight and other anthropometric measures (body mass index, body composition). Report a rapid or unexplained weight loss or decreased body fat.

Interventions
- For patients who are medically able to begin exercise, implement appropriate resistive exercises and aerobic training to maintain muscle strength and aerobic capacity during cancer chemotherapy or to help restore function after chemotherapy.
- Because of potential arrhythmias and bleeding problems, use caution during aerobic exercise and endurance conditioning. Terminate exercise if patient exhibits untoward symptoms (chest pain, shortness of breath, unusual fatigue) or displays other criteria for exercise termination (see Appendix L).

Patient/Client-Related Instruction
- Advise patient and family/caregivers that fatigue and weakness are likely and may be severe. Implement assistive devices (walker, cane, wheelchair) as needed to help maintain mobility and prevent falls.
- Instruct patient to report other bothersome side effects such as severe or skin reactions (rash, hair loss, facial swelling, changes in skin pigmentation or hair color) or GI problems (nausea, vomiting, diarrhea, indigestion).

Pharmacokinetics

Absorption: Well absorbed following oral administration; crushing tablet and ingesting food ↑ absorption.
Distribution: unknown.
Protein Binding: >99%.
Metabolism and Excretion: Mostly metabolized by the liver (primarily by the CYP3A4 enzyme system, minor amounts by CYP1A2 and CYP2C8) followed by elimination in feces; <4% excreted by the kidneys.
Half-life: 30.9 hr.

TIME/ACTION PROFILE (blood levels)

ROUTE	ONSET	PEAK	DURATION
PO	PO	2–4 hr	24 hr

Contraindications/Precautions

Contraindicated in: Severe hepatic impairment; History of hemoptysis, cerebral or GI bleeding in preceding 6 mo; Risk/history of arterial thrombotic events, including MI, angina, or ischemic stroke within preceding 6 mo; Concurrent use of strong CYP3A4 inhibitors (if concurrent use is necessary, consider dose ↓ of pazopanib); Concurrent use of strong CYP3A4 inducers (may ↓ effectiveness); Concurrent use of drugs that have narrow therapeutic windows and that are metabolized by CYP3A4, CYP2D6, or CYP2C8 enzyme systems; OB: May cause fetal harm, avoid use during pregnancy; Lactation: Avoid use during breast-feeding.
Use Cautiously in: Congenital prolonged QTc interval or concurrent medications/diseases that prolong QTc (may ↑ risk of torsades de pointes); Electrolyte abnormalities (correct prior to use; may ↑ risk of potentially serious arrhythmia); Patients at risk for gastrointestinal perforation/fistula; Surgery, interruption of therapy recommended; Hypertension, control before therapy is initiated; Hypothyroidism (may worsen condition); Concurrent use of inducers of the CYP3A4 enzyme system, consider alternate concurrent medication with little or no enzyme induction potential or avoid pazopanib; Moderate hepatic impairment (dose ↓ recommended); Geri: May be more sensitive to drug effects, consider age-related ↓ in cardiac, renal, and hepatic function, concurrent disease states, and drug therapy; OB: Women with childbearing potential; Pedi: Safety and effectiveness not established.

Interactions

Drug-Drug: Concurrent use of **strong CYP3A4 inhibitors**, including **ketoconazole, ritonavir** and **clarithromycin,** may ↑ levels and should be avoided; if required, dose of pazopanib should be ↓ to 400 mg daily or more if necessary; Concurrent use of **strong CYP3A4 inducers**, including **rifampin**, may ↓ levels and effectiveness and should be avoided; Concurrent use with **drugs with narrow therapeutic windows that are metabolized by CYP3A4, CYP2D6, or CYP2C8** may ↑ levels of such drugs and the risk of toxicity/adverse reactions is not recommended.

Route/Dosage

PO (Adults): 800 mg once daily; *strong inhibitors or CYP3A4*—400 mg once daily; further reductions may be necessary.

Hepatic Impairment

PO (Adults): *Moderate hepatic impairment*—200 mg once daily.

Availability

Tablets: 200 mg

pegaptanib (peg-ap-ta-nib)

Macugen

Classification
Therapeutic: ocular agents
Pharmacologic: vascular endothelial growth-factor antagonists

Indications

Neovascular (wet) age-related macular degeneration.

Action

Acts as an antagonist of vascular endothelial growth factor (VEGF). VEGF may be responsible for the formation of incompetent, leaky blood vessels associated with macular degeneration. **Therapeutic Effects:** Decreased rate of loss of visual acuity.

Adverse Reactions/Side Effects

EENT: cataract, blurred vision, conjunctival bleeding, irritation/pain, ↑ intraocular pressure, ocular inflammation, infection (rare), retinal detachment (rare), traumatic cataract formation (rare). **Misc:** Anaphylaxis, angioedema.

PHYSICAL THERAPY IMPLICATIONS

Examination and Evaluation

- Monitor signs of anaphylaxis and angioedema, including pulmonary symptoms (tightness in the throat and chest, wheezing, cough, dyspnea) or skin reactions (rash, pruritus, urticaria, facial swelling). Notify physician immediately if these reactions occur.

Patient/Client-Related Instruction

- Advise patient about the likelihood of vision disturbances, including blurred vision, cloudy vision, and eye inflammation. Instruct patient to report severe or unexpected vision problems.

Pharmacokinetics

Absorption: Slowly absorbed into systemic circulation after intravitreous administration.
Distribution: Unknown.
Metabolism and Excretion: Metabolized by exonucleases and endonucleases.
Half-life: 10 days (plasma).

TIME/ACTION PROFILE

ROUTE	ONSET	PEAK	DURATION
intravitreal	unknown	unknown	6 wk

Contraindications/Precautions

Contraindicated in: Ocular/periocular infections.
Use Cautiously in: OB: Use only if maternal benefit outweighs fetal risk; Lactation/Pedi: Safety not established.

Interactions

Drug-Drug: None known.

Route/Dosage

Intravitreal (Adults): 0.3 mg q 6 wk.

Availability

Solution for intravitreous injection: 0.3 mg/mL in 1-mL single use glass syringes.

pegaspargase
(peg-ah-**spar**-jase)
Oncaspar, PEG-l-asparaginase

Classification
Therapeutic: antineoplastics
Pharmacologic: enzymes

Indications

Treatment (usually with other agents) of acute lymphoblastic leukemia (ALL) in patients who have had a previous hypersensitivity reaction to native asparaginase.

Action

Consists of L-asparaginase bound to polyethylene glycol (PEG). This compound depletes asparagine, which leukemic cells cannot synthesize. Normal cells are able to produce their own asparagine and are less susceptible to the effects of asparaginase. Binding to PEG renders asparaginase less antigenic and therefore less likely to induce hypersensitivity reactions.
Therapeutic Effects: Death of leukemic cells.

Adverse Reactions/Side Effects

CNS: SEIZURES, headache, malaise. **GI:** PANCREATITIS, abdominal pain, abnormal liver function tests, anorexia, diarrhea, lip edema, nausea, vomiting. **Derm:** jaundice. **Endo:** hyperglycemia. **F and E:** peripheral edema. **Hemat:** decreased fibrinogen disseminated intravascular coagulation, hemolytic anemia, increased thromboplastin, leukopenia, pancytopenia, thrombocytopenia. **Local:** injection site hypersensitivity, injection site pain, thrombosis. **MS:** arthralgia, myalgia, pain in extremities. **Neuro:** paresthesia. **Misc:** chills, hypersensitivity reactions, night sweats.

PHYSICAL THERAPY IMPLICATIONS

Examination and Evaluation

- Be alert for new seizures or increased seizure activity, especially at the onset of drug treatment. Document the number, duration, and severity of seizures, and report these findings immediately to the physician or nursing staff.
- Watch for signs of pancreatitis, including upper abdominal pain (especially after eating), indigestion, weight loss, oily stools. Report these signs to the physician or nursing staff immediately.
- Monitor signs of hypersensitivity reactions, including pulmonary symptoms (tightness in the throat and chest, wheezing, cough, dyspnea) or skin reactions (rash, pruritus, urticaria). Notify physician or nursing staff immediately if these reactions occur.
- Report signs of blood dyscrasias, including leukopenia (fever, sore throat, signs of infection), thrombocytopenia (bruising, nose bleeds, bleeding gums), or hemolytic anemia (unusual fatigue, shortness of breath, dizziness, headache, coldness in hands and feet, pale skin, chest pain).
- Assess peripheral edema using girth measurements, volume displacement, and measurement of pitting edema (See Appendix N). Report increased swelling in feet and ankles or a sudden increase in body weight due to fluid retention.
- Be alert for signs of hyperglycemia, including confusion, drowsiness, flushed/dry skin, fruit-like breath odor, rapid/deep breathing, polyuria, loss of appetite, and unusual thirst. Patients with diabetes mellitus should check blood glucose levels frequently.
- Assess signs of paresthesia (numbness, tingling) or muscle twitching. Perform objective tests including electroneuromyography and sensory testing to document any drug-related neuropathic changes.
- Assess any joint, muscle, or extremity pain to rule out musculoskeletal pathology; that is, try to determine if pain is drug-induced rather than caused by anatomical or biomechanical problems.
- Monitor IV injection site for pain, swelling, and irritation. Report prolonged or excessive injection site reactions to the physician.

Interventions

- For patients who are medically able to begin exercise, implement appropriate resistive exercises and aerobic training to maintain muscle strength and aerobic capacity during cancer chemotherapy, or to help restore function after chemotherapy.

Patient/Client-Related Instruction

- Advise patient to guard against infection (frequent hand washing, etc.), and to avoid crowds and contact with persons with contagious diseases.
- Instruct patient to report other troublesome side effects such as severe or prolonged headache, malaise, chills, night sweats, or GI problems (nausea, vomiting, diarrhea, loss of appetite, abdominal pain).

Pharmacokinetics

Absorption: IV administration results in complete bioavailability.
Distribution: Unknown.
Metabolism and Excretion: Metabolized by serum proteases and in the reticuloendothelial system.
Half-life: 5.7 days (less in patients with previous hypersensitivity to native L-asparaginase).

TIME/ACTION PROFILE (hematologic effects)

ROUTE	ONSET	PEAK	DURATION
IV	rapid	unknown	14 days

Contraindications/Precautions

Contraindicated in: Pancreatitis or history of pancreatitis; History of previous hemorrhagic reaction to asparaginase therapy; Previous hypersensitivity reactions to pegaspargase.
Use Cautiously in: History of previous hypersensitivity reactions to other drugs; Patients with childbearing potential; OB: Pregnancy or lactation (safety not established).

Interactions

Drug-Drug: May alter response to **anticoagulants** or **antiplatelet agents**. May alter the response to other **drugs that are metabolized by the liver**.

Route/Dosage

IM, IV (Adults Up to 21 yr and Children with Body Surface Area ≥0.6 m^2): 2500 IU/m^2 q 14 days (usually in combination with other agents).
IM, IV (Children with Body Surface Area <0.6 m^2): 82.5 IU/kg q 14 days (usually in combination with other agents).

Availability

Injection: 750 IU/mL.

pegfilgrastim (peg-fil-**gras**-tim)

Neulasta

Classification
Therapeutic: colony-stimulating factors

Indications

To decrease the incidence of infection (febrile neutropenia) in patients with nonmyeloid malignancies receiving myelosuppressive antineoplastics associated with a high risk of febrile neutropenia.

Action

Filgrastim is a glycoprotein that binds to and stimulates neutrophils to divide and differentiate. Also activates mature neutrophils. Binding to a polyethylene glycol molecule prolongs its effects. **Therapeutic Effects:** Decreased incidence of infection in patients who are neutropenic from chemotherapy.

Adverse Reactions/Side Effects

Resp: ADULT RESPIRATORY DISTRESS SYNDROME (ARDS).
GI: SPLENIC RUPTURE. **Hemat:** SICKLE CELL CRISIS, leukocytosis.
MS: medullary bone pain. **Misc:** ALLERGIC REACTION, INCLUDING ANAPHYLAXIS.

PHYSICAL THERAPY IMPLICATIONS

Examination and Evaluation

- Assess respiration, and notify physician immediately if patient exhibits signs of respiratory distress syndrome. Signs include severe shortness of breath, rapid labored breathing, cyanosis, confusion, extreme tiredness, cough, and fever. Monitor pulse oximetry and perform pulmonary function tests (See Appendices I, J, K) to quantify suspected changes in ventilation and respiratory function.
- Monitor signs of allergic reactions and anaphylaxis, including pulmonary symptoms (tightness in the throat and chest, wheezing, cough, dyspnea) or skin reactions (rash, pruritus, urticaria). Notify physician or nursing staff immediately if these reactions occur.
- Be alert for signs of red blood cell abnormalities such as sickle cell crisis and increased white blood cell counts (leukocytosis). Signs include including fever, weakness, weight loss, loss of appetite, dizziness, fainting, dyspnea, bleeding/bruising, or pain or tingling in the arms, legs, or abdomen. Report these signs to the physician or nursing staff immediately.
- Watch for signs of spleen rupture, including pain and tenderness in the upper left abdomen, lightheadedness, dizziness, and confusion. Report these signs to the physician or nursing staff immediately.
- Assess any bone pain to rule out musculoskeletal pathology; that is, try to determine if pain is drug induced rather than caused by fracture or biomechanical problems.

Interventions

- For patients who are medically able to begin exercise, implement appropriate resistive exercises and aerobic training to maintain muscle strength and aerobic capacity during cancer chemotherapy or to help restore function after chemotherapy.

Patient/Client-Related Instruction

- Instruct patient to guard against infection (frequent hand washing, etc.), and to avoid crowds and contact with persons with contagious diseases.

Pharmacokinetics

Absorption: Well absorbed following SC administration.
Distribution: Unknown.
Metabolism and Excretion: Unknown.
Half-life: 15–80 hr.

TIME/ACTION PROFILE

ROUTE	ONSET	PEAK	DURATION
SC	unknown	unknown	unknown

Contraindications/Precautions

Contraindicated in: Hypersensitivity to filgrastim or *Escherichia coli*–derived proteins.
Use Cautiously in: Patients with sickle cell disease (increased risk of sickle cell crisis); Concurrent use of lithium; Malignancy with myeloid characteristics; Pregnancy, lactation, or children (safety not established; 6 mg fixed dose should not be used in infants, children, and smaller adolescents weighing <45 kg; use in pregnancy only if potential benefits to mother justifies potential risk to the fetus).

Interactions

Drug-Drug: Simultaneous use with **antineoplastics** may have adverse effects on rapidly proliferating neutrophils; avoid use for 24 hr before and 24 hr following chemotherapy. **Lithium** may potentiate the release of neutrophils; concurrent use should be undertaken cautiously.

Route/Dosage

SC (Adults): 6 mg per chemotherapy cycle.

Availability

Solution for SC injection: 6 mg/0.6 mL in prefilled syringes.

pegloticase (peg-loe-ti-kase)

Krystexxa

Classification
Therapeutic: antigout agents
Pharmacologic: enzymes

Indications

Treatment of chronic gout in adults who have not responded to/cannot tolerate xanthine oxidase inhibitors, including allopurinol.

Action

Consists of recombinant uricase covalently bonded to monomethoxypoly (ethylene glycol) [mPEG]); uricase catalyzes the oxidation of uric acid to allantoin, a water-soluble by-product that is readily excreted in urine. **Therapeutic Effects:** ↓ serum uric acid levels with resultant ↓ in attacks of gout and its sequelae.

Adverse Reactions/Side Effects

CV: chest pain. **EENT:** nasopharyngitis. **GI:** nausea, constipation, vomiting. **Derm:** contusion/ecchymoses. **Metab:** gout flare. **Misc:** ALLERGIC REACTIONS, INCLUDING ANAPHYLAXIS, INFUSION REACTIONS.

PHYSICAL THERAPY IMPLICATIONS

Examination and Evaluation

- Monitor signs of allergic reactions and anaphylaxis, including pulmonary symptoms (tightness in the throat and chest, wheezing, cough dyspnea) or skin reactions (rash, pruritus, urticaria). Be especially alert for allergy-like responses that occur during and after administration (infusion related reactions). Notify physician or nursing staff immediately of any signs of hypersensitivity.
- If treating gouty arthritis, periodically assess impairments (pain, range of motion), functional ability, and disability to help document whether drug therapy is successful. Report any increase in symptoms that occur when initiating drug therapy (gout flare).
- Monitor any chest pain and attempt to determine if pain is drug-induced or caused by cardiovascular dysfunction (e.g., angina that occurs during exercise). Report severe or unexplained chest pain.

Interventions

- If treating arthritic conditions, implement appropriate manual therapy techniques, physical agents, therapeutic exercises, and orthotic/assistive devices to reduce pain, improve function, and augment the effects of drug therapy.

Patient/Client-Related Instruction

- Instruct patient and family/caregivers to report other troublesome side effects such as severe or prolonged irritation of the nose or pharynx, skin reactions (contusions, bruising), and GI problems (nausea, vomiting, constipation).

Pharmacokinetics

Absorption: IV administration results in complete bioavailability.
Distribution: Unknown.
Metabolism and Excretion: Unknown.
Half-life: Unknown.

TIME/ACTION PROFILE (effects on serum uric acid)

ROUTE	ONSET	PEAK	DURATION
IV	rapid	within 24 hr	>300 hr

Contraindications/Precautions

Contraindicated in: Glucose-6-phosphate dehydrogenase (G6PD) deficiency (risk of hemolysis and methemoglobinemia). Lactation: Breast-feeding is not recommended.
Use Cautiously in: Congestive heart failure (may ↑ risk of exacerbation); Retreatment after a drug-free interval (↑ risk of allergic reactions, monitor carefully); Geri: Elderly patients may be more sensitive to drug effects; OB: Use during pregnancy only if clearly needed; Pedi: Safe and effective use in children <18 yr not established.

Interactions

Drug-Drug: May interfere with the action of other **PEG-containing therapies.**

Route/Dosage

IV (Adults): 8 mg q 2 wk.

Availability

Injection for IV infusion (requires dilution): 8 mg/1 mL

pegvisomant (peg-vis-oh-mant)

Somavert

Classification
Therapeutic: hormones
Pharmacologic: growth hormones

Indications

Treatment of acromegaly in patients who do not respond to or are not candidates for surgery, radiation, or other medical therapies.

Action

Binds to growth hormone (GH) receptor sites on cell surfaces, blocking the effects of endogenous growth hormone. Bound to polyethylene glycol (PEG) to reduce clearance and increase duration of action.
Therapeutic Effects: Decreased manifestations of acromegaly and normalized insulin-like growth factor-1 (IGF-1) levels.

Adverse Reactions/Side Effects

CV: hypertension, peripheral edema. **GI:** ↑ LFTs.
MS: back pain. **Endo:** growth hormone deficiency, ↑ glucose tolerance. **Derm:** lipohypertrophy.

PHYSICAL THERAPY IMPLICATIONS

Examination and Evaluation

- Assess blood pressure periodically (See Appendix F). Report a sustained increase in blood pressure (hypertension) to the physician.
- Assess peripheral edema using girth measurements, volume displacement, and measurement of pitting edema (See Appendix N). Report increased swelling in feet and ankles or a sudden increase in body weight due to fluid retention.
- Monitor signs of increased glucose tolerance, as indicated by weakness, malaise, irritability, and fatigue. Patients with diabetes mellitus should check blood glucose levels frequently.
- Assess any back pain to rule out musculoskeletal pathology; that is, try to determine if pain is drug induced rather than caused by anatomic or biomechanical problems.
- Periodically assess body weight and other anthropometric measures (body mass index, body composition). Report a rapid or unexplained weight gain or increased body fat.

Interventions

- Do not apply physical agents (heat, cold, electrotherapeutic modalities) or massage at or near the injection site; these interventions will alter drug absorption from subcutaneous tissues.

Patient/Client-Related Instruction

- Instruct patient to report signs of liver dysfunction, including loss of appetite, abdominal pain, severe nausea and vomiting, yellow skin or eyes, skin rashes, flu-like symptoms, and muscle/joint pain. Periodic liver function tests (LFTs) may be needed to monitor hepatic function.

Pharmacokinetics

Absorption: 57% absorbed following SC administration.
Distribution: Does not distribute extensively into tissues.
Metabolism and Excretion: Unknown.
Half-life: 6 days.

TIME/ACTION PROFILE (effects on IGF-1)

ROUTE	ONSET	PEAK	DURATION
SC	within 2 wk	4–6 wk	unknown

Contraindications/Precautions

Contraindicated in: Hypersensitivity; Latex allergy (vial stopper contains latex).
Use Cautiously in: Diabetes mellitus; Patients with growth hormone–secreting tumors; Lactation/Pedi: Safety not established; OB: Use only if clearly needed.

Interactions

Drug-Drug: Patients receiving **opioid analgesics** often require ↑ doses of pegvisomant to normalize IGF-1.

P

Route/Dosage

Subcut (Adults): *Loading dose*—40 mg; *maintenance dose*—10 mg daily; further adjustments in increments/decrements of 5 mg are made based on monitoring of IGF-1 levels (not to exceed 30 mg/day).

Availability

Lyophilized powder for reconstitution: 10-, 15-, and 20-mg vials with diluent (sterile water for injection).

pemetrexed (pe-me-**treks**-ed)

Alimta

Classification

Therapeutic: antineoplastics

Pharmacologic: antimetabolites, folate antagonists

Indications

Malignant pleural mesothelioma (with cisplatin) when tumor is unresectable or patient is not a candidate for surgery. Local advanced or metastatic non–small-cell lung cancer in previously treated patients.

Action

Disrupts folate-dependent metabolic processes involved in thymidine and purine synthesis. Converted intracellularly to polyglutamate form which increases duration of action. **Therapeutic Effects:** Decreases growth and spread of mesothelioma.

Adverse Reactions/Side Effects

Resp: pharyngitis. **CV:** chest pain. **GI:** constipation, nausea, stomatitis, vomiting, anorexia, diarrhea, esophagitis, mouth pain. **Derm:** desquamation, rash. **Hemat:** anemia, leukopenia, thrombocytopenia. **Neuro:** neuropathy. **Misc:** fever, infection.

PHYSICAL THERAPY IMPLICATIONS

Examination and Evaluation

- Watch for signs of leukopenia (fever, sore throat, signs of infection), thrombocytopenia (bruising, nose bleeds, bleeding gums), or unusual weakness and fatigue that might be due to anemia. Report these signs to the physician or nursing staff.
- Assess numbness, tingling, or weakness that might indicate peripheral neuropathy. Establish baseline electroneuromyographic values using EMG and nerve conduction at the beginning of drug treatment whenever possible. Periodically reexamine these values to document drug-induced changes in peripheral nerve function.
- Monitor any chest pain, and assess heart rate (HR) and blood pressure (BP) whenever patient experiences symptoms (See Appendices F, G). Refer patients with abnormal HR or BP responses or prolonged and persistent chest pain to the physician for further evaluation.

Interventions

- For patients who are medically able to begin exercise, implement appropriate resistive exercises and aerobic training to maintain muscle strength and aerobic capacity during cancer chemotherapy or to help restore function after chemotherapy.

Patient/Client-Related Instruction

- Instruct patient to decrease risk of infections (frequent hand washing, etc.), and to avoid contact with persons with contagious diseases.
- Advise patient about the likelihood of GI reactions, including nausea, vomiting, diarrhea, constipation, loss of appetite, heartburn, and pain/inflammation in or around the mouth. Instruct patient to report severe or prolonged GI problems.
- Advise patient that rash, exfoliation, and other skin reactions are likely. Report severe or unexpected skin reactions to the physician.
- Instruct patient and family/caregivers to report other side effects such as severe or prolonged fever, upper respiratory tract inflammation, or signs of infection.

Pharmacokinetics

Absorption: IV administration results in complete bioavailability.

Distribution: Unknown.

Metabolism and Excretion: Minimal metabolism; 70–90% excreted unchanged in urine.

Half-life: 3.5 hr (normal renal function).

TIME/ACTION PROFILE (hematologic effects)

ROUTE	ONSET	PEAK	DURATION
IV	unknown	8–15 days	21 days

Contraindications/Precautions

Contraindicated in: Hypersensitivity; CCr <45 mL/min; **OB:** Pregnancy, lactation.

Use Cautiously in: Concurrent use of NSAIDs (avoid those with short half-lives); CCr 45–80 mL/min; 3rd-space fluid accumulation (ascites, pleural effusions); consider drainage prior to therapy; Hepatic impairment (dosage alteration recommended); Pedi: Children (safety not established).

Interactions

Drug-Drug: NSAIDs, especially those with short half-lives, ↑ blood levels and risk of toxicity; avoid for 2 days before, day of, and 2 days after treatment. **Probenecid** ↑ blood levels. Concurrent use of **nephrotoxic agents** ↑ risk of nephrotoxicity.

Route/Dosage

IV (Adults): *Mesothelioma*—500 mg/m^2 on day 1 of each 21-day cycle (with cisplatin); concurrent hydration, folic acid, vitamin B_{12}, pretreatment with dexamethasone required. Dose adjustments for hematologic, nonhematologic toxicities and neurotoxicity recommended. *Non–small-cell lung cancer*—500 mg/m^2 on day 1 of each 21-day cycle (pretreatment with corticosteroids, folic acid, and vitamin B_{12} recommended). Dose adjustments for hematologic, nonhematologic toxicities and neurotoxicity recommended.

Availability

lyophilized powder for IV infusion: 500 mg/vial.

penbutolol (pen-byoo-toe-lole)

Levatol

Classification
Therapeutic: antihypertensives
Pharmacologic: beta blockers

Indications

Management of hypertension.

Action

Blocks stimulation of $beta_1$ (myocardial) and $beta_2$ (pulmonary, vascular, and uterine)–adrenergic receptor sites. Also has intrinsic sympathomimetic activity (ISA), which may produce less bradycardia. **Therapeutic Effects:** Decreased heart rate and blood pressure.

Adverse Reactions/Side Effects

CNS: fatigue, weakness, anxiety, depression, dizziness, drowsiness, insomnia, memory loss, mental status changes, nervousness, nightmares. **EENT:** blurred vision, dry eyes, nasal stuffiness. **Resp:** bronchospasm, wheezing. **CV:** ARRHYTHMIAS, BRADYCARDIA, CHF, PULMONARY EDEMA, orthostatic hypotension, peripheral vasoconstriction. **GI:** constipation, diarrhea, nausea. **GU:** erectile dysfunction, decreased libido. **Derm:** itching, rashes. **Endo:** hyperglycemia, hypoglycemia. **MS:** arthralgia, back pain, muscle cramps. **Neuro:** paresthesia. **Misc:** drug-induced lupus syndrome.

PHYSICAL THERAPY IMPLICATIONS

Examination and Evaluation

- Assess heart rate, ECG, and heart sounds, especially during exercise (See Appendices G, H). Report immediately an unusually slow heart rate (bradycardia) or signs of other arrhythmias, including palpitations, chest discomfort, shortness of breath, fainting, and fatigue/weakness.
- Assess routinely for signs of CHF and pulmonary edema, including dyspnea, rales/crackles, weight gain, peripheral edema, and jugular venous distention. Report these signs to the physician immediately.
- Assess blood pressure (BP) periodically and compare to normal values (See Appendix F) to help document antihypertensive effects.
- Assess BP when patient assumes a more upright position (lying to standing, sitting to standing, lying to sitting). Document orthostatic hypotension and contact physician when systolic BP falls >20 mm Hg, or diastolic BP falls >10 mm Hg.
- Assess symptoms of bronchospasm (wheezing, coughing, tightness in chest). Perform pulmonary function tests to quantify suspected changes in ventilation and respiration (See Appendices I, J, K). Repeated or prolonged bronchoconstriction may require a change in dose or medication (e.g., switch to a more cardioselective beta blocker).
- Monitor signs of peripheral vasoconstriction, such as extreme coldness in the hands and feet, cyanosis, and muscle cramping. Notify physician of severe or prolonged signs of vasoconstriction.
- Assess any back pain, joint pain, or muscle cramps to rule out musculoskeletal pathology; that is, try to determine if pain is drug induced rather than caused by anatomic or biomechanical problems.
- Assess signs of paresthesia (numbness, tingling), and perform objective tests, including electroneuromyography and sensory testing to document any drug-related neuropathic changes.
- Monitor mood and personality changes, including depression, anxiety, memory loss, or other changes in behavior. Notify physician if these changes become problematic.
- Assess dizziness and drowsiness that might affect gait, balance, and other functional activities (See Appendix C). Report balance problems and functional limitations to the physician, and caution the patient and family/caregivers to guard against falls and trauma.
- Monitor excessive fatigue or weakness. Beta blockers often cause some degree of fatigue and weakness, but any sudden or severe change in muscle strength or energy levels should be reported.
- Be alert for signs of hypoglycemia (weakness, malaise, irritability, fatigue) or hyperglycemia (drowsiness, fruity breath, increased urination, unusual thirst). Medication may mask some signs of hypoglycemia, but dizziness and sweating may still occur. Patients with diabetes mellitus should check blood glucose levels frequently.
- Monitor signs of drug-induced lupus syndrome, including increased BP, fever, joint pain, skin rashes, and redness/irritation of the eye (uveitis). Notify physician promptly if these signs appear.

P

Interventions

- Because of an increased risk of cardiac arrhythmias (bradycardia, others), use caution during aerobic exercise and endurance conditioning Terminate exercise if patient exhibits untoward symptoms (chest pain, shortness of breath, unusual fatigue), or displays other criteria for exercise termination (See Appendix L).
- Establish aerobic exercise workloads that account for the effects of beta blockers on heart rate. Some heart rate guidelines may not be appropriate because beta blockers typically decrease maximal HR by 20–30 bpm. Use other guidelines such as rating of perceived exertion (RPE, modified Borg scale) to determine exercise workloads.
- To minimize orthostatic hypotension, patient should move slowly when assuming a more upright position.

Patient/Client-Related Instruction

- Remind patients to take medication as directed to control hypertension even if they are asymptomatic.
- Counsel patients about additional interventions to help control BP, including regular exercise, weight loss, sodium restriction, stress reduction, moderation of alcohol consumption, and smoking cessation.
- Instruct patient or family/caregivers to report other troublesome side effects such as severe or prolonged insomnia, nightmares, blurred vision, dry eyes, stuffy nose, sexual problems (decreased libido, erectile dysfunction), skin reactions (rash, itching), or GI problems (nausea, constipation, diarrhea).

Pharmacokinetics

Absorption: Well absorbed after oral administration.
Distribution: Moderate CNS penetration; crosses the placenta.
Protein Binding: 80–98%.
Metabolism and Excretion: Mostly metabolized by the liver.
Half-life: 5 hr.

TIME/ACTION PROFILE (cardiovascular effects)

ROUTE	ONSET	PEAK	DURATION
PO	1 hr	1.5–3 hr*	Up to 24 hr

*After single dose; full effect not seen until several weeks of therapy.

Contraindications/Precautions

Contraindicated in: Uncompensated CHF; Pulmonary edema; Cardiogenic shock; Bradycardia or heart block.
Use Cautiously in: Renal impairment; Hepatic impairment (lower doses may be necessary); Pulmonary disease (including asthma); Diabetes mellitus (may mask signs of hypoglycemia); Thyrotoxicosis (may mask symptoms); Patients with a history of severe allergic reactions (intensity of reactions may be increased); Geriatric patients (increased sensitivity to beta blockers; initial dosage reduction recommended); Pregnancy, lactation, or children (safety not established; all agents cross the placenta and may cause fetal/neonatal bradycardia, hypotension, hypoglycemia, or respiratory depression).

Interactions

Drug-Drug: General anesthesia, IV phenytoin, and **verapamil** may cause additive myocardial depression. Additive bradycardia may occur with **digoxin**. Additive hypotension may occur with other **antihypertensives**, acute ingestion of **alcohol**, or **nitrates**. Concurrent use with **amphetamines, cocaine, ephedrine, epinephrine, norepinephrine, phenylephrine,** or **pseudoephedrine** may result in unopposed alpha-adrenergic stimulation (excessive hypertension, bradycardia). Concurrent administration of **thyroid preparations** ↓ effectiveness. May alter the effectiveness of **insulins** or **oral hypoglycemic agents** (dosage adjustments may be necessary). May ↓ the effectiveness of **beta-adrenergic bronchodilators** and **theophylline**. May ↓ the beneficial $beta_1$-cardiovascular effects of **dopamine** or **dobutamine**. Use cautiously within 14 days of **MAO inhibitors** (may result in hypertension). Concurrent **NSAIDs** may ↓ antihypertensive action.

Route/Dosage

PO (Adults): 20 mg once daily.

Availability

Tablets: 20 mg.

penciclovir (pen-**sye**-kloe-veer)

Denavir

Classification
Therapeutic: antivirals (topical)
Pharmacologic: nucleoside analogues

Indications

Recurrent herpes labialis (cold sores).

Action

Inhibits viral DNA synthesis and replication. **Therapeutic Effects:** Death of herpes virus. Decreases lesion duration and pain. Active against herpes viruses.

Adverse Reactions/Side Effects

CNS: headache. **Local:** application site reactions.

PHYSICAL THERAPY IMPLICATIONS

Examination and Evaluation

- Assess skin and mucosal lesions to help document whether drug therapy is successful in controlling infection. Report any local irritation or inflammation at the application site.

Interventions

- Avoid contact with cutaneous or mucosal lesions when treating patient.
- Always wash hands thoroughly and disinfect equipment (whirlpools, electrotherapeutic devices, treatment tables, and so forth) to help prevent the spread of infection. Employ universal precautions as indicated for specific patients.

Patient/Client-Related Instruction

- Advise patient to apply medication as directed. Penciclovir should not be used more frequently or longer than prescribed.
- Remind patient that penciclovir does not cure herpes infections. The virus lies dormant in nerve cells, and this drug will not prevent the spread of infection to others.
- Instruct patient and family/caregivers to report other troublesome side effects, including severe or prolonged headache.

Pharmacokinetics

Absorption: Not absorbed following topical use.
Distribution: Unknown.
Metabolism and Excretion: Converted intracellularly to active triphosphate form; excreted in urine.
Half-life: 2–2.5 hr.

TIME/ACTION PROFILE

ROUTE	ONSET	PEAK	DURATION
topical	unknown	unknown	unknown

Contraindications/Precautions

Contraindicated in: Hypersensitivity to penciclovir or other components of the formulation.
Use Cautiously in: Pregnancy, lactation, or children (safety not established).

Interactions

Drug-Drug: None significant.

Route/Dosage

PO (Adults): Apply 1% cream q 2 hr for 4 days while awake.

Availability

Cream: 1% in 2-g tubes.

penicillamine (pen-i-sil-a-meen)

Cuprimine, Depen

Classification
Therapeutic: antidotes, antirheumatics (disease-modifying antirheumatic drugs, DMARDs), antiurolithics
Pharmacologic: chelating agents

Indications

Progressive rheumatoid arthritis resistant to conventional therapy. Management of copper deposition in Wilson's disease. Management of recurrent cystine calculi. **Unlabeled Use:** Adjunct in the treatment of heavy metal poisoning.

Action

Antirheumatic effect, probably resulting from enhanced lymphocyte function. Chelates heavy metals, including copper, mercury, lead, and iron, into complexes that are excreted by the kidneys. Forms a soluble complex with cystine that is readily excreted by the kidneys. **Therapeutic Effects:** Decreased disease progression in rheumatoid arthritis. Decreased copper deposition in Wilson's disease. Decreased cystine renal calculi formation.

Adverse Reactions/Side Effects

EENT: blurred vision, eye pain. **Resp:** coughing, shortness of breath, wheezing. **GI:** altered taste, anorexia, cholestatic jaundice, diarrhea, drug-induced pancreatitis, dyspepsia, epigastric pain, hepatic dysfunction, nausea, oral ulceration, vomiting. **GU:** proteinuria. **Derm:** pemphigus, ecchymoses, hives, itching, rashes, wrinkling. **Hemat:** APLASTIC ANEMIA, anemia, eosinophilia, leukopenia, thrombocytopenia, thrombocytosis. **MS:** arthralgia, migratory polyarthritis. **Neuro:** myasthenia gravis syndrome. **Misc:** GOODPASTURE'S SYNDROME (GLOMERULONEPHRITIS AND INTRA-ALVEOLAR HEMORRHAGE), allergic reactions, fever, lymphadenopathy, systemic lupus erythematosus–like syndrome.

PHYSICAL THERAPY IMPLICATIONS

Examination and Evaluation

- Monitor any unusual weakness and fatigue that might be due to aplastic anemia. Report signs of anemia or other blood dyscrasias such as leukopenia (fever, sore throat, signs of infection), or thrombocytopenia (bleeding gums, bruising, petechiae, blood in stools, urine, or emesis).
- Be alert for signs of Goopasture's syndrome, including renal dysfunction (hematuria, increased frequency, burning sensation while urinating, cloudy urine, decreased urine output, edema and hypertension due to fluid retention), pulmonary symptoms (dry cough, dyspnea, coughing up blood), and generalized weakness and fatigue. Notify physician immediately of these signs.
- Assess any new or increased joint pain to rule out musculoskeletal pathology; that is, try to determine if pain is drug induced rather than caused by arthritis or anatomic and biomechanical problems.
- If treating rheumatoid arthritis, periodically assess patient's impairments (pain, range of motion),

functional ability, and disability to help document whether antirheumatic drug therapy is successful.

- Be alert for early signs of myasthenia gravis syndrome, such as drooping eyelids, facial muscle weakness, and difficulty swallowing and speaking. Report these signs to the physician immediately, and monitor other muscle groups for signs of unusual weakness and fatigue, especially after repeated contraction.
- Monitor signs of drug-induced lupus-like syndrome, including increased blood pressure, fever, joint pain, skin rashes, and redness/irritation of the eye (uveitis). Notify physician promptly if these signs appear.

Interventions

- If treating rheumatoid arthritis, implement appropriate manual therapy techniques, physical agents, therapeutic exercises, and orthotic/assistive devices to reduce pain, improve function, and augment the effects of antirheumatic drug therapy.
- Help patients with arthritis explore other nonpharmacologic methods to reduce chronic arthritis pain, such as relaxation techniques, exercise, counseling, and so forth.

Patient/Client-Related Instruction

- Advise patient about the likelihood of GI reactions such as nausea, vomiting, diarrhea, loss of appetite, and heartburn. Instruct patient to report severe or prolonged GI problems, or signs of hepatic toxicity (abdominal pain, severe nausea and vomiting, yellow skin or eyes, fever, sore throat, malaise, weakness, facial edema, lethargy, unusual bleeding or bruising), or pancreatitis (upper abdominal pain after eating, indigestion, weight loss, oily stools).
- Advise patient that skin reactions such as rash, itching, hives, pruritus, and blistering are likely. Report severe or unexpected skin reactions to the physician.
- Advise patient to guard against infection (frequent hand washing, etc.), and to avoid crowds and contact with persons with contagious diseases.
- Instruct patient to report any vision problems or eye pain.

Pharmacokinetics

Absorption: Well absorbed after oral administration.
Distribution: Crosses the placenta.
Metabolism and Excretion: Some excreted in urine as heavy metal–penicillamine complex, some excreted in urine as cystine-penicillamine complex, some metabolized by the liver.
Half-life: 1–7.5 hr (4–6 days during long-term use).

TIME/ACTION PROFILE

ROUTE	ONSET	PEAK	DURATION
PO (antirheumatic)	2–3 mo	unknown	1–3 mo
PO (Wilson's disease)	1–3 mo	unknown	unknown

Contraindications/Precautions

Contraindicated in: Hypersensitivity; Cross-sensitivity with penicillin may exist; Patients currently receiving gold salts, antimalarials, antineoplastics, oxyphenbutazone, or phenylbutazone; Concurrent use of iron supplements; OB: Pregnancy (penicillamine should be avoided in pregnant patients with rheumatoid arthritis or cystinuria); OB: Lactation.
Use Cautiously in: Renal impairment (↑ risk of adverse renal reactions in patients with rheumatoid arthritis); History of aplastic anemia due to penicillamine; Patients requiring surgery (may impair wound healing); Geri: Geriatric patients (↑ risk of hematologic toxicity, skin rash and taste abnormality; dose reduction recommended); OB: Pregnancy (for patients with Wilson's disease, limit daily dose to <1 g. If cesarean section is planned, decrease daily dose to 250 mg for last 6 wk of pregnancy and until incision is healed).

Interactions

Drug-Drug: ↑ risk of adverse hematologic effects with **antineoplastics, immunosuppressants**, or **gold salts** (avoid concurrent use). Concurrent administration of **iron supplements** ↓ absorption of penicillamine. May ↓ serum **digoxin** levels.
Drug-Food: May ↑ requirements for **pyridoxine** (vitamin B_6).

Route/Dosage

PO (Adults): *Antirheumatic*—125–250 mg/day as a single dose; may be slowly increased up to 1.5 g/day. *Chelating agent (Wilson's disease)*—250 mg qid. *Antiurolithic*—500 mg qid.
PO (Children >6 mo): *Chelating agent (Wilson's disease)*—250 mg/day as a single dose; older children may receive the adult dose. *Antiurolithic*—7.5 mg/kg qid.

Availability

Capsules: 125 mg, 250 mg. **Tablets:** 250 mg.

penicillin G (pen-i-**sil**-in gee)
Pfizerpen

procaine penicillin G
(proe-**kane** pen-i-sil-in gee)
✱ Ayercillin, Wycillin

benzathine penicillin G
(**benz**-a-theen pen-i-**sil**-in gee)
Bicillin L-A, ✱ Megacillin, Permapen

Classification
Therapeutic: anti-infectives
Pharmacologic: penicillins

Indications

Treatment of a wide variety of infections, including Pneumococcal pneumonia, Streptococcal pharyngitis, Syphilis, Gonorrhea strains. Treatment of enterococcal infections (requires the addition of an aminoglycoside). Prevention of rheumatic fever. Should not be used as a single agent to treat anthrax. **Unlabeled Use:** Treatment of Lyme disease, prevention of recurrent *Streptococcal pneumoniae* septicemia in children with sickle-cell disease.

Action

Bind to bacterial cell wall, resulting in cell death. **Therapeutic Effects:** Bactericidal action against susceptible bacteria. **Spectrum:** Active against Most gram-positive organisms, including many streptococci (*Streptococcus pneumoniae*, group A beta-hemolytic streptococci), staphylococci (non–penicillinase-producing strains), and *Bacillus anthracis*; Some gram-negative organisms, such as *Neisseria meningitidis* and *N. gonorrhoeae* (only penicillin-susceptible strains); Some anaerobic bacteria and spirochetes, including *Borrelia burgdorferi*.

Adverse Reactions/Side Effects

CNS: SEIZURES. **GI:** diarrhea, epigastric distress, nausea, vomiting, pseudomembranous colitis. **GU:** interstitial nephritis. **Derm:** rash, urticaria. **Hemat:** eosinophilia, leukopenia. **Local:** pain at IM site, phlebitis at IV site. **Misc:** ALLERGIC REACTIONS, INCLUDING ANAPHYLAXIS AND SERUM SICKNESS, superinfection.

PHYSICAL THERAPY IMPLICATIONS

Examination and Evaluation

- Watch for seizures; notify physician immediately if patient develops or increases seizure activity.
- Monitor signs of allergic reactions and anaphylaxis, including pulmonary symptoms (tightness in the throat and chest, wheezing, cough dyspnea) or skin reactions (rash, prurits, urticaria). Notify physician or nursing staff immediately if these reactions occur.
- Assess muscle aches and joint pain (arthralgia) that may be caused by serum sickness. Notify physician if these symptoms seem to be drug related rather than caused by musculoskeletal injury or if muscle and joint pain are accompanied by allergy-like reactions (fever, rashes, etc.)
- Monitor signs of eosinophilia (fatigue, weakness, myalgia) or leukopenia (fever, sore throat, signs of infection); report these signs to the physician.
- Monitor injection site for pain, swelling, and irritation. Report prolonged or excessive injection site reactions to the physician.

Interventions

- Always wash hands thoroughly and disinfect equipment (whirlpools, electrotherapeutic devices, treatment tables, and so forth) to help prevent the spread of infection. Use universal precautions or isolation procedures as indicated for specific patients.

Patient/Client-Related Instruction

- Instruct patient to notify physician immediately if signs of the following occur:
  - Pseudomembranous colitis (diarrhea, abdominal pain, fever, pus or mucus in stools) or other severe or prolonged GI problems (nausea, vomiting, heartburn).
  - Superinfection (black, furry overgrowth on tongue; vaginal itching or discharge; loose or foul-smelling stools).
  - Interstitial nephritis (blood in urine, decreased urine output, weight gain from fluid retention).
- Instruct patient and family/caregivers to report other troublesome side effects such as severe or prolonged skin problems (rash, itching) or GI problems (nausea, vomiting, diarrhea, heartburn).

Pharmacokinetics

Absorption: Variably absorbed from the GI tract. *Procaine and benzathine penicillin G*—IM absorption is delayed and prolonged and results in sustained therapeutic blood levels.
Distribution: Widely distributed, although CNS penetration is poor in the presence of normal (uninflamed) meninges. Crosses the placenta and enters breast milk.
Protein Binding: 60%.
Metabolism and Excretion: Minimally metabolized by the liver, excreted mainly unchanged by the kidneys.
Half-life: 30–60 min.

TIME/ACTION PROFILE (blood levels)

ROUTE	ONSET	PEAK	DURATION
penicillin G IM benzathine	rapid	0.25–0.5 hr	4–6 hr
penicillin IM procaine	delayed	12–24 hr	3 wk
penicillin IM	delayed	1–4 hr	12 hr
penicillin G IV	rapid	end of infusion	4–6 hr

Contraindications/Precautions

Contraindicated in: Previous hypersensitivity to penicillins (cross-sensitivity exists with cephalosporins and other beta-lactam antibiotics); Hypersensitivity to procaine or benzathine (procaine and benzathine preparations only); Some products may contain tartrazine and should be avoided in patients with known hypersensitivity.

P

Use Cautiously in: Severe renal insufficiency (dosage reduction recommended); OB: Although safety not established, has been used safely; Lactation: Safety not established; Geri: Consider decreased body mass, age-related decrease in renal/hepatic/cardiac function, intercurrent diseases and drug therapy.

Interactions

Drug-Drug: Penicillin may ↓ effectiveness of oral contraceptive agents. **Probenecid** ↓ renal excretion and ↑ blood levels of penicillin (therapy may be combined for this purpose). **Neomycin** may ↓ absorption of penicillin. Concurrent use with **methotrexate** ↓ methotrexate elimination and ↑ risk of serious toxicity.

Route/Dosage

Aqueous Penicillin G

IM, IV (Adults): *Most infections*—1–5 million units q 4–6 hr.

IM, IV (Children): 8333–16,667 units/kg q 4 hr; 12,550–25,000 units/kg q 6 hr; up to 250,000 units/kg/day in divided doses; some infections may require up to 300,000 units/kg/day.

IV (Infants >7 days): 75,000 units/kg/day in divided doses every 8 hr; *meningitis*—200,000–300,000 units/kg/day in divided doses q 6 hr.

IV (Infants <7 days): 50,000 units/kg/day in divided doses q 12 hr; *Streptococcus B meningitis*—100,000–150,000 units/kg/day in divided doses.

Benzathine Penicillin G

IM (Adults): *Streptococcal infections/erysipeloid*—1.2 million units single dose. *Primary, secondary, and early latent syphilis*—2.4 million units single dose. *Tertiary and late latent syphilis (not neurosyphilis)*—2.4 million units once weekly for 3 wk. *Prevention of rheumatic fever*—1.2 million units q 3–4 wk.

IM (Children >27 kg): *Streptococcal infections/erysipeloid*—900,000–1.2 million units (single dose). *Primary, secondary, and early latent syphilis*—up to 2.4 million units single dose. *Late latent or latent syphilis of undetermined duration*—50,000 units/kg weekly for 3 wk. *Prevention of rheumatic fever*—1.2 million units q 2–3 wk.

IM (Children <27 kg): *Streptococcal infections/erysipeloid*—300,000–600,000 units single dose. *Primary, secondary, and early latent syphilis*—up to 2.4 million units single dose. *Late latent or latent syphilis of undetermined duration*—50,000 units/kg weekly for 3 wk. *Prevention of rheumatic fever*—1.2 million units q 2–3 wk.

Procaine Penicillin G

IM (Adults): *Moderate or severe infections*—600,000–1.2 million units/day, single dose or 2 divided doses. *Neurosyphilis*—2.4 million units/day with 500 mg probenecid PO qid for 10–14 days.

IM (Children): *Congenital syphilis*—50,000 units/kg/day for 10–14 days.

Availability (generic available)

Penicillin G Potassium

Powder for injection: 5 million units/vial, 20 million units/vial. **Premixed (frozen) solution for injection:** 1 million units/50 mL, 2 million units/50 mL, 3 million units/50 mL.

Penicillin G Sodium

Powder for injection: 5 million units/vial.

Procaine Penicillin G

Suspension for IM injection: 600,000 units/mL in 1- and 2-mL prefilled syringes.

Benzathine Penicillin G

Suspension for IM injection: 600,000 units/mL in 1-, 2-, and 4-mL prefilled syringes.

penicillin V (pen-i-sil-in vee)

✱ Apo-Pen VK, Beepen-VK, ✱ Nadopen-V, ✱ Novo-Pen-VK, ✱ Pen-Vee, Pen-Vee K, ✱ PVF K, Veetids

Classification

Therapeutic: anti-infectives
Pharmacologic: penicillins

Indications

Treatment of a wide variety of infections, including Pneumococcal pneumonia, Streptococcal pharyngitis, Syphilis, Gonorrhea strains. Treatment of enterococcal infections (requires the addition of an aminoglycoside). Prevention of rheumatic fever. Should not be used as a single agent to treat anthrax. **Unlabeled Use:** Treatment of Lyme disease, prevention of recurrent *Streptococcal pneumoniae* septicemia in children with sickle-cell disease.

Action

Bind to bacterial cell wall, resulting in cell death. **Therapeutic Effects:** Bactericidal action against susceptible bacteria. **Spectrum:** Active against most gram-positive organisms, including many streptococci (*Streptococcus pneumoniae*, group A beta-hemolytic streptococci), staphylococci (non–penicillinase-producing strains), and *Bacillus anthracis*. Some gram-negative organisms, such as *Neisseria meningitidis* and *N. gonorrhoeae)* (only penicillin-susceptible strains, some anaerobic bacteria and spirochetes, including *Borrelia burgdorferi*.

Adverse Reactions/Side Effects

CNS: SEIZURES. **GI:** diarrhea, epigastric distress, nausea, vomiting, pseudomembranous colitis. **GU:** interstitial nephritis. **Derm:** rash, urticaria. **Hemat:** eosinophilia, leukopenia. **Misc:** ALLERGIC REACTIONS, INCLUDING ANAPHYLAXIS AND SERUM SICKNESS, superinfection.

PHYSICAL THERAPY IMPLICATIONS

Examination and Evaluation

- Watch for seizures; notify physician immediately if patient develops or increases seizure activity.
- Monitor signs of allergic reactions and anaphylaxis, including pulmonary symptoms (tightness in the throat and chest, wheezing, cough dyspnea) or skin reactions (rash, pruritus, urticaria). Notify physician or nursing staff immediately if these reactions occur.
- Assess muscle aches and joint pain (arthralgia) that may be caused by serum sickness. Notify physician if these symptoms seem to be drug related rather than caused by musculoskeletal injury or if muscle and joint pain are accompanied by allergy-like reactions (fever, rashes, etc.)
- Monitor signs of eosinophilia (fatigue, weakness, myalgia) or leukopenia (fever, sore throat, signs of infection); report these signs to the physician.

Interventions

- Always wash hands thoroughly and disinfect equipment (whirlpools, electrotherapeutic devices, treatment tables, and so forth) to help prevent the spread of infection. Employ universal precautions or isolation procedures as indicated for specific patients.

Patient/Client-related Instruction

- Instruct patient to notify physician immediately if signs of the following occur:
  - Pseudomembranous colitis (diarrhea, abdominal pain, fever, pus or mucus in stools) or other severe or prolonged GI problems (nausea, vomiting, heartburn).
  - Euperinfection (black, furry overgrowth on tongue; vaginal itching or discharge; loose or foul-smelling stools).
  - Interstitial nephritis (blood in urine, decreased urine output, weight gain from fluid retention).
- Instruct patient and family/caregivers to report other troublesome side effects such as severe or prolonged skin problems (rash, itching) or GI problems (nausea, vomiting, diarrhea, heartburn).

Pharmacokinetics

Absorption: Variably absorbed from the GI tract. *Penicillin V*—resists acid degradation in the GI tract.
Distribution: Widely distributed, although CNS penetration is poor in the presence of normal (uninflamed) meninges. Crosses the placenta and enters breast milk.
Protein Binding: 60%.
Metabolism and Excretion: Minimally metabolized by the liver, excreted mainly unchanged by the kidneys.
Half-life: 30–60 min.

TIME/ACTION PROFILE (blood levels)

ROUTE	ONSET	PEAK	DURATION
penicillin V PO	rapid	0.5–1 hr	4–6 hr

Contraindications/Precautions

Contraindicated in: Previous hypersensitivity to penicillins (cross-sensitivity exists with cephalosporins and other beta-lactam antibiotics); Some products may contain tartrazine and should be avoided in patients with known hypersensitivity.
Use Cautiously in: Severe renal insufficiency (dosage reduction recommended); OB: Although safety not established, has been used safely; Lactation: Safety not established; Geri: Consider decreased body mass, age-related decrease in renal/hepatic/cardiac function, intercurrent diseases and drug therapy.

P

Interactions

Drug-Drug: Penicillin may ↓ effectiveness of oral contraceptive agents. **Probenecid** ↓ renal excretion and ↑ blood levels of penicillin (therapy may be combined for this purpose). **Neomycin** may ↓ absorption of penicillin. Concurrent use with **methotrexate** ↓ methotrexate elimination and ↑ risk of serious toxicity.

Route/Dosage

250 mg = 400,000 units.
PO (Adults and Children ≥12 yr): *Most infections*—125–500 mg q 6–8 hr. *Rheumatic fever prevention*—125–250 mg q 12 hr.
PO (Children <12 yr): *Lyme disease*—50 mg/kg/day in 4 divided doses (unlabeled); prevention of *S. pneumoniae* sepsis in children with sickle cell disease—125 mg twice daily.

Availability (generic available)

Tablets: 250 mg, 500 mg. **Oral solution:** 125 mg/5 mL, 250 mg/5 mL.

pentamidine (pen-tam-i-deen)

NebuPent, Pentam 300, Pentacarinat, Pneumopent

Classification
Therapeutic: antiprotozoals

Indications

IV: Treatment of *Pneumocystis carinii* pneumonia (PCP). **Inhalation:** Prevention of PCP in AIDS or HIV-positive patients who have had PCP or who have a

peripheral CD4 lymphocyte count of ≤200/mm^3.
Unlabeled Use: Inhalation: Treatment of PCP.

Action

Appears to disrupt DNA or RNA synthesis in protozoa. Also has a direct toxic effect on pancreatic islet cells.
Therapeutic Effects: Death of susceptible protozoa.

Adverse Reactions/Side Effects

For parenteral form, unless otherwise indicated
CNS: anxiety, headache, confusion, dizziness, hallucinations. **EENT: inhalation:** burning in throat. **Resp: inhalation:** bronchospasm, cough. **CV:** ARRHYTHMIAS, HYPOTENSION. **GI:** PANCREATITIS, abdominal pain, anorexia, drug-induced hepatitis, nausea, unpleasant metallic taste, vomiting. **GU:** nephrotoxicity. **Derm:** pallor, rash. **Endo:** HYPOGLYCEMIA, hyperglycemia. **F and E:** hyperkalemia, hypocalcemia. **Hemat:** anemia, leukopenia, thrombocytopenia. **Local: IV**—phlebitis, pruritus, urticaria at IV site; **IM**—sterile abscesses at IM sites. **Misc:** ALLERGIC REACTIONS, INCLUDING ANAPHYLAXIS, STEVENS-JOHNSON SYNDROME, chills, fever.

PHYSICAL THERAPY IMPLICATIONS

Examination and Evaluation

- Assess heart rate, ECG, and heart sounds, especially during exercise (see Appendixes G, H). Report any rhythm disturbances or symptoms of cardiac dysfunction, including palpitations, chest discomfort, shortness of breath, fainting, and fatigue/weakness.
- Monitor signs of allergic reactions and anaphylaxis, including pulmonary symptoms (tightness in the throat and chest, wheezing, cough, dyspnea) or skin reactions associated with Stevens-Johnson syndrome (exfoliation, rash, dermatitis, pruritus, urticaria). Notify physician or nursing staff immediately if these reactions occur.
- Monitor signs of pancreatitis, including upper abdominal pain (especially after eating), indigestion, weight loss, oily stools. Report these signs to the physician immediately.
- Monitor signs of hypoglycemia (weakness, malaise, irritability, fatigue) or hyperglycemia (drowsiness, fruity breath, increased urination, unusual thirst). Notify physician about glycemic problems, especially severe hypoglycemia that might lead to dizziness, syncope, coma, and seizures.
- Assess blood pressure (BP) periodically and compare to normal values (See Appendix F). Report low BP (hypotension), especially if patient experiences dizziness, fatigue, or other symptoms.
- Monitor signs of leukopenia (fever, sore throat, signs of infection), thrombocytopenia (bruising, nose bleeds, and bleeding gums), or unusual weakness and fatigue that might be due to anemia, coagulation disorders, or other blood dyscrasias. Report these signs to the physician.
- Assess symptoms of bronchospasm (wheezing, coughing, tightness in chest), especially when this drug is inhaled. Perform pulmonary function tests to quantify suspected changes in ventilation and respiration (See Appendix I).
- Monitor signs of electrolyte imbalances such as high plasma potassium levels (hyperkalemia) or low calcium levels (hypocalcemia), including bradycardia, fatigue, weakness, numbness, and tingling, muscle cramps, and muscle hyperexcitability and tetany. Notify physician of these signs.
- Monitor severe or prolonged confusion, anxiety, hallucinations, or other changes in mood or behavior. Notify physician if these changes become problematic.
- Monitor IV injection site for pain, swelling, and irritation. Report prolonged or excessive injection site reactions to the physician.

Interventions

- Because of the risk of arrhythmias and abnormal BP responses, use extreme caution during aerobic exercise and other forms of therapeutic exercise. Assess exercise tolerance frequently (BP, heart rate, fatigue levels), and terminate exercise immediately if any untoward responses occur (See Appendix L).

Patient/Client-Related Instruction

- Advise patient to report signs of nephrotoxicity (blood or pus in urine, decreased urine output, weight gain from fluid retention, fatigue).
- Advise patient about the likelihood of GI reactions (nausea, vomiting, loss of appetite, abdominal pain). Instruct patient to report severe or prolonged GI problems, signs of drug-induced hepatitis, including yellow skin or eyes, abdominal pain, severe nausea and vomiting, fever, sore throat, malaise, weakness, and facial edema.
- Instruct patient to report other untoward side effects such as severe or prolonged headache, chills, fever, skin rash, or GI problems (nausea, diarrhea, unpleasant taste, loss of appetite).

Pharmacokinetics

Absorption: Minimal systemic absorption occurs following inhalation.
Distribution: Widely and extensively distributed but does not cross the blood-brain barrier. Concentrates in liver, kidneys, lungs, and spleen, with prolonged storage in some tissues.
Metabolism and Excretion: 1–30% excreted unchanged by the kidneys. Remainder of metabolic fate unknown.
Half-life: 6.4–9.4 hr (increased in renal impairment).

TIME/ACTION PROFILE (blood levels)

ROUTE	ONSET	PEAK	DURATION
IV	unknown	end of infusion	24 hr
inhalation	unknown	unknown	unknown

Contraindications/Precautions

Contraindicated in: History of previous anaphylactic reaction to pentamidine.
Use Cautiously in: Hypotension; Hypertension; Hypoglycemia; Hyperglycemia; Hypocalcemia; Leukopenia; Thrombocytopenia; Anemia; Renal impairment (dose reduction required); Diabetes mellitus; Liver impairment; Cardiovascular disease; Bone marrow depression, previous antineoplastic therapy, or radiation therapy; OB: Pregnancy or lactation (safety not established during pregnancy; breast-feeding not recommended).

Interactions

Interactions listed for parenteral administration
Drug-Drug: Concurrent use with **erythromycin** IV may ↑ risk of potentially fatal arrhythmias. Additive nephrotoxicity with other **nephrotoxic agents**, including **aminoglycosides, amphotericin B,** and **vancomycin**. Additive bone marrow depression with **antineoplastics** or previous **radiation therapy**. ↑ risk of pancreatitis with **didanosine**. ↑ risk of nephrotoxicity, hypocalcemia, and hypomagnesemia with **foscarnet**.

Route/Dosage

IV (Adults and Children): 4 mg/kg once daily for 14–21 days (longer treatment may be required in AIDS patients; some patients may respond to 3 mg/kg/day).
Inhalation (Adults): *NebuPent, Pentacarinat*—300 mg q 4 wk, using a Respirgard II jet nebulizer (150 mg q 2 wk has also been used). *Pneumopent*—60 mg q 24–72 hr for 5 doses over a 2-wk period, then q 2 wk using a Fisoneb ultrasonic nebulizer.
Inhaln (Children >5 yr): *NebuPent, Pentacarinat*—300 mg q 4 wk, using a Respirgard II jet nebulizer (for patients who cannot tolerate trimethoprim/sulfamethoxazole; unlabeled).

Availability (generic available)

Injection: 300 mg/vial. **Solution for aerosol use (NebuPent, Pentacarinat):** 300 mg/vial. **Solution for aerosol use (Pneumopent):** 60 mg/vial.

HIGH ALERT

pentazocine (pen-taz-oh-seen)

Talwin, Talwin NX

Classification
Therapeutic: opioid analgesics
Pharmacologic: opioid agonists/antagonists

Schedule IV

Indications

Moderate-to-severe pain. Also used for Analgesia during labor, Sedation prior to surgery; Supplementation in balanced anesthesia.

Action

Binds to opiate receptors in the CNS. Alters perception of and response to painful stimuli, while producing generalized CNS depression. Has partial antagonist properties, which may result in opioid withdrawal in physically dependent patients. **Therapeutic Effects:** Decrease in moderate to severe pain.

Adverse Reactions/Side Effects

CNS: dizziness, euphoria, hallucinations, headache, sedation, confusion, dysphoria, floating feeling, unusual dreams. **EENT:** blurred vision, diplopia, miosis (high doses). **Resp:** respiratory depression. **CV:** hypertension, hypotension, palpitations. **GI:** nausea, constipation, dry mouth, ileus, vomiting. **GU:** urinary retention. **Derm:** clammy feeling, sweating. **Local:** severe tissue damage at subcut sites. **Misc:** physical dependence, psychologic dependence, tolerance.

P

PHYSICAL THERAPY IMPLICATIONS

Examination and Evaluation

- Assess symptoms of respiratory depression, including decreased respiratory rate, confusion, bluish color of the skin and mucous membranes (cyanosis), and difficult, labored breathing (dyspnea). Monitor pulse oximetry and perform pulmonary function tests (See Appendix I) to quantify suspected changes in ventilation and respiratory function. Excessive respiratory depression requires emergency care.
- Be alert for excessive sedation or changes in mood and behavior (euphoria, dysphoria, confusion, hallucinations). Notify physician or nurse immediately if patient is unconscious or extremely difficult to arouse.
- Use appropriate pain scales (visual analogue scales, others) to document whether this drug is successful in helping manage the patient's pain.
- Assess blood pressure (BP) and compare to normal values (See Appendix F). Report changes in BP, either a problematic decrease in BP (hypotension) or a sustained increase in BP (hypertension).
- Assess dizziness and drowsiness that might affect gait, balance, and other functional activities (See Appendix C). Report balance problems and functional limitations to the physician and nursing staff, and caution the patient and family/caregivers to guard against falls and trauma.
- Monitor injection site for pain, swelling, and irritation. Report prolonged or excessive injection-site reactions to the physician.

Interventions

- Implement appropriate manual therapy techniques, physical agents, and therapeutic exercises to reduce pain and help wean patient off opioid analgesics as soon as possible.
- Because of the risk of abnormal BP responses, use caution during aerobic exercise and other forms of therapeutic exercise. Assess exercise tolerance frequently (BP, heart rate, fatigue levels), and terminate exercise immediately if any untoward responses occur (see Appendix L).
- Help patient explore other nonpharmacologic methods to reduce chronic pain, such as relaxation techniques, exercise, counseling, and so forth.
- Guard against falls and trauma (hip fractures, head injury). Implement fall-prevention strategies (See Appendix E), especially if patient exhibits sedation, dizziness, or blurred vision.
- To minimize orthostatic hypotension, patient should move slowly when assuming a more upright position.

Patient/Client-Related Instruction

- Advise patient that opioid analgesics are usually more effective if given before pain becomes severe; emphasize that adequate pain control will allow better participation in physical therapy.
- Educate patient about the dangers of opioid overdose; encourage patient to adhere to proper dosing schedule.
- Emphasize that the risk of physical addiction (tolerance and dependence) is usually minimal during short-term treatment of pain. Advise patient that addiction is more likely during excessive or inappropriate use of opioid analgesics.
- Advise patient to avoid alcohol and other CNS depressants because of the increased risk of sedation and decreased CNS function.
- Advise patient to increase fluid intake and dietary fiber to avoid constipation. Laxatives may also be helpful in patients susceptible to fecal impaction (e.g., people with spinal cord injury).
- Instruct patient to report other troublesome side effects such as severe or prolonged headache, urinary retention, unusual dreams, heart palpitations, excessive sweating, vision disturbances, or GI problems (nausea, vomiting, dry mouth).

Pharmacokinetics

Absorption: Well absorbed following oral, IM, and SC administration. Small amount (0.5 mg) of naloxone in tablets included to prevent parenteral abuse.

Distribution: Widely distributed. Crosses the placenta.

Metabolism and Excretion: Mostly metabolized by the liver. Small amounts excreted unchanged by the kidneys.

Half-life: 2–3 hr.

TIME/ACTION PROFILE (analgesia)

ROUTE	ONSET	PEAK	DURATION
PO	15–30 min	60–90 min	3 hr
IM, SC	15–20 min	30–60 min	2–3 hr
IV	2–3 min	15–30 min	2–3 hr

Contraindications/Precautions

Contraindicated in: Hypersensitivity; Patients who are physically dependent on opioids (may precipitate withdrawal).

Use Cautiously in: Head trauma; History of drug abuse; ↑ intracranial pressure; Severe renal, hepatic, or pulmonary disease; Hypothyroidism; Adrenal insufficiency; Alcoholism; Debilitated patients or patients with severe liver impairment (dose reduction recommended); Geri: Appears on Beers' list and is associated with ↑ risk of falls. Geriatric patients are more susceptible to adverse CNS effects; dose reduction recommended; Undiagnosed abdominal pain; Prostatic hyperplasia; Patients who have recently received opioid agonists; OB: Pregnancy (has been used during labor but may cause respiratory depression in the newborn); Lactation or children (safety not established).

Interactions

Drug-Drug: Use with caution in patients receiving **MAO inhibitors** (may result in unpredictable reactions—↓ initial dose of pentazocine to 25% of usual dose). Additive CNS depression with **alcohol, antihistamines**, and **sedative/hypnotics**. May precipitate withdrawal in patients who are physically dependent on **opioid analgesic agonists**. May ↓ analgesic effects of other **opioids**.

Drug-Natural: Concomitant use of **kava, valerian,** or **chamomile** can ↑ CNS depression.

Route/Dosage

PO (Adults): 50–100 mg q 3–4 hr (not to exceed 600 mg/day).

SC, IV, IM (Adults): 30 mg q 3–4 hr (not to exceed 30 mg/dose IV or 60 mg/dose IM or SC; not to exceed 360 mg/day SC, IV, or IM). *Obstetrical use*—20 mg IV or 30 mg IM when contractions become regular; may repeat q 2–3 hr for 2–3 doses.

Availability

Tablets: 50 mg (with 0.5 mg naloxone), 50 mg. **Injection:** 30 mg/mL. ***In combination with:*** acetaminophen (Talacen) or aspirin (Talwin compound). See Appendix B.

pentobarbital
(pen-toe-**bar**-bi-tal)
Nembutal, Novopentobarb, Nova Rectal

Classification
Therapeutic: anticonvulsants, sedative/hypnotics
Pharmacologic: barbiturates

Schedule II (oral and parenteral), III (rectal)

Indications
Hypnotic agent (short-term). Preoperative sedation and other situations in which sedation is required. Treatment of seizures. **Unlabeled Use: IV:** Induction of coma in selected patients with cerebral ischemia and management of increased intracranial pressure (high doses).

Action
Depresses the CNS, probably by potentiating gamma-aminobutyric acid (GABA), an inhibitory neurotransmitter. Produces all levels of CNS depression, including the sensory cortex, motor activity, and altered cerebellar function. Anticonvulsant effect due to decreased synaptic transmission and increased seizure threshold. May decrease cerebral blood flow, cerebral edema, and intracranial pressure (IV only). **Therapeutic Effects:** Sedation and/or induction of sleep.

Adverse Reactions/Side Effects
CNS: drowsiness, hangover, lethargy, delirium, excitation, mental depression, vertigo. **Resp:** respiratory depression. **IV:** LARYNGOSPASM, bronchospasm. **CV: IV:** hypotension. **GI:** constipation, diarrhea, nausea, vomiting. **Derm:** rashes, urticaria. **Local:** phlebitis at IV site. **MS:** arthralgia, myalgia, neuralgia. **Misc:** HYPERSENSITIVITY REACTIONS, INCLUDING ANGIOEDEMA AND SERUM SICKNESS, physical dependence, psychologic dependence.

PHYSICAL THERAPY IMPLICATIONS

Examination and Evaluation
- Monitor signs of hypersensitivity reactions such as angioedema and serum sickness. Signs include laryngeal spasm and bronchospasm (tightness in the throat and chest, wheezing, cough, dyspnea) and skin reactions (rash, pruritus, urticaria, swelling in the face). Notify physician or nursing staff immediately if these reactions occur.
- Document the number, duration, and severity of seizures to help document whether this drug is effective in reducing seizure activity.
- Assess any breathing problems, and report signs of respiratory depression such as shortness of breath, reduced pulse oximetry values, cyanosis, and labored or difficult breathing. Severe respiratory depression requires emergency care.
- Assess dizziness and vertigo that might affect gait, balance, and other functional activities (See Appendix C). Report balance problems and functional limitations to the physician and nursing staff, and caution the patient and family/caregivers to guard against falls and trauma.
- Monitor excitation, delirium, drowsiness, lethargy, mental depression, or symptoms resembling a "hangover." Repeated or excessive symptoms may require change in dose or medication.
- Assess blood pressure after IV administration and compare to normal values (See Appendix F). Report low blood pressure (hypotension), especially if patient experiences dizziness or syncope.
- Assess any muscle, nerve, or joint pain to rule out neuromusculoskeletal pathology; that is, try to determine if pain is drug induced rather than caused by anatomic or neurologic problems.
- Assess injection site during and after IV administration, and report signs of phlebitis (local pain, swelling, inflammation).

Interventions
- Guard against falls and trauma (hip fractures, head injury, and so forth), especially if drowsiness, vertigo, or syncope affects gait and balance. Implement fall-prevention strategies, especially if balance is impaired (See Appendix E).
- To minimize orthostatic hypotension, patient should move slowly when assuming a more upright position.

Patient/Client-Related Instruction
- Advise patient to avoid alcohol and other CNS depressants because of the increased risk of sedation and adverse effects.
- Advise patients on prolonged antiseizure therapy not to discontinue medication without their physician. This drug can cause tolerance and dependence, and abrupt withdrawal may cause increased seizures and other withdrawal reactions.
- Advise patient about the risk of daytime drowsiness and decreased attention and mental focus. Use care if driving or in other activities that require strong concentration and fast responses.
- Instruct patient and family/caregivers to report other troublesome side effects such as severe or prolonged skin reactions (rash, itching), or GI problems (nausea, vomiting, diarrhea, constipation).

P

Pharmacokinetics

Absorption: Well absorbed following all routes.
Distribution: Widely distributed; highest concentrations in brain and liver. Crosses the placenta; small amounts enter breast milk.
Metabolism and Excretion: Metabolized by the liver. Minimal renal excretion.
Half-life: Children: 25 hr; Adults: 35–50 hr.

TIME/ACTION PROFILE (sedation)

ROUTE	ONSET	PEAK	DURATION*
PO	15–60 min	3–4 hr	1–4 hr
rectal	15–60 min	unknown	1–4 hr
IM	10–25 min	unknown	1–4 hr
IV	immediate	1 min	15 min

*Noted as hypnotic effect; sedative effects are longer lasting.

Contraindications/Precautions

Contraindicated in: Hypersensitivity; Some products contain tartrazine, alcohol, or propylene glycol and should be avoided in patients with known hypersensitivity or intolerance; Comatose patients or those with preexisting CNS depression (unless used to induce coma); Uncontrolled severe pain; Pregnancy or lactation.
Use Cautiously in: Hepatic dysfunction; Severe renal impairment; Patients who may be suicidal or who may have been addicted to drugs previously; Geriatric or debilitated patients (initial dosage reduction recommended); Hypovolemic shock; Hypnotic use should be short-term (chronic use may lead to dependence).

Interactions

Drug-Drug: Additive CNS depression with other **CNS depressants**, including **alcohol, antihistamines, opioids,** and other **sedative/hypnotics**. May induce hepatic enzymes, which metabolize other drugs, ↓ their effectiveness, including **oral contraceptives, warfarin, carbamazepine, chloramphenicol, cyclosporine, dacarbazine, doxycycline, corticosteroids, tricyclic antidepressants,** and **quinidine**. May ↑ the risk of hepatic toxicity of **acetaminophen**. **MAO inhibitors, valproic acid,** or **divalproex** may ↓ the metabolism of pentobarbital, ↑ sedation.
Drug-Natural: Concomitant use of **kava, valerian, skullcap, chamomile,** or **hops** can ↑ CNS depression. **St. John's wort** may ↓ effects.

Route/Dosage

PO (Adults): *Sedative*—20 mg tid–qid. *Hypnotic/preoperative sedative*—100 mg.
PO (Children): *Sedative*—2–6 mg/kg/day. *Preoperative sedative*—2–6 mg/kg (up to 100 mg/dose).
IM (Adults): *Hypnotic/preoperative sedative*—150–200 mg.
IM (Children): *Sedative*—2–6 mg/kg/day in divided doses. *Preoperative sedative*—2–6 mg/kg (up to 100 mg/dose).
IV (Adults): *Hypnotic/anticonvulsant*—100 mg initially; additional small doses may be given q min up to 500 mg total. *Induction of coma*—5–7 mg/kg, then 3–4 mg/kg q 3–4 hr dose adjusted by serum level (unlabeled).
IV (Children): *Sedative*—1–3 mg/kg to a maximum of 100 mg until asleep. *Conscious sedation*—Initial 2 mg/kg; may repeat q 5–10 min with 1–2 mg/kg until adequate sedation achieved. Maximum total dose 6 mg/kg or 150–200 mg. *Induction of coma*—10–15 mg/kg slowly over 1–2 hr, followed by a maintenance infusion of 1–3 mg/kg/hr.
Rect (Adults): *Sedative*—30 mg bid–qid. *Hypnotic*—120–200 mg at bedtime.
Rect (Children): *Sedative*—2 mg/kg (60 mg/m^2) tid.
Rect (Children 12–14 yr): *Preoperative sedative/hypnotic*—60–120 mg.
Rect (Children 5–12 yr): *Preoperative sedative/hypnotic*—60 mg.
Rect (Children 1–4 yr): *Preoperative sedative/hypnotic*—30–60 mg.
Rect (Children 2 mo–1 yr): *Preoperative sedative/hypnotic*—30 mg.

Availability (generic available)

Capsules: 50 mg, 100 mg. **Elixir:** 20 mg/5 mL. **Suppositories:** 25 mg, 30 mg, 50 mg, 60 mg, 120 mg, 200 mg. **Injection:** 50 mg/mL in 2-mL ampules, prefilled syringes, and 20- and 50-mL vials.

pentosan (pen-toe-san)

Elmiron

Classification

Therapeutic: agents for interstitial cystitis
Pharmacologic: heparin-like compounds

Indications

Management symptoms (bladder pain/discomfort) of chronic interstitial cystitis (IC).

Action

Adheres to uroepithelium, providing a protective barrier against irritating solutes in urine; has anticoagulant and fibrinolytic properties. **Therapeutic Effects:** ↓ pain and discomfort in chronic IC.

Adverse Reactions/Side Effects

CNS: dizziness, headache. **EENT:** epistaxis. **GI:** abdominal pain, diarrhea, dyspepsia, gum bleeding, ↑ liver enzymes, nausea, rectal bleeding. **Derm:** alopecia, ecchymosis, rash. **Hemat:** bleeding, ↑ bleeding time.

PHYSICAL THERAPY IMPLICATIONS

Examination and Evaluation

- Assess for signs of bleeding and increased bleeding time, including bleeding gums, nosebleeds, and rectal bleeding. Notify physician if this drug causes increased bleeding.

- Monitor signs of interstitial cystitis, including chronic pelvic pain, persistent urge to urinate, and painful sexual intercourse. Document whether this drug is successful in reducing these symptoms.
- Assess dizziness that might affect gait, balance, and other functional activities (see Appendix C). Report balance problems and functional limitations to the physician, and caution the patient and family/caregivers to guard against falls and trauma.

Interventions

- Use caution with any physical interventions that could increase bleeding, including wound débridement, chest percussion, joint mobilization, and application of local heat.

Patient/Client-Related Instruction

- Instruct patient to report other bothersome side effects such as severe or prolonged headache, skin reactions (rash, bruising, hair loss), or GI problems (nausea, diarrhea, abdominal pain, indigestion).

Pharmacokinetics

Absorption: 6% absorbed following oral administrations.
Distribution: Distributes into uroepithelium of the genitourinary tract with less found in liver, spleen, lung, skin, periosteum, and bone marrow.
Metabolism and Excretion: Metabolized by saturable enzyme systems in liver, spleen, and kidney. Majority (58–84%) excreted in feces as unchanged (unabsorbed drug). Metabolites of absorbed drug are renally excreted; minimal renal excretion of unchanged drug.
Half-life: 27 hr.

TIME/ACTION PROFILE (↓ symptoms)

ROUTE	ONSET	PEAK	DURATION
PO	within 4 wk–6 mo	unknown	unknown

Contraindications/Precautions

Contraindicated in: Hypersensitivity.
Use Cautiously in: Underlying coagulopathy, concurrent medications that ↑ bleeding risk, history of aneurysms. Thrombocytopenia, hemophilia, GI ulceration/bleeding, polyps, diverticula; History of heparin-induced thrombocytopenia; risk of bleeding may be ↑ hepatic insufficiency; OB: Use in pregnancy only if clearly needed; Lactation: Use cautiously in breast-feeding women; Pedi: safe and effective use in children <16 yr has not been established.

Interactions

Drug-Drug: Concurrent use of **coumarin anticoagulants, heparins, t-PA, streptokinase,** high-dose **aspirin,** or **NSAIDs** may ↑ risk of bleeding.

Route/Dosage

PO (Adults): 100 mg tid.

Availability

Capsules: 100 mg.

pentostatin (pen-toe-stah-tin)

Nipent

Classification
Therapeutic: antineoplastics
Pharmacologic: enzyme inhibitors

Indications

Treatment of hairy-cell leukemia in patients with active disease.

Action

Inhibits adenine deaminase (ADA), an enzyme that blocks the synthesis of DNA, especially in T cells of the lymphoid system. **Therapeutic Effects:** Decreased signs and symptoms of hairy-cell leukemia (recovery of hematologic parameters, organomegaly, and lymphadenopathy).

Adverse Reactions/Side Effects

CNS: CNS toxicity, fatigue, headache, weakness. **EENT:** epistaxis, keratoconjunctivitis, pharyngitis, rhinitis, sinusitis, vision changes. **Resp:** PULMONARY TOXICITY, bronchitis, dyspnea, pneumonia, cough, pulmonary edema. **CV:** MI, angina pectoris, arrhythmias, thrombophlebitis. **GI:** anorexia, diarrhea, hepatotoxicity, nausea, vomiting, constipation, flatulence, abdominal pain, stomatitis. **GU:** renal toxicity. **Derm:** itching, skin rash, dry skin. **Hemat:** anemia, leukopenia, thrombocytopenia. **MS:** arthralgia, myalgia. **Misc:** ALLERGIC REACTIONS, INCLUDING ANAPHYLAXIS, fever, flu-like syndrome, weight loss.

PHYSICAL THERAPY IMPLICATIONS

Examination and Evaluation

- Continually monitor for signs of MI, including sudden chest pain, pain radiating into the arm or jaw, shortness of breath, dizziness, sweating, anxiety, and nausea. Seek immediate medical assistance if patient develops these signs.
- Monitor signs of allergic reactions and anaphylaxis, including pulmonary symptoms (wheezing, cough, dyspnea) or skin reactions (rash, pruritus, urticaria). Notify physician or nursing staff immediately if these reactions occur.
- Assess pulmonary function periodically by measuring lung volumes, breath sounds, and respiratory

rate (See Appendices I, J, K). Notify physician or nursing staff immediately if patient experiences signs of bronchitis, pneumonia, pulmonary edema, or pulmonary toxicity. These signs include dry cough, dyspnea, abnormal breath sounds, tightness in the throat and chest, shortness of breath, fever, and cyanosis.

- Assess heart rate, ECG, and heart sounds, especially during exercise (See Appendices G, H). Report any rhythm disturbances or symptoms of increased arrhythmias, including palpitations, chest discomfort, shortness of breath, fainting, and fatigue/weakness.
- Watch for signs of leukopenia (fever, sore throat, signs of infection), thrombocytopenia (bruising, nose bleeds, bleeding gums), or unusual weakness and fatigue that might be due to anemia. Report these signs to the physician or nursing staff.
- Monitor signs of CNS neurotoxicity, including confusion, agitation, severe headache, hearing loss, visual disturbances, and decreased consciousness. Notify physician or nursing staff, especially if patient becomes unresponsive or difficult to arouse.
- Watch for signs of renal toxicity, including hematuria, increased urinary frequency, cloudy urine, and decreased urine output. Report these signs to the physician or nursing staff.
- Monitor signs of thrombophlebitis, especially at the IV injection site. Signs include localized pain, redness, or swelling in the affected area. Report these signs to the physician or nursing staff.
- Assess any muscle or joint pain to rule out musculoskeletal pathology; that is, try to determine if pain is drug-induced rather than caused by anatomical or biomechanical problems.
- Periodically assess body weight and other anthropometric measures (body mass index, body composition). Report a rapid or unexplained weight loss or decreased body fat.

Interventions

- For patients who are medically able to begin exercise, implement appropriate resistive exercises and aerobic training to maintain muscle strength and aerobic capacity during cancer chemotherapy, or to help restore function after chemotherapy.
- Because of the risk of cardiac and pulmonary problems, use extreme caution during aerobic exercise and other forms of therapeutic exercise. Assess exercise tolerance frequently (blood pressure, heart rate, respiratory symptoms, fatigue levels), and terminate exercise immediately if any untoward responses occur (See Appendix L).

Patient/Client-related Instruction

- Advise patient and family or caregiver about the signs of MI, pulmonary toxicity, and allergic reactions (see above under Examination and Evaluation), and to seek immediate medical assistance if these signs develop.
- Because of immunosuppressant effects, advise patient to decrease risk of infections (frequent hand washing, etc.) and avoid contact with persons with contagious diseases.
- Advise patient about the likelihood of GI reactions, including nausea, vomiting, diarrhea, constipation, loss of appetite, abdominal pain, and inflammation in or around the mouth. Instruct patient to report severe or prolonged GI reactions, and to also report signs of hepatotoxicity, including anorexia, abdominal pain, severe nausea and vomiting, yellow skin or eyes, fever, sore throat, malaise, weakness, facial edema, lethargy, and unusual bleeding or bruising.
- Advise patient and family/caregivers that fatigue and weakness are likely and may be severe. Functional abilities may be limited, and patient may need to use assistive devices during ambulation.
- Instruct patient to report other problematic side effects such as severe or prolonged nasopharyngeal inflammation, nose bleeds, eye irritation, fever, flu-like symptoms, or skin reactions (rash, itching, dry skin).

Pharmacokinetics

Absorption: IV administration results in complete bioavailability.
Distribution: Highest in the kidneys; minimal penetration into the CNS.
Metabolism and Excretion: 90% renally excreted.
Half-life: 6 hr (increased in renal impairment).

TIME/ACTION PROFILE (clinical response)

ROUTE	ONSET	PEAK	DURATION
IV	4.7 mo	unknown	>7.7 mo (range 1.4–35.1 mo)*

*Inhibition of adenine deaminase lasts for >1 wk after administration.

Contraindications/Precautions

Contraindicated in: Hypersensitivity to pentostatin or mannitol; Concurrent use of fludarabine (↑ risk of potentially fatal pulmonary toxicity).
Use Cautiously in: Cardiovascular disease, seizures, or preexisting renal, hepatic, or pulmonary disease or other chronic debilitating illness; Patients with childbearing potential; Pregnancy, lactation, or children (safety not established).

Interactions

Drug-Drug: Risk of fatal pulmonary toxicity is ↑ by concurrent use of **fludarabine**. Effects of **vidarabine** are ↑ by pentostatin, which may result in ↑ toxicity of both agents.

Route/Dosage

IV (Adults): 4 mg/m^2 q other week.

Availability
Powder for injection: 10 mg/vial.

pentoxifylline (pen-tox-if-i-lin)
Trental

Classification
Therapeutic: blood viscosity reducing agent

Indications
Management of symptomatic peripheral vascular disease (intermittent claudication).

Action
↑ the flexibility of RBCs by increasing levels of cyclic adenosine monophosphate (cAMP). ↓ blood viscosity by inhibiting platelet aggregation and decreasing fibrinogen. **Therapeutic Effects:** ↑ blood flow.

Adverse Reactions/Side Effects
CNS: agitation, dizziness, drowsiness, headache, insomnia, nervousness. **EENT:** blurred vision. **Resp:** dyspnea. **CV:** angina, arrhythmias, edema, flushing, hypotension. **GI:** abdominal discomfort, belching, bloating, diarrhea, dyspepsia, flatus, nausea, vomiting. **Neuro:** tremor.

PHYSICAL THERAPY IMPLICATIONS

Examination and Evaluation
- Assess patient's walking distance and pain-free walking time. Document an increase in walking distance and time as an indication that this drug is helping reduce intermittent claudication.
- Assess heart rate, ECG, and heart sounds, especially during exercise (See Appendices G, H). Report any rhythm disturbances or signs of arrhythmias, including palpitations, chest discomfort, shortness of breath, dyspnea, fainting, and fatigue/weakness.
- Assess blood pressure (BP) periodically and compare to normal values (See Appendix F). Report low BP (hypotension), especially if patient experiences dizziness, fatigue, or other symptoms.
- Assess peripheral edema using girth measurements, volume displacement, and measurement of pitting edema (See Appendix N). Report increased swelling in feet and ankles due to peripheral vasodilation.
- Monitor personality changes, including agitation or nervousness. Notify physician if these changes become problematic.
- Assess dizziness or drowsiness that might affect gait, balance, and other functional activities (See Appendix C). Report balance problems and functional limitations to the physician, and caution the patient and family/caregivers to guard against falls and trauma.

Interventions
- Implement therapeutic exercises and ambulation activities to augment the effects of drug therapy and promote increased walking distance. Patients should attempt to walk as long as possible after the onset of leg pain and progressively increase the time spent walking before stopping due to claudication.
- Because of the risk of arrhythmias and abnormal BP responses, use caution during aerobic exercise and other forms of therapeutic exercise. Assess exercise tolerance frequently (BP, heart rate, fatigue levels), and terminate exercise immediately if any untoward cardiac responses occur (See Appendix L).

Patient/Client-Related Instruction
- Instruct patient to report other bothersome side effects such as severe or prolonged headache, sleep loss, blurred vision, tremor, or GI problems (nausea, vomiting, diarrhea, abdominal pain, belching, bloating, indigestion, flatulence).

Pharmacokinetics
Absorption: Well absorbed following oral administration.
Distribution: Bound to RBC membrane. Enters breast milk.
Metabolism and Excretion: Metabolized by RBCs and the liver.
Half-life: 25–50 min.

TIME/ACTION PROFILE (improvement in blood flow)

ROUTE	ONSET	PEAK	DURATION
PO	2–4 wk	8 wk	8 hr

Contraindications/Precautions
Contraindicated in: Hypersensitivity; Intolerance to other xanthine derivatives (caffeine and theophylline).
Use Cautiously in: Coronary artery or cerebrovascular disease; Renal disease (lower doses may be used); Geriatric patients (increased risk of adverse reactions); Pregnancy, lactation, or children (safety not established).

Interactions
Drug-Drug: Additive hypotension may occur with **antihypertensives** and **nitrates**. May ↑ the risk of bleeding with **warfarin, heparin, aspirin, NSAIDs, cefoperazone, cefotetan, valproic acid, clopidogrel, ticlopidine, eptifibatide, tirofiban,** or **thrombolytic agents**. May ↑ the risk of **theophylline** toxicity. **Smoking** may ↓ the beneficial effects of pentoxifylline.

P

Drug-Natural: Increased bleeding risk with **anise, arnica, asafoetida, chamomile, clove, dong quai, fenugreek, feverfew, garlic, ginger, ginkgo, Panax ginseng, licorice**, and others.

Route/Dosage

PO (Adults): 400 mg tid; if GI or CNS side effects occur, ↓ dose to 400 mg bid.

Availability (generic available)

Controlled-release tablets: 400 mg. **Extended-release tablets:** 400 mg.

perindopril (per-in-do-pril)

Aceon, 🍁Coversyl

Classification

Therapeutic: antihypertensives
Pharmacologic: angiotnsin-converting enzyme (ACE) inhibitors

Indications

Alone or with other agents in the management of hypertension. Reduction of risk of death from cardiovascular causes or nonfatal myocardial infarction in patients with stable coronary artery disease.

Action

ACE inhibitors block the conversion of angiotensin I to the vasoconstrictor angiotensin II. ACE inhibitors also prevent the degradation of bradykinin and other vasodilatory prostaglandins. ACE inhibitors also increase plasma renin levels and reduce aldosterone levels. Net result is systemic vasodilation. **Therapeutic Effects:** Lowering of blood pressure in patients with hypertension. ↓ risk of death from cardiovascular causes or myocardial infarction in patients with stable coronary artery disease.

Adverse Reactions/Side Effects

CNS: dizziness, headache, weakness. **Resp:** <u>cough</u>. **CV:** <u>hypotension</u>. **GI:** diarrhea, dyspepsia. **GU:** impaired renal function. **Derm:** rashes. **F and E:** hyperkalemia. **MS:** back pain. **Misc:** ANGIOEDEMA.

PHYSICAL THERAPY IMPLICATIONS

Examination and Evaluation

- Watch for signs of angioedema, including rashes, raised patches of red or white skin (welts), burning/itching skin, swelling in the face, and difficulty breathing. Notify physician immediately of these signs.
- Assess blood pressure periodically and compare to normal values (See Appendix F) to help document antihypertensive effects. Report low blood pressure (hypotension), especially if patient experiences dizziness or syncope.
- Monitor symptoms of high plasma potassium levels (hyperkalemia), including bradycardia, fatigue, weakness, numbness, and tingling. Notify physician because severe cases can lead to life-threatening arrhythmias and paralysis.
- Watch for signs of impaired renal function, including decreased urine output, cloudy urine, or sudden weight gain due to fluid retention. Report these signs to the physician.
- Assess dizziness that might affect gait, balance, and other functional activities (See Appendix C). Report balance problems and functional limitations to the physician, and caution the patient and family/caregivers to guard against falls and trauma.
- Assess any back pain to rule out musculoskeletal pathology; that is, try to determine if pain is drug induced rather than caused by anatomic or biomechanical problems.

Interventions

- Avoid physical therapy interventions that cause systemic vasodilation (large whirlpool, Hubbard tank). Additive effects of this drug and the intervention may cause a dangerous fall in blood pressure.
- To minimize orthostatic hypotension, patient should move slowly when assuming a more upright position.
- Use caution during aerobic exercise and other forms of therapeutic exercise in patient with stable coronary artery disease. Assess exercise tolerance frequently (blood pressure, heart rate, fatigue levels), and terminate exercise immediately if any untoward responses occur (see Appendix L).

Patient/Client-Related Instruction

- Remind patients to take medication as directed to control hypertension and other cardiac conditions even if they are asymptomatic.
- Counsel patients about additional interventions to help control blood pressure and cardiac dysfunction, including regular exercise, weight loss, sodium restriction, stress reduction, moderation of alcohol consumption, and smoking cessation.
- Instruct patient to notify physician of a prolonged dry cough; drug therapy may need to be altered to resolve this side effect.
- Instruct patient or family/caregivers to report other troublesome side effects such as severe or prolonged headache, skin rash, or GI problems (diarrhea, indigestion).

Pharmacokinetics

Absorption: 25% bioavailability as perindoprilat following oral administration.
Distribution: Crosses the placenta; may enter breast milk.

Metabolism and Excretion: Converted by the liver to perindoprilat, the active metabolite; primarily excreted in urine.
Half-life: *Perindoprilat:* 3–10 hr (increased in renal impairment).

TIME/ACTION PROFILE (plasma concentrations)

ROUTE	ONSET	PEAK	DURATION
PO	within 1–2 hr	3–7 hr	up to 24 hr

Contraindications/Precautions

Contraindicated in: Hypersensitivity; Pregnancy; History of angioedema with previous use of ACE inhibitors.
Use Cautiously in: Renal impairment, hypovolemia, hyponatremia, elderly patients, concurrent diuretic therapy (initial dosage reduction recommended); Black patients (monotherapy for hypertension less effective, may require additional therapy; higher risk of angioedema); Surgery/anesthesia (hypotension may be exaggerated); Women of childbearing potential; Lactation/Pedi: Safety not established.
Exercise Extreme Caution in: Family history of angioedema.

Interactions

Drug-Drug: Excessive hypotension may occur with concurrent use of **diuretics**. Additive hypotension with other **antihypertensives**. ↑ risk of hyperkalemia with concurrent use of **potassium supplements, potassium-containing salt substitutes, angiotensin II receptor antagonists**, and **potassium-sparing diuretics**. Antihypertensive response may be blunted by **NSAIDs**. ↑ levels and may increase the risk of **lithium** toxicity.

Route/Dosage

Hypertension

PO (Adults): 4 mg once daily; may be slowly increased up to 16 mg/day in 1–2 divided doses (should not exceed 8 mg/day in elderly patients) (initiate therapy at 2–4 mg/day (in 1–2 divided doses) in patients receiving diuretics).

Stable Coronary Artery Disease

PO (Adults): 4 mg once daily for 2 wk; may be increased, if tolerated, to 8 mg once daily. *Elderly patients*—2 mg once daily for 1 wk; may be increased, if tolerated, to 4 mg once daily for 1 wk; then, increase as tolerated to 8 mg once daily.

Renal Impairment

PO (Adults): *CCr 30–60 mL/min*—Initiate therapy at 2 mg once daily, may be slowly titrated up to 8 mg/day in 1–2 divided doses.

Availability

Tablets: 2 mg, 4 mg, 8 mg.

permethrin (per-meth-rin)

Acticin, Elimite, Nix

Classification
Therapeutic: pediculicides

Indications

1% lotion: Eradication of *Pediculus humanus capitis* (head lice and their eggs): Prevention of infestation of head lice during epidemics. **5% cream:** Eradication of *Sarcoptes scabiei* (scabies).

Action

Causes repolarization and paralysis in lice by disrupting sodium transport in normal nerve cells.
Therapeutic Effects: Death of parasites.

Adverse Reactions/Side Effects

Derm: burning, itching, rash, redness, stinging, swelling. **Neuro:** numbness, tingling.

PHYSICAL THERAPY IMPLICATIONS

Examination and Evaluation

- Monitor symptoms such as itching scalp to help document drug effectiveness.

Interventions

- Avoid contact with infected areas or wear protective gloves when treating patient.
- Always wash hands thoroughly and disinfect bedding and equipment (whirlpools, electrotherapeutic devices, treatment tables, and so forth) to help prevent the spread of infection.

Patient/Client-Related Instruction

- Advise patient to report any increased local sensitivity to this drug (pain, burning, itching, stinging, swelling, numbness, tingling).
- Instruct patient about proper hygiene; e.g., clean or discard infected clothing, not share combs and hats with others, thoroughly wash and dry the scalp, and so forth.
- Advise patient to apply the drug as directed; that is, apply the drug topically for the recommended period of time before washing off.

Pharmacokinetics

Absorption: Small amounts (<2%) systemically absorbed. Remains on hair for 10 days.
Distribution: Unknown.

Metabolism and Excretion: Rapidly inactivated by enzymes.
Half-life: Unknown.

TIME/ACTION PROFILE (pediculicidal action)

ROUTE	ONSET	PEAK	DURATION
topical	10 min	unknown	14 days

Contraindications/Precautions

Contraindicated in: Hypersensitivity to permethrin, pyrethrins (insecticides or veterinary pesticides), chrysanthemums, or isopropyl alcohol.
Use Cautiously in: Pregnancy or lactation; Children <2 yr (1% lotion); Children <2 mo (5% cream).

Interactions

Drug-Drug: No significant interactions.

Route/Dosage

Head Lice (Treatment and Prevention)

Topical (Adults and Children >2 yr): 1% lotion applied to the hair, left on for 10 min, then rinsed, for 1 application.

Scabies

Topical (Adults and Children): Massage 5% cream into all skin surfaces. Leave on for 8–14 hr, then wash off.
Topical (Infants >2 mo): Massage 5% cream into hairline, scalp, neck, temple, and forehead. Leave on for 8–14 hr, then wash off.

Availability (generic available)

Liquid cream rinse (lotion): 1% in 60-mL containers OTC. **Cream:** 5% in 60-g tube.

perphenazine (per-fen-a-zeen)

Apo-Perphenazine, PMS Perphenazine, Trilafon

Classification
Therapeutic: antiemetics, antipsychotics (conventional)
Pharmacologic: phenothiazines

Indications

Schizophrenia. Nausea and vomiting. **Unlabeled Use:** Other psychotic disorders, bipolar disorder. Treatment of intractable hiccups (IV only).

Action

Alters the effects of dopamine in the CNS. Possesses significant anticholinergic and alpha-adrenergic blocking activity. Blocks dopamine in the chemoreceptor trigger zone (CTZ). **Therapeutic Effects:** Diminished signs and symptoms of psychoses. Decreased nausea, vomiting, or hiccups.

Adverse Reactions/Side Effects

CNS: NEUROLEPTIC MALIGNANT SYNDROME, extrapyramidal reactions, sedation, tardive dyskinesia. **EENT:** blurred vision, dry eyes, lens opacities. **CV:** hypotension, tachycardia. **GI:** constipation, dry mouth, anorexia, ileus, weight gain. **GU:** discoloration of urine, urinary retention. **Derm:** photosensitivity, pigment changes, rashes. **Endo:** galactorrhea, amenorrhea. **Hemat:** AGRANULOCYTOSIS, leukopenia. **Metab:** hyperthermia. **Misc:** allergic reactions.

PHYSICAL THERAPY IMPLICATIONS

Examination and Evaluation

- Monitor and report signs of neuroleptic malignant syndrome (hyperthermia, diaphoresis, generalized muscle rigidity, altered mental status, tachycardia, changes in blood pressure [BP], incontinence). Symptoms typically occur within 4–14 days after initiation of drug therapy, but can occur at any time during drug use.
- Watch for signs of agranulocytosis and leukopenia, including fever, sore throat, mucosal lesions, and other signs of infection. Report these signs to the physician or nursing staff immediately.
- Assess motor function, and be alert for extrapyramidal symptoms. Report these symptoms immediately, especially tardive dyskinesia, because this problem may be irreversible. Common extrapyramidal symptoms include:
  - Tardive dyskinesia (uncontrolled rhythmic movement of mouth, face, and extremities, lip smacking or puckering, puffing of cheeks, uncontrolled chewing, rapid or worm-like movements of tongue).
  - Pseudoparkinsonism (shuffling gait, rigidity, tremor, pill-rolling motion, loss of balance control, difficulty speaking or swallowing, mask-like face).
  - Akathisia (restlessness or desire to keep moving).
  - Other dystonias and dyskinesias (dystonic muscle spasms, twisting motions, twitching, inability to move eyes, weakness of arms or legs).
- Monitor signs of hypersensitivity reactions, including pulmonary symptoms (laryngeal edema, wheezing, dyspnea) or skin reactions (rash, pruritus, urticaria). Notify physician or nursing staff immediately if these reactions occur.
- Assess BP periodically and compare to normal values (See Appendix F). Report low BP (hypotension), especially if patient experiences dizziness or syncope.
- Assess heart rate, ECG, and heart sounds, especially during exercise (See Appendices G, H). Report a rapid heart rate (tachycardia) or signs of other arrhythmias, including palpitations, chest discomfort, shortness of breath, fainting, and fatigue/weakness.

- If used to control nausea and vomiting, monitor the frequency, severity, and duration of GI problems to help document drug effectiveness.
- Periodically assess body weight and other anthropometric measures (body mass index, body composition). Report a rapid or unexplained weight gain or increased body fat.

Interventions

- Guard against falls and trauma (hip fractures, head injury, and so forth) caused by drowsiness, blurred vision, or extrapyramidal symptoms; implement fall-prevention strategies (See Appendix E).
- Because of the risk of tachycardia and abnormal BP responses, use caution during aerobic exercise and other forms of therapeutic exercise. Assess exercise tolerance frequently (BP, heart rate, fatigue levels), and terminate exercise immediately if any untoward responses occur (See Appendix L).
- To minimize orthostatic hypotension, patient should move slowly when assuming a more upright position.
- This drug impairs body temperature regulation; use care during exercise, and during other activities that increase body temperature (hot whirlpools, saunas, and so forth).
- Causes photosensitivity; use care if administering UV treatments. Advise patient to avoid direct sunlight and use sunscreens and protective clothing.
- Help patient and family/caregivers explore nonpharmacologic methods (exercise, counseling, support groups) to reduce schizophrenic episodes and behavioral problems.

Patient/Client-Related Instruction

- Advise patient to avoid alcohol and other CNS depressants because of the increased risk of sedation and adverse effects.
- Instruct patient to report other problematic side effects such as severe or prolonged blurred vision, excessive sedation, dry eyes, vision problems, urinary retention, nipple discharge, menstrual disturbances, skin reactions (rash, changes in pigmentation), or GI problems (constipation, dry mouth, loss of appetite).

Pharmacokinetics

Absorption: Absorption from tablet is poor (approximately 20%) and variable; may be better with oral liquid formulations; well absorbed following IM administration.
Distribution: Widely distributed; high concentrations in the CNS; crosses the placenta and enters breast milk.
Protein Binding: ≥90%.
Metabolism and Excretion: Highly metabolized by the liver and GI mucosa; some conversion to active compounds.
Half-life: 8.4–12.3 hr.

TIME/ACTION PROFILE (PO, IM = antipsychotic effect*; IV = antiemetic effect)

ROUTE	ONSET	PEAK	DURATION
PO	2–6 hr	unknown	6–12 hr
IM	2–6 hr	unknown	6–12 hr
IV	rapid	unknown	unknown

*Optimal antipsychotic response may not occur for several weeks.

Contraindications/Precautions

Contraindicated in: Hypersensitivity (cross-sensitivity with other phenothiazines may occur); Hypersensitivity to bisulfites (injection only); Known alcohol intolerance (concentrate only); Angle-closure glaucoma; Preexisting bone marrow depression or blood dyscrasias; Severe liver or cardiovascular disease; Intestinal obstruction; Lactation: Recommend discontinue drug or bottle-feed.
Use Cautiously in: Geri: Geriatric, emaciated, or debilitated patients ($\frac{1}{2}$–$\frac{1}{3}$ of usual initial dose recommended); ↑ risk of mortality in elderly patients treated for dementia-related psychosis; Diabetes mellitus; Respiratory disease; Prostatic hyperplasia; CNS tumors; History of seizure disorder; OB/Pedi: Safety not established.

Interactions

Drug-Drug: Additive hypotension with **antihypertensives**, acute ingestion of **alcohol,** or **nitrates**. Additive CNS depression with **MAO inhibitors** or other **CNS depressants**, including **alcohol, antihistamines, opioid analgesics, sedative/hypnotics**, and **general anesthetics**. Additive anticholinergic effects with other **drugs possessing anticholinergic properties,** including **antihistamines, antidepressants, atropine, disopyramide, haloperidol**, and **other phenothiazines**. Hypotension and tachycardia may occur with **epinephrine**. ↑ risk of agranulocytosis with other agents that cause bone marrow suppression, including **antithyroid agents**. ↑ risk of extrapyramidal reactions with **lithium**. May mask **lithium** toxicity. **Antacids** or **lithium** may ↓ absorption of perphenazine. May ↓ antiparkinson effect of **levodopa** or **bromocriptine**.
Drug-Natural: ↑ anticholinergic effects with **angel's trumpet, jimson weed**, and **scopolia**.

Route/Dosage

PO (Adults): *Schizophrenia*—2–16 mg bid–qid (not to exceed 64 mg/day). *Nausea/vomiting*—8–16 mg/day in divided doses (not to exceed 24 mg/day).

IM (Adults): *Psychoses*—5–10 mg initially; may repeat q 6 hr (not to exceed 15–30 mg/day). *Nausea/vomiting*—5 mg initially; may be increased to 10 mg if needed.
IV (Adults): *Severe nausea/vomiting/hiccups*—1 mg at 1- to 2-min intervals to a total of 5 mg or as an infusion at a rate not to exceed 0.5 mg/min (not to exceed 5 mg total dose).

Availability (generic available)

Tablets: 2 mg, 4 mg, 8 mg, 16 mg. **Syrup:** 2 mg/5 mL. **Oral concentrate:** 16 mg/5 mL. **Injection:** 5 mg/mL in 1-mL ampules. ***In combination with:*** amitriptyline (Etrafon, Triavil). See Appendix B.

phenazopyridine

(fen-az-oh-**peer**-i-deen)

Azo-Standard, Baridium, Geridium, Phenazo, Prodium, Pyridiate, Pyridium, Pyridium Plus, Urodine, Urogesic, UTI Relief

Classification
Therapeutic: nonopioid analgesics
Pharmacologic: urinary tract analgesics

Indications

Provides relief from the following urinary tract symptoms, which may occur in association with infection or following urologic procedures: Pain, Itching, Burning, Urgency, Frequency.

Action

Acts locally on the urinary tract mucosa to produce analgesic or local anesthetic effects. Has no antimicrobial activity. **Therapeutic Effects:** Diminished urinary tract discomfort.

Adverse Reactions/Side Effects

CNS: headache, vertigo. **GI:** hepatotoxicity, nausea. **GU:** bright-orange urine, renal failure. **Derm:** rash. **Hemat:** hemolytic anemia, methemoglobinemia.

PHYSICAL THERAPY IMPLICATIONS

Examination and Evaluation

- Be alert for signs of liver toxicity, including anorexia, abdominal pain, severe nausea and vomiting, yellow skin or eyes, skin rashes, flu-like symptoms, and muscle/joint pain. Report these signs to the physician immediately.
- Monitor signs of hemolytic anemia (unusual fatigue, shortness of breath, dizziness, headache, pale skin, chest pain, coldness in hands and feet) and methemoglobinemia (bluish coloring of the skin, lips fingernails; headache; shortness of breath; lack of energy). Notify physician immediately if these signs occur.
- Monitor signs of renal failure, including decreased urine output, increased blood pressure, muscle cramps/twitching, edema/weight gain from fluid retention, yellowish brown skin, and confusion that progresses to seizures and coma. Report these signs to the physician immediately.
- Assess pain and other urinary tract symptoms (burning, itching, urinary frequency) to document whether this drug is successful in helping manage the patient's pain.
- Assess vertigo that might affect gait, balance, and other functional activities. Report balance problems and functional limitations to the physician and nursing staff, and caution the patient and family/caregivers to guard against falls and trauma.

Patient/Client-Related Instruction

- Instruct patient and family/caregivers to report other troublesome side effects such as severe or prolonged headache, nausea, or skin rash.

Pharmacokinetics

Absorption: Appears to be well absorbed following oral administration.
Distribution: Unknown. Small amounts cross the placenta.
Metabolism and Excretion: Rapidly excreted unchanged in the urine.
Half-life: Unknown.

TIME/ACTION PROFILE (urinary analgesia)

ROUTE	ONSET	PEAK	DURATION
PO	unknown	5–6 hr	6–8 hr

Contraindications/Precautions

Contraindicated in: Hypersensitivity; Glomerulonephritis; Severe hepatitis, uremia, or renal failure; Renal insufficiency; G6PD deficiency.
Use Cautiously in: Hepatitis; Pregnancy or lactation (safety not established).

Interactions

Drug-Drug: None significant.

Route/Dosage

PO (Adults): 200 mg tid for 2 days.
PO (Children): 4 mg/kg tid for 2 days.

Availability (generic available)

Tablets: 95 mg OTC, 100 mg, 100 mg OTC, 200 mg OTC, 200 mg.

phenelzine (fen-el-zeen)
Nardil

Classification
Therapeutic: antidepressants
Pharmacologic: monoamine oxidase (MAO) inhibitors

Indications

Treatment of neurotic or atypical depression (usually reserved for patients who do not tolerate or respond to other modes of therapy [e.g., tricyclic antidepressants, SSRIs, SSNRIs, or electroconvulsive therapy]).

Action

Inhibits the enzyme monoamine oxidase, resulting in an accumulation of various neurotransmitters (dopamine, epinephrine, norepinephrine, and serotonin) in the body. **Therapeutic Effects:** Improved mood in depressed patients.

Adverse Reactions/Side Effects

CNS: SEIZURES, dizziness, drowsiness, fatigue, headache, hyperreflexia, insomnia, tremor, twitching, weakness, euphoria, paresthesia, restlessness. **EENT:** blurred vision, glaucoma, nystagmus. **CV:** HYPERTENSIVE CRISIS, edema, orthostatic hypotension. **GI:** constipation, dry mouth, abdominal pain, liver function test elevation, nausea, vomiting. **GU:** sexual dysfunction, urinary retention. **Derm:** pruritus, rashes. **F and E:** hypernatremia. **Endo:** weight gain.

PHYSICAL THERAPY IMPLICATIONS

Examination and Evaluation

- Be alert for new seizures or increased seizure activity, especially at the onset of drug treatment. Document the number, duration, and severity of seizures, and report these findings immediately to the physician.
- Measure blood pressure (BP) periodically and compare to normal values (See Appendix F). Immediately report a large, rapid increase in BP (hypertensive crisis). Signs and symptoms of hypertensive crisis include chest pain, tachycardia or bradycardia, severe headache, nausea, vomiting, neck stiffness, sweating, and enlarged pupils. The risk of hypertensive crisis is increased when this drug is taken with other antidepressants, excessive caffeine, other drugs that increase BP, or foods that contain tyramine (e.g., fermented wines, cheeses).
- Be alert for increased depression and suicidal thoughts and ideology, especially when initiating drug treatment or in children and teenagers. Notify physician or mental health professional immediately if patient exhibits worsening depression.
- Be alert for anxiety, euphoria, severe restlessness, or other alterations in mental status. Notify health care professional if these symptoms become problematic.
- Assess BP when patient assumes a more upright position (lying to standing, sitting to standing, lying to sitting). Document orthostatic hypotension and contact physician when systolic BP falls >20 mm Hg or diastolic BP falls >10 mm Hg.
- Assess peripheral edema using girth measurements, volume displacement, and measurement of pitting edema (See Appendix N). Report increased swelling in feet and ankles or a sudden increase in body weight due to sodium retention (hypernatremia) and fluid retention.
- Assess paresthesias (numbness, tingling), tremor, or increased reflex activity. Perform objective tests including electroneuromyography and sensory testing to document any drug-related neuropathic changes.
- Assess dizziness and drowsiness that might affect gait, balance, and other functional activities (See Appendix C). Report balance problems and functional limitations to the physician, and caution the patient and family/caregivers to guard against falls and trauma.
- Periodically assess body weight and other anthropometric measures (body mass index, body composition). Report a rapid or unexplained weight gain.

Interventions

- Guard against falls and trauma (hip fractures, head injury, and so forth), and implement fall prevention strategies in patients with dizziness, blurred vision, or other conditions that affect balance (See Appendix E).
- To minimize orthostatic hypotension, patient should move slowly when assuming a more upright position.
- Help patient explore nonpharmacologic methods to reduce depression (exercise, counseling, support groups, and so forth).

Patient/Client-Related Instruction

- Advise patient that antidepressant effects may not occur immediately; it may take 2 wk or more before an improvement in mood is observed.
- Advise patient to avoid alcohol and other CNS depressants because of the increased risk of sedation and adverse effects.
- Instruct patient to report other troublesome side effects such as severe or prolonged headache, sleep loss, vision disturbances, sexual dysfunction, urinary retention, skin reactions (rash, itching), or GI problems (nausea, vomiting, constipation, dry mouth, abdominal pain).

Pharmacokinetics

Absorption: Well absorbed from the GI tract.
Distribution: Crosses the placenta and probably enters breast milk.
Metabolism and Excretion: Metabolized by the liver; excreted in urine as metabolites and unchanged drug.
Half-life: 12 hr.

TIME/ACTION PROFILE (antidepressant effect)

ROUTE	ONSET	PEAK	DURATION
PO	2–4 wk	3–6 wk	2 wk

Contraindications/Precautions

Contraindicated in: Hypersensitivity; Liver disease; Severe renal disease; Pheochromocytoma; Heart failure; Patients undergoing elective surgery requiring general anesthesia (should be discontinued at least 10 days before surgery); Excessive consumption of caffeine; Concurrent use of meperidine, SSRI antidepressants, SSNRI antidepressants, tricyclic antidepressants, tetracyclic antidepressants, nefazodone, trazodone, procarbazine, selegiline, linezolid, carbamazepine, cyclobenzaprine, bupropion, buspirone, sympathomimetics, other MAO inhibitors, dextromethorphan, narcotics, alcohol, general anesthetics, diuretics, or tryptophan; Concurrent use of foods containing high concentrations of tyramine (see Appendix L); Lactation.
Use Cautiously in: Patients who may be suicidal or have a history of drug dependency; Pedi: May ↑ risk of suicide attempt/ideation, especially during first 1–2 mo of treatment or with dose adjustments; Schizophrenia; Bipolar disorder; Seizure disorders; Diabetes (↑ risk of hypoglycemia); Geri: Geriatric patients (↑ risk of adverse reactions); Pregnancy (safety not established); Children (safety and effectiveness not established).

Interactions

Drug-Drug: Serious, potentially fatal adverse reactions may occur with concurrent use of other **antidepressants (SSRIs, SSNRIs, bupropion, tricyclics, tetracyclics, nefazodone, trazodone), carbamazepine, cyclobenzaprine, sibutramine, procarbazine,** or **selegiline**. Avoid using within 2 wk of each other (wait 5 wk from end of **fluoxetine** therapy). Hypertensive crisis may occur with **amphetamines, methyldopa, levodopa, dopamine, epinephrine, norepinephrine, reserpine, methylphenidate,** or **vasoconstrictors**. Hypertension or hypotension, coma, seizures, respiratory depression, and death may occur with **meperidine** (avoid using within 2–3 wk of MAO inhibitor therapy). Concurrent use with **dextromethorphan** may produce psychosis or bizarre behavior. Hypertension may occur with concurrent use of **buspirone**; avoid using within 2 wk of each other. Additive hypotension may occur with **antihypertensives, spinal anesthesia, opioids,** or **barbiturates**. Additive hypoglycemia may occur with **insulins** or **oral hypoglycemic agents**. Risk of seizures may be ↑ with **tramadol**.
Drug-Natural: Serious, potentially fatal adverse effects (serotonin syndrome) may occur with concomitant use of **St. John's wort** and **SAMe**. Hypertensive crises may occur with large amounts of **caffeine**-containing herbs (**cola nut, guarana,** or **malt**). Insomnia, headache, tremor, hypomania may occur with **ginseng**. Hypertensive crises, disorientation, and memory impairment may occur with **tryptophan** or supplements containing **tyrosine** or **phenylalanine**.
Drug-Food: Hypertensive crisis may occur with ingestion of foods containing high concentrations of **tyramine** (see Appendix L). Consumption of foods or beverages with high **caffeine** content increases the risk of hypertension and arrhythmias.

Route/Dosage

PO (Adults): 15 mg tid; increase to 60–90 mg/day in divided doses; after maximal benefit achieved, gradually reduce to smallest effective dose (15 mg/day or every other day).

Availability

Tablets: 15 mg Rx.

phenobarbital
(fee-noe-**bar**-bi-tal)
✱ Ancalixir, Luminal, Solfoton

Classification
Therapeutic: anticonvulsants, sedative/hypnotics
Pharmacologic: barbiturates

Schedule IV

Indications

Anticonvulsant in tonic-clonic (grand mal), partial, and febrile seizures in children. Preoperative sedative and in other situations in which sedation may be required. Hypnotic (short-term). **Unlabeled Use:** Prevention/treatment of hyperbilirubinemia in neonates.

Action

Produces all levels of CNS depression. Depresses the sensory cortex, decreases motor activity, and alters cerebellar function. Inhibits transmission in the nervous system and raises the seizure threshold. Capable of inducing (speeding up) enzymes in the liver that metabolize drugs, bilirubin, and other compounds. **Therapeutic Effects:** Anticonvulsant activity. Sedation.

Adverse Reactions/Side Effects

CNS: hangover, delirium, depression, drowsiness, excitation, lethargy, vertigo. **Resp:** respiratory depression. **IV:** LARYNGOSPASM, bronchospasm. **CV: IV:** hypotension. **GI:** constipation, diarrhea, nausea, vomiting. **Derm:** photosensitivity, rashes, urticaria. **Local:** phlebitis at IV site. **MS:** arthralgia, myalgia, neuralgia. **Misc:** HYPERSENSITIVITY REACTIONS, INCLUDING ANGIOEDEMA AND SERUM SICKNESS, physical dependence, psychological dependence.

PHYSICAL THERAPY IMPLICATIONS

Examination and Evaluation

- Monitor signs of hypersensitivity reactions, including skin problems (rashes, raised patches of red or white skin, burning/itching skin), fever, swelling in the face, difficulty breathing, muscle aches (myalgia), and joint pain (arthralgia). Notify physician or nursing staff immediately because these symptoms may indicate serious reactions such as angioedema and serum sickness.
- Assess symptoms of bronchospasm and laryngospasm (wheezing, coughing, tightness in chest), especially after IV administration. Perform pulmonary function tests (See Appendices I, J, K) to document suspected changes in ventilation and respiratory function, or if patient exhibits signs of respiratory depression (dyspnea, hypoxia).
- Monitor daytime drowsiness and "hangover" symptoms (headache, nausea, irritability, dysphoria, lethargy, vertigo). Repeated or excessive symptoms may require change in dose or medication.
- Be alert for depression, delirium, excitation, or other alterations in mood or behavior. Notify physician promptly if these symptoms develop (See Appendix D).
- In patients with seizures, document the number, duration, and severity of seizures to help document antiseizure drug effects.
- Assess blood pressure after IV administration and compare to normal values (See Appendix F). Report low blood pressure (hypotension), especially if patient experiences dizziness or syncope.
- Assess IV injection site, and report excessive or prolonged local pain, swelling, and inflammation.

Interventions

- Guard against falls and trauma (hip fractures, head injury, and so forth), especially if drowsiness and vertigo carry over into the daytime. Implement fall-prevention strategies, especially if balance is impaired (See Appendix E).
- If treating insomnia, help patient explore nonpharmacologic methods to induce sleep, such as relaxation techniques, reduced caffeine intake, and so forth.
- Causes photosensitivity; use care if administering UV treatments. Advise patient to avoid direct sunlight and use sunscreens and protective clothing.

Patient/Client-Related Instruction

- Advise patient to avoid alcohol and other CNS depressants because of the increased risk of sedation and adverse effects.
- When treating insomnia, remind patient that this drug is typically recommended for only short-term use (2 wk or less). Long-term use can cause tolerance and physical/psychologic dependence.
- Advise patients on prolonged (antiseizure) therapy not to discontinue medication without consulting their physician. Abrupt withdrawal may cause increased seizures.
- Instruct patient or family/caregivers to report other troublesome side effects such as severe or prolonged skin reactions (rash, hives) or GI problems (nausea, vomiting, diarrhea, constipation).

P

Pharmacokinetics

Absorption: Absorption is slow but relatively complete (70–90%).
Distribution: Unknown.
Metabolism and Excretion: 75% metabolized by the liver, 25% excreted unchanged by the kidneys.
Half-life: Neonates: 1.8–8.3 days; Infants: 0.8–5.5 days; Children: 1.5–3 days; Adults: 2–6 days.

TIME/ACTION PROFILE (sedation*)

ROUTE	ONSET	PEAK	DURATION
PO	30–60 min	unknown	>6 hr
IM, SC	10–30 min	unknown	4–6 hr
IV	5 min	30 min	4–6 hr

*Full anticonvulsant effects occur after 2–3 wk of chronic dosing unless a loading dose has been used.

Contraindications/Precautions

Contraindicated in: Hypersensitivity; Comatose patients or those with preexisting CNS depression; Severe respiratory disease with dyspnea or obstruction; Uncontrolled severe pain; Known alcohol intolerance (elixir only); Lactation: Discontinue drug or bottle-feed.
Use Cautiously in: Hepatic dysfunction; Severe renal impairment; History of suicide attempt or drug abuse; Hypnotic use should be short-term. Chronic use may lead to dependence; OB: Chronic use during pregnancy results in drug dependency in the infant; may result in coagulation defects and fetal malformation; acute use at term may result in respiratory depression in the newborn; Geri: Initial dose reduction recommended;

Hypnotic use should be short term. Chronic use may lead to dependence.

Interactions

Drug-Drug: Additive CNS depression with other **CNS depressants**, including **alcohol, antihistamines, opioid analgesics**, and other **sedative/hypnotics**. May induce hepatic enzymes that metabolize other drugs, ↓ their effectiveness, including **hormonal contraceptives, warfarin, chloramphenicol, cyclosporine, dacarbazine, corticosteroids, tricyclic antidepressants, felodipine, clonazepam, carbamazepine, verapamil, theophylline, metronidazole**, and **quinidine**. May ↑ risk of hepatic toxicity of **acetaminophen. MAO inhibitors, valproic acid**, or **divalproex** may ↓ metabolism of phenobarbital, ↑ sedation. **Rifampin** may ↑ metabolism of and ↓ effects of phenobarbital. May ↑ risk of hematologic toxicity with **cyclophosphamide**.
Drug-Natural: Concomitant use of **kava, valerian, chamomile, or hops** can ↑ CNS depression. **St. John's wort** may ↓ effects.

Route/Dosage

Status Epilepticus

IV (Adults and Children >1 mo): 15–18 mg/kg in a single or divided dose, maximum loading dose 20 mg/kg.
IV (Neonates): 15–20 mg/kg in a single or divided dose.

Maintenance Anticonvulsant

IV, PO (Adults and Children >12 yr): 1–3 mg/kg/day as a single dose or 2 divided doses.
IV, PO (Children 5–12 yr): 4–6 mg/kg/day in 1–2 divided doses.
IV, PO (Children 1–5 yr): 6–8 mg/kg/day in 1–2 divided doses.
IV, PO (Infants): 5–6 mg/kg/day in 1–2 divided doses.
IV, PO (Neonates): 3–4 mg/kg/day once daily; may need to increase up to 5 mg/kg/day by 2nd week of therapy.

Sedation

PO, IM (Adults): 30–120 mg/day in 2–3 divided doses. *Preoperative sedation*—100–200 mg IM 1–1.5 hr before the procedure.
PO (Children): 2 mg/kg 3 times daily. *Preoperative sedation*—1–3 mg/kg PO/IM/IV 1–1.5 hr before the procedure.

Hypnotic

PO, SC, IV, IM (Adults): 100–320 mg at bedtime.
IV, IM, SC (Children): 3–5 mg/kg at bedtime.

Hyperbilirubinemia

PO (Adults): 90–180 mg/day in 2–3 divided doses.
PO (Children <12 yr): 3–8 mg/kg/day in 2–3 divided doses, doses up to 12 mg/kg/day have been used.

Availability (generic available)

Tablets: 8 mg, 15 mg, 30 mg, 60 mg, 100 mg. **Capsules:** 15 mg. **Elixir:** 20 mg/5 mL. **Injection:** 30 mg/mL in 1-mL prefilled syringes, 60 mg/mL in 1-mL prefilled syringes, 65 mg/mL in 1-mL vials, 130 mg/mL in 1-mL prefilled syringes, 1-mL vials, and 1-mL ampules. ***In combination with:*** phenytoin. See Appendix B.

phentermine (fen-ter-meen)

Adipex-P, Banobese, Fastin, Ionamin, Obi-Nix, OBY-CAP, Phentercot, Phentride, T-Diet, Teramine, Zantryl

Classification
Therapeutic: weight control agents
Pharmacologic: appetite suppressants

Schedule IV

Indications

Short-term treatment of obesity in conjunction with other interventions (dietary restriction, exercise); used to produce and maintain weight loss in patients with a BMI ≥30 kg/m^2 or ≥27 kg/m^2 in the presence of other risk factors (diabetes, hypertension, hyperlipidemia).

Action

Decreases hunger by altering the chemical control of nerve impulse transmission in the appetite control center of the hypothalamus. **Therapeutic Effects:** Appetite suppression with resultant weight loss.

Adverse Reactions/Side Effects

CNS: CNS stimulation, confusion, dizziness, dysphoria, euphoria, headache, insomnia, mental depression, restlessness. **EENT:** blurred vision. **CV:** hypertension, palpitations, tachycardia. **GI:** constipation, diarrhea, dry mouth, nausea, unpleasant taste, vomiting. **GU:** changes in libido, erectile dysfunction.

PHYSICAL THERAPY IMPLICATIONS

Examination and Evaluation

- Periodically assess body weight and other anthropometric measures (body mass index, body composition) to document whether drug therapy is successful in promoting weight loss.
- Be alert for signs of excessive CNS effects, including hyperactivity, restlessness, tremor, confusion, hallucinations, depression, or other changes in mood and behavior. Report these signs to the physician.
- Assess heart rate, ECG, and heart sounds, especially during exercise (See Appendices G, H). Report fast heart rate (tachycardia), or symptoms of other arrhythmias, including palpitations, chest

discomfort, shortness of breath, fainting, and fatigue/weakness.

- Assess blood pressure (BP) and compare to normal values (See Appendix F). Report a sustained increase in BP (hypertension).
- Assess dizziness that might affect gait, balance, and other functional activities (See Appendix C). Report balance problems and functional limitations to the physician, and caution the patient and family/caregivers to guard against falls and trauma.

Interventions

- Because of the risk of arrhythmias and abnormal BP responses, use caution during aerobic exercise and other forms of therapeutic exercise. Assess exercise tolerance frequently (BP, heart rate, fatigue levels), and terminate exercise immediately if any untoward responses occur (See Appendix L).

Patient/Client-Related Instruction

- Make sure the patient has discussed use of this drug with his/her physician. Advise patient about the potential cardiac and CNS risks, and counsel patient about other interventions (diet, exercise) that can help achieve and maintain weight loss.
- Instruct patient and family/caregivers to report other troublesome side effects, including severe or prolonged headache, blurred vision, sleep loss, sexual problems (changes in libido, erectile dysfunction), or GI problems (nausea, vomiting, constipation, diarrhea, unpleasant taste, dry mouth).

Pharmacokinetics

Absorption: Unknown.
Distribution: Unknown.
Metabolism and Excretion: Metabolized by the liver.
Half-life: 19–24 hr.

TIME/ACTION PROFILE (appetite suppression)

ROUTE	ONSET	PEAK	DURATION
PO—hydrochloride	unknown	unknown	4 hr*
PO—resin complex	unknown	unknown	12–14 hr

*For 8-mg tablets, increase to 12–14 hr for 30-mg capsules or 37.5-mg tablets.

Contraindications/Precautions

Contraindicated in: Hypersensitivity or known intolerance to sympathomimetic amines; Cardiovascular disease; Hyperthyroidism; Moderate-to-severe hypertension; History of drug abuse; Agitation; Glaucoma; Concurrent or recent (within 14 days) MAO inhibitor therapy; Concurrent SSRI antidepressants.
Use Cautiously in: Mild hypertension; Diabetes mellitus; Pregnancy, lactation, or children <12 yr (safety not established).

Interactions

Drug-Drug: Concurrent use with **MAO inhibitors** may result in hypertensive crisis (do not use within 14 days of MAO inhibitors). ↑ risk of adverse CNS events with **alcohol**. Concurrent use with **SSRI antidepressants** is not recommended. May ↓ **insulin** requirements in diabetic patients.

Route/Dosage

PO (Adults): *Phentermine hydrochloride tablets or capsules*—8 mg tid or 15–37.5 mg once daily; *Phentermine resin complex capsules*—15–30 mg once daily.

Availability (generic available)

Phentermine hydrochloride tablets: 8 mg, 37.5 mg. **Phentermine hydrochloride capsules:** 15 mg, 18.75 mg, 30 mg, 37.5 mg. **Phentermine resin complex capsules:** 15 mg, 30 mg.

P

phentolamine (fen-tole-a-meen)

Regitine, ✤Rogitine

Classification
Therapeutic: agents for pheochromocytoma
Pharmacologic: alpha-adrenergic blockers

Indications

IV: Control of blood pressure during surgical removal of a pheochromocytoma. **IV, Infiltration:** Prevention and treatment of dermal necrosis and sloughing following extravasation of norepinephrine, phenylephrine, or dopamine. **Unlabeled Use: IM, IV:** Treatment of hypertension associated with pheochromocytoma or adrenergic (sympathetic) excess, such as administration of phenylephrine, tyramine-containing foods in patients on MAO inhibitor therapy, or clonidine withdrawal.

Action

Produces incomplete and short-lived blockade of alpha-adrenergic receptors located primarily in smooth muscle and exocrine glands. Induces hypotension by direct relaxation of vascular smooth muscle and by alpha blockade. **Therapeutic Effects:** Reduction of blood pressure in situations in which hypertension is due to adrenergic (sympathetic) excess. When infiltrated locally, reverses vasoconstriction caused by norepinephrine or dopamine.

Adverse Reactions/Side Effects

With parenteral use

CNS: CEREBROVASCULAR SPASM, dizziness, weakness. **EENT:** nasal stuffiness. **CV:** HYPOTENSION, MI, angina, arrhythmias, tachycardia. **GI:** abdominal pain, diarrhea, nausea, vomiting, aggravation of peptic ulcer. **Derm:** flushing.

PHYSICAL THERAPY IMPLICATIONS

Examination and Evaluation

- Continually monitor for signs of MI, including sudden chest pain, pain radiating into the arm or jaw, shortness of breath, dizziness, sweating, anxiety, and nausea. Seek immediate medical assistance if patient develops these signs.
- Be alert for signs of cerebrovascular spasm, including sudden severe headache, confusion, nausea, vomiting, dizziness, paralysis, numbness, speech problems, and visual disturbances. Report these signs to the physician or nursing staff immediately.
- Assess blood pressure (BP) periodically and compare to normal values (See Appendix F). Report low BP (hypotension), especially if patient experiences dizziness, fatigue, or other symptoms.
- Assess heart rate, ECG, and heart sounds, especially during exercise (See Appendices G, H). Report any rhythm disturbances or symptoms of increased arrhythmias, including palpitations, chest pain, shortness of breath, fainting, and fatigue/weakness.

Interventions

- Because of the risk of MI, cerebrovascular spasm, and abnormal BP responses, use extreme caution during aerobic exercise and other forms of therapeutic exercise. Assess exercise tolerance frequently (BP, heart rate, fatigue levels), and terminate exercise immediately if any untoward responses occur (See Appendix L).
- To minimize orthostatic hypotension, patient should move slowly when assuming a more upright position.

Patient/Client-Related Instruction

- Advise patient and family or caregiver about the signs of MI and cerebrovascular spasm (see above under Examination and Evaluation), and to seek immediate medical assistance if these signs develop.
- Instruct patient or family/caregivers to report other bothersome side effects such as severe or prolonged nasal stuffiness, skin reactions (flushing), or GI problems (diarrhea, nausea, vomiting, abdominal pain, peptic ulcer).

Pharmacokinetics

Absorption: Well absorbed following IM administration.
Distribution: Unknown.
Metabolism and Excretion: 10% excreted unchanged by kidneys.
Half-life: Unknown.

TIME/ACTION PROFILE (alpha-adrenergic blockade)

ROUTE	ONSET	PEAK	DURATION
IM	unknown	20 min	30–45 min
IV	immediate	2 min	15–30 min

Contraindications/Precautions

Contraindicated in: Hypersensitivity; Coronary or cerebral arteriosclerosis; Renal impairment.
Use Cautiously in: Peptic ulcer disease; Geri: Geriatric patients (more susceptible to hypotensive effects; dose reduction recommended); OB/Geri: Pregnancy or lactation (safety not established).

Interactions

Drug-Drug: Antagonizes the effects of **alpha-adrenergic stimulants**. May ↓ pressor response to **ephedrine** or **phenylephrine**. Severe hypotension may occur with concurrent use of **epinephrine** or **methoxamine**. Use with **guanadrel** may result in exaggerated hypotension and bradycardia. ↓ peripheral vasoconstriction from high doses of **dopamine**.

Route/Dosage

Hypertension Associated with Pheochromocytoma—Before/During Surgery

IV (Adults): 5 mg given 1–2 hr preoperatively, repeated as necessary. May be infused at a rate of 0.5–1 mg/min during surgery.
IV, IM (Children): 1 mg or 0.1 mg/kg (3 mg/m^2) given 1–2 hr preoperatively, repeated IV as necessary during surgery.

Prevention of Dermal Necrosis During Infusion of Norepinephrine, Phenylephrine, or Dopamine

IV (Adults): Add 10 mg phentolamine to every 1000 mL of fluid containing norepinephrine.

Treatment of Dermal Necrosis Following Extravasation of Norepinephrine, Phenylephrine, or Dopamine

Infiltrate: (Adults): 5–10 mg.
Infiltrate: (Children): 0.1–0.2 mg/kg (up to 10 mg).

Availability (generic available)

Powder for injection: 5 mg/vial.

HIGH ALERT

phenylephrine (fen-il-ef-rin)

Neo-Synephrine

Classification

Therapeutic: vasopressors
Pharmacologic: adrenergics, vasopressors

Indications

Management of hypotension associated with shock that may persist after adequate fluid replacement. Management of hypotension associated with anesthesia. Management of paroxysmal supraventricular tachycardia. **Anesthesia adjunct:** Prolongation of the duration of spinal anesthesia, Localization of the effect of regional anesthesia.

Action

Constricts blood vessels by stimulating alpha-adrenergic receptors. **Therapeutic Effects:** Increased blood pressure. Restoration of normal sinus rhythm.

Adverse Reactions/Side Effects

CNS: anxiety, dizziness, headache, insomnia, nervousness, restlessness, trembling, weakness. **Resp:** dyspnea, respiratory distress. **CV:** ARRHYTHMIAS, bradycardia, chest pain, hypertension, tachycardia, vasoconstriction. **Derm:** blanching, pallor, piloerection, sweating. **Local:** phlebitis, sloughing at IV sites. **Neuro:** tremor.

PHYSICAL THERAPY IMPLICATIONS

Examination and Evaluation

- Assess heart rate, ECG, and heart sounds, especially during exercise (See Appendices G, H). Although intended to treat certain arrhythmias, this drug can unmask or precipitate new arrhythmias (proarrhythmic effect). Report any rhythm disturbances or symptoms of increased arrhythmias, including palpitations, chest pain, shortness of breath, fainting, and fatigue/weakness.
- Assess blood pressure when patient is lying down. Compare to normal values (See Appendix F), and report a sustained increase in blood pressure (hypertension) to the physician.
- Monitor signs of peripheral vasoconstriction, such as extreme coldness in the hands and feet, cyanosis, and muscle cramping. Notify physician of severe or prolonged signs of vasoconstriction.
- Assess symptoms of respiratory distress including dyspnea, shortness of breath, and cyanosis. Monitor pulse oximetry and perform pulmonary function tests (See Appendix I) to quantify suspected changes in ventilation and respiratory function. Excessive respiratory depression requires emergency care.
- Monitor and report signs of CNS toxicity, including nervousness, anxiety, restlessness, sleep loss, and trembling/tremors. Sustained or severe CNS signs may indicate overdose or excessive use of this drug.
- Assess dizziness that might affect gait, balance, and other functional activities (See Appendix C). Report balance problems and functional limitations to the physician and nursing staff, and caution the patient and family/caregivers to guard against falls and trauma.
- Assess administration site and report signs of irritation, skin damage, or phlebitis (local pain, swelling, inflammation).

Interventions

- Because of the risk of cardiovascular stimulation, use caution during aerobic exercise and endurance conditioning. Assess exercise tolerance frequently (blood pressure, heart rate, fatigue levels), and terminate exercise immediately if any untoward responses occur (See Appendix L).
- If used to prolong regional or spinal anesthesia, be sure that sensation has returned to the affected areas before applying manual techniques or physical agents (heat, cold, electrotherapeutic devices).

Patient/Client-Related Instruction

- Instruct patient and family/caregivers to report other troublesome side effects such as severe or prolonged headache or skin reactions (pallor, blanching, increased sweating).

Pharmacokinetics

Absorption: Well absorbed from IM sites.
Distribution: Unknown.
Metabolism and Excretion: Metabolized by the liver and other tissues.
Half-life: 2.5 hr.

TIME/ACTION PROFILE (vasopressor effects)

ROUTE	ONSET	PEAK	DURATION
IV	immediate	unknown	15–20 min
IM	10–15 min	unknown	0.5–2 hr
SC	10–15 min	unknown	50–60 min

Contraindications/Precautions

Contraindicated in: Uncorrected fluid volume deficits; Tachyarrhythmias; Pheochromocytoma; Angle-closure glaucoma; Acute pancreatitis; Hepatitis; Hypersensitivity to bisulfites.
Use Cautiously in: Occlusive vascular diseases; Cardiovascular disease; Diabetes mellitus; OB: Pregnancy and lactation (safety not established).
Exercise Extreme Caution in: Geri: Geriatric patients are more likely to experience adverse reactions, which result in hallucinations, convulsions, CNS depression, and death; Hyperthyroidism; Bradycardia; Partial heart block; Severe cardiovascular disease.

Interactions

Drug-Drug: Use with **general anesthetics** may result in myocardial irritability; use with extreme caution. Use with **MAO inhibitors, ergot alkaloids (ergonovine, methylergonovine), or oxytocics** results in severe hypertension. **Alpha-adrenergic blockers (phentolamine)** may antagonize vasopressor effects. **Atropine** blocks bradycardia from phenylephrine and enhances pressor effects.

Route/Dosage

Hypotension

SC, IM (Adults): 2–5 mg.
SC, IM (Children): 0.1 mg/kg/dose q 1–2 hr as needed; maximum dose 5 mg.
IV (Adults): 0.2 mg (range 0.1–0.5 mg); may be repeated q 10–15 min *or* as an infusion at 100–180 mcg/min initially, 40–60 mcg/min maintenance.
IV (Children): 5–20 mcg/kg/dose q 10–15 min as needed or 0.1–0.5 mcg/kg/min infusion, titrate to effect.

Hypotension During Spinal Anesthesia

SC, IM (Adults): 2–3 mg has been used 3–4 min before spinal anesthesia to prevent hypotension.
IM, SC (Children): 0.5–1 mg/25 lb body weight.
IV (Adults): 0.2 mg; may repeat q 10–15 min and may be increased by 0.1–0.2 mg/dose (not to exceed 0.5 mg/dose).

Antiarrhythmic (PSVT)

IV (Adults): 0.25–0.5 mg over 20–30 sec (single doses not to exceed 1 mg).
IV (Children): 5–10 mcg/kg over 20–30 sec.

Vasoconstrictor for Regional Anesthesia

Local: (Adults): Add 1 mg to every 20 mL of local anesthetic (yields a 1:20,000 solution).

Prolongation of Spinal Anesthesia

Spinal: (Adults): 2–5 mg added to anesthetic solution.

Availability

Injection: 1% (10 mg/mL) in 1-mL ampules.

phenytoin (fen-i-toyn)

Dilantin, Phenytek

Classification
Therapeutic: antiarrhythmics (group IB), anticonvulsants
Pharmacologic: hydantoins

Indications

Treatment/prevention of tonic-clonic (grand mal) seizures and complex partial seizures. **Unlabeled Use:** As an antiarrhythmic, particularly for ventricular arrhythmias associated with digoxin toxicity, prolonged QT interval, and surgical repair of congenital heart diseases in children. Management of neuropathic pain, including trigeminal neuralgia.

Action

Limits seizure propagation by altering ion transport. May also decrease synaptic transmission. Antiarrhythmic properties as a result of shortening the action potential and ↓ automaticity. **Therapeutic Effects:** Diminished seizure activity. Termination of ventricular arrhythmias.

Adverse Reactions/Side Effects

Most listed are for chronic use of phenytoin
CNS: ataxia, agitation, confusion, dizziness, drowsiness, dysarthria, dyskinesia, extrapyramidal syndrome, headache, insomnia, weakness. **EENT:** diplopia, nystagmus. **CV:** hypotension (↑ with IV phenytoin), tachycardia. **GI:** gingival hyperplasia, nausea, constipation, drug-induced hepatitis, vomiting. **Derm:** hypertrichosis, rash, exfoliative dermatitis, pruritus. **Hemat:** AGRANULOCYTOSIS, APLASTIC ANEMIA, leukopenia, megaloblastic anemia, thrombocytopenia. **MS:** osteomalacia. **Misc:** ALLERGIC REACTIONS, INCLUDING STEVENS-JOHNSON SYNDROME, fever, lymphadenopathy.

PHYSICAL THERAPY IMPLICATIONS

Examination and Evaluation

- Be alert for phenytoin hypersensitivity syndrome (fever, skin rash, lymphadenopathy). Rash usually occurs within the first 2 wk of therapy. Hypersensitivity syndrome usually occurs at 3–8 wk but may occur up to 12 wk after initiation of therapy. Report these signs immediately because this syndrome may lead to renal failure, rhabdomyolysis, or hepatic necrosis.
- Monitor other skin reactions (itching/burning skin, hives, exfoliation, dermatitis). Notify physician immediately about because certain skin reactions may indicate serious hypersensitivity reactions (Stevens-Johnson syndrome).
- Be alert for signs of agranulocytosis (fever, sore throat, mucosal lesions, signs of infection), aplastic anemia (unusual fatigue, weakness, dizziness, pallor), thrombocytopenia (bruising, nose bleeds, bleeding gums), or fatigue and poor health that might be due to other anemias and blood dyscrasias. Report these signs to the physician immediately. Periodic blood tests may be needed to monitor WBC and RBC counts.
- Document the number, duration, and severity of seizures to help determine if this drug is effective in reducing seizure activity.
- Assess dizziness that might affect gait, balance, and other functional activities (See Appendix C). Report balance problems and functional limitations to the physician and nursing staff, and caution the patient and family/caregivers to guard against falls and trauma.
- Monitor daytime drowsiness, confusion, or agitation. Repeated or excessive symptoms may require change in dose or medication.
- Assess gait and motor function and document any signs of incoordination, ataxia, or other motor

symptoms that might indicate extrapyramidal syndrome such as involuntary movements of the jaw, limbs, Parkinson-like symptoms, and other dystonias and dyskinesias. Report these signs to the physician.

- If treating neuropathic pain, use visual analogue scales and other appropriate pain scales to assess the patient's pain and help document effects of drug therapy.
- If treating arrhythmias, assess heart rate, ECG, and heart sounds, especially during exercise (See Appendices G, H). Document whether this drug helps reduce ventricular arrhythmias and other rhythm disturbances and decreases the symptoms of arrhythmias (palpitations, chest discomfort, shortness of breath, fainting, fatigue/weakness).
- Assess blood pressure after IV administration and compare to normal values (See Appendix F). Report low blood pressure (hypotension), especially if patient experiences dizziness or syncope.
- Assess any bone pain or muscle weakness that might indicate osteomalacia. Pain typically occurs as a dull ache in the lower spine, pelvis, or legs. Report signs of osteomalacia to the physician for possible treatment (vitamin D supplements, increased exposure to UV light).

Interventions

- Guard against falls and trauma (hip fractures, head injury, and so forth), especially if drowsiness, dizziness, or motor problems (ataxia, dyskinesias) affect gait and balance. Implement fall-prevention strategies, especially if balance is impaired (See Appendix E).
- To minimize orthostatic hypotension, patient should move slowly when assuming a more upright position.
- Because of the risk of tachycardia and other arrhythmias, use caution during aerobic exercise and other forms of therapeutic exercise. Assess exercise tolerance frequently (blood pressure, heart rate, fatigue levels), and terminate exercise immediately if any untoward responses occur (See Appendix L).

Patient/Client-Related Instruction

- Advise patient to avoid alcohol and other CNS depressants because of the increased risk of sedation and adverse effects.
- Advise patients on prolonged antiseizure therapy not to discontinue medication without consulting their physician. Abrupt withdrawal may cause increased seizures.
- Advise patient about the risk of daytime drowsiness and decreased attention and mental focus. Use care if driving or in other activities that require strong concentration and fast responses.
- Advise patient about the likelihood of GI reactions such as constipation and vomiting. Instruct patient to report severe or prolonged GI problems or signs of drug-induced hepatitis, including yellow skin or eyes, abdominal pain, severe nausea and vomiting, fever, sore throat, malaise, weakness, and facial edema.
- Encourage patient and family/caregivers to perform rigorous oral hygiene and teeth cleansing to reduce gingival hyperplasia.
- Instruct patient and family/caregivers to report other troublesome side effects such as severe or prolonged headache, insomnia, fever, swollen/tender lymph nodes, visual problems (double vision, nystagmus), or skin reactions (rash, itching, dermatitis).

Pharmacokinetics

Absorption: Absorbed slowly from the GI tract. Bioavailability differs among products; the Dilantin and Phenytek preparations are considered to be "extended" products. Other products are considered to be prompt release.

Distribution: Distributes into CSF and other body tissues and fluids. Enters breast milk; crosses the placenta, achieving similar maternal/fetal levels. Preferentially distributes into fatty tissue.

Protein Binding: Adults 90–95%; decreased protein binding in neonates (up to 20% free fraction available), infants (up to 15% free), and patients with hyperbilirubinemia, hypoalbuminemia, severe renal dysfunction, or uremia.

Metabolism and Excretion: Mostly metabolized by the liver; minimal amounts excreted in the urine.

Half-life: 22 hr (range 7–42 hr).

TIME/ACTION PROFILE (anticonvulsant effect)

ROUTE	ONSET	PEAK	DURATION
PO	2–24 hr (1 wk)*	1.5–3 hr	6–12 hr
PO-ER	2–24 hr (1 wk)	4–12 hr	12–36 hr
IV	0.5–1 hr (1 wk)	rapid	12–24 hr

*( ) = time required for onset of action without a loading dose.

Contraindications/Precautions

Contraindicated in: Hypersensitivity; Hypersensitivity to propylene glycol (phenytoin injection only); Alcohol intolerance (phenytoin injection and liquid only); Sinus bradycardia, sinoatrial block, 2nd- or 3rd-degree heart block, or Stokes-Adams syndrome (phenytoin injection only).

Use Cautiously in: Hepatic or renal disease (↑ risk of adverse reactions; dose reduction recommended for hepatic impairment); Patients with severe cardiac or respiratory disease (use of IV phenytoin may result in an ↑ risk of serious adverse reactions); OB: Safety not established; may result in fetal hydantoin syndrome if used chronically or hemorrhage in the newborn if used at term; Lactation: Safety not established; Pedi: Suspension contains sodium benzoate, a metabolite of benzyl alcohol that can cause potentially fatal gasping syndrome in neonates; Geri: Use of IV phenytoin may result in an ↑ risk of serious adverse reactions.

Interactions

Drug-Drug: Disulfiram, acute ingestion of **alcohol, amiodarone, ethosuximide, isoniazid, chloramphenicol, sulfonamides, fluoxetine, gabapentin, H_2 antagonists, benzodiazepines, omeprazole, ketoconazole, fluconazole, estrogens, succinimides, halothane, methylphenidate, phenothiazines, salicylates, ticlopidine, tolbutamide, topiramate, trazodone, felbamate,** and **cimetidine** may ↑ phenytoin blood levels. **Barbiturates, carbamazepine, reserpine,** and chronic ingestion of **alcohol** may ↓ phenytoin blood levels. Phenytoin may ↓ the effects of **amiodarone, benzodiazepines, carbamazepine, chloramphenicol, corticosteroids, disopyramide, warfarin, felbamate, doxycycline, lamotrigine, oral contraceptives, paroxetine, propafenone, rifampin, ritonavir, quinidine, tacrolimus, theophylline, topiramate, tricyclic antidepressants, zonisamide, methadone, cyclosporine,** and **estrogens**. IV phenytoin and **dopamine** may cause additive hypotension. Additive CNS depression with other **CNS depressants**, including **alcohol, antihistamines, antidepressants, opioids,** and **sedative/hypnotics**. **Antacids** may ↓ absorption of orally administered phenytoin. ↑ systemic clearance of antileukemic drugs **teniposide** and **methotrexate,** which has been associated with a worse event–free survival, phenytoin use is not recommended in children undergoing chemotherapy for acute lymphocytic leukemia. **Calcium** and **sucralfate** ↓ phenytoin absorption.

Drug-Food: Phenytoin may ↓ absorption of **folic acid**. Concurrent administration of **enteral tube feedings** may ↓ phenytoin absorption.

Route/Dosage

IM administration is not recommended due to erratic absorption and pain on injection.

Anticonvulsant

PO (Adults): Loading dose of 15–20 mg/kg as extended capsules in 3 divided doses given every 2–4 hr; maintenance dose 5–6 mg/kg/day given in 1–3 divided doses; usual dosing range = 200–1200 mg/day.

PO (Children 10–16 yr): 6–7 mg/kg/day in 2–3 divided doses.

PO (Children 7–9 yr): 7–8 mg/kg/day in 2–3 divided doses.

PO (Children 4–6 yr): 7.5–9 mg/kg/day in 2–3 divided doses.

PO (Children 0.5–3 yr): 8–10 mg/kg/day in 2–3 divided doses.

PO (Neonates up to 6 months): 5–8 mg/kg/day in 2 divided doses; may require q 8 hr dosing.

IV (Adults): *Status epilepticus loading dose*—15–20 mg/kg. Rate not to exceed 25–50 mg/min. *Maintenance dose*—same as PO dosing above.

IV (Children): *Status epilepticus loading dose*—15–20 mg/kg at 1–3 mg/kg/min. *Maintenance dose*—same as PO dosing above.

Antiarrhythmic

IV (Adults): 50–100 mg q 10–15 min until arrhythmia is abolished, or a total of 15 mg/kg has been given, or toxicity occurs.

PO (Adults): Loading dose: 250 mg QID for 1 day, then 250 mg bid for 2 days, then maintenance at 300–400 mg/day in divided doses 1–4 times/day.

IV (Children): 1.25 mg/kg q 5 min; may repeat up to total loading dose of 15 mg/kg. *Maintenance dose*—5–10 mg/kg/day in 2–3 divided doses IV or PO.

Availability (generic available)

Chewable tablets: 50 mg Rx. **Oral suspension:** 125 mg/5 mL Rx. **Extended-release capsules:** 30 mg Rx, 100 mg Rx, 200 mg Rx, 300 mg Rx. **Injection:** 50 mg/mL Rx.

pimecrolimus

(pim-eck-roe-**lee**-mus)

Elidel

Classification

Therapeutic: immunosuppressants (topical)

Pharmacologic: calcineurin inhibitors

Indications

Short-term and intermittent long-term management of mild-to-moderate atopic dermatitis unresponsive to or in patients intolerant of conventional treatment.

Action

Inhibits T-cell and mast cell activation by interfering with production of inflammatory cytokines. **Therapeutic Effects:** ↓ severity of atopic dermatitis.

Adverse Reactions/Side Effects

Local: burning. **Misc:** ↑ risk of lymphoma/skin cancer.

PHYSICAL THERAPY IMPLICATIONS

Examination and Evaluation

- Assess the area being treated to help document whether drug therapy is successful in resolving skin conditions.
- Monitor any new or increased skin reactions at the site of application, including burning, rash, or

other suspicious skin lesions that might indicate skin cancer or lymphoma. Report severe or unusual skin reactions to the physician.

Patient/Client-Related Instruction

- Check that the patient and family or caregivers understand topical application procedures and adhere to the recommended dosing schedule.

Pharmacokinetics

Absorption: Minimally absorbed through intact skin.
Distribution: Local distribution after topical administration.
Metabolism and Excretion: Systemic metabolism and excretion is negligible with local application.
Half-life: Not applicable.

TIME/ACTION PROFILE (improvement in symptoms)

ROUTE	ONSET	PEAK	DURATION
topical	within 6 days	unknown	unknown

Contraindications/Precautions

Contraindicated in: Hypersensitivity; Should not be applied to areas of active cutaneous viral infections (increased risk of dissemination); Concurrent use of occlusive dressings; Netherton's syndrome (increased absorption of pimecrolimus); Lactation: Discontinue breast-feeding.
Use Cautiously in: Possible risk of cancer. Do not use as first-line therapy; Clinical infection at treatment site (infection should be treated/cleared prior to use); Skin papillomas (warts); allow treatment/resolution prior to use; Natural/artificial sunlight (minimize exposure); OB: Use only if clearly needed; Pedi: Use only if other treatments have failed; safety not established in children <2 yr.

Interactions

Drug-Drug: None significant as systemic absorption is negligible.

Route/Dosage

Topical (Adults and Children ≥2 yr): Apply thin film twice daily; rub in gently and completely.

Availability

Cream: 1% in 30-g, 60-g, and 100-g tubes.

pimozide (pi-moe-zide)

Orap

Classification
Therapeutic: antipsychotics (conventional)
Pharmacologic: diphenylbutyl piperidines

Indications

Suppression of motor and vocal tics in Tourette's disorder with severe, compromising symptoms in patients with an unfavorable response to haloperidol. Second-line treatment after failure with atypical antipsychotics. **Unlabeled Use:** Psychotic disorders that fail to respond to standard treatment.

Action

Blocks dopamine receptors in the CNS. Increases brain turnover of dopamine, blocks calcium channels, and may antagonize opiate receptors. **Therapeutic Effects:** Decreased tics in patients with Tourette's disorder.

Adverse Reactions/Side Effects

CNS: NEUROLEPTIC MALIGNANT SYNDROME, mood/behavior effects, weakness, drowsiness. **EENT:** blurred vision, dry eyes. **CV:** ARRHYTHMIAS (PROLONGED QTC INTERVAL), hypotension. **GI:** constipation, dry mouth, ↓ appetite, nausea, vomiting, weight loss. **GU:** ↓ libido, erectile dysfunction. **Derm:** skin discoloration. **Endo:** galactorrhea (women). **Hemat:** blood dyscrasias. **Neuro:** akathisia, parkinsonism, dystonic reactions, tardive dyskinesia, akinesia.

PHYSICAL THERAPY IMPLICATIONS

Examination and Evaluation

- Be alert for signs of neuroleptic malignant syndrome, including hyperthermia, diaphoresis, generalized muscle rigidity, altered mental status, tachycardia, changes in blood pressure (BP), and incontinence. Symptoms typically occur within 4–14 days after initiation of drug therapy, but can occur at any time during drug use. Report these signs to the physician immediately.
- Assess heart rate, ECG, and heart sounds, especially during exercise (See Appendices G, H). Report any rhythm disturbances or symptoms of increased arrhythmias, including palpitations, chest discomfort, shortness of breath, fainting, and fatigue/weakness.
- Assess BP periodically and compare to normal values (See Appendix F). Report low BP (hypotension), especially if patient experiences dizziness, fatigue, or other symptoms.
- Assess motor function, and be alert for extrapyramidal symptoms. Report these symptoms immediately, especially tardive dyskinesia, because this problem may be irreversible. Common extrapyramidal symptoms include:
  - Tardive dyskinesia (uncontrolled rhythmic movement of mouth, face, and extremities, lip smacking or puckering, puffing of cheeks, uncontrolled chewing, rapid or worm-like movements of tongue).

P

  - Pseudoparkinsonism (shuffling gait, rigidity, tremor, pill-rolling motion, loss of balance control, difficulty speaking or swallowing, mask-like face).
  - Akathisia (restlessness or desire to keep moving).
  - Other dystonias and dyskinesias (dystonic muscle spasms, twisting motions, twitching, inability to move eyes, weakness of arms or legs).
- Monitor unusual weakness and fatigue that might be due to anemia, or other symptoms such as fever, sore throat, mucosal lesions, or signs of infection that might be due to other blood dyscrasias. Notify physician if these signs occur.
- Periodically assess body weight and other anthropometric measures (body mass index, body composition). Report a rapid or unexplained weight loss or decreased body fat.

Interventions
- Guard against falls and trauma (hip fractures, head injury, and so forth) caused by drowsiness, blurred vision, or extrapyramidal symptoms; implement fall prevention strategies (See Appendix E).
- Because of the risk of arrhythmias and abnormal BP responses, use caution during aerobic exercise and other forms of therapeutic exercise. Assess exercise tolerance frequently (BP, heart rate, fatigue levels), and terminate exercise immediately if any untoward responses occur (See Appendix L).
- To minimize orthostatic hypotension, patient should move slowly when assuming a more upright position.
- Help patient and family/caregivers explore nonpharmacologic methods (exercise, counseling, support groups) to reduce schizophrenic episodes.

Patient/Client-Related Instruction
- Advise patient to avoid alcohol and other CNS depressants because of the increased risk of sedation and adverse effects.
- Instruct patient to report other problematic side effects such as severe or prolonged blurred vision, dry eyes, sexual dysfunction (decreased libido, erectile dysfunction), nipple discharge in women, or GI problems (nausea, vomiting, constipation, dry mouth, loss of appetite).

Pharmacokinetics
Absorption: 50% absorbed following oral administration.
Distribution: Unknown.
Metabolism and Excretion: Undergoes extensive first-pass hepatic metabolism, at least partly by P4503A4 (CYP3A4) and CYP1A2 enzyme systems. Some metabolites have CNS activity.
Half-life: 29–111 hr.

TIME/ACTION PROFILE (blood levels)

ROUTE	ONSET	PEAK	DURATION
PO	unknown	6–8 hr	unknown

Contraindications/Precautions
Contraindicated in: Hypersensitivity (cross-sensitivity with other antipsychotics may occur); Concurrent use of agents that may be causing the motor and vocal tics; Congenital long QT syndrome (↑ risk of serious arrhythmias); Recent MI, heart failure; Concurrent use of agents that prolong the QT interval, including dofetilide, sotalol, quinidine, other Class IA or III antiarrhythmics, thioridazine, chlorpromazine, droperidol, sparfloxacin, moxifloxacin, mefloquine, pentamidine, arsenic trioxide, levomethadyl acetate, dolasetron, tacrolimus, ziprasidone, erythromycin, citalopram, escitalopram, clarithromycin and azithromycin (↑ risk of serious arrhythmias); Concurrent use of CYP3A4 enzyme inhibitors, including erythromycin, clarithromycin, azithromycin, itraconazole, ketoconazole, ritonavir, saquinavir, indinavir, nelfinavir, nefazodone, zileuton, and fluvoxamine (↑ risk of serious arrhythmias); CNS depression or comatose state; Motor or vocal tics not caused by Tourette's disorder; Hypokalemia or hypomagnesemia (↑ risk of serious arrhythmias).
Use Cautiously in: History of breast cancer; Angle-closure glaucoma; History of paralytic ileus; Hepatic or renal impairment; Prostatic hyperplasia; History of seizures (threshold may be lowered); Hypokalemia (↑ risk of arrhythmias); OB/Lactation: Safety not established, discontinue drug or bottle-feed; Pedi/Geri: ↑ sensitivity; ↑ risk of mortality in elderly patients treated for dementia-related psychosis.

Interactions
Drug-Drug: Concurrent use of **macrolide anti-infectives (erythromycin, clarithromycin, azithromycin), dofetilide, sotalol, quinidine, other Class IA or III antiarrhythmics, thioridazine, chlorpromazine, droperidol, sparfloxacin, gemifloxacin, moxifloxacin, mefloquine, pentamidine, arsenic trioxide, dolasetron, citalopram, escitalopram, tacrolimus,** and **ziprasidone** ↑ the risk of serious ventricular arrhythmias and should be avoided; similar effects may occur with **tricyclic antidepressants, disopyramide,** or **procainamide.** Blood levels and risk of cardiac arrhythmias are ↑ by concurrent use of **ritonavir**; concurrent use is contraindicated. Metabolism of pimozide may be impaired by **azole antifungals**; concurrent use of **itraconazole, fluvoxamine,** and **ketoconazole** is contraindicated. ↑ risk of CNS depression with **alcohol** or other **CNS depressants. Amphetamines, methylphenidate,** or **pemoline** may provoke tics that cannot be treated with pimozide; discontinue these before initiating therapy with pimozide. Blocks the effects of

amphetamines. Concurrent use with **MAO inhibitors** ↑ risk of sedative, hypotensive, and anticholinergic adverse reactions. Concurrent use with **fluoxetine** may result in bradycardia.
Drug-Natural: Concomitant use of **kava, valerian,** or **chamomile** can ↑ CNS depression. See **sedative** drug-drug interactions above. **St. John's wort** may affect pimozide levels and effectiveness; avoid concurrent use.
Drug-Food: Grapefruit juice ↑ risks of arrhythmias.

Route/Dosage

Tourette's Disorder

PO (Adults): 1–2 mg/day in divided doses; may be ↑ gradually as needed and tolerated up to 0.2 mg/kg/day or 10 mg/day, whichever is less.
PO (Children >12 yr): 0.05 mg/kg/day as a single bedtime dose; may be ↑ every 3rd day as needed and tolerated up to 0.2 mg/kg/day or 10 mg/day, whichever is less.
PO (Geriatric Patients): Use lower initial doses and more gradual titration.

Psychotic Disorders (Unlabeled)

PO (Adults): 2–4 mg/day as a single morning dose; may be ↑ by 2–4 mg/day at weekly intervals as needed and tolerated (usual dose is 6 mg/day, range 2–12 mg/day); up to 0.3 mg/kg/day or 20 mg/day, whichever is less.

Availability

Tablets: 1 mg, 2 mg, 4 mg, 10 mg.

pindolol (pin-doe-lole)

Novo-Pindol, Syn-Pindolol, Visken

Classification
Therapeutic: antihypertensives
Pharmacologic: beta blockers

Indications

Management of hypertension. **Unlabeled Use:** Management of angina pectoris.

Action

Blocks stimulation of $beta_1$ (myocardial) and $beta_2$ (pulmonary, vascular, and uterine)–adrenergic receptor sites. Has intrinsic sympathomimetic activity (ISA), which may produce less bradycardia. **Therapeutic Effects:** ↓ heart rate and blood pressure.

Adverse Reactions/Side Effects

CNS: fatigue, weakness, anxiety, depression, dizziness, drowsiness, insomnia, memory loss, mental status changes, nervousness, nightmares. **EENT:** blurred vision, dry eyes, nasal stuffiness. **Resp:** bronchospasm, wheezing. **CV:** ARRHYTHMIAS, BRADYCARDIA, CHF, PULMONARY EDEMA, orthostatic hypotension, peripheral vasoconstriction. **GI:** constipation, diarrhea, nausea. **GU:** erectile dysfunction, decreased libido. **Derm:** itching, rashes. **Endo:** hyperglycemia, hypoglycemia. **MS:** arthralgia, back pain, muscle cramps. **Neuro:** paresthesia. **Misc:** drug-induced lupus syndrome.

PHYSICAL THERAPY IMPLICATIONS

Examination and Evaluation

- Assess heart rate, ECG, and heart sounds, especially during exercise (See Appendices G, H). Report immediately an unusually slow heart rate (bradycardia) or signs of other arrhythmias, including palpitations, chest discomfort, shortness of breath, fainting, and fatigue/weakness.
- Assess routinely for signs of CHF and pulmonary edema, including dyspnea, rales/crackles, weight gain, peripheral edema, and jugular venous distention. Report these signs to the physician immediately.
- Assess blood pressure (BP) periodically and compare to normal values (See Appendix F) to help document antihypertensive effects.
- Assess BPe when patient assumes a more upright position (lying to standing, sitting to standing, lying to sitting). Document orthostatic hypotension and contact physician when systolic BP falls >20 mm Hg, or diastolic BP falls >10 mm Hg.
- Assess exercise tolerance and episodes of angina pectoris. Document improvements in these variables, but also report any decline in exercise tolerance or increased frequency/severity of anginal attacks.
- Assess symptoms of bronchospasm (wheezing, coughing, tightness in chest). Perform pulmonary function tests to quantify suspected changes in ventilation and respiration (See Appendices I, J, K). Repeated or prolonged bronchoconstriction may require a change in dose or medication (e.g., switch to a more cardioselective beta blocker).
- Monitor signs of peripheral vasoconstriction, such as extreme coldness in the hands and feet, cyanosis, and muscle cramping. Notify physician of severe or prolonged signs of vasoconstriction.
- Assess any back pain, joint pain, or muscle cramps to rule out musculoskeletal pathology; that is, try to determine if pain is drug induced rather than caused by anatomic or biomechanical problems.
- Assess signs of paresthesia (numbness, tingling), and perform objective tests, including

P

electroneuromyography and sensory testing to document any drug-related neuropathic changes.

- Monitor mood and personality changes, including depression, anxiety, memory loss, or other changes in behavior. Notify physician if these changes become problematic.
- Assess dizziness and drowsiness that might affect gait, balance, and other functional activities (See Appendix C). Report balance problems and functional limitations to the physician, and caution the patient and family/caregivers to guard against falls and trauma.
- Monitor excessive fatigue or weakness. Beta blockers often cause some degree of fatigue and weakness, but any sudden or severe change in muscle strength or energy levels should be reported.
- Be alert for signs of hypoglycemia (weakness, malaise, irritability, fatigue) or hyperglycemia (drowsiness, fruity breath, increased urination, unusual thirst). Medication may mask some signs of hypoglycemia, but dizziness and sweating may still occur. Patients with diabetes mellitus should check blood glucose levels frequently.
- Monitor signs of drug-induced lupus syndrome, including increased BP, fever, joint pain, skin rashes, and redness/irritation of the eye (uveitis). Notify physician promptly if these signs appear.

Interventions

- Design and implement aerobic exercise and endurance training programs to improve coronary perfusion, reduce angina, and improve myocardial pumping ability.
- Because of an increased risk of arrhythmias, CHF, and pulmonary edema, use caution during aerobic exercise and endurance conditioning. Terminate exercise if patient exhibits untoward symptoms (chest pain, shortness of breath, unusual fatigue), or displays other criteria for exercise termination (See Appendix L).
- Establish aerobic exercise workloads that account for the effects of beta blockers on heart rate. Some heart rate guidelines may not be appropriate because beta blockers typically decrease maximal HR by 20–30 bpm. Use other guidelines such as rating of perceived exertion (RPE, modified Borg scale) to determine exercise workloads.
- To minimize orthostatic hypotension, patient should move slowly when assuming a more upright position.

Patient/Client-Related Instruction

- Remind patients to take medication as directed to control hypertension even if they are asymptomatic.
- Counsel patients about additional interventions to help control BP and cardiac dysfunction, such as regular exercise, weight loss, sodium restriction, stress reduction, moderation of alcohol consumption, and smoking cessation.
- Instruct patient or family/caregivers to report other troublesome side effects such as severe or prolonged insomnia, nightmares, blurred vision, dry eyes, stuffy nose, sexual problems (decreased libido, erectile dysfunction), skin reactions (rash, itching), or GI problems (nausea, constipation, diarrhea).

Pharmacokinetics

Absorption: Well absorbed following oral administration.
Distribution: Moderate CNS penetration. Crosses the placenta; enters breast milk.
Metabolism and Excretion: Partially metabolized by the liver; 50% excreted unchanged by the kidneys.
Half-life: 3–4 hr.

TIME/ACTION PROFILE (cardiovascular effects)

ROUTE	ONSET	PEAK	DURATION
PO	7 days	2 wk	8–24 hr

Contraindications/Precautions

Contraindicated in: Uncompensated CHF; Pulmonary edema; Cardiogenic shock; Bradycardia or heart block.
Use Cautiously in: Renal impairment; Hepatic impairment; Geriatric patients (↑ sensitivity to beta blockers; initial dosage reduction recommended); Pulmonary disease (including asthma); Diabetes mellitus (may mask signs of hypoglycemia); Thyrotoxicosis (may mask symptoms); Patients with a history of severe allergic reactions (intensity of reactions may be increased); Pregnancy, lactation, or children (safety not established; may cause fetal/neonatal bradycardia, hypotension, hypoglycemia, or respiratory depression).

Interactions

Drug-Drug: General anesthesia, IV phenytoin, and **verapamil** may cause additive myocardial depression. Additive bradycardia may occur with **digoxin**. Additive hypotension may occur with other **antihypertensives**, acute ingestion of **alcohol,** or **nitrates**. Concurrent use with **amphetamines, cocaine, ephedrine, epinephrine, norepinephrine, phenylephrine**, or **pseudoephedrine** may result in unopposed alpha-adrenergic stimulation (excessive hypertension, bradycardia). Concurrent **thyroid preparations** administration may ↓ effectiveness. May alter the effectiveness of **insulin** or **oral hypoglycemic agents** (dosage adjustments may be necessary). May ↓ the effectiveness of **beta-adrenergic bronchodilators** and **theophylline**. May ↓ the beneficial beta cardiovascular effects of **dopamine** or **dobutamine.** Use cautiously within 14 days of **MAO inhibitors** (may result in hypertension). Concurrent **NSAIDs** may ↓ antihypertensive action.

Route/Dosage

PO (Adults): 5 mg bid initially; may be increased by 10 mg/day q 2–3 wk as needed (up to 45–60 mg/day).

Availability (generic available)

Tablets: 5 mg, 10 mg, 15 mg.

pioglitazone (pi-oh-glit-a-zone)

Actos

Classification

Therapeutic: antidiabetics (oral)
Pharmacologic: thiazolidinediones

Indications

Management of type 2 diabetes mellitus; may also be used with a sulfonylurea, metformin, or insulin when the combination of diet, exercise, and metformin does not achieve glycemic control.

Action

Improves sensitivity to insulin by acting as an agonist at receptor sites involved in insulin responsiveness and subsequent glucose production and utilization. Requires insulin for activity. **Therapeutic Effects:** ↓ insulin resistance, resulting in glycemic control without hypoglycemia.

Adverse Reactions/Side Effects

CV: edema. **GI:** hepatitis, ↑ liver enzymes. **Hemat:** anemia. **Misc:** fractures (arm, hand, foot) in female patients.

PHYSICAL THERAPY IMPLICATIONS

Examination and Evaluation

- Assess peripheral edema using girth measurements, volume displacement, and measurement of pitting edema (See Appendix N). Report increased swelling in feet and ankles or a sudden increase in body weight due to fluid retention. Also report signs of pulmonary edema such as dyspnea and abnormal breath sounds (rales/crackles; See Appendix K).
- Assess any pain that might indicate fractures, especially in the arms, hand, and feet in women. Protect and support any suspected fracture sites, and report the problem to the physician for further evaluation.
- Monitor signs of drug-induced hepatitis, including anorexia, abdominal pain, severe nausea and vomiting, yellow skin or eyes, skin rashes, flu-like symptoms, and muscle/joint pain. Report these signs to the physician.
- Be alert for signs of hypoglycemia, especially during and after exercise. Common neuromuscular signs include anxiety; restlessness; tingling in hands, feet, lips, or tongue; chills; cold sweats; confusion; difficulty in concentration; drowsiness; excessive hunger; headache; irritability; nervousness; tremor; weakness; unsteady gait. Report persistent or repeated episodes of hypoglycemia to the physician.
- Monitor signs of anemia, including unusual fatigue, shortness of breath with exertion, and bruising. Notify physician immediately if these signs occur.
- Assess blood pressure periodically (See Appendix F). A sudden or sustained increase in blood pressure (hypertension) may indicate problems in diabetes management and should be reported to the physician.

Interventions

- Implement aerobic exercise and endurance training programs to maintain optimal body weight, improve insulin sensitivity, and reduce the risk of macrovascular disease (heart attack, stroke) and microvascular problems (reduced blood flow to tissues and organs that causes poor wound healing, neuropathy, retinopathy, and nephropathy).

Patient/Client-Related Instruction

- Encourage patient to monitor blood glucose before and after exercise and to adjust food intake to maintain normal glycemic levels.
- Emphasize the importance of adhering to nutritional guidelines and the need for periodic assessment of glycemic control (serum glucose and glycosylated hemoglobin levels) throughout the management of diabetes mellitus.
- Advise patient about symptoms of hyperglycemia (confusion, drowsiness; flushed, dry skin; fruit-like breath odor; rapid, deep breathing, polyuria; loss of appetite; unusual thirst). Drug dosages may need to be adjusted to prevent repeated episodes of hyperglycemia.

Pharmacokinetics

Absorption: Well absorbed following oral administration.
Distribution: Unknown.
Protein Binding: >99% bound to plasma proteins. Active metabolites are also highly (>99 %) bound.
Metabolism and Excretion: Extensively metabolized by the liver; at least 2 metabolites have pharmacologic activity. Minimal renal excretion of unchanged drug.
Half-life: *Pioglitazone*—3–7 hr; *total pioglitazone (pioglitazone plus metabolites)*—16–24 hr.

TIME/ACTION PROFILE (effects on blood glucose)

ROUTE	ONSET	PEAK	DURATION
PO	30 min	2–4 hr	24 hr

Contraindications/Precautions

Contraindicated in: Hypersensitivity; Diabetic ketoacidosis; Clinical evidence of active liver disease or ↑ ALT (>2.5 times upper limit of normal); OB: Pregnancy or lactation (not recommended for use during pregnancy or lactation; insulin should be used); Pedi: Children <18 yr or type 1 diabetes (requires insulin for activity).

Use Cautiously in: Edema; CHF (avoid use in moderate-to-severe CHF); Hepatic impairment; Women (may ↑ distal upper and lower limb fractures); Women with childbearing potential (may restore ovulation and risk of pregnancy).

Interactions

Drug-Drug: May ↓ efficacy of **hormonal contraceptives**. Pioglitazone is metabolized by the **CYP4503A4** enzyme system. Concurrent use of drugs that alter the activity of this system may result in drug-drug interactions. **Ketoconazole** may ↑ effects of pioglitazone. Concurrent use with **insulin** may ↑ risk of CHF (consider predisposing factors).

Drug-Natural: Glucosamine may worsen blood glucose control. **Chromium**, and **coenzyme Q 10** may produce ↑ hypoglycemic effects.

Route/Dosage

PO (Adults): 15–30 mg once daily; may be increased to 45 mg/day if needed. Doses greater than 30 mg have not been evaluated in combination with insulin and other antidiabetics.

Availability

Tablets: 15 mg, 30 mg, 45 mg. ***In combination with:*** Metformin (Actoplus Met), glimepiride (Duetact). See Appendix B.

piperacillin/tazobactam

(pi-**per**-a-sil-in/taye-zoe-**bak**-tam)

Zosyn

Classification

Therapeutic: anti-infectives

Pharmacologic: extended spectrum penicillins

Indications

Appendicitis and peritonitis. Skin and skin structure infections. Gynecologic infections. Community-acquired and nosocomial pneumonia caused by piperacillin-resistant, beta-lactamase–producing bacteria.

Action

Piperacillin: Binds to bacterial cell wall membrane, causing cell death. Spectrum is extended compared with other penicillins. **Tazobactam:** Inhibits beta-lactamase, an enzyme that can destroy penicillins.

Therapeutic Effects: Death of susceptible bacteria.

Spectrum: Active against piperacillin-resistant, beta-lactamase–producing *Bacteroides fragilis*, *E. coli*, *Acinetobacter baumannii*, *Klebsiella pneumoniae*, *Pseudomonas aeruginosa*, *Staphylococcus aureus*, *Haemophilus influenzae*.

Adverse Reactions/Side Effects

CNS: SEIZURES (HIGHER DOSES), confusion, dizziness, headache, insomnia, lethargy. **GI:** PSEUDOMEMBRANOUS COLITIS, diarrhea, constipation, drug-induced hepatitis, nausea, vomiting. **GU:** interstitial nephritis. **Derm:** rashes (↑ in cystic fibrosis patients), urticaria. **Hemat:** bleeding, leukopenia, neutropenia, thrombocytopenia. **Local:** pain, phlebitis at IV site. **Misc:** HYPERSENSITIVITY REACTIONS, INCLUDING ANAPHYLAXIS AND SERUM SICKNESS, fever (↑ in cystic fibrosis patients), superinfection.

PHYSICAL THERAPY IMPLICATIONS

Examination and Evaluation

- Watch for seizures; notify physician immediately if patient develops or increases seizure activity.
- Monitor signs of pseudomembranous colitis, including diarrhea, abdominal pain, fever, pus or mucus in stools, and other severe or prolonged GI problems (nausea, vomiting, heartburn). Notify physician or nursing staff immediately of these signs.
- Monitor signs of allergic reactions and anaphylaxis, including pulmonary symptoms (tightness in the throat and chest, wheezing, cough dyspnea) or skin reactions (rash, pruritus, urticaria). Notify physician or nursing staff immediately if these reactions occur.
- Assess muscle aches and joint pain (arthralgia) that may be caused by serum sickness. Notify physician if these symptoms seem to be drug-related rather than caused by musculoskeletal injury, or if muscle and joint pain are accompanied by allergyc-like reactions (fever, rashes, etc.)
- Monitor signs of blood dyscrasias such as leukopenia and neutropenia (fever, sore throat, signs of infection) or thrombocytopenia (bruising, nose bleeds, and bleeding gums). Report these signs to the physician.
- Assess dizziness and confusion that might affect gait, balance, and other functional activities (See Appendices C, D). Report balance problems and functional limitations to the physician and nursing staff, and caution the patient and family/caregivers to guard against falls and trauma.
- Monitor injection site for pain, swelling, and irritation. Report prolonged or excessive injection site reactions to the physician.

Interventions

- Always wash hands thoroughly and disinfect equipment (whirlpools, electrotherapeutic devices, treatment tables, and so forth) to help prevent the spread of infection. Use universal precautions or isolation procedures as indicated for specific patients.

Patient/Client-Related Instruction

- Instruct patient to notify physician immediately if signs of the following occur:
  - Superinfection (black, furry overgrowth on tongue; vaginal itching or discharge; loose or foul-smelling stools).
  - Interstitial nephritis (blood in urine, decreased urine output, weight gain from fluid retention).
- Advise patient about the likelihood of GI reactions (diarrhea, nausea, vomiting). Instruct patient to report severe or prolonged GI problems or signs of drug-induced hepatitis (yellow skin or eyes, abdominal pain, severe nausea and vomiting, fever, sore throat, malaise, weakness, facial edema).
- Instruct patient and family/caregivers to report other troublesome side effects such as severe or prolonged headache, insomnia, lethargy, fever, or skin problems (rash, itching).

Pharmacokinetics

Absorption: Piperacillin is well absorbed (80%) from IM sites.
Distribution: Widely distributed. Enter CSF well only when meninges are inflamed. Cross the placenta and enter breast milk in low concentrations.
Metabolism and Excretion: Piperacillin (68%) and tazobactam (80%) are mostly excreted unchanged by the kidneys.
Half-life: 0.7–1.2 hr.

TIME/ACTION PROFILE (piperacillin blood levels)

ROUTE	ONSET	PEAK	DURATION
IV	rapid	end of infusion	4–6 hr

Contraindications/Precautions

Contraindicated in: Hypersensitivity to penicillins, beta-lactams, cephalosporins, or tazobactam (cross-sensitivity may occur).
Use Cautiously in: Renal impairment (dosage reduction or ↑ interval recommended if CCr <40 mL/min); Sodium restriction; Pedi: Children (safety and efficacy not established); OB: Pregnancy and lactation (safety not established).

Interactions

Drug-Drug: Probenecid ↓ renal excretion and ↑ blood levels. May alter excretion of **lithium**. **Potassium-losing diuretics, corticosteroids,** or **amphotericin B** may ↑ risk of hypokalemia. ↑ risk of hepatotoxicity with other **hepatotoxic agents**. May ↓ half-life of **aminoglycosides** in patients with renal impairment. May ↑ levels and risk of toxicity from **methotrexate**.

Route/Dosage

Contains 2.79 mEq (64 mg) sodium/g of piperacillin; dose below expressed as combined piperacillin/tazobactam content.
IV (Adults): *Most infections*—3.375 g q 6 hr. *Nosocomial pneumonia*—4, 5 g q 6 hr.

Renal Impairment

IV (Adults): *CCr 20–40 ml/min*—2.25 g q 6 hr (3.375 g q 6 hr for nosocomial pneumonia); *CCr <20 mL/min*—2.25 g q 8 hr (2.25 g q 6 hr for nosocomial pneumonia); *Hemodialysis*—2.25 g q 12 h (2.25 g q 8 hr for nosocomial pneumonia).

Availability

Powder for injection: 2-g piperacillin/0.25-g tazobactam vials and 50-mL premixed frozen containers, 3-g piperacillin/0.375-g tazobactam vials and 50-mL premixed frozen containers, 4-g piperacillin/0.5-g tazobactam vials and 50-mL premixed frozen containers, 36-g piperacillin/4.5-g tazobactam bulk vials.

pirbuterol (peer-byoo-ter-ole)

Maxair

Classification
Therapeutic: bronchodilators
Pharmacologic: adrenergics

Indications

Management of reversible airway disease due to intermittent asthma or COPD (quick-relief agent).

Action

Results in the accumulation of cyclic adenosine monophosphate (cAMP) at beta-adrenergic receptors. Produces bronchodilation. Inhibits the release of mediators of immediate hypersensitivity reactions from mast cells. Relatively selective for $beta_2$ (pulmonary)–adrenergic receptor sites with less effect on $beta_1$ (cardiac)–adrenergic receptors. **Therapeutic Effects:** Bronchodilation.

Adverse Reactions/Side Effects

CNS: nervousness, restlessness, tremor, headache, insomnia. **Resp:** PARADOXICAL BRONCHOSPASM. **CV:** angina, arrhythmias, hypertension, tachycardia. **GI:** nausea, vomiting. **Endo:** hyperglycemia.

PHYSICAL THERAPY IMPLICATIONS

Examination and Evaluation

- Watch for signs of paradoxical bronchospasm, including wheezing, cough, dyspnea, shortness of breath, and tightness in chest and throat. These signs are more common at higher doses or during excessive use of the inhaler. If condition occurs, advise patient to withhold medication and notify physician or other health care professional immediately.
- Assess pulmonary function at rest and during exercise (See Appendices I, J, K) to document effectiveness of medication in controlling bronchospasm.
- Assess blood pressure (BP) periodically and compare to normal values (See Appendix F). Report a sustained increase in BP (hypertension).
- Assess heart rate, ECG, and heart sounds, especially during exercise (See Appendices G, H). Report a rapid heart rate (tachycardia) or signs of other arrhythmias, including palpitations, chest discomfort, shortness of breath, fainting, and fatigue/weakness.
- Monitor and report signs of CNS toxicity, including nervousness, restlessness, or tremor. Sustained or severe CNS signs may indicate overdose or excessive use of this drug.
- Be alert for signs of hyperglycemia, including confusion, drowsiness, flushed/dry skin, fruit-like breath odor, rapid/deep breathing, polyuria, loss of appetite, and unusual thirst. Patients with diabetes mellitus should check blood glucose levels frequently.

Interventions

- When implementing airway clearance techniques or respiratory muscle training, attempt to intervene when the airway is maximally bronchodilated. Peak responses typically occur about 1.5 hr after inhalation.
- Because of the risk of cardiovascular stimulation, use caution during aerobic exercise and endurance conditioning. Cardiac effects should be minimal at lower doses or occasional inhaled use. Cardiovascular effects such as arrhythmias, angina pectoris, or increased BP may occur at higher doses or during excessive use, and are caused by inadvertent stimulation of beta receptors on the heart.

Patient/Client-Related Instruction

- Advise patient not to exceed the recommended dose or frequency of inhalations. Contact physician immediately if bronchospasm is not relieved by medication or is accompanied by diaphoresis, dizziness, or other symptoms.
- Counsel patient on proper use of inhaler; observe use of this device whenever possible to ensure proper technique.
- Instruct patient and family/caregivers to report other troublesome side effects such as severe or prolonged headache, sleep loss, or GI problems (nausea, vomiting).

Pharmacokinetics

Absorption: Minimal systemic absorption occurs following inhalation.
Distribution: Unknown.
Metabolism and Excretion: Metabolized by the liver.
Half-life: 2 hr.

TIME/ACTION PROFILE (bronchodilation)

ROUTE	ONSET	PEAK	DURATION
inhalation	within 5 min	1.5 hr	6–8 hr

Contraindications/Precautions

Contraindicated in: Hypersensitivity to adrenergic amines; Known hypersensitivity or intolerance to fluorocarbons.
Use Cautiously in: Cardiac disease; Hypertension; Hyperthyroidism; Diabetes; Glaucoma; Elderly patients (more susceptible to adverse reactions; may require dosage reduction); Excessive use may lead to tolerance and paradoxical bronchospasm (inhaler); Pregnancy (near term), lactation, and children <2 yr (safety not established).

Interactions

Drug-Drug: Concurrent use with other **adrenergics** will have ↑ adrenergic side effects. Use with **MAO inhibitors** may lead to hypertensive crisis. **Beta blockers** may ↓ therapeutic effect.
Drug-Natural: Use with caffeine-containing herbs **(cola nut, guarana, mate, tea, coffee)** ↑ stimulant effect.

Route/Dosage

Inhalation (Adults): 1–2 inhalations q 4–6 hr (not to exceed 12 inhalations/day).

Availability

Inhalation aerosol: 200 mcg/spray (≥300 inhalations/25.6-g canister).

piroxicam (peer-ox-i-kam)

Apo-Piroxicam, Feldene, Novo-Pirocam, Nu-Pirox, PMS-Piroxicam

Classification
Therapeutic: antirheumatics, nonsteroidal anti-inflammatory agents
Pharmacologic: enolic acids (oxicams)

Indications

Management of inflammatory disorders, including Rheumatoid arthritis, Osteoarthritis. **Unlabeled Use:** Management of dysmenorrhea.

Action

Inhibits prostaglandin synthesis. **Therapeutic Effects:** Suppression of pain and inflammation.

Adverse Reactions/Side Effects

CNS: drowsiness, headache, dizziness. **EENT:** blurred vision, tinnitus. **CV:** edema. **GI:** DRUG-INDUCED HEPATITIS, GI BLEEDING, discomfort, dyspepsia, nausea, vomiting, anorexia, constipation, diarrhea, flatulence. **GU:** renal failure. **Derm:** EXFOLIATIVE DERMATITIS, STEVENS-JOHNSON SYNDROME, TOXIC EPIDERMAL NECROLYSIS, rashes. **Hemat:** blood dyscrasias, prolonged bleeding time. **Misc:** ALLERGIC REACTIONS, INCLUDING ANAPHYLAXIS.

PHYSICAL THERAPY IMPLICATIONS

Examination and Evaluation

- Monitor signs of GI bleeding, including abdominal pain, vomiting blood, blood in stools, or black, tarry stools. Report these signs to the physician immediately.
- Be alert for signs of drug-induced hepatitis, including anorexia, abdominal pain, severe nausea and vomiting, yellow skin or eyes, skin rashes, flu-like symptoms, and muscle/joint pain. Report these signs to the physician immediately.
- Monitor signs of allergic reactions and anaphylaxis, including pulmonary symptoms (laryngeal edema, wheezing, cough, dyspnea) or skin reactions (rash, pruritus, urticaria). Be especially alert for exfoliation, dermatitis, and other severe skin reactions that might indicate serious hypersensitivity reactions (Stevens-Johnson syndrome, toxic epidermal necrolysis). Notify physician immediately if these reactions occur.
- Assess pain and other variables (range of motion, muscle strength) to document whether this drug is successful in helping manage the patient's pain and decreasing impairments.
- Assess blood pressure (BP) periodically and compare to normal values (See Appendix F). NSAIDs can increase BP in certain patients.
- Be alert for signs of prolonged bleeding time such as bleeding gums, nosebleeds, and unusual or excessive bruising. Report these signs to the physician.
- Monitor unusual weakness and fatigue that might be due to anemia, or other symptoms such as fever, sore throat, mucosal lesions, or signs of infection that might be due to other blood dyscrasias. Notify physician if these signs occur.
- Assess peripheral edema using girth measurements, volume displacement, and measurement of pitting edema (See Appendix N). Report increased swelling in feet and ankles or a sudden increase in body weight due to fluid retention.
- Monitor signs of renal failure, including decreased urine output, increased BP, muscle cramps/twitching, edema/weight gain from fluid retention, yellowish brown skin, and confusion that progresses to seizures and coma. Report these signs immediately to the physician.
- Assess dizziness and drowsiness that might affect gait, balance, and other functional activities (See Appendix C). Report balance problems and functional limitations to the physician, and caution the patient and family/caregivers to guard against falls and trauma.

Interventions

- Implement appropriate manual therapy techniques, physical agents, and therapeutic exercises to reduce pain and decrease the need for piroxicam and other NSAIDs.
- If treating arthritic conditions, recommend orthotic and assistive devices as needed to reduce pain, improve function, and augment the effects of drug therapy.
- Use caution with any physical interventions that could increase bleeding, including wound débridement, chest percussion, joint mobilization, and application of local heat.
- Help patient explore other nonpharmacologic methods to reduce chronic pain, such as relaxation techniques, exercise, counseling, and so forth.

Patient/Client-Related Instruction

- Advise patient that analgesics are usually more effective if given before pain becomes severe; emphasize that adequate pain control will allow better participation in physical therapy.
- Inform patient that NSAIDs may impair bone and cartilage healing. Advise patient to consult physician about NSAID use, especially after fractures, spinal fusion, and other bone surgeries.
- Caution patient about the use of over-the-counter products that contain NSAIDs or acetaminophen while taking prescription doses of piroxicam. Use of multiple NSAIDs increases the risk of toxicity and overdose.
- Instruct patient to report excessive or prolonged headache or ringing/buzzing in the ears (tinnitus); these signs may indicate drug toxicity.
- Advise patient about the risks of gastric irritation. Instruct patient to notify physician of GI reactions such as severe or prolonged nausea, vomiting, constipation, diarrhea, indigestion, flatulence, abdominal pain, and loss of appetite.
- Advise patient to reduce alcohol intake because alcohol increases the risk of gastric toxicity.

- Instruct patient and family/caregivers to report other troublesome side effects such as severe or prolonged vision disturbances or skin reactions (rash, hives, itching).

Pharmacokinetics

Absorption: Well absorbed from the GI tract.
Distribution: Unknown. Enters breast milk in small amounts.
Metabolism and Excretion: Mostly metabolized by the liver. Minimal amounts excreted unchanged by the kidneys.
Half-life: 50 hr.

TIME/ACTION PROFILE

ROUTE	ONSET	PEAK	DURATION
PO (analgesic effect)	1 hr	unknown	48–72 hr
PO (anti-inflammatory effect)	7–12 days	2–3 wk*	Unknown

*May take up to 12 wk.

Contraindications/Precautions

Contraindicated in: Hypersensitivity; Cross-sensitivity may exist with other NSAIDs, including aspirin; Active GI bleeding or ulcer disease; OB: Lactation; Perioperative pain from coronary artery bypass graft (CABG) surgery.
Use Cautiously in: Cardiovascular disease or risk factors for cardiovascular disease (may ↑ risk of serious cardiovascular thrombotic events, myocardial infarction, and stroke, especially with prolonged use); Severe hepatic disease; History of ulcer disease; Geri: Appears on Beers' list. Geriatric patients are at increased risk for GI bleeding, edema, renal failure; Renal impairment (dosage reduction recommended); OB/Pedi: Pregnancy or children (safety not established; avoid use during 2nd half of pregnancy).

Interactions

Drug-Drug: Concurrent use with **aspirin** ↓ piroxicam blood levels and may ↓ effectiveness. ↑ risk of bleeding with **anticoagulants, cefoperazone, cefotetan, heparin, ticlopidine, clopidogrel, eptifibatide, tirofiban, thrombolytic agents**, and **valproic acid**. ↑ adverse GI side effects with **aspirin, corticosteroids**, and other **NSAIDs**. **Probenecid** ↑ blood levels and may increase toxicity. May ↓ response to **antihypertensives** or **diuretics**. May ↑ serum levels and risk of toxicity from **lithium**. May ↑ risk of hypoglycemia from **insulin** or **oral hypoglycemic agents**. ↑ risk of adverse renal effects with **gold compounds, cyclosporine**, or chronic use of **acetaminophen**. May ↑ risk of hematologic toxicity from **antineoplastics** or **radiation therapy**.
Drug-Natural: ↑ anticoagulant effect and bleeding risk with **arnica, chamomile, clove, dong quai, fenugreek, feverfew, garlic, ginger, ginkgo, *Panax ginseng***, and others.

Route/Dosage

PO (Adults): *Anti-inflammatory*—10–20 mg/day; may be given as single dose or 2 divided doses. *Anti-dysmenorrheal*—40 mg initially, then 20 mg/day.
PO (Geriatric Patients): 10 mg/day initially.

Availability (generic available)

Capsules: 10 mg, 20 mg. **Suppositories:** 10 mg, 20 mg.

pitavastatin (pit-av-a-**stat**-in)

Livalo

Classification
Therapeutic: lipid-lowering agents
Pharmacologic: HMG CoA reductase inhibitors (statins)

Indications

Treatment of primary hyperlipidemia and mixed dyslipidemia (adjunctive therapy to diet); to reduce elevated total cholesterol (TC), low-density lipoprotein cholesterol (LDL-C), apolipoprotein B (Apo B), and triglycerides (TG); and to increase high-density lipoprotein cholesterol (HDL-C).

Action

Inhibits 3-hydroxy-3-methylglutaryl coenzyme A (HMG CoA) reductase, an enzyme which is responsible for catalyzing an early step in cholesterol synthesis
Therapeutic Effects: Lowering of TC, LDL-C, Apo B, and TG; increasing HDL-CI conjunction with multiple risk factor interventions, lowering of cardiovascular risk.

Adverse Reactions/Side Effects

GI: constipation, diarrhea, ↑ liver enzymes.
Derm: pruritus, rash, urticaria. **MS:** RHABDOMYOLYSIS, arthralgia, myalgia, myositis, back pain, extremity pain, myalgia. **Misc:** hypersensitivity reactions.

PHYSICAL THERAPY IMPLICATIONS

Examination and Evaluation

- Assess any muscle pain, tenderness, or weakness, especially if accompanied by fever, malaise, and dark-colored urine. Advise patient that these symptoms may represent drug-induced myopathy, and that myopathy can progress to severe muscle damage (rhabdomyolysis). Report any unexplained musculoskeletal symptoms to the physician immediately, and suspend exercise and gait training until these symptoms can be evaluated.
- Assess any back, joint, or extremity pain to rule out musculoskeletal pathology; that is, try to determine if pain is drug-induced rather than caused by anatomical or biomechanical problems.
- Monitor signs of hypersensitivity reactions, including pulmonary symptoms (tightness in the throat

and chest, wheezing, cough, dyspnea) or skin reactions (rash, pruritus, urticaria). Notify physician immediately if these reactions occur.

Interventions

- In patients with drug-induced myopathy, implement gradual strengthening and other therapeutic exercises to facilitate recovery from muscle pain and weakness. Use caution during early stages to avoid fatigue of affected muscles, and implement assistive devices (walker, cane, crutches) as needed to prevent falls and assist mobility. Increase exercise intensity as tolerated; recovery from myopathy typically takes 4–6 wk, but can be longer in older patients or people with comorbidities.
- Design and implement aerobic exercise and endurance training programs to improve cardiovascular function and help reduce the risk of coronary heart disease.

Patient/Client-Related Instruction

- Remind patients to take medication as directed to control hyperlipidemia even though they are asymptomatic.
- Counsel patients about additional interventions to help control lipid disorders and improve cardiovascular health, including dietary modification, regular exercise, moderation of alcohol consumption, and smoking cessation.
- Instruct patient to report other bothersome side effects such as severe or prolonged skin reactions (rash, hives, itching) or GI problems (constipation, diarrhea).

Pharmacokinetics

Absorption: Well absorbed (51%) following oral administration.
Distribution: unknown.
Protein Binding: >99%.
Metabolism and Excretion: Mostly metabolized by the liver; 15% excreted in urine, 79% excreted in feces mostly as metabolites.
Half-life: 12 hr.

TIME/ACTION PROFILE (effect on lipids)

ROUTE	ONSET	PEAK	DURATION
PO	within 4 wk	4 wk	unknown

Contraindications/Precautions

Contraindicated in: Hypersensitivity; Active liver disease, including unexplained elevations in liver function tests; Concurrent use of cyclosporine or lopinavir/ritonavir; Severe renal impairment (CCr <30 mL/min); OB: Pregnancy or women who may become pregnant Lactation: Breast-feeding should be avoided.

Use Cautiously in: Renal impairment (↑ risk of myopathy, dosage reduction recommended for CCr 30–<60 mL/min); Hypothyroidism, concurrent use of fibrates or lipid-lowering doses of niacin (↑ risk of myopathy); Geri: ↑ risk of myopathy (age >65 yr); History of alcohol abuse or moderate alcohol consumption (↑ risk of liver damage); Pedi: Safe and effective use in children not established.

Interactions

Drug-Drug: Concurrent use with **lopinavir/ritonavir** or **cyclosporine** should be avoided due to increased levels and risk of toxicity/adverse reactions. **Erythromycin** ↑ blood levels and risk of toxicity; daily dose should not exceed 1 mg. **Rifampin** ↑ blood levels and risk of toxicity; daily dose should not exceed 2 mg. Concurrent use with **fibrates** or lipid-lowering dose of **niacin** ↑ risk of adverse skeletal muscle effects (consider lower dose of pitavastatin with niacin). **Alcohol** may ↑ risk of liver toxicity.

Route/Dosage

PO (Adults): 2 mg once daily initially; may be increased up to 4 mg depending on response. *With erythromycin*—daily dose should not exceed 1 mg; with *rifampin*—daily dose should not exceed 2 mg.

Renal Impairment

PO (Adults): *CCr 30–<60 mL/min*—1 mg once daily initially, may be increased up to 2 mg daily.

Availability

Tablets: 1 mg, 2 mg, 4 mg

plerixafor (pler-ix-a-fore)

Mozobil

Classification
Therapeutic: none assigned
Pharmacologic: hematopoietic stem cell mobilizers

Indications

Mobilizes hematopoietic stem cells to peripheral blood for collection and use in autologous transplantation in patients with non-Hodgkin's lymphoma and multiple myeloma; used in combination with granulocyte-colony stimulation factor (G-CSF).

Action

Inhibits the CXCR-4 chemokine receptor, blocking its binding ability. Inhibition decreases adherence of stem cells to bone marrow, freeing them up to mobilize to peripheral blood. **Therapeutic Effects:** Mobilization of stem cells to peripheral blood allowing collection.

Adverse Reactions/Side Effects

CNS: dizziness, fatigue, headache, insomnia.
GI: SPLENIC RUPTURE, diarrhea, nausea, vomiting, abdominal distention/pain, constipation, dry mouth, dyspepsia, flatulence. **Derm:** erythema, sweating. **Hemat:** leukemia/tumor cell mobilization, thrombocytopenia. **Local:** injection site reactions. **MS:** musculoskeletal pain. **Neuro:** oral hypoesthesia.

PHYSICAL THERAPY IMPLICATIONS

Examination and Evaluation

- Watch for signs of spleen rupture, including pain and tenderness in the upper left abdomen, lightheadedness, dizziness, and confusion. Report these signs to the physician or nursing staff immediately.
- Monitor signs of thrombocytopenia such as bruising, nose bleeds and bleeding gums. Report these signs to the physician or nursing staff immediately.
- Assess any muscle or joint pain to rule out musculoskeletal pathology; that is, try to determine if pain is drug induced rather than caused by anatomic or biomechanical problems.
- Assess dizziness that might affect gait, balance, and other functional activities (See Appendix C). Report balance problems and functional limitations to the physician and nursing staff, and caution the patient and family/caregivers to guard against falls and trauma.
- Monitor subcutaneous injection site for pain, swelling, and irritation. Report prolonged or excessive injection site reactions to the physician.

Interventions

- For patients who are medically able to begin exercise, implement appropriate resistive exercises and aerobic training to maintain muscle strength and aerobic capacity during cancer chemotherapy or to help restore function after chemotherapy.

Patient/Client-Related Instruction

Instruct patient to report other bothersome side effects such as severe or prolonged headache, sleep loss, numbness around the mouth, skin reactions (flushing, increased sweating), or GI problems (nausea, vomiting, diarrhea, constipation, abdominal pain, indigestion, flatulence).

Pharmacokinetics

Absorption: Well absorbed following SC administration.
Distribution: Largely confined to extravascular fluid space.
Metabolism and Excretion: Not metabolized by the liver; 70% unchanged in urine.
Half-life: 5.3 hr.

TIME/ACTION PROFILE (mobilization of cells)

ROUTE	ONSET	PEAK	DURATION
SC	rapid	10–14 hr*	unknown

*With G-CSF pretreatment.

Contraindications/Precautions

Contraindicated in: Leukemia; OB/Lactation: Pregnancy, lactation.
Use Cautiously in: Renal impairment (dose reduction required if CCr ≤50 mL/min); Geri: Consider age-related decrease in renal function and greater sensitivity to drug effects; OB: Women with childbearing potential; Pedi: Safety and effectiveness in children have not been established.

Interactions

Drug-Drug: None noted.

Route/Dosage

SC (Adults): *Following pretreatment with G-CSF for 4 days*—0.24 mg/kg once daily for up to 4 days (not to exceed 40 mg/day); use actual body weight to calculate dose.

Renal Impairment

SC (Adults): *Following pretreatment with G-CSF for 4 days*—0.16 mg/kg once daily for up to 4 days (not to exceed 27 mg/day).

Availability

Solution for SC injection: 20 mg/mL in 1.2-mL vials.

porfimer (pore-fim-er)

Photofrin

Classification
Therapeutic: antineoplastics
Pharmacologic: photosensitizers

Indications

Part of photodynamic therapy (PDT) for Esophageal cancer that has completely or partially obstructed the esophagus and cannot be treated with Nd:YAG laser therapy, Reduction of obstruction and palliation of symptoms in patients with completely or partially obstructive endobronchial non–small-cell lung cancer, Microinvasive endobronchial non–small-cell lung cancer when surgery or radiation are not options, High-grade dysplasia due to Barrett's esophagus in patients who are unable to have esophagectomy.

Action

Porfimer is retained by the tumor, which is then treated with a laser light. When porfimer absorbs the light, a photochemical reaction occurs, causing cellular damage. Thromboxane A is also produced, causing additional local tumor necrosis. **Therapeutic Effects:** Shrinkage of esophageal or endobronchial tumors.

Adverse Reactions/Side Effects

CNS: insomnia, anxiety, confusion, weakness. **Resp:** RESPIRATORY INSUFFICIENCY, dyspnea, mucositis reaction, pharyngitis, pleural effusion, pneumonia, cough, tracheoesophageal fistula. **CV:** HEART FAILURE, atrial fibrillation, chest pain, edema, hypertension, hypotension, tachycardia. **GI:** ESOPHAGEAL RUPTURE, GI BLEEDING, abdominal pain, constipation, nausea, vomiting, anorexia, diarrhea, dyspepsia, eructation, esophageal tumor bleeding, esophageal stricture. **Derm:** photosensitivity. **F and E:** dehydration. **Hemat:** anemia. **Misc:** fever, pain, moniliasis, urinary tract infection, weight loss.

PHYSICAL THERAPY IMPLICATIONS

Examination and Evaluation

- Monitor respiration, and report signs of respiratory insufficiency, pleural effusion, or pneumonia. Signs include shortness of breath, dyspnea, rapid/shallow breathing, chest pain, fever, and cyanosis. Monitor pulse oximetry and perform pulmonary function tests (See Appendces I, J, K) to quantify suspected changes in ventilation and respiratory function. Excessive respiratory depression requires emergency care.
- Monitor signs of GI bleeding, including abdominal pain, vomiting blood, blood in stools, or black, tarry stools. Report these signs to the physician immediately.
- Be alert for signs of esophageal rupture, including chest and abdominal pain, nausea, vomiting blood, rapid breathing, and shock. Request emergency care if these signs occur.
- Assess signs of heart failure, including dyspnea, rales/crackles, peripheral edema, jugular venous distention, and exercise intolerance. Report these signs to the physician immediately.
- Assess heart rate, ECG, and heart sounds, especially during exercise (See Appendices G, H). Report any rhythm disturbances or symptoms of increased arrhythmias, including palpitations, chest discomfort, shortness of breath, fainting, and fatigue/weakness.
- Assess blood pressure (BP) and compare to normal values (See Appendix F). Report changes in BP, either a problematic decrease in BP (hypotension) or a sustained increase in BP (hypertension).
- Assess peripheral edema using girth measurements, volume displacement, and measurement of pitting edema (See Appendix N). Report increased swelling in feet and ankles or a sudden increase in body weight due to fluid retention.
- Monitor signs of anemia, including unusual fatigue, shortness of breath with exertion, pallor, and bruising. Notify physician if these signs occur.
- Be alert for confusion, agitation, sleep loss, or other alterations in mental status. Notify physician promptly if these symptoms develop (See Appendix D).
- Assess any muscle or joint pain to rule out musculoskeletal pathology; that is, try to determine if pain is drug induced rather than caused by anatomic or biomechanical problems.

Interventions

- For patients who are medically able to begin exercise, implement appropriate resistive exercises and aerobic training to maintain muscle strength and aerobic capacity during cancer chemotherapy or to help restore function after chemotherapy.
- Because of the risk of cardiovascular and respiratory problems, use caution during aerobic exercise and other forms of therapeutic exercise. Assess exercise tolerance frequently (BP, heart rate, fatigue levels), and terminate exercise immediately if any untoward responses occur (See Appendix L).
- Make sure patient maintains adequate fluid intake to avoid dehydration, especially during exercise.
- Causes photosensitivity; use care if administering UV treatments. Advise patient to avoid direct sunlight and use sunscreens and protective clothing.

Patient/Client-Related Instruction

- Advise patient about the likelihood of GI problems such as nausea, vomiting, diarrhea, constipation, indigestion, belching, loss of appetite, and abdominal pain. Instruct patient to notify physician or nursing staff about severe of unexpected GI reactions.
- Instruct patient and family/caregivers to report other troublesome side effects such as severe or prolonged cough, fever, weight loss, and urinary tract or vaginal infections.

Pharmacokinetics

Absorption: IV administration results in complete bioavailability.
Distribution: Retained for a longer period by tumors, skin, and reticuloendothelial tissue.
Protein Binding: 90%.
Metabolism and Excretion: Unknown.
Half-life: 250 hr.

TIME/ACTION PROFILE (antitumor effect)

ROUTE	ONSET	PEAK	DURATION
IV	rapid*	unknown	unknown

*After laser light treatment.

Contraindications/Precautions

Contraindicated in: History of porphyria or hypersensitivity to porphyrins; Tracheobronchial or bronchoesophageal fistulas or tumors with potential to erode into a major blood vessel or the trachea; Not suitable for acute treatment of patients with severe respiratory distress due to obstructive endobrachial lesion; Esophageal or gastric varices, or esophageal ulcers >1 cm in diameter; Should not be used within 4 wk of radiation therapy.

Use Cautiously in: Direct sunlight or bright indoor light (photosensitivity will occur); Pregnancy, lactation, or children (contraception should be practiced; safety not established).

Interactions

Drug-Drug: Photosensitizing effect may be ↑ by concurrent use of **tetracyclines, sulfonamides, phenothiazines, sulfonylurea oral hypoglycemic agents**, or **thiazide diuretics**. The effects of photodynamic therapy may be altered by **calcium channel blockers, corticosteroids, ethanol, mannitol, dimethyl sulfoxide, beta carotene, vasoconstrictors**, or **agents that affect clotting**.

Route/Dosage

IV (Adults): 2 mg/kg followed 40–50 hr later by laser light therapy. A 2nd session of laser light therapy may be given 96–120 hr after porfimer and may be preceded by gentle tumor débridement. Up to 3 treatments may be given; 30-day minimum interval between treatments.

Availability

Lyophilized for injection (requires reconstitution): 75 mg/vial.

posaconazole

(poe-sa-**kon**-a-zole)

Noxafil

Classification

Therapeutic: antifungals

Pharmacologic: triazoles

Indications

Prevention of invasive *Aspergillus* and *Candida* infections in severely immunocompromised patients. Treatment of oropharyngeal candidiasis (including candidiasis unresponsive to itraconazole or fluconazole).

Action

Blocks ergosterol synthesis, a major component of fungal plasma membrane. **Therapeutic Effects:** Fungistatic/fungicidal action against susceptible fungi.

Adverse Reactions/Side Effects

GI: HEPATOCELLULAR DAMAGE, diarrhea, nausea, vomiting. **Endo:** adrenal insufficiency.
Metab: ALLERGIC RECTIONS.

PHYSICAL THERAPY IMPLICATIONS

Examination and Evaluation

- Be alert for signs of hepatotoxicity, including anorexia, abdominal pain, severe nausea and vomiting, yellow skin or eyes, fever, sore throat, malaise, weakness, facial edema, lethargy, and unusual bleeding or bruising. Report these signs to the physician or nursing staff immediately.
- Monitor signs of allergic reactions, including pulmonary symptoms (tightness in the throat and chest, wheezing, cough, dyspnea) or skin reactions (rash, pruritus, urticaria). Notify physician or nursing staff immediately if these reactions occur.
- Monitor and report signs of adrenal insufficiency, including hypotension, weight loss, weakness, nausea, vomiting, anorexia, lethargy, confusion, and restlessness.

Interventions

- Always wash hands thoroughly and disinfect equipment (whirlpools, electrotherapeutic devices, treatment tables, and so forth) to help prevent the spread of infection. Use universal precautions or isolation procedures as indicated for specific patients.

Patient/Client-Related Instruction

- Advise patient to take this drug as directed for the full course of treatment even if feeling better.
- Instruct patient to report other troublesome side effects such as prolonged or severe nausea, vomiting, or diarrhea.

Pharmacokinetics

Absorption: Well absorbed following oral administration; absorption is optimized by food.
Distribution: Extensive extravascular distribution and penetration into body tissues.
Protein Binding: >98%.
Metabolism and Excretion: Some metabolism via UDP glucuronidation; 66% eliminated unchanged in feces, 13% in urine (mostly as metabolites).
Half-life: 35 hr.

TIME/ACTION PROFILE (blood levels)

ROUTE	ONSET	PEAK	DURATION
PO	unknown	3–5 hr	8 hr

Contraindications/Precautions

Contraindicated in: Hypersensitivity; Concurrent use of pimozide or quinidine (↑ risk of serious arrhythmias); Concurrent use of ergot alkaloids (↑ risk of ergotism).

Use Cautiously in: History of/predisposition to QTc prolongation, including congenital QTc prolongation, concurrent medications which prolong QTc, high cumulative anthracycline history, or electrolyte abnormalities (hypokalemia, hypomagnesemia); correct preexisting abnormalities prior to administration; Hypersensitivity to other azole antifungals; Hepatic impairment; Severe diarrhea, vomiting, or renal impairment (monitor for breakthrough fungal infections); OB: Use only in pregnancy or lactation if maternal benefit outweighs risk to child; Pedi: Safe use in children <13 yr not established.

Interactions

Drug-Drug: Posaconazole inhibits the CYP3A4 enzyme systems and should be expected to interact with other drugs affected by this system. **Rifabutin, phenytoin**, and **cimetidine** ↓ levels and may ↓ antifungal effectiveness; avoid concurrent use. ↑ **cyclosporine, sirolimus**, and **tacrolimus** levels and risk of toxicity; ↓ dose initially and monitor levels frequently. ↑ **rifabutin** levels; avoid concurrent use of **phenytoin** and **midazolam**; monitor for excess clinical effect and dose accordingly. ↑ levels and risk of toxicity from **ergot alkaloids**, including **ergotamine** and **dihydroergotamine**; concurrent administration is contraindicated. ↑ levels and risk of neurotoxicity of **vinca alkaloids**, including **vincristine** and **vinblastine**; consider dose adjustment. ↑ levels and risk of toxicity of **HMG CoA reductase inhibitors (statins)**; consider ↓ statin dose. May ↑ levels and risk of adverse cardiovascular reactions to **calcium channel blockers**; consider dosage reduction.

Route/Dosage

PO (Adults): 200 mg tid.

Availability

Oral suspension (cherry): 40 mg/mL in 105-mL bottles.

pralatrexate (praye-la-**treks**-ate)

Folotyn

Classification

Therapeutic: antineoplastics

Pharmacologic: folic acid analogues

Indications

Treatment relapsed/refractory peripheral T-cell lymphoma.

Action

Interferes with folic acid metabolism by acting as a folate analogue metabolic inhibitor that competitively inhibits dihydrofolate reductase; also acts as a competitive inhibitor for polyglutamylation by the enzyme folylpolyglutamyl synthetase. Results is inhibition of DNA synthesis. **Therapeutic Effects:** Death of rapidly replication cells, particularly malignant ones.

Adverse Reactions/Side Effects

CNS: fatigue. **EENT:** epistaxis, pharyngolaryngeal pain. **Resp:** dyspnea, cough. **CV:** edema, tachycardia. **GI:** mucositis, nausea, abdominal pain, anorexia, constipation, diarrhea, vomiting, liver function abnormalities. **Derm:** pruritus, rash. **F and E:** dehydration, hypokalemia. **Hemat:** NEUTROPENIA, THROMBOCYTOPENIA, anemia. **MS:** back pain, extremity pain. **Misc:** SEPSIS, fever, night sweats

PHYSICAL THERAPY IMPLICATIONS

Examination and Evaluation

- Watch for signs of neutropenia (fever, sore throat, mucosal lesions, other signs of infection), thrombocytopenia (bruising, nose bleeds, bleeding gums), or unusual weakness and fatigue that might be due to anemia. Report these signs to the physician or nursing staff immediately.
- Be alert for signs of infection and sepsis, including high fever (>101.3 F), tachycardia, rapid/shallow breathing, abrupt change in mental status, decreased urine output, and severe hypotension. Report these signs to the physician or nursing staff immediately.
- Assess any breathing problems, and report severe or prolonged cough or difficult, labored breathing.
- Assess peripheral edema using girth measurements, volume displacement, and measurement of pitting edema (See Appendix N). Report increased swelling in feet and ankles or a sudden increase in body weight due to fluid retention.
- Assess any back pain or extremity pain to rule out musculoskeletal pathology; that is, try to determine if pain is drug induced rather than caused by anatomic or biomechanical problems.
- Monitor and report any muscle weakness, aches, or cramps that might indicate low potassium levels (hypokalemia).
- Assess dizziness (See Appendix C) that might affect gait, balance, and other functional activities. Report balance problems and functional limitations to the physician and nursing staff, and caution the patient and family/caregivers to guard against falls and trauma.

Interventions

- For patients with cancer who are medically able to begin exercise, implement appropriate resistive exercises and aerobic training to maintain muscle

strength and aerobic capacity during cancer chemotherapy or to help restore function after chemotherapy.
- Make sure patient maintains adequate fluid intake to avoid dehydration, especially during exercise.

Patient/Client-Related Instruction

- Instruct patient to guard against infection (frequent hand washing, etc.), and to avoid crowds and contact with persons with contagious diseases.
- Advise patient and family/caregivers that fatigue and weakness are likely and may be severe. Implement assistive devices (walker, cane, wheelchair) as needed to help maintain mobility and prevent falls.
- Advise patient about the likelihood of GI reactions such as nausea, vomiting, diarrhea, constipation, abdominal pain, loss of appetite, and inflammation of mucous membranes. Instruct patient to report severe or prolonged GI problems or signs of hepatic toxicity (abdominal pain, severe nausea and vomiting, yellow skin or eyes, fever, sore throat, malaise, weakness, facial edema, lethargy, unusual bleeding or bruising).
- Instruct patient or family/caregivers to report other troublesome side effects, including severe or prolonged nosebleeds, pain in the throat and pharynx, fever, night sweats, or skin reactions (rash, itching).

Pharmacokinetics

Absorption: IV administration results in complete bioavailability.
Distribution: unknown
Metabolism and Excretion: Some metabolism by the liver; 34% excreted unchanged in urine.
Half-life: 12–18 hr.

TIME/ACTION PROFILE (effects on blood counts)

ROUTE	ONSET	PEAK	DURATION
IV	45 days*	unknown	unknown

*Median time to 1st response.

Contraindications/Precautions

Contraindicated in: OB: Avoid use during pregnancy; Lactation: Breast-feeding should be avoided.
Use Cautiously in: Moderate-to-severe renal impairment; Geri: Consider age-related decrease in renal function; OB: Patients with childbearing potential; Pedi: Safe and effective use in children has not been established.

Interactions

Drug-Drug: Probenecid, **NSAIDs**, and **trimethoprim/sulfamethoxazole** may ↓ clearance and ↑ blood levels and the risk of toxicity.

Route/Dosage

IV (Adults): 30 mg/m^2 once weekly for 6 wk in 7-wk cycles (supplemental intramuscular vitamin B_{12} 1 mg q 8–10 wk and folic acid 1–1.25 mg orally on a daily basis is required); if adverse reactions occur, dose may be decreased to 20 mg/m^2.

Availability

Solution for intravenous injection: 20 mg/mL in 1- and 2-mL vials.

pramipexole (pra-mi-peks-ole)

Mirapex

Classification

Therapeutic: antiparkinson agents
Pharmacologic: dopamine agonists

Indications

Management of idiopathic Parkinson's disease. Restless leg syndrome.

Action

Stimulates dopamine receptors in the striatum of the brain. **Therapeutic Effects:** Decreased tremor and rigidity in Parkinson's disease. Decreased leg restlessness.

Adverse Reactions/Side Effects

CNS: SLEEP ATTACKS, amnesia, dizziness, drowsiness, hallucinations, weakness, abnormal dreams, confusion, dyskinesia, extrapyramidal syndrome, headache, insomnia. **CV:** orthostatic hypotension. **GI:** constipation, dry mouth, dyspepsia, nausea, tooth disease. **GU:** urinary frequency. **MS:** leg cramps. **Neuro:** hypertonia, unsteadiness/falling.

PHYSICAL THERAPY IMPLICATIONS

Examination and Evaluation

- Be aware that pramipexole can cause sudden, unexpected episodes of falling asleep (sleep attacks). Use caution during activities where patient might fall asleep suddenly.
- Assess gait and motor function to help determine antiparkinson effects, especially when starting drug therapy or during dosing changes or addition of other antiparkinson drugs. Motor function should be assessed at different times of the day, such as when drugs are reaching peak therapeutic levels (i.e., 30–60 min after oral dose), as well as when drug effects are minimal (just before the next dose).
- Document increased motor side effects such as involuntary movements (dyskinesias), increased muscle tone, fluctuations in response (on-off phenomenon, end-of-dose akinesia), or other abnormal movement patterns (extrapyramidal syndrome). Notify physician because increased motor side effects might require dose adjustment or a change in medication regimen.
- Monitor confusion, hallucinations, memory loss, and other psychologic problems. Repeated or

excessive symptoms may require change in dose or medication.

- Assess dizziness, drowsiness, and unsteadiness that affects gait, balance, and other functional activities (See Appendix C). Report balance problems and functional limitations to the physician, and caution the patient and family/caregivers to guard against falls and trauma.
- Assess blood pressure (BP) when patient assumes a more upright position (lying to standing, sitting to standing, lying to sitting). Document orthostatic hypotension and contact physician when systolic BP falls >20 mm Hg, or diastolic BP falls >10 mm Hg.
- If used to treat restless leg syndrome, assess the severity and frequency of restless episodes (i.e., an intense need to get up and move around) and lower extremity symptoms such as crawling, tingling, cramping, aching, burning, creeping, and similar sensations. Document whether drug therapy is effective in reducing these symptoms.

Interventions

- Implement therapeutic exercises (coordination exercises, gait training, cardiovascular conditioning) to complement the effects of drug therapy and help achieve optimal function.
- Guard against falls and trauma (hip fractures, head injury, and so forth). Implement fall- prevention strategies (See Appendix E), especially if patient exhibits Parkinson's symptoms (postural instability, rigidity) combined with drug side effects (dizziness, unsteadiness, dyskinesias).
- To minimize orthostatic hypotension, patient should move slowly when assuming a more upright position.

Patient/Client-Related Instruction

- Advise patient and family or caregiver about the possibility of sleep attacks (see above under Examination and Evaluation).
- Advise patient to avoid alcohol because of the increased risk of sedation and adverse effects.
- Advise patient about the likelihood of GI reactions such as nausea, constipation, indigestion, and dry mouth. Instruct patient to report severe or prolonged GI problems.
- Instruct patient to report other troublesome side effects such as severe or prolonged headaches, sleep loss, nightmares, leg cramps, urinary retention, and tooth disease.

Pharmacokinetics

Absorption: >90% absorbed following oral administration.
Distribution: Widely distributed.
Metabolism and Excretion: 90% excreted unchanged in urine.
Half-life: 8 hr (increased in geriatric patients and patients with renal impairment).

TIME/ACTION PROFILE (blood levels)

ROUTE	ONSET	PEAK	DURATION
PO	unknown	2 hr	8 hr

Contraindications/Precautions

Contraindicated in: Hypersensitivity.
Use Cautiously in: Geri: ↑ risk of hallucinations; Renal impairment (↑ dosing interval recommended if CCr <60 mL/min); OB/Lactation/Pedi: Safety not established.

Interactions

Drug-Drug: Concurrent **levodopa** ↑ risk of hallucinations and dyskinesia. Effectiveness may be ↑ by **cimetidine**. Effectiveness may be ↓ by **dopamine antagonists**, including **butyrophenones, metoclopramide, phenothiazines,** or **thioxanthenes**.

Route/Dosage

PO (Adults): *Parkinson's disease* —0.125 mg tid initially; may be increased q 5–7 days (range 1.5–4.5 mg/day in 3 divided doses). *Restless leg syndrome*— 0.125 mg once daily 1–3 hr before bedtime. May be increased at 4- to 7-day intervals to 0.25 mg, then up to 0.5 mg.

Renal Impairment

PO (Adults): *Parkinson's disease—CCr 35–59 mL/min*—0.125 mg bid initially, may be increased q 5–7 days up to 1.5 mg bid; *CCr 15–34 mL/min*—0.125 mg once daily initially, may be increased q 5–7 days up to 1.5 mg once daily. *Restless leg syndrome*—0.125 mg once daily 1–3 hr before bedtime. May be increased at 14-day intervals to 0.25 mg, then up to 0.5 mg.

Availability (generic available)

Tablets: 0.125 mg, 0.25 mg, 0.5 mg, 0.75 mg, 1 mg, 1.5 mg.

HIGH ALERT

pramlintide (pram-lin-tide)

Symlin

Classification

Therapeutic: antidiabetics
Pharmacologic: hormones

Indications

Used with mealtime insulin in the management of diabetics whose blood sugar cannot be controlled by optimal

P

insulin therapy; can be used with other agents (sulfonylureas, metformin).

Action

Acts as a synthetic analogue of amylin, an endogenous pancreatic hormone that helps to control postprandial hyperglycemia; effects include slowed gastric emptying, suppression of glucagon secretion, and regulation of food intake. **Therapeutic Effects:** Improved control of postprandial hyperglycemia.

Adverse Reactions/Side Effects

Noted for concurrent use with insulin
CNS: dizziness, fatigue, headache. **Resp:** cough.
GI: nausea, abdominal pain, anorexia, vomiting.
Endo: HYPOGLYCEMIA. **Derm:** local allergy. **MS:** arthralgia.
Misc: injection-site reactions, systemic allergic reactions.

PHYSICAL THERAPY IMPLICATIONS

Examination and Evaluation

- Be alert for signs of hypoglycemia, especially during and after exercise. Common neuromuscular symptoms include anxiety; restlessness; tingling in hands, feet, lips, or tongue; chills; cold sweats; confusion; difficulty in concentration; drowsiness; excessive hunger; headache; irritability; nervousness; tremor; weakness; unsteady gait. Report repeated or severe hypoglycemic episodes to the physician.
- Monitor signs of systemic allergic reactions, including pulmonary symptoms (tightness in the throat and chest, wheezing, cough, dyspnea) or skin reactions (rash, pruritus, urticaria). Notify physician immediately if these reactions occur.
- Assess any joint pain to rule out musculoskeletal pathology; that is, try to determine if pain is drug induced rather than caused by anatomic or biomechanical problems.
- Assess dizziness that might affect gait, balance, and other functional activities (See Appendix C). Report balance problems and functional limitations to the physician, and caution the patient and family/caregivers to guard against falls and trauma.
- Assess injection site for redness, swelling, or local allergic reactions. Make sure patient understands the need to rotate injections sites to prevent local damage.

Interventions

- Implement aerobic exercise and endurance training programs to maintain optimal body weight, improve insulin sensitivity, and reduce the risk of macrovascular disease (heart attack, stroke) and microvascular problems (reduced blood flow to tissues and organs that causes poor wound healing, neuropathy, retinopathy, and nephropathy).
- Provide a source of oral glucose (fruit juice, glucose gels/tablets, etc.) to treat mild hypoglycemia. Call for emergency assistance if symptoms persist or in cases of severe hypoglycemia. Emergency treatment typically consists of IV glucose, glucagon, or epinephrine.
- Do not apply physical agents (heat, cold, electrotherapeutic modalities) or massage at or near the injection site; these interventions will alter drug absorption from subcutaneous tissues.

Patient/Client-Related Instruction

- Encourage patient to monitor blood glucose before and after exercise, and to adjust medications accordingly based on exercise duration and intensity.
- Emphasize the importance of adhering to nutritional guidelines, and the need for periodic assessment of glycemic control (serum glucose and glycosylated hemoglobin levels) throughout the management of diabetes mellitus.
- Advise patient about symptoms of hyperglycemia (confusion, drowsiness; flushed, dry skin; fruit-like breath odor; rapid, deep breathing; polyuria; loss of appetite; unusual thirst). Medication dosages may need to be adjusted to prevent repeated episodes of hyperglycemia.
- Instruct patient and family/caregivers to report other troublesome side effects such as severe or prolonged headache, cough, or GI problems (nausea, vomiting, abdominal pain, loss of appetite).

Pharmacokinetics

Absorption: 30–40% absorbed following SC administration.
Distribution: Does not appear to significantly cross the placenta.
Metabolism and Excretion: Metabolized by the kidneys; major metabolite has pharmacologic properties similar to the parent compound.
Half-life: 48 min.

TIME/ACTION PROFILE (effect on blood sugar*)

ROUTE	ONSET	PEAK	DURATION
SC	rapid	20 min	3 hr

*Blood level.

Contraindications/Precautions

Contraindicated in: Hypersensitivity; Inability to identify hypoglycemia; Gastroparesis or need for medications to stimulate gastric motility; Poor compliance with current insulin regimen or self-monitoring; HbA1c >9%; Recurring severe hypoglycemia within the last 6 mo, requiring treatment; Pedi: Children.
Use Cautiously in: OB/Lactation: Use only if maternal benefit outweighs potential risks to fetus/newborn.

Interactions

Drug-Drug: ↑ likelihood of hypoglycemia with short-acting **insulin**; reduce dose of short-acting premeal insulin by 50%. Avoid concurrent use with other agents that ↓ GI motility, including **atropine** and other **anticholinergics**. Avoid concurrent use with other agents that ↓ GI absorption of nutrients, including **α-glucosidase inhibitors,** including **acarbose** and **miglitol**. May delay oral absorption of concurrently administered drugs; if prompt absorption is desired, administer 1 hr before or 2 hr after pramlintide.

Route/Dosage

Insulin-Using Type 2 Diabetes

SC (Adults): 60 mcg, immediately prior to major meals initially; if no significant nausea occurs, dose may be increased to 120 mcg.

Type 1 Diabetes

SC (Adults): 15 mcg, immediately prior to major meals initially; if no significant nausea occurs, dose may be increased by 15 mcg q 3 days up to 60 mcg.

Availability

Injection: 0.6 mg/mL in 5-mL vials.

prasugrel (pra-soo-grel)

Effient

Classification

Therapeutic: antiplatelet agents

Pharmacologic: thienopyridines

Indications

Reduction of thrombotic cardiovascular events (including stent thrombosis) in patients with acute coronary syndrome who will be managed with PCI, including patients with unstable angina or non–ST-elevation myocardial infarction (NSTEMI). Reduction of thrombotic cardiovascular events (including stent thrombosis) in patients with STEMI when managed with either primary/delayed PCI.

Action

Acts by irreversibly binding its active metabolite to the $P2Y_{12}$ class of ADP receptors on platelets; inhibiting platelet activation and aggregation. **Therapeutic Effects:** Decreased thrombotic event, including cardiovascular death, nonfatal myocardial infarction (MI), and nonfatal stroke.

Adverse Reactions/Side Effects

CNS: dizziness, fatigue, headache. **Resp:** cough, dyspnea. **CV:** atrial fibrillation, bradycardia, hypertension, hypotension, peripheral edema. **GI:** diarrhea, nausea. **Derm:** rash. **Hemat:** BLEEDING, THROMBOTIC THROMBOCYTOPENIC PURPURA, leukopenia. **Metab:** hyperlipidemia. **MS:** back pain, extremity pain. **Misc:** fever, noncardiac chest pain

PHYSICAL THERAPY IMPLICATIONS

Examination and Evaluation

- Be alert for signs of bleeding, including bleeding gums, nosebleeds, unusual bruising, hematuria, blood in stools, and a fall in hematocrit or blood pressure. Notify physician or nursing staff immediately if these signs occur.
- Monitor signs of thrombotic thrombocytopenic purpura, such as purplish spots on the skin, decreased consciousness, fatigue, weakness, shortness of breath on exertion, and tachycardia. Report these signs to the physician or nursing staff immediately.
- Assess heart rate, ECG, and heart sounds, especially during exercise (See Appendices G, H). Report an unusually slow heart rate (bradycardia) or signs of other arrhythmias, including palpitations, chest discomfort, shortness of breath, fainting, and fatigue/weakness.
- Assess blood pressure periodically and compare to normal values (See Appendix F). Report low blood pressure (hypotension), especially if patient experiences dizziness or syncope.
- Assess peripheral edema using girth measurements, volume displacement, and measurement of pitting edema (See Appendix N). Report increased swelling in feet and ankles or a sudden increase in body weight due to fluid retention.
- Watch for signs of leukopenia, including fever, sore throat, mucosal lesions, or other signs of infection. Report these signs to the physician or nursing staff.
- Assess any breathing problems, and report severe or prolonged cough or difficult, labored breathing.
- Assess any back pain or extremity pain to rule out musculoskeletal pathology; that is, try to determine if pain is drug induced rather than caused by anatomic or biomechanical problems.
- Assess dizziness that might affect gait, balance, and other functional activities (See Appendix C). Report balance problems and functional limitations to the physician and nursing staff, and caution the patient and family/caregivers to guard against falls and trauma.

Interventions

- Use caution with any physical interventions that could increase bleeding, including wound débridement, chest percussion, joint mobilization, and application of local heat.
- Use caution during aerobic exercise in patients at risk for MI, stroke, or other cardiovascular events. Assess exercise tolerance frequently (blood pressure,

P

heart rate, fatigue levels), and terminate exercise immediately if any untoward responses occur (See Appendix L).

Patient/Client-Related Instruction

- Remind patients to take medication as directed to reduce the risk of heart attack and stroke even if they are asymptomatic.
- Counsel patients about additional interventions to help reduce the risk of cardiovascular pathology, including regular exercise, weight loss, sodium restriction, stress reduction, moderation of alcohol consumption, and smoking cessation.
- Advise patient that this drug may cause problems in fat metabolism, including increased cholesterol. Remind patient that periodic blood tests may be needed to monitor plasma lipids.
- Instruct patient or family/caregivers to report other bothersome side effects such as severe or prolonged headache, fatigue, chest pain, fever, skin rash, or GI problems (nausea, diarrhea).

Pharmacokinetics

Absorption: Well absorbed following oral administration (79%), then rapidly converted to an active metabolite.
Distribution: Unknown.
Protein Binding: *Active metabolite*—98%.
Metabolism and Excretion: Active metabolite is metabolized to 2 inactive compounds; 68% excreted in the urine and 27% in feces as inactive metabolites.
Half-life: *Active metabolite*—7 hr (range 2–15 hr).

TIME/ACTION PROFILE (effect on platelet function)

ROUTE	ONSET	PEAK	DURATION
PO	within 1 hr	2 hr	5–9 days*

*Following discontinuation.

Contraindications/Precautions

Contraindicated in: Hypersensitivity; Active pathologic bleeding; History of transient ischemic attack or stroke.
Use Cautiously in: Patients about to undergo coronary artery bypass grafting (CABG) (↑ risk of bleeding; discontinue at least 7 days prior to surgery). Premature discontinuation (↑ risk of stent thrombosis, MI, and death). Body weight <60 kg, propensity to bleed, severe hepatic impairment, concurrent use of medications that ↑ the risk of bleeding (↑ risk of bleeding). Hypotension in the setting of recent coronary angiography, PCI, CABG, or other surgical procedure (suspect bleeding but do not discontinue prasugrel). Geri: Use in patients ≥75 yr of age generally not recommended (↑ risk of fatal/intracranial bleeding and questionable benefit, except in high-risk patients such as those with diabetes or prior MI). OB: Use only if potential benefit to mother justifies potential risk to fetus. Lactation: Use only if potential benefit to the mother justifies potential risk to nursing infant. Pedi: Safety and effectiveness not established.

Interactions

Drug-Drug: ↑ risk of bleeding with **warfarin** and **NSAIDs.**

Route/Dosage

Aspirin 75–325 mg/daily should be taken concurrently.
PO (Adults ≥60 kg): 60 mg initially as a loading dose, then 10 mg once daily.
PO (Adults <60 kg): Consider maintenance dose of 5 mg once daily.

Availability

Tablets: 5 mg, 10 mg.

pravastatin (prav-a-**stat**-in)

Pravachol

Classification
Therapeutic: lipid-lowering agents
Pharmacologic: HMG-CoA reductase inhibitors (statins)

Indications

Adjunctive management of primary hypercholesterolemia and mixed dyslipidemias. Primary prevention of coronary heart disease (myocardial infarction, coronary revascularization, cardiovascular mortality) in asymptomatic patients with increased total and low-density lipoprotein (LDL) cholesterol and decreased high-density lipoprotein (HDL) cholesterol. Secondary prevention of myocardial infarction, coronary revascularization, stroke, and overall mortality in patients with clinically evident coronary heart disease.

Action

Inhibits 3-hydroxy-3-methylglutaryl coenzyme A (HMG CoA) reductase, an enzyme which is responsible for catalyzing an early step in the synthesis of cholesterol. **Therapeutic Effects:** Lowering of total and LDL cholesterol and triglycerides. Slightly increases HDL cholesterol. Slows the progression of coronary atherosclerosis with resultant decrease in coronary heart disease–related events.

Adverse Reactions/Side Effects

CNS: dizziness, headache, insomnia, weakness. **EENT:** rhinitis. **Resp:** bronchitis. **CV:** chest pain, peripheral edema. **GI:** abdominal cramps, constipation, diarrhea, flatus, heartburn, altered taste, drug-induced hepatitis, dyspepsia, elevated liver enzymes, nausea, pancreatitis. **GU:** erectile dysfunction. **Derm:** rashes, pruritus. **MS:** RHABDOMYOLYSIS, arthralgia, arthritis, myalgia, myositis. **Misc:** hypersensitivity reactions.

PHYSICAL THERAPY IMPLICATIONS

Examination and Evaluation

- Assess any joint pain, or muscle pain, tenderness, or weakness, especially if accompanied by fever, malaise, and dark-colored urine. Advise patient that these symptoms may represent drug-induced myopathy and that myopathy can progress to severe muscle damage (rhabdomyolysis). Report any unexplained musculoskeletal symptoms to the physician immediately, and suspend exercise and gait training until these symptoms can be evaluated.
- Monitor signs of hypersensitivity reactions, including pulmonary symptoms (tightness in the throat and chest, wheezing, cough, dyspnea) or skin reactions (rash, pruritus, urticaria). Notify physician immediately if these reactions occur.
- Assess dizziness that might affect gait, balance, and other functional activities (See Appendix C). Report balance problems and functional limitations to the physician, and caution the patient and family/caregivers to guard against falls and trauma.
- Assess peripheral edema using girth measurements, volume displacement, and measurement of pitting edema (See Appendix N). Report increased swelling in feet and ankles or a sudden increase in body weight due to fluid retention.
- Monitor any chest pain and attempt to determine if pain is drug induced or caused by cardiovascular dysfunction (e.g., angina that occurs during exercise). Notify physician about suspected cardiac dysfunction.
- Monitor symptoms of bronchitis, including cough, production of sputum, shortness of breath, and wheezing. Report prolonged or severe symptoms to the physician.

Interventions

- In patients with drug-induced myopathy, implement gradual strengthening and other therapeutic exercises to facilitate recovery from muscle pain and weakness. Use caution during early stages to avoid fatigue of affected muscles, and implement assistive devices (walker, cane, crutches) as needed to prevent falls and assist mobility. Increase exercise intensity as tolerated; recovery from myopathy typically takes 4–6 wk but can be longer in older patients or people with comorbidities.
- Design and implement aerobic exercise and endurance training programs to improve cardiovascular function and help reduce the risk of coronary heart disease.

Patient/Client-Related Instruction

- Remind patients to take medication as directed to control hyperlipidemia even though they are asymptomatic.
- Counsel patients about additional interventions to help control lipid disorders and improve cardiovascular health, including dietary modification, regular exercise, moderation of alcohol consumption, and smoking cessation.
- Instruct patient to report signs of drug-induced hepatitis (anorexia, abdominal pain, severe nausea and vomiting, yellow skin or eyes, skin rashes, flu-like symptoms) or pancreatitis (upper abdominal pain after eating, indigestion, weight loss, oily stools)
- Instruct patient to report other prolonged or severe GI reactions, including nausea, constipation, diarrhea, heartburn, altered taste, abdominal cramps, or flatulence.
- Advise patient to consult physician if erectile dysfunction or other sexual problems occur.
- Instruct patient and family/caregivers to report other troublesome side effects such as severe or prolonged headache, sleep loss, or nasal inflammation (rhinitis).

Pharmacokinetics

Absorption: Poorly and variably absorbed following oral administration.
Distribution: Unknown.
Metabolism and Excretion: Extensively metabolized by the liver, most during 1st pass; excreted in bile and feces. 20% excreted unchanged by the kidneys.
Half-life: 1.3–2.7 hr.

TIME/ACTION PROFILE (cholesterol-lowering effect)

ROUTE	ONSET	PEAK	DURATION
PO	days	2–4 wk	unknown

Contraindications/Precautions

Contraindicated in: Hypersensitivity; Active liver disease or unexplained persistent elevations in AST & ALT; OB: Pregnancy or lactation.
Use Cautiously in: History of liver disease; Alcoholism; Renal impairment; Pedi: Children <8 yr (safety not established); Women of childbearing age.

Interactions

Drug-Drug: Cholesterol-lowering effect may be ↑ with **bile acid sequestrants (cholestyramine, colestipol)**. Bioavailability may be ↓ by **bile acid sequestrants**. Risk of myopathy is ↑ by concurrent **amiodarone, cyclosporine, gemfibrozil, clofibrate, clarithromycin, erythromycin, nefazodone,** large doses of **niacin, nelfinavir, verapamil,** and **azole antifungals** (combined use with clofibrate or

P

gemfibrozil not recommended). May ↑ effects of **warfarin**. Levels may be significantly ↑ by **azole antifungals** (temporarily discontinue HMG CoA reductase inhibitor; effect is less than with other statins). **Saquinavir** and **ritonavir** may ↓ levels and effectiveness.
Drug-Food: Grapefruit juice ↑ blood levels and the risk of rhabdomyolysis.

Route/Dosage

PO (Adults): 10–20 mg once daily at bedtime; may be adjusted at 4-wk intervals as needed (usual range 10–40 mg/day).
PO (Children 14-18 yr): 40 mg once daily.
PO (Children 8-13 yr): 20 mg once daily.
PO (Geriatric Patients): 10–20 mg once daily at bedtime; may be adjusted at 4-wk intervals as needed (usual range 10–20 mg/day).

Hepatic Impairment

Renal Impairment

PO (Adults): 10–20 mg once daily at bedtime; may be adjusted at 4-wk intervals as needed (usual range 10–20 mg/day).

Availability (generic available)

Tablets: 10 mg, 20 mg, 40 mg, 80 mg.

prazosin (pra-zoe-sin)

Minipress

Classification
Therapeutic: antihypertensives
Pharmacologic: peripherally acting antiadrenergics

Indications

Mild-to-moderate hypertension. **Unlabeled Use:** Management of urinary outflow obstruction in patients with benign prostatic hyperplasia.

Action

Dilates both arteries and veins by blocking postsynaptic $alpha_1$-adrenergic receptors. ↓ contractions in smooth muscle of prostatic capsule. **Therapeutic Effects:** Lowering of blood pressure. ↓ cardiac preload and afterload. ↓ symptoms of prostatic hyperplasia (urinary urgency, urinary hesitancy, nocturia).

Adverse Reactions/Side Effects

CNS: dizziness, headache, weakness, drowsiness, mental depression, syncope. **EENT:** blurred vision. **CV:** 1st-dose orthostatic hypotension, palpitations, angina, edema. **GI:** abdominal cramps, diarrhea, dry mouth, nausea, vomiting. **GU:** erectile dysfunction, priapism.

PHYSICAL THERAPY IMPLICATIONS

Examination and Evaluation

- Assess blood pressure (BP) periodically and compare to normal values (See Appendix F). Document whether drug therapy is successful in controlling hypertension. Also, be alert for a fall in BP and related symptoms (dizziness, syncope) that occurs when the patient changes position (orthostatic hypotension), especially after the initial dose. Document orthostatic hypotension and contact physician when systolic BP falls >20 mm Hg or diastolic BP falls >10 mm Hg.
- If treating benign prostate hypertrophy (BPH), monitor signs such as difficulty starting a urine stream, painful urination, weak urine flow, feeling that the bladder is not completely empty, frequent nighttime urination, and an urge to urinate again soon after urinating. Document any change in BPH symptoms to help determine the effects of drug therapy.
- Assess heart rate, ECG, and heart sounds, especially during exercise (See Appendices G, H). Report any rhythm disturbances or symptoms of increased arrhythmias, including palpitations, chest pain, shortness of breath, fainting, and fatigue/weakness.
- Assess dizziness and weakness that might affect gait, balance, and other functional activities (See Appendix C). Report balance problems and functional limitations to the physician, and caution the patient and family/caregivers to guard against falls and trauma.
- Be alert for signs of mental depression or other changes in mood and behavior. Notify physician if these changes become problematic.
- Assess peripheral edema using girth measurements, volume displacement, and measurement of pitting edema (See Appendix N). Report increased swelling in feet and ankles or a sudden increase in body weight due to fluid retention.

Interventions

- Because of the risk of palpitations and abnormal BP responses, use caution during aerobic exercise and other forms of therapeutic exercise. Assess exercise tolerance frequently (BP, heart rate, fatigue levels), and terminate exercise immediately if any untoward responses occur (See Appendix L).
- Avoid physical therapy interventions that cause systemic vasodilation (large whirlpool, Hubbard tank). Additive effects of this drug and the intervention may cause a dangerous fall in BP.
- To minimize orthostatic hypotension, advise patient to move slowly when assuming a more upright position.

Patient/Client-Related Instruction

- Remind patients to take medication as directed to control hypertension even if they are asymptomatic.
- Counsel patients about additional interventions to help control BP, such as regular exercise, weight loss, sodium restriction, stress reduction, moderation of alcohol consumption, and smoking cessation.
- When treating BPH, advise patient that urinary symptoms (retention, dribbling, hesitancy, urgency) should improve, and to contact the physician if these symptoms continue to worsen.
- Instruct patient or family/caregivers to report other bothersome side effects such as severe or prolonged headache, drowsiness, blurred vision, sexual dysfunction, or GI problems (diarrhea, nausea, vomiting, abdominal cramps, dry mouth).

Pharmacokinetics

Absorption: 60% absorbed following oral administration.
Distribution: Widely distributed.
Protein Binding: 97%.
Metabolism and Excretion: Extensively metabolized by the liver. Minimal (5–10%) renal excretion of unchanged drug.
Half-life: 2–3 hr.

TIME/ACTION PROFILE (antihypertensive effects)

ROUTE	ONSET	PEAK	DURATION
PO	2 hr	2–4 hr*	10 hr

*Following single dose; maximal antihypertensive effects occur after 3–4 wk of chronic dosing.

Contraindications/Precautions

Contraindicated in: Hypersensitivity.
Use Cautiously in: Renal insufficiency (increased sensitivity to effects; dosage reduction may be required); Pregnancy, lactation, or children (safety not established); Angina pectoris; When adding diuretics (reduce dose of prazosin).

Interactions

Drug-Drug: Additive hypotension with acute ingestion of **alcohol**, other **antihypertensives**, or **nitrates**. Antihypertensive effects may be decreased by **NSAIDs**.

Route/Dosage

Hypertension

PO (Adults): 1 mg bid–tid (give 1st dose at bedtime) for initial 3 days of therapy, then increase gradually to maintenance dose of 6–15 mg/day in 2–3 divided doses (not to exceed 20–40 mg/day).
PO (Children): 50–400 mcg (0.05–0.4 mg)/kg/day in 2–3 divided doses (not to exceed 7 mg/dose or 15 mg/day).

Benign Prostatic Hyperplasia

PO (Adults): 1–5 mg twice daily.

Availability (generic available)

Capsules: 1 mg, 2 mg, 5 mg. **Tablets:** 1 mg, 2 mg, 5 mg. ***In combination with:*** polythiazide (Minizide). See Appendix B.

prednicarbate

(pred-ni-**kar**-bate)
Dermatop

Classification
Therapeutic: anti-inflammatories (steroidal), immune modifiers
Pharmacologic: corticosteroids (topical)

Indications

Management of inflammation and pruritus associated with various allergic/immunologic skin problems.

Action

Suppresses normal immune response and inflammation. **Therapeutic Effects:** Suppression of dermatologic inflammation and immune processes.

Adverse Reactions/Side Effects

Derm: allergic contact dermatitis, atrophy, burning, dryness, edema, pruritus, hypertrichosis, hypopigmentation, irritation, maceration. **Misc:** adrenal suppression (use of occlusive dressings, long-term therapy).

PHYSICAL THERAPY IMPLICATIONS

Examination and Evaluation

- Assess the area being treated to help document whether drug therapy is successful in resolving skin conditions.
- Monitor any new or increased reactions at the site of application, including inflammation, irritation, infection, burning, swelling, exfoliation, and rash. Report severe or prolonged skin reactions to the physician.
- Report signs of adrenal suppression, including hypotension, weight loss, weakness, nausea, vomiting, anorexia, lethargy, confusion, and restlessness.

Interventions

- Protect skin from breakdown, especially over bony prominences.

Patient/Client-Related Instruction

- Advise patients on long-term treatment to consult physician before stopping this medication. Stopping the medication suddenly may result in adrenocortical shock (severe hypotension, hypoglycemia,

P

weakness, vomiting). If these signs appear, notify physician immediately; may be life threatening.
- Check that the patient and family or caregivers understand topical application procedures and adhere to the recommended dosing schedule.

Pharmacokinetics

Absorption: Minimal. Prolonged use on large surface areas or large amounts applied or use of occlusive dressings may ↑ systemic absorption.
Distribution: Remains primarily at site of action.
Metabolism and Excretion: Usually metabolized in skin.
Half-life: Unknown.

TIME/ACTION PROFILE (response depends on condition being treated)

ROUTE	ONSET	PEAK	DURATION
topical	mins–hrs	hrs–days	hrs–days

Contraindications/Precautions

Contraindicated in: Hypersensitivity or known intolerance to corticosteroids or components of vehicles (ointment or cream base, preservative, alcohol); Untreated bacterial or viral infections.
Use Cautiously in: Hepatic dysfunction; Diabetes mellitus, cataracts, glaucoma, or tuberculosis (use of large amounts of high-potency agents may worsen condition); Patients with preexisting skin atrophy; Pregnancy, lactation, or children (chronic high-dose usage may result in adrenal suppression in mother, growth suppression in children; children may be more susceptible to adrenal and growth suppression).

Interactions

Drug-Drug: None significant.

Route/Dosage

Topical (Adults and Children ≥12 yr): Apply to affected area bid.

Availability

Cream: 0.1%.

prednisolone (pred-nis-oh-lone)

Flo-Pred, Orapred, Pediapred, Prelone

Classification
Therapeutic: anti-inflammatories (steroidal) (intermediate-acting), immune modifiers
Pharmacologic: corticosteroids

Indications

Used systemically and locally in a wide variety of chronic diseases including Inflammatory, Allergic, Hematologic, Neoplastic, Autoimmune disorders. Suitable for alternate-day dosing in the management of chronic illness. Replacement therapy in adrenal insufficiency. **Unlabeled Use:** Adjunctive therapy of hypercalcemia. Adjunctive management of nausea and vomiting from chemotherapy.

Action

In pharmacologic doses, suppresses inflammation and the normal immune response. Has numerous intense metabolic effects (see Adverse Reactions and Side Effects). Suppresses adrenal function at chronic doses of 5 mg/day. Has minimal mineralocorticoid activity.
Therapeutic Effects: Suppression of inflammation and modification of the normal immune response. Replacement therapy in adrenal insufficiency.

Adverse Reactions/Side Effects

Adverse reactions/side effects are much more common with high-dose/long-term therapy
CNS: depression, euphoria, headache, increased intracranial pressure (children only), personality changes, psychoses, restlessness. **EENT:** cataracts, increased intraocular pressure. **CV:** hypertension. **GI:** PEPTIC ULCERATION, anorexia, nausea, vomiting. **Derm:** acne, decreased wound healing, ecchymoses, fragility, hirsutism, petechiae. **Endo:** adrenal suppression, hyperglycemia. **F and E:** fluid retention (long-term high doses), hypokalemia, hypokalemic alkalosis. **Hemat:** THROMBOEMBOLISM, thrombophlebitis. **Metab:** weight gain, weight loss. **MS:** muscle wasting, osteoporosis, aseptic necrosis of joints, muscle pain. **Misc:** cushingoid appearance (moon face, buffalo hump), increased susceptibility to infection.

PHYSICAL THERAPY IMPLICATIONS

Examination and Evaluation

- Monitor signs of thrombophlebitis (lower extremity swelling, warmth, erythema, tenderness) and thromboembolism (shortness of breath, chest pain, cough, bloody sputum). Notify physician immediately, and request objective tests (Doppler ultrasound, lung scan, others) if thrombosis is suspected.
- Monitor and report signs of peptic ulcer, including heartburn, nausea, vomiting blood, tarry stools, and loss of appetite.
- Assess signs of increased intracranial pressure in children, including changes in mood and behavior, decreased consciousness, headache, lethargy, seizures, and vomiting. Notify physician immediately of these signs.
- Assess any muscle or joint pain. Report persistent or increased musculoskeletal pain to determine presence of bone or joint pathology (aseptic necrosis, fracture).
- Assess muscle strength periodically to determine degree of muscle wasting during long- term use.
- Measure blood pressure periodically and compare to normal values (See Appendix F). Report a sustained increase in blood pressure (hypertension) to the physician.

- Assess peripheral edema using girth measurements, volume displacement, and measurement of pitting edema (See Appendix N). Report increased swelling in feet and ankles or a sudden increase in body weight due to fluid retention.
- Monitor personality changes, including depression, euphoria, restlessness, hallucinations, and psychosis. Notify physician if these changes become problematic.
- Be alert for signs of low potassium levels (hypokalemia) and metabolic acidosis, including hyperventilation, cardiac arrhythmias, dizziness, and confusion. Notify physician immediately if these signs occur.
- Report signs of adrenal suppression, including hypotension, weight loss, weakness, nausea, vomiting, anorexia, lethargy, confusion, and restlessness.
- Monitor signs of hyperglycemia (confusion; drowsiness; flushed, dry skin; fruit-like breath odor; rapid, deep breathing; polyuria; loss of appetite; unusual thirst). Insulin dosages may need to be adjusted to prevent repeated episodes of hyperglycemia.
- Periodically assess body weight and other anthropometric measures (body mass index, body composition). Report a rapid or unexplained weight gain or weight loss.

Interventions

- Implement resistive exercises and weight-bearing activities to minimize muscle wasting and osteoporosis. Use caution to prevent musculoskeletal damage in patients with preexisting muscle and bone loss.
- Protect skin from breakdown, especially over bony prominences.

Patient/Client-Related Instruction

- Advise patient that wound healing may be delayed; instruct patient to check skin regularly and report any nonhealing sores.
- Advise patient that corticosteroids cause immunosuppression and may mask symptoms of infection. Instruct patient to avoid people with known contagious illnesses and to report possible infections immediately.
- Advise patients on long-term treatment to consult physician before stopping this medication. Stopping the medication suddenly may result in adrenocortical shock (severe hypotension, hypoglycemia, weakness, vomiting). If these signs appear, notify physician immediately; may be life threatening.
- Instruct patient to report any loss of vision that might indicate cataracts or increased intraocular pressure.
- Advise patient about possible Cushingoid appearance, including puffiness in the face (moon face), increased fat in the torso, thin arms and legs, abdominal skin striations, bruising, and deposition of fat at the posterior base of the neck (buffalo hump). Discuss possible effects on body image, and help patient explore coping mechanisms.
- Instruct patient and family/caregivers to report other troublesome side effects such as severe or prolonged headache, GI reactions (nausea, vomiting, loss of appetite), or skin reactions (acne, hair growth).

Pharmacokinetics

Absorption: Well absorbed following oral administration. Sodium phosphate salt is rapidly absorbed following IM administration. Acetate and tebutate salts are slowly but completely absorbed following IM administration. Absorption from local sites (intra-articular, intralesional) is slow but complete.
Distribution: Widely distributed, crosses the placenta, and probably enters breast milk.
Metabolism and Excretion: Metabolized mostly by the liver.
Half-life: 2.1–3.5 hr (plasma), 18–36 hr (tissue); adrenal suppression lasts 1.25–1.5 days.

TIME/ACTION PROFILE (anti-inflammatory activity)

ROUTE	ONSET	PEAK	DURATION
PO	unknown	1–2 hr	1.25–1.5 days
IM, IV (phosphate)	rapid	1 hr	unknown
IM (acetate)	slow	unknown	unknown

Contraindications/Precautions

Contraindicated in: Active untreated infections (may be used in patients being treated for tuberculous meningitis); Lactation (avoid chronic use); Known alcohol or bisulfite hypersensitivity or intolerance (some products contain these; avoid in susceptible patients).
Use Cautiously in: Chronic treatment (leads to adrenal suppression; use lowest possible dose for shortest period of time); Pedi: chronic use will result in decreased growth; use lowest possible dose for shortest period of time; Stress (surgery, infections); supplemental doses may be needed; Potential infections may mask signs (fever, inflammation); Neonates (oral solution and syrup contain benzoic acid, a metabolite of benzyl alcohol that can cause potentially fatal gasping syndrome); OB: safety not established.

Interactions

Drug-Drug: Additive hypokalemia with **thiazide** and **loop diuretics, amphotericin B, piperacillin,** or **ticarcillin**. Hypokalemia may ↑ risk of **digitalis glycoside** toxicity. May ↑ requirement for **insulin** or **oral hypoglycemic agents. Phenytoin,**

P

phenobarbital, and **rifampin** stimulate metabolism; may ↓ effectiveness. **Oral contraceptives** may block metabolism. ↑ risk of adverse GI effects with **NSAIDs** (including **aspirin**). At chronic doses that suppress adrenal function, may ↓ antibody response to and ↑ risk of adverse reactions from **live-virus vaccines**. May ↑ risk of tendon rupture from **fluoroquinolones**. Concurrent use may inhibit the response to **somatrem** or **somatropin** at doses of 2.5–3.75 mg/m²/day of prednisolone.

Route/Dosage

PO (Adults): *Most uses*—5–60 mg/day as a single dose or in divided doses. *Multiple sclerosis*—200 mg/day for 7 days, then 80 mg every other day for 1 mo. *Asthma exacerbations*—120–180 mg/day in divided doses tid–qid for 48 hr, then 60–80 mg/day in 2 divided doses.

PO (Children): *Anti–inflammatory/immunosuppressive*—0.1–2 mg/kg/day in 1–4 divided doses. *Nephrotic syndrome*——2 mg/kg/day (60 mg/m²/day) in 1–3 divided doses daily (maximum dose 80 mg/day) until urine is protein free for 4–6 wk, followed by 2 mg/kg/dose (40 mg/m²/dose) every other day in the morning, gradually taper off over 4–6 wk. *Asthma exacerbations*—1 mg/kg q 6 hr for 48 hr, then 1–2 mg/kg/day (maximum 60 mg/day) divided bid.

Availability (generic available)

Tablets: 5 mg. **Orally disintegrating tablets (grape flavor):** 10 mg, 15 mg, 30 mg. **Syrup:** 5 mg/5 mL, 15 mg/5 mL.

prednisone (pred-ni-sone)

Sterapred

Classification

Therapeutic: anti-inflammatories (steroidal) (intermediate acting), immune modifiers
Pharmacologic: corticosteroids

Indications

Used systemically and locally in a wide variety of chronic diseases, including Inflammatory, Allergic, Hematologic, Neoplastic, Autoimmune disorders. Suitable for alternate-day dosing in the management of chronic illness. **Unlabeled Use:** Adjunctive therapy of hypercalcemia. Adjunctive management of nausea and vomiting from chemotherapy.

Action

In pharmacologic doses, suppresses inflammation and the normal immune response. Has numerous intense metabolic effects (see Adverse Reactions and Side Effects). Suppresses adrenal function at chronic doses of 5 mg/day. Replaces endogenous cortisol in deficiency states. Has minimal mineralocorticoid activity.

Therapeutic Effects: Suppression of inflammation and modification of the normal immune response.

Adverse Reactions/Side Effects

Adverse reactions/side effects are much more common with high-dose/long-term therapy

CNS: depression, euphoria, headache, increased intracranial pressure (children only), personality changes, psychoses, restlessness. **EENT:** cataracts, increased intraocular pressure. **CV:** hypertension. **GI:** PEPTIC ULCERATION, anorexia, nausea, vomiting. **Derm:** acne, decreased wound healing, ecchymoses, fragility, hirsutism, petechiae. **Endo:** adrenal suppression, hyperglycemia. **F and E:** fluid retention (long-term high doses), hypokalemia, hypokalemic alkalosis. **Hemat:** THROMBOEMBOLISM, thrombophlebitis. **Metab:** weight gain, weight loss. **MS:** muscle wasting, osteoporosis, aseptic necrosis of joints, muscle pain. **Misc:** cushingoid appearance (moon face, buffalo hump), increased susceptibility to infection.

PHYSICAL THERAPY IMPLICATIONS

Examination and Evaluation

- Monitor signs of thrombophlebitis (lower extremity swelling, warmth, erythema, tenderness) and thromboembolism (shortness of breath, chest pain, cough, bloody sputum). Notify physician immediately, and request objective tests (Doppler ultrasound, lung scan, others) if thrombosis is suspected.
- Monitor and report signs of peptic ulcer, including heartburn, nausea, vomiting blood, tarry stools, and loss of appetite.
- Assess signs of increased intracranial pressure in children, including changes in mood and behavior, decreased consciousness, headache, lethargy, seizures, and vomiting. Notify physician immediately of these signs.
- Assess any muscle or joint pain. Report persistent or increased musculoskeletal pain to determine presence of bone or joint pathology (aseptic necrosis, fracture).
- Assess muscle strength periodically to determine degree of muscle wasting during long- term use.
- Measure blood pressure periodically and compare to normal values (See Appendix F). Report a sustained increase in blood pressure (hypertension) to the physician.
- Assess peripheral edema using girth measurements, volume displacement, and measurement of pitting edema (See Appendix N). Report increased swelling in feet and ankles or a sudden increase in body weight due to fluid retention.
- Monitor personality changes, including depression, euphoria, restlessness, hallucinations, and psychosis. Notify physician if these changes become problematic.

- Be alert for signs of low potassium levels (hypokalemia) and metabolic acidosis, including hyperventilation, cardiac arrhythmias, dizziness, and confusion. Notify physician immediately if these signs occur.
- Report signs of adrenal suppression, including hypotension, weight loss, weakness, nausea, vomiting, anorexia, lethargy, confusion, and restlessness.
- Monitor signs of hyperglycemia (confusion; drowsiness; flushed, dry skin; fruit-like breath odor; rapid, deep breathing; polyuria; loss of appetite; unusual thirst). Insulin dosages may need to be adjusted to prevent repeated episodes of hyperglycemia.
- Periodically assess body weight and other anthropometric measures (body mass index, body composition). Report a rapid or unexplained weight gain or weight loss.

Interventions

- Implement resistive exercises and weight-bearing activities to minimize muscle wasting and osteoporosis. Use caution to prevent musculoskeletal damage in patients with preexisting muscle and bone loss.
- Protect skin from breakdown, especially over bony prominences.

Patient/Client-Related Instruction

- Advise patient that wound healing may be delayed; instruct patient to check skin regularly and report any nonhealing sores.
- Advise patient that corticosteroids cause immunosuppression and may mask symptoms of infection. Instruct patient to avoid people with known contagious illnesses and to report possible infections immediately.
- Advise patients on long-term treatment to consult physician before stopping this medication. Stopping the medication suddenly may result in adrenocortical shock (severe hypotension, hypoglycemia, weakness, vomiting). If these signs appear, notify physician immediately; may be life threatening.
- Instruct patient to report any loss of vision that might indicate cataracts or increased intraocular pressure.
- Advise patient about possible cushingoid appearance, including puffiness in the face (moon face), increased fat in the torso, thin arms and legs, abdominal skin striations, bruising, and deposition of fat at the posterior base of the neck (buffalo hump). Discuss possible effects on body image, and help patient explore coping mechanisms.
- Instruct patient and family/caregivers to report other troublesome side effects such as severe or prolonged headache, GI reactions (nausea, vomiting, loss of appetite), or skin reactions (acne, hair growth).

Pharmacokinetics

Absorption: Well absorbed after oral administration.
Distribution: Widely distributed; crosses the placenta and probably enters breast milk.
Metabolism and Excretion: Converted by the liver to prednisolone, which is then metabolized by the liver.
Half-life: 3.4–3.8 hr (plasma), 18–36 hr (tissue); adrenal suppression lasts 1.25–1.5 days.

TIME/ACTION PROFILE (anti-inflammatory activity)

ROUTE	ONSET	PEAK	DURATION
PO	hrs	unknown	1.25–1.5 days

Contraindications/Precautions

Contraindicated in: Active untreated infections (may be used in patients being treated for tuberculous meningitis); Some products contain alcohol and should be avoided in patients with known intolerance; Lactation: Avoid chronic use.
Use Cautiously in: Chronic treatment (leads to adrenal suppression; use lowest possible dose for shortest period of time); Pedi: Chronic use will result in decreased growth; use lowest possible dose for shortest period of time; Stress (surgery, infections); supplemental doses may be needed; Potential infections may mask signs (fever, inflammation); OB: Safety not established.

Interactions

Drug-Drug: Additive hypokalemia with **thiazide** and **loop diuretics**, **amphotericin B**, **piperacillin**, or **ticarcillin**. Hypokalemia may ↑ risk of **digitalis glycoside** toxicity. May ↑ requirement for **insulins** or **oral hypoglycemic agents. Phenytoin, phenobarbital,** and **rifampin** stimulate metabolism; may ↓ effectiveness. **Oral contraceptives** may block metabolism. ↑ risk of adverse GI effects with **NSAIDs** (including aspirin). At chronic doses that suppress adrenal function, may ↓ antibody response to and ↑ the risk of adverse reactions from **live virus vaccines**. May ↑ risk of tendon rupture from **fluoroquinolones**.

Route/Dosage

PO (Adults): *Most uses*—5–60 mg/day as a single dose or in divided doses. *Multiple sclerosis*—200 mg/day for 1 wk, then 80 mg every other day for 1 mo. *Adjunctive therapy of* Pneumocystis carinii *pneumonia in AIDS patients*—40 mg twice daily for 5 days, then 40 mg once daily for 5 days, then 20 mg once daily for 10 days.
PO (Children): *Nephrotic syndrome*—2 mg/kg/day initially given in 1–3 divided doses (maximum 80 mg/day) until urine is protein free for 4–6 wk. Maintenance dose of 2 mg/kg/day every other day in

the morning, gradually taper off after 4–6 wk. *Asthma exacerbation*—1 mg/kg q 6 hr for 48 hr, then 1–2 mg/kg/day (maximum 60 mg/day) in divided doses twice daily.

Availability (generic available)

Tablets: 1 mg, 2.5 mg, 5 mg, 10 mg, 20 mg, 50 mg. **Oral solution:** 5 mg/5 mL, 5 mg/1 mL.

pregabalin (pre-gab-a-lin)

Lyrica

Classification

Therapeutic: analgesics, anticonvulsants
Pharmacologic: gamma-aminobutyric acid (GABA) analogues, nonopioid analgesics

Schedule V

Indications

Pain due to diabetic peripheral neuropathy, postherpetic neuralgia, fibromyalgia. Adjunctive therapy of partial-onset seizures in adults.

Action

Binds to calcium channels in CNS tissues which regulate neurotransmitter release. Does not bind to opioid receptors. **Therapeutic Effects:** Decreased neuropathic or postherpetic pain. Decreased partial-onset seizures.

Adverse Reactions/Side Effects

CNS: dizziness, drowsiness, impaired attention/concentration/thinking. **CV:** edema. **EENT:** blurred vision. **GI:** dry mouth, abdominal pain, constipation, ↑ appetite, vomiting. **Hemat:** ↓ platelet count. **Metab:** weight gain. **Misc:** allergic reactions, fever.

PHYSICAL THERAPY IMPLICATIONS

Examination and Evaluation

- Assess pain using visual analogue scales and other appropriate pain scales when this drug is used to treat neuropathic pain or other pain syndromes (fibromyalgia, postherpetic neuralgia). Document any changes in pain to help determine the effects of drug therapy.
- If used to treat seizures, document the number, duration, and severity of seizures to help determine if this drug is effective in reducing seizure activity.
- Monitor and report drowsiness, concentration difficulties, or other cognitive impairments. Repeated or excessive symptoms may require change in dose or medication.
- Assess peripheral edema using girth measurements, volume displacement, and measurement of pitting edema (See Appendix N). Report increased swelling in feet and ankles or a sudden increase in body weight due to fluid retention.
- Assess dizziness that might affect gait, balance, and other functional activities (See Appendix C). Report balance problems and functional limitations to the physician, and caution the patient and family/caregivers to guard against falls and trauma.
- Monitor signs of allergic reactions, including pulmonary symptoms (tightness in the throat and chest, wheezing, cough, dyspnea) or skin reactions (rash, pruritus, urticaria). Notify physician if these reactions occur.
- Periodically assess body weight and other anthropometric measures (body mass index, body composition). Report a substantial or unexplained weight gain or increase in body fat.

Interventions

- Guard against falls and trauma (hip fractures, head injury, and so forth), especially if gait and balance are affected by drowsiness or dizziness. Implement fall-prevention strategies, especially if balance is impaired (See Appendix E).
- If treating neuropathic pain or other pain syndromes, implement appropriate interventions (physical agents, manual techniques, therapeutic exercise) to manage pain and reduce the need for drug therapy. Help patient also explore other nonpharmacologic methods to reduce chronic pain, such as relaxation techniques, imagery, counseling, and so forth.

Patient/Client-Related Instruction

- Advise patient to avoid alcohol and other CNS depressants because of the increased risk of sedation and adverse effects.
- Advise patients on prolonged antiseizure therapy not to discontinue medication without consulting their physician. Abrupt withdrawal may cause increased seizures.
- Advise patient about the risk of daytime drowsiness and decreased attention and mental focus. Use care if driving or in other activities that require strong concentration or fast responses.
- Instruct patient to report other troublesome side effects such as severe or prolonged fever, blurred vision, or GI problems (vomiting, constipation, abdominal pain, dry mouth).

Pharmacokinetics

Absorption: Well absorbed (90%) following oral administration.
Distribution: Probably crosses the blood-brain barrier.
Metabolism and Excretion: Minimally metabolized, 90% excreted unchanged in urine.
Half-life: 6 hr.

TIME/ACTION PROFILE (decreased post–herpetic pain)

ROUTE	ONSET	PEAK	DURATION
PO	unknown	2–4 wk	unknown

Contraindications/Precautions

Contraindicated in: Myopathy (known/suspected); OB: Lactation.

Use Cautiously in: Renal impairment (dose alteration recommended for CCr <60 mL/min); Geri: Elderly patients (consider age-related decrease in renal function; CHF; History of drug dependence/drug-seeking behavior; Pedi: Children (safety not established); OB: Use only if maternal benefit outweighs fetal risk; may also have ↑ risk of male-mediated teratogenicity).

Interactions

Drug-Drug: Concurrent use with **thiazolidinediones (pioglitazone, rosiglitazone)** may ↑ risk of fluid retention. ↑ risk of CNS depression with other **CNS depressants,** including **opioids, alcohol, benzodiazepines,** or other **sedatives/hypnotics.**

Route/Dosage

PO (Adults): *Diabetic neuropathic pain*—50 mg tid, increased over 7 days up to 100 mg tid; *Partial-onset seizures*—150 mg/day initially in 2–3 divided doses, may be gradually increased to 600 mg/day; *Postherpetic neuralgia*—75 mg bid or 50 mg tid initially, may be increased over 7 days to 300 mg/day in 2–3 divided doses, after 2–4 wk may be increased to 600 mg/day in 2–3 divided doses; Fibromyalgia—75 mg bid initially, may be increased to 150 mg bid within 1 wk based on efficacy and tolerability. May be increased to 225 bid.

Renal Impairment

PO (Adults): *CCr 30–60 mL/min*—75–300 mg/day in 2–3 divided doses; *CCr 15–30 mL/min*—25–150 mg/day in 1–2 divided doses; *CCr <15 mL/min*—25–75 mg/day as a single daily dose.

Availability

Capsules: 25 mg, 50 mg, 75 mg, 100 mg, 150 mg, 200 mg, 225 mg, 300 mg.

primidone (pri-mi-done)

Apo-Primidone, Myidone, Mysoline, PMS-Primidone, Sertan

Classification

Therapeutic: anticonvulsants

Pharmacologic: barbiturate analogue

Indications

Management of tonic-clonic, complex partial, and focal seizures. **Unlabeled Use:** Management of essential (familial) tremor.

Action

↓ neuronal excitability. ↑ the threshold of electric stimulation of the motor cortex. **Therapeutic Effects:** Prevention of seizures.

Adverse Reactions/Side Effects

CNS: ataxia, drowsiness, vertigo, excitement (increased in children). **EENT:** visual changes. **Resp:** dyspnea. **CV:** edema, orthostatic hypotension. **GI:** anorexia, drug-induced hepatitis, nausea, vomiting. **Derm:** alopecia, rash. **Hemat:** blood dyscrasias, megaloblastic anemia. **Misc:** folic acid deficiency.

PHYSICAL THERAPY IMPLICATIONS

Examination and Evaluation

- Document the number, duration, and severity of seizures to help document whether this drug is effective in reducing seizure activity.
- Be alert for signs of megaloblastic anemia (unusual fatigue, weakness, dizziness, pallor) or signs of fever, infection, and poor health that might be due to other blood dyscrasias or folic acid deficiency. Report these signs to the physician immediately.
- Assess dizziness and vertigo that might affect gait, balance, and other functional activities (See Appendix C). Report balance problems and functional limitations to the physician, and caution the patient and family/caregivers to guard against falls and trauma.
- Assess peripheral edema using girth measurements, volume displacement, and measurement of pitting edema (See Appendix N). Report increased swelling in feet and ankles or a sudden increase in body weight due to fluid retention.
- Assess blood pressure (BP) when patient assumes a more upright position (lying to standing, sitting to standing, lying to sitting). Document orthostatic hypotension and contact physician when systolic BP falls >20 mm Hg, or diastolic BP falls >10 mm Hg.
- Monitor daytime drowsiness or excitement. Repeated or excessive symptoms may require change in dose or medication.

Interventions

- Guard against falls and trauma (hip fractures, head injury, and so forth), especially if drowsiness or vertigo affects gait and balance. Implement fall-prevention strategies, especially if balance is impaired (See Appendix E).

P

- To minimize orthostatic hypotension, patient should move slowly when assuming a more upright position.

Patient/Client-Related Instruction

- Advise patient to avoid alcohol and other CNS depressants because of the increased risk of sedation and adverse effects.
- Advise patients on prolonged antiseizure therapy not to discontinue medication without consulting their physician. Abrupt withdrawal may cause increased seizures.
- Advise patient about the risk of daytime drowsiness and decreased attention and mental focus. Use care if driving or in other activities that require strong concentration and fast responses.
- Advise patient about the likelihood of GI reactions such as nausea, vomiting, and loss of appetite. Instruct patient to report severe or prolonged GI problems or signs of drug-induced hepatitis, including yellow skin or eyes, abdominal pain, severe nausea and vomiting, fever, sore throat, malaise, weakness, and facial edema.
- Instruct patient and family/caregivers to report other troublesome side effects such as severe or prolonged respiratory problems (difficult, labored breathing), visual problems (double vision, nystagmus), or skin reactions (rash, hair loss).

Pharmacokinetics

Absorption: 80–100% absorbed from the GI tract when administered orally.
Distribution: Widely distributed. Crosses the placenta and enters breast milk.
Metabolism and Excretion: Converted to phenobarbital and another active anticonvulsant compound (PEMA) by the liver.
Half-life: 3–7 hr.

TIME/ACTION PROFILE (anticonvulsant effect)

ROUTE	ONSET	PEAK	DURATION
PO	4–7 days	7–10 days	8–12 hr

Contraindications/Precautions

Contraindicated in: Hypersensitivity to primidone or phenobarbital; Porphyria.
Use Cautiously in: Severe liver disease (dosage adjustment required); Pregnancy and lactation (safety not established; may cause hemorrhage in the newborn).

Interactions

Drug-Drug: Induces liver enzymes and may hasten metabolism and ↓ the effectiveness of other drugs metabolized by the liver, including **hormonal contraceptives, chloramphenicol, acebutolol, propranolol, metoprolol, timolol, doxycycline, corticosteroids, tricyclic antidepressants, phenothiazines, phenylbutazone**, and **quinidine**. Additive CNS depression with other **CNS depressants**, including **alcohol, antihistamines, opioid analgesics**, and **sedative/hypnotics**. Concurrent use with **phenobarbital** may lead to phenobarbital toxicity.
Drug-Natural: Concomitant use of **kava, valerian, skullcap, chamomile**, or **hops** can ↑ CNS depression. See **sedative drug-drug** interactions above.
St. John's wort may affect primidone levels and effectiveness; avoid use.
Drug-Food: ↓ the absorption of **folic acid**.

Route/Dosage

PO (Adults and Children >8 yr): Initial dose of 100–125 mg hs for 3 days, then 100–125 mg bid for 3 days, then 100–125 mg tid for 3 days, then maintenance dose of 250 mg tid–qid (not to exceed 2 g/day).
PO (Children <8 yr): Initial dose of 50 mg hs for 3 days, then 50 mg bid for next 3 days, then 100 mg bid for 3 days, then maintenance dose of 125–250 mg tid (10–25 mg/kg/day).

Availability (generic available)

Tablets: 50 mg, 125 mg, 250 mg. **Oral suspension:** 250 mg/5 mL. **Chewable tablets:** 125 mg.

probenecid (proe-ben-e-sid)

Benuryl, Probalan

Classification
Therapeutic: antigout agents, uricosurics
Pharmacologic: benzoic acids derivatives

Indications

Prevention of recurrences of gouty arthritis. Treatment of hyperuricemia secondary to thiazide therapy. Used to increase and prolong serum levels of penicillin and related anti-infectives.

Action

Inhibits renal tubular reabsorption of uric acid, thus promoting its renal excretion. **Therapeutic Effects:** Reduction of serum uric acid levels.

Adverse Reactions/Side Effects

CNS: headache, dizziness. **GI:** nausea, vomiting, abdominal pain, diarrhea, drug-induced hepatitis, sore gums. **GU:** uric acid stones, urinary frequency. **Derm:** flushing, rashes. **Hemat:** APLASTIC ANEMIA, anemia.

PHYSICAL THERAPY IMPLICATIONS

Examination and Evaluation

- Monitor signs of anemia, including unusual fatigue, shortness of breath with exertion, pallor, and bruising. Notify physician immediately if these signs occur.

- Periodically assess patient's impairments (pain, range of motion), functional ability, and disability to help determine if gout symptoms are reduced by drug therapy.
- Assess dizziness that might affect gait, balance, and other functional activities (See Appendix C). Report balance problems and functional limitations to the physician, and caution the patient and family/caregivers to guard against falls and trauma.

Interventions

- Implement appropriate manual therapy techniques, physical agents, therapeutic exercises, and orthotic/assistive devices to reduce pain, improve function, and augment the effects of antigout drug therapy.

Patient/Client-Related Instruction

- Advise patient about the likelihood of GI reactions such as nausea, vomiting, diarrhea, abdominal pain, and sore gums. Instruct patient to report severe or prolonged GI problems or signs of drug-induced hepatitis (yellow skin or eyes, abdominal pain, severe nausea and vomiting, fever, sore throat, malaise, weakness, facial edema).
- Instruct patient to report other untoward side effects such as severe or prolonged headache, urinary frequency, pain associated with kidney stones, or skin reactions (rash, flushing).

Pharmacokinetics

Absorption: Well absorbed following oral administration.
Distribution: Crosses the placenta.
Protein Binding: 75–95%.
Metabolism and Excretion: Mostly metabolized by the liver; 10% excreted unchanged in the urine.
Half-life: 4–17 hr.

TIME/ACTION PROFILE (effects on serum uric acid levels)

ROUTE	ONSET	PEAK	DURATION
PO	30 min	2–4 hr	8 hr

Contraindications/Precautions

Contraindicated in: Hypersensitivity; Chronic high-dose salicylate therapy; Children <2 yr.
Use Cautiously in: Peptic ulcer; Blood dyscrasias; Uric acid kidney stones; Renal impairment (dosage reduction recommended; may not be effective if CCr ≤30 mL/min); Pregnancy or lactation (has been used safely during pregnancy; safety during lactation not established).

Interactions

Drug-Drug: ↑ blood levels of **acyclovir, allopurinol, barbiturates, benzodiazepines, cephalosporins, clofibrate, dapsone, dyphylline, methotrexate, NSAIDs, pantothenic acid, penicillamine, penicillins, rifampin, sulfonamides, sulfonylurea oral hypoglycemic agents**, or **zidovudine**. Large doses of **salicylates** may ↓ uricosuric activity.

Route/Dosage

PO (Adults and Children >50 kg): *Hyperuricemia*—250 mg bid for 1 wk; increase to 500 mg bid, then may increase by 500 mg/day every 4 wk (not to exceed 3 g/day). *Augmentation of penicillin/cephalosporins*—500 mg qid. *Single-dose therapy of gonorrhea*—1 g with amoxicillin or penicillin.
PO (Children 2–14 yr and ≤50 kg): 25 mg/kg (700 mg/m^2) initially; then 10 mg/kg (300 mg/m^2) qid.

Availability

Tablets: 0.5 g.

P

procainamide
(proe-**kane**-ah-mide)
Pronestyl

Classification
Therapeutic: antiarrhythmics (class IA)
Pharmacologic: membrane stabilizers

Indications

Treatment of a variety of ventricular and atrial arrhythmias, including Atrial premature contractions, Premature ventricular contractions, Ventricular tachycardia, Paroxysmal atrial tachycardia. Maintenance of normal sinus rhythm after conversion from atrial fibrillation or flutter.

Action

Decreases myocardial excitability. Slows conduction velocity. May depress myocardial contractility.
Therapeutic Effects: Suppression of arrhythmias.

Adverse Reactions/Side Effects

CNS: SEIZURES, confusion, dizziness. **CV:** ASYSTOLE, HEART BLOCK, VENTRICULAR ARRHYTHMIAS, hypotension. **GI:** diarrhea, anorexia, bitter taste, nausea, vomiting. **Derm:** rashes. **Hemat:** AGRANULOCYTOSIS, eosinophilia, leukopenia, thrombocytopenia. **Misc:** chills, drug-induced systemic lupus syndrome, fever.

PHYSICAL THERAPY IMPLICATIONS

Examination and Evaluation

- Be alert for new seizures or increased seizure activity. Document the number, duration, and severity of seizures, and report these findings to the physician immediately.

- Monitor cardiac symptoms at rest and during exercise. Seek immediate medical assistance if symptoms of asystole or heart block develop, including sudden chest pain, pain radiating into the arm or jaw, shortness of breath, dizziness, sweating, anxiety, nausea, and loss of consciousness.
- Assess heart rate, ECG, and heart sounds, especially during exercise (See Appendices G, H). Although intended to treat certain arrhythmias, this drug can unmask or precipitate new arrhythmias (proarrhythmic effect). Report any rhythm disturbances or symptoms of increased arrhythmias, including palpitations, chest pain, shortness of breath, fainting, and fatigue/weakness.
- Assess blood pressure periodically and compare to normal values (See Appendix F). Report low blood pressure (hypotension), especially if patient experiences dizziness or syncope.
- Monitor signs of blood dyscrasias including agranulocytosis and leukopenia (fever, sore throat, mucosal lesions, signs of infection), eosinophilia (fatigue, weakness, myalgia), or thrombocytopenia (bruising, nose bleeds, bleeding gums). Report these signs to the physician immediately.
- Be alert for early signs of myasthenia gravis syndrome, such as drooping eyelids, facial muscle weakness, and difficulty swallowing and speaking. Report these signs to the physician immediately, and monitor other muscle groups for signs of unusual weakness and fatigue, especially after repeated contraction.
- Assess dizziness that might affect gait, balance, and other functional activities (See Appendix C). Report balance problems and functional limitations to the physician, and caution the patient and family/caregivers to guard against falls and trauma.

Interventions

- Because of the risk of serious cardiac arrhythmias, use extreme caution during aerobic exercise and other forms of therapeutic exercise. Assess exercise tolerance frequently (blood pressure, heart rate, fatigue levels), and terminate exercise immediately if any untoward responses occur (See Appendix L).

Patient/Client-Related Instruction

- Advise patient and family or caregivers about the signs of cardiac arrest and arrhythmias (see above under Examination and Evaluation) and to seek immediate medical assistance if these signs develop
- Instruct patient and family/caregivers to report other side effects such as severe or prolonged confusion, chills, fever, skin rash, or GI problems (nausea, vomiting diarrhea, loss of appetite, bitter taste).

Pharmacokinetics

Absorption: Well absorbed (75–90%) following IM administration. Sustained-release oral preparation is more slowly absorbed.

Distribution: Rapidly and widely distributed.

Metabolism and Excretion: Converted by the liver to *N*-acetylprocainamide (NAPA), an active antiarrhythmic compound. Remainder (40–70%) excreted unchanged by the kidneys.

Half-life: 2.5–4.7 hr (NAPA—7 hr); prolonged in renal impairment.

TIME/ACTION PROFILE (antiarrhythmic effects)

ROUTE	ONSET	PEAK	DURATION
IV	immediate	25–60 min	3–4 hr
IM	10–30 min	15–60 min	3–4 hr

Contraindications/Precautions

Contraindicated in: Hypersensitivity; AV block; Myasthenia gravis; Hypersensitivity to tartrazine (FDC yellow dye #5; present in some oral products).

Use Cautiously in: MI or cardiac glycoside toxicity; CHF, renal or hepatic insufficiency, geriatric patients (dose reduction or ↑ dosing intervals recommended); Pregnancy, lactation, or children (safety not established).

Interactions

Drug-Drug: May have additive or antagonistic effects with other **antiarrhythmics**. Additive neurologic toxicity (confusion, seizures) with **lidocaine**. **Antihypertensives** and **nitrates** may potentiate hypotensive effect. Potentiates **neuromuscular blocking agents**. May partially antagonize the therapeutic effects of **anticholinesterase agents** in myasthenia gravis. ↑ risk of arrhythmias with **pimozide**. Additive anticholinergic effects with other **drugs possessing anticholinergic properties**, including **antihistamines, antidepressants, atropine, haloperidol,** and **phenothiazines**. Effects of procainamide may be ↑ by **cimetidine, quinidine,** or **trimethoprim**.

Route/Dosage

IM (Adults): 50 mg/kg/day in divided doses q 3–6 hr.

IV (Adults): 100 mg q 5 min until arrhythmia is abolished or 1000 mg have been given; wait at least 10 min until further dosing *or* loading infusion of 500–600 mg over 30–60 min followed by maintenance infusion of 1–4 mg/min.

Availability

Injection: 100 mg/mL in 10-mL vials, 500 mg/mL in 2-mL vials.

procarbazine

(proe-**kar**-ba-zeen)

Matulane, ✽Natulan

Classification

Therapeutic: antineoplastics

Pharmacologic: alkylating agents

Indications

Treatment of Hodgkin's disease (with other treatment modalities). **Unlabeled Use:** Other lymphomas, Brain and lung tumors, Multiple myeloma, Malignant melanoma, Polycythemia vera.

Action

Appears to inhibit DNA, RNA, and protein synthesis (cell-cycle S-phase–specific). **Therapeutic Effects:** Death of rapidly replicating cells, particularly malignant ones.

Adverse Reactions/Side Effects

CNS: SEIZURES, confusion, dizziness, drowsiness, hallucinations, headache, mania, mental depression, nightmares, psychosis, syncope, tremor. **EENT:** nystagmus, photophobia, retinal hemorrhage. **Resp:** cough, pleural effusions. **CV:** edema, hypotension, tachycardia. **GI:** nausea, vomiting, anorexia, diarrhea, dry mouth, dysphagia, hepatic dysfunction, stomatitis. **GU:** gonadal suppression. **Derm:** alopecia, photosensitivity, pruritus, rashes. **Endo:** gynecomastia. **Hemat:** anemia, leukopenia, thrombocytopenia. **Neuro:** neuropathy, paresthesia. **Misc:** ascites, secondary malignancy.

PHYSICAL THERAPY IMPLICATIONS

Examination and Evaluation

- Be alert for new seizures or increased seizure activity. Document the number, duration, and severity of seizures, and report these findings immediately to the physician or nursing staff.
- Assess heart rate, ECG, and heart sounds, especially during exercise (See Appendices G, H). Report a rapid heart rate (tachycardia) or signs of other arrhythmias, including palpitations, chest discomfort, shortness of breath, fainting, and fatigue/weakness.
- Assess blood pressure (BP) periodically and compare to normal values (See Appendix F). Report low BP (hypotension), especially if patient experiences dizziness or syncope.
- Assess peripheral edema using girth measurements, volume displacement, and measurement of pitting edema (See Appendix N). Report increased swelling in feet and ankles or a sudden increase in body weight due to fluid retention.
- Monitor prolonged cough or other signs of pleural effusion such as chest pain, shortness of breath, and abnormal breath sounds (See Appendices J, K). Notify physician if breathing becomes compromised.
- Watch for signs of leukopenia (fever, sore throat, signs of infection), thrombocytopenia (bruising, nose bleeds, bleeding gums), or unusual weakness and fatigue that might be due to anemia. Report these signs to the physician or nursing staff.
- Monitor signs of paresthesia and peripheral neuropathy (numbness, tingling, muscle weakness). Establish baseline electroneuromyographic values using EMG and nerve conduction at the beginning of drug treatment whenever possible. Periodically reexamine these values to document drug-induced changes in peripheral nerve function.
- Monitor and report signs of CNS toxicity, including confusion, mania, tremor, hallucinations, or psychosis.
- Assess dizziness and drowsiness that might affect gait, balance, and other functional activities (See Appendix C). Report balance problems and functional limitations to the physician and nursing staff, and caution the patient and family/caregivers to guard against falls and trauma.
- Monitor signs of malignancy, including a change in bowel or bladder habits, nonhealing sores, unusual bleeding or discharge, a lump in the breast or other parts of the body, chronic indigestion or difficulty in swallowing, obvious changes in a wart or mole, and persistent coughing or hoarseness. Report these signs to the physician immediately.

Interventions

- For patients who are medically able to begin exercise, implement appropriate resistive exercises and aerobic training to maintain muscle strength and aerobic capacity during cancer chemotherapy or to help restore function after chemotherapy.
- Because of the risk of arrhythmias and abnormal BP responses, use caution during aerobic exercise and other forms of therapeutic exercise Assess exercise tolerance frequently (BP, heart rate, fatigue levels), and terminate exercise immediately if any untoward responses occur (See Appendix L).
- Causes photosensitivity; use care if administering UV treatments. Advise patient to avoid direct sunlight and use sunscreens and protective clothing.

Patient/Client-Related Instruction

- Advise patient to guard against infection (frequent hand washing, etc.), and to avoid crowds and contact with persons with contagious diseases.
- Advise patient about the likelihood of GI reactions, including nausea, vomiting, diarrhea, difficulty swallowing, loss of appetite, and inflammation in or around the mouth. Instruct patient or family and caregivers to report severe or prolonged GI problems, and also to report signs of liver dysfunction, including abdominal pain, severe nausea and vomiting, yellow skin or eyes, fever, sore throat, malaise,

weakness, facial edema, lethargy, and unusual bleeding or bruising.

- Advise patient that hair loss and other skin reactions (rash, itching) are likely, but to report other severe or unexpected skin reactions to the physician.
- Instruct patient to report other troublesome side effects including severe or prolonged headache, nightmares, vision disturbances, and breast enlargement in men (gynecomastia).

Pharmacokinetics

Absorption: Well absorbed following oral administration.
Distribution: Widely distributed; crosses the blood-brain barrier.
Metabolism and Excretion: Metabolized by the liver; <5% excreted unchanged by the kidneys; some respiratory elimination as methane and carbon dioxide.
Half-life: 1 hr.

TIME/ACTION PROFILE (effects on blood counts)

ROUTE	ONSET	PEAK	DURATION
PO	14 days	2–8 weeks	28 days or more (up to 6 weeks)

Contraindications/Precautions

Contraindicated in: Hypersensitivity; Pregnancy or lactation; Alcoholism; Severe renal or liver impairment; Pheochromocytoma; CHF.
Use Cautiously in: Patients with childbearing potential; Infections; Decreased bone marrow reserve; Other chronic debilitating illnesses; Headaches; Psychiatric illness; Liver impairment; Cardiovascular disease.

Interactions

Drug-Drug: Concurrent use with **sympathomimetics,** including **methylphenidate,** may produce life-threatening hypertension (avoid concurrent use during and for 14 days following procarbazine). Deep coma and death may result from concurrent use of **opioid analgesics;** avoid **meperidine**. Use small incremental doses of other agents and titrate to effect. ↑ bone marrow depression may occur with other **antineoplastics** or **radiation therapy**. Seizures and hyperpyrexia may occur with concurrent use of **MAO inhibitors, tricyclic antidepressants, SSRI antidepressants** (should not be used within 5 wk of **fluoxetine**), or **carbamazepine**. May ↓ serum **digoxin** levels. Concurrent use with **levodopa** may result in flushing and hypertension. ↑ CNS depression with other **CNS depressants**, including **alcohol, antidepressants, antihistamines, opioid analgesics, phenothiazines**, and **sedative/hypnotics**. Disulfiram-like reaction may occur with **alcohol**. **Cigarette smoking** may ↑ the risk of secondary lung cancer.
Drug-Food: Ingestion of foods high in **tyramine** content (see Appendix L) may result in hypertension. Ingestion of foods high in **caffeine** content may result in arrhythmias.

Route/Dosage

PO (Adults): 2–4 mg/kg/day as a single dose or in divided doses for 1 wk, then 4–6 mg/kg/day until response is obtained; then maintenance dose of 1–2 mg/kg/day. Dosage should be rounded off to the nearest 50 mg.
PO (Children): 50 mg/m^2/day for 7 days, then 100 mg/m^2/day; maintenance dose of 50 mg/m^2/day.

Availability

Capsules: 50 mg.

prochlorperazine

(proe-klor-**per**-a-zeen)
Compazine, Stemetil, Ultrazine

Classification
Therapeutic: antiemetics, antipsychotics
Pharmacologic: phenothiazines

Indications

Management of nausea and vomiting. Treatment of psychoses. Treatment of anxiety.

Action

Alters the effects of dopamine in the CNS. Possesses significant anticholinergic and alpha-adrenergic blocking activity. Depresses the chemoreceptor trigger zone (CTZ) in the CNS. **Therapeutic Effects:** Diminished nausea and vomiting. Diminished signs and symptoms of psychoses or anxiety.

Adverse Reactions/Side Effects

CNS: NEUROLEPTIC MALIGNANT SYNDROME, extrapyramidal reactions, sedation, tardive dyskinesia. **EENT:** blurred vision, dry eyes, lens opacities. **CV:** ECG changes, hypotension, tachycardia. **GI:** constipation, dry mouth, anorexia, drug-induced hepatitis, ileus. **GU:** pink or reddish brown discoloration of urine, urinary retention. **Derm:** photosensitivity, pigment changes, rashes. **Endo:** galactorrhea. **Hemat:** AGRANULOCYTOSIS, leukopenia. **Metab:** hyperthermia. **Misc:** allergic reactions.

PHYSICAL THERAPY IMPLICATIONS

Examination and Evaluation

- Monitor and report immediately signs of neuroleptic malignant syndrome, including hyperthermia, diaphoresis, generalized muscle rigidity, altered mental status, tachycardia, changes in blood pressure (BP), and incontinence. Symptoms typically occur within 4–14 days after initiation of drug therapy, but can occur at any time during drug use.
- Watch for signs of agranulocytosis and leukopenia, including fever, sore throat, mucosal lesions, and

other signs of infection. Report these signs to the physician or nursing staff immediately.

- Assess motor function, and be alert for extrapyramidal symptoms. Report these symptoms immediately, especially tardive dyskinesia, because this problem may be irreversible. Common extrapyramidal symptoms include:
  - Tardive dyskinesia (uncontrolled rhythmic movement of mouth, face, and extremities, lip smacking or puckering, puffing of cheeks, uncontrolled chewing, rapid or worm-like movements of tongue).
  - Pseudoparkinsonism (shuffling gait, rigidity, tremor, pill-rolling motion, loss of balance control, difficulty speaking or swallowing, mask-like face).
  - Akathisia (restlessness or desire to keep moving).
  - Other dystonias and dyskinesias (dystonic muscle spasms, twisting motions, twitching, inability to move eyes, weakness of arms or legs).
- Monitor signs of allergic reactions, including pulmonary symptoms (tightness in the throat and chest, wheezing, dyspnea) or skin reactions (rash, pruritus, urticaria). Notify physician or nursing staff immediately if these reactions occur.
- Assess heart rate, ECG, and heart sounds, especially during exercise (See Appendices G, H). Report a rapid heart rate (tachycardia) or signs of other arrhythmias, including palpitations, chest discomfort, shortness of breath, fainting, and fatigue/weakness.
- Assess BP periodically, and compare to normal values (See Appendix F). Report low BP (hypotension), especially if patient experiences dizziness or syncope.
- If used to control nausea and vomiting, monitor the frequency, severity, and duration of GI problems to help document drug effectiveness.

Interventions

- Guard against falls and trauma (hip fractures, head injury, and so forth) caused by drowsiness, blurred vision, or extrapyramidal symptoms; implement fall-prevention strategies (See Appendix E).
- Because of the risk of ECG changes and abnormal BP responses, use caution during aerobic exercise and other forms of therapeutic exercise Assess exercise tolerance frequently (BP, heart rate, fatigue levels), and terminate exercise immediately if any untoward responses occur (See Appendix L).
- To minimize orthostatic hypotension, patient should move slowly when assuming a more upright position.
- This drug impairs body temperature regulation; use care during exercise and during other activities that increase body temperature (hot whirlpools, saunas, and so forth).
- Causes photosensitivity; use care if administering UV treatments. Advise patient to avoid direct sunlight and use sunscreens and protective clothing.
- Help patient and family/caregivers explore nonpharmacologic methods (exercise, counseling, support groups) to reduce schizophrenic episodes and behavioral problems.

Patient/Client-Related Instruction

- Advise patient to avoid alcohol and other CNS depressants because of the increased risk of sedation and adverse effects.
- Advise patient about the likelihood of GI problems such as constipation, dry mouth, and loss of appetite. Instruct patient to report severe or prolonged GI reactions, and also to report signs of drug-induced hepatitis, including abdominal pain, severe nausea and vomiting, yellow skin or eyes, skin rashes, flu-like symptoms, and muscle/joint pain.
- Instruct patient to report other problematic side effects such as severe or prolonged vision disturbances, dry eyes, excessive sedation, urinary retention, nipple discharge, or skin reactions (rash, changes in pigmentation).

Pharmacokinetics

Absorption: Absorption from tablet is variable; may be better with oral liquid formulations. Well absorbed after IM administration.
Distribution: Widely distributed, high concentrations in the CNS. Crosses the placenta and probably enters breast milk.
Protein Binding: ≥90%.
Metabolism and Excretion: Highly metabolized by the liver and GI mucosa. Converted to some compounds with antipsychotic activity.
Half-life: Unknown.

TIME/ACTION PROFILE (antiemetic effect)

ROUTE	ONSET	PEAK	DURATION
PO	30–40 min	unknown	3–4 hr
PO-ER	30–40 min	unknown	10–12 hr
Rect	60 min	unknown	3–4 hr
IM	10–20 min	10–30 min	3–4 hr
IV	rapid (min)	10–30 min	3–4 hr

Contraindications/Precautions

Contraindicated in: Hypersensitivity; Cross-sensitivity with other phenothiazines may exist; Angle-closure glaucoma; Bone marrow depression; Severe liver or cardiovascular disease; Hypersensitivity to bisulfites or benzyl alcohol (some parenteral products); Pedi: Children <2 yr or 9.1 kg.

P

Use Cautiously in: Geri: Geriatric or debilitated patients (dose reduction recommended); ↑ risk of mortality in elderly patients treated for dementia-related psychosis; Diabetes mellitus; Respiratory disease; Prostatic hypertrophy; CNS tumors; Epilepsy; Intestinal obstruction; OB/Lactation: Safety not established.

Interactions

Drug-Drug: Additive hypotension with **antihypertensives, nitrates**, or acute ingestion of **alcohol**. Additive CNS depression with other **CNS depressants**, including **alcohol, antidepressants, antihistamines, opioid analgesics, sedative/hypnotics**, or **general anesthetics**. Additive anticholinergic effects with other **drugs possessing anticholinergic properties**, including **antihistamines**, some **antidepressants, atropine, haloperidol**, and other **phenothiazines. Lithium** ↑ risk of extrapyramidal reactions. May mask early signs of **lithium** toxicity. ↑ risk of agranulocytosis with **antithyroid agents**. ↓ beneficial effects of **levodopa. Antacids** may ↓ absorption.

Drug-Natural: Concomitant use of **kava-kava, valerian, chamomile**, or **hops** can ↑ CNS depression. ↑ anticholinergic effects with **angel's trumpet, jimson weed**, and **scopolia**.

Route/Dosage

Pediatric dose should not exceed 10 mg on the 1st day and then should not exceed 20 mg/day in children 2–5 yr or 25 mg/day in children 6–12 yr.

Antiemetic

PO (Adults and Children ≥12 yr): 5–10 mg tid–qid; may also be given as 15–30 mg once daily *or* 10 mg bid as ER capsules (up to 40 mg/day).

PO (Children 18–39 kg): 2.5 mg tid *or* 5 mg bid (not to exceed 15 mg/day).

PO (Children 14–17 kg): 2.5 mg bid–tid (not to exceed 10 mg/day).

PO (Children 9–13 kg): 2.5 mg 1–2 times daily (not to exceed 7.5 mg/day).

IM (Adults and Children ≥12 yr): 5–10 mg q 3–4 hr as needed. *Nausea/vomiting associated with surgery*—5–10 mg; may be repeated once.

IM (Children 2–12 yr): 132 mcg (0.132 mg)/kg; usually only 1 dose is required.

IV (Adults and Children ≥12 yr): 2.5–10 mg (not to exceed 40 mg/day). *Nausea/vomiting associated with surgery*—5–10 mg; may be repeated once.

IM (Children 2–12 yr): 132 mcg (0.132 mg)/kg; usually only 1 dose is required.

IV (Adults and Children ≥12 yr): 2.5–10 mg (not to exceed 40 mg/day). *Nausea/vomiting associated with surgery*—5–10 mg; may be repeated once.

Rect (Adults): 25 mg bid.

Rect (Children 18–39 kg): 2.5 mg tid or 5 mg bid (not to exceed 15 mg/day).

Rect (Children 14–17 kg): 2.5 mg bid–tid (not to exceed 10 mg/day).

Rect (Children 9–13 kg): 2.5 mg 1–2 times daily (not to exceed 7.5 mg/day).

Antipsychotic

PO (Adults and Children ≥12 yr): 5–10 mg tid–qid; may be increased q 2–3 days (up to 150 mg/day).

PO (Children 2–12 yr): 2.5 mg bid–tid.

IM (Adults): 10–20 mg q 2–4 hr for up to 4 doses, then 10–20 mg q 4–6 hr (up to 200 mg/day).

IM (Children 2–12 yr): 132 mcg (0.132 mg)/kg (not to exceed 10 mg/dose).

IV (Adults and Children ≥12 yr): 2.5–10 mg (up to 40 mg/day).

Rect (Adults): 10 mg tid–qid; may be increased by 5–10 mg q 2–3 days as needed.

Antianxiety

PO (Adults and Children ≥12 yr): 5 mg tid–qid (not to exceed 20 mg/day or longer than 12 wk); may also be given as 15 mg once daily or 10 mg bid as ER capsules.

IM (Adults and Children ≥12 yr): 5–10 mg q 3–4 hr as needed (up to 40 mg/day).

IM (Children 2–12 yr): 132 mcg (0.132 mg)/kg.

IV (Adults): 2.5–10 mg (up to 40 mg/day).

Availability (generic available)

Tablets: 5 mg, 10 mg, 25 mg. **Syrup (fruit flavor):** 5 mg/5 mL (edisylate), 5 mg/5 mL (mesylate). **Extended-release capsules:** 10 mg, 15 mg, 30 mg. **Injection:** 5 mg/mL (edisylate), 5 mg/mL (mesylate). **Suppositories:** 2.5 mg, 5 mg, 25 mg.

progesterone (proe-**jes**-te-rone)

Crinone, Endometrin, Prochieve, Prometrium

Classification
Therapeutic: hormones
Pharmacologic: progestins

Indications

Secondary amenorrhea and abnormal uterine bleeding due to hormonal imbalance. **Prometrium:** Prevention of cell overgrowth in the uterine lining in postmenopausal women who have not had a hysterectomy (with estrogen). Part of assisted reproductive technology (ART) in the management of infertility (4% and 8% vaginal gel). **Endometrin:** Support of embryo implantation and early pregnancy.
Unlabeled Use: Corpus luteum dysfunction.

Action

Produces Secretory changes in the endometrium; Increase in basal body temperature; Histologic changes in vaginal epithelium; Relaxation of uterine smooth muscle; Mammary alveolar tissue growth; Pituitary inhibition; Withdrawal bleeding in the presence of estrogen. **Therapeutic Effects:** Restoration of hormonal balance with control of uterine bleeding. Successful outcome in assisted reproduction.

Adverse Reactions/Side Effects

CNS: depression. **EENT:** retinal thrombosis.
CV: PULMONARY EMBOLISM, THROMBOEMBOLISM, thrombophlebitis. **GI:** gingival bleeding, hepatitis. **GU:** cervical erosions. **Derm:** chloasma, melasma, rashes.
Endo: amenorrhea, breakthrough bleeding, breast tenderness, changes in menstrual flow, galactorrhea, spotting. **F and E:** edema. **Local:** irritation or pain at IM injection site. **Misc:** ALLERGIC REACTIONS, INCLUDING ANAPHYLAXIS AND ANGIOEDEMA, weight gain, weight loss.

PHYSICAL THERAPY IMPLICATIONS

Examination and Evaluation

- Monitor signs of thrombophlebitis (localized pain, swelling, warmth, erythema, tenderness) and pulmonary embolism (shortness of breath, chest pain, cough, bloody sputum). Notify physician immediately, and request objective tests (Doppler ultrasound, lung scan, others) if thromboembolism is suspected.
- Monitor signs of allergic reactions, including anaphylaxis and angioedema. Signs include pulmonary symptoms (tightness in the chest and throat, wheezing, cough, dyspnea) or skin reactions (rash, pruritus, urticaria, swelling in the face). Notify physician immediately if these reactions occur.
- Assess peripheral edema using girth measurements, volume displacement, and measurement of pitting edema (See Appendix N). Report increased swelling in feet and ankles or a sudden increase in body weight due to fluid retention.
- Report signs of drug-induced hepatitis, including anorexia, abdominal pain, severe nausea and vomiting, yellow skin or eyes, skin rashes, flu-like symptoms, and muscle/joint pain.
- Monitor and report depression or other changes in mood and behavior.
- Periodically assess body weight and other anthropometric measures (body mass index, body composition). Report a rapid or sustained weight loss or gain, or a substantial change in lean body mass.
- Monitor IM injection site for pain, swelling, and irritation. Report prolonged or excessive injection site reactions to the physician.

Interventions

- Because of the risk of thromboembolism, use caution during aerobic exercise and other forms of therapeutic exercise. Assess exercise tolerance frequently (blood pressure, heart rate, fatigue levels), and terminate exercise immediately if any untoward responses occur (See Appendix L).

Patient/Client-Related Instruction

- Caution patient and family/caregivers about risks of thromboembolism, and review warning signs of a pulmonary embolism (sudden shortness of breath, dyspnea, bloody sputum, cough).
- Caution patient that cigarette smoking may increase the risk of infarction and thromboembolic disease, especially for women older than 35.
- Advise women about possible changes in menstrual function. Instruct patient to notify the physician about any abnormal bleeding.
- Instruct patient to report other troublesome side effects such as visual problems, bleeding gums, or skin disorders (rash, discoloration).

Pharmacokinetics

Absorption: Micronization increases oral and vaginal absorption.
Distribution: Enters breast milk.
Protein Binding: ≥90%.
Metabolism and Excretion: Metabolized by the liver; 50–60% eliminated by kidneys; 10% eliminated in feces.
Half-life: Several minutes.

TIME/ACTION PROFILE (blood levels)

ROUTE	ONSET	PEAK	DURATION
PO	unknown	2–4 hr	unknown
vaginal	unknown	34.8–55 hr	unknown
IM	unknown	19.6–28 hr	unknown

Contraindications/Precautions

Contraindicated in: Hypersensitivity; Hypersensitivity to parabens or sesame oil (IM suspension only); Thromboembolic disease; Cerebrovascular disease; Severe liver disease; Breast or genital cancer; Porphyria; Missed abortion; OB: Pregnancy (except corpus luteum dysfunction).
Use Cautiously in: History of liver disease; Renal disease; Cardiovascular disease; Seizure disorders; Mental depression.

Interactions

Drug-Drug: May ↓ effectiveness of **bromocriptine** when used concurrently for galactorrhea and amenorrhea.

Route/Dosage

PO (Adults): *Secondary amenorrhea*— 400 mg once daily in the evening for 10 days; *prevention of postmenopausal estrogen-induced endometrial*

P

hyperplasia—200 mg once daily at bedtime for 14 days on days 8–21 of a 28-day cycle or on days 12–25 of a 30-day cycle; if patient currently receives ≥1.25 mg/day of estrogen, then a daily of dose of 300 mg of progesterone as 100 mg 2 hr after breakfast and 200 mg at bedtime is used; further adjustments may be required.

Vaginal (Adults): *Secondary amenorrhea*—45 mg (1 applicatorful of 4% gel) once every other day for up to 6 doses, may be increased to 90 mg (1 applicatorful of 8% gel) once every other day for up to 6 doses; *Corpus luteum insufficiency or assisted reproduction technology*—For luteal phase support: 90 mg (1 applicatorful of 8% gel) once daily; for in vitro fertilization: 90 mg (1 applicatorful of 8% gel) once daily beginning within 24 hr of embryo transfer and continued through day 30 posttransfer (if pregnancy occurs, treatment may be continued for up to 10–12 wk); *Partial or complete ovarian failure*—90 mg (1 applicatorful of 8% gel) bid while undergoing donor oocyte transfer (if pregnancy occurs, treatment may be continued for up to 10–12 wk); *Support of embryo implantation and early pregnancy*—100-mg insert bid or tid for up to 10 wk.

IM (Adults): *Secondary amenorrhea*—100–150 mg (single dose) or 5–10 mg daily for 6–8 days given 8–10 days before expected menstrual period; *Dysfunctional uterine bleeding*—5–10 mg daily for 6 days; *Corpus luteum insufficiency*—12.5 mg/day at onset of ovulation for 2 wk; may continue until 11th wk of gestation (unlabeled).

Availability (generic available)

Micronized capsules (Prometrium): 100 mg, 200 mg. **Bioadhesive vaginal gel (Crinone, Prochieve):** 4%, 8%. **Vaginal tablets (Endometrin):** 100 mg. **Injection:** 50 mg/mL in 10-mL vials.

promethazine

(proe-**meth**-a-zeen)

Antinaus, Histanil, Pentazine, Phenadoz, Phenergan, Promacot, Promet, Prorex

Classification

Therapeutic: antiemetics, antihistamines, sedative/hypnotics

Pharmacologic: phenothiazines

Indications

Treatment of various allergic conditions and motion sickness. Preoperative sedation. Treatment and prevention of nausea and vomiting. Adjunct to anesthesia and analgesia.

Action

Blocks the effects of histamine. Has inhibitory effect on the chemoreceptor trigger zone in the medulla, resulting in antiemetic properties. Alters the effects of dopamine in the CNS. Possesses significant anticholinergic activity. Produces CNS depression by indirectly decreased stimulation of the CNS reticular system.

Therapeutic Effects: Relief of symptoms of histamine excess usually seen in allergic conditions. Diminished nausea or vomiting. Sedation.

Adverse Reactions/Side Effects

CNS: NEUROLEPTIC MALIGNANT SYNDROME, <u>confusion</u>, <u>disorientation</u>, <u>sedation</u>, dizziness, extrapyramidal reactions, fatigue, insomnia, nervousness. **EENT:** blurred vision, diplopia, tinnitus. **CV:** bradycardia, hypertension, hypotension, tachycardia. **GI:** constipation, drug-induced hepatitis, dry mouth. **Derm:** photosensitivity, severe tissue necrosis upon infiltration at IV site, rashes. **Hemat:** blood dyscrasias.

PHYSICAL THERAPY IMPLICATIONS

Examination and Evaluation

- Monitor and report signs of neuroleptic malignant syndrome, including hyperthermia, diaphoresis, generalized muscle rigidity, altered mental status, tachycardia, changes in blood pressure (BP), and incontinence. Symptoms typically occur within 4–14 days after initiation of drug therapy, but can occur at any time during drug use.
- Assess motor function, and be alert for extrapyramidal reactions. Report these symptoms immediately, especially tardive dyskinesia, because this problem may be irreversible. Common extrapyramidal symptoms include:
  - Tardive dyskinesia (uncontrolled rhythmic movement of mouth, face, and extremities, lip smacking or puckering, puffing of cheeks, uncontrolled chewing, rapid or worm-like movements of tongue).
  - Pseudoparkinsonism (shuffling gait, rigidity, tremor, pill-rolling motion, loss of balance control, difficulty speaking or swallowing, mask-like face).
  - Akathisia (restlessness or desire to keep moving).
  - Other dystonias and dyskinesias (dystonic muscle spasms, twisting motions, twitching, inability to move eyes, weakness of arms or legs).
- Assess heart rate, ECG, and heart sounds, especially during exercise (See Appendices G, H). Report any rhythm disturbances or symptoms of increased arrhythmias, including palpitations, chest discomfort, shortness of breath, fainting, and fatigue/weakness.
- Assess BP and compare to normal values (See Appendix F). Report changes in BP, either a

problematic decrease in BP (hypotension) or a sustained increase in BP (hypertension).

- Monitor unusual weakness and fatigue that might be due to anemia or other symptoms such as fever, sore throat, mucosal lesions, or signs of infection that might be due to other blood dyscrasias. Notify physician if these signs occur.
- Assess dizziness and drowsiness that might affect gait, balance, and other functional activities (See Appendix C). Report balance problems and functional limitations to the physician and nursing staff, and caution the patient and family/caregivers to guard against falls and trauma.
- Monitor changes in mood and behavior, including confusion, disorientation, and nervousness. Notify physician if these changes become problematic.
- If used to control nausea and vomiting, monitor the frequency, severity, and duration of GI problems to help document drug effectiveness.
- Monitor IV injection site for local damage and necrosis. Report injection site reactions to the physician.

Interventions

- Guard against falls and trauma (hip fractures, head injury, and so forth) caused by drowsiness, blurred vision, or extrapyramidal symptoms; implement fall-prevention strategies (See Appendix E).
- Because of the risk of arrhythmias and abnormal BP responses, use caution during aerobic exercise and other forms of therapeutic exercise. Assess exercise tolerance frequently (BP, heart rate, fatigue levels), and terminate exercise immediately if any untoward responses occur (See Appendix L).
- Causes photosensitivity; use care if administering UV treatments. Advise patient to avoid direct sunlight and use sunscreens and protective clothing.

Patient/Client-Related Instruction

- Advise patient to avoid alcohol and other CNS depressants because of the increased risk of sedation and adverse effects.
- Instruct patient to report signs of drug-induced hepatitis, including anorexia, abdominal pain, nausea and vomiting, yellow skin or eyes, skin rashes, flu-like symptoms, and muscle/joint pain.
- Instruct patient to report other problematic side effects such as vision disturbances, sleep loss, ringing/buzzing in the ears (tinnitus), excessive sedation, dry mouth, or skin rash.

Pharmacokinetics

Absorption: Well absorbed after oral (88%) and IM administration; rectal administration may be less reliable.

Distribution: Widely distributed; crosses the blood-brain barrier and the placenta.

Protein Binding: 65–90%.

Metabolism and Excretion: Metabolized by the liver.

Half-life: 9–16 hr.

TIME/ACTION PROFILE (noted as antihistaminic effects; sedative effects last 2–8 hr)

ROUTE	ONSET	PEAK	DURATION
PO, IM	20 min	unknown	4–12 hr
rectal	20 min	unknown	4–12 hr
IV	3–5 min	unknown	4–12 hr

Contraindications/Precautions

Contraindicated in: Hypersensitivity; Comatose patients; Prostatic hypertrophy; Bladder neck obstruction; Some products contain alcohol or bisulfites and should be avoided in patients with known intolerance; Angle-closure glaucoma; Pedi: May cause fatal respiratory depression in children <2 yr.

Use Cautiously in: IV administration, may cause severe injury to tissue; Hypertension; Cardiovascular disease; Impaired liver function; Prostatic hypertrophy; Glaucoma; Asthma; Sleep apnea; Epilepsy; Underlying bone marrow depression; Pedi: For children >2 yr, use lowest effective dose, avoid concurrent respiratory depressants; OB: Has been used safely during labor; avoid chronic use during pregnancy; Lactation: Safety not established; may cause drowsiness in infant; Geri: Appears on Beers' list. Geriatric patients are sensitive to anticholinergic effects and have increased risk for side effects.

Interactions

Drug-Drug: Additive CNS depression with other **CNS depressants**, including **alcohol**, other **antihistamines**, **opioid analgesics**, and other **sedative/hypnotics**. Neuroleptic malignant syndrome can occur when used concurrently with **antipsychotics**. Additive anticholinergic effects with other **drugs possessing anticholinergic properties**, including other **antihistamines**, **antidepressants**, **atropine**, **haloperidol**, other **phenothiazines**, **quinidine**, and **disopyramide**. May precipitate seizures when used with **drugs that lower seizure threshold**. Concurrent use with **MAO inhibitors** may result in ↑ sedation and anticholinergic side effects.

Route/Dosage

Antihistamine

PO (Adults): 6.25–12.5 mg tid and 25 mg hs.

PO (Children ≥2 yr): 0.1 mg/kg/dose (not to exceed 12.5 mg) q 6 hr during the day and 0.5 mg/kg/dose (not to exceed 25 mg) hs.

P

IM, IV, Rect (Adults): 25 mg; may repeat in 2 hr.
Rect (Children ≥2 yr): 0.125 mg/kg q 4–6 hr *or* 0.5 mg/kg hs.

Antivertigo (Motion Sickness)

PO (Adults): 25 mg 30–60 min before departure; may be repeated in 8–12 hr.
PO, Rect (Children ≥2 yr): 0.5 mg/kg (not to exceed 25 mg) 30–60 min before departure; may be given q 12 hr as needed.

Sedation

PO, Rectal, IM, IV (Adults): 25–50 mg; may repeat q 4–6 hr if needed.
PO, Rectal, IM (Children >2 yr): 0.5–1 mg/kg (not to exceed 50 mg) q 6 hr as needed.

Sedation During Labor

IM, IV (Adults): 50 mg in early labor; when labor is established, additional doses of 25–75 mg may be given 1–2 times at 4-hr intervals (24-hr dose should not exceed 100 mg).

Antiemetic

PO, Rectal, IM, IV (Adults): 12.5–25 mg q 4 hr as needed; initial PO dose should be 25 mg.
PO, Rectal, IM, IV (Children ≥2 yr): 0.25–1 mg/kg (not to exceed 25 mg) q 4–6 hr.

Availability (generic available)

Tablets: 10 mg OTC, 12.5 mg, 12.5 mg OTC, 25 mg, 25 mg OTC, 50 mg, 50 mg OTC. **Syrup (cherry flavor):** 3.25 mg/120 mL, 6.25 mg/5 mL, 10 mg/5 mL OTC, 25 mg/5 mL. **Injection:** 25 mg/mL in 1-mL ampules and 1- and 10-mL vials, 50 mg/mL in 1-mL ampules and 10-mL vials. **Suppositories:** 2.5 mg, 5 mg, 12.5 mg, 25 mg. ***In combination with:*** codeine, dextromethorphan, phenylephrine, and/or pseudoephedrine in a variety of cough and cold preparations. See Appendix B.

propafenone (proe-**paf**-e-nown)

Rythmol

Classification
Therapeutic: antiarrhythmics (class IC)
Pharmacologic: membrane stabilizers

Indications

Treatment of life-threatening ventricular arrhythmias, including ventricular tachycardia. Prolongs the time to recurrence of symptomatic paroxysmal atrial arrhythmias, including paroxysmal atrial fibrillation/flutter (PAF) and paroxysmal supraventricular tachycardia (PSVT). **Unlabeled Use:** Single-dose treatment for atrial fibrillation.

Action

Slows conduction in cardiac tissue by altering transport of ions across cell membranes. **Therapeutic Effects:** Suppression of ventricular arrhythmias.

Adverse Reactions/Side Effects

CNS: dizziness, shaking, weakness. **EENT:** blurred vision. **CV:** SUPRAVENTRICULAR ARRHYTHMIA, VENTRICULAR ARRHYTHMIAS, conduction disturbances, angina, bradycardia, hypotension. **GI:** altered taste, constipation, nausea, vomiting, diarrhea, dry mouth. **Derm:** rash. **MS:** joint pain.

PHYSICAL THERAPY IMPLICATIONS

Examination and Evaluation

- Assess heart rate, ECG, and heart sounds, especially during exercise (See Appendices G, H). Although intended to treat certain arrhythmias, this drug can unmask or precipitate new arrhythmias (proarrhythmic effect). Report any rhythm disturbances or symptoms of increased arrhythmias, including palpitations, chest pain, shortness of breath, fainting, and fatigue/weakness.
- Assess blood pressure periodically and compare to normal values (See Appendix F). Report low blood pressure (hypotension), especially if patient experiences dizziness or syncope.
- Assess any joint pain to rule out musculoskeletal pathology; that is, try to determine if pain is drug induced rather than caused by anatomic or biomechanical problems.
- Assess dizziness and weakness that might affect gait, balance, and other functional activities (See Appendix C). Report balance problems and functional limitations to the physician, and caution the patient and family/caregivers to guard against falls and trauma.

Interventions

- Because of the risk of CHF and arrhythmias, use extreme caution during aerobic exercise and other forms of therapeutic exercise. Assess exercise tolerance frequently (blood pressure, heart rate, fatigue levels), and terminate exercise immediately if any untoward responses occur (See Appendix L).

Patient/Client-Related Instruction

- Advise patient and family or caregivers about the signs of arrhythmias (see above under Examination and Evaluation) and to seek immediate medical assistance if these signs develop
- Instruct patient and family/caregivers to report other side effects such as severe or prolonged shaking, blurred vision, skin rash, or GI problems (nausea, vomiting, diarrhea, constipation, altered taste, dry mouth).

Pharmacokinetics

Absorption: Although well absorbed following oral administration, undergoes rapid hepatic metabolism (bioavailability 3–11%).
Distribution: Widely distributed; crosses the placenta.
Metabolism and Excretion: Extensively metabolized by the liver (CYP1A2, CYP2D6, and CYP3A4 enzyme systems); some metabolites have antiarrhythmic activity. >90% of patients are considered extensive metabolizers. Others metabolize propafenone more slowly.
Half-life: 2–10 hr in extensive metabolizers; 10–32 hr in slow metabolizers.

TIME/ACTION PROFILE (antiarrhythmic effects)

ROUTE	ONSET	PEAK	DURATION
PO	hrs–days	4–5 days*	hrs

*Chronic dosing.

Contraindications/Precautions

Contraindicated in: Hypersensitivity; Cardiogenic shock; Conduction disorders, including sick sinus syndrome and AV block (without a pacemaker); Bradycardia; Severe hypotension; Concurrent quinidine or amiodarone; Nonallergic bronchospasm; Electrolyte disturbances; Uncontrolled CHF.
Use Cautiously in: Severe hepatic or renal impairment (dose reduction may be necessary); Geri: Lower doses may be necessary due to age-related decrease in renal/hepatic/cardiovascular function, concurrent chronic illnesses and medications); OB/Pedi: Pregnancy, lactation, or children (safety not established).

Interactions

Drug-Drug: Any **inhibitors of the CYP1A2, CYP2D6, or CYP3A4 enzyme systems** may ↑ levels, including **desipramine, paroxetine, ritonavir, sertraline, ketoconazole, saquinavir, erythromycin** (blood level monitoring recommended). **Quinidine** is a strong inhibitor of CYP2D6 and significantly ↑ levels of propafenone; concurrent use is not recommended. Propafenone is also an inhibitor of CYP2D6 and may ↑ levels of **desipramine, imipramine, haloperidol,** and **venlafaxine**. Significantly ↑ serum **digoxin** levels (blood level monitoring recommended; ↓ dose may be required). ↑ blood levels of **metoprolol** and **propranolol** (↓ dose may be required). Concurrent use of **local anesthetics** may ↑ risk of CNS adverse reactions. ↑ effects of **warfarin** (↓ warfarin dose if necessary; monitor prothrombin time). Concurrent with **amiodarone** can adversely effect conduction/repolarization and should be avoided. May ↑ risk of CNS adverse reactions with **lidocaine**. May ↑ **cyclosporine** through blood levels and risk of nephrotoxicity. **Rifampin** may ↓ serum levels and effectiveness of propafenone. **Cimetidine** may ↑ serum levels.
Drug-Food: Grapefruit juice may ↑ levels.

Route/Dosage

PO (Adults): 150 mg q 8 hr; may be gradually increased at 3- to 4-day intervals as required up to 300 mg q 8–12 hr. *Single dose treatment of atrial fibrillation (unlabeled)*—450 or 600 mg.

Availability (generic available)

Tablets: 150 mg, 225 mg, 300 mg.

propantheline
(proe-**pan**-the-leen)
✱ Probanthel, Pro-Banthine

Classification
Therapeutic: antiulcer agents
Pharmacologic: anticholinergics, antimuscarinics

Indications

Adjunctive therapy in the treatment of peptic ulcer disease.
Unlabeled Use: Antisecretory or antispasmodic agent.

Action

Competitively inhibits the muscarinic action of acetylcholine, resulting in decreased GI secretions.
Therapeutic Effects: Reduction of signs and symptoms of peptic ulcer disease.

Adverse Reactions/Side Effects

CNS: confusion, dizziness, drowsiness, excitement. **EENT:** blurred vision, mydriasis, photophobia. **CV:** tachycardia, orthostatic hypotension, palpitations. **GI:** constipation, dry mouth. **GU:** urinary hesitancy, urinary retention. **Derm:** rash. **Misc:** decreased sweating.

PHYSICAL THERAPY IMPLICATIONS

Examination and Evaluation

- Assess heart rate, ECG, and heart sounds, especially during exercise (See Appendices G, H). Report a rapid heart rate (tachycardia) or signs of other arrhythmias, including palpitations, chest discomfort, shortness of breath, fainting, and fatigue/weakness.
- Assess blood pressure (BP) when patient assumes a more upright position (lying to standing, sitting to standing, lying to sitting). Document orthostatic hypotension and contact physician when systolic BP falls >20 mm Hg, or diastolic BP falls >10 mm Hg.

- If used to treat peptic ulcer, monitor any changes in symptoms such as decreased abdominal pain and improved appetite to help document whether drug therapy is successful.
- Be alert for decreased sweating and increased body temperature (hyperthermia), especially during exercise. Notify physician of a prolonged or persistent elevation in body temperature.
- Monitor signs of urine retention (difficult urination, painful or distended abdomen). Excessive urinary retention may require dose adjustment by physician.
- Monitor and report excessive confusion, excitement, or other alterations in mental status.
- Assess dizziness and drowsiness that might affect gait, balance, and other functional activities (See Appendix C). Report balance problems and functional limitations to the physician, and caution the patient and family/caregivers to guard against falls and trauma.

Interventions

- Because of the risk of arrhythmias and impaired thermoregulation, use caution during aerobic exercise and other forms of therapeutic exercise. Assess exercise tolerance frequently (BP, heart rate, fatigue levels), and terminate exercise immediately if any untoward responses occur (See Appendix L).
- To minimize orthostatic hypotension, patient should move slowly when assuming a more upright position.

Patient/Client-Related Instruction

- Instruct patient and family/caregivers to report other troublesome side effects such as severe or prolonged vision problems, skin rash, or GI problems (constipation, dry mouth).

Pharmacokinetics

Absorption: Incompletely absorbed from the GI tract.
Distribution: Distribution not known. Does not cross the blood-brain barrier.
Metabolism and Excretion: Inactivated in the upper small intestine.
Half-life: Unknown.

TIME/ACTION PROFILE (anticholinergic effects)

ROUTE	ONSET	PEAK	DURATION
PO	30–60 min	2–6 hr	6 hr

Contraindications/Precautions

Contraindicated in: Hypersensitivity; Angle-closure glaucoma; Tachycardia secondary to cardiac insufficiency or thyrotoxicosis; Myasthenia gravis.
Use Cautiously in: Geriatric patients or patients of small stature (dosage reduction required); Prostatic hypertrophy; Chronic renal, cardiac, or pulmonary disease; Patients who may have intra-abdominal infections; Geri: Appears on Beers' list. Geriatric patients have increased sensitivity to anticholinergics; Pregnancy, lactation, or children (safety not established).

Interactions

Drug-Drug: Additive anticholinergic effects with other **drugs possessing anticholinergic properties,** including **antihistamines, antidepressants, atropine, haloperidol, phenothiazines, quinidine,** and **disopyramide.** May alter the absorption of other **orally administered drugs** by slowing motility of the GI tract. **Antacids** and **adsorbent antidiarrheals** ↓ the absorption of anticholinergics (avoid taking within 2–3 hr of propantheline). May ↑ GI mucosal lesions in patients taking **solid oral potassium chloride supplements.**
Drug-Natural: ↑ anticholinergic effects with **angel's trumpet, jimson weed,** and **scopolia.**

Route/Dosage

PO (Adults): 15 mg tid, 30 mg hs.
PO (Geriatric Patients, Patients with Mild Symptoms, or Small Stature): 7.5 mg tid–qid.
PO (Children): 0.375 mg/kg (10 mg/m^2) qid.

Availability (generic available)

Tablets: 7.5 mg, 15 mg.

propofol (proe-poe-fol)

Diprivan

Classification
Therapeutic: general anesthetics

Indications

Induction of general anesthesia in children >3 yr and adults. Maintenance of balanced anesthesia when used with other agents in children >2 mo and adults. Initiation and maintenance of monitored anesthesia care (MAC). Sedation of intubated, mechanically ventilated patients in intensive care units (ICUs).

Action

Short-acting hypnotic. Mechanism of action is unknown. Produces amnesia. Has no analgesic properties. **Therapeutic Effects:** Induction and maintenance of anesthesia.

Adverse Reactions/Side Effects

CNS: dizziness, headache. **Resp:** APNEA, cough. **CV:** bradycardia, hypotension, hypertension. **GI:** abdominal cramping, hiccups, nausea, vomiting. **Derm:** flushing. **Local:** burning, pain, stinging, coldness, numbness, tingling at IV site. **MS:** involuntary muscle movements, perioperative myoclonia. **GU:** discoloration of urine (green). **Misc:** PROPOFOL INFUSION SYNDROME, fever.

PHYSICAL THERAPY IMPLICATIONS*

**Implications refer primarily to any residual effects that occur typically within 24 hr after anesthesia.*

Examination and Evaluation

- Assess respiration and notify physician immediately if patient exhibits any interruption in respiratory rate (apnea) or signs of respiratory depression, including decreased respiratory rate, confusion, bluish color of the skin and mucous membranes (cyanosis), and difficult, labored breathing (dyspnea). Monitor pulse oximetry and perform pulmonary function tests (See Appendices I, J, K) to quantify suspected changes in ventilation and respiratory function. Apnea or excessive respiratory depression requires emergency care.
- Assess heart rate, ECG, and heart sounds, especially during long-term (>24 hr) administration to children or critically ill patients. Be especially alert for an unusually slow heart rate (bradycardia) that can progress to asystole. Bradycardia and other arrhythmias may indicate propofol infusion syndrome, a potentially fatal event accompanied by metabolic acidosis, rhabdomyolysis, and renal failure. Report these signs to the physician or nursing staff immediately.
- Assess blood pressure (BP) and compare to normal values (See Appendix F). Report changes in BP, either a problematic decrease in BP (hypotension) or a sustained increase in BP (hypertension).
- Be alert for residual muscle rigidity and involuntary muscle movements. Report any sustained or problematic changes in muscle tone or excitability.
- If used during mechanical ventilation, observe whether the patient is adequately sedated and the chest wall is relaxed and compliant with ventilation. Notify physician or nursing staff if the patient is agitated or appears to be resisting mechanical ventilation.
- Assess residual dizziness that might affect gait, balance, and other functional activities (See Appendix C). Report balance problems and functional limitations to the physician and nursing staff, and caution the patient and family/caregivers to guard against falls and trauma.
- Monitor injection site for pain, swelling, and irritation. Report prolonged or excessive injection-site reactions to the physician.

Interventions

- Because of the risk of respiratory depression, arrhythmias, and abnormal BP responses, use caution during aerobic exercise and other forms of therapeutic exercise. Assess exercise tolerance frequently (BP, heart rate, respiratory rate, fatigue levels), and terminate exercise immediately if any untoward responses occur (see Appendix L).
- To minimize orthostatic hypotension, patient should move slowly when assuming a more upright position.

Patient/Client-Related Instruction

- Advise patient to avoid alcohol or other CNS depressants for 24 hr after anesthesia.
- Instruct patient to report other troublesome side effects such as severe or prolonged headache, cough, fever, skin reactions (flushing), or GI problems (nausea, vomiting, hiccups, abdominal cramps).

Pharmacokinetics

Absorption: Administered IV only, resulting in complete absorption.
Distribution: Rapidly and widely distributed. Crosses the blood-brain barrier well; rapidly redistributed to other tissues. Crosses the placenta and enters breast milk.
Protein Binding: 95–99%.
Metabolism and Excretion: Rapidly metabolized by the liver.
Half-life: 3–12 hr (blood-brain equilibration half-life 2.9 min).

TIME/ACTION PROFILE (loss of consciousness)

ROUTE	ONSET	PEAK	DURATION*
IV	40 sec	unknown	3–5 min

*Time to recovery is 8 min (up to 19 min if opioid analgesics have been used).

Contraindications/Precautions

Contraindicated in: Hypersensitivity to propofol, soybean oil, egg lecithin, or glycerol; OB: Labor and delivery.
Use Cautiously in: Cardiovascular disease; Lipid disorders (emulsion may have detrimental effect); Increased intracranial pressure; Cerebrovascular disorders; Geri: Geriatric (>60 yr), debilitated, or hypovolemic patients (lower induction and maintenance dosage reduction recommended); Lactation: Pedi: Children <3 yr (for induction of anesthesia), children <2 mo (maintenance of anesthesia), or lactation (safety not established).

Interactions

Drug-Drug: Additive CNS and respiratory depression with **alcohol, antihistamines, opioid analgesics,** and **sedative/hypnotics** (dose reduction may be required). **Theophylline** may antagonize the CNS effects of propofol. Propofol may ↑ the serum concentrations of **alfentanil**. Cardiorespiratory instability can occur when used with **acetazolamide**. Serious bradycardia can occur with concurrent use of **fentanyl** in children. ↑ risk of hypertriglyceridemia with **intravenous fat emulsion**.

Route/Dosage

General Anesthesia

IV (Adults <55 yr): *Induction*—40 mg q 10 sec until induction achieved (2–2.5 mg/kg total). *Maintenance*—100–200 mcg/kg/min. Rates of 150–200 mcg/kg/min are usually required during first 10–15 min after induction, then decreased by 30–50% during first 30 min of maintenance. Rates of 50–100 mcg/kg/min are associated with optimal recovery time. May also be given intermittently in increments of 25–50 mg.

IV (Geriatric Patients, Cardiac patients, Debilitated Patients, or Hypovolemic Patients): *Induction*—20 mg q 10 sec until induction achieved (1–1.5 mg/kg total). *Maintenance*—50–100 mcg/kg/min (dose in cardiac anesthesia ranges from 50–150 mcg/kg/min depending on concurrent use of opioid).

IV (Adults Undergoing Neurosurgical Procedures): *Induction*—20 mg q 10 sec until induction achieved (1–2 mg/kg total). *Maintenance*—100–200 mcg/kg/min.

IV (Children ≥3 yr–16 yr): *Induction*—2.5–3.5 mg/kg; use lower dose for children ASA III or IV.

IV (Children 2 mo–16 yr): *Maintenance*—125–300 mcg/kg/min (following first 30 min of maintenance; rate should be decreased if possible); younger children may require larger infusion rates compared to older children.

Monitored Anesthesia Care (MAC) Sedation

IV (Adults <55 yr): *Initiation*—100–150 mcg/kg/min infusion *or* 0.5 mg/kg as slow injection. *Maintenance*—25–75 mcg/kg/min infusion or incremental boluses of 10–20 mg.

IV (Geriatric Patients, Debilitated Patients, or ASA III/IV Patients): *Initiation*—Use slower infusion or injection rates. *Maintenance*—20% less than the usual adult infusion dose; rapid/repeated bolus dosing should be avoided.

ICU Sedation

IV (Adults): 5 mcg/kg/min for a minimum of 5 min. Additional increments of 5–10 mcg/kg/min over 5–10 min may be given until desired response is obtained. (Range 5–50 mcg/kg/min.) Dose should be reassessed every 24 hr.

Availability (generic available)

Injection: 10 mg/mL in 20-, 50-, and 100-mL infusion vials.

propoxyphene hydrochloride

(pro-**pox**-i-feen hye-droe-**klor**-ide)
Darvon

Classification
Therapeutic: opioid analgesics
Pharmacologic: opioid agonists

Indications

Mild-to-moderate pain.

Action

Binds to opiate receptors in the CNS. Alters the perception of and response to painful stimuli, while producing generalized CNS depression. **Therapeutic Effects:** Decrease in pain.

Adverse Reactions/Side Effects

CNS: disorientation, dizziness, weakness, dysphoria, euphoria, headache, insomnia, paradoxical excitement, sedation. **EENT:** blurred vision. **CV:** hypotension. **GI:** nausea, abdominal pain, constipation, vomiting. **Derm:** rash. **Misc:** physical dependence, psychologic dependence, tolerance.

PHYSICAL THERAPY IMPLICATIONS

Examination and Evaluation

- Be alert for excessive sedation or changes in mood and behavior (euphoria, dysphoria, disorientation, excitement). Notify physician or nurse immediately if patient is unconscious or extremely difficult to arouse.
- Use appropriate pain scales (visual analogue scales, others) to document whether this drug is successful in helping manage the patient's pain.
- Assess blood pressure periodically and compare to normal values (See Appendix F). Report low blood pressure (hypotension), especially if patient experiences dizziness, fainting, or other symptoms.
- Assess dizziness that might affect gait, balance, and other functional activities (See Appendix C). Report balance problems and functional limitations to the physician and nursing staff, and caution the patient and family/caregivers to guard against falls and trauma.

Interventions

- Implement appropriate manual therapy techniques, physical agents, and therapeutic exercises to reduce pain and help wean patient off opioid analgesics as soon as possible.
- Because of the risk of hypotension, use caution during aerobic exercise and other forms of therapeutic exercise. Assess exercise tolerance frequently (blood pressure, heart rate, fatigue levels), and terminate exercise immediately if any untoward responses occur (See Appendix L).

- Help patient explore other nonpharmacologic methods to reduce chronic pain, such as relaxation techniques, exercise, counseling, and so forth.
- Guard against falls and trauma (hip fractures, head injury). Implement fall-prevention strategies (See Appendix E), especially if patient exhibits sedation, dizziness, or blurred vision.
- To minimize orthostatic hypotension, patient should move slowly when assuming a more upright position.

Patient/Client-Related Instruction

- Advise patient that opioid analgesics are usually more effective if given before pain becomes severe; emphasize that adequate pain control will allow better participation in physical therapy.
- Educate patient about the dangers of opioid overdose; encourage patient to adhere to proper dosing schedule.
- Emphasize that the risk of physical addiction (tolerance and dependence) is usually minimal during short-term treatment of pain. Advise patient that addiction is more likely during excessive or inappropriate use of opioid analgesics.
- Advise patient to avoid alcohol and other CNS depressants because of the increased risk of sedation and decreased CNS function.
- Advise patient to increase fluid intake and dietary fiber to avoid constipation. Laxatives may also be helpful in patients susceptible to fecal impaction (e.g., people with spinal cord injury).
- Instruct patient to report other troublesome side effects such as severe or prolonged headache, sleep loss, vision disturbances, skin rash, or GI problems (nausea, vomiting, abdominal pain).

Pharmacokinetics

Absorption: Well absorbed following oral administration.
Distribution: Widely distributed. Probably crosses the placenta. Enters breast milk in small amounts.
Metabolism and Excretion: Mostly metabolized by the liver. Some conversion to norpropoxyphene, a toxic metabolite. This metabolite accumulates in elderly patients and patients with decreased renal function.
Half-life: 6–12 hr.

TIME/ACTION PROFILE (analgesic effect)

ROUTE	ONSET	PEAK	DURATION
PO	15–60 min	2–3 hr	4–6 hr

Contraindications/Precautions

Contraindicated in: Hypersensitivity; OB/Lactation/Pedi: Safety not established.
Use Cautiously in: Head trauma; Increased intracranial pressure; Severe renal, hepatic, or pulmonary disease; Hypothyroidism; Adrenal insufficiency; Alcoholism; Undiagnosed abdominal pain; Prostatic hyperplasia; Geri: Appears on Beers' list. Elderly or debilitated patients require reduced dosages.

Interactions

Drug-Drug: Use with extreme caution in patients receiving **MAO inhibitors** (may result in unpredictable, severe, and potentially fatal reactions—decrease initial dose to 25% of usual dose). ↑ CNS depression with **alcohol**, **antidepressants**, and **sedative/hypnotics**. **Smoking** ↑ metabolism and may ↓ analgesic effectiveness. Administration of **partial-antagonist opioid analgesics** may precipitate withdrawal in physically dependent patients. **Nalbuphine**, **buprenorphine**, or **pentazocine** may ↓ analgesia.
Drug-Natural: Concomitant use of **kava**, **valerian**, or **chamomile** can ↑ CNS depression.

Route/Dosage

PO (Adults): 65 mg q 4 hr as needed (not to exceed 390 mg/day as hydrochloride). 100 mg propoxyphene napsylate = 65 mg propoxyphene hydrochloride.

Availability (generic available)

Capsules: 65 mg. **Tablets:** 65 mg. ***In combination with:*** nonopioid analgesics and caffeine: See Appendix B.

P

HIGH ALERT

propranolol (proe-pran-oh-lole)

Apo-Propranolol, Betachron E-R, Inderal, Inderal LA, InnoPran XL, Novopranol, PMS Propranolol

Classification
Therapeutic: antianginals, antiarrhythmics (class II), antihypertensives, vascular headache suppressants
Pharmacologic: beta blockers

Indications

Management of hypertension, angina, arrhythmias, hypertrophic cardiomyopathy, thyrotoxicosis, essential tremors, pheochromocytoma. Also used in the prevention and management of MI and the prevention of vascular headaches. **Unlabeled Use:** Also used to manage alcohol withdrawal, aggressive behavior, antipsychosis-associated akathisia, situational anxiety, and esophageal varices. Posttraumatic stress disorder (PTSD) (Ongoing clinical trials at National Institute for Mental Health [NIMH].).

Action

Blocks stimulation of $beta_1$ (myocardial) and $beta_2$ (pulmonary, vascular, and uterine)–adrenergic receptor sites. **Therapeutic Effects:** Decreased heart rate and blood pressure. Suppression of arrhythmias. Prevention of MI.

Adverse Reactions/Side Effects

CNS: fatigue, weakness, anxiety, dizziness, drowsiness, insomnia, memory loss, mental depression, mental status changes, nervousness, nightmares. **EENT:** blurred vision, dry eyes, nasal stuffiness. **Resp:** bronchospasm, wheezing. **CV:** ARRHYTHMIAS, BRADYCARDIA, CHF, PULMONARY EDEMA, orthostatic hypotension, peripheral vasoconstriction. **GI:** constipation, diarrhea, nausea. **GU:** erectile dysfunction, decreased libido. **Derm:** itching, rashes. **Endo:** hyperglycemia, hypoglycemia (increased in children). **MS:** arthralgia, back pain, muscle cramps. **Neuro:** paresthesia. **Misc:** drug-induced lupus syndrome.

PHYSICAL THERAPY IMPLICATIONS

Examination and Evaluation

- Assess heart rate, ECG, and heart sounds, especially during exercise (See Appendices G, H). Report immediately an unusually slow heart rate (bradycardia) or signs of other arrhythmias, including palpitations, chest discomfort, shortness of breath, fainting, and fatigue/weakness.
- Assess routinely for signs of CHF and pulmonary edema, including dyspnea, rales/crackles, weight gain, peripheral edema, and jugular venous distention. Report these signs to the physician immediately.
- Assess blood pressure (BP) periodically and compare to normal values (See Appendix F) to help document antihypertensive effects.
- Assess BP when patient assumes a more upright position (lying to standing, sitting to standing, lying to sitting). Document orthostatic hypotension and contact physician when systolic BP falls >20 mm Hg, or diastolic BP falls >10 mm Hg.
- Assess exercise tolerance and episodes of angina pectoris. Document improvements in these variables, but also report any decline in exercise tolerance or increased frequency/severity of anginal attacks.
- Monitor signs of peripheral vasoconstriction, such as extreme coldness in the hands and feet, cyanosis, and muscle cramping. Notify physician of severe or prolonged signs of vasoconstriction.
- Assess symptoms of bronchospasm (wheezing, coughing, tightness in chest). Perform pulmonary function tests to quantify suspected changes in ventilation and respiration (See Appendices I, J, K). Repeated or prolonged bronchoconstriction may require a change in dose or medication (e.g., switch to a more cardioselective beta blocker).
- Assess signs of paresthesia (numbness, tingling) or muscle twitching. Perform objective tests, including electroneuromyography and sensory testing to document any drug-related neuropathic changes.
- Assess any back pain, joint pain, or muscle cramping to rule out musculoskeletal pathology; that is, try to determine if pain is drug induced rather than caused by anatomic or biomechanical problems.
- Be alert for signs of hypoglycemia (weakness, malaise, irritability, fatigue) or hyperglycemia (drowsiness, fruity breath, increased urination, unusual thirst). Medication may mask some signs of hypoglycemia, but dizziness and sweating may still occur. Patients with diabetes mellitus should check blood glucose levels frequently.
- Assess dizziness and drowsiness that might affect gait, balance, and other functional activities (See Appendix C). Report balance problems and functional limitations to the physician, and caution the patient and family/caregivers to guard against falls and trauma.
- Monitor excessive fatigue or weakness. Beta blockers often cause some degree of fatigue and weakness, but any sudden or severe change in muscle strength or energy levels should be reported.
- Monitor mood and personality changes, including depression, anxiety, nervousness, memory loss, or other changes in behavior. Notify physician if these changes become problematic.
- Monitor signs of drug-induced lupus syndrome, including increased BP, fever, joint pain, skin rashes, and redness/irritation of the eye (uveitis). Notify physician promptly if these signs appear.
- If used to prevent vascular headaches, monitor the incidence and severity of attacks to document whether this drug is successful in helping manage the patient's pain.
- If used to treat essential tremors, document any change in tremors and motor function to help determine if this drug is successful in reducing tremors.

Interventions

- Because of an increased risk of cardiac arrhythmias, CHF, and pulmonary edema, use caution during aerobic exercise and endurance conditioning. Likewise, monitor patients closely during treatment of other cardiac problems (angina, cardiomyopathy, recent MI). Terminate exercise if patient exhibits untoward symptoms (chest pain, shortness of breath, unusual fatigue), or displays other criteria for exercise termination (See Appendix L).
- Establish aerobic exercise workloads that account for the effects of beta blockers on heart rate (HR). Some heart rate guidelines may not be appropriate because beta blockers typically decrease maximal HR by 20–30 bpm. Use other guidelines such as rating of perceived exertion (RPE, modified Borg scale) to determine exercise workloads.

- To minimize orthostatic hypotension, patient should move slowly when assuming a more upright position.

Patient/Client-Related Instruction

- Remind patients to take medication as directed to control hypertension and other cardiac conditions even if they are asymptomatic.
- Counsel patients about additional interventions to help control BP and cardiac dysfunction, including regular exercise, weight loss, sodium restriction, stress reduction, moderation of alcohol consumption, and smoking cessation.
- Instruct patient or family/caregivers to report other troublesome side effects such as severe or prolonged insomnia, nightmares, dry eyes, blurred vision, stuffy nose, sexual problems (decreased libido, erectile dysfunction), skin reactions (rash, itching), or GI problems (nausea, constipation, diarrhea).

Pharmacokinetics

Absorption: Well absorbed but undergoes extensive 1st-pass hepatic metabolism.
Distribution: Moderate CNS penetration. Crosses the placenta; enters breast milk.
Protein Binding: 93%.
Metabolism and Excretion: Almost completely metabolized by the liver.
Half-life: 3.4–6 hr.

TIME/ACTION PROFILE (cardiovascular effects)

ROUTE	ONSET	PEAK	DURATION
PO	30 min	60–90 min*	6–12 hr
PO-ER	unknown	6 hr	24 hr
IV	immediate	1 min	4–6 hr

*Following single dose, full effect not seen until several weeks of therapy.

Contraindications/Precautions

Contraindicated in: Uncompensated CHF; Pulmonary edema; Cardiogenic shock; Bradycardia or heart block.
Use Cautiously in: Renal or hepatic impairment; pulmonary disease (including asthma); diabetes mellitus (may mask signs of hypoglycemia); thyrotoxicosis (may mask symptoms); history of severe allergic reactions (may ↑ intensity of response); OB: Crosses the placenta and may cause fetal/neonatal bradycardia, hypotension, hypoglycemia, or respiratory depression. May also ↓ blood supply to the placenta, ↑ the risk for premature birth or fetal death, and cause intrauterine growth retardation. May ↑ risk of cardiac and pulmonary complications in the infant during the neonatal time frame. Lactation: Appears in breast milk; use formula if propranolol must be taken; Pedi: ↑ risk of hypoglycemia, especially during periods of fasting such as before surgery, during prolonged exertion, or with coexisting renal insufficiency; Geri: ↑ sensitivity to all beta blockers; initial dose reduction and careful titration recommended.

Interactions

Drug-Drug: General anesthesia, IV phenytoin, and **verapamil** may cause additive myocardial depression. Additive bradycardia may occur with **digoxin**. Additive hypotension may occur with other **antihypertensives**, acute ingestion of **alcohol**, or **nitrates**. Concurrent use with **amphetamines, cocaine, ephedrine, epinephrine, norepinephrine, phenylephrine**, or **pseudoephedrine** may result in unopposed alpha-adrenergic stimulation (excessive hypertension, bradycardia). Concurrent **thyroid** administration may ↓ effectiveness. May alter the effectiveness of **insulin** or **oral hypoglycemics** (dose adjustments may be necessary). May ↓ effectiveness of **beta-adrenergic bronchodilators** and **theophylline**. May ↓ beneficial beta cardiovascular effects of **dopamine** or **dobutamine**. Use cautiously within 14 days of **MAO inhibitor** therapy (may result in hypertension). **Cimetidine** may ↑ blood levels and toxicity. Concurrent **NSAIDs** may ↓ antihypertensive action. **Smoking** ↑ metabolism and ↓ effects; smoking cessation may ↑ effects.

Route/Dosage

PO (Adults): *Antianginal*—80–320 mg/day in 2–4 divided doses or once daily as extended/sustained-release capsules. *Antihypertensive*—40 mg bid initially; may be increased as needed (usual range 120–240 mg/day; doses up to 1 g/day have been used); *or* 80 mg once daily as extended/sustained-release capsules, increased as needed up to 120 mg. *InnoPran XL* dosing form is designed to be given once daily hs. *Antiarrhythmic*—10–30 mg tid–qid. *Prevention of MI*—180–240 mg/day in divided doses. *Hypertrophic cardiomyopathy*—20–40 mg tid–qid. *Adjunct therapy of pheochromocytoma*—20 mg tid to 40 mg tid–qid concurrently with alpha-blocking therapy, started 3 days before surgery is planned. *Vascular headache prevention*—20 mg qid *or* 80 mg/day as extended/sustained-release capsules; may be increased as needed up to 240 mg/day. *Management of tremor*—40 mg bid; may be increased up to 120 mg/day (up to 320 mg has been used).
PO (Children): *Antihypertensive/antiarrhythmic*—0.5–1 mg/kg/day in 2–4 divided doses; may be increased as needed (usual range for maintenance dose is 2–4 mg/kg/day in 2 divided doses).
IV (Adults): *Antiarrhythmic*—1–3 mg; may be repeated after 2 min and again in 4 hr if needed.

IV (Children): *Antiarrhythmic*—10–100 mcg (0.01–0.1 mg)/kg (up to 1 mg/dose); may be repeated q 6–8 hr if needed.

Availability (generic available)

Oral solution: 4 mg/mL, 8 mg/mL. **Tablets:** 10 mg, 20 mg, 40 mg, 60 mg, 80 mg. **Sustained-release capsules (Inderal LA):** 60 mg, 80 mg, 120 mg, 160 mg. **Extended-release capsules:** 60 mg, 80 mg, 120 mg, 160 mg **Injection:** 1 mg/mL. ***In combination with:*** hydrochlorothiazide (Inderide). See Appendix B.

propylthiouracil

(proe-pil-thye-oh-**yoor**-a-sil)

✱Propyl-Thyracil, PTU

Classification

Therapeutic: antithyroid agents

Pharmacologic: thioamide derivatives

Indications

Palliative treatment of hyperthyroidism. Adjunct in the control of hyperthyroidism in preparation for thyroidectomy or radioactive iodine therapy.

Action

Inhibits the synthesis of thyroid hormones. **Therapeutic Effects:** ↓ signs and symptoms of hyperthyroidism.

Adverse Reactions/Side Effects

CNS: drowsiness, headache, vertigo. **GI:** nausea, vomiting, diarrhea, drug-induced hepatitis, loss of taste. **Derm:** rash, skin discoloration, urticaria. **Endo:** hypothyroidism. **Hemat:** AGRANULOCYTOSIS, leukopenia, thrombocytopenia. **MS:** arthralgia. **Misc:** fever, lymphadenopathy, parotitis.

PHYSICAL THERAPY IMPLICATIONS

Examination and Evaluation

- Monitor signs of agranulocytosis and leukopenia (fever, sore throat, mucosal lesions, signs of infection) and thrombocytopenia (bruising, nose bleeds, bleeding gums). Report these signs to the physician immediately.
- Monitor and report signs of excessive or inadequate dosing. Inadequate doses of propylthiouracil mimic hyperthyroidism, as indicated by nervousness, weight loss, muscle wasting, tachycardia, and heat intolerance. Excessive doses mimic hypothyroidism, as indicated by lethargy, weight gain, bradycardia, and cold intolerance.
- Assess vertigo that might affect gait, balance, and other functional activities. Report balance problems and functional limitations to the physician, and caution the patient and family/caregivers to guard against falls and trauma.
- Assess any joint pain to rule out musculoskeletal pathology; that is, try to determine if pain is drug induced rather than caused by anatomic or biomechanical problems.

Interventions

- Use caution during aerobic exercise and endurance conditioning in patients with symptoms of hyperthyroidism because of the risk of arrhythmias. Assess heart rate and exercise tolerance frequently, and terminate exercise immediately if any untoward responses occur (See Appendix L).
- Guard against falls and trauma. Implement fall-prevention strategies (See Appendix E), especially if patient exhibits vertigo or other impairments that affect gait and balance.

Patient/Client-Related Instruction

- Advise patient about the likelihood of GI reactions such as nausea, vomiting, diarrhea, loss of taste, and inflammation of the salivary glands (parotitis). Instruct patient to report severe or prolonged GI problems, or signs of drug-induced hepatitis (yellow skin or eyes, abdominal pain, severe nausea and vomiting, fever, sore throat, malaise, weakness, facial edema).
- Instruct patient to report other troublesome side effects including severe or prolonged headache, fever, swollen lymph nodes, or skin reactions (rash, hives, discoloration).

Pharmacokinetics

Absorption: Rapidly absorbed from the GI tract.
Distribution: Concentrates in the thyroid gland; crosses the placenta and enters breast milk in low concentrations.
Metabolism and Excretion: Metabolized by the liver.
Half-life: 1–2 hr.

TIME/ACTION PROFILE (effects on clinical thyroid status)

ROUTE	ONSET	PEAK	DURATION
PO	10–21 days*	6–10 wk	wks

*Effects on serum thyroid hormone concentration may occur within 60 min of a single dose.

Contraindications/Precautions

Contraindicated in: Hypersensitivity.
Use Cautiously in: ↓ bone marrow reserve; Pregnancy (may be used safely; however, fetus may develop thyroid problems); Lactation (safety not established).

Interactions

Drug-Drug: Additive bone marrow depression with **antineoplastics** or **radiation therapy**. Additive antithyroid effects with **lithium, potassium iodide,** or **sodium iodide.** ↑ risk of agranulocytosis with **phenothiazines.**

Route/Dosage

PO (Adults): *Thyrotoxic crisis*—200–400 mg q 4 hr during the first 24 hr. *Hyperthyroidism*—300–900 mg once daily or in 2–4 divided doses initially (up to 1.2 g/day); maintenance dose 50–600 mg/day once daily or in 2–4 divided doses.
PO (Children >10 yr): 50–300 mg/day given once daily or in 2–4 divided doses.
PO (Children 6–10 yr): 50–150 mg/day given once daily or in 2–4 divided doses.
PO (Neonates): 10 mg/kg/day in divided doses.

Availability (generic available)

Tablets: 50 mg, 100 mg.

pseudoephedrine

(soo-doe-e-**fed**-rin)
Balminil Decongestant Syrup, Cenafed, Congestaid, Decofed, Dimetapp Maximum Strength 12-Hour Non-Drowsy Extentabs, Dimetapp Decongestant Pediatric, Drixoral 12 Hour Non-Drowsy Formula, Efidac 24, Eltor 120, Genafed, Halofed, Kid Kare, Medi-First Sinus Decongestant, PediaCare Infants' Decongestant Drops, Pediatric Nasal Decongestant, Simply Stuffy, Sinustop , Robidrine, Silfedrine, Sudafed, Sudafed Children's Non-Drowsy, Sudafed 12 Hour, Sudafed Non-Drowsy Maximum Strength, Sudodrin, Triaminic Allergy Congestion Softchews, Unifed

Classification
Therapeutic: allergy, cold, and cough remedies, nasal drying agents/decongestants
Pharmacologic: sympathomimetics

Indications

Symptomatic management of nasal congestion associated with acute viral upper respiratory tract infections. Used in combination with antihistamines in the management of allergic conditions. Used to open obstructed eustachian tubes in chronic otic inflammation or infection.

Action

Stimulates alpha- and beta-adrenergic receptors. Produces vasoconstriction in the respiratory tract mucosa (alpha-adrenergic stimulation) and possibly bronchodilation ($beta_2$-adrenergic stimulation). **Therapeutic Effects:** Reduction of nasal congestion, hyperemia, and swelling in nasal passages.

Adverse Reactions/Side Effects

CNS: SEIZURES, anxiety, nervousness, dizziness, drowsiness, excitability, fear, hallucinations, headache, insomnia, restlessness, weakness. **Resp:** respiratory difficulty. **CV:** CARDIOVASCULAR COLLAPSE, palpitations, hypertension, tachycardia. **GI:** anorexia, dry mouth. **GU:** dysuria. **Misc:** diaphoresis.

PHYSICAL THERAPY IMPLICATIONS

Examination and Evaluation

- Be alert for new seizures or increased seizure activity, especially at the onset of drug treatment. Document the number, duration, and severity of seizures, and report these findings to the physician immediately.
- Watch for a sudden fall in blood pressure and related signs (dizziness, syncope, loss of consciousness) that might indicate cardiovascular collapse. Seek immediate medical assistance if patient develops these signs.
- Assess heart rate, ECG, and heart sounds, especially during exercise (See Appendixes G, H). Report a rapid heart rate (tachycardia) or signs of other arrhythmias, including palpitations, chest discomfort, shortness of breath, fainting, and fatigue/weakness.
- Assess blood pressure periodically and compare to normal values (See Appendix F). Report a sustained increase in blood pressure (hypertension) to the physician.
- Watch for signs of respiratory difficulties, including dyspnea, chest pain, shortness of breath, and cyanosis. Monitor pulse oximetry and perform pulmonary function tests (See Appendices I, J, K) to quantify suspected changes in ventilation and respiratory function.
- Monitor and report signs of CNS toxicity, including anxiety, nervousness, restlessness, fear, and hallucinations. Sustained or severe CNS signs may indicate overdose or excessive use of this drug.

Interventions

- Because of the risk of cardiovascular stimulation, use caution during aerobic exercise and endurance conditioning. Assess exercise tolerance frequently (blood pressure, heart rate, fatigue levels), and terminate exercise immediately if any untoward responses occur (See Appendix L).

Patient/Client-Related Instruction

- Remind patients that over-the-counter cold/flu products may contain pseudoephedrine. Patients should consult their physician or pharmacist to determine if these products can increase their risk of cardiovascular disease.
- Because of the risk of cardiovascular and CNS stimulation, caution patient to avoid taking more than the recommended dose. Instruct patient to contact their physician if nasal symptoms do not improve within 7 days, if fever is present, or if cardiovascular or CNS abnormalities arise (see above under Examination and Evaluation).
- Instruct patient and family/caregivers to report other troublesome side effects such as severe or prolonged headache, sleep loss, problems with urination, excessive sweating, or GI problems (dry mouth, loss of appetite).

Pharmacokinetics

Absorption: Well absorbed after oral administration.
Distribution: Appears to enter the CSF; probably crosses the placenta and enters breast milk.
Metabolism and Excretion: Partially metabolized by the liver. 55–75% excreted unchanged by the kidneys (depends on urine pH).
Half-life: Children: 3.1 hr; Adults: 9–16 hr (depends on urine pH).

TIME/ACTION PROFILE (decongestant effects)

ROUTE	ONSET	PEAK	DURATION
PO	15–30 min	unknown	4–6 hr
PO-ER	60 min	unknown	12 hr

Contraindications/Precautions

Contraindicated in: Hypersensitivity to sympathomimetic amines; Hypertension, severe coronary artery disease; Concurrent MAO inhibitor therapy; Known alcohol intolerance (some liquid products).
Use Cautiously in: Hyperthyroidism; Diabetes mellitus; Prostatic hyperplasia; Ischemic heart disease; Glaucoma; Neonates (some products contain a metabolite of benzyl alcohol, avoid use); Pregnancy or lactation (safety not established).

Interactions

Drug-Drug: Concurrent use with **MAO inhibitors** may cause hypertensive crisis. Additive adrenergic effects with other **adrenergics**. Concurrent use with **beta blockers** may result in hypertension or bradycardia. **Drugs that acidify the urine** may ↓ effectiveness. **Phenothiazines** and **tricyclic antidepressants** potentiate pressor effects. **Drugs that alkalinize the urine (sodium bicarbonate, high-dose antacid therapy)** may intensify effectiveness.
Drug-Food: Foods that acidify the urine may ↓ effectiveness. **Foods that alkalinize the urine** may intensify effectiveness.

Route/Dosage

PO (Adults and Children >12 yr): 60 mg q 6 hr as needed (not to exceed 240 mg/day) *or* 120 mg of extended-release preparation q 12 hr *or* 240 mg extended-release preparation q 24 hr.
PO (Children 6–12 yr): 30 mg q 6 hr as needed (not to exceed 120 mg/day).
PO (Children 2–5 yr): 15 mg q 6 hr (not to exceed 60 mg/day).
PO (Children <2 yr): 4 mg/kg/day in divided doses q 6 hr.

Availability (generic available)

Tablets: 30 mg OTC, 60 mg OTC. **Extended-release tablets:** 120 mg OTC. **Controlled-release tablets:** 240 mg OTC. **Capsules:** 60 mg OTC. **Extended-release capsules:** 240 mg OTC. **Softgel capsules:** 30 mg OTC. **Liquid (grape and others):** 15 mg/5 mL OTC, 30 mg/5 mL OTC. **Drops (cherry and fruit flavor):** 7.5 mg/0.8 mL OTC. ***In combination with:*** antihistamines, acetaminophen, cough suppressants, and expectorants OTC. See Appendix B.

pyrazinamide

(peer-a-**zin**-a-mide)

PMS Pyrazinamide, Tebrazid

Classification

Therapeutic: antituberculars
Pharmacologic: nicotinic acid derivatives

Indications

Used in combination with other agents in the treatment of active tuberculosis.

Action

Mechanism not known. **Therapeutic Effects:** Bacteriostatic action against susceptible mycobacteria.
Spectrum: Active against mycobacteria only.

Adverse Reactions/Side Effects

GI: HEPATOTOXICITY, anorexia, diarrhea, nausea, vomiting. **GU:** dysuria. **Derm:** acne, itching, photosensitivity, skin rash. **Hemat:** anemia, thrombocytopenia. **Metab:** hyperuricemia. **MS:** arthralgia, gouty arthritis.

PHYSICAL THERAPY IMPLICATIONS

Examination and Evaluation

- Be alert for signs of hepatotoxicity, including anorexia, abdominal pain, severe nausea and vomiting, yellow skin or eyes, fever, sore throat, malaise, weakness, facial edema, lethargy, and unusual bleeding or bruising. Report these signs immediately to the physician.

- Assess any joint pain or arthritic symptoms to rule out musculoskeletal pathology; that is, try to determine if pain is drug induced rather than caused by anatomic or biomechanical problems.
- Monitor signs of blood dyscrasias such as thrombocytopenia (bruising, nose bleeds, and bleeding gums), or unusual weakness and fatigue that might be due to anemia. Report these signs to the physician.

Interventions

- Always wash hands thoroughly and disinfect equipment (whirlpools, electrotherapeutic devices, treatment tables, and so forth) to help prevent the spread of infection. Use universal precautions or isolation procedures as indicated for specific patients.
- Causes photosensitivity; use care if administering UV treatments.

Patient/Client-Related Instruction

- Advise patient about photosensitivity and to use sunscreens, protective clothing, and avoid prolonged sun exposure. Advise patient to also report any rashes or other skin reactions.
- Instruct patient and family/caregivers to report other troublesome side effects such as severe or prolonged skin problems (rash, acne, itching), GI problems (diarrhea, nausea, vomiting, loss of appetite), or difficult/painful urination.

Pharmacokinetics

Absorption: Well absorbed after oral administration.
Distribution: Widely distributed. Reaches high concentrations in the CNS (same as plasma). Excreted in breast milk.
Metabolism and Excretion: Mostly metabolized by the liver. Metabolite (pyrazinoic acid) has antimycobacterial activity; 3–4% excreted unchanged by the kidneys.
Half-life: *Pyrazinamide*—9.5 hr. *Pyrazinoic acid*—12 hr. Both are prolonged in renal impairment.

TIME/ACTION PROFILE (blood levels)

ROUTE	ONSET	PEAK	DURATION
PO	unknown	1–2 hr (4–5 hr*)	24 hr

*For pyrazinoic acid.

Contraindications/Precautions

Contraindicated in: Hypersensitivity; Cross-sensitivity with ethionamide, isoniazid, niacin, or nicotinic acid may exist; Severe liver impairment; Concurrent use with rifampin.
Use Cautiously in: Gout; Diabetes mellitus; Acute intermittent porphyria; Pregnancy (safety not established).

Interactions

Drug-Drug: Concurrent use with **rifampin** may result in life-threatening hepatotoxicity and should be avoided. May ↓ blood levels and effectiveness of **cyclosporine**. May ↓ effectiveness of **antigout agents**.

Route/Dosage

PO (Adults and Children): 15–30 mg/kg/day as a single dose. Up to 60 mg/kg/day has been used in isoniazid-resistant tuberculosis (not to exceed 2 g/day as a single dose or 3 g/day in divided doses). May also be given as 50–70 mg/kg 2–3 times weekly (not to exceed 2 g/dose on daily regimen, 3 g/dose for 3-times-weekly regimen, or 4 g/dose for twice-weekly regimen). *Patients with HIV*—20–30 mg/kg/day for first 2 mo of therapy; further dosing depends on regimen employed.

Availability (generic available)

Tablets: 500 mg.

pyridoxine (peer-i-**dox**-een)

Beesix, Doxine, Nestrex, Pyri, Rodex, Vitabee 6

OTHER NAMES:

Viatmin B_6

Classification

Therapeutic: vitamins
Pharmacologic: water-soluble vitamins

Indications

Treatment and prevention of pyridoxine deficiency (may be associated with poor nutritional status or chronic debilitating illnesses). Treatment of pyridoxine-dependent seizures in infants. Treatment and prevention of neuropathy, which may develop from isoniazid, penicillamine, or hydralazine therapy. Management of isoniazid overdose >10 g.

Action

Required for amino acid, carbohydrate, and lipid metabolism. Used in the transport of amino acids, formation of neurotransmitters, and synthesis of heme. **Therapeutic Effects:** Prevention of pyridoxine deficiency. Prevention or reversal of neuropathy associated with hydralazine, penicillamine, or isoniazid therapy.

P

Adverse Reactions/Side Effects

Adverse reactions listed are seen with excessive doses only

Neuro: sensory neuropathy, paresthesia. **Misc:** pyridoxine-dependency syndrome.

PHYSICAL THERAPY IMPLICATIONS

Examination and Evaluation

- Be alert for signs of sensory neuropathy and paresthesias (numbness, tingling). Establish baseline electroneuromyographic values using EMG and nerve conduction at the beginning of drug treatment whenever possible, and reexamine these values periodically to document changes in peripheral nerve function.
- In infants receiving large doses, watch for signs of pyridoxine-dependency syndrome. Signs include CNS excitability (irritability, aggravated startle response, seizures) and GI distress (distension, vomiting, diarrhea). Notify physician or nursing staff if these signs occur.

Patient/Client-Related Instruction

- Encourage patient to consult with a nutritionist for dietary sources of pyroxidine and other vitamins. Explain that the best source of vitamins is a well-balanced diet with foods from the four basic food groups.

Pharmacokinetics

Absorption: Well absorbed from the GI tract.
Distribution: Stored in liver, muscle, and brain. Crosses the placenta and enters breast milk.
Metabolism and Excretion: Converted in RBCs to pyridoxal phosphate and another active metabolite. Amounts in excess of requirements are excreted unchanged by the kidneys.
Half-life: 15–20 days.

TIME/ACTION PROFILE

ROUTE	ONSET	PEAK	DURATION
PO, IM, IV	unknown	unknown	unknown

Contraindications/Precautions

Contraindicated in: Hypersensitivity to pyridoxine or any component.
Use Cautiously in: Parkinson's disease (treatment with levodopa only); Pregnancy (chronic ingestion of large doses may produce pyridoxine-dependency syndrome in newborn).

Interactions

Drug-Drug: Interferes with the therapeutic response to **levodopa** when used without carbidopa. Requirements are increased by **isoniazid, hydralazine, chloramphenicol, penicillamine, estrogens,** and **immunosuppressants.** Decreases serum levels of **phenobarbital** and **phenytoin.**

Route/Dosage

Prevention of Deficiency (Recommended Daily Allowance)

PO (Adults and Children >14 yr): 1.2–1.7 mg/day (larger doses required with cycloserine, ethionamide, hydralazine, immunosuppressants, isoniazid, penicillamine, and estrogen-containing oral contraceptives).
PO (Children 9–13 yr): 1 mg/day (larger doses required with cycloserine, ethionamide, hydralazine, immunosuppressants, isoniazid, and penicillamine).
PO (Children 1–8 yr): 0.5–0.6 mg/day (larger doses required with cycloserine, ethionamide, hydralazine, immunosuppressants, isoniazid, and penicillamine).
PO (Infants 6–12 m): 0.3 mg/day.
PO (Infants <6 mo): 0.1 mg/day.

Treatment of Deficiency

PO (Adults): 2.5–10 mg/day until clinical signs are corrected, then 2–5 mg/day.
PO (Children): 5–25 mg/day for 3 wk, then 1.5–2.5 mg/day.

Pyridoxine-Dependent Seizures

PO, IM, IV (Neonates and Infants): 10–100 mg initially then 50–100 mg/day orally.

Drug-Induced Neuritis

PO (Adults): Treatment-100–300 mg/day; *Prophylaxis*—25–100 mg/day.
PO (Children): Treatment-10–50 mg/day; *Prophylaxis*—1–2 mg/kg/day.

Isoniazid Overdose (>10 g)

IM, IV (Adults and Children): Amount in milligrams equal to amount of isoniazid ingested given as 1–4 g IV, then 1 g IM q 30 min.

Availability (generic available)

Tablets: 20 mg OTC, 25 mg OTC, 50 mg OTC, 100 mg OTC, 250 mg OTC, 500 mg OTC. **Extended-release tablets:** 100 mg OTC, 200 mg OTC, 500 mg OTC. **Extended-release capsules:** 150 mg OTC. **Injection:** 100 mg/mL in 10- and 30-mL vials. ***In combination with:*** vitamins, minerals, and trace elements in a variety of multivitamin preparations OTC.

pyrimethamine

(peer-i-**meth**-a-meen)
Daraprim

Classification
Therapeutic: antimalarials, antiprotozoals
Pharmacologic: folic acid antagonist

Indications

Used in combination with other antimalarials in the treatment of chloroquine-resistant malaria. Used in combination with a sulfonamide in the treatment of toxoplasmosis. **Unlabeled Use:** Used in combination with other agents (sulfonamides, dapsone) in the treatment of *Pneumocystis carinii* pneumonia.

Action

Binds to an enzyme in the protozoa, which results in depletion of folic acid. **Therapeutic Effects:** Death and arrested growth of susceptible organisms (protozoa).

Adverse Reactions/Side Effects

CNS: SEIZURES (HIGH DOSES), headache, insomnia, lightheadedness, malaise, mental depression. **Resp:** dry throat, pulmonary eosinophilia. **CV:** ARRHYTHMIAS (LARGE DOSES). **GI:** atrophic glossitis (high doses), anorexia, diarrhea, nausea. **GU:** hematuria. **Derm:** abnormal pigmentation, dermatitis. **Hemat:** megaloblastic anemia (high doses), pancytopenia, thrombocytopenia. **Misc:** fever.

PHYSICAL THERAPY IMPLICATIONS

Examination and Evaluation

- Be alert for new seizures or increased seizure activity, especially at the onset of drug treatment. Document the number, duration, and severity of seizures, and report these findings immediately to the physician.
- Assess heart rate, ECG, and heart sounds, especially during exercise (See Appendices G, H). Report any rhythm disturbances or symptoms of cardiac dysfunction, including palpitations, chest discomfort, shortness of breath, fainting, and fatigue/weakness.
- Monitor signs of thrombocytopenia (bruising, nose bleeds, bleeding gums) or unusual weakness and fatigue that might be due to megaloblastic anemia or other blood dyscrasias. Report these signs to the physician.
- Assess any breathing problems, and report difficult, labored breathing or abnormal breath sounds (rales, crackles). Notify physician because these may be signs of pulmonary eosinophilia.
- Monitor severe or prolonged malaise, mental depression, or other changes in mood or behavior. Notify physician if these changes become problematic.
- If treating malaria, monitor any changes in symptoms (decreased fever, chills, sweating) to help document whether antimalarial drug therapy is successful.

Interventions

- Because of the risk of arrhythmias, use caution during aerobic exercise and other forms of therapeutic exercise. Assess exercise tolerance frequently (blood pressure, heart rate, fatigue levels), and terminate exercise immediately if any untoward responses occur (See Appendix L).

Patient/Client-Related Instruction

- Remind patient to take this drug as directed when treating malaria even if patient is asymptomatic.
- Instruct patient to report other untoward side effects such as severe or prolonged headache, fever, sleep loss, throat irritation, bloody urine, skin reactions (hyperpigmentation, dermatitis), GI problems (nausea, diarrhea, loss of appetite), or changes in the tongue resulting in a smooth and tender/painful tongue surface (atrophic glossitis).

Pharmacokinetics

Absorption: Well absorbed after oral administration.
Distribution: Widely distributed with high concentrations achieved in blood cells, kidneys, lungs, liver, and spleen. Some enters CSF (13–26% of serum levels). Crosses the placenta and enters breast milk.
Metabolism and Excretion: Mostly metabolized by the liver. 20–30% excreted unchanged by the kidneys.
Half-life: 4 days (shortened in patients with AIDS).

TIME/ACTION PROFILE (blood levels)

ROUTE	ONSET	PEAK	DURATION
PO	unknown	3 hr	2 wk*

*Suppressive levels.

Contraindications/Precautions

Contraindicated in: Hypersensitivity; First 14–16 wk of pregnancy; Megaloblastic anemia caused by folate deficiency; Concurrent folate antagonist therapy (because of risk of megaloblastic anemia); Tablets contain lactose and potato starch and should be avoided in patients with known hypersensitivity/intolerance.
Use Cautiously in: History of seizures (high doses); Underlying anemia or bone marrow depression; Impaired liver function; G6PD deficiency; OB: Pregnancy >16 wk (may require concurrent leucovorin); OB: Lactation (large doses to mother may cause folic acid deficiency in infant).

Interactions

Drug-Drug: ↑ risk of bone marrow depression with other **bone marrow depressants**, including **antineoplastics**, **proguanil**, or **radiation therapy**. ↑ risk of megaloblastic anemia with folate antagonists (**methotrexate**); concurrent use should be avoided.

P

Route/Dosage

Treatment of Malaria

PO (Adults and Children >10 yr): 50 mg/day for 2 days, then 25 mg once weekly in combination with other agents.
PO (Children 4–10 yr): 25 mg daily for 2 days, then 12.5 mg once weekly in combination with other agents.

Toxoplasmosis

PO (Adults): 50–200 mg/day for 1–2 days, followed by 25–50 mg/day for 2–6 wk; given with a sulfonamide.
PO (Children): 1 mg/kg/day for 1–3 days, then 0.5 mg/kg/day for 4–6 wk; given with a sulfonamide.

Toxoplasmosis in AIDS Patients

PO (Adults): 100–200 mg/day for 1–2 days, followed by 50–100 mg/day for 3–6 wk, then 25–50 mg/day for life; given with clindamycin or sulfadiazine.

Availability

Tablets: 25 mg. ***In combination with:*** sulfadoxine (Fansidar) Rx. See Appendix B.

quazepam (kway-ze-pam)
Doral

Classification
Therapeutic: sedative/hypnotics
Pharmacologic: benzodiazepines

Schedule IV

Indications
Short-term (up to 4 wk) management of insomnia.

Action
Depresses the CNS, probably by potentiating gamma-aminobutyric acid (GABA), an inhibitory neurotransmitter. **Therapeutic Effects:** Relief of insomnia.

Adverse Reactions/Side Effects
CNS: abnormal thinking, behavior changes, daytime drowsiness, confusion, dizziness, hallucinations, headache, insomnia, nervousness, sleep driving, slurred speech, weakness. **EENT:** blurred vision. **CV:** palpitations. **GI:** abdominal pain, constipation, diarrhea, dry mouth, nausea, vomiting. **GU:** urinary frequency, urinary hesitancy. **Derm:** itching, skin rash. **MS:** muscle spasm. **Neuro:** ataxia, trembling. **Misc:** allergic reactions, changes in libido, physical dependence, psychologic dependence, tolerance.

PHYSICAL THERAPY IMPLICATIONS

Examination and Evaluation
- Monitor daytime drowsiness, short-term memory deficits, slurred speech, and "hangover" symptoms (headache, nausea, malaise, irritability, dysphoria). Repeated or excessive symptoms may require change in dose or medication.
- Assess any muscle spasms to rule out musculoskeletal pathology; that is, try to determine if symptoms are drug induced rather than caused by anatomic or biomechanical problems.
- Monitor signs of allergic reactions, including pulmonary symptoms (tightness in the throat and chest, wheezing, cough, dyspnea) or skin reactions (rash, pruritus, urticaria). Notify physician immediately if these reactions occur.
- Assess dizziness or ataxia that might affect gait, balance, and other functional activities (See Appendix C). Report balance problems and functional limitations to the physician, and caution the patient and family/caregivers to guard against falls and trauma.
- Report any behavioral or personality changes such as confusion, nervousness, hallucinations, or expression of abnormal thoughts.

Interventions
- Guard against falls and trauma (hip fractures, head injury, and so forth). Implement fall-prevention strategies, especially in older adults or if drowsiness and dizziness carry over into the daytime (See Appendix E).
- Help patient explore nonpharmacologic methods to improve sleep, such as relaxation techniques, regular exercise, avoid caffeine, and so forth.

Patient/Client-Related Instruction
- Instruct patients on prolonged treatment not to discontinue medication without consulting their physician. Long-term use can cause tolerance and physical/psychologic dependence, and increased sleep problems (rebound insomnia) can occur when the drug is suddenly discontinued.
- Advise patient to avoid alcohol and other CNS depressants because of the increased risk of sedation and adverse effects.
- Caution patient and family/caregivers to guard against complex motor behaviors that can occur while asleep, including driving a car (sleep driving).
- Instruct patient to report other bothersome side effects including severe or prolonged headache, blurred vision, palpitations, problems with urination, change in libido, skin reactions (rash, itching), or GI problems (nausea, vomiting, constipation, diarrhea, dry mouth, abdominal pain).

Pharmacokinetics
Absorption: Well absorbed after oral administration.
Distribution: Unknown.
Protein Binding: >95%.
Metabolism and Excretion: Mostly metabolized by the liver. Two metabolites have CNS-depressant activity (2-oxoquazepam and *N*-desalkylflurazepam).
Half-life: *Quazepam*—39 hr (increased in geriatric patients); *2-oxoquazepam*—39 hr; N-*desalkylflurazepam*—70–75 hr.

TIME/ACTION PROFILE (sedation)

ROUTE	ONSET	PEAK	DURATION
PO	30 min	2 hr	8 hr

Contraindications/Precautions
Contraindicated in: Hypersensitivity; Cross-sensitivity with other benzodiazepines may exist; Preexisting CNS depression; Severe uncontrolled pain; Angle-closure glaucoma; OB: Pregnancy or lactation.
Use Cautiously in: Hepatic dysfunction; Very small or debilitated patients (dose reduction may be necessary); Geri: Long-acting benzodiazepines cause prolonged sedation in the elderly. Appears on Beers' list and is

Q

associated with increased risk of falls (↓ dose required or consider short-acting benzodiazepine.); History of suicide attempt or drug abuse; Children <18 yr (safety not established).

Interactions

Drug-Drug: Additive CNS depression with **alcohol, antihistamines, antidepressants, MAO inhibitors,** other **sedative/hypnotics,** or **opioid analgesics. Cimetidine** or **hormonal contraceptives** may ↓ metabolism and increase effects of quazepam. May ↓ efficacy of **levodopa. Rifampin** or cigarette smoking **(nicotine)** ↑ metabolism and may ↓ effectiveness. **Drug-Natural: St. John's wort** may affect quazepam levels and effectiveness; avoid use. Concomitant use of **kava, valerian, chamomile, or hops** can ↑ CNS depression.

Route/Dosage

PO (Adults): 15 mg hs; some patients may require 7.5 mg.

Availability

Tablets: 7.5 mg, 15 mg.

quetiapine (kwet-eye-a-peen)

Seroquel, Seroquel XR

Classification

Therapeutic: antipsychotics, mood stabilizers

Pharmacologic: dibenzothiazeprine derivatives

Indications

Schizophrenia. Depressive episodes with bipolar disorder. Acute manic episodes associated with bipolar I disorder (as monotherapy or with lithium or divalproex). Maintenance treatment of bipolar I disorder (with lithium or divalproex).

Action

Probably acts by serving as an antagonist of dopamine and serotonin. Also antagonizes histamine H_1 receptors and $alpha_1$-adrenergic receptors. **Therapeutic Effects:** Decreased manifestations of psychoses, depression, or acute mania.

Adverse Reactions/Side Effects

CNS: NEUROLEPTIC MALIGNANT SYNDROME, SEIZURES, <u>dizziness</u>, cognitive impairment, extrapyramidal symptoms, sedation, tardive dyskinesia. **EENT:** ear pain, rhinitis, pharyngitis. **Resp:** cough, dyspnea. **CV:** palpitations, peripheral edema, orthostatic hypotension. **GI:** anorexia, constipation, dry mouth, dyspepsia. **Derm:** sweating. **Hemat:** leukopenia. **Metab:** <u>weight gain</u>, hyperglycemia. **Misc:** flu-like syndrome.

PHYSICAL THERAPY IMPLICATIONS

Examination and Evaluation

- Monitor and immediately report signs of neuroleptic malignant syndrome, including hyperthermia, diaphoresis, generalized muscle rigidity, decreased cognition, tachycardia, changes in blood pressure (BP), and incontinence. Symptoms typically occur within 4–14 days after initiation of drug therapy, but can occur at any time during drug use.
- Be alert for new seizures or increased seizure activity, especially at the onset of drug treatment. Document the number, duration, and severity of seizures, and report these findings immediately to the physician.
- Assess motor function, and be alert for extrapyramidal symptoms. Report these symptoms immediately, especially tardive dyskinesia, because this problem may be irreversible. Common extrapyramidal symptoms include:
  - Tardive dyskinesia (uncontrolled rhythmic movement of mouth, face, and extremities, lip smacking or puckering, puffing of cheeks, uncontrolled chewing, rapid or worm-like movements of tongue).
  - Pseudoparkinsonism (shuffling gait, rigidity, tremor, pill-rolling motion, loss of balance control, difficulty speaking or swallowing, mask-like face).
  - Akathisia (restlessness or desire to keep moving).
  - Other dystonias and dyskinesias (dystonic muscle spasms, twisting motions, twitching, inability to move eyes, weakness of arms or legs).
- Assess BP when patient assumes a more upright position (lying to standing, sitting to standing, lying to sitting). Document orthostatic hypotension and contact physician when systolic BP falls >20 mm Hg, or diastolic BP falls >10 mm Hg.
- Monitor any cardiac palpitations, prolonged cough, or difficult, labored breathing. Report these symptoms if they become problematic.
- Assess peripheral edema using girth measurements, volume displacement, and measurement of pitting edema (See Appendix N). Report increased swelling in feet and ankles or a sudden increase in body weight due to fluid retention.
- Watch for signs of leukopenia, including fever, sore throat, mucosal lesions, and other signs of infection. Report these signs to the physician.
- Be alert for signs of hyperglycemia, including confusion, drowsiness, flushed/dry skin, fruit-like breath odor, rapid/deep breathing, polyuria, loss of appetite, and unusual thirst. Patients with diabetes mellitus should check blood glucose levels frequently.

- Assess dizziness and drowsiness that might affect gait, balance, and other functional activities (See Appendix C). Report balance problems and functional limitations to the physician and nursing staff, and caution the patient and family/caregivers to guard against falls and trauma.
- Periodically assess body weight and other anthropometric measures (body mass index, body composition). Report a substantial weight gain or increased body fat.

Interventions

- Guard against falls and trauma (hip fractures, head injury, and so forth) caused by drowsiness, dizziness, or extrapyramidal symptoms; implement fall prevention strategies (See Appendix E).
- To minimize orthostatic hypotension, patient should move slowly when assuming a more upright position.
- Help patient and family/caregivers explore nonpharmacologic methods (exercise, counseling, support groups) to reduce schizophrenic or manic episodes.

Patient/Client-Related Instruction

- Advise patient to avoid alcohol and other CNS depressants because of the increased risk of sedation and adverse effects.
- Instruct patient to report other problematic side effects such as severe or prolonged ear pain, blurred vision, nasopharyngeal irritation, excessive sweating, flu-like symptoms (chills, fever, body aches), or GI problems (constipation, indigestion, dry mouth, loss of appetite).

Pharmacokinetics

Absorption: Well absorbed after oral administration.
Distribution: Widely distributed.
Metabolism and Excretion: Extensively metabolized by the liver (mostly by P450 CYP3A4 enzyme system); <1% excreted unchanged in the urine.
Half-life: 6 hr.

TIME/ACTION PROFILE (antipsychotic effects)

ROUTE	ONSET	PEAK	DURATION
PO	unknown	unknown	8–12 hr
PO-XR	unknown	unknown	unknown

Contraindications/Precautions

Contraindicated in: Hypersensitivity; Lactation: Discontinue drug or bottle-feed.
Use Cautiously in: Cardiovascular disease, cerebrovascular disease, dehydration or hypovolemia (↑ risk of hypotension); History of seizures, Alzheimer's dementia; Diabetes (may ↑ risk of hyperglycemia); Patients at risk for aspiration pneumonia; Pedi: May ↑ risk of suicide attempt/ideation, especially during early treatment or dose adjustment; risk may be greater in children or adolescents; Hepatic impairment (dose ↓ may be necessary); Hypothyroidism (may be exacerbated); History of suicide attempt; OB/Pedi: Safety not established; Geri: May require ↓ doses; ↑ risk of mortality in elderly patients treated for dementia-related psychosis.

Interactions

Drug-Drug: ↑ CNS depression may occur with **alcohol, antihistamines, opioid analgesics,** and **sedative/hypnotics**. ↑ risk of hypotension with acute ingestion of **alcohol** or **antihypertensives**. **Phenytoin** and **thioridazine** ↑ clearance and ↓ effectiveness of quetiapine (dose change may be necessary); similar effects may occur with **carbamazepine, barbiturates, rifampin,** or **corticosteroids**. Effects may be ↑ by **ketoconazole, itraconazole, fluconazole, protease inhibitors** or **erythromycin**, as well as by other **agents that inhibit the cytochrome P450 CYP3A4 enzyme.**

Route/Dosage

PO (Adults): *Schizophrenia*—25 mg bid initially, ↑ by 25–50 mg bid–tid over 3 days, up to 300–400 mg/day in 2–3 divided doses by the 4th day (not to exceed 800 mg/day); or 300 mg once daily as extended-release tablets, ↑ by 300 mg/day, up to 400–800 mg/day (not to exceed 800 mg/day). Elderly patients or patients with hepatic impairment should be started on immediate-release product and converted to extended-release product once effective dose is reached. *Bipolar mania*—Immediate–release: 50 mg twice daily on day 1, ↑ dose by 100 mg/day up to 200 mg bid on day 4, then may ↑ in ≤200 mg/day increments up to 400 mg bid on day 6 if required; Extended-release: 300 mg once daily on day 1, then 600 mg once daily on day 2, then 400–800 mg once daily starting on day 3. *Bipolar depression*—Immediate–release or extended-release: 50 mg once daily hs on day 1, then 100 mg daily hs on day 2, then 200 mg daily hs on day 3, then 300 mg daily hs thereafter. *Bipolar maintenance*—Continue at the dose required to maintain symptom remission (usual dosage: 400–800 mg/day given as once daily dose [extended-release] or in 2 divided doses (immediate-release).

Availability

Tablets: 25 mg, 50 mg, 100 mg, 200 mg, 300 mg, 400 mg. **Extended-release Tablets:** 50 mg, 150 mg, 200 mg, 300 mg, 400 mg.

Q

quinapril (kwin-a-pril)

Accupril

Classification

Therapeutic: antihypertensives

Pharmacologic: angiotensin-converting enzyme (ACE) inhibitors

Indications

Alone or with other agents in the management of hypertension. Management of heart failure.

Action

ACE inhibitors block the conversion of angiotensin I to the vasoconstrictor angiotensin II. ACE inhibitors also prevent the degradation of bradykinin and other vasodilatory prostaglandins. ACE inhibitors also increase plasma renin levels and reduce aldosterone levels. Net result is systemic vasodilation. **Therapeutic Effects:** Lowering of blood pressure in hypertensive patients. ↓ afterload and symptoms in patients with heart failure.

Adverse Reactions/Side Effects

CNS: dizziness, fatigue, headache. **Resp:** cough. **CV:** hypotension, chest pain. **GI:** abdominal pain, diarrhea, nausea, vomiting. **GU:** impaired renal function. **Derm:** rashes. **F and E:** hyperkalemia. **MS:** back pain, myalgia. **Resp:** dyspnea. **Misc:** ANGIOEDEMA.

PHYSICAL THERAPY IMPLICATIONS

Examination and Evaluation

- Monitor signs of angioedema, including rashes, raised patches of red or white skin (welts), burning/itching skin, swelling in the face, and difficulty breathing. Notify physician of these signs immediately.
- Assess blood pressure periodically and compare to normal values (See Appendix F) to help document antihypertensive effects.
- Assess signs and symptoms of CHF (dyspnea, rales/crackles, peripheral edema, jugular venous distention, exercise intolerance) to help document whether drug therapy is effective in reducing these symptoms.
- Watch for signs of impaired renal function, including decreased urine output, cloudy urine, or sudden weight gain due to fluid retention. Report these signs to the physician.
- Monitor symptoms of high plasma potassium levels (hyperkalemia), including bradycardia, fatigue, weakness, numbness, and tingling. Notify physician because severe cases can lead to life-threatening arrhythmias and paralysis.
- Assess any back pain or muscle pain to rule out musculoskeletal pathology; that is, try to determine if pain is drug induced rather than caused by anatomic or biomechanical problems.
- Assess dizziness that might affect gait, balance, and other functional activities (See Appendix C). Report balance problems and functional limitations to the physician, and caution the patient and family/caregivers to guard against falls and trauma.

Interventions

- Implement aerobic exercise and cardiac conditioning programs to augment drug therapy and maintain or improve cardiovascular pump function in patients with heart failure and other cardiac conditions.
- Avoid physical therapy interventions that cause systemic vasodilation (large whirlpool, Hubbard tank). Additive effects of this drug and the intervention may cause a dangerous fall in blood pressure.
- To minimize orthostatic hypotension, patient should move slowly when assuming a more upright position.

Patient/Client-Related Instruction

- Remind patients to take medication as directed to control hypertension and other cardiac conditions even if they are asymptomatic.
- Instruct patients with heart failure to weigh themselves every day, and to call their physician if they gain 3 lb or more in 1 day or more than 5 lb in 1 week. Sudden weight gain may indicate fluid build-up due to worsening heart failure.
- Counsel patients about additional interventions to help control blood pressure and cardiac dysfunction, including regular exercise, weight loss, sodium restriction, stress reduction, moderation of alcohol consumption, and smoking cessation.
- Instruct patient to notify physician of a prolonged dry cough; drug therapy may need to be altered to resolve this side effect.
- Instruct patient or family/caregivers to report other troublesome side effects such as severe or prolonged headache, chest pain, skin rash, or GI problems (nausea, vomiting, diarrhea, abdominal pain).

Pharmacokinetics

Absorption: 60% absorbed following oral administration (high-fat meal may decrease absorption).
Distribution: Crosses the placenta; enters breast milk.
Protein Binding: 97%.
Metabolism and Excretion: Converted by the liver, GI mucosa, and tissue to quinaprilat, the active metabolite: 96% eliminated by the kidneys.
Half-life: *Quinapril*— 0.8 hr; *Quinaprilat*—3 hr (increased in renal impairment).

TIME/ACTION PROFILE (effect on blood pressure—single dose*)

ROUTE	ONSET	PEAK	DURATION
PO	within 1 hr	2–4 hr	up to 24 hr

*Full effects may not be noted for several weeks.

Contraindications/Precautions

Contraindicated in: Hypersensitivity; History of angioedema with previous use of ACE inhibitors; OB: Potential for injury or death of fetus. If pregnancy occurs, discontinue immediately. Lactation: Discontinue or use formula.
Use Cautiously in: Patients with renal impairment, hypovolemia, hyponatremia, and concurrent diuretic therapy— initial dosage reduction recommended; Black patients (monotherapy for hypertension less effective, may require additional therapy; higher risk for angioedema); Surgery/anesthesia (hypotension may be exaggerated); Women of childbearing potential; Pedi: Safety not established children <6 yr; Geri: Initial dosage reduction recommended.
Exercise Extreme Caution in: Family history of angioedema.

Interactions

Drug-Drug: Excessive hypotension may occur with concurrent use of **diuretics**. Additive hypotension with other **antihypertensive agents.** ↑risk of hyperkalemia with concurrent use of **potassium supplements, potassium-sparing diuretics, potassium-containing salt substitutes,** or **angiotensin II receptor antagonists**. Antihypertensive response may be blunted by **NSAIDs**. ↑ levels and may ↑ the risk of **lithium** toxicity. May ↓ absorption of **tetracycline, doxycycline,** and **fluoroquinolone** antibiotics (due to magnesium in tablets).

Route/Dosage

Hypertension

PO (Adults): 10–20 mg once daily initially, may be titrated every 2 wk up to 80 mg/day in single or 2 divided daily doses (initiate therapy at 5 mg/day in patients receiving diuretics).

Renal Impairment

PO (Adults): *CCr >60 mL/min*—Initiate therapy at 10 mg/day; *CCr 30–60 mL/min*—Initiate therapy at 5 mg/day; *CCr 10–30 mL/min*—Initiate therapy at 2.5 mg/day.

Heart Failure

PO (Adults): 5 mg twice initially, may be titrated at weekly intervals up to 20 mg twice daily.

Renal Impairment

PO (Adults): *CCr 30–60 mL/min*—Initiate therapy at 5 mg/day; if tolerated, increase to 5 mg twice daily on following day. *CCr 10–30 mL/min*—Initiate therapy at 2.5 mg/day; if tolerated, increase to 2.5 mg twice daily on following day.

Availability (generic available)

Tablets: 5 mg, 10 mg, 20 mg, 40 mg. ***In combination with:*** hydrochlorothiazide (Accuretic, Quinaretic). See Appendix B.

quinidine (kwin-i-deen)

quinidine gluconate

Apo-Quin-G

quinidine sulfate

Apo-Quinidine

Classification
Therapeutic: antiarrhythmics (class IA)
Pharmacologic: membrane stabilizers

Indications

Restoration and maintenance of sinus rhythm in patients with atrial fibrillation or flutter. Prevention of recurrent ventricular arrhythmias. Treatment of malaria.

Action

Decrease myocardial excitability. Slow conduction velocity. **Therapeutic Effects:** Suppression of arrhythmias.

Adverse Reactions/Side Effects

CNS: dizziness, confusion, fatigue, headache, syncope, vertigo. **EENT:** blurred vision, diplopia, mydriasis, photophobia, tinnitus. **CV:** HYPOTENSION, TORSADES DE POINTES, arrhythmias, palpitations, tachycardia. **GI:** anorexia, abdominal cramping, diarrhea, nausea, vomiting, drug-induced hepatitis. **Derm:** rash. **Hemat:** AGRANULOCYTOSIS, hemolytic anemia, thrombocytopenia. **Neuro:** ataxia, tremor. **Misc:** fever.

PHYSICAL THERAPY IMPLICATIONS

Examination and Evaluation

- Assess heart rate, ECG, and heart sounds, especially during exercise (See Appendices G, H). Although intended to treat certain arrhythmias, this drug can unmask or precipitate new arrhythmias (proarrhythmic effect). Report any rhythm disturbances or symptoms of increased arrhythmias, including palpitations, chest pain, shortness of breath, fainting, and fatigue/weakness.

- Assess blood pressure periodically and compare to normal values (See Appendix F). Report low blood pressure (hypotension), especially if patient experiences dizziness or syncope.
- Monitor signs of blood dyscrasias including agranulocytosis (fever, sore throat, mucosal lesions, other signs of infection), thrombocytopenia (bruising, nose bleeds, bleeding gums), or hemolytic anemia (unusual fatigue, shortness of breath, dizziness, headache, coldness in your hands and feet, pale skin, chest pain). Report these signs to the physician immediately.
- Assess dizziness or ataxia that might affect gait, balance, and other functional activities (See Appendix C). Report balance problems and functional limitations to the physician, and caution the patient and family/caregivers to guard against falls and trauma.

Interventions

- Because of the risk of serious cardiac arrhythmias, use extreme caution during aerobic exercise and other forms of therapeutic exercise. Assess exercise tolerance frequently (blood pressure, heart rate, fatigue levels), and terminate exercise immediately if any untoward responses occur (See Appendix L).

Patient/Client-Related Instruction

- Advise patient and family/caregivers about the signs of cardiac arrhythmias (see above under Examination and Evaluation), and to seek immediate medical assistance if these signs develop.
- Advise patient about the likelihood of GI reactions such as nausea, vomiting, diarrhea, and loss of appetite. Instruct patient to report severe or prolonged GI problems, or signs of drug-induced hepatitis (yellow skin or eyes, abdominal pain, severe nausea and vomiting, fever, sore throat, malaise, weakness, facial edema).
- Instruct patient and family/caregivers to report other side effects such as severe or prolonged headache, confusion, vision problems, ringing/buzzing in the ears (tinnitus), tremor, fatigue, fever, or skin rash.

Pharmacokinetics

Absorption: Bioavailability of oral formulations is 70–80%. Extended-release preparations are absorbed slowly following oral administration.
Distribution: Widely distributed. Cross the placenta; enter breast milk.
Metabolism and Excretion: Metabolized by the liver; 5–20% excreted unchanged by the kidneys.
Half-life: 6–8 hr (increased in CHF or severe liver impairment).

TIME/ACTION PROFILE (antiarrhythmic effects)

ROUTE	ONSET	PEAK	DURATION
PO (sulfate)	30 min	1–1.5 hr	6–8 hr
PO (sulfate-ER)	unknown	4 hr	8–12 hr
PO (gluconate)	unknown	3–4 hr	6–8 hr
IV	1–5 min	rapid	6–8 hr

Contraindications/Precautions

Contraindicated in: Hypersensitivity; Conduction defects (in the absence of a pacemaker); Myasthenia gravis.
Use Cautiously in: CHF (dose reduction recommended); Severe liver disease (dose reduction recommended); Hypokalemia or hypomagnesemia (↑ risk of torsades de pointes); Bradycardia (↑ risk of torsades de pointes); Renal impairment; OB/Lactation/Pedi: Safety not established; extended-release preparations should not be used in children.

Interactions

Drug-Drug: May ↑ risk of QT interval prolongation when used with **tricyclic antidepressants, erythromycin, clarithromycin, haloperidol, sotalol**, or **fluoroquinolones**. ↑ serum **digoxin** levels and may cause toxicity (dose reduction recommended). **Phenytoin, phenobarbital, carbamazepine**, or **rifampin** may ↑ metabolism and ↓ effectiveness. **Cimetidine, diltiazem, verapamil, amiodarone, ketoconazole, itraconazole**, and **protease inhibitors** ↓ metabolism and may ↑ blood levels. Excretion is delayed and effects ↑ by drugs that alkalinize the urine, including **carbonic anhydrase inhibitors, thiazide diuretics**, and **sodium bicarbonate**. Potentiates the effects of **neuromuscular blocking agents** and **warfarin**. Additive hypotension with **antihypertensives, nitrates**, and acute ingestion of **alcohol**. May ↑ **procainamide, haloperidol, mexiletine**, or **tricyclic antidepressant** levels and risk of toxicity. May antagonize **anticholinesterase therapy** in patients with myasthenia gravis. Additive anticholinergic effects may occur with **agents having anticholinergic properties** (including **antihistamines, tricyclic antidepressants**).
Drug-Food: Grapefruit juice ↑ serum levels and effect (avoid concurrent use). **Foods that alkalinize the urine** may ↑ serum quinidine levels and the risk of toxicity.

Route/Dosage

Quinidine Gluconate (62% Quinidine)

PO (Adults): 324–972 mg q 8–12 hr.
IV (Adults): 200–400 mg given at a rate ≤10 mg/min until arrhythmia is suppressed, QRS complex widens, bradycardia or hypotension occurs.

Quinidine Sulfate (83% Quinidine)

PO (Adults): *Atrial/ventricular arrhythmias*—200–400 mg q 4–6 hr; may be ↑ to achieve therapeutic response (not to exceed 3–4 g/day).
PO (Children): 6 mg/kg 4–5 times daily.

Availability (generic available)

Quinidine Gluconate

Extended-release tablets: 324 mg. **Solution for Injection:** 80 mg/mL in 10-mL vials.

Quinidine Sulfate

Tablets: 200 mg, 300 mg. **Extended-release tablets:** 300 mg.

quinupristin/dalfopristin

(kwin-oo-**pris**-tin/dal-foe-**pris**-tin)
Synercid

Classification
Therapeutic: anti-infectives
Pharmacologic: streptogramins

Indications

Treatment of serious or life-threatening infections associated with vancomycin-resistant *Enterococcus faecium* (VREF). Complicated skin/skin structure infections caused by *Staphylococcus aureus* (methicillin, susceptible) or *Streptococcus pyogenes*.

Action

Quinupristin inhibits the late phase of protein synthesis at the level of the bacterial ribosome; dalfopristin inhibits the early phase. **Therapeutic Effects:** Bacteriostatic effect against susceptible organisms. **Spectrum:** Active against vancomycin-resistant and multidrug-resistant strains of *E. faecium*, *S. aureus* (methicillin-susceptible), and *S. pyogenes*. Not active against *E. faecalis*.

Adverse Reactions/Side Effects

CNS: headache. **CV:** thrombophlebitis. **GI:** PSEUDOMEMBRANOUS COLITIS, diarrhea, nausea, vomiting.
Derm: pruritus, rash.
Local: edema/inflammation/pain at infusion site, infusion-site reactions. **Misc:** ALLERGIC REACTIONS, INCLUDING ANAPHYLAXIS, pain.

PHYSICAL THERAPY IMPLICATIONS

Examination and Evaluation

- Monitor signs of pseudomembranous colitis, including diarrhea, abdominal pain, fever, pus or mucus in stools, and other severe or prolonged GI problems (nausea, vomiting, heartburn). Notify physician or nursing staff immediately of these signs.
- Monitor signs of allergic reactions and anaphylaxis, including pulmonary symptoms (tightness in the throat and chest, wheezing, cough, dyspnea) or skin reactions (rash, pruritus, urticaria). Notify physician or nursing staff immediately if these reactions occur.
- Assess any signs of thrombophlebitis, including localized pain, redness, or swelling in the affected area. Report these signs to the physician.
- Monitor injection site for pain, swelling, and irritation. Report prolonged or excessive injection site reactions to the physician.

Interventions

- Always wash hands thoroughly and disinfect equipment (whirlpools, electrotherapeutic devices, treatment tables, and so forth) to help prevent the spread of infection. Use universal precautions or isolation procedures as indicated for specific patients.

Patient/Client-Related Instruction

- Advise patient about the likelihood of GI reactions such as nausea, vomiting, and diarrhea. Instruct patient to report severe or prolonged GI problems.
- Instruct patient and family/caregivers to report other troublesome side effects such as severe or prolonged headache, pain, or skin reactions (rash, itching).

Pharmacokinetics

Absorption: IV administration results in complete bioavailability.
Distribution: Unknown.
Protein Binding: Moderate.
Metabolism and Excretion: Both are converted to compounds with additional anti-infective activity; parent drugs and metabolites are mostly excreted in feces (75–77%); 15% of quinupristin and 17% of dalfopristin excreted in urine.
Half-life: *Quinupristin*—0.85 hr; *dalfopristin*—0.7 hr.

TIME/ACTION PROFILE

ROUTE	ONSET	PEAK	DURATION
IV	rapid	end of infusion	8–12 hr

Contraindications/Precautions

Contraindicated in: Hypersensitivity.
Use Cautiously in: Concurrent use of other drugs metabolized by the cytochrome P450 3A4 enzyme system (serious interactions may occur; see Drug-Drug Interactions); Hepatic impairment (dose adjustment may be necessary); Patients with a history of GI disease, especially colitis; Pregnancy, lactation, or children <16 yr (safety not established).

Interactions

Drug-Drug: Inhibits the cytochrome P450 3A4 drug metabolizing enzyme system; inhibits metabolism of **cyclosporine, midazolam,** and **nifedipine** and ↑ risk of toxicity (careful monitoring required). Similar effects may be expected with concurrent use of **delavirdine, nevirapine, indinavir, ritonavir, vinca alkaloids, docetaxel, paclitaxel, diazepam, verapamil, diltiazem, HMG CoA reductase inhibitors, tacrolimus, methylprednisolone, carbamazepine, quinidine, lidocaine**, and **disopyramide**.

Route/Dosage

IV (Adults): *Vancomycin-resistant* E. faecium—7.5 mg/kg q 8 hr for at least 7 days; *Complicated skin/skin structure infections*—7.5 mg/kg q 12 hr for at least 7 days.

Availability

Powder for injection: 500 mg (150 mg quinupristin and 350 mg dalfopristin in 10-mL vials), 600 mg (180 mg quinupristin and 420 mg dalfopristin in 10-mL vials).

rabeprazole (ra-bep-ra-zole)

Aciphex, ✱Pariet

Classification

Therapeutic: antiulcer agents

Pharmacologic: proton-pump inhibitors

Indications

Gastroesophageal reflux disease (GERD). Duodenal ulcers (including combination therapy with clarithromycin and amoxicillin to eradicate *Helicobacter pylori* and prevent recurrence). Pathologic hypersecretory conditions, including Zollinger-Ellison syndrome.

Action

Binds to an enzyme in the presence of acidic gastric pH, preventing the final transport of hydrogen ions into the gastric lumen. **Therapeutic Effects:** Diminished accumulation of acid in the gastric lumen, with lessened acid reflux. Healing of duodenal ulcers and esophagitis. ↓ acid secretion in hypersecretory conditions.

Adverse Reactions/Side Effects

CNS: dizziness, headache, malaise. **GI:** abdominal pain, constipation, diarrhea, nausea. **Derm:** photosensitivity, rash. **MS:** neck pain. **Misc:** allergic reactions, chills, fever.

PHYSICAL THERAPY IMPLICATIONS

Examination and Evaluation

- Monitor improvements in GI symptoms (gastritis, heartburn, and so forth) to help determine if drug therapy is successful.
- Monitor signs of allergic reactions, including pulmonary symptoms (tightness in the throat and chest, wheezing, cough, dyspnea) or skin reactions (rash, pruritus, urticaria). Notify physician immediately if these reactions occur.
- Assess dizziness that might affect gait, balance, and other functional activities (See Appendix C). Report balance problems and functional limitations to the physician, and caution the patient and family/caregivers to guard against falls and trauma.
- Monitor any neck pain to rule out musculoskeletal pathology; that is, attempt to determine if pain is drug induced rather than caused by anatomic or biomechanical problems.

Interventions

- In cases of NSAID-induced gastritis, implement appropriate manual therapy techniques, physical agents, and therapeutic exercises to reduce pain and decrease the need for aspirin and other NSAIDs.
- Causes photosensitivity; use care if administering UV treatments. Advise patient to avoid direct sunlight and use sunscreens and protective clothing.

Patient/Client-Related Instruction

- Advise patient to avoid alcohol and foods that may cause an increase in GI irritation.
- Instruct patient to report bothersome or prolonged side effects, including headache, chills, fever, malaise, or GI effects (nausea, diarrhea, constipation, abdominal pain).

Pharmacokinetics

Absorption: Delayed-release tablet is designed to allow rabeprazole, which is not stable in gastric acid, to pass through the stomach intact. Subsequently 52% is absorbed after oral administration.
Distribution: Unknown.
Protein Binding: 96.3%.
Metabolism and Excretion: Mostly metabolized by the liver (hepatic cytochrome P450 3A and 2C19 enzyme systems); 10% excreted in feces; remainder excreted in urine as inactive metabolites.
Half-life: 1–2 hr.

TIME/ACTION PROFILE (acid suppression)

ROUTE	ONSET	PEAK	DURATION
PO	within 1 hr	unknown	24 hr*

*Suppression continues to increase over the 1st week of therapy.

Contraindications/Precautions

Contraindicated in: Hypersensitivity to rabeprazole or related drugs (benzimidazoles).
Use Cautiously in: Severe hepatic impairment (dose reduction may be necessary); Geri: ↑ risk of hip fractures in patients using high doses for >1 yr; OB/Lactation/Pedi: Pregnancy, lactation, or children <12 yr (breast-feeding not recommended; use in pregnancy only if needed; safety not established).

Interactions

Drug-Drug: Rabeprazole is metabolized by the CYP450 enzyme system and may interact with other drugs metabolized by this system. May ↓ absorption of drugs requiring acid pH, including **ketoconazole, itraconazole, atazanavir, ampicillin esters, iron salts**, and **digoxin**. ↑ blood levels of **digoxin**. May ↑ the risk of bleeding with **warfarin** (monitor INR/PT).

Route/Dosage

PO (Adults): *GERD, duodenal ulcers*—20 mg once daily; *prevention of duodenal ulcer recurrence*—20 mg bid for 7 days with amoxicillin, 1000 mg bid for 7 days, and clarithromycin 500 mg bid for 7 days;

R

hypersecretory conditions—60 mg once daily initially, may be adjusted as needed and continued as necessary; doses up to 100 mg daily or 60 mg bid have been used.
PO (Children ≥12 yr): *GERD*—20 mg once daily.

Availability
Delayed-release tablets: 20 mg.

raloxifene (ra-lox-i-feen)
Evista

Classification
Therapeutic: bone resorption inhibitors
Pharmacologic: selective estrogen receptor modulators

Indications
Treatment and prevention of osteoporosis in postmenopausal women. Reduction of the risk of breast cancer in postmenopausal women with osteoporosis and those at high risk for invasive breast cancer.

Action
Binds to estrogen receptors, producing estrogen-like effects on bone, resulting in reduced resorption of bone and decreased bone turnover. **Therapeutic Effects:** Prevention of osteoporosis in patients at risk. ↓ risk of breast cancer.

Adverse Reactions/Side Effects
CV: STROKE, deep vein thrombosis, pulmonary embolism, retinal vein thrombosis. **MS:** leg cramps. **Misc:** hot flashes.

PHYSICAL THERAPY IMPLICATIONS

Examination and Evaluation
- Be alert for signs of stroke, including sudden severe headache, confusion, nausea, vomiting, paralysis, numbness, speech problems, and visual disturbances. Seek immediate medical assistance if these signs occur.
- Monitor signs of deep vein thrombosis (localized pain, swelling, warmth, erythema, tenderness) and pulmonary embolism (shortness of breath, chest pain, cough, bloody sputum). Notify physician immediately, and request objective tests (Doppler ultrasound, lung scan, others) if thromboembolism is suspected.
- Watch for any changes in vision such as cloudy or blurred vision that might indicate retinal vein thrombosis. Report these changes to the physician immediately.
- Assess leg cramps to rule out musculoskeletal pathology; that is, try to determine if pain is drug induced rather than caused by anatomic or biomechanical problems.

Interventions
- Because of the risk of stroke and pulmonary embolism, use caution during aerobic exercise and other forms of therapeutic exercise. Assess exercise tolerance frequently (blood pressure, heart rate, fatigue levels), and terminate exercise immediately if any untoward responses occur (See Appendix L).
- Institute weight bearing and resistance exercises as tolerated to maintain or increase bone mineral density. Start with low-impact or aquatic programs in patients with extensive demineralization, and increase exercise intensity slowly to prevent fractures.
- Protect against falls and fractures (See Appendix E). Modify home environment (remove throw rugs, improve lighting, etc.) and provide assistive devices (cane, walker) or other protective devices as needed to improve balance and prevent falls.
- For patients with cancer who are medically able to begin exercise, implement appropriate resistive exercises and aerobic training to maintain muscle strength and aerobic capacity during cancer chemotherapy or to help restore function after chemotherapy.

Patient/Client-Related Instruction
- Advise patient and family or caregiver about the signs of stroke and pulmonary embolism (see above under Examination and Evaluation), and to seek immediate medical assistance if these signs develop.
- Instruct patient to report other troublesome side effects such as severe or prolonged hot flashes.

Pharmacokinetics
Absorption: Although well absorbed (>60%), after oral administration, extensive 1st-pass metabolism results in 2% bioavailability.
Distribution: Highly bound to plasma proteins; remainder of distribution unknown.
Protein Binding: Highly bound to plasma proteins.
Metabolism and Excretion: Extensively metabolized by the liver; undergoes enterohepatic cycling; excreted primarily in feces.
Half-life: 27.7 hr.

TIME/ACTION PROFILE (effects on bone turnover)

ROUTE	ONSET	PEAK	DURATION
PO	unknown	3 mo	unknown

Contraindications/Precautions
Contraindicated in: Hypersensitivity; History of thromboembolic events; OB: Women with childbearing potential; OB/Pedi: Pregnancy, lactation, or children.
Use Cautiously in: Potential immobilization (increased risk of thromboembolic events); History of stroke or transient ischemic attack; Atrial fibrillation; Hypertension; Cigarette smoking.

Interactions

Drug-Drug: Cholestyramine ↓ absorption (avoid concurrent use). May alter effects of **warfarin** and other **highly protein-bound drugs**. Concurrent systemic **estrogen** therapy is not recommended.

Route/Dosage

PO (Adults): 60 mg once daily.

Availability

Tablets: 60 mg.

raltegravir (ral-teg-ra-veer)

Isentress

Classification

Therapeutic: antiretrovirals
Pharmacologic: integrase strand transfer inhibitors (INSTIs)

Indications

HIV infection (with other antiretrovirals) in patients who are failing other treatments as evidenced by continued viral replication and resistance to other agents.

Action

Inhibits HIV-1 integrase, which is required for viral replication. **Therapeutic Effects:** Evidence of decreased viral replication and reduced viral load with slowed progression of HIV and its sequelae.

Adverse Reactions/Side Effects

CNS: headache, dizziness, fatigue, weakness. **CV:** myocardial infarction. **GI:** diarrhea, abdominal pain, gastritis, hepatitis, vomiting. **GU:** renal failure/impairment. **Hemat:** anemia, neutropenia. **Metab:** lipodystrophy. **Misc:** hypersensitivity reactions, immune reconstitution syndrome, fever.

PHYSICAL THERAPY IMPLICATIONS

Examination and Evaluation

- Seek immediate medical assistance if symptoms of MI develop, including sudden chest pain, pain radiating into the arm or jaw, shortness of breath, dizziness, sweating, anxiety, and nausea.
- Monitor signs of hypersensitivity reactions, including pulmonary symptoms (tightness in the throat and chest, wheezing, cough, dyspnea) or skin reactions (rash, hives, itching). Notify physician immediately if these signs occur.
- Be alert for signs of an unusually aggressive immune reaction to opportunistic infection (immune reconstitution syndrome). Signs include fever, pain, warmth and redness and swelling at the site of infection. Notify physician of these signs immediately.
- Assess dizziness or weakness that might affect gait, balance, and other functional activities (See Appendix C). Report balance problems and functional limitations to the physician and nursing staff, and caution the patient and family/caregivers to guard against falls and trauma.
- Monitor signs of renal failure, including decreased urine output, increased blood pressure, muscle cramps/twitching, edema/weight gain from fluid retention, yellowish brown skin, and confusion that progresses to seizures and coma. Report these signs to the physician immediately.
- Monitor signs of anemia (unusual fatigue, shortness of breath with exertion, bruising) and neutropenia (fever, sore throat, signs of infection). Notify physician immediately if these signs occur.

Interventions

- Implement resistive exercises and other therapeutic exercises as needed to maintain muscle strength and function and prevent muscle wasting associated with HIV infection and AIDS.
- Because of the risk of MI, use extreme caution during aerobic exercise and other forms of therapeutic exercise. Assess exercise tolerance frequently (blood pressure, heart rate, fatigue levels), and terminate exercise immediately if any untoward responses occur (See Appendix L).

Patient/Client-Related Instruction

- Emphasize the importance of taking raltegravir as directed even if the patient is asymptomatic, and that this drug must always be used in combination with other antiretroviral drugs. Do not take more than prescribed amount, and do not stop taking without consulting health care professional.
- Inform patient that raltegravir does not cure HIV or AIDS or prevent associated or opportunistic infections. Raltegravir does not reduce the risk of transmission of HIV to others through sexual contact or blood contamination. Caution patient to use a condom, and to avoid sharing needles or donating blood to prevent spreading the AIDS virus to others.
- Inform patient that redistribution and accumulation of body fat may occur, causing central obesity, thin arms and legs, dorsocervical fat enlargement (buffalo hump), breast enlargement, and other symptoms that resemble Cushing's syndrome (moon face, striations on abdominal skin). Discuss possible effects on body image, and help patient explore coping mechanisms.
- Advise patient about the likelihood of GI reactions (vomiting, diarrhea, gastritis, abdominal pain). Instruct patient to report severe or prolonged GI problems or signs of drug-induced hepatitis (yellow

skin or eyes, abdominal pain, severe nausea and vomiting, fever, sore throat, malaise, weakness, facial edema).
- Instruct patient to report other troublesome side effects such as prolonged or severe headache or fever.

Pharmacokinetics

Absorption: Well absorbed following oral administration.
Distribution: Unknown.
Distribution: Unknown.
Metabolism and Excretion: Mostly metabolized by the uridine diphosphate glucuronosyltransferase (UGT) A1A enzyme system; 23% excreted in urine as parent drug and metabolite.
Half-life: 9 hr.

TIME/ACTION PROFILE (blood levels)

ROUTE	ONSET	PEAK	DURATION
PO	unknown	3 hr	12 hr

Contraindications/Precautions

Contraindicated in: OB: Lactation (breast-feeding not recommended in HIV-infected patients).
Use Cautiously in: Geri: Choose dose carefully, considering concurrent disease states, drug therapy, and age-related ↓ in hepatic and renal function; Concurrent use of medications associated with rhabdomyolysis/ myopathy (may increase risk); OB: Use in pregnancy only if maternal benefit outweighs fetal risk; Pedi: Safe use in children <16 yr not established.

Interactions

Drug-Drug: Concurrent use with **strong inducers of the UGT A1A enzyme system,** including **rifampin,** may ↓ blood levels and effectiveness. Concurrent use with **strong inhibitors of the UGT A1A enzyme system** may ↑ blood levels. ↑ risk of rhabdomyolysis/myopathy **HMG CoA reductase inhibitors.**

Route/Dosage

PO (Adults): 400 mg bid.

Availability

Tablets: 400 mg.

ramelteon (ra-mel-tee-on)

Rozerem

Classification
Therapeutic: sedative/hypnotics
Pharmacologic:melatonin receptor agonist

Indications

Treatment of insomnia characterized by difficult sleep onset.

Action

Activates melatonin receptors, which promotes maintenance of circadian rhythm, a part of the sleep-wake cycle. **Therapeutic Effects:** Easier onset of sleep.

Adverse Reactions/Side Effects

CNS: abnormal thinking, behavior changes, dizziness, fatigue, hallucinations, headache, insomnia (worsened), sleep driving. **GI:** nausea. **Endo:** ↑ prolactin levels, ↓ testosterone levels. **Misc:** ANGIOEDEMA.

PHYSICAL THERAPY IMPLICATIONS

Examination and Evaluation

- Be alert for signs of angioedema, including rashes, raised patches of red or white skin (welts), burning/ itching skin, swelling in the face, and difficulty breathing. Notify physician immediately of these signs.
- Monitor daytime drowsiness, hallucinations, behavior changes, and "drugged" feelings. Repeated or excessive symptoms may require change in dose or medication.

Interventions

- Guard against falls and trauma (hip fractures, head injury, and so forth). Implement fall-prevention strategies, especially in older adults or if drowsiness and fatigue carry over into the daytime (See Appendix E).
- Help patient explore non pharmacologic methods to improve sleep, such as relaxation techniques, regular exercise, avoid caffeine, and so forth.

Patient/Client-Related Instruction

- Advise patient about the risk of daytime drowsiness and decreased attention and mental focus. Use care if driving or in other activities that require strong concentration.
- Caution patient and family/caregivers that "sleepwalking" and other complex activities, including driving a car (sleep driving), may occur while completely asleep. Care should be taken to monitor such activities and prevent access to motor vehicles while under the influence of this drug.
- Advise patient to avoid alcohol and other CNS depressants because of the increased risk of sedation and adverse effects.
- Instruct patient and family/caregivers to report other troublesome side effects such as severe or prolonged headache, nausea, abnormal thoughts, worsening insomnia, or decreased libido (due to changes in prolactin or testosterone).

Pharmacokinetics

Absorption: Well absorbed (84%), but bioavailability is low (1.8%) due to extensive 1st-pass liver metabolism. Absorption in increased by a high-fat meal.
Distribution: Widely distributed to body tissues.
Metabolism and Excretion: Extensively metabolized by the liver; mainly by CYP1A2 enzyme system. Metabolites are excreted mostly in urine (88%); 4% excreted in feces.
Half-life: 1–2.6 hr.

TIME/ACTION PROFILE (blood levels)

ROUTE	ONSET	PEAK	DURATION
PO	rapid	30–90 min	unknown

Contraindications/Precautions

Contraindicated in: Hypersensitivity; History of angioedema with previous use; Severe hepatic impairment; Concurrent use of fluvoxamine; OB: Lactation; Pedi: Safety not established.
Use Cautiously in: Depression or history of suicidal ideation; Moderate hepatic impairment; Concurrent use of CYP3A4 inhibitors, such as ketoconazole; Concurrent use of CYP2C9 inhibitors, such as fluconazole; OB: Use only if maternal benefit outweighs fetal risk.

Interactions

Drug-Drug: Blood levels and effects are ↑ by **fluvoxamine**, potent inhibitor of the CYP1A2 enzyme system; concurrent use is contraindicated. Levels and effects may be ↓ by **rifampin**, an inducer of CYP enzymes. Concurrent use of CYP3A4 inhibitors, such as **ketoconazole,** may ↑ levels and effects; use cautiously. Concurrent use of CYP2C9 inhibitors, such as **fluconazole,** may ↑ levels and effects; use cautiously. ↑ risk of excessive CNS depression with other CNS depressants, including **alcohol, benzodiazepines, opioids**, and other **sedative/hypnotics.**

Route/Dosage

PO (Adults): 8 mg within 30 min of going to bed.

Availability

Tablets: 8 mg.

ramipril (ram-i-pril)

Altace

Classification
Therapeutic: antihypertensives
Pharmacologic: ACE inhibitors

Indications

Alone or with other agents in the management of hypertension. Reduction of risk of myocardial infarction, stroke, or death from cardiovascular causes in patients at least 55 years of age who are at high-risk of developing a major cardiovascular event because of a history of coronary artery disease, stroke, peripheral vascular disease, or diabetes that is accompanied by at least 1 other cardiovascular risk factor. Reduction of risk of death, heart failure–related hospitalizations and progression of heart failure in patients with signs of heart failure following myocardial infarction.

Action

Angiotensin-converting enzyme (ACE) inhibitors block the conversion of angiotensin I to the vasoconstrictor angiotensin II. ACE inhibitors also prevent the degradation of bradykinin and other vasodilatory prostaglandins. ACE inhibitors also increase plasma renin levels and reduce aldosterone levels. Net result is systemic vasodilation. **Therapeutic Effects:** Lowering of blood pressure in hypertensive patients. ↓ risk of myocardial infarction, stroke, or death from cardiovascular causes in high-risk patients. Increased survival and decreased heart failure progression after myocardial infarction.

Adverse Reactions/Side Effects

CNS: dizziness, fatigue, headache, vertigo, weakness. **Resp:** <u>cough</u>. **CV:** <u>hypotension</u>, chest pain. **GI:** diarrhea, nausea, vomiting. **GU:** impaired renal function. **Derm:** rashes. **F and E:** hyperkalemia.
Misc: ANGIOEDEMA.

PHYSICAL THERAPY IMPLICATIONS

Examination and Evaluation

- Monitor signs of angioedema, including rashes, raised patches of red or white skin (welts), burning/itching skin, swelling in the face, and difficulty breathing. Notify physician of these signs immediately.
- Assess blood pressure periodically and compare to normal values (See Appendix F) to help document antihypertensive effects. Report low blood pressure (hypotension), especially if patient experiences dizziness or syncope.
- Assess signs and symptoms of CHF (dyspnea, rales/crackles, peripheral edema, jugular venous distention, exercise intolerance) to help document whether drug therapy is effective in reducing these symptoms.
- Watch for signs of impaired renal function, including decreased urine output, cloudy urine, or sudden weight gain due to fluid retention. Report these signs to the physician.
- Monitor signs of high plasma potassium levels (hyperkalemia), including bradycardia, fatigue, weakness, numbness, and tingling. Notify physician

because severe cases can lead to life-threatening arrhythmias and paralysis.

- Assess dizziness and vertigo that might affect gait, balance, and other functional activities (See Appendix C). Report balance problems and functional limitations to the physician, and caution the patient and family/caregivers to guard against falls and trauma.

Interventions

- Implement aerobic exercise and cardiac conditioning programs to augment drug therapy and maintain or improve cardiovascular pump function in patients with heart failure and other cardiac conditions.
- Use caution during aerobic exercise and other forms of therapeutic exercise in patient with coronary artery disease, diabetes mellitus, or other cardiovascular risk factors. Assess exercise tolerance frequently (blood pressure, heart rate, fatigue levels), and terminate exercise immediately if any untoward responses occur (See Appendix L).
- Avoid physical therapy interventions that cause systemic vasodilation (large whirlpool, Hubbard tank). Additive effects of this drug and the intervention may cause a dangerous fall in blood pressure.
- To minimize orthostatic hypotension, patient should move slowly when assuming a more upright position.

Patient/Client-Related Instruction

- Remind patients to take medication as directed to control hypertension and other cardiac conditions even if they are asymptomatic.
- Instruct patients with heart failure to weigh themselves every day, and call their physician if they gain 3 lb or more in 1 day or more than 5 lb in 1 wk. Sudden weight gain may indicate fluid build-up due to worsening heart failure.
- Counsel patients about additional interventions to help control blood pressure and cardiac dysfunction, including regular exercise, weight loss, sodium restriction, stress reduction, moderation of alcohol consumption, and smoking cessation.
- Instruct patient to notify physician of a prolonged dry cough; drug therapy may need to be altered to resolve this side effect.
- Instruct patient or family/caregivers to report other troublesome side effects such as severe or prolonged headache, chest pain, skin rash, or GI problems (nausea, vomiting, diarrhea).

Pharmacokinetics

Absorption: 50–60% absorbed following oral administration.

Distribution: Crosses the placenta; may enter breast milk.

Metabolism and Excretion: Converted by the liver to ramiprilat, the active metabolite; 60% excreted in urine; 40% in feces.

Half-life: *Ramiprilat:* 13–17 hr (increased in renal impairment).

TIME/ACTION PROFILE (effect on blood pressure—single dose*)

ROUTE	ONSET	PEAK	DURATION
PO	within 1–2 hr	3–6 hr	24 hr

*Full effects may not be noted for several weeks

Contraindications/Precautions

Contraindicated in: Hypersensitivity; History of angioedema with previous use of ACE inhibitors; OB: Potential for injury or death of fetus. If pregnancy occurs, discontinue immediately; Lactation: Discontinue drug or use formula.

Use Cautiously in: Black patients (monotherapy for hypertension less effective, may require additional therapy; higher risk of angioedema); Surgery/anesthesia (hypotension may be exaggerated); Women of childbearing potential; Renal impairment (especially renal artery stenosis), hypovolemia, hyponatremia, concurrent diuretic therapy—initial dose reduction recommended; Pedi: Safety not established; Geri: Initial dose reduction recommended.

Exercise Extreme Caution in: Family history of angioedema.

Interactions

Drug-Drug: Excessive hypotension may occur with concurrent use of **diuretics**. Additive hypotension with other **antihypertensive agents**. ↑ risk of hyperkalemia with concurrent use of **potassium supplements**, **potassium-sparing diuretics, potassium-containing salt substitutes**, or **angiotensin II receptor antagonists**. Antihypertensive response may be blunted by **NSAIDs**. ↑ levels and may ↑ the risk of **lithium** toxicity.

Route/Dosage

Hypertension

PO (Adults): 2.5 mg once daily slowly may be increased up to 20 mg/day in 1–2 divided doses (initiate therapy at 1.25 mg/day in patients receiving diuretics).

Heart Failure Post–Myocardial Infarction

PO (Adults): 1.25–2.5 mg bid initially; may be increased slowly up to 5 mg bid.

Reduction in Risk of MI, Stroke, and Death from Cardiovascular Causes

PO (Adults): 2.5 mg once daily for 1 wk, then 5 mg once daily for 3 wk, then increased as tolerated to 10 mg once daily (can also be given in 2 divided doses).

Renal Impairment

PO (Adults): *CCr <40 mL/min*—Initiate therapy at 1.25 mg once daily; may be slowly titrated up to 5 mg/day in 1–2 divided doses.

Availability (generic available)

Capsules: 1.25 mg, 2.5 mg, 5 mg, 10 mg.

ranibizumab (ran-i-bi-zoo-mab)

Lucentis

Classification

Therapeutic: ocular agents

Pharmacologic: monoclonal antibodies

Indications

Treatment of neovascular (wet) macular degeneration.

Action

Binds to vascular endothelial growth factor A (VEGF-A) receptor sites, preventing the binding of endogenous VEGF-A, resulting in ↓ endothelial proliferation, vascular leakage, and new vessel formation. **Therapeutic Effects:** ↓ progression of visual loss.

Adverse Reactions/Side Effects

EENT: conjunctival hemorrhage, eye pain, ↑ intraocular pressure, intraocular inflammation, vitreal floaters, endophthalmitis, retinal detachment.
CV: arterial thromboembolic events.

PHYSICAL THERAPY IMPLICATIONS

Examination and Evaluation

- Monitor any eye pain, conjunctival hemorrhage, or other eye problems. Be alert for balance or mobility deficits that may indicate worsening vision. Report these findings to the physician.

Interventions

- Guard against falls and trauma. Implement fall-prevention strategies, especially if patient exhibits blurred vision or other visual impairments (See Appendix E).

Patient/Client-Related Instruction

- Instruct patient to report any loss of vision that might indicate increased intraocular pressure or other vision problems.

Pharmacokinetics

Absorption: Intravitreal injection results in complete local bioavailability. Very low serum levels are achieved.
Distribution: Unknown.
Metabolism and Excretion: Unknown.
Half-life: 9 days (intravitreal).

TIME/ACTION PROFILE

ROUTE	ONSET	PEAK	DURATION
intravitreal	unknown	after injection	1 mo

Contraindications/Precautions

Contraindicated in: Hypersensitivity; Ocular/periocular infections.
Use Cautiously in: OB: Use only in pregnancy if clearly needed, use cautiously during lactation; Pedi: Safe use in children not established.

Interactions

Drug-Drug: ↑ risk of serious intraocular inflammation with **verteporfin**.

Route/Dosage

Intravitreal (Adults): 0.5 mg (0.05 mL) once monthly; after 4 mo, injections may be given q 1–3 mo.

Availability

Solution for intravitreal injection: each vial delivers 0.5 mg (0.05 mL).

ranitidine (ra-ni-ti-deen)

Apo-Ranitidine, Zantac, Zantac-C, Zantac 75

Classification

Therapeutic: antiulcer agents

Pharmacologic: histamine H_2 antagonists

Indications

Short-term treatment of active duodenal ulcers and benign gastric ulcers. Maintenance therapy for duodenal and gastric ulcers after healing of active ulcer(s). Management of gastric hypersecretory states (Zollinger-Ellison syndrome). Treatment of and maintenance therapy for erosive esophagitis. Treatment of gastroesophageal reflux disease (GERD). Heartburn, acid indigestion, and sour stomach (OTC use). **IV:** Prevention and treatment of stress-induced upper GI bleeding in critically ill patients.

Action

Inhibits the action of histamine at the H_2 receptor site located primarily in gastric parietal cells, resulting in inhibition of gastric acid secretion. **Therapeutic Effects:** Healing and prevention of ulcers. Decreased symptoms of gastroesophageal reflux. Decreased secretion of gastric acid.

Adverse Reactions/Side Effects

CNS: confusion, dizziness, drowsiness, hallucinations, headache. **CV:** ARRHYTHMIAS. **GI:** constipation, diarrhea, nausea. **GU:** decreased sperm count, erectile dysfunction. **Endo:** gynecomastia. **Hemat:** AGRANULOCYTOSIS, APLASTIC ANEMIA, anemia, neutropenia, thrombocytopenia. **Local:** pain at IM site. **Misc:** hypersensivity reactions, vasculitis.

PHYSICAL THERAPY IMPLICATIONS

Examination and Evaluation

- Assess heart rate, ECG, and heart sounds, especially during exercise (See Appendices G, H). Report any rhythm disturbances or symptoms of increased arrhythmias, including palpitations, chest discomfort, shortness of breath, fainting, and fatigue/weakness.
- Report signs of agranulocytosis and neutropenia (fever, sore throat, mucosal lesions, signs of infection, bruising), aplastic anemia (unusual fatigue, weakness), or thrombocytopenia (bruising, bleeding gums, nose bleeds).
- Monitor signs of hypersensitivity reactions, including pulmonary symptoms (tightness in the throat or chest, wheezing, cough, dyspnea) or skin reactions (rash, pruritus, urticaria). Notify physician or nursing staff immediately if these reactions occur.
- Be alert for signs of vasculitis, including fatigue, weakness, muscle pain, joint pain, numbness, fever, loss of appetite, and weight loss. Report these signs to the physician.
- Assess dizziness and drowsiness that might affect gait, balance, and other functional activities (See Appendix C). Report balance problems and functional limitations to the physician and nursing staff, and caution the patient and family/caregivers to guard against falls and trauma.
- Monitor other CNS symptoms such as confusion, hallucinations, and headache. Excessive or prolonged CNS symptoms may require a reduction in dose.
- Monitor IM injection site for pain, swelling, and irritation. Report prolonged or excessive injection site reactions to the physician.

Interventions

- Use caution during aerobic exercise and endurance conditioning because of an increased risk of cardiac arrhythmias. Terminate exercise if patient exhibits untoward symptoms (chest pain, shortness of breath, etc.), or displays other criteria for exercise termination (See Appendix L).

Patient/Client-Related Instruction

- Advise patient to avoid alcohol and foods that may cause an increase in GI irritation.
- Instruct patient to report troublesome GI effects such as severe or prolonged constipation, diarrhea, or nausea.
- Advise men to consult their physician if they experience erectile dysfunction or breast enlargement (gynecomastia).

Pharmacokinetics

Absorption: 50% absorbed after PO administration.
Distribution: Enters breast milk and cerebrospinal fluid.
Metabolism and Excretion: Metabolized by the liver, mostly on first pass; 30% excreted unchanged by the kidneys after parenteral administration.
Half-life: Neonates (on ECMO): 6.6 hr; Infants: 3.5 hr; Children: 1.8–2 hr; Adults: 2–2.5 hr (increased in renal impairment to 4.8 hr).

TIME/ACTION PROFILE

ROUTE	ONSET	PEAK	DURATION
PO	unknown	1–3 hr	8–12 hr
IM	unknown	15 min	8–12 hr
IV	unknown	15 min	8–12 hr

Contraindications/Precautions

Contraindicated in: Hypersensitivity; Syrup contains alcohol and should be avoided in patients with known intolerance.
Use Cautiously in: Phenylketonuric patients (effervescent tablets and granules contain phenylalanine); Geri: Geriatric patients are more susceptible to adverse CNS reactions, including dizziness and confusion; dosage reduction recommended; Renal impairment (more susceptible to adverse CNS reactions; increased dosage interval recommended if CCr <50 mL/min); Hepatic impairment; Acute porphyria (may precipitate an attack); Pregnancy; Lactation: Passes into breast milk and can cause decreased stomach acid in the infant.

Interactions

Drug-Drug: ↓ absorption of **ketoconazole** and **itraconazole**. **Antacids** and **sucralfate** ↓ absorption of ranitidine. **Clarithromycin** ↑ ranitidine levels.

Route/Dosage

PO (Adults): *Short-term treatment of active ulcers*—150 mg bid or 300 mg once daily hs. *Duodenal ulcer prophylaxis*—150 mg once daily hs. *GERD*—150 mg bid. *Erosive esophagitis*—150 mg qid initially, then 150 mg bid as maintenance. *Gastric hypersecretory conditions*—150 mg bid initially; up to 6 g/day have been used. *OTC use*—75 mg when symptoms occur (up to bid).
PO (Children 1 mo-16 yr): *Treatment of active ulcers*—2–4 mg/kg/day divided bid, maximum 300 mg/day. *GERD and erosive esophagitis*—4–10 mg/kg/day

divided bid, maximum 300 mg/day for GERD, 600 mg/day for erosive esophagitis.
PO (Neonates): 2 mg/kg/day divided q 12 hr.
IV, IM (Adults): 50 mg q 6–8 hr (not to exceed 400 mg/day). *Continuous IV infusion*—6.25 mg/hr. *Gastric hypersecretory conditions*—1 mg/kg/hr; may be increased by 0.5 mg/kg/hr (not to exceed 2.5 mg/kg/hr).
IV, IM (Children 1 mo—16 yr): *Treatment of active ulcers*—2–4 mg/kg/day divided q 6–8 hr, maximum 200 mg/day. *Continuous infusion*—1 mg/kg/dose followed by 0.08–0.17 mg/kg/hr.
IV (Neonates): 1.5 mg/kg/dose load, then in 12 hr start maintenance of 1.5–2 mg/kg/day divided q 12 hr. *Continuous IV infusion*—1.5 mg/kg/dose load followed by 0.04–0.08 mg/kg/hr infusion.

Renal Impairment
PO (Adults): *CCr10–50 mL/min*—reduce dose to 50% of dose recommended for indication; *CCr <10 mL/min*—reduce dose to 25% of dose recommended for indication; further reductions may be necessary if there is coexistent hepatic impairment.

Availability (generic available)
Tablets: 75 mg OTC, 150 mg, 300 mg. **Effervescent tablets (EFFERdose):** 25 mg, 150 mg. **Capsules:** 150 mg, 300 mg. **Syrup (peppermint flavor):** 15 mg/mL. **Solution for injection:** 25 mg/mL in 2-, 6-, and 40-mL vials. **Premixed infusion:** 50 mg/50 mL 0.45% NaCl.

ranolazine (ra-nole-a-zeen)
Ranexa
Classification
Therapeutic: antianginals
Pharmacologic: piperazine derivative

Indications
Chronic angina pectoris not adequately controlled by conventional antianginals (amlodipine, beta blockers, nitrates).

Action
Does not decrease blood pressure or heart rate; remainder of mechanism is not known. **Therapeutic Effects:** Decreased frequency of angina.

Adverse Reactions/Side Effects
CNS: dizziness, headache. **EENT:** tinnitus. **CV:** palpitations, QTc prolongation. **GI:** abdominal pain, constipation, dry mouth, nausea, vomiting.

PHYSICAL THERAPY IMPLICATIONS

Examination and Evaluation
- Assess heart rate, ECG, and heart sounds, especially during exercise (See Appendices G, H). Report any rhythm disturbances or symptoms of increased arrhythmias, including palpitations, chest pain, shortness of breath, fainting, and fatigue/weakness.
- Assess dizziness that might affect gait, balance, and other functional activities (See Appendix C). Report balance problems and functional limitations to the physician and nursing staff, and caution the patient and family/caregivers to guard against falls and trauma.

Interventions
- Design and implement aerobic exercise and endurance training programs to increase coronary perfusion and reduce angina.
- Because of an increased risk of cardiac arrhythmias, use caution during aerobic exercise and endurance conditioning. Terminate exercise if patient exhibits untoward symptoms (chest pain, shortness of breath, unusual fatigue), or displays other criteria for exercise termination (See Appendix L).

Patient/Client-Related Instruction
- Remind patients to take medication as directed to control angina even if they are asymptomatic.
- Counsel patients about additional interventions to help control angina and cardiac dysfunction such as regular exercise, weight loss, sodium restriction, stress reduction, moderation of alcohol consumption, and smoking cessation.
- Instruct patient or family/caregivers to report other troublesome side effects such as severe or prolonged headache, ringing/buzzing in the ears (tinnitus), or GI problems (nausea, vomiting, constipation, dry mouth, abdominal pain).

Pharmacokinetics
Absorption: Highly variable.
Distribution: Unknown.
Metabolism and Excretion: Metabolized in the gut (P-glycoprotein) and by the liver (primarily CYP3A and less by CYP2D6); <5% excreted unchanged in urine and feces.
Half-life: 7 hr.

TIME/ACTION PROFILE (blood levels)

ROUTE	ONSET	PEAK	DURATION
PO	unknown	2–5 hr	12 hr

R

Contraindications/Precautions

Contraindicated in: Hypersensitivity; Preexisting QTc prolongation or concurrent use of other medications causing QTc prolongation; Potent inhibitors of CYP3A (ketoconazole, verapamil, diltiazem); Hepatic impairment; Lactation.

Use Cautiously in: Geri: Patients >75 yr (↑ risk of adverse reactions; Severe renal impairment [may ↑ blood pressure]); OB: Pregnancy (use only when use outweighs risk to fetus); Pedi: Children (safety not established).

Interactions

Drug-Drug: ↑ blood levels of **simvastatin** and its active metabolite. Partially inhibits CYP2D6 enzyme system; may ↓ metabolism and increase effects of **tricyclic antidepressants** and **antipsychotics**; dosage adjustments may be necessary. Inhibits P-glycoprotein (P-gp) which may lead to ↑ **digoxin** levels; dosage adjustment may be required.

Route/Dosage

PO (Adults): 500 mg bid initially; may be increased to 1000 mg bid.

Availability

Extended-release tablet: 500 mg.

rasagiline (ras-aj-i-leen)

Azilect

Classification

Therapeutic: antiparkinson agents

Pharmacologic: monoamine oxidase type B inhibitors

Indications

Parkinson's disease (monotherapy and adjunctive to levodopa).

Action

Irreversibly inactivates monoamine oxidase (MAO) by binding to it at type B (brain sites); inactivation of MAO leads to increased amounts of dopamine available in the CNS. Differs from selegiline by its nonamphetamine characteristics. **Therapeutic Effects:** Improvement in symptoms of Parkinson's disease, allowing increase in function.

Adverse Reactions/Side Effects

CNS: depression, dizziness, hallucinations, malaise, vertigo. **EENT:** conjunctivitis, rhinitis. **Resp:** asthma. **CV:** chest pain, orthostatic hypotension (may ↑ levodopa-induced hypotension), syncope. **GI:** anorexia, dizziness, dyspepsia, gastroenteritis, vomiting. **GU:** albuminuria, ↓ libido. **Derm:** alopecia, ecchymosis, ↑ melanoma risk, rash. **Endo:** weight loss. **Hemat:** leukopenia. **MS:** arthralgia, arthritis, neck pain. **Neuro:** dyskinesia (may ↑ levodopa-induced dyskinesia), paresthesia. **Misc:** allergic reactions, flu-like syndrome, ↑ fall risk, fever.

PHYSICAL THERAPY IMPLICATIONS

Examination and Evaluation

- Assess patient's gait and motor function to help determine antiparkinson effects, especially when starting drug therapy, or during dosing changes or addition of other antiparkinson drugs. Motor function should be assessed at different times of the day, such as when drugs are reaching peak therapeutic levels (i.e., 30–60 min after oral dose), as well as when drug effects are minimal (just before the next dose).
- Document increased side effects such as involuntary movements (dyskinesias), especially if used with levodopa. Notify physician because increased side effects might require dose adjustment or a change in medication regimen.
- Assess blood pressure (BP) when patient assumes a more upright position (lying to standing, sitting to standing, lying to sitting). Document orthostatic hypotension and contact physician when systolic BP falls >20 mm Hg or diastolic BP falls >10 mm Hg.
- Monitor hallucinations, malaise, depression, and other psychologic problems. Repeated or excessive symptoms may require change in dose or medication.
- Assess dizziness, vertigo, or syncope that might affect gait, balance, and other functional activities (See Appendix C). Report balance problems and functional limitations to the physician, and caution the patient and family/caregivers to guard against falls and trauma.
- Assess signs of paresthesia (numbness, tingling). Perform objective tests, including electroneuromyography and sensory testing to document any drug-related neuropathic changes.
- Assess symptoms of asthma, such as wheezing, dyspnea, coughing, chest pain, and tightness in the throat and chest. Perform pulmonary function tests to quantify suspected changes in ventilation and respiration (See Appendixes I, J, K).
- Monitor signs of blood dyscrasias such as leukopenia (fever, sore throat, signs of infection). Report these signs to the physician.
- Monitor signs of allergic reactions, including pulmonary symptoms (tightness in the throat and chest, wheezing, cough, dyspnea) or skin reactions (rash, pruritus, urticaria). Notify physician immediately if these reactions occur.
- Assess any joint or neck pain to rule out musculoskeletal pathology; that is, try to determine if pain is

drug induced rather than caused by anatomic or biomechanical problems.

- Report any suspicious skin lesions to the physician; this drug can increase melanoma risk.

Interventions

- Implement therapeutic exercises (coordination exercises, gait training, cardiovascular conditioning) to complement the effects of drug therapy and help achieve optimal function.
- Guard against falls and trauma (hip fractures, head injury, and so forth). Implement fall-prevention strategies (See Appendix E), especially if patient exhibits Parkinson symptoms (postural instability, rigidity) combined with drug side effects (dizziness, vertigo, dyskinesias).

Patient/Client-Related Instruction

- Because of an increased risk of melanoma, advise patient to check skin regularly and use sunscreens, protective clothing, and avoid prolonged sun exposure. Advise patient to report any suspicious skin lesions.
- Instruct patient to report other bothersome side effects such as severe or prolonged eye irritation, nasal inflammation, weight loss, decreased libido, fever, flu-like symptoms, skin reactions (rash, bruising, hair loss), or GI problems (vomiting, indigestion, cramping, loss of appetite).

Pharmacokinetics

Absorption: 36% absorbed following oral administration.

Distribution: Readily crosses the blood-brain barrier.

Metabolism and Excretion: Extensively metabolized by the liver (CYP1A2 enzyme) to an inactive metabolite); less than 1% excreted in urine.

Half-life: 1.3 hr; does not correlate with duration of MAO-B inhibition.

TIME/ACTION PROFILE

ROUTE	ONSET	PEAK	DURATION
PO	rapid	1 hr	40 days*

*Recovery of MAO-B function.

Contraindications/Precautions

Contraindicated in: Hypersensitivity; Concurrent meperidine, tramadol, propoxyphene, methadone, sympathomimetic amines, dextromethorphan, mirtazapine, cyclobenzaprine, cocaine or St. John's wort; Moderate to severe hepatic impairment; Elective surgery requiring general anesthesia; allow 14 days after discontinuation; Pheochromocytoma.

Use Cautiously in: Mild hepatic impairment (↑ blood levels); OB: Pregnancy and lactation, use only if maternal benefit outweighs fetal risk; may inhibit lactation; Pedi: Safety in children has not been established.

Interactions

Drug-Drug: ciprofloxacin and other **inhibitors of the CYP1A2 enzyme** ↑ rasagiline levels; dose adjustment is recommended. **Meperidine** has resulted in life-threatening reactions when used with other MAO inhibitors; wait at least 14 days after discontinuation of rasagiline to initiate meperidine. Similar reactions may occur with **tramadol, methadone,** and **propoxyphene**; concurrent use should be avoided. Concurrent use with **dextromethorphan** may result in psychosis/bizarre behavior and should be avoided. Risk of adverse reactions in ↑ with **mirtazapine** and **cyclobenzaprine**; concurrent use should be avoided. Hypertensive crisis may occur with **sympathomimetic amines,** including **amphetamines, cold products,** and some **weight loss products** containing **vasoconstrictors** such as **pseudoephedrine, phenylephrine,** or **ephedrine**; avoid concurrent use. Risk of CNS toxicity is ↑ with **tricyclic antidepressants, SSRI antidepressants, NSRI antidepressants,** and other **MAO inhibitors**; rasagiline should be discontinued at least 14 days prior to initiation of antidepressants (**fluoxetine** should be discontinued at least 5 wk prior to rasagiline therapy). Hypertensive crisis may also occur when rasagiline is used with **other MAO inhibitors**; allow at least 14 days between usages.

Drug-Natural: Risk of toxicity is ↑ with **St. John's wort.**

Drug-Food: Ingestion of **tyramine-rich foods or beverages** may result in life-threatening hypertensive crisis.

Route/Dosage

PO (Adults): *Monotherapy*—1 mg daily; *adjunct therapy*—0.5 mg daily, may be increased to 1 mg daily; *concurrent ciprofloxacin or other CYP1A2 inhibitors*—0.5 mg daily.

Hepatic Impairment

PO (Adults): *Mild hepatic impairment*—1 mg daily; *adjunct therapy*—0.5 mg daily; may be increased to 1 mg daily.

Availability

Tablets: 0.5 mg, 1 mg.

rasburicase (ras-**byoor**-i-kase)

Elitek

Classification

Therapeutic: antigout agents, antihyperuricemics

Pharmacologic: enzymes

R

Indications
Initial management of increased uric acid levels in children with leukemia, lymphoma, or other malignancies who are being treated with antineoplastics which are expected to produce hyperuricemia.

Action
An enzyme which promotes the conversion of uric acid to allantoin, an inactive, water-soluble compound. Produced by recombinant DNA technology. **Therapeutic Effects:** Decreased sequelae of hyperuricemia (nephropathy, arthropathy).

Adverse Reactions/Side Effects
CNS: headache. **Resp:** respiratory distress.
GI: abdominal pain, constipation, diarrhea, nausea, vomiting, mucositis. **Derm:** rash. **Hemat:** HEMOLYSIS, METHEMOGLOBINEMIA, neutropenia. **Misc:** HYPERSENSITIVITY REACTIONS, INCLUDING ANAPHYLAXIS, fever, sepsis.

PHYSICAL THERAPY IMPLICATIONS

Examination and Evaluation
- Monitor signs of hypersensitivity reactions and anaphylaxis, including pulmonary symptoms (tightness in the throat and chest, wheezing, cough dyspnea) or skin reactions (rash, pruritus, urticaria). Notify physician or nursing staff immediately of any signs of hypersensitivity.
- Be alert for signs of hemolysis (unusual fatigue, shortness of breath, dizziness, headache, coldness in your hands and feet, pale/yellow skin, chest pain), methemoglobinemia (bluish coloring of the skin, lips fingernails; headache; lack of energy), and neutropenia (fever, sore throat, signs of infection). Report these signs to the physician or nursing staff immediately.
- Assess symptoms of respiratory distress, including shortness of breath, dyspnea, and cyanosis. Monitor pulse oximetry and perform pulmonary function tests (See Appendices I, J, K) to quantify suspected changes in ventilation and respiratory function. Excessive respiratory depression requires emergency care.

Interventions
- For patients who are medically able to begin exercise, implement appropriate resistive exercises and aerobic training to maintain muscle strength and aerobic capacity during cancer chemotherapy or to help restore function after chemotherapy.

Patient/Client-Related Instruction
- Instruct patient and family/caregivers to report other troublesome side effects such as severe or prolonged headache, fever, skin rash, or GI problems (nausea, vomiting, diarrhea, constipation, abdominal pain, inflammation in/around the mouth).

Pharmacokinetics
Absorption: IV administration results in complete bioavailability.
Distribution: Unknown.
Metabolism and Excretion: Unknown.
Half-life: 18 hr.

TIME/ACTION PROFILE (decrease in uric acid)

ROUTE	ONSET	PEAK	DURATION
IV	rapid	unknown	4–24 hr

Contraindications/Precautions
Contraindicated in: G6PD deficiency; Previous allergic reaction, hemolysis, or methemoglobinemia from rasburicase; Lactation.
Use Cautiously in: OB: Pregnancy (use only if clearly needed).

Interactions
Drug-Drug: None known.

Route/Dosage
IV (Children): 0.15 or 0.2 mg/kg daily as a single dose for 5 days.

Availability
Lyophilized powder for reconstitution: 1.5 mg/vial in cartons of 3 vials with specific diluent Rx.

HIGH ALERT

remifentanil (rem-i-fen-ta-nil)
Ultiva

Classification
Therapeutic: opioid analgesics
Pharmacologic: opioid agonists

Schedule II

Indications
Analgesic supplement to general anesthesia; usually with other agents (ultra–short-acting barbiturates, neuromuscular blockers, and inhalation anesthetics) to produce balanced anesthesia. Induction/maintenance of anesthesia (with oxygen or oxygen/nitrous oxide and a neuromuscular blocker). Analgesic component for monitored anesthesia care (MAC).

Action
Binds to opiate receptors in the CNS, altering the response to and perception of pain. Produces CNS depression. **Therapeutic Effects:** Supplement in anesthesia. Decreased pain.

Adverse Reactions/Side Effects
CNS: confusion, paradoxical excitation/delirium, postoperative depression, postoperative drowsiness.

EENT: blurred/double vision. **Resp:** APNEA, LARYNGOSPASM, allergic bronchospasm, respiratory depression. **CV:** arrhythmias, bradycardia, circulatory depression, hypotension. **GI:** biliary spasm, nausea/vomiting (↑ in children). **Derm:** facial itching. **MS:** skeletal and thoracic muscle rigidity, shivering (↑ in children).

PHYSICAL THERAPY IMPLICATIONS*

**Implications refer primarily to any residual effects that occur typically within 24 hr after anesthesia.*

Examination and Evaluation

- Assess respiration, and notify physician immediately if patient exhibits any interruption in respiratory rate (apnea) or signs of respiratory depression, including decreased respiratory rate, confusion, bluish color of the skin and mucous membranes (cyanosis), and difficult, labored breathing (dyspnea). Monitor pulse oximetry and perform pulmonary function tests (See Appendix I) to quantify suspected changes in ventilation and respiratory function. Apnea or excessive respiratory depression requires emergency care.
- Monitor signs of laryngeal spasm and allergic bronchospasm, including tightness in the throat and chest, wheezing, cough, and severe shortness of breath. Notify physician or nursing staff immediately if these reactions occur.
- Be alert for excessive sedation or changes in mood and behavior (confusion, excitation, delirium). Notify physician or nursing staff immediately if patient is unconscious or extremely difficult to arouse.
- Use appropriate pain scales (visual analogue scales, others) to document whether this drug is successful in helping manage the patient's pain.
- Assess blood pressure periodically and compare to normal values (See Appendix F). Report low blood pressure (hypotension) or signs of circulatory depression, including dizziness, fainting, weakness, pallor, and light-headedness.
- Assess heart rate, ECG, and heart sounds, especially during exercise (See Appendices G, H). Report slow heart rate (bradycardia) or symptoms of other arrhythmias, including palpitations, chest discomfort, shortness of breath, fainting, and fatigue/weakness.
- Be alert for residual muscle rigidity and decreased thoracic and limb movements after rapid IV administration. Report a sustained increase in muscle tone.

Interventions

- Implement appropriate manual therapy techniques, physical agents, and therapeutic exercises to reduce pain and help wean patient off opioid analgesics as soon as possible.
- Because of the risk of respiratory depression and hypotension, use caution during aerobic exercise and other forms of therapeutic exercise. Assess exercise tolerance frequently (blood pressure, heart rate, respiratory rate, fatigue levels), and terminate exercise immediately if any untoward responses occur (See Appendix L).
- Guard against falls and trauma (hip fractures, head injury). Implement fall-prevention strategies (See Appendix E), especially if patient exhibits sedation, dizziness, or blurred vision.
- To minimize orthostatic hypotension, patient should move slowly when assuming a more upright position.

Patient/Client-Related Instruction

- Advise patient to avoid alcohol and other CNS depressants because of the increased risk of sedation and decreased CNS function.
- Instruct patient to report other troublesome side effects such as severe or prolonged facial itching, vision disturbances, shivering, or GI problems (nausea, vomiting, indigestion).

R

Pharmacokinetics

Absorption: IV administration results in complete bioavailability.
Distribution: Widely distributed.
Metabolism and Excretion: Metabolized by blood and tissue esterases, metabolites are excreted by the kidneys.
Half-life: 3–10 min.

TIME/ACTION PROFILE (analgesia*)

ROUTE	ONSET	PEAK	DURATION
IV	rapid	3–5 min	5–10 min

*Respiratory depression may last longer than analgesia.

Contraindications/Precautions

Contraindicated in: Hypersensitivity; cross-sensitivity with other opioid analgesic agents may occur; Known intolerance; Not to be given epidurally or intrathecally (because of glycine in the formulation).
Use Cautiously in: Geriatric, debilitated, or critically ill patients (↓ starting dose of remifentanil by 50% in patients >65 yr); Morbidly obese patients (determine dose by ideal body weight [IBW] if >30% over IBW); Diabetics; Severe pulmonary or hepatic disease; CNS tumors; ↑ intracranial pressure; Head trauma; Adrenal insufficiency; Undiagnosed abdominal pain; Hypothyroidism; Alcoholism; Cardiac disease (arrhythmias); Morbidly obese patients; **OB, Pedi:** Pregnancy,

lactation, and children <2 yr (safety not established in younger age groups for some agents).

Interactions

Drug-Drug: Avoid use in patients who have received **MAO inhibitors** within the previous 14 days (may produce unpredictable, potentially fatal reactions). ↑ CNS and respiratory depression with other **CNS depressants**, including **alcohol, antihistamines, antidepressants**, other **sedative/hypnotics**, and other **opioids**. ↑ risk of hypotension with **benzodiazepines**. **Nalbuphine, buprenorphine,** or **pentazocine** may ↓ analgesia.

Route/Dosage

Induction of Anesthesia

IV (Adults): 0.5–1 mcg/kg/min continuous infusion (an initial dose of 1 mcg/kg may be given over 30–60 sec).

Maintenance of Anesthesia

IV (Adults): *With nitrous oxide 66%*—0.4 mcg/kg/min (range 0.1–2 mcg/kg/min); *with isoflurane (0.4–1.5 MAC) or propofol (100–200 mcg/kg/min)*—0.25 mcg/kg/min (range 0.05–2 mcg/kg/min). Supplemental bolus doses of 1 mcg/kg may be given.

IV (Children 1–12 yr): *With halothane 0.3–1.5 MAC, sevoflurane 0.3–1.5 MAC or isoflurane 0.4–1.5 MAC*—0.25 mcg/kg/min (range 0.05–1.3 mcg/kg/min); supplemental doses of 1 mcg/kg may be given.

IV (Infants birth–2 mo): *With nitrous oxide 70%*—0.4 mcg/kg/min (range 0.4–1 mcg/kg/min); supplemental doses of 1 mcg/kg may be given.

Continuation as an Analgesic in Immediately Postoperative Period

IV (Adults): 0.1 mcg/kg/min (range 0.025–0.2 mcg/kg/min).

Monitored Anesthesia Care (Remifentanil Alone)

IV (Adults): *Single IV dose*—1 mcg/kg given 90 sec before local anesthetic or *continuous infusion*—0.1 mcg/kg/min beginning 5 min before local anesthetic, then 0.05 mcg/kg/min after local anesthetic (range 0.025–0.2 mcg/kg/min).

Monitored Anesthesia Care (Remifentanil + Midazolam)

IV (Adults ≥2 yr): *Single IV dose*—0.5 mcg/kg given 90 sec before local anesthetic or *continuous infusion*—0.05 mcg/kg/min beginning 5 min before local anesthetic, then 0.025 mcg/kg/min after local anesthetic (range 0.025–0.2 mcg/kg/min).

Coronary Artery Bypass Surgery

IV (Adults): *Induction and maintenance of anesthesia*—1 mcg/kg/min (range for maintenance 0.125–4 mcg/kg/min; *continuation as an analgesic into ICU*—1 mcg/kg/min (range 0.05–1 mcg/kg/min).

Availability

Powder for injection: 1-mg, 2-mg, and 5-mg vials Rx.

repaglinide (re-pag-li-nide)

Gluconorm, Prandin

Classification

Therapeutic: antidiabetics

Pharmacologic: meglitinides

Indications

Type 2 diabetes mellitus, with diet and exercise; may be used with metformin, rosiglitazone, or pioglitazone.

Action

Stimulates the release of insulin from pancreatic beta cells by closing potassium channels, which results in the opening of calcium channels in beta cells. This is followed by release of insulin. **Therapeutic Effects:** Lowering of blood glucose levels.

Adverse Reactions/Side Effects

CV: angina, chest pain. **Endo:** HYPOGLYCEMIA, hyperglycemia.

PHYSICAL THERAPY IMPLICATIONS

Examination and Evaluation

- Be alert for signs of hypoglycemia, especially during and after exercise. Common neuromuscular signs include anxiety; restlessness; tingling in hands, feet, lips, or tongue; chills; cold sweats; confusion; difficulty in concentration; drowsiness; excessive hunger; headache; irritability; nervousness; tremor; weakness; unsteady gait. Be alert for signs of hypoglycemia, especially during and after exercise. Report episodes of severe hypoglycemia to the physician immediately.
- Monitor symptoms of angina pectoris or chest pain at rest and during exercise. Report these symptoms to the physician.
- Assess blood pressure periodically (See Appendix F). A sudden or sustained increase in blood pressure (hypertension) may indicate problems in diabetes management, and should be reported to the physician.

Interventions

- Implement aerobic exercise and endurance training programs to maintain optimal body weight, improve insulin sensitivity, and reduce the risk of macrovascular disease (heart attack, stroke) and microvascular problems (reduced blood flow to tissues and organs that causes poor wound healing, neuropathy, retinopathy, and nephropathy).

- Because of the risk of angina pectoris, use caution during aerobic exercise and other forms of therapeutic exercise. Assess exercise tolerance frequently (blood pressure, heart rate, fatigue levels), and terminate exercise immediately if any untoward responses occur (See Appendix L).
- Provide a source of oral glucose (fruit juice, glucose gels/tablets, etc.) to treat mild hypoglycemia. Call for emergency assistance if symptoms persist or in cases of severe hypoglycemia. Emergency treatment typically consists of IV glucose, glucagon, or epinephrine.

Patient/Client-Related Instruction

- Encourage patient to monitor blood glucose before and after exercise, and to adjust food intake to maintain normal glycemic levels.
- Emphasize the importance of adhering to nutritional guidelines and the need for periodic assessment of glycemic control (serum glucose and glycosylated hemoglobin levels) throughout the management of diabetes mellitus.
- Advise patient about symptoms of hyperglycemia (confusion, drowsiness; flushed, dry skin; fruit-like breath odor; rapid, deep breathing, polyuria; loss of appetite; unusual thirst). Drug dosages may need to be adjusted to prevent repeated episodes of hyperglycemia.

Pharmacokinetics

Absorption: Well absorbed (56%) following oral administration.
Distribution: Unknown.
Protein Binding: >98%.
Metabolism and Excretion: Mostly metabolized by the liver; metabolites are excreted primarily in feces.
Half-life: 1 hr.

TIME/ACTION PROFILE

ROUTE	ONSET	PEAK	DURATION
PO	within 30 min	60–90 min	<4 hr

Contraindications/Precautions

Contraindicated in: Hypersensitivity; Lactation: Lactation; Diabetic ketoacidosis; Insulin-dependent diabetes.
Use Cautiously in: Impaired liver function (longer dosing intervals may be necessary); Severe renal impairment (dose reduction recommended); Geri: Consider age-related ↓ in renal/hepatic/cardiovascular function; OB/Pedi: Safety not established; insulin recommended to control diabetes during pregnancy.

Interactions

Drug-Drug: Ketoconazole, miconazole, gemfibrozil, itraconazole, and **erythromycin** may ↓ metabolism and ↑ risk of hypoglycemia. Effects may also be ↑ by **NSAIDs, hormonal contraceptives, simvastatin, sulfonamides, chloramphenicol, warfarin, probenecid, MAO inhibitors**, and **beta blockers**. Effects may be ↓ by **corticosteroids, phenothiazines, thyroid preparations, estrogens, hormonal contraceptives, phenytoin, nicotinic acid, sympathomimetics, isoniazid**, and **calcium channel blockers**.
Drug-Natural: Glucosamine may worsen blood glucose control. **Chromium** and **coenzyme Q10** may produce ↑ hypoglycemic effects.

Route/Dosage

PO (Adults): 0.5–4 mg taken before meals (not to exceed 16 mg/day).

Renal Impairment

PO (Adults): *Severe renal impairment*—start with 0.5 mg/day and titrate carefully.

Availability

Tablets: 0.5 mg, 1 mg, 2 mg. ***In combination with:*** metformin (PrandiMet). See Appendix B.

reserpine (re-ser-peen)

Novoreserpine, Reserfia

Classification
Therapeutic: antihypertensives
Pharmacologic: peripherally acting antiadrenergics

Indications

Used in combination with other antihypertensives in the management of hypertension.

Action

Depletes stores of norepinephrine and inhibits uptake in postganglionic adrenergic nerve endings. **Therapeutic Effects:** Lowering of blood pressure.

Adverse Reactions/Side Effects

CNS: depression, drowsiness, lethargy, anxiety, headache, nervousness, nightmares. **EENT:** nasal stuffiness, blurred vision, conjunctival congestion, miosis. **CV:** bradycardia, angina, arrhythmias, edema. **GI:** diarrhea, cramps, dry mouth, GI bleeding, nausea, vomiting. **GU:** erectile dysfunction. **Derm:** flushing. **Endo:** galactorrhea, gynecomastia. **F and E:** sodium and water retention.

PHYSICAL THERAPY IMPLICATIONS

Examination and Evaluation

- Assess blood pressure periodically and compare to normal values (See Appendix F). Document whether

drug therapy is successful in controlling hypertension.
- Assess heart rate, ECG, and heart sounds, especially during exercise (See Appendices G, H). Report any rhythm disturbances or symptoms of increased arrhythmias, including palpitations, chest pain, shortness of breath, fainting, and fatigue/weakness.
- Assess dizziness and weakness that might affect gait, balance, and other functional activities (See Appendix C). Report balance problems and functional limitations to the physician, and caution the patient and family/caregivers to guard against falls and trauma.
- Be alert for signs of depression, anxiety, lethargy, nervousness, or other changes in mood and behavior. Notify physician if these changes become problematic.
- Assess peripheral edema using girth measurements, volume displacement, and measurement of pitting edema (See Appendix N). Report increased swelling in feet and ankles or a sudden increase in body weight due to sodium and water retention.

Interventions

- Because of the risk of arrhythmias, use caution during aerobic exercise and other forms of therapeutic exercise. Assess exercise tolerance frequently (blood pressure, heart rate, fatigue levels), and terminate exercise immediately if any untoward responses occur (See Appendix L).
- Avoid physical therapy interventions that cause systemic vasodilation (large whirlpool, Hubbard tank). Additive effects of this drug and the intervention may cause a dangerous fall in blood pressure.
- To minimize orthostatic hypotension, advise patient to move slowly when assuming a more upright position.

Patient/Client-Related Instruction

- Remind patients to take medication as directed to control hypertension even if they are asymptomatic.
- Counsel patients about additional interventions to help control blood pressure, such as regular exercise, weight loss, sodium restriction, stress reduction, moderation of alcohol consumption, and smoking cessation.
- Instruct patient or family/caregivers to report other bothersome side effects such as severe or prolonged headache, drowsiness, nightmares, vision disturbances, nasal congestion, skin flushing, sexual dysfunction, nipple discharge, breast enlargement in men (gynecomastia), or GI problems (diarrhea, nausea, vomiting, cramps, dry mouth, GI bleeding).

Pharmacokinetics

Absorption: 40–50% absorbed after oral administration.
Distribution: Widely distributed. Crosses the placenta and enters breast milk.
Protein Binding: Highly protein bound.
Metabolism and Excretion: Metabolized by the liver. At least 50% lost in feces as unabsorbed drug after oral administration. Small amounts excreted unchanged by the kidneys.
Half-life: 11 days.

TIME/ACTION PROFILE (antihypertensive effect)

ROUTE	ONSET	PEAK	DURATION
PO	several days–3 wk	3–6 wk	1–6 wk

Contraindications/Precautions

Contraindicated in: Hypersensitivity; Active gastrointestinal disease; Severe renal insufficiency; Mental depression; Electroconvulsive therapy.
Use Cautiously in: History of peptic ulcer disease, ulcerative colitis, or gallstones; Geri: Appears on Beers' list. Geriatric patients are at increased risk of depression, erectile dysfunction, sedation, and orthostatic hypertension at doses above 0.25 mg; Pregnancy, lactation, or children (safety not established; not recommended for use in children).

Interactions

Drug-Drug: Additive hypotension with other **antihypertensives**, **nitrates**, or acute ingestion of **alcohol**. ↑ risk of arrhythmias with **digoxin, quinidine, procainamide**, or other **antiarrhythmics**. Excitement and hypertension may result from concurrent **MAO inhibitor** therapy. May ↓ the therapeutic response to **ephedrine** or **levodopa**. May ↑ responsiveness to **direct-acting adrenergic amines (dopamine, dobutamine, metaraminol, phenylephrine**). Additive CNS depression with other **CNS depressants**, including **alcohol, antihistamines, antidepressants, opioid analgesics**, or **sedative/hypnotics**. Effectiveness may be ↓ by concurrent **NSAIDs**.
Drug-Natural: Also see **sedative** interaction. Concomitant use of **kava, valerian, skullcap, chamomile**, or **hops** can ↑ CNS depression.

Route/Dosage

PO (Adults): 100–250 mcg (0.1–0.25 mg)/day is usual maintenance dose; may be given in an initial dose in patients not receiving other antihypertensives of 500 mcg (0.5 mg) daily for 1–2 wk, then reduce to maintenance dose.

Availability (generic available)

Tablets: 0.1 mg, 0.25 mg, 1 mg. ***In combination with:*** thiazide diuretics and/or hydralazine. See Appendix B.

retapamulin (re-ta-pam-yoo-lin)

Altabax

Classification

Therapeutic: anti-infectives

Pharmacologic: pleuromutilins

Indications

Topical treatment of impetigo caused by methicillin-susceptible *Staphylococcus aureus* or *Streptococcus pyogenes*.

Action

Interferes with bacterial protein synthesis at the level of the 50S ribosome. **Therapeutic Effects:** Bacteriostatic action against susceptible organisms.

Adverse Reactions/Side Effects

Derm: application site irritation.

PHYSICAL THERAPY IMPLICATIONS

Examination and Evaluation

- Assess the area being treated to help determine if drug therapy is successful in resolving skin conditions.
- Monitor any new or increased skin reactions at the site of application, including rash, itching, burning, or other suspicious skin lesions. Report severe or unusual skin reactions to the physician.

Interventions

- Always wash hands thoroughly and disinfect equipment (whirlpools, electrotherapeutic devices, treatment tables, and so forth) to help prevent the spread of infection. Use universal precautions or isolation procedures as indicated for specific patients.

Patient/Client-Related Instruction

- Check that the patient and family or caregivers understand topical application procedures, and adhere to the recommended dosing schedule.
- Instruct patient with skin lesions to avoid itching or scratching the affected area. Patients should avoid contact with other individuals (e.g., other athletes) during the active phase of the infection.

Pharmacokinetics

Absorption: Minimal systemic absorption.
Distribution: Unknown.
Metabolism and Excretion: Small amounts absorbed are extensively metabolized.
Half-life: Unknown.

TIME/ACTION PROFILE

ROUTE	ONSET	PEAK	DURATION
topical	unknown	unknown	12 hr

Contraindications/Precautions

Contraindicated in: No contraindications.
Use Cautiously in: OB: Use only in pregnancy when maternal benefit outweighs fetal risk; safe use during lactation not established; Pedi: Safe use in children <9 mo not established.

Interactions

Drug-Drug: None.

Route/Dosage

Topical (Adults and Children ≥9 mo): Apply thin layer to affected area (up to 100 cm^2 in adults or 2% total body area in children) bid for 5 days.

Availability

Ointment: 10 mg/g in 5-, 10-, and 15-g tubes.

HIGH ALERT

reteplase (re-te-plase)

Retavase

Classification

Therapeutic: thrombolytics

Pharmacologic: plasminogen activators

R

Indications

Acute myocardial infarction (MI). **Unlabeled Use:** Occluded central venous access devices. Deep venous thrombosis (DVT). Acute peripheral arterial thrombosis.

Action

Directly converts plasminogen to plasmin, which then degrades clot-bound fibrin. **Therapeutic Effects:** Lysis of thrombi in coronary arteries, with improvement of ventricular function, and reduced risk of heart failure or death. Restoration of cannula or catheter function. Restoration of blood flow following lysis of peripheral venous or arterial thrombi.

Adverse Reactions/Side Effects

CNS: INTRACRANIAL HEMORRHAGE. **EENT:** epistaxis, gingival bleeding. **Resp:** bronchospasm, hemoptysis. **CV:** reperfusion arrhythmias, hypotension, RECURRENT ISCHEMIA/THROMBOEMBOLISM. **GI:** GI BLEEDING, nausea, RETROPERITONEAL BLEEDING, vomiting. **GU:** GU TRACT BLEEDING. **Derm:** ecchymoses, flushing, urticaria.

Hemat: BLEEDING. **Local:** hemorrhage at injection site, phlebitis at injection site. **MS:** musculoskeletal pain. **Misc:** ALLERGIC REACTIONS, INCLUDING ANAPHYLAXIS, fever.

PHYSICAL THERAPY IMPLICATIONS

Examination and Evaluation

- Watch for signs of bleeding and hemorrhage, including bleeding gums, nosebleeds, unusual bruising, coughing up blood, black/tarry stools, hematuria, or a fall in hematocrit or blood pressure. Be especially alert for signs of intracranial bleeds, including sudden severe headache, confusion, nausea, vomiting, paralysis, numbness, speech problems, and visual disturbances. Notify physician or nursing staff immediately if these signs occur.
- Be alert for signs of recurrent cardiac ischemia (chest pain, pain radiating into the arm or jaw, shortness of breath, dizziness, sweating, anxiety) or recurrent peripheral arterial thrombosis (pain, cramping, coldness, cyanosis in the affected limb). Notify physician or nursing staff immediately if these signs occur.
- Monitor signs of recurrent thromboembolism and pulmonary embolism, including shortness of breath, chest pain, cough, and bloody sputum. Notify physician immediately, and request objective tests (Doppler ultrasound, lung scan, others) if PE is suspected.
- Monitor signs of allergic reactions or anaphylaxis, including pulmonary symptoms (tightness in the throat and chest, wheezing, cough, dyspnea) or skin reactions (rash, pruritus, urticaria). Notify physician or nursing staff immediately if these reactions occur.
- Assess heart rate, ECG, and heart sounds when cardiac perfusion is restored (see Appendixes G, H). Report any rhythm disturbances or symptoms of increased arrhythmias, including palpitations, chest discomfort, shortness of breath, fainting, and fatigue/weakness.
- Assess blood pressure, especially for the first few days after infusion. Report low blood pressure (hypotension), especially if patient experiences dizziness or syncope.
- Assess any muscle of joint pain to rule out musculoskeletal pathology or hemorrhage; that is, try to determine if pain is drug-induced rather than caused by anatomical or biomechanical problems. Be especially concerned about back pain that could indicate retroperitoneal bleeding.
- Assess injection site during and after IV administration, and report signs of bleeding or phlebitis (local pain, swelling, inflammation).

Interventions

- Use caution with any physical interventions that could increase bleeding, including wound débridement, chest percussion, joint mobilization, and application of local heat.
- Use extreme caution during aerobic exercise in patients with recent MI. Assess exercise tolerance frequently (blood pressure, heart rate, fatigue levels), and terminate exercise immediately if any untoward responses occur (See Appendix L).
- For patients with DVT, recommend or implement other physical methods to decrease DVT and prevent recurrent thromboembolism, including graduated compression stockings and intermittent pneumatic compression pumps.

Patient/Client-Related Instruction

- Instruct patient to immediately report signs of GI bleeding, including abdominal pain, vomiting blood, blood in stools, or black, tarry stools.
- Instruct patient or family/caregivers to report other troublesome side effects, including severe or prolonged fever, bronchospasm, skin reactions (bruising, flushing, hives), or GI problems (nausea, vomiting).

Pharmacokinetics

Absorption: Complete after IV administration. Intracoronary administration or administration into occluded catheters or cannulae has a more localized effect.
Distribution: Unknown.
Metabolism and Excretion: Cleared primarily by the liver and kidneys.
Half-life: 13–16 min.

TIME/ACTION PROFILE (fibrinolysis)

ROUTE	ONSET	PEAK	DURATION
IV	30 min	30–90 min	48 hr

Contraindications/Precautions

Contraindicated in: Active internal bleeding; History of cerebrovascular accident; Recent (within 2 mo) intracranial or intraspinal injury or trauma; Intracranial neoplasm, arteriovenous malformation, or aneurysm; Severe uncontrolled hypertension; Known bleeding tendencies; Hypersensitivity.
Use Cautiously in: Recent (within 10 days) major surgery, trauma, GI or GU bleeding; Left heart thrombus; Severe hepatic or renal disease; Hemorrhagic ophthalmic conditions; Septic phlebitis; Previous puncture of a noncompressible vessel; Subacute bacterial endocarditis or acute pericarditis; Geriatric patients (>75 yr; ↑ risk of intracranial bleeding); Pregnancy, lactation, or children (safety not established).
Exercise Extreme Caution in: Patients receiving concurrent anticoagulant therapy (↑ risk of intracranial bleeding).

Interactions

Drug-Drug: Aspirin, other **NSAIDs**, **warfarin**, **heparin** and **heparin-like agents**, **abciximab**, **eptifibatide**, **tirofiban**, **clopidogrel**, **ticlopidine**, or **dipyridamole**—

concurrent use ↑ risk of bleeding, although these agents are frequently used together or in sequence. Effects may be ↓ by **antifibrinolytic agents**, including **aminocaproic acid** or **tranexamic acid**.
Drug-Natural: ↑ anticoagulant effect and bleeding risk with **anise, arnica, chamomile, clove, dong quai, fenugreek, feverfew, garlic, ginger, ginkgo,** ***Panax ginseng*****, licorice**, and others.

Route/Dosage
IV (Adults): 10 units, followed 30 min later by an additional 10 units.

Availability
Powder for injection: 10.8 units (18.8 mg)/vial.

ribavirin (rye-ba-**vye**-rin)
Copegus, Rebetol, Virazole

Classification
Therapeutic: antivirals
Pharmacologic: nucleoside analogues

Indications
Inhalation: Treatment of severe lower respiratory tract infections caused by the respiratory syncytial virus (RSV) in infants and young children. **PO:** *Rebetol*—with interferon alfa-2b (*Intron A*) or peginterferon alfa-2b (*PEG-Intron*) in the treatment of chronic hepatitis C in patients who have failed previous therapy. **PO:** *Copegus*—with peginterferon alfa-2a (Pegasys) in the treatment of chronic hepatitis C in patients who have failed previous therapy. **Unlabeled Use:** Early (within 24 hr of symptoms) secondary treatment of influenza A or B in young adults.

Action
Inhibits viral DNA and RNA synthesis and subsequent replication. Must be phosphorylated intracellularly to be active. **Therapeutic Effects: Inhalation:** Virustatic action. **PO:** Decreased progression and sequelae of chronic hepatitis C.

Adverse Reactions/Side Effects

Inhalation
CNS: dizziness, faintness. **EENT:** blurred vision, conjunctivitis, erythema of the eyelids, ocular irritation, photosensitivity. **CV:** CARDIAC ARREST, hypotension. **Derm:** rash. **Hemat:** hemolytic anemia (with interferon alpha-2b), reticulocytosis.

Oral (may reflect combination with interferon)
CNS: emotional lability (↑ in children), fatigue (↓ in children), impaired concentration (↓ in children), insomnia (↓ in children), irritability (↓ in children). **EENT:** dry mouth. **Resp:** dyspnea (↓ in children). **GI:** anorexia (↑ in children), dyspepsia (↓ in children), vomiting (↑ in children). **Hemat:** hemolytic anemia. **Derm:** pruritus (↓ in children). **MS:** arthralgia (↓ in children). **Misc:** fever (↑ in children).

PHYSICAL THERAPY IMPLICATIONS

Examination and Evaluation
- Be alert for signs of cardiac arrest, and seek immediate medical assistance if the patient collapses, loses consciousness, stops breathing, and lacks a pulse.
- Monitor signs of hemolytic anemia, including unusual weakness and fatigue, dizziness, jaundice, and abdominal pain. Report these signs to the physician immediately.
- Assess blood pressure periodically and compare to normal values (See Appendix F). Report low blood pressure (hypotension), especially if patient experiences dizziness or faintness.
- Assess any breathing problems, and report difficult or labored breathing (dyspnea).
- Assess any joint pain to rule out musculoskeletal pathology; that is, try to determine if pain is drug induced rather than caused by anatomic or biomechanical problems.
- Assess dizziness that might affect gait, balance, or other functional activities (See Appendix C). Report balance problems and functional limitations to the physician and nursing staff, and caution the patient and family/caregivers to guard against falls and trauma.
- Be alert for emotional outbursts, impaired concentration, irritability, and fatigue. Notify physician if these symptoms develop.

Interventions
- Always wash hands thoroughly and disinfect equipment (whirlpools, electrotherapeutic devices, treatment tables, and so forth) to help prevent the spread of infection. Employ universal precautions as indicated for specific patients.

Patient/Client-Related Instruction
- Instruct patient and family/caregivers to report other troublesome side effects, including severe or prolonged fever, vision problems, skin problems (rash, itching), or GI problems (vomiting, indigestion, loss of appetite).

Pharmacokinetics
Absorption: Systemic absorption occurs following nasal and oral inhalation. Rapidly and extensively

R

absorbed following oral administration, but undergoes 1st-pass hepatic metabolism (64% bioavailability).
Distribution: 70% of inhaled drug is deposited in the respiratory tract. Appears to concentrate in the respiratory tract and red blood cells. Enters breast milk.
Metabolism and Excretion: Eliminated from the respiratory tract by distribution across membranes, macrophages, and ciliary motion. Metabolized primarily by the liver; metabolites are renally excreted.
Half-life: *Inhalation*—9.5 hr (40 days in RBCs); *oral*—43.6 hr (single dose); 12 days (multiple dose).

TIME/ACTION PROFILE (blood levels)

ROUTE	ONSET	PEAK	DURATION
inhalation	unknown	end of inhalation	unknown
PO	unknown	1.7–3 hr	12 hr

Contraindications/Precautions
Contraindicated in: Hypersensitivity; **Inhalation:** Patients receiving mechanically assisted ventilation; **Oral:** OB: Pregnancy or lactation; OB: Male partners of pregnant patients; CCr <50 mL/min; Significant/unstable cardiovascular disease; Hemoglobinopathies; Autoimmune hepatitis or hepatic decompensation before/during treatment (for combined therapy with interferon alfa-2b or peginterferon alfa-2a); Concurrent use of didanosine, stavudine, or zidovudine.
Use Cautiously in: **PO:** Sarcoidosis (may exacerbate condition); Anemia (dose reduction/discontinuation may be required); Any preexisting cardiac disease; OB: Patients with childbearing potential.

Interactions
Drug-Drug: **Oral:** May ↓ the antiretroviral action of **stavudine** and **zidovudine**. May ↑ hematologic toxicity of **zidovudine**. May ↑ blood levels and risk of toxicity of **didanosine**. Although used together in the management of hepatitis, concurrent use with **interferon alpha-2b** ↑ risk of hemolytic anemia.

Route/Dosage
Inhalation (Infants and Young Children): 300 mL of 20 mg/mL solution delivered via mist for 12–18 hr/day.

Rebetol (with interferon alfa-2b or peginterferon alfa-2b)
PO (Adults >75 kg): 600 mg in the morning, then 600 mg in the evening for 6 mo.
PO (Adults ≤75 kg and children >61 kg): 400 mg in the morning, then 600 mg in the evening for 6 mo.
PO (Children 50–61 kg): 400 mg in the morning and evening.
PO (Children 37–49 kg): 200 mg in the morning and 400 mg in the evening.
PO (Children 25–36 kg): 200 mg in the morning and evening.

Copegus—viral genotype 1 or 4 (with peginterferon alfa-2a)
PO (Adults ≥75 kg): 600 mg bid for 48 wk.
PO (Adults <75 kg): 500 mg bid for 48 wk.

Copegus—viral genotype 2 or 4 (with peginterferon alfa-2a)
PO (Adults): 400 mg bid for 24 wk.

Availability
Powder for reconstitution for aerosol use: 6 g/vial. **Capsules (Rebetol):** 200 mg. **Tablets (Copegus):** 200 mg, 400 mg. ***In combination with:*** Rebetol with interferon alfa-2b (Intron A) as combination therapy for chronic hepatitis C (Rebetron). See Appendix B; *Copegus* is intended for combined therapy with pegylated interferon alfa-2a (Pegasys).

rifabutin (rif-a-byoo-tin)
Mycobutin

Classification
Therapeutic: agents for atypical mycobacterium
Pharmacologic: rifamycins

Indications
Prevention of disseminated *Mycobacterium avium* complex (MAC) disease in patients with advanced HIV infection. **Unlabeled Use:** Treatment of *Helicobacter pylori* ulcer disease which has failed on other regimens (with pantoprazole and amoxicillin).

Action
Appears to inhibit DNA-dependent RNA polymerase in susceptible organisms. **Therapeutic Effects:** Antimycobacterial action against susceptible organisms.
Spectrum: Active against *M. avium* and most strains of *M. tuberculosis*.

Adverse Reactions/Side Effects
EENT: brown-orange discoloration of tears, ocular disturbances. **Resp:** dyspnea. **CV:** chest pain, chest pressure. **GI:** PSEUDOMEMBRANOUS COLITIS, brown-orange discoloration of saliva, altered taste, drug-induced hepatitis. **GU:** brown-orange discoloration of urine. **Derm:** rash, skin discoloration. **Hemat:** hemolysis, neutropenia, thrombocytopenia. **MS:** arthralgia, myositis. **Misc:** brown-orange discoloration of body fluids, flu-like syndrome.

PHYSICAL THERAPY IMPLICATIONS

Examination and Evaluation

- Monitor signs of pseudomembranous colitis, including diarrhea, abdominal pain, fever, pus or mucus in stools, and other severe or prolonged GI problems (nausea, vomiting, heartburn). Notify physician or nursing staff immediately of these signs.
- Assess any joint pain or muscle pain and inflammation to rule out musculoskeletal pathology; that is, try to determine if pain is drug induced rather than caused by anatomic or biomechanical problems.
- Monitor any chest pain, chest pressure, or difficult, labored breathing. Attempt to determine if pain is drug induced or caused by cardiovascular dysfunction (e.g., angina that occurs during exercise).
- Monitor signs of neutropenia (fever, sore throat, signs of infection) or thrombocytopenia (bruising, nose bleeds, and bleeding gums). Report these signs to the physician.

Interventions

- Always wash hands thoroughly and disinfect equipment (whirlpools, electrotherapeutic devices, treatment tables, and so forth) to help prevent the spread of infection. Use universal precautions or isolation procedures as indicated for specific patients.

Patient/Client-Related Instruction

- Advise patient about possible discoloration of skin, tears, saliva, and other body fluids. Instruct patient to notify physician if discoloration becomes troublesome or if skin rashes or other skin reactions become problematic.
- Instruct patient to report signs of drug-induced hepatitis, including anorexia, abdominal pain, severe nausea and vomiting, yellow skin or eyes, fever, sore throat, malaise, weakness, facial edema, lethargy, and unusual bleeding or bruising.
- Instruct patient to report other troublesome side effects such as vision problems, altered taste, or flu-like symptoms.

Pharmacokinetics

Absorption: Well absorbed following oral administration (50–85%). Absorption is decreased in HIV-positive patients (20%).
Distribution: Widely distributed to body tissues and fluids.
Metabolism and Excretion: Mostly metabolized by the liver; <5% excreted unchanged by the kidneys.
Half-life: 45 hr.

TIME/ACTION PROFILE (blood levels)

ROUTE	ONSET	PEAK	DURATION
PO	rapid	2–4 hr	24 hr

Contraindications/Precautions

Contraindicated in: Hypersensitivity. Cross-sensitivity with other rifamycins (rifampin) may occur; Active tuberculosis; Concurrent ritonavir or delavirdine.
Use Cautiously in: OB/Lactation/Pedi: Safety not established.

Interactions

Drug-Drug: ↑ metabolism and may ↓ the effectiveness of other drugs, including **amprenavir, efavirenz, indinavir, nelfinavir, nevirapine, saquinavir** (dosage adjustment may be necessary), **delavirdine** (concurrent use should be avoided), **corticosteroids, disopyramide, quinidine, opioid analgesics, oral hypoglycemic agents, warfarin, estrogens, estrogen-containing contraceptives, phenytoin, verapamil, fluconazole, quinidine, tocainide, theophylline, zidovudine**, and **chloramphenicol**. **Ritonavir** ↑ blood levels of rifabutin (concurrent use is contraindicated); similar effects occur with **efavirenz** and **nevirapine**.

Route/Dosage

PO (Adults): 300 mg once daily. If GI upset occurs, may give as 150 mg bid with food. *H. pylori*—300 mg/day (unlabeled).

Availability

Capsules: 150 mg.

R

rifampin (rif-am-pin)

Rifadin, Rimactane, ✱Rofact

Classification
Therapeutic: antituberculars
Pharmacologic: rifamycins

Indications

Active tuberculosis (with other agents). Elimination of meningococcal carriers. **Unlabeled Use:** Prevention of disease caused by *Haemophilus influenzae* type B in close contacts.

Action

Inhibits RNA synthesis by blocking RNA transcription in susceptible organisms. **Therapeutic Effects:** Bactericidal action against susceptible organisms. **Spectrum:** Broad spectrum notable for activity against *Mycobacterium* spp., *Staphylococcus aureus, H. influenzae, Legionella pneumophila, Neisseria meningitidis.*

Adverse Reactions/Side Effects

CNS: ataxia, confusion, drowsiness, fatigue, headache, weakness. **EENT:** red discoloration of tears.

GI: abdominal pain, diarrhea, flatulence, heartburn, nausea, vomiting, drug-induced hepatitis, red discoloration of saliva. **GU:** red discoloration of urine.
Hemat: hemolytic anemia, thrombocytopenia.
MS: arthralgia, myalgia. **Misc:** red discoloration of all body fluids, flu-like syndrome.

PHYSICAL THERAPY IMPLICATIONS

Examination and Evaluation

- Assess ataxia or incoordination that might affect gait, balance, and other functional activities. Report balance problems and functional limitations to the physician, and caution the patient and family/caregivers to guard against falls and trauma (See Appendix E).
- Monitor signs of thrombocytopenia (bruising, nose bleeds, and bleeding gums) or hemolytic anemia (unusual weakness and fatigue, dizziness, jaundice, abdominal pain). Report these signs to the physician.
- Assess any joint pain or muscle pain to rule out musculoskeletal pathology; that is, try to determine if pain is drug induced versus pain caused by anatomic or biomechanical problems.
- Monitor confusion, drowsiness, fatigue, or weakness. Notify physician if these symptoms become problematic.

Interventions

- Always wash hands thoroughly and disinfect equipment (whirlpools, electrotherapeutic devices, treatment tables, and so forth) to help prevent the spread of infection. Use universal precautions or isolation procedures as indicated for specific patients.

Patient/Client-Related Instruction

- Advise patient about possible discoloration of tears, saliva, urine, and other body fluids. Instruct patient to notify physician if discoloration becomes troublesome.
- Advise patient about the likelihood of GI reactions (nausea, vomiting, diarrhea, flatulence, abdominal pain, heartburn). Instruct patient to report severe or prolonged GI problems, or signs of drug-induced hepatitis (loss of appetite, yellow skin or eyes, severe nausea and vomiting, fever, sore throat, malaise, weakness, facial edema).
- Instruct patient to report other troublesome side effects such as severe or prolonged headache or flu-like symptoms.

Pharmacokinetics

Absorption: Well absorbed following oral administration.
Distribution: Widely distributed; enters CSF. Crosses placenta; enters breast milk.
Metabolism and Excretion: Mostly metabolized by the liver; 60% eliminated in feces via biliary elimination.
Half-life: 3 hr.

TIME/ACTION PROFILE (blood levels)

ROUTE	ONSET	PEAK	DURATION
PO	rapid	2–4 hr	12–24 hr
IV	rapid	end of infusion	12–24 hr

Contraindications/Precautions

Contraindicated in: Hypersensitivity; Concurrent indinavir, nelfinavir, pyrazinamide, or saquinavir.
Use Cautiously in: History of liver disease; Concurrent use of other hepatotoxic agents; Pregnancy or lactation.

Interactions

Drug-Drug: ↑ risk of hepatotoxicity with other **hepatotoxic agents**, including **alcohol, ketoconazole, isoniazid, pyrazinamide** (concurrent use with **pyrazinamide** may result in potentially fatal hepatotoxicity and should be avoided). Rifampin significantly ↓ blood levels of **delavirdine, indinavir, nelfinavir**, and **saquinavir**; concurrent use is contraindicated. Rifampin stimulates liver enzymes, which may ↑ metabolism and ↓ effectiveness of other drugs, including **ritonavir, nevirapine**, and **efavirenz** (dosage adjustment may be necessary), **corticosteroids, disopyramide, quinidine, opioid analgesics, oral hypoglycemic agents, warfarin, estrogens, phenytoin, verapamil, fluconazole, ketoconazole, itraconazole, quinidine, tocainide, theophylline, chloramphenicol**, and **hormonal contraceptive agents**.

Route/Dosage

Tuberculosis

PO, IV (Adults): 600 mg/day or 10 mg/kg/day (up to 600 mg/day) single dose; may also be given 2–3 times weekly.
PO, IV (Children): 10–20 mg/kg/day single dose (not to exceed 600 mg/day); may also be given 2–3 times weekly.

Asymptomatic Carriers of Meningococcus

PO, IV (Adults): 600 mg q 12 hr for 2 days.
PO, IV (Children ≥1 mo): 10 mg/kg q 12 hr for 2 days.
PO (Infants <1 mo): 5 mg/kg q 12 hr for 2 days.

Prevention of *H. influenzae* Type B Infection

PO (Adults): 600 mg/day for 4 days.
PO (Children): 20 mg/kg/day for 4 days.

Availability (generic available)

Capsules: 150 mg, 300 mg. **Powder for injection:** 600 mg/vial. ***In combination with:*** isoniazid (Rifamate); isoniazid and pyrazinamide (Rifater). See Appendix B.

rifapentine (rif-a-**pen**-teen)
Priftin

Classification
Therapeutic: antituberculars
Pharmacologic: rifamycins

Indications

Treatment of pulmonary tuberculosis: Must be used in combination with other agents.

Action

Inhibits DNA-dependent RNA polymerase. **Therapeutic Effects:** Bactericidal action against intracellular and extracellular susceptible strains of *Mycobacterium tuberculosis*.

Adverse Reactions/Side Effects

CNS: dizziness, headache. **Resp:** hemoptysis. **CV:** hypertension. **GI:** PSEUDOMEMBRANOUS COLITIS, anorexia, diarrhea, dyspepsia, increased liver enzymes, nausea, vomiting. **GU:** hematuria, proteinuria, pyuria, urinary casts. **Derm:** acne, pruritus, rash. **Hemat:** anemia, leukopenia, lymphopenia, neutropenia, thrombocytosis. **MS:** arthralgia. **Misc:** pain.

PHYSICAL THERAPY IMPLICATIONS

Examination and Evaluation

- Monitor signs of pseudomembranous colitis, including diarrhea, abdominal pain, fever, pus or mucus in stools, and other severe or prolonged GI problems (nausea, vomiting, heartburn). Notify physician or nursing staff immediately of these signs.
- Monitor any chest pain or breathing problems, and instruct patient to immediately report coughing up blood (hemoptysis).
- Assess any joint or muscle pain to rule out musculoskeletal pathology; that is, try to determine if pain is drug induced rather than caused by anatomic or biomechanical problems.
- Assess dizziness that might affect gait, balance, and other functional activities (See Appendix C). Report balance problems and functional limitations to the physician and nursing staff, and caution the patient and family/caregivers to guard against falls and trauma.
- Monitor signs of leukopenia or neutropenia (fever, sore throat, signs of infection), thrombocytosis (headache, chest pain, dizziness, fainting, vision problems, numbness/tingling in the hands and feet), or unusual weakness and fatigue that might be due to anemia. Report these signs to the physician.
- Assess blood pressure periodically and report a sustained increase in BP (hypertension) (See Appendix F).

Interventions

- Always wash hands thoroughly and disinfect equipment (whirlpools, electrotherapeutic devices, treatment tables, and so forth) to help prevent the spread of infection. Use universal precautions or isolation procedures as indicated for specific patients.

Patient/Client-Related Instruction

- Advise patient about the likelihood of GI reactions such as diarrhea, nausea, vomiting, loss of appetite, abdominal pain, and indigestion. Instruct patient to report severe or prolonged GI problems.
- Instruct patient to report other troublesome side effects such as severe or prolonged headache, skin problems (acne, rash, itching), or blood in the urine.

Pharmacokinetics

Absorption: 70% absorbed following oral administration.
Distribution: Widely distributed in body tissues and fluids.
Protein Binding: *Rifapentine*—97.7%; *desacetyl rifapentine*—93.2%.
Metabolism and Excretion: Mostly metabolized by the liver; 17% excreted by the kidneys; some conversion to another active compound (25-desacetyl rifapentine).
Half-life: 13 hr (rifapentine and desacetyl rifapentine).

TIME/ACTION PROFILE (blood levels)

ROUTE	ONSET	PEAK	DURATION
PO	unknown	5–6 hr	unknown

Contraindications/Precautions

Contraindicated in: Hypersensitivity to rifapentine or other rifamycins (rifampin or rifabutin).
Use Cautiously in: History of liver disease; Pregnancy, lactation, or children <12 yr (safety not established).
Exercise Extreme Caution in: Concurrent protease inhibitor therapy.

Interactions

Drug-Drug: ↑ metabolism and may ↓ activity of **phenytoin, disopyramide, mexiletine, quinidine, tocainide, chloramphenicol, clarithromycin, dapsone, doxycycline, fluoroquinolones, warfarin, fluconazole, itraconazole, ketoconazole,** some **sedative/hypnotics (benzodiazepines** and

R

barbiturates), some **beta blockers**, some **calcium channel blockers, corticosteroids, digoxin, clofibrate, hormonal contraceptives, haloperidol, protease inhibitors (indinavir, ritonavir, nelfinavir, saquinavir), sulfonylurea oral hypoglycemic agents, cyclosporine, tacrolimus, levothyroxine,** some **opioids, progestins, quinine, reverse transcriptase inhibitors (delavirdine, zidovudine), sildenafil, theophylline**, some **reverse transcriptase inhibitors**, and **tricyclic antidepressants**; dosage adjustments may be necessary. **Antacids** ↓ absorption.
Drug-Food: Food ↑ absorption.

Route/Dosage

Must be used in combination with other antituberculars.
PO (Adults): *Intensive phase*—600 mg twice weekly (not less than 72 hr between doses) for 2 mo; *continuation phase*—600 mg once weekly for 4 mo.

Availability

Tablets: 150 mg.

rifaximin (ri-fax-i-min)

Xifaxan

Classification
Therapeutic: anti-infectives
Pharmacologic: rifamycins

Indications

Travelers' diarrhea due to noninvasive strains of *Escherichia coli*.

Action

Inhibits bacterial RNA synthesis by binding to bacterial DNA-dependent RNA polymerase. **Therapeutic Effects:** Decreased severity of travelers' diarrhea. **Spectrum:** *E. coli* (enterotoxigenic and enteroaggregative strains).

Adverse Reactions/Side Effects

CNS: dizziness. **GI:** PSEUDOMEMBRANOUS COLITIS.

PHYSICAL THERAPY IMPLICATIONS

Examination and Evaluation

- Monitor signs of pseudomembranous colitis, including diarrhea, abdominal pain, fever, pus or mucus in stools, and other severe or prolonged GI problems (nausea, vomiting, heartburn). Notify physician or nursing staff immediately of these signs.
- Assess dizziness that might affect gait, balance, and other functional activities (See Appendix C). Report balance problems and functional limitations to the physician and nursing staff, and caution the patient and family/caregivers to guard against falls and trauma.

Interventions

- Always wash hands thoroughly and disinfect equipment (whirlpools, electrotherapeutic devices, treatment tables, and so forth) to help prevent the spread of infection. Use universal precautions or isolation procedures as indicated for specific patients.

Pharmacokinetics

Absorption: Poorly absorbed (<0.4%), action is primarily in GI tract.
Distribution: 80–90% concentrated in gut.
Metabolism and Excretion: Almost exclusively excreted unchanged in feces.
Half-life: 6 hr.

TIME/ACTION PROFILE

ROUTE	ONSET	PEAK	DURATION
PO	unknown	unknown	unknown

Contraindications/Precautions

Contraindicated in: Hypersensitivity to rifaximin or other rifamycins; Diarrhea with fever or bloody stools; Diarrhea caused by other infections agents; Lactation.
Use Cautiously in: Pregnancy (use only benefits outweigh risk to fetus); Children <12 yr (safety not established).

Interactions

Drug-Drug: Although rifaximin induces the CYP3A4 enzyme system, since it is not absorbed, drug interactions are unlikely.

Route/Dosage

PO (Adults and Children ≥12 yr): 200 mg tid for 3 days.

Availability

Tablets: 200 mg.

rilonacept (ri-lon-a-sept)

Arcalyst

Classification
Therapeutic: orphan drugs
Pharmacologic: fusion proteins, interleukin antagonists

Indications

Treatment of cryopyrin-associated periodic syndromes (CAPS), including familial cold autoinflammatory syndrome (FCAS) and Muckle-Wells syndrome (MWS).

Action

Modulates cryopyrin by blocking interleukin-1 beta (IL-1ß), preventing its interaction with surface receptors. **Therapeutic Effects:** ↓ inflammatory manifestations of CAPS, including fever, rash, arthralgia, myalgia, fatigue, and conjunctivitis.

Adverse Reactions/Side Effects

Resp: upper respiratory tract infections, cough. **Local:** injection site reactions. **Metab:** changes in lipid profile. **Neuro:** hypoesthesia. **Misc:** SERIOUS LIFE-THREATENING INFECTIONS, hypersensitivity reactions.

PHYSICAL THERAPY IMPLICATIONS

Examination and Evaluation

- Report any signs of infection, including upper respiratory tract infections. Signs of respiratory infection include cough, fever, nasal congestion, sneezing, runny nose, and sore throat.
- Assess pain and other variables (range of motion, muscle strength) to document whether this drug is successful in helping manage muscle or joint pain associated with autoinflammatory conditions.
- Assess any changes in sensation, including decreased sensitivity to touch (hypoesthesia) Perform objective tests including electroneuromyography and sensory testing to document any drug-related neuropathic changes.
- Monitor signs of hypersensitivity reactions, including pulmonary symptoms (tightness in the throat and chest, wheezing, cough, dyspnea) or skin reactions (rash, pruritus, urticaria). Notify physician or nursing staff immediately if these reactions occur.
- Assess the subcutaneous injection site for pain, swelling, and irritation. Report prolonged or excessive injection site reactions to the physician.

Interventions

- Implement appropriate manual therapy techniques, physical agents, therapeutic exercises, and orthotic/assistive devices to reduce pain, improve function, and augment the effects of drug therapy.
- Do not apply massage or physical agents (heat, cold, electrotherapeutic modalities) at or near the subcutaneous application site. These interventions can alter drug absorption from subcutaneous tissues.
- Help patients explore other nonpharmacologic methods to reduce chronic musculoskeletal pain, such as relaxation techniques, exercise, counseling, and so forth.

Patient/Client-Related Instruction

- Advise patient to guard against infection (frequent hand washing, etc.), and to avoid crowds and contact with persons with contagious diseases.
- Advise patient that this drug may cause problems in fat metabolism. Remind patient that periodic blood tests may be needed to monitor plasma lipid profile.

Pharmacokinetics

Absorption: Absorbed following subcutaneous administration.
Distribution: Unknown.
Metabolism and Excretion: Unknown.
Half-life: Unknown.

TIME/ACTION PROFILE (improvement in symptoms)

ROUTE	ONSET	PEAK	DURATION
SC	within several days	unknown	unknown

Contraindications/Precautions

Contraindicated in: Active or chronic infections; OB: May cause fetal harm.
Use Cautiously in: Patients at risk of infections; Lactation: Use cautiously; Pedi: Safety and effectiveness have not been established in children <12 yr.

Interactions

Drug-Drug: May ↓ the antibody response to and ↑ adverse reactions from **live vaccines**; vaccination should take place prior to initiation of treatment. Concurrent use with **TNF inhibitors** ↑ risk of serious infections and is not recommended. **Medications that are substrates of the CYP450 enzyme system**, especially those with narrow therapeutic indices such as **warfarin**, should be monitored carefully as enzyme activity may ↑ (normalize) as a result of treatment.

Route/Dosage

SC (Adults ≥18 yr): 320 mg initially, followed by 160 mg weekly.
SC (Children and Adolescents 12–17 yr): 4.4 mg/kg (not to exceed 320 mg) initially, followed by 2.2 mg/kg (not to exceed 160 mg) weekly.

Availability

Powder for subcutaneous administration (requires reconstitution): 220 mg/20-mL vial.

riluzole (ril-yoo-zole)

Rilutek

Classification

Therapeutic: agents for amyotrophic lateral sclerosis
Pharmacologic: glutamate antagonist

Indications

Treatment of patients with amyotrophic lateral sclerosis (ALS).

Action

Action may be related to inhibition of glutamate release, inactivation of sodium channels, or interference with neurotransmitter binding at receptor sites. **Therapeutic Effects:** Extended survival or time to tracheostomy in ALS patients.

Adverse Reactions/Side Effects

CNS: dizziness, weakness, headache. **Resp:** decreased lung function. **CV:** hypertension, peripheral edema. **GI:** abdominal pain, anorexia, diarrhea, dyspepsia, flatulence, nausea, vomiting. **Metab:** weight loss. **MS:** arthralgia, back pain. **Neuro:** circumoral paresthesia.

PHYSICAL THERAPY IMPLICATIONS

Examination and Evaluation

- Assess breathing and notify physician or nursing staff if patient exhibits signs of decreased lung function (dyspnea, shortness of breath, cyanosis). Monitor pulse oximetry and perform pulmonary function tests (See Appendices I, J, K) to quantify suspected changes in ventilation and respiratory function.
- Assess blood pressure (BP) and compare to normal values (See Appendix F). Report a sustained increase in BP (hypertension).
- Assess peripheral edema using girth measurements, volume displacement, and measurement of pitting edema (See Appendix N). Report increased swelling in feet and ankles or a sudden increase in body weight due to fluid retention.
- Assess any back pain or joint pain to rule out musculoskeletal pathology; that is, try to determine if pain is drug induced rather than caused by anatomic or biomechanical problems.
- Be alert for dizziness or weakness that might affect transfers or other functional activities. Report balance problems to the physician and nursing staff, and caution the patient and family/caregivers to guard against falls and trauma.

Interventions

- Implement therapeutic exercises (range of motion, resistive training, aerobic activities, respiratory muscle training) as tolerated to compliment the effects of drug therapy and help maintain pulmonary and musculoskeletal function.

Patient/Client-Related Instruction

- Instruct patient and family/caregivers to report other troublesome side effects, including severe or prolonged headache, numbness around the mouth, or GI problems (nausea, vomiting, diarrhea, indigestion, loss of appetite, flatulence, abdominal pain).

Pharmacokinetics

Absorption: Well absorbed (90%) after oral administration, but bioavailability is 50%.
Distribution: Readily penetrates brain.
Protein Binding: 96%.
Metabolism and Excretion: Highly metabolized by the liver (some metabolites are pharmacologically active); 2% excreted unchanged in urine.
Half-life: 12 hr (after multiple doses).

TIME/ACTION PROFILE

ROUTE	ONSET	PEAK	DURATION
PO	unknown	unknown	unknown

Contraindications/Precautions

Contraindicated in: Severe hypersensitivity.
Use Cautiously in: Hepatic or renal impairment; Female and Japanese patients (decreased metabolism); Pregnancy, lactation, or children (safety not established).

Interactions

Drug-Drug: Effects may be ↑ by **amitriptyline, caffeine, fluoroquinolones,** or **theophylline**. Effects may be ↓ by cigarette smoke **(nicotine), rifampin,** or **omeprazole**.
Drug-Natural: St. John's wort may ↓ riluzole levels and effectiveness.
Drug-Food: Effects may be ↓ by **charcoal-broiled foods. High-fat meals** decrease absorption.

Route/Dosage

PO (Adults): 50 mg q 12 hr.

Availability

Tablets: 50 mg.

rimantadine (ri-man-ti-deen)

Flumadine

Classification
Therapeutic: antivirals

Indications

Prevention and treatment of influenza A infection in high-risk adults. Prevention of influenza A infection in high-risk children. **Unlabeled Use:** Treatment of influenza A infection in children.

Action

Diminishes replication of influenza A virus by inhibiting uncoating of the virus. **Therapeutic Effects:** When given prophylactically, prevents infection with influenza A virus. When administered within 48 hr of onset of infections, ↓ the duration of fever and other associated symptoms.

Adverse Reactions/Side Effects

CNS: SEIZURES, agitation, dizziness, fatigue, headache, impaired concentration, insomnia, mental depression. **EENT:** tinnitus. **Resp:** dyspnea. **GI:** abdominal pain, anorexia, diarrhea, dry mouth, dyspepsia, nausea, vomiting. **Derm:** rash.

PHYSICAL THERAPY IMPLICATIONS

Examination and Evaluation

- Be alert for new seizures or increased seizure activity, especially at the onset of drug treatment. Document the number, duration, and severity of seizures, and report these findings immediately to the physician.
- Be alert for agitation, impaired concentration, mental depression, or other abnormal behaviors. Notify the physician promptly if these symptoms develop.
- Assess any breathing problems, and report difficult or labored breathing (dyspnea).
- Assess dizziness that might affect gait, balance, or other functional activities (See Appendix C). Report balance problems and functional limitations to the physician and nursing staff, and caution the patient and family/caregivers to guard against falls and trauma.

Interventions

- Always wash hands thoroughly and disinfect equipment (whirlpools, electrotherapeutic devices, treatment tables, and so forth) to help prevent the spread of infection. Employ universal precautions as indicated for specific patients.

Patient/Client-Related Instruction

- Instruct patient and family/caregivers to report other troublesome side effects, including severe or prolonged headache, insomnia, skin rash, ringing/buzzing in the ears (tinnitus), or GI problems (nausea, vomiting, diarrhea, abdominal pain, indigestion, loss of appetite).

Pharmacokinetics

Absorption: Well absorbed after oral administration.
Distribution: Unknown.
Metabolism and Excretion: Mostly metabolized by the liver; <25% excreted unchanged in urine.
Half-life: 25 hr (range 13–65 hr).

TIME/ACTION PROFILE (blood levels)

ROUTE	ONSET	PEAK	DURATION
PO	rapid	6 hr	n/a

Contraindications/Precautions

Contraindicated in: Hypersensitivity to rimantadine or amantadine; Lactation.
Use Cautiously in: History of seizures; Geri: Geriatric patients or patients with severe hepatic or renal disease (dosage reduction recommended if CCr ≤10 mL/min); OB: Pregnancy (safety not established).

Interactions

Drug-Drug: Cimetidine may ↑ blood levels. May interfere with efficacy of **intranasal influenza virus vaccine:** do not administer within 48 hr before or 2 wk after.

Route/Dosage

PO (Adults and Children >10 yr): 100 mg bid.
PO (Geriatric Patients and Patients with Severe Hepatic or Renal Impairment [CCr <10 mL/min]): 100 mg daily.
PO (Children <10 yr): 5 mg/kg/day as a single dose (not to exceed 150 mg/day).

Availability

Tablets: 100 mg. **Syrup (raspberry):** 50 mg/5 mL.

R

risedronate (ris-ed-roe-nate)

Actonel

Classification
Therapeutic: bone resorption inhibitors
Pharmacologic: bisphosphonates

Indications

Prevention and treatment of postmenopausal and corticosteroid-induced osteoporosis. Treatment of Paget's disease in men and women. Treatment of osteoporosis in men.

Action

Inhibits bone resorption by binding to bone hydroxyapatite, which inhibits osteoclast activity. **Therapeutic Effects:** Reversal of the progression of osteoporosis with decreased fractures and other sequelae. Reduced bone turnover and resorption; normalization of serum alkaline phosphatase with reduced complications of Paget's disease.

Adverse Reactions/Side Effects

CNS: weakness. **EENT:** amblyopia, conjunctivitis, dry eyes, eye pain/inflammation, tinnitus. **CV:** chest pain, edema. **GI:** abdominal pain, diarrhea, belching, colitis, constipation, dysphagia, esophagitis, esophageal ulcer, gastric ulcer, nausea. **Derm:** rash. **MS:** arthralgia, musculoskeletal pain, osteonecrosis (primarily of jaw). **Misc:** flu-like syndrome.

PHYSICAL THERAPY IMPLICATIONS

Examination and Evaluation

- Assess any muscle or joint pain. Report persistent or increased musculoskeletal pain to determine presence of bone or joint pathology, including fracture. Be especially aware of possible mouth and jaw pain due to osteonecrosis of the jaw.
- Assess peripheral edema using girth measurements, volume displacement, and measurement of pitting edema (See Appendix N). Report increased swelling in feet and ankles or a sudden increase in body weight due to fluid retention.

Interventions

- Institute weight-bearing and resistance exercises as tolerated to maintain or increase bone mineral density. Start with low-impact or aquatic programs in patients with extensive demineralization, and increase exercise intensity slowly to prevent fractures.
- Protect against falls and fractures (See Appendix E). Modify home environment (remove throw rugs, improve lighting, etc.) and provide assistive devices (cane, walker) or other protective devices as needed to improve balance and prevent falls.

Patient/Client-Related Instruction

- Encourage patient to modify behaviors that increase the risk of osteoporosis (stop smoking, reduce alcohol consumption).
- Advise patient about the benefits of proper diet in sustaining bone mineralization. If necessary, refer patient for nutritional counseling about supplemental calcium and vitamin D.
- Instruct patient on the importance of taking this drug exactly as directed and to remain upright for 30 min following dose to facilitate passage to stomach and minimize risk of esophageal irritation.
- Instruct patient to notify physician about any vision disturbances or eye pain and inflammation.
- Instruct patient to report other troublesome side effects such as severe or prolonged weakness, chest pain, skin rash, buzzing/ringing in the ears (tinnitus), flu-like symptoms, new/worsening heartburn, or other GI problems (nausea, diarrhea, constipation, difficulty swallowing, belching, abdominal pain).

Pharmacokinetics

Absorption: Rapidly but poorly absorbed following oral administration (0.63% bioavailability).
Distribution: 60% of absorbed dose distributes to bone.
Metabolism and Excretion: 40% of absorbed dose is excreted unchanged by kidneys; unabsorbed drug is excreted in feces.
Half-life: *Initial*—1.5 hr; *terminal*—220 hr (reflects dissociation from bone).

TIME/ACTION PROFILE (effects on serum alkaline phosphatase)

ROUTE	ONSET	PEAK	DURATION
PO	within days	30 days	up to 16 mo

Contraindications/Precautions

Contraindicated in: Hypersensitivity; Hypocalcemia; Lactation; Severe renal impairment (CCr <30 mL/min).
Use Cautiously in: History of upper GI disorders; Other disturbances of bone or mineral metabolism (correct abnormalities before initiating therapy); Dietary deficiencies (supplemental vitamin D and calcium may be required); Concurrent dental surgery (may ↑ risk of jaw osteonecrosis); OB/Pedi: Safety not established; use in pregnancy only if potential benefit justifies potential risks.

Interactions

Drug-Drug: Concurrent use with **NSAIDs** or **aspirin** ↑ risk of GI irritation. Absorption is ↓ by **calcium supplements** or **antacids**.
Drug-Food: Food ↓ absorption (administer at least 30 min before breakfast).

Route/Dosage

PO (Adults): *Postmenopausal osteoporosis*—5 mg daily, *or* 35 mg once weekly, *or* 75 mg taken on 2 consecutive days for a total of 2 tablets each month, *or* 150 mg once monthly; *Osteoporosis in men*—35 mg once weekly; *Glucocorticoid-induced osteoporosis*—5 mg daily; *Paget's disease*—30 mg daily for 2 mo; retreatment may be considered after 2 mo off therapy.

Availability

Tablets: 5 mg, 30 mg, 35 mg, 75 mg, 150 mg. ***In combination with:*** calcium carbonate.

risperidone (ris-per-i-done)

Risperdal, Risperdal M-TAB, Risperdal Consta

Classification

Therapeutic: antipsychotics, mood stabilizers
Pharmacologic: benzisoxazoles

Indications

Schizophrenia in adults and adolescents age 13–17 yr. Bipolar mania (oral only) in adults and children 10–17 yr in adults and children 10–17 yr; can be used with lithium or valproate (adults only). Treatment of irritability associated with autistic disorder in children age 5–16 yr.

Action

May act by antagonizing dopamine and serotonin in the CNS. **Therapeutic Effects:** Decreased symptoms of psychoses, bipolar mania, or autism.

Adverse Reactions/Side Effects

CNS: NEUROLEPTIC MALIGNANT SYNDROME, aggressive behavior, dizziness, extrapyramidal reactions, headache, increased dreams, increased sleep duration, insomnia, sedation, fatigue, impaired temperature regulation, nervousness, tardive dyskinesia. **EENT:** pharyngitis, rhinitis, visual disturbances. **Resp:** cough, dyspnea. **CV:** arrhythmias, orthostatic hypotension, tachycardia. **GI:** constipation, diarrhea, dry mouth, nausea, abdominal pain, anorexia, dyspepsia, increased salivation, vomiting, weight gain, weight loss, polydipsia. **GU:** decreased libido, dysmenorrhea/menorrhagia, difficulty urinating, polyuria. **Derm:** itching/skin rash, dry skin, increased pigmentation, increased sweating, photosensitivity, seborrhea. **Endo:** galactorrhea, hyperglycemia. **MS:** arthralgia, back pain.

PHYSICAL THERAPY IMPLICATIONS

Examination and Evaluation

- Monitor and report signs of neuroleptic malignant syndrome, including hyperthermia, diaphoresis, generalized muscle rigidity, altered mental status, tachycardia, changes in blood pressure (BP), and incontinence. Symptoms typically occur within 4–14 days after initiation of drug therapy, but can occur at any time during drug use.
- Assess motor function, and be alert for extrapyramidal symptoms. Report these symptoms immediately, especially tardive dyskinesia, because this problem may be irreversible. Common extrapyramidal symptoms include:
  - Tardive dyskinesia (uncontrolled rhythmic movement of mouth, face, and extremities, lip smacking or puckering, puffing of cheeks, uncontrolled chewing, rapid or worm-like movements of tongue).
  - Pseudoparkinsonism (shuffling gait, rigidity, tremor, pill-rolling motion, loss of balance control, difficulty speaking or swallowing, mask-like face).
  - Akathisia (restlessness or desire to keep moving).
  - Other dystonias and dyskinesias (dystonic muscle spasms, twisting motions, twitching, inability to move eyes, weakness of arms or legs).
- Assess heart rate, ECG, and heart sounds, especially during exercise (See Appendices G, H). Report a rapid heart rate (tachycardia) or signs of other arrhythmias, including palpitations, chest discomfort, shortness of breath, fainting, and fatigue/weakness.
- Assess BP when patient assumes a more upright position (lying to standing, sitting to standing, lying to sitting). Document orthostatic hypotension and contact physician when systolic BP falls >20 mm Hg or diastolic BP falls >10 mm Hg.
- Report any troublesome respiratory problems, including severe or prolonged cough, nasopharyngeal irritation, or difficult/labored breathing.
- Be alert for signs of hyperglycemia, including confusion, drowsiness, flushed/dry skin, fruit-like breath odor, rapid/deep breathing, polyuria, loss of appetite, and unusual thirst. Patients with diabetes mellitus should check blood glucose levels frequently.
- Monitor personality changes, including nervousness, aggressive behavior, and depression. Notify physician if these changes become problematic.
- Assess dizziness and drowsiness that might affect gait, balance, and other functional activities (See Appendix C). Report balance problems and functional limitations to the physician, and caution the patient and family/caregivers to guard against falls and trauma.
- If used to control behavioral problems in children, document any changes in irritability or combative behavior to help determine drug efficacy and appropriate dosing.
- Assess any back pain or joint pain to rule out musculoskeletal pathology; that is, try to determine if pain is drug induced rather than caused by anatomic or biomechanical problems.
- Periodically assess body weight and other anthropometric measures (body mass index, body composition). Report a substantial weight gain or weight loss.

Interventions

- Guard against falls and trauma (hip fractures, head injury, and so forth) caused by drowsiness, dizziness, blurred vision, or extrapyramidal symptoms; implement fall-prevention strategies (See Appendix E).
- Because of the risk of arrhythmias and abnormal BP responses, use caution during aerobic exercise and other forms of therapeutic exercise. Assess exercise tolerance frequently (BP, heart rate, fatigue levels), and terminate exercise immediately if any untoward responses occur (See Appendix L).
- To minimize orthostatic hypotension, patient should move slowly when assuming a more upright position.
- This drug impairs body temperature regulation; use care during exercise, and during other activities that increase body temperature (hot whirlpools, saunas, and so forth).

- Causes photosensitivity; use care if administering UV treatments. Advise patient to avoid direct sunlight and use sunscreens and protective clothing.
- Help patient and family/caregivers explore nonpharmacologic methods (exercise, counseling, support groups) to reduce schizophrenic episodes and behavioral problems.

Patient/Client-Related Instruction

- Advise patient to avoid alcohol and other CNS depressants because of the increased risk of sedation and adverse effects.
- Instruct patient to report other problematic side effects such as severe or prolonged headache, vision disturbances, sleep disturbances, urinary retention, decreased libido, nipple discharge, menstrual disorders, skin reactions (rash, itching, increased pigmentation, excessive sweating, oily discharge), or GI problems (nausea, vomiting, diarrhea, constipation, abdominal pain, loss of appetite, dry mouth, indigestion).

Pharmacokinetics

Absorption: 70% after administration of tablets, solution, or orally disintegrating tablets. Following IM administration, small initial release of drug, followed by 3-wk lag; the rest of release starts at 3 wk and lasts 4–6 wk.
Distribution: Unknown.
Metabolism and Excretion: Extensively metabolized by the liver. Metabolism is genetically determined; extensive metabolizers (most patients) convert risperidone to 9-hydroxyrisperidone rapidly. Poor metabolizers (6–8% of whites) convert it more slowly. The 9-hydroxyrisperidone is an antipsychotic compound. Risperidone and its active metabolite are renally eliminated.
Half-life: *Extensive metabolizers*—3 hr for risperidone, 21 hr for 9-hydroxyrisperidone. *Poor metabolizers*—20 hr for risperidone, 30 hr for 9-hydroxyrisperidone.

TIME/ACTION PROFILE (clinical effects)

ROUTE	ONSET	PEAK	DURATION
PO	1–2 wk	unknown	up to 6 wk*
IM	3 wk	4–6 wk	up to 6 wk*

*After discontinuation.

Contraindications/Precautions

Contraindicated in: Hypersensitivity; Lactation: Discontinue drug or bottle-feed.
Use Cautiously in: Debilitated patients, patients with renal or hepatic impairment (initial dose reduction recommended); Underlying cardiovascular disease (may be more prone to arrhythmias and hypotension); History of seizures; History of suicide attempt or drug abuse; Diabetes or risk factors for diabetes (may worsen glucose control); Patients at risk for aspiration; OB/Pedi: Safety not established; Geri: Initial dose reduction recommended. ↑ risk of mortality in elderly patients treated for dementia-related psychosis.

Interactions

Drug-Drug: May ↓ the antiparkinsonian effects of **levodopa** or other **dopamine agonists. Carbamazepine, phenytoin, rifampin, phenobarbital,** and other **enzyme inducers** ↑ metabolism and may ↓ effectiveness; dose adjustments may be necessary. **Fluoxetine** and paroxetine ↑ blood levels and may ↑ effects; dose adjustments may be necessary. **Clozapine** ↓ metabolism and may ↑ effects of risperidone. ↑ CNS depression may occur with other **CNS depressants**, including **alcohol, antihistamines, sedative/hypnotics**, or **opioid analgesics**.
Drug-Natural: Kava, valerian, or chamomile can ↑ CNS depression.

Route/Dosage

Schizophrenia

PO (Adults): 1 mg bid, increased by 1–2 mg/day no more frequently than q 24 hr to 4–8 mg daily.
PO (Children 13–17 yr): 0.5 mg once daily; increased by 0.5–1 mg no more frequently than q 24 hr to 3 mg daily. May administer half the daily dose bid if drowsiness persists.
IM (Adults): 25 mg q 2 wk; some patients may require larger dose of 37.5 or 50 mg q 2 wk.

Bipolar Mania

PO (Adults): 2–3 mg/day as a single daily dose; dose may be increased at 24-hr intervals by 1 mg (range 1–5 mg/day).
PO (Children 13–17 yr): 0.5 mg once daily; increased by 0.5–1.0 mg no more frequently than q 24 hr to 2.5 mg daily. May administer half the daily dose bid if drowsiness persists.
PO (Geriatric Patients or Debilitated Patients): Start with 0.5 mg bid; increase by 0.5 mg bid, up to 1.5 mg bid; then increase at weekly intervals if necessary. May also be given as a single daily dose after initial titration.

Irritability Associated with Autistic Disorder

PO (Children 5–16 yr weighing <20 kg): 0.25 mg/day initially. After at least 4 days of therapy, may increase to 0.50 mg/day. Dose increases in increments of 0.25 mg/day may be considered at 2 wk or longer intervals. May be given as a single or divided dose.
PO (Children 5–16 yr weighing >20 kg): 0.50 mg/day initially. After at least 4 days of therapy, may increase to 1 mg/day. Dose increases in increments of 0.5 mg/day

may be considered at 2 wk or longer intervals. May be given as a single or divided dose.

Renal Impairment

Hepatic Impairment

PO (Adults): Start with 0.5 mg bid; increase by 0.5 mg bid, up to 1.5 mg bid; then increase at weekly intervals if necessary. May also be given as a single daily dose after initial titration.

Availability (generic available)

Tablets: 0.25 mg, 0.5 mg, 1 mg, 2 mg, 3 mg, 4 mg. **Orally disintegrating tablets (Risperdal M-Tabs):** 0.5 mg, 1 mg, 2 mg, 3 mg, 4 mg. **Oral solution:** 1 mg/mL in 30-mL bottles. **Microspheres for injection (Risperdal Consta) (requires specific diluent for suspension):** 12.5 mg/vial kit, 25 mg/vial kit, 37.5 mg/vial kit , 50 mg/vial kit.

ritonavir (ri-toe-na-veer)

Norvir

Classification

Therapeutic: antiretrovirals

Pharmacologic: protease inhibitors

Indications

HIV infection (with other antiretrovirals).

Action

Inhibits the action of HIV protease and prevents the cleavage of viral polyproteins. **Therapeutic Effects:** Increased CD4 cell counts and decreased viral load with subsequent slowed progression of HIV infection and its sequelae.

Adverse Reactions/Side Effects

CNS: SEIZURES, abnormal thinking, weakness, dizziness, headache, malaise, somnolence, syncope. **EENT:** pharyngitis, throat irritation. **Resp:** ANGIOEDEMA, bronchospasm. **CV:** heart block, orthostatic hypotension, vasodilation. **GI:** abdominal pain, altered taste, anorexia, diarrhea, nausea, vomiting, constipation, dyspepsia, flatulence. **GU:** renal insufficiency. **Derm:** rash, skin eruptions, sweating, urticaria. **Endo:** hyperglycemia. **F and E:** dehydration. **Metab:** hyperlipidemia. **MS:** increased creatine phosphokinase, myalgia. **Neuro:** circumoral paresthesia, peripheral paresthesia. **Misc:** HYPERSENSITIVITY REACTIONS, INCLUDING STEVENS-JOHNSON SYNDROME AND ANAPHYLAXIS, fat redistribution, fever.

PHYSICAL THERAPY IMPLICATIONS

Examination and Evaluation

- Be alert for new seizures or increased seizure activity, especially at the onset of drug treatment. Document the number, duration, and severity of seizures, and report these findings immediately to the physician.
- Monitor signs of hypersensitivity reactions and anaphylaxis, including pulmonary symptoms (tightness in the throat and chest, wheezing, cough, dyspnea) or skin reactions (rash, hives, itching, raised patches of red or white skin, burning, acne, exfoliation, abnormal sweating). Notify physician immediately, especially about skin responses that may indicate serious allergic reactions such as Stevens-Johnson syndrome and angioedema.
- Assess heart rate, ECG, and heart sounds, especially during exercise (See Appendices G, H). Report any rhythm disturbances or symptoms of heart block including palpitations, chest discomfort, shortness of breath, fainting, and fatigue/weakness.
- Assess blood pressure (BP) when patient assumes a more upright position (lying to standing, sitting to standing, lying to sitting). Document orthostatic hypotension and contact the physician when systolic BP falls >20 mm Hg or diastolic BP falls >10 mm Hg.
- Assess symptoms of bronchospasm (wheezing, coughing, tightness in chest) or other prolonged or severe respiratory problems (difficult or labored breathing). Perform pulmonary function tests to quantify suspected changes in ventilation and respiration (See Appendices I, J, K).
- Be alert for signs of peripheral paresthesia and neuropathy (numbness, tingling). Establish baseline electroneuromyographic values using EMG and nerve conduction at the beginning of drug treatment whenever possible, and re-examine these values periodically to document drug-induced changes in nerve and muscle function.
- Assess any muscle pain to rule out musculoskeletal pathology; that is, try to determine if pain is drug induced rather than caused by anatomic or biomechanical problems. Report any sudden or progressive increase in muscle pain or weakness that might indicate myopathy.
- Be alert for signs of hyperglycemia, including confusion, drowsiness, flushed/dry skin, fruit-like breath odor, rapid/deep breathing, polyuria, loss of appetite, and unusual thirst. Patients with diabetes mellitus should check blood glucose levels frequently.

R

- Assess dizziness or syncope that might affect gait, balance, and other functional activities (See Appendix C). Report balance problems and functional limitations to the physician and nursing staff, and caution the patient and family/caregivers to guard against falls and trauma.
- Monitor personality changes, including abnormal thinking, somnolence, and increased thoughts of suicide. Notify physician if these changes become problematic.

Interventions

- Implement resistive exercises and other therapeutic exercises as needed to maintain muscle strength and function, and prevent muscle wasting associated with HIV infection and AIDS.
- Design and implement aerobic exercise and endurance training programs to help prevent heart disease associated with drug-related hyperlipidemia and other problems with lipid and glucose metabolism.
- Because of the risk of heart block and other arrhythmias, use caution during aerobic exercise and other forms of therapeutic exercise. Assess exercise tolerance frequently (BP, heart rate, fatigue levels), and terminate exercise immediately if any untoward responses occur (See Appendix L).
- To minimize orthostatic hypotension, patient should move slowly when assuming a more upright position.
- Make sure that fluid intake is adequate during and after exercise; this drug increases the risk of dehydration.

Patient/Client-Related Instruction

- Emphasize the importance of taking ritonavir as directed even if the patient is asymptomatic and that this drug must always be used in combination with other antiretroviral drugs. Do not take more than prescribed amount and do not stop taking without consulting health care professional.
- Inform patient that ritonavir does not cure HIV or AIDS or prevent associated or opportunistic infections. Ritonavir does not reduce the risk of transmission of HIV to others through sexual contact or blood contamination. Caution patient to use a condom, and avoid sharing needles or donating blood to prevent spreading the AIDS virus to others.
- Advise patient that this drug may cause problems in fat and glucose metabolism (hyperlipidemia and hyperglycemia, respectively). Remind patient that periodic blood tests may be needed to monitor plasma lipids and glucose tolerance.
- Inform patient that redistribution and accumulation of body fat may occur, causing central obesity, thin arms and legs, dorsocervical fat enlargement (buffalo hump), breast enlargement, and other symptoms that resemble Cushing syndrome (moon face, striations on abdominal skin). Discuss possible effects on body image, and help patient explore coping mechanisms.
- Instruct patient to report signs of kidney insufficiency, including hematuria, increased urinary frequency, cloudy urine, decreased urine output, and sudden weight gain due to fluid retention.
- Instruct patient to report other troublesome side effects such as prolonged or severe headache, fever, upper respiratory tract irritation, skin reactions (rash, hives, sweating, acne), or GI problems (diarrhea, nausea, vomiting, constipation, flatulence, heartburn, loss of appetite).

Pharmacokinetics

Absorption: Appears to be well absorbed after oral administration.
Distribution: Poor CNS penetration.
Protein Binding: 98–99%.
Metabolism and Excretion: Highly metabolized by the liver (by P450 CYP3A and CYP2D6 enzymes); one metabolite has antiretroviral activity; 3.5% excreted unchanged in urine.
Half-life: 3–5 hr.

TIME/ACTION PROFILE (blood levels)

ROUTE	ONSET	PEAK	DURATION
PO	rapid	4 hr*	12 hr

*Nonfasting.

Contraindications/Precautions

Contraindicated in: Hypersensitivity; Concurrent use of alfuzosin, amiodarone, dihydroergotamine, ergotamine, ergonovine, flecainide, fluticasone, lovastatin, meperidine, methylergonovine, midazolam, pimozide, propafenone, quinidine, simvastatin, St. John's wort, triazolam, or voriconazole; Hypersensitivity or intolerance to alcohol or castor oil (present in capsules and liquid).
Use Cautiously in: Impaired hepatic function, history of hepatitis; Diabetes mellitus; Hemophilia (↑ risk of bleeding); Structural heart disease, conduction abnormalities, ischemic heart disease, or heart failure (↑ risk of heart block); OB/Lactation/Pedi: Pregnancy, lactation, or children <12 yr (safety not established; breast-feeding not recommended in HIV-infected patients).

Interactions

Drug-Drug: Produces large ↑ in blood levels and effects of **amiodarone, alfuzosin, flecainide, fluticasone (inhalation), meperidine, pimozide, propafenone**, and **quinidine**; concurrent use should be avoided. Ergot toxicity may occur with concurrent use of **ergonovine, ergotamine methylergonovine**, or **dihydroergotamine**; concurrent use should be avoided. ↑ risk of rhabdomyolysis with **lovastatin** or **simvastatin**; concurrent use should be avoided. ↑ blood levels and the risk of excessive sedation and/or respiratory depression from **midazolam** and **triazolam**; concurrent use should be avoided. ↑ blood levels of **maraviroc**; ↓ maraviroc dose to 150 mg bid. ↑ blood levels of **clarithromycin**; ↓ clarithromycin dose if CCr <60 mL/min. ↑ blood levels of **rifabutin**; ↓ rifabutin dose to 150 mg every other day or 3 times weekly. May lead to ↓ antifungal effects of **voriconazole**; concurrent use should be avoided. May also ↑ blood levels and effects of some **opioid analgesics (alfentanil, fentanyl, hydrocodone, oxycodone)**, **tramadol**; some **NSAIDs (diclofenac, ibuprofen, indomethacin)**; some **antiarrhythmics (disopyramide, lidocaine, mexiletine)**; many **antidepressants (amitriptyline, clomipramine, desipramine, imipramine, nortriptyline, nefazodone, sertraline, trazodone, fluoxetine, paroxetine, venlafaxine)**; some **antiemetics (dronabinol, ondansetron)**; some **beta blockers (metoprolol, pindolol, propranolol, timolol)**; many **calcium channel blockers (amlodipine, diltiazem, felodipine, isradipine, nicardipine, nifedipine, nimodipine, nisoldipine, verapamil)**; some **antineoplastics (etoposides, paclitaxel, tamoxifen, vinblastine, vincristine)**; some **corticosteroids (dexamethasone, prednisone)**, most **HMG CoA reductase inhibitors**; some **immunosuppressants (cyclosporine, tacrolimus)**; some **antipsychotics (chlorpromazine, haloperidol, perphenazine, risperidone, thioridazine)**; and also **quinidine**, **saquinavir**, **methamphetamine**, and **warfarin**. Dosage ↓ may be necessary. ↓ blood levels and effects of **hormonal contraceptives, zidovudine, bupropion**, and **theophylline**; dose alteration or alternative therapy may be necessary. Levels may be ↑ by **clarithromycin** or **fluoxetine**. ↑ risk of heart block with **beta blockers, verapamil, diltiazem, digoxin**, or **atazanavir**. May ↑ concentrations of phosphodiesterase type 5 inhibitors (PDE5) causing hypotension, visual changes, priapism; ↓ starting doses not to exceed 25 mg within 48 hr for **sildenafil**, 2.5 mg q 72 hr for **vardenafil** and 10 mg q 72 hr for **tadalafil**. **Drug-Natural: St. John's wort** ↓ levels and may promote resistance; concurrent use not recommended. **Drug-Food: Food** ↑ absorption.

Route/Dosage

PO (Adults): 300 mg bid for 1 day, then 400 mg bid for 3 days, then 500 mg bid for 1 day, then 600 mg bid as maintenance.
PO (Children): 250 mg/m² bid initially; increase by 50 mg/m² bid q 2–3 days up to 400 mg/m² bid (if unable to get up to 400 mg/m² bid, additional antiretroviral therapy is required).

Availability

Capsules: 100 mg. **Oral solution:** 600 mg/7.5 mL (80 mg/mL) in 240-mL bottles.

rituximab (ri-tux-i-mab)

Rituxan

Classification
Therapeutic: antineoplastics
Pharmacologic: monoclonal antibodies

Indications

Treatment of low-grade or follicular, CD20-positive, B-cell non-Hodgkin's lymphoma alone, with, or following treatment with cyclophosphamide, vincristine, and prednisolone (CVP). Moderately to severely active rheumatoid arthritis with methotrexate in patients who have had an inadequate response to one of more TNF antagonist therapies.

Action

Binds to the CD20 antigen on the surface of lymphoma cells, preventing the activation process for cell-cycle initiation and differentiation. **Therapeutic Effects:** Death of lymphoma cells. Reduced signs and symptoms of rheumatoid arthritis.

Adverse Reactions/Side Effects

CNS: PROGRESSIVE MULTIFOCAL LEUKOENCEPHALOPATHY, headache. **Resp:** bronchospasm, cough, dyspnea. **CV:** ARRHYTHMIAS, hypotension, peripheral edema. **GI:** abdominal pain, altered taste, dyspepsia. **Derm:** MUCOCUTANEOUS SKIN REACTIONS, flushing, urticaria. **Endo:** hyperglycemia. **F and E:** hypocalcemia. **Hemat:** ANEMIA, NEUTROPENIA, THROMBOCYTOPENIA. **MS:** arthralgia, back pain. **Misc:** ALLERGIC REACTIONS, INCLUDING ANAPHYLAXIS AND ANGIOEDEMA, infections, INFUSION REACTIONS, TUMOR LYSIS SYNDROME, fever/chills/rigors (infusion related).

PHYSICAL THERAPY IMPLICATIONS

Examination and Evaluation

- Monitor signs of allergic reactions including anaphylaxis and angioedema. Reactions include pulmonary symptoms (tightness in the throat and chest, wheezing, cough, dyspnea) and skin reactions (rash, pruritus, urticaria, burning skin, swelling in the face). Be especially alert for these signs after drug infusion (infusion reactions). Notify physician or nursing staff immediately if these reactions occur.

- Monitor and report signs of progressive multifocal leukoencephalopathy, including headache, confusion, seizures, and loss of vision. Early recognition and adjustment of drug dosage is important in resolving this syndrome.
- Assess heart rate (HR), ECG, and heart sounds, especially during exercise (see Appendixes G, H). Report any rhythm disturbances or symptoms of increased arrhythmias, including palpitations, chest discomfort, shortness of breath, fainting, and fatigue/weakness.
- Monitor neuromuscular signs of electrolyte imbalances that might indicate tumor lysis syndrome. Signs include severe muscle weakness or paralysis due to increased plasma potassium (hyperkalemia), or muscle hyperexcitability and tetany due to phosphate and calcium imbalances (hyperphosphatemia and hypocalcemia). Notify physician or nursing staff immediately if these signs occur.
- Monitor and report skin or mucocutaneous reactions, including inflammation, swelling, and burning pain of the skin and mucous membranes.
- Monitor signs of bone marrow suppression, including neutropenia (fever, sore throat, signs of infection), thrombocytopenia (bruising, nose bleeds, and bleeding gums), or unusual weakness and fatigue that might be due to anemia or other blood dyscrasias. Notify physician of these signs immediately.
- If treating rheumatoid arthritis, periodically assess patient's impairments (pain, range of motion), functional ability, and disability to help determine if antirheumatic drug therapy is successful.
- Assess any increased joint or back pain to rule out musculoskeletal pathology; that is, try to determine if pain is drug induced rather than caused by anatomic or biomechanical problems.
- Assess blood pressure (BP) periodically. Report a problematic decrease in BP (hypotension; See Appendix F), especially if dizziness and syncope occurs.
- Report signs of bronchospasm (wheezing, coughing, tightness in chest) or other prolonged or severe respiratory problems (difficult or labored breathing). Perform pulmonary function tests and monitor breath sounds to quantify suspected changes in ventilation and respiration (See Appendices I, J, K).
- Monitor signs of hyperglycemia (drowsiness, fruity breath, increased urination, unusual thirst). Patients with diabetes mellitus should check blood glucose levels frequently.
- Assess peripheral edema using girth measurements, volume displacement, and measurement of pitting edema (See Appendix N). Report increased swelling in feet and ankles or a sudden increase in body weight due to fluid retention.

Interventions

- For patients who are medically able to begin exercise, implement appropriate resistive exercises and aerobic training to maintain muscle strength and aerobic capacity during cancer chemotherapy, or to help restore function after chemotherapy.
- If treating rheumatoid arthritis, implement appropriate manual therapy techniques, physical agents, therapeutic exercises, and orthotic/assistive devices to reduce pain, improve function, and augment the effects of antirheumatic drug therapy.
- Help patients with arthritis explore other nonpharmacologic methods to reduce chronic pain (relaxation techniques, exercise, counseling, and so forth).
- Use caution during aerobic exercise and endurance conditioning because of potential adverse changes in BP and HR. Terminate exercise if patient exhibits untoward symptoms (chest pain, shortness of breath, etc.), or displays other criteria for exercise termination (See Appendix L).

Patient/Client-Related Instruction

- Make sure patient and family or caregivers understand the need to immediately report skin reactions or signs of allergic responses as listed above (see Examination and Evaluation).
- Advise patient to guard against infection (frequent hand washing, etc.), and to avoid crowds and contact with persons with contagious diseases.
- Instruct patient or family/caregivers to report other bothersome side effects such as severe or prolonged headache, indigestion, altered taste, abdominal pain, chills, fever, or other signs of infection.

Pharmacokinetics

Absorption: IV administration results in complete bioavailability.
Distribution: Binds specifically to CD20 binding sites on lymphoma cells.
Metabolism and Excretion: Unknown.
Half-life: 59.8–174 hr (depending on tumor burden).

TIME/ACTION PROFILE (B-cell depletion)

ROUTE	ONSET	PEAK	DURATION
IV	within 14 days	3–4 wk	6–9 mo*

*Duration of depletion after 4 wk of treatment.

Contraindications/Precautions

Contraindicated in: Hypersensitivity to murine (mouse) proteins; OB: Can pass placental barrier potentially causing fetal B-cell depletion. Give only if clearly needed; Lactation: Potential for immunosuppression in infant. Discontinue nursing.
Use Cautiously in: Preexisting bone marrow depression; Hepatitis B infection (may reactivate infection during and for several months after treatment); Systemic lupus

erythematosus (may cause fatal progressive multifocal leukoencephalopathy); HIV infection (may increase risk of HIV-associated lymphoma); Pedi: Safety not established.

Interactions

Drug-Drug: None known.

Route/Dosage

Relapsed or refractory, low-grade or follicular, CD20-positive, B-cell Non-Hodgkin's lymphoma

IV (Adults): 375 mg/m^2 once weekly for 4–8 doses.

Retreatment therapy

IV (Adults): 375 mg/m^2 once weekly for 4 doses.

Previously untreated follicular, CD20-positive, B-cell Non-Hodgkin's lymphoma

IV (Adults): 375 mg/m^2 given on day 1 of each cycle of CVP for up to 8 doses.

Previously untreated low-grade, CD20-positive, B-cell Non-Hodgkin's lymphoma

IV (Adults): For patients who have not progressed following 6–8 cycles of CVP chemotherapy, 375 mg/m^2 given once weekly for 4 doses given every 6 mo for up to 16 doses.

Diffuse large B-cell Non-Hodgkin's lymphoma

IV (Adults): 375 mg/m^2 given on day 1 of each cycle of CVP for up to 8 infusions.

Rheumatoid arthritis

IV (Adults): Two 1000 mg separated by 2 wk.

Availability

Solution for injection (requires dilution): 10 mg/mL in 100-mg and 500-mg vials.

rizatriptan (riz-a-trip-tan)

Maxalt, Maxalt-MLT

Classification

Therapeutic: vascular headache suppressants

Pharmacologic: 5-HT$_1$ agonists

Indications

Acute treatment of migraine headache.

Action

Acts as an agonist at specific 5-HT$_1$ receptor sites in intracranial blood vessels and sensory trigeminal nerves. **Therapeutic Effects:** Cranial vessel vasoconstriction with associated decrease in release of neuropeptides and resultant decrease in migraine headache.

Adverse Reactions/Side Effects

CNS: dizziness, drowsiness, weakness. **CV:** CORONARY ARTERY VASOSPASM, MI, VENTRICULAR FIBRILLATION, VENTRICULAR TACHYCARDIA, chest pain, myocardial ischemia. **GI:** dry mouth, nausea. **Misc:** HYPERSENSITIVITY REACTIONS, INCLUDING ANGIOEDEMA, toxic epidermal necrolysis, pain.

PHYSICAL THERAPY IMPLICATIONS

Examination and Evaluation

- Continually monitor for signs of coronary artery vasospasm and MI, including sudden chest pain, pain radiating into the arm or jaw, shortness of breath, dizziness, sweating, anxiety, and nausea. Seek immediate medical assistance if patient develops these signs.
- Assess heart rate, ECG, and heart sounds, especially during exercise (See Appendices G, H). Report any rhythm disturbances or symptoms of increased arrhythmias, including palpitations, chest discomfort, shortness of breath, dizziness, fainting, and fatigue/weakness.
- Monitor signs of allergic reactions and angioedema, including pulmonary symptoms (tightness in the throat and chest, wheezing, cough, dyspnea) or skin reactions (rash, pruritus, urticaria, swelling in the face). Be especially alert for severe skin reactions that might indicate toxic epidermal necrosis. Notify physician immediately if these reactions occur.
- Assess the frequency and severity of headaches, and document whether drug therapy is successful in decreasing the severity of migraine headache attacks.
- Assess any muscle pain to rule out musculoskeletal pathology; that is, try to determine if pain is drug induced rather than caused by anatomic or biomechanical problems.
- Watch for dizziness and drowsiness that affects gait, balance, and other functional activities (See Appendix C). Report balance problems and functional limitations to the physician, and caution the patient and family/caregivers to guard against falls and trauma.

Interventions

- Because of the risk of MI and arrhythmias, use extreme caution during aerobic exercise and other forms of therapeutic exercise. Assess exercise tolerance frequently (blood pressure, heart rate, respiration, fatigue levels), and terminate exercise immediately if any untoward responses occur (See Appendix L).

R

- Implement appropriate interventions (manual techniques, physical agents, therapeutic exercise) to manage headache pain and reduce the need for drug therapy. Help patient also explore other nonpharmacologic methods to reduce chronic headache pain (relaxation techniques, imagery, and so forth).
- If a headache occurs and drug treatment is needed during a rehabilitation session, allow patient to recover in a quiet, darkened room to allow the drug to achieve maximal effects.

Patient/Client-Related Instruction

- Advise patient and family or caregiver about the signs of MI (see above under Examination and Evaluation), and to seek immediate medical assistance if these signs develop.
- Advise the patient to bring this drug to each therapy session; this drug is most effective when taken at the first signs of a migraine attack.
- Advise patient to adhere to the correct dosing schedule, and to not exceed the recommended frequency and number of doses per 24-hr period.
- Instruct patient to report other troublesome side effects such as severe or prolonged weakness or GI problems (nausea, dry mouth).

Pharmacokinetics

Absorption: Completely absorbed after oral administration, but 1st-pass metabolism results in 45% bioavailability.
Distribution: Unknown.
Metabolism and Excretion: Primarily metabolized by monoamine oxidase-A (MAO-A); minor conversion to an active compound; 14% excreted unchanged in urine.
Half-life: 2–3 hr.

TIME/ACTION PROFILE (blood levels)

ROUTE	ONSET	PEAK	DURATION
PO	30 min	1–1.5 hr	unknown

Contraindications/Precautions

Contraindicated in: Hypersensitivity; Ischemic or vasospastic cardiovascular, cerebrovascular, or peripheral vascular syndromes; History of significant cardiovascular disease; Uncontrolled hypertension; Should not be used within 24 hr of other 5-HT_1 agonists or ergot-type compounds (dihydroergotamine); Basilar or hemiplegic migraine; Concurrent MAO-A inhibitor therapy or within 2 wk of discontinuing MAO-A inhibitor therapy; Phenylketonuria (orally disintegrating tablet contains aspartame).
Use Cautiously in: Severe renal impairment, especially in patients on dialysis; Moderate hepatic impairment; Pregnancy, lactation, or children <18 yr (safety not established).
Exercise Extreme Caution in: Cardiovascular risk factors (hypertension, hypercholesterolemia, cigarette smoking, obesity, diabetes, strong family history, menopausal women or men >40 yr); use only if cardiovascular status has been evaluated and determined to be safe and first dose is administered under supervision.

Interactions

Drug-Drug: Concurrent use with **MAO-A inhibitors** ↑ blood levels and adverse reactions (concurrent use or use within 2 wk or MAO inhibitor is contraindicated). Concurrent use with other **5-HT agonists** or **ergot-type compounds (dihydroergotamine)** may result in ↑ vasoactive properties (avoid use within 24 hr of each other). **Propranolol** ↑ blood levels and risk of adverse reactions (dosage reduction recommended). Concurrent use with **SSRI antidepressants** may result in weakness, hyperreflexia, and incoordination.
Drug-Natural: ↑ risk of serotonergic side effects, including serotonin syndrome with **St. John's wort** and **SAMe.**

Route/Dosage

PO (Adults): 5–10 mg (use 5-mg dose in patients receiving propranolol); may be repeated in 2 hr; not to exceed 3 doses/24 hr. Dose is same for both types of tablets.

Availability

Tablets: 5 mg, 10 mg. **Orally disintegrating tablets (Maxalt-MLT) (peppermint flavor):** 5 mg, 10 mg.

roflumilast (row-floo-mi-last)

Daliresp

Classification

Therapeutic: agents for COPD.
Pharmacologic: phosphodiesterase inhibitors.

Indications

To ↓ the risk of exacerbations in severe COPD patients that have a history of chronic bronchitis with exacerbations.

Action

Roflumilast and 1 active metabolite (roflumilast N-oxide) act as selective inhibitors of phosphodiesterase-4 (PDE4), responsible for breaking down 3′,5′-adenosine monophosphate (cAMP). Resulting intracellular accumulation of cAMP in lung tissue. Reduces cells (neutrophils, eosinophils and total cells) in sputum. **Therapeutic Effects:** ↓ exacerbations in COPD patients.

Adverse Reactions/Side Effects

CNS: SUICIDAL THOUGHTS, anxiety, depression, dizziness, headache, insomnia. **GI:** diarrhea, abdominal pain, ↓ appetite, dyspepsia, gastritis, nausea, vomiting. **Metab:** weight loss. **MS:** muscle spasms. **Neuro:** tremor.

PHYSICAL THERAPY IMPLICATIONS

Examination and Evaluation

- Be alert for suicidal thoughts and ideology; notify physician immediately if patient exhibits suicidal behaviors, depression, anxiety, or other adverse changes in mood and behavior.
- Perform pulmonary function tests periodically (See Appendices I, J, K) to document effects of drug therapy on ventilation and respiratory function.
- Monitor any muscle spasms or tremor. Report any neuromuscular problems that affect gait or other functional activities.
- Assess dizziness that might affect gait, balance, and other functional activities (See Appendix C). Report balance problems and functional limitations to the physician and nursing staff, and caution the patient and family/caregivers to guard against falls and trauma.
- Periodically assess body weight and other anthropometric measures (body mass index, body composition). Report a rapid or unexplained weight loss or decreased body fat.

Interventions

- When implementing airway clearance techniques or respiratory muscle training, attempt to intervene when the airway is maximally bronchodilated. Peak responses typically occur about 1 hr after oral administration.

Patient/Client-Related Instruction

- Advise patient to not exceed the recommended dose or frequency of administration. Contact physician if COPD exacerbations are not adequately controlled by the current medication regimen, or if respiratory symptoms continue to worsen.
- Instruct patient and family/caregivers to report other troublesome side effects, including severe or prolonged headache, sleep loss, or GI problems (nausea, vomiting, diarrhea, indigestion, abdominal pain, decreased appetite).

Pharmacokinetics

Absorption: Well absorbed following oral administration.
Distribution: Parent drug and metabolites probably enter breast milk.
Protein Binding: *Roflumilast*—99%; *roflumilast N-oxide*—97%.
Metabolism and Excretion: Mostly metabolized (87.5%), primarily by CYP3A4 and CYP1A2 enzyme systems. 1 metabolite, roflumilast N-oxide, is pharmacologically active. Inactive metabolites excreted in urine.
Half-life: *Roflumilast*—17 hr; *roflumilast N-oxide*—30 hr.

TIME/ACTION PROFILE (blood levels)

ROUTE	ONSET	PEAK	DURATION
PO	unknown	1 (4–13*)	24 hr

*For roflumilast N-oxide.

Contraindications/Precautions

Contraindicated in: Acute bronchospasm. Moderate-to-severe hepatic impairment; Concurrent use of strong inducers of CYP3A4 and CYP1A2 enzyme systems; Lactation: Avoid breast-feeding.
Use Cautiously in: History of depression/suicidal thoughts; OB: Use only if potential maternal benefit justifies potential risk to the fetus; Pedi: Safe and effective use in children has not been established.

Interactions

Drug-Drug: Strong inducers of the CYP3A4 and CYP1A2 enzyme systems, including **rifampicin, phenobarbital, carbamazepine**, and **phenytoin,** ↓ blood levels and effectiveness; concurrent use should be avoided; Blood levels and risk of adverse reactions ↑ by concurrent use of **inhibitors of the CYP3A4 enzyme system and dual inhibitors of the CP3A4 and CYP1A2 enzyme systems,** including **erythromycin, ketoconazole, fluvoxamine, enoxacin,** and **cimetidine; Gestodene** and **ethinyl estradiol** may also ↑ levels and risk of adverse reactions; risk should be considered.

Route/Dosage

PO (Adults): 500 mcg once daily.

Availability

Tablets: 500 mcg.

romidepsin (roe-mi-dep-sin)

Istodax

Classification
Therapeutic: antineoplastics
Pharmacologic: enzyme inhibitors

Indications

Treatment of cutaneous T-cell lymphoma (CTCL) that has not responded to at least one prior systemic therapy.

Action

Acts as an inhibitor of histone deacetylase (HDAC). HDACs modulate gene expression and transcription factors. Inhibition results in cell cycle arrest and apoptosis; **Therapeutic Effects:** ↓ extent and spread of CTCL.

Adverse Reactions/Side Effects

CNS: fatigue. **CV:** ECG changes. **GI:** anorexia, nausea, vomiting. **Hemat:** ANEMIA, LEUKOPENIA, THROMBOCYTOPENIA.

PHYSICAL THERAPY IMPLICATIONS

Examination and Evaluation

- Watch for signs of leukopenia (fever, sore throat, other signs of infection), thrombocytopenia (bruising, nose bleeds, bleeding gums), or unusual weakness and fatigue that might be due to anemia. Report these signs to the physician or nursing staff immediately.
- Assess heart rate, ECG, and heart sounds, especially during exercise (See Appendices G, H). Report any rhythm disturbances or symptoms of increased arrhythmias, including palpitations, chest discomfort, shortness of breath, fainting, and fatigue/weakness.

Interventions

- For patients who are medically able to begin exercise, implement appropriate resistive exercises and aerobic training to maintain muscle strength and aerobic capacity during cancer chemotherapy or to help restore function after chemotherapy.
- Because of potential ECG changes, use caution during aerobic exercise and other forms of therapeutic exercise. Assess exercise tolerance frequently (blood pressure, heart rate, fatigue levels), and terminate exercise immediately if any untoward responses occur (See Appendix L).

Patient/Client-Related Instruction

- Advise patient and family/caregivers that fatigue and weakness are likely, and may be severe. Implement assistive devices (walker, cane, wheelchair) as needed to help maintain mobility and prevent falls.
- Instruct patient to report severe or prolonged GI problems, such as nausea, vomiting, and loss of appetite.

Pharmacokinetics

Absorption: IV administration results in complete bioavailability.
Distribution: Unknown.
Protein Binding: 92–94%.
Metabolism and Excretion: Extensively metabolized, mostly by the CYP3A4 enzyme system
Half-life: 3 hr.

TIME/ACTION PROFILE (response)

ROUTE	ONSET	PEAK	DURATION
IV	2 mo	4–6 mo	25–33 mo

Contraindications/Precautions

Contraindicated in: OB: Pregnancy (may cause fetal harm); Lactation: Avoid use.
Use Cautiously in: Congenital long QT syndrome, history of significant cardiovascular disease, concurrent antiarrhythmics or other medications that cause significant QT prolongation (↑ risk of arrhythmias); Electrolyte abnormalities (correct magnesium and potassium abnormalities prior to use); Moderate-to-severe hepatic impairment or end-stage renal disease; Geri: Elderly patients may be more sensitive to drug effects; Pedi: Safe and effective use in children has not been established.

Interactions

Drug-Drug: May ↑ risk of bleeding with **warfarin** or **NSAIDs;** May ↓ effectiveness of **estrogen-containing contraceptives** (competes with β-estradiol for binding to estrogen receptors); **Strong CYP3A4 inhibitors,** including **ketoconazole, itraconazole, clarithromycin, atazanavir, indinavir, nefazodone, nelfinavir, ritonavir, saquinavir, telithromycin,** and **voriconazole,** may ↑ levels and risk of toxicity; avoid concurrent use; **Strong CYP3A4 inducers,** including **dexamethasone, carbamazepine, phenytoin, rifampin, rifabutin, rifapentine,** and **Phenobarbital,** may ↓ levels and effectiveness; avoid concurrent use; **Drugs that inhibit P-gp,** including **amiodarone, atorvastatin, cyclosporine, dipyridamole, ketoconazole, nelfinavir, quinidine, quinine, reserpine, saquinavir, spironolactone, tacrolimus,** and **verapamil,** may ↑ levels and the risk of toxicity; use cautiously

Route/Dosage

IV (Adults): 14 mg/m^2 on days 1, 8, and 15 of a 28-day cycle, cycle may be repeated every 28 days depending on benefit and patient tolerance; dose may be ↓ to 10 mg/m^2 if adverse reactions occur.

Availability

Lyophilized powder for injection (requires reconstitution): 20 mg/vial (contains povidone; enclosed diluent contains propylene glycol and dehydrated alcohol).

romiplostim (roe-mi-**ploe**-stim)

Nplate

Classification

Therapeutic: antithrombocytopenics
Pharmacologic: thrombopoietin receptor agonists

Indications

Treatment of thrombocytopenia associated with chronic immune (idiopathic) thrombocytopenic purpura that has not responded to corticosteroids, immunoglobulins, or splenectomy where there is risk of bleeding.

Action

Acts as thrombopoietin (TPO) receptor agonist.
Therapeutic Effects: Improved platelet count with decreased sequelae of thrombocytopenia (bleeding).

Adverse Reactions/Side Effects

CNS: dizziness, insomnia, headache. **GI:** abdominal pain, dyspepsia. **Hemat:** bone marrow fibrosis, thrombosis/thromboembolism (dose related). **MS:** extremity pain, myalgia, arthralgia, shoulder pain. **Neuro:** paresthesia.

PHYSICAL THERAPY IMPLICATIONS

Examination and Evaluation

- Monitor abnormal blood coagulation, including venous thrombosis (lower extremity swelling, warmth, erythema, tenderness), arterial thrombosis (extreme coldness in the hands and feet, cyanosis, muscle cramping), and pulmonary embolism (shortness of breath, chest pain, cough, bloody sputum). Notify physician immediately, and request objective tests (Doppler ultrasound, others) if thrombosis is suspected.
- Monitor signs of anemia caused by bone marrow fibrosis. Signs include unusual fatigue, shortness of breath with exertion, pallor, and bruising. Notify physician immediately if these signs occur.
- Assess any muscle, joint, or extremity pain to rule out musculoskeletal pathology; that is, try to determine if pain is drug induced rather than caused by anatomic or biomechanical problems.
- Assess signs of paresthesia (numbness, tingling). Perform objective tests, including electroneuromyography and sensory testing to document any drug-related neuropathic changes.
- Assess dizziness that might affect gait, balance, and other functional activities (See Appendix C). Report balance problems and functional limitations to the physician, and caution the patient and family/caregivers to guard against falls and trauma.

Interventions

- Because of the risk of thromboembolism, use caution during aerobic exercise and other forms of therapeutic exercise. Assess exercise tolerance frequently (blood pressure, heart rate, fatigue levels), and terminate exercise immediately if any untoward responses occur (See Appendix L).
- If administered via local (subcutaneous) injection, do not apply massage or physical agents (heat, cold, electrotherapeutic modalities) at or near the application site. These interventions can affect drug absorption from subcutaneous tissues.

Patient/Client-Related Instruction

- Caution patient and family/caregivers about risks of thromboembolism, and review warning signs of these problems (see above under Evaluation and Examination).
- Instruct patient to report other troublesome side effects such as severe or prolonged headache, sleep loss, or GI problems (indigestion, abdominal pain).

Pharmacokinetics

Absorption: Well absorbed following subcutaneous administration.
Distribution: Binds to specific cellular receptors.
Metabolism and Excretion: Unknown.
Half-life: 1–34 days.

TIME/ACTION PROFILE

ROUTE	ONSET	PEAK	DURATION
SC	unknown	1 wk	2 wk

Contraindications/Precautions

Contraindicated in: None noted.
Use Cautiously in: Hepatic or renal impairment; Geri: Elderly patients may be more sensitive to effects, escalate dose cautiously, consider concurrent disease states, age-related decreases in organ function and drug therapy; OB: May cause fetal harm, enroll in registry; avoid use during lactation; Pedi: Safe use in children <18 yr not established.

Interactions

Drug-Drug: Drugs affecting platelet function should be avoided.

Route/Dosage

SC (Adults): 1 mcg/kg weekly; increase by 1 mcg/kg weekly to achieve and maintain platelet count of $\geq 50 \times 10^9$/L up to 10 mcg/kg.

Availability

Single-use vial (requires reconstitution): 250 mcg, 500 mcg.

ropinirole (roe-pin-i-role)

Requip, Requip XL

Classification
Therapeutic: antiparkinson agents
Pharmacologic: dopamine agonists

R

Indications

Management of signs and symptoms of idiopathic Parkinson's disease. Restless legs syndrome (immediate-release only).

Action

Stimulates dopamine receptors in the brain. **Therapeutic Effects:** Decreased tremor and rigidity in Parkinson's disease. Decreased leg restlessness.

Adverse Reactions/Side Effects

CNS: SLEEP ATTACKS, dizziness, syncope, confusion, drowsiness, fatigue, hallucinations, headache, ↑ dyskinesia, weakness. **EENT:** abnormal vision. **CV:** orthostatic hypotension, peripheral edema. **GI:** constipation, dry mouth, dyspepsia, nausea, vomiting. **Derm:** increased sweating.

PHYSICAL THERAPY IMPLICATIONS

Examination and Evaluation

- Be aware that ropinirole can cause sudden, unexpected episodes of falling asleep (sleep attacks). Use caution during activities in which patient might fall asleep suddenly.
- Assess gait and motor function to help determine antiparkinson effects, especially when starting drug therapy or during dosing changes or addition of other antiparkinson drugs. Motor function should be assessed at different times of the day, such as when drugs are reaching peak therapeutic levels (i.e., 30–60 min after oral dose), as well as when drug effects are minimal (just before the next dose).
- Document increased motor side effects such as involuntary movements (dyskinesias), fluctuations in response (on-off phenomenon, end-of-dose akinesia), or other abnormal movement patterns. Notify physician because increased motor side effects might require dose adjustment or a change in medication regimen.
- Monitor confusion, hallucinations, and other psychologic problems. Repeated or excessive symptoms may require change in dose or medication.
- Assess dizziness, drowsiness, and syncope that affects gait, balance, and other functional activities (See Appendix C). Report balance problems and functional limitations to the physician, and caution the patient and family/caregivers to guard against falls and trauma.
- Assess blood pressure (BP) when patient assumes a more upright position (lying to standing, sitting to standing, lying to sitting). Document orthostatic hypotension and contact physician when systolic BP falls >20 mm Hg, or diastolic BP falls >10 mm Hg.
- Assess peripheral edema using girth measurements, volume displacement, and measurement of pitting edema (See Appendix N). Report increased swelling in feet and ankles or a sudden increase in body weight due to fluid retention.
- If used to treat restless leg syndrome, assess the severity and frequency of restless episodes (i.e., an intense need to get up and move around) and lower extremity symptoms such as crawling, tingling, cramping, aching, burning, creeping, and similar sensations. Document whether drug therapy is effective in reducing these symptoms.

Interventions

- Implement therapeutic exercises (coordination exercises, gait training, cardiovascular conditioning) to complement the effects of drug therapy and help achieve optimal function.
- Guard against falls and trauma (hip fractures, head injury, and so forth). Implement fall- prevention strategies (See Appendix E), especially if patient exhibits Parkinson's symptoms (postural instability, rigidity) combined with drug side effects (dizziness, dyskinesias).
- To minimize orthostatic hypotension, patient should move slowly when assuming a more upright position.

Patient/Client-Related Instruction

- Advise patient and family or caregiver about the possibility of sleep attacks (see above under Examination and Evaluation).
- Advise patient to avoid alcohol because of the increased risk of sedation and adverse effects.
- Advise patient about the likelihood of GI reactions such as nausea, vomiting, constipation, indigestion, and dry mouth. Instruct patient to report severe or prolonged GI problems.
- Instruct patient to report other troublesome side effects such as severe or prolonged headaches, vision disturbances, or increased sweating.

Pharmacokinetics

Absorption: 55% absorbed following oral administration.
Distribution: Widely distributed.
Metabolism and Excretion: Extensively metabolized by the liver (by cytochrome P450 CYP1A2 enzyme system); <10% excreted unchanged in urine.
Half-life: 6 hr.

TIME/ACTION PROFILE

ROUTE	ONSET	PEAK	DURATION
PO	unknown	unknown	8 hr

Contraindications/Precautions

Contraindicated in: Hypersensitivity.
Use Cautiously in: Geri: ↑ risk of hallucinations in patients >65 yr; Hepatic impairment (slower titration may be required); Severe cardiovascular disease;

OB/Lactation/Pedi: Safety not established; may inhibit lactation.

Interactions

Drug-Drug: Drugs that alter the activity of cytochrome P450 CYP1A2 enzyme system may affect the activity of ropinirole. Effects may be ↑ by **estrogens**. Effects may be ↓ by **phenothiazines, butyrophenones, thioxanthenes,** or **metoclopramide.** May ↑ effects of **levodopa** (may allow dose reduction of levodopa).

Route/Dosage

PO (Adults): *Parkinson's disease*—Immediate-release: 0.25 mg tid for 1 wk, then 0.5 mg tid for 1 wk, then 0.75 mg tid for 1 wk, then 1 mg tid for 1 wk; then may ↑ by 1.5 mg/day every week, up to 9 mg/day; then may ↑ by up to 3 mg/day every week up to 24 mg/day; Extended-release: 2 mg once daily for 1–2 wk; may ↑ by 2 mg/day every week up to 24 mg/day. *Restless legs syndrome*—0.25 mg once daily initially, 1–3 hr before bedtime. After 2 days, ↑ to 0.5 mg once daily and to 1 mg once daily by the end of first week of dosing, then ↑ by 0.5 mg weekly, up to 4 mg/day as needed/tolerated.

Availability (generic available)

Tablets: 0.25 mg, 0.5 mg, 1 mg, 2 mg, 3 mg, 4 mg, 5 mg. **Extended-release tablets:** 2 mg, 3 mg, 4 mg, 8 mg.

ropivacaine (roe-piv-i-kane)

Naropin

Classification

Therapeutic: epidural local anesthetics, anesthetics (topical/local)

Indications

Local or regional anesthesia for surgery. Acute pain management.

Action

Local anesthetics inhibit initiation and conduction of sensory nerve impulses by altering the influx of sodium and efflux of potassium in neurons, slowing or stopping pain transmission. **Therapeutic Effects:** Decreased pain or induction of anesthesia; low doses have minimal effect on sensory or motor function; higher doses may produce complete motor blockade.

Adverse Reactions/Side Effects

CNS: SEIZURES, anxiety, dizziness, headache, rigors. **CV:** CARDIOVASCULAR COLLAPSE, arrhythmias, bradycardia, chest pain, hypertension, hypotension, tachycardia. **GI:** nausea, vomiting. **GU:** urinary retention. **Derm:** pruritus. **F and E:** hypokalemia, metabolic acidosis. **Hemat:** anemia. **Neuro:** circumoral tingling/numbness, paresthesia. **Resp:** dyspnea. **Misc:** allergic reactions, fever.

PHYSICAL THERAPY IMPLICATIONS

Examination and Evaluation

- Be alert for new seizures or increased seizure activity. Document the number, duration, and severity of seizures, and report these findings to the physician immediately.
- Monitor cardiac symptoms at rest and during exercise, and be alert for signs of severe cardiac insufficiency due to cardiac arrest (cardiovascular collapse). Seek immediate medical assistance if symptoms of cardiac arrest develop, including sudden chest pain, pain radiating into the arm or jaw, shortness of breath, dizziness, sweating, anxiety, and nausea.
- Assess heart rate, ECG, and heart sounds, especially during exercise (See Appendices G, H). Report any rhythm disturbances or symptoms of increased arrhythmias, including palpitations, chest discomfort, shortness of breath, fainting, and fatigue/weakness.
- Be alert for other signs of systemic toxicity including anxiety, confusion, nervousness, tremor, headache, blurred or double vision, nausea, vomiting, slurred speech, ringing in ears, tremors, twitching, difficulty breathing, hypotension, severe dizziness or fainting, and unusually slow heart rate. Report these signs to the physician or nursing staff immediately.
- Assess blood pressure (BP) and compare to normal values (See Appendix F). Report changes in BP, either a problematic decrease in BP (hypotension) or a sustained increase in BP (hypertension).
- Monitor signs of allergic reactions, including pulmonary symptoms (laryngeal edema, bronchospasm, wheezing, cough, dyspnea) or skin reactions (rash, pruritus, urticaria). Notify physician or nursing staff immediately if these reactions occur.
- Monitor signs of anemia, including unusual fatigue, shortness of breath with exertion, and bruising. Notify physician immediately if these signs occur.
- Monitor signs of metabolic acidosis including headache, lethargy, stupor, seizures, vision disturbances, increased respiration, cardiac arrhythmias, weakness, and GI symptoms (nausea, vomiting, abdominal pain). Notify physician immediately if these signs occur.

R

- Monitor and report any muscle weakness, aches, or cramps that might indicate low potassium levels (hypokalemia).
- Assess signs of paresthesia (numbness, tingling) or numbness around the mouth. Perform objective tests, including electroneuromyography and sensory testing to document any drug-related neuropathic changes.
- Assess dizziness that might affect gait, balance, and other functional activities (See Appendix C). Report balance problems and functional limitations to the physician and nursing staff, and caution the patient and family/caregivers to guard against falls and trauma.

Interventions

- Because of the risk of arrhythmias and cardiac arrest, use extreme caution during aerobic exercise and other forms of therapeutic exercise. Assess exercise tolerance frequently (BP, heart rate, fatigue levels), and terminate exercise immediately if any untoward responses occur (See Appendix L).
- Assess sensation to the affected area before applying physical agents (heat, cold, electrotherapy) or manual techniques. Use caution until the residual effects of local anesthesia have been resolved.

Patient/Client-Related Instruction

- Advise patient and family or caregivers about the signs of cardiac arrest (see above under Examination and Evaluation), and to seek immediate medical assistance if these signs develop.
- Instruct patient and family/caregivers to report other bothersome side effects such as severe or prolonged headache, anxiety, urinary retention, skin problems (rash, itching), or GI reactions (nausea, vomiting).

Pharmacokinetics

Absorption: Systemic absorption follows epidural administration, but amount absorbed depends on dose.
Distribution: If systemic absorption occurs, this agent is widely distributed and crosses the placenta.
Metabolism and Excretion: Small amounts that may reach systemic circulation are mostly metabolized by the liver; < 1% excreted unchanged in the urine.
Half-life: 4.2 hr (after epidural use).

TIME/ACTION PROFILE (analgesia)

ROUTE	ONSET	PEAK	DURATION
epidural	10–30 min	unknown	2–8 hr*

*Duration of anesthetic block.

Contraindications/Precautions

Contraindicated in: Hypersensitivity; cross-sensitivity with other amide local anesthetics may occur (bupivacaine, lidocaine, mepivacaine, prilocaine).

Use Cautiously in: Concurrent use of other local anesthetics; Liver disease; Concurrent use of anticoagulants (including low-dose heparin and low-molecular-weight heparins/heparinoids) ↑ the risk of spinal/epidural hematomas; Pedi: Safety not established.

Interactions

Drug-Drug: Additive toxicity may occur with concurrent use of other **amide local anesthetics** (including **lidocaine**, **mepivacaine**, and **prilocaine**). **Fluvoxamine**, **amiodarone**, **ciprofloxacin**, and **propofol** may ↑ the effects of ropivacaine.

Route/Dosage

Surgical Anesthesia

Epidural (Adults): *Lumbar epidural*—15–30 mL of 0.5% solution, or 15–25 mL of 0.75% solution, or 15–20 mL of 1% solution; *Lumbar epidural for cesarean section*—20–30 mL of 0.5% solution or 15–20 mL of 0.75% solution; *Thoracic epidural*—5–15 mL of 0.5–0.75% solution.
Major nerve block: (Adults): 35–50 mL of 0.5% solution or 10–40 mL of 0.75% solution.
Field block: (Adults): 1–40 mL of 0.5% solution.

Labor Pain

Epidural (Adults): *Lumbar epidural*—10–20 mL of 0.2% solution initially, then continuous infusion of 6–14 mL/hr of 0.2% solution with incremental injection of 10–15 mL/hr of 0.2% solution.

Postoperative Pain

Epidural (Adults): *Lumbar or thoracic epidural*—Continuous infusion of 6–14 mL/hr of 0.2% solution.
Infiltration (minor nerve block): (Adults): 1–100 mL of 0.2% solution or 1–40 mL of 0.5% solution.

Availability

Solution for injection (preservative-free): 0.2%, 0.5%, 0.75%, 1%.

rosiglitazone

(roe-zi-**glit**-a-zone)
Avandia

Classification
Therapeutic: antidiabetics
Pharmacologic: thiazolidinediones

Indications

Type 2 diabetes mellitus (with diet and exercise); may be used with metformin, sulfonylureas, or insulin.

Action

Improves sensitivity to insulin by acting as an agonist at receptor sites involved in insulin responsiveness and subsequent glucose production and utilization.

Requires insulin for activity. **Therapeutic Effects:** Decreased insulin resistance, resulting in glycemic control without hypoglycemia.

Adverse Reactions/Side Effects

CV: CHF, edema. **EENT:** new onset and worsening diabetic macular edema. **Derm:** urticaria. **GI:** hepatitis, ↑ liver enzymes. **Hemat:** anemia. **Metab:** LACTIC ACIDOSIS, ↑ total cholesterol, LDL and HDL, weight gain. **Misc:** angioedema (rare), fractures (arm, hand, foot) in female patients.

PHYSICAL THERAPY IMPLICATIONS

Examination and Evaluation

- Assess signs of congestive heart failure, including dyspnea, rales/crackles, peripheral edema, jugular venous distention, and exercise intolerance. Report these signs to the physician immediately.
- Monitor signs of lactic acidosis, especially during exercise. Signs include confusion, lethargy, stupor, shallow rapid breathing, tachycardia, hypotension, nausea, and vomiting. Notify physician immediately if these signs occur.
- Assess any pain that might indicate fractures, especially in the arms, hand, and feet in women. Protect and support any suspected fracture sites, and report the problem to the physician for further evaluation.
- Monitor signs of drug-induced hepatitis, including anorexia, abdominal pain, severe nausea and vomiting, yellow skin or eyes, skin rashes, flu-like symptoms, and muscle/joint pain. Report these signs to the physician.
- Be alert for signs of hypoglycemia, especially during and after exercise. Common neuromuscular signs include anxiety; restlessness; tingling in hands, feet, lips, or tongue; chills; cold sweats; confusion; difficulty in concentration; drowsiness; excessive hunger; headache; irritability; nervousness; tremor; weakness; unsteady gait. Report persistent or repeated episodes of hypoglycemia to the physician.
- Monitor signs of anemia, including unusual fatigue, shortness of breath with exertion, and bruising. Notify physician immediately if these signs occur.
- Monitor signs of angioedema, including rashes, raised patches of red or white skin (welts), burning/itching skin, swelling in the face, and difficulty breathing. Notify physician immediately of these signs.
- Periodically assess body weight and report a rapid or sustained weight gain. Advise patient that this drug may cause problems in fat metabolism, and that periodic blood tests may be needed to monitor plasma lipids.
- Assess blood pressure periodically (See Appendix F). A sudden or sustained increase in blood pressure (hypertension) may indicate problems in diabetes management and should be reported to the physician.

Interventions

- Implement aerobic exercise and endurance training programs to maintain optimal body weight, improve insulin sensitivity, and reduce the risk of macrovascular disease (heart attack, stroke) and microvascular problems (reduced blood flow to tissues and organs that causes poor wound healing, neuropathy, retinopathy, and nephropathy).
- Because of the risk of CHF and lactic acidosis, use extreme caution during aerobic exercise and other forms of therapeutic exercise. Assess exercise tolerance frequently (blood pressure, heart rate, fatigue levels), and terminate exercise immediately if any untoward responses occur (See Appendix L).

Patient/Client-Related Instruction

- Encourage patient to monitor blood glucose before and after exercise and to adjust food intake to maintain normal glycemic levels.
- Emphasize the importance of adhering to nutritional guidelines and the need for periodic assessment of glycemic control (serum glucose and glycosylated hemoglobin levels) throughout the management of diabetes mellitus.
- Instruct patient to report any vision disturbances, especially signs of macular edema (blurry or decreased central vision with peripheral vision intact).
- Advise patient about symptoms of hyperglycemia (confusion, drowsiness; flushed, dry skin; fruit-like breath odor; rapid, deep breathing, polyuria; loss of appetite; unusual thirst). Drug dosages may need to be adjusted to prevent repeated episodes of hyperglycemia.

Pharmacokinetics

Absorption: Well absorbed (99%) following oral administration.
Distribution: Unknown.
Protein Binding: 99.8% bound to plasma proteins.
Metabolism and Excretion: Entirely metabolized by the liver.
Half-life: 3.2–3.6 hr (increased in liver disease).

TIME/ACTION PROFILE (effects on blood glucose)

ROUTE	ONSET	PEAK	DURATION
PO	unknown	unknown	12–24 hr

Contraindications/Precautions

Contraindicated in: Hypersensitivity; Diabetic ketoacidosis; Clinical evidence of active liver disease or increased ALT (>2.5 times upper limit of normal);

R

Renal disease or dysfunction (creatinine over 1.5 mg/dL in males or 1.4 mg/dL in females; OB/Lactation: Potential for fetal or infant harm. Insulin monotherapy should be used; Pedi: Safety and effectiveness not established.

Use Cautiously in: Edema; CHF (avoid use in moderate to severe CHF unless benefits outweigh risks); Concurrent use with insulin (may increase risk of adverse cardiovascular reactions); Hepatic impairment; OB: May restore ovulation and risk of pregnancy in premenopausal women; Geri: Dose reduction and careful titration recommended due to age-related decline in renal function. Avoid maximum dose. Should not be given to patients older than 80 yr.

Interactions

Drug-Drug: Concurrent use with **rifampin** ↓ levels and may ↓ effectiveness. **Gemfibrozil** ↑ levels and may ↑ risk of hypoglycemia (↓ dose of rosiglitazone).

Drug-Natural: Glucosamine may worsen blood glucose control. **Chromium** and **coenzyme Q10** may produce additive hypoglycemic effects.

Route/Dosage

PO (Adults): 4 mg as a single dose once daily or 2 mg twice daily; after 8 wk, may be increased if necessary to 8 mg once daily or 4 mg bid.

Availability

Tablets: 2 mg, 4 mg, 8 mg. ***In combination with:*** metformin (Avandamet), glimepiride (Avandaryl). See Appendix B.

rosuvastatin
(roe-**soo**-va-sta-tin)
Crestor

Classification
Therapeutic: lipid-lowering agents
Pharmacologic: HMG CoA reductase inhibitors (statins)

Indications

Adjunctive management of primary hypercholesterolemia and mixed dyslipidemias.

Action

Inhibits 3-hydroxy-3-methylglutaryl coenzyme A (HMG CoA) reductase, an enzyme which is responsible for catalyzing an early step in the synthesis of cholesterol.

Therapeutic Effects: Lowering of total and LDL cholesterol and triglycerides. Slightly increases HDL cholesterol. Slows the progression of coronary atherosclerosis.

Adverse Reactions/Side Effects

CNS: weakness. **GI:** abdominal pain, constipation, nausea. **Derm:** rash. **Metab:** RHABDOMYOLYSIS, myalgia.

PHYSICAL THERAPY IMPLICATIONS

Examination and Evaluation

- Assess any joint pain or muscle pain, tenderness, or weakness, especially if accompanied by fever, malaise, and dark-colored urine. Advise patient that these symptoms may represent drug-induced myopathy, and that myopathy can progress to severe muscle damage (rhabdomyolysis). Report any unexplained musculoskeletal symptoms to the physician immediately, and suspend exercise and gait training until these symptoms can be evaluated.

Interventions

- In patients with drug-induced myopathy, implement gradual strengthening and other therapeutic exercises to facilitate recovery from muscle pain and weakness. Use caution during early stages to avoid fatigue of affected muscles, and implement assistive devices (walker, cane, crutches) as needed to prevent falls and assist mobility. Increase exercise intensity as tolerated; recovery from myopathy typically takes 4–6 wk, but can be longer in older patients or people with comorbidities.
- Design and implement aerobic exercise and endurance training programs to improve cardiovascular function and help reduce the risk of coronary heart disease.

Patient/Client-Related Instruction

- Remind patients to take medication as directed to control hyperlipidemia even though they are asymptomatic.
- Counsel patients about additional interventions to help control lipid disorders and improve cardiovascular health, including dietary modification, regular exercise, moderation of alcohol consumption, and smoking cessation.
- Instruct patient and family/caregivers to report other troublesome side effects such as severe or prolonged skin rash or GI problems such as nausea, constipation, and abdominal pain.

Pharmacokinetics

Absorption: 20% absorbed following oral administration.

Distribution: Unknown.

Metabolism and Excretion: 10% metabolized, 90% excreted unchanged in feces.

Half-life: 19 hr.

TIME/ACTION PROFILE (effect on lipids)

ROUTE	ONSET	PEAK	DURATION
PO	unknown	2–4 wk	unknown

Contraindications/Precautions

Contraindicated in: Hypersensitivity; Active liver disease or unexplained persistent elevations in AST & ALT; OB: Pregnancy or lactation.

Use Cautiously in: History of liver disease; Alcoholism; Renal impairment; Patients of Asian ancestry (may have ↑ blood levels and ↑ risk of rhabdomyolysis); Concurrent use of gemfibrozil, azole antifungals, protease inhibitors, niacin, cyclosporine, amiodarone, or verapamil (higher risk of myopathy/rhabdomyolysis); OB: Women of childbearing age; Pedi: Children (safety not established).

Interactions

Drug-Drug: Antacids ↓ absorption (administer 2 hr after rosuvastatin). **Cyclosporine** ↑ levels and risk of toxicity (dosage adjustment required). ↑ levels of **norgestrel** and **ethinyl estradiol**. Concurrent use of **fibrates** or **niacin** (↑ risk of rhabdomyolysis; avoid **gemfibrozil** if possible). May ↑ risk of bleeding with **warfarin** (monitor INR).

Drug-Food: Grapefruit juice ↑ blood levels and the risk of rhabdomyolysis.

Route/Dosage

PO (Adults): 10 mg once daily initially (range 5–20 mg initially); dose may be adjusted at 2- to 4-wk intervals, some patients may require up to 40 mg/day, however this dose is associated with ↑ risk of rhabdomyolysis; *Patients of Asian ancestry*—initial dose should be 5 mg; *concurrent cyclosporine therapy*—not to exceed 5 mg once daily; *concurrent gemfibrozil therapy*—not to exceed 10 mg once daily (avoid if possible).

Renal Impairment

PO (Adults): *CCr <30 mL/min*—5 mg once daily initially, may be increased to but not exceed 10 mg/day.

Availability

Tablets: 5 mg, 10 mg, 20 mg, 40 mg.

rotigotine transdermal system
(ro-ti-goe-teen)

Neupro

Classification

Therapeutic: antiparkinson agents

Pharmacologic: dopamine agonists

Indications

Symptomatic management of early-stage idiopathic Parkinson's disease.

Action

Acts as an agonist of dopamine in the CNS, primarily at D2 receptor sites. **Therapeutic Effects:** Improvement in symptoms of Parkinson's disease.

Adverse Reactions/Side Effects

CNS: DROWSINESS, insomnia, confusion, dizziness, hallucinations, headache, malaise, sudden sleep attacks. **CV:** peripheral edema, postural hypotension, syncope. **GI:** nausea, vomiting, anorexia, dry mouth, dyspepsia, ↑ liver enzymes. **GU:** urinary incontinence. **Derm:** application site reactions, ↑ risk of melanoma, ↑ sweating, pruritus, purpura. **Metab:** weight gain. **MS:** leg pain. **Neuro:** abnormal gait, ataxia, dyskinesia, hypertonia, hypoesthesia, neuralgia, paresthesia. **Misc:** fever.

PHYSICAL THERAPY IMPLICATIONS

Examination and Evaluation

- Be aware that rotigotine can cause severe drowsiness and sudden, unexpected episodes of falling asleep (sleep attacks). Use caution during activities where patient might fall asleep suddenly.
- Assess gait and motor function to help determine antiparkinson effects, especially when starting drug therapy or during dosing changes or addition of other antiparkinson drugs. Motor function should be assessed at different times of the day, such as when drugs are reaching peak therapeutic levels (i.e., 15–18 hr after applying the patch), as well as when drug effects are minimal (just before applying the next patch).
- Document increased side effects such as involuntary movements (dyskinesias) or fluctuations in response (on-off phenomenon, end-of-dose akinesia). Notify physician because increased side effects might require dose adjustment or a change in medication regimen.
- Monitor confusion, hallucinations, and other psychological problems. Repeated or excessive symptoms may require change in dose or medication.
- Assess blood pressure (BP) when patient assumes a more upright position (lying to standing, sitting to standing, lying to sitting). Document orthostatic hypotension and contact physician when systolic BP falls >20 mm Hg or diastolic BP falls >10 mm Hg.
- Assess peripheral edema using girth measurements, volume displacement, and measurement of pitting edema (See Appendix N). Report increased swelling in feet and ankles or a sudden increase in body weight due to fluid retention.
- Assess any nerve pain or signs of paresthesia (numbness, tingling). Perform objective tests,

R

including electroneuromyography and sensory testing to document any drug-related neuropathic changes.

- Assess dizziness and syncope that might affect gait, balance, and other functional activities (See Appendix C). Report balance problems and functional limitations to the physician, and caution the patient and family/caregivers to guard against falls and trauma.
- Periodically assess body weight and other anthropometric measures (body mass index, body composition). Report a rapid or unexplained weight gain or increased body fat.
- Monitor transdermal application site for skin reactions (rash, irritation, dermatitis). Report prolonged or excessive application site reactions to the physician.
- Report any suspicious skin lesions to the physician; this drug can increase melanoma risk.

Interventions

- Implement therapeutic exercises (coordination exercises, gait training, cardiovascular conditioning) to complement the effects of drug therapy and help achieve optimal function.
- Guard against falls and trauma (hip fractures, head injury, and so forth). Implement fall- prevention strategies (See Appendix E), especially if patient exhibits Parkinson's symptoms (postural instability, rigidity) combined with drug side effects (dizziness, ataxia, dyskinesias).
- To minimize orthostatic hypotension, patient should move slowly when assuming a more upright position.
- Avoid touching the transdermal application site, and do not apply massage or physical agents (heat, cold, electrotherapeutic modalities) at or near the application site.

Patient/Client-Related Instruction

- Advise patient and family/caregivers to follow instructions for transdermal (patch) application.
- Advise patient to avoid alcohol because of the increased risk of sedation and adverse effects.
- Because of an increased risk of melanoma, advise patient to check skin regularly and use sunscreens, protective clothing, and avoid prolonged sun exposure. Advise patient to report any suspicious skin lesions.
- Advise patient about the likelihood of GI reactions such as nausea, vomiting, loss of appetite, indigestion, and dry mouth. Instruct patient to report severe or prolonged GI problems.
- Instruct patient to report other bothersome side effects such as severe or prolonged headaches, fever, urinary incontinence, leg pain, sleep loss, and skin reactions (sweating, itching, bruising).

Pharmacokinetics

Absorption: 45% absorbed from patch over 24 hr.
Distribution: Unknown.
Metabolism and Excretion: Mostly metabolized and excreted in urine as metabolites (71%); 11% excreted in feces.
Half-life: Biphasic: initial half-life 3 hr; terminal half-life 5–7 hr.

TIME/ACTION PROFILE

ROUTE	ONSET	PEAK	DURATION
transdermal	1–3 hr	15–18 hr (range 4–27 hr)	24 hr

Contraindications/Precautions

Contraindicated in: Hypersensitivity to rotigotine or sulfites; OB: Lactation.
Use Cautiously in: Severe cardiovascular disease (may ↑ risk of postural hypotension); Severe hepatic impairment; Geri: Skin changes in patients >80 yr may result in higher blood levels; OB: use only if maternal benefits outweigh risk to fetus; Pedi: Safe use in children not established.

Interactions

Drug-Drug: Concurrent use of **dopamine antagonists**, including some **antipsychotics** or **metoclopramide**, may ↓ effectiveness.

Route/Dosage

Transdermal (Adults): 2 mg/24 hr initially; may increase by 2 mg/24 hr weekly, up to 6 mg/24 hr.

Availability

Transdermal system: 2 mg/24 hr (contains 4.5 mg rotigotine/10 cm^2), 4 mg/24 hr (contains 9 mg rotigotine/20 cm^2), 6 mg/24 hr (contains 13.5 mg rotigotine/30 cm^2).

rufinamide (roo-fin-a-mide)

Banzol

Classification
Therapeutic: anticonvulsants
Pharmacologic: triazoles

Indications

Adjunctive treatment of seizures associated with Lennox-Gastaut syndrome in patients older than 4 yr.

Action

Although antiepileptic mechanism is unknown, rufinamide modulates the activity of sodium channels, prolonging the inactive state of the channel. **Therapeutic Effects:** Decreased incidence and severity of seizures associated with Lennox-Gastaut syndrome.

Adverse Reactions/Side Effects

CNS: dizziness, fatigue, headache, somnolence, ↑ suicidal thoughts/behavior. **EENT:** diplopia. **CV:** QT prolongation. **GI:** nausea, changes in appetite. **GU:** urinary frequency. **Derm:** rash. **Hemat:** anemia. **Neuro:** ataxia, coordination abnormalities, gait disturbances. **Misc:** MULTI-ORGAN HYPERSENSITIVITY REACTIONS, hypersensitivity reactions (↑ children).

PHYSICAL THERAPY IMPLICATIONS

Examination and Evaluation

- Monitor signs of hypersensitivity reactions involving multiple organs and systems. Common signs include fever, skin rash, other skin reactions (itching, welts, dermatitis), hepatitis (anorexia, abdominal pain, severe nausea and vomiting, yellow skin or eyes, fever, sore throat, malaise, weakness, facial edema, lethargy, unusual bleeding or bruising), and pulmonary symptoms (tightness in the throat and chest, wheezing, cough, dyspnea). Notify physician immediately if these reactions occur.
- Document the number, duration, and severity of seizures to help determine if this drug is effective in reducing seizure activity.
- Assess heart rate, ECG, and heart sounds, especially during exercise (See Appendices G, H). Report any rhythm disturbances or symptoms of increased arrhythmias, including palpitations, chest discomfort, shortness of breath, fainting, and fatigue/weakness.
- Monitor signs of anemia, including unusual fatigue, shortness of breath with exertion, and bruising. Notify physician immediately if these signs occur.
- Assess dizziness that might affect gait, balance, and other functional activities (See Appendix C). Report balance problems and functional limitations to the physician, and caution the patient and family/caregivers to guard against falls and trauma.
- Monitor any behavioral changes or evidence of suicidal thoughts and behaviors. Notify physician or other mental health care professional immediately of these behaviors.
- Assess gait and motor function and document any signs of incoordination, ataxia, or gait disturbances. Report these signs to the physician.

Interventions

- Guard against falls and trauma (hip fractures, head injury, and so forth), especially if drowsiness, dizziness, or motor problems affect gait and balance. Implement fall prevention strategies, especially if balance is impaired (See Appendix E).

Patient/Client-Related Instruction

- Advise patient to avoid alcohol and other CNS depressants because of the increased risk of sedation and adverse effects.
- Advise patients on prolonged antiseizure therapy not to discontinue medication without consulting their physician. Abrupt withdrawal may cause increased seizures.
- Advise patient about the risk of daytime drowsiness and decreased attention and mental focus. Use care if driving or in other activities that require strong concentration and fast responses.
- Instruct patient and family/caregivers to report other troublesome side effects such as severe or prolonged headache, double vision, skin rash, urinary frequency, or GI problems (nausea, change in appetite).

Pharmacokinetics

Absorption: 85% absorbed following oral administration; food enhances absorption.
Distribution: Evenly distributed between erythrocytes and plasma.
Metabolism and Excretion: Extensively metabolized; metabolites are primarily renally excreted.
Half-life: 6–10 hr.

TIME/ACTION PROFILE

ROUTE	ONSET	PEAK	DURATION
PO	unknown	4–6 hr	12 hr

Contraindications/Precautions

Contraindicated in: Hypersensitivity; Familial short QT syndrome; Severe hepatic impairment.
Use Cautiously in: History of suicidal thoughts or behavior; Mild-to-moderate hepatic impairment.

Interactions

Drug-Drug: Potent inducers of the CYP450 enzyme, including **carbamazepine**, **phenytoin**, **primidone**, and **Phenobarbital,** ↑ clearance and may ↓ blood levels. **Valproate** ↓ clearance and may ↑ blood levels; valproate should be started at a low dose in patients stabilized on rufinamide. In patients stabilized on valproate, rufinamide should be started at a low dose. May ↓ blood levels and effectiveness of **hormonal contraceptives**. May ↑ blood levels of **phenytoin**.

Route/Dosage

PO (Adults): 400–800 mg/day in 2 divided doses; increase by 400–800 mg q 2 days until a maximum daily dose of 3200 mg/day (1600 mg bid) is reached.
PO (Children ≥4 yr): 10 mg/kg/day in 2 divided doses; ↑ by 10 mg/kg q 2 days until a maximum daily dose of 45 mg/kg/day or 3200 mg/day given in 2 divided doses, whichever is less, is reached.

Availability

Tablets: 200 mg.

salmeterol (sal-met-er-ole)

Serevent

Classification

Therapeutic: bronchodilators

Pharmacologic: adrenergics

Indications

Long-term control of reversible airway obstruction due to asthma and for maintenance treatment of asthma and prevention of bronchospasm. Prevention of exercise-induced asthma. Maintenance treatment to prevent bronchospasm in COPD, including chronic bronchitis and emphysema.

Action

Produces accumulation of cyclic adenosine monophosphate (cAMP) at $beta_2$-adrenergic receptors. Relatively specific for beta (pulmonary) receptors. **Therapeutic Effects:** Bronchodilation.

Adverse Reactions/Side Effects

CNS: headache, nervousness. **CV:** palpitations, tachycardia. **GI:** abdominal pain, diarrhea, nausea. **MS:** muscle cramps/soreness. **Neuro:** trembling. **Resp:** paradoxical bronchospasm, cough.

PHYSICAL THERAPY IMPLICATIONS

Examination and Evaluation

- Assess pulmonary function at rest and during exercise (See Appendices I, J, K) to document effectiveness of medication in controlling bronchospasm.
- Watch for signs of paradoxical bronchospasm (wheezing, cough, dyspnea, tightness in chest and throat), especially at higher doses or during excessive use of the inhaler. If condition occurs, advise patient to withhold medication and notify physician or other health care professional immediately.
- Assess heart rate, ECG, and heart sounds, especially during exercise (See Appendices G, H). Report a rapid heart rate (tachycardia) or signs of other arrhythmias, including palpitations, chest discomfort, shortness of breath, fainting, and fatigue/weakness.
- Monitor and report signs of CNS toxicity, including nervousness or trembling. Sustained or severe CNS signs may indicate overdose or excessive use of this drug.
- Assess any muscle cramps or soreness. Report severe or prolonged musculoskeletal symptoms.

Interventions

- When implementing airway clearance techniques or respiratory muscle training, attempt to intervene when the airway is maximally bronchodilated. Peak responses typically occur about 3–4 hr after inhalation.
- Because of the risk of cardiovascular stimulation, use caution during aerobic exercise and endurance conditioning. Cardiac effects should be minimal at lower doses or occasional inhaled use. Cardiovascular effects such as arrhythmias, angina pectoris, or increased blood pressure (BP) may occur at higher doses or during excessive use, and are caused by inadvertent stimulation of beta receptors on the heart.

Patient/Client-Related Instruction

- Advise patient not to exceed the recommended dose or frequency of inhalations. Contact physician immediately if bronchospasm is not relieved by medication or is accompanied by diaphoresis, dizziness, or other symptoms.
- Counsel patient on proper use of inhaler; observe use of this device whenever possible to ensure proper technique.
- Instruct patient and family/caregivers to report severe or prolonged headache or GI problems (nausea, diarrhea, abdominal pain).

Pharmacokinetics

Absorption: Minimal systemic absorption follows inhalation.

Distribution: Action is primarily local.

Metabolism and Excretion: Unknown.

Half-life: 3–4 hr.

TIME/ACTION PROFILE (bronchodilation)

ROUTE	ONSET	PEAK	DURATION
inhalation	10–25 min	3–4 hr	12 hr*

*9 hr in adolescents.

Contraindications/Precautions

Contraindicated in: Hypersensitivity; Acute attack of asthma (onset of action is delayed).

Use Cautiously in: Cardiovascular disease (including angina and hypertension); Convulsive disorders; Diabetes; Glaucoma; Hyperthyroidism; Pheochromocytoma; Excessive use (may lead to tolerance and paradoxical bronchospasm); OB/Lactation/Pedi: Pregnancy, lactation, or children <4 yr (dry powder inhalation may be used in children 4–12 yr; aerosol inhalation may be used in children >12 yr; may inhibit contractions during labor).

Interactions

Drug-Drug: Beta blockers may ↓ therapeutic effects of salmeterol. **MAO inhibitors** and **tricyclic antidepressants** potentiate cardiovascular effects. ↑ levels and ↑ risk

S

of cardiovascular effects when used with potent CYP3A4 inhibitors (e.g., **ketoconazole, itraconazole, ritonavir, atazanavir, clarithromycin, indinavir, nefazodone, nelfinavir, or saquinavir**); concurrent use is not recommended.

Drug-Natural: Use with caffeine-containing herbs **(cola nut, guarana, mate, tea, coffee)** ↑ stimulant effect.

Route/Dosage

Inhalation (Adults and Children ≥4 yr): Diskus—50 mcg (1 inhalation as dry powder) bid (approximately 12 hr apart); Inhaler—42 mcg (2 puffs) bid (12 hr apart); *Exercise-induced bronchospasm*—Inhaler: 42 mcg (2 puffs) 30–60 min before exercise.

Availability

Powder for inhalation (Serevent Diskus): 50 mcg/blister. **Aerosol for oral inhalation (Serevent Inhaler):** 25 mcg/actuation (delivers 21 mcg/inhalation) 6.5 g (60 inhalations), 13 g (120 inhalations). ***In combination with:*** fluticasone (Advair Diskus). See Appendix B.

salsalate (sal-sa-late)

Amigesic, Anaflex, Disalcid, Marthritic, Mono-Gesic, Salflex, Salgesic, Salsitab

Classification

Therapeutic: antipyretics, nonopioid analgesics
Pharmacologic: salicylates

Indications

Inflammatory disorders, including Rheumatoid arthritis, Osteoarthritis. Mild-to-moderate pain. Fever.

Action

Produce analgesia and reduce inflammation and fever by inhibiting the production of prostaglandins.

Therapeutic Effects: Analgesia. Reduction of inflammation. Reduction of fever.

Adverse Reactions/Side Effects

EENT: tinnitus. **GI:** GI BLEEDING, dyspepsia, epigastric distress, nausea, abdominal pain, anorexia, hepatotoxicity, vomiting. **Derm:** EXFOLIATIVE DERMATITIS, STEVENS-JOHNSON SYNDROME, TOXIC EPIDERMAL NECROLYSIS. **Misc:** ALLERGIC REACTIONS, INCLUDING ANAPHYLAXIS AND LARYNGEAL EDEMA.

PHYSICAL THERAPY IMPLICATIONS

Examination and Evaluation

- Monitor signs of GI bleeding, including abdominal pain, vomiting blood, blood in stools, or black, tarry stools. Report these signs to the physician immediately.
- Monitor signs of allergic reactions and anaphylaxis, including pulmonary symptoms (laryngeal edema, wheezing, cough, dyspnea) or skin reactions (rash, pruritus, urticaria, dermatitis, exfoliation). Be especially alert for severe skin reactions that may indicate Stevens-Johnson syndrome or toxic epidermal necrosis. Notify physician immediately if these reactions occur. Allergic reactions are more common in people with asthma, nasal polyps, or aspirin-induced allergies.
- Assess pain and other variables (range of motion, muscle strength) to document whether this drug is successful in helping manage the patient's pain and decreasing impairments.
- Assess blood pressure (BP) periodically and compare to normal values (See Appendix F). Salicylates and other NSAIDs can increase BP in certain patients.
- Be alert for signs of hepatotoxicity, including anorexia, abdominal pain, severe nausea and vomiting, yellow skin or eyes, fever, sore throat, malaise, weakness, facial edema, lethargy, and unusual bleeding or bruising. Report these signs to the physician immediately.

Interventions

- Implement appropriate manual therapy techniques, physical agents, and therapeutic exercises to reduce pain and decrease the need for salicylates and other NSAIDs.
- Help patient explore other nonpharmacologic methods to reduce chronic pain, such as relaxation techniques, exercise, counseling, and so forth.

Patient/Client-Related Instruction

- Advise patient that analgesics are usually more effective if given before pain becomes severe; emphasize that adequate pain control will allow better participation in physical therapy.
- Advise patient about the risks of gastric irritation. Instruct patient to notify health care professional of GI effects such as severe or prolonged nausea, vomiting, heartburn, indigestion, loss of appetite, and abdominal pain.
- Advise patient to reduce alcohol intake because alcohol increases the risk of gastric toxicity.
- Inform patient that salicylates and other NSAIDs may impair bone and cartilage healing. Advise patient to consult physician about salicylate use, especially after fractures, spinal fusion, and other bone surgeries.
- Instruct patient to report excessive or prolonged headache or ringing/buzzing in the ears (tinnitus); these signs may indicate salicylate toxicity.
- Caution patient about the use of over-the-counter products that contain aspirin, other NSAIDs, or acetaminophen while taking high doses of

salicylates. Use of multiple NSAIDs increases the risk of toxicity and overdose.

Pharmacokinetics

Absorption: Splits into 2 molecules of salicylic acid after oral administration; absorbed in the small intestine.
Distribution: Rapidly and widely distributed; crosses the placenta and enters breast milk.
Metabolism and Excretion: Extensively metabolized by the liver; inactive metabolites excreted by the kidneys. Amount excreted unchanged by the kidneys depends on urine pH; as pH increases, amount excreted unchanged increases from 2–3% up to 80%.
Half-life: 2–3 hr for low doses; up to 15–30 hr with larger doses because of saturation of liver metabolism.

TIME/ACTION PROFILE

ROUTE	ONSET	PEAK	DURATION
PO	5–30 min	1–3 hr	3–6 hr

Contraindications/Precautions

Contraindicated in: Hypersensitivity to aspirin or other salicylates; Cross-sensitivity with other NSAIDs may exist (less with nonaspirin salicylates); Perioperative pain from coronary artery bypass graft (CABG) surgery; Pedi: May increase the risk of Reye's syndrome in children or adolescents with viral infections.
Use Cautiously in: Cardiovascular disease or risk factors for cardiovascular disease (may ↑ risk of serious cardiovascular thrombotic events, myocardial infarction, and stroke, especially with prolonged use); History of GI bleeding or ulcer disease; Chronic alcohol use/abuse; Severe hepatic disease; OB: Salicylates may have adverse effects on fetus and mother and should be avoided during pregnancy, especially during the 3rd trimester; Lactation: Safety not established; Geri: ↑ risk of adverse reactions, especially GI bleeding; more sensitive to toxic levels).

Interactions

Drug-Drug: May ↑ activity of **penicillins, phenytoin, methotrexate, valproic acid, oral hypoglycemic agents,** and **sulfonamides.** May ↓ beneficial effects of **probenecid** or **sulfinpyrazone. Urinary acidification** ↑ reabsorption and may ↑ serum salicylate levels. **Alkalinization of the urine** or the ingestion of large amounts of **antacids** ↑ excretion and ↓ serum salicylate levels. May blunt the therapeutic response to **diuretics** or other **antihypertensives.** ↑ risk of GI irritation with **NSAIDs.**
Drug-Food: Foods capable of acidifying the urine (See Appendix L) may ↑ serum salicylate levels.

Route/Dosage

PO (Adults): 1 g 3 tid initially; further titration may be required.

Availability

Tablets: 500 mg, 750 mg.

samarium Sm 153 lexidronam

(sa-**mar**-ee-yum leks-i-**droe**-nam)
Quadramet

Classification
Therapeutic: nonopioid analgesics
Pharmacologic: radiopharmaceuticals

Indications

Treatment of bone pain in patients with confirmed osteoblastic skeletal metastases that enhance on radionuclide bone scan. **Unlabeled Use:** Ankylosing spondylitis, Paget's disease, rheumatoid arthritis.

Action

Preferentially taken up by bone tumors and metastatic bone lesions, where selective irradiation takes place.
Therapeutic Effects: Decreased pain from bony metastases.

Adverse Reactions/Side Effects

CV: arrhythmias, hypertension. **Hemat:** anemia, neutropenia, thrombocytopenia. **MS:** transient increase in bone pain.

PHYSICAL THERAPY IMPLICATIONS

Examination and Evaluation

- Assess heart rate, ECG, and heart sounds, especially during exercise (See Appendices G, H). Report any rhythm disturbances or symptoms of increased arrhythmias, including palpitations, chest discomfort, shortness of breath, fainting, and fatigue/weakness.
- Assess blood pressure (BP) and compare to normal values (See Appendix F). Report a sustained increase in BP (hypertension).
- Be alert for neutropenia (fever, sore throat, signs of infection), thrombocytopenia (bruising, nose bleeds, and bleeding gums), or unusual weakness and fatigue that might be due to anemia. Notify physician or nursing staff of these symptoms.
- Assess musculoskeletal pain and other variables (range of motion, muscle strength) to document whether this drug is successful in helping manage the patient's pain and decreasing impairments.

S

Monitor any transient increase in bone pain, and report a sustained or severe increase in musculoskeletal pain.

Interventions

- Implement appropriate manual therapy techniques, physical agents, and therapeutic exercises to reduce pain and decrease the need for analgesic drugs.
- Because of the risk of arrhythmias and abnormal BP responses, use caution during aerobic exercise and other forms of therapeutic exercise. Assess exercise tolerance frequently (BP, heart rate, fatigue levels), and terminate exercise immediately if any untoward responses occur (See Appendix L).
- Help patient explore other nonpharmacologic methods to reduce chronic pain, such as relaxation techniques, exercise, counseling, and so forth.

Pharmacokinetics

Absorption: IV administration results in complete bioavailability.
Distribution: Taken up and is selectively retained by metastatic bone lesions.
Metabolism and Excretion: Unbound drug is excreted in urine.
Half-life: 65 min (radioactivity).

TIME/ACTION PROFILE (pain relief)

ROUTE	ONSET	PEAK	DURATION
IV	1–2 wk	unknown	unknown

Contraindications/Precautions

Contraindicated in: Hypersensitivity; Pregnancy or lactation.
Use Cautiously in: Women with childbearing potential; Diminished bone marrow reserve or other chronic debilitating illness (allow recovery from previous treatments); Patients with a life expectancy <6 mo; Children <16 yr (safety not established).

Interactions

Drug-Drug: Additive bone marrow toxicity with **antineoplastics** or previous **radiation therapy**.

Route/Dosage

IV (Adults): 1 millicuries (mCi)/kg.

Availability

Radioactive Injection: 1850 megabecquerels/mL (50 mCi/mL) in 2-mL fill- and 3-mL fill-vials.

sapropterin (sap-roe-**ter**-in)

Kuvan

Classification
Therapeutic: antihyperphenylalaninemics
Pharmacologic: synthetic BH4

Indications

To reduce phenylalanine (Phe) levels in patients with hyperphenylalaninemia (HPA) caused by tetrahydrobiopterin (BH4)-responsive phenylketonuria (PKU); used with a Phe-restricted diet.

Action

Acts as a synthetic form of the cofactor (BH4) for the enzyme phenylalanine hydroxylase (PAH). PAH converts phenylalanine to tyrosine. In PKU patients, activity of PAH is deficient. BH4 helps to activate PAH and thus reduce Phe levels. **Therapeutic Effects:** Preservation of brain function by lowering Phe levels.

Adverse Reactions/Side Effects

CNS: headache. **EENT:** pharyngolaryngeal pain.
GI: abdominal pain, diarrhea, nausea, vomiting.
Hemat: neutropenia.

PHYSICAL THERAPY IMPLICATIONS

Examination and Evaluation

- Assess any pain in the laryngeal or pharyngeal areas. Report severe or prolonged pharyngeal or laryngeal pain.
- Monitor signs of neutropenia, including fever, sore throat, and signs of infection. Report these signs to the physician.

Patient/Client-Related Instruction

- Instruct patient to report other bothersome side effects such as severe or prolonged headache or GI problems (nausea, vomiting, diarrhea, abdominal pain).

Pharmacokinetics

Absorption: Well absorbed following oral administration; food increases absorption.
Distribution: Unknown.
Metabolism and Excretion: Unknown.
Half-life: 6.7 hr.

TIME/ACTION PROFILE (effect on Phe levels)

ROUTE	ONSET	PEAK	DURATION
PO	within 24 hr	up to 1 mo	unknown

Contraindications/Precautions

Contraindicated in: Lactation: Should not be used if breast-feeding.
Use Cautiously in: Hepatic or renal impairment; Concurrent use of levodopa; OB: Use during pregnancy only if clearly needed; Pedi: Safety and effectiveness in children <4 yr not established.

Interactions

Drug-Drug: Concurrent use of **medications known to inhibit folate metabolism,** including **methotrexate,** can ↓ BH4 levels; use cautiously. Concurrent use of **medications known to affect nitric**

oxide–mediated vasorelaxation, including **sildenafil, vardenafil,** or **tadalafil** could ↑ risk of hypotension. Concurrent use of **levodopa,** may ↑ risk of seizures, overstimulation, and irritability; use cautiously.

Route/Dosage

PO (Adults): 10 mg/kg once daily, titrated on the basis of Phe levels (range 5–20 mg/kg/day).

Availability

Tablets: 100 mg.

saquinavir (sa-kwin-a-vir)

Invirase

Classification
Therapeutic: antiretrovirals
Pharmacologic: protease inhibitors

Indications

HIV infection with ritonavir (may also add other antiretrovirals).

Action

Inhibits the action of HIV protease and prevents the cleavage of viral polyproteins. **Therapeutic Effects:** Slowing of the progression of HIV infection and its sequelae. Increased CD4 cell counts and decreased viral load.

Adverse Reactions/Side Effects

CNS: SEIZURES, confusion, headache, mental depression, psychic disorders, weakness. **CV:** thrombophlebitis. **GI:** abdominal discomfort, diarrhea, increased liver enzymes, jaundice, nausea. **Derm:** photosensitivity, severe cutaneous reactions. **Endo:** hyperglycemia. **Hemat:** acute myeloblastic leukemia, hemolytic anemia, thrombocytopenia. **Neuro:** ataxia. **Misc:** STEVENS-JOHNSON SYNDROME.

PHYSICAL THERAPY IMPLICATIONS

Examination and Evaluation

- Be alert for new seizures or increased seizure activity, especially at the onset of drug treatment. Document the number, duration, and severity of seizures, and report these findings immediately to the physician.
- Monitor rashes or other skin reactions (hives, acne, abnormal sweating, exfoliation). Notify physician immediately because certain skin reactions may indicate serious hypersensitivity reactions (Stevens-Johnson syndrome).
- Assess any signs of thrombophlebitis, including localized pain, redness, or swelling in the affected area. Report these signs to the physician, and avoid exercising the affected extremity while awaiting further tests and evaluation.
- Assess weakness or ataxia that might affect gait, balance, and other functional activities. Report balance problems and functional limitations to the physician, and caution the patient and family/caregivers to guard against falls and trauma.
- Monitor signs of thrombocytopenia (bruising, nose bleeds and bleeding gums), hemolytic anemia (weakness, fatigue, dizziness, jaundice, abdominal pain), or unusual weakness and fatigue that might be due to other anemias and leukemias. Report these signs to the physician.
- Monitor confusion, headache, mental depression, personality changes, and increased thoughts of suicide. Notify physician if these changes become problematic.

Interventions

- Implement resistive exercises and other therapeutic exercises as needed to maintain muscle strength and function, and prevent muscle wasting associated with HIV infection and AIDS.
- Design and implement aerobic exercise and endurance training programs to help prevent heart disease associated with drug-related hyperlipidemia and other problems with lipid and glucose metabolism.
- Causes photosensitivity; use care if administering UV treatments.

Patient/Client-Related Instruction

- Emphasize the importance of taking saquinavir as directed even if the patient is asymptomatic, and that this drug must always be used in combination with other antiretroviral drugs. Do not take more than prescribed amount, and do not stop taking without consulting health care professional.
- Inform patient that saquinavir does not cure HIV or AIDS or prevent associated or opportunistic infections. Saquinavir does not reduce the risk of transmission of HIV to others through sexual contact or blood contamination. Caution patient to use a condom, and to avoid sharing needles or donating blood to prevent spreading the AIDS virus to others.
- Advise patient about photosensitivity, and to use sunscreens, protective clothing, and avoid prolonged sun exposure. Advise patient to also report any rashes or other skin reactions.
- Advise patient about symptoms of hyperglycemia (confusion, drowsiness; flushed, dry skin; fruit-like breath odor; rapid, deep breathing, polyuria; loss of appetite; unusual thirst). Patients with diabetes should check blood glucose levels frequently.

Pharmacokinetics

Absorption: Incompletely absorbed after oral administration; rapidly undergoes extensive 1st-pass hepatic metabolism. Absorption of Invirase and Fortovase is not the same; products are not interchangeable.
Distribution: Distributes into tissues, but CNS penetration is poor.
Protein Binding: 98%.
Metabolism and Excretion: Mostly metabolized by the liver. <1% excreted unchanged in urine.
Half-life: 13 hr.

TIME/ACTION PROFILE (blood levels)

ROUTE	ONSET	PEAK	DURATION
PO	unknown	unknown	8 hr

Contraindications/Precautions

Contraindicated in: Hypersensitivity; Concurrent dihydroergotamine (or other ergot derivatives), midazolam, rifabutin, rifampin, lovastatin, simvastatin, and triazolam; OB: Lactation (breast-feeding not recommended in HIV infection).
Use Cautiously in: Diabetes mellitus (may exacerbate hyperglycemia; hyperglycemia may progress to ketoacidosis); Hemophilia (↑ risk of bleeding); Hepatic impairment (may exacerbate liver dysfunction caused by hepatitis B or C or other causes); **OB, Pedi:** Pregnancy or children <16 yr (safety not established).

Interactions

Drug-Drug: **Rifampin** and **rifabutin** significantly ↓ saquinavir levels; concurrent use is contraindicated. **Dihydroergotamine** and **ergotamine** (↑ risk of vasoconstriction); **midazolam** and **triazolam** (↑ CNS depression); **lovastatin** and **simvastatin** (↑ risk of myopathy); concurrent use is contraindicated. Coadministration with **clarithromycin** significantly ↑ saquinavir levels and ↓ clarithromycin levels. Saquinavir levels are also significantly ↑ by **indinavir, delavirdine, nelfinavir, ritonavir,** and **ketoconazole** (dose adjustments may be necessary). **Carbamazepine, phenobarbital, phenytoin, nevirapine,** and **dexamethasone** may ↓ saquinavir levels. Concurrent use with proton pump inhibitors may ↑ saquinavir levels. May ↑ serum cortisol levels with **fluticasone.** May ↑ serum **trazodone** levels.
Drug-Natural: St. John's wort ↓ levels and effectiveness; may promote development of drug resistance.
Drug-Food: Grapefruit juice ↑ serum levels and effects. Food significantly ↑ the absorption of saquinavir. **Garlic** can significantly ↓ levels.

Route/Dosage

Invirase

PO (Adults): 600 mg tid within 2 hr of a meal *or* 1000 mg bid.

Availability

Invirase

Capsules: 200 mg. **Tablets:** 500 mg.

sargramostim

(sar-**gram**-oh-stim)
Leukine

OTHER NAMES:
rHu GM-CSF (recombinant human granulocyte/macrophage colony-stimulating factor)

Classification
Therapeutic: colony-stimulating factors
Pharmacologic: biologic response modifiers

Indications

Acceleration of bone marrow recovery after Autologous bone marrow transplantation in patients with non-Hodgkin's lymphoma, acute lymphoblastic leukemia, or Hodgkin's disease, Allogenic bone marrow transplantation from HLA-matched donors. Management of bone marrow transplant failure or engraftment delay. After induction chemotherapy for acute myelogenous leukemia (AML) in patients ≥55 yr. Mobilization and after transplant of autologous peripheral blood progenitor cells (PBPCs); increases harvest by leukapheresis.

Action

Consists of a glycoprotein produced by recombinant DNA technique that is capable of binding to and stimulating the production, division, differentiation, and activation of granulocytes and macrophages.
Therapeutic Effects: Accelerated recovery of bone marrow after autologous bone marrow transplantation, resulting in decreased risk of infection and other complications.

Adverse Reactions/Side Effects

CNS: headache, malaise, weakness. **Resp:** dyspnea. **CV:** pericardial effusion, peripheral edema, transient supraventricular tachycardia. **GI:** diarrhea. **Derm:** itching, rash. **MS:** arthralgia, bone pain, myalgia. **Misc:** chills, fever, 1st-dose reaction.

PHYSICAL THERAPY IMPLICATIONS

Examination and Evaluation

- Assess heart rate, ECG, and heart sounds, especially during exercise (See Appendices G, H). Report any rhythm disturbances or symptoms of increased arrhythmias, including palpitations, chest discomfort, shortness of breath, fainting, and fatigue/weakness.

- Assess peripheral edema using girth measurements, volume displacement, and measurement of pitting edema (See Appendix N). Report increased swelling in feet and ankles or a sudden increase in body weight due to fluid retention.
- Be alert for signs of pericardial effusion, including chest pain, dyspnea, shortness of breath when reclining, dry cough, low grade fever, fainting, dizziness, tachycardia, and a feeling of anxiety. Report these signs to the physician.
- Assess any bone, joint, or muscle pain to rule out musculoskeletal pathology; that is, try to determine if pain is drug induced rather than caused by anatomic or biomechanical problems.

Interventions

- For patients with cancer who are medically able to begin exercise, implement appropriate resistive exercises and aerobic training to maintain muscle strength and aerobic capacity during cancer chemotherapy, or to help restore function after chemotherapy.
- Because of the risk of arrhythmias and pericardial effusion, use caution during exercise, and terminate exercise if patient exhibits untoward symptoms (chest pain, severe shortness of breath, fatigue), or displays other criteria for exercise termination (See Appendix L).

Patient/Client-Related Instruction

- Instruct patient or family/caregivers to report other troublesome side effects, including severe or prolonged headache, chills, fever, diarrhea, or skin problems (rash, itching).

Pharmacokinetics

Absorption: After IV administration, absorption is essentially complete. Well absorbed after subcut administration.
Distribution: Unknown.
Metabolism and Excretion: Unknown.
Half-life: Unknown.

TIME/ACTION PROFILE (noted as effects on blood counts)

ROUTE	ONSET	PEAK	DURATION
SC, IV	rapid	unknown	3–7 days

Contraindications/Precautions

Contraindicated in: Presence of ≥10% leukemic myeloid blast cells in bone marrow or peripheral blood; Hypersensitivity to granulocyte/macrophage colony-stimulating factor (GM-CSF), yeast products, or additives (mannitol, tromethamine, or sucrose); Products containing benzyl alcohol should not be used in newborns.

Use Cautiously in: Preexisting fluid retention, CHF, or pulmonary infiltrates; Preexisting cardiac disease; Myeloid malignancies; Previous extensive radiation or chemotherapy (response may be limited); OB: Pregnancy (use only if clearly needed); Lactation or children (safety not established).

Interactions

Drug-Drug: Lithium or **corticosteroids** may potentiate myeloproliferative effects of sargramostim (concurrent use should be undertaken cautiously).

Route/Dosage

After Bone Marrow Transplantation

IV (Adults): 250 mcg/m²/day for 21 days.

Failure/Delay of Engraftment after Bone Marrow Transplantation

IV (Adults): 250 mcg/m²/day for 14 days; may be repeated after a 7-day rest between courses; if results are inadequate, a 3rd course at 500 mcg/m²/day for 14 days may be given after a 7-day rest.

After Chemotherapy for AML

IV (Adults): 250 mcg/m²/day started around day 11 or 4 days after induction if day 10 bone marrow is hypoplastic with <5% blast cells and continued until absolute neutrophil count (ANC) >1500 cells/mm³ for 3 consecutive days (not to exceed 42 days); if adverse reactions occur, ↓ dose by 50% or temporarily discontinue.

Mobilization of PBPCs

IV, SC (Adults): 250 mcg/m²/day continued throughout collection of PBPCs.

After PBPC Transplantation

IV, SC (Adults): 250 mcg/m²/day continued until ANC >1500 cells/mm³ for 3 consecutive days.

Availability

Powder for injection: 250 mcg/vial, 500 mcg/vial.

saxagliptin (saks-a-glip-tin)

Onglyza

Classification
Therapeutic: antidiabetics
Pharmacologic: dipeptidyl peptidase-4 inhibitors

Indications

Adjunct with diet and exercise to improve glycemic control in adults with type 2 diabetes mellitus.

Action

Acts as a competitive inhibitor of dipeptidyl peptidase-4 (DPP4) which slows inactivation of incretin hormones,

S

thereby increasing their concentrations and reducing fasting and postprandial glucose concentrations; **Therapeutic Effects:** Improved control of blood glucose.

Adverse Reactions/Side Effects

CNS: headache. **CV:** peripheral edema (↑ with thiazolidinediones). **GI:** abdominal pain, vomiting. **Hemat:** ↓ lymphocyte count. **Endo:** hypoglycemia (↑ with sulfonylureas). **Misc:** hypersensitivity reactions, including urticaria and facial edema.

PHYSICAL THERAPY IMPLICATIONS

Examination and Evaluation

- Monitor signs of hypersensitivity reactions, including pulmonary symptoms (tightness in the throat and chest, wheezing, cough, dyspnea) and skin reactions (rash, pruritus, urticaria, burning skin, exfoliation, swelling in the face). Notify physician immediately of these signs.
- Be alert for signs of hypoglycemia, especially during and after exercise. Common neuromuscular signs include anxiety; restlessness; tingling in hands, feet, lips, or tongue; chills; cold sweats; confusion; difficulty in concentration; drowsiness; excessive hunger; headache; irritability; nervousness; tremor; weakness; unsteady gait. Report persistent or repeated episodes of hypoglycemia to the physician.
- Assess blood pressure periodically (See Appendix F). A sudden or sustained increase in blood pressure (hypertension) may indicate problems in diabetes management and should be reported to the physician.
- Assess peripheral edema using girth measurements, volume displacement, and measurement of pitting edema (See Appendix N). Report increased swelling in feet and ankles or a sudden increase in body weight due to fluid retention.

Interventions

- Implement aerobic exercise and endurance training programs to maintain optimal body weight, improve insulin sensitivity, and reduce the risk of macrovascular disease (heart attack, stroke) and microvascular problems (reduced blood flow to tissues and organs that causes poor wound healing, neuropathy, retinopathy, and nephropathy).

Patient/Client-Related Instruction

- Encourage patient to monitor blood glucose before and after exercise, and to adjust food intake to maintain normal glycemic levels.
- Emphasize the importance of adhering to nutritional guidelines and the need for periodic assessment of glycemic control (serum glucose and glycosylated hemoglobin levels) throughout the management of diabetes mellitus.
- Advise patient about symptoms of hyperglycemia (confusion, drowsiness; flushed, dry skin; fruit-like breath odor; rapid, deep breathing, polyuria; loss of appetite; unusual thirst). Drug dosages may need to be adjusted to prevent repeated episodes of hyperglycemia.
- Instruct patient to report other troublesome side effects such as severe or prolonged headache or GI problems (vomiting, abdominal pain).

Pharmacokinetics

Absorption: Well absorbed following oral administration.
Distribution: Unknown.
Metabolism and Excretion: Metabolized by the liver via the P450 3A4/5 (CYP3A4/5) enzyme system, with conversion to 5-hydroxysaxagliptin, a pharmacologically active metabolite; 24% of saxagliptin is excreted unchanged in urine, 36% of hydroxysaxagliptin is excreted unchanged in urine, 22% is eliminated in feces as unabsorbed drug/metabolites excreted in bile.
Half-life: *Saxagliptin*—2.5 hr; *5-hydroxysaxagliptin*—3.1 hr

TIME/ACTION PROFILE (DDP-4 inhibition)

ROUTE	ONSET	PEAK	DURATION
PO	unknown	2 hr (4 hr for 5-hydroxysaxagliptin)*	24 hr

*Blood levels.

Contraindications/Precautions

Contraindicated in: Type 1 diabetes; Diabetic ketoacidosis.
Use Cautiously in: Geri: May be more sensitive to effects; consider age-related ↓ in renal function; OB: Use only if clearly needed; Lactation: Use cautiously; Pedi: Safety and effectiveness not established.

Interactions

Drug-Drug: Strong **CYP3A4/5 inhibitors,** including **ketoconazole, atazanavir, clarithromycin, indinavir, itraconazole, nefazodone, nelfinavir, ritonavir, saquinavir,** and **telithromycin,** ↑ blood levels; daily dose should not exceed 2.5 mg; ↑ risk of hypoglycemia with **sulfonylureas.**

Route/Dosage

PO (Adults): 2.5–5 mg once daily; *Strong P450 3A4/5 (CYP3A4/5) inhibitors*—2.5 mg once daily.

Renal Impairment

PO (Adults): *CCr ≤50 mL/min*—2.5 mg once daily.

Availability

Tablets: 2.5 mg, 5 mg
In combination with: metformin XR (Kombiglyze XR). See Appendix B.

scopolamine (skoe-**pol**-a-meen)

Isopto Hyoscine, Transderm-Scop, ✱Transderm-V

Classification
Therapeutic: antiemetics
Pharmacologic: anticholinergics

Indications

Transdermal: Prevention of motion sickness. Management of nausea and vomiting associated with opioid analgesia or general anesthesia/recovery from anesthesia. **IM, IV, SC:** Preoperatively to produce amnesia and to decrease salivation and excessive respiratory secretions.

Action

Inhibits the muscarinic activity of acetylcholine. Corrects the imbalance of acetylcholine and norepinephrine in the CNS, which may be responsible for motion sickness. **Therapeutic Effects:** Reduction of nausea and vomiting. Preoperative amnesia and decreased secretions.

Adverse Reactions/Side Effects

CNS: drowsiness, confusion. **EENT:** blurred vision, mydriasis, photophobia. **CV:** tachycardia, palpitations. **GI:** dry mouth, constipation. **GU:** urinary hesitancy, urinary retention. **Derm:** decreased sweating.

PHYSICAL THERAPY IMPLICATIONS

Examination and Evaluation

- Assess heart rate, ECG, and heart sounds, especially during exercise (See Appendices G, H). Report a rapid heart rate (tachycardia) or signs of other arrhythmias, including palpitations, chest discomfort, shortness of breath, fainting, and fatigue/weakness.
- Be alert for decreased sweating and increased body temperature (hyperthermia), especially during exercise. Notify physician of a prolonged or persistent elevation in body temperature.
- Monitor any improvements in symptoms (nausea, vomiting, dizziness) to help document the effects of this drug.
- Monitor signs of urine retention (difficult urination, painful or distended abdomen). Excessive urinary retention may require dose adjustment by physician.

Interventions

- Because of the risk of arrhythmias and impaired thermoregulation, use caution during aerobic exercise and other forms of therapeutic exercise. Assess exercise tolerance frequently (blood pressure, heart rate, fatigue levels), and terminate exercise immediately if any untoward responses occur (See Appendix L).

Patient/Client-Related Instruction

- Instruct patient and family/caregivers to report other troublesome side effects such as severe or prolonged confusion, drowsiness, vision problems or GI problems (constipation, dry mouth).

Pharmacokinetics

Absorption: Well absorbed following IM, SC, and transdermal administration.
Distribution: Crosses the placenta and blood-brain barrier.
Metabolism and Excretion: Mostly metabolized by the liver.
Half-life: 8 hr.

TIME/ACTION PROFILE (antiemetic, sedative properties)

ROUTE	ONSET	PEAK	DURATION
PO, IM, SC	30 min	1 hr	4–6 hr
IV	10 min	1 hr	2–4 hr
Transdermal	4 hr	unknown	72 hr

Contraindications/Precautions

Contraindicated in: Hypersensitivity; Hypersensitivity to bromides (injection only); Angle-closure glaucoma; Acute hemorrhage; Tachycardia secondary to cardiac insufficiency or thyrotoxicosis.
Use Cautiously in: OB/Geri: Geriatric patients, infants, and children (↑ risk of adverse reactions); Possible intestinal obstruction; Prostatic hyperplasia; Chronic renal, hepatic, pulmonary, or cardiac disease; OB: Pregnancy or lactation (safety not established; to minimize exposure to fetus, apply 1 hr prior to cesarean section.

Interactions

Drug-Drug: ↑ anticholinergic effects with **antihistamines, antidepressants, quinidine,** or **disopyramide.** ↑ CNS depression with **alcohol, antidepressants, antihistamines, opioid analgesics,** or **sedative/hypnotics.** May alter the absorption of other **orally administered drugs** by slowing motility of the GI tract. May ↑ GI mucosal lesions in patients taking oral **wax-matrix potassium chloride preparations. Drug-Natural:** ↑ anticholinergic effects with **jimson weed** and **scopolia.**

Route/Dosage

Transdermal (Adults): *Motion sickness*—1.5 mg Transderm-Scop system delivers 1 mg over 72 hr; apply 4 hr prior to travel (US product); *Recovery from anesthesia/surgery*—1.5 mg Transderm-Scop system delivers 1 mg over 72 hr; apply evening before surgery or 1 hr prior to cesarean section.

IM, IV, SC (Adults): *Antiemetic/anticholinergic*—0.3–0.6 mg; *antisecretory effect*—0.2–0.6 mg; *amnestic effect*—0.32–0.65 mg; *sedation*—0.6 mg tid–qid.
IM, IV, SC (Children): *Antiemetic/anticholinergic*—6 mcg/kg or 0.2 mg/m².
IM (Children 8–12 yr): *Antisecretory*—0.3 mg.
IM (Children 3–8 yr): *Antisecretory*—0.2 mg.
IM (Children 7 mo–3 yr): *Antisecretory*—0.15 mg.
IM (Children 4–7 mo): *Antisecretory*—0.1 mg.

Availability (generic available)

Transdermal therapeutic system: Transderm-Scop—1.5 mg scopolamine/patch releases 0.5 mg scopolamine over 3 days in packs of 4 units, Transderm-V—1.5 mg scopolamine/patch releases 1 mg scopolamine over 3 days.
Injection: 0.3 mg/mL in 1-mL vials, 0.4 mg/mL in 0.5-mL ampules and 1-mL vials, 0.86 mg/mL in 0.5-mL ampules, 1 mg/mL in 1-mL vials.

secobarbital

(see-koe-**bar**-bi-tal)

Novosecobarb, Seconal

Classification
Therapeutic: sedative/hypnotics
Pharmacologic: barbiturates

Schedule II

Indications

Short-term treatment of insomnia. Adjunctive agent for anesthesia.

Action

Produces CNS depression through gamma-aminobutyric acid (GABA)–like effects. **Therapeutic Effects:** Induction of sleep, sedation, or anesthesia.

Adverse Reactions/Side Effects

CNS: abnormal thinking, behavior changes, delirium, excess sedation, excitation, hallucinations, mental depression, vertigo, sleep disorders, sleep—driving. **Resp:** respiratory depression. **GI:** nausea, vomiting. **Derm:** photosensitivity, rashes, urticaria. **MS:** arthralgia, myalgia. **Neuro:** neuralgia. **Misc:** physical dependence, psychologic dependence.

PHYSICAL THERAPY IMPLICATIONS

Examination and Evaluation

- Assess symptoms of respiratory depression (dyspnea, cyanosis). Monitor pulse oximetry and perform pulmonary function tests (See Appendices I, J, K) to quantify suspected changes in ventilation and respiratory function. Excessive respiratory depression requires emergency care.
- Monitor daytime drowsiness. Repeated or excessive drowsiness may require change in dose or medication.
- Assess dizziness and vertigo that might affect gait, balance, and other functional activities (See Appendix C). Report balance problems and functional limitations to the physician and nursing staff, and caution the patient and family/caregivers to guard against falls and trauma.
- Report any personality and behavioral changes, including excitation, hallucinations, mental depression, delirium, or expression of abnormal thoughts.
- Assess any muscle, joint, or nerve pain to rule out musculoskeletal pathology; that is, try to determine if pain is drug induced rather than caused by biomechanical or neurophysiologic problems.

Interventions

- Guard against falls and trauma (hip fractures, head injury, and so forth), especially if drowsiness and vertigo carry over into the daytime. Implement fall prevention strategies, especially if balance is impaired (See Appendix E).
- Causes photosensitivity; use care if administering UV treatments. Advise patient to avoid direct sunlight and use sunscreens and protective clothing.
- Help patient explore nonpharmacologic methods to induce sleep, such as relaxation techniques, reduced caffeine intake, and so forth.

Patient/Client-Related Instruction

- Advise patient to avoid alcohol and other CNS depressants because of the increased risk of sedation and adverse effects.
- Remind patient that this drug is typically recommended for only occasional use as a preoperative sedative or short-term use (2 wk or less) to treat insomnia. Long-term use can cause tolerance and dependence.
- Advise patient about the risk of daytime drowsiness and decreased attention and mental focus. Use care if driving or in other activities that require strong concentration.
- Caution patient and family/caregivers about the risk of other bizarre or complex somnolent behaviors, such as driving while asleep.
- Instruct patient or family/caregivers to report other severe or prolonged side effects such as sleep disorders, skin reactions (rash, hives), or GI problems (nausea, vomiting).

Pharmacokinetics

Absorption: Well absorbed following oral administration.
Distribution: Widely distributed; highest concentration in brain and liver. Crosses the placenta; small amounts enter breast milk.
Metabolism and Excretion: Metabolized by the liver.

Protein Binding: 55%.
Half-life: 30 hr.

TIME/ACTION PROFILE (hypnotic effect)

ROUTE	ONSET	PEAK	DURATION
PO	10–15 min	2–4 hr	6–8 hr

Contraindications/Precautions

Contraindicated in: Hypersensitivity; Preexisting CNS depression; Uncontrolled severe pain; Porphyria; OB: Pregnancy or lactation.

Use Cautiously in: Hepatic or renal impairment; Geri: Appears on Beers' list. Geriatric patients are at ↑ risk for side effects (dose reduction recommended); Chronic obstructive pulmonary disease; Prolonged use (may lead to physical and psychologic dependence).

Interactions

Drug-Drug: Additive CNS depression with **alcohol, antihistamines, antidepressants, opioid analgesics,** and other **sedative/hypnotics. Valproates** may ↓ metabolism and ↑ CNS depression. Stimulates hepatic enzymes, which metabolize other drugs, resulting in ↓ effectiveness of **hormonal contraceptives, chloramphenicol, cyclosporine, corticosteroids, dacarbazine, levothyroxine,** and **quinidine.**

Drug-Natural: See **sedative/hypnotic drug-drug** interactions above. **St. John's wort** may ↓ secobarbital levels and effect. Concomitant use of **kava, valerian, chamomile,** or **hops** can ↑ CNS depression.

Route/Dosage

PO (Adults): *Preoperative sedation*—200–300 mg 1–2 hr before surgery; *bedtime hypnotic*—100 mg.

PO (Children): *Preoperative sedation*—2–6 mg/kg (not to exceed 100 mg).

Availability

Capsules: 100 mg. ***In combination with:*** amobarbital (Tuinal).

selegiline (se-lee-ji-leen)

Apo-Selegiline, Carbex, Eldepryl, Gen-Selegiline, Nu-Selegiline, Novo-Selegiline, SD-Deprenyl, Zelapar

Classification
Therapeutic: antiparkinson agents
Pharmacologic: monoamine oxidase type B inhibitors

Indications

Management of Parkinson's disease (with levodopa or levodopa/carbidopa) in patients who fail to respond to levodopa/carbidopa alone.

Action

Following conversion by MAO to its active form, selegiline inactivates MAO by irreversibly binding to it at type B (brain) sites. Inactivation of MAO leads to increased amounts of dopamine available in the CNS. **Therapeutic Effects:** Increased response to levodopa/dopamine therapy in Parkinson's disease.

Adverse Reactions/Side Effects

CNS: confusion, dizziness, fainting, hallucinations, insomnia, vivid dreams. **GI:** <u>nausea</u>, abdominal pain, dry mouth.

PHYSICAL THERAPY IMPLICATIONS

Examination and Evaluation

- Assess gait and motor function to help determine antiparkinson effects, especially when starting drug therapy, or during dosing changes or addition of other antiparkinson drugs. Motor function should be assessed at different times of the day, such as when drugs are reaching peak therapeutic levels (i.e., 30–60 min after oral dose), as well as when drug effects are minimal (just before the next dose).
- Document increased motor side effects such as involuntary movements (dyskinesias), fluctuations in response (on-off phenomenon, end-of-dose akinesia), or other abnormal movement patterns. Notify physician because increased motor side effects might require dose adjustment or a change in medication regimen.
- Monitor confusion, hallucinations, and other psychologic problems. Repeated or excessive symptoms may require change in dose or medication.
- Assess dizziness and fainting that affects gait, balance, and other functional activities (see Appendix C). Report balance problems and functional limitations to the physician, and caution the patient and family/caregivers to guard against falls and trauma.

Interventions

- Implement therapeutic exercises (coordination exercises, gait training, cardiovascular conditioning) to complement the effects of drug therapy and help achieve optimal function.
- Guard against falls and trauma (hip fractures, head injury, and so forth). Implement fall-prevention strategies (See Appendix E), especially if patient exhibits Parkinson's symptoms (postural instability, rigidity) combined with drug side effects (dizziness, fainting).

Patient/Client-Related Instruction

- Advise patient to avoid alcohol because of the increased risk of sedation and adverse effects.
- Instruct patient to report other troublesome side effects such as severe or prolonged sleep loss, vivid dreams, or GI reactions (nausea, abdominal pain, dry mouth).

S

Pharmacokinetics

Absorption: Appears to be well absorbed following oral administration.
Distribution: Widely distributed.
Metabolism and Excretion: Metabolism involves some conversion to amphetamine and methamphetamine. 45% excreted in urine as metabolites.
Half-life: Unknown; orally disintegrating tablets 1.3 hr.

TIME/ACTION PROFILE (onset of beneficial effects in Parkinson's disease)

ROUTE	ONSET	PEAK	DURATION
PO	2–3 days	40–90 min	unknown
Orally disintegrating	5 min	10–15 min	unknown

Contraindications/Precautions

Contraindicated in: Hypersensitivity; Concurrent meperidine or opioid analgesic therapy (possible fatal reactions); Concurrent use of SSRIs or tricyclic antidepressants.
Use Cautiously in: Doses >10 mg/day (↑ risk of hypertensive reactions with tyramine-containing foods and some medications); History of peptic ulcer disease.

Interactions

Drug-Drug: Concurrent use with **meperidine** or other **opioid analgesics** may possibly result in a potentially fatal reaction (excitation, sweating, rigidity, and hypertension; or hypotension and coma). Serotonin syndrome (confusion, agitation, hyperpyrexia, hypertension, seizures) may occur with concurrent use of **nefazolone** or **SSRI antidepressants** (fluoxetine should be discontinued 5 wk prior to selegiline, **venlafaxine** should be discontinued 7 days before selegiline, other agents should be discontinued 2 wk before selegiline). Selegiline should be discontinued 2 wk before **SSRIs** are initiated. Concurrent use with **tricyclic antidepressants** may result in asystole, diaphoresis, hypertension, syncope, behavioral changes, altered consciousness, hyperpyrexia, tremors, muscle rigidity, and seizures (avoid concurrent use; discontinue selegiline 2 wk before initiating tricyclic antidepressant therapy). May initially ↑ risk of side effects of **levodopa/carbidopa** (dosage of levodopa/carbidopa may need to be ↓ by 10–30%).
Drug-Food: Doses >10 mg/day may produce hypertensive reactions with **tyramine-containing foods**.

Route/Dosage

PO (Adults): 5 mg bid, with breakfast and lunch (some patients may require further dividing of doses—2.5 mg qid).
PO (Adults): *Orally disintegrating tablets*—1.25 mg once daily for at least 6 wk. After 6 wk, may ↑ to 2.5 mg if effect not achieved and patient is tolerating medication.

Availability (generic available)

Capsules: 5 mg. **Tablets:** 5 mg. **Orally-disintegrating tablets:** 1.25 mg.

selegiline transdermal
(se-**lee**-ji-leen)
Emsam

Classification
Therapeutic: antidepressants
Pharmacologic: monoamine oxidase type B inhibitors

Indications

Major depressive disorder.

Action

Following conversion by MAO to its active form, selegiline inactivates MAO by irreversibly binding to it at type B (brain) sites; this results in higher levels of monoamine neurotransmitters in the brain (dopamine, serotonin, norepinephrine). **Therapeutic Effects:** Decreased symptoms of depression.

Adverse Reactions/Side Effects

CNS: insomnia, abnormal thinking, agitation, amnesia, worsening of mania/hypomania. **EENT:** tinnitus. **Resp:** ↑ cough. **CV:** HYPERTENSIVE CRISIS, chest pain, orthostatic hypotension, peripheral edema. **GI:** diarrhea, altered taste, anorexia, constipation, flatulence, gastroenteritis, vomiting. **GU:** dysmenorrhea, metrorrhagia, urinary frequency. **Derm:** application-site reactions, acne, ecchymoses, pruritus, sweating. **MS:** myalgia, neck pain, pathologic fracture. **Neuro:** paresthesia.

PHYSICAL THERAPY IMPLICATIONS

Examination and Evaluation

- Measure blood pressure (BP) periodically and compare to normal values (See Appendix F). Immediately report a large, rapid increase in BP (hypertensive crisis). Signs and symptoms of hypertensive crisis include chest pain, tachycardia or bradycardia, severe headache, nausea, vomiting, neck stiffness, sweating, and enlarged pupils. The risk of hypertensive crisis is increased when this drug is taken with other antidepressants, excessive caffeine, other drugs that increase BP, or foods that contain tyramine (e.g., fermented wines, cheeses).
- Be alert for increased depression, especially in the initial period of drug therapy and in children and teenagers. Notify physician or mental health

professional immediately if patient exhibits worsening depression or other changes in mood and behavior.

- Be alert for agitation, memory problems, abnormal thoughts, or other alterations in mental status. Notify health care professional if these symptoms become problematic.
- Assess BP when patient assumes a more upright position (lying to standing, sitting to standing, lying to sitting). Document orthostatic hypotension and contact the physician when systolic BP falls >20 mm Hg, or diastolic BP falls >10 mm Hg.
- Assess peripheral edema using palpation, girth measurements, and volume displacement. Report increased swelling in feet and ankles or other signs of edema caused by fluid retention.
- Assess any muscle or neck pain, or pain that might indicate fractures. Protect and support any suspected fracture sites, and report the problem to the physician for further evaluation.
- Assess paresthesias (numbness, tingling), and perform objective tests, including electroneuromyography and sensory testing to document any drug-related neuropathic changes.
- Monitor transdermal application site for skin reactions (rash, irritation, dermatitis). Report prolonged or excessive application site reactions to the physician.

Interventions

- To minimize orthostatic hypotension, patient should move slowly when assuming a more upright position.
- Avoid touching the transdermal application site, and do not apply massage or physical agents (heat, cold, electrotherapeutic modalities) at or near the application site.
- Help patient explore nonpharmacologic methods to reduce depression, such as exercise, counseling, support groups, and so forth.

Patient/Client-Related Instruction

- Advise patient and family/caregivers to follow instructions for transdermal (patch) application.
- Advise patient that antidepressant effects may not occur immediately; it may take 2 wk or more before an improvement in mood is observed.
- Advise patient to avoid alcohol and other CNS depressants because of the increased risk of sedation and adverse effects.
- Instruct patient to report other troublesome side effects such as severe or prolonged headache, cough, ringing/buzzing in the ears (tinnitus), menstrual problems, urinary frequency, sleep loss, skin problems (acne, bruising, sweating, itching), or GI problems (constipation, diarrhea, vomiting, flatulence, loss of appetite, abdominal pain, altered taste).

Pharmacokinetics

Absorption: 25–30% of patch content is transdermally absorbed; blood levels are higher than those following oral administration because there is less 1st-pass hepatic metabolism.
Distribution: Rapidly distributes to all body tissues; crosses the blood-brain barrier.
Metabolism and Excretion: Mostly metabolized by the liver, primarily by the CYP2A6, CYP2C9, and CYP3A4/5 enzyme systems. 10% excreted in urine as metabolites, 2% in feces; negligible renal excretion of unchanged drug.
Half-life: 18–25 hr.

TIME/ACTION PROFILE

ROUTE	ONSET	PEAK	DURATION
transdermal	unknown	2 or more weeks	2 wk (after discontinuation)

Contraindications/Precautions

Contraindicated in: Hypersensitivity; Pheochromocytoma; Concurrent selective serotonin reuptake inhibitors (fluoxetine, paroxetine citalopram, escitalopram, and others), nonselective serotonin reuptake inhibitors (venlafaxine, duloxetine), tricyclic antidepressants (amitriptyline, imipramine, and others), carbamazepine, oxcarbazepine, amphetamines, vasoconstrictors (ephedrine, pseudoephedrine), bupropion, meperidine, tramadol, methadone, propoxyphene, dextromethorphan, mirtazapine cyclobenzaprine, other MAO inhibitors (isocarboxazid, phenelzine, tranylcypromine), oral selegiline, sympathomimetic amines, amphetamines, cocaine or local anesthetics with vasoconstrictors; St. John's wort; Alcohol.
Use Cautiously in: Elective surgery within 10 days; benzodiazepines, mivacurium, rapacuronium, fentanyl, morphine, and codeine may be used cautiously; May ↑ risk of suicide attempt/ideation, especially during early treatment or dose adjustment; risk may be greater in children or adolescents (safe use in children <12 yr not established); History of mania; Dosing at 9 mg/24 hr or 12 mg/24 hr requires dietary modification (avoid foods containing large amounts of tyramine); Geri: May be more susceptible to orthostatic hypotension; OB: Use only if benefit outweighs risk to the fetus; Lactation: Safety not established; Pedi: Safe use in children and adolescents not established.

Interactions

Drug-Drug: Concurrent **selective serotonin reuptake inhibitors (fluoxetine, paroxetine, citalopram, escitalopram,** and others), **nonselective serotonin**

S

reuptake inhibitors (venlafaxine, duloxetine), tricyclic antidepressants (amitriptyline, imipramine, and others), **carbamazepine, oxcarbazepine, amphetamines, vasoconstrictors (ephedrine, pseudoephedrine, phenylpropanolamine), bupropion, meperidine, tramadol, methadone, propoxyphene, dextromethorphan, mirtazapine, cyclobenzaprine,** other MAO inhibitors (**isocarboxazid, phenelzine, tranylcypromine**), oral **selegiline, sympathomimetic amines, amphetamines, cocaine,** or **local anesthetics with vasoconstrictors;** these may all ↑ risk of hypertensive crisis. (**Fluoxetine** should not be used within 2 wk of initiating therapy.) **Drug-Natural: St. John's wort** may ↑ risk of hypertensive crisis.

Route/Dosage

Transdermal (Adults): 6 mg/24 hr, if necessary, may be increased at 2-wk intervals in increments of 3 mg, up to 12 mg/24 hr.

Availability

Transdermal patch: 6 mg/24 hr, 9 mg/24 hr, 12 mg/24 hr.

sertaconazole

(ser-ta-**kon**-a-zole)

Ertaczo

Classification

Therapeutic: antifungals

Pharmacologic: imidazoles

Indications

Topical treatment of interdigital tinea pedis in immunocompetent patients >12 yr.

Action

Inhibits synthesis of ergosterol, a component of fungal cell membrane, resulting in cytoplasmic leakage and fungal cell death. **Therapeutic Effects:** Resolution of fungal infection. **Spectrum:** Active against *Trichophyton rubrum*, *T. mentagrophytes*, *Epidermophyton floccosum*.

Adverse Reactions/Side Effects

Derm: application site reactions, burning, contact dermatitis, dry skin, tenderness.

PHYSICAL THERAPY IMPLICATIONS

Examination and Evaluation

- Assess healing of skin lesions to help document drug effectiveness.

Interventions

- Avoid contact with cutaneous lesions when treating patient.
- Always wash hands thoroughly and disinfect equipment (whirlpools, electrotherapeutic devices, treatment tables, and so forth) to help prevent the spread of infection.

Patient/Client-Related Instruction

- Advise patient to report any increased local sensitivity to this drug (pain, burning, itching, swelling).
- Instruct patient about proper hygiene; e.g., thoroughly wash and dry the affected area, wear clean socks and ventilated shoes for tinea pedis, and so forth.
- Advise patient to apply the drug as directed for the full course of treatment even if feeling better.
- Inform patient that full therapeutic response may take up to 4 wk.
- Advise patient to seek medical help if infections persist or recur after the full treatment. Recurrent fungal infections may be a sign of systemic illness.

Pharmacokinetics

Absorption: Minimal systemic absorption.
Distribution: Unknown.
Metabolism and Excretion: Unknown.
Half-life: Unknown.

TIME/ACTION PROFILE

ROUTE	ONSET	PEAK	DURATION
topical	within 2 wk	unknown	unknown

Contraindications/Precautions

Contraindicated in: Hypersensitivity to sertaconazole or other imidazoles.
Use Cautiously in: Children <12 yr, lactation (safety not established); Pregnancy (use only if clearly needed).

Interactions

Drug-Drug: None noted.

Route/Dosage

Topical (Adults and Children >12 yr): Apply bid for 4 wk.

Availability

2% cream: 15-g tube, 30-g tube.

sertraline (ser-tra-leen)

Zoloft

Classification

Therapeutic: antidepressants

Pharmacologic: selective serotonin reuptake inhibitors (SSRIs)

Indications

Major depressive disorder. Panic disorder. Obsessive-compulsive disorder (OCD). Posttraumatic stress disorder (PTSD). Social anxiety disorder (social phobia). Premenstrual dysphoric disorder (PMDD). **Unlabeled Use:** Generalized anxiety disorder (GAD).

Action

Inhibits neuronal uptake of serotonin in the CNS, thus potentiating the activity of serotonin. Has little effect on norepinephrine or dopamine. **Therapeutic Effects:** Antidepressant action. Decreased incidence of panic attacks. Decreased obsessive and compulsive behavior. Decreased feelings of intense fear, helplessness, or horror. Decreased social anxiety. Decrease in premenstrual dysphoria.

Adverse Reactions/Side Effects

CNS: NEUROLEPTIC MALIGNANT SYNDROME, SUICIDAL THOUGHTS, dizziness, drowsiness, fatigue, headache, insomnia, agitation, anxiety, confusion, emotional lability, impaired concentration, manic reaction, nervousness, weakness, yawning. **EENT:** pharyngitis, rhinitis, tinnitus, visual abnormalities. **CV:** chest pain, palpitations. **GI:** diarrhea, dry mouth, nausea, abdominal pain, altered taste, anorexia, constipation, dyspepsia, flatulence, ↑ appetite, vomiting. **GU:** sexual dysfunction, menstrual disorders, urinary disorders, urinary frequency. **Derm:** ↑ sweating, hot flashes, rash. **F and E:** hyponatremia. **MS:** back pain, myalgia. **Neuro:** tremor, hypertonia, hypoesthesia, paresthesia, twitching. **Misc:** SEROTONIN SYNDROME, fever, thirst.

PHYSICAL THERAPY IMPLICATIONS

Examination and Evaluation

- Watch for signs of neuroleptic malignant syndrome, including hyperthermia, diaphoresis, generalized muscle rigidity, altered mental status, tachycardia, changes in blood pressure (BP), and incontinence. Symptoms typically occur within 4–14 days after initiation of drug therapy but can occur at any time during drug use. Report these signs to the physician immediately.
- Monitor and report signs of serotonin syndrome, including hyperthermia, rigidity, myoclonus, and autonomic instability with fluctuating vital signs and extreme agitation that may proceed to delirium and coma. Patients should not take sertraline with other drugs that increase serotonin levels (e.g., MAO inhibitors).
- Be alert for increased depression and suicidal thoughts and ideology, especially when initiating drug treatment, and in children and teenagers. Notify physician or other mental health care professional immediately if patient exhibits worsening depression.
- Inform physician if patient demonstrates other mood changes such as increased anxiety, agitation, impaired memory, impaired concentration, emotional lability, manic reactions, or confusion (See Appendix D).
- Monitor symptoms of chest pain and palpitations, especially during exercise. Report severe or prolonged cardiac symptoms.
- Assess any back pain or muscle pain to rule out musculoskeletal pathology; that is, try to determine if pain is drug-induced rather than caused by anatomic or biomechanical problems.
- Assess paresthesias (numbness, tingling), tremor, twitching, or changes in muscle tone. Perform objective tests, including electroneuromyography and sensory testing to document any drug-related neuropathic changes.
- Assess dizziness and drowsiness that might affect gait, balance, and other functional activities (See Appendix C). Report balance problems and functional limitations to the physician, and caution the patient and family/caregivers to guard against falls and trauma.

Interventions

- Guard against falls and trauma (hip fractures, head injury, and so forth), and implement fall-prevention strategies (See Appendix E).
- To minimize orthostatic hypotension, patient should move slowly when assuming a more upright position.
- Help patient explore nonpharmacologic methods (exercise, counseling, support groups, and so forth) to reduce depression and other psychologic disorders.

Patient/Client-Related Instruction

- Advise patient that antidepressant effects may not occur immediately; it may take 2 wk or more before an improvement in mood is observed.
- Advise patient to avoid alcohol and other CNS depressants because of the increased risk of sedation and adverse effects.
- Instruct patient to report severe or prolonged GI problems, including nausea, vomiting, diarrhea, constipation, abdominal pain, indigestion, flatulence, dry mouth, altered taste, or changes in appetite.
- Instruct patient to report other problematic side effects such as severe or prolonged headache, vision disturbances, ringing/buzzing in the ears (tinnitus), upper respiratory tract irritation, urinary frequency, menstrual disorders, sexual dysfunction, skin reactions (rash, hot flashes, excessive sweating), and flu-like symptoms (fever, malaise).

Pharmacokinetics

Absorption: Appears to be well absorbed after oral administration.

S

Distribution: Extensively distributed throughout body tissues.
Protein Binding: 98%.
Metabolism and Excretion: Extensively metabolized by the liver; one metabolite has some antidepressant activity; 14% excreted unchanged in feces.
Half-life: 24 hr.

TIME/ACTION PROFILE (antidepressant effect)

ROUTE	ONSET	PEAK	DURATION
PO	within 2–4 wk	unknown	Unknown

Contraindications/Precautions

Contraindicated in: Hypersensitivity; Concurrent MAO inhibitor therapy (may result in serious, potentially fatal reactions); Concurrent pimozide; Oral concentrate contains alcohol; avoid in patients with known intolerance.
Use Cautiously in: Severe hepatic or renal impairment; Patients with a history of mania; History of suicide attempt; May ↑ risk of suicide attempt/ideation, especially during early treatment or dose adjustment; this risk appears to be greater in adolescents or children; OB/Lactation: Pregnancy or lactation; Pedi: May ↑ risk of suicide attempt/ideation, especially during dose early treatment or dose adjustment; risk may be greater in children or adolescents.

Interactions

Drug-Drug: Serious, potentially fatal reactions (hyperthermia, rigidity, myoclonus, autonomic instability, with fluctuating vital signs and extreme agitation, which may proceed to delirium and coma) may occur with concurrent **MAO inhibitors.** MAO inhibitors should be stopped at least 14 days before sertraline therapy. Sertraline should be stopped at least 14 days before MAO inhibitor therapy. May ↑ **pimozide** levels and the risk of potentially life-threatening cardiovascular reactions. Drugs that affect serotonergic neurotransmitter systems, including **linezolid, tramadol,** and **triptans,** ↑ risk of serotonin syndrome. May ↑ sensitivity to **adrenergics** and ↑ the risk of serotonin syndrome. Concurrent use with **alcohol** is not recommended. May ↑ levels/effects of **warfarin, phenytoin, tricyclic antidepressants,** some **benzodiazepines (alprazolam), clozapine,** or **tolbutamide.** ↑ risk of bleeding with **NSAIDS, aspirin, clopidogrel,** or **warfarin. Cimetidine** ↑ blood levels and effects.
Drug-Natural: ↑ risk of serotonergic side effects, including serotonin syndrome with **St. John's wort** and **SAMe.**

Route/Dosage

Depression/OCD

PO (Adults): 50 mg/day as a single dose in the morning or evening initially; after several weeks may be ↑ at weekly intervals up to 200 mg/day, depending on response.
PO (Children 13–17 yr): *OCD*—50 mg once daily.
PO (Children 6–12 yr): *OCD*—25 mg once daily.

Panic Disorder

PO (Adults): 25 mg/day initially; may ↑ after 1 wk to 50 mg/day.

PTSD

PO (Adults): 25 mg once daily for 7 days, then ↑ to 50 mg once daily; may then be ↑ if needed at intervals of at least 7 days (range 50–200 mg once daily).

Social Anxiety Disorder

PO (Adults): 25 mg once daily initially, then 50 mg once daily; may be ↑ at weekly intervals up to 200 mg/day.

PMDD

PO (Adults): 50 mg/day initially either daily or daily during luteal phase of cycle. Daily dosing may be titrated upward in 50-mg increments at the beginning of a cycle. In luteal phase-only dosing, a 50-mg/day titration step for 3 days at the beginning of each luteal phase dosing period should be used (range 50–150 mg/day).

Availability (generic available)

Tablets: 25 mg, 50 mg, 100 mg. **Capsules:** 50 mg, 100 mg. **Oral concentrate (12% alcohol):** 20 mg/mL in 60-mL bottles.

sevelamer (se-vel-a-mer)

Renagel, Renvela

Classification
Therapeutic: electrolyte modifiers
Pharmacologic: phosphate binders

Indications

Reduction of serum phosphate levels in patients with hyperphosphatemia associated with end-stage renal disease.

Action

A polymer that binds phosphate in the GI tract, preventing its absorption. **Therapeutic Effects:** Decreased serum phosphate levels and reduction in the consequences of hyperphosphatemia (ectopic calcification, secondary hyperparathyroidism with osteitis fibrosa).

Adverse Reactions/Side Effects

GI: diarrhea, dyspepsia, vomiting, constipation, flatulence, nausea.

PHYSICAL THERAPY IMPLICATIONS

Interventions

- Implement therapeutic exercises (resistive training, aerobic exercises, gait training) as tolerated to complement the effects of drug therapy and help maintain function in patients with end-stage renal disease.

Patient/Client-Related Instruction

- Advise patient about the likelihood of GI reactions such as nausea, vomiting, diarrhea, constipation, indigestion, and flatulence. Instruct patient to report severe or prolonged GI problems.

Pharmacokinetics

Absorption: Not absorbed; action is local (in GI tract).
Distribution: Unknown.
Metabolism and Excretion: Eliminated in feces.
Half-life: Unknown.

TIME/ACTION PROFILE (decrease in serum phosphate levels)

ROUTE	ONSET	PEAK	DURATION
PO	5 days	2 wk	unknown

Contraindications/Precautions

Contraindicated in: Hypersensitivity; Hypophosphatemia; Bowel obstruction.
Use Cautiously in: Dysphagia, swallowing disorders, severe GI motility disorders, or major GI tract surgery; OB/Lactation/Pedi: Safety not established.

Interactions

Drug-Drug: Concurrent **anticonvulsants** or **antiarrhythmics;** sevelamer may affect absorption; administer 1 hr before or 3 hr after. May ↓ absorption of other drugs and ↓ effectiveness, especially **drugs whose efficacy is dependent on tightly controlled blood levels.**

Route/Dosage

PO (Adults): 800–1600 mg with each meal.

Availability

Tablets: 400 mg, 800 mg.

sibutramine (si-byoo-tra-meen)

Meridia

Classification

Therapeutic: weight-control agents
Pharmacologic: appetite suppressants

Schedule IV

Indications

Treatment of obesity in patients with body mass index ≥30 kg/m^2 (or ≥27 kg/m^2 in patients with diabetes, hypertension, or other risk factors) in conjunction with other interventions (dietary restriction, exercise); used to produce and maintain weight loss.

Action

Acts as an inhibitor of the reuptake of serotonin, norepinephrine, and dopamine; increases the satiety-producing effects of serotonin. **Therapeutic Effects:** Decreased hunger with resultant weight loss in obese patients.

Adverse Reactions/Side Effects

CNS: SEIZURES, <u>headache</u>, <u>insomnia</u>, CNS stimulation, dizziness, drowsiness, emotional lability, nervousness. **EENT:** laryngitis/pharyngitis, rhinitis, sinusitis. **CV:** hypertension, palpitations, tachycardia, vasodilation. **GI:** <u>anorexia</u>, <u>constipation</u>, <u>dry mouth</u>, altered taste, dyspepsia, increased appetite, nausea. **GU:** dysmenorrhea. **Derm:** increased sweating, rash.

PHYSICAL THERAPY IMPLICATIONS

Examination and Evaluation

- Be alert for new seizures or increased seizure activity, especially at the onset of drug treatment. Document the number, duration, and severity of seizures, and report these findings to the physician immediately.
- Be alert for signs of excessive CNS stimulation, including nervousness, hyperactivity, restlessness, tremor, hallucinations, mania, irritability, or disordered thoughts. Report these signs to the physician.
- Assess heart rate, ECG, and heart sounds, especially during exercise (See Appendices G, H). Report fast heart rate (tachycardia) or symptoms of other arrhythmias, including palpitations, chest discomfort, shortness of breath, fainting, and fatigue/weakness.
- Assess blood pressure (BP) and compare to normal values (See Appendix F). Report a sustained increase in BP (hypertension).
- Assess dizziness and drowsiness that might affect gait, balance, and other functional activities (See Appendix C). Report balance problems and functional limitations to the physician and nursing staff, and caution the patient and family/caregivers to guard against falls and trauma.

Interventions

- Implement therapeutic exercises (aerobic activities, resistive training) to complement the effects of drug therapy and help achieve optimal weight control.
- Because of the risk of arrhythmias and abnormal BP responses, use caution during aerobic exercise and other forms of therapeutic exercise. Assess exercise tolerance frequently (BP, heart rate, fatigue levels), and terminate exercise immediately if any untoward responses occur (See Appendix L).

S

Patient/Client-Related Instruction

- Instruct patient and family/caregivers to report other troublesome side effects, including severe or prolonged headache, sleep loss, skin problems (rash, sweating); nasal/pharyngeal/laryngeal irritation, menstrual abnormalities, or GI problems (nausea, constipation, altered taste, dry mouth, change in appetite).

Pharmacokinetics

Absorption: 77% absorbed, then rapidly undergoes extensive 1st-pass hepatic metabolism (via the P450 3A4 metabolic pathway) to active metabolites (M1 and M2).
Distribution: Widely and rapidly distributed; high concentrations in liver and kidneys.
Metabolism and Excretion: Active metabolites are extensively metabolized to inactive metabolites that are mostly excreted by the kidneys.
Half-life: *M1 metabolite*—14 hr; *M2 metabolite*—16 hr.

TIME/ACTION PROFILE (appetite suppression/weight loss)

ROUTE	ONSET	PEAK	DURATION
PO	days	4 wk	unknown

Contraindications/Precautions

Contraindicated in: Hypersensitivity; Anorexia nervosa; Concurrent use of other centrally acting appetite suppressants, MAO inhibitors, SSRIs, sumatriptan, naratriptan, zolmitriptan, dihydroergotamine, dextromethorphan, meperidine, pentazocine, fentanyl, lithium, or tryptophan; Organic causes of obesity (untreated hypothyroidism); Severe hepatic/renal impairment; Uncontrolled/poorly controlled hypertension; History of coronary artery disease, CHF, arrhythmias, or stroke; Excessive consumption of alcohol; Pregnancy or lactation.
Use Cautiously in: History of seizures; Angle-closure glaucoma; Geriatric patients; Children <16 yr (safety not established).

Interactions

Drug-Drug: Concurrent use of **other centrally acting appetite suppressants, MAO inhibitors, SSRIs, naratriptan, frovatriptan, rizatriptan, zolmitriptan, sumatriptan, dihydroergotamine, dextromethorphan, meperidine, pentazocine, fentanyl, lithium,** or **tryptophan** may result in potentially fatal serotonin syndrome (avoid concurrent use; allow 2 wk between use of MAO inhibitors and sibutramine). Concurrent use of **decongestants** may ↑ the risk of hypertension. **Drugs that affect the P450 3A4 enzyme system** may alter the effects of sibutramine. **Ketoconazole, cimetidine,** and **erythromycin** ↓ metabolism and may ↑ blood levels and effects.

Route/Dosage

PO (Adults): 10 mg once daily; may be increased to 15 mg/day after 4 wk. Patients who do not tolerate an initial dose of 10 mg/day may be started on 5 mg/day.

Availability

Capsules: 5 mg, 10 mg, 15 mg.

sildenafil (sil-den-a-fil)

Revatio, Viagra

Classification
Therapeutic: vasodilator
Pharmacologic: phosphodiesterase type 5 inhibitors

Indications

Viagra: Erectile dysfunction. *Revatio:* Pulmonary hypertension.

Action

Viagra: Enhances effects of nitric oxide released during sexual stimulation. Nitric oxide activates guanylate cyclase, which produces increased levels of cyclic guanosine monophosphate (cGMP). cGMP produces smooth muscle relaxation of the corpus cavernosum, which promotes increased blood flow and subsequent erection. Sildenafil inhibits the enzyme phosphodiesterase type 5 (PDE5); PDE5 inactivates cGMP. *Revatio:* Produces vasodilation of the pulmonary vascular bed. **Therapeutic Effects:** *Viagra:* Enhanced blood flow to the corpus cavernosum and erection sufficient to allow sexual intercourse. Requires sexual stimulation. *Revatio:* Improved exercise tolerance.

Adverse Reactions/Side Effects

CNS: headache, dizziness, insomnia. **EENT:** HEARING LOSS, VISION LOSS, epistaxis, nasal congestion. **CV:** MI, SUDDEN DEATH, CARDIOVASCULAR COLLAPSE. **GI:** dyspepsia, diarrhea. **GU:** priapism, urinary tract infection. **Derm:** flushing, rash. **MS:** myalgia. **Neuro:** paresthesias.

PHYSICAL THERAPY IMPLICATIONS

Examination and Evaluation

- Monitor cardiac symptoms at rest and during exercise, and be alert for signs of severe cardiac insufficiency due to myocardial infarction (MI) or cardiovascular collapse. Seek immediate medical assistance if symptoms of cardiac arrest develop, including sudden chest pain, pain radiating into the arm or jaw, shortness of breath, dizziness, sweating, anxiety, and nausea.
- Be alert for sudden loss of vision or hearing, and seek emergency care for any changes in vision or hearing.
- For patients with pulmonary hypertension, assess exercise tolerance and other symptoms (shortness

of breath, fatigue, dizziness, chest pain, peripheral edema) to help document whether drug therapy is effective in reducing these symptoms.

- Assess any muscle pain to rule out musculoskeletal pathology; that is, try to determine if pain is drug induced rather than caused by anatomic or biomechanical problems.
- Assess signs of paresthesia (numbness, tingling). Perform objective tests, including electroneuromyography and sensory testing to document any drug-related neuropathic changes.
- Assess dizziness that might affect gait, balance, and other functional activities (See Appendix C). Report balance problems and functional limitations to the physician, and caution the patient and family/caregivers to guard against falls and trauma.

Interventions

- Because of the risk of MI and cardiovascular collapse, use extreme caution during aerobic exercise and other forms of therapeutic exercise. Assess exercise tolerance frequently (blood pressure, heart rate, fatigue levels), and terminate exercise immediately if any untoward responses occur (See Appendix L).

Patient/Client-Related Instruction

- Advise patient and family or caregivers about the signs of cardiac arrest (see above under Examination and Evaluation), and to seek immediate medical assistance if these signs develop.
- Instruct patient to notify health care professional promptly if erection lasts longer than 4 hr or if they experience a sudden decrease or loss of vision or hearing.
- Instruct patient and family/caregivers to report other bothersome side effects such as severe or prolonged headache, sleep loss, nose bleeds, nasal congestion, urinary tract infections, skin problems (rash, flushing), or GI reactions (diarrhea, indigestion).

Pharmacokinetics

Absorption: Rapidly absorbed (40%) after oral administration.
Distribution: Widely distributed to tissues; negligible amount in semen.
Protein Binding: 96%.
Metabolism and Excretion: Mostly metabolized by the liver (by P450 3A4 enzyme system); 1 metabolite is active and accounts for 20% or more of drug effect. Metabolites excreted mostly (80%) in feces; 13% excreted in urine.
Half-life: 4 hr (for sildenafil and active metabolite).

TIME/ACTION PROFILE (vasodilation, ability to produce erection)

ROUTE	ONSET	PEAK	DURATION
PO	within 1 hr	30–120 min	up to 4 hr

Contraindications/Precautions

Contraindicated in: Hypersensitivity; Concurrent organic nitrate therapy (nitroglycerin, isosorbide mononitrate, isosorbide dinitrate), ritonavir, ketoconazole and itraconazole; Pulmonary veno-occlusive disease; **Viagra:** OB/Pedi: Newborns, women, children.
Use Cautiously in: Serious underlying cardiovascular disease (including history of MI, stroke, or serious arrhythmia within 6 mo), cardiac failure, or coronary artery disease with unstable angina; History of CHF, coronary artery disease, uncontrolled hypertension (BP >170/110 mmHg) or hypotension (BP <90/50 mmHg), dehydration, autonomic dysfunction, or severe left ventricular outflow obstruction; Concurrent treatment with antihypertensives or glipizide; Renal impairment (CCr 30 mL/min, hepatic impairment; all result in ↑ blood levels; ↓ dose required); Anatomic penile deformity (angulation, cavernosal fibrosis, Peyronie's disease); Conditions associated with priapism (sickle cell anemia, multiple myeloma, leukemia); Bleeding disorders or active peptic ulceration; History of sudden severe vision loss or nonarteritic ischemic optic neuropathy (NAION); may ↑ risk of recurrence; Retinitis pigmentosa; Concurrent bosentan, erythromycin, or saquinavir (↓ dose recommended); Alpha-adrenergic blockers (patients should be on stable dose of alpha blockers before starting sildenafil); Geri: ↑ blood levels and may require lower doses; consider age-related decrease in cardiac, hepatic, and renal function as well as concurrent drug therapy and chronic disease states.); Lactation: Lactation; Pedi: ***Revatio***—Safe use in pediatric patients with pulmonary hypertension not established; May ↑ risk of bleeding with **warfarin.**

Interactions

Drug-Drug: ↑ risk of hypotension with **nitrates** in any form or **ritonavir**; concurrent use is contraindicated because of the risk of serious and potentially fatal hypotension. Blood levels and effects, including the risk of hypotension, may be ↑ by **enzyme inhibitors,** including **cimetidine, erythromycin, tacrolimus, ketoconazole, itraconazole,** and **protease inhibitor antiretrovirals,** including **nelfinavir, indinavir, saquinavir** (initial dose of sildenafil for erectile dysfunction should be ↓ to 25 mg). ↑ risk of hypotension with **alpha-adrenergic blockers** and acute ingestion of **alcohol. Rifampin, bosentan, barbiturates, carbamazepine, phenytoin,**

S

efavirenz, nevirapine, rifampin, or **rifabutin** may ↓ blood levels and effects; dose adjustments may be necessary in the treatment of pulmonary arterial hypertension. ↑ levels of **bosentan.** Use cautiously with **glipizide.**

Route/Dosage

Revatio (for pulmonary arterial hypertension)

PO (Adults): 20 mg tid; dose adjustments may be necessary for concurrent bosentan, barbiturates, carbamazepine, phenytoin, efavirenz, nevirapine, rifampin, or rifabutin.

Viagra (for erectile dysfunction)

PO (Adults): 50 mg taken 1 hr before sexual activity (range 25–100 mg taken 30 min–4 hr before sexual activity); not more than once daily; *Concurrent use with alpha-blocker antihypertensives*—do not use 50–100 mg dose within 4 hr of alpha blocker, 25 mg dose may be taken anytime.

PO (Geriatric Patients ≥65 yr or with concurrent enzyme inhibitors): 25 mg taken 1 hr before sexual activity (range 25–100 mg taken 30 min–4 hr before sexual activity); not more than once daily.

Hepatic/Renal Impairment

PO (Adults): 25 mg taken 1 hr before sexual activity (range 25–100 mg taken 30 min–4 hr before sexual activity); not more than once daily.

Availability

Tablets (Viagra): 25 mg, 50 mg, 100 mg. **Tablets (Revatio):** 20 mg.

silodosin (sil-oh-doe-sin)

Rapaflo

Classification

Therapeutic: benign prostatic hyperplasia (BPH) agents

Pharmacologic: alpha-adrenergic blockers

Indications

Treatment of the signs/symptoms or BPH.

Action

Blocks postsynaptic $alpha_1$-adrenergic receptors. ↓ contractions in the smooth muscle of the prostatic capsule. **Therapeutic Effects:** ↓ signs and symptoms of BPH (urinary urgency, hesitancy, nocturia).

Adverse Reactions/Side Effects

CNS: dizziness, headache. **CV:** orthostatic hypotension. **GI:** diarrhea. **GU:** retrograde ejaculation.

PHYSICAL THERAPY IMPLICATIONS

Examination and Evaluation

- Monitor signs of BPH such as difficulty starting a urine stream, painful urination, weak urine flow, feeling that the bladder is not completely empty, frequent nighttime urination, and an urge to urinate again soon after urinating. Document any change in BPH symptoms to help assess the effects of drug therapy.
- Assess blood pressure (BP) when patient assumes a more upright position (lying to standing, sitting to standing, lying to sitting). Document orthostatic hypotension and contact the physician when systolic BP falls >20 mm Hg, or diastolic BP falls >10 mm Hg.
- Assess dizziness that might affect gait, balance, and other functional activities (see Appendix C). Report balance problems and functional limitations to the physician, and caution the patient and family/caregivers to guard against falls and trauma.

Interventions

- Avoid physical therapy interventions that cause systemic vasodilation (large whirlpool, Hubbard tank). Additive effects of this drug and the intervention may cause a dangerous fall in blood pressure
- To minimize orthostatic hypotension, advise patient to move slowly when assuming a more upright position.

Patient/Client-Related Instruction

- Advise patient that urinary symptoms (retention, dribbling, hesitancy, urgency) should improve, and to contact the physician if these symptoms continue to worsen.
- Instruct patient or family/caregivers to report other bothersome side effects such as severe or prolonged headache, diarrhea, or problems with ejaculation.

Pharmacokinetics

Absorption: 32% absorbed following oral administration.

Distribution: Unknown.

Protein Binding: 97%.

Metabolism and Excretion: Extensively metabolized (CYP3A4, UGT2B7, and other metabolic pathways involved); 33.5% excreted in urine and 54.9% in feces.

Half-life: 13.3 hr.

TIME/ACTION PROFILE (effect on symptoms of BPH)

ROUTE	ONSET	PEAK	DURATION
PO	rapid	24 hr	24 hr*

*Following discontinuation.

Contraindications/Precautions

Contraindicated in: Not indicated for use in women or children; Severe renal impairment (CrCl <30 mL/min);

Severe hepatic impairment (Child-Pugh score of 10 or greater); Concurrent use of strong CYP3A4 inhibitors or P-glycoprotein (P-gp) inhibitors.
Use Cautiously in: Moderate inhibitors of the CYP3A4 enzyme system; Cataract surgery (may cause Intraoperative Floppy Iris Syndrome); Moderate renal impairment (lower dose recommended); Geri: Increased risk of orthostatic hypotension; Pedi: Safety and effectiveness have not been established.

Interactions

Drug-Drug: Strong inhibitors of CYP3A4 (including **ketoconazole, clarithromycin, itraconazole,** and **ritonavir**) ↓ metabolism, ↑ blood levels, and risk of toxicity; concurrent use is contraindicated. Concurrent use with **moderate CYP3A4 inhibitors** (including **diltiazem, erythromycin,** and **verapamil**) may ↑ silodosin levels; use cautiously. Concurrent use with **antihypertensives** (including **calcium channel blockers** and **thiazides**), other **alpha blockers,** and **phosphodiesterase type 5 inhibitors** (including **sildenafil** and **tadalafil**) ↑ the risk of dizziness and orthostatic hypotension. **P-gp inhibitors,** including **cyclosporine**), may ↑ levels; concurrent use not recommended.

Route/Dosage

PO (Adults): 8 mg once daily.

Renal Impairment

PO (Adults CCr 30–50 mL/min): 4 mg once daily.

Availability

Capsules: 4 mg, 8 mg.

silver sulfadiazine

(sil-ver sul-fa-dye-a-zeen)

✱Flamazine, Flint SSD, Sildimac, Silvadene, Thermazene

Classification

Therapeutic: anti-infectives (topical)
Pharmacologic: sulfonamides

Indications

Prevention and treatment of wound sepsis in patients with 2nd- and 3rd-degree burns. **Unlabeled Use:** Management of Minor skin infections, Dermal ulcers.

Action

Splits to produce bactericidal concentrations of silver and sulfadiazine. Action is at level of cell membrane and cell wall. **Therapeutic Effects:** Bactericidal action against organisms found in burns. **Spectrum:** Broad spectrum includes activity against many gram-negative and gram-positive bacteria, anaerobes, and some yeast.

Pharmacokinetics

Absorption: Small amounts of silver are systemically absorbed following topical application. Up to 10% of sulfadiazine is absorbed.
Distribution: Unknown.
Metabolism and Excretion: Absorbed sulfadiazine is excreted unchanged by the kidneys.
Half-life: Unknown.

TIME/ACTION PROFILE (anti-infective action)

ROUTE	ONSET	PEAK	DURATION
topical	on contact	unknown	as long as applied

Contraindications/Precautions

Contraindicated in: Hypersensitivity (cross-sensitivity with sulfonamides may occur); Infants <2 mo (risk of kernicterus); Pregnancy near term (increased risk of

Adverse Reactions/Side Effects

Derm: burning, itching, pain, rash, skin discoloration, skin necrosis. **Hemat:** leukopenia.

PHYSICAL THERAPY IMPLICATIONS

Examination and Evaluation

- Assess the size, depth, color, drainage, and periwound area to document whether drug therapy is successful in decreasing infection and promoting wound healing.
- Monitor any new or increased skin reactions at the site of application, including rash, burning, itching, pain, and necrosis. Report any suspicious skin reactions to the physician.
- Be alert for signs of leukopenia, including fever, sore throat, and signs of infection. Report these signs to the physician.

Interventions

- Implement wound care procedures (whirlpool, pulsed lavage, gentle débridement) as needed to cleanse burns and ulcers. Make sure the drug is reapplied and dressings are changed according to the recommended procedures.
- When indicated, use appropriate physical agents (ultrasound, electric stimulation, ultraviolet light) to facilitate wound healing and augment drug effects.

S

Patient/Client-Related Instruction

- Check that the patient and family or caregivers understand topical application and wound care procedures and adhere to the recommended dosing schedule.
- Instruct patient and family/caregivers about prevention of other types of skin ulcers and the need for visual inspection to prevent recurrence or development of new ulcers.

kernicterus in infant); G6PD deficiency; Porphyria.
Use Cautiously in: Impaired hepatic or renal function; Children (safety not established).

Interactions
Drug-Drug: Silver may inactivate concurrently applied topical **proteolytic enzymes (fibrinolysin, desoxyribonuclease).**

Route/Dosage
Topical (Adults and Children >1 mo): Apply 1% cream 1–2 times daily in layer 1.5-mm thick.

Availability (generic available)
Cream: 10 mg/g in 20-, 25-, 50-, 85-, 400-, 1000-g containers.

simvastatin (sim-va-**stat**-in)
Zocor

Classification
Therapeutic: lipid-lowering agents
Pharmacologic: HMG-CoA reductase inhibitors (statin)

Indications
Adjunctive management of primary hypercholesterolemia and mixed dyslipidemias. Secondary prevention of myocardial infarction, coronary revascularization, stroke, and cardiovascular mortality in patients with clinically evident coronary heart disease.

Action
Inhibits 3-hydroxy-3-methylglutaryl coenzyme A (HMG CoA) reductase, an enzyme which is responsible for catalyzing an early step in the synthesis of cholesterol. **Therapeutic Effects:** Lowering of total and LDL cholesterol and triglycerides. Slightly increases HDL cholesterol. Slows the progression of coronary atherosclerosis with resultant decrease in coronary heart disease–related events.

Adverse Reactions/Side Effects
CNS: dizziness, headache, insomnia, weakness.
GI: abdominal cramps, constipation, diarrhea, flatus, heartburn, altered taste, drug-induced hepatitis, dyspepsia, elevated liver enzymes, nausea, pancreatitis.
GU: erectile dysfunction. **Derm:** rashes, pruritus.
MS: RHABDOMYOLYSIS, arthralgia, myalgia, myositis.
Misc: hypersensitivity reactions.

PHYSICAL THERAPY IMPLICATIONS

Examination and Evaluation
- Assess any joint pain, muscle pain, tenderness, or weakness, especially if accompanied by fever, malaise, and dark-colored urine. Advise patient that these symptoms may represent drug-induced myopathy and that myopathy can progress to severe muscle damage (rhabdomyolysis). Report any unexplained musculoskeletal symptoms to the physician immediately, and stop exercise and gait training until these symptoms can be assessed.
- Monitor signs of hypersensitivity reactions, including pulmonary symptoms (tightness in the throat and chest, wheezing, cough, dyspnea) or skin reactions (rash, pruritus, urticaria). Notify physician if these reactions occur.
- Assess dizziness that might affect gait, balance, and other functional activities (See Appendix C). Report balance problems and functional limitations to the physician, and caution the patient and family/caregivers to guard against falls and trauma.

Interventions
- In patients with drug-induced myopathy, implement gradual strengthening and other therapeutic exercises to facilitate recovery from muscle pain and weakness. Use caution during early stages to avoid fatigue of affected muscles, and implement assistive devices (walker, cane, crutches) as needed to prevent falls and assist mobility. Increase exercise intensity as tolerated; recovery from myopathy typically takes 4–6 wk, but can be longer in older patients or people with comorbidities.
- Design and implement aerobic exercise and endurance training programs to improve cardiovascular function and help reduce the risk of coronary heart disease.

Patient/Client-Related Instruction
- Remind patients to take medication as directed to control hyperlipidemia even though they are asymptomatic.
- Counsel patients about additional interventions to help control lipid disorders and improve cardiovascular health, including dietary modification, regular exercise, moderation of alcohol consumption, and smoking cessation.
- Instruct patient to report signs of drug-induced hepatitis (anorexia, abdominal pain, severe nausea and vomiting, yellow skin or eyes, skin rashes, flu-like symptoms) or pancreatitis (upper abdominal pain after eating, indigestion, weight loss, oily stools)
- Instruct patient to report other prolonged or severe GI reactions, including nausea, constipation, diarrhea, heartburn, abdominal cramps, altered taste, or flatulence.
- Advise patient to consult physician if erectile dysfunction or other sexual problems occur.
- Instruct patient and family/caregivers to report other troublesome side effects such as severe or prolonged headache, sleep loss, or skin reactions (rash, itching).

Pharmacokinetics

Absorption: 85% absorbed, but rapidly metabolized.
Distribution: Unknown.
Protein Binding: 95%.
Metabolism and Excretion: Extensively metabolized by the liver, most during 1st pass; excreted in bile and feces; 13% excreted unchanged by the kidneys.
Half-life: Unknown.

TIME/ACTION PROFILE (cholesterol-lowering effect)

ROUTE	ONSET	PEAK	DURATION[†]
PO	days	2–4 wk	unknown

[†]After discontinuation

Contraindications/Precautions

Contraindicated in: Hypersensitivity; Active liver disease or unexplained persistent elevations in AST & ALT; OB/Lactation: Pregnancy or lactation.
Use Cautiously in: History of liver disease; Alcoholism; Renal impairment; Concurrent use of gemfibrozil, azole antifungals, protease inhibitors, niacin, cyclosporine, amiodarone, or verapamil (↑ risk of myopathy/rhabdomyolysis); OB: Women of childbearing age; Pedi: Children <10 yr (safety not established).

Interactions

Drug-Drug: Cholesterol-lowering effect may be ↑ with **bile acid sequestrants (cholestyramine, colestipol).** Bioavailability may be ↓ by **bile acid sequestrants.** Risk of myopathy is ↑ by concurrent **amiodarone, verapamil, cyclosporine, gemfibrozil, clofibrate, erythromycin,** large doses of **niacin, ritonavir, azole,** or **antifungals** (combined use with **clofibrate** or **gemfibrozil** not recommended). May slightly ↑ serum **digoxin** levels. May ↑ risk of bleeding with **warfarin.** Levels may be significantly ↑ by **azole** and **antifungals** (temporarily discontinue **HMG CoA reductase inhibitor**).
Drug-Food: Grapefruit juice ↑ blood levels ↑ risk of rhabdomyolysis.

Route/Dosage

PO (Adults): 5–80 mg once daily in the evening.
Geriatric patients, patients with LDL <190 mg/dL, or patients receiving cyclosporine—5 mg/day initially. ↑ at 4-wk intervals (not to exceed 10 mg/day in patients receiving cyclosporine or 20 mg/day in patients receiving amiodarone or verapamil) up to 40 mg/day.
PO (Children and adolescents 10–17 yr): 10 mg/day initially; may be increased at 4-wk intervals up to 40 mg/day (not to exceed 10 mg/day in patients receiving cyclosporine or 20 mg/day in patients receiving amiodarone or verapamil).

Renal Impairment

PO (Adults): *Severe renal impairment*—5 mg/day initially, titrate carefully.

Availability (generic available)

Tablets: 5 mg, 10 mg, 20 mg, 40 mg, 80 mg.
In combination with: ezetimibe (Vytorin); niacin (Simcor). See Appendix B.

sinecatechins (sin-e-**kat**-e-kins)
Veregen

Classification
Therapeutic: antivirals
Pharmacologic: botanical agents

Indications

Treatment of external genital and perianal warts (*Condylomata acuminata* caused by human papillomavirus [HPV]) in immunocompetent patients 18 yr and older.

Action

Beneficial effects may be due to antioxidant properties; made from extract of green tea. **Therapeutic Effects:** Regression of warts

Adverse Reactions/Side Effects

Local: <u>burning</u>, <u>edema</u>, <u>erythema</u>, <u>induration</u>, <u>pain/discomfort</u>, <u>pruritus</u>, <u>erosion/ulceration</u>, <u>vesicular rash</u>, bleeding , desquamation, discharge, irritation, phimosis, rash, regional lymphadenitis, scar.

PHYSICAL THERAPY IMPLICATIONS

Examination and Evaluation

- Monitor any new or increased skin reactions at the site of application, including pain, inflammation, irritation, bleeding, burning, swelling, exfoliation, and rash. Report severe or prolonged skin reactions to the physician.

Patient/Client-Related Instruction

- Check that the patient and family or caregivers understand topical application procedures and adhere to the recommended dosing schedule.

Pharmacokinetics

Absorption: Minimal systemic absorption (less than that of a cup of green tea).
Distribution: Unknown.
Metabolism and Excretion: Unknown.
Half-life: Unknown.

S

TIME/ACTION PROFILE

ROUTE	ONSET	PEAK	DURATION
topical	unknown	unknown	unknown

Contraindications/Precautions

Contraindicated in: Not to be used for urethral, intra-vaginal, cervical, rectal, or intra-anal human papilloma viral disease or on open wounds.
Use Cautiously in: Safe and effective use in immunosuppressed patients has not been established; OB: Use during pregnancy only if potential maternal benefit justifies potential risk to the fetus; Pedi: Safe and effective use in patients <18 yr has not been established.

Interactions

Drug-Drug: None noted.

Route/Dosage

PO (Adults>18 yr): apply to warts tid for up to 16 wk.

Availability

15% Ointment: 15-g tubes.

sipuleucel (si-pyoo-**loo**-sel)

Provenge

Classification
Therapeutic: antineoplastics
Pharmacologic: autologous cellular immunotherapies

Indications

Asymptomatic/minimally symptomatic metastatic castrate-resistant (hormone refractory) prostate cancer.

Action

Autologous immunotherapy produced by collecting peripheral mononuclear cells during leukapheresis. Cells include antigen-presenting cells (APCs), which are activated during a culture period with prostatic acid phosphatase (PAP, an antigen found in prostatic cancer tissue) linked to granulocyte/macrophage colony-stimulating factor (GM-CSF, which activates immune cells). Induces an immune response against prostatic acid phosphatase. **Therapeutic Effects:** ↓ spread of prostate cancer.

Adverse Reactions/Side Effects

CNS: fatigue, headache, dizziness, insomnia. **Resp:** dyspnea. **CV:** hypertension, peripheral edema. **GI:** constipation, diarrhea, nausea, vomiting. **GU:** hematuria. **Derm:** flushing, rash, sweating. **Hemat:** anemia. **MS:** back pain, joint pain, extremity pain, muscle spasms, musculoskeletal pain. **Neuro:** paresthesia, tremor. **Misc:** chills, fever, acute infusion reactions, citrate toxicity.

PHYSICAL THERAPY IMPLICATIONS

Examination and Evaluation

- Report allergy-like responses such as wheezing, laryngeal edema, urticaria, and other skin reactions that occur during and after administration (infusion-related events).
- Assess blood pressure (BP) and compare to normal values (See Appendix F). Report a sustained increase in BP (hypertension).
- Assess peripheral edema using girth measurements, volume displacement, and measurement of pitting edema (See Appendix N). Report increased swelling in feet and ankles or a sudden increase in body weight due to fluid retention.
- Monitor signs of anemia, including unusual fatigue, shortness of breath with exertion, bruising, and pale skin. Notify physician immediately if these signs occur.
- Assess any breathing problems, and report signs of difficult or labored breathing (dyspnea).
- Watch for signs of citrate toxicity and related low calcium levels (hypocalcemia). Signs include headache, lethargy, weakness, cramping, and muscle hyperexcitability and tetany. Notify physician immediately if these signs occur.
- Assess signs of paresthesia (numbness, tingling) or tremor. Perform objective tests, including electroneuromyography and sensory testing to document any drug-related neuropathic changes.
- Assess any back, joint, or extremity pain or muscle spasms to rule out musculoskeletal pathology; that is, try to determine if pain is drug-induced rather than caused by anatomic or biomechanical problems.
- Assess dizziness that might affect gait, balance, and other functional activities (See Appendix C). Report balance problems and functional limitations to the physician and nursing staff, and caution the patient and family/caregivers to guard against falls and trauma.

Interventions

- For patients who are medically able to begin exercise, implement appropriate resistive exercises and aerobic training to maintain muscle strength and aerobic capacity during cancer chemotherapy or to help restore function after chemotherapy.

Patient/Client-Related Instruction

- Instruct patient or family/caregivers to report other side effects such as severe or prolonged headache, fatigue, sleep loss, chills, fever, bloody urine, skin reactions (rash, flushing, excessive sweating), or GI problems (nausea, vomiting, diarrhea, constipation).

Pharmacokinetics

Absorption: IV administration results in complete bioavailability.
Distribution: Unknown.
Metabolism and Excretion: Unknown.
Half-life: Unknown.

TIME/ACTION PROFILE

ROUTE	ONSET	PEAK	DURATION
IV	unknown	unknown	unknown

Contraindications/Precautions

Contraindicated in: None noted.
Use Cautiously in: Intended for autologous use only.

Interactions

Drug-Drug: Concurrent use of **immunosuppressants** may alter safety/efficacy.

Route/Dosage

IV (Adults): 1 dose q 2 wk for a total of 3 doses.

Availability

Suspension for IV infusion: minimum of 50 million autologous CD54$^+$ cells activated with PAP–GM-CSF suspended in 250 mL lactated Ringer's injection.

sirolimus (sir-oh-li-mus)

Rapamune

Classification
Therapeutic: immunosuppressants
Pharmacologic: macrolides

Indications

Prevention of organ rejection in allogenic kidney transplantation (with corticosteroids and cyclosporine). Sirolimus is also eluted from the Cypher coronary stent used in angioplasty procedures.

Action

Inhibits T-lymphocyte activation/proliferation, which occurs as a response to antigenic and cytokine stimulation; antibody production is also inhibited.
Therapeutic Effects: Decreased incidence and severity of organ rejection.

Adverse Reactions/Side Effects

Reflects combined therapy with corticosteroids and cyclosporine

CNS: insomnia. **Resp:** interstitial lung disease.
CV: edema, hypotension. **GI:** hepatic toxicity. **GU:** renal impairment. **Derm:** acne, rash, thrombocytopenic purpura. **F and E:** hypokalemia. **Hemat:** leukopenia, thrombocytopenia, anemia. **Metab:** hyperlipidemia. **MS:** arthralgias. **Neuro:** tremor. **Misc:** ↑ risk of infection, ↑ risk of lymphoma, ↑ risk of lymphocele, mucosal herpes simplex infections, ↓ wound healing, lymphocele.

PHYSICAL THERAPY IMPLICATIONS

Examination and Evaluation

- Assess any breathing problems or signs of interstitial lung disease such as dry cough, wheezing, chest pain, shortness of breath, and difficult or labored breathing. Monitor pulse oximetry and perform pulmonary function tests (See Appendices I, J, K) to quantify suspected changes in ventilation and respiratory function.
- Be alert for signs of hepatic toxicity, including anorexia, abdominal pain, severe nausea and vomiting, yellow skin or eyes, fever, sore throat, malaise, weakness, facial edema, lethargy, and unusual bleeding or bruising. Report these signs to the physician immediately.
- Assess blood pressure periodically and compare to normal values (See Appendix F). Report low blood pressure (hypotension), especially if patient experiences dizziness or syncope.
- Assess peripheral edema using girth measurements, volume displacement, and measurement of pitting edema (See Appendix N). Report increased swelling in feet and ankles or a sudden increase in body weight due to fluid retention.
- Monitor any muscle weakness, aches, or cramps that might indicate low potassium levels (hypokalemia).
- Monitor signs of lymphoma, including swollen lymph glands, unexplained weight loss, fatigue, weakness, fever, night sweats, dyspnea, cough, and abdominal pain/bloating. Report these signs to the physician immediately.
- Watch for signs of renal impairment, including decreased urine output, cloudy urine, and sudden weight gain due to fluid retention. Report these signs to the physician.
- Assess any joint pain to rule out musculoskeletal pathology; that is, try to determine if pain is drug induced rather than caused by anatomic or biomechanical problem.

Interventions

- Implement appropriate strengthening, aerobic, and other therapeutic exercises to improve function and promote recovery following organ transplants.
- Because of the risk of interstitial lung disease, use caution during aerobic exercise and other forms of therapeutic exercise. Assess exercise tolerance frequently (blood pressure, heart rate, fatigue

S

levels), and terminate exercise immediately if any untoward responses occur (See Appendix L).

Patient/Client-Related Instruction

- Because of immunosuppressant effects, advise patient to guard against infection (frequent hand washing, etc.), and to avoid crowds and contact with persons with contagious diseases.
- Advise patient that wound healing may be delayed; instruct patient to check skin regularly and report any nonhealing sores.
- Advise patient that this drug may cause problems in fat metabolism (hyperlipidemia). Remind patient that periodic blood tests may be needed to monitor plasma lipids.
- Instruct patient to report other bothersome side effects such as severe or prolonged tremor, sleep loss, infections, or skin reactions (rash, acne, bruising).

Pharmacokinetics

Absorption: Rapidly absorbed following oral administration (14% bioavailability).
Distribution: Concentrates in erythrocytes; distributes to heart, intestines, kidneys, liver, lungs, muscle, spleen, and testes in high concentrations.
Protein Binding: 92%.
Metabolism and Excretion: Extensively metabolized (some metabolism by P450 3A4 system); 91% excreted in feces.
Half-life: 62 hr.

TIME/ACTION PROFILE (blood levels)

ROUTE	ONSET	PEAK	DURATION
PO	Rapid	1–2 hr	24 hr

Contraindications/Precautions

Contraindicated in: Hypersensitivity; Alcohol intolerance/sensitivity (solution contains ethanol); Concurrent ketoconazole, voriconazole, itraconazole, erythromycin, telithromycin, clarithromycin, rifampin, rifabutin or grapefruit juice; Severe hepatic impairment; OB/Lactation: Pregnancy and lactation.
Use Cautiously in: Mild-to-moderate hepatic impairment; OB: Women with childbearing potential; Pedi: Children <13 yr (safety not established).

Interactions

Drug-Drug: Cyclosporine (modified) greatly ↑ blood levels (administer sirolimus 4 hr after cyclosporine). Drugs which inhibit the CYP3A4 enzyme system may be expected to ↑ blood levels and the risk of adverse reactions. **Ketoconazole, voriconazole, itraconazole, clarithromycin, erythromycin,** and **telithromycin** significantly ↑ blood levels (concurrent use is contraindicated). Blood levels are also ↑ by **diltiazem** and **verapamil** (monitor sirolimus levels and adjust dose as necessary) and may be ↑ by **nicardipine, verapamil, clotrimazole, fluconazole, troleandomycin, metoclopramide, cimetidine, danazol,** and **protease inhibitor antiretrovirals. Rifampin** and **rifabutin** ↑ metabolism by stimulating the CYP3A4 enzyme system and significantly ↓ blood levels. Blood levels may also be ↓ by **carbamazepine, phenobarbital, phenytoin,** and **rifapentine.** Risk of renal impairment may be ↑ by concurrent use of other **nephrotoxic agents.** Concurrent use with **tacrolimus** and **corticosteroids** in lung transplantation may ↑ risk of anastomotic dehiscence; fatalities have been reported (not approved for this use). Concurrent use with **tacrolimus and corticosteroids** in liver transplantation may ↑ risk of hepatic artery thrombosis; fatalities have been reported (not approved for this use). May ↓ antibody response to and ↑ risk of adverse reactions to **live-virus vaccines** (avoid vaccination).
Drug-Natural: Concomitant use with **echinacea** and **melatonin** may interfere with immunosuppression. **St. John's wort** may ↑ blood levels and the risk of toxicity.
Drug-Food: Grapefruit juice ↓ CYP3A4 metabolism and ↑ levels; do not use as a diluent and avoid concurrent ingestion.

Route/Dosage

PO (Adults and Children ≥13 yr): 6-mg loading dose, followed by 2 mg/day maintenance dose. *Dosing following cyclosporine withdrawal*—Patients at low-to-moderate risk for rejection after transplantation may be withdrawn from cyclosporine over 4–8 wk beginning 2–4 mo after transplant. Thereafter, sirolimus dose should be titrated upward to maintain a whole blood trough level of 12–14 ng/mL. Clinical assessment should also be used to gauge dose. Dose changes can be made at 7- to 14-day intervals. The following formula may also be used: sirolimus maintenance dose = current dose x (target concentration/current concentration). If a large increase is needed, a loading dose may be given and blood levels reassessed 3–4 days later. Loading dose may be calculated by the following formula: sirolimus loading dose = 3 × (new maintenance dose-current maintenance dose). Loading doses >40 mg should be spread over 2 days.
PO (Adults and Children ≥13 yr and <40 kg): 3 mg/m^2 loading dose, followed by 1 mg/m^2/day maintenance dose. *See adjustments above for doses following cyclosporine withdrawal.*

Hepatic Impairment

PO (Adults and Children ≥13 yr and <40 kg): Decrease maintenance dose by 33%; loading dose is unchanged.

Availability

Tablet: 1 mg, 2 mg. **Oral solution:** 1 mg/mL in 60-mL bottles (with oral syringes).

sitagliptin (sit-a-glip-tin)
Januvia

Classification
Therapeutic: antidiabetics
Pharmacologic: enzyme inhibitors

Indications
Adjunct to diet and exercise to improve glycemic control in patients with type 2 diabetes mellitus; may be used as monotherapy or combination therapy with metformin and a thiazolidinedione and/or a sulfonylurea.

Action
Inhibits the enzyme dipeptidyl peptidase-4 (DPP-4), which slows the inactivation of incretin hormones, resulting in increased levels of active incretin hormones. These hormones are released by the intestine throughout the day, and are involved in regulation of glucose homeostasis. Increased/prolonged incretin levels increase insulin release and decrease glucagon levels. **Therapeutic Effects:** Improved control of blood glucose.

Adverse Reactions/Side Effects
CNS: headache. **GI:** nausea, diarrhea. **Resp:** upper respiratory tract infection, nasopharyngitis.
Misc: hypersensitivity reactions including anaphylaxis, angioedema, and exfoliative skin conditions (Stevens-Johnson syndrome), rash, urticaria.

PHYSICAL THERAPY IMPLICATIONS

Examination and Evaluation
- Monitor signs of hypersensitivity reactions (anaphylaxis, angioedema, Stevens-Johnson syndrome), including pulmonary symptoms (tightness in the throat and chest, wheezing, cough, dyspnea) and skin reactions (rash, pruritius, urticaria, burning skin, exfoliation, swelling in the face). Notify physician immediately of these signs.
- Be alert for signs of hypoglycemia, especially during and after exercise. Common neuromuscular signs include anxiety; restlessness; tingling in hands, feet, lips, or tongue; chills; cold sweats; confusion; difficulty in concentration; drowsiness; excessive hunger; headache; irritability; nervousness; tremor; weakness; unsteady gait. Report persistent or repeated episodes of hypoglycemia to the physician.
- Monitor symptoms of upper respiratory tract infection and inflammation including cough, production of mucus, wheezing, chest discomfort, shortness of breath, fatigue, chills, and fever. Report severe or prolonged symptoms to the physician.
- Assess blood pressure periodically (See Appendix F). A sudden or sustained increase in blood pressure (hypertension) may indicate problems in diabetes management and should be reported to the physician.

Interventions
- Implement aerobic exercise and endurance training programs to maintain optimal body weight, improve insulin sensitivity, and reduce the risk of macrovascular disease (heart attack, stroke) and microvascular problems (reduced blood flow to tissues and organs that causes poor wound healing, neuropathy, retinopathy, and nephropathy).

Patient/Client-Related Instruction
- Encourage patient to monitor blood glucose before and after exercise and to adjust food intake to maintain normal glycemic levels.
- Emphasize the importance of adhering to nutritional guidelines and the need for periodic assessment of glycemic control (serum glucose and glycosylated hemoglobin levels) throughout the management of diabetes mellitus.
- Advise patient about symptoms of hyperglycemia (confusion, drowsiness; flushed, dry skin; fruit-like breath odor; rapid, deep breathing, polyuria; loss of appetite; unusual thirst). Drug dosages may need to be adjusted to prevent repeated episodes of hyperglycemia.
- Instruct patient to report other troublesome side effects such as severe or prolonged headache or GI problems (nausea, diarrhea).

Pharmacokinetics
Absorption: 87% absorbed following oral administration.
Distribution: Unknown.
Metabolism and Excretion: 79% excreted unchanged in urine, minor metabolism.
Half-life: 12.4 hr.

TIME/ACTION PROFILE

ROUTE	ONSET	PEAK	DURATION
PO	rapid	1–4 hr	24 hr

Contraindications/Precautions
Contraindicated in: Type 1 diabetes mellitus; Diabetic ketoacidosis; hypersensitivity.
Use Cautiously in: Renal impairment (dose reduction required for CCr <50 mL/min; Geri: Consider age-related decrease in renal function when determining dose; OB/Lactation: Use in pregnancy only if clearly needed; use cautiously in lactation; Pedi: Safe use in children not established.

S

Interactions

Drug-Drug: May slightly ↑ serum digoxin levels; monitoring recommended.

Route/Dosage

PO (Adults): 100 mg once daily.

Renal Impairment

PO (Adults): *CC 30–<50 mL/min*—50 mg once daily; *CC <30 mL/min*—25 mg once daily.

Availability

Tablets: 25 mg, 50 mg, 100 mg. ***In combination with:*** metformin (Janumet). See Appendix B.

solifenacin (soe-li-**fen**-a-sin)

VESIcare

Classification

Therapeutic: urinary tract antispasmodics

Pharmacologic: anticholinergics

Indications

Overactive bladder with symptoms (urge incontinence, urgency, frequency).

Action

Acts as a muscarinic (cholinergic) receptor antagonist; antagonizes bladder smooth muscle contraction. **Therapeutic Effects:** Decreased symptoms of overactive bladder.

Adverse Reactions/Side Effects

EENT: blurred vision. **GI:** constipation, dry mouth, dyspepsia, nausea.

PHYSICAL THERAPY IMPLICATIONS

Examination and Evaluation

- Monitor signs of urine retention (difficult urination, painful or distended abdomen). Excessive urinary retention may require dose adjustment by physician.

Interventions

- When appropriate, implement pelvic floor muscle–strengthening activities and other therapeutic exercises to help maintain bladder control.

Patient/Client-Related Instruction

- Advise patient to increase fluid intake and dietary fiber to avoid constipation. Laxatives may also be helpful in patients susceptible to fecal impaction.
- Instruct patient and family/caregivers to report other troublesome side effects such as severe or prolonged blurred vision or GI problems (nausea, dry mouth, indigestion).

Pharmacokinetics

Absorption: Well absorbed (90%).
Distribution: Unknown.
Protein Binding: 98%.
Metabolism and Excretion: Extensively metabolized by the CYP3A4 enzyme system. 69% excreted in urine as metabolites, 22% in feces.
Half-life: 45–68 hr.

TIME/ACTION PROFILE

ROUTE	ONSET	PEAK	DURATION
PO	unknown	3–8 hr	24 hr

Contraindications/Precautions

Contraindicated in: Hypersensitivity; Urinary retention; Gastric retention; Uncontrolled angle-closure glaucoma; Severe hepatic impairment; Lactation.

Use Cautiously in: Concurrent use of CYP3A4 inhibitors (use lower dose/clinical monitoring may be necessary); Moderate hepatic impairment (lower dose recommended); Renal impairment (dose should not exceed 5 mg/day if CCr < 30 mL/min); Bladder outflow obstruction; GI obstructive disorders, severe constipation or ulcerative colitis; Myasthenia gravis; Angle-closure glaucoma; Children (safety not established); Pregnancy (use only if maternal benefit outweighs fetal risk).

Interactions

Drug-Drug: Drugs that induce or inhibit the CYP3A4 enzyme system may significantly alter blood levels of solifenacin; **ketoconazole** ↑ blood levels and risk of toxicity (do not exceed 5 mg/day).

Route/Dosage

PO (Adults): 5 mg once daily, may be ↑ to 10 mg once daily; *hepatic impairment/severe renal impairment, concurrent use of ketoconazole or other inhibitors of CYP3A4*—dose should not exceed 5 mg/day.

Availability

Tablets: 5 mg, 10 mg.

somatropin (recombinant) (soe-ma-**troe**-pin)

Humatrope

Classification

Therapeutic: hormones

Pharmacologic: growth hormones

Indications

Growth failure in children due to deficiency of growth hormone. Growth failure in children with idiopathic short stature (non–growth hormone–deficient short stature). Short stature associated with Turner's syndrome. SHOX (short stature homeobox-containing gene) deficiency. Growth hormone deficiency in adults as a result of pituitary disease, hypothalamic disease, surgery, radiation or trauma.

Action

Produce growth (skeletal and cellular). Metabolic actions include Increased protein synthesis, Increased carbohydrate metabolism, Lipid mobilization, Retention of sodium, phosphorus, and potassium. Somatropin has the same amino acid sequence as naturally occurring growth hormone and is produced by recombinant DNA techniques. Growth hormone enhances GI tract mucosal transport of water, electrolytes, and nutrients. **Therapeutic Effects:** Increased skeletal growth in children with growth hormone deficiency. Replacement of somatropin in deficient adults. Increased bone density in adult growth hormone–deficient patients.

Adverse Reactions/Side Effects

CV: edema of the hands and feet. **Endo:** hyperglycemia, hypothyroidism, insulin resistance. **Local:** pain at injection site, local lipoatrophy, or lipodystrophy with SC use. **MS:** arthralgia.

PHYSICAL THERAPY IMPLICATIONS

Examination and Evaluation

- Periodically assess height and weight in children to help document the effects of drug therapy.
- Assess edema in the hands and feet using girth measurements, volume displacement, and measurement of pitting edema (See Appendix N). Report increased swelling, especially if ROM and function are compromised.
- Assess any joint pain to rule out musculoskeletal pathology; that is, try to determine if pain is drug-induced rather than caused by anatomic or biomechanical problems.
- Be alert for signs of hyperglycemia and insulin resistance, including confusion, drowsiness, flushed/dry skin, fruit-like breath odor, rapid/deep breathing, polyuria, loss of appetite, and unusual thirst. Patients with diabetes mellitus should check blood glucose levels frequently.
- Monitor any decrease in metabolism that might indicate hypothyroidism. Common signs include bradycardia, lethargy, cold intolerance, weight gain, and muscle weakness. Report these signs to the physician.
- Monitor subcutaneous injection site for bruising or decreased local fat accumulation (lipoatrophy, lipodystrophy). Report prolonged or excessive injection site reactions to the physician.

Interventions

- Design and implement therapeutic exercise programs to capitalize on growth hormone effects and increase muscle strength and bone mineral density in children and adults.
- Do not apply physical agents (heat, cold, electrotherapeutic modalities) or massage over the injection site; these interventions can alter drug absorption from subcutaneous tissues.

Patient/Client-Related Instruction

- Advise patient and family/caregivers to adhere to recommended dosing schedule. Emphasize that growth hormones must not be used to increase athletic performance, and that administration to people without growth hormone deficiency or after epiphyseal closure may result in acromegaly (coarsening of facial features; enlarged hands, feet, and internal organs; increased blood glucose; hypertension).

Pharmacokinetics

Absorption: Well absorbed.
Distribution: Localize to highly perfused organs (liver, kidneys).
Metabolism and Excretion: Broken down in renal cells to amino acids that are recirculated; some liver metabolism.
Half-life: *SC*—3.8 hr; *IM*—4.9 hr.

TIME/ACTION PROFILE (growth)

ROUTE	ONSET	PEAK	DURATION
IM, SC	within 3 mo	unknown	12–48 hr

Contraindications/Precautions

Contraindicated in: Closure of epiphyses; Active neoplasia; Hypersensitivity to growth hormone, *m*-cresol, or glycerin preservative; Acute critical illness (therapy should not be initiated) or respiratory failure; Diabetic retinopathy; Prader-Willi syndrome with obesity and respiratory impairment (risk of fatal complications; can be used only if growth hormone deficiency is documented).
Use Cautiously in: Growth hormone deficiency due to intracranial lesion; Coexisting adrenocorticotropic hormone (ACTH) deficiency; Diabetes (may cause insulin resistance); Geriatric patients (↑ sensitivity, ↑ risk of adverse reactions); Thyroid dysfunction; Pregnancy or lactation (safety not established).

Interactions

Drug-Drug: Excessive **corticosteroid** use (equivalent to 10–15 mg/m^2/day) may ↓ response to growth hormone.

Route/Dosage

SC (Adults): 0.006 mg/kg/day (up to 0.0125 mg/kg/day) or 0.2 mg/day starting dose (without consideration of body weight) then gradually increase by

0.1–0.2 mg/day q 1–2 mo until clinical response achieved.
IM, SC (Children): *Growth hormone deficiency*—0.18 mg/kg (0.54 unit/kg)/wk given in divided doses on 3 alternating days or 6–7 days/wk (maximum: 0.3 mg/kg or 0.9 unit/kg/wk). *Turner's syndrome*—0.375 mg/kg (1.125 unit/kg)/wk divided into 3, 6, or 7 daily doses. *Idiopathic short stature*—0.37 mg/kg/wk divided into 6–7 daily doses. *SHOX deficiency*—0.35 mg/kg/wk divided into 7 daily doses.

Availability

Powder for injection: 5-mg/vial, 6-mg, 12-mg, and 24-mg cartridge kits.

somatropin (recombinant)

(soe-ma-**troe**-pin)
Norditropin

Classification
Therapeutic: hormones
Pharmacologic: growth hormones

Indications

Growth failure in children due to deficiency of growth hormone. Growth hormone deficiency in adults as a result of pituitary disease, hypothalamic disease, surgery, radiation, or trauma.

Action

Produce growth (skeletal and cellular). Metabolic actions include increased protein synthesis, ↑ carbohydrate metabolism, Lipid mobilization, Retention of sodium, phosphorus, and potassium. Somatropin has the same amino acid sequence as naturally occurring growth hormone and is produced by recombinant DNA techniques. Growth hormone enhances GI tract mucosal transport of water, electrolytes, and nutrients.
Therapeutic Effects: ↑ skeletal growth in children with growth hormone deficiency. Replacement of somatropin in deficient adults. ↑ bone density in adult growth hormone–deficient patients.

Adverse Reactions/Side Effects

CV: edema of the hands and feet. **Endo:** hyperglycemia, hypothyroidism, insulin resistance. **Local:** pain at injection site, local lipoatrophy or lipodystrophy with SC use. **MS:** arthralgia.

PHYSICAL THERAPY IMPLICATIONS

Examination and Evaluation

- Periodically assess height and weight in children to help document the effects of drug therapy.
- Assess edema in the hands and feet using girth measurements, volume displacement, and measurement of pitting edema (See Appendix N). Report increased swelling, especially if ROM and function are compromised.
- Assess any joint pain to rule out musculoskeletal pathology; that is, try to determine if pain is drug induced rather than caused by anatomic or biomechanical problems.
- Be alert for signs of hyperglycemia and insulin resistance, including confusion, drowsiness, flushed/dry skin, fruit-like breath odor, rapid/deep breathing, polyuria, loss of appetite, and unusual thirst. Patients with diabetes mellitus should check blood glucose levels frequently.
- Monitor any decrease in metabolism that might indicate hypothyroidism. Common signs include bradycardia, lethargy, cold intolerance, weight gain, and muscle weakness. Report these signs to the physician.
- Monitor subcutaneous injection site for bruising or decreased local fat accumulation (lipoatrophy, lipodystrophy). Report prolonged or excessive injection site reactions to the physician.

Interventions

- Design and implement therapeutic exercise programs to capitalize on growth hormone effects and increase muscle strength and bone mineral density in children and adults.
- Do not apply physical agents (heat, cold, electrotherapeutic modalities) or massage over the injection site; these interventions can alter drug absorption from subcutaneous tissues.

Patient/Client-Related Instruction

- Advise patient and family/caregivers to adhere to recommended dosing schedule. Emphasize that growth hormones must not be used to increase athletic performance, and that administration to people without growth hormone deficiency or after epiphyseal closure may result in acromegaly (coarsening of facial features; enlarged hands, feet, and internal organs; increased blood glucose; hypertension).

Pharmacokinetics

Absorption: Well absorbed.
Distribution: Localize to highly perfused organs (liver, kidneys).
Metabolism and Excretion: Broken down in renal cells to amino acids that are recirculated; some liver metabolism.
Half-life: *SC*—3.8 hr.

TIME/ACTION PROFILE (growth)

ROUTE	ONSET	PEAK	DURATION
IM, SC	within 3 mo	unknown	12–48 hr

Contraindications/Precautions

Contraindicated in: Closure of epiphyses; Active neoplasia; Hypersensitivity to growth hormone or phenol preservative; Acute critical illness (therapy should not be initiated) or respiratory failure; Diabetic retinopathy; Prader-Willi syndrome with obesity and respiratory impairment (risk of fatal complications; can be used only if growth hormone deficiency is documented).

Use Cautiously in: Growth hormone deficiency due to intracranial lesion; Coexisting adrenocorticotropic hormone (ACTH) deficiency; Diabetes (may cause insulin resistance); Geriatric patients (↑ sensitivity, ↑ risk of adverse reactions; Thyroid dysfunction; Pregnancy or lactation (safety not established).

Interactions

Drug-Drug: Excessive **corticosteroid** use (equivalent to 10–15 mg/m²/day) may ↓ response to growth hormone.

Route/Dosage

SC (Adults): 0.004 mg/kg/day, may be increased to 0.016 mg/kg/day after 6 wk or 0.2 mg/day starting dose (without consideration of body weight), then gradually increase by 0.1–0.2 mg/day q 1–2 mo until clinical response achieved.

SC (Children): 0.024–0.034 mg/kg/day given 6–7 times weekly.

Availability

Cartridges for injection (using NordiPen): 5 mg/1.5 mL (orange), 10 mg/1.5 mL (blue), 15 mg/1.5 mL (green).

Prefilled pens for injection (Nordiflex): 5 mg/1.5 mL (orange), 10 mg/1.5 mL (blue), 15 mg/1.5mL (green).

somatropin (recombinant)

(soe-ma-**troe**-pin)

Nutropin, Nutropin AQ, Nutropin Depot

Classification

Therapeutic: hormones

Pharmacologic: growth hormones

Indications

Growth failure in children due to deficiency of growth hormone. Growth failure in children with idiopathic short stature (non–growth-hormone–deficient short stature). Short stature associated with Turner's syndrome. Growth failure associated with chronic renal insufficiency. Growth hormone deficiency in adults as a result of pituitary disease, hypothalamic disease, surgery, radiation or trauma.

Action

Produce growth (skeletal and cellular). Metabolic actions include ↑ protein synthesis; ↑ carbohydrate metabolism; Lipid mobilization; Retention of sodium, phosphorus, and potassium. Somatropin has the same amino acid sequence as naturally occurring growth hormone and is produced by recombinant DNA techniques. Growth hormone enhances GI tract mucosal transport of water, electrolytes, and nutrients.

Therapeutic Effects: ↑ skeletal growth in children with growth hormone deficiency. Replacement of somatropin in deficient adults. ↑ bone density in adult growth hormone–deficient patients.

Adverse Reactions/Side Effects

CV: edema of the hands and feet. **Endo:** hyperglycemia, hypothyroidism, insulin resistance. **Local:** pain at injection site, local lipoatrophy, or lipodystrophy with SC use. **MS:** arthralgia.

PHYSICAL THERAPY IMPLICATIONS

Examination and Evaluation

- Periodically assess height and weight in children to help document the effects of drug therapy.
- Assess edema in the hands and feet using girth measurements, volume displacement, and measurement of pitting edema (See Appendix N). Report increased swelling, especially if ROM and function are compromised.
- Assess any joint pain to rule out musculoskeletal pathology; that is, try to determine if pain is drug induced rather than caused by anatomic or biomechanical problems.
- Be alert for signs of hyperglycemia and insulin resistance, including confusion, drowsiness, flushed/dry skin, fruit-like breath odor, rapid/deep breathing, polyuria, loss of appetite, and unusual thirst. Patients with diabetes mellitus should check blood glucose levels frequently.
- Monitor any decrease in metabolism that might indicate hypothyroidism. Common signs include bradycardia, lethargy, cold intolerance, weight gain, and muscle weakness. Report these signs to the physician.
- Monitor subcutaneous injection site for bruising or decreased local fat accumulation (lipoatrophy, lipodystrophy). Report prolonged or excessive injection site reactions to the physician.

Interventions

- Design and implement therapeutic exercise programs to capitalize on growth hormone effects and increase muscle strength and bone mineral density in children and adults.
- Do not apply physical agents (heat, cold, electrotherapeutic modalities) or massage over the injection site; these interventions can alter drug absorption from subcutaneous tissues.

Patient/Client-Related Instruction

- Advise patient and family/caregivers to adhere to recommended dosing schedule. Emphasize that growth hormones must not be used to increase athletic performance, and that administration to people without growth hormone deficiency or after epiphyseal closure may result in acromegaly (coarsening of facial features; enlarged hands, feet, and internal organs; increased blood glucose; hypertension).

Pharmacokinetics

Absorption: Well absorbed.
Distribution: Localize to highly perfused organs (liver, kidneys).
Metabolism and Excretion: Broken down in renal cells to amino acids that are recirculated; some liver metabolism.
Half-life: *Subcut*—3.8 hr.

TIME/ACTION PROFILE (growth)

ROUTE	ONSET	PEAK	DURATION
IM, SC	within 3 mo	unknown	12–48 hr

Contraindications/Precautions

Contraindicated in: Closure of epiphyses; Active neoplasia; Hypersensitivity to growth hormone or benzyl alcohol preservative; Acute critical illness (therapy should not be initiated) or respiratory failure; Diabetic retinopathy; Prader-Willi syndrome with obesity and respiratory impairment (risk of fatal complications; can be used only if growth hormone deficiency is documented).
Use Cautiously in: Growth hormone deficiency due to intracranial lesion; Coexisting adrenocorticotropic hormone (ACTH) deficiency; Diabetes (may cause insulin resistance); Geriatric patients (↑ sensitivity, ↑ risk of adverse reactions; Thyroid dysfunction; Neonates (diluent contains benzyl alcohol and may cause fatal gasping syndrome); Pregnancy or lactation (safety not established).

Interactions

Drug-Drug: Excessive **corticosteroid** use (equivalent to 10–15 mg/m^2/day) may ↓ response to growth hormone.

Route/Dosage

SC (Children): *Growth hormone deficiency or idiopathic short stature*—0.3 mg/kg/wk divided into daily doses. Pubertal patients with growth hormone deficiency may require up to 0.7 mg/kg/wk. *Chronic renal insufficiency*—0.35 mg/kg/wk given as daily injections. *Turner's syndrome*— up to 0.375 mg/kg/wk in 3–7 divided doses.
SC (Adults): initially 0.006 mg/kg daily; may be increased up to 0.025 mg/kg/day in patients <35 yr or 0.0125 mg/kg in patients >35 yr or 0.2 mg/day starting dose (without consideration of body weight) then gradually ↑ by 0.1–0.2 mg/day q 1–2 mo until clinical response achieved.

Availability

Nutropin

Powder for injection: 5-mg (15 units)/vial, 10-mg (30 units)/vial.

Nutropin AQ

Solution for injection (AQ): 10 mg (30 units)/mL in 2-mL vial or 10 mg (30 units)/mL in 2-mL pen cartridge.

somatropin (recombinant)

(soe-ma-**troe**-pin)
Saizen

Classification
Therapeutic: hormones
Pharmacologic: growth hormones

Indications

Growth failure in children due to inadequate secretion of growth hormone. Growth hormone deficiency in adults as a result of pituitary disease, hypothalamic disease, surgery, radiation, or trauma.

Action

Produce growth (skeletal and cellular). Metabolic actions include ↑ protein synthesis, ↑ carbohydrate metabolism, Lipid mobilization, Retention of sodium, phosphorus, and potassium. Somatropin has the same amino acid sequence as naturally occurring growth hormone and is produced by recombinant DNA techniques. Growth hormone enhances GI tract mucosal transport of water, electrolytes, and nutrients.
Therapeutic Effects: ↑ skeletal growth in children with growth hormone deficiency. Replacement of somatropin in deficient adults. ↑ bone density in adult growth hormone–deficient patients.

Adverse Reactions/Side Effects

CV: edema of the hands and feet. **Derm:** exacerbation of preexisting psoriasis. **Endo:** hyperglycemia, hypothyroidism, insulin resistance. **Local:** pain at injection site, local lipoatrophy, or lipodystrophy with SC use. **MS:** arthralgia, musculoskeletal pain, swelling, stiffness.

PHYSICAL THERAPY IMPLICATIONS

Examination and Evaluation

- Periodically assess height and weight in children to help document the effects of drug therapy.
- Assess edema in the hands and feet using girth measurements, volume displacement, and

measurement of pitting edema (See Appendix N). Report increased swelling, especially if ROM and function are compromised.

- Assess any joint pain or musculoskeletal pain, swelling, or stiffness to rule out musculoskeletal pathology; that is, try to determine if pain is drug induced rather than caused by anatomic or biomechanical problems.
- Be alert for signs of hyperglycemia and insulin resistance, including confusion, drowsiness, flushed/dry skin, fruit-like breath odor, rapid/deep breathing, polyuria, loss of appetite, and unusual thirst. Patients with diabetes mellitus should check blood glucose levels frequently.
- Monitor any decrease in metabolism that might indicate hypothyroidism. Common signs include bradycardia, lethargy, cold intolerance, weight gain, and muscle weakness. Report these signs to the physician.
- Monitor skin reactions in patients with preexisting psoriasis, and report any increase in symptoms such as scaly patches and red, itching, burning, dry, and cracked skin.
- Monitor subcutaneous injection site for bruising or decreased local fat accumulation (lipoatrophy, lipodystrophy). Report prolonged or excessive injection site reactions to the physician.

Interventions

- Design and implement therapeutic exercise programs to capitalize on growth hormone effects and increase muscle strength and bone mineral density in children and adults.
- Do not apply physical agents (heat, cold, electrotherapeutic modalities) or massage over the injection site; these interventions can alter drug absorption from subcutaneous tissues.

Patient/Client-Related Instruction

- Advise patient and family/caregivers to adhere to recommended dosing schedule. Emphasize that growth hormones must not be used to increase athletic performance, and that administration to people without growth hormone deficiency or after epiphyseal closure may result in acromegaly (coarsening of facial features; enlarged hands, feet, and internal organs; increased blood glucose; hypertension).

Pharmacokinetics

Absorption: Well absorbed.
Distribution: Localize to highly perfused organs (liver, kidneys).
Metabolism and Excretion: Broken down in renal cells to amino acids that are recirculated; some liver metabolism.
Half-life: *SCt*—3.8 hr; *IM*—4.9 hr.

TIME/ACTION PROFILE (growth)

ROUTE	ONSET	PEAK	DURATION
IM, SC	within 3 mo	unknown	12–48 hr

Contraindications/Precautions

Contraindicated in: Closure of epiphyses; Active neoplasia; Hypersensitivity to growth hormone or benzyl alcohol preservative; Acute critical illness (therapy should not be initiated) or respiratory failure; Diabetic retinopathy; Prader-Willi syndrome with obesity and respiratory impairment (risk of fatal complications; can be used only if growth hormone deficiency is documented).
Use Cautiously in: Growth hormone deficiency due to intracranial lesion; Coexisting adrenocorticotropic hormone (ACTH) deficiency; Diabetes (may cause insulin resistance); Geriatric patients (↑ sensitivity, ↑ risk of adverse reactions; Thyroid dysfunction; Neonates (diluent contains benzyl alcohol and may cause fatal gasping syndrome); Pregnancy or lactation (safety not established).

Interactions

Drug-Drug: Excessive **corticosteroid** use (equivalent to 10–15 mg/m^2/day) may ↓ response to growth hormone.

Route/Dosage

SC, IM (Adults): initially 0.005 mg/kg/day, may be increased to 0.01 mg/kg/day after 4 wk.
SC, IM (Children): 0.06 mg (0.18 unit/kg) 3 times weekly.

Availability

Powder for injection: 5-mg (15 units)/vial, 8.8-mg (26.4 units)/vial, 8.8-mg (26.4 units)/vial in click-easy device.

S

somatropin (recombinant)

(soe-ma-**troe**-pin)
Serostim

Classification
Therapeutic: hormones
Pharmacologic: growth hormones

Indications

Treatment of HIV-associated wasting.

Action

Produce growth (skeletal and cellular). Metabolic actions include ↑ protein synthesis, ↑ carbohydrate metabolism, Lipid mobilization, Retention of sodium,

phosphorus, and potassium. Somatropin has the same amino acid sequence as naturally occurring growth hormone and is produced by recombinant DNA techniques. Growth hormone enhances GI tract mucosal transport of water, electrolytes, and nutrients.
Therapeutic Effects: ↓ wasting in patients with AIDS.

Adverse Reactions/Side Effects

CV: edema of the hands and feet. **Endo:** hyperglycemia, hypothyroidism, insulin resistance. **Local:** pain at injection site, local lipoatrophy or lipodystrophy with SC use. **MS:** arthralgia, carpal tunnel syndrome.

PHYSICAL THERAPY IMPLICATIONS

Examination and Evaluation

- Assess edema in the hands and feet using girth measurements, volume displacement, and measurement of pitting edema (See Appendix N). Report increased swelling, especially if ROM and function are compromised, or if patient exhibits signs of carpal tunnel syndrome (numbness, tingling, and weakness in median nerve distribution to the hand).
- Assess any joint pain to rule out musculoskeletal pathology; that is, try to determine if pain is drug induced rather than caused by anatomic or biomechanical problems.
- Be alert for signs of hyperglycemia and insulin resistance, including confusion, drowsiness, flushed/dry skin, fruit-like breath odor, rapid/deep breathing, polyuria, loss of appetite, and unusual thirst. Patients with diabetes mellitus should check blood glucose levels frequently.
- Monitor any decrease in metabolism that might indicate hypothyroidism. Common signs include bradycardia, lethargy, cold intolerance, weight gain, and muscle weakness. Report these signs to the physician.
- Monitor subcutaneous injection site for bruising or decreased local fat accumulation (lipoatrophy, lipodystrophy). Report prolonged or excessive injection site reactions to the physician.

Interventions

- Design and implement therapeutic exercise programs to capitalize on growth hormone effects and increase muscle strength and decrease muscle wasting in patients with AIDs.
- Do not apply physical agents (heat, cold, electrotherapeutic modalities) or massage over the injection site; these interventions can alter drug absorption from subcutaneous tissues.

Patient/Client-Related Instruction

- Advise patient and family/caregivers to adhere to recommended dosing schedule. Emphasize that growth hormones must not be used to increase athletic performance, and that administration to people without growth hormone deficiency or after epiphyseal closure may result in acromegaly (coarsening of facial features; enlarged hands, feet, and internal organs; increased blood glucose; hypertension).

Pharmacokinetics

Absorption: Well absorbed.
Distribution: Localize to highly perfused organs (liver, kidneys).
Metabolism and Excretion: Broken down in renal cells to amino acids that are recirculated; some liver metabolism.
Half-life: *SC*—4.28 ± 2.15 hr.

TIME/ACTION PROFILE

ROUTE	ONSET	PEAK	DURATION
SC	unknown	unknown	unknown

Contraindications/Precautions

Contraindicated in: Closure of epiphyses; Active neoplasia; Hypersensitivity to growth hormone; Acute critical illness (therapy should not be initiated) or respiratory failure; Diabetic retinopathy; Prader-Willi syndrome with obesity and respiratory impairment (risk of fatal complications; can be used only if growth hormone deficiency is documented).
Use Cautiously in: Growth hormone deficiency due to intracranial lesion; Coexisting adrenocorticotropic hormone (ACTH) deficiency; Diabetes (may cause insulin resistance); Geriatric patients (↑ sensitivity, ↑ risk of adverse reactions; Thyroid dysfunction; Pregnancy or lactation (safety not established).

Interactions

Drug-Drug: Excessive **corticosteroid** use (equivalent to 10–15 mg/m²/day) may ↓ response to growth hormone.

Route/Dosage

SC (Adults): *>55 kg*—6 mg once daily; *45–55 kg*—5 mg once daily; *35–45 kg*—4 mg once daily; *<35 kg*—0.1 mg/kg once daily.
SC (Children): 0.04–0.07 mg/kg/day.

Availability

Powder for injection: 4-mg (12 units)/vial, 5-mg (15 units)/vial, 6-mg (18 units)/vial.

somatropin (recombinant)

(soe-ma-**troe**-pin)
Tev-Tropin

Classification
Therapeutic: hormones
Pharmacologic: growth hormones

Indications
Growth failure in children due to inadequate secretion growth hormone.

Action
Produce growth (skeletal and cellular). Metabolic actions include ↑ protein synthesis, ↑ carbohydrate metabolism, Lipid mobilization, Retention of sodium, phosphorus, and potassium. Somatropin has the same amino acid sequence as naturally occurring growth hormone and is produced by recombinant DNA techniques. Growth hormone enhances GI tract mucosal transport of water, electrolytes, and nutrients. **Therapeutic Effects:** ↑ skeletal growth in children with growth hormone deficiency.

Adverse Reactions/Side Effects
CV: edema of the hands and feet. **Endo:** hyperglycemia, hypothyroidism, insulin resistance. **Local:** pain at injection site, local lipoatrophy, or lipodystrophy with SC use. **MS:** arthralgia.

PHYSICAL THERAPY IMPLICATIONS

Examination and Evaluation
- Periodically assess height and weight in children to help document the effects of drug therapy.
- Assess edema in the hands and feet using girth measurements, volume displacement, and measurement of pitting edema (See Appendix N). Report increased swelling, especially if ROM and function are compromised.
- Assess any joint pain to rule out musculoskeletal pathology; that is, try to determine if pain is drug induced rather than caused by anatomic or biomechanical problems.
- Be alert for signs of hyperglycemia and insulin resistance, including confusion, drowsiness, flushed/dry skin, fruit-like breath odor, rapid/deep breathing, polyuria, loss of appetite, and unusual thirst. Patients with diabetes mellitus should check blood glucose levels frequently.
- Monitor any decrease in metabolism that might indicate hypothyroidism. Common signs include bradycardia, lethargy, cold intolerance, weight gain, and muscle weakness. Report these signs to the physician.
- Monitor subcutaneous injection site for bruising or decreased local fat accumulation (lipoatrophy, lipodystrophy). Report prolonged or excessive injection site reactions to the physician.

Interventions
- Design and implement therapeutic exercise programs to capitalize on growth hormone effects and increase muscle strength and function in children.
- Do not apply physical agents (heat, cold, electrotherapeutic modalities) or massage over the injection site; these interventions can alter drug absorption from subcutaneous tissues.

Patient/Client-Related Instruction
- Advise patient and family/caregivers to adhere to recommended dosing schedule. Emphasize that growth hormones must not be used to increase athletic performance, and that administration to people without growth hormone deficiency or after epiphyseal closure may result in acromegaly (coarsening of facial features; enlarged hands, feet, and internal organs; increased blood glucose; hypertension).

Pharmacokinetics
Absorption: Well absorbed (70%).
Distribution: Localize to highly perfused organs (liver, kidneys).
Metabolism and Excretion: Broken down in renal cells to amino acids that are recirculated; some liver metabolism.
Half-life: *SC*—2.7 hr.

TIME/ACTION PROFILE (growth)

ROUTE	ONSET	PEAK	DURATION
SC	within 3 mo	unknown	unknown

Contraindications/Precautions
Contraindicated in: Closure of epiphyses; Active neoplasia; Hypersensitivity to growth hormone or *m*-cresol preservative; Acute critical illness (therapy should not be initiated) or respiratory failure; Diabetic retinopathy; Prader-Willi syndrome with obesity and respiratory impairment (risk of fatal complications; can be used only if growth hormone deficiency is documented).
Use Cautiously in: Growth hormone deficiency due to intracranial lesion; Coexisting adrenocorticotropic hormone (ACTH) deficiency; Diabetes (may cause insulin resistance); Geriatric patients (↑ sensitivity, ↑ risk of adverse reactions; Thyroid dysfunction; Neonates (diluent contains benzyl alcohol and may cause fatal gasping syndrome); Pregnancy or lactation (safety not established).

Interactions
Drug-Drug: Excessive **corticosteroid** use (equivalent to 10–15 mg/m^2/day) may ↓ response to growth hormone.

Route/Dosage
SC (Children): up to 0.1 mg/kg (0.3 units/kg) 3 times weekly.

S

Availability

Powder for injection: 5-mg (15 units)/vial.

somatropin (recombinant)

(soe-ma-**troe**-pin)

Zorbtive

Classification

Therapeutic: hormones

Pharmacologic: growth hormones

Indications

Treatment of short bowel syndrome in patients receiving specialized nutritional support.

Action

Produce growth (skeletal and cellular). Metabolic actions include ↑ protein synthesis; ↑carbohydrate metabolism; Lipid mobilization; Retention of sodium, phosphorus, and potassium. Somatropin has the same amino acid sequence as naturally occurring growth hormone and is produced by recombinant DNA techniques. Growth hormone enhances GI tract mucosal transport of water, electrolytes, and nutrients. **Therapeutic Effects:** Enhanced GI absorption of water, electrolytes, and nutrients in short bowel syndrome.

Adverse Reactions/Side Effects

CV: edema of the hands and feet. **CNS:** fever, malaise, dizziness. **Derm:** swelling of hands and feet. **Endo:** hyperglycemia, hypothyroidism, insulin resistance. **GI:** flatulence, vomiting. **Local:** pain at injection site, local lipoatrophy, or lipodystrophy with SC use. **MS:** arthralgia, musculoskeletal pain.

PHYSICAL THERAPY IMPLICATIONS

Examination and Evaluation

- Monitor body weight and other symptoms (weakness, fatigue, malaise) to help document whether this drug is successful in enhancing GI absorption of nutrients, water, and electrolytes.
- Assess edema in the hands and feet using girth measurements, volume displacement, and measurement of pitting edema (See Appendix N). Report increased swelling, especially if ROM and function are compromised.
- Assess any joint pain or muscle pain to rule out musculoskeletal pathology; that is, try to determine if pain is drug induced rather than caused by anatomic or biomechanical problems.
- Be alert for signs of hyperglycemia and insulin resistance, including confusion, drowsiness, flushed/dry skin, fruit-like breath odor, rapid/deep breathing, polyuria, loss of appetite, and unusual thirst. Patients with diabetes mellitus should check blood glucose levels frequently.
- Monitor any decrease in metabolism that might indicate hypothyroidism. Common signs include bradycardia, lethargy, cold intolerance, weight gain, and muscle weakness. Report these signs to the physician.
- Assess dizziness that might affect gait, balance, and other functional activities (See Appendix C). Report balance problems and functional limitations to the physician, and caution the patient and family/caregivers to guard against falls and trauma.
- Monitor subcutaneous injection site for bruising or decreased local fat accumulation (lipoatrophy, lipodystrophy). Report prolonged or excessive injection site reactions to the physician.

Interventions

- Do not apply physical agents (heat, cold, electrotherapeutic modalities) or massage over the injection site; these interventions can alter drug absorption from subcutaneous tissues.

Patient/Client-Related Instruction

- Advise patient and family/caregivers to adhere to recommended dosing schedule. Emphasize that growth hormones must not be used to increase athletic performance, and that administration to people without growth hormone deficiency or after epiphyseal closure may result in acromegaly (coarsening of facial features; enlarged hands, feet, and internal organs; increased blood glucose; hypertension).
- Instruct patient and family/caregivers to report other troublesome side effects such as severe or prolonged fever or GI problems (vomiting, flatulence).

Pharmacokinetics

Absorption: Well absorbed.

Distribution: Localize to highly perfused organs (liver, kidneys).

Metabolism and Excretion: Broken down in renal cells to amino acids that are recirculated; some liver metabolism.

Half-life: *SC*—4.28 ± 2.15 hr.

TIME/ACTION PROFILE

ROUTE	ONSET	PEAK	DURATION
SC	unknown	unknown	unknown

Contraindications/Precautions

Contraindicated in: Closure of epiphyses; Active neoplasia; Hypersensitivity to growth hormone or benzyl alcohol; Acute critical illness (therapy should not be initiated) or respiratory failure; Diabetic retinopathy; Prader-Willi syndrome with obesity and respiratory impairment (risk of fatal complications; can be used only if growth hormone deficiency is documented).

Use Cautiously in: Growth hormone deficiency due to intracranial lesion; Coexisting adrenocorticotropic hormone (ACTH) deficiency; Diabetes (may cause insulin resistance); Geriatric patients (↑ sensitivity, ↑ risk of adverse reactions; Thyroid dysfunction; Pregnancy or lactation (safety not established).

Interactions

Drug-Drug: Excessive **corticosteroid** use (equivalent to 10–15 mg/m²/day) may ↓ response to growth hormone.

Route/Dosage

SC (Adults): 0.1 mg/kg/day for 4 wk (not to exceed 8 mg/dose), dose may be stopped for 5 days and resumed at half dose for fluid retention or arthralgias.

Availability

Powder for injection: 8.8 mg (26.4 units) multidose vials.

sorafenib (sor-a-fen-ib)

Nexavar

Classification

Therapeutic: antineoplastics

Pharmacologic: enzyme inhibitors

Indications

Advanced renal cell carcinoma. Unresectable hepatocellular carcinoma.

Action

Inhibits tumor growth by inhibiting multikinase enzyme, some of which are involved in angiogenesis. **Therapeutic Effects:** Decreased growth and spread of advanced renal cell carcinoma.

Adverse Reactions/Side Effects

CNS: depression, fatigue, weakness. **Resp:** hoarseness. **CV:** hypertension, myocardial ischemia. **GI:** ↑ increased lipase/amylase, constipation, diarrhea, dyspepsia, dysphagia, mucositis/stomatitis, nausea, vomiting, anorexia. **GU:** erectile dysfunction. **Derm:** acne, erythema, exfoliative dermatitis, flushing, hand-foot skin reaction, pruritus, rash, dry skin. **F and E:** hypophosphatemia. **Hemat:** anemia, bleeding, leukopenia, thrombocytopenia, lymphopenia. **MS:** arthralgia, myalgia. **Neuro:** neuropathy. **Misc:** weight loss.

PHYSICAL THERAPY IMPLICATIONS

Examination and Evaluation

- Monitor signs of leukopenia (fever, sore throat, signs of infection), thrombocytopenia (bruising, nose bleeds, bleeding gums), or unusual weakness and fatigue that might be due to anemia, coagulation disorders, or other blood dyscrasias. Report these signs to the physician or nursing staff.
- Assess blood pressure (BP) and compare to normal values (See Appendix F). Report a sustained increase in BP (hypertension).
- Monitor and report any chest pain that might indicate myocardial ischemia.
- Assess any muscle or joint pain to rule out musculoskeletal pathology; that is, try to determine if pain is drug induced rather than caused by anatomic or biomechanical problems.
- Be alert for signs of peripheral neuropathy (numbness, tingling, decreased muscle strength). Establish baseline electroneuromyographic values using EMG and nerve conduction at the beginning of drug treatment whenever possible, and reexamine these values periodically to document drug-induced changes in peripheral nerve function.
- Monitor signs of low phosphate levels (hypophosphatemia), including skeletal muscle dysfunction or weakness, respiratory muscle weakness, and mental status changes such as irritability and confusion that progresses to delirium and coma. Report these signs to the physician.
- Periodically assess body weight and other anthropometric measures (body mass index, body composition). Report a rapid or unexplained weight loss or decreased body fat.

Interventions

- For patients who are medically able to begin exercise, implement appropriate resistive exercises and aerobic training to maintain muscle strength and aerobic capacity during cancer chemotherapy or to help restore function after chemotherapy.

Patient/Client-Related Instruction

- Advise patient to guard against infection (frequent hand washing, etc.), and to avoid crowds and contact with persons with contagious diseases.
- Advise patient and family/caregivers that fatigue and weakness are likely and may be severe. Functional abilities may be limited, and patient may need to use assistive devices during ambulation.
- Advise patient about the likelihood of GI reactions such as nausea, vomiting, constipation, diarrhea, loss of appetite, indigestion, difficulty swallowing, and irritation in/around the mouth. Instruct patient to report severe or prolonged GI problems.
- Instruct patient to report other bothersome side effects such as severe or prolonged depression, hoarseness, erectile dysfunction, skin reactions

S

(rash, acne, itching, flushing, exfoliative dermatitis, dry skin), or hand-foot skin reactions (pain, redness, and dry, scaly skin on the palms of the hands and soles of the feet).

Pharmacokinetics

Absorption: 38–49% absorbed following oral administration; absorption decreased by high fat meals.
Distribution: Unknown.
Protein Binding: 95% bound to plasma proteins.
Metabolism and Excretion: Mostly metabolized by the liver (CYP3A4 and UGT1A9 systems); some metabolites are pharmacologically active. Absorbed drug is eliminated in feces (51%); of absorbed drug, 77% is excreted in feces and 19% is renally eliminated.
Half-life: 25–48 hr.

TIME/ACTION PROFILE (blood levels)

ROUTE	ONSET	PEAK	DURATION
PO	unknown	3 hr	12 hr

Contraindications/Precautions

Contraindicated in: Hypersensitivity; OB/Lactation: Pregnancy or lactation.
Use Cautiously in: History of cardiovascular disease; Drugs that affect the CYP3A4 or UGT1A9 systems; may result in significant interactions; OB: Childbearing potential; Pedi: Safety not established.

Interactions

Drug-Drug: May ↑ risk of bleeding with **warfarin.** Metabolism is ↑ by and blood levels ↓ by **inducers of CYP3A4,** including **rifampin, phenytoin, phenobarbital, carbamazepine,** and **dexamethasone.** ↑ blood levels and may ↑ effects of **irinotecan, docetaxel,** and **doxorubicin.**
Drug-Natural: Metabolism is ↑ by and blood levels ↓ by **St. John's wort.**

Route/Dosage

PO (Adults): 400 mg bid; dose reduction recommended for skin toxicity and/or neuropathy.

Availability

Tablets: 200 mg.

sotalol (soe-ta-lole)

Betapace, Betapace AF, Sorine, Sotacor

Classification

Therapeutic: antiarrhythmics (classes II and III)
Pharmacologic: beta blockers

Indications

Management of life-threatening ventricular arrhythmias. **Betapace AF:** Maintenance of normal sinus rhythm in patients with highly symptomatic atrial fibrillation/atrial flutter (AFIB/AFL) who are currently in sinus rhythm.

Action

Blocks stimulation of beta$_1$ (myocardial) and beta$_2$ (pulmonary, vascular, and uterine)–adrenergic receptor sites. **Therapeutic Effects:** Suppression of arrhythmias.

Adverse Reactions/Side Effects

CNS: fatigue, weakness, anxiety, dizziness, drowsiness, insomnia, memory loss, mental depression, mental status changes, nervousness, nightmares. **EENT:** blurred vision, dry eyes, nasal stuffiness. **Resp:** bronchospasm, wheezing. **CV:** ARRHYTHMIAS, BRADYCARDIA, CHF, PULMONARY EDEMA, orthostatic hypotension, peripheral vasoconstriction. **GI:** constipation, diarrhea, nausea. **GU:** erectile dysfunction, decreased libido. **Derm:** itching, rashes. **Endo:** hyperglycemia, hypoglycemia. **MS:** arthralgia, back pain, muscle cramps. **Neuro:** paresthesia. **Misc:** drug-induced lupus syndrome.

PHYSICAL THERAPY IMPLICATIONS

Examination and Evaluation

- Assess heart rate, ECG, and heart sounds, especially during exercise (See Appendices G, H). Although intended to treat certain arrhythmias, this drug can unmask or precipitate new arrhythmias (proarrhythmic effect). Report immediately an abnormally slow heart rate (bradycardia) or symptoms of other arrhythmias, including palpitations, chest pain, shortness of breath, fainting, and fatigue/weakness.
- Assess routinely for signs of CHF and pulmonary edema, including dyspnea, rales/crackles, weight gain, peripheral edema, and jugular venous distention. Report these signs to the physician immediately.
- Assess symptoms of bronchospasm (wheezing, coughing, tightness in chest). Perform pulmonary function tests to quantify suspected changes in ventilation and respiration (See Appendices I, J, K). Repeated or prolonged bronchoconstriction may require a change in dose or medication (e.g., switch to a more cardioselective beta blocker).
- Assess blood pressure (BP)when patient assumes a more upright position (lying to standing, sitting to standing, lying to sitting). Document orthostatic hypotension and contact physician when systolic BP falls >20 mm Hg or diastolic BP falls >10 mm Hg.
- Monitor signs of peripheral vasoconstriction, such as extreme coldness in the hands and feet, cyanosis, and muscle cramping. Notify physician of severe or prolonged signs of vasoconstriction.
- Be alert for signs of hypoglycemia (weakness, malaise, irritability, fatigue) or hyperglycemia (drowsiness, fruity breath, increased urination,

unusual thirst). Medication may mask some signs of hypoglycemia, but dizziness and sweating may still occur. Patients with diabetes mellitus should check blood glucose levels frequently.

- Assess any back or joint pain to rule out musculoskeletal pathology; that is, try to determine if pain is drug induced rather than caused by anatomic or biomechanical problems.
- Assess signs of paresthesia (numbness, tingling) or muscle cramping. Perform objective tests, including electroneuromyography and sensory testing to document any drug-related neuropathic changes.
- Assess dizziness and drowsiness that might affect gait, balance, and other functional activities (See Appendix C). Report balance problems and functional limitations to the physician, and caution the patient and family/caregivers to guard against falls and trauma.
- Monitor mood and personality changes, including depression, anxiety, memory loss, or other changes in behavior. Notify physician if these changes become problematic.
- Monitor excessive fatigue or weakness. Beta blockers often cause some degree of fatigue and weakness, but any sudden or severe change in muscle strength or energy levels should be reported.
- Monitor signs of drug-induced lupus syndrome, including increased BP, fever, joint pain, skin rashes, and redness/irritation of the eye (uveitis). Notify physician promptly if these signs appear.

Interventions

- Because of an increased risk of cardiac arrhythmias, CHF, and pulmonary edema, use extreme caution during aerobic exercise and endurance conditioning. Terminate exercise if patient exhibits untoward symptoms (chest pain, shortness of breath, unusual fatigue), or displays other criteria for exercise termination (See Appendix L).
- Establish aerobic exercise workloads that account for the effects of beta blockers on heart rate (HR). Some heart rate guidelines may not be appropriate because beta blockers typically decrease maximal HR by 20–30 bpm. Use other guidelines such as rating of perceived exertion (RPE, modified Borg scale) to determine exercise workloads.
- To minimize orthostatic hypotension, patient should move slowly when assuming a more upright position.

Patient/Client-Related Instruction

- Remind patients to take medication as directed to control cardiac function even if they are asymptomatic.
- Counsel patients about additional interventions to help control cardiac arrhythmias, including regular exercise, caffeine restriction, stress reduction, moderation of alcohol consumption, and smoking cessation.
- Instruct patient or family/caregivers to report other troublesome side effects such as severe or prolonged insomnia, nightmares, blurred vision, dry eyes, stuffy nose, sexual problems (decreased libido, erectile dysfunction), skin reactions (rash, itching), or GI problems (nausea, constipation, diarrhea).

Pharmacokinetics

Absorption: Well absorbed following oral administration.
Distribution: Crosses the placenta; enters breast milk.
Metabolism and Excretion: Elimination is mostly renal.
Half-life: 12 hr (increased in renal impairment).

TIME/ACTION PROFILE (antiarrhythmic effects)

ROUTE	ONSET	PEAK	DURATION
PO	hrs	2–3 days	8–12 hr

Contraindications/Precautions

Contraindicated in: Hypersensitivity; Uncompensated CHF; Pulmonary edema; Asthma; Cardiogenic shock; Congenital or acquired long QT syndromes; Sinus bradycardia, 2nd- and 3rd-degree AV block (unless a functioning pacemaker is present); CCr <40 mL/min in patients who are being treated with Betapace AF.
Use Cautiously in: Renal impairment (increased dosing interval recommended if CCr ≤60 mL/min for patients with ventricular arrhythmias); Hepatic impairment; Hypokalemia (increased risk of serious arrhythmias); Geriatric patients (increased sensitivity to beta blockers; initial dosage reduction recommended); Other pulmonary pathology; Diabetes mellitus (may mask signs of hypoglycemia); Thyrotoxicosis (may mask symptoms); Patients with a history of severe allergic reactions (intensity of reactions may be increased); Pregnancy, lactation, or children (safety not established; may cause fetal/neonatal bradycardia, hypotension, hypoglycemia, or respiratory depression).

Interactions

Drug-Drug: Concurrent use with other **class 1A antiarrhythmics** is not recommended due to increased risk of arrhythmias. **General anesthesia, IV phenytoin,** and **verapamil** may cause additive myocardial depression. Concurrent use with other **calcium channel blockers** may ↑ the risk of adverse cardiovascular reactions. Additive bradycardia may occur with **digoxin.** Additive hypotension may occur with other **antihypertensives,** acute ingestion of **alcohol, or nitrates.** Concurrent use with **amphetamines, cocaine, ephedrine, epinephrine, norepinephrine, phenylephrine,** or **pseudoephedrine** may result in unopposed

S

alpha-adrenergic stimulation (excessive hypertension, bradycardia). Concurrent **thyroid** administration may ↓ effectiveness. May alter the effectiveness of **insulin** or **oral hypoglycemic agents** (dosage adjustments may be necessary). May ↓ the effectiveness of **beta-adrenergic bronchodilators** and **theophylline.** May ↓ the beneficial $beta_1$ cardiovascular effects of **dopamine** or **dobutamine.** Discontinuation of **clonidine** in patients receiving sotalol may result in excessive rebound hypertension. Use cautiously within 14 days of **MAO inhibitors** (may result in hypertension).

Route/Dosage

Ventricular arrhythmias

PO (Adults): 80 mg bid; may be gradually ↑ (usual maintenance dose is 160–320 mg/day in 2–3 divided doses; some patients may require up to 480–640 mg/day).

Renal Impairment

PO (Adults): *CCr 30–59 mL/min*—initial dose of 80 mg, with subsequent doses given q 24 hr; *CCr <10 mL/min—29 ml/min*—initial dose of 80 mg, with subsequent doses given q 36–48 hr.

Atrial fibrillation/atrial flutter

PO (Adults): 80 mg twice daily; may be ↑ during careful monitoring to 120 mg bid if necessary.

Renal Impairment

PO (Adults): *CCr 40–60 mL/min*—80 mg once daily.

Availability (generic available)

Tablets: 80 mg, 120 mg, 160 mg, 240 mg.
Tablets (Betapace AF): 80 mg, 120 mg, 160 mg.

spinosad (spy-no-sad)

Natroba

Classification
Therapeutic: pediculocides

Indications

Treatment of head lice in adults and children >4 yr.

Action

Causes neuronal hyperexcitation in insects, resulting paralysis and death of lice. **Therapeutic Effects:** Eradication of head lice.

Adverse Reactions/Side Effects

EENT: ocular erythema. **Local:** erythema.

PHYSICAL THERAPY IMPLICATIONS

Examination and Evaluation

- Monitor symptoms such as itching scalp to help document drug effectiveness.
- Watch for and report excessive redness, warmth, and irritation in the scalp and eyes.

Interventions

- Avoid contact with infected areas or wear protective gloves when treating patient.
- Always wash hands thoroughly and disinfect bedding and equipment (whirlpools, electrotherapeutic devices, treatment tables, and so forth) to help prevent the spread of infection.

Patient/Client-Related Instruction

- Advise patient to report any increased local sensitivity to this drug.
- Instruct patient about proper hygiene; e.g., clean or discard infected clothing, not share combs and hats with others, thoroughly wash and dry the scalp, and so forth.
- Advise patient to apply the drug as directed; that is, apply the drug topically for the recommended period of time before washing off.

Pharmacokinetics

Absorption: Undetectable systemic absorption follows topical use.
Distribution: Unknown.
Metabolism and Excretion: Unknown.
Half-life: Unknown

TIME/ACTION PROFILE

ROUTE	ONSET	PEAK	DURATION
topical	within min	unknown	unknown

Contraindications/Precautions

Contraindicated in: Pedi: Children <6 mo (↑ risk of benzyl alcohol absorption).
Use Cautiously in: OB: Use in pregnancy only if clearly needed; Lactation: use with caution; Pedi: Safe and effective use in children <4 yr not established.

Interactions

Drug-Drug: None noted.

Route/Dosage

Topical (Adults and Children >4 yr): Apply amount necessary to wet scalp, leave in place for 10 min, then rinse; may be repeated after 7 days if live lice are still seen.

Availability

Topical suspension: 0.9% in 120-mL bottles

spironolactone

(speer-oh-no-**lak**-tone)
Aldactone, Novospiroton

Classification
Therapeutic: diuretics, potassium-sparing diuretics
Pharmacologic: aldosterone antagonists

Indications

Management of primary hyperaldosteronism. Management of edema associated with congestive heart failure, cirrhosis, and nephrotic syndrome. Management of essential hypertension. Treatment of hypokalemia (counteracts potassium loss caused by other diuretics).

Action

Causes loss of sodium bicarbonate and calcium while saving potassium and hydrogen ions by antagonizing aldosterone. **Therapeutic Effects:** Weak diuretic and antihypertensive responses when compared with other diuretics. Conservation of potassium.

Adverse Reactions/Side Effects

CNS: dizziness, clumsiness, headache. **CV:** arrhythmias. **GI:** GI irritation. **GU:** erectile dysfunction, dysuria. **Endo:** gynecomastia (in males), breast tenderness, deepening of voice, increased hair growth (in females). **F and E:** hyperkalemia, hyponatremia, hyperchloremic metabolic acidosis. **Hemat:** agranulocytosis. **MS:** muscle cramps. **Misc:** allergic reactions.

PHYSICAL THERAPY IMPLICATIONS

Examination and Evaluation

- Monitor signs of fluid, electrolyte, or acid-base imbalances, including dizziness, clumsiness, drowsiness, headache, blurred vision, confusion, hypotension, or muscle cramps and weakness. Report excessive or prolonged symptoms to the physician.
- Assess dizziness and clumsiness that might affect gait, balance, and other functional activities (See Appendix C). Report balance problems and functional limitations to the physician, and caution the patient and family/caregivers to guard against falls and trauma.
- Assess heart rate, ECG, and heart sounds, especially during exercise (See Appendices G, H). Report any rhythm disturbances or symptoms of increased arrhythmias, including palpitations, chest discomfort, shortness of breath, fainting, and fatigue/weakness.
- Assess blood pressure periodically and compare to normal values (See Appendix F) to help document antihypertensive effects.
- When used to treat edema, help determine drug effects by assessing peripheral edema using girth measurements, volume displacement, and measurement of pitting edema (See Appendix N). Also monitor signs of pulmonary edema such as dyspnea and rales/crackles (See Appendix K). Document whether peripheral and pulmonary symptoms are controlled adequately by diuretic therapy.
- Monitor signs of allergic reactions, including pulmonary symptoms (tightness in the throat and chest, wheezing, cough, dyspnea) or skin reactions (rash, pruritus, urticaria). Notify physician immediately if these reactions occur.

Interventions

- Implement fall-prevention strategies, especially in older adults or if patient exhibits sedation, dizziness, clumsiness, or other impairments that affect gait and balance (See Appendix E).
- Use caution during aerobic exercise, especially in hot environments. Increased sweating will cause fluid and electrolyte loss, and may exaggerate arrhythmias and diuretic side effects (dizziness, muscle cramps, and so forth).
- To minimize orthostatic hypotension, patient should move slowly when assuming a more upright position.

Patient/Client-Related Instruction

- Remind patients to take medication as directed to control hypertension and other cardiac conditions even if they are asymptomatic.
- Counsel patients about additional interventions to help control blood pressure and cardiac dysfunction, such as regular exercise, weight loss, sodium restriction, stress reduction, moderation of alcohol consumption, and smoking cessation.
- Instruct patient or family and caregivers to report other troublesome side effects such as severe or prolonged GI irritation, or problems related to sexual function and gender appearance such as erectile dysfunction and breast growth in men, or abnormal hair growth and deepening voice in women.

Pharmacokinetics

Absorption: >90% absorbed.
Distribution: Crosses the placenta; enters breast milk.
Protein Binding: >90%.
Metabolism and Excretion: Converted by the liver to its active diuretic compound (canrenone).
Half-life: 78–84 min (spironolactone); 13–24 hr (canrenone).

TIME/ACTION PROFILE (diuretic effect)

ROUTE	ONSET	PEAK	DURATION
PO	unknown	1–3 hr	2–3 days*

*Multiple doses.

Contraindications/Precautions

Contraindicated in: Hypersensitivity; Anuria; Acute renal insufficiency; Significant renal impairment (CCr <30 mL/min); Hyperkalemia.

S

Use Cautiously in: Hepatic dysfunction; Geriatric or debilitated patients or patients with diabetes mellitus (increased risk of hyperkalemia); **OB/Lactation:** May cause endocrine dysfunction in infants. Is tumorigenic and should not be given to nursing mothers. Alternative method of feeding should be used if spironolactone is essential.

Interactions

Drug-Drug: ↑ hypotension with acute ingestion of **alcohol,** other **antihypertensive agents,** or **nitrates.** Use with **indomethacin, potassium supplements, angiotensin II receptor antagonists, angiotensin converting enzyme inhibitors,** or **cyclosporine** ↑ risk of hyperkalemia. ↓ **lithium** excretion. Antihypertensive and diuretic effectiveness may be ↓ by **NSAIDs.** May ↑ the effects of **digoxin.** ↓ hypoprothrombinemic effect of **oral anticoagulants.**

Route/Dosage

PO (Adults): 25–400 mg/day as a single dose or 2 divided doses. *Congestive heart failure*—12.5–25 mg/day (unlabeled).

PO (Children >1 mo): *Diuretic, hypertension*—1.5–3.3 mg/kg/day (60 mg/m^2/day) as a single dose or 2–4 divided doses. *Diagnosis of primary aldosteronism*—100–400 mg/m^2/day in 1–2 divided doses.

PO (Neonates): 1–3 mg/kg/day divided q 12–24 hr.

Availability (generic available)

Tablets: 25 mg, 50 mg, 100 mg. ***In combination with:*** hydrochlorothiazide (Aldactazide, [Novo-Spirozine], Spirozide). See Appendix B.

stavudine (stav-yoo-deen)

d4T, Zerit, Zerit XR

Classification

Therapeutic: antiretrovirals

Pharmacologic: nucleoside reverse transcriptase inhibitors

Indications

HIV infection unresponsive or intolerant to conventional therapy.

Action

Converted intracellularly to stavudine triphosphate, which inhibits viral DNA synthesis and replication. **Therapeutic Effects:** Virustatic action against HIV. Decreased viral load and increased cell count. Not curative, but may slow progression of HIV infection and decrease the incidence and severity of its sequelae.

Adverse Reactions/Side Effects

CNS: headache, insomnia, weakness. **GI:** HEPATIC TOXICITY, PANCREATITIS, anorexia, diarrhea. **F and E:** LACTIC ACIDOSIS. **Hemat:** anemia. **MS:** arthralgia, myalgia. **Neuro:** peripheral neuropathy.

PHYSICAL THERAPY IMPLICATIONS

Examination and Evaluation

- Be alert for signs of liver toxicity, including anorexia, abdominal pain, abdominal swelling (ascites), severe nausea and vomiting, yellow skin or eyes, fever, sore throat, malaise, weakness, facial edema, lethargy, and unusual bleeding or bruising. Notify physician of these signs immediately.
- Monitor signs of pancreatitis, including upper abdominal pain (especially after eating), indigestion, weight loss, and oily stools. Report these signs to the physician immediately.
- Monitor signs of lactic acidosis, including confusion, lethargy, stupor, shallow rapid breathing, tachycardia, hypotension, nausea, and vomiting. Notify physician immediately if these signs occur.
- Assess any weakness, muscle pain, or joint pain to rule out musculoskeletal pathology; that is, try to determine if pain is drug induced rather than caused by anatomic or biomechanical problems.
- Be alert for signs of peripheral neuropathy (numbness, tingling, decreased muscle strength). Establish baseline electroneuromyographic values using EMG and nerve conduction at the beginning of drug treatment whenever possible, and reexamine these values periodically to document drug-induced changes in peripheral nerve function.
- Monitor any unusual weakness, fatigue, or pallor that might be due to anemia and other blood dyscrasias. Report these signs to the physician.

Interventions

- Implement resistive exercises and other therapeutic exercises as tolerated to maintain muscle strength and function, and prevent muscle wasting associated with HIV infection and AIDS.
- Because of the risk of lactic acidosis, use caution during aerobic exercise and other forms of therapeutic exercise. Assess exercise tolerance frequently (blood pressure, heart rate, fatigue levels), and terminate exercise immediately if any untoward responses occur (See Appendix L).

Patient/Client-Related Instruction

- Emphasize the importance of taking stavudine as directed even if the patient is asymptomatic, and that this drug must always be used in combination with other antiretroviral drugs. Do not take more than prescribed amount, and do not stop taking without consulting health care professional.
- Inform patient that stavudine does not cure HIV or AIDS or prevent associated or opportunistic infections. Stavudine does not reduce the risk of transmission of HIV to others through sexual contact or

blood contamination. Caution patient to use a condom, and to avoid sharing needles or donating blood to prevent spreading the AIDS virus to others.

- Instruct patient to report other troublesome side effects such as prolonged or severe headache, sleep loss, or GI problems (diarrhea, loss of appetite).

Pharmacokinetics

Absorption: Well absorbed after oral administration (78–80% bioavailability). XR formulation produces less fluctuation in levels.
Distribution: Crosses the blood-brain barrier; enters RBCs and plasma equally.
Metabolism and Excretion: Converted intracellularly to stavudine triphosphate, which is the active drug; 40% excreted unchanged in urine; 50% nonrenally eliminated.
Half-life: *Adults*—1–1.6 hr; *children*—0.9–1.1 hr; *adults with renal impairment*—4.8 hr; *intracellular half-life*—3.5 hr.

TIME/ACTION PROFILE (blood levels)

ROUTE	ONSET	PEAK	DURATION
PO	unknown	0.5–1.5 hr	12 hr
PO-XR	unknown	3 hr	24 hr

Contraindications/Precautions

Contraindicated in: Hypersensitivity.
Use Cautiously in: Patients with a history of alcohol abuse; Patients with a history of liver disease or hepatic impairment; Renal impairment (dosage reduction and/or increased dosing interval recommended if CCr <50 mL/min); History of peripheral neuropathy; Pregnancy or lactation (safety not established; breast-feeding should be avoided by HIV-infected mothers because of transmission of the virus in breast milk; concurrent use with didanosine during pregnancy may increase the risk of fetal lactic acidosis).

Interactions

Drug-Drug: Use cautiously with **drugs causing peripheral neuropathy (chloramphenicol, cisplatin, dapsone, didanosine, ethambutol, ethionamide, hydralazine, isoniazid, lithium, metronidazole, nitrofurantoin, phenytoin, vincristine, or zalcitabine)**. Concurrent use with **didanosine** may ↑ risk of pancreatitis. Concurrent use with **zidovudine** is not recommended because of possible antiretroviral antagonism.

Route/Dosage

PO (Adults ≥60 kg): 40 mg bid *or* 100 mg once daily as XR capsules.
PO (Adults <60 kg): 30 mg bid *or* 75 mg once daily as XR capsules.
PO (Children at least 14 days old and <30 kg): 1 mg/kg q 12 hr (not to exceed 40 mg q 12 hr).
PO (Infants birth–13 days): 0.5 mg/kg q 12 hr.

Renal Impairment

PO (Adults ≥60 kg): *CCr 26–50 mL/min*—20 mg q 12 hr; *CCr 10–25 mL/min*—20 mg q 24 hr.
PO (Adults <60 kg): *CCr 26–50 mL/min*—15 mg q 12 hr; *CCr 10–25 mL/min*—15 mg q 24 hr.

Availability

Capsules: 15 mg, 20 mg, 30 mg, 40 mg. **Powder for oral solution (fruit flavored):** 1 mg/mL (after reconstitution) in 200-mL bottle. **Extended-release capsules:** 37.5 mg, 50 mg, 75 mg, 100 mg.

HIGH ALERT

streptokinase

(strep-toe-**kye**-nase)
Kabbikinase, Streptase

Classification
Therapeutic: thrombolytics
Pharmacologic: plasminogen activators

S

Indications

Acute myocardial infarction (MI). Pulmonary embolism (PE). Deep vein thrombosis (DVT). Acute peripheral arterial thrombosis. Occluded arteriovenous cannulae.

Action

Combines with plasminogen to form activator complexes, then converts plasminogen to plasmin, which is then able to degrade clot-bound fibrin. **Therapeutic Effects:** Lysis of thrombi in coronary arteries, with preservation of ventricular function. Lysis of pulmonary emboli and subsequent restoration of blood flow. Restoration of cannula patency and function.

Adverse Reactions/Side Effects

CNS: INTRACRANIAL HEMORRHAGE. **EENT:** epistaxis, gingival bleeding. **Resp:** bronchospasm, hemoptysis. **CV:** reperfusion arrhythmias, hypotension, RECURRENT ISCHEMIA/THROMBOEMBOLISM. **GI:** GI BLEEDING, hepatotoxicity, nausea, RETROPERITONEAL BLEEDING, vomiting. **GU:** GU TRACT BLEEDING. **Derm:** ecchymoses, flushing, urticaria. **Hemat:** BLEEDING. **Local:** hemorrhage at injection site, phlebitis at injection site. **MS:** musculoskeletal pain. **Misc:** ALLERGIC REACTIONS, INCLUDING ANAPHYLAXIS, fever.

PHYSICAL THERAPY IMPLICATIONS

Examination and Evaluation

- Assess for signs of bleeding and hemorrhage, including bleeding gums, nosebleeds, unusual bruising, coughing up blood, black/tarry stools, hematuria, and a fall in hematocrit or blood pressure. Be especially alert for signs of intracranial bleeds, including sudden severe headache, confusion, nausea, vomiting, paralysis, numbness, speech problems, visual disturbances. Notify physician or nursing staff immediately if these signs occur.

- Be alert for signs of recurrent cardiac ischemia (chest pain, pain radiating into the arm or jaw, shortness of breath, dizziness, sweating, anxiety) or recurrent peripheral arterial thrombosis (pain, cramping, coldness, cyanosis in the affected limb). Notify physician or nursing staff immediately if these signs occur.
- Monitor signs of recurrent thromboembolism and PE such as shortness of breath, chest pain, cough, and bloody sputum. Notify physician immediately, and request objective tests (Doppler ultrasound, lung scan, others) if PE is suspected.
- Watch for signs of allergic reactions and anaphylaxis, including pulmonary symptoms (tightness in the throat and chest, wheezing, cough, dyspnea) or skin reactions (rash, pruritus, urticaria). Notify physician or nursing staff immediately if these reactions occur.
- Assess heart rate, ECG, and heart sounds when cardiac perfusion is restored (See Appendices G, H). Report any rhythm disturbances or symptoms of increased arrhythmias, including palpitations, chest discomfort, shortness of breath, fainting, and fatigue/weakness.
- Assess blood pressure, especially for the first few days after infusion. Report low blood pressure (hypotension), especially if patient experiences dizziness or syncope.
- Assess any muscle of joint pain to rule out musculoskeletal pathology or hemorrhage; that is, try to determine if pain is drug induced rather than caused by anatomic or biomechanical problems. Be especially concerned about back pain that could indicate retroperitoneal bleeding.
- Watch for signs of hepatotoxicity, including anorexia, abdominal pain, severe nausea and vomiting, yellow skin or eyes, fever, sore throat, malaise, weakness, facial edema, lethargy, and unusual bleeding or bruising. Report these signs to the physician or nursing staff.
- Assess injection site during and after IV administration, and report signs of bleeding or phlebitis (local pain, swelling, inflammation).

Interventions

- Use caution with any physical interventions that could increase bleeding, including wound débridement, chest percussion, joint mobilization, and application of local heat.
- Use extreme caution during aerobic exercise in patients with recent MI. Assess exercise tolerance frequently (blood pressure, heart rate, fatigue levels, neurologic signs), and terminate exercise immediately if any untoward responses occur (See Appendix L).
- For patients with DVT, recommend or implement other physical methods to decrease DVT and prevent recurrent thromboembolism, including graduated compression stockings and intermittent pneumatic compression pumps.

Patient/Client-Related Instruction

- Instruct patient to immediately report signs of GI bleeding, including abdominal pain, vomiting blood, blood in stools, or black, tarry stools.
- Instruct patient or family/caregivers to report other problematic side effects such as severe or prolonged fever, skin reactions (flushing, hives), or GI problems (nausea, vomiting).

Pharmacokinetics

Absorption: Complete after IV administration. Administration into occluded cannulae has a more localized effect.
Distribution: Streptokinase appears to cross the placenta minimally, if at all. Remainder of distribution for streptokinase is not known.
Metabolism and Excretion: Rapidly cleared from circulation by antibodies and other unknown mechanisms.
Half-life: Initial half-life (due to clearance by antibodies)—18 min, then 83 min.

TIME/ACTION PROFILE (fibrinolysis)

ROUTE	ONSET	PEAK	DURATION
IV	immediate	rapid	4 hr (up to 12 hr)

Contraindications/Precautions

Contraindicated in: Active internal bleeding; History of cerebrovascular accident; Recent (within 2 mo) intracranial or intraspinal injury or trauma; Intracranial neoplasm, arteriovenous malformation, or aneurysm; Severe uncontrolled hypertension; Known bleeding tendencies; Hypersensitivity; cross-sensitivity with anistreplase and streptokinase may occur.
Use Cautiously in: Recent (within 10 days) major surgery, trauma, GI or GU bleeding; Left heart thrombus; Severe hepatic or renal disease; Hemorrhagic ophthalmic conditions; Septic phlebitis; Previous puncture of a noncompressible vessel; Subacute bacterial endocarditis or acute pericarditis; Recent streptococcal infection or previous therapy with anistreplase or streptokinase (within 5 days–6 mo); may produce resistance because of antibody formation; increased dosage requirements may be encountered (anistreplase and streptokinase only); Previous therapy with

streptokinase or anistreplase (within 12 mo); may produce resistance because of antibody formation; Geriatric patients (>75 yr; increased risk of intracranial bleeding); Pregnancy, lactation, or children (safety not established).
Exercise Extreme Caution in: Patients receiving warfarin therapy; Early postpartum period (10 days).

Interactions

Drug-Drug: Aspirin, other **NSAIDs, warfarin, heparin** and **heparin-like agents, abciximab, eptifibatide, tirofiban, clopidogrel, ticlopidine,** or **dipyridamole**—concurrent use ↑ risk of bleeding, although these agents are frequently used together or in sequence. Effects may be ↓ by **antifibrinolytic agents,** including **aminocaproic acid** or **tranexamic acid.**
Drug-Natural: ↑ anticoagulant effect and bleeding risk with **anise, arnica, chamomile, clove, dong quai, fenugreek, feverfew, garlic, ginger, ginkgo,** ***Panax ginseng*****, licorice,** and others.

Route/Dosage

Myocardial Infarction

IV (Adults): 1.5 million IU given as a continuous infusion over up to 60 min.
Intracoronary: (Adults): 20,000 IU bolus followed by 2000 IU/min infusion for 60 min.

Deep Venous Thrombosis, Pulmonary Emboli, Arterial Emboli, or Other Thromboses

IV (Adults): 250,000 IU loading dose, followed by 100,000 IU/hr for 24 hr for pulmonary emboli, 72 hr for recurrent pulmonary emboli or deep vein thrombosis.

Occluded Arteriovenous Cannulae

IV (Adults): 250,000 IU/2 mL instilled into occluded catheter.

Availability

Powder for injection: 250,000 IU/vial, 600,000 IU/vial, 750,000 IU/vial, 1,500,000 IU/vial.

streptomycin
(strep-toe-**mye**-sin)

Classification
Therapeutic: anti-infectives
Pharmacologic: aminoglycosides

Indications

In combination with other agents in the management of active tuberculosis. In combination with other agents in the management of serious enterococcal or gram-negative infections.

Action

Inhibits protein synthesis in bacteria at level of 30S ribosome. **Therapeutic Effects:** Bactericidal action. **Spectrum:** Notable for activity against. Enterococci (synergy with a penicillin is required). Also active against *Mycobacterium*.

Adverse Reactions/Side Effects

EENT: ototoxicity (vestibular and cochlear).
GU: nephrotoxicity. **F and E:** hypomagnesemia.
MS: muscle paralysis (high parenteral doses).
Misc: hypersensitivity reactions.

PHYSICAL THERAPY IMPLICATIONS

Examination and Evaluation

- Monitor signs of hypersensitivity reactions, including pulmonary symptoms (tightness in the throat and chest, wheezing, cough dyspnea) or skin reactions (rash, pruritus, urticaria). Notify physician or nursing staff immediately if these reactions occur.
- Report any muscle weakness or paralysis that occurs following injection of high doses.
- Monitor signs of ototoxicity, including hearing loss, tinnitus, and balance problems (See Appendix E for fall assessment and prevention). Report these signs, and caution the patient and family/caregivers to guard against falls and trauma.
- Monitor signs of low magnesium levels (hypomagnesemia), such as lethargy, irritability, insomnia, muscle tremors, and confusion. Notify physician of these signs.

Interventions

- Always wash hands thoroughly and disinfect equipment (whirlpools, electrotherapeutic devices, treatment tables, and so forth) to help prevent the spread of infection. Use universal precautions or isolation procedures as indicated for specific patients.

Patient/Client-Related Instruction

- Advise patient to report signs of nephrotoxicity, including blood or pus in urine, decreased urine output, fatigue, and weight gain from fluid retention.

Pharmacokinetics

Absorption: Well absorbed after IM and intraperitoneal administration. Negligible absorption when administered orally.
Distribution: Widely distributed throughout extracellular fluid; crosses the placenta; small amounts enter breast milk. Poor penetration into CSF.

S

Metabolism and Excretion: Excretion is >90% renal.
Half-life: 2–4 hr (increased in renal impairment).

TIME/ACTION PROFILE (blood levels†)

ROUTE	ONSET	PEAK	DURATION
IM	rapid	30–90 min	N/A

*All parenterally administered aminoglycosides.

Contraindications/Precautions

Contraindicated in: Hypersensitivity; Cross-sensitivity among aminoglycosides may occur.
Use Cautiously in: Renal impairment (dosage adjustments necessary; blood level monitoring useful in preventing ototoxicity and nephrotoxicity); Hearing impairment; Geriatric patients and premature infants (difficulty in assessing auditory and vestibular function; age-related renal impairment); Neuromuscular diseases such as myasthenia gravis; Obese patients (dosage should be based on ideal body weight); Neonates (increased risk of neuromuscular blockade; difficulty in assessing auditory and vestibular function; immature renal function); Pregnancy (may cause congenital deafness); Lactation (safety not established).

Interactions

Drug-Drug: Inactivated by **penicillins** and **cephalosporins** when coadministered to patients with renal insufficiency. Possible respiratory paralysis after **inhalation anesthetics** or **neuromuscular blockers.** ↑ incidence of ototoxicity with **loop diuretics.** ↑ incidence of nephrotoxicity with other **nephrotoxic drugs.**

Route/Dosage

IM (Adults): *Tuberculosis*—1 g/day initially, ↓ to 1 g 2–3 times weekly; *other infections*—250 mg–1 g q 6 hr or 500 mg–2 g q 12 hr.
IM (Children): *Tuberculosis*—20 mg/kg/day (not to exceed 1 g/day); *other infections*—5–10 mg/kg q 6 hr or 10–20 mg/kg q 12 hr.

Renal Impairment

IM (Adults): 1 g initially; further dosing determined by blood level monitoring and assessment of renal function.

Availability (generic available)

Injection: 500 mg/ml Rx, 1 g Rx.

streptozocin (strep-toe-zoe-sin)

Zanosar

Classification
Therapeutic: antineoplastics
Pharmacologic: antitumor antibiotics

Indications

Metastatic islet cell carcinoma of the pancreas.
Unlabeled Use: Metastatic carcinoid tumor, Hodgkin's disease, Pancreatic adenocarcinoma, Colorectal cancer.

Action

Inhibits DNA synthesis by cross-linking DNA strands (cell-cycle phase–nonspecific). **Therapeutic Effects:** Death of rapidly replicating cells, particularly malignant ones.

Adverse Reactions/Side Effects

CNS: confusion, lethargy, mental depression.
GI: DRUG-INDUCED HEPATITIS, nausea, vomiting, diarrhea, duodenal ulcer. **GU:** nephrotoxicity, gonadal suppression, proteinuria. **F and E:** hypophosphatemia.
Hemat: anemia, leukopenia, thrombocytopenia, eosinophilia. **Local:** phlebitis at IV site, injection-site reactions. **Metab:** HYPOGLYCEMIA (FIRST DOSE), hyperglycemia. **Misc:** fever.

PHYSICAL THERAPY IMPLICATIONS

Examination and Evaluation

- Watch for signs of drug-induced hepatitis, including anorexia, abdominal pain, severe nausea and vomiting, yellow skin or eyes, skin rashes, flu-like symptoms, and muscle/joint pain. Report these signs to the physician or nursing staff immediately.
- Be alert for signs of hypoglycemia, especially after the first dose. Common neuromuscular signs include anxiety; restlessness; tingling in hands, feet, lips, or tongue; chills; cold sweats; confusion; difficulty in concentration; drowsiness; nightmares or trouble sleeping; excessive hunger; headache; irritability; nervousness; tremor; weakness; unsteady gait. Notify physician or nursing staff immediately of any hypoglycemic reactions.
- Be alert for signs of hyperglycemia, including confusion, drowsiness, flushed/dry skin, fruit-like breath odor, rapid/deep breathing, polyuria, loss of appetite, and unusual thirst. Patients with diabetes mellitus should check blood glucose levels frequently.
- Watch for signs of leukopenia (fever, sore throat, signs of infection), thrombocytopenia (bruising, nose bleeds, bleeding gums), or unusual weakness and fatigue that might be due to anemia. Report these signs to the physician or nursing staff.
- Monitor signs of low phosphate levels (hypophosphatemia), including skeletal muscle dysfunction or weakness, respiratory muscle weakness, and mental status changes such as irritability and confusion that progresses to delirium and coma. Report these signs to the physician.
- Monitor and report signs of nephrotoxicity, including hematuria, increased urinary frequency, cloudy urine, and decreased urine output.
- Monitor and report signs of CNS toxicity, including confusion, decreased alertness, or severe lethargy.

- Assess IV site during and after IV administration, and report signs of phlebitis or other injection site reactions (local pain, swelling, inflammation).

Interventions

- For patients who are medically able to begin exercise, implement appropriate resistive exercises and aerobic training to maintain muscle strength and aerobic capacity during cancer chemotherapy or to help restore function after chemotherapy.

Patient/Client-Related Instruction

- Advise patient to guard against infection (frequent hand washing, etc.), and to avoid crowds and contact with persons with contagious diseases.
- Instruct patient to report other troublesome side effects, including severe or prolonged fever or GI problems (nausea, vomiting, diarrhea, stomach pain).

Pharmacokinetics

Absorption: Administered IV only, resulting in complete bioavailability.
Distribution: Rapidly distributed. High concentrations in liver, pancreas, kidneys, and intestine. Probably crosses the placenta. Active metabolite enters the CSF.
Metabolism and Excretion: Highly metabolized in liver and kidneys. 10–20% excreted unchanged by the kidneys. Small amounts excreted in expired air (5%) and feces (1%).
Half-life: 35–40 min.

TIME/ACTION PROFILE

ROUTE	ONSET	PEAK	DURATION
IV (effects on blood counts)	unknown	1–2 wk	unknown
IV (tumor response)	17 days	35 days	unknown

Contraindications/Precautions

Contraindicated in: Hypersensitivity.
Use Cautiously in: Underlying or preexisting renal disease (dosage reduction recommended); Liver disease; Geriatric patients (consider ↓ body mass, age-related ↓ in renal/hepatic/cardiac function as well as intercurrent illness and drug therapies; Patients with childbearing potential; Active infections; ↓ bone marrow reserve; Other chronic debilitating illnesses; Pregnancy, lactation, or children (safety not established).

Interactions

Drug-Drug: ↑ myelosuppression with other **antineoplastics.** ↑ risk of nephrotoxicity with other **nephrotoxic agents (aminoglycoside antibiotics).** Toxicity may be ↑ by concurrent **phenytoin** therapy. May ↑ toxicity of **doxorubicin.** May ↓ antibody response to **live-virus vaccines** and ↑ risk of adverse reactions.

Route/Dosage

IV (Adults): 500 mg/m²/day for 5 days q 4–6 wk *or* 1 g/m²/wk for 2 wk; then may be ↑ (not to exceed 1.5 g/m²/dose) and given weekly for 4–6 doses.

Availability

Powder for injection: 1 g/vial.

strontium-89 chloride
(stron-tee-um klor-ide)
Metastron

Classification
Therapeutic: nonopioid analgesics
Pharmacologic: radiopharmaceuticals

Indications

Treatment of bone pain in patients with painful skeletal metastases.

Action

Preferentially taken up by bone tumors and metastatic bone lesions, where selective irradiation takes place.
Therapeutic Effects: Decreased pain from bony metastases. Because of delayed onset, adequate analgesia should be provided until effects of strontium are evident.

Adverse Reactions/Side Effects

Hemat: anemia, neutropenia, thrombocytopenia.
MS: transient increase in bone pain.

PHYSICAL THERAPY IMPLICATIONS

Examination and Evaluation

- Monitor signs of neutropenia (fever, sore throat, signs of infection), thrombocytopenia (bruising, nose bleeds, and bleeding gums), or unusual weakness and fatigue that might be due to anemia. Report these signs to the physician or nursing staff.
- Assess any bone pain, and report bone pain that does not resolve spontaneously.

Interventions

- For patients who are medically able to begin exercise, implement appropriate resistive exercises and aerobic training to maintain muscle strength and aerobic capacity during cancer chemotherapy or to help restore function after chemotherapy.
- Implement appropriate manual therapy techniques, physical agents, and therapeutic exercises as indicated to help reduce bone pain and decrease the need for analgesic medications.

- Implement assistive devices (walker, cane, wheelchair) as needed to help protect metastatic bone lesions and prevent fractures.

Pharmacokinetics

Absorption: IV administration results in complete bioavailability.
Distribution: Selectively localized in and retained by metastatic bone lesions. Excreted in breast milk.
Metabolism and Excretion: 67% excreted in urine, 33% in feces.
Half-life: (physical half-life) 50.5 days.

TIME/ACTION PROFILE (pain relief)

ROUTE	ONSET	PEAK	DURATION
IV	7–20 days	variable	6 mo (range 4–12 mo)

Contraindications/Precautions

Contraindicated in: Lactation; Pregnancy.
Use Cautiously in: Women with childbearing potential; Children <18 yr (safety not established); Patients with platelet counts <60,000 mm^3 or WBCs <2400 mm^3; Diminished bone marrow reserve or other chronic debilitating illness; Patients with a life expectancy <1–3 wk.

Interactions

Drug-Drug: Additive bone marrow toxicity with **antineoplastics** or previous **radiation therapy.** **Calcium-containing medications** may decrease bone uptake and effectiveness of strontium (discontinue 2 wk prior to strontium; may resume 2 wk after strontium).

Route/Dosage

IV (Adults): 148 megabecquerels (4 millicuries) or 1.5–2.2 megabecquerels/kg (40–60 microcuries/kg), not to be repeated sooner than 90 days.

Availability

Radioactive injection: 10.9–22.6 mg/mL (148 megabecquerels or 4 millicuries) in 10-mL vials, 13.4–20.1 mg/mL (150 megabecquerels or 4.05 millicuries) in 10-mL vials.

HIGH ALERT

succinylcholine

(sux-sin-il-**koe**-leen)
Anectine, Quelicin

Classification
Therapeutic: neuromuscular blocking agents—depolarizing

Indications

Used during surgical procedures to produce skeletal muscle paralysis after induction of anesthesia and provision of opioid analgesics.

Action

Prevents neuromuscular transmission by blocking the effect of acetylcholine at the myoneural junction. Has agonist activity initially, producing fasciculation. Causes the release of histamine. Has no analgesic or anxiolytic effects. **Therapeutic Effects:** Skeletal muscle paralysis.

Adverse Reactions/Side Effects

Most adverse reactions to succinylcholine are extensions of pharmacologic effects
Resp: APNEA, bronchospasm. **CV:** arrhythmias, bradycardia, hypotension. **F and E:** HYPERKALEMIA. **MS:** RHABDOMYOLYSIS, muscle fasciculation. **Misc:** MALIGNANT HYPERTHERMIA, myoglobinemia (↑ in children), myoglobinuria (↑ in children), tachyphylaxis.

PHYSICAL THERAPY IMPLICATIONS

Examination and Evaluation

- Assess respiration, and notify physician or nursing staff immediately if patient exhibits any interruption in respiratory rate (apnea) or signs of respiratory failure (rapid labored breathing, cyanosis, confusion, irritability, sleepiness, headache, oxygen desaturation).
- Monitor symptoms of high plasma potassium levels (hyperkalemia), including bradycardia, fatigue, weakness, numbness, and tingling. Notify physician or nursing staff immediately because severe cases can lead to life-threatening arrhythmias and paralysis.
- Be alert for a rapid rise in body temperature, especially if accompanied by muscle rigidity and stiffness. These may be signs of malignant hyperthermia, and the physician or nursing staff should be notified immediately.
- Assess any muscle pain, tenderness, or weakness, especially if accompanied by fever, malaise, and dark-colored urine. These symptoms may indicate myopathy that can progress to severe muscle damage (rhabdomyolysis). Report any unexplained musculoskeletal symptoms to the physician or nursing staff immediately.
- Assess symptoms of bronchospasm (wheezing, coughing, tightness in chest) or decreased respiratory muscle function. Perform pulmonary function tests to quantify suspected changes in ventilation and respiration (See Appendix I).
- Assess heart rate, ECG, and heart sounds, especially during exercise (See Appendices G, H). Report any rhythm disturbances or symptoms of increased arrhythmias, including palpitations, chest discomfort, shortness of breath, fainting, and fatigue/weakness.
- Assess blood pressure periodically and compare to normal values (See Appendix F). Report low blood pressure (hypotension), especially if patient experiences dizziness, fatigue, or other symptoms

- Be alert for a sudden increase in muscle contraction that might indicate a rapid decrease in drug effectiveness (tachyphylaxis).

Interventions

- Design and implement therapeutic exercises (resistive training, gait training) as needed to help resolve any residual weakness or myopathy caused by this drug. Begin exercises at low intensity and progress the exercise regimen slowly to avoid fatigue or excessive stress to damaged muscles.

Pharmacokinetics

Absorption: Well absorbed after deep IM administration.
Distribution: Widely distributed into extracellular fluid. Crosses the placenta in small amounts.
Metabolism and Excretion: 90% metabolized by pseudocholinesterase in plasma. 10% excreted unchanged by the kidneys.
Half-life: Unknown.

TIME/ACTION PROFILE (skeletal muscle paralysis)

ROUTE	ONSET	PEAK	DURATION
IM	up to 3 min	unknown	10–30 min
IV	0.5–1 min	1–2 min	4–10 min

Contraindications/Precautions

Contraindicated in: Hypersensitivity to succinylcholine or parabens; Plasma pseudocholinesterase deficiency; Children and neonates (continuous infusions); Personal history of malignant hyperthermia.
Use Cautiously in: Familial history of malignant hyperthermia; History of pulmonary disease, renal or liver impairment; Major trauma, burns, or underlying myopathy (↑ risk of rhabdomyolysis and hyperkalemia, especially in children or adolescents); Glaucoma; Electrolyte disturbances; Patients receiving digoxin; Fractures or muscular spasm; Myasthenia gravis or myasthenic syndromes; Geriatric or debilitated patients; Has been used in pregnant women undergoing cesarean section; Neonates and children (↑ risk of malignant hyperthermia).

Interactions

Drug-Drug: Concurrent administration of **echothiophate, isofluorphate,** or **demecarium** (eyedrops) reduces pseudocholinesterase activity and intensifies paralysis. Intensity and/or duration of paralysis may be prolonged by pretreatment with **general anesthesia, aminoglycosides, polymyxin B, colistin, clindamycin, lidocaine, quinidine, procainamide, beta blockers, lithium, cyclophosphamide, phenelzine, potassium-losing diuretics,** and **magnesium salts.** ↑ risk of adverse cardiovascular reactions with **opioid analgesics** or **digoxin.**

Route/Dosage

IV route is preferred, but deep IM injection may be used in children and patients without vascular access.

Test Dose

IV (Adults): 5–10 mg (0.1 mg/kg); then assess respiratory function.

Short Procedures

IV (Adults): 0.6 mg/kg (range 0.3–1.1 mg/kg) up to 150 mg total dose; additional doses depend on response; maintenance: 0.04–0.07 mg/kg q 5–10 min as needed.
IV (Children): 1–2 mg/kg, up to 150 mg; additional doses depend on response; maintenance: 0.3–0.6 mg/kg q 5–10 min as needed (continuous infusion not recommended in children or neonates because of the risk of malignant hyperthermia).

Prolonged Procedures

IV (Adults): 2.5 mg/min infusion (range 0.5–10 mg/min).

Intramuscular Dosing

IM (Adults): same as IV.
IM (Children): 2.5–4 mg/kg (total dose not to exceed 150 mg).

Availability

Injection: 20 mg/mL in 10-mL vials, 50 mg/mL in 10-mL vials, 100 mg/mL in 10- and 20-mL vials. **Powder for injection:** 100 mg/vial. **Powder for infusion:** 500 mg/vial, 1 g/vial.

sucralfate (soo-kral-fate)

Carafate, ✱Sulcrate

Classification
Therapeutic: antiulcer agents
Pharmacologic: GI protectants

Indications

Short-term management of duodenal ulcers. Maintenance (preventive) therapy of duodenal ulcers. **Unlabeled Use:** Management of gastric ulcer or gastroesophageal reflux. Prevention of gastric mucosal injury caused by high-dose aspirin or other NSAIDs in patients with rheumatoid arthritis or in high-stress situations (e.g., intensive care unit). **Suspension:** Mucositis/stomatitis/rectal or oral ulcerations from various etiologies.

Action

Aluminum salt of sulfated sucrose reacts with gastric acid to form a thick paste, which selectively adheres to the ulcer surface. **Therapeutic Effects:** Protection of ulcers, with subsequent healing.

Adverse Reactions/Side Effects

CNS: dizziness, drowsiness. **GI:** constipation, diarrhea, dry mouth, gastric discomfort, indigestion, nausea. **Derm:** pruritus, rashes.

PHYSICAL THERAPY IMPLICATIONS

Examination and Evaluation

- Assess dizziness and drowsiness that might affect gait, balance, and other functional activities (See Appendix C). Report balance problems and functional limitations to the physician, and caution the patient and family/caregivers to guard against falls and trauma.

Patient/Client-Related Instruction

- Advise patient to avoid alcohol and foods that may cause an increase in GI irritation.
- Instruct patient to report troublesome side effects such as severe or prolonged skin reactions (rash, itching) or GI problems (nausea, diarrhea, constipation, gastric pain, indigestion, dry mouth).

Pharmacokinetics

Absorption: Systemic absorption is minimal (<5%).
Distribution: Unknown.
Metabolism and Excretion: >90% is eliminated in the feces.
Half-life: 6–20 hr.

TIME/ACTION PROFILE (mucosal protectant effect)

ROUTE	ONSET	PEAK	DURATION
PO	1–2 hr	unknown	6 hr

Contraindications/Precautions

Contraindicated in: Hypersensitivity.
Use Cautiously in: Renal failure (accumulation of aluminum can occur).

Interactions

Drug-Drug: May ↓ the absorption of **phenytoin, fat-soluble vitamins,** or **tetracycline.** Concurrent **antacids, cimetidine,** or **ranitidine** ↓ the effectiveness of sucralfate. ↓ absorption of **fluoroquinolones** (separate administration by 2 hr).

Route/Dosage

Treatment of Ulcers

PO (Adults): 1 g qid, 1 hr before meals and hs; or 2 g bid, on waking and hs.

Prevention of Ulcers

PO (Adults): 1 g bid, 1 hr before a meal.

Gastroesophageal Reflux

PO (Adults): 1 g qid, 1 hr before meals and hs (unlabeled).
PO (Children): 40–80 mg/kg/day divided q 6 hr, 1 hr before meals and hs (unlabeled).

Stomatitis

PO (Adults and Children): 5–10 mL of suspension swish and spit or swish and swallow qid.

Proctitis

Rect (Adults): 2 g of suspension given as an enema once or twice daily.

Availability (generic available)

Tablets: 1 g. **Oral suspension:** 500 mg/5 mL.

HIGH ALERT

sufentanil (soo-**fen**-ta-nil)

Sufenta

Classification

Therapeutic: opioid analgesics, analgesic adjuncts
Pharmacologic: opioid agonists

Schedule II

Indications

IV: Analgesic supplement to general anesthesia; usually with other agents (ultra–short-acting barbiturates, neuromuscular blockers, and inhalation anesthetics) to produce balanced anesthesia in patients who are intubated and ventilated. Induction/maintenance of anesthesia (with oxygen or oxygen/nitrous oxide and a neuromuscular blocker). **Epidural:** Obstetric pain during labor and vaginal delivery (in combination with bupivacaine). **Unlabeled Use: Epidural:** Postoperative pain.

Action

Binds to opioid receptors in the CNS, altering the response to and perception of pain. Produces CNS depression. **Therapeutic Effects:** Supplement in anesthesia. ↓ pain.

Adverse Reactions/Side Effects

CNS: confusion, paradoxical excitation/delirium, postoperative depression, postoperative drowsiness. **EENT:** blurred/double vision. **Resp:** APNEA, CARDIAC ARREST, LARYNGOSPASM, allergic bronchospasm, respiratory depression. **CV:** arrhythmias, bradycardia, circulatory depression, hypotension. **GI:** biliary spasm, nausea/vomiting, constipation. **Derm:** facial itching. **MS:** skeletal and thoracic muscle rigidity. **Misc:** ALLERGIC REACTIONS, INCLUDING ANAPHYLAXIS.

PHYSICAL THERAPY IMPLICATIONS

Examination and Evaluation

- Assess respiration, and notify physician immediately if patient exhibits any interruption in respiratory rate (apnea) or signs of respiratory depression, including decreased respiratory rate, confusion, bluish color of the skin and mucous membranes (cyanosis), and difficult, labored breathing (dyspnea). Monitor pulse oximetry and perform pulmonary function tests (See Appendix I) to quantify suspected changes in ventilation and respiratory function. Apnea or excessive respiratory depression requires emergency care.

- Continually monitor for signs of cardiac arrest, including sudden chest pain, pain radiating into the arm or jaw, shortness of breath, dizziness, sweating, anxiety, nausea, and loss of consciousness. Seek immediate medical assistance if patient develops these signs.
- Monitor signs of laryngeal spasm and allergic bronchospasm, including tightness in the throat and chest, wheezing, cough, and severe shortness of breath. Notify physician or nursing staff immediately if these reactions occur.
- Be alert for other signs of allergic reactions and anaphylaxis, including skin reactions such as rash, pruritus, and urticaria. Notify physician or nursing staff immediately if these reactions occur.
- Be alert for excessive sedation or changes in mood and behavior (confusion, depression, excitation, delirium). Notify physician or nursing staff immediately if patient is unconscious or extremely difficult to arouse.
- Use appropriate pain scales (visual analogue scales, others) to document whether this drug is successful in helping manage the patient's pain.
- Assess blood pressure periodically and compare to normal values (See Appendix F). Report low blood pressure (hypotension) or signs of circulatory depression, including dizziness, fainting, weakness, pallor, and light-headedness.
- Assess heart rate, ECG, and heart sounds, especially during exercise (See Appendices G, H). Report slow heart rate (bradycardia) or symptoms of other arrhythmias, including palpitations, chest discomfort, shortness of breath, fainting, and fatigue/weakness.
- Be alert for residual muscle rigidity and decreased thoracic and limb movements. Report a sustained increase in muscle tone.

Interventions

- Implement appropriate manual therapy techniques, physical agents, and therapeutic exercises to reduce pain and help wean patient off opioid analgesics as soon as possible.
- Because of the risk of cardiac arrest, arrhythmias, and respiratory depression, use extreme caution during aerobic exercise and other forms of therapeutic exercise. Assess exercise tolerance frequently (blood pressure, heart rate, respiratory rate, fatigue levels), and terminate exercise immediately if any untoward responses occur (See Appendix L).
- To minimize orthostatic hypotension, patient should move slowly when assuming a more upright position.

Patient/Client-Related Instruction

- Advise patient to avoid alcohol and other CNS depressants because of the increased risk of sedation and decreased CNS function.
- Instruct patient to report other troublesome side effects such as severe or prolonged facial itching, vision disturbances, or GI problems (nausea, vomiting, indigestion, constipation).

Pharmacokinetics

Absorption: IV administration results in complete bioavailability.
Distribution: Does not readily penetrate adipose tissue; crosses the placenta, enters breast milk.
Metabolism and Excretion: Mostly metabolized by the liver; some metabolism in small intestine; ↓ in neonates, further ↓ in neonates with cardiovascular disease.
Half-life: 2.7 hr (↑ during cardiopulmonary bypass; ↑ in neonates, further ↑ in neonates with cardiovascular disease).

TIME/ACTION PROFILE (analgesia*)

ROUTE	ONSET	PEAK	DURATION
epidural	unknown	unknown	70–90 min
IV	within 1 min	unknown	5 min

*Respiratory depression may last longer than analgesia.

Contraindications/Precautions

Contraindicated in: Hypersensitivity; cross-sensitivity among agents may occur; Known intolerance.
Use Cautiously in: Geriatric, debilitated, or critically ill patients; Diabetic patients; Severe pulmonary or hepatic disease; CNS tumors; Increased intracranial pressure; Head trauma; Adrenal insufficiency; Undiagnosed abdominal pain; Hypothyroidism; Alcoholism; Cardiac disease (arrhythmias); Pregnancy, lactation, and children (clearance is ↓ in neonates and further ↓ in neonates with cardiovascular disease, adjust dose accordingly; has been used during labor and cesarean section—drowsiness may occur in infant).

Interactions

Drug-Drug: Avoid use in patients who have received **MAO inhibitors** within the previous 14 days (may produce unpredictable, potentially fatal reactions). ↑ CNS and respiratory depression with other **CNS depressants,** including **alcohol, antihistamines,**

S

antidepressants, other **sedative/hypnotics,** and other **opioids.** ↑ risk of hypotension with **benzodiazepines. Cimetidine, erythromycin,** or other **agents that decrease hepatic metabolism** may prolong duration of recovery. **Nalbuphine, buprenorphine,** or **pentazocine** may ↓ analgesia.

Route/Dosage

Low-Dose Anesthesia Adjunct

IV (Adults): 0.5–2 mcg/kg initially; supplemental doses of 10–25 mcg may be given as needed (not to exceed 1 mcg/kg/hr when administered with nitrous oxide and oxygen).

Moderate-Dose Anesthesia Adjunct

IV (Adults): 2–8 mcg/kg initiallyl; supplemental doses of 10–50 mcg may be given as needed (not to exceed 1 mcg/kg/hr when administered with nitrous oxide and oxygen).

Primary Anesthesia (with 100% Oxygen)

IV (Adults): 8–30 mcg/kg initially; supplemental doses of 25–50 mcg may be given as needed or a continuous infusion may be used.
IV (Children): *Cardiovascular surgery*—10–25 mcg/kg initially, followed by maintenance doses of up to 25–50 mcg; clearance in neonates is ↓ and more ↓ in neonates with cardiovascular disease, adjust dose accordingly.

Obstetric Analgesia

Epidural (Adults): 10–15 mcg in combination with 10 mL of 0.0125% bupivacaine; may be repeated after 1 hr for 2 additional doses.

Postoperative Pain (unlabeled)

Epidural (Adults): 30–60 mcg in 10 mL of 0.9% sodium chloride; additional doses of 25 mcg may be given hourly if needed.

Availability (generic available)

Injection: 50 mcg/mL in 1-, 2-, and 5-mL ampules.

sulconazole (sul-kon-a-zole)

Exelderm

Classification
Therapeutic: antifungals (topical)
Pharmacologic: imidazoles

Indications

Treatment of a variety of cutaneous fungal infections, including tinea pedis (athlete's foot), tinea cruris (jock itch), tinea corporis (ringworm), and tinea versicolor.

Action

Affects the synthesis of the fungal cell wall. **Therapeutic Effects:** ↓ in symptoms of fungal infection.

Adverse Reactions/Side Effects

Local: burning, itching, local hypersensitivity reactions, redness, stinging.

PHYSICAL THERAPY IMPLICATIONS

Examination and Evaluation

- Assess healing of skin lesions to help document drug effectiveness.

Interventions

- Avoid contact with cutaneous lesions when treating patient.
- Always wash hands thoroughly and disinfect equipment (whirlpools, electrotherapeutic devices, treatment tables, and so forth) to help prevent the spread of infection.

Patient/Client-Related Instruction

- Advise patient to report any increased local sensitivity to this drug (pain, burning, itching, swelling).
- Instruct patient about proper hygiene; e.g., thoroughly wash and dry the affected area, wear clean socks and ventilated shoes for tinea pedis, and so forth.
- Advise patient to apply the drug as directed for the full course of treatment even if feeling better.
- Inform patient that early relief of cutaneous symptoms may be seen in 2–3 days. Full therapeutic response may take 2–3 wk for tinea cruris, tinea corporis, and tinea versicolor and 4 wk for tinea pedis.
- Advise patient to seek medical help if infections persist or recur after the full treatment. Recurrent fungal infections may be a sign of systemic illness.

Pharmacokinetics

Absorption: Absorption through intact skin is minimal.
Distribution: Distribution after topical administration is primarily local.
Metabolism and Excretion: Systemic metabolism and excretion not known following local application.
Half-life: Not applicable.

TIME/ACTION PROFILE

ROUTE	ONSET	PEAK	DURATION
topical	unknown	unknown	unknown

Contraindications/Precautions

Contraindicated in: Hypersensitivity to active ingredients, additives, preservatives, or bases.
Use Cautiously in: Nail and scalp infections (may require additional systemic therapy); OB/Lactation: Safety not established.

Interactions

Drug-Drug: Not known.

Route/Dosage

Topical (Adults): Apply once or twice daily (twice daily for tinea pedis). Patients with tinea corporis, tinea cruris, or tinea versicolor should be treated for 3 wk. Patients with tinea pedis should be treated for 4 wk.

Availability

Cream: 1% (15 g, 30 g, 60 g). **Solution:** 1% (30 mL).

sulfasalazine

(sul-fa-**sal**-a-zeen)

Azulfidine, Azulfidine EN-tabs, PMS-Sulfasalazine, ✱Salazopyrin, S.A.S

Classification

Therapeutic: antirheumatics (disease-modifying antirheumatic drugs, DMARDs), gastrointestinal anti-inflammatories—therapeutic

Indications

Inflammatory bowel diseases, including Ulcerative colitis, Proctitis, Proctosigmoiditis. Rheumatoid arthritis unresponsive or intolerant to salicylates and/or NSAIDs.

Action

Locally acting anti-inflammatory action in the colon, where activity is probably a result of inhibition of prostaglandin synthesis. **Therapeutic Effects:** Reduction in the symptoms of inflammatory bowel disease.

Adverse Reactions/Side Effects

CNS: headache. **Resp:** pneumonitis. **GI:** anorexia, diarrhea, nausea, vomiting, drug-induced hepatitis. **GU:** crystalluria, oligospermia, orange-yellow discoloration of urine. **Derm:** rashes, exfoliative dermatitis, photosensitivity, yellow discoloration. **Hemat:** AGRANULOCYTOSIS, APLASTIC ANEMIA, blood dyscrasias, eosinophilia, megaloblastic anemia, thrombocytopenia. **Neuro:** peripheral neuropathy. **Misc:** hypersensitivity reactions, including SERUM SICKNESS AND STEVENS-JOHNSON SYNDROME, fever.

PHYSICAL THERAPY IMPLICATIONS

Examination and Evaluation

- Monitor and report signs of agranulocytosis (fever, sore throat, mucosal lesions, signs of infection), thrombocytopenia (bruising, nose bleeds, bleeding gums), or any unusual weakness and fatigue that might be due to aplastic anemia or other anemias. Periodic blood tests may be needed to monitor WBC and RBC counts.
- Monitor signs of hypersensitivity reactions, especially signs of serum sickness (muscle aches, joint pains, fever, skin rash) or Stevens-Johnson syndrome (hives, acne, abnormal sweating, exfoliation). Notify physician immediately if these reactions occur.
- If treating rheumatoid arthritis, periodically assess patient's impairments (pain, range of motion), functional ability, and disability to help document whether antirheumatic drug therapy is successful.
- Assess any breathing problems or signs of pneumonitis such as dry cough, wheezing, chest pain, shortness of breath, and difficult or labored breathing. Monitor pulse oximetry and perform pulmonary function tests (See Appendices I, J, K) to quantify suspected changes in ventilation and respiratory function.
- Be alert for signs of peripheral neuromyopathy (numbness, tingling, decreased muscle strength). Establish baseline electroneuromyographic values at the beginning of drug treatment whenever possible, and reexamine these values periodically to document drug-induced changes in peripheral nerve function.
- If treating inflammatory bowel diseases, monitor any changes in symptoms (decreased abdominal pain, decreased diarrhea, improved appetite) to help document whether drug therapy is successful.

Interventions

- Implement appropriate manual therapy techniques, physical agents, therapeutic exercises, and orthotic/assistive devices to reduce pain, improve function, and augment the effects of anti-rheumatic drug therapy.
- Help patient explore other nonpharmacologic methods to reduce chronic arthritis pain, such as relaxation techniques, exercise, counseling, and so forth.
- Causes photosensitivity; use care if administering UV treatments. Advise patient to avoid direct sunlight and use sunscreens and protective clothing.

Patient/Client-Related Instruction

- Advise patient about the likelihood of GI reactions such as nausea, vomiting, diarrhea, and loss of appetite. Instruct patient to report severe or prolonged GI problems, or signs of drug-induced hepatitis such as yellow skin or eyes, abdominal pain, severe nausea and vomiting, fever, sore throat, malaise, weakness, and facial edema.
- Advise patient to guard against infection (frequent hand washing, etc.), and to avoid crowds and contact with persons with contagious diseases.

S

- Instruct patient to report other untoward side effects such as severe or prolonged headache or skin reactions (rash, dermatitis, yellow discoloration).

Pharmacokinetics

Absorption: 10–15% absorbed after oral administration.
Distribution: Widely distributed; crosses the placenta and enters breast milk.
Protein Binding: 99%.
Metabolism and Excretion: Split by intestinal bacteria into sulfapyridine and 5-aminosalicylic acid. Some absorbed sulfasalazine is excreted by bile back into intestines; 15% excreted unchanged by the kidneys. Sulfapyridine also excreted mostly by the kidneys.
Half-life: 6 hr.

TIME/ACTION PROFILE (blood levels)

ROUTE	ONSET	PEAK	DURATION
PO	1 hr	1.5–6 hr	6–12 hr

Contraindications/Precautions

Contraindicated in: Hypersensitivity reactions to sulfonamides, salicylates, or sulfasalazine; Cross-sensitivity with furosemide, sulfonylurea hypoglycemic agents, or carbonic anhydrase inhibitors may exist; G6PD deficiency; Hypersensitivity to bisulfites (mesalamine enema only); Urinary tract or intestinal obstruction; Porphyria; Children <2 yr.
Use Cautiously in: Severe hepatic or renal impairment; Renal impairment; History of porphyria; Pregnancy (has been used safely); Lactation (safety not established).

Interactions

Drug-Drug: May ↑ action/risk of toxicity from **oral hypoglycemic agents, phenytoin, methotrexate, zidovudine,** or **warfarin.** ↑ risk of drug-induced hepatitis with other **hepatotoxic agents.** ↑ risk of crystalluria with **methenamine.** May ↓ metabolism and ↑ effects/toxicity of **mercaptopurine** or **thioguanine.**
Drug-Food: May ↓ **iron** and **folic acid** absorption.

Route/Dosage

Inflammatory bowel disease

PO (Adults): 1 g q 6–8 hr (may start with 500 mg q 6–12 hr), followed by maintenance dose of 500 mg q 6 hr.
PO (Children >2 yr): *Initial*—6.7–10 mg/kg q 4 hr *or* 10–15 mg/kg q 6 hr *or* 13.3–20 mg/kg q 8 hr. *Maintenance*—7.5 mg/kg q 6 hr (not to exceed 2 g/day).

Rheumatoid arthritis

PO (Adults): 500 mg–1 g/day (as delayed-release tablets) for 1 wk, then increase by 500 mg/day q wk up to 2 g/day in 2 divided doses; if no benefit seen after 12 wk, increase to 3 g/day in 2 divided doses.
PO (Children ≥6 yr): 30–50 mg/kg/day in 2 divided doses (as delayed-release tablets); initiate therapy at ¼–1/3 of planned maintenance dose and increase q 7 days until maintenance dose is reached (not to exceed 2 g/day).

Availability (generic available)

Tablets: 500 mg. **Delayed-release (enteric-coated) tablets (Azulfidine EN-tabs):** 500 mg. **Oral suspension:** 250 mg/5 mL. **Rectal suspension:** 3 g.

sulfinpyrazone

(sul-fin-**peer**-a-zone)
Antazone, Anturan, Anturane, Apo-Sulfinpyrazone, Novopyrazone

Classification
Therapeutic: antigout agents
Pharmacologic: uricosurics

Indications

Management (long-term) of gout.

Action

Decreases serum uric acid levels by decreasing renal reabsorption and subsequently increasing urinary excretion. **Therapeutic Effects:** Reduction in serum uric acid levels.

Adverse Reactions/Side Effects

GI: GI BLEEDING, nausea, vomiting, abdominal pain.
Derm: rash. **Hemat:** blood dyscrasias. **Misc:** fever.

PHYSICAL THERAPY IMPLICATIONS

Examination and Evaluation

- Watch for signs of GI bleeding, including abdominal pain, vomiting blood, blood in stools, or black, tarry stools. Report these signs to the physician immediately.
- Assess pain and other variables (range of motion, gait, other functional activities) to document whether this drug is successful in helping manage the patient's pain and decreasing impairments related to gout.
- Watch for signs of leukopenia (fever, sore throat, signs of infection), thrombocytopenia (bruising, nose bleeds, bleeding gums), or unusual weakness and fatigue that might be due to anemia or other blood dyscrasias. Report these signs to the physician.

Interventions

- Implement appropriate physical agents, therapeutic exercises, orthoses, and assistive devices to reduce gout pain and compliment the effects of drug therapy.

Patient/Client-Related Instruction

- Instruct patient to immediately report signs of GI bleeding, including abdominal pain, vomiting blood, blood in stools, or black, tarry stools.
- Instruct patient and family/caregivers to report other troublesome side effects such as severe or prolonged fever, skin rash, or GI problems (nausea, vomiting, abdominal pain).

Pharmacokinetics

Absorption: Well absorbed following oral administration.
Distribution: Distribution to tissues not known.
Protein Binding: 98–99%.
Metabolism and Excretion: Mostly metabolized by the liver. Converted to compounds with uricosuric (parahydroxy-sulfinpyrazone) and antiplatelet activity (sulfide metabolite).
Half-life: 3 hr (1 hr for parahydroxy-sulfinpyrazone; up to 13 hr for sulfide metabolite).

TIME/ACTION PROFILE (hypouricemic effects)

ROUTE	ONSET	PEAK	DURATION
PO	unknown	unknown	4–10 hr

Contraindications/Precautions

Contraindicated in: Hypersensitivity; Cross-sensitivity with oxyphenbutazone and phenylbutazone may exist.
Use Cautiously in: History of blood dyscrasias; History of GI bleeding; History of kidney stones; Neoplastic disease or radiation therapy (↑ risk of uric acid stone formation); Acute attacks of gout.

Interactions

Drug-Drug: ↑ risk of bleeding with **aspirin,** other **NSAIDs, anticoagulants, cefoperazone, cefotetan, clopidogrel, eptifibatide, tirofiban, ticlopidine, valproic acid,** or **thrombolytic agents.** ↓ blood levels and may ↓ effectiveness of **nitrofurantoin, theophylline,** or **verapamil.** Uricosuric effect may be ↓ by **salicylates** or **niacin.** Concurrent use of **antineoplastics** ↑ risk of uric acid kidney stones.
Drug-Natural: ↑ bleeding risk with **anise, arnica, chamomile, clove, feverfew, garlic, ginger, ginkgo, *Panax ginseng*,** and others.

Route/Dosage

Hypouricemic

PO (Adults): 100–200 mg bid initially; may be ↑ by 200 mg/day q 2 days up to 800 mg/day in 2 divided doses (usual range 200–400 mg/day).

Availability (generic available)

Capsules: 100 mg. **Tablets:** 100 mg, 200 mg.

sulfisoxazole (sul-fi-sox-a-zole)

Apo-Sulfisoxazole, Gantrisin, ✱Novo-Soxazole, ✱Sulfizole

Classification
Therapeutic: anti-infectives
Pharmacologic: sulfonamides

Indications

PO: Treatment of urinary tract infections, acute otitis media, meningitis, nocardiosis, and, in combination with other anti-infectives, malaria and toxoplasmosis. Prophylaxis for meningococcal meningitis for sensitive strains in family groups or large closed populations.
Unlabeled Use: Prevention of recurrent otitis media.

Action

Interferes with bacterial folic acid synthesis. **Therapeutic Effects:** Bacteriostatic action against susceptible bacteria. **Spectrum:** Notable for activity against some gram-positive pathogens, including streptococci and staphylococci, *Clostridium perfringens*, *C. tetani*, *Nocardia asteroides*. Active against some gram-negative pathogens, including *Enterobacter*, *Escherichia coli*, *Klebsiella*, *Proteus mirabilis*, *P. vulgaris*, *Salmonella*, *Shigella*.

Adverse Reactions/Side Effects

CNS: ataxia, confusion, dizziness, drowsiness, mental depression, psychosis, restlessness. **GI:** nausea, diarrhea, anorexia, hepatitis, vomiting. **GU:** crystalluria. **Derm:** rash, exfoliative dermatitis, photosensitivity. **Hemat:** agranulocytosis, aplastic anemia, eosinophilia, thrombocytopenia. **Neuro:** peripheral neuropathy. **Misc:** HYPERSENSITIVITY REACTIONS, INCLUDING SERUM SICKNESS AND STEVENS-JOHNSON SYNDROME, fever, superinfection.

PHYSICAL THERAPY IMPLICATIONS

Examination and Evaluation

- Monitor signs of hypersensitivity reactions, including serum sickness (muscle aches, joint pain, fatigue) and Stevens-Johnson syndrome (exfoliation, rash, hives, acne, abnormal sweating). Notify physician immediately because these signs may indicate serious hypersensitivity reactions
- Monitor signs of blood dyscrasias, including agranulocytosis (fever, sore throat, mucosal lesions, signs of infection), thrombocytopenia (bruising, nose bleeds, bleeding gums), and aplastic anemia or eosinophilia (unusual fatigue, weakness, myalgia). Report these signs to the physician.

S

- Monitor signs of peripheral neuropathy (numbness, tingling). Perform objective tests (nerve conduction, monofilaments) to document any neuropathic changes.
- Assess dizziness, drowsiness, or ataxia that might affect gait, balance, and other functional activities (See Appendix C). Report balance problems and functional limitations to the physician and nursing staff, and caution the patient and family/caregivers to guard against falls and trauma.
- Be alert for confusion, restlessness, mental depression, psychosis, or other alterations in mental status. Notify health care professional promptly if these symptoms develop.

Interventions

- Always wash hands thoroughly and disinfect equipment (whirlpools, electrotherapeutic devices, treatment tables, and so forth) to help prevent the spread of infection. Employ universal precautions or isolation procedures as indicated for specific patients.
- Causes photosensitivity; use care if administering UV treatments.

Patient/Client-Related Instruction

- Advise patient about photosensitivity, and to use sunscreens, protective clothing, and avoid prolonged sun exposure. Advise patient to also report any rashes or other skin reactions.
- Advise patient about the likelihood of GI reactions such as nausea, vomiting, diarrhea, and loss of appetite. Instruct patient to report severe or prolonged GI problems, or signs of hepatitis (yellow skin or eyes, abdominal pain, severe nausea and vomiting, fever, sore throat, malaise, weakness, facial edema).
- Instruct patient and family/caregivers to report other troublesome side effects such as severe or prolonged fever or signs of superinfection (black, furry overgrowth on tongue, vaginal itching or discharge, loose or foul-smelling stools).

Pharmacokinetics

Absorption: Well absorbed following oral administration.
Distribution: Widely distributed. Crosses the placenta; enters breast milk.
Metabolism and Excretion: Mostly metabolized by the liver.
Half-life: 5–8 hr.

TIME/ACTION PROFILE (blood levels)

ROUTE	ONSET	PEAK	DURATION
PO	1 hr	2–4 hr	4–6 hr

Contraindications/Precautions

Contraindicated in: Hypersensitivity to sulfonamides (cross-sensitivity with furosemide, thiazide diuretics, sulfonylurea oral hypoglycemic agents, and carbonic anhydrase inhibitors may exist); Porphyria; Pregnant women at term (may cause kernicterus in the infant); G6PD deficiency; Known alcohol intolerance (oral suspension only); Infants <2 mo (unless with pyrimethamine for congenital toxoplasmosis).
Use Cautiously in: Renal impairment (dosage reduction may be recommended); Hepatic impairment.

Interactions

Drug-Drug: May enhance the action and ↑ the risk of toxicity from **oral hypoglycemic agents, methotrexate, phenytoin, zidovudine,** or **warfarin.** ↑ risk of crystalluria with **methenamine.** ↑ risk of drug-induced hepatitis with other **hepatotoxic agents.**

Route/Dosage

PO (Adults): 2–4 g initially, then 750 mg–1.5 g q 4 hr or 1–2 g q 6 hr (not to exceed 12 g/day).
PO (Children >2 mo): 75 mg/kg (2 g/m^2) initially, then 25 mg (667 mg/m^2) q 4 hr or 37.5 mg/kg (1 g/m^2) q 6 hr (not to exceed 6 g/day).

Availability (generic available)

Tablets: 500 mg. **Oral suspension (raspberry flavor):** 500 mg/5 mL in 16-oz bottle.

sumatriptan (soo-ma-trip-tan)

Imitrex, Imitrex Statdose

Classification

Therapeutic: vascular headache suppressants
Pharmacologic: 5-HT$_1$ agonists

Indications

Acute treatment of migraine attacks. **SC:** Acute treatment of cluster headache episodes.

Action

Acts as a selective agonist of 5-HT$_1$ at specific vascular serotonin receptor sites, causing vasoconstriction in large intracranial arteries. **Therapeutic Effects:** Relief of acute attacks of migraine.

Adverse Reactions/Side Effects

All adverse reactions are less common after oral administration

CNS: dizziness, vertigo, anxiety, drowsiness, fatigue, feeling of heaviness, feeling of tightness, headache, malaise, strange feeling, tight feeling in head, weakness. **EENT:** alterations in vision, nasal sinus discomfort, throat discomfort. **CV:** MI, angina, chest pressure, chest tightness, coronary vasospasm, ECG changes, transient hypertension. **GI:** abdominal discomfort, dysphagia. **Derm:** tingling, warm sensation, burning sensation, cool sensation, flushing. **Local:** injection-site reaction. **MS:** jaw discomfort, muscle cramps, myalgia, neck pain, neck stiffness. **Neuro:** numbness.

PHYSICAL THERAPY IMPLICATIONS

Examination and Evaluation

- Continually monitor for signs of coronary artery vasospasm and MI, including sudden chest pain, pain radiating into the arm or jaw, shortness of breath, dizziness, sweating, anxiety, and nausea. Seek immediate medical assistance if patient develops these signs.
- Assess heart rate, ECG, and heart sounds, especially during exercise (See Appendices G, H). Report any rhythm disturbances or symptoms of increased arrhythmias, including palpitations, chest discomfort, shortness of breath, dizziness, fainting, and fatigue/weakness.
- Assess the frequency and severity of headaches, and document whether drug therapy is successful in decreasing migraine or cluster headache attacks.
- Assess any muscle pain, cramps, jaw discomfort, or neck pain and stiffness to rule out musculoskeletal pathology; that is, try to determine if pain is drug induced rather than caused by anatomic or biomechanical problems.
- Assess signs of paresthesia (numbness, tingling). Perform objective tests, including electroneuromyography and sensory testing to document any drug-related neuropathic changes.
- Monitor excessive drowsiness, anxiety, or strange sensations such as tightness or heaviness. Notify physician if these symptoms become problematic.
- Watch for dizziness and vertigo that affects gait, balance, and other functional activities (See Appendix C). Report balance problems and functional limitations to the physician, and caution the patient and family/caregivers to guard against falls and trauma.
- Monitor SC injection site for pain, swelling, and irritation. Report prolonged or excessive injection site reactions to the physician.

Interventions

- Because of the risk of MI and arrhythmias, use extreme caution during aerobic exercise and other forms of therapeutic exercise. Assess exercise tolerance frequently (blood pressure, heart rate, respiration, fatigue levels), and terminate exercise immediately if any untoward responses occur (See Appendix L).
- Implement appropriate interventions (manual techniques, physical agents, therapeutic exercise) to manage headache pain and reduce the need for drug therapy. Help patient also explore other nonpharmacologic methods to reduce chronic headache pain (relaxation techniques, imagery, and so forth).
- If a headache occurs and drug treatment is needed during a rehabilitation session, allow patient to recover in a quiet, darkened room to allow the drug to achieve maximal effects.

Patient/Client-Related Instruction

- Advise patient and family or caregiver about the signs of MI (see above under Examination and Evaluation) and to seek immediate medical assistance if these signs develop.
- Advise the patient to bring this drug to each therapy session; this drug is most effective when taken at the first signs of a migraine attack. Make sure patients understand the correct administration techniques for intranasal inhalation or SC injection.
- Advise patient to adhere to the correct dosing schedule, and to not exceed the recommended frequency and number of doses per 24-hr period.
- Instruct patient to report other troublesome side effects such as severe or prolonged headache, drowsiness, altered vision, skin reactions (tingling, warmth, other strange sensations), or GI problems (abdominal discomfort, swallowing difficulties).

Pharmacokinetics

Absorption: Well absorbed (97%) after SC administration. Absorption after oral administration is incomplete and significant amounts undergo substantial hepatic metabolism, resulting in poor bioavailability (14%). Well absorbed after intranasal administration.
Distribution: Does not cross the blood-brain barrier. Remainder of distribution not known.
Metabolism and Excretion: Mostly metabolized (80%) by the liver.
Half-life: 2 hr.

TIME/ACTION PROFILE (relief of migraine)

ROUTE	ONSET	PEAK	DURATION
PO	within 30 min	2–4 hr	up to 24 hr
SC	30 min	up to 2 hr	up to 24 hr
nasal	within 60 min	2 hr	unknown

Contraindications/Precautions

Contraindicated in: Hypersensitivity; Patients with ischemic heart disease or signs and symptoms of ischemic heart disease, Prinzmetal's angina, or uncontrolled hypertension; Concurrent MAO inhibitor therapy; Geri: Excessive risk of cardiovascular complications.
Use Cautiously in: Patients with childbearing potential; OB/Lactation/Pedi: Safety not established.
Exercise Extreme Caution in: Cardiovascular risk factors (hypertension, hypercholesterolemia, smoking, obesity, diabetes, family history, menopausal women

S

or men >40 yr); use only if cardiovascular status has been evaluated and determined to be safe and first dose is administered under supervision.

Interactions

Drug-Drug: The risk of vasospastic reactions may be ↑ by concurrent use of **ergotamine** or **dihydroergotamine** (avoid within 24 hr of each other). Concurrent use with **lithium, MAO inhibitors** (do not use within 2 wk of discontinuing MAO inhibitor), or **SSRI antidepressants** (may cause weakness, hyperreflexia, and incoordination). ↑ serotonin levels and serotonin syndrome may occur when used concurrently with **SSRI and SNRI antidepressants.**
Drug-Natural: ↑ risk of serotonergic side effects, including serotonin syndrome with **St. John's wort** and **SAMe.**

Route/Dosage

PO (Adults): 25 mg initially; if response is inadequate at 2 hr, up to 100 mg may be given (initial doses of 25–50 mg may be more effective than 25 mg).
If headache recurs, doses may be repeated q 2 hr (not to exceed 300 mg/day). If PO therapy is to follow SC injection, additional PO sumatriptan may be taken q 2 hr (not to exceed 200 mg/day).
SC (Adults): 6 mg; may repeat after 1 hr (not to exceed 12 mg in 24 hr).
Intranasal (Adults): Single dose of 5, 10, or 20 mg in one nostril; may be repeated in 2 hr, not to exceed 40 mg/24 hr or treatment of >5 episodes/mo.

Hepatic Impairment

PO (Adults): 25 mg initially; if response is inadequate at 2 hr, up to 50 mg may be given (initial doses of 25–50 mg may be more effective than 25 mg). If headache recurs, doses may be repeated q 2 hr (not to exceed 300 mg/day). If PO therapy is to follow SC injection, additional PO sumatriptan may be taken q 2 hr (not to exceed 200 mg/day); no single oral dose should exceed 50 mg.

Availability

Tablets: 25 mg, 50 mg, 100 mg. **Injection:** 4 mg/0.5-mL prefilled syringes (for use in Statdose system), 6 mg/0.5-mL prefilled syringes (for use in STAT dose system) or vials. **Nasal spray:** 5 mg/nasal spray device (delivers 5 mg/spray) (box of 6), 20 mg/nasal spray device (delivers 20 mg/spray) (box of 6). ***In combination with:*** naproxen (Treximet). See Appendix B.

sunitinib (soo-ni-ti-nib)

Sutent

Classification
Therapeutic: antineoplastics
Pharmacologic: enzyme inhibitors

Indications

Gastrointestinal stromal tumor which has progressed on or intolerance to imatinib. Advanced renal cell carcinoma.

Action

Inhibits multiple receptor tyrosine kinases, which are enzymes implicated in tumor growth, abnormal vascular growth, and tumor metastases. **Therapeutic Effects:** Decreased tumor spread.

Adverse Reactions/Side Effects

CNS: fatigue, dizziness, headache. **CV:** CHF, hypertension, peripheral edema, thromboembolic events.
GI: diarrhea, dyspepsia, nausea, stomatitis, vomiting, altered taste, anorexia, constipation, ↑ lipase/amylase, ↑ liver enzymes, oral pain. **Derm:** alopecia, hand-foot syndrome, hair color change, rash, skin discoloration.
Endo: adrenal insufficiency, hypothyroidism.
F and E: dehydration, hypophosphatemia.
Hemat: HEMORRHAGE, anemia, lymphopenia, neutropenia, thrombocytopenia. **Metab:** hyperuricemia. **MS:** arthralgia, back pain, limb pain, myalgia. **Misc:** fever.

PHYSICAL THERAPY IMPLICATIONS

Examination and Evaluation

- Assess for signs of bleeding and hemorrhage (bleeding gums; nosebleed; unusual bruising; black, tarry stools; hematuria; fall in hematocrit or blood pressure). Notify physician or nursing staff immediately if these signs occur.
- Assess signs of congestive heart failure, including dyspnea, rales/crackles, peripheral edema, jugular venous distention, and exercise intolerance. Report these signs to the physician or nursing staff immediately.
- Monitor signs of leukopenia (fever, sore throat, signs of infection), thrombocytopenia (bruising, nose bleeds, bleeding gums), or unusual weakness and fatigue that might be due to anemia or other blood dyscrasias. Report these signs to the physician or nursing staff.
- Assess blood pressure (BP) and compare to normal values (See Appendix F). Report a sustained increase in BP (hypertension).
- Assess peripheral edema using girth measurements, volume displacement, and measurement of pitting edema (See Appendix N). Report increased swelling in feet and ankles or a sudden increase in body weight due to fluid retention.
- Monitor signs of thromboembolic events, including venous thrombosis (lower extremity swelling, warmth, erythema, tenderness) and arterial thrombosis (extreme coldness in the hands and feet, cyanosis, muscle cramping). Notify physician immediately, and request objective tests (Doppler ultrasound, others) if thrombosis is suspected.

- Assess any muscle, joint, back, or limb pain to rule out musculoskeletal pathology; that is, try to determine if pain is drug-induced rather than caused by anatomic or biomechanical problems.
- Monitor signs of low phosphate levels (hypophosphatemia), including skeletal muscle dysfunction or weakness, respiratory muscle weakness, and mental status changes such as irritability and confusion that progresses to delirium and coma. Report these signs to the physician.
- Report signs of adrenal insufficiency, including hypotension, weight loss, weakness, nausea, vomiting, anorexia, lethargy, confusion, and restlessness.
- Monitor and report a decrease in metabolism that might indicate hypothyroidism. These signs typically include bradycardia, lethargy, cold intolerance, weight gain, and muscle weakness.
- Assess dizziness that might affect gait, balance, and other functional activities (See Appendix C). Report balance problems and functional limitations to the physician and nursing staff, and caution the patient and family/caregivers to guard against falls and trauma.

Interventions

- For patients who are medically able to begin exercise, implement appropriate resistive exercises and aerobic training to maintain muscle strength and aerobic capacity during cancer chemotherapy, or to help restore function after chemotherapy.
- Because of the risk of CHF and hemorrhage, use caution during aerobic exercise and other forms of therapeutic exercise. Assess exercise tolerance frequently (BP, heart rate, fatigue levels), and terminate exercise immediately if any untoward responses occur (See Appendix L).
- Make sure patient maintains adequate fluid intake to avoid dehydration, especially during exercise.

Patient/Client-Related Instruction

- Advise patient to guard against infection (frequent hand washing, etc.), and to avoid crowds and contact with persons with contagious diseases.
- Advise patient and family/caregivers that fatigue and weakness are likely and may be severe. Functional abilities may be limited, and patient may need to use assistive devices during ambulation.
- Advise patient about the likelihood of GI reactions such as nausea, vomiting, constipation, diarrhea, loss of appetite, altered taste, indigestion, oral pain, and irritation in/around the mouth. Instruct patient to report severe or prolonged GI problems.
- Instruct patient to report other bothersome side effects such as severe or prolonged headache, fever, skin reactions (rash, discoloration, hair loss), or hand-foot syndrome (pain, redness, and dry, scaly skin on the palms of the hands and soles of the feet).

Pharmacokinetics

Absorption: Well absorbed following oral administration.
Distribution: Unknown.
Protein Binding: *Sunitinib*—95%; *primary active metabolite*— 90%.
Metabolism and Excretion: Metabolized by the CYP3A4 enzyme system to its primary active metabolite. This metabolite is further metabolized by CYP3A4. Excretion is primarily fecal.
Half-life: *Sunitinib*—40–60 hr; *primary active metabolite*— 80–110 hr.

TIME/ACTION PROFILE (blood levels)

ROUTE	ONSET	PEAK	DURATION
PO	unknown	6–12 hr	24 hr

S

Contraindications/Precautions

Contraindicated in: Hypersensitivity; OB: Pregnancy, lactation; Concurrent use of ketoconazole or St. John's wort.
Use Cautiously in: Hepatic/renal impairment; OB: Childbearing potential; Pedi: Children (safety not established).

Interactions

Drug-Drug: Ketoconazole and other **inhibitors of the CYP3A4 enzyme system** may ↑ levels and the risk of toxicity; dosage may need to be ↓ (avoid ketoconazole). **Rifampin** and other **inducers of the CYP3A4 enzyme system** may ↓ levels and effectiveness; dose may need to be ↑.
Drug-Natural: St. John's wort may ↓ levels and effectiveness; avoid concurrent use.

Route/Dosage

PO (Adults): 50 mg once daily for 4 wk, followed by 2-wk rest; alteration of dose is based on safety/tolerability and is made in 12.5-mg increments/decrements.

Availability

Capsules: 12.5 mg, 25 mg, 50 mg.

tacrolimus (oral, IV)
(ta-**kroe**-li-mus)
Prograf

tacrolimus (topical)
(ta-**kroe**-li-mus)
Protopic

Classification
Therapeutic: immunosuppressants
Pharmacologic: macrolides

Indications
Oral, IV: Prevention of organ rejection in patients who have undergone allogenic liver, kidney, or heart transplantation (used concurrently with corticosteroids).
Topical: Moderate-to-severe atopic dermatitis in nonimmunocompromised patients who do not respond to or cannot tolerate alternative, conventional therapies.

Action
Inhibits T-lymphocyte activation. **Therapeutic Effects:** Prevention of transplanted organ rejection (oral, IV). Improvement in signs/symptoms of atopic dermatitis (topical).

Adverse Reactions/Side Effects
CNS: SEIZURES, dizziness, headache, insomnia, tremor, abnormal dreams, agitation, anxiety, confusion, emotional lability, depression, hallucinations, psychoses, somnolence. **EENT:** abnormal vision, amblyopia, tinnitus. **Resp:** cough, pleural effusion, asthma, bronchitis, pharyngitis, pneumonia, pulmonary edema. **CV:** hypertension, peripheral edema, QTc prolongation. **GI:** GI BLEEDING, abdominal pain, anorexia, ascites, constipation, diarrhea, dyspepsia, ↑ liver function studies, nausea, vomiting, cholangitis, cholestatic jaundice, dysphagia, flatulence, ↑ appetite, oral thrush. **GU:** nephrotoxicity, urinary tract infection. **Derm:** pruritus, rash, alopecia, herpes simplex, hirsutism, sweating, photosensitivity. **Endo:** hyperglycemia. **F and E:** hyperkalemia, hyperlipidemia, hypokalemia, hypomagnesemia, hypophosphatemia, hyperphosphatemia, hyperuricemia, hypocalcemia, hyponatremia, metabolic acidosis, metabolic alkalosis. **Hemat:** anemia, leukocytosis, leukopenia, thrombocytopenia, coagulation defects. **MS:** arthralgia, hypertonia, leg cramps, muscle spasm, myalgia, myasthenia, osteoporosis. **Neuro:** paresthesia, neuropathy. **Misc:** ALLERGIC REACTIONS, INCLUDING ANAPHYLAXIS, fever, generalized pain, abnormal healing, chills, ↑ risk of lymphoma/skin cancer.

PHYSICAL THERAPY IMPLICATIONS

Examination and Evaluation
- Be alert for new seizures or increased seizure activity, especially at the onset of drug treatment. Document the number, duration, and severity of seizures, and report these findings to the physician immediately.
- Be alert for signs of allergic reactions and anaphylaxis, including pulmonary symptoms (tightness in the throat and chest, wheezing, cough, dyspnea) or skin reactions (rash, pruritus, urticaria). Notify physician or nursing staff immediately if these reactions occur.
- Monitor signs of GI bleeding, including abdominal pain, vomiting blood, blood in stools, or black, tarry stools. Report these signs to the physician or nursing staff immediately.
- Assess any breathing problems or signs of pulmonary dysfunction (pneumonia, pulmonary edema, pleural effusion). Signs include cough, shortness of breath, chest pain, labored breathing, fever, and abnormal breath sounds. Monitor pulse oximetry and perform pulmonary function tests (See Appendices I, J, K) to quantify suspected changes in ventilation and respiratory function.
- Assess blood pressure (BP) periodically and compare to normal values (See Appendix F). Report a sustained increase in BP (hypertension).
- Assess heart rate, ECG, and heart sounds, especially during exercise (See Appendices G, H). Report any ECG abnormalities or signs of arrhythmias, including palpitations, chest discomfort, shortness of breath, fainting, and fatigue/weakness.
- Assess peripheral edema using girth measurements, volume displacement, and measurement of pitting edema (See Appendix N). Report increased swelling in feet and ankles or a sudden increase in body weight due to fluid retention.
- If applied topically to treat dermatitis, monitor any changes in skin lesions to help document the effects of drug therapy.
- Monitor signs of leukopenia (fever, sore throat, mucosal lesions, signs of infection, bruising), thrombocytopenia (bruising, nose bleeds, bleeding gums), or unusual weakness, fatigue, or coagulation abnormalities that might be due to anemia or other blood dyscrasias. Periodic blood tests may be needed to monitor WBC and RBC counts.
- Be alert for signs of increased white blood cell counts (leukocytosis), including fever, weakness, weight loss, loss of appetite, dizziness, fainting, dyspnea, bleeding/bruising, or pain or tingling in the arms, legs, or abdomen. Report these signs to the physician or nursing staff immediately.

- Monitor signs of lymphoma (swollen lymph glands, unexplained weight loss, fatigue, weakness, fever, night sweats, dyspnea, cough, abdominal pain/bloating) or suspicious skin lesions that might indicate skin cancer. Report these signs to the physician immediately.
- Be alert for signs of hyperglycemia, including confusion, drowsiness, flushed/dry skin, fruit-like breath odor, rapid/deep breathing, polyuria, loss of appetite, and unusual thirst. Patients with diabetes mellitus should check blood glucose levels frequently.
- Watch for signs of renal toxicity (decreased urine output, cloudy urine, sudden weight gain due to fluid retention) or urinary tract infection (blood in the urine, increased nighttime urination, pain and burning during urination). Report these signs to the physician.
- Be alert for signs of paresthesia and neuropathy, including numbness, tingling, and muscle weakness. Establish baseline electroneuromyographic values at the beginning of drug treatment whenever possible, and reexamine these values periodically to document drug-induced changes in peripheral nerve function.
- Monitor neuromuscular signs of acid-base imbalance (acidosis, alkalosis) or electrolyte imbalances (hypocalcemia, hypokalemia, hyperkalemia, hypomagnesemia, hypophosphatemia, hyponatremia), including headache, lethargy, irritability, insomnia, confusion, weakness, cramping, tremors, and changes in muscle excitability. Notify physician immediately if these signs occur.
- Monitor personality changes, including depression, anxiety, agitation, emotional instability, confusion, hallucinations, and psychosis. Notify physician if these changes become problematic.
- Assess any joint or muscle pain or muscle spasms to rule out musculoskeletal pathology; that is, try to determine if pain is drug induced rather than caused by anatomic or biomechanical problems.
- Assess dizziness that might affect gait, balance, and other functional activities (See Appendix C). Report balance problems and functional limitations to the physician and nursing staff, and caution the patient and family/caregivers to guard against falls and trauma.

Interventions

- Implement appropriate strengthening, aerobic, and other therapeutic exercises to improve function and promote recovery following organ transplants.
- Because of the risk of arrhythmias and abnormal BP responses, use caution during aerobic exercise and other forms of therapeutic exercise. Assess exercise tolerance frequently (BP, heart rate, fatigue levels), and terminate exercise immediately if any untoward responses occur (See Appendix L).
- Causes photosensitivity; use care if administering UV treatments. Advise patient to avoid direct sunlight and use sunscreens and protective clothing.

Patient/Client-Related Instruction

- Because of immunosuppressant effects, advise patient to guard against infection (frequent hand washing, etc.), and to avoid crowds and contact with persons with contagious diseases.
- If applied topically, check that the patient and family or caregivers understand topical application procedures and adhere to the recommended dosing schedule.
- Advise patient that wound healing may be delayed; instruct patient to check skin regularly and report any nonhealing sores.
- Advise patient that this drug may cause problems in fat metabolism (hyperlipidemia). Remind patient that periodic blood tests may be needed to monitor plasma lipids.
- Instruct patient to report other bothersome side effects such as severe or prolonged headache, sleep loss, abnormal dreams, ringing/buzzing in the ears (tinnitus), vision disturbances, infections, chills, fever, skin reactions (rash, itching, changes in hair growth, increased sweating), or GI problems (nausea, vomiting, diarrhea, constipation, flatulence, indigestion, difficulty swallowing, changes in appetite, abdominal pain).

Pharmacokinetics

Absorption: Absorption following oral administration is erratic and incomplete (5–67%). Minimal following topical use.
Distribution: Crosses the placenta and enters breast milk.
Protein Binding: 99%.
Metabolism and Excretion: 99% metabolized by the liver; <1% excreted unchanged in the urine.
Half-life: *Liver transplant patients*—11.7 hr; *healthy volunteers*—21.2 hr.
Protein Binding: 99%.

TIME/ACTION PROFILE (immunosuppression)

ROUTE	ONSET	PEAK	DURATION
PO	rapid	1.3–3.2 hr*	12 hr
IV	rapid	unknown	8–12 hr
topical	unknown	1–2 wk	unknown

*Blood level.

Contraindications/Precautions

Contraindicated in: Hypersensitivity to tacrolimus or to castor oil (a component in the injection); Lactation: Enters breast milk, posing risk to fetus.
Use Cautiously in: Renal or hepatic impairment (dosage reduction may be required; if oliguria occurs, wait 48 hr before initiating tacrolimus); Concurrent use with cyclosporine should be avoided; Exposure to

sunlight/UV light (may ↑ risk of malignant skin changes); OB: Hyperkalemia and renal impairment may occur in the newborn; use only if benefit to mother justifies risk to the fetus.

Interactions

Drug-Drug: Risk of nephrotoxicity is ↑ by concurrent use of **aminoglycosides, amphotericin B, cisplatin,** or **cyclosporine** (allow 24 hr to pass after stopping cyclosporine before starting tacrolimus). Concurrent use of **potassium-sparing diuretics, ACE inhibitors,** or **angiotensin II receptor antagonists** ↑ risk of hyperkalemia. The following drugs ↑ tacrolimus blood levels: **azole antifungals, bromocriptine, calcium channel blockers, chloramphenicol, cimetidine, clarithromycin, cyclosporine, danazol, erythromycin, lansoprazole, magnesium/aluminum hydroxide, methylprednisolone, omeprazole, nefazodone, metoclopramide, protease inhibitors,** and **voriconazole. Phenobarbital, phenytoin, caspofungin, sirolimus, carbamazepine,** and **rifamycins** may ↓ tacrolimus blood levels. **Vaccinations** may be less effective if given concurrently with tacrolimus (avoid use of live-virus vaccines).
Drug-Natural: Concomitant use with **astragalus, echinacea,** and **melatonin** may interfere with immunosuppression. **St. John's wort** may ↓ tacrolimus blood levels.
Drug-Food: Food ↓ the rate and extent of GI absorption. **Grapefruit juice** ↑ absorption.

Route/Dosage

Because of the potential risk for anaphylaxis, the IV route of administration of tacrolimus should be reserved for those patients unable to take the drug orally.

Kidney Transplantation

PO (Adults): *Initial dose*—0.2 mg/kg/day in 2 divided doses; titrate to achieve recommended blood concentration.
PO (Children): 0.15–0.4 mg/kg/day in 2 divided doses.
IV (Adults): *Initial dose*—0.03–0.1 mg/kg/day as a continuous infusion; titrate dose to achieve recommended blood concentration.
IV (Children): 0.03–0.15 mg/kg/day.

Liver Transplantation

PO (Adults): *Initial dose*—0.1–0.15 mg/kg/day in 2 divided doses; titrate to achieve recommended blood concentration.
PO (Children): *Initial dose*—0.15–0.2 mg/kg/day in 2 divided doses; titrate to achieve recommended blood concentration.
IV (Adults and Children): Same as for kidney transplant.

Heart Transplantation

PO (Adults): *Initial dose*—0.075 mg/kg/day in 2 divided doses; titrate to achieve recommended blood concentration.
IV (Adults): *Initial dose*—0.01 mg/kg/day as a continuous infusion; titrate dose to achieve recommended blood concentration.
Topical (Adults): Apply 0.03% or 0.1% ointment twice daily. Discontinue when signs/symptoms of atopic dermatitis resolve.
Topical (Children ≥2–15 yr): Apply 0.03% ointment twice daily. Discontinue when signs/symptoms of atopic dermatitis resolve.

Availability

Capsules: 0.5 mg, 1 mg, 5 mg. **Injection:** 5 mg/mL. **Ointment:** 0.03% in 30-g, 60-g, and 100-g tubes, 0.1% in 30-g, 60-g, and 100-g tubes.

tadalafil (ta-daye-la-fil)

Cialis

Classification
Therapeutic: vasodilator
Pharmacologic: phosphodiesterase type 5 inhibitors

T

Indications

Erectile dysfunction.

Action

Increases cyclic guanosine monophosphate (cGMP) levels by inhibiting phosphodiesterase type 5 (PDE5), an enzyme responsible for the breakdown of cGMP. cGMP produces smooth muscle relaxation of the corpus cavernosum, which in turn promotes increased blood flow and subsequent erection. **Therapeutic Effects:** Enhanced blood flow to the corpus cavernosum and erection sufficient to allow sexual intercourse. Requires sexual stimulation.

Adverse Reactions/Side Effects

CNS: <u>headache</u>. **EENT:** HEARING LOSS, VISION LOSS, nasal congestion. **CV:** hypotension. **GI:** dyspepsia. **GU:** priapism. **Derm:** <u>flushing</u>. **MS:** back pain, limb pain, myalgia.

PHYSICAL THERAPY IMPLICATIONS

Examination and Evaluation

- Be alert for sudden loss of vision or hearing, and seek emergency care for any changes in vision or hearing.

- Assess blood pressure periodically and compare to normal values (See Appendix F). Report low blood pressure (hypotension), especially if patient experiences dizziness, fatigue, or other symptoms.
- Assess any muscle, back, or limb pain to rule out musculoskeletal pathology; that is, try to determine if pain is drug induced rather than caused by anatomic or biomechanical problems.

Interventions

- To minimize orthostatic hypotension, patient should move slowly when assuming a more upright position.

Patient/Client-Related Instruction

- Instruct patient to notify health care professional promptly if erection lasts longer than 4 hr or if they experience a sudden decrease or loss of vision or hearing.
- Instruct patient to report other bothersome side effects such as severe or prolonged headache, nasal congestion, skin flushing, or indigestion.

Pharmacokinetics

Absorption: Well absorbed following oral administration.
Distribution: Extensive tissue distribution; penetrates semen.
Protein Binding: 94%.
Metabolism and Excretion: Mostly metabolized by the liver (mainly CYP3A4 enzyme system); metabolites are excreted in feces (61%) and urine (36%).
Half-life: 17.5 hr.

TIME/ACTION PROFILE (improved erectile function)

ROUTE	ONSET	PEAK	DURATION
PO	rapid	0.5–6 hr	36

Contraindications/Precautions

Contraindicated in: Hypersensitivity; Concurrent use of nitrates; Unstable angina, recent history of stroke, life-threatening heart failure within 6 mo, uncontrolled hypertension, arrhythmias, stroke within 6 mo, or MI within 90 days; Any other cardiovascular pathology precluding sexual activity; Known hereditary degenerative retinal disorders; Severe hepatic impairment; Congenital or acquired QT prolongation or concurrent use of class IA or III antiarrhythmics; Pedi: Women, children, or newborns.
Use Cautiously in: Left ventricular outflow obstruction; Penile deformity; Underlying conditions predisposing to priapism, including sickle cell anemia, multiple myeloma, or leukemia; Bleeding disorders or active peptic ulcer disease; Strong inhibitors of the CYP3A4 enzyme system; Alpha-adrenergic blockers (patients should be on stable dose of alpha blockers before starting tadalafil); History of sudden severe vision loss or nonarteritic ischemic optic neuropathy (NAION); may ↑ risk of recurrence; Geri: May experience more side effects.

Interactions

Drug-Drug: Concurrent use of **nitrates** may cause serious, life-threatening hypotension and is contraindicated. ↑ risk of hypotension with **alpha-adrenergic blockers** and acute ingestion of **alcohol.** Strong inhibitors of CYP3A4, including **ritonavir, ketoconazole,** and **itraconazole,** ↑ effects and the risk of adverse reactions (dosage adjustments recommended). Similar effects may be expected of other **inhibitors of CY3A4.**

Route/Dosage

PO (Adults): 10 mg prior to sexual activity (range 5–20 mg; not to exceed one dose/24 hr) *or* 2.5 mg once daily (max: 5 mg/day); *Concurrent use of CYP3A4 inhibitors, including itraconazole, ketoconazole, and ritonavir*—single dose should not exceed 10 mg in any 72-hr period; for once daily dose regimen, daily dose should not exceed 2.5 mg.

Renal Impairment

PO (Adults): *CCr 31–50 mL/min*—Initial dose should not exceed 5 mg/day; maximum dose should not exceed 10 mg in 48 hr (no adjustment required for once daily use); *CCr <30 mL/min*—maximum dose 5 mg (once daily dose regimen not recommended).

Hepatic Impairment

PO (Adults): *Mild or moderate hepatic impairment (Child-Pugh class A or B)*—Daily dose should not exceed 10 mg (once daily dose regimen not recommended).

Availability

Tablets: 2.5 mg, 5 mg, 10 mg, 20 mg.

tamoxifen (ta-mox-i-fen)

Alpha-Tamoxifen, Med Tamoxifen, ✱Nolvadex-D, Novo-Tamoxifen, Soltamox, ✱Tamofen, ✱Tamone, ✱Tamoplex

Classification
Therapeutic: antineoplastics
Pharmacologic: antiestrogens

Indications

Adjuvant therapy of breast cancer after surgery and radiation (delays recurrence). Palliative or adjunctive treatment of advanced breast cancer. Prevention of breast cancer in high-risk patients. Treatment of ductal carcinoma in situ following breast surgery and radiation. McCune-Albright syndrome with precocious puberty in girls 2–10 yr.

Action

Competes with estrogen for binding sites in breast and other tissues. Reduces DNA synthesis and estrogen response. **Therapeutic Effects:** Suppression of tumor growth. Reduced incidence of breast cancer in high-risk patients. Delayed puberty in McCune-Albright syndrome.

Adverse Reactions/Side Effects

CNS: confusion, depression, headache, weakness. **EENT:** blurred vision. **CV:** PULMONARY EMBOLISM, STROKE, edema. **GI:** nausea, vomiting. **GU:** UTERINE MALIGNANCIES, vaginal bleeding. **F and E:** hypercalcemia. **Hemat:** leukopenia, thrombocytopenia. **Metab:** hot flashes. **MS:** bone pain. **Misc:** tumor flare.

PHYSICAL THERAPY IMPLICATIONS

Examination and Evaluation

- Be alert for signs of stroke (sudden severe headache, confusion, nausea, vomiting, paralysis, numbness, speech problems, visual disturbances), especially during exercise. Seek immediate medical assistance if these signs occur.
- Monitor signs of pulmonary embolism, including shortness of breath, chest pain, cough, and bloody sputum. Notify physician immediately, and request objective tests (Doppler ultrasound, lung scan, others) if thromboembolism is suspected.
- Be alert for signs of uterine malignancy, including abnormal uterine bleeding, vaginal discharge, abdominal pain, bloating, unexplained weight loss, or a change in bowel or bladder habits. Report these signs to the physician immediately.
- Report signs of leukopenia (fever, sore throat, signs of infection) or thrombocytopenia (bruising, nose bleeds, bleeding gums).
- Assess peripheral edema using girth measurements, volume displacement, and measurement of pitting edema (See Appendix N). Report increased swelling in feet and ankles or a sudden increase in body weight due to fluid retention.
- Assess any bone pain or other musculoskeletal pain. Suggest additional tests (radiography, MRI) as needed to rule out fracture.
- Monitor and report depression, confusion, or other changes in mood and behavior.
- Report signs of high calcium levels (hypercalcemia), including muscle pain, weakness, joint pain, confusion, and lethargy.

Interventions

- For patients who are medically able to begin exercise, implement appropriate resistive exercises and aerobic training to maintain muscle strength and aerobic capacity during cancer chemotherapy, or to help restore function after chemotherapy.
- Because of the risk of stroke and pulmonary embolism, use caution during aerobic exercise and other forms of therapeutic exercise. Assess exercise tolerance frequently (blood pressure, heart rate, fatigue levels), and terminate exercise immediately if any untoward responses occur (See Appendix L).

Patient/Client-Related Instruction

- Advise patient and family or caregiver about the signs of stroke and pulmonary embolism (see above under Examination and Evaluation), and to seek immediate medical assistance if these signs develop.
- Instruct patient to report other troublesome side effects such as blurred vision, headaches, hot flashes, or GI problems (nausea, vomiting).

Pharmacokinetics

Absorption: Absorbed after oral administration.
Distribution: Widely distributed.
Metabolism and Excretion: Mostly metabolized by the liver. Slowly eliminated in the feces. Minimal amounts excreted in the urine.
Half-life: 7 days.

TIME/ACTION PROFILE (tumor response)

ROUTE	ONSET	PEAK	DURATION
PO	4–10 wk	several mos	several weeks

Contraindications/Precautions

Contraindicated in: Hypersensitivity; Concurrent warfarin therapy with history of deep vein thrombosis (patients at high risk for breast cancer only); Pregnancy or lactation.
Use Cautiously in: ↓ bone marrow reserve; Women with childbearing potential.

Interactions

Drug-Drug: Estrogens and **aminoglutethimide** may ↓ effectiveness of concurrently administered tamoxifen. Blood levels are ↑ by **bromocriptine.** May ↑ the anticoagulant effect of **warfarin.** Risk of thromboembolic events is ↑ by concurrent use of other **antineoplastics.**

Route/Dosage

Treatment of Breast Cancer

PO (Adults): 10–20 mg bid; doses of 20 mg/day may be taken as a single dose.

Prevention of Breast Cancer/Ductal Carcinoma in Situ

PO (Adults): 20 mg once daily for 5 yr.

McCune-Albright Syndrome

PO (Children [girls] 2–10 yr): 20 mg once daily for up to 1 yr.

Availability (generic available)

Tablets: 10 mg, 20 mg. **Enteric-coated tablets:** 20 mg. **Oral Solution (Soltamox) (sugar-free licorice and aniseed taste and smell):** 10 mg/5 mL.

tamsulosin (tam-**soo**-loe-sin)

Flomax

Classification

Therapeutic: none assigned

Pharmacologic: peripherally acting antiadrenergics

Indications

Management of outflow obstruction in male patients with prostatic hyperplasia.

Action

Decreases contractions in smooth muscle of the prostatic capsule by preferentially binding to alpha$_1$-adrenergic receptors. **Therapeutic Effects:** Decreased symptoms of prostatic hyperplasia (urinary urgency, hesitancy, nocturia).

Adverse Reactions/Side Effects

CNS: dizziness, headache. **EENT:** rhinitis.
CV: orthostatic hypotension. **GU:** retrograde/diminished ejaculation.

PHYSICAL THERAPY IMPLICATIONS

Examination and Evaluation

- Monitor signs of benign prostatic hyperplasia (BPH) such as difficulty starting a urine stream, painful urination, weak urine flow, feeling that the bladder is not completely empty, frequent nighttime urination, and an urge to urinate again soon after urinating. Document any change in BPH symptoms to help assess the effects of drug therapy.
- Assess blood pressure (BP) when patient assumes a more upright position (lying to standing, sitting to standing, lying to sitting). Document orthostatic hypotension and contact the physician when systolic BP falls >20 mm Hg or diastolic BP falls >10 mm Hg.
- Assess dizziness that might affect gait, balance, and other functional activities (See Appendix C). Report balance problems and functional limitations to the physician, and caution the patient and family/caregivers to guard against falls and trauma.

Interventions

- Avoid physical therapy interventions that cause systemic vasodilation (large whirlpool, Hubbard tank). Additive effects of this drug and the intervention may cause a dangerous fall in BP.
- To minimize orthostatic hypotension, advise patient to move slowly when assuming a more upright position.

Patient/Client-Related Instruction

- Advise patient that urinary symptoms (retention, dribbling, hesitancy, urgency) should improve, and to contact the physician if these symptoms continue to worsen.
- Instruct patient or family/caregivers to report other bothersome side effects such as severe or prolonged headache, nasal irritation, or problems with ejaculation.

Pharmacokinetics

Absorption: Slowly absorbed after oral administration.
Distribution: Widely distributed.
Protein Binding: 94–99%.
Metabolism and Excretion: Extensively metabolized by the liver; <10% excreted unchanged in urine.
Half-life: 14 hr.

TIME/ACTION PROFILE (increase in urine flow)

ROUTE	ONSET	PEAK	DURATION
PO	unknown	2 wk	unknown

Contraindications/Precautions

Contraindicated in: Hypersensitivity.
Use Cautiously in: Patients at risk for prostate carcinoma (symptoms may be similar).

Interactions

Drug-Drug: Cimetidine may ↑ blood levels and the risk of toxicity. ↑ risk of hypotension with other peripherally acting antiadrenergics (**doxazosin, prazosin, terazosin**); concurrent use should be avoided.

Route/Dosage

PO (Adults): 0.4 mg once daily after a meal; may be increased after 2–4 wk to 0.8 mg/day.

Availability

Capsules: 0.4 mg.

tapentadol (ta-**pen**-ta-dol)

Nucynta

Classification

Therapeutic: analgesics (centrally acting), opioid analgesics

Pharmacologic: opioid agonists

Schedule II

Indications

Management of moderate-to-severe acute pain in patients ≥18 yr.

Action

Acts as μ-opioid receptor agonist. Also inhibits the reuptake of norepinephrine. **Therapeutic Effects:** ↓ in pain severity.

Adverse Reactions/Side Effects

CNS: SEIZURES, dizziness, headache, somnolence.
Resp: RESPIRATORY DEPRESSION. **GI:** nausea, vomiting.

PHYSICAL THERAPY IMPLICATIONS

Examination and Evaluation

- Assess symptoms of respiratory depression, including decreased respiratory rate, confusion, bluish color of the skin and mucous membranes (cyanosis), and difficult, labored breathing (dyspnea). Monitor pulse oximetry and perform pulmonary function tests (See Appendix I) to quantify suspected changes in ventilation and respiratory function. Excessive respiratory depression requires emergency care.
- Be alert for new seizures or increased seizure activity, especially at the onset of drug treatment. Document the number, duration, and severity of seizures, and report these findings immediately to the physician.
- Be alert for excessive sedation or somnolence. Notify physician or nurse immediately if patient is unconscious or extremely difficult to arouse.
- Use appropriate pain scales (visual analogue scales, others) to document whether this drug is successful in helping manage the patient's pain.
- Assess dizziness that might affect gait, balance, and other functional activities (See Appendix C). Report balance problems and functional limitations to the physician and nursing staff, and caution the patient and family/caregivers to guard against falls and trauma.

Interventions

- Implement appropriate manual therapy techniques, physical agents, and therapeutic exercises to reduce pain and help wean patient off opioid analgesics as soon as possible.
- Because of the risk of respiratory depression, use caution during aerobic exercise and other forms of therapeutic exercise. Assess exercise tolerance frequently (blood pressure, heart rate, respiratory rate, fatigue levels), and terminate exercise immediately if any untoward responses occur (See Appendix L).
- Help patient explore other nonpharmacologic methods to reduce chronic pain, such as relaxation techniques, exercise, counseling, and so forth.

Patient/Client-Related Instruction

- Advise patient that opioid analgesics are usually more effective if given before pain becomes severe; emphasize that adequate pain control will allow better participation in physical therapy.
- Educate patient about the dangers of opioid overdose; encourage patient to adhere to proper dosing schedule.
- Emphasize that the risk of physical addiction (tolerance and dependence) is usually minimal during short-term treatment of pain. Advise patient that addiction is more likely during excessive or inappropriate use of opioid analgesics.
- Advise patient to avoid alcohol and other CNS depressants because of the increased risk of sedation and decreased CNS function.
- Instruct patient to report other troublesome side effects such as severe or prolonged headache or GI problems (nausea, vomiting).

Pharmacokinetics

Absorption: 32% absorbed following oral administration.
Distribution: Widely distributed.
Metabolism and Excretion: Undergoes extensive 1st-pass hepatic metabolism (97%); metabolites have no analgesic activity; metabolized drug is 99% renally excreted.
Half-life: 4 hr.

TIME/ACTION PROFILE (analgesic effect)

ROUTE	ONSET	PEAK	DURATION
PO	unknown	1 hr	4–6 hr

Contraindications/Precautions

Contraindicated in: Significant respiratory depression in unmonitored settings or where resuscitative equipment is not readily available; Paralytic ileus; Severe hepatic impairment; Concurrent MAO inhibitors or use of MAO inhibitors in the preceding 2 wk; Lactation: Lactation; Pedi: Safe use in children <18 yr not established; not recommended.
Use Cautiously in: Conditions associated with hypoxia, hypercapnea, or decreased respiratory reserve, including asthma, chronic obstructive pulmonary disease, cor pulmonale, extreme obesity, sleep apnea syndrome, myxedema, kyphoscoliosis, CNS depression, use of other CNS depressants, or coma (↑ risk of further respiratory depression); use smallest effective dose; Geri: Elderly or debilitated patients (↑ risk of respiratory depression); consider age-related ↓ in hepatic, renal, and cardiovascular function, concurrent disease states, and drug therapy (initial dose should be lower); History of substance abuse or addiction disorder; History or ↑ risk of seizures; OB: Use in pregnancy only if potential benefit justifies potential risk to the fetus.

Interactions

Drug-Drug: Concurrent **MAO inhibitors** or use of MAO inhibitors in the preceding 2 wk can result in potentially life-threatening adverse cardiovascular reactions due to additive effects on norepinephrine levels. Concurrent use of other **CNS depressants,**

T

including **sedative/hypnotics, alcohol, antihistamines, antidepressants, phenothiazines,** and other **opioids,** ↑ risk of further CNS depression; consider dose ↓ of 1 or both agents. ↑ risk of serotonin syndrome with **SNRIs, SSRIs, triptans, tricyclic antidepressants,** and **MAO inhibitors.**

Route/Dosage

PO (Adults): 50, 75, or 100 mg initially, then every 4–6 hr as needed and tolerated. If pain control is not achieved within 1st hour of 1st dose, an additional dose may be given. Doses should not exceed 700 mg on the 1st day or 600 mg/day thereafter.

Hepatic Impairment

PO (Adults): *Moderate hepatic impairment*—50 mg every 8 hr initially, then titrate to maintain analgesia without intolerable side effects.

Availability

Immediate-release tablets: 50 mg, 75mg, 100 mg.

tegaserod (te-gas-er-od)

Zelnorm

Classification

Therapeutic: anti-irritable bowel syndrome agents

Pharmacologic: 5-HT_4 agonists

Indications

Short-term treatment of irritable bowel syndrome (IBS) in women whose primary symptom is constipation in patients younger than 55 yr. Chronic idiopathic constipation in patients younger than 55 yr for whom no other treatment has provided satisfactory relief and/or who had satisfactory improvement previously with tegaserod. Only available under an emergency investigational new drug (IND) process. To qualify, patients must have a condition characterized as immediately life threatening or requiring hospitalization. Physicians would need to make the request for emergency use through the FDA.

Action

Acts as a partial agonist of 5-hydroxytryptamine (5-HT, serotonin) at the 5-HT_4 receptor site. Agonist activity causes the release of other neurotransmitters and results in increased peristalsis, increased intestinal secretion, and decreased visceral sensitivity. **Therapeutic Effects:** Decreased constipation.

Adverse Reactions/Side Effects

CNS: headache. **GI:** diarrhea.

PHYSICAL THERAPY IMPLICATIONS

Examination and Evaluation

- Monitor GI symptoms (constipation, abdominal pain, bloating, cramps) to help document whether drug therapy is successful in reducing these symptoms.

Patient/Client-Related Instruction

- Advise patient to avoid alcohol and foods that may increase GI irritation and constipation.
- Instruct patient to report other bothersome side effects such as severe or prolonged headache or diarrhea.

Pharmacokinetics

Absorption: 10% absorbed following oral administration.
Distribution: Extensively distributed to tissues.
Protein Binding: 98% bound to plasma proteins.
Metabolism and Excretion: 66% excreted unchanged in feces; remainder is metabolized in the GI tract and by the liver. Metabolites are renally excreted.
Half-life: 11 hr.

TIME/ACTION PROFILE

ROUTE	ONSET	PEAK	DURATION
PO	unknown	1 hr*	1–2wk†

*Blood levels.
†Return of symptoms following discontinuation.

Contraindications/Precautions

Contraindicated in: Hypersensitivity; Moderate-to-severe hepatic impairment; Severe renal impairment; History of bowel obstruction, gallbladder disease, sphincter of Oddi dysfunction, or intra-abdominal adhesions; Concurrent or frequent diarrhea; Exclusion criteria for emergency access include history, current diagnosis, or symptoms of CV disease, Presence of CV risk factors, Uncompensated depression or anxiety, Suicidal ideation or behavior.
Use Cautiously in: Mild hepatic impairment; Geri: Safety not established; OB: Pregnancy, lactation, or children <18 yr (safety not established).

Interactions

Drug-Drug: None known.

Route/Dosage

PO (Adults): 6 mg bid before meals.

Availability

Tablets: 2 mg, 6 mg.

telbivudine (tel-bi-vu-deen)

Tyzek

Classification

Therapeutic: antivirals

Pharmacologic: nucleoside analogues

Indications

Management of Chronic Hepatitis B with evidence of currently active disease.

Action

Converted intracellularly to the triphosphate active metabolite which inhibits DNA polymerase by acting as a nucleoside analogue. Result is inhibition of viral replication. **Therapeutic Effects:** ↓ progression of Chronic Hepatitis B infection.

Adverse Reactions/Side Effects

CV: fatigue, headache. **GI:** ↑ hepatomegaly. **Hemat:** neutropenia. **Metab:** LACTIC ACIDOSIS. **MS:** myopathy. **Misc:** fever.

PHYSICAL THERAPY IMPLICATIONS

Examination and Evaluation

- Be alert for signs of lactic acidosis, including confusion, lethargy, stupor, shallow rapid breathing, tachycardia, hypotension, nausea, and vomiting. Notify physician immediately if these signs occur.
- Assess any musculoskeletal pain, muscle tenderness, or weakness, especially if accompanied by fever, malaise, and dark-colored urine. These symptoms may represent drug-induced myopathy, and that myopathy can progress to severe muscle damage (rhabdomyolysis). Report any unexplained musculoskeletal symptoms to the physician immediately.
- Monitor signs of enlarged liver (hepatomegaly) that can progress to liver dysfunction and liver failure. Signs of liver disease include anorexia, abdominal pain, abdominal swelling (ascites), severe nausea and vomiting, yellow skin or eyes, fever, sore throat, malaise, weakness, facial edema, lethargy, and unusual bleeding or bruising. Notify physician of these signs immediately.
- Monitor signs of neutropenia, including fever, sore throat, mucosal lesions, signs of infection, bruising, and bleeding. Report these signs to the physician.

Interventions

- Implement resistive exercises and other therapeutic exercises as tolerated to maintain muscle strength and function and prevent muscle wasting associated with hepatitis B infection.
- Because of the risk of lactic acidosis and myopathy, use caution during aerobic exercise and other forms of therapeutic exercise. Assess exercise tolerance frequently (blood pressure, heart rate, fatigue levels), and terminate exercise immediately if any untoward responses occur (See Appendix L).

Patient/Client-Related Instruction

- Emphasize the importance of taking telbivudine as directed even if the patient is asymptomatic. Do not take more than prescribed amount, and do not stop taking without consulting health care professional.
- Inform patient that telbivudine does not cure hepatitis B or reduce the risk of transmission of hepatitis to other people. Caution patient to use a condom, and toavoid sharing needles or donating blood to prevent spreading the hepatitis B virus to others.
- Instruct patient to report other troublesome side effects such as prolonged or severe headache, fever, or fatigue.

Pharmacokinetics

Absorption: Rapidly absorbed following oral administration; bioavailability unknown.
Distribution: Widely distributed into tissues.
Metabolism and Excretion: Excreted entirely as unchanged drug; no metabolism.
Half-life: *Effective*—15 hr; *elimination half–life*—40–49 hr.

TIME/ACTION PROFILE (blood levels)

ROUTE	ONSET	PEAK	DURATION*
PO	unknown	1–4 hr	24 hr

*Patients with normal renal function.

Contraindications/Precautions

Contraindicated in: Hypersensitivity; OB: Lactation.
Use Cautiously in: Moderate-to-severe renal impairment (dosage modification recommended for CCR <50 mL/min); Discontinuation of medication (may result in exacerbation of hepatitis B); Geri: Consider age-related ↓ in renal function; OB: Use only in pregnancy if maternal benefit outweighs fetal risk; Pedi: Safe use in children >16 yr not established.

Interactions

Drug-Drug: Drugs that alter renal function may alter blood levels and effectiveness.

Route/Dosage

PO (Adults and Children ≥16 yr): 600 mg daily.

Renal Impairment

PO (Adults and Children ≥16 yr): *CCr 30–49 mL/min*—600 mg once q 48 hr; *CCr <30 mL/min (not on dialysis)*—600 mg once q 72 hr; *End-stage renal disease*—600 mg once q 96 hr.

Availability

Tablets: 600 mg.

telithromycin
(tel-i-thro-**mye**-sin)
Ketek

Classification
Therapeutic: anti-infectives
Pharmacologic: ketolides

Indications

Community-acquired pneumonia.

Action

Blocks bacterial protein synthesis at the level of the 50S ribosomal subunit. **Therapeutic Effects:** Resolution of infection. **Spectrum:** Active against the following organisms: *Staphylococcus aureus* (methicillin and erythromycin-susceptible strains only), *Streptococcus pneumoniae* (including multidrug-resistant strains), *Haemophilus influenzae*, *Moraxella catarrhalis*, *Chlamydophila pneumoniae*, and *Mycoplasma pneumoniae*.

Adverse Reactions/Side Effects

CNS: loss of consciousness. **EENT:** visual disturbances. **CV:** arrhythmias, QTc prolongation. **GI:** PSEUDOMEMBRANOUS COLITIS, diarrhea, hepatitis, HEPATIC FAILURE, nausea. **Neuro:** exacerbation of myasthenia gravis.

PHYSICAL THERAPY IMPLICATIONS

Examination and Evaluation

- Monitor signs of pseudomembranous colitis, including diarrhea, abdominal pain, fever, pus or mucus in stools, and other severe or prolonged GI problems (nausea, vomiting, heartburn). Notify physician or nursing staff immediately of these signs.
- Be alert for signs of hepatitis and liver failure, including yellow skin or eyes, abdominal pain, severe nausea and vomiting, fever, sore throat, malaise, weakness, and facial edema. Report these signs to the physician immediately.
- Monitor level of alertness and report any loss of consciousness immediately.
- Assess heart rate, ECG, and heart sounds, especially during exercise (See Appendices G, H). Report any rhythm disturbances or symptoms of increased arrhythmias, including palpitations, chest discomfort, shortness of breath, fainting, and fatigue/weakness.
- Be alert for signs of myasthenia gravis syndrome, such as drooping eyelids, facial muscle weakness, and difficulty swallowing and speaking. Report these signs to the physician immediately, and monitor other muscle groups for signs of unusual weakness and fatigue, especially after repeated contraction.

Interventions

- Always wash hands thoroughly and disinfect equipment (whirlpools, electrotherapeutic devices, treatment tables, and so forth) to help prevent the spread of infection. Use universal precautions or isolation procedures as indicated for specific patients.
- Because of the risk of arrhythmias, use caution during aerobic exercise and other forms of therapeutic exercise. Assess exercise tolerance frequently (blood pressure, heart rate, fatigue levels), and terminate exercise immediately if any untoward responses occur (See Appendix L).

Patient/Client-Related Instruction

- Instruct patient to report any visual disturbances (e.g., blurred vision or double vision) or severe or prolonged GI reactions (diarrhea, nausea).

Pharmacokinetics

Absorption: 57% absorbed following oral administration; unaffected by food.
Distribution: Concentrates in bronchial mucosa, epithelial lining fluid, and alveolar macrophages.
Metabolism and Excretion: 70% metabolized by the liver (50% by CYP3A4), 13% excreted unchanged in urine, 7% excreted unchanged via biliary/intestinal elimination.
Half-life: 10 hr.

TIME/ACTION PROFILE (blood levels)

ROUTE	ONSET	PEAK	DURATION
PO	rapid	1 hr	24 hr

Contraindications/Precautions

Contraindicated in: Hypersensitivity; History of hepatitis or jaundice associated with use of telithromycin; Hypersensitivity to macrolides (erythromycin, azithromycin, clarithromycin); Concurrent use of pimozide, ergot alkaloids, simvastatin, lovastatin, atorvastatin, or rifampin; Congenital QTc prolongation, uncorrected hypokalemia or hypomagnesemia, bradycardia, concurrent use of class IA (quinidine, procainamide) or class III antiarrhythmics (dofetilide); Myasthenia gravis; Lactation: Excreted in breast milk; consider alternative to breast-feeding.
Use Cautiously in: CCr <30 mL/min (dosage not established); Concurrent use of midazolam and other benzodiazepines; OB: Use only if benefits outweigh risks to fetus; Pedi: Safety not established.

Interactions

Drug-Drug: Blood levels are ↑ by **ketoconazole** and **itraconazole.** ↑ levels and risk of myopathy from **simvastatin, lovastatin,** and **atorvastatin;** avoid concurrent use. ↑ levels and risk of excessive sedation with **midazolam;** careful titration is required. Similar effects may occur with **triazolam.** ↑ levels of **metoprolol;** use caution in patients with CHF. May also ↑ levels, effects and risk of toxicity from **ergot derivatives (ergotamine, dihydroergotamine)**; concurrent use not recommended; similar effects may occur with **carbamazepine, cyclosporine, tacrolimus, sirolimus, hexobarbital,** or **phenytoin. Rifampin** ↓ levels and effectiveness; avoid concurrent use. Similar effects may occur with **phenytoin, carbamazepine,** or **phenobarbital.**

Route/Dosage

PO (Adults): *Community-acquired pneumonia*—800 mg once daily for 7–10 days.

Availability

Tablets: 300 mg, 400 mg.

telmisartan (tel-mi-**sar**-tan)

Micardis

Classification

Therapeutic: antihypertensives

Pharmacologic: angiotensin II receptor antagonists

Indications

Alone or with other agents in the management of hypertension.

Action

Blocks the vasoconstrictor and aldosterone-secreting effects of angiotensin II at various receptor sites, including vascular smooth muscle and the adrenal glands. **Therapeutic Effects:** Lowering of blood pressure in hypertensive patients.

Adverse Reactions/Side Effects

CNS: dizziness, fatigue, headache. **CV:** hypotension. **EENT:** sinusitis. **F and E:** hyperkalemia. **GI:** abdominal pain, diarrhea, dyspepsia. **GU:** impaired renal function. **MS:** back pain, myalgia. **Misc:** ANGIOEDEMA.

PHYSICAL THERAPY IMPLICATIONS

Examination and Evaluation

- Watch for signs of angioedema, including rashes, raised patches of red or white skin (welts), burning/itching skin, swelling in the face, and difficulty breathing. Report these signs to the physician immediately.
- Assess blood pressure periodically and compare to normal values (See Appendix F) to help document antihypertensive effects.
- Monitor signs of high plasma potassium levels (hyperkalemia), including bradycardia, fatigue, weakness, numbness, and tingling. Notify physician because severe cases can lead to life-threatening arrhythmias and paralysis.
- Watch for and report signs of impaired renal function, including decreased urine output, cloudy urine, or sudden weight gain due to fluid retention.
- Assess any muscle pain or back pain to rule out musculoskeletal pathology; that is, try to determine if pain is drug induced rather than caused by anatomic or biomechanical problems.
- Assess dizziness that might affect gait, balance, and other functional activities (See Appendix C). Report balance problems and functional limitations to the physician, and caution the patient and family/caregivers to guard against falls and trauma.

Interventions

- Avoid physical therapy interventions that cause systemic vasodilation (large whirlpool, Hubbard tank). Additive effects of this drug and the intervention may cause a dangerous fall in blood pressure.
- To minimize orthostatic hypotension, patient should move slowly when assuming a more upright position.

Patient/Client-Related Instruction

- Remind patients to take medication as directed to control hypertension even if they are asymptomatic.
- Counsel patients about additional interventions to help control blood pressure, including regular exercise, weight loss, sodium restriction, stress reduction, moderation of alcohol consumption, and smoking cessation.
- Instruct patient or family/caregivers to report other troublesome side effects such as severe or prolonged headache, nasal inflammation, or GI problems (diarrhea, indigestion, abdominal pain).

Pharmacokinetics

Absorption: 42–58% absorbed following oral administration (bioavailability increased in patients with hepatic impairment).

Distribution: Crosses the placenta.

Protein Binding: 99.5%.

Metabolism and Excretion: Excreted mostly unchanged in feces via biliary excretion.

Half-life: 24 hr.

TIME/ACTION PROFILE (antihypertensive effect)

ROUTE	ONSET	PEAK	DURATION
PO	within 3 hr*	4 wks†	24 hr†

*After single dose.

†Chronic dosing.

Contraindications/Precautions

Contraindicated in: Hypersensitivity; Bilateral renal artery stenosis; OB: Potential for injury or death of fetus. If pregnancy occurs, discontinue immediately; Lactation: Discontinue drug or use formula.

Use Cautiously in: Volume- or salt-depleted patients or patients receiving large doses of diuretics (correct deficits before initiating therapy); Black patients (may not be as effective); Impaired renal function caused by primary renal disease or heart failure (may worsen renal function); Obstructive biliary disorders or hepatic impairment; Women of childbearing potential; Pedi: Safety not established for children <18 yr.

Interactions

Drug-Drug: Additive hypotensive effects with other **antihypertensives.** Excessive hypotension may occur with concurrent use of **diuretics.** ↑ risk of hyperkalemia with concurrent use of **potassium supplements, potassium-containing salt substitutes, angiotensin-converting enzyme inhibitors,** or **potassium-sparing diuretics.** May ↑ serum **digoxin** levels. Antihypertensive effects may be blunted by **NSAIDs.**

Route/Dosage

PO (Adults): 40 mg once daily (volume-depleted patients should start with 20 mg); may be titrated up to 80 mg/day.

Availability

Tablets: 20 mg, 40 mg, 80 mg. ***In combination with:*** hydrochlorothiazide (Micardis HCT). See Appendix B.

temazepam (tem-**az**-a-pam)

Restoril

Classification

Therapeutic: sedative/hypnotics

Pharmacologic: benzodiazepines

Schedule IV

Indications

Short-term management of insomnia (<4 wk).

Action

Acts at many levels in the CNS, producing generalized depression. Effects may be mediated by gamma-aminobutyric acid (GABA), an inhibitory neurotransmitter. **Therapeutic Effects:** Relief of insomnia.

Adverse Reactions/Side Effects

CNS: abnormal thinking, behavior changes, hangover, dizziness, drowsiness, hallucinations, lethargy, paradoxic excitation, sleep driving. **EENT:** blurred vision. **GI:** constipation, diarrhea, nausea, vomiting. **Derm:** rashes. **Misc:** physical dependence, psychologic dependence, tolerance.

PHYSICAL THERAPY IMPLICATIONS

Examination and Evaluation

- Monitor daytime drowsiness, short-term memory deficits, and "hangover" symptoms (headache, nausea, lethargy, irritability, dysphoria). Repeated or excessive symptoms may require change in dose or medication.
- Assess dizziness that might affect gait, balance, and other functional activities (See Appendix C). Report balance problems and functional limitations to the physician, and caution the patient and family/caregivers to guard against falls and trauma.
- Report any behavioral or personality changes such as excessive excitation, hallucinations, or expression of abnormal thoughts.

Interventions

- Guard against falls and trauma (hip fractures, head injury, and so forth). Implement fall-prevention strategies, especially in older adults or if drowsiness and dizziness carry over into the daytime (See Appendix E).
- Help patient explore nonpharmacologic methods to improve sleep, such as relaxation techniques, regular exercise, avoid caffeine, and so forth.

Patient/Client-Related Instruction

- Instruct patients on prolonged treatment not to discontinue medication without consulting their physician. Long-term use can cause tolerance and physical/psychologic dependence, and increased sleep problems (rebound insomnia) can occur when the drug is suddenly discontinued.
- Advise patient to avoid alcohol and other CNS depressants because of the increased risk of sedation and adverse effects.
- Caution patient and family/caregivers to guard against complex motor behaviors that can occur while asleep, including driving a car.
- Instruct patient to report other bothersome side effects including severe or prolonged blurred vision, skin rash, or GI problems (nausea, vomiting, constipation, diarrhea).

Pharmacokinetics

Absorption: Well absorbed after oral administration.
Distribution: Widely distributed; crosses blood-brain barrier. Probably crosses the placenta and enters breast milk. Accumulation of drug occurs with chronic dosing.
Protein Binding: 96%.
Metabolism and Excretion: Metabolized by the liver.
Half-life: 10–20 hr.

TIME/ACTION PROFILE (sedation)

ROUTE	ONSET	PEAK	DURATION
PO	30 min	2–3 hr	6–8 hr

Contraindications/Precautions

Contraindicated in: Hypersensitivity; Cross-sensitivity with other benzodiazepines may exist; Preexisting CNS depression; Severe uncontrolled pain; Angle-closure glaucoma; Impaired respiratory function; Sleep apnea; OB: Neonates born to mothers taking temazepam may experience withdrawal effects; Lactation: Infants may become sedated. Discontinue drug or bottle-feed.
Use Cautiously in: Preexisting hepatic dysfunction; History of suicide attempt or drug addiction;

Geri: Elderly patients have increased sensitivity to benzodiazepines. Appears on Beers' list and is associated with increased risk of falls (↓ dose required).

Interactions

Drug-Drug: ↑ CNS depression with **alcohol, antidepressants, antihistamines, opioid analgesics,** and other **sedative/hypnotics.** May ↓ efficacy of **levodopa. Rifampin** or **smoking** ↑ metabolism and may ↓ effectiveness of temazepam. **Probenecid** may prolong effects of temazepam. Sedative effects may be ↓ by **theophylline.**
Drug-Natural: Concomitant use of **kava, valerian, skullcap, chamomile,** or **hops** can ↑ CNS depression.

Route/Dosage

PO (Adults): 15–30 mg at bedtime initially if needed; some patients may require only 7.5 mg.
PO (Geriatric Patients or Debilitated Patients): 7.5 mg hs.

Availability (generic available)

Capsules: 7.5 mg, 15 mg, 22.5 mg, 30 mg.

temozolomide

(te-mo-**zole**-oh-mide)
Temodar

Classification
Therapeutic: antineoplastics
Pharmacologic: alkylating agents

Indications

Refractory anaplastic astrocytoma progressing despite treatment with a nitrosourea and procarbazine. Glioblastoma multiforme (with or after radiation).

Action

Temozolomide is not active until converted at physiologic pH to 3-methyl-(triazen-1-yl)imidazole-4-carboxamide (MTIC), which alkylates DNA, disrupting its synthesis. **Therapeutic Effects:** Death of rapidly replicating cells, especially malignant ones, resulting in regression or slowed tumor growth.

Adverse Reactions/Side Effects

CNS: SEIZURES, fatigue, headache, abnormal coordination, anxiety, depression, dizziness, drowsiness, mental status changes, weakness. **EENT:** abnormal vision, diplopia. **Resp:** cough. **CV:** peripheral edema. **GI:** nausea, vomiting, abdominal pain, anorexia, constipation, diarrhea, dysphagia. **Derm:** pruritus, rash. **Endo:** adrenal hypercorticism. **Hemat:** leukopenia, thrombocytopenia, anemia. **Metab:** ↑ weight. **MS:** abnormal gait, back pain. **Neuro:** hemiparesis, myalgia. **Misc:** breast pain (women), fever, secondary malignancies (rare).

PHYSICAL THERAPY IMPLICATIONS

Examination and Evaluation

- Be alert for new seizures or increased seizure activity, especially at the onset of drug treatment. Document the number, duration, and severity of seizures, and report these findings to the physician or nursing staff immediately.
- Instruct patient to report signs of leukopenia (fever, sore throat, signs of infection), thrombocytopenia (bruising, nose bleeds, and bleeding gums), or unusual weakness and fatigue that might be due to anemia. Report these signs to the physician or nursing staff.
- Assess coordination problems, gait abnormalities, or hemiparesis that affects balance and functional activities. Report balance problems and functional limitations to the physician and nursing staff, and caution the patient and family/caregivers to guard against falls and trauma.
- Assess any back or muscle pain to rule out musculoskeletal pathology; that is, try to determine if pain is drug induced rather than caused by anatomic or biomechanical problems.
- Assess dizziness and drowsiness that might affect gait, balance, and other functional activities (See Appendix C). Report balance problems and functional limitations to the physician and nursing staff, and caution the patient and family/caregivers to guard against falls and trauma.
- Assess peripheral edema using girth measurements, volume displacement, and measurement of pitting edema (See Appendix N). Report increased swelling in feet and ankles or a sudden increase in body weight due to fluid retention.
- Monitor changes in mood or behavior such as anxiety, depression, or other alterations in mental status. Notify health care professional promptly if these symptoms develop.
- Monitor signs of increased adrenal cortex activity (adrenal hypercorticism). Signs include cushingoid appearance, including puffiness in the face (moon face), increased abdominal fat, thin arms and legs, abdominal skin striations, changes in skin pigmentation, bruising, and deposition of fat behind the base of the neck (buffalo hump). Report these signs to the physician or nursing staff.
- Periodically assess body weight and other anthropometric measures (body mass index, body composition). Report a rapid or unexplained weight gain or increased body fat.

T

Interventions

- For patients who are medically able to begin exercise, implement appropriate resistive exercises and aerobic training to maintain muscle strength and aerobic capacity during cancer chemotherapy or to help restore function after chemotherapy.

Patient/Client-Related Instruction

- Advise patient and family/caregivers that fatigue and weakness are likely and may be severe. Implement assistive devices (walker, cane, wheelchair) as needed to help maintain mobility and prevent falls.
- Advise patient about the likelihood of GI reactions, including nausea, vomiting, diarrhea, constipation, abdominal pain, difficulty swallowing, and loss of appetite. Severe or unusual GI problems should be reported to the physician.
- Advise patient that hair loss and other skin reactions (rash, pruritus) are likely. Report severe or unexpected skin reactions to the physician.
- Advise patient to guard against infection (frequent hand washing, etc.), and to avoid crowds and contact with persons with contagious diseases.
- Instruct patient and family/caregivers to report other troublesome side effects such as severe or prolonged headache, cough, vision disturbances, fever, or breast pain.

Pharmacokinetics

Absorption: Rapidly converted to MTIC, the active metabolite.
Distribution: Unknown.
Metabolism and Excretion: Further metabolism results in the formation of methylhydrazine, which is responsible for most activity.
Half-life: 1.8 hr.

TIME/ACTION PROFILE (effect on blood counts)

ROUTE	ONSET	PEAK	DURATION
PO (WBC)	unknown	28 days (range 1–44 days)	14 days
PO (platelets)	unknown	26 days (range 21–40 days)	14 days

Contraindications/Precautions

Contraindicated in: Hypersensitivity to temozolomide or dacarbazine (DTIC); OB: Pregnancy or lactation.
Use Cautiously in: Severe hepatic or renal impairment; Geri: Geriatric patients and women (↑ risk of myelosuppression); Active infection; Decreased bone marrow reserve; Other chronic debilitating illness; OB: Patients with childbearing potential; Pedi: Children (safety not established).

Interactions

Drug-Drug: ↑ bone marrow depression may occur with other **antineoplastics** or **radiation therapy.** May ↓ the antibody response to **live-virus vaccines** and ↑ risk of adverse reactions.

Route/Dosage

PO (Adults): *Anaplastic astrocytoma*—150 mg/m^2/day for 5 consecutive days of each 28-day treatment cycle; doses adjusted on the basis of blood counts; *Glioblastoma multiforme*—75 mg/m^2/day for 42 consecutive days concurrently with radiation initially, then starting 4 wks after last dose, maintenance dose of 150 mg/m^2/day for 5 consecutive days of 1 28-day treatment cycle, then 200 mg/m^2 for 5 consecutive days of each 28-day treatment cycle for 5 cycles; doses adjusted on the basis of blood counts. Concurrent prophylaxis against *Pneumocystis carnii* pneumonia is required during first 42 days of regimen.

Availability

Capsules: 5 mg, 20 mg, 100 mg, 250 mg.

temsirolimus

(tem-sir-**oh**-li-mus)
Torisel

Classification
Therapeutic: antineoplastics
Pharmacologic: enzyme inhibitors

Indications

Advanced renal cell carcinoma.

Action

Binds to an intracellular protein. The resultant complex inhibits an enzyme, mTOR (mammalian target of rapamycin). Inhibition of this enzyme arrests cell growth in the G1 phase. **Therapeutic Effects:** Decreased spread of renal cell carcinoma.

Adverse Reactions/Side Effects

CNS: weakness. **EENT:** conjunctivitis.
CV: hypertension, venous thromboembolism.
Resp: INTERSTITIAL LUNG DISEASE. **GI:** BOWEL PERFORATION, anorexia, ↑ liver enzymes, mucositis, nausea.
GU: RENAL FAILURE. **Derm:** rash, abnormal wound healing.
Endo: hyperglycemia. **F and E:** edema, hypophosphatemia. **Hemat:** anemia, leukopenia, lymphopenia, thrombocytopenia. **Metab:** hyperlipidemia, hypertriglyceridemia. **Misc:** hypersensitivity reactions, including anaphylaxis, ↑ risk of infections.

PHYSICAL THERAPY IMPLICATIONS

Examination and Evaluation

- Assess any breathing problems or signs of interstitial lung disease such as dry cough, wheezing, chest pain, shortness of breath, and difficult or labored breathing. Monitor pulse oximetry and perform pulmonary function tests (See Appendices I, J, K) to quantify suspected changes in ventilation and respiratory function.

- Monitor signs of kidney failure, including decreased urine output, increased blood pressure (BP), muscle cramps/twitching, edema/weight gain from fluid retention, yellowish brown skin, and confusion that progresses to seizures and coma. Report these signs to the physician or nursing staff immediately.
- Be alert for signs of bowel perforation, including sudden severe abdominal pain accompanied by nausea, vomiting, chills, and fever. Report these signs to the physician or nursing staff immediately.
- Monitor signs of hypersensitivity reactions or anaphylaxis, including pulmonary symptoms (tightness in the throat and chest, wheezing, cough, dyspnea) or skin reactions (rash, pruritus, urticaria). Notify physician or nursing staff immediately if these reactions occur.
- Monitor signs of venous thrombosis (lower extremity swelling, warmth, erythema, tenderness) and thromboembolism (shortness of breath, chest pain, cough, bloody sputum). Notify physician immediately, and request objective tests (Doppler ultrasound, lung scan, others) if thrombosis is suspected.
- Assess BP and compare to normal values (See Appendix F). Report a sustained increase in BP (hypertension).
- Assess peripheral edema using girth measurements, volume displacement, and measurement of pitting edema (See Appendix N). Report increased swelling in feet and ankles or a sudden increase in body weight due to fluid retention.
- Be alert for signs of leukopenia (fever, sore throat, other signs of infection), thrombocytopenia (bruising, nose bleeds, bleeding gums), or unusual weakness and fatigue that might be due to anemia or other blood dyscrasias. Report these signs to the physician or nursing staff immediately.
- Be alert for signs of hyperglycemia, including confusion, drowsiness, flushed/dry skin, fruit-like breath odor, rapid/deep breathing, polyuria, loss of appetite, and unusual thirst. Patients with diabetes mellitus should check blood glucose levels frequently.
- Monitor signs of low phosphate levels (hypophosphatemia), including skeletal muscle dysfunction or weakness, respiratory muscle weakness, and mental status changes such as irritability and confusion that progresses to delirium and coma. Report these signs to the physician or nursing staff.

Interventions

- For patients who are medically able to begin exercise, implement appropriate resistive exercises and aerobic training to maintain muscle strength and aerobic capacity during cancer chemotherapy, or to help restore function after chemotherapy.
- Because of the risk of pulmonary toxicity and blood dyscrasias, use caution during aerobic exercise and other forms of therapeutic exercise. Assess exercise tolerance frequently (BP, heart rate, respiratory symptoms, fatigue levels), and terminate exercise immediately if any untoward responses occur (See Appendix L).

Patient/Client-Related Instruction

- Instruct patient to guard against infection (frequent hand washing, etc.), and to avoid crowds and contact with persons with contagious diseases.
- Advise patient and family/caregivers that fatigue and weakness are likely and may be severe. Implement assistive devices (walker, cane, wheelchair) as needed to help maintain mobility and prevent falls.
- Advise patient that this drug may cause problems in fat metabolism (hyperlipidemia, hypertriglyceridemia). Remind patient that periodic blood tests may be needed to monitor plasma lipids.
- Instruct patient to report other troublesome side effects such as prolonged or severe eye irritation, skin reactions (rash, delayed wound healing), or GI problems (nausea, loss of appetite, irritation in/around the mouth).

Pharmacokinetics

Absorption: IV administration results in complete bioavailability.
Distribution: Temsirolimus and sirolimus partition extensively in formed blood elements.
Metabolism and Excretion: Mostly metabolized by the liver to sirolimus, an active metabolite; primarily eliminated in feces.
Half-life: *Temsirolimus*—17.3 hr; *sirolimus*—54.6 hr.

TIME/ACTION PROFILE

ROUTE	ONSET	PEAK	DURATION
IV	unknown	end of infusion	1 wk

Contraindications/Precautions

Contraindicated in: OB: Pregnancy and lactation.
Use Cautiously in: Hypersensitivity to temsirolimus, sirolimus, or polysorbate 80; Perioperative patients (may impair wound healing); OB: Patients which childbearing potential; Pedi: Safe use in children not established.

Interactions

Drug-Drug: Concurrent use of strong **CYP3A4 enzyme inhibitors,** including **ketoconazole, itraconazole, voriconazole, clarithromycin, telithromycin, atazanavir, indinavir, nelfinavir, ritonavir,** or **saquinavir,** ↑ blood levels and ↑ risk of

toxicity; consider ↓ dose to 12.5 mg weekly. Concurrent use of strong **inducers of the CYP3A4 enzyme system**, including **dexamethasone, phenytoin, phenobarbital, carbamazepine, rifampin, rifabutin**, or **rifampicin**, may ↓ blood levels and ↓ efficacy; consider ↑ dose to 50 mg weekly. Concurrent use with **sunitinib** ↑ risk of toxicity (rash, gout, cellulitis). May ↓ antibody response to and ↑ risk of adverse reactions from **live-virus vaccines**; avoid current use.
Drug-Natural: St. John's wort may ↓ blood levels; avoid concurrent use.
Drug-Food: Grapefruit juice may ↑ blood levels and ↑ risk of toxicity.

Route/Dosage
IV (Adults): 25 mg once weekly; dose modification is required for bone marrow toxicity or concurrent use of agents affecting the CYP3A4 enzyme system (pretreatment with antihistamine is recommended).

Availability
Concentrated solution for IV infusion (must be diluted): 25 mg/1 mL in 1-mL vial (comes with a diluent containing polysorbate 80, polyethylene glycol 400, and dehydrated alcohol).

HIGH ALERT

tenecteplase (te-nek-te-plase)
TNKase

Classification
Therapeutic: thrombolytics
Pharmacologic: plasminogen activators

Indications
Reduction of mortality associated with acute myocardial infarction.

Action
Converts plasminogen to plasmin, which is then able to degrade fibrin present in clots. Directly activates plasminogen. **Therapeutic Effects:** Lysis of thrombi in coronary arteries, with preservation of myocardium and resultant decrease in mortality.

Adverse Reactions/Side Effects
Adverse reactions are frequently sequelae of underlying disease
CV: ARRTHYTHMIAS, CARDIOGENIC SHOCK, CARDIAC TAMPONADE, EMBOLISM, HEART FAILURE, MYOCARDIAL INFARCTION, MYOCARDIAL RUPTURE, PERICARDITIS, PERICARDIAL EFFUSION, PULMONARY EDEMA, RECURRENT MYOCARDIAL ISCHEMIA, THROMBOSIS, hypotension. **GI:** nausea, vomiting. **Hemat:** BLEEDING. **Misc:** allergic reactions, including anaphylaxis, fever.

PHYSICAL THERAPY IMPLICATIONS

Examination and Evaluation
- Watch for signs of bleeding and hemorrhage, including bleeding gums, nosebleeds, unusual bruising, coughing up blood, black/tarry stools, hematuria, or a fall in hematocrit or blood pressure. Be especially alert for signs of intracranial bleeds, including sudden severe headache, confusion, nausea, vomiting, paralysis, numbness, speech problems, and visual disturbances. Notify physician or nursing staff immediately if these signs occur.
- Be alert for signs of recurrent cardiac ischemia and MI (chest pain, pain radiating into the arm or jaw, shortness of breath, dizziness, sweating, anxiety) or recurrent peripheral arterial thrombosis (pain, cramping, coldness, cyanosis in the affected limb). Notify physician or nursing staff immediately if these signs occur.
- Assess signs of heart failure and pulmonary edema, including dyspnea, rales/crackles, peripheral edema, jugular venous distention, and exercise intolerance. Report these signs to the physician or nursing staff immediately.
- Assess heart rate, ECG, and heart sounds, especially for the first few days after infusion (See Appendices G, H). Report immediately any rhythm disturbances, or symptoms of increased arrhythmias (palpitations, chest discomfort, shortness of breath, fainting, fatigue/weakness).
- Assess blood pressure, especially for the first few days after infusion. Report low blood pressure (hypotension), especially if patient experiences dizziness or syncope.
- Monitor signs of allergic reactions and anaphylaxis, including pulmonary symptoms (tightness in the throat and chest, wheezing, cough, dyspnea) or skin reactions (rash, pruritus, urticaria). Notify physician or nursing staff immediately if these reactions occur.
- Assess injection site during and after IV administration, and report signs of bleeding or phlebitis (local pain, swelling, inflammation).

Interventions
- Use caution with any physical interventions that could increase bleeding, including wound débridement, chest percussion, joint mobilization, and application of local heat.
- Use extreme caution during aerobic exercise in patients with recent MI. Assess exercise tolerance frequently (blood pressure, heart rate, fatigue levels), and terminate exercise immediately if any untoward responses occur (See Appendix L).

Patient/Client-Related Instruction
- Instruct patient to immediately report signs of GI bleeding, including abdominal pain,

vomiting blood, blood in stools, or black, tarry stools.

- Instruct patient or family/caregivers to report other problematic side effects such as severe or prolonged fever or GI problems (nausea, vomiting).

Pharmacokinetics

Absorption: IV administration results in complete bioavailability.
Distribution: Unknown.
Metabolism and Excretion: Mostly metabolized by the liver.
Half-life: *Initial phase*—20–24 min; *terminal phase*—90–130 min.

TIME/ACTION PROFILE (fibrinolysis)

ROUTE	ONSET	PEAK	DURATION
IV	rapid	unknown	unknown

Contraindications/Precautions

Contraindicated in: Active internal bleeding; History of cerebrovascular accident; Recent (within 2 mo) intracranial or intraspinal surgery or trauma; Intracranial neoplasm, arteriovenous malformation, or aneurysm; Severe uncontrolled hypertension; Known bleeding diathesis; Hypersensitivity.
Use Cautiously in: Recent major surgery, trauma, GI, or GU bleeding; Cerebrovascular disease; Hypertension (BP ≥180 mm Hg and or diastolic ≥110 mm Hg); Presence or high likelihood of left heart thrombus; Subacute bacterial endocarditis or acute pericarditis; Hemostatic defect, especially those associated with severe hepatic or renal disease; Severe hepatic dysfunction; Geriatric patients (increased risk of intracranial bleeding); Hemorrhagic ophthalmic conditions; Septic phlebitis or occluded AV cannula at infected site; Concurrent warfarin therapy or recent therapy with glycoprotein (GP) IIb/IIIa inhibitors (abciximab, eptifibatide, tirofiban); Pregnancy, lactation, or children (safety not established).

Interactions

Drug-Drug: Aspirin, NSAIDs, warfarin, heparin and heparin-like agents, abciximab, eptifibatide, tirofiban, clopidogrel, ticlopidine, or **dipyridamole**—concurrent use may increase the risk of bleeding, although these agents are frequently used together or in sequence. Risk of bleeding may be increased by concurrent use of **cefotetan, cefoperazone,** or **valproic acid.**

Route/Dosage

IV (Adults <60 kg): 30 mg.
IV (Adults ≥60 kg and <70 kg): 35 mg.
IV (Adults ≥70 kg and <80 kg): 40 mg.
IV (Adults ≥80 kg and <90 kg): 45 mg.
IV (Adults ≥90 kg): 50 mg.

Availability

Powder for injection: 50 mg/vial with 10-mL syringe and TwinPak Dual Cannula Device and 10-mL vial of sterile water for injection.

HIGH ALERT

teniposide (ten-ip-oh-side)

Vumon, VM-26

Classification
Therapeutic: antineoplastics
Pharmacologic: podophyllotoxin derivatives

Indications

Induction therapy for refractory acute lymphoblastic leukemia in children (in combination with other agents). **Unlabeled Use:** Neuroblastoma, adult non-Hodgkin's lymphoma.

Action

Damages DNA prior to mitosis (cycle-dependent and phase-specific). **Therapeutic Effects:** Death of rapidly replicating cells, particularly malignant ones.

Adverse Reactions/Side Effects

CNS: acute CNS depression. **CV:** hypotension.
GI: diarrhea, mucositis, nausea, vomiting.
Derm: alopecia, rashes. **Endo:** gonadal suppression.
Hemat: neutropenia, anemia, leukopenia, thrombocytopenia. **Local:** phlebitis at IV site. **Neuro:** peripheral neurotoxicity. **Misc:** ALLERGIC REACTIONS, INCLUDING ANAPHYLAXIS, fever.

PHYSICAL THERAPY IMPLICATIONS

Examination and Evaluation

- Monitor signs of allergic reactions and anaphylaxis, including pulmonary symptoms (tightness in the throat and chest, wheezing, cough, dyspnea) or skin reactions (rash, pruritus, urticaria). Notify physician or nursing staff immediately if these reactions occur.
- Assess levels of arousal, attention, and cognitive functioning using appropriate scales (See Appendix D). Report decreased cognitive function that might indicate acute CNS depression.
- Assess blood pressure periodically and compare to normal values (See Appendix F). Report low blood pressure (hypotension), especially if patient experiences dizziness or syncope.
- Watch for signs of leukopenia (fever, sore throat, signs of infection), thrombocytopenia (bruising,

nose bleeds, bleeding gums), or unusual weakness and fatigue that might be due to anemia. Report these signs to the physician or nursing staff.

- Be alert for signs of peripheral neuropathy (numbness, tingling, decreased muscle strength). Establish baseline electroneuromyographic values using EMG and nerve conduction at the beginning of drug treatment whenever possible, and reexamine these values periodically to document drug-induced changes in peripheral nerve function.
- Monitor IV injection site for pain, swelling, and inflammation (phlebitis). Report phlebitis or other prolonged or excessive injection-site reactions to the physician or nursing staff.

Interventions

- For patients who are medically able to begin exercise, implement appropriate resistive exercises and aerobic training to maintain muscle strength and aerobic capacity during cancer chemotherapy or to help restore function after chemotherapy.

Patient/Client-Related Instruction

- Instruct patient to guard against infection (frequent hand washing, etc.), and to avoid crowds and contact with persons with contagious diseases.
- Advise patient about the likelihood of GI reactions, including nausea, vomiting, diarrhea, and irritation in or around the mouth. Instruct patient or family and caregivers to report other severe or unexpected GI problems.
- Advise patient that hair loss and skin rashes are likely. Instruct patient to report severe or unexpected skin problems.
- Instruct patient or family/caregivers to report other bothersome side effects such as severe or prolonged fever.

Pharmacokinetics

Absorption: IV administration results in complete bioavailability.
Distribution: Limited distribution into the CSF (may be increased in patients with brain tumors).
Protein Binding: >99%.
Metabolism and Excretion: 44% excreted by the kidneys. 10% or less is eliminated in feces.
Half-life: 5 hr.

TIME/ACTION PROFILE (effects on blood counts)

ROUTE	ONSET	PEAK	DURATION
IV	unknown	16–18 days	15 days

Contraindications/Precautions

Contraindicated in: Hypersensitivity to teniposide or polyoxyethylated castor oil; Pregnancy or lactation; Preparations containing benzyl alcohol should be avoided in newborns.
Use Cautiously in: Patients with Down syndrome (more susceptible to the myelosuppressive effects; initial dose of 1st course of therapy should be reduced by 50%); Patients with hepatic impairment, childbearing potential, active infections, ↓ bone marrow reserve, or other chronic debilitating illnesses.

Interactions

Drug-Drug: Myelosuppression may be ↑ by **sodium salicylate, tolbutamide, sulfamethizole,** other **antineoplastics,** or **radiation therapy.**

Route/Dosage

Several regimens have been used. These are examples.
IV (Children): Teniposide 165 mg/m² in combination with cytarabine 300 mg/m² twice weekly for 8–9 doses. Another regimen uses teniposide 250 mg/m² in combination with vincristine 1.5 mg/m² weekly for 4–8 wk with prednisone 40 mg/m²/day for 28 days.

Availability

Injection: 10 mg/mL in 5-mL ampules.

tenofovir (te-noe-foe-veer)

Viread

Classification
Therapeutic: antiretrovirals
Pharmacologic: nucleoside reverse transcriptase inhibitors

Indications

HIV infection (with other antiretrovirals). Chronic hepatitis B.

Action

Active drug (tenofovir) is phosphorylated intracellularly; tenofovir diphosphate inhibits HIV reverse transcriptase resulting in disruption of DNA synthesis.
Therapeutic Effects: Slowed progression of HIV infection and decreased occurrence of sequelae. Increased CD4 cell count and decreased viral load. Decreased progression/sequelae of chronic hepatitis B infection.

CNS: depression, headache, weakness. **GI:** HEPATOMEGALY (with steatosis), diarrhea, nausea, abdominal pain, anorexia, vomiting, flatulence. **GU:** renal impairment. **F and E:** LACTIC ACIDOSIS, hypophosphatemia. **Derm:** rash. **MS:** ↓ bone mineral density.

PHYSICAL THERAPY IMPLICATIONS

Examination and Evaluation

- Be alert for signs of enlarged, fatty liver (hepatomegaly with steatosis) that can progress to liver dysfunction and liver failure. Signs of liver disease include anorexia, abdominal pain, abdominal swelling (ascites), severe nausea and vomiting, yellow skin or eyes, fever, sore throat, malaise, weakness, facial edema, lethargy, and unusual bleeding or bruising. Notify physician of these signs immediately.

- Monitor signs of lactic acidosis, including confusion, lethargy, stupor, shallow rapid breathing, tachycardia, hypotension, nausea, and vomiting. Notify physician immediately if these signs occur.
- Assess signs of low phosphate levels (hypophosphatemia), including skeletal muscle dysfunction or weakness, respiratory muscle weakness, and mental status changes such as irritability and confusion that progresses to delirium and coma. Report these signs to the physician.

Interventions

- Implement resistive exercises and other therapeutic exercises as tolerated to maintain bone mineral density, increase muscle strength and function, and prevent muscle wasting associated with HIV infection and AIDS.
- Because of the risk of lactic acidosis, use caution during aerobic exercise and other forms of therapeutic exercise. Assess exercise tolerance frequently (blood pressure, heart rate, fatigue levels), and terminate exercise immediately if any untoward responses occur (See Appendix L).

Patient/Client-Related Instruction

- Emphasize the importance of taking tenofovir as directed even if the patient is asymptomatic, and that this drug must always be used in combination with other antiretroviral drugs. Do not take more than prescribed amount, and do not stop taking without consulting health care professional.
- Inform patient that tenofovir does not cure HIV or AIDS or prevent associated or opportunistic infections. Tenofovir does not reduce the risk of transmission of HIV to others through sexual contact or blood contamination. Caution patient to use a condom and avoid sharing needles or donating blood to prevent spreading the AIDS virus to others.
- Instruct patient to report signs of kidney impairment, including bloody urine, increased urinary frequency, cloudy urine, decreased urine output, and edema/fluid retention.
- Instruct patient to report other troublesome side effects such as prolonged or severe headache, depression, skin rash, or GI problems (diarrhea, nausea, vomiting, flatulence, abdominal pain, loss of appetite).

Pharmacokinetics

Absorption: Tenofovir disoproxil fumarate is a prodrug, which is split into tenofovir, the active component.
Distribution: Absorption is enhanced by food.
Metabolism and Excretion: 70–80% excreted unchanged in urine by glomerular filtration and active tubular secretion.
Half-life: Unknown.

TIME/ACTION PROFILE (blood levels)

ROUTE	ONSET	PEAK	DURATION
PO	unknown	2 hr*	24 hr

*When taken with food.

Contraindications/Precautions

Contraindicated in: Hypersensitivity; Lactation: HIV-infected women should not breast-feed.
Use Cautiously in: Coinfection with HIV and chronic hepatitis B; Obesity, women, prolonged nucleoside exposure (may be risk factors for lactic acidosis/hepatomegaly); Renal impairment (use cautiously if CCr <60 mL/min); History of pathologic bone fractures or at risk for osteopenia; OB: Has been used safely; Pedi: Safety not established.

Interactions

Drug-Drug: Concurrent use with **didanosine** results in ↑ blood levels of didanosine (tenofovir should be given 2 hr before or 1 hr after didanosine). Blood levels may be ↑ by **cidofovir, acyclovir, ganciclovir,** or **valganciclovir.** Risk of renal toxicity ↑ by other **nephrotoxic agents.** Combination therapy with **atazanavir** may lead to ↓ virologic response and possible resistance to atazanavir (small amounts of **ritonavir** may be added to boost blood levels); may also ↑ tenofovir levels. **Lopinavir/ritonavir** may ↑ levels. Concurrent use with **adefovir** for chronic hepatitis B infection should be avoided.

Route/Dosage

PO (Adults): 300 mg once daily.

Renal Impairment

PO (Adults): *CCr 30–49 mL/min*—300 mg every 48 hr; *CCr 10–29 mL/min*—300 mg every 72–96 hr; *Hemodialysis patients*—300 mg every 7 days following dialysis.

Availability

Tablets: 300 mg. ***In combination with:*** emtricitabine (Truvada); efavirenz and emtricitabine (Atripla). See Appendix B.

terazosin (ter-ay-zoe-sin)

Hytrin

Classification
Therapeutic: antihypertensives
Pharmacologic: peripherally acting antiadrenergics

T

Indications

Mild-to-moderate hypertension (alone or with other agents). Urinary outflow obstruction in patients with prostatic hyperplasia.

Action

Dilates both arteries and veins by blocking postsynaptic alpha$_1$-adrenergic receptors. ↓ contractions in smooth muscle of the prostatic capsule. **Therapeutic Effects:** Lowering of blood pressure. ↓ symptoms of prostatic hyperplasia (urinary urgency, hesitancy, nocturia).

Adverse Reactions/Side Effects

CNS: dizziness, headache, weakness, drowsiness, nervousness. **EENT:** nasal congestion, blurred vision, conjunctivitis, sinusitis. **Resp:** dyspnea. **CV:** first-dose orthostatic hypotension, arrhythmias, chest pain, palpitations, peripheral edema, tachycardia.
GI: nausea, abdominal pain, diarrhea, dry mouth, vomiting. **GU:** erectile dysfunction, urinary frequency. **Derm:** pruritus. **Metab:** weight gain. **MS:** arthralgia, back pain, extremity pain. **Neuro:** paresthesia.
Misc: fever.

PHYSICAL THERAPY IMPLICATIONS

Examination and Evaluation

- Assess blood pressure (BP) periodically and compare to normal values (See Appendix F). Document whether drug therapy is successful in controlling hypertension. Also, be alert for a fall in BP and related symptoms (dizziness, syncope) that occurs when the patient changes position (orthostatic hypotension), especially after the initial doses. Document orthostatic hypotension and contact physician when systolic BP falls >20 mm Hg or diastolic BP falls >10 mm Hg.
- If treating benign prostate hypertrophy (BPH), monitor signs such as difficulty starting a urine stream, painful urination, weak urine flow, feeling that the bladder is not completely empty, frequent nighttime urination, and an urge to urinate again soon after urinating. Document any change in BPH symptoms to help determine the effects of drug therapy.
- Assess heart rate, ECG, and heart sounds, especially during exercise (See Appendices G, H). Report any rhythm disturbances or symptoms of increased arrhythmias, including palpitations, chest discomfort, shortness of breath, fainting, and fatigue/weakness.
- Assess peripheral edema using girth measurements, volume displacement, and measurement of pitting edema (See Appendix N). Report increased swelling in feet and ankles or a sudden increase in body weight due to fluid retention.
- Assess dizziness and weakness that might affect gait, balance, and other functional activities (See Appendix C). Report balance problems and functional limitations to the physician, and caution the patient and family/caregivers to guard against falls and trauma.
- Assess any breathing problems, and report signs of difficult or labored breathing.
- Be alert for signs of depression, nervousness, or other changes in mood and behavior. Notify health care professional if these changes become problematic.
- Assess any back or joint pain to rule out musculoskeletal pathology; that is, try to determine if pain is drug induced rather than caused by anatomic or biomechanical problems.
- Assess signs of paresthesia including numbness, tingling, and muscle weakness. Perform objective tests, including electroneuromyography and sensory testing to document any drug-related neuropathic changes.
- Periodically assess body weight and other anthropometric measures (body mass index, body composition). Report a rapid or unexplained weight gain or increased body fat.

Interventions

- Because of the risk of arrhythmias and abnormal BP responses, use caution during aerobic exercise and other forms of therapeutic exercise. Assess exercise tolerance frequently (BP, heart rate, fatigue levels), and terminate exercise immediately if any untoward responses occur (See Appendix L).
- Avoid physical therapy interventions that cause systemic vasodilation (large whirlpool, Hubbard tank). Additive effects of this drug and the intervention may cause a dangerous fall in blood pressure
- To minimize orthostatic hypotension, advise patient to move slowly when assuming a more upright position.

Patient/Client-Related Instruction

- Remind patients to take medication as directed to control hypertension even if they are asymptomatic.
- Counsel patients about additional interventions to help control BP, such as regular exercise, weight loss, sodium restriction, stress reduction, moderation of alcohol consumption, and smoking cessation.
- When treating BPH, advise patient that urinary symptoms (retention, dribbling, hesitancy, urgency) should improve, and to contact the physician if these symptoms continue to worsen.
- Instruct patient or family/caregivers to report other bothersome side effects such as severe or prolonged headache, drowsiness, fever, vision disturbances, nasal irritation/congestion, increased urinary frequency, sexual dysfunction, skin reactions (rash, itching), or GI problems (diarrhea, nausea, vomiting, dry mouth, abdominal pain).

Pharmacokinetics

Absorption: Well absorbed after oral administration.
Distribution: Unknown.
Metabolism and Excretion: 50% metabolized by the liver, 10% excreted unchanged by the kidneys, 20% excreted unchanged in feces, 40% eliminated in bile.
Half-life: 12 hr.

TIME/ACTION PROFILE

ROUTE	ONSET*†	PEAK†	DURATION*
PO—hypertension	15 min	6–8 wk	24 hr
PO—prostatic hyperplasia	2–6 wk	unknown	Unknown

*After single dose.
†After multiple oral dosing.

Contraindications/Precautions

Contraindicated in: Hypersensitivity.
Use Cautiously in: Dehydration, volume or sodium depletion, ↑ risk of hypotension; Pregnancy, lactation, or children (safety not established).

Interactions

Drug-Drug: ↑ hypotension with other **antihypertensives,** acute ingestion of **alcohol,** or **nitrates. NSAIDs, sympathomimetics,** or **estrogens** may ↓ effects of antihypertensive therapy.

Route/Dosage

The first dose should be taken at bedtime.

Hypertension

PO (Adults): 1 mg initially, then slowly increase up to 5 mg/day (usual range 1–5 mg/day); may be given as single dose or in 2 divided doses (not to exceed 20 mg/day).

Benign Prostatic Hyperplasia

PO (Adults): 1 mg hs; gradually may be increased up to 5–10 mg/day.

Availability (generic available)

Tablets: 1 mg, 2 mg, 5 mg, 10 mg.

terbinafine (systemic)

(ter-bin-a-feen)
Lamisal

terbinafine (topical)

(ter-bin-a-feen)
✱Apo-Terbinafine, Lamisil AT, ✱Novo-Terbinafine, ✱PMS-Terbinafine

Classification
Therapeutic: antifungals
Pharmacologic: allylamines

Indications

Systemic: Onychomycosis (fungal nail infection). Tinea capitis.
Topical: Treatment of a variety of cutaneous fungal infections, including tinea pedis (athlete's foot), tinea cruris (jock itch), and tinea corporis (ringworm).

Action

Interferes with fungal cell wall synthesis (ergosterol biosynthesis) by inhibiting the enzyme squalene epoxidase. **Therapeutic Effects:** Fungal cell death. **Spectrum:** Active against dermatophytes and other fungi.

Adverse Reactions/Side Effects

CNS: headache. **Resp:** cough, nasopharyngitis. **CV:** CHF. **GI:** HEPATOTOXICITY, anorexia, diarrhea, nausea, stomach pain, vomiting, altered taste. **Derm:** TOXIC EPIDERMAL NECROLYSIS, itching, rash. **Hemat:** neutropenia, pancytopenia. **Misc:** STEVENS-JOHNSON SYNDROME, pyrexia. **Local:** burning, itching, local hypersensitivity reactions, redness, stinging.

PHYSICAL THERAPY IMPLICATIONS

Examination and Evaluation

- Be alert for signs of hepatotoxicity, including anorexia, abdominal pain, severe nausea and vomiting, yellow skin or eyes, fever, sore throat, malaise, weakness, facial edema, lethargy, and unusual bleeding or bruising. Notify physician of these signs immediately.
- Monitor rashes or other severe skin reactions such as exfoliation, hives, itching, raised patches of red or white skin (welts), burning, acne, and abnormal sweating Notify physician immediately because certain skin responses may indicate serious hypersensitivity reactions (toxic epidermal necrolysis, Stevens-Johnson syndrome).
- Monitor other signs of allergic reactions and anaphylaxis, including pulmonary symptoms such as tightness in the throat and chest, wheezing, cough, and dyspnea. Notify physician immediately if these reactions occur.
- Assess signs of congestive heart failure (dyspnea, rales/crackles, peripheral edema, jugular venous distention, exercise intolerance). Report these signs to the physician.
- Monitor signs of neutropenia (fever, sore throat, signs of infection), thrombocytopenia (bruising, nose bleeds, and bleeding gums), or unusual weakness and fatigue that might be due to anemias or other blood dyscrasias. Notify physician of these signs.
- For cutaneous or nail infections, assess healing of lesions to help document drug effectiveness.

T

Interventions

- Avoid contact with cutaneous lesions when treating patient.
- Always wash hands thoroughly and disinfect equipment (whirlpools, electrotherapeutic devices, treatment tables, and so forth) to help prevent the spread of infection. Use universal precautions or isolation procedures as indicated for specific patients.

Patient/Client-Related Instruction

- Advise patient to take or apply this drug as directed for the full course of treatment even if feeling better.
- Advise patient to report any increased local sensitivity to topical application of this drug (pain, burning, itching, swelling).
- Instruct patients with cutaneous infections about proper hygiene; e.g., thoroughly wash and dry the affected area, wear clean socks and ventilated shoes for tinea pedis, and so forth.
- Inform patient that early relief of cutaneous symptoms may be seen in 2–3 days. Full therapeutic response may take up to 1 wk.
- Advise patient to seek medical help if infections persist or recur after the full treatment. Recurrent fungal infections may be a sign of systemic illness.
- Instruct patient on systemic doses to report other troublesome side effects such as prolonged or severe headache, cough, nasal irritation, skin problems (rash, itching), or GI reactions (diarrhea, nausea, vomiting, loss of appetite, abdominal pain).

Pharmacokinetics

Absorption: 70–80% absorbed after oral administration.
Distribution: Extensively distributed; penetrates dermis and epidermis; concentrates in stratum corneum, hair, scalp, and nails. Enters breast milk.
Protein Binding: 99%.
Metabolism and Excretion: Extensively metabolized by the liver.
Half-life: *Plasma*—22 days; longer from skin and nails.

TIME/ACTION PROFILE (antifungal tissue levels)

ROUTE	ONSET	PEAK	DURATION
PO	several days	days–wks	several wks
topical	unknown	unknown	unknown

Contraindications/Precautions

Contraindicated in: Hypersensitivity; Chronic or active liver disease; CHF of left ventricular dysfunction.
Use Cautiously in: *Systemic:* History of alcoholism; Renal impairment (dose reduction recommended for CCr <50 mL/min); OB/Lactation: Pregnancy, lactation (safety not established). *Topical:* Nail and scalp infections (may require additional systemic therapy); OB/Lactation: Safety not established.

Interactions

Drug-Drug: Alcohol or other **hepatotoxic agents** may ↑ risk of hepatotoxicity. **Rifampin** and other **drugs that induce hepatic drug-metabolizing enzymes** may ↓ effectiveness. **Cimetidine** and other **drugs that inhibit hepatic drug-metabolizing enzymes** may ↑ effectiveness.
Drug-Natural: ↑ **caffeine** levels and side effects with caffeine-containing herbs (**cola nut, guarana, mate, tea, coffee**).

Route/Dosage

PO (Adults): 250 mg once daily for 6 wk for fingernail infection or 12 wk for toenail infection.
PO (Children ≥4 yr– ≥35 kg): 250 mg/day for 6 wk.
PO (Children ≥4 yr– 25–35 kg): 187.5 mg/day for 6 wk.
PO (Children ≥4 yr–<25 kg): 125 mg/day for 6 wk.
Topical (Adults and Children ≥12 yr): Apply bid for 1 wk for tinea pedis. Apply once daily for 1 wk for tinea cruris or tinea corporis.

Availability (generic available)

Tablets: 250 mg. **Oral granules:** 125-mg packets, 187.5-mg packets.
Cream: 1% OTC. **Gel:** 1% OTC. **Spray liquid:** 1% OTC.

terbutaline (ter-byoo-ta-leen)

Brethaire, Bricanyl

Classification
Therapeutic: bronchodilators
Pharmacologic: adrenergics

Indications

Management of reversible airway disease due to asthma or COPD; inhalation and SC used for short-term control and oral agent as long-term control. **Unlabeled Use:** Management of preterm labor (tocolytic).

Action

Results in the accumulation of cyclic adenosine monophosphate (cAMP) at beta-adrenergic receptors. Produces bronchodilation. Inhibits the release of mediators of immediate hypersensitivity reactions from mast cells. Relatively selective for $beta_2$ (pulmonary)–adrenergic receptor sites, with less effect on $beta_1$ (cardiac)–adrenergic receptors. **Therapeutic Effects:** Bronchodilation.

Adverse Reactions/Side Effects

CNS: nervousness, restlessness, tremor, headache, insomnia. **Resp:** PARADOXICAL BRONCHOSPASM (EXCESSIVE USE OF INHALERS). **CV:** angina, arrhythmias, hypertension, tachycardia. **GI:** nausea, vomiting. **Endo:** hyperglycemia.

PHYSICAL THERAPY IMPLICATIONS

Examination and Evaluation

- Watch for signs of paradoxical bronchospasm (wheezing, cough, dyspnea, tightness in chest and throat), especially at higher or excessive doses. If condition occurs, advise patient to withhold medication and notify physician or other health care professional immediately.
- Assess pulmonary function at rest and during exercise (See Appendices I, J, K) to document effectiveness of medication in controlling bronchospasm.
- Assess blood pressure (BP) periodically and compare to normal values (See Appendix F). Report a sustained increase in BP (hypertension) to the physician.
- Assess heart rate, ECG, and heart sounds, especially during exercise (See Appendices G, H). Report a rapid heart rate (tachycardia) or signs of other arrhythmias, including palpitations, chest discomfort, shortness of breath, fainting, and fatigue/weakness.
- Be alert for signs of hyperglycemia, including confusion, drowsiness, flushed/dry skin, fruit-like breath odor, rapid/deep breathing, polyuria, loss of appetite, and unusual thirst. Patients with diabetes mellitus should check blood glucose levels frequently.
- Monitor and report signs of CNS toxicity, including nervousness, restlessness, tremor, or hyperactivity. Sustained or severe CNS signs may indicate overdose or excessive use of this drug.

Interventions

- When implementing airway clearance techniques or respiratory muscle training, attempt to intervene when the airway is maximally bronchodilated. Peak responses typically occur 1–2 hr after inhalation, 2–3 hr after oral administration, and 0.5-1 hr after SC injection.
- Because of the risk of cardiovascular stimulation, use caution during aerobic exercise and endurance conditioning. Cardiac effects should be minimal at lower oral doses or occasional inhaled use. Cardiovascular effects such as arrhythmias, angina pectoris, or increased BP may occur at higher doses or during excessive use, and are caused by inadvertent stimulation of beta receptors on the heart.

Patient/Client-Related Instruction

- Advise patient to not exceed the recommended dose or frequency of inhalations. Contact physician immediately if bronchospasm is not relieved by medication or is accompanied by diaphoresis, dizziness, or other symptoms.
- Counsel patient on proper use of inhaler; observe use of this device whenever possible to ensure proper technique.
- Instruct patient and family/caregivers to report other bothersome side effects such as severe or prolonged headache, sleep loss, or GI problems (nausea, vomiting).

Pharmacokinetics

Absorption: 35–50% absorbed following oral administration but rapidly undergoes 1st-pass metabolism. Well absorbed following SC administration. Minimal absorption occurs following inhalation.
Distribution: Enters breast milk.
Metabolism and Excretion: Partially metabolized by the liver; 60% excreted unchanged by the kidneys following SC administration.
Half-life: Unknown.

TIME/ACTION PROFILE (bronchodilation)

ROUTE	ONSET	PEAK	DURATION
PO	within 60–120 min	within 2–3 hr	4–8 hr
Inhalation	5–30 min	1–2 hr	3–6 hr
SC	within 15 min	within 0.5–1 hr	1.5–4 hr

Contraindications/Precautions

Contraindicated in: Hypersensitivity to adrenergic amines; Known hypersensitivity or intolerance to fluorocarbons (inhalation only).
Use Cautiously in: Cardiac disease; Hypertension; Hyperthyroidism; Diabetes; Glaucoma; Geri: Geriatric patients (more susceptible to adverse reactions; may require dose reduction); Excessive use may lead to tolerance and paradoxical bronchospasm (inhaler); OB/Pedi: Pregnancy (near term), lactation, and children <2 yr (safety not established).

Interactions

Drug-Drug: Concurrent use with other **adrenergics** (sympathomimetic) will have additive adrenergic side effects. Use with **MAO inhibitors** may lead to hypertensive crisis. **Beta blockers** may negate therapeutic effect.
Drug-Natural: Use with caffeine-containing herbs **(cola nut, guarana, mate, tea, coffee)** ↑ stimulant effect.

Route/Dosage

PO (Adults and Children >15 yr): *Bronchodilation*—2.5–5 mg tid, given q 6 hr (not to exceed 15 mg/24 hr). *Tocolysis*—2.5 mg q 4–6 hr until delivery (unlabeled).
PO (Children 12–15 yr): 2.5 mg tid (given q 6 hr).
Inhaln (Adults and Children ≥12 yr): 2 inhalations (200 mcg/spray) q 4–6 hr.

SC (Adults): *Bronchodilation*—250 mcg; may repeat in 15–30 min (not to exceed 500 mcg/4 hr). *Tocolysis*—250 mcg q 1 hr until contractions stop (unlabeled).
IV (Adults): *Tocolysis*—10 mcg/min infusion; increase by 5 mcg/min q 10 min until contractions stop (not to exceed 80 mcg/min). After contractions have stopped for 30 min, decrease infusion rate to lowest effective amount and maintain for 4–8 hr (unlabeled).

Availability (generic available)

Tablets: 2.5 mg, 5 mg. **Injection:** 1 mg/mL. **Inhalation aerosol:** 200 mcg/spray (≥300 inhalations/10.5-g canister), 500 mcg/spray.

terconazole (ter-kon-a-zole)

Terazol-3, Terazol-7

Classification
Therapeutic: antifungals (vaginal)
Pharmacologic: triazoles

Indications

Treatment of vulvovaginal candidiasis.

Action

Affects the permeability of the fungal cell wall, allowing leakage of cellular contents. Not active against bacteria. **Therapeutic Effects:** Inhibited growth and death of susceptible *Candida*, with ↓ in accompanying symptoms of vulvovaginitis (vaginal burning, itching, discharge).

Adverse Reactions/Side Effects

GI: abdominal pain. **GU:** dysmenorrhea, irritation, itching, vulvovaginal burning. **Misc:** fever.

PHYSICAL THERAPY IMPLICATIONS

Examination and Evaluation

- Monitor patient's symptoms to help document drug effectiveness.

Interventions

- Always wash hands thoroughly and disinfect equipment (whirlpools, electrotherapeutic devices, treatment tables, and so forth) to help prevent the spread of infection.

Patient/Client-Related Instruction

- Advise patient to report any increased local sensitivity to this drug (pain, burning, itching, swelling) or other adverse reactions (fever, abdominal pain, menstrual problems).
- Therapeutic response for vaginal infections is usually seen after 1 wk. Advise patient that application is typically continued throughout the full course of therapy even if feeling better. Therapy should be continued during menstrual period.
- Advise patient to seek medical help if infections persist or recur after the full treatment. Recurrent fungal infections may be a sign of systemic illness.

Pharmacokinetics

Absorption: 5–16% is systemically absorbed following intravaginal administration.
Distribution: Unknown. Action is primarily local.
Metabolism and Excretion: Negligible with local application.
Half-life: Not applicable.

TIME/ACTION PROFILE (plasma concentrations)

ROUTE	ONSET	PEAK	DURATION
intravaginal	unknown	6.6 hr	unknown

Contraindications/Precautions

Contraindicated in: Hypersensitivity to active ingredients, additives, or preservatives.
Use Cautiously in: OB/Lactation: Safety not established.

Interactions

Drug-Drug: Not known.

Route/Dosage

Vag (Adults): *Vaginal cream*—1 applicatorful (5 g) of 0.4% cream hs for 7 days *or* 1 applicatorful (5 g) of 0.8% cream hs for 3 days. *Vaginal suppositories*—1 suppository (80 mg) hs for 3 days.

Availability (generic available)

Vaginal cream: 0.4% Rx, 0.8% Rx. **Vaginal suppositories:** 80 mg Rx.

teriparatide (ter-i-par-a-tide)

Forteo

Classification
Therapeutic: hormones
Pharmacologic: parathyroid hormones (rDNA origin)

Indications

Treatment of osteoporosis in postmenopausal women at high risk for fractures. To increase bone mass in men with osteoporosis at high risk for fractures. Most useful for those have failed or are intolerant to other osteoporosis therapies.

Action

Regulates calcium and phosphate metabolism in bone and kidney by binding to specific cell receptors; stimulates osteoblastic activity. ↑ serum calcium and ↓ serum phosphorus. **Therapeutic Effects:** ↑ bone mineral density with reduced risk of fractures.

Adverse Reactions/Side Effects

CV: orthostatic hypotension. **MS:** muscle spasms.

PHYSICAL THERAPY IMPLICATIONS

Examination and Evaluation

- Assess blood pressure (BP) when patient assumes a more upright position (lying to standing, sitting to standing, lying to sitting). Document orthostatic hypotension and contact the physician when systolic BP falls >20 mm Hg, or diastolic BP falls >10 mm Hg.
- Assess any muscle spasms to rule out musculoskeletal pathology; that is, try to determine if pain is drug induced rather than caused by anatomic or biomechanical problems.

Interventions

- Institute weight-bearing and resistance exercises as tolerated to maintain or increase bone mineral density. Start with low impact or aquatic programs in patients with extensive demineralization, and increase exercise intensity slowly to prevent fractures.
- Protect against falls and fractures (See Appendix E). Modify home environment (remove throw rugs, improve lighting, etc.) and provide assistive devices (cane, walker) or other protective devices as needed to improve balance and prevent falls.
- To minimize orthostatic hypotension, patient should move slowly when assuming a more upright position.

Patient/Client-Related Instruction

- Advise patient about the benefits of proper diet in sustaining bone mineralization. If necessary, refer patient for nutritional counseling about supplemental calcium and vitamin D.
- Encourage patient to modify behaviors that increase the risk of osteoporosis (stop smoking, reduce alcohol consumption).

Pharmacokinetics

Absorption: Extensively absorbed after SC administration.
Distribution: Unknown.
Metabolism and Excretion: Metabolized by the liver; metabolites renally excreted.
Half-life: 1 hr (after SC use).

TIME/ACTION PROFILE (effects on serum calcium)

ROUTE	ONSET	PEAK	DURATION
SC	2 hr	4–6 hr	16–24 hr

Contraindications/Precautions

Contraindicated in: Hypersensitivity; Paget's disease of the bone or other metabolic bone disease; Unexplained ↑ alkaline phosphatase; Pedi: Pediatric or young adult patients; Previous radiation therapy, history of bone metastases, or skeletal malignancy; Preexisting hypercalcemia; OB/Lactation: Pregnancy or lactation.
Use Cautiously in: Concurrent **digoxin.**

Interactions

Drug-Drug: Transient hypercalcemia may ↑ the risk of **digoxin** toxicity.

Route/Dosage

SC (Adults): 20 mcg once daily.

Availability

Prefilled pen delivery device (FORTEO pen): delivers 20 mcg/day.

tesamorelin (tes-a-**moe**-rel-in)

Egrifta

Classification
Therapeutic: none assigned
Pharmacologic: growth hormone–releasing factor analogues

Indications

Reduction of excess abdominal fat (lipodystrophy) seen in HIV-infected patients.

Action

Acts as an analogue of human growth hormone–releasing factor (GRF, GHRH), resulting in endogenous production of growth hormone (GH), which has anabolic and lipolytic properties. **Therapeutic Effects:** Reduction of abdominal adipose tissue in HIV-infected patients.

Adverse Reactions/Side Effects

CV: peripheral edema. **Endo:** glucose intolerance. **Local:** erythema, hemorrhage, irritation, pain, pruritus. **MS:** arthralgia, carpal tunnel syndrome, extremity pain, myalgia. **Misc:** hypersensitivity reactions.

PHYSICAL THERAPY IMPLICATIONS

Examination and Evaluation

- Periodically assess body weight, abdominal girth, and other anthropometric measures (body mass index, body composition). Document whether this drug is successful in helping decrease abdominal fat.
- Monitor signs of hypersensitivity reactions, including pulmonary symptoms (tightness in the throat and chest, wheezing, cough, dyspnea) or skin

reactions (rash, pruritus, urticaria). Notify physician immediately if these reactions occur.

- Assess peripheral edema using girth measurements, volume displacement, and measurement of pitting edema (See Appendix N). Report increased swelling in feet and ankles or a sudden increase in body weight due to fluid retention.
- Assess any muscle, joint, or extremity pain to rule out musculoskeletal pathology; that is, try to determine if pain is drug induced rather than caused by anatomic or biomechanical problems.
- Watch for symptoms of carpal tunnel syndrome, including pain, numbness, tingling, and weakness in the median nerve distribution to the hand. Assess these symptoms using EMG and nerve conduction, and reexamine these values periodically to document drug-induced changes in median nerve function.
- Be alert for signs of glucose intolerance and subsequent hyperglycemia, including confusion, drowsiness, flushed/dry skin, fruit-like breath odor, rapid/deep breathing, polyuria, loss of appetite, and unusual thirst. Patients with diabetes mellitus should check blood glucose levels frequently.
- Monitor subcutaneous injection site for pain, redness, itching, and hemorrhage. Report prolonged or excessive injection site reactions to the physician.

Interventions

- Implement resistive exercises and other therapeutic exercises as needed to maintain muscle strength and function and prevent muscle wasting associated with HIV infection and AIDS.
- Design and implement aerobic exercise and endurance training programs to help prevent heart disease associated with drug-related hyperlipidemia and other problems with lipid and glucose metabolism.
- Do not apply physical agents (heat, cold, electrotherapeutic modalities) or massage over the injection site; these interventions can alter drug absorption from subcutaneous tissues.

Patient/Client-Related Instruction

- Check that patient and family/caregivers understand administration techniques and use appropriate safety precautions (maintain sterility, do not share needles, and so forth).

Pharmacokinetics

Absorption: <4% absorbed following subcutaneous administration.
Distribution: Unknown.
Metabolism and Excretion: Unknown.
Half-life: 26–38 min.

TIME/ACTION PROFILE (effect on visceral adipose tissue)

ROUTE	ONSET	PEAK	DURATION
SC	within 3 mo	10–12 mo	3 mo*

*Following discontinuation.

Contraindications/Precautions

Contraindicated in: Hypersensitivity to tesamorelin or mannitol; Any pathology that alters the hypothalamic-pituitary axis, including hypophysectomy, hypopituitarism, pituitary surgery/tumor, cranial irradiation/trauma; OB: may cause fetal harm; Lactation: Breast-feeding should be avoided by HIV-infected patients.
Use Cautiously in: Acute critical illness (may ↑ risk of serious complications; consider discontinuation); Preexisting malignancy (disease should be inactive or treatment completed); Nonmalignant neoplasms (carefully consider benefit); Persistently elevated insulin-like growth factor (IGF-1; may require discontinuation); Diabetes mellitus (may cause glucose intolerance); Pedi: Safe and effective use in children not established.

Interactions

Drug-Drug: May alter the clearance and actions of drugs known to be metabolized by the CYPP450 enzyme system, including **corticosteroids, androgens, estrogens** and **progestins** (including **hormonal contraceptives**), **anticonvulsants,** and **cyclosporine,** careful monitoring for efficacy and/or toxicity recommended; Inhibits the conversion of **cortisone acetate** and **prednisone** to active forms; patients on replacement therapy may need ↑ maintenance/stress doses

Route/Dosage

SC (Adults): 2 mg once daily.

Availability

Lyophilized powder for SC administration (requires reconstitution): 1 mg/vial.

testosterone cypionate

(tes-**tos**-ter-one sip-**eye**-oh-nate)
Depo-Testosterone

Classification
Therapeutic: hormones
Pharmacologic: androgens

Schedule III

Indications

Hypogonadism in androgen-deficient men.

Action

Responsible for the normal growth and development of male sex organs. Maintenance of male secondary sex characteristics: Growth and maturation of the prostate, seminal vesicles, penis, scrotum; Development of male hair distribution; Vocal cord thickening; Alterations in body musculature and fat distribution. **Therapeutic Effects:** Correction of hormone deficiency in male hypogonadism.

Adverse Reactions/Side Effects

EENT: deepening of voice. **CV:** edema. **GI:** cholestatic jaundice, drug-induced hepatitis, liver function test elevation, nausea, vomiting. **GU:** change in libido, erectile dysfunction, priapism, prostatic enlargement. **Endo:** gynecomastia, hirsutism, oligospermia, hypercholesterolemia. **F and E:** hypercalcemia, hyperkalemia, hyperphosphatemia. **Derm:** male pattern baldness. **Local:** pain at injection site.

PHYSICAL THERAPY IMPLICATIONS

Examination and Evaluation

- Watch for signs of hepatoxicity and drug-induced hepatitis, including anorexia, abdominal pain, severe nausea and vomiting, yellow skin or eyes, fever, sore throat, malaise, weakness, facial edema, lethargy, and unusual bleeding or bruising. Report these signs to the physician.
- Assess peripheral edema using girth measurements, volume displacement, and measurement of pitting edema (See Appendix N). Report increased swelling in feet and ankles or a sudden increase in body weight due to fluid retention.
- Monitor signs of electrolyte imbalances, including high plasma potassium levels (bradycardia, fatigue, weakness, numbness, tingling), high calcium levels (muscle pain and weakness, joint pain, confusion, lethargy), or high phosphate levels (ectopic calcification). Notify physician because severe cases can lead to life-threatening arrhythmias and paralysis.
- Periodically assess body weight and other anthropometric measures (body mass index, body composition). A rapid or unexplained weight gain or increase in muscle mass may indicate androgen abuse.
- Monitor personality changes, including irritability and increased aggression. Aggressive behaviors ("roid rage") may indicate inappropriate or excessive androgen use.
- Monitor IM injection site for pain, swelling, and irritation. Report prolonged or excessive injection site reactions to the physician.

Interventions

- Design and implement resistive exercise programs to capitalize on androgen effects and increase muscle strength in androgen-deficient men.
- Do not apply physical agents (heat, cold, electrotherapeutic modalities) or massage over the injection site; these interventions can alter drug absorption from subcutaneous tissues.

Patient/Client-Related Instruction

- Advise patient against use of testosterone and other androgens to artificially increase muscle mass and enhance athletic performance. Androgen abuse is not safe and can cause liver damage, cardiovascular disease, and other serious side effects.
- Advise patient about risk of breast enlargement, persistent erections, erectile dysfunction, changes in libido, and other masculinization effects (male pattern baldness, increased body hair, deepening voice). Notify physician if these side effects become persistent or troublesome.
- Instruct men to report signs of prostate enlargement, including difficulty urinating and increased urge to urinate.
- Advise patient that this drug may cause problems in fat metabolism (hypercholesterolemia). Remind patient that periodic blood tests may be needed to monitor plasma lipids.
- Instruct patient or family/caregivers to report other bothersome side effects such as severe or prolonged GI problems (nausea, vomiting).

Pharmacokinetics

Absorption: Well absorbed from IM sites; absorbed slowly.
Distribution: Crosses the placenta.
Protein Binding: 98%.
Metabolism and Excretion: Metabolized by the liver; 90% eliminated in urine as metabolites.
Half-life: 8 days.

TIME/ACTION PROFILE (androgenic effects*)

ROUTE	ONSET	PEAK	DURATION
IM	unknown	unknown	2–4 wk

*Response is highly variable among individuals; may take months.

Contraindications/Precautions

Contraindicated in: Hypersensitivity; OB: Pregnancy and lactation; Male patients with breast or prostate cancer; Severe liver, renal, or cardiac disease; Patients with known hypersensitivity to benzyl alcohol.
Use Cautiously in: Benign prostatic hyperplasia; Hypercalcemia; Geriatric patients (↑ risk of prostatic hyperplasia/carcinoma); Males <12 yr (safety and effectiveness not established).

Interactions

Drug-Drug: May ↑ action of **warfarin, oral hypoglycemic agents,** and **insulin.** Concurrent use with **corticosteroids** may ↑ risk of edema formation.

Route/Dosage

IM (Adults): *Replacement therapy*—50–400 mg q 2–4 wk.

Availability (generic available)

Injection (in oil): 100 mg/mL in 10-mL vials, 200 mg/mL in 1- and 10-mL vials.

tetrabenazine

(tet-ra-**ben**-a-zeen)

Xenazine

Classification

Therapeutic: antichoreas

Pharmacologic: reversible monoamine depleters

Indications

Treatment of chorea due to Huntington's disease.

Action

Acts as a reversible inhibitor of the vesicle monoamine transporter type 2 (VMAT-2); which inhibits the reuptake of serotonin, norepinephrine, and dopamine into vesicles in presynaptic neurons. **Therapeutic Effects:** ↓ chorea due to Huntington's disease.

Adverse Reactions/Side Effects

CNS: anxiety, fatigue, insomnia, depression, sedation/somnolence, cognitive defects, dizziness, headache. **Resp:** shortness of breath. **CV:** hypotension, QTc prolongation. **GI:** nausea, dysphagia. **Neuro:** akathisia, balance difficulty, dysarthria, parkinsonism, unsteady gait. **Misc:** NEUROLEPTIC MALIGNANT SYNDROME.

PHYSICAL THERAPY IMPLICATIONS

Examination and Evaluation

- Be alert for signs of neuroleptic malignant syndrome, including hyperthermia, diaphoresis, generalized muscle rigidity, altered mental status, tachycardia, changes in blood pressure (BP), and incontinence. Report these signs to the physician or nursing staff immediately.
- Document the incidence and severity of involuntary movements related to chorea (rapid jerky motions, other dyskinesias) to help document whether this drug is successful in reducing these symptoms. Notify physician of changes in abnormal movements to help find an optimal dose of this drug to control chorea.
- Assess BP periodically and compare to normal values (See Appendix F). Report low BP (hypotension), especially if patient experiences dizziness, fatigue, or other symptoms.
- Assess heart rate, ECG, and heart sounds, especially during exercise (See Appendices G, H). Report any rhythm disturbances or symptoms of increased arrhythmias, including palpitations, chest discomfort, shortness of breath, fainting, and fatigue/weakness.
- Assess dizziness, Parkinson-like symptoms, severe restlessness (akathisia), or other motor problems that affect gait, balance, and functional activities. Report balance problems and functional limitations to the physician and nursing staff, and caution the patient and family/caregivers to guard against falls and trauma.
- Monitor anxiety, depression, decreased cognition, and other psychologic problems. Repeated or excessive symptoms may require change in dose or medication.

Interventions

- Implement therapeutic exercises (coordination exercises, gait training) to complement the effects of drug therapy and help achieve optimal function.
- Because of the risk of arrhythmias and abnormal BP responses, use caution during aerobic exercise and other forms of therapeutic exercise. Assess exercise tolerance frequently (BP, heart rate, fatigue levels), and terminate exercise immediately if any untoward responses occur (See Appendix L).
- Guard against falls and trauma (hip fractures, head injury, and so forth). Implement fall- prevention strategies (See Appendix E), especially if patient exhibits motor problems (Parkinson symptoms, postural instability, rigidity) combined with drug side effects (dizziness, balance deficits).

Patient/Client-Related Instruction

- Advise patient to avoid alcohol because of the increased risk of sedation and adverse effects.
- Instruct patient to report other troublesome side effects such as severe or prolonged headache, shortness of breath, sleep loss, vivid dreams, or GI reactions (nausea, difficulty swallowing).

Pharmacokinetics

Absorption: At least 75% absorbed following oral administration.

Distribution: Crosses the blood-brain barrier.

Metabolism and Excretion: Rapidly and extensively metabolized by the liver; CYP2D6 plays a large role in the metabolic process. Metabolites are renally excreted. Two metabolites, α-dihydrotetrabenazine (α-HTBZ) and β-HTBZ, bind to VMAT-2 and are pharmacologically active.

Half-life: α-HTBZ—4–8 hr; β-HTBZ—2–4 hr.

TIME/ACTION PROFILE (blood levels)

ROUTE	ONSET	PEAK	DURATION
PO	unknown	1–1.5 hr	12–18 hr*

*Return of symptoms following discontinuation.

Contraindications/Precautions

Contraindicated in: Hepatic impairment; Concurrent use of reserpine or MAO inhibitors; Patients who are actively suicidal or have untreated depression; Lactation: Breast-feeding.

Use Cautiously in: History of/propensity for depression or history of psychiatric illness; history of suicidality; Poor CYP2D6 metabolizers; initial dose reduction required; Concurrent use of CYP2D6 inhibitors; dose modification required; Recent history of myocardial infarction or unstable heart disease; OB: Use during pregnancy only when potential benefit justifies potential risk to the fetus; Pedi: Safe and effective use in children has not been established.

Interactions

Drug-Drug: Blood levels are ↑ by drugs that inhibit the CYP2D6 enzyme system, including **fluoxetine, paroxetine,** and **quinidine;** initial dose reduction of tetrabenazine recommended. **Reserpine** binds to VMAT-2 and depletes monoamines in the CNS; avoid concurrent use; wait 3 wk after discontinuing to initiate tetrabenazine. Concurrent use of **MAO inhibitors** ↑ risk of serious adverse reactions and is contraindicated. Concurrent use with **neuroleptic drugs** or **dopamine antagonists,** including **haloperidol, chlorpromazine, risperidone,** and **olanzapine,** may ↑ risk of QTc prolongation, neuroleptic malignant syndrome, and extrapyramidal disorders. Concurrent use of **alcohol** or other **CNS depressants** may ↑ risk of CNS depression.

Route/Dosage

PO (Adults): 12.5 mg/day for 1 wk initially, ↑ by 12.5 weekly up to 37.5–50 mg/day in 3 divided doses; *concurrent use of strong inhibitors or CYP2D6 or poor CYP2D6 metabolizers*—start with initial dose of 6.25 mg, titrate carefully.

Availability

Tablets: 12.5 mg, 25 mg.

tetracycline (tet-ra-**sye**-kleen)

chromycin, Apo-Tetra, Novotetra, Nu-Tetra, Panmycin, Sumycin, Robitet, Tetracyn

Classification

Therapeutic: anti-infectives

Indications

Treatment of various infections due to unusual organisms, including *Mycoplasma, Chlamydia, Rickettsia, Borrelia burgdorferi*. Treatment of gonorrhea and syphilis in penicillin-allergic patients. Prevention of exacerbations of chronic bronchitis. Treatment of acne.

Action

Inhibits bacterial protein synthesis at the level of the 30S bacterial ribosome. **Therapeutic Effects:** Bacteriostatic action against susceptible bacteria. **Spectrum:** Includes activity against some gram-positive pathogens: *Bacillus anthracis, Clostridium perfringens, C. tetani, Listeria monocytogenes, Nocardia, Propionibacterium acnes, Actinomyces israelii*. Active against some gram-negative pathogens: *Haemophilus influenzae, Legionella pneumophila, Yersinia enterocolitica, Y. pestis, Neisseria gonorrhoeae, N. meningitidis*. Also active against several other pathogens, including *Mycoplasma, Treponema pallidum, Chlamydia, Rickettsia, B. burgdorferi*.

Adverse Reactions/Side Effects

CNS: benign intracranial hypertension (increased in children), dizziness. **GI:** diarrhea, nausea, vomiting, esophagitis, hepatotoxicity, pancreatitis. **Derm:** photosensitivity, rashes. **Hemat:** blood dyscrasias. **Misc:** hypersensitivity reactions, superinfection.

PHYSICAL THERAPY IMPLICATIONS

Examination and Evaluation

- Monitor signs of hypersensitivity reactions or anaphylaxis, including pulmonary symptoms (tightness in the throat and chest, wheezing, cough dyspnea) or skin reactions (rash, angioedema, pruritus, urticaria). Notify physician or nursing staff immediately if these reactions occur.
- Monitor signs of leukopenia (fever, sore throat, signs of infection), thrombocytopenia (bruising, nose bleeds, and bleeding gums), or unusual weakness and fatigue that might be due to anemia or other blood dyscrasias. Report these signs to the physician immediately.
- Monitor and report signs of benign intracranial hypertension, especially in children. Signs include dizziness, headache, tinnitus, nausea, and disturbed vision (e.g., blurry or double vision).
- Assess dizziness that might affect gait, balance, and other functional activities (See Appendix C). Report balance problems and functional limitations to the physician, and caution the patient and family/caregivers to guard against falls and trauma.

Interventions

- Always wash hands thoroughly and disinfect equipment (whirlpools, electrotherapeutic devices, treatment tables, and so forth) to help prevent the spread of infection. Use universal precautions or isolation procedures as indicated for specific patients.

- Because of the risk of intracranial hypertension, avoid activities that might increase intracranial pressure such as elevating the feet above the head (Trendelenburg's position) or holding breath and straining during a bowel movement (Valsalva's maneuver).
- Causes photosensitivity; use care if administering UV treatments.

Patient/Client-Related Instruction

- Instruct patient to notify physician immediately of signs of superinfection, including black, furry overgrowth on tongue, vaginal itching or discharge, and loose or foul-smelling stools.
- Advise patient about the likelihood of GI reactions (nausea, vomiting, diarrhea, heartburn). Instruct patient to report severe or prolonged GI problems, signs of liver toxicity (yellow skin or eyes, abdominal pain, severe nausea and vomiting, fever, sore throat, malaise, weakness, facial edema), or pancreatitis (upper abdominal pain after eating, indigestion, weight loss, oily stools).
- Advise patient about photosensitivity, and to use sunscreens, protective clothing, and avoid prolonged sun exposure. Advise patient to also report any rashes or other skin reactions.

Pharmacokinetics

Absorption: 60–80% absorbed after oral administration.
Distribution: Widely distributed, some CSF and good bone penetration; crosses the placenta and enters breast milk.
Metabolism and Excretion: Excreted mostly unchanged by the kidneys.
Half-life: 6–12 hr.

TIME/ACTION PROFILE (blood levels)

ROUTE	ONSET	PEAK	DURATION
PO	1–2 hr	2–4 hr	6–12 hr

Contraindications/Precautions

Contraindicated in: Hypersensitivity; Some products contain alcohol or bisulfites and should be avoided in patients with known hypersensitivity or intolerance; Children <8 yr (permanent staining of teeth); Pregnancy (risk of permanent staining of teeth in infant if used during last half of pregnancy); Lactation.
Use Cautiously in: Cachectic or debilitated patients; Renal disease; Nephrogenic diabetes insipidus.

Interactions

Drug-Drug: May enhance the effect of **warfarin.** May ↓ effectiveness of **estrogen-containing oral contraceptives. Antacids, calcium, iron,** and **magnesium** form insoluble compounds (chelates) and ↓ absorption of tetracycline. **Sucralfate** may bind to tetracycline and prevent its absorption from the GI tract. **Cholestyramine** or **colestipol** ↓ absorption. **Adsorbent antidiarrheal agents** may ↓ absorption. **Barbiturates, phenytoin,** or **carbamazepine** may ↓ activity of doxycycline.
Drug-Food: Calcium in foods or **dairy products** ↓ absorption by forming insoluble compounds (chelates).

Route/Dosage

PO (Adults): 250–500 mg q 6 hr or 500 mg–1 g q 12 hr. *Chronic treatment of acne*—500 mg–2 g/day for 3 wk, then decreased to 125 mg–1 g/day.
PO (Children ≥8 yr): 6.25–12.5 mg/kg q 6 hr or 12.5–25 mg/kg q 12 hr.

Availability (generic available)

Capsules: 250 mg, 500 mg. **Oral suspension (fruit flavors):** 125 mg/5 mL.

thalidomide (tha-lid-oh-mide)

Thalomid

Classification

Therapeutic: immunosuppressants

Indications

Cutaneous manifestations of moderate-to-severe erythema nodosum leprosum (ENL). Prevention (maintenance) and suppression of recurrent ENL. Newly diagnosed multiple myeloma (with dexamethasone). **Unlabeled Use:** Behçet's syndrome. HIV-associated wasting syndrome. Aphthous stomatitis (including HIV associated). Crohn's disease.

Action

May suppress excess levels of tumor necrosis factor-alpha (TNF-alpha) in patients with ENL and alter leukocyte migration by altering characteristics of cell surfaces. **Therapeutic Effects:** ↓ skin lesions in ENL and prevention of recurrence.

Adverse Reactions/Side Effects

CNS: dizziness, drowsiness. **CV:** bradycardia, edema, orthostatic hypotension, thromboembolic events (↑ risk with dexamethasone in multiple myeloma). **GI:** constipation. **Derm:** rash, photosensitivity. **Hemat:** neutropenia. **Neuro:** peripheral neuropathy. **Misc:** SEVERE BIRTH DEFECTS, hypersensitivity reactions, increased HIV viral load.

PHYSICAL THERAPY IMPLICATIONS

Examination and Evaluation

- Monitor signs of hypersensitivity reactions or anaphylaxis, including pulmonary symptoms (tightness in the throat and chest, wheezing, cough, dyspnea) or skin reactions (rash, pruritus, urticaria). Notify physician or nursing staff immediately if these reactions occur.

- Assess heart rate, especially during exercise (See Appendix G). Report bradycardia or symptoms of increased arrhythmias, including palpitations, chest discomfort, shortness of breath, fainting, and fatigue/weakness.
- Assess blood pressure (BP) when patient assumes a more upright position (lying to standing, sitting to standing, lying to sitting). Document orthostatic hypotension when systolic BP falls >20 mm Hg or diastolic BP falls >10 mm Hg.
- Assess peripheral edema using girth measurements, volume displacement, and measurement of pitting edema (See Appendix N). Report increased swelling in feet and ankles or a sudden increase in body weight due to fluid retention.
- Monitor signs of venous thrombosis (lower extremity swelling, warmth, erythema, tenderness) and thromboembolism (shortness of breath, chest pain, cough, bloody sputum). Notify physician immediately, and request objective tests (Doppler ultrasound, lung scan, others) if thrombosis is suspected.
- Be alert for signs of neutropenia including fever, sore throat, and other signs of infection. Report these signs to the physician or nursing staff.
- Be alert for signs of peripheral neuropathy (numbness, tingling, decreased muscle strength). Establish baseline electroneuromyographic values at the beginning of drug treatment whenever possible, and reexamine these values periodically to document drug-induced changes in peripheral nerve function.
- If treating erythema nodosum leprosum, assess the number, size, and redness of skin nodules to help determine if drug treatment is successful in suppressing cutaneous lesions.
- Assess dizziness and drowsiness that might affect gait, balance, and other functional activities (See Appendix C). Report balance problems and functional limitations to the physician and nursing staff, and caution the patient and family/caregivers to guard against falls and trauma.

Interventions

- For patients who are medically able to begin exercise, implement appropriate resistive exercises and aerobic training to maintain or restore muscle strength and aerobic capacity during various conditions such as newly diagnosed multiple myeloma, HIV wasting syndrome, and Crohn's disease.
- Because of potential cardiac problems (bradycardia, orthostatic hypotension, thromboembolism), use caution during aerobic exercise and endurance conditioning. Terminate exercise if patient exhibits untoward symptoms (chest pain, shortness of breath, etc.), or displays other criteria for exercise termination (See Appendix L).
- Causes photosensitivity; use care if administering UV treatments. Advise patient to avoid direct sunlight and use sunscreens and protective clothing.

Patient/Client-Related Instruction

- Advise patient about the risk of severe birth defects. Women of childbearing age who are sexually active must use two methods of reliable contraception for 1 mo prior to, during, and for 1 mo following discontinuation of this drug. For men, a latex condom must be used even if a successful vasectomy has been performed.
- Advise patient to guard against infection (frequent hand washing, etc.), and to avoid crowds and contact with persons with contagious diseases.
- Instruct patient or family/caregivers to report other bothersome side effects such as severe or prolonged constipation or skin rashes.

Pharmacokinetics

Absorption: 67–93% absorbed following oral administration.
Distribution: Crosses the placenta; highly protein bound.
Protein Binding: Highly bound.
Metabolism and Excretion: Hydrolyzed in plasma to multiple metabolites.
Half-life: 5–7 hr.

TIME/ACTION PROFILE (dermatologic effects)

ROUTE	ONSET	PEAK	DURATION
PO	48 hr	1–2 mo	unknown

Contraindications/Precautions

Contraindicated in: Pregnancy; OB: Women with childbearing potential (unless specific conditions are met); Sexually mature men (unless specific conditions are met); OB: Lactation; Hypersensitivity.
Use Cautiously in: Pedi: Children <12 yr (safety not established).

Interactions

Drug-Drug: ↑ CNS depression with concurrent use of **barbiturates, sedative/hypnotics, alcohol, chlorpromazine, reserpine,** or other **CNS depressants.** Concurrent use of **agents that may cause peripheral neuropathy** ↑ risk of peripheral neuropathy.
Drug-Natural: Concomitant use with **echinacea,** and **melatonin** may interfere with immunosuppression.

Route/Dosage

ENL

PO (Adults ≥50 kg): 100–300 mg/day initially; up to 400 mg/day has been used, depending on previous response. Every 3–6 mo attempts should be made to taper and discontinue in decrements of 50 mg q 2–4 wk. **PO (Adults <50 kg):** 100 mg/day initially; up to 400 mg/day has been used, depending on previous response. Every 3–6 mo attempts should be made to taper and discontinue in decrements of 50 mg q 2–4 wk.

Multiple Myeloma

PO (Adults): 200 mg daily in 28-day treatment cycles. Dexamethasone 40 mg is administered on days 1–4, 9–12, 17–20.

Availability

Capsules: 50 mg, 100 mg, 150 mg, 200 mg.

theophylline (thee-off-i-lin)

✱Apo-Theo LA, Elixophyllin, ✱Novo-Theophyl SR, ✱PMS-Theophylline, ✱Pulmophylline, Quibron-T, Theochron, Theo-24, Uniphyl

Classification

Therapeutic: bronchodilators
Pharmacologic: xanthines

Indications

Long-term control of reversible airway obstruction caused by asthma or COPD.

Action

Inhibit phosphodiesterase, producing increased tissue concentrations of cyclic adenosine monophosphate (cAMP). Increased levels of cAMP result in Bronchodilation, CNS stimulation, Positive inotropic and chronotropic effects, Diuresis, Gastric acid secretion. **Therapeutic Effects:** Bronchodilation.

Adverse Reactions/Side Effects

CNS: SEIZURES, anxiety, headache, insomnia, irritability. **CV:** ARRHYTHMIAS, tachycardia, angina, palpitations. **GI:** nausea, vomiting, anorexia. **Neuro:** tremor.

PHYSICAL THERAPY IMPLICATIONS

Examination and Evaluation

- Be alert for new seizures or increased seizure activity, especially at the onset of drug treatment. Document the number, duration, and severity of seizures, and report these findings to the physician immediately.
- Assess heart rate, ECG, and heart sounds, especially during exercise (See Appendices G, H). Report a rapid heart rate (tachycardia) or signs of other arrhythmias, including palpitations, chest pain, shortness of breath, fainting, and fatigue/weakness.
- Assess pulmonary function periodically by measuring lung volumes, breath sounds, respiratory rate, and other symptoms (wheezing, dyspnea, shortness of breath) (See Appendixes I, J, K). Report changes in pulmonary function to help document the effects of drug therapy in treating or preventing bronchoconstriction.
- Monitor and report signs of CNS toxicity, including tremor, anxiety, irritability, or other changes in mood or behavior. Sustained or severe CNS signs may indicate overdose or excessive use of this drug.

Interventions

- Because of the risk of cardiovascular stimulation, use caution during aerobic exercise and endurance conditioning. Assess exercise tolerance frequently (blood pressure, heart rate, fatigue levels), and terminate exercise immediately if any untoward responses occur (See Appendix L).

Patient/Client-Related Instruction

- Because of the risk of cardiovascular and CNS stimulation, caution patient to avoid taking more than the recommended dose. Instruct patient to contact physician immediately if bronchospasm is not relieved by medication or worsens after treatment.
- Advise patient to minimize intake of caffeine or other xanthine-containing foods or beverages (colas, coffee, tea, chocolate) and to reduce intake of charcoal-broiled foods.
- Instruct patient and family/caregivers to report other troublesome side effects such as severe or prolonged headache, sleep loss, skin rash, or GI problems (nausea, vomiting, loss of appetite).

Pharmacokinetics

Absorption: Well absorbed from PO dosage forms; absorption from extended-release dosage forms is slow but complete.
Distribution: Widely distributed; crosses the placenta and into breast milk; does not distribute into adipose tissue.
Metabolism and Excretion: 90% metabolized by the liver to several metabolites (including the active metabolites, caffeine and 3-methylxanthine); metabolites are renally excreted; 10% excreted unchanged by the kidneys.
Half-life: *Theophylline*—Premature infants: 20–30 hr; Term infants: 11–25 hr; Children 1–4 yr: 3.4 hr; Children 6–17 yr: 3.7 hr; Adults: 9–10 hr (↑ in patients >60 yr, patients with congestive heart failure or liver disease; ↓ in cigarette smokers).

TIME/ACTION PROFILE (bronchodilation)

ROUTE	ONSET*	PEAK	DURATION
PO	rapid	1–2 hr	6 hr
PO-ER	delayed	4–8 hr	8–24 hr
IV	rapid	end of infusion	6–8 hr

*Provided that a loading dose has been given and steady-state blood levels exist.

Contraindications/Precautions

Contraindicated in: Hypersensitivity to aminophylline or theophylline.
Use Cautiously in: Cardiac arrhythmias; Reduce dose in patients with heart failure, liver disease, or hypothyroidism; Peptic ulcer disease; Seizure disorders; OB/Lactation: Safety not established; Pedi/Geri: Dosage reduction required for patients >60 yr and <1 yr.

Interactions

Drug-Drug: Additive CV and CNS side effects with **adrenergics (sympathomimetic).** May ↓ the therapeutic effect of **lithium** and **phenytoin.** Smoking, **barbiturates, carbamazepine, phenytoin, nevirapine,** and **rifampin** may ↑ metabolism and may ↓ effectiveness. **Erythromycin, beta blockers, clarithromycin, calcium channel blockers, cimetidine, hormonal contraceptives, disulfiram, doxycycline, estrogens, fluvoxamine, isoniazid, ketoconazole, mexiletine, nefazodone, protease inhibitors, quinidine,** some **fluoroquinolones,** and large doses of **allopurinol** ↓ metabolism and may lead to toxicity.
Drug-Natural: Caffeine-containing herbs (**cola nut, guarana, mate, tea, coffee**) may ↑ serum levels and risk of CNS and CV side effects. ↓ serum levels and effectiveness with **St. John's wort.**
Drug-Food: Excessive regular intake of **charcoal-broiled foods** may ↓ effectiveness.

Route/Dosage

Dose should be determined by theophylline serum level monitoring. Loading dose should be decreased or eliminated if theophylline preparation has been used in preceding 24 hr. Aminophylline is 80% theophylline (100 mg aminophylline = 80 mg theophylline). Extended-release (controlled-release, sustained-release) products may be given q 8–24 hr, depending upon the formulation.
PO (Adults Healthy, Nonsmoking): *Loading dose*—5 mg/kg, followed by 10 mg/kg/day divided q 8–12 hr (not to exceed 900 mg/day).
PO (Adults with Congestive Heart Failure, Cor Pulmonale, or Liver Dysfunction): *Loading dose*—5 mg/kg, followed by 5 mg/kg/day divided q 8–12 hr (not to exceed 400 mg/day).
PO (Children 12–16 yr, Nonsmoking): *Loading dose*—5 mg/kg, followed by 13 mg/kg/day divided q 8–12 hr.
PO (Children 9–12 yr, Adolescent and Adult Smokers < 50 yr): *Loading dose*—5 mg/kg, followed by 16 mg/kg/day divided q 8–12 hr.
PO (Children 1–9 yr): *Loading dose*—5 mg/kg, followed by 20–24 mg/kg/day divided q 8–12 hr.
PO (Infants 6 mo–1 yr): *Loading dose*—5 mg/kg, followed by 12–18 mg/kg/day divided q 6–8 hr.
PO (Infants 6 wk–6 mo): *Loading dose*—5 mg/kg, followed by 10 mg/kg/day divided q 6–8 hr.
PO (Neonates up to 6 wk): *Loading dose*—4 mg/kg, followed by 4 mg/kg/day divided q 12 hr.
IV (Adults and Children): See aminophylline monograph for IV doses.

Availability

Sustained-release tablets (8–12 hr): 300 mg Rx. **Extended-release tablets (12–24 hr):** 100 mg Rx, 200 mg Rx, 300 mg Rx, 450 mg Rx. **Controlled-release tablets (24 hr):** 400 mg Rx, 600 mg Rx. **Extended-release capsules (12 hr):** 125 mg Rx, 200 mg Rx, 300 mg Rx. **Extended-release capsules (24 hr):** 100 mg Rx, 200 mg Rx, 300 mg Rx, 400 mg Rx. **Elixir (orange/raspberry, mixed fruit, and other flavors):** 80 mg/15 ml Rx. **Injection (with dextrose):** 0.8 mg/mL Rx, 1.6 mg/mL Rx, 2 mg/mL Rx, 3.2 mg/mL Rx, 4 mg/mL Rx.

thiethylperazine

(thye-eth-il-**per**-a-zeen)
Norzine, Torecan

Classification
Therapeutic: antiemetics
Pharmacologic: phenothiazines

T

Indications

Management of nausea and vomiting.

Action

Alters the effects of dopamine in the CNS. Depresses the chemoreceptive trigger zone (CTZ) and vomiting center in the CNS. **Therapeutic Effects:** Diminished nausea and vomiting.

Adverse Reactions/Side Effects

CNS: NEUROLEPTIC MALIGNANT SYNDROME, sedation, cerebral vascular spasm, extrapyramidal reactions, headache, restlessness, tardive dyskinesia. **EENT:** dry eyes, blurred vision, lens opacities, tinnitus. **CV:** hypotension (following IM use), peripheral edema. **GI:** constipation, dry mouth, altered taste, anorexia, drug-induced hepatitis, ileus. **GU:** urinary retention. **Derm:** photosensitivity, pigment changes, rashes. **Endo:** galactorrhea. **Hemat:** AGRANULOCYTOSIS, leukopenia. **Metab:** hyperthermia. **Neuro:** trigeminal neuralgia. **Misc:** allergic reactions.

PHYSICAL THERAPY IMPLICATIONS

Examination and Evaluation

- Monitor and report signs of neuroleptic malignant syndrome (hyperthermia, diaphoresis, generalized muscle rigidity, altered mental status, tachycardia, changes in blood pressure [BP], incontinence). Symptoms typically occur within 4–14 days after initiation of drug therapy, but can occur at any time during drug use.

- Monitor signs of agranulocytosis and leukopenia including fever, sore throat, mucosal lesions, signs of infection, and bruising. Report these signs to the physician immediately.
- Monitor the frequency, severity, and duration of GI problems (nausea, vomiting) to help document drug effectiveness in controlling these symptoms.
- Assess motor function, and be alert for extrapyramidal reactions. Report these symptoms immediately, especially tardive dyskinesia, because this problem may be irreversible. Common extrapyramidal symptoms include:
  - Tardive dyskinesia (uncontrolled rhythmic movement of mouth, face, and extremities, lip smacking or puckering, puffing of cheeks, uncontrolled chewing, rapid or worm-like movements of tongue).
  - Pseudoparkinsonism (shuffling gait, rigidity, tremor, pill-rolling motion, loss of balance control, difficulty speaking or swallowing, mask-like face).
  - Akathisia (restlessness or desire to keep moving).
  - Other dystonias and dyskinesias (dystonic muscle spasms, twisting motions, twitching, inability to move eyes, weakness of arms or legs).
- Assess BP periodically and compare to normal values (See Appendix F). Report low BP (hypotension), especially if patient experiences dizziness, fatigue, or other symptoms.
- Assess peripheral edema using girth measurements, volume displacement, and measurement of pitting edema (See Appendix N). Report increased swelling in feet and ankles or a sudden increase in body weight due to fluid retention.
- Monitor any facial pain consistent with trigeminal neuralgia; that is, sharp or electric-like pain radiating into the cheek, jaw, teeth, gums, lips, and sometimes the eye and forehead. Notify physician and discuss possible physical interventions to control this pain.

Interventions

- Guard against falls and trauma (hip fractures, head injury, and so forth) caused by drowsiness, blurred vision, or extrapyramidal symptoms; implement fall prevention strategies (See Appendix E).
- Because of an increased risk of hyperthermia, use caution during aerobic exercise, especially in hot environments. Carefully monitor the patient's exercise tolerance and terminate exercise if any untoward effects occur (See Appendix L).
- Causes photosensitivity; use care if administering UV treatments. Advise patient to avoid direct sunlight and use sunscreens and protective clothing.

Patient/Client-Related Instruction

- Advise patient to avoid alcohol and other CNS depressants because of the increased risk of sedation and adverse effects.
- Advise patient about the likelihood of GI problems such as constipation, loss of appetite, altered taste, and dry mouth. Instruct patient to report severe of prolonged GI problems or signs of drug-induced hepatitis (abdominal pain, severe nausea and vomiting, yellow skin or eyes, skin rashes, flu-like symptoms, muscle/joint pain).
- Instruct patient to report other problematic side effects such as severe or prolonged headache, vision disturbances, excessive sedation, ringing/buzzing in the ears (tinnitus), urinary retention, nipple discharge, or skin problems (rash, pigment changes).

Pharmacokinetics

Absorption: Well absorbed following oral, rectal, or IM administration.
Distribution: Widely distributed; high concentrations in the CNS. Crosses the placenta and probably enters breast milk.
Protein Binding: ≥90%.
Metabolism and Excretion: Highly metabolized by the liver and GI mucosa.
Half-life: Unknown.

TIME/ACTION PROFILE (antiemetic effect)

ROUTE	ONSET	PEAK	DURATION
PO	30 min	unknown	4 hr
IM	unknown	unknown	unknown

Contraindications/Precautions

Contraindicated in: Hypersensitivity; Hypersensitivity to bisulfites (IM); Hypersensitivity to aspirin or tartrazine (tablets); Cross-sensitivity with other phenothiazines may occur; Angle-closure glaucoma; Bone marrow depression; Severe liver or cardiovascular disease; Pregnancy.
Use Cautiously in: Geriatric or debilitated patients (dosage reduction recommended); Diabetes mellitus; Respiratory disease; Prostatic hyperplasia; CNS tumors; Epilepsy; Intestinal obstruction; Children <12 yr or lactation (safety not established).

Interactions

Drug-Drug: Additive hypotension with **antihypertensives,** acute ingestion of **alcohol,** or **nitrates.** Additive CNS depression with other **CNS depressants,** including **alcohol, antihistamines, opioid analgesics, sedative/hypnotics,** or **general anesthetics.** Additive anticholinergic effects with other **drugs possessing anticholinergic properties,** including **antihistamines, antidepressants, atropine, disopyramide, haloperidol,** and other **phenothiazines.** May ↓ the beneficial effects of **levodopa.** May block alpha-adrenergic effects of **epinephrine,** resulting in severe hypotension and tachycardia.

Route/Dosage

PO, IM (Adults): 10 mg 1–3 times daily.

Availability

Tablets: 10 mg. **Injection:** 5 mg/mL in 2-mL ampules.

HIGH ALERT

thioguanine (thye-oh-gwon-een)

Lanvis

OTHER NAMES:
6-thioguanine

Classification
Therapeutic: antineoplastics
Pharmacologic: antimetabolites

Indications

Induction and consolidation of remission in acute nonlymphocytic leukemia (in combination with other agents).

Action

Incorporated into DNA and RNA, subsequently disrupting synthesis (cell-cycle S phase–specific). **Therapeutic Effects:** Death of rapidly replicating cells, especially malignant ones. Immunosuppressive properties.

Adverse Reactions/Side Effects

EENT: loss of vibratory sense. **GI:** diarrhea, hepatotoxicity, jaundice, nausea, stomatitis, vomiting, anorexia, hepatic veno-occlusive disease. **GU:** gonadal suppression. **Derm:** dermatitis, rash. **Hemat:** anemia, leukopenia, thrombocytopenia, pancytopenia. **Metab:** hyperuricemia. **Neuro:** unsteady gait.

PHYSICAL THERAPY IMPLICATIONS

Examination and Evaluation

- Watch for signs of leukopenia (fever, sore throat, signs of infection), thrombocytopenia (bruising, nose bleeds, bleeding gums), or unusual weakness and fatigue that might be due to anemia or other blood dyscrasias. Report these signs to the physician.
- Monitor vibratory sensation. Report loss of vibratory sense or other sensory dysfunction.
- Assess gait, and notify physician and family/caregivers if patient is not safe when ambulating independently.

Interventions

- For patients who are medically able to begin exercise, implement appropriate resistive exercises and aerobic training to maintain muscle strength and aerobic capacity during cancer chemotherapy or to help restore function after chemotherapy.
- Provide gait training and balance activities. Guard against falls and trauma due to unsteady gait (See Appendix E).

Patient/Client-Related Instruction

- Advise patient to decrease risk of infections (frequent hand washing, etc.) and avoid contact with persons with contagious diseases.
- Advise patient about the likelihood of GI reactions, including nausea, vomiting, diarrhea, and inflammation in or around the mouth. Instruct patient to report severe or prolonged GI problems, and to also report signs of hepatotoxicity such as anorexia, abdominal pain, severe nausea and vomiting, yellow skin or eyes, fever, sore throat, malaise, weakness, facial edema, lethargy, and unusual bleeding or bruising.
- Advise patient that rashes, dermatitis, and other skin reactions are likely. Report severe or unexpected skin reactions to the physician.

T

Pharmacokinetics

Absorption: Variable and incomplete (average, 30%) following oral administration.
Distribution: Probably does not enter the CSF. Crosses the placenta.
Metabolism and Excretion: Highly metabolized by the liver.
Half-life: 11 hr.

TIME/ACTION PROFILE (effect on blood counts)

ROUTE	ONSET	PEAK	DURATION
PO	7–10 days	14 days	21 days

Contraindications/Precautions

Contraindicated in: Hypersensitivity; Pregnancy or lactation; Tumors with demonstrated resistance to thioguanine or mercaptopurine (usually complete cross-resistance).
Use Cautiously in: Patients with childbearing potential; Infections; Decreased bone marrow reserve; Other chronic debilitating illnesses; Patients with thiopurine methyltransferase (TPMT) enzyme deficiency (substantial dosage reductions are required to avoid hematologic adverse events).

Interactions

Drug-Drug: ↑ bone marrow depression with other **antineoplastics** or **radiation therapy. Sulfasalazine,**

olsalazine, and **mesalamine** may ↓ metabolism and ↑ effects.

Route/Dosage

Many other protocols are used.

PO (Adults and Children): *Induction*—2 mg/kg (75–100 mg/m^2) per day, rounded off to nearest 20 mg given as single dose; after 4 wk may increase to 3 mg/kg. *Maintenance*—2–3 mg/kg (100 mg/m^2) per day.

Availability

Tablets: 40 mg.

thioridazine

(thye-oh-**rid**-a-zeen)

Apo-Thioridazine, Mellaril, Mellaril-S, Novo-Ridazine, PMS Thioridazine

Classification

Therapeutic: antipsychotics

Pharmacologic: phenothiazines

Indications

Treatment of refractory schizophrenia. Considered 2nd-line treatment after failure with atypical antipsychotics.

Action

Alters the effects of dopamine in the CNS. Possesses significant anticholinergic and alpha-adrenergic blocking activity. **Therapeutic Effects:** Diminished signs and symptoms of psychoses.

Adverse Reactions/Side Effects

CNS: NEUROLEPTIC MALIGNANT SYNDROME, sedation, extrapyramidal reactions, tardive dyskinesia. **EENT:** blurred vision, dry eyes, lens opacities, pigmentary retinopathy (high doses). **CV:** ARRHYTHMIAS, QTC PROLONGATION, hypotension, tachycardia. **GI:** constipation, dry mouth, anorexia, drug-induced hepatitis, ileus, weight gain. **GU:** urinary retention, priapism. **Derm:** photosensitivity, pigment changes, rashes. **Endo:** galactorrhea, amenorrhea. **Hemat:** AGRANULOCYTOSIS, leukopenia. **Metab:** hyperthermia. **Misc:** allergic reactions.

PHYSICAL THERAPY IMPLICATIONS

Examination and Evaluation

- Watch for signs of neuroleptic malignant syndrome, including hyperthermia, diaphoresis, generalized muscle rigidity, altered mental status, tachycardia, changes in blood pressure (BP), and incontinence. Symptoms typically occur within 4–14 days after initiation of drug therapy, but can occur at any time during drug use. Report these signs to the physician or nursing staff immediately.
- Assess heart rate, ECG, and heart sounds, especially during exercise (See Appendices G, H). Report immediately a rapid heart rate (tachycardia) or signs of other arrhythmias, including palpitations, chest discomfort, shortness of breath, fainting, and fatigue/weakness.
- Monitor signs of agranulocytosis and leukopenia, including fever, sore throat, mucosal lesions, and other signs of infection. Report these signs to the physician or nursing staff immediately.
- Assess motor function, and be alert for extrapyramidal symptoms. Report these symptoms immediately, especially tardive dyskinesia, because this problem may be irreversible. Common extrapyramidal symptoms include:
  - Tardive dyskinesia (uncontrolled rhythmic movement of mouth, face, and extremities, lip smacking or puckering, puffing of cheeks, uncontrolled chewing, rapid or worm-like movements of tongue).
  - Pseudoparkinsonism (shuffling gait, rigidity, tremor, pill-rolling motion, loss of balance control, difficulty speaking or swallowing, mask-like face).
  - Akathisia (restlessness or desire to keep moving).
  - Other dystonias and dyskinesias (dystonic muscle spasms, twisting motions, twitching, inability to move eyes, weakness of arms or legs).
- Monitor signs of allergic reactions, including pulmonary symptoms (laryngeal edema, wheezing, dyspnea) or skin reactions (rash, pruritus, urticaria). Notify physician or nursing staff immediately if these reactions occur.
- Assess BP periodically, and compare to normal values (See Appendix F). Report low BP (hypotension), especially if patient experiences dizziness or syncope.
- Periodically assess body weight and other anthropometric measures (body mass index, body composition). Report a rapid or unexplained weight gain or increased body fat.

Interventions

- Guard against falls and trauma (hip fractures, head injury, and so forth) caused by drowsiness, blurred vision, or extrapyramidal symptoms; implement fall-prevention strategies (See Appendix E).
- Because of the risk of arrhythmias and abnormal BP responses, use caution during aerobic exercise and other forms of therapeutic exercise. Assess exercise tolerance frequently (BP, heart rate, fatigue levels), and terminate exercise immediately if any untoward responses occur (See Appendix L).
- To minimize orthostatic hypotension, patient should move slowly when assuming a more upright position.
- This drug impairs body temperature regulation; use care during exercise, and during other activities

that increase body temperature (hot whirlpools, saunas, and so forth).

- Causes photosensitivity; use care if administering UV treatments. Advise patient to avoid direct sunlight and use sunscreens and protective clothing.
- Help patient and family/caregivers explore nonpharmacologic methods (exercise, counseling, support groups) to reduce schizophrenic episodes.

Patient/Client-Related Instruction

- Advise patient to avoid alcohol and other CNS depressants because of the increased risk of sedation and adverse effects.
- Advise patient about the likelihood of GI reactions, including constipation, dry mouth, and loss of appetite. Instruct patient to report severe or prolonged GI problems, and to also report signs of drug-induced hepatitis such as abdominal pain, severe nausea and vomiting, yellow skin or eyes, fever, sore throat, malaise, weakness, facial edema, lethargy, and unusual bleeding or bruising.
- Instruct patient to report other problematic side effects such as prolonged or severe vision problems, excessive sedation, dry eyes, urinary retention, painful/sustained erections, nipple discharge, menstrual disturbances, or skin reactions (rash, changes in pigmentation).

Pharmacokinetics

Absorption: Absorption from tablets is variable; may be better with oral liquid formulations.
Distribution: Widely distributed, high concentrations in the CNS. Crosses the placenta and enters breast milk.
Protein Binding: ≥90%.
Metabolism and Excretion: Highly metabolized by the liver and GI mucosa.
Half-life: 21–24 hr.

TIME/ACTION PROFILE (antipsychotic effects)

ROUTE	ONSET	PEAK	DURATION
PO	unknown	unknown	8–12 hr

Contraindications/Precautions

Contraindicated in: Hypersensitivity; Cross-sensitivity with other phenothiazines may exist; Angle-closure glaucoma; Bone marrow depression; Severe liver or cardiovascular disease; Known alcohol intolerance (concentrate only); Concurrent fluvoxamine, propranolol, pindolol, fluoxetine, other agents known to inhibit the CYP450 2D6 enzyme, or agents known to prolong the QTc interval (risk of life-threatening arrhythmias); Hypokalemia (correct prior to use); QTc interval >450 msec.
Use Cautiously in: Debilitated patients; Glaucoma; Urinary retention; Diabetes mellitus; Patients with risk factors for electrolyte imbalance (dehydration, diuretic therapy); Respiratory disease; Prostatic hyperplasia; CNS tumors; Epilepsy; Intestinal obstruction; OB/Lactation: Safety not established. Recommend discontinue drug or bottle feed; Geri: May be at ↑ risk for extrapyramidal and CNS adverse effects; appears on Beers' list; ↑ risk of mortality in elderly patients treated for dementia-related psychosis.

Interactions

Drug-Drug: Concurrent **fluvoxamine, propranolol, pindolol, fluoxetine,** other **agents known to inhibit the CYP450 2D6 enzyme,** or **agents known to prolong the QTc interval** (risk of life-threatening arrhythmias). **Diuretics** ↑ the risk of electrolyte imbalance and arrhythmias. Additive hypotension with other **antihypertensives, nitrates,** and acute ingestion of **alcohol.** Additive CNS depression with other **CNS depressants,** including **alcohol, antihistamines, opioid analgesics, sedative/hypnotics,** and **general anesthetics.** Additive anticholinergic effects with other **drugs possessing anticholinergic properties,** including **antihistamines, antidepressants, atropine, haloperidol,** other **phenothiazines,** and **disopyramide. Lithium** ↓ blood levels of thioridazine. Thioridazine may mask early signs of **lithium** toxicity and ↑ the risk of extrapyramidal reactions. ↑ risk of agranulocytosis with **antithyroid agents.** Concurrent use with **epinephrine** may result in severe hypotension and tachycardia. May ↓ the effectiveness of **levodopa.**

Route/Dosage

PO (Adults and Children >12 yr): 50–100 mg tid initially; may be gradually ↑ to a maintenance dose of up to 800 mg/day.
PO (Children): 0.5 mg/kg/day in divided doses initially; may be gradually ↑ to a maintenance dose of up to 3 mg/kg/day.

Availability (generic available)

Tablets: 10 mg, 15 mg, 25 mg, 50 mg, 100 mg, 150 mg, 200 mg. **Oral suspension:** 10 mg/5 mL, 25 mg/5 mL, 100 mg/5 mL. **Concentrated oral solution:** 30 mg/mL, 100 mg/mL.

HIGH ALERT

thiotepa (thye-oh-tep-a)

Thioplex

Classification

Therapeutic: antineoplastics
Pharmacologic: alkylating agents

T

Indications

Bladder Instillation: Management/prophylaxis of superficial tumors of the bladder after local resection. **IV:** Breast and ovarian cancer (palliative). **Intracavitary Instillation:** Prevention of recurrent malignant effusions in pleura, pericardium, or peritoneum.

Action

Disrupts protein, DNA, and RNA synthesis by cross-linking strands of DNA and RNA (cell-cycle phase–nonspecific). **Therapeutic Effects:** Death of rapidly replicating cells, particularly malignant ones. Has immunosuppressive properties.

Adverse Reactions/Side Effects

CNS: dizziness, headache, blurred vision. **EENT:** throat tightness. **GI:** anorexia, nausea, stomatitis, vomiting. **GU:** gonadal suppression, dysuria, urinary retention. **Derm:** alopecia, hives, pruritus, rash. **Hemat:** anemia, leukopenia, thrombocytopenia. **Local:** pain at IV site, pain at site of intracavitary instillation. **Metab:** hyperuricemia. **Misc:** allergic reactions, fever, fatigue, weakness.

PHYSICAL THERAPY IMPLICATIONS

Examination and Evaluation

- Watch for signs of leukopenia (fever, sore throat, signs of infection), thrombocytopenia (bruising, nose bleeds, bleeding gums), or unusual weakness and fatigue that might be due to anemia. Report these signs to the physician or nursing staff immediately.
- Monitor signs of allergic reactions, including pulmonary symptoms (tightness in the throat and chest, wheezing, cough, dyspnea) or skin reactions (rash, pruritus, urticaria). Notify physician or nursing staff immediately if these reactions occur.
- Assess dizziness that might affect gait, balance, and other functional activities (See Appendix C). Report balance problems and functional limitations to the physician and nursing staff, and caution the patient and family/caregivers to guard against falls and trauma.
- Assess IV site during and after IV administration, and report signs of phlebitis or other injection-site reactions (local pain, swelling, inflammation). Also report prolonged or severe pain that might occur if this drug is administered into the bladder or other body cavity.

Interventions

- For patients who are medically able to begin exercise, implement appropriate resistive exercises and aerobic training to maintain muscle strength and aerobic capacity during cancer chemotherapy or to help restore function after chemotherapy.

Patient/Client-Related Instruction

- Instruct patient to guard against infection (frequent hand washing, etc.), and to avoid crowds and contact with persons with contagious diseases.
- Advise patient and family/caregivers that fatigue and weakness are likely, and may be severe. Implement assistive devices (walker, cane, wheelchair) as needed to help maintain mobility and prevent falls.
- Advise patient about the likelihood of GI problems (nausea, vomiting, loss of appetite, irritation in/around the mouth) or skin reactions (rash, hair loss, itching, hives). Instruct patient to report excessive or unusual GI problems or skin reactions.
- Instruct patient or family/caregivers to report other side effects such as severe or prolonged headache, blurred vision, throat tightness, fever, or problems with urination (urine retention, difficult/painful urination).

Pharmacokinetics

Absorption: Variably absorbed following instillation (10–100%).

Distribution: Unknown.

Metabolism and Excretion: Extensively metabolized (primarily to active metabolite, TEPA).

Half-life: Thiotepa, 2.4 hr; TEPA, 15.7–17.6 hr.

TIME/ACTION PROFILE (noted as effects on blood counts; effects after intracavitary administration are highly variable)

ROUTE	ONSET	PEAK	DURATION
IV	10 days (up to 30 days)	14 days	21 days

Contraindications/Precautions

Contraindicated in: Hypersensitivity; Pregnancy or lactation.

Use Cautiously in: Patients with childbearing potential; Active infections; ↓ bone marrow reserve; Other chronic debilitating illnesses; Severe hepatic or renal disease.

Interactions

Drug-Drug: ↑ bone marrow depression with other **antineoplastics** or **radiation therapy.** May prolong apnea after **succinylcholine.**

Route/Dosage

Bladder Instillation

Intravesical: (Adults): 60 mg retained for 2 hr weekly for 4 wk; course may be repeated 2–3 times cautiously (bone marrow depression may occur).

Palliative Therapy of Breast, Ovarian Cancer

IV (Adults): 300–400 mcg/kg q 1–4 wk or 200 mcg/kg daily for 4–5 days q 2–4 wk.

Malignant Effusions

Intracavitary: (Adults): 600–800 mcg/kg q 1–4 wk (range 70–800 mcg/kg).

Availability (generic available)

Injection: 15 mg/vial.

thiothixene (thye-oh-thiks-een)

Navane

Classification

Therapeutic: antipsychotics (conventional)
Pharmacologic: thioxanthenes

Indications

Schizophrenia. Considered 2nd-line treatment after failure with atypical antipsychotics. **Unlabeled Use:** Other psychotic disorders, bipolar disorder.

Action

Alters the effect of dopamine in the CNS. **Therapeutic Effects:** Diminished signs and symptoms of psychoses.

Adverse Reactions/Side Effects

CNS: NEUROLEPTIC MALIGNANT SYNDROME, extrapyramidal reactions, sedation, tardive dyskinesia, seizures. **EENT:** blurred vision, dry eyes, lens opacities. **CV:** hypotension, tachycardia, nonspecific ECG changes. **GI:** constipation, dry mouth, anorexia, ileus, nausea. **GU:** urinary retention. **Derm:** photosensitivity, pigment changes, rashes. **Endo:** breast enlargement, galactorrhea. **Hemat:** leukocytosis, leukopenia. **Metab:** hyperpyrexia. **Misc:** allergic reactions.

PHYSICAL THERAPY IMPLICATIONS

Examination and Evaluation

- Watch for signs of neuroleptic malignant syndrome, including hyperthermia, diaphoresis, generalized muscle rigidity, altered mental status, tachycardia, changes in blood pressure (BP), and incontinence. Symptoms typically occur within 4–14 days after initiation of drug therapy, but can occur at any time during drug use. Report these signs to the physician immediately.
- Assess motor function, and be alert for extrapyramidal symptoms. Report these symptoms immediately, especially tardive dyskinesia, because this problem may be irreversible. Common extrapyramidal symptoms include:
  - Tardive dyskinesia (uncontrolled rhythmic movement of mouth, face, and extremities, lip smacking or puckering, puffing of cheeks, uncontrolled chewing, rapid or worm-like movements of tongue).
  - Pseudoparkinsonism (shuffling gait, rigidity, tremor, pill-rolling motion, loss of balance control, difficulty speaking or swallowing, mask-like face).
  - Akathisia (restlessness or desire to keep moving).
  - Other dystonias and dyskinesias (dystonic muscle spasms, twisting motions, twitching, inability to move eyes, weakness of arms or legs).
- Be alert for new seizures or increased seizure activity, especially at the onset of drug treatment. Document the number, duration, and severity of seizures, and report these findings to the physician immediately.
- Assess heart rate, ECG, and heart sounds, especially during exercise (See Appendices G, H). Report immediately a rapid heart rate (tachycardia) or signs of other arrhythmias, including palpitations, chest discomfort, shortness of breath, fainting, and fatigue/weakness.
- Assess BP periodically and compare to normal values (See Appendix F). Report low BP (hypotension), especially if patient experiences dizziness or syncope.
- Watch for signs of leukocytosis and leukopenia, including fever, sore throat, mucosal lesions, and other signs of infection. Report these signs to the physician immediately.
- Monitor signs of allergic reactions, including pulmonary symptoms (laryngeal edema, wheezing, dyspnea) or skin reactions (rash, pruritus, urticaria). Notify physician immediately if these reactions occur.

Interventions

- Guard against falls and trauma (hip fractures, head injury, and so forth) caused by drowsiness, blurred vision, or extrapyramidal symptoms; implement fall prevention strategies (See Appendix E).
- Because of the risk of arrhythmias and abnormal BP responses, use caution during aerobic exercise and other forms of therapeutic exercise. Assess exercise tolerance frequently (BP, heart rate, fatigue levels), and terminate exercise immediately if any untoward responses occur (See Appendix L).
- To minimize orthostatic hypotension, patient should move slowly when assuming a more upright position.
- This drug impairs body temperature regulation; use care during exercise, and during other activities that increase body temperature (hot whirlpools, saunas, and so forth).
- Causes photosensitivity; use care if administering UV treatments. Advise patient to avoid direct sunlight and use sunscreens and protective clothing.
- Help patient and family/caregivers explore non-pharmacologic methods (exercise, counseling, support groups) to reduce schizophrenic episodes and other mood disorders.

T

Patient/Client-Related Instruction

- Advise patient to avoid alcohol and other CNS depressants because of the increased risk of sedation and adverse effects.
- Instruct patient to report other problematic side effects such as severe or prolonged nausea, vision problems, excessive sedation, dry eyes, urinary retention, nipple discharge, breast enlargement, skin reactions (rash, changes in pigmentation), or GI problems (nausea, dry mouth, constipation, loss of appetite).

Pharmacokinetics

Absorption: Well absorbed following oral administration.

Distribution: Widely distributed; crosses the placenta.

Metabolism and Excretion: Mainly metabolized by the liver.

Half-life: 30 hr.

TIME/ACTION PROFILE (antipsychotic effects)

ROUTE	ONSET	PEAK	DURATION
PO	days–wks	unknown	unknown
IM	1–6 hr	unknown	unknown

Contraindications/Precautions

Contraindicated in: Hypersensitivity to thiothixene or other phenothiazines (cross-sensitivity may occur); Circulatory collapse; Blood dyscrasias; Central nervous system depression.

Use Cautiously in: Geri: Geriatric or debilitated patients (initial dose reduction may be required); ↑ risk of mortality in elderly patients treated for dementia-related psychosis; Diabetes mellitus; Respiratory disease; Prostatic hypertrophy; CNS tumors; Epilepsy; Intestinal obstruction; OB/Lactation/Pedi: Safety not established. Discontinue drug or bottle-feed.

Interactions

Drug-Drug: Additive hypotension with **antihypertensives,** acute ingestion of **alcohol,** and **nitrates.** Additive hypotension may occur if **epinephrine** is given to treat hypotension. Additive CNS depression with other **CNS depressants,** including **alcohol, antihistamines, antidepressants, opioid analgesics,** and **sedative/hypnotics.** Additive anticholinergic effects with other **drugs having anticholinergic properties,** including **antihistamines, antidepressants, quinidine,** or **disopyramide.** May ↓ the effectiveness of **levodopa.** ↑ risk of cardiac effects with **quinidine.**

Drug-Natural: Concomitant use of **kava, valerian, skullcap, chamomile,** or **hops** can ↑ CNS depression.

Route/Dosage

PO (Adults): *Mild conditions*—2 mg tid (up to 15 mg/day if necessary; *severe conditions*—5 mg bid [up to 20–30 mg/day]; not to exceed 60 mg/day).

Availability (generic available)

Capsules: 1 mg, 2 mg, 5 mg, 10 mg, 20 mg. **Concentrated oral solution:** 5 mg/mL in 30- and 120-mL containers.

thyroid (thye-royd)

Armour thyroid, Thyrar, Thyroid Strong, Westhroid

Classification

Therapeutic: hormones

Pharmacologic: thyroid preparations

Indications

Thyroid supplementation in hypothyroidism. Treatment or suppression of euthyroid goiters and thyroid cancer. Diagnostic agent for suppression tests to differentiate mild hyperthyroidism from thyroid gland autonomy.

Action

Replacement of or supplementation to endogenous thyroid hormones. Principal effect is increasing metabolic rate of body tissues: Promote gluconeogenesis, ↑ utilization and mobilization of glycogen stores, Stimulate protein synthesis, Promote cell growth and differentiation, Aid in the development of the brain and CNS. Contains T_3 (triiodothyronine) and T_4 (thyroxine) activity. **Therapeutic Effects:** Replacement in deficiency states with restoration of normal hormonal balance.

Adverse Reactions/Side Effects

Usually only seen when excessive doses cause iatrogenic hyperthyroidism

CNS: insomnia, irritability, headache. **CV:** arrhythmias, tachycardia, angina pectoris. **GI:** abdominal cramps, diarrhea, vomiting. **Derm:** hyperhidrosis. **Endo:** hyperthyroidism, menstrual irregularities. **Metab:** weight loss, heat intolerance. **MS:** accelerated bone maturation in children.

PHYSICAL THERAPY IMPLICATIONS

Examination and Evaluation

- Monitor and report signs of excessive or inadequate dosing. Excessive doses mimic hyperthyroidism, as indicated by nervousness, weight loss, muscle wasting, tachycardia, and heat intolerance. Inadequate doses mimic hypothyroidism, as indicated by lethargy, weight gain, bradycardia, and cold intolerance.
- Assess heart rate, ECG, and heart sounds, especially during exercise (See Appendices G, H). Report any rhythm disturbances or symptoms of increased

arrhythmias, including palpitations, chest discomfort, shortness of breath, fainting, and fatigue/weakness.

- Assess episodes of angina pectoris at rest and during exercise. Attempt to determine if pain is drug related, or caused by cardiovascular dysfunction (e.g., angina that occurs during exercise).
- Assess height in children periodically; inform physician of delayed growth that might indicate premature skeletal maturation and closure of epiphyseal plates.
- Monitor and report signs of CNS toxicity, including irritability and sleep loss. Sustained or severe CNS signs are typically consistent with hyperthyroidism, and may require an adjustment in drug dose.

Interventions

- Because of the risk of arrhythmias and angina, use caution during aerobic exercise and endurance conditioning. Assess heart rate and exercise tolerance frequently, and terminate exercise immediately if any untoward responses occur (See Appendix L).

Patient/Client-Related Instruction

- Caution patient about the risk of increased sweating (hyperhidrosis), and advise patient about proper skin care (thoroughly cleanse and dry the affected areas; apply astringent powders if necessary).
- Instruct patient to report other troublesome side effects, including severe or prolonged headache, menstrual irregularities, or GI problems (nausea, vomiting, abdominal cramps).

Pharmacokinetics

Absorption: Levothyroxine is variably (50–80%) absorbed from the GI tract. Liothyronine is well absorbed.
Distribution: Distributed into most body tissues. Thyroid hormones do not readily cross the placenta; minimal amounts enter breast milk.
Metabolism and Excretion: Metabolized by the liver and other tissues. Thyroid hormone undergoes enterohepatic recirculation and is excreted in the feces via the bile.
Half-life: T_3 *(liothyronine)*—1–2 days; T_4 *(thyroxine)*—6–7 days.

TIME/ACTION PROFILE

ROUTE	ONSET	PEAK	DURATION
Levothyroxine PO	unknown	1–3 wk	1–3 wk
Liothyronine PO	unknown	24–72 hr	72 hr

Contraindications/Precautions

Contraindicated in: Hypersensitivity; Recent MI; Hyperthyroidism; Hypersensitivity to beef (Thyrar product).
Use Cautiously in: Cardiovascular disease (initiate therapy with lower doses); Severe renal insufficiency; Uncorrected adrenocortical disorders; Geri: Geriatric patients are extremely sensitive to thyroid hormones; initial dosage should be reduced.

Interactions

Drug-Drug: Bile acid sequestrants ↓ absorption of orally administered thyroid preparations. Alters the effectiveness of **warfarin** (INR will ↑ with thyroid hormone supplementation). May ↑ requirement for **insulin** or **oral hypoglycemic agents** in diabetics. Concurrent **estrogen** therapy may ↑ thyroid replacement requirements. ↑ cardiovascular effects with **adrenergics** (sympathomimetics).
Drug-Food: Foods or supplements containing high amounts of calcium, iron, magnesium, or zinc may bind thyroid hormones and prevent complete absorption.

Route/Dosage

Each 1 gr = 60 mg and is equivalent to approximately 100 mcg of levothyroxine (T_4) or 25 mcg of liothyronine (T_3).

Thyroid

PO (Adults and Children): *Hypothyroidism*—60 mg/day; ↑ q 4 wk by 30 mg; usual maintenance dose is 60–120 mg/day. *Myxedema/hypothyroidism with cardiovascular disease*—15 mg/day initially; ↑ by 30 mg/day q 2 wk, then may ↑ by 30–60 mg q 2 wk; usual maintenance dose is 60–120 mg/day.
PO (Geriatric Patients): 7.5–15 mg/day initially; may double dose q 6–8 wk until desired effect is obtained.

Availability

Tables (regular): 15 mg, 30 mg, 60 mg, 90 mg, 120 mg, 180 mg, 240 mg, 300 mg.

tiagabine (tye-ag-a-been)

Gabitril

Classification
Therapeutic: anticonvulsants

Indications

Adjunctive treatment of partial seizures.

Action

Enhances the activity of gamma-aminobutyric acid, an inhibitory neurotransmitter. **Therapeutic Effects:** ↓ frequency of seizures.

T

Adverse Reactions/Side Effects

CNS: dizziness, drowsiness, nervousness, weakness, cognitive impairment, confusion, difficulty concentrating, hallucinations, headache, mental depression, personality disorder. **EENT:** abnormal vision, ear pain, tinnitus. **Resp:** dyspnea, epistaxis. **CV:** chest pain, edema, hypertension, palpitations, syncope, tachycardia. **GI:** abdominal pain, gingivitis, nausea, stomatitis. **GU:** dysmenorrhea, dysuria, metrorrhagia, urinary incontinence. **Derm:** alopecia, dry skin, rash, sweating. **Metab:** weight gain, weight loss. **MS:** arthralgia, neck pain. **Neuro:** ataxia, tremors. **Misc:** allergic reactions, chills, lymphadenopathy.

PHYSICAL THERAPY IMPLICATIONS

Examination and Evaluation

- Document the number, duration, and severity of seizures to help determine if this drug is effective in reducing seizure activity.
- Assess dizziness, ataxia, or tremors that might affect gait, balance, and other functional activities (See Appendix C). Report balance problems and functional limitations to the physician, and caution the patient and family/caregivers to guard against falls and trauma.
- Monitor daytime drowsiness, confusion, hallucinations, cognitive impairment, concentration problems, mental depression, or other changes in personality. Repeated or excessive symptoms may require change in dose or medication.
- Monitor signs of allergic reactions, including pulmonary symptoms (tightness in the throat and chest, wheezing, cough, dyspnea) or skin reactions (rash, pruritus, urticaria). Notify physician if these reactions occur.
- Assess blood pressure (BP) and compare to normal values (See Appendix F). Report a sustained increase in BP (hypertension).
- Assess heart rate, ECG, and heart sounds, especially during exercise (See Appendices G, H). Report rapid heart rate (tachycardia) or signs of other arrhythmias, including palpitations, chest discomfort, shortness of breath, fainting, and fatigue/weakness.
- Assess peripheral edema using girth measurements, volume displacement, and measurement of pitting edema (See Appendix N). Report increased swelling in feet and ankles or a sudden increase in body weight due to fluid retention.
- Assess any joint pain or neck pain to rule out musculoskeletal pathology; that is, try to determine if pain is drug induced rather than caused by anatomic or biomechanical problems.
- Periodically assess body weight and other anthropometric measures (body mass index, body composition). Report a rapid or unexplained weight loss or weight gain.

Interventions

- Guard against falls and trauma (hip fractures, head injury, and so forth), especially if dizziness or ataxia affect gait and balance. Implement fall-prevention strategies, especially if balance is impaired (See appendix E).

Patient/Client-Related Instruction

- Advise patient to avoid alcohol and other CNS depressants because of the increased risk of sedation and adverse effects.
- Advise patients on prolonged antiseizure therapy not to discontinue medication without consulting their physician. Abrupt withdrawal may cause increased seizures.
- Advise patient about the risk of daytime drowsiness and decreased attention and mental focus. Use care if driving or in other activities that require strong concentration and fast responses.
- Instruct patient and family/caregivers to report other troublesome side effects such as severe or prolonged headache, double vision, ringing/buzzing in the ears (tinnitus), nosebleeds, swollen/tender glands, chills, menstrual irregularities, urinary problems, GI problems (nausea, abdominal pain, inflammation in/around the mouth), or skin reactions (rash, dry skin, hair loss, increased sweating).

Pharmacokinetics

Absorption: 90% absorbed following oral administration.
Distribution: Unknown.
Protein Binding: 96%.
Metabolism and Excretion: Mostly metabolized by the liver; 2% excreted unchanged in urine.
Half-life: *Without enzyme-inducing antiepileptic drugs*—7–9 hr; *with enzyme-inducing antiepileptic drugs*—4–7 hr.

TIME/ACTION PROFILE (blood levels)

ROUTE	ONSET	PEAK	DURATION
PO	unknown	45 min	unknown

Contraindications/Precautions

Contraindicated in: Hypersensitivity.
Use Cautiously in: Hepatic impairment (↓ dose/↑ interval may be necessary); Patients receiving concurrent non–enzyme-inducing antiepileptic drug therapy such as valproates (may require lower doses and/or slower titration); Using tiagabine for off-label uses or other conditions leading to increased levels (may ↑ risk of new onset seizures); OB/Pedi: Pregnancy, lactation, or children <12 yr (safety not established).

Interactions

Drug-Drug: Carbamazepine, phenytoin, primidone, and **phenobarbital** induce metabolism and ↓ blood levels; although concurrent therapy is usually necessary, adjustments may be required when altering regimens.

Route/Dosage

PO (Adults >18 yr): 4 mg once daily initially for 1 wk; may ↑ by 4–8 mg/day at weekly intervals, up to 56 mg/day in 2–4 divided doses.
PO (Children 12–18 yr): 4 mg once daily initially for 1 wk; may ↑ by 4 mg/day after 1 wk, then may ↑ by 4–8 mg/day at weekly intervals, up to 32 mg/day in 2–4 divided doses.

Availability

Tablets: 2 mg, 4 mg, 12 mg, 16 mg, 20 mg.

ticarcillin/clavulanate

(tye-kar-**sil**-in/klav-yoo-**lan**-ate)
Timentin

Classification
Therapeutic: anti-infectives
Pharmacologic: extended-spectrum penicillins

Indications

Treatment of Skin and skin structure infections; Bone and joint infections; Septicemia; Lower respiratory tract, Intra-abdominal, gynecologic, and urinary tract infections.

Action

Binds to bacterial cell wall membrane, causing cell death. Addition of clavulanate enhances resistance to beta-lactamase, an enzyme that can inactivate penicillins. **Therapeutic Effects:** Bactericidal action. **Spectrum:** Similar to penicillin but extended to include several gram-negative aerobic pathogens, notably: *Pseudomonas aeruginosa*, *Escherichia coli*, *Citrobacter*, *Enterobacter*, *Haemophilus influenzae*, *Klebsiella*, *Serratia marcescens*. Active against some anaerobic bacteria, including bacteroides.

Adverse Reactions/Side Effects

CNS: SEIZURES (HIGH DOSES), confusion, lethargy. **CV:** CHF, arrhythmias. **GI:** PSEUDOMEMBRANOUS COLITIS, diarrhea, nausea. **GU:** hematuria (children only). **Derm:** rashes, urticaria. **F and E:** hypokalemia, hypernatremia. **Hemat:** bleeding, blood dyscrasias, increased bleeding time. **Local:** phlebitis. **Metab:** metabolic alkalosis. **Misc:** HYPERSENSITIVITY REACTIONS, INCLUDING ANAPHYLAXIS, superinfection.

PHYSICAL THERAPY IMPLICATIONS

Examination and Evaluation

- Watch for seizures; notify physician immediately if patient develops or increases seizure activity.
- Assess signs of congestive heart failure (CHF), such as dyspnea, rales/crackles, peripheral edema, jugular venous distention, and exercise intolerance. Report these signs to the physician immediately.
- Monitor signs of pseudomembranous colitis, including diarrhea, abdominal pain, fever, pus or mucus in stools, and other severe or prolonged GI problems (nausea, vomiting, heartburn). Notify physician or nursing staff immediately of these signs.
- Monitor signs of hypersensitivity reactions and anaphylaxis, including pulmonary symptoms (tightness in the throat and chest, wheezing, cough dyspnea) or skin reactions (rash, pruritus, urticaria). Notify physician or nursing staff immediately if these reactions occur.
- Assess heart rate, ECG, and heart sounds, especially during exercise (See Appendices G, H). Report any rhythm disturbances or symptoms of increased arrhythmias, including palpitations, chest discomfort, shortness of breath, fainting, and fatigue/weakness.
- Monitor any unusual bleeding (bruising, nose bleeds, bleeding gums) that might indicate thrombocytopenia. Also monitor signs of other blood dyscrasias such as leukopenia and neutropenia (fever, sore throat, signs of infection). Report these signs to the physician.
- Monitor neuromuscular signs of acid-base and electrolyte imbalances (alkalosis, hypokalemia, hypernatremia), including headache, lethargy, weakness, cramping, and muscle hyperexcitability and tetany. Notify physician immediately if these signs occur.
- Assess confusion that might affect gait, balance, and other functional activities (See Appendix D). Report balance problems and functional limitations to the physician and nursing staff, and caution the patient and family/caregivers to guard against falls and trauma.
- Monitor IV injection site for pain, swelling, and irritation. Report prolonged or excessive injection site reactions to the physician.

Interventions

- Because of the risk of CHF and arrhythmias, use caution during aerobic exercise and other forms of therapeutic exercise. Assess exercise tolerance frequently (blood pressure, heart rate, fatigue levels), and terminate exercise immediately if any untoward responses occur (See Appendix L).
- Always wash hands thoroughly and disinfect equipment (whirlpools, electrotherapeutic devices, treatment tables, and so forth) to help prevent the spread of infection. Employ universal precautions or isolation procedures as indicated for specific patients.

Patient/Client-Related Instruction

- Instruct patient to notify physician immediately of signs of superinfection, including black, furry overgrowth on tongue, vaginal itching or discharge, and loose or foul-smelling stools.
- Instruct children and family/caregivers to report blood in the urine (hematuria).
- Instruct patient and family/caregivers to report other troublesome side effects such as severe or prolonged lethargy or skin problems (rash, itching).

Pharmacokinetics

Absorption: IV administration results in complete bioavailability.
Distribution: Widely distributed. Enters CSF well when meninges are inflamed. Crosses the placenta; enters breast milk in low concentrations.
Metabolism and Excretion: 10% of ticarcillin is metabolized by the liver; 90% excreted unchanged by the kidneys. Clavulanate is metabolized by the liver.
Half-life: *Ticarcillin*—1.1 hr (increased in renal impairment); *clavulanate*—1.1 hr.

TIME/ACTION PROFILE (blood levels)

ROUTE	ONSET	PEAK	DURATION
IV	rapid	end of infusion	4–6 hr

Contraindications/Precautions

Contraindicated in: Hypersensitivity to penicillins (cross-sensitivity with cephalosporins may occur).
Use Cautiously in: Renal impairment (dose reduction and/or ↑ interval required if CCr <60 mL/min); CHF (due to high sodium content); Pedi: Children <3 mo (safety and effectiveness not established); OB/Lactation: Safety not established.

Interactions

Drug-Drug: Probenecid ↓ renal excretion and ↑ blood levels.

Route/Dosage

Ticarcillin/clavulanate contains 4.51–6 mEq sodium/g and 0.15 mEq potassium/g of ticarcillin/clavulanate. 3 g ticarcillin plus 100 mg clavulanate labeled as 3.1 g combined potency. Dosing is based on ticarcillin component.
IV (Adults and Children >16 yr): 3 g ticarcillin q 4–6 hr.
IV (Children 3 mo–16 yr): *<60 kg*—Mild-to-moderate infection: 50 mg ticarcillin/kg q 6 hr; severe infection: 50 mg ticarcillin/kg q 4 hr. *≥60 kg*—Mild-to-moderate infection: 3 g ticarcillin q 6 hr; severe infection: 3 g ticarcillin q 4 hr.

Renal Impairment

IV (Adults): Give loading dose of 3 g ticarcillin × 1 dose, followed by maintenance dose based on CCr. *CCr 30–60 mL/min*—2 g ticarcillin q 4 hr; *10–30 mL/min*—2 g ticarcillin q 8 hr; *CCr < 10 mL/min*—2 g ticarcillin q 12 hr; *CCr < 10 mL/min with hepatic dysfunction*—2 g ticarcillin q 24 hr; *Peritoneal dialysis*—3 g ticarcillin q 12 hr; *Hemodialysis*—2 g ticarcillin q 12 hr supplemented with 3 g ticarcillin after each dialysis session.

Availability

Powder for injection: 3.1-g vials, 31-g vials.
Premixed infusion: 3.1 g/100 mL.

ticlopidine (tye-**kloe**-pi-deen)

Ticlid

Classification
Therapeutic: antiplatelet agents
Pharmacologic: platelet aggregation inhibitors

Indications

Prevention of stroke in patients who have had a completed thrombotic stroke or precursors to stroke and are unable to tolerate aspirin. **Unlabeled Use:** Prevention of early restenosis in intracoronary stents.

Action

Inhibits platelet aggregation by altering the function of platelet membranes. Prolongs bleeding time.
Therapeutic Effects: ↓ incidence of stroke in high-risk patients.

Adverse Reactions/Side Effects

CNS: dizziness, headache, weakness. **EENT:** epistaxis, tinnitus. **GI:** diarrhea, abnormal liver function tests, anorexia, GI fullness, GI pain, nausea, vomiting.
GU: hematuria. **Derm:** rashes, ecchymoses, pruritus, urticaria. **Hemat:** AGRANULOCYTOSIS, APLASTIC ANEMIA, INTRACEREBRAL BLEEDING, NEUTROPENIA, bleeding, thrombocytopenia. **Metab:** hypercholesterolemia, hypertriglyceridemia.

PHYSICAL THERAPY IMPLICATIONS

Examination and Evaluation

- Assess for signs of bleeding and hemorrhage, including bleeding gums, nosebleeds, unusual bruising, black/tarry stools, hematuria, and a fall in hematocrit or blood pressure. Be especially alert for signs of intracranial bleeds, including sudden severe headache, confusion, nausea, vomiting, paralysis, numbness, speech problems, and visual disturbances. Notify physician or nursing staff immediately if these signs occur.
- Watch for signs of neutropenia or agranulocytosis (fever, sore throat, mucosal lesions, other signs of infection), thrombocytopenia (bruising, nose bleeds, bleeding gums), or unusual weakness and

fatigue that might be due to aplastic anemia or other blood dyscrasias. Report these signs to the physician or nursing staff immediately.

- Assess dizziness and weakness that might affect gait, balance, and other functional activities (See Appendix C). Report balance problems and functional limitations to the physician and nursing staff, and caution the patient and family/caregivers to guard against falls and trauma.

Interventions

- Use caution with any physical interventions that could increase bleeding, including wound débridement, chest percussion, joint mobilization, and application of local heat.
- Use caution during aerobic exercise in patients with a history of stroke or who are at risk for stroke. Assess exercise tolerance frequently (blood pressure, heart rate, fatigue levels, neurological signs), and terminate exercise immediately if any untoward responses occur (See Appendix L).

Patient/Client-Related Instruction

- Instruct patient to immediately report signs of GI bleeding, including abdominal pain, vomiting blood, blood in stools, or black, tarry stools.
- Remind patients to take medication as directed to reduce the risk of stroke even if they are asymptomatic.
- Counsel patients about additional interventions to help reduce the risk of stroke and other cardiovascular pathology, including regular exercise, weight loss, sodium restriction, stress reduction, moderation of alcohol consumption, and smoking cessation.
- Advise patient that this drug may cause problems in fat metabolism, including increased cholesterol and triglycerides. Remind patient that periodic blood tests may be needed to monitor plasma lipids.
- Instruct patient or family/caregivers to report other troublesome side effects such as severe or prolonged headache, ringing/buzzing in the ears (tinnitus), skin reactions (rash, itching, hives), or GI problems (nausea, vomiting, diarrhea, gastric pain, loss of appetite).

Pharmacokinetics

Absorption: >80% absorbed after oral administration.
Distribution: Unknown.
Protein Binding: 98%.
Metabolism and Excretion: Extensively metabolized by the liver; minimal excretion of unchanged drug by the kidneys.
Half-life: *Single dose*—12.6 hr; *multiple dosing*—4–5 days.

TIME/ACTION PROFILE (effect on platelet function)

ROUTE	ONSET	PEAK	DURATION
PO	within 4 days	8–11 days	2 wk

Contraindications/Precautions

Contraindicated in: Hypersensitivity; Bleeding disorders; Active bleeding; Severe liver disease.
Use Cautiously in: Risk of bleeding (trauma, surgery, history of ulcer disease); Renal or hepatic impairment (dosage adjustments may be necessary); Geri: Appears on Beers' list. Geriatric patients have increased sensitivity to ticlopidine; Pregnancy, lactation, or children <18 yr (safety not established).

Interactions

Drug-Drug: Aspirin potentiates the effect of ticlopidine on platelets (concurrent use not recommended). ↑ risk of bleeding with **heparins, warfarin, tirofiban, eptifibatide, clopidogrel,** or **thrombolytic agents. Cimetidine** ↓ metabolism of ticlopidine and may ↑ the risk of toxicity. Ticlopidine ↓ metabolism of **theophylline** and ↑ the risk of toxicity.
Drug-Food: Absorption of ticlopidine is ↑ by taking with **food.**

Route/Dosage

PO (Adults): 250 mg bid with food.

Availability

Tablets: 250 mg.

tigecycline (tye-ge-**sye**-kleen)

Tygacil

Classification
Therapeutic: anti-infectives
Pharmacologic: glycylcyclines

Indications

Complicated skin/skin structure infections or complicated intra-abdominal infections caused by susceptible bacteria.

Action

Inhibits bacterial protein synthesis by binding to the 30S ribosomal subunit. **Therapeutic Effects:** Resolution of infection. **Spectrum:** Active against the following gram-positive bacteria: *Enterococcus faecalis* (vancomycin-susceptible strains only), *Staphylococcus aureus, Streptococcus agalactiae, S. anginosus,* and *S. pyogenes.* Also active against these gram-positive organisms: *Citrobacter freundii, Enterobacter cloacae, Escherichia coli, Klebsiella oxytoca,*

T

and *K. pneumoniae*. Additionally active against the following anaerobes: *Bacteroides fragilis, B. thetaiotaomicron, B. uniformis, B. vulgatus, Clostridium perfringens,* and *Peptostreptococcus micros*.

Adverse Reactions/Side Effects

CNS: somnolence. **CV:** changes in heart rate, vasodilation. **GI:** PSEUDOMEMBRANOUS COLITIS, nausea, vomiting, altered taste, anorexia, dry mouth, jaundice. **GU:** ↑ creatinine. **Endo:** hyperglycemia. **F and E:** hypocalcemia, hyponatremia. **Local:** injection site reactions. **Misc:** allergic reactions.

PHYSICAL THERAPY IMPLICATIONS

Examination and Evaluation

- Monitor signs of pseudomembranous colitis, including diarrhea, abdominal pain, fever, pus or mucus in stools, and other severe or prolonged GI problems (nausea, vomiting, heartburn). Notify physician or nursing staff immediately of these signs.
- Monitor signs of allergic reactions, including pulmonary symptoms (tightness in the throat and chest, wheezing, cough, dyspnea) or skin reactions (rash, pruritus, urticaria). Notify physician or nursing staff immediately if these reactions occur.
- Assess heart rate, ECG, and heart sounds, especially during exercise (See Appendices G, H). Report any rhythm disturbances or symptoms of increased arrhythmias, including palpitations, chest discomfort, shortness of breath, fainting, and fatigue/weakness.
- Monitor signs of electrolyte imbalances such as low calcium or low sodium levels (hypocalcemia, hyponatremia, respectively). Signs include headache, lethargy, weakness, cramping, and muscle hyperexcitability and tetany. Notify physician immediately if these signs occur.
- Monitor level of alertness and report any severe or prolonged sleepiness or somnolence.
- Monitor IV injection site for pain, swelling, and irritation. Report prolonged or excessive injection site reactions to the physician.

Interventions

- Always wash hands thoroughly and disinfect equipment (whirlpools, electrotherapeutic devices, treatment tables, and so forth) to help prevent the spread of infection. Use universal precautions or isolation procedures as indicated for specific patients.
- Because of the risk of arrhythmias, use caution during aerobic exercise and other forms of therapeutic exercise. Assess exercise tolerance frequently (blood pressure, heart rate, fatigue levels), and terminate exercise immediately if any untoward responses occur (See Appendix L).

Patient/Client-Related Instruction

- Advise patient and family/caregivers about symptoms of hyperglycemia (confusion, drowsiness; flushed, dry skin; fruit-like breath odor; rapid, deep breathing, polyuria; loss of appetite; unusual thirst). Insulin dosages may need to be adjusted to prevent repeated episodes of hyperglycemia.
- Advise patient about the likelihood of GI reactions such as nausea, vomiting, loss of appetite, and altered taste. Instruct patient to report severe or prolonged GI problems.

Pharmacokinetics

Absorption: IV administration results in complete bioavailability.
Distribution: Widely distributed with good penetration into gallbladder, lung and colon; crosses the placenta.
Metabolism and Excretion: Minimal metabolism; primary route of elimination is biliary/fecal excretion of unchanged drug and metabolites (59%), 33% renal (22% unchanged).
Half-life: 27.1 hr (after 1 dose); 42.4 hr (after multiple doses).

TIME/ACTION PROFILE (blood levels)

ROUTE	ONSET	PEAK	DURATION
IV	rapid	end of infusion	12 hr

Contraindications/Precautions

Contraindicated in: Hypersensitivity; Pedi: Children <18 yr.
Use Cautiously in: Complicated intra-abdominal infections due to perforation; Severe hepatic impairment (reduced maintenance dose recommended); Geri: Older patients may be more sensitive to adverse effects; OB: Use in pregnancy only when potential maternal benefit outweighs fetal risk; use cautiously during lactation.

Interactions

Drug-Drug: May ↓ the effectiveness of **hormonal contraceptives.** Effects on **warfarin** are unknown (monitoring recommended).

Route/Dosage

IV (Adults >18 yr): 100 mg initially, then 50 mg every 12 hr for 5–14 days.

Hepatic Impairment

IV (Adults >18 yr): *Child-Pugh C*—100 mg initially, then 25 mg every 12 hr.

Availability

Lyophilized powder for reconstitution: 50 mg/5-mL vial.

tiludronate (tye-loo-droe-nate)

Skelid

Classification

Therapeutic: bone resorption inhibitors

Pharmacologic: bisphosphonates

Indications

Management of Paget's disease of the bone in patients with Serum alkaline phosphatase ≥2 times the upper limit of normal, Symptoms, Risk for complications.

Action

Inhibits resorption of bone by inhibiting osteoclast activity. **Therapeutic Effects:** ↓ progression of Paget's disease.

Adverse Reactions/Side Effects

CNS: anxiety, drowsiness, fatigue, insomnia, nervousness, syncope, vertigo, weakness. **EENT:** cataracts, conjunctivitis, glaucoma, pharyngitis, rhinitis, sinusitis. **Resp:** bronchitis. **CV:** chest pain, dependent edema, hypertension, peripheral edema. **GI:** abdominal pain, anorexia, constipation, diarrhea, dry mouth, dysphagia, esophageal ulcer, esophagitis, flatulence, gastric ulcer, gastritis, nausea, tooth disorder, vomiting. **GU:** urinary tract infection. **Derm:** flushing, increased sweating, pruritus, rash, skin disorder. **Endo:** hyperparathyroidism. **F and E:** hypocalcemia. **MS:** musculoskeletal pain, arthrosis, involuntary muscle contractions, osteonecrosis (primarily of jaw), pathological fractures. **Neuro:** paresthesia. **Misc:** infection.

PHYSICAL THERAPY IMPLICATIONS

Examination and Evaluation

- Assess any joint pain, muscle pain, or muscle spasms. Report persistent or increased musculoskeletal pain to determine presence of bone or joint pathology, including fracture. Be especially aware of possible mouth and jaw pain due to osteonecrosis of the jaw.
- Assess peripheral edema using girth measurements, volume displacement, and measurement of pitting edema (See Appendix N). Report increased swelling in feet and ankles or a sudden increase in body weight due to fluid retention.
- Assess blood pressure (BP) and compare to normal values (See Appendix F). Report a sustained increase in BP (hypertension).
- Assess vertigo, syncope, and drowsiness that might affect gait, balance, and other functional activities. Report balance problems and functional limitations to the physician, and caution the patient and family/caregivers to guard against falls and trauma.
- Assess signs of paresthesia (numbness, tingling) or muscle twitching. Perform objective tests, including electroneuromyography and sensory testing, to document any drug-related neuropathic changes.
- Monitor neuromuscular signs of low calcium levels (hypocalcemia), including headache, lethargy, weakness, cramping, and muscle hyperexcitability and tetany. Notify physician immediately if these signs occur.
- Be alert for signs of hyperparathyroidism, including excessive urination, fatigue, malaise, mental symptoms (depression, forgetfulness), GI problems (abdominal pain, nausea, vomiting, loss of appetite), kidney stones, and fragile bones. Report these signs to the physician.
- Monitor and report anxiety, nervousness, or other changes in mood and behavior.

Interventions

- Institute weight-bearing and resistance exercises as tolerated to maintain or increase bone mineral density. Start with low impact or aquatic programs in patients with extensive demineralization, and increase exercise intensity slowly to prevent fractures.
- Protect against falls and fractures (See Appendix E). Modify home environment (remove throw rugs, improve lighting, etc.) and provide assistive devices (cane, walker) or other protective devices as needed to improve balance and prevent falls.

Patient/Client-Related Instruction

- Encourage patient to modify behaviors that increase the risk of osteoporosis (stop smoking, reduce alcohol consumption).
- Advise patient about the benefits of proper diet in sustaining bone mineralization. If necessary, refer patient for nutritional counseling about supplemental calcium and vitamin D.
- Instruct patient on the importance of taking this drug exactly as directed, and to remain upright for 30 min following dose to facilitate passage to stomach and minimize risk of esophageal irritation.
- Instruct patient to notify physician about any vision disturbances or eye pain and inflammation.
- Instruct patient to report other side effects such as severe or prolonged headache, bronchitis, nasal/sinus irritation, difficulty swallowing, urinary tract infection, skin reactions (rash, itching, sweating, flushing), retrosternal pain, new/worsening heartburn, or other GI problems (nausea, vomiting, diarrhea, constipation, flatulence, abdominal pain).

Pharmacokinetics

Absorption: Rapidly but poorly absorbed following oral administration (6% bioavailability).

T

Distribution: Distributes to bone and soft tissue; subsequently is slowly released from bone.
Protein Binding: 90% protein binding.
Metabolism and Excretion: Excreted mostly in urine.
Half-life: 150 hr.

TIME/ACTION PROFILE (blood levels)

ROUTE	ONSET	PEAK	DURATION
PO	unknown	within 2 hr	unknown

Contraindications/Precautions

Contraindicated in: Hypersensitivity; Severe renal impairment (CCr <30 mL/min).
Use Cautiously in: Dental surgery (may ↑ risk of jaw osteonecrosis); OB/Lactation/Pedi: Safety not established.

Interactions

Drug-Drug: Absorption is ↓ by concurrent administration of **calcium supplements, aspirin**, or **aluminum-** or **magnesium-containing antacids.** Bioavailability is ↑ by concurrent administration of **indomethacin.**
Drug-Food: Food ↓ absorption.

Route/Dosage

PO (Adults): 400 mg/day taken with 8 oz of plain water only, for 3 mo.

Availability

Tablets: 400 mg.

timolol (tim-oh-lole)

Apo-Timol, Blocadren, Novo-Timol

Classification
Therapeutic: antihypertensives, vascular headache suppressants
Pharmacologic: beta blockers

Indications

Hypertension (alone or with other agents). Prevention of MI. Prevention of migraine headaches. **Unlabeled Use:** Ventricular arrhythmias. Essential tremor. Anxiety.

Action

Blocks stimulation of beta$_1$ (myocardial)– and beta$_2$ (pulmonary, vascular, and uterine)–adrenergic receptor sites. **Therapeutic Effects:** Decreased heart rate and blood pressure. Prevention of MI. ↓ frequency of migraine headache.

Adverse Reactions/Side Effects

CNS: fatigue, weakness, anxiety, depression, dizziness, drowsiness, insomnia, memory loss, mental status changes, nervousness, nightmares. **EENT:** blurred vision, dry eyes, nasal stuffiness. **Resp:** bronchospasm, wheezing. **CV:** ARRHYTHMIAS, BRADYCARDIA, CHF, PULMONARY EDEMA, orthostatic hypotension, peripheral vasoconstriction. **GI:** constipation, diarrhea, nausea. **GU:** erectile dysfunction, decreased libido. **Derm:** itching, rashes. **Endo:** hyperglycemia, hypoglycemia. **MS:** arthralgia, back pain, muscle cramps. **Neuro:** paresthesia. **Misc:** ANAPHYLAXIS (RARE).

PHYSICAL THERAPY IMPLICATIONS

Examination and Evaluation

- Assess heart rate, ECG, and heart sounds, especially during exercise (See Appendices G, H). Although sometimes used to treat certain arrhythmias, this drug can unmask or precipitate new arrhythmias (proarrhythmic effect). Report an unusually slow heart rate (bradycardia) or signs of other arrhythmias, including palpitations, chest discomfort, shortness of breath, fainting, and fatigue/weakness.
- Assess routinely for signs of CHF and pulmonary edema, including dyspnea, rales/crackles, weight gain, peripheral edema, and jugular venous distention. Report these signs to the physician immediately.
- Assess blood pressure (BP) periodically and compare to normal values (See Appendix F) to help document antihypertensive effects.
- Assess BP when patient assumes a more upright position (lying to standing, sitting to standing, lying to sitting). Document orthostatic hypotension and contact physician when systolic BP falls >20 mm Hg, or diastolic BP falls >10 mm Hg.
- Watch for signs of peripheral vasoconstriction, such as extreme coldness in the hands and feet, cyanosis, and muscle cramping. Notify physician of severe or prolonged signs of vasoconstriction.
- Assess any back pain, joint pain, or muscle cramps to rule out musculoskeletal pathology; that is, try to determine if pain is drug induced rather than caused by anatomic or biomechanical problems.
- Assess signs of paresthesia (numbness, tingling), and perform objective tests, including electroneuromyography and sensory testing, to document any drug-related neuropathic changes.
- Monitor mood and personality changes, including depression, anxiety, nervousness, memory loss, or other changes in mental status. Notify physician if these changes become problematic
- Assess dizziness and drowsiness that might affect gait, balance, and other functional activities (See Appendix C). Report balance problems and functional limitations to the physician, and caution the patient and family/caregivers to guard against falls and trauma.
- Monitor excessive fatigue or weakness. Beta blockers often cause some degree of fatigue and weakness,

but any sudden or severe change in muscle strength or energy levels should be reported.

- Be alert for signs of hypoglycemia (weakness, malaise, irritability, fatigue) or hyperglycemia (drowsiness, fruity breath, increased urination, unusual thirst). Medication may mask some signs of hypoglycemia, but dizziness and sweating may still occur. Patients with diabetes mellitus should check blood glucose levels frequently.
- If used to prevent migraine headaches, monitor the incidence and severity of attacks to document whether this drug is successful in helping manage the patient's pain.
- Although rare, be alert for signs of hypersensitivity reactions or anaphylaxis, including pulmonary symptoms (tightness in the throat and chest, wheezing, cough, dyspnea) or skin reactions (rash, pruritus, urticaria). Notify physician immediately if these reactions occur.

Interventions

- Because of an increased risk of cardiac arrhythmias, CHF, and pulmonary edema, use caution during aerobic exercise and endurance conditioning. Likewise, monitor patients closely during treatment of other cardiac problems (ventricular arrhythmias, MI prevention). Terminate exercise if patient exhibits untoward symptoms (chest pain, shortness of breath, unusual fatigue), or displays other criteria for exercise termination (See Appendix L).
- Establish aerobic exercise workloads that account for the effects of beta blockers on heart rate (HR). Some HR guidelines may not be appropriate because beta blockers typically decrease maximal HR by 20–30 bpm. Use other guidelines such as rating of perceived exertion (RPE, modified Borg scale) to determine exercise workloads.
- To minimize orthostatic hypotension, patient should move slowly when assuming a more upright position.

Patient/Client-Related Instruction

- Remind patients to take medication as directed to control hypertension and other cardiac conditions even if they are asymptomatic.
- Counsel patients about additional interventions to help control BP and cardiac dysfunction (regular exercise, weight loss, sodium restriction, stress reduction, moderation of alcohol consumption, and smoking cessation).
- Instruct patient or family/caregivers to report other troublesome side effects such as severe or prolonged insomnia, nightmares, vision disturbances, dry eyes, stuffy nose, sexual problems (decreased libido, erectile dysfunction), skin reactions (rash, itching), or GI problems (nausea, constipation, diarrhea).

Pharmacokinetics

Absorption: Well absorbed after oral administration.
Distribution: Enters breast milk.
Metabolism and Excretion: Extensively metabolized by the liver.
Half-life: 3–4 hr.

TIME/ACTION PROFILE (cardiovascular effects)

ROUTE	ONSET	PEAK	DURATION
PO	unknown	1–2 hr*	12–24 hr

*After single dose, full effect is not seen until several weeks of therapy.

Contraindications/Precautions

Contraindicated in: Uncompensated CHF; Pulmonary edema; Cardiogenic shock; Bradycardia or heart block.

Use Cautiously in: Renal impairment; Hepatic impairment; Geriatric patients (increased sensitivity to beta blockers; initial dosage reduction recommended, consider age-related ↓ in body mass, renal/hepatic/cardiac function); Pulmonary disease (including asthma); Diabetes mellitus (may mask signs of hypoglycemia); Thyrotoxicosis (may mask symptoms); Patients with a history of severe allergic reactions (intensity of reactions may be ↑); Pregnancy, lactation, or children (safety not established; all agents cross the placenta and may cause fetal/neonatal bradycardia, hypotension, hypoglycemia, or respiratory depression).

Interactions

Drug-Drug: General anesthesia, IV phenytoin, and **verapamil** may ↑ myocardial depression. ↑ bradycardia may occur with **digoxin.** ↑ hypotension may occur with other **antihypertensives,** acute ingestion of **alcohol,** or **nitrates.** Concurrent use with **amphetamines, cocaine, ephedrine, epinephrine, norepinephrine, phenylephrine,** or **pseudoephedrine** may result in unopposed alpha-adrenergic stimulation (excessive hypertension, bradycardia). Concurrent **thyroid** administration may ↓ effectiveness. May alter the effectiveness of **insulins** or **oral antidiabetics** (dosage adjustments may be necessary). May ↓ effectiveness of **bronchodilators** and **theophylline.** May beneficial cardiovascular effects of **dopamine** or **dobutamine.** Use cautiously within 14 days of **MAO inhibitor** therapy (may result in hypertension). **Cimetidine** may ↑ toxicity. Concurrent **NSAIDs** may ↓ antihypertensive action.

Route/Dosage

PO (Adults): *Antihypertensive*—10 mg bid initially; may be increased q 7 days as needed (usual maintenance dose is 10–20 mg bid; up to 60 mg/day).

T

Prevention of MI—10 mg bid, starting 1–4 wk after MI. *Prevention of vascular headache*—10 mg bid initially, may be given as a single daily dose; may be increased up to 10 mg in the morning and 20 mg in the evening.

Availability (generic available)

Tablets: 5 mg, 10 mg, 20 mg.

tinidazole (ti-nid-a-zole)

Tindamax

Classification

Therapeutic: antiprotozoals

Pharmacologic: imidazoles

Indications

Bacterial vaginosis; Trichomoniasis; Giardiasis; Amebiasis.

Action

Interaction with protozoa results in release of a free nitro radical that has antiprotozoal activity. **Therapeutic Effects:** Resolution of protozoal infections. **Spectrum:** Active against *Trichomonas vaginalis*, *Giardia duodenalis* (also known as *G. lamblia*), and *Entamoeba histolytica*.

Adverse Reactions/Side Effects

CNS: dizziness, headache, malaise. **GI:** constipation, dyspepsia, metallic/bitter taste, vomiting. **Hemat:** transient leukopenia/neutropenia.

PHYSICAL THERAPY IMPLICATIONS

Examination and Evaluation

- Assess dizziness that might affect gait, balance, and other functional activities (See Appendix C). Report balance problems and functional limitations to the physician, and caution the patient and family/caregivers to guard against falls and trauma.
- Monitor signs of leukopenia/neutropenia, including fever, sore throat, and signs of infection. Notify physician if these signs do not improve spontaneously.

Interventions

- Always wash hands thoroughly and disinfect equipment (whirlpools, electrotherapeutic devices, treatment tables, and so forth) to help prevent the spread of infection. Use universal precautions or isolation procedures as indicated for specific patients.

Patient/Client-Related Instruction

- Advise patient to report bothersome side effects such as severe or prolonged headache or GI reactions (nausea, vomiting, constipation, indigestion, altered taste).

Pharmacokinetics

Absorption: Rapidly and completely absorbed following oral administration.

Distribution: Extensively distributed; crosses placenta and blood-brain barrier, enters breast milk.

Metabolism and Excretion: Mostly metabolized (CYP3A4 enzyme system); 20–25% excreted unchanged in urine, 12% excreted in feces.

Half-life: 12–14 hr.

TIME/ACTION PROFILE (blood levels)

ROUTE	ONSET	PEAK	DURATION
PO	rapid	2 hr	24 hr

Contraindications/Precautions

Contraindicated in: Hypersensitivity; cross sensitivity with other imidazoles may occur; 1st trimester of pregnancy; Lactation.

Use Cautiously in: CNS pathology; History of blood dyscrasia; Hemodialysis (removes significant amount of tinidazole; supplement postdialysis with additional 50% of dose); Hepatic impairment; Unrecognized candidiasis (requires concurrent antifungal therapy); Children younger than 3 yr (safety not established).

Interactions

Drug-Drug: ↑ risk of bleeding with **warfarin.** Disulfiram-like reaction may occur with **alcohol** or **propylene glycol; disulfiram** should be avoided for at least 2 wk before tinidazole. May ↑ level of **lithium, cyclosporine, tacrolimus, fluorouracil,** and **intravenous fosphenytoin** (observe/monitor for toxicity if administered concurrently). **Drugs that induce to CYP450 liver enzyme system (phenobarbital, rifampin, phenytoin, or fosphenytoin)** may ↓ levels and effectiveness. **Drugs that inhibit to CYP450 liver enzyme system (cimetidine or ketoconazole)** may ↑ levels. **Oxytetracycline** may ↓ effectiveness. Absorption is ↓ by **cholestyramine;** separate dosing.

Route/Dosage

PO (Adults): *Bacterial vaginosis*—1 g for 5 days; *Trichomoniasis and giardiasis*—2 g single dose; *Intestinal amebiasis*—2 g/day for 3 days; *Amebic liver abscess*—2 g/day for 3–5 days.

PO (Children older than 3 yr): *Giardiasis*—50 mg/kg (up to 2 g) single dose; *Intestinal amebiasis*—50 mg/kg/day for 3 days; *Amebic liver abscess*—50 mg/kg/day for 3–5 days.

Availability

Tablets: 250 mg, 500 mg.

HIGH ALERT

tinzaparin (tin-zah-par-in)
Innohep

Classification
Therapeutic: anticoagulants
Pharmacologic: antithrombotics

Indications

Treatment of acute symptomatic deep vein thrombosis (DVT) with or without pulmonary embolism (with warfarin). **Unlabeled Use:** Systemic anticoagulation for other diagnoses.

Action

Potentiates the inhibitory effect of antithrombin on factor X and thrombin. **Therapeutic Effects:** Prevention of thrombus formation.

Adverse Reactions/Side Effects

GI: increased liver function tests. **Hemat:** BLEEDING, thrombocytopenia. **Local:** ecchymoses, hematoma, local irritation, pain. **Misc:** hypersensitivity reactions.

PHYSICAL THERAPY IMPLICATIONS

Examination and Evaluation

- Watch for signs of bleeding and hemorrhage, including bleeding gums, nosebleeds, unusual bruising, black/tarry stools, hematuria, or a fall in hematocrit or blood pressure. Notify physician or nursing staff immediately if tinzaparin causes excessive anticoagulation.
- Monitor symptoms of DVT (pain, swelling, warmth, redness) to determine if drug therapy is effective in preventing or reducing venous thrombosis. Request or administer objective tests (Doppler ultrasound) if symptoms increase.
- In patients with DVT, watch for signs of pulmonary embolism, including shortness of breath, chest pain, cough, and bloody sputum. Notify physician or nursing staff immediately if these signs occur.
- Be alert for acute arterial or venous thrombosis caused by heparin-induced thrombocytopenia (HIT). Although the risk of HIT is lower compared with traditional heparin, tinzaparin may initiate an immune reaction in certain patients where antibodies attack circulating platelets. Although most cases of HIT are minor and asymptomatic, some patients may experience life- or limb-threatening platelet clots, resulting in myocardial infarction, ischemic stroke, acute leg ischemia, or venous thromboembolism. HIT can occur during and up to several weeks after heparin therapy. Any signs of increased clotting should be reported immediately.
- Monitor signs of hypersensitivity reactions, including pulmonary symptoms (tightness in the throat and chest, wheezing, cough, dyspnea) or skin reactions (rash, pruritus, urticaria). Notify physician or nursing staff immediately if these reactions occur.
- Assess injection site for pain, swelling, irritation, or bruising. Report prolonged or excessive injection site reactions to the physician or nursing staff.

Interventions

- Use caution with any physical interventions that could increase bleeding, including wound débridement, chest percussion, joint mobilization, and application of local heat.
- Recommend or implement other physical methods to decrease DVT and prevent thromboembolism, including graduated compression stockings and intermittent pneumatic compression pumps.
- Implement early mobilization and ambulation to reduce the risk of new or increased DVT. Early ambulation appears to be safe in patients with DVT if the patient is adequately heparinized (INR values in acceptable range), does not have an active pulmonary embolism, or have other risk factors that contraindicate ambulation.
- Use caution during aerobic exercise and other forms of therapeutic exercise in patients with unstable angina or MI. Assess exercise tolerance frequently (blood pressure, heart rate, fatigue levels), and terminate exercise immediately if any untoward responses occur (See Appendix L).
- Do not apply physical agents (heat, cold, electrotherapeutic modalities) or massage over the injection site; these interventions can alter drug absorption from subcutaneous tissues.

Patient/Client-Related Instruction

- Instruct patient to immediately report signs of GI bleeding, including abdominal pain, vomiting blood, blood in stools, or black, tarry stools.

Pharmacokinetics

Absorption: Well absorbed following SC administration.
Distribution: Unknown.
Metabolism and Excretion: Partially metabolized; elimination is primarily renal.
Half-life: 3.9 hr.

TIME/ACTION PROFILE

ROUTE	ONSET	PEAK	DURATION
SC	Rapid		24 hr

Contraindications/Precautions

Contraindicated in: Hypersensitivity, including hypersensitivity to bisulfites (contains metabisulfite),

T

benzyl alcohol, or pork products; Active major bleeding; History of heparin-induced thrombocytopenia.
Use Cautiously in: Geri: Geriatric patients (may have ↑ sensitivity); Renal insufficiency; Diabetic retinopathy; Concurrent use of platelet inhibitors, oral anticoagulants, or thrombolytics (↑ risk of bleeding); OB: Pregnancy (benzyl alcohol in formulation may cause gasping syndrome in neonate; use during pregnancy only if clearly needed); Pedi: Lactation or children (safety not established).
Exercise Extreme Caution in: Spinal/epidural anesthesia or spinal puncture (↑ risk of spinal/epidural hematoma that may lead to long-term or permanent paralysis; Bacterial endocarditis; Severe uncontrolled hypertension; Congenital/acquired bleeding disorders, including hepatic failure and amyloidosis; Active ulcerative/angiodysplastic GI disease; Shortly after brain/spinal/ophthalmologic surgery; Hemorrhagic stroke.

Interactions

Drug-Drug: Concurrent use of **platelet inhibitors, warfarin,** or **thrombolytics** (↑ risk of bleeding).

Route/Dosage

SC (Adults): 175 anti-Xa IU/kg once daily for at least 6 days and until therapeutic anticoagulation is achieved with warfarin (INR >2 for 2 consecutive days).

Availability

Solution for injection: 20,000 anti-Xa units/mL in 2-mL vials.

tioconazole (tye-oh-**kon**-a-zole)

1-Day, Monistat-1 Day, Vagistat-1

Classification
Therapeutic: antifungals (vaginal)
Pharmacologic: imidazoles

Indications

Treatment of vulvovaginal candidiasis.

Action

Affects the permeability of the fungal cell wall, allowing leakage of cellular contents. Not active against bacteria. **Therapeutic Effects:** Inhibited growth and death of susceptible *Candida*, with ↓ in accompanying symptoms of vulvovaginitis (vaginal burning, itching, discharge).

Adverse Reactions/Side Effects

GU: irritation, vulvovaginal burning.

PHYSICAL THERAPY IMPLICATIONS

Examination and Evaluation

- Monitor patient's symptoms to help document drug effectiveness.

Interventions

- Always wash hands thoroughly and disinfect equipment (whirlpools, electrotherapeutic devices, treatment tables, and so forth) to help prevent the spread of infection.

Patient/Client-Related Instruction

- Advise patient to report any increased local sensitivity to this drug (pain, burning, itching, swelling).
- Therapeutic response for vaginal infections is usually seen after 1 wk. Advise patient that application is typically continued throughout the full course of therapy even if feeling better. Therapy should be continued during menstrual period.
- Advise patient to seek medical help if infections persist or recur after the full treatment. Recurrent fungal infections may be a sign of systemic illness.

Pharmacokinetics

Absorption: Minimal through intact skin.
Distribution: Unknown. Action is primarily local.
Metabolism and Excretion: Negligible with local application.
Half-life: Not applicable.

TIME/ACTION PROFILE

ROUTE	ONSET	PEAK	DURATION
intravaginal	unknown	unknown	unknown

Contraindications/Precautions

Contraindicated in: Hypersensitivity to active ingredients, additives, or preservatives; OB/Lactation: Safety not established.
Use Cautiously in: Patients with recurrent vulvovaginal yeast infections.

Interactions

Drug-Drug: Not known.

Route/Dosage

Vag (Adults and Children ≥12 yr): *Vaginal ointment*—1 applicatorful (4.6 g) hs as a single dose.

Availability

Vaginal ointment: 6.5% OTC.

tiotropium (tye-o-**trope**-ee-yum)

Spiriva

Classification
Therapeutic: bronchodilators
Pharmacologic: anticholinergics

Indications

Long-term maintenance treatment of bronchospasm due to COPD.

Action

Acts an anticholinergic by selectively and reversibly inhibiting M_3 receptors in smooth muscle of airways. **Therapeutic Effects:** ↓ incidence and severity of bronchospasm.

Adverse Reactions/Side Effects

EENT: glaucoma. **Resp:** paradoxical bronchospasm. **CV:** ↑ heart rate. **GI:** dry mouth, constipation. **GU:** urinary difficulty, urinary retention. **Misc:** HYPERSENSITIVITY REACTIONS, INCLUDING ANGIOEDEMA.

PHYSICAL THERAPY IMPLICATIONS

Examination and Evaluation

- Be alert for signs of hypersensitivity reactions and angioedema, including pulmonary symptoms (tightness in the throat and chest, wheezing, cough, dyspnea) or skin reactions (rash, pruritus, urticaria, swelling in the face). Notify physician immediately if these reactions occur.
- Assess pulmonary function at rest and during exercise (See Appendices I, J, K) to document effectiveness of medication in controlling bronchospasm in COPD.
- Monitor signs of paradoxical bronchospasm (wheezing, cough, dyspnea, tightness in chest and throat), especially at higher or excessive doses. If condition occurs, advise patient to withhold medication and notify physician immediately.
- Assess heart rate, ECG, and heart sounds, especially during exercise (See Appendices G, H). Report a rapid heart rate (tachycardia) or signs of other arrhythmias, including palpitations, chest discomfort, shortness of breath, fainting, and fatigue/weakness.
- Monitor and report any vision disturbances that might indicate glaucoma, such as blurred vision, tunnel vision, halos around lights, and so forth.

Interventions

- Design and implement appropriate aerobic exercise and respiratory muscle training programs to maintain optimal cardiovascular and pulmonary function. Work with patient and family/caregivers to find forms of exercise (e.g., swimming) that can help improve respiratory function without triggering bronchoconstrictive attacks.
- When implementing airway clearance techniques or respiratory muscle training, attempt to intervene when the airway is maximally bronchodilated. Peak responses typically occur 5 min after inhalation.

Patient/Client-Related Instruction

- Advise patient to not exceed the recommended dose or frequency of inhalations. Contact physician immediately if bronchospasm is not relieved by medication or is accompanied by diaphoresis, dizziness, or other symptoms.
- Counsel patient on proper use of inhaler; observe use of this device whenever possible to ensure proper technique.
- Instruct patient and family/caregivers to report troublesome side effects such as severe or prolonged problems with urination or GI problems (constipation, dry mouth).

Pharmacokinetics

Absorption: 19.5% absorbed following inhalation.
Distribution: Extensive tissue distribution; due to route of administration, ↑ concentrations occur in lung.
Metabolism and Excretion: 74% excreted unchanged in urine; 25% of absorbed drug is metabolized.
Half-life: 5–6 days.

TIME/ACTION PROFILE (bronchodilation)

ROUTE	ONSET	PEAK	DURATION
inhalation	Rapid	5 min	24 hr

Contraindications/Precautions

Contraindicated in: Hypersensitivity to tiotropium, atropine, or their derivatives; Concurrent ipratropium. **Use Cautiously in:** Angle-closure glaucoma, prostatic hyperplasia, bladder neck obstruction (may worsen condition); CCr ≤50 mL/min (monitor closely); Pregnancy, lactation or children (safety not established).

Interactions

Drug-Drug: Should not be used concurrently with **ipratropium** due to risk of additive anticholinergic effects.

Route/Dosage

Inhalation (Adults): 18 mcg once daily.

Availability

Dry powder capsules for inhalation: 18 mcg.

tipranavir (ti-pran-a-veer)

Aptivus

Classification

Therapeutic: antiretrovirals
Pharmacologic: protease inhibitors

Indications

Advanced HIV disease resistant to more than one protease inhibitor (must be used with ritonavir).

T

Action

Inhibits processing of viral polyproteins, preventing formation of mature virions. **Therapeutic Effects:** ↓ viral load and sequelae of HIV infection.

Adverse Reactions/Side Effects

CV: INTRACRANIAL HEMORRHAGE, fatigue, headache. **GI:** HEPATOTOXICITY, abdominal pain, diarrhea, nausea, vomiting. **Derm:** rash (↑ in women and peds). **Endo:** hyperglycemia. **Metab:** ↑ cholesterol, ↑ triglycerides. **Misc:** allergic reactions, bleeding, fat redistribution, fever, immune reconstitution syndrome.

PHYSICAL THERAPY IMPLICATIONS

Examination and Evaluation

- Be alert for signs of intracranial hemorrhage, including sudden severe headache, confusion, nausea, vomiting, paralysis, numbness, speech problems, visual disturbances, and loss of consciousness. Seek immediate medical assistance if patient exhibits these signs.
- Monitor signs of hepatotoxicity, including anorexia, abdominal pain, severe nausea and vomiting, yellow skin or eyes, fever, sore throat, malaise, weakness, facial edema, lethargy, and unusual bleeding or bruising. Notify physician immediately if these signs occur.
- Monitor signs of hyperglycemia, including confusion, drowsiness, flushed/dry skin, fruit-like breath odor, rapid/deep breathing, polyuria, loss of appetite, and unusual thirst. Patients with diabetes mellitus should check blood glucose levels frequently.
- Be alert for signs of an unusually aggressive immune reaction to opportunistic infection (immune reconstitution syndrome). Signs include fever, pain, warmth and redness and swelling at the site of infection. Notify physician of these signs immediately.
- Monitor other signs of allergic reactions, including pulmonary symptoms (tightness in the throat and chest, wheezing, cough, dyspnea) or skin reactions (rash, pruritus, urticaria). Notify physician or nursing staff immediately if these reactions occur.

Interventions

- Implement resistive exercises and other therapeutic exercises as needed to maintain muscle strength and function and prevent muscle wasting associated with HIV infection and AIDS.
- Design and implement aerobic exercise and endurance training programs to help prevent heart disease associated with drug-related hyperlipidemia and other problems with lipid and glucose metabolism.

Patient/Client-Related Instruction

- Emphasize the importance of taking tipranavir as directed even if the patient is asymptomatic, and that this drug must always be used in combination with other antiretroviral drugs. Do not take more than prescribed amount and do not stop taking without consulting health care professional.
- Inform patient that tipranavir does not cure HIV or AIDS or prevent associated or opportunistic infections. Tipranavir does not reduce the risk of transmission of HIV to others through sexual contact or blood contamination. Caution patient to use a condom and avoid sharing needles or donating blood to prevent spreading the AIDS virus to others.
- Advise patient that this drug may cause problems in fat metabolism, including hyperlipidemia and hypertriglyceridemia. Remind patient that periodic blood tests may be needed to monitor plasma lipids.
- Advise patient about possible changes in body composition such as increased abdominal fat with thin arms and legs. Discuss possible effects on body image, and help patient explore coping mechanisms.
- Instruct patient and family/caregivers to report other bothersome side effects such as severe or prolonged headache, fatigue, fever, bleeding, skin rash, or GI reactions (nausea, vomiting, diarrhea, abdominal pain).

Pharmacokinetics

Absorption: Well absorbed following oral administration.
Distribution: Unknown.
Protein Binding: >99.9%.
Metabolism and Excretion: Rapidly and extensively metabolized (primarily by CYP3A4), requiring coadministration with ritonavir as a metabolic inhibitor to achieve therapeutic blood levels; eliminated mostly in feces, minimal renal excretion.
Half-life: 5.5–6 hr.

TIME/ACTION PROFILE (blood levels*)

ROUTE	ONSET	PEAK	DURATION
PO	rapid	2 hr	12 hr

*With ritonavir.

Contraindications/Precautions

Contraindicated in: Hypersensitivity; Moderate-to-severe hepatic impairment (Child-Pugh Class B or C); Concurrent use of some antiarrhythmics (amiodarone, flecainide, propafenone, quinidine), ergot derivatives, midazolam (oral) or triazolam.
Use Cautiously in: Known sulfonamide allergy (contains sulfa moiety); Preexisting liver disease (may ↑ risk of hepatotoxicity); History of or risk factors for diabetes (may cause hyperglycemia); Hemophilia (may ↑ risk of bleeding).

Interactions

Drug-Drug: ↑ blood levels and risk of toxicity from some **antiarrhythmics (amiodarone, flecainide,**

propafenone, quinidine), ergot derivatives (dihydroergotamine, ergonovine, ergotamine, methylergonovine), midazolam (oral), and **triazolam.** Concurrent use with **ritonavir** may lead to intracranial hemorrhage. **Antacids** ↓ absorption (separate dosing). **Hormonal contraceptives** may ↑ risk of rash. May ↓ effectiveness of **hormonal contraceptives.** ↑ risk of bleeding with **antiplatelets, anticoagulants,** or **vitamin E.**

Route/Dosage

PO (Adults): 500 mg bid with ritonavir 200 mg bid.
PO (Children ≥2 yr): 14 mg/kg (max: 500 mg/dose) bid with ritonavir 6 mg/kg (max: 200 mg/dose) bid; if intolerance develops, may ↓ dose to tipranavir 12 mg/kg bid with ritonavir 5 mg/kg bid.

Availability

Capsules: 250 mg. **Oral solution (butter mint-butter toffee):** 100 mg/mL (contains vitamin E 116 international units/mL).

HIGH ALERT

tirofiban (tye-roe-**fye**-ban)

Aggrastat

Classification

Therapeutic: antiplatelet agents

Pharmacologic: glycoprotein IIb/IIIa inhibitors

Indications

Treatment of acute coronary syndrome (unstable angina/non–Q-wave MI), including patients who will be managed medically and those who will undergo percutaneous transluminal angioplasty (PCTA) or atherectomy. Used concurrently with aspirin and heparin.

Action

Decreases platelet aggregation by reversibly antagonizing the binding of fibrinogen to the glycoprotein IIb/IIIa binding site on platelet surfaces. **Therapeutic Effects:** Inhibition of platelet aggregation resulting in ↓ incidence of new MI, death, or refractory ischemia with the need for repeat cardiac procedures.

Adverse Reactions/Side Effects

Noted for patients receiving heparin and aspirin in addition to tirofiban

CNS: dizziness, headache. **CV:** bradycardia, coronary dissection, edema, vasovagal reaction. **GI:** nausea. **Derm:** hives, rash. **Hemat:** BLEEDING, thrombocytopenia. **MS:** leg pain. **Misc:** fever, hypersensitivity reactions, pelvic pain, sweating.

PHYSICAL THERAPY IMPLICATIONS

Examination and Evaluation

- Watch for signs of bleeding and hemorrhage, including bleeding gums, nosebleeds, unusual bruising, black/tarry stools, hematuria, or a fall in hematocrit or blood pressure. Notify physician or nursing staff immediately if tirofiban causes excessive anticoagulation.
- Monitor signs of hypersensitivity reactions, including pulmonary symptoms (tightness in the throat and chest, wheezing, cough, dyspnea) or skin reactions (rash, pruritus, urticaria). Notify physician or nursing staff immediately if these reactions occur.
- Assess heart rate, ECG, and heart sounds, especially during exercise (See Appendices G, H). Report an unusually slow heart rate (bradycardia) or signs of other arrhythmias, including palpitations, chest discomfort, shortness of breath, fainting, and fatigue/weakness.
- Assess peripheral edema using girth measurements, volume displacement, and measurement of pitting edema (See Appendix N). Report increased swelling in feet and ankles or a sudden increase in body weight due to fluid retention.
- Assess any pelvic or leg pain to rule out musculoskeletal pathology; that is, try to determine if pain is drug induced rather than caused by anatomic or biomechanical problems.
- Assess dizziness that might affect gait, balance, and other functional activities (See Appendix C). Report balance problems and functional limitations to the physician and nursing staff, and caution the patient and family/caregivers to guard against falls and trauma.

Interventions

- Use caution with any physical interventions that could increase bleeding, including wound débridement, chest percussion, joint mobilization, and application of local heat.
- Because of the risk of cardiac arrhythmias (bradycardia) and a vasovagal response, use caution during aerobic exercise and endurance conditioning. Assess exercise tolerance frequently (blood pressure, heart rate, fatigue levels), and terminate exercise immediately if any untoward responses occur (See Appendix L).

Patient/Client-Related Instruction

- Instruct patient to immediately report signs of GI bleeding, including abdominal pain, vomiting blood, blood in stools, or black, tarry stools.
- Remind patients to take medication as directed to reduce the risk of coronary infarction even if they are asymptomatic.

T

- Counsel patients about additional interventions to help reduce the risk of heart disease, including regular exercise, weight loss, sodium restriction, stress reduction, moderation of alcohol consumption, and smoking cessation.
- Instruct patient or family/caregivers to report other problematic side effects such as severe or prolonged headache, fever, nausea, or skin reactions (rash, hives, excessive sweating).

Pharmacokinetics

Absorption: IV administration results in complete bioavailability.
Distribution: Unknown.
Metabolism and Excretion: Excreted mostly unchanged by the kidneys (65%); 25% excreted unchanged in feces.
Half-life: 2 hr.

TIME/ACTION PROFILE (effects on platelet function)

ROUTE	ONSET	PEAK	DURATION
IV	Rapid	30 min*	brief†

*>90% inhibition of platelet aggregation at end of initial 30-min infusion.
†Inhibition is reversible following cessation of infusion.

Contraindications/Precautions

Contraindicated in: Hypersensitivity; Active internal bleeding or history of bleeding within previous 30 days; History of intracranial hemorrhage, intracranial neoplasm, arteriovenous malformation or aneurysm; History of thrombocytopenia during previous tirofiban therapy; History of hemorrhagic stroke or other stroke within 30 days; Major surgical procedure or severe physical trauma within 30 days; History, symptoms, or other findings associated with aortic aneurysm; Severe hypertension (systolic BP >180 mm Hg and/or diastolic BP >110 mm Hg); Concurrent use of other glycoprotein IIb/IIIa receptor antagonists; Acute pericarditis; Lactation.
Use Cautiously in: Platelet count <150,000/mm^3; Hemorrhagic retinopathy; Female patients and geriatric patients (↑ risk of bleeding); Severe renal insufficiency (↓ rate of infusion by 50% if CCr <30 mL/min); Pregnancy or children (safety not established; use in pregnancy only if clearly needed).

Interactions

Drug-Drug: Aspirin, other **NSAIDs, warfarin, heparin** and **heparin-like agents, abciximab, eptifibatide, clopidogrel, ticlopidine,** or **dipyridamole**—concurrent use may ↑ risk of bleeding, although these agents are frequently used together or in sequence. Risk of bleeding may be ↑ by concurrent use of **cefotetan, cefoperazone, or valproic acid.**
Drug-Natural: ↑ anticoagulant effect and bleeding risk with **anise, arnica, chamomile, clove, dong quai, fenugreek, feverfew, garlic, ginger, ginkgo,** ***Panax ginseng*****, licorice,** and others.

Route/Dosage

IV (Adults): 0.4 mcg/kg/min for 30 min, then 0.1 mcg/kg/min, continued throughout angiography and for 12–24 hr after angioplasty or atherectomy.

Renal Impairment

IV (Adults): *CCr <30 mL/min*—0.2 mcg/kg/min for 30 min, then 0.05 mcg/kg/min, continued throughout angiography and for 12–24 hr after angioplasty or atherectomy.

Availability

Concentrated solution for IV infusion (dilute before use): 12.5 mg/50 mL (250 mcg/mL) in 50-mL vials. **Premixed solution for infusion:** 5 mg/100 mL (50 mcg/mL) in 100-mL single-dose containers, 12.5 mg/250 mL (50 mcg/mL) in 250-mL single-dose containers.

tizanidine (tye-zan-i-deen)

Zanaflex

Classification
Therapeutic: antispasticity agents (centrally acting)
Pharmacologic: adrenergics

Indications

Increased muscle tone associated with spasticity due to multiple sclerosis or spinal cord injury.

Action

Acts as an agonist at central alpha-adrenergic receptor sites. Reduces spasticity by ↑ presynaptic inhibition of motor neurons. **Therapeutic Effects:** ↓ spasticity, allowing better function.

Adverse Reactions/Side Effects

CNS: anxiety, depression, dizziness, sedation, weakness, dyskinesia, hallucinations, nervousness. **EENT:** blurred vision, pharyngitis, rhinitis. **CV:** hypotension, bradycardia. **GI:** abdominal pain, diarrhea, dry mouth, dyspepsia, constipation, hepatocellular injury, increased liver enzymes, vomiting. **GU:** urinary frequency. **Derm:** rash, skin ulcers, sweating.
MS: back pain, myasthenia, paresthesia. **Misc:** fever, speech disorder.

PHYSICAL THERAPY IMPLICATIONS

Examination and Evaluation

- Assess patient's spasticity, ROM, functional ability, and posture (e.g., head control and trunk stability), especially when beginning tizanidine treatment or during dose adjustments. Communicate with physician, family/caregivers, and other health professionals to determine if dosage is helping achieve desired functional outcomes.

- Be alert for symptoms such as back pain, muscle weakness, paresthesia, or dyskinesia. Differentiate whether these symptoms are caused by neuromuscular pathology versus drug induced.
- Assess dizziness that might affect gait, balance, and other functional activities (See Appendix C). Report balance problems and functional limitations to the physician, and caution the patient and family/caregivers to guard against falls and trauma.
- Monitor CNS symptoms such as anxiety, nervousness, depression, sedation, speech problems, and hallucinations. Report these problems; excessive or prolonged CNS symptoms may require a reduction in dose.
- Assess blood pressure periodically and compare to normal values (See Appendix F). Report low blood pressure (hypotension), especially if patient experiences dizziness, fatigue, or other symptoms.
- Assess heart rate, ECG, and heart sounds, especially during exercise (See Appendices G, H). Report slow heart rate (bradycardia) or symptoms of other arrhythmias, including palpitations, chest discomfort, shortness of breath, fainting, and fatigue/weakness.

Interventions

- Implement aggressive therapeutic exercises (neuromuscular reeducation, postural stabilization, gait training, other task-specific training) to help patient adjust to reduced spasticity and tone.
- Because of the risk of hypotension and bradycardia, use caution during aerobic exercise and other forms of therapeutic exercise. Assess exercise tolerance frequently (blood pressure, heart rate, fatigue levels), and terminate exercise immediately if any untoward responses occur (See Appendix L).
- Guard against falls and trauma due to sedation, dizziness, or abnormally low tone in the trunk and lower extremities. Implement fall prevention strategies, especially if patient exhibits excessive sedation, dizziness, or other impairments that affect gait and balance (See Appendix E).
- To minimize orthostatic hypotension, patient should move slowly when assuming a more upright position.

Patient/Client-Related Instruction

- Advise patient to avoid alcohol and other CNS depressants because of the increased risk of sedation and adverse effects.
- Instruct patient or family/caregivers to report other troublesome side effects such as severe or prolonged fever, nasopharyngeal inflammation, blurred vision, increased urination, skin reactions (rash, ulcers, increased sweating), or GI problems (vomiting, diarrhea, constipation, indigestion, abdominal pain).

Pharmacokinetics

Absorption: Completely absorbed after oral administration but rapidly metabolized, resulting in 40% bioavailability.
Distribution: Widely distributed.
Metabolism and Excretion: 95% metabolized by the liver.
Half-life: 2.5 hr.

TIME/ACTION PROFILE (reduced muscle tone)

ROUTE	ONSET	PEAK	DURATION
PO	unknown	1–2 hr	3–6 hr

Contraindications/Precautions

Contraindicated in: Hypersensitivity.
Use Cautiously in: Renal impairment; Geri: Geriatric patients; Concurrent antihypertensive therapy; OB/Pedi: Pregnancy, lactation, or children (safety not established).
Exercise Extreme Caution in: Impaired hepatic function.

Interactions

Drug-Drug: Blood levels and effects ↑ by concurrent use of **hormonal contraceptives** or **alcohol.** ↑ risk of hypotension with **$alpha_2$-adrenergic agonist antihypertensives** (avoid concurrent use). ↑ CNS depression may occur with **alcohol** or other **CNS depressants,** including some **antidepressants, sedative/hypnotics, antihistamines,** and **opioid analgesics.** Concurrent CYP1A2 inhibitors (**ciprofloxacin, fluvoxamine,** and others) may ↑ levels and risk of hypotension and excessive sedation.

Route/Dosage

PO (Adults): 4 mg q 6–8 hr initially (no more than 3 doses/24 hr); increase by 2–4 mg/dose up to 8 mg/dose or 24 mg/day (not to exceed 36 mg/day). Some patients may tolerate bid dosing.

Availability (generic available)

Tablets: 2 mg, 4 mg. **Capsules:** 2 mg, 4 mg, 6 mg.

tobramycin (toe-bra-**mye**-sin)

Nebcin, TOBI

Classification
Therapeutic: anti-infectives
Pharmacologic: aminoglycosides

Indications

Treatment of serious gram-negative bacillary infections and infections caused by staphylococci when penicillins or other less toxic drugs are contraindicated. **Ophthalmic:** Treatment of localized infections due to susceptible organisms. **Inhalation:** Management of cystic fibrosis patients with *Pseudomonas aeruginosa*.

Action

Inhibits protein synthesis in bacteria at level of 30S ribosome. **Therapeutic Effects:** Bactericidal action. **Spectrum:** Most aminoglycosides notable for activity against: *Pseudomonas aeruginosa*, *Klebsiella pneumoniae*, *Escherichia coli*, *Proteus*, *Serratia*, *Acinetobacter*, *Staphylococcus aureus*. In treatment of enterococcal infections, synergy with a penicillin is required.

Adverse Reactions/Side Effects

EENT: ototoxicity (vestibular and cochlear), Ophthalmic only: burning, stinging, blurred vision (ointment only). **Inhalation only:** tinnitus, voice alteration. **GU:** nephrotoxicity. **F and E:** hypomagnesemia. **MS:** muscle paralysis (high parenteral doses). **Misc:** hypersensitivity reactions.

PHYSICAL THERAPY IMPLICATIONS

Examination and Evaluation

- Monitor signs of hypersensitivity reactions, including pulmonary symptoms (tightness in the throat and chest, wheezing, cough dyspnea) or skin reactions (rash, pruritus, urticaria). Notify physician or nursing staff immediately if these reactions occur.
- Report any muscle weakness or paralysis that occurs following injection of high doses.
- Monitor signs of ototoxicity, including hearing loss, tinnitus, and balance problems (See Appendix E for fall assessment and prevention). Report these signs, and caution the patient and family/caregivers to guard against falls and trauma.
- Monitor signs of low magnesium levels (hypomagnesemia), such as lethargy, irritability, insomnia, muscle tremors, and confusion. Notify physician of these signs.

Interventions

- Always wash hands thoroughly and disinfect equipment (whirlpools, electrotherapeutic devices, treatment tables, and so forth) to help prevent the spread of infection. Employ universal precautions or isolation procedures as indicated for specific patients.

Patient/Client-Related Instruction

- Advise patient to report signs of nephrotoxicity, including blood or pus in urine, decreased urine output, fatigue, and weight gain from fluid retention.
- Advise patient to report any vision disturbances or eye pain and inflammation that occurs during local (ophthalmologic) administration.

Pharmacokinetics

Absorption: Well absorbed after IM administration. IV administration results in complete bioavailability. Low absorption follows administration by inhalation.
Distribution: Widely distributed throughout extracellular fluid; crosses the placenta; small amounts enter breast milk. Poor penetration into CSF.
Metabolism and Excretion: Excretion is >90% renal.
Half-life: Neonates: 2–11 hr; Infants: 3–5 hr; Children: 1–3 hr; Adolescents: 0.5–2.5 hr; Adults: 2–4 hr (↑ in renal impairment to 5–70 hr).

TIME/ACTION PROFILE (blood levels*)

ROUTE	ONSET	PEAK	DURATION
IM	rapid	30–90 min	6–24 hr
IV	rapid	end of infusion†	6–24 hr

*All parenterally administered aminoglycosides.
†Postdistribution peak occurs 30 min after the end of a 30-min infusion and 15 min after the end of a 1-hr infusion.

Contraindications/Precautions

Contraindicated in: Hypersensitivity; Most parenteral products contain bisulfites and should be avoided in patients with known intolerance; Cross-sensitivity among aminoglycosides may occur.
Use Cautiously in: Renal impairment (dosage adjustments necessary; blood level monitoring useful in preventing ototoxicity and nephrotoxicity); Hearing impairment; Geriatric patients and premature infants (difficulty in assessing auditory and vestibular function; age-related renal impairment); Neonates (↑ risk of neuromuscular blockade; difficulty in assessing auditory and vestibular function; immature renal function); Neuromuscular diseases such as myasthenia gravis; Obese patients (dosage should be based on ideal body weight); Pregnancy (may cause congenital deafness); Lactation.

Interactions

Drug-Drug: Inactivated by **penicillins** and **cephalosporins** when coadministered to patients with renal insufficiency. Possible respiratory paralysis after **inhalation anesthetics** or **neuromuscular blockers.** ↑ incidence of ototoxicity with **loop diuretics.** ↑ incidence of nephrotoxicity with other **nephrotoxic drugs.**

Route/Dosage

IM, IV (Adults): 3–6 mg/kg/day in 3 divided doses, or 4–6.6 mg/kg once daily.
IM, IV (Children >5 yr): 6–7.5 mg/kg/day divided q 8 hr, up to 13 mg/kg/day divided q 6–8 hr in cystic

fibrosis patients (dosing interval may vary from q 6 hr–q 24 hr, depending on clinical situation).
IM, IV (Children 1 mo–5 yr): 7.5 mg/kg/day divided q 8 hr, up to 13 mg/kg/day divided q 6–8 hr in cystic fibrosis.
IM, IV (Neonates): *Preterm <1000 g*—3.5 mg/kg/dose q 24 hr *0–4 wk;, <1200 g*—2.5 mg/kg/dose q 18 hr; *Postnatal age <7 days*—2.5 mg/kg/dose q 12 hr; *Postnatal age >7 days, 1200–2000 g*—2.5 mg/kg/dose q 8–12 hr; *Postnatal age >7 days, >2000 g*—2.5 mg/kg/dose q 8 hr.
Inhalation (Adults and Children): Standard dose: 40–80 mg bid–tid times/day; High dose: 300 mg bid for 28 days, then off for 28 days, then repeat cycle.
Ophthalmic (Adults and Children >2 mo): Apply 0.5-inch ribbon into the affected eye bid–tid, for severe infections, apply q 3–4 hr.

Renal Impairment

IM, IV (Adults): 1 mg/kg initially, further dosing determined by blood level monitoring and assessment of renal function.

Availability (generic available)

Injection: 10 mg/mL, 40 mg/mL, 1.2-g vial.
Ophthalmic solution: 3 mg/mL in 5-mL container.
Ophthalmic ointment: 3 mg/g in 3.5-g tube.
Nebulizer solution: 300 mg/5 mL in 5-mL ampules.

tocainide (toe-**kay**-nide)

Tonocard

Classification
Therapeutic: antiarrhythmics (class IB)

Indications

Life-threatening ventricular arrhythmias, including multifocal and unifocal premature ventricular contractions and ventricular tachycardia.

Action

Suppresses automaticity of conduction tissue and spontaneous depolarization of the ventricles during diastole. Has little or no effect on heart rate.
Therapeutic Effects: Suppression of arrhythmias.

Adverse Reactions/Side Effects

CNS: SEIZURES, changes in mood, drowsiness, hallucinations, headache, restlessness, tremor, coma, dizziness, mental depression, paranoia. **EENT:** blurred vision, thirst, tinnitus. **Resp:** PULMONARY FIBROSIS, pneumonia. **CV:** SINUS ARREST, CHF, arrhythmias, bradycardia, hypotension, palpitations, tachycardia, angina, conduction disturbances, hypertension. **GI:** anorexia, diarrhea, nausea, vomiting, abdominal discomfort, constipation, drug-induced hepatitis, dyspepsia, dysphagia. **GU:** urinary retention. **Derm:** alopecia, flushing, rashes, sweating. **Hemat:** AGRANULOCYTOSIS, leukopenia, neutropenia, thrombocytopenia. **MS:** arthralgia, myalgia. **Neuro:** myasthenia gravis, numbness.

PHYSICAL THERAPY IMPLICATIONS

Examination and Evaluation

- Be alert for new seizures or increased seizure activity. Document the number, duration, and severity of seizures, and report these findings immediately to the physician.
- Monitor cardiac symptoms at rest and during exercise. Seek immediate medical assistance if symptoms of sinus arrest develop, including sudden chest pain, pain radiating into the arm or jaw, shortness of breath, dizziness, sweating, anxiety, nausea, and loss of consciousness.
- Assess signs of congestive heart failure including dyspnea, rales/crackles, peripheral edema, jugular venous distention, and exercise intolerance. Report these signs to the physician immediately.
- Assess any breathing problems or signs of pulmonary fibrosis or pneumonia such as dry cough, wheezing, chest pain, shortness of breath, fever, and difficult or labored breathing. Monitor pulse oximetry and perform pulmonary function tests (See Appendices I, J, K) to quantify suspected changes in ventilation and respiratory function. Report any pulmonary dysfunction to the physician.
- Monitor signs of blood dyscrasias including agranulocytosis, neutropenia, and leukopenia (fever, sore throat, mucosal lesions, signs of infection) or thrombocytopenia (bruising, nose bleeds, bleeding gums). Report these signs to the physician immediately.
- Assess heart rate, ECG, and heart sounds, especially during exercise (See Appendices G, H). Although intended to treat certain arrhythmias, this drug can unmask or precipitate new arrhythmias (proarrhythmic effect). Report any rhythm disturbances or symptoms of increased arrhythmias, including palpitations, chest pain, shortness of breath, fainting, and fatigue/weakness.
- Assess blood pressure (BP) and compare to normal values (See Appendix F). Report a sustained increase in BP (hypertension).
- Be alert for early signs of myasthenia gravis syndrome, such as drooping eyelids, facial muscle weakness, and difficulty swallowing and speaking. Report these signs to the physician immediately, and monitor other muscle groups for signs of

T

unusual weakness and fatigue, especially after repeated contraction.

- Assess any joint or muscle pain to rule out musculoskeletal pathology; that is, try to determine if pain is drug induced rather than caused by anatomic or biomechanical problems.
- Be alert for changes in mood and behavior, including restlessness, paranoia, hallucinations, mental depression, and excessive drowsiness that can progress to coma. These signs may indicate CNS toxicity and should be reported to physician or other health care professional.
- Assess dizziness that might affect gait, balance, and other functional activities (See Appendix C). Report balance problems and functional limitations to the physician, and caution the patient and family/caregivers to guard against falls and trauma.

Interventions

- Because of the risk of serious cardiovascular and pulmonary problems, use extreme caution during aerobic exercise and other forms of therapeutic exercise. Assess exercise tolerance frequently (BP, heart rate, fatigue levels), and terminate exercise immediately if any untoward responses occur (See Appendix L).

Patient/Client-Related Instruction

- Advise patient and family or caregivers about the signs of cardiac arrest, arrhythmias, and CHF (see above under Examination and Evaluation), and to seek immediate medical assistance if these signs develop
- Advise patient about the likelihood of GI reactions such as nausea, vomiting, diarrhea, constipation, indigestion, difficulty swallowing, and abdominal pain. Instruct patient to report severe or prolonged GI problems, or signs of drug-induced hepatitis (yellow skin or eyes, abdominal pain, severe nausea and vomiting, fever, sore throat, malaise, weakness, facial edema).
- Instruct patient and family/caregivers to report other side effects such as severe or prolonged headache, vision problems, ringing/buzzing in the ears (tinnitus), numbness, urinary retention, or skin reactions (rash, sweating, flushing, hair loss).

Pharmacokinetics

Absorption: Well absorbed after oral administration.
Distribution: Widely distributed; crosses the blood-brain barrier.
Metabolism and Excretion: Partially metabolized by the liver. 30–50% excreted unchanged by the kidneys.
Half-life: 11–23 hr.

TIME/ACTION PROFILE (antiarrhythmic effects)

ROUTE	ONSET	PEAK	DURATION
PO	30–60 min	0.5–2 hr	8–12 hr

Contraindications/Precautions

Contraindicated in: Hypersensitivity; Advanced heart block.
Use Cautiously in: CHF; Geriatric patients or hepatic or renal impairment (dosage reduction recommended); Pregnancy, lactation, or children (safety not established).

Interactions

Drug-Drug: Additive cardiac effects with other **antiarrhythmics.** Concurrent use with **metoprolol** may result ↑ the risk of adverse cardiovascular reactions. **Cimetidine** or **rifampin** may ↓ blood levels of tocainide.

Route/Dosage

PO (Adults): 400 mg q 8 hr initially; usual maintenance dose 1.2–1.8 g/day in divided doses q 8–12 hr.

Availability

Tablets: 400 mg, 600 mg, 400 mg.

tocilizumab (toe-si-liz-oo-mab)

Actemra

Classification
Therapeutic: antirheumatics, immunosuppressants
Pharmacologic: interleukin antagonists

Indications

Treatment of adults with moderately to severely active rheumatoid arthritis who have not responded to one or more tumor necrosis factor (TNF) antagonist therapies (may be used alone or with methotrexate or other disease-modifying antirheumatic drugs [DMARDs]).

Action

Acts as in inhibitor of interleukin-6 (IL-6) receptors by binding to them. IL-6 is a mediator of various inflammatory processes. **Therapeutic Effects:** Slowed progression of rheumatoid arthritis

Adverse Reactions/Side Effects

CNS: headache, dizziness. **EENT:** nasopharyngitis. **Resp:** upper respiratory tract infections. **CV:** hypertension. **GI:** GASTROINTESTINAL PERFORATION, ↑ liver enzymes. **Derm:** rash. **Hemat:** NEUTROPENIA, THROMBOCYTOPENIA. **Metab:** ↑ lipids. **Misc:** SERIOUS INFECTIONS, INCLUDING TUBERCULOSIS, DISSEMINATED FUNGAL INFECTIONS, AND INFECTIONS WITH OPPORTUNISTIC PATHOGENS; HYPERSENSITIVITY REACTIONS, INCLUDING ANAPHYLAXIS, infusion reactions.

PHYSICAL THERAPY IMPLICATIONS

Examination and Evaluation

- Monitor signs of hypersensitivity reactions and anaphylaxis, including pulmonary symptoms (tightness in the throat and chest, wheezing, cough, dyspnea) or skin reactions (rash, pruritus, urticaria). Be especially alert for allergy-like responses that occur during and after administration (infusion reactions). Notify physician or nursing staff immediately of any signs of hypersensitivity.

- Watch for signs of infection, especially tuberculosis, pulmonary fungal infections, or other respiratory infections. Signs include fatigue, chills, fever, night sweats, loss of appetite, and pulmonary pathology (persistent cough, coughing up blood, chest pain when breathing and coughing). Report these signs to the physician or nursing staff immediately.
- Monitor and report signs of neutropenia (fever, sore throat, other signs of infection) or thrombocytopenia (bruising, nose bleeds, bleeding gums). Periodic blood tests may be needed to monitor WBC and RBC counts.
- Watch for signs of GI perforation, including severe abdominal pain, nausea, vomiting, chills, and fever. Report these signs to the physician or nursing staff immediately.
- Assess blood pressure (BP) periodically and compare to normal values (See Appendix F). Report a sustained increase in BP (hypertension).
- Periodically assess impairments (pain, range of motion), functional ability, and disability to help document whether antirheumatic drug therapy is successful.
- Assess dizziness that might affect gait, balance, and other functional activities (See Appendix C). Report balance problems and functional limitations to the physician and nursing staff, and caution the patient and family/caregivers to guard against falls and trauma.

Interventions

- Implement appropriate manual therapy techniques, physical agents, therapeutic exercises, and orthotic/assistive devices to reduce pain, improve function, and augment the effects of antirheumatic drug therapy.
- Help patients with arthritis explore other nonpharmacologic methods to reduce chronic arthritis pain, such as relaxation techniques, exercise, counseling, and so forth.

Patient/Client-Related Instruction

- Instruct patient to guard against infection (frequent hand washing, etc.), and to avoid crowds and contact with persons with contagious diseases.
- Advise patient that this drug may cause problems in fat metabolism (hyperlipidemia, hypercholesterolemia). Remind patient that periodic blood tests may be needed to monitor plasma lipids.
- Instruct patient to report other troublesome side effects, including severe or prolonged headache, nasal/pharyngeal irritation, or skin rashes.

Pharmacokinetics

Absorption: IV administration results in complete bioavailability.
Distribution: Unknown.
Metabolism and Excretion:
Half-life: *4 mg/kg dose*—up to 11 days; *8 mg/kg*—up to 13 days.

TIME/ACTION PROFILE (improvement)

ROUTE	ONSET	PEAK	DURATION
IV	within 1 mo	4 mo	unknown

Contraindications/Precautions

Contraindicated in: Serious infections; Patients at risk for GI perforation, including patients with diverticulitis; Active hepatic disease/impairment; Absolute neutrophil count (ANC) <2000/mm^3 (<500/mm^3 while on therapy) or platelet count below 100,000/mm^3 (<50,000/mm^3 while on therapy). Lactation: Not recommended during breast-feeding.
Use Cautiously in: Renal or hepatic impairment; Patients with tuberculosis risk factors. Geri: ↑ risk of adverse reactions. OB: Use only if potential benefit justifies potential risk to fetus. Pedi: Safety and effectiveness not established.

Interactions

Drug-Drug: May alter the activity of CYP450 enzymes; the effects of the following drugs should be monitored: **cyclosporine, theophylline, warfarin, hormonal contraceptives, atorvastatin,** and **lovastatin.** Other drugs which are substrates for this system should also be monitored; effect may persist for several weeks after discontinuation; May ↓ antibody response to and ↑ risk of adverse reactions to **live-virus vaccines;** do not administer concurrently.

Route/Dosage

PO (Adults): 4 mg/kg; may be ↑ to 8 mg/kg based on clinical response; dose reductions are recommended for ↑ liver enzymes, neutropenia, and thrombocytopenia.

Availability

Solution for IV infusion (requires dilution): 20 mg/mL

HIGH ALERT

tolazamide (tole-a-za-mide)

Tolamide, Tolinase

Classification
Therapeutic: antidiabetics
Pharmacologic: sulfonylureas

T

Indications

Control of blood sugar in type 2 diabetes mellitus when diet therapy fails. Requires some pancreatic function.

Action

Lowers blood sugar by stimulating the release of insulin from the pancreas and increasing the sensitivity to insulin at receptor sites. May also decrease hepatic glucose production. **Therapeutic Effects:** Lowering of blood sugar in diabetic patients.

Adverse Reactions/Side Effects

CNS: dizziness, drowsiness, headache, weakness. **GI:** constipation, cramps, diarrhea, drug-induced hepatitis, dyspepsia, increased appetite, nausea, vomiting. **Derm:** photosensitivity, rashes. **Endo:** hypoglycemia. **F and E:** hyponatremia. **Hemat:** APLASTIC ANEMIA, agranulocytosis, leukopenia, pancytopenia, thrombocytopenia.

PHYSICAL THERAPY IMPLICATIONS

Examination and Evaluation

- Monitor signs of aplastic anemia (fatigue, weakness, shortness of breath with exertion, tachycardia, dizziness, headache), agranulocytosis (fever, sore throat, mucosal lesions, signs of infection, bruising), thrombocytopenia (bruising, nose bleeds, and bleeding gums), or unusual weakness and fatigue that might be due to other blood dyscrasias. Report these signs to the physician immediately.
- Be alert for signs of hypoglycemia, especially during and after exercise. Common neuromuscular signs include anxiety; restlessness; tingling in hands, feet, lips, or tongue; chills; cold sweats; confusion; difficulty in concentration; drowsiness; excessive hunger; headache; irritability; nervousness; tremor; weakness; unsteady gait. Report persistent or repeated episodes of hypoglycemia to the physician.
- Assess any dizziness (See Appendix C) or drowsiness that might impair gait, balance, and other complex motor tasks (driving a car). Report balance problems and functional limitations to the physician, and caution the patient and family/caregivers to guard against falls and trauma.
- Monitor signs of low sodium levels (hyponatremia), including headache, confusion, lethargy, irritability, decreased consciousness, and neuromuscular abnormalities (muscle weakness and cramps). Report severe or prolonged signs to the physician.
- Assess blood pressure periodically (See Appendix F). A sudden or sustained increase in blood pressure (hypertension) may indicate problems in diabetes management, and should be reported to the physician.

Interventions

- Implement aerobic exercise and endurance training programs to maintain optimal body weight, improve insulin sensitivity, and reduce the risk of macrovascular disease (heart attack, stroke) and microvascular problems (reduced blood flow to tissues and organs that causes poor wound healing, neuropathy, retinopathy, and nephropathy).
- Provide a source of oral glucose (fruit juice, glucose gels/tablets, etc.) to treat mild hypoglycemia. Call for emergency assistance if symptoms persist or in cases of severe hypoglycemia. Emergency treatment typically consists of IV glucose, glucagon, or epinephrine.
- Causes photosensitivity; use care if administering UV treatments.

Patient/Client-Related Instruction

- Encourage patient to monitor blood glucose before and after exercise and to adjust food intake to maintain normal glycemic levels.
- Emphasize the importance of adhering to nutritional guidelines and the need for periodic assessment of glycemic control (serum glucose and glycosylated hemoglobin levels) throughout the management of diabetes mellitus.
- Advise patient about symptoms of hyperglycemia (confusion, drowsiness; flushed, dry skin; fruit-like breath odor; rapid, deep breathing, polyuria; loss of appetite; unusual thirst). Drug dosages may need to be adjusted to prevent repeated episodes of hyperglycemia.
- Instruct patient to report severe or prolonged GI problems (diarrhea, constipation, cramps) or signs of drug-induced hepatitis (anorexia, abdominal pain, severe nausea and vomiting, yellow skin or eyes, skin rashes, flu-like symptoms, muscle/joint pain).
- Advise patient about photosensitivity, and to use sunscreens, protective clothing, and avoid prolonged sun exposure. Advise patient to also report any rashes or other skin reactions.

Pharmacokinetics

Absorption: Well absorbed following oral administration.
Distribution: Unknown.
Protein Binding: 94%.
Metabolism and Excretion: Mostly metabolized by the liver; some conversion to metabolites with hypoglycemic activity.
Half-life: 7 hr.

TIME/ACTION PROFILE (hypoglycemic activity)

ROUTE	ONSET	PEAK	DURATION
PO	60 min	3–4 hr	10–20 hr

Contraindications/Precautions

Contraindicated in: Hypersensitivity; Hypersensitivity to sulfonamides (cross-sensitivity may occur); Type 1 diabetes (as monotherapy); Diabetic coma or

ketoacidosis; Severe renal, hepatic, thyroid, or other endocrine disease; Uncontrolled infection, serious burns, or trauma.
Use Cautiously in: Severe cardiovascular disease; Geriatric patients (↑ sensitivity; dosage reduction may be required); Hepatic or renal impairment (↑ risk of hypoglycemia); Infection, stress, or changes in diet may alter requirements for control of blood sugar; Impaired thyroid, pituitary, or adrenal function; Malnutrition, high fever, prolonged nausea, or vomiting; Pregnancy or lactation (safety not established; insulin recommended during pregnancy).

Interactions

Drug-Drug: Ingestion of **alcohol** may result in disulfiram-like reaction. Effectiveness may be decreased by concurrent use of **diuretics, corticosteroids, phenothiazines, hormonal contraceptives, estrogens, thyroid preparations, phenytoin, nicotinic acid,** sympathomimetics (**adrenergics**), and **isoniazid. Alcohol, androgens (testosterone), chloramphenicol, clofibrate, MAO inhibitors, NSAIDs** (except diclofenac), **salicylates, sulfonamides,** and **warfarin** may ↑ the risk of hypoglycemia. Concurrent use with **warfarin** may alter the response to both agents (↑ effects of both initially, then ↓ activity; close monitoring recommended during any changes in dosage). **Beta blockers** may mask the signs and symptoms of hypoglycemia.
Drug-Natural: Glucosamine may worsen blood glucose control. **Fenugreek, chromium,** and **coenzyme Q10** may produce additive hypoglycemic effects.

Route/Dosage

PO (Adults): 100–250 mg/day (range 100–1000 mg/day; doses >500 mg/day should be given as divided doses).
PO (Geriatric Patients or Malnourished, Underweight Patients): 100 mg/day initially.

Availability (generic available)

Tablets: 100 mg, 250 mg, 500 mg.

tolbutamide (tole-byoo-ta-mide)

*Apo-Tolbutamide, *Mobenol, *Novo-Butamide, Orinase, Tol-Tab

Classification
Therapeutic: antidiabetics
Pharmacologic: sulfonylureas

Indications

PO: Control of blood sugar in type 2 diabetes mellitus when diet therapy fails. Requires some pancreatic function. **IV:** Diagnosis of pancreatic islet cell adenomas.

Action

Lowers blood sugar by stimulating the release of insulin from the pancreas and increasing the sensitivity to insulin at receptor sites. May also ↓ hepatic glucose production. **Therapeutic Effects:** Lowering of blood sugar in diabetic patients. Pronounced and prolonged hypoglycemic effect diagnostic of pancreatic islet cell adenoma.

Adverse Reactions/Side Effects

CNS: dizziness, drowsiness, headache, weakness.
GI: constipation, cramps, diarrhea, drug-induced hepatitis, heartburn, increased appetite, nausea, vomiting. **Derm:** <u>photosensitivity</u>, rashes. **Endo:** <u>hypoglycemia</u>. **F and E:** hyponatremia. **Hemat:** APLASTIC ANEMIA, agranulocytosis, leukopenia, pancytopenia, thrombocytopenia.

PHYSICAL THERAPY IMPLICATIONS

Examination and Evaluation

- Monitor signs of aplastic anemia (fatigue, weakness, shortness of breath with exertion, tachycardia, dizziness, headache), agranulocytosis (fever, sore throat, mucosal lesions, signs of infection, bruising), thrombocytopenia (bruising, nose bleeds, and bleeding gums), or unusual weakness and fatigue that might be due to other blood dyscrasias. Report these signs to the physician immediately.
- Be alert for signs of hypoglycemia, especially during and after exercise. Common neuromuscular signs include anxiety; restlessness; tingling in hands, feet, lips, or tongue; chills; cold sweats; confusion; difficulty in concentration; drowsiness; excessive hunger; headache; irritability; nervousness; tremor; weakness; unsteady gait. Report persistent or repeated episodes of hypoglycemia to the physician.
- Assess any dizziness (See Appendix C) or drowsiness that might impair gait, balance, and other complex motor tasks (driving a car). Report balance problems and functional limitations to the physician, and caution the patient and family/caregivers to guard against falls and trauma.
- Monitor signs of low sodium levels (hyponatremia), including headache, confusion, lethargy, irritability, decreased consciousness, and neuromuscular abnormalities (muscle weakness and cramps). Report severe or prolonged signs to the physician.
- Assess blood pressure periodically (See Appendix F). A sudden or sustained increase in blood pressure (hypertension) may indicate problems in diabetes management and should be reported to the physician.

Interventions

- Implement aerobic exercise and endurance training programs to maintain optimal body weight, improve insulin sensitivity, and reduce the risk of macrovascular disease (heart attack, stroke) and microvascular problems (reduced blood flow to tissues and organs that causes poor wound healing, neuropathy, retinopathy, and nephropathy).
- Provide a source of oral glucose (fruit juice, glucose gels/tablets, etc.) to treat mild hypoglycemia. Call for emergency assistance if symptoms persist or in cases of severe hypoglycemia. Emergency treatment typically consists of IV glucose, glucagon, or epinephrine.
- Causes photosensitivity; use care if administering UV treatments.

Patient/Client-Related Instruction

- Encourage patient to monitor blood glucose before and after exercise and to adjust food intake to maintain normal glycemic levels.
- Emphasize the importance of adhering to nutritional guidelines and the need for periodic assessment of glycemic control (serum glucose and glycosylated hemoglobin levels) throughout the management of diabetes mellitus.
- Advise patient about symptoms of hyperglycemia (confusion, drowsiness; flushed, dry skin; fruit-like breath odor; rapid, deep breathing, polyuria; loss of appetite; unusual thirst). Drug dosages may need to be adjusted to prevent repeated episodes of hyperglycemia.
- Instruct patient to report severe or prolonged GI problems (diarrhea, constipation, heartburn, cramps) or signs of drug-induced hepatitis (anorexia, abdominal pain, severe nausea and vomiting, yellow skin or eyes, skin rashes, flu-like symptoms, muscle/joint pain).
- Advise patient about photosensitivity and to use sunscreens, protective clothing, and avoid prolonged sun exposure. Advise patient to also report any rashes or other skin reactions.

Pharmacokinetics

Absorption: Well absorbed following oral administration; IV administration results in complete bioavailability.
Distribution: Unknown.
Protein Binding: 96%.
Metabolism and Excretion: Mostly metabolized by the liver.
Half-life: 7 hr (range 4–25 hr).

TIME/ACTION PROFILE (hypoglycemic activity)

ROUTE	ONSET	PEAK	DURATION
PO	60 min	4–6 hr	6–12 hr
IV*	rapid	30–45 min	120–210 min

*Normal subjects.

Contraindications/Precautions

Contraindicated in: Hypersensitivity (cross-sensitivity with sulfonamides may occur); Type 1 diabetes; Diabetic coma or ketoacidosis; Severe renal, hepatic, thyroid, or other endocrine disease; Uncontrolled infection, serious burns, or trauma.
Use Cautiously in: Severe cardiovascular disease; Geriatric patients (↑ sensitivity; dosage reduction may be required); Hepatic or renal impairment (↑ risk of hypoglycemia); Infection, stress, or changes in diet may alter requirements for control of blood sugar; Impaired thyroid, pituitary, or adrenal function; Malnutrition, high fever, prolonged nausea, or vomiting; Pregnancy or lactation (safety not established; insulin recommended during pregnancy).

Interactions

Drug-Drug: Ingestion of **alcohol** may result in disulfiram-like reaction. Effectiveness may be decreased by concurrent use of **diuretics, corticosteroids, phenothiazines, hormonal contraceptives, estrogens, thyroid preparations, phenytoin, nicotinic acid, sympathomimetics,** and **isoniazid. Alcohol, androgens (testosterone), chloramphenicol, clofibrate, MAO inhibitors, NSAIDs** (except diclofenac), **salicylates,** and **sulfonamides** may ↑ the risk of hypoglycemia. Concurrent use with **warfarin** may alter the response to both agents (↑ effects of both initially, then ↓ activity; close monitoring recommended during any changes in dosage). **Beta blockers** may mask the signs and symptoms of hypoglycemia.
Drug-Natural: Glucosamine may worsen blood glucose control. **Fenugreek, chromium,** and **coenzyme Q10** may produce additive hypoglycemic effects.

Route/Dosage

PO (Adults): 1000–2000 mg/day in single or divided doses; then adjusted to maintenance dose of 250–2000 mg/day (some patients may require up to 3000 mg/day).
IV (Adults): 1 g as part of the Fajan test.

Availability (generic available)

Tablets: 500 mg. **Powder for injection:** 1 g with 20 mL diluent.

tolcapone (tole-ka-pone)

Tasmar

Classification

Therapeutic: antiparkinson agents
Pharmacologic: catechol-O-methyltransferase inhibitors

Indications

Management of Parkinson's disease with carbidopa/levodopa in patients without severe movement abnormalities who do not respond to other treatments.

Action

Acts as a selective and reversible inhibitor of the enzyme catechol-*O*-methyltransferase. Inhibition of this enzyme prevents the breakdown of levodopa, greatly increasing its availability to the CNS. **Therapeutic Effects:** Prolongs duration of response to levodopa without end-of-dose motor fluctuations. ↓ signs and symptoms of Parkinson's disease.

Adverse Reactions/Side Effects

CNS: headache, sleep disorder, hallucinations, syncope. **CV:** orthostatic hypotension. **GI:** HEPATOTOXICITY, HEPATIC FAILURE, constipation, diarrhea, anorexia, elevated liver enzymes, nausea, vomiting. **GU:** hematuria, yellow discoloration of urine. **Derm:** increased sweating. **Neuro:** dyskinesia, dystonia.

PHYSICAL THERAPY IMPLICATIONS

Examination and Evaluation

- Be alert for signs of hepatotoxicity and liver failure, including anorexia, abdominal pain, severe nausea and vomiting, yellow skin or eyes, fever, sore throat, malaise, weakness, facial edema, lethargy, and unusual bleeding or bruising. Notify physician of these signs immediately.
- Assess gait and motor function to help determine antiparkinson effects, especially when starting drug therapy or during dosing changes or addition of other antparkinson drugs. Motor function should be assessed at different times of the day, such as when drugs are reaching peak therapeutic levels (i.e., 30–60 min after oral dose), as well as when drug effects are minimal (just before the next dose).
- Document increased motor side effects such as involuntary movements (dyskinesias), changes in muscle tone (dystonia), fluctuations in response (on-off phenomenon, end-of-dose akinesia), or other abnormal movement patterns. Notify physician because increased motor side effects might require dose adjustment or a change in medication regimen.
- Monitor hallucinations and other psychologic problems. Repeated or excessive symptoms may require change in dose or medication.
- Assess blood pressure (BP) when patient assumes a more upright position (lying to standing, sitting to standing, lying to sitting). Document orthostatic hypotension and contact physician when systolic BP falls >20 mm Hg, or diastolic BP falls >10 mm Hg.

Interventions

- Implement therapeutic exercises (coordination exercises, gait training, cardiovascular conditioning) to complement the effects of drug therapy and help achieve optimal function.
- Guard against falls and trauma (hip fractures, head injury, and so forth). Implement fall-prevention strategies (See Appendix E), especially if patient exhibits Parkinson's symptoms (postural instability, rigidity) combined with drug side effects (dyskinesias, fainting).
- To minimize orthostatic hypotension and syncope, patient should move slowly when assuming a more upright position.

Patient/Client-Related Instruction

- Advise patient to avoid alcohol because of the increased risk of sedation and adverse effects.
- Advise patient about the likelihood of GI reactions such as nausea, vomiting, diarrhea, and constipation. Instruct patient to report severe or prolonged GI problems.
- Instruct patient to report other troublesome side effects such as severe or prolonged headaches, sleep disorders, bloody or discolored urine, fainting, or increased sweating.

Pharmacokinetics

Absorption: Rapidly absorbed following oral administration with 65% bioavailability.
Distribution: Unknown.
Protein Binding: >99% bound to plasma proteins.
Metabolism and Excretion: Mostly metabolized by the liver; <0.5% excreted unchanged in urine.
Half-life: 2–3 hr.

TIME/ACTION PROFILE (blood levels)

ROUTE	ONSET	PEAK	DURATION
PO	unknown	1.7 hr	8 hr

Contraindications/Precautions

Contraindicated in: Hypersensitivity; Concurrent MAO inhibitor therapy; Clinical evidence of liver disease.
Use Cautiously in: Severe renal impairment (safety not established if CCr <25 mL/min); OB: Pregnancy or lactation (safety not established).

Interactions

Drug-Drug: Concurrent use with **MAO inhibitors** is not recommended; both agents inhibit the metabolic pathways of catecholamines. May ↑ the effects of **methyldopa, apomorphine, dobutamine,** or **isoproterenol;** dose reduction may be necessary. ↑ the bioavailability of **levodopa** by twofold; this is a desired effect.

Route/Dosage

PO (Adults): 100 mg tid; may be cautiously increased to 200 mg tid if benefit is justified.

T

Availability

Tablets: 100 mg, 200 mg.

tolnaftate (tol-naf-tate)

✱ Pitrex, Podactin, Q-Naftate, Tinactin, Ting

Classification

Therapeutic: antifungals (topical)
Pharmacologic: thiocarbamates

Indications

Treatment of a variety of cutaneous fungal infections, including tinea pedis (athlete's foot), tinea cruris (jock itch), and tinea corporis (ringworm).

Indications

Distorts the hyphae and stunts mycelial growth in fungi.

Action

Therapeutic Effects: ↓ in symptoms of fungal infection.

Adverse Reactions/Side Effects

Local: burning, itching, local hypersensitivity reactions, redness, stinging.

PHYSICAL THERAPY IMPLICATIONS

Examination and Evaluation

- Assess healing of skin lesions to help document drug effectiveness.

Interventions

- Avoid contact with cutaneous lesions when treating patient.
- Always wash hands thoroughly and disinfect equipment (whirlpools, electrotherapeutic devices, treatment tables, and so forth) to help prevent the spread of infection.

Patient/Client-Related Instruction

- Advise patient to report any increased local sensitivity to this drug (pain, burning, itching, swelling).
- Instruct patient about proper hygiene; e.g., thoroughly wash and dry the affected area, wear clean socks and ventilated shoes for tinea pedis, and so forth.
- Advise patient to apply the drug as directed for the full course of treatment even if feeling better.
- Inform patient that early relief of cutaneous symptoms may be seen in 2–3 days. Full therapeutic response may take 2 wk for tinea cruris and tinea corporis and 4 wk for tinea pedis.
- Advise patient to seek medical help if infections persist or recur after the full treatment. Recurrent fungal infections may be a sign of systemic illness.

Pharmacokinetics

Absorption: Absorption through intact skin is minimal.
Distribution: Distribution after topical administration is primarily local.
Metabolism and Excretion: Systemic metabolism and excretion not known following local application.
Half-life: Not applicable.

TIME/ACTION PROFILE

ROUTE	ONSET	PEAK	DURATION
Topical	24–72 hr	unknown	unknown

Contraindications/Precautions

Contraindicated in: Hypersensitivity to active ingredients, additives, preservatives, or bases; Some products contain alcohol and should be avoided in patients with known intolerance.
Use Cautiously in: Nail and scalp infections (may require additional systemic therapy); OB/Lactation: Safety not established.

Interactions

Drug-Drug: Not known.

Route/Dosage

Topical (Adults and Children ≥2 yr): Apply bid for up to 2 wk for tinea cruris and for up to 4 wk for tinea pedis or tinea corporis.

Availability (generic available)

Cream: 1% OTC. **Powder:** 1% OTC. **Solution:** 1% OTC. **Spray liquid:** 1% OTC. **Spray powder:** 1% OTC.

tolterodine (tol-ter-oh-deen)

Detrol, Detrol LA

Classification

Therapeutic: urinary tract antispasmodics
Pharmacologic: anticholinergics

Indications

Treatment of overactive bladder function that results in urinary frequency, urgency, or urge incontinence.

Action

Acts as a competitive muscarinic receptor antagonist resulting in inhibition of cholinergically mediated bladder contraction. **Therapeutic Effects:** ↓ urinary frequency, urgency, and urge incontinence.

Adverse Reactions/Side Effects

CNS: <u>headache</u>, <u>dizziness</u>. **EENT:** blurred vision, dry eyes. **GI:** <u>dry mouth</u>, constipation, dyspepsia.

PHYSICAL THERAPY IMPLICATIONS

Examination and Evaluation

- Assess dizziness that might affect gait, balance, and other functional activities (See Appendix C). Report balance problems and functional limitations to the physician, and caution the patient and family/caregivers to guard against falls and trauma.

- Monitor signs of urine retention (difficult urination, painful or distended abdomen). Excessive urinary retention may require dose adjustment by physician.

Interventions

- When appropriate, implement pelvic floor muscle strengthening activities and other therapeutic exercises to help maintain bladder control.

Patient/Client-Related Instruction

- Advise patient to increase fluid intake and dietary fiber to avoid constipation. Laxatives may also be helpful in patients susceptible to fecal impaction.
- Instruct patient and family/caregivers to report other troublesome side effects such as severe or prolonged headache, blurred vision, dry eyes, or GI problems (dry mouth, indigestion).

Pharmacokinetics

Absorption: Well absorbed (77%) following oral administration.
Distribution: Unknown.
Protein Binding: 96.3%.
Metabolism and Excretion: Extensively metabolized by the liver; 1 metabolite (5-hydroxymethyltolterodine) is active; other metabolites are excreted in urine.
Half-life: *Tolterodine*—1.9–3.7 hr; *5-hydroxymethyltolterodine*—2.9–3.1 hr.

TIME/ACTION PROFILE (effects on bladder function)

ROUTE	ONSET	PEAK	DURATION
PO	unknown	unknown	12 hr

Contraindications/Precautions

Contraindicated in: Urinary retention; Gastric retention; Uncontrolled angle-closure glaucoma; Lactation.
Use Cautiously in: GI obstructive disorders, including pyloric stenosis (increased risk of gastric retention); Significant bladder outflow obstruction (↑ risk of urinary retention); Controlled angle-closure glaucoma; Significant hepatic impairment (lower doses recommended); Impaired renal function; Pregnancy (safe use not established; use only if potential maternal benefit justifies potential risk to fetus); Children (safety not established).

Interactions

Drug-Drug: Erythromycin, clarithromycin, ketoconazole, itraconazole, and **miconazole** may inhibit metabolism and ↑ effects of tolterodine.

Route/Dosage

PO (Adults): 2 mg bid as tablets; may be lowered depending on response *or* 2–4 mg once daily as extended-release capsules.
PO (Adults with Impaired Hepatic Function or Concurrent Enzyme Inhibitors): 1 mg bid.

Availability

Tablets: 1 mg, 2 mg, **Extended-release capsules:** 2 mg, 4 mg.

topiramate (toe-peer-i-mate)

Topamax

Classification
Therapeutic: anticonvulsants, mood stabilizers

Indications

Seizures including: partial-onset, primary generalized tonic-clonic, seizures due to Lennox-Gastaut syndrome. Prevention of migraine headache in adults. **Unlabeled Use:** Adjunct in treatment of bipolar disorder.

Action

Action may be due to Blockade of sodium channels in neurons, Enhancement of gamma-aminobutyrate (GABA), an inhibitory neurotransmitter, Prevention of activation of excitatory receptors. **Therapeutic Effects:** ↓ incidence of seizures. ↓ incidence/severity of migraine headache.

T

Adverse Reactions/Side Effects

CNS: INCREASED SEIZURES, dizziness, drowsiness, fatigue, impaired concentration/memory, nervousness, psychomotor slowing, speech problems, sedation, aggressive reaction, agitation, anxiety, cognitive disorders, confusion, depression, malaise, mood problems. **EENT:** abnormal vision, diplopia, nystagmus, acute myopia/secondary angle closure glaucoma. **GI:** nausea, abdominal pain, anorexia, constipation, dry mouth. **GU:** kidney stones. **Derm:** oligohidrosis (↑ in children). **F and E:** hyperchloremic metabolic acidosis. **Hemat:** leukopenia. **Metab:** weight loss, hyperthermia (↑ in children). **Neuro:** ataxia, paresthesia, tremor. **Misc:** SUICIDE ATTEMPT, fever.

PHYSICAL THERAPY IMPLICATIONS

Examination and Evaluation

- Document the number, duration, and severity of seizures to help determine if this drug is effective in reducing seizure activity. Report an increase in seizure activity to the physician immediately.
- Be alert for suicidal thoughts and ideology; notify physician immediately if patient exhibits signs of depression or other changes in mood and behavior.
- Assess dizziness or ataxia that might affect gait, balance, and other functional activities (See Appendix C). Report balance problems and

functional limitations to the physician, and caution the patient and family/caregivers to guard against falls and trauma.

- Monitor daytime drowsiness, nervousness, agitation, confusion, aggressive behavior, cognitive impairment, memory loss, or difficulty concentrating. Repeated or excessive symptoms may require change in dose or medication.
- Assess signs of paresthesia (numbness, tingling) or tremor. Perform objective tests including electroneuromyography and sensory testing to document any drug-related neuropathic changes.
- Monitor signs of metabolic acidosis, including headache, lethargy, stupor, seizures, vision disturbances, increased respiration, cardiac arrhythmias, weakness, and GI symptoms (nausea, vomiting, abdominal pain). Notify physician immediately if these signs occur.
- Be alert for signs of leukopenia, including fever, sore throat, mucosal lesions, and signs of infection. Report these signs to the physician.
- Monitor and report signs of kidney stones, including severe pain in the side and back, pain on urination, bloody urine, and a persistent urge to urinate.
- Periodically assess body weight and other anthropometric measures (body mass index, body composition). Report a rapid or unexplained weight loss or decrease in body fat.
- If used to prevent migraine headaches, document the frequency and severity of migraines to determine if this drug is successful in helping manage this condition.
- If treating bipolar disorder, monitor any changes in the patient's mood or behavior. Report manic symptoms (excitement, agitation) or symptoms of depression (sadness, apathy, loss of energy).

Interventions

- Guard against falls and trauma (hip fractures, head injury, and so forth), especially if dizziness or ataxia affects gait and balance. Implement fall-prevention strategies, especially if balance is impaired (See Appendix E).

Patient/Client-Related Instruction

- Advise patient to avoid alcohol and other CNS depressants because of the increased risk of sedation and adverse effects.
- Advise patients on prolonged antiseizure therapy not to discontinue medication without consulting their physician. Abrupt withdrawal may cause increased seizures.
- Advise patient about the risk of daytime drowsiness and decreased attention and mental focus. Use care if driving or in other activities that require strong concentration and fast responses.
- Instruct patient and family/caregivers to report other troublesome side effects such as severe or prolonged fever, vision problems, inadequate sweating, or GI problems (nausea, constipation, abdominal pain, loss of appetite, dry mouth).

Pharmacokinetics

Absorption: Well absorbed (80%) after oral administration.

Distribution: Unknown.

Metabolism and Excretion: 70% excreted unchanged in urine.

Half-life: 21 hr.

TIME/ACTION PROFILE (blood levels*)

ROUTE	ONSET	PEAK	DURATION
PO	unknown	2 hr	12 hr

*After single dose.

Contraindications/Precautions

Contraindicated in: Hypersensitivity; Lactation: Lactation.

Use Cautiously in: All patients (may ↑ risk of suicidal thoughts/behaviors); Renal impairment (dosage reduction recommended if CCr <70 mL/min/1.73 m^2); Hepatic impairment; Dehydration; OB: Use only if maternal benefit outweighs fetal risk; Pedi: Children are more prone to oligohidrosis and hyperthermia; safety in children <2 yr not established; Geri: Consider age-related ↓ in renal/hepatic impairment, concurrent disease states and drug therapy.

Interactions

Drug-Drug: Blood levels and effects may be ↓ by **phenytoin, carbamazepine,** or **valproic acid.** May ↑ blood levels and effects of **phenytoin** or **amitriptyline.** May ↓ blood levels and effects of **hormonal contraceptives, risperidone, lithium,** or **valproic acid.** ↑ risk of CNS depression with **alcohol** or other **CNS depressants. Carbonic anhydrase inhibitors (acetazolamide)** may ↑ risk of kidney stones. Concurrent use with **valproic acid** may ↑ risk of hyperammonemia/encephalopathy.

Route/Dosage

Epilepsy (monotherapy)

PO (Adults and children ≥10 yr): *Seizures/migraine prevention*—50 mg/day initially; gradually ↑ over 6 wk to 400 mg/day in 2 divided doses.

Epilepsy (adjunctive therapy)

PO (Adults and Children ≥17 yr): 25–50 mg/day ↑ by 25–50 mg/day at weekly intervals up to 200–400 mg/day in 2 divided doses (200–400 mg/day in 2 divided doses for partial seizures and 400 mg/day in 2 divided doses for primary generalized tonic/clonic seizures).

Renal Impairment

PO (Adults): *CCr <70 mL/min*—50% of the usual dose.

PO (Children 2–17 yr): *Seizures*—5–9 mg/kg/day in 2 divided doses; initiate with 25 mg (or less based in 1–3 mg/kg) nightly for 7 days then ↑ at 1- to 2-wk intervals in increments of 1–3 mg/kg/day in 2 divided doses; titration should be based on clinical outcome.

Migraine prevention

PO (Adults): 25 mg at night initially; ↑ by 25 mg/day at weekly intervals up to target dose of 100 mg/day in 2 divided doses.

Availability

Sprinkle capsules: 15 mg, 25 mg. **Tablets:** 25 mg, 50 mg, 100 mg, 200 mg.

HIGH ALERT

topotecan (toe-poe-**tee**-kan)

Hycamtin

Classification

Therapeutic: antineoplastics

Pharmacologic: enzyme inhibitors

Indications

IV: Metastatic ovarian cancer that has not responded to previous chemotherapy. Small-cell lung cancer unresponsive to 1st-line therapy. **PO:** Relapsed small-cell lung cancer in patients with a complete or partial prior response and who are at least 45 days from the end of 1st-line chemotherapy. Stage IV-B persistent or recurrent cervical cancer not amenable to treatment with surgery or radiation (with cisplatin).

Action

Interferes with DNA synthesis by inhibiting the enzyme topoisomerase. **Therapeutic Effects:** Death of rapidly replicating cells, particularly malignant ones.

Adverse Reactions/Side Effects

CNS: headache, fatigue, weakness. **Resp:** dyspnea. **GI:** abdominal pain, diarrhea, nausea, vomiting, anorexia, constipation, increased liver enzymes, stomatitis. **Derm:** alopecia. **Hemat:** anemia, leukopenia, thrombocytopenia. **MS:** arthralgia.

PHYSICAL THERAPY IMPLICATIONS

Examination and Evaluation

- Watch for signs of leukopenia (fever, sore throat, signs of infection), thrombocytopenia (bruising, nose bleeds, bleeding gums), or unusual weakness and fatigue that might be due to anemia. Report these signs to the physician.
- Assess respiratory symptoms such as difficult or labored breathing. Monitor pulse oximetry and perform pulmonary function tests (See Appendix I) to quantify suspected changes in ventilation and respiratory function.
- Assess any joint pain to rule out musculoskeletal pathology; that is, try to determine if pain is drug induced rather than caused by anatomic or biomechanical problems.

Interventions

- For patients who are medically able to begin exercise, implement appropriate resistive exercises and aerobic training to maintain muscle strength and aerobic capacity during cancer chemotherapy, or to help restore function after chemotherapy.

Patient/Client-Related Instruction

- Advise patient to guard against infection (frequent hand washing, etc.), and to avoid crowds and contact with persons with contagious diseases.
- Advise patient about the likelihood of GI reactions (nausea, vomiting, diarrhea, constipation, loss of appetite, irritation in/around the mouth). Instruct patient or family and caregivers to also report signs of hepatotoxicity, including anorexia, abdominal pain, severe nausea and vomiting, yellow skin or eyes, fever, sore throat, malaise, weakness, facial edema, lethargy, and unusual bleeding or bruising.
- Advise patient and family/caregivers that fatigue and weakness are likely and may be severe. Functional abilities may be limited, and patient may need to use assistive devices during ambulation.
- Advise patient that hair loss is likely. Instruct patient to report severe or unexpected skin problems.
- Instruct patient or family/caregivers to report other bothersome side effects such as severe or prolonged headache.

Pharmacokinetics

Absorption: IV administration results in complete bioavailability.

Distribution: Unknown.

Metabolism and Excretion: 30% excreted in urine; small amounts metabolized by the liver.

Half-life: *PO*—3–6 hr; *IV*—2–3 hr.

TIME/ACTION PROFILE (effects on WBCs)

ROUTE	ONSET	PEAK	DURATION
PO	unknown	1–2 hr	24 hr
IV	within days	11 days	7 days

Contraindications/Precautions

Contraindicated in: Hypersensitivity; Pregnancy or lactation; Preexisting severe myelosuppression.

Use Cautiously in: Impaired renal function (reduce dose if CCr <40 mL/min); Platelet count

T

<25,000 cells/mm^3 (reduce dose); Patients with childbearing potential.

Interactions

Drug-Drug: Neutropenia is prolonged by concurrent use of **filgrastim** (do not use until day 6; 24 hr following completion of topotecan). ↑ myelosuppression with other **antineoplastics** (especially **cisplatin**) or **radiation therapy.** May ↓ antibody response to and ↑ risk of adverse reactions from **live-virus vaccines.**

Route/Dosage

PO (Adults): 2.3 mg/m^2/day for 5 days repeated every 21 days (round calculated oral dose to nearest 0.25 mg and prescribe the minimum number of 1 mg and 0.25 mg capsules with the same number of capsules prescribed for each of the 5 days.

IV (Adults): *Ovarian and Small Cell Lung Cancer*—1.5 mg/m^2/day for 5 days starting on day 1 of a 21-day course; *Cervical Cancer*—75 mg/m^2 on days 1, 2, and 3 followed by cisplatin on day 1 and repeated every 21 days.

Renal Impairment

PO (Adults): *Ovarian and Small-Cell Lung Cancer—CCr 30–49 mL/min*—1.8 mg/m^2/day starting on day 1 of a 21-day course.

IV (Adults): *CCr 20–39 mL/min*—0.75mg/m^2/day for 5 days starting on day 1 of a 21-day course.

Cervical Cancer—Administer at standard doses only if serum creatinine is ≤1.5 mg/dL. Do not administer if serum creatinine is >1.5 mg/dL.

Availability

Capsules: 0.25 mg, 1 mg. **Lyophilized powder for injection:** 4 mg/vial.

toremifene (tore-em-i-feen)

Fareston

Classification

Therapeutic: antineoplastics

Pharmacologic: antiestrogens

Indications

Management of metastatic breast cancer in postmenopausal women with estrogen receptor–positive or unknown tumors.

Action

Exerts antiestrogenic effects by competing for estrogen-binding sites found in breast cancers. **Therapeutic Effects:** Regression of breast cancer.

Adverse Reactions/Side Effects

CNS: depression, dizziness, headache, lethargy. **EENT:** blurred vision, cataracts, corneal keratopathy, dry eyes, glaucoma. **CV:** CHF, MI, PULMONARY EMBOLISM, angina, arrhythmias, edema, thrombophlebitis. **GI:** nausea, elevated liver enzymes, vomiting. **GU:** vaginal discharge, vaginal bleeding. **Derm:** sweating. **F and E:** hypercalcemia. **Hemat:** anemia. **Misc:** hot flashes, tumor flare.

PHYSICAL THERAPY IMPLICATIONS

Examination and Evaluation

- Be alert for signs of myocardial infarction (MI), including sudden chest pain, pain radiating into the arm or jaw, shortness of breath, dizziness, sweating, anxiety, and nausea. Seek immediate medical assistance if patient develops these signs.
- Monitor signs of pulmonary embolism (PE) such as shortness of breath, chest pain, cough, and bloody sputum. Notify physician immediately, and request objective tests (Doppler ultrasound, lung scan, others) if thromboembolism is suspected.
- Assess signs of congestive heart failure (CHF), including dyspnea, rales/crackles, peripheral edema, jugular venous distention, and exercise intolerance. Report these signs to the physician or nursing staff.
- Assess heart rate, ECG, and heart sounds, especially during exercise (See Appendices G, H). Report any rhythm disturbances or symptoms of increased arrhythmias, including palpitations, chest discomfort, shortness of breath, fainting, and fatigue/weakness.
- Assess peripheral edema using girth measurements, volume displacement, and measurement of pitting edema (See Appendix N). Report increased swelling in feet and ankles or a sudden increase in body weight due to fluid retention.
- Monitor signs of thrombophlebitis, including localized pain, redness, warmth, and swelling in the affected area. Report these signs to the physician or nursing staff.
- Monitor signs of anemia, including unusual fatigue, shortness of breath with exertion, bruising, and pale skin. Notify physician or nursing staff if these signs occur.
- Assess any muscle, bone, or nerve pain at or near the tumor site. Increased pain at the onset of drug treatment may indicate tumor enlargement (tumor flare), and should be reported to the physician.
- Monitor and report depression, lethargy, or other changes in mood and behavior.
- Report signs of high calcium levels (hypercalcemia), including muscle pain, weakness, joint pain, confusion, and lethargy.
- Assess dizziness that might affect gait, balance, and other functional activities (See Appendix C). Report balance problems and functional limitations to the physician and nursing staff, and caution the patient and family/caregivers to guard against falls and trauma.

Interventions

- For patients who are medically able to begin exercise, implement appropriate resistive exercises and aerobic training to maintain muscle strength and aerobic capacity during cancer chemotherapy or to help restore function after chemotherapy.
- Because of the risk of MI, CHF, and PE, use extreme caution during aerobic exercise and other forms of therapeutic exercise. Assess exercise tolerance frequently (blood pressure, heart rate, fatigue levels), and terminate exercise immediately if any untoward responses occur (See Appendix L).

Patient/Client-Related Instruction

- Instruct patient and family or caregiver to seek immediate medical assistance if patient exhibits signs of MI, CHF, or PE (indicated above under Examination and Evaluation).
- Instruct patient to report other troublesome side effects such as prolonged or severe headaches, vision problems, hot flashes, vaginal discharge/bleeding, skin reactions (sweating), or GI problems (nausea, vomiting).

Pharmacokinetics

Absorption: Well absorbed following oral administration.
Distribution: Widely distributed; 99% bound to plasma proteins.
Protein Binding: 99.5%.
Metabolism and Excretion: Extensively metabolized; undergoes enterohepatic circulation.
Half-life: 5 days.

TIME/ACTION PROFILE (blood levels)

ROUTE	ONSET	PEAK	DURATION
PO	unknown	3 hr	4–6 wk*

*Steady-state blood levels occur after 4–6 wk.

Contraindications/Precautions

Contraindicated in: Hypersensitivity; Pregnancy or lactation; History of thromboembolic disease.
Use Cautiously in: Bone metastases (↑ risk of hypercalcemia); Preexisting endometrial hyperplasia (long-term treatment should be avoided).

Interactions

Drug-Drug: Concurrent use of **agents that decrease urinary excretion of calcium (thiazide diuretics)** may ↑ the risk of hypercalcemia. May ↑ the effect of **warfarin.**

Route/Dosage

PO (Adults): 60 mg once daily.

Availability

Tablets: 60 mg.

torsemide (tore-se-mide)

Demadex

Classification
Therapeutic: antihypertensives
Pharmacologic: loop diuretics

Indications

Edema due to CHF; Hepatic or renal disease; Hypertension.

Action

Inhibits the reabsorption of sodium and chloride from the loop of Henle and distal renal tubule. ↑ renal excretion of water, sodium, chloride, magnesium, hydrogen, and calcium. Effectiveness persists in impaired renal function. **Therapeutic Effects:** Diuresis and subsequent mobilization of excess fluid (edema, pleural effusions). ↓ blood pressure.

Adverse Reactions/Side Effects

CNS: dizziness, headache, nervousness. **EENT:** hearing loss, tinnitus. **CV:** hypotension. **GI:** constipation, diarrhea, dry mouth, dyspepsia, nausea, vomiting. **GU:** excessive urination. **Derm:** photosensitivity, rash. **Endo:** hyperglycemia, hyperuricemia. **F and E:** <u>dehydration</u>, hypocalcemia, <u>hypochloremia</u>, <u>hypokalemia</u>, <u>hypomagnesemia</u>, <u>hyponatremia</u>, <u>hypovolemia</u>, <u>metabolic alkalosis</u>. **MS:** arthralgia, muscle cramps, myalgia. **Misc:** increased BUN.

PHYSICAL THERAPY IMPLICATIONS

Examination and Evaluation

- Monitor signs of metabolic acidosis, including headache, lethargy, stupor, seizures, vision disturbances, increased respiration, cardiac arrhythmias, weakness, nausea, vomiting, and abdominal pain. Notify physician immediately if these signs occur.
- Monitor neuromuscular signs of fluid and electrolyte imbalances (hypocalcemia, hypokalemia, hyponatremia, hypovolemia, hypomagnesemia), including muscle aches, cramping, hyperexcitability, tremors, and tetany. Notify physician immediately if these signs occur.
- Assess blood pressure periodically and compare to normal values (See Appendix F) to help document antihypertensive effects. Report low blood pressure (hypotension), especially if patient experiences dizziness or syncope.
- When used to treat edema, help determine drug effects by assessing peripheral edema using girth measurements, volume displacement, and measurement of pitting edema (See Appendix N). Also monitor signs of pulmonary edema such as dyspnea and

T

rales/crackles (See Appendix K). Document whether peripheral and pulmonary symptoms are controlled adequately by diuretic therapy.

- Be alert for signs of hyperglycemia, including confusion, drowsiness, flushed/dry skin, fruit-like breath odor, rapid/deep breathing, polyuria, loss of appetite, and unusual thirst. Patients with diabetes mellitus should check blood glucose levels frequently.
- Assess any muscle or joint pain to rule out musculoskeletal pathology; that is, try to determine if pain is drug-induced rather than caused by anatomical or biomechanical problems.
- Assess dizziness that might affect gait, balance, and other functional activities (See Appendix C). Report balance problems and functional limitations to the physician, and caution the patient and family/caregivers to guard against falls and trauma.

Interventions

- Implement fall-prevention strategies, especially in older adults or if patient exhibits sedation, dizziness, blurred vision, or other impairments that affect gait and balance (See Appendix E).
- Use caution during aerobic exercise, especially in hot environments. Increased sweating will cause fluid and electrolyte loss, and may exaggerate metabolic acidosis and diuretic side effects (dizziness, muscle cramps, and so forth).
- To minimize orthostatic hypotension, patient should move slowly when assuming a more upright position.
- Causes photosensitivity; use care if administering UV treatments. Advise patient to avoid direct sunlight and use sunscreens and protective clothing.

Patient/Client-Related Instruction

- Remind patients to take medication as directed to control hypertension and other cardiac conditions even if they are asymptomatic.
- Counsel patients about additional interventions to help control blood pressure and cardiac dysfunction, such as regular exercise, weight loss, sodium restriction, stress reduction, moderation of alcohol consumption, and smoking cessation.
- Remind patient and family/caregivers that diuretics typically increase urine output. Any unusual problems such as excessive or painful urination or blood in the urine should be reported to the physician.
- Instruct patient to report other bothersome side effects, including severe or prolonged headache, skin rash, hearing loss, ringing/buzzing in the ears (tinnitus), or GI problems (nausea, vomiting, diarrhea, constipation, indigestion, dry mouth).

Pharmacokinetics

Absorption: 80% absorbed after oral administration.
Distribution: Widely distributed.
Protein Binding: ≥99%.
Metabolism and Excretion: 80% metabolized by liver, 20% excreted in urine.
Half-life: 3.5 hr.

TIME/ACTION PROFILE (diuretic effect)

ROUTE	ONSET	PEAK	DURATION
PO	within 60 min	60–120 min	6–8 hr
IV	within 10 min	within 60 min	6–8 hr

Contraindications/Precautions

Contraindicated in: Hypersensitivity; Cross-sensitivity with thiazides and sulfonamides may occur; Hepatic coma or anuria.
Use Cautiously in: Severe liver disease (may precipitate hepatic coma; concurrent use with potassium-sparing diuretics may be necessary); Electrolyte depletion; Geri: Geriatric patients may have ↑ risk of side effects, especially hypotension and electrolyte imbalance, at usual doses; Diabetes mellitus; ↑ azotemia; OB/Lactation/Pedi: Safety not established.

Interactions

Drug-Drug: ↑ hypotension with **antihypertensives, nitrates,** or acute ingestion of **alcohol.** ↑ risk of hypokalemia with other **diuretics, amphotericin B, stimulant laxatives,** and **corticosteroids.** Hypokalemia may ↑ risk of **digoxin** toxicity and ↑ risk of arrhythmia in patients taking drugs that prolong the QT interval. ↓ **lithium** excretion, may cause **lithium** toxicity. ↑ risk of ototoxicity with **aminoglycosides. NSAIDS** ↓ effects of torsemide. ↑ risk of **salicylate** toxicity (with use of high-dose **salicylate** therapy). ↓ effects of torsemide when given at same time as **cholestyramine.**

Route/Dosage

Congestive Heart Failure

PO, IV (Adults): 10–20 mg once daily; dose may be doubled until desired effect is obtained (maximum daily dose = 200 mg).

Chronic Renal Failure

PO, IV (Adults): 20 mg once daily; dose may be doubled until desired effect is obtained (maximum daily dose = 200 mg).

Hepatic Cirrhosis

PO, IV (Adults): 5–10 mg once daily (with aldosterone antagonist or potassium-sparing diuretic); dose may be doubled until desired effect is obtained (maximum daily dose = 40 mg).

Hypertension

PO, IV (Adults): 2.5–5 mg once daily, may be increased to 10 mg once daily after 4–6 wk (if still not effective, add another agent).

Availability (generic available)

Tablets: 5 mg Rx, 10 mg Rx, 20 mg Rx, 100 mg Rx.
Injection: 10 mg/mL Rx.

tositumomab (I 131 tositumomab)

(to-si-**too**-mo-mab)
Bexxar

Classification
Therapeutic: antineoplastics
Pharmacologic: monoclonal antibodies (radiolabled monoclonal antibodies)

Indications

CD20-positive, follicular, non-Hodgkin's lymphoma refractory to rituximab and in relapse.

Action

Binds to CD20 antigens on the surface of specific lymphocytes producing antibody-mediated cytotoxicity and cell death due to ionizing radiation. **Therapeutic Effects:** Sustained depletion of CD20 lymphocytes, with ↓ progression of lymphoma.

Adverse Reactions/Side Effects

CNS: dizziness, drowsiness, headache, weakness. **CV:** edema, hypotension. **GI:** abdominal pain, diarrhea, nausea, vomiting. **Endo:** hypothyroidism. **Hemat:** NEUTROPENIA, THROMBOCYTOPENIA, anemia. **Metab:** weight loss. **MS:** arthralgia, back pain, myalgia, neck pain. **Misc:** hypersensitivity reactions, including anaphylaxis, infusional toxicity, fever, secondary malignancies.

PHYSICAL THERAPY IMPLICATIONS

Examination and Evaluation

- Watch for signs of neutropenia (fever, sore throat, signs of infection), thrombocytopenia (bruising, nose bleeds, bleeding gums), or unusual weakness and fatigue that might be due to anemia. Notify physician or nursing staff immediately of these signs.
- Monitor signs of allergic reactions, including anaphylaxis. Reactions include pulmonary symptoms (tightness in the throat and chest, wheezing, cough, dyspnea) and skin reactions (rash, pruritus, urticaria). Be especially alert for these signs after drug infusion (infusion toxicity). Notify physician or nursing staff immediately if these reactions occur.
- Assess any increased joint, muscle, neck, or back pain to rule out musculoskeletal pathology; that is, try to determine if pain is drug induced rather than caused by anatomic or biomechanical problems.
- Assess blood pressure periodically. Report a problematic decrease in blood pressure (hypotension, See Appendix F), especially if dizziness and syncope occurs.
- Assess peripheral edema using girth measurements, volume displacement, and measurement of pitting edema (See Appendix N). Report increased swelling in feet and ankles or a sudden increase in body weight due to fluid retention.
- Assess dizziness and drowsiness that might affect gait, balance, and other functional activities (See Appendix C). Report balance problems and functional limitations to the physician and nursing staff, and caution the patient and family/caregivers to guard against falls and trauma.
- Monitor signs of hypothyroidism such as bradycardia, lethargy, cold intolerance, weight gain, and muscle weakness. Notify physician of these signs.
- Be alert for signs of secondary malignancies, including a change in bowel or bladder habits, nonhealing sores, unusual bleeding or discharge, a lump in the breast or other parts of the body, chronic indigestion or difficulty in swallowing, obvious changes in a wart or mole, and persistent coughing or hoarseness. Report these signs to the physician immediately.
- Periodically assess body weight and other anthropometric measures (body mass index, body composition). Report a rapid or unexplained weight loss or decreased body fat.

Interventions

- For patients who are medically able to begin exercise, implement appropriate resistive exercises and aerobic training to maintain muscle strength and aerobic capacity during cancer chemotherapy, or to help restore function after chemotherapy.

Patient/Client-Related Instruction

- Advise patient to guard against infection (frequent hand washing, etc.), and to avoid crowds and contact with persons with contagious diseases.
- Instruct patient or family/caregivers to report other bothersome side effects such as severe or prolonged headache, fever, or GI problems (nausea, vomiting, diarrhea, abdominal pain).

Pharmacokinetics

Absorption: IV administration results in complete bioavailability.
Distribution: Unknown.
Metabolism and Excretion: Excreted primarily by kidneys.
Half-life: Unknown.

TIME/ACTION PROFILE (depletion of lymphocytes)

ROUTE	ONSET	PEAK	DURATION
IV	unknown	7 wk	12 wk

Contraindications/Precautions

Contraindicated in: Hypersensitivity to murine (mouse) proteins; Pregnancy or lactation; Intolerance to thyroid blocking agents (these agents are required concurrently).
Use Cautiously in: >25% lymphoma marrow involvement, platelet count <100,000 cells/mm^3, neutrophil count <15,000 cells/mm^3 (safety not established); Presence of human antimouse antibodies (HAMA; ↑ risk of serious hypersensitivity, including anaphylaxis); Impaired renal function; Children (safety not established).

Interactions

Drug-Drug: May ↓ response to and ↑ risk of adverse reactions to **live-virus vaccines. Anticoagulants** or **agents interfering with platelet function** may ↑ risk of bleeding.

Route/Dosage

Pretreatment with thyroid blocking agents and premedication to prevent infusional reactions is required.
IV (Adults): *Dosimetric step*—tositumomab 450 mg and iodine I 131 tositumomab (containing 5 mCi I-131 and 35 mg tositumomab), followed 7–14 days later by therapeutic step. *Therapeutic step*—tositumomab 450 mg and iodine I 131 tositumomab (dose calculated by formulae and information provided with packaging); administer only if biodistribution is not altered.

Availability

These products are shipped only to practitioners who are participating in certification or are certified in preparation and administration of Bexxar. Dosimetric packaging is shipped from separate sites and must arrive simultaneously.
Tositumomab for injection: Package contains 2 225-mg vials and 1 35-mg vial; concentration 14 mg/mL. **I 131 tositumomab for injection:** 1 or 2 single-use vials containing not <20 mL of iodine I 131 tositumomab at nominal protein and activity concentrations of 1.1 mg/mL and 5.6 mCi/mL at calibration. Refer to product specification sheet for more specific information.

tramadol (tram-a-dol)

Ralivia, Ultram, Ultram ER

Classification
Therapeutic: analgesics (centrally acting)
Pharmacologic: opioid agonists

Indications

Moderate-to-moderately severe pain.

Action

Binds to mu-opioid receptors. Inhibits reuptake of serotonin and norepinephrine in the CNS.
Therapeutic Effects: ↓ pain.

Adverse Reactions/Side Effects

CNS: SEIZURES, dizziness, headache, somnolence, anxiety, CNS stimulation, confusion, coordination disturbance, euphoria, malaise, nervousness, sleep disorder, weakness. **EENT:** visual disturbances. **CV:** vasodilation. **GI:** constipation, nausea, abdominal pain, anorexia, diarrhea, dry mouth, dyspepsia, flatulence, vomiting. **GU:** menopausal symptoms, urinary retention/frequency. **Derm:** pruritus, sweating. **Neuro:** hypertonia. **Misc:** physical dependence, psychological dependence, tolerance.

PHYSICAL THERAPY IMPLICATIONS

Examination and Evaluation

- Watch for new seizures or increased seizure activity, especially at the onset of drug treatment. Document the number, duration, and severity of seizures, and report these findings immediately to the physician or nursing staff.
- Be alert for excessive sedation or somnolence. Notify physician or nurse immediately if patient is unconscious or extremely difficult to arouse.
- Monitor other changes in mood and behavior, including euphoria, confusion, malaise, nervousness, and anxiety. Notify physician if these changes become problematic.
- Use appropriate pain scales (visual analogue scales, others) to document whether this drug is successful in helping manage the patient's pain.
- Assess any incoordination or increased muscle tone. Report any coordination problems or hypertonia that might impair function or increase the risk of falls.
- Assess dizziness that might affect gait, balance, and other functional activities (See Appendix C). Report balance problems and functional limitations to the physician and nursing staff, and caution the patient and family/caregivers to guard against falls and trauma.

Interventions

- Implement appropriate manual therapy techniques, physical agents, and therapeutic exercises to reduce pain and help wean patient off centrally acting analgesics as soon as possible.
- Help patient explore other nonpharmacologic methods to reduce chronic pain, such as relaxation techniques, exercise, counseling, and so forth.

- Guard against falls and trauma (hip fractures, head injury). Implement fall-prevention strategies (See Appendix E), especially if patient exhibits sedation, dizziness, or blurred vision.

Patient/Client-Related Instruction

- Advise patient that centrally acting analgesics are usually more effective if given before pain becomes severe; emphasize that adequate pain control will allow better participation in physical therapy.
- Educate patient about the dangers of overdose; encourage patient to adhere to proper dosing schedule.
- Emphasize that the risk of physical addiction (tolerance and dependence) is usually minimal during short-term treatment of pain. Advise patient that addiction is more likely during excessive or inappropriate use of centrally acting analgesics.
- Advise patient to avoid alcohol and other CNS depressants because of the increased risk of sedation and decreased CNS function.
- Advise patient to increase fluid intake and dietary fiber to avoid constipation. Laxatives may also be helpful in patients susceptible to fecal impaction (e.g., people with spinal cord injury).
- Instruct patient to report other troublesome side effects such as severe or prolonged headache, vision disturbances, urinary retention or frequency, menopausal problems, skin reactions (itching, excessive sweating), or GI problems (nausea, vomiting, diarrhea, indigestion, dry mouth, loss of appetite, abdominal pain, flatulence).

Pharmacokinetics

Absorption: 75% absorbed after oral administration.
Distribution: Crosses the placenta; enters breast milk.
Metabolism and Excretion: Mostly metabolized by the liver; 1 metabolite has analgesic activity; 30% is excreted unchanged in urine.
Half-life: *Tramadol*—5–9 hr, *ER*—7.9 hr; *active metabolite*—5–9 hr, *ER*—8.8 hr (both are ↑ in renal or hepatic impairment).

TIME/ACTION PROFILE (analgesia)

ROUTE	ONSET	PEAK	DURATION
PO	1 hr	2–3 hr	4–6 hr
ER		12 hr	24 hr

Contraindications/Precautions

Contraindicated in: Hypersensitivity; Cross-sensitivity with opioids may occur; Patients who are acutely intoxicated with alcohol, sedative/hypnotics, centrally acting analgesics, opioid analgesics, or psychotropic agents; Patients who are physically dependent on opioid analgesics (may precipitate withdrawal); OB/Lactation: Not recommended for use; CCr <30 mL/min or severe hepatic impairment (Child-Pugh Class C), *ER formulation only*.
Use Cautiously in: Geri: Not to exceed 300 mg/day in patients >75 yr; Patients with a history of epilepsy or risk factors for seizures; Renal impairment (↑ dosing interval recommended if CCr <30 mL/min); Hepatic impairment (↑ dosing interval recommended in patients with cirrhosis); Patients receiving MAO inhibitors or CNS depressants; Patients who are suicidal; ↑ intracranial pressure or head trauma; Patients with a history of opioid dependence or who have recently received large doses of opioids; Pedi: Children <16 yr (safety not established).

Interactions

Drug-Drug: ↑ risk of CNS depression when used concurrently with other **CNS depressants,** including **alcohol, antihistamines, sedative/hypnotics, opioid analgesics, anesthetics,** or **psychotropic agents.** ↑ risk of seizures with high doses of **penicillins, cephalosporins, phenothiazines, opioid analgesics,** or **antidepressants. Carbamazepine** ↑ metabolism and ↓ effectiveness of tramadol (↑ doses may be required). Use cautiously in patients who are receiving **MAO inhibitors** (↑ risk of adverse reactions). Effectiveness may be altered by concurrent **quinidine.** ↑ risk of serotonin syndrome when used concurrently with **SSRI and SNRI antidepressants, TCAs, MAO inhibitors** and **5-HT$_1$ agonists.**
Drug-Natural: Concomitant use of **kava, valerian,** or **chamomile** can ↑ CNS depression.

Route/Dosage

PO (Adults ≥18 yr): *Rapid titration*—50–100 mg q 4–6 hr (not to exceed 400 mg/day or 300 mg in patients >75 yr). *Gradual titration*—25 mg/day initially, increase by 25 mg/day every 3 days to 100 mg/day, then increase by 50 mg/day every 3 days up to 200 mg/day *or* extended-release 100 mg/day; may be ↑ by 100-mg increments every 5 days based on pain level and tolerability, not to exceed 300 mg/day.

Renal Impairment

PO (Adults): *CCr <30 mL/min*—increase dosing to q 12 hr (not to exceed 200 mg/day).

Hepatic Impairment

PO (Adults): 50 mg q 12 hr.

Availability (generic available)

Tablets: 50 mg. **Extended-release tablets:** 100 mg, 200 mg, 300 mg. ***In combination with:*** acetaminophen (Ultracet). See Appendix B.

T

trandolapril (tran-doe-la-pril)

Mavik

Classification

Therapeutic: antihypertensives

Pharmacologic: angiotensin-converting enzyme (ACE) inhibitors

Indications

Alone or with other agents in the management of hypertension. Reduction of risk of death and heart-failure–related hospitalizations in patients with left ventricular systolic dysfunction or heart failure symptoms following myocardial infarction.

Action

ACE inhibitors block the conversion of angiotensin I to the vasoconstrictor angiotensin II. ACE inhibitors also prevent the degradation of bradykinin and other vasodilatory prostaglandins. ACE inhibitors also ↑ plasma renin levels and reduce aldosterone levels. Net result is systemic vasodilation.

Therapeutic Effects: Lowering of blood pressure in hypertensive patients. ↑ survival after myocardial infarction.

Adverse Reactions/Side Effects

CNS: weakness. **Resp:** cough. **CV:** hypotension. **Endo:** hyperuricemia. **GI:** diarrhea, dyspepsia. **GU:** impaired renal function. **Derm:** rashes. **F and E:** hyperkalemia, hypocalcemia. **MS:** myalgia. **Misc:** ANGIOEDEMA.

PHYSICAL THERAPY IMPLICATIONS

Examination and Evaluation

- Monitor signs of angioedema, including rashes, raised patches of red or white skin (welts), burning/itching skin, swelling in the face, and difficulty breathing. Report these signs to the physician immediately.
- Assess blood pressure periodically and compare to normal values (See Appendix F) to help document antihypertensive effects. Report low blood pressure (hypotension), especially if patient experiences dizziness or syncope.
- Assess signs and symptoms of CHF, including dyspnea, rales/crackles, peripheral edema, jugular venous distention, and exercise intolerance. Document whether drug therapy is effective in reducing these symptoms.
- Monitor signs of impaired renal function, including decreased urine output, cloudy urine, or sudden weight gain due to fluid retention. Report these signs to the physician.
- Watch for signs of electrolyte imbalances (hypocalcemia, hyperkalemia), including headache, lethargy, weakness, cramping, muscle pain, and muscle hyperexcitability and tetany. Notify physician immediately if these signs occur.

Interventions

- Implement aerobic exercise and cardiac conditioning programs to augment drug therapy and maintain or improve cardiovascular pump function in patients with heart failure and other cardiac conditions.
- Use caution during aerobic exercise and other forms of therapeutic exercise in patients recovering from myocardial infarction. Assess exercise tolerance frequently (blood pressure, heart rate, fatigue levels), and terminate exercise immediately if any untoward responses occur (See Appendix L).
- Avoid physical therapy interventions that cause systemic vasodilation (large whirlpool, Hubbard tank). Additive effects of this drug and the intervention may cause a dangerous fall in blood pressure.
- To minimize orthostatic hypotension, patient should move slowly when assuming a more upright position.

Patient/Client-Related Instruction

- Remind patients to take medication as directed to control hypertension and other cardiac conditions even if they are asymptomatic.
- Instruct patients with heart failure to weigh themselves every day, and to call their physician if they gain 3 lb or more in 1 day or more than 5 lb in 1 wk. Sudden weight gain may indicate fluid buildup due to worsening heart failure.
- Counsel patients about additional interventions to help control blood pressure and cardiac dysfunction, including regular exercise, weight loss, sodium restriction, stress reduction, moderation of alcohol consumption, and smoking cessation.
- Instruct patient to notify physician of a prolonged dry cough; drug therapy may need to be altered to resolve this side effect.
- Instruct patient or family/caregivers to report other troublesome side effects such as severe or prolonged headache, rash, or GI problems (diarrhea, indigestion).

Pharmacokinetics

Absorption: 70% bioavailability as trandolaprilat following oral administration.

Distribution: Crosses the placenta; enters breast milk.

Protein Binding: 80%.

Metabolism and Excretion: Converted by the liver to trandolaprilat, the active metabolite; 33% excreted in urine, 66% in feces.

Half-life: *Trandolapril:* 6 hr; *Trandolaprilat:* 10 hr (increased in renal impairment).

TIME/ACTION PROFILE (antihypertensive effect)

ROUTE	ONSET	PEAK	DURATION
PO	within 1–2 hr*	within 1 wk†	up to 24 hr†

*After single dose.
†Chronic dosing.

Contraindications/Precautions

Contraindicated in: Hypersensitivity; History of angioedema with previous use of ACE inhibitors; OB: Potential for injury or death of fetus. If pregnancy occurs, discontinue immediately. Lactation: Discontinue drug or use formula.

Use Cautiously in: Black patients (monotherapy for hypertension less effective, may require additional therapy; higher risk of angioedema); Surgery/anesthesia (hypotension may be exaggerated); Women of childbearing potential; Renal impairment), hypovolemia, hyponatremia, concurrent diuretic therapy, and Geri: Initial dosage reduction recommended; Pedi: Safety not established.

Exercise Extreme Caution in: Family history of angioedema.

Interactions

Drug-Drug: Excessive hypotension may occur with concurrent use of **diuretics.** Additive hypotension with other **antihypertensive agents.** ↑ risk of hyperkalemia with concurrent use of **potassium supplements, potassium-containing salt substitutes, angiotensin II receptor antagonists,** and **potassium-sparing diuretics.** Antihypertensive response may be blunted by **NSAIDs.** ↑ levels and may increase the risk of **lithium** toxicity.

Route/Dosage

PO (Adults): *Hypertension*—mg once daily (2 mg in black patients). May be increased weekly up to 4 mg once daily; bid dosing may be necessary in some patients (initiate therapy with 0.5 mg/day in patients receiving diuretics). *Heart failure post-MI or left ventricular dysfunction post-MI*—Initiate therapy at 1 mg once daily; titrate up to 4 mg once daily if possible.

Renal Impairment

PO (Adults): *CCr <30 mL/min*—Initiate therapy at 0.5 mg once daily; may be slowly titrated upward (max dose = 4 mg/day).

Hepatic Impairment

PO (Adults): Initiate therapy at 0.5 mg once daily; may be slowly titrated upward (max dose = 4 mg/day).

Availability (generic available)

Tablets: 1 mg, 2 mg, 4 mg. ***In combination with:*** verapamil (Tarka). See Appendix B.

tranexamic acid
(tran-eks-**am**-ik **as**-id)
Cyklokapron

Classification
Therapeutic: hemostatic agents
Pharmacologic: antifibrinolytics, plasminogen inactivators

Indications

Prevention or reduction of hemorrhage following dental surgery in hemophiliacs.

Action

Inhibits activation of plasminogen, thereby preventing the conversion of plasminogen to plasmin. **Therapeutic Effects:** ↓ bleeding following dental surgery in hemophiliacs. Reduced need for replacement therapy.

Adverse Reactions/Side Effects

CNS: dizziness. **EENT:** visual abnormalities.
CV: hypotension, thromboembolism, thrombosis.
GI: diarrhea, nausea, vomiting.

PHYSICAL THERAPY IMPLICATIONS

Examination and Evaluation

- Be alert for bleeding gums, nosebleeds, or other unusual bleeding or bruising that might indicate inadequate drug effects. Report signs of bleeding to the physician immediately.
- Monitor increased blood coagulation, including venous thrombosis (lower extremity swelling, warmth, erythema, tenderness) or arterial thrombosis (extreme coldness in the hands and feet, cyanosis, muscle cramping). Watch for pulmonary embolism (shortness of breath, chest pain, cough, bloody sputum) or arterial thrombosis that could lead to MI or stroke. Notify physician immediately, and request objective tests (Doppler ultrasound, others) if thrombosis is suspected.
- Assess blood pressure and compare to normal values (See Appendix F). Report low blood pressure (hypotension), especially if patient develops dizziness or syncope.
- Assess dizziness that might affect gait, balance, and other functional activities (See Appendix C). Report balance problems and functional limitations to the physician, and caution the patient and family/caregivers to guard against falls and trauma.

Patient/Client-Related Instruction

- Instruct patient to report other troublesome side effects such as severe or prolonged vision abnormalities or GI problems (nausea, vomiting, diarrhea).

Pharmacokinetics

Absorption: 30–50% absorbed following oral administration.
Distribution: Penetrates readily into joint fluid and synovial membranes.
Metabolism and Excretion: 95% excreted unchanged in urine.
Half-life: 2 hr (↑ in renal impairment); 3 hr in joint fluid.

TIME/ACTION PROFILE (blood levels)

ROUTE	ONSET	PEAK	DURATION
PO	unknown	3 hr	7–8 hr*
IV	unknown	unknown	7–8 hr

*Antifibrinolytic concentration in plasma; tissue levels persist for 17 hr.

Contraindications/Precautions

Contraindicated in: Hypersensitivity; Active intravascular clotting; Acquired defective color vision; Subarachnoid hemorrhage.
Use Cautiously in: Renal impairment (↑ dosing interval is recommended if serum creatinine >1.36 mg/dL); Hematuria originating in the upper urinary tract; Conditions associated with ↑ thrombus formation; Pregnancy or lactation (safety not established).

Interactions

Drug-Drug: Concurrent use of **clotting factor complexes** may ↑ the risk of thrombotic complications (give tranexamic acid 8 hr following clotting factor replacement therapy).

Route/Dosage

PO (Adults and Children): 25 mg/kg tid–qid, beginning the day before surgery, then tid–qid for 2–8 days postop.
IV (Adults and Children): 10 mg/kg just prior to surgery with appropriate replacement therapy, then tid–qid for 2–8 days.

Renal Impairment

PO (Adults and Children): *Serum creatinine 1.36–2.83 mg/dL*—15 mg/kg bid; *serum creatinine 2.83–5.66 mg/dL*—15 mg/kg daily; *serum creatinine >5.66 mg/dL*—15 mg/kg q 48 hr or 7.5 mg/kg once daily.

Renal Impairment

IV (Adults and Children): *Serum creatinine 1.36–2.83 mg/dL*—10 mg/kg bid; *serum creatinine 2.83–5.66 mg/dL*— 10 mg/kg daily; *serum creatinine >5.66 mg/dL*— 10 mg/kg q 48 hr or 5 mg/kg once daily.

Availability

Tablets: 500 mg. **Solution for injection:** 100 mg/mL in 5-mL ampules, 100 mg/mL in 10-mL ampules.

tranylcypromine

(tran-il-**sip**-roe-meen)
Parnate

Classification
Therapeutic: antidepressants
Pharmacologic: monoamine oxidase (MAO) inhibitors

Indications

Treatment of major depressive episode without melancholia (usually reserved for patients who do not tolerate or respond to other modes of therapy [e.g., tricyclic antidepressants, SSRIs, SSNRIs, or electroconvulsive therapy]).

Action

Inhibits the enzyme monoamine oxidase, resulting in an accumulation of various neurotransmitters (dopamine, epinephrine, norepinephrine, and serotonin) in the body. **Therapeutic Effects:** Improved mood in depressed patients.

Adverse Reactions/Side Effects

CNS: SEIZURES, confusion, dizziness, drowsiness, headache, insomnia, restlessness, tremor, paresthesia, weakness. **EENT:** blurred vision, tinnitus.
CV: HYPERTENSIVE CRISIS, edema, orthostatic hypotension, tachycardia. **GI:** abdominal pain, anorexia, constipation, diarrhea, dry mouth, hepatitis, nausea.
GU: sexual dysfunction, urinary retention.
Hemat: AGRANULOCYTOSIS, leukopenia, thrombocytopenia.
Derm: alopecia, rashes. **MS:** muscle spasm.

PHYSICAL THERAPY IMPLICATIONS

Examination and Evaluation

- Be alert for new seizures or increased seizure activity, especially at the onset of drug treatment. Document the number, duration, and severity of seizures, and report these findings to the physician immediately.
- Measure blood pressure (BP) periodically and compare to normal values (See Appendix F). Immediately report a large, rapid increase in BP (hypertensive crisis). Signs and symptoms of hypertensive crisis include chest pain, tachycardia or bradycardia, severe headache, nausea, vomiting, neck stiffness, sweating, and enlarged pupils. The risk of hypertensive crisis is increased when this drug is taken with other antidepressants, excessive caffeine, other drugs that increase BP, or foods that contain tyramine (e.g., fermented wines, cheeses).
- Watch for signs of agranulocytosis and leukopenia (fever, sore throat, mucosal lesions, other signs of infection) and thrombocytopenia (bruising, nose bleeds, bleeding gums). Report these signs to the physician immediately.

- Be alert for increased depression and suicidal thoughts and ideology, especially when initiating drug treatment or in children and teenagers. Notify physician or mental health professional immediately if patient exhibits worsening depression.
- Be alert for restlessness, confusion, or other alterations in mood and behavior (See Appendix D). Notify health care professional if these symptoms become problematic.
- Assess BP when patient assumes a more upright position (lying to standing, sitting to standing, lying to sitting). Document orthostatic hypotension and contact physician when systolic BP falls >20 mm Hg, or diastolic BP falls >10 mm Hg.
- Assess heart rate, ECG, and heart sounds, especially during exercise (See Appendices G, H). Report a rapid heart rate (tachycardia) or signs of other arrhythmias, including palpitations, chest discomfort, shortness of breath, fainting, and fatigue/weakness.
- Assess peripheral edema using girth measurements, volume displacement, and measurement of pitting edema (see Appendix N). Report increased swelling in feet and ankles or a sudden increase in body weight due to fluid retention.
- Assess paresthesias (numbness, tingling), tremor, or muscle spasms. Perform objective tests, including electroneuromyography and sensory testing, to document any drug-related neuromyopathic changes.
- Assess dizziness and drowsiness that might affect gait, balance, and other functional activities (See Appendix C). Report balance problems and functional limitations to the physician and nursing staff, and caution the patient and family/caregivers to guard against falls and trauma.

Interventions

- Guard against falls and trauma (hip fractures, head injury, and so forth), and implement fall prevention strategies in patients with dizziness or other conditions that affect balance (See Appendix E).
- Because of the risk of abnormal BP responses and cardiac arrhythmias, use caution during aerobic exercise and endurance conditioning. Assess exercise tolerance frequently (BP, heart rate, fatigue levels), and terminate exercise immediately if any untoward responses occur (See Appendix L).
- To minimize orthostatic hypotension, patient should move slowly when assuming a more upright position.
- Help patient explore nonpharmacologic methods to reduce depression (exercise, counseling, support groups, and so forth).

Patient/Client-Related Instruction

- Advise patient that antidepressant effects may not occur immediately; it may take 2 wk or more before an improvement in mood is observed.
- Advise patient to avoid alcohol and other CNS depressants because of the increased risk of sedation and adverse effects.
- Instruct patient to report severe or prolonged GI problems (nausea, constipation, diarrhea, dry mouth), or signs of drug-induced hepatitis (anorexia, abdominal pain, severe nausea and vomiting, yellow skin or eyes, skin rashes, flu-like symptoms, muscle/joint pain).
- Instruct patient to report other troublesome side effects such as severe or prolonged headache, sleep loss, blurred vision, ringing/buzzing in the ears (tinnitus), sexual dysfunction, urinary retention, or skin reactions (rash, hair loss).

Pharmacokinetics

Absorption: Unknown.
Distribution: Crosses the placenta and enters breast milk.
Metabolism and Excretion: Unknown.
Half-life: 90–190 min.

TIME/ACTION PROFILE (antidepressant effect)

ROUTE	ONSET	PEAK	DURATION
PO	2 days–3 wk	2–3 wk	3–5 days

Contraindications/Precautions

Contraindicated in: Hypersensitivity; Liver disease; Cerebrovascular disease; Cardiovascular disease; Hypertension; Pheochromocytoma; Patients undergoing elective surgery requiring general anesthesia (should be discontinued at least 10 days before surgery); History of headache; Excessive consumption of caffeine; Concurrent use of meperidine, SSRI antidepressants, SSNRI antidepressants, tricyclic antidepressants, tetracyclic antidepressants, nefazodone, trazodone, procarbazine, selegiline, linezolid, carbamazepine, cyclobenzaprine, bupropion, buspirone, sympathomimetics, other MAO inhibitors, dextromethorphan, narcotics, alcohol, general anesthetics, diuretics, antihistamines, or tryptophan; Concurrent use of foods containing high concentrations of tyramine; Lactation.
Use Cautiously in: Patients who may be suicidal or have a history of drug dependency; Pedi: May ↑ risk of suicide attempt/ideation especially during first 1–2 mo of treatment or with dose adjustments; Hyperthyroidism; Schizophrenia; Bipolar disorder; Seizure disorders; Renal dysfunction; Diabetes (↑ risk of hypoglycemia); Geri: Geriatric patients (↑ risk of adverse reactions);

Pregnancy (safety not established); Children (safety and effectiveness not established).

Interactions

Drug-Drug: Serious, potentially fatal adverse reactions may occur with concurrent use of other **antidepressants (SSRIs, SSNRIs, bupropion, tricyclics, tetracyclics, nefazodone, trazodone), carbamazepine, cyclobenzaprine, sibutramine, procarbazine,** or **selegiline.** Avoid using within 2 wk of each other (wait 5 wk from end of **fluoxetine** therapy). Hypertensive crisis may occur with **amphetamines, methyldopa, levodopa, dopamine, epinephrine, norepinephrine, reserpine, methylphenidate,** or **vasoconstrictors.** Hypertension or hypotension, coma, seizures, respiratory depression, and death may occur with **meperidine** (avoid using within 2–3 wk of MAO inhibitor therapy). Concurrent use with **dextromethorphan** may produce psychosis or bizarre behavior. Hypertension may occur with concurrent use of **buspirone;** avoid using within 2 wk of each other. Additive hypotension may occur with **antihypertensives, spinal anesthesia, opioids,** or **barbiturates.** Additive hypoglycemia may occur with **insulins** or **oral hypoglycemic agents.** Risk of seizures may be ↑ with **tramadol.**
Drug-Natural: Serious, potentially fatal adverse effects (serotonin syndrome) may occur with concomitant use of **St. John's wort** and **SAMe.** Hypertensive crises may occur with large amounts of **caffeine**-containing herbs **(cola nut, guarana,** or **malt).** Insomnia, headache, tremor, hypomania may occur with **ginseng.** Hypertensive crises, disorientation, and memory impairment may occur with **tryptophan** or supplements containing **tyrosine** or **phenylalanine.**
Drug-Food: Hypertensive crisis may occur with ingestion of foods containing high concentrations of **tyramine.** Consumption of foods or beverages with high **caffeine** content increases the risk of hypertension and arrhythmias.

Route/Dosage

PO (Adults): 30 mg/day in 2 divided doses (morning and afternoon); after 2 wk can increase by 10 mg/day, at 1- to 3-wk intervals, up to 60 mg/day.

Availability

Tablets: 10 mg Rx.

HIGH ALERT

trastuzumab (traz-**too**-zoo-mab)

Herceptin

Classification

Therapeutic: antineoplastics
Pharmacologic: monoclonal antibodies

Indications

1st-line treatment of metastatic breast cancer (with paclitaxel) that displays overexpression of the human epidermal growth factor receptor 2 (HER2) protein. Treatment of metastatic breast cancer (as monotherapy) that displays overexpression of the human epidermal growth factor receptor 2 (HER2) protein in patients who have already received other chemotherapy regimens. Adjuvant treatment of HER2 overexpressing node-positive or node-negative breast cancer (to be used with alone after multimodality anthracycline-based therapy or as part of 1 of the following regimens: doxorubicin, cyclophosphamide, and either paclitaxel or docetaxel; with docetaxel and carboplatin).

Action

A monoclonal antibody that binds to HER2 sites in breast cancer tissue and inhibits proliferation of cells that overexpress HER2 protein. **Therapeutic Effects:** Regression of breast cancer and metastases.

Adverse Reactions/Side Effects

CNS: dizziness, headache, insomnia, weakness, depression. **Resp:** INTERSTITIAL PNEUMONITIS, PULMONARY EDEMA, PULMONARY FIBROSIS, dyspnea, increased cough, pharyngitis, rhinitis, sinusitis. **CV:** ARRHYTHMIAS, CHF, hypertension, tachycardia. **GI:** abdominal pain, anorexia, diarrhea, nausea, vomiting. **Derm:** rash, acne, herpes simplex. **F and E:** edema. **Hemat:** anemia, leukopenia. **MS:** back pain, arthralgia, bone pain. **Neuro:** neuropathy, paresthesia, peripheral neuritis. **Misc:** HYPERSENSITIVITY REACTIONS, chills, fever, infection, flu-like syndrome.

PHYSICAL THERAPY IMPLICATIONS

Examination and Evaluation

- Assess heart rate, ECG, and heart sounds, especially during exercise (See Appendices G, H). Report any rhythm disturbances or symptoms of increased arrhythmias, including palpitations, chest discomfort, shortness of breath, fainting, and fatigue/weakness.
- Assess signs of congestive heart failure, including dyspnea, rales/crackles, peripheral edema, jugular venous distention, and exercise intolerance. Report these signs to the physician immediately.
- Assess any breathing problems that might indicate pulmonary edema, pulmonary fibrosis, or interstitial pneumonitis. Signs include cough, wheezing, chest pain, fever, shortness of breath, and difficult or labored breathing Monitor pulse oximetry and perform pulmonary function tests (See Appendices I, J, K) to quantify suspected changes in ventilation and respiratory function.
- Be alert for signs of hypersensitivity reactions. Reactions include pulmonary symptoms (tightness in the throat and chest, wheezing, cough, dyspnea)

and skin reactions (rash, pruritus, urticaria). Notify physician or nursing staff immediately if these reactions occur.

- Assess blood pressure (BP) and compare to normal values (See Appendix F). Report a sustained increase in BP (hypertension).
- Assess peripheral edema using girth measurements, volume displacement, and measurement of pitting edema (See Appendix N). Report increased swelling in feet and ankles or a sudden increase in body weight due to fluid retention.
- Monitor signs of leukopenia (fever, sore throat, signs of infection) or unusual weakness and fatigue that might be due to anemia. Notify physician of these signs immediately.
- Be alert for signs of paresthesias and peripheral neuropathy (numbness, tingling, decreased muscle strength). Establish baseline electroneuromyographic values using EMG and nerve conduction at the beginning of drug treatment whenever possible, and reexamine these values periodically to document drug-induced changes in peripheral nerve function.
- Assess any increased joint pain or back pain to rule out musculoskeletal pathology; that is, try to determine if pain is drug induced rather than caused by anatomic or biomechanical problems.
- Assess dizziness that might affect gait, balance, and other functional activities (See Appendix C). Report balance problems and functional limitations to the physician and nursing staff, and caution the patient and family/caregivers to guard against falls and trauma.

Interventions

- For patients who are medically able to begin exercise, implement appropriate resistive exercises and aerobic training to maintain muscle strength and aerobic capacity during cancer chemotherapy or to help restore function after chemotherapy.
- Because of the risk of arrhythmias, CHF, and respiratory disorders, use extreme caution during aerobic exercise and other forms of therapeutic exercise. Assess exercise tolerance frequently (BP, heart rate, fatigue levels), and terminate exercise immediately if any untoward responses occur (See Appendix L).

Patient/Client-Related Instruction

- Advise patient to guard against infection (frequent hand washing, etc.), and to avoid crowds and contact with persons with contagious diseases.
- Instruct patient or family/caregivers to report other bothersome side effects such as severe or prolonged headache, depression, sleep loss, nasal/pharyngeal irritation, flu-like symptoms (fever, chills), skin reactions (rash, acne, herpes eruptions), or GI problems (nausea, vomiting, diarrhea, abdominal pain, loss of appetite).

Pharmacokinetics

Absorption: IV administration results in complete bioavailability.
Distribution: Binds to HER2 proteins.
Metabolism and Excretion: Unknown.
Half-life: 10-mg dose—1.7 days; 500-mg dose—12 days.

TIME/ACTION PROFILE (blood levels)

ROUTE	ONSET	PEAK	DURATION
IV	unknown	unknown	unknown

Contraindications/Precautions

Contraindicated in: None known.
Use Cautiously in: Preexisting pulmonary conditions; Hypersensitivity to trastuzumab, Chinese hamster ovary cell proteins, or other components of the product; Hypersensitivity to benzyl alcohol (use sterile water for injection instead of bacteriostatic water, which accompanies the vial); Geri: May have ↑ risk of cardiac dysfunction; OB/Lactation: Use during pregnancy only if clearly needed; not recommended for use during lactation; Pedi: Safety not established.
Exercise Extreme Caution in: Patients with preexisting cardiac dysfunction.

Interactions

Drug-Drug: Concurrent **anthracycline (daunorubicin, doxorubicin,** or **idarubicin)** therapy may ↑ risk of cardiotoxicity. Blood levels are ↑ by concurrent **paclitaxel.**

Route/Dosage

Adjuvant Treatment of Breast Cancer

IV (Adults): *During and following paclitaxel, docetaxel, or docetaxel/carboplatin*—4 mg/kg initially, then 2 mg/kg weekly during chemotherapy for the first 12 wk (paclitaxel or docetaxel) or 18 wk (docetaxel/carboplatin); 1 wk after the last weekly dose, give 6 mg/kg q 3 wk; *As single agent within 3 wk following completion of multimodality, anthracycline-based chemotherapy regimens*—8 mg/kg initially, then 6 mg/kg q 3 wk.

Metastatic Breast Cancer

IV (Adults): 4 mg/kg initially, then 2 mg/kg weekly until disease progresses.

Availability

Lyophilized powder for injection: 440 mg/vial with 30 mL bacteriostatic water for injection (contains benzyl alcohol).

T

trazodone (traz-oh-done)

Classification
Therapeutic: antidepressants

Indications

Major depression. **Unlabeled Use:** Insomnia, chronic pain syndromes, including diabetic neuropathy, and anxiety.

Action

Alters the effects of serotonin in the CNS. **Therapeutic Effects:** Antidepressant action, which may develop only over several weeks.

Adverse Reactions/Side Effects

CNS: drowsiness, confusion, dizziness, fatigue, hallucinations, headache, insomnia, nightmares, slurred speech, syncope, weakness. **EENT:** blurred vision, tinnitus. **CV:** hypotension, arrhythmias, chest pain, hypertension, palpitations, QT interval prolongation, tachycardia. **GI:** dry mouth, altered taste, constipation, diarrhea, excess salivation, flatulence, nausea, vomiting. **GU:** hematuria, erectile dysfunction, priapism, urinary frequency. **Derm:** rashes. **Hemat:** anemia, leukopenia. **MS:** myalgia. **Neuro:** tremor.

PHYSICAL THERAPY IMPLICATIONS

Examination and Evaluation

- Assess blood pressure (BP) and compare to normal values (See Appendix F). Report changes in BP, either a sustained increase in BP (hypertension) or a problematic decrease in BP (hypotension) that results in dizziness and syncope.
- Assess heart rate, ECG, and heart sounds, especially during exercise (See Appendices G, H). Report a rapid heart rate (tachycardia) or signs of other arrhythmias, including palpitations, chest discomfort, shortness of breath, fainting, and fatigue/weakness.
- Watch for signs of leukopenia (fever, sore throat, signs of infection) or unusual weakness and fatigue that might be due to anemia. Report these signs to the physician.
- Be alert for increased depression and suicidal thoughts and ideology, especially when initiating drug treatment, and in children and teenagers. Notify physician or mental health professional immediately if patient exhibits worsening depression.
- Be alert for confusion, slurred speech, hallucinations, or other alterations in mood and behavior (See Appendix D). Notify physician if these symptoms become problematic.
- Assess dizziness and drowsiness that might affect gait, balance, and other functional activities (See Appendix C). Report balance problems and functional limitations to the physician, and caution the patient and family/caregivers to guard against falls and trauma.
- Assess any muscle pain or tremor to rule out musculoskeletal pathology; that is, try to determine if pain is drug induced rather than caused by anatomic or biomechanical problems.
- If used to treat chronic pain syndromes or neuropathy, assess pain levels periodically to help document drug efficacy.

Interventions

- Guard against falls and trauma (hip fractures, head injury, and so forth), and implement fall-prevention strategies (See Appendix E).
- Because of the risk of cardiac arrhythmias and changes in BP, use caution during aerobic exercise and endurance conditioning Assess exercise tolerance frequently (BP, heart rate, fatigue levels), and terminate exercise immediately if any untoward responses occur (See Appendix L).
- To minimize orthostatic hypotension, patient should move slowly when assuming a more upright position.
- Help patient explore nonpharmacologic methods (exercise, counseling, support groups, and so forth) to reduce depression and other psychologic disorders.

Patient/Client-Related Instruction

- Advise patient that antidepressant effects may not occur immediately; it may take 2 wk or more before an improvement in mood is observed.
- Advise patient to avoid alcohol and other CNS depressants because of the increased risk of sedation and adverse effects.
- Instruct patient to report severe or prolonged GI problems, including nausea, vomiting, diarrhea, constipation, flatulence, dry mouth, excessive salivation, or a change in taste.
- Instruct patient to report other problematic side effects such as severe of prolonged headache, sleep disturbances, blurred vision, buzzing/ringing in the ears (tinnitus), urinary frequency, bloody urine, sexual problems (erectile dysfunction, sustained/painful erections), or skin rash.

Pharmacokinetics

Absorption: Well absorbed after oral administration.
Distribution: Widely distributed.
Protein Binding: 89–95%.
Metabolism and Excretion: Extensively metabolized by the liver (CYP3A4 enzyme system); minimal excretion of unchanged drug by the kidneys.
Half-life: 5–9 hr.

TIME/ACTION PROFILE (antidepressant effect)

ROUTE	ONSET	PEAK	DURATION
PO	1–2 wk	2–4 wk	wks

Contraindications/Precautions

Contraindicated in: Hypersensitivity; Recovery period after MI; Concurrent electroconvulsive therapy.
Use Cautiously in: Cardiovascular disease; Suicidal behavior; May ↑ risk of suicide attempt/ideation, especially during early treatment or dose adjustment; Severe hepatic or renal disease (dose reduction recommended); Lactation: Discontinue drug or bottle feed; Pedi: Suicide risk may be greater in children and adolescents; safe use not established; Geri: Initial dose reduction recommended.

Interactions

Drug-Drug: May ↑ **digoxin** or **phenytoin** serum levels. ↑ CNS depression with other **CNS depressants,** including **alcohol, opioid analgesics,** and **sedative/hypnotics.** ↑ hypotension with **antihypertensives,** acute ingestion of **alcohol,** or **nitrates.** Concurrent use with **fluoxetine** ↑ levels and risk of toxicity from trazodone. **Drugs that inhibit the CYP3A4 enzyme system,** including **ritonavir indinavir** and **ketoconazole,** ↑ levels and the risk of toxicity. **Drugs that induce the CYP3A4 enzyme system,** including **carbamazepine,** ↓ levels and may ↓ effectiveness. Do note use within 14 days of **MAOI** therapy. May ↑ prothrombin time (PT) with **warfarin.**
Drug-Natural: Concomitant use of **kava, valerian,** or **chamomile** can ↑ CNS depression. ↑ risk of serotonergic side effects, including serotonin syndrome, with **St. John's wort** and **SAMe.**

Route/Dosage

PO (Adults): *Depression*—150 mg/day in 3 divided doses; ↑ by 50 mg/day q 3–4 days until desired response (not to exceed 400 mg/day in outpatients or 600 mg/day in hospitalized patients). *Insomnia*—25–100 mg hs.
PO (Geriatric Patients): 75 mg/day in divided doses initially; may be ↑ q 3–4 days.

Availability (generic available)

Tablets: 50 mg, 100 mg, 150 mg, 300 mg.

treprostinil (tre-pros-ti-nil)

Remodulin

Classification
Therapeutic: vasodilators
Pharmacologic: prostacyclins

Indications

Treatment of pulmonary arterial hypertension in patients with New York Heart Association (NYHA) class II–IV symptoms.

Action

Treprostinil is a prostacyclin that produces direct vasodilation of pulmonary and systemic arterial vascular beds. Also inhibits platelet aggregation. **Therapeutic Effects:** ↓ exercise-associated symptoms in patients with pulmonary arterial hypertension.

Adverse Reactions/Side Effects

CNS: dizziness, <u>headache</u>. **CV:** <u>vasodilation</u>, hypotension, edema. **GI:** <u>diarrhea</u>, <u>nausea</u>. **Derm:** <u>rash</u>, pruritus, flushing. **Local:** <u>infusion site pain/reaction</u>. **MS:** <u>jaw pain</u>.

PHYSICAL THERAPY IMPLICATIONS

Examination and Evaluation

- Assess signs and symptoms of CHF (dyspnea, rales/crackles, jugular venous distention, exercise intolerance) to help document whether drug therapy is effective in reducing these symptoms.
- Assess peripheral edema using girth measurements, volume displacement, and measurement of pitting edema (See Appendix N). Report increased swelling in feet and ankles due to vasodilation.
- Assess blood pressure periodically and compare to normal values (See Appendix F). Report low blood pressure (hypotension), especially if patient experiences dizziness, fatigue, or other symptoms.
- Assess any jaw pain to rule out musculoskeletal pathology; that is, try to determine if pain is drug induced rather than caused by anatomic or biomechanical problems.
- Assess dizziness that might affect gait, balance, and other functional activities (See Appendix C). Report balance problems and functional limitations to the physician and nursing staff, and caution the patient and family/caregivers to guard against falls and trauma.
- Monitor subcutaneous injection site for pain, swelling, and irritation. Report prolonged or excessive injection site reactions to the physician.

Interventions

- Design and implement aerobic exercise and endurance training programs as tolerated to help improve myocardial pumping ability.
- Use caution during aerobic exercise and endurance conditioning. Terminate exercise if patient exhibits untoward symptoms (chest pain, shortness of breath, unusual fatigue), or displays other criteria for exercise termination (See Appendix L).
- Avoid physical therapy interventions that cause systemic vasodilation (large whirlpool, Hubbard tank). Additive effects of this drug and the intervention may cause a dangerous fall in blood pressure.

T

- Do not apply physical agents (heat, cold, electrotherapeutic modalities) or massage at or near the injection site; these interventions will alter drug absorption from subcutaneous tissues.
- To minimize orthostatic hypotension, patient should move slowly when assuming a more upright position.

Patient/Client-Related Instruction

- Counsel patients about additional interventions to help cardiac dysfunction, including regular exercise, weight loss, sodium restriction, stress reduction, moderation of alcohol consumption, and smoking cessation.
- Instruct patient or family/caregivers to report other troublesome side effects such as severe or prolonged headache, skin problems (rash, itching, flushing), or GI problems (nausea, diarrhea).

Pharmacokinetics

Absorption: Rapidly and completely (near 100%) absorbed following SC administration.
Distribution: Unknown.
Protein Binding: 91%.
Metabolism and Excretion: Extensively metabolized by the liver, metabolites are renally excreted; minimal excretion of unchanged drug in urine.
Half-life: 4 hr.

TIME/ACTION PROFILE (clinical improvement)

ROUTE	ONSET	PEAK	DURATION
SC	unknown	1 wk	unknown

Contraindications/Precautions

Contraindicated in: Known hypersensitivity.
Use Cautiously in: Renal impairment; Hepatic impairment (dose reduction recommended in mild-to-moderate hepatic insufficiency; data not available for severe hepatic insufficiency); Avoid abrupt discontinuation or rapid dosage reduction; Pregnancy (use only if clearly needed); Lactation or children ≤16 yr.

Interactions

Drug-Drug: ↑ risk of hypotension with **antihypertensives, diuretics,** or **vasodilators.** Risk of bleeding may be ↑ by concurrent use of **anticoagulants.**

Route/Dosage

SC (Adults): 1.25 ng/kg/min; may be reduced to 0.625 ng/kg/min if intolerance occurs. Increments of no more than 1.25 ng/kg/min may be made weekly for the first 4 wk, and then no more than 2.5 ng/kg/min weekly for the remainder of therapy up to 40 ng/kg/min. Avoid abrupt discontinuation or rapid ↓ in dosing. Infusion rate may be calculated with the following formula: **Infusion rate** (mL/hr) = **Dose** (ng/kg/min) × **weight** (kg) × **[0.00006/treprostinil dose strength concentration** (mg/mL)**]**.

Availability

Solution for continuous SC administration (no dilution required): 1 mg/mL in 20-mL vials, 2.5 mg/mL in 20-mL vials, 5 mg/mL in 20-mL vials, 10 mg/mL in 20-mL vials.

HIGH ALERT

tretinoin (oral) (tret-i-noyn)

Vesanoid

tretinoin (topical) (tret-i-noyn)

Altinac, Avita, Retin-A, Retin-A Micro, Renova, ✱Stieva-A, Vitamin A Acid

Classification
Therapeutic: antineoplastics (oral)
Therapeutic: antiacne agents (topical)
Pharmacologic: retinoids

Indications

Oral: Induction of remission in acute promyelocytic leukemia in patients who cannot receive anthracyclines due to lack of response, intolerance, or the presence of a contraindication.
Topical: Management of acne vulgaris. Decreased facial dermal effects of photoaging (used with sun avoidance; 0.05% water-in-oil cream formulation only).

Action

Oral: Causes maturation of promyelocytes derived from the leukemic clone. **Therapeutic Effects:** Repopulation with normal hematopoietic cells in patients who achieve remission.
Topical: ↓ the formation of microcomedones and stimulates turnover of follicular epithelium.
Therapeutic Effects: ↓ acne formation with improved skin appearance. ↓ skin roughness, hyperpigmentation, and wrinkling due to photoaging.

Adverse Reactions/Side Effects (Oral)

CNS: SEIZURES, anxiety, confusion, depression, dizziness, fatigue, headache, insomnia, malaise, pseudotumor cerebri, weakness, agitation, cerebral hemorrhage, hallucinations, intracranial hypertension. **EENT:** altered visual acuity, ocular disorders, visual disturbances, visual field defects, earache, hearing loss. **Resp:** asthma, laryngeal edema. **CV:** CARDIAC FAILURE, MI, STROKE, arrhythmias, chest discomfort, edema, hypertension, hypotension, peripheral edema, phlebitis. **GI:** GI BLEEDING, abdominal distention, abdominal pain, anorexia, constipation, diarrhea, dry mouth, dyspepsia, hepatosplenomegaly, mucositis, nausea, ulcer, vomiting. **GU:** renal insufficiency, acute renal failure, dysuria, enlarged prostate, renal tubular necrosis, urinary frequency. **Derm:** alopecia, cellulitis, dry skin, facial edema, flushing, increased sweating, pallor, pruritus, rash, skin changes. **F and E:** acidosis, fluid imbalance. **Hemat:** disseminated intravascular coagulation, hemorrhage, leukocytosis. **Metab:** weight gain, weight loss. **MS:** bone inflammation, bone pain, flank pain, myalgia. **Neuro:** paresthesias. **Misc:** fever, infections, pain, hypothermia, retinoic acid–acute promyelocytic leukemia syndrome, shivering.

Adverse Reactions/Side Effects (Topical)

Derm: photosensitivity, redness, blistering, edema, crusting, hyperpigmentation, hypopigmentation.

PHYSICAL THERAPY IMPLICATIONS*

**Implications refer primarily to oral/systemic use for cancer*

Evaluation and Examination

- Continually monitor for signs of stroke (sudden severe headache, confusion, nausea, vomiting, paralysis, numbness, speech problems, visual disturbances) and MI or cardiac failure (sudden chest pain, pain radiating into the arm or jaw, shortness of breath, dizziness, sweating, anxiety, nausea, loss of consciousness). Seek immediate medical assistance if patient develops these signs.
- Be alert for seizures and other signs of neurotoxicity (anxiety, confusion, hallucinations, dizziness, depression, changes in vision or hearing). Notify physician immediately if these signs occur.
- Monitor signs of GI bleeding, including abdominal pain, vomiting blood, blood in stools, or black, tarry stools. Report these signs to the physician immediately.
- Assess blood pressure (BP) and compare to normal values (See Appendix F). Report changes in BP, either a problematic decrease in BP (hypotension) or a sustained increase in BP (hypertension).
- Assess heart rate, ECG, and heart sounds, especially during exercise (See Appendices G, H). Report any rhythm disturbances or symptoms of increased arrhythmias, including palpitations, chest discomfort, shortness of breath, fainting, and fatigue/weakness.
- Monitor unusual weakness, fatigue, or abnormal bleeding (bleeding gums, nosebleeds, abnormal bruising) that might be due to leukemias including acute promyelocytic leukemia (APL) syndrome.
- Assess any breathing problems, and report signs of pulmonary edema (dyspnea, rales/crackles, shortness of breath).
- Assess any muscle or bone pain to rule out musculoskeletal pathology; that is, try to determine if pain is drug induced rather than caused by anatomical or biomechanical problems.
- Be alert for signs of paresthesias (numbness, tingling, decreased muscle strength). Establish baseline electroneuromyographic values at the beginning of drug treatment whenever possible, and reexamine these values periodically to document drug-induced changes in peripheral nerve function.
- Monitor signs of acidosis or fluid imbalance, including confusion, lethargy, stupor, shallow rapid breathing, tachycardia, and hypotension. Notify physician immediately if these signs occur.
- Assess peripheral edema using girth measurements, volume displacement, and measurement of pitting edema (See Appendix N). Report increased swelling in feet and ankles or a sudden increase in body weight due to fluid retention.
- Monitor injection site for pain and irritation. Report prolonged or excessive injection-site reactions to the physician.

Interventions

- For patients who are medically able to begin exercise, implement appropriate resistive exercises and aerobic training to maintain muscle strength and aerobic capacity during cancer chemotherapy or to help restore function after chemotherapy.
- Because of an increased risk of cardiovascular events (MI, stroke, cardiac failure), use extreme caution during aerobic exercise and endurance conditioning. Terminate exercise if patient exhibits untoward symptoms (chest pain, shortness of breath, etc.) or displays other criteria for exercise termination (See Appendix L).
- Causes photosensitivity; use care if administering UV treatments. Advise patient to avoid direct sunlight and use sunscreens and protective clothing.

Patient/Client-Related Instruction

- Advise patient to guard against infection (frequent hand washing, etc.), and to avoid crowds and contact with persons with contagious diseases.
- Advise patient that fatigue and weakness are likely and may be severe. Functional abilities may be limited, and patient may need to use assistive devices during ambulation.
- Advise patient that rashes and other skin reactions (cellulitis, sweating, hair loss, redness, change in pigmentation) are likely, especially during topical application. Report severe or unexpected skin reactions to the physician.
- Instruct patient to report signs of renal insufficiency, including difficult urination, increased frequency, cloudy urine, and decreased urine output.
- Instruct patient to report severe or prolonged fever or flu-like symptoms (chills, muscle aches).

T

Pharmacokinetics
Absorption: Well absorbed following oral administration. Minimal systemic absorption occurs with limited topical surface-area application.
Distribution: Crosses the placenta; remainder of distribution unknown.
Protein Binding: >95%.
Metabolism and Excretion: Oral doses are metabolized by the liver; metabolites are renally excreted. <5% of dose applied to skin is excreted in urine.
Half-life: Oral: 0.5–2 hr. Topical: Unknown

TIME/ACTION PROFILE (complete remission)

ROUTE	ONSET	PEAK	DURATION
PO	unknown	40–50 days	unknown
Topical (acne)	2–3 wk	6 wk	unknown
Topical (photoaging)	within 24 wk	unknown	2 mo

Contraindications/Precautions
Contraindicated in: Hypersensitivity to tretinoin or parabens; Pregnancy or lactation.
Use Cautiously in: Oral: Women of childbearing potential. **Topical:** Areas around the mouth, eyes, angles of the nose, or other mucous membranes; Pregnancy, lactation, or children (safe use not established); Safety/effectiveness in patients ≥50 yr, with a history of skin cancer or with moderately pigmented skin or for longer than 48 wk not established.

Interactions
Drug-Drug: Oral: Rifampin, corticosteroids, phenobarbital, and **pentobarbital** ↑ metabolism and may ↓ effectiveness. **Cimetidine, cyclosporine, diltiazem, erythromycin, ketoconazole,** and **verapamil** ↓ metabolism and may ↑ effects. **Topical:** Concurrent use with **keratolytic agents** (benzoyl peroxide, salicylic acid, sulfur, or resorcinol) ↑ risk of excessive skin irritation. ↑ risk of photosensitivity with other **photosensitizing agents.** Risk of irritation ↑ by other **topical skin-care products** (aftershave, cover-up, make-up, perfumes, colognes). ↑ absorption of **topical minoxidil.**
Drug-Natural: St. John's wort may ↑ metabolism and ↓ effectiveness.
Drug-Food: Absorption is ↑ by **food.**

Route/Dosage
PO (Adults): 45 mg/m^2/day in 2 divided doses; treatment should be continued for 30 days after a complete remission has been achieved or for a total of 90 days, whichever is first.

Acne
Topical (Adults and Adolescents >12 yr): Apply once daily hs.

Photoaging
Topical (Adults): *Renova*—Apply a thin film once daily hs; if irritation occurs, lower concentration or less frequent application may be tried.

Availability
Capsules: 10 mg.
Cream: 0.025% in 20- and 45-g containers, 0.05% in 20- and 45-g containers, 0.1% in 20- and 45-g containers. **Gel:** 0.025% in 15- and 45-g containers, 0.01% in 15- and 45-g containers. **Gel microsphere formulation:** 0.1% in 20- and 45-g containers, 0.04% in 20- and 45-g containers. **Liquid:** 0.05% in 30-mL containers. ***In combination with:*** 0.01% tretinoin with 2% mequinol topical solution (Solage). See Appendix B.

triamcinolone (systemic)
(trye-am-**sin**-oh-lone)
✱Amcort, Aristospan, Kenalog, Trivaris

Classification
Therapeutic: anti-inflammatories (steroidal) (intermediate-acting), immunosuppressants
Pharmacologic: corticosteroids

Indications
Used systemically and locally in a wide variety of chronic diseases, including Inflammatory, Allergic, Hematologic, Neoplastic, Autoimmune disorders. Suitable for alternate-day dosing in the management of chronic illness. Replacement therapy in adrenal insufficiency.

Action
In pharmacologic doses, suppresses inflammation and the normal immune response. Has numerous intense metabolic effects (see Adverse Reactions and Side Effects). Suppresses adrenal function at chronic doses of 4 mg/day. Has negligible mineralocorticoid activity.
Therapeutic Effects: Suppression of inflammation and modification of the normal immune response. Replacement therapy in adrenal insufficiency.

Adverse Reactions/Side Effects
Adverse reactions/side effects are much more common with high-dose/long-term therapy
CNS: depression, euphoria, headache, increased intracranial pressure (children only), personality changes, psychoses, restlessness. **EENT:** cataracts, increased intraocular pressure. **CV:** hypertension. **GI:** PEPTIC ULCERATION, anorexia, nausea, vomiting. **Derm:** acne, decreased wound healing, ecchymoses, fragility, hirsutism, petechiae. **Endo:** adrenal suppression,

hyperglycemia. **F and E:** fluid retention (long-term high doses), hypokalemia, hypokalemic alkalosis. **Hemat:** THROMBOEMBOLISM, thrombophlebitis. **Metab:** weight gain, weight loss. **MS:** muscle wasting, osteoporosis, aseptic necrosis of joints, muscle pain. **Misc:** cushingoid appearance (moon face, buffalo hump), increased susceptibility to infection.

PHYSICAL THERAPY IMPLICATIONS

Examination and Evaluation

- Monitor signs of thrombophlebitis (lower extremity swelling, warmth, erythema, tenderness) and thromboembolism (shortness of breath, chest pain, cough, bloody sputum). Notify physician immediately, and request objective tests (Doppler ultrasound, lung scan, others) if thrombosis is suspected.
- Monitor and report signs of peptic ulcer, including heartburn, nausea, vomiting blood, tarry stools, and loss of appetite.
- Assess signs of increased intracranial pressure in children, including changes in mood and behavior, decreased consciousness, headache, lethargy, seizures, and vomiting. Notify physician immediately of these signs.
- Assess any muscle or joint pain. Report persistent or increased musculoskeletal pain to determine presence of bone or joint pathology (aseptic necrosis, fracture).
- Assess muscle strength periodically to determine degree of muscle wasting during long- term use.
- Measure blood pressure periodically and compare to normal values (See Appendix F). Report a sustained increase in blood pressure (hypertension) to the physician.
- Assess peripheral edema using girth measurements, volume displacement, and measurement of pitting edema (See Appendix N). Report increased swelling in feet and ankles or a sudden increase in body weight due to fluid retention.
- Monitor personality changes, including depression, euphoria, restlessness, hallucinations, and psychosis. Notify physician if these changes become problematic.
- Be alert for signs of low potassium levels (hypokalemia) and metabolic acidosis, including hyperventilation, cardiac arrhythmias, dizziness, and confusion. Notify physician immediately if these signs occur.
- Report signs of adrenal suppression, including hypotension, weight loss, weakness, nausea, vomiting, anorexia, lethargy, confusion, and restlessness.
- Monitor signs of hyperglycemia (confusion; drowsiness; flushed, dry skin; fruit-like breath odor; rapid, deep breathing; polyuria; loss of appetite; unusual thirst). Insulin dosages may need to be adjusted to prevent repeated episodes of hyperglycemia.
- Periodically assess body weight and other anthropometric measures (body mass index, body composition). Report a rapid or unexplained weight gain or weight loss.

Interventions

- Implement resistive exercises and weight-bearing activities to minimize muscle wasting and osteoporosis. Use caution to prevent musculoskeletal damage in patients with preexisting muscle and bone loss.
- Protect skin from breakdown, especially over bony prominences.

Patient/Client-Related Instruction

- Advise patient that wound healing may be delayed; instruct patient to check skin regularly and report any nonhealing sores.
- Advise patient that corticosteroids cause immunosuppression and may mask symptoms of infection. Instruct patient to avoid people with known contagious illnesses and to report possible infections immediately.
- Advise patients on long-term treatment to consult physician before stopping this medication. Stopping the medication suddenly may result in adrenocortical shock (severe hypotension, hypoglycemia, weakness, vomiting). If these signs appear, notify physician immediately; may be life-threatening.
- Instruct patient to report any loss of vision that might indicate cataracts or increased intraocular pressure.
- Advise patient about possible cushingoid appearance, including puffiness in the face (moon face), increased fat in the torso, thin arms and legs, abdominal skin striations, bruising, and deposition of fat at the posterior base of the neck (buffalo hump). Discuss possible effects on body image, and help patient explore coping mechanisms.
- Instruct patient and family/caregivers to report other troublesome side effects such as severe or prolonged headache, GI reactions (nausea, vomiting, loss of appetite), or skin reactions (acne, hair growth).

Pharmacokinetics

Absorption: Well absorbed following oral administration. Acetonide salt is slowly but completely absorbed following IM administration. Absorption of hexacetonide salt from local sites (intra-articular, intralesional) is slow but complete.
Distribution: Widely distributed, crosses the placenta, and probably enters breast milk.
Metabolism and Excretion: Metabolized mostly by the liver.

T

Half-life: 2–>5 hr (plasma), 18–36 hr (tissue).

TIME/ACTION PROFILE (anti-inflammatory activity)

ROUTE	ONSET	PEAK	DURATION
PO	unknown	1–2 hr	2.25 days
IM (acetonide)	24–48 hr	unknown	1–6 wk

Contraindications/Precautions

Contraindicated in: Active untreated infections (may be used in patients being treated for tuberculous meningitis); Lactation: Avoid chronic use; Some products contain tartrazine and should be avoided in patients with known hypersensitivity; Pedi: Products containing benzyl alcohol should not be used in neonates.

Use Cautiously in: Chronic treatment (will lead to adrenal suppression; use lowest possible dose for shortest period of time); Pedi: Chronic use will result in decreased growth; use lowest possible dose for shortest period of time; Hypothyroidism; Cirrhosis; Ulcerative colitis; Stress (surgery, infections); supplemental doses may be needed; Potential infections may mask signs (fever, inflammation); OB: Safety not established.

Interactions

Drug-Drug: Additive hypokalemia with **thiazide, loop diuretics,** or **amphotericin B.** Hypokalemia may ↑ risk of **digitalis glycoside** toxicity. May ↑ requirement for **insulin** or **oral hypoglycemic agents. Phenytoin, phenobarbital,** and **rifampin** stimulate metabolism; may ↓ effectiveness. **Oral contraceptives** may block metabolism. ↑ risk of adverse GI effects with **NSAIDs** (including **aspirin**). At chronic doses that suppress adrenal function, may ↓ the antibody response to and ↑ the risk of adverse reactions from **live-virus vaccines.**

Route/Dosage

IM (Adults): *Triamcinolone acetonide*—40–80 mg q 4 wk.

Intra-articular: (Adults): *Triamcinolone hexacetonide*—2–20 mg q 3–4 wk (dose depends on size of joint to be injected, amount of inflammation, and amount of fluid present).

IM (Children): *Triamcinolone acetonide*—40 mg q 4 wk or 30–200 mcg/kg (1–6.25 mg/m^2) q 1–7 days.

Availability (generic available)

Suspension for injection (acetonide): 10 mg/mL, 40 mg/mL, 80 mg/mL. **Suspension for injection (hexacetonide):** 5 mg/mL, 20 mg/mL.

triamterene (trye-am-ter-een)

Dyrenium

Classification

Therapeutic: diuretics (potassium-sparing)

Indications

Counteracts potassium loss caused by other diuretics. Used with other agents to treat edema or hypertension.

Action

Inhibition of sodium resorption in the kidney, while saving potassium and hydrogen ions. **Therapeutic Effects:** Weak diuretic and antihypertensive response when compared with other diuretics. Conservation of potassium.

Adverse Reactions/Side Effects

CNS: dizziness. **CV:** arrhythmias. **GI:** nausea, vomiting. **GU:** erectile dysfunction, bluish urine, nephrolithiasis. **Derm:** photosensitivity. **F and E:** hyperkalemia, hyponatremia. **Hemat:** blood dyscrasias. **MS:** muscle cramps. **Misc:** allergic reactions.

PHYSICAL THERAPY IMPLICATIONS

Examination and Evaluation

- Monitor signs of fluid or electrolyte imbalances (hyperkalemia, hyponatremia), including dizziness, drowsiness, headache, blurred vision, confusion, hypotension, or muscle cramps and weakness. Report excessive or prolonged symptoms to the physician.
- Assess dizziness that might affect gait, balance, and other functional activities (See Appendix C). Report balance problems and functional limitations to the physician, and caution the patient and family/caregivers to guard against falls and trauma.
- Assess heart rate, ECG, and heart sounds, especially during exercise (See Appendices G, H). Report any rhythm disturbances or symptoms of increased arrhythmias, including palpitations, chest discomfort, shortness of breath, fainting, and fatigue/weakness.
- Assess blood pressure periodically and compare to normal values (See Appendix F) to help document antihypertensive effects.
- When used to treat edema, help determine drug effects by assessing peripheral edema using girth measurements, volume displacement, and measurement of pitting edema (See Appendix N). Also monitor signs of pulmonary edema such as dyspnea and rales/crackles (See Appendix K). Document whether peripheral and pulmonary symptoms are controlled adequately by diuretic therapy.
- Monitor signs of allergic reactions, including pulmonary symptoms (tightness in the throat and chest, wheezing, cough, dyspnea) or skin reactions (rash, pruritus, urticaria). Notify physician immediately if these reactions occur.

Interventions

- Implement fall-prevention strategies, especially in older adults or if patient exhibits sedation, dizziness, blurred vision, or other impairments that affect gait and balance (See Appendix E).

- Use caution during aerobic exercise, especially in hot environments. Increased sweating will cause fluid and electrolyte loss, and may exaggerate arrhythmias and diuretic side effects (dizziness, muscle cramps, and so forth).
- To minimize orthostatic hypotension, patient should move slowly when assuming a more upright position.
- Causes photosensitivity; use care if administering UV treatments.

Patient/Client-Related Instruction

- Remind patients to take medication as directed to control hypertension and other cardiac conditions even if they are asymptomatic.
- Counsel patients about additional interventions to help control blood pressure and cardiac dysfunction, such as regular exercise, weight loss, sodium restriction, stress reduction, moderation of alcohol consumption, and smoking cessation.
- Instruct patient to report signs of leukopenia (fever, sore throat, signs of infection), thrombocytopenia (bruising, nose bleeds, and bleeding gums), or unusual weakness and fatigue that might be due to anemia or other blood dyscrasias.
- Advise patient about photosensitivity, and to use sunscreens, protective clothing, and avoid prolonged sun exposure. Instruct patient to also report any rashes or other skin reactions.
- Instruct patient or family and caregivers to report other troublesome side effects such as severe or prolonged GI problems (nausea, vomiting), erectile dysfunction, or signs of kidney stones (severe pain in the back and side, increased urge to urinate, blood in the urine).

Pharmacokinetics

Absorption: 30–70% absorbed.
Distribution: Widely distributed.
Metabolism and Excretion: 80% metabolized by the liver, some excretion of unchanged drug.
Half-life: 1.7–2.5 hr.

TIME/ACTION PROFILE (diuretic effect)

ROUTE	ONSET	PEAK	DURATION
PO	2–4 hr*†	1–several days†	7–9 hr*

*Single dose.
†Multiple doses.

Contraindications/Precautions

Contraindicated in: Hypersensitivity; Hyperkalemia; Concurrent use of potassium supplements or other potassium-sparing agents.

Use Cautiously in: Hepatic dysfunction; Patients with diabetes mellitus (↑ risk of hyperkalemia); Renal insufficiency; History of gout or kidney stones; Pregnancy, lactation, or children (safety not established).

Interactions

Drug-Drug: ↑ hypotension with acute ingestion of **alcohol**, other **antihypertensive agents**, or **nitrates.** Use with **ACE inhibitors, indomethacin, angiotensin II receptor antagonists potassium supplements**, or **cyclosporine** ↑ risk of hyperkalemia. ↓ **lithium** excretion. Effectiveness may be ↓ by **NSAIDs.** ↓ the effects of **folic acid** (leucovorin should be used). May ↑ risk of toxicity from **amantadine.**

Route/Dosage

PO (Adults): 25–100 mg/day (not to exceed 300 mg/day).
PO (Children): 2–4 mg/kg/day (120 mg/m2/day) in divided doses given daily or every other day (not to exceed 6 mg/kg/day or 300 mg/day).

Availability

Capsules: 50 mg, 100 mg. **Tablets:** 50 mg, 100 mg. ***In combination with:*** hydrochlorothiazide (Apo-Triazide, Dyazide, Maxzide, [Novo-Triamzide]). See Appendix B.

T

triazolam (trye-az-oh-lam)

Apo-Triazo, Gen-Triazolam, Halcion, Novo-Triolam, Nu-Triazo

Classification
Therapeutic: sedative/hypnotics
Pharmacologic: benzodiazepines

Schedule IV

Indications

Short-term management of insomnia.

Action

Acts at many levels in the CNS, producing generalized depression. Effects may be mediated by gamma-aminobutyric acid (GABA), an inhibitory neurotransmitter. **Therapeutic Effects:** Relief of insomnia.

Adverse Reactions/Side Effects

CNS: abnormal thinking, behavior changes, dizziness, excessive sedation, hangover, headache, anterograde amnesia, confusion, hallucinations, sleep driving, lethargy, mental depression, paradoxical excitation. **EENT:** blurred vision. **GI:** constipation, diarrhea, nausea, vomiting. **Derm:** rashes. **Misc:** physical dependence, psychologic dependence, tolerance.

PHYSICAL THERAPY IMPLICATIONS

Examination and Evaluation

- Monitor daytime drowsiness, anxiety, short-term memory deficits, and "hangover" symptoms (headache, blurred vision, nausea, irritability, lethargy, dysphoria). Repeated or excessive symptoms may require change in dose or medication.
- Watch for other behavioral or personality changes such as confusion, nervousness, excitation, decreased concentration, hallucinations, or expression of abnormal thoughts. Notify physician if these changes become problematic.
- Assess dizziness that might affect gait, balance, and other functional activities (See Appendix C). Report balance problems and functional limitations to the physician, and caution the patient and family/caregivers to guard against falls and trauma.

Interventions

- Guard against falls and trauma (hip fractures, head injury, and so forth). Implement fall-prevention strategies, especially in older adults or if drowsiness and dizziness carry over into the daytime (See Appendix E).
- Help patient explore nonpharmacologic methods to improve sleep, such as relaxation techniques, regular exercise, avoid caffeine, and so forth.

Patient/Client-Related Instruction

- Instruct patients on prolonged treatment not to discontinue medication without consulting their physician. Long-term use can cause tolerance and physical/psychologic dependence, and increased sleep problems (rebound insomnia) can occur when the drug is suddenly discontinued.
- Advise patient to avoid alcohol and other CNS depressants because of the increased risk of sedation and adverse effects.
- Caution patient and family/caregivers to guard against complex motor behaviors that can occur while asleep, including driving a car.
- Instruct patient to report severe or prolonged skin rash or GI problems (nausea, vomiting, diarrhea, constipation).

Pharmacokinetics

Absorption: Well absorbed following oral administration.
Distribution: Widely distributed, crosses blood-brain barrier. Probably crosses the placenta and enters breast milk.
Protein Binding: 89%.
Metabolism and Excretion: Metabolized by the liver.
Half-life: 1.6–5.4 hr.

TIME/ACTION PROFILE (sedation)

ROUTE	ONSET	PEAK	DURATION
PO	15–30 min	6–8 hr	unknown

Contraindications/Precautions

Contraindicated in: Hypersensitivity; Cross-sensitivity with other benzodiazepines may occur; Preexisting CNS depression; Uncontrolled severe pain; OB/Pedi: Pregnancy, lactation, or children.
Use Cautiously in: Preexisting hepatic dysfunction (dose reduction recommended); History of suicide attempt or drug addiction; Geri: Elderly patients have ↑ sensitivity to benzodiazepines. Appears on Beers' list and is associated with ↑ risk of falls (↓ dose required); Debilitated patients (initial dose reduction recommended).

Interactions

Drug-Drug: **Cimetidine, erythromycin, fluconazole, itraconazole, ketoconazole, indinavir, nelfinavir, ritonavir, or saquinavir** may ↓ metabolism and enhance actions of triazolam; combination should be avoided. Additive CNS depression with **alcohol, antidepressants, antihistamines,** and **opioid analgesics.** May ↓ effectiveness of **levodopa.** May ↑ toxicity of **zidovudine. Isoniazid** may ↓ excretion and ↑ effects of triazolam. Sedative effects may be ↓ by **theophylline.**
Drug-Natural: Concomitant use of **kava, valerian, chamomile,** or **hops** can ↑ CNS depression.
Drug-Food: Grapefruit juice significantly ↑ blood levels and effects.

Route/Dosage

PO (Adults): 125–250 mcg (up to 500 mcg) hs.
PO (Geriatric Patients or Debilitated Patients): 125 mcg hs initially; may be ↑ as needed.

Availability (generic available)

Tablets: 125 mcg, 250 mcg.

trifluoperazine

(trye-floo-oh-**pair**-a-zeen)
Apo-Trifluoperazine, Novo-Flurazine, PMS-Trifluoperazine, ✱ Solazine, Stelazine, ✱ Terfluzine

Classification
Therapeutic: antipsychotics (conventional)
Pharmacologic: phenothiazines

Indications

Schizophrenia, nonpsychotic anxiety. Considered 2nd-line treatment after failure with atypical antipsychotics.
Unlabeled Use: Other psychotic disorders; bipolar disorder.

Action

Alters the effects of dopamine in the CNS. Possesses significant anticholinergic and alpha-adrenergic blocking activity. **Therapeutic Effects:** Diminished signs and symptoms of psychoses.

Adverse Reactions/Side Effects

CNS: *NEUROLEPTIC MALIGNANT SYNDROME*, extrapyramidal reactions, sedation, tardive dyskinesia. **EENT:** dry eyes, blurred vision, lens opacities. **CV:** hypotension, tachycardia. **GI:** constipation, anorexia, dry mouth, hepatitis, ileus. **GU:** urinary retention, priapism. **Derm:** photosensitivity, pigment changes, rashes. **Endo:** galactorrhea, amenorrhea. **Hemat:** *AGRANULOCYTOSIS*, leukopenia. **Metab:** hyperthermia. **Misc:** allergic reactions.

PHYSICAL THERAPY IMPLICATIONS

Examination and Evaluation

- Be alert for signs of neuroleptic malignant syndrome, including hyperthermia, diaphoresis, generalized muscle rigidity, altered mental status, tachycardia, changes in blood pressure (BP), and incontinence. Symptoms typically occur within 4–14 days after initiation of drug therapy, but can occur at any time during drug use. Report these signs to the physician immediately.
- Watch for signs of agranulocytosis and leukopenia, including fever, sore throat, mucosal lesions, and other signs of infection. Report these signs to the physician immediately.
- Assess motor function, and be alert for extrapyramidal symptoms. Report these symptoms immediately, especially tardive dyskinesia, because this problem may be irreversible. Common extrapyramidal symptoms include:
  - Tardive dyskinesia (uncontrolled rhythmic movement of mouth, face, and extremities, lip smacking or puckering, puffing of cheeks, uncontrolled chewing, rapid or worm-like movements of tongue).
  - Pseudoparkinsonism (shuffling gait, rigidity, tremor, pill-rolling motion, loss of balance control, difficulty speaking or swallowing, mask-like face).
  - Akathisia (restlessness or desire to keep moving).
  - Other dystonias and dyskinesias (dystonic muscle spasms, twisting motions, twitching, inability to move eyes, weakness of arms or legs).
- Monitor signs of allergic reactions, including pulmonary symptoms (laryngeal edema, wheezing, dyspnea) or skin reactions (rash, pruritus, urticaria). Notify physician immediately if these reactions occur.
- Assess heart rate, ECG, and heart sounds, especially during exercise (See Appendices G, H). Report a rapid heart rate (tachycardia) or signs of other arrhythmias, including palpitations, chest discomfort, shortness of breath, fainting, and fatigue/weakness.
- Assess BP periodically and compare to normal values (See Appendix F). Report low BP (hypotension), especially if patient experiences dizziness or syncope.

Interventions

- Guard against falls and trauma (hip fractures, head injury, and so forth) caused by drowsiness, blurred vision, or extrapyramidal symptoms; implement fall-prevention strategies (See Appendix E).
- Because of the risk of tachycardia and abnormal BP responses, use caution during aerobic exercise and other forms of therapeutic exercise. Assess exercise tolerance frequently (BP, heart rate, fatigue levels), and terminate exercise immediately if any untoward responses occur (See Appendix L).
- To minimize orthostatic hypotension, patient should move slowly when assuming a more upright position.
- This drug impairs body temperature regulation; use care during exercise, and during other activities that increase body temperature (hot whirlpools, saunas, and so forth).
- Causes photosensitivity; use care if administering UV treatments. Advise patient to avoid direct sunlight and use sunscreens and protective clothing.
- Help patient and family/caregivers explore nonpharmacologic methods (exercise, counseling, support groups) to reduce schizophrenic episodes and mood disorders.

Patient/Client-Related Instruction

- Advise patient to avoid alcohol and other CNS depressants because of the increased risk of sedation and adverse effects.
- Advise patient about the likelihood of GI problems such as constipation, loss of appetite, and dry mouth. Instruct patient to report severe or prolonged GI reactions, and to also report signs of drug-induced hepatitis, including anorexia, abdominal pain, severe nausea and vomiting, yellow skin or eyes, skin rashes, flu-like symptoms, and muscle/joint pain.
- Instruct patient to report other problematic side effects such as severe or prolonged vision disturbances, dry eyes, excessive sedation, urinary retention, painful/sustained erections, nipple discharge, menstrual disturbances, or skin reactions (rash, changes in pigmentation).

Pharmacokinetics

Absorption: Absorption from tablets is variable; may be better with oral liquid formulations. Well absorbed following IM administration.

T

Distribution: Widely distributed, high concentrations in the CNS. Crosses the placenta and enters breast milk.
Protein Binding: ≥90%.
Metabolism and Excretion: Highly metabolized by the liver.
Half-life: Unknown.

TIME/ACTION PROFILE (antipsychotic effects)

ROUTE	ONSET	PEAK	DURATION
PO	unknown	unknown	12–24 hr
IM	unknown	unknown	4–6 hr

Contraindications/Precautions

Contraindicated in: Hypersensitivity; Cross-sensitivity with other phenothiazines may exist; Hypersensitivity to bisulfites (oral concentrate only); Angle-closure glaucoma; Bone marrow depression; Severe liver or cardiovascular disease; Lactation: Discontinue drug or bottle-feed.
Use Cautiously in: Geri: Geriatric or debilitated patients (dose reduction recommended); ↑ risk of mortality in elderly patients treated for dementia-related psychosis; OB: Safety not established; may cause adverse effects in the newborn; Diabetes mellitus; Respiratory disease; Prostatic hyperplasia; CNS tumors; Epilepsy; Intestinal obstruction.

Interactions

Drug-Drug: Additive hypotension with **antihypertensives,** acute ingestion of **alcohol,** or **nitrates.** Additive CNS depression with other **CNS depressants,** including **alcohol, antihistamines, opioids, sedative/hypnotics,** and **general anesthetics.** Additive anticholinergic effects with other **drugs having anticholinergic properties,** including **antihistamines, antidepressants,** other **phenothiazines, quinidine,** and **disopyramide.** Acute encephalopathy may occur with **lithium.** May decrease the effectiveness of **levodopa.** ↑ risk of agranulocytosis with **antithyroid drugs. Lithium** ↓ absorption and may increase risk of extrapyramidal reactions.

Route/Dosage

PO (Adults): *Psychoses*—2–5 mg 1–2 times daily (up to 40 mg/day). *Anxiety*—1–2 mg bid (not to exceed 6 mg/day or treatment longer than 12 wk).
PO (Children 6–12 yr): 1 mg once or twice daily (up to 15 mg/day).
IM (Adults): 1–2 mg q 4–6 hr (up to 10 mg/day).
IM (Children): 1 mg once or twice daily.

Availability (generic available)

Tablets: 1 mg, 2 mg, 5 mg, 10 mg, 20 mg. **Syrup:** 1 mg/mL, 10 mg/mL. **Oral solution:** 10 mg/mL in 60-mL bottles Rx. **Injection:** 2 mg/mL in 10-mL vials.

trihexyphenidyl

(trye-heks-ee-**fen**-i-dil)
Apo-Trihex, Artane, PMS-Trihexyphenidyl, Trihexane, Trihexy

Classification
Therapeutic: antiparkinson agents
Pharmacologic: anticholinergics

Indications

Adjunct in the management of parkinsonian syndrome of many causes, including drug-induced parkinsonism.

Action

Inhibits the action of acetylcholine, resulting in Decreased sweating and salivation, Mydriasis (pupillary dilation), Increased heart rate. Also has spasmolytic action on smooth muscle. Inhibits cerebral motor centers and blocks efferent impulses. **Therapeutic Effects:** Diminished signs and symptoms of parkinsonian syndrome (tremors, rigidity).

Adverse Reactions/Side Effects

CNS: dizziness, nervousness, confusion, drowsiness, headache, psychoses, weakness. **EENT:** blurred vision, mydriasis. **CV:** orthostatic hypotension, tachycardia. **GI:** dry mouth, nausea, constipation, vomiting. **GU:** urinary hesitancy, urinary retention. **Derm:** decreased sweating.

PHYSICAL THERAPY IMPLICATIONS

Examination and Evaluation

- Assess patient's gait and motor function to help document antiparkinson effects, especially when starting drug therapy or during dosing changes or addition of other antiparkinson drugs. Motor function should be assessed at different times of the day, such as when drugs are reaching therapeutic levels (i.e., 2–3 hr after oral dose), as well as when drug effects are minimal (just before the next dose).
- Assess heart rate, ECG, and heart sounds, especially during exercise (See Appendices G, H). Report fast heart rate (tachycardia) or signs of other arrhythmias, including palpitations, chest discomfort, shortness of breath, fainting, and fatigue/weakness.
- Assess blood pressure (BP) when patient assumes a more upright position (lying to standing, sitting to standing, lying to sitting). Document orthostatic hypotension and contact the physician when systolic BP falls >20 mm Hg, or diastolic BP falls >10 mm Hg.
- Report confusion, nervousness, psychosis, and other psychologic problems. Repeated or excessive symptoms may require change in dose or medication.
- Assess dizziness and drowsiness that might affect gait, balance, and other functional activities

(See Appendix C). Report balance problems and functional limitations to the physician, and caution the patient and family/caregivers to guard against falls and trauma.

Interventions

- Implement therapeutic exercises (coordination exercises, gait training, cardiovascular conditioning) to complement the effects of drug therapy and help achieve optimal function.
- Because of the risk of arrhythmias and abnormal BP responses, use caution during aerobic exercise and other forms of therapeutic exercise. Assess exercise tolerance frequently (BP, heart rate, fatigue levels), and terminate exercise immediately if any untoward responses occur (See Appendix L).
- Guard against falls and trauma (hip fractures, head injury, and so forth). Implement fall- prevention strategies (See Appendix E), especially if patient exhibits Parkinson's symptoms (postural instability, rigidity) combined with drug side effects (dizziness, blurred vision, weakness).
- To minimize orthostatic hypotension, patient should move slowly when assuming a more upright position.

Patient/Client-Related Instruction

- Instruct patient to report other bothersome side effects, including severe or prolonged headache, vision problems, decreased sweating, urinary problems (hesitancy, retention), or GI problems (nausea, vomiting, constipation, dry mouth).

Pharmacokinetics

Absorption: Well absorbed following oral administration.
Distribution: Unknown.
Metabolism and Excretion: Excreted mostly in urine.
Half-life: 3.7 hr.

TIME/ACTION PROFILE (antiparkinson effects)

ROUTE	ONSET	PEAK	DURATION
PO	1 hr	2–3 hr	6–12 hr
PO-ER	unknown	unknown	12–24 hr

Contraindications/Precautions

Contraindicated in: Hypersensitivity; Angle-closure glaucoma; Acute hemorrhage; Tachycardia secondary to cardiac insufficiency; Thyrotoxicosis; Known alcohol intolerance (elixir only).
Use Cautiously in: Geriatric and very young patients (↑ risk of adverse reactions); Intestinal obstruction or infection; Prostatic hyperplasia; Chronic renal, hepatic, pulmonary, or cardiac disease; Pregnancy, lactation, or children (safety not established).

Interactions

Drug-Drug: Additive anticholinergic effects with other **drugs having anticholinergic properties,** including ↑ the risk of psychoses. Additive CNS depression with other **CNS depressants,** including **alcohol, antihistamines, opioids,** and **sedative/hypnotics.** Anticholinergics may alter the absorption of other **orally administered drugs** by slowing motility of the GI tract. **Antacids** may ↓ absorption.
Drug-Natural: ↑ effects with **angel's trumpet** and **jimson weed** and **scopolia.**

Route/Dosage

PO (Adults): 1–2 mg/day initially; increase by 2 mg q 3–5 days. Usual maintenance dose is 6–10 mg/day in 3 divided doses (up to 15 mg/day). Extended-release (Artane Sequels) preparations may be given q 12 hr after daily dose has been determined using conventional tablets or liquid.

Availability (generic available)

Tablets: 2 mg, 5 mg. **Elixir (lime-mint flavor):** 2 mg/5 mL. **Extended-release capsules:** 5 mg.

trimethoprim/sulfamethoxazole

(trye-**meth**-oh-prim/
sul-fa-meth-**ox**-a-zole)
Apo-Sulfatrim, Apo-Sulfatrim DS, Bactrim, Bactrim DS, Cofatrim, Cotrim, Cotrim DS, Novo-Trimel, Novo-Trimel DS, Nu-Cotrimox, Nu-Cotrimox DS, Roubac, Septra, Septra DS, SMZ/TMP, Sulfatrim, Sulfatrim DS, TMP/SMX, TMP/SMZ

Classification

Therapeutic: anti-infectives, antiprotozoals
Pharmacologic: folate antagonists, sulfonamides

T

Indications

Treatment of: Bronchitis, *Shigella* enteritis, Otitis media, *Pneumocystis carinii* pneumonia (PCP), Urinary tract infections, Traveler's diarrhea. Prevention of PCP in HIV-positive patients. **Unlabeled Use:** Biliary tract infections, osteomyelitis, burn and wound infections, chlamydial infections, endocarditis, gonorrhea, intra-abdominal infections, nocardiosis, rheumatic fever prophylaxis, sinusitis, eradication of meningococcal carriers, prophylaxis of urinary tract infections, and an alternative agent in the treatment of chancroid. Prevention of bacterial infections in immunosuppressed patients.

Action

Combination inhibits the metabolism of folic acid in bacteria at two different points. **Therapeutic Effects:** Bactericidal action against susceptible bacteria. **Spectrum:** Active against many strains of gram-positive aerobic pathogens, including, *Streptococcus pneumoniae*, *Staphylococcus aureus*, Group A beta-hemolytic streptococci, *Nocardia*, *Enterococcus*. Has activity against many aerobic gram-negative pathogens, such as *Acinetobacter*, *Enterobacter*, *Klebsiella pneumoniae*, *Escherichia coli*, *Proteus mirabilis*, *Shigella*, *Haemophilus influenzae*, including ampicillin-resistant strains. *P. carinii* (a protozoa). Not active against *Pseudomonas aeruginosa*.

Adverse Reactions/Side Effects

CNS: fatigue, hallucinations, headache, insomnia, mental depression. **GI:** PSEUDOMEMBRANOUS COLITIS, HEPATIC NECROSIS, nausea, vomiting, diarrhea, stomatitis, hepatitis, cholestatic jaundice. **GU:** crystalluria. **Derm:** TOXIC EPIDERMAL NECROLYSIS, rashes, photosensitivity. **Hemat:** AGRANULOCYTOSIS, APLASTIC ANEMIA, hemolytic anemia, leukopenia, megaloblastic anemia, thrombocytopenia. **Local:** phlebitis at IV site. **Misc:** ALLERGIC REACTIONS, INCLUDING ERYTHEMA MULTIFORME, STEVENS-JOHNSON SYNDROME, fever.

PHYSICAL THERAPY IMPLICATIONS

Examination and Evaluation

- Monitor signs of allergic reactions, including pulmonary symptoms (tightness in the throat and chest, wheezing, cough, dyspnea) or skin reactions (rash, pruritus, urticaria, dermatitis, exfoliation). Notify physician immediately, especially about severe skin reactions that might indicate Stevens-Johnson syndrome, toxic epidermal necrosis, or erythema mutiforme.
- Watch for signs of pseudomembranous colitis, including diarrhea, abdominal pain, fever, pus or mucus in stools, or other severe or prolonged GI problems (nausea, cramps, vomiting). Report these signs to the physician immediately.
- Be alert for signs of hepatic necrosis, including anorexia, abdominal pain, severe nausea and vomiting, yellow skin or eyes, fever, sore throat, malaise, weakness, facial edema, lethargy, and unusual bleeding or bruising. Report these signs to the physician immediately.
- Monitor signs of agranulocytosis (fever, sore throat, mucosal lesions, signs of infection), aplastic anemia (fatigue, shortness of breath with exertion, pale skin), thrombocytopenia (bruising, nose bleeds, bleeding gums), or unusual weakness, fatigue, infection, or other symptoms that might be due to other blood dyscrasias. Report these signs to the physician immediately.
- Monitor signs of mental depression, hallucinations, or other changes in mood and behavior. Notify physician if these changes become problematic.
- Assess IV site during and after IV administration, and report signs of phlebitis and venous thrombosis (local pain, swelling, inflammation).

Interventions

- Always wash hands thoroughly and disinfect equipment (whirlpools, electrotherapeutic devices, treatment tables, and so forth) to help prevent the spread of infection. Employ universal precautions or isolation procedures as indicated for specific patients.
- Causes photosensitivity; use care if administering UV treatments. Advise patient to avoid direct sunlight and use sunscreens and protective clothing.

Patient/Client-Related Instruction

- Instruct patient and family/caregivers to report other troublesome side effects such as severe or prolonged headache, fever, skin rash, or GI reactions (nausea, vomiting, diarrhea, inflammation in/around the mouth).

Pharmacokinetics

Absorption: Well absorbed from the GI tract.
Distribution: Widely distributed. Crosses the blood-brain barrier and placenta and enters breast milk.
Metabolism and Excretion: Some metabolism by the liver (20%); remainder excreted unchanged by the kidneys.
Half-life: *Trimethoprim*—6–11 hr; *sulfamethoxazole*—9–12 hr, both prolonged in renal failure.

TIME/ACTION PROFILE (blood levels)

ROUTE	ONSET	PEAK	DURATION
PO	rapid	2–4 hr	6–12 hr
IV	rapid	end of infusion	6–12 hr

Contraindications/Precautions

Contraindicated in: Hypersensitivity to sulfonamides or trimethoprim; Megaloblastic anemia secondary to folate deficiency; Severe renal impairment; Pregnancy, lactation, or children <2 mo (can cause kernicterus in neonates).
Use Cautiously in: Impaired hepatic or renal function (dosage reduction required if CCr <30 mL/min); HIV-positive patients (increased incidence of adverse reactions).

Interactions

Drug-Drug: May ↑ half-life, ↓ clearance, and exaggerate folic acid deficiency caused by **phenytoin.** May ↑ effects of **sulfonylurea oral antidiabetics, phenytoin, digoxin, thiopental,** and **warfarin.** May ↑ toxicity of **methotrexate.** ↑ risk of thrombocytopenia from **thiazide diuretics** (↑ in geriatric patients).

↓ efficacy of **cyclosporine (decreases serum concentrations)** and ↑ risk of nephrotoxicity.

Route/Dosage

(TMP = trimethoprim; SMX = sulfamethoxazole). Dosing based on TMP content.

Bacterial Infections

PO, IV (Adults and Children >2 mo): *Mild-to-moderate infections*—6–12 mg TMP/kg/day divided q 12 hr; *Serious infection/*Pneumocystis—15–20 mg TMP/kg /day/divided q 6–8 hr.
PO (Adults): *Urinary tract infection/chronic bronchitis*—1 double-strength tablet (160 mg TMP/800 mg SMX) q 12 hr for 10–14 days.

Urinary Tract Infection Prophylaxis

PO, IV (Adults and Children >2 mo): 2 mg TMP/kg/dose daily or 5 mg TMP/kg/dose twice weekly.
***P. carinii* Pneumonia (Prevention)**
PO (Adults): 1 double-strength tablet (160 mg TMP/800 mg SMX) daily (may also be given 3 times weekly).
PO (Children >1 mo): 150 mg TMP/m^2/day divided q 12 hr on 3 consecutive days/wk (not to exceed 320 mg TMP/1600 mg SMX per day).

Availability (generic available)

Tablets: 20 mg TMP/100 mg SMX, 80 mg TMP/400 mg SMX, 160 mg TMP/800 mg SMX. **Oral suspension (cherry, grape flavors):** 40 mg TMP/200 mg SMX/5 mL. **Solution for injection:** 16 mg TMP/80 mg SMX/mL in 5-, 10-, and 30-mL vials.

trimipramine
(trye-mip-ra-meen)
Surmontil

Classification
Therapeutic: antidepressants
Pharmacologic: tricyclic antidepressants

Indications

Treatment of depression, often in conjunction with psychotherapy.

Action

Potentiates the effect of serotonin and norepinephrine in the CNS. Has significant anticholinergic properties, including sedation. **Therapeutic Effects:** Antidepressant action.

Adverse Reactions/Side Effects

CNS: lethargy, sedation. **EENT:** blurred vision, dry eyes, dry mouth. **CV:** ARRHYTHMIAS, hypotension, ECG changes. **GI:** constipation, hepatitis, paralytic ileus, increased appetite, weight gain. **GU:** urinary retention, ↓ libido. **Derm:** photosensitivity. **Endo:** changes in blood glucose, gynecomastia. **Hemat:** blood dyscrasias.

PHYSICAL THERAPY IMPLICATIONS

Examination and Evaluation

- Assess heart rate, ECG, and heart sounds, especially during exercise (See Appendices G, H). Report any rhythm disturbances or symptoms of increased arrhythmias, including palpitations, chest discomfort, shortness of breath, fainting, and fatigue/weakness.
- Assess blood pressure periodically and compare to normal values (See Appendix F). Report low blood pressure (hypotension), especially if patient experiences dizziness or syncope.
- Watch for signs of leukopenia (fever, sore throat, signs of infection), thrombocytopenia (bruising, nose bleeds, bleeding gums), or unusual weakness and fatigue that might be due to anemia or other blood dyscrasias. Report these signs to the physician.
- Be alert for increased depression and suicidal thoughts and ideology, especially when initiating drug treatment or in children and teenagers. Notify physician or mental health professional immediately if patient exhibits worsening depression.
- Monitor other alterations in mental status including lethargy and sedation. Notify physician if these symptoms become problematic.
- Watch for signs of hypoglycemia (weakness, malaise, irritability, fatigue) or hyperglycemia (drowsiness, fruity breath, increased urination, unusual thirst). Patients with diabetes mellitus should check blood glucose levels frequently.
- Periodically assess body weight and other anthropometric measures (body mass index, body composition). Report a rapid or unexplained weight gain or increased body fat.

Interventions

- Guard against falls and trauma (hip fractures, head injury, and so forth), and implement fall prevention strategies (See Appendix E).
- Because of the risk of cardiac arrhythmias and abnormal BP responses, use caution during aerobic exercise and endurance conditioning. Assess exercise tolerance frequently (blood pressure, heart rate, fatigue levels), and terminate exercise immediately if any untoward responses occur (See Appendix L).
- To minimize orthostatic hypotension, patient should move slowly when assuming a more upright position.

- Causes photosensitivity; use care if administering UV treatments. Advise patient to avoid direct sunlight and use sunscreens and protective clothing.
- Help patient explore nonpharmacologic methods to reduce depression (exercise, counseling, support groups, and so forth).

Patient/Client-Related Instruction

- Advise patient that antidepressant effects may not occur immediately; it may take 2 wk or more before an improvement in mood is observed.
- Advise patient to avoid alcohol and other CNS depressants because of the increased risk of sedation and adverse effects.
- Advise patient that this medication should be tapered at the completion of long-term therapy. Abrupt discontinuation may cause nausea, vomiting, diarrhea, headache, trouble sleeping with vivid dreams, and irritability
- Instruct patient to report severe or prolonged constipation, or signs of liver dysfunction and hepatitis (yellow skin or eyes, abdominal pain, severe nausea and vomiting, fever, sore throat, malaise, weakness, facial edema).
- Instruct patient to report other problematic side effects such as severe or prolonged dry eyes/mouth, blurred vision, urinary retention, decreased libido, or increased breast growth in men (gynecomastia).

Pharmacokinetics

Absorption: Well absorbed following oral administration.
Distribution: Unknown.
Metabolism and Excretion: Mostly metabolized by the liver.
Half-life: 7–30 hr.

TIME/ACTION PROFILE

ROUTE	ONSET	PEAK	DURATION
PO	2–3 wk (up to 30 days)	2–6 wk	days–wks

Contraindications/Precautions

Contraindicated in: Hypersensitivity; cross-sensitivity may occur with other tricyclic antidepressants; Recovery phase following MI; Concurrent MAO inhibitor therapy; wait 2 wk following cessation to initiate trimipramine in lower doses initially; Angle-closure glaucoma.
Use Cautiously in: History or symptoms compatible with bipolar disease (may precipitate mixed/manic episodes); May ↑ risk of suicide attempt/ideation, especially during early treatment or dose adjustment; Pedi: risk may be greater in children and adolescents; Prostatic hyperplasia (↑ risk of urinary retention); History of seizures (may ↓ threshold); Hepatic impairment; Electroshock therapy (may ↑ risk of adverse reactions); ↑ intraocular pressure; Hyperthyroidism (↑ risk of cardiovascular toxicity); OB: Use only if clearly needed and maternal benefits outweigh risks to fetus; Lactation: May cause sedation in infant; Pedi: Safety not established; Geri: ↑ risk of adverse reactions, including falls secondary to sedative and anticholinergic affects.
Exercise Extreme Caution in: Preexisting cardiovascular disease.

Interactions

Drug-Drug: Concurrent **MAO inhibitors** may result in hyperpyretic reactions, convulsive crises, and death. **Guanethidine** or **similar agents** (effects may be negated by trimipramine). Trimipramine is metabolized in the liver by the cytochrome P450 2D6 enzyme, and its action may be affected by drugs that compete for metabolism by this enzyme, including **other antidepressants, phenothiazines, carbamazepine, class 1C antiarrhythmics,** including **propafenone,** and **flecainide;** when used concurrently, dose of one or the other or both may be necessary. Concurrent use of other drugs that inhibit the activity of the enzyme, including **cimetidine, quinidine, amiodarone,** and **ritonavir,** may result in ↑ effects of trimipramine. Concurrent use with **SSRI antidepressants** may result in toxicity and should be avoided (fluoxetine should be stopped 5 wk before starting trimipramine). Concurrent use with **clonidine** may result in hypertensive crisis and should be avoided. Concurrent use with **levodopa** may result in delayed or absorption of levodopa or hypertension. Blood levels and effects may be ↓ by **rifamycins (rifampin, rifapentine,** and **rifabutin**). Concurrent use with **moxifloxacin** ↑ risk of adverse cardiovascular reactions. ↑ CNS depression with other **CNS depressants,** including **alcohol, antihistamines, clonidine, opioids,** and **sedative/hypnotics. Barbiturates** may alter blood levels and effects. ↑ adrenergic and anticholinergic side effects with other **agents having adrenergic** or **anticholinergic properties.** Levels and risk of toxicity may be ↑ by **phenothiazines** or **oral contraceptives.** Nicotine may ↑ metabolism and alter effects.
Drug-Natural: St. John's wort may ↓ serum concentrations and efficacy. Concomitant use of **kava-kava, valerian,** or **chamomile** can ↑ CNS depression. ↑ anticholinergic effects with **jimson weed** and **scopolia.**

Route/Dosage

PO (Adults): 75 mg/day in divided doses or as a single daily dose hs; may be increased up to 150 mg/day; not to exceed 200 mg/day (300 mg/day in hospitalized patients). *Adolescent and elderly patients*—50 mg/day, may gradually ↑ up to 100 mg/day.

Availability

Capsules: 25 mg, 50 mg, 100 mg.

triprolidine (trye-proe-li-deen)

Classification
Therapeutic: antihistamines

Indications
Symptomatic relief of allergic symptoms caused by histamine release or symptoms associated with the common cold. Most useful in management of nasal allergies and allergic dermatoses. Available only in combination with a decongestant.

Action
Antagonizes the effects of histamine at peripheral histamine-1 (H_1) receptors, including pruritus and urticaria. Also has a drying effect on the nasal mucosa. **Therapeutic Effects:** Relief of symptoms associated with histamine excess usually seen in allergic conditions or with the common cold.

Adverse Reactions/Side Effects
CNS: sedation, dizziness, excitation (higher in children). **EENT:** blurred vision. **CV:** arrhythmias, hypertension, hypotension, palpitations. **GI:** dry mouth, constipation. **GU:** urinary hesitancy, urinary retention.

PHYSICAL THERAPY IMPLICATIONS

Examination and Evaluation
- Assess blood pressure (BP) and compare to normal values (See Appendix F). Report changes in BP, either a sustained increase in BP (hypertension) or a problematic decrease in BP (hypotension) that results in dizziness and syncope.
- Assess heart rate, ECG, and heart sounds, especially during exercise (See Appendices G, H). Report any rhythm disturbances or symptoms of increased arrhythmias, including palpitations, chest discomfort, shortness of breath, fainting, and fatigue/weakness.
- Monitor symptoms of nasal allergies (sneezing, rhinitis, itching eyes, cough) or allergic skin reactions (rash, hives, itching) to help document benefits of this drug in treating these disorders.
- Assess dizziness and drowsiness that might affect gait, balance, and other functional activities (See Appendix C). Report balance problems and functional limitations to the physician, and caution the patient and family/caregivers to guard against falls and trauma.
- Monitor signs of increased excitation, especially in children. Severe or problematic excitation may require a change in dose or drug.

Interventions
- Guard against falls and trauma (hip fractures, head injury, and so forth). Implement fall- prevention strategies, especially in older adults or if balance is impaired (See Appendix E).
- Because of an increased risk of arrhythmias and abnormal BP responses, use caution during aerobic exercise and other forms of therapeutic exercise. Assess exercise tolerance frequently (BP, heart rate, fatigue levels), and terminate exercise immediately if any untoward responses occur (See Appendix L).

Patient/Client-Related Instruction
- Advise patient about the risk of daytime drowsiness and decreased attention and mental focus. These problems can be severe in certain people. Use care if driving or in other activities that require quick reactions and strong concentration.
- Advise patient to avoid alcohol and other CNS depressants because of the increased risk of sedation and adverse effects.
- Instruct patient to report other troublesome side effects such as severe or prolonged constipation, dry mouth, blurred vision, or problems with urination (hesitancy, retention).

Pharmacokinetics
Absorption: Well absorbed following oral administration.
Distribution: Widely distributed. Minimal amounts excreted in breast milk. Crosses the blood-brain barrier.
Metabolism and Excretion: Extensively metabolized by the liver.
Half-life: 3–3.3 hr.

TIME/ACTION PROFILE (antihistaminic effects)

ROUTE	ONSET	PEAK	DURATION
PO	15–60 min	1–2 hr	4–8 hr

Contraindications/Precautions
Contraindicated in: Hypersensitivity; Angle-closure glaucoma; Acute attacks of asthma; Lactation; Known alcohol intolerance (some liquids).
Use Cautiously in: Geriatric patients (increased risk of adverse reactions); Liver disease; Prostatic hyperplasia; Pregnancy (safety not established).

Interactions
Drug-Drug: Additive CNS depression with other **CNS depressants,** including **alcohol, opioid analgesics,** and **sedative/hypnotics.** Additive anticholinergic effects with other **drugs possessing anticholinergic properties,** including **antidepressants, atropine,**

haloperidol, phenothiazines, quinidine, and **disopyramide. MAO inhibitors** intensify and prolong anticholinergic effects of **antihistamines.**
Drug-Natural: Concomitant use of **kava, valerian, skullcap, chamomile,** or **hops** can ↑ CNS depression. ↑ anticholinergic effects with **angel's trumpet, jimson weed,** and **scopolia.**

Route/Dosage

PO (Adults): 2.5 mg q 4–6 hr (not to exceed 10 mg/24 hr).
PO (Children 6–12 yr): 1.25 mg q 4–6 hr (not to exceed 5 mg/24 hr).
PO (Children 4–6 yr): 938 mcg q 4–6 hr (not to exceed 3.744 mg/24 hr).
PO (Children 2–4 yr): 0.625 mg q 4–6 hr (not to exceed 2.5 mg/24 hr).
PO (Children 4 mo–2 yr): 313 mcg q 4–6 hr (not to exceed 1.252 mg/24 hr).

Availability

Syrup, oral solution, or tablets: in combination only (see below). ***In combination with:*** pseudoephedrine, with or without acetaminophen, guaifenesin, dextromethorphan, or codeine Rx, OTC. See Appendix B.

triptorelin (trip-to-**rel**-in)

Trelstar Depot

Classification
Therapeutic: antineoplastics
Pharmacologic: hormones

Indications

Palliative treatment of advanced prostate cancer when orchiectomy or estrogen administration are contraindicated or unacceptable.

Action

A synthetic analogue of luteinizing hormone–releasing hormone (LHRH); Initially causes a transient ↑ in testosterone; however, with continuous administration, testosterone levels are ↓. Reduces gonadotropins, testosterone, and estradiol. **Therapeutic Effects:** ↓ testosterone levels and resultant ↓ in spread of prostate cancer.

Adverse Reactions/Side Effects

CNS: dizziness, emotional lability, fatigue, headache, insomnia. **CV:** hypertension. **GI:** diarrhea, vomiting. **GU:** erectile dysfunction, urinary retention, urinary tract infection. **Derm:** pruritus. **Hemat:** anemia. **Local:** injection site pain. **MS:** musculoskeletal pain. **Misc:** ALLERGIC REACTIONS, INCLUDING ANAPHYLAXIS AND ANGIOEDEMA.

PHYSICAL THERAPY IMPLICATIONS

Examination and Evaluation

- Monitor signs of allergic reactions and anaphylaxis or angioedema, including pulmonary symptoms (tightness in the throat and chest, wheezing, cough, dyspnea) or skin reactions (rash, raised patches of red or white skin, burning/itching skin, swelling in the face). Notify physician or nursing staff immediately if these reactions occur.
- Assess blood pressure periodically and compare to normal values (See Appendix F). Report a sustained increase in blood pressure (hypertension).
- Assess any joint or muscle to rule out musculoskeletal pathology; that is, try to determine if pain is drug induced rather than caused by anatomic or biomechanical problems.
- Monitor signs of anemia, including unusual fatigue, shortness of breath with exertion, and bruising, and pale skin. Notify physician immediately if these signs occur.
- Monitor personality or behavioral changes, including emotional instability or difficulty sleeping. Notify physician if these changes become problematic.
- Assess dizziness that might affect gait, balance, and other functional activities (See Appendix C). Report balance problems and functional limitations to the physician and nursing staff, and caution the patient and family/caregivers to guard against falls and trauma.
- Monitor IM injection site for pain, swelling, and irritation. Report prolonged or excessive injection site reactions to the physician.

Interventions

- For patients who are medically able to begin exercise, implement appropriate resistive exercises and aerobic training to maintain muscle strength and aerobic capacity during cancer chemotherapy or to help restore function after chemotherapy.

Patient/Client-Related Instruction

- Instruct patient to report problems with urination, including urinary retention or signs of a urinary tract infection (blood in the urine, increased nighttime urination, pain and burning during urination).
- Instruct patient or family/caregivers to report other troublesome side effects such as severe or prolonged headache, erectile dysfunction, skin reactions (itching, redness), or GI problems (diarrhea, vomiting).

Pharmacokinetics

Absorption: Well absorbed following IM administration.
Distribution: Unknown.

Metabolism and Excretion: Unknown.
Half-life: 3 hr.

TIME/ACTION PROFILE (effects on hormone levels)

ROUTE	ONSET	PEAK	DURATION
IM	unknown	1 hr*	4 wk

*Blood level of triptorelin.

Contraindications/Precautions

Contraindicated in: Hypersensitivity to triptorelin or similar agents; Pregnancy, lactation, or children.
Use Cautiously in: Metastatic vertebral lesions and/or upper or lower urinary tract obstruction (symptoms may transiently worsen following initiation of therapy); Renal or hepatic impairment (may need dosage adjustment).

Interactions

Drug-Drug: Concurrent use of **hyperprolactinemic drugs** should be avoided (may ↓ number of drug receptor sites).

Route/Dosage

IM (Adults): 3.75 mg monthly.

Availability

Suspension for IM injection (Depot): 3.75 mg/vial.

T

ulipristal (yoo-li-pris-tal)

Ella

Classification

Therapeutic: contraceptive hormones (emergency)

Pharmacologic: progesterone agonists/antagonists

Indications

Prevention of pregnancy following unprotected intercourse or known/suspected contraceptive failure; not intended for routine use.

Action

Binds to progesterone receptors. Delays follicular rupture, thereby inhibiting/delaying ovulation. Changes in endometrial environment may also contribute to action. **Therapeutic Effects:** Prevention of pregnancy.

Adverse Reactions/Side Effects

CNS: headache, dizziness, fatigue. **GI:** abdominal pain, nausea. **GU:** altered menstrual cycle, dysmenorrhea.

PHYSICAL THERAPY IMPLICATIONS

Examination and Evaluation

- Assess dizziness or fatigue that might affect gait, balance, and other functional activities (See Appendix C). Report any persistent balance problems and functional limitations to the physician, and caution the patient and family/caregivers to guard against falls and trauma.

Patient/Client-Related Instruction

- Instruct patient to report other troublesome side effects such as prolonged or severe headache, menstrual problems, or GI reactions (nausea, abdominal pain).

Pharmacokinetics

Absorption: Well absorbed following oral administration.
Distribution: Unknown.
Protein Binding: >94%.
Metabolism and Excretion: Mostly metabolized by CYP3A4 enzyme system; 1 metabolite (monodemethyl-ulipristal) pharmacologically active.
Half-life: *Uliprostal*—32 hr; *monodemethyl-ulispristal*—27 hr.

TIME/ACTION PROFILE

ROUTE	ONSET	PEAK*	DURATION
PO	unknown	ulipristal—0.9 hr; monodemethyl-ulispristal—1 hr	unknown

*Blood level.

Contraindications/Precautions

Contraindicated in: Pregnancy or termination of existing pregnancy. Lactation: Not recommended during breast-feeding.
Use Cautiously in: Repeated use; regular contraception should be continued/instituted and additional method should be used during current cycle.

Interactions

Drug-Drug: Effectiveness may be ↓ by **drugs that induce the CYP3A4 enzyme system,** including **barbiturates, bosentan, carbamazepine, oxcarbazepine, phenytoin, topiramate, felbamate, griseofulvin,** and **rifampin;** Effects may be ↑ **drugs that inhibit the CYP3A4 enzyme system,** including **itraconazole** and **ketoconazole;** Efficacy of **hormonal contraceptives** may be ↓ during current cycle.
Drug-Natural: Effectiveness may be ↓ by **St. John's wort.**

Route/Dosage

PO (Adults): 1 tablet as soon as possible within 120 hr (5 days) after unprotected intercourse or known/suspected contraceptive failure. If vomiting occurs within 3 hr, dose may be repeated.

Availability

Tablet: 30 mg.

U

HIGH ALERT

urokinase (yoor-oh-kye-nase)

Abbokinase

Classification

Therapeutic: thrombolytics

Pharmacologic: plasminogen activators

Indications

Pulmonary embolism (PE). **Unlabeled Use:** Deep venous thrombosis (DVT). Acute peripheral arterial thrombosis. Acute ischemic stroke. Acute myocardial infarction (MI). Occluded central venous access devices.

Action

Directly converts plasminogen to plasmin, which then degrades clot-bound fibrin. **Therapeutic Effects:** Lysis of pulmonary emboli. Lysis of thrombi in coronary arteries, with improvement of ventricular function, and reduced risk of heart failure or death. Lysis of thrombi causing ischemic stroke, reducing risk of neurologic sequelae. Restoration of cannula or catheter function.

Adverse Reactions/Side Effects

CNS: INTRACRANIAL HEMORRHAGE. **EENT:** epistaxis, gingival bleeding. **Resp:** bronchospasm, hemoptysis. **CV:** reperfusion arrhythmias, hypotension, RECURRENT ISCHEMIA/THROMBOEMBOLISM. **GI:** GI BLEEDING, nausea, RETROPERITONEAL BLEEDING, vomiting. **GU:** GU TRACT BLEEDING. **Derm:** ecchymoses, flushing, urticaria. **Hemat:** BLEEDING. **Local:** hemorrhage at injection site, phlebitis at injection site. **MS:** musculoskeletal pain. **Misc:** ALLERGIC REACTIONS, INCLUDING ANAPHYLAXIS, fever.

PHYSICAL THERAPY IMPLICATIONS

Examination and Evaluation

- Assess for signs of bleeding and hemorrhage, including bleeding gums, nosebleeds, unusual bruising, coughing up blood, black/tarry stools, hematuria, or a fall in hematocrit or blood pressure. Be especially alert for signs of intracranial bleeds, including sudden severe headache, confusion, nausea, vomiting, paralysis, numbness, speech problems, visual disturbances. Notify physician or nursing staff immediately if these signs occur.
- Monitor signs of recurrent thromboembolism and PE, including shortness of breath, chest pain, cough, and bloody sputum. Notify physician immediately, and request objective tests (Doppler ultrasound, lung scan, others) if PE is suspected.
- Be alert for signs of recurrent cardiac ischemia (chest pain, pain radiating into the arm or jaw, shortness of breath, dizziness, sweating, anxiety), cerebral ischemia (sudden dizziness, vertigo, slurred speech, incoordination, numbness), or peripheral arterial thrombosis (pain, cramping, coldness, and cyanosis in the affected limb). Notify physician or nursing staff immediately if these signs occur.
- Monitor signs of allergic reactions or anaphylaxis, including pulmonary symptoms (tightness in the throat and chest, bronchospasm, wheezing, cough, dyspnea) or skin reactions (rash, pruritus, urticaria). Notify physician or nursing staff immediately if these reactions occur.
- Assess heart rate, ECG, and heart sounds when cardiac perfusion is restored (See Appendices G, H). Report any rhythm disturbances or symptoms of increased arrhythmias, including palpitations, chest discomfort, shortness of breath, fainting, and fatigue/weakness.
- Assess blood pressure, especially for the first few days after infusion. Report low blood pressure (hypotension), especially if patient experiences dizziness or syncope.
- Assess any muscle of joint pain to rule out musculoskeletal pathology or hemorrhage; that is, try to determine if pain is drug induced rather than caused by anatomic or biomechanical problems. Be especially concerned about back pain that could indicate retroperitoneal bleeding.
- Assess injection site during and after IV administration, and report signs of bleeding or phlebitis (local pain, swelling, inflammation).

Interventions

- Use caution with any physical interventions that could increase bleeding, including wound débridement, chest percussion, joint mobilization, and application of local heat.
- Use extreme caution during aerobic exercise in patients with recent MI or ischemic stroke. Assess exercise tolerance frequently (blood pressure, heart rate, fatigue levels, neurological signs), and terminate exercise immediately if any untoward responses occur (See Appendix L).
- For patients with DVT, recommend or implement other physical methods to decrease DVT and prevent recurrent thromboembolism, including graduated compression stockings and intermittent pneumatic compression pumps.

Patient/Client-Related Instruction

- Instruct patient to immediately report signs of GI bleeding, including abdominal pain, vomiting blood, blood in stools, or black, tarry stools.
- Instruct patient or family/caregivers to report other troublesome side effects such as severe or prolonged fever, skin reactions (rash, itching, discoloration), or GI problems (nausea, vomiting).

Pharmacokinetics

Absorption: Complete after IV administration. Intracoronary administration or administration into occluded catheters or cannulae has a more localized effect.
Distribution: Unknown.
Metabolism and Excretion: Rapidly metabolized by the liver.
Half-life: Up to 20 min.

TIME/ACTION PROFILE (fibrinolysis)

ROUTE	ONSET	PEAK	DURATION
IV	immediate	rapid	up to 12 hr

Contraindications/Precautions

Contraindicated in: Active internal bleeding; History of cerebrovascular accident; Recent (within 2 mo) intracranial or intraspinal injury or trauma; Intracranial neoplasm, arteriovenous malformation, or aneurysm; Severe uncontrolled hypertension; Known bleeding tendencies; Hypersensitivity.
Use Cautiously in: Recent (within 10 days) major surgery, trauma, GI or GU bleeding; Left heart thrombus; Severe hepatic or renal disease; Hemorrhagic ophthalmic conditions; Septic phlebitis; Previous puncture

of a noncompressible vessel; Subacute bacterial endocarditis or acute pericarditis; Geriatric patients (>75 yr; ↑ risk of intracranial bleeding); Pregnancy, lactation, or children (safety not established).
Exercise Extreme Caution in: Patients receiving concurrent anticoagulant therapy (↑ risk of intracranial bleeding).

Interactions

Drug-Drug: Aspirin, other **NSAIDs, warfarin, heparin** and **heparin-like agents, abciximab, eptifibatide, tirofiban, clopidogrel, ticlopidine,** or **dipyridamole**—concurrent use ↑ risk of bleeding, although these agents are frequently used together or in sequence. Effects may be ↓ by **antifibrinolytic agents,** including **aminocaproic acid** or **tranexamic acid.**
Drug-Natural: ↑ anticoagulant effect and bleeding risk with **anise, arnica, chamomile, clove, dong quai, fenugreek, feverfew, garlic, ginger, ginkgo,** Panax ginseng, **licorice,** and others.

Route/Dosage

Pulmonary Emboli

IV (Adults): 4400 IU/kg loading dose, followed by 4400 IU/kg/hr for 12 hr.

Acute Peripheral Arterial Thrombosis

IV (Adults): 240,000 IU/hr for 2–4 hr or until blood flow is restored.
IV (Adults): 120,000 IU/hr for up to a maximum of 48 hr.
IV (Adults): 120,000 IU/hr for 2 hr, followed by 60,000 IU/hr until blood flow is restored.

Occluded Venous Catheters

IV (Adults): 5,000 IU/mL instilled into catheter (volume equal to the volume of the catheter); attempt aspiration q 5 min; repeat dosing of urokinase may be necessary.

Availability

Powder for injection: 250,000 IU/vial.

ursodiol (er-soe-dye-ole)

Actigall, Urso 250, Urso Forte

Classification
Therapeutic: gallstone dissolution agents

Indications

Gallbladder stone dissolution and prevention; Primary biliary cirrhosis. **Unlabeled Use:** Biliary atresia TPN-induced cholestasis.

Action

↓ cholesterol content of bile and bile stones by suppressing cholesterol synthesis and secretion from the liver and inhibits intestinal absorption of cholesterol. **Therapeutic Effects:** Gallstone dissolution and reduction in gallstone formation.↓ progression of liver disease and improvement in liver function tests.

Adverse Reactions/Side Effects

CNS: anxiety, depression, fatigue, headache, sleep disorder. **Derm:** hair thinning, pruritus, rash.
GI: abdominal/biliary pain, constipation, diarrhea, flatulence↑ liver enzymes nausea, stomatitis, vomiting.
Neuro: arthralgias, myalgia. **Resp:** cough, rhinitis.

PHYSICAL THERAPY IMPLICATIONS

Examination and Evaluation

- Watch for changes in mood and behavior, including anxiety and depression. Notify physician if these changes become problematic.
- Assess any muscle or joint pain to rule out musculoskeletal pathology; that is, try to determine if pain is drug induced rather than caused by anatomic or biomechanical problems.

Patient/Client-Related Instruction

- Advise patient about the likelihood of GI problems, including nausea, vomiting, diarrhea, constipation, abdominal pain, flatulence, and irritation in or around the mouth. Instruct patient to report severe or prolonged GI reactions.
- Instruct patient and family/caregivers to report other troublesome side effects such as severe or prolonged headache, cough, nasal irritation, or skin reactions (rash, itching, thinning hair).

Pharmacokinetics

Absorption: 90%.
Distribution: Only small quantities are found in the systemic circulation; sites of action include the liver, bile, and gut lumen.
Protein Binding: 70%.
Metabolism and Excretion: Undergoes extensive enterohepatic recycling; excreted in feces via bile.
Half-life: 100 hr.

TIME/ACTION PROFILE

ROUTE	ONSET	PEAK	DURATION
PO	unknown	unknown	unknown

Contraindications/Precautions

Contraindicated in: Patients requiring cholecystectomy; Calcified cholesterol stones, radiopaque stones, bile pigment stones, or stones >20 mm.
Use Cautiously in: Chronic liver disease.

U

Interactions

Drug-Drug: Bile acid sequestering agents (cholestyramine, colestipol) and aluminum based anatacids may decrease effects by reducing absorption. Estrogens, oral. contraceptives, and clofibrate (and perhaps other lipid-lowering drugs) may counteract effectiveness by increasing hepatic cholesterol secretion and encouraging cholesterol gallstone formation.

Route/Dosage

PO (Adults): *Gallstone dissolution*—Initial 8–10 mg/kg/day in 2–3 divided doses; maintenance: 250 mg/day hs for 6 mo–1 yr; *Gallstone prevention*—300 mg bid; *Primary biliary cirrhosis*—13–15 mg/kg/day in 2–4 divided doses.
PO (Children and Infants): *TPN-induced cholestasis*—30 mg/kg/day in 2–3 divided doses.
PO (Infants): *Biliary atresia*—10–15 mg/kg/day.

Availability (generic available)

Capsules: 300 mg **Tablets:** 250 mg; 500 mg.

ustekinumab

(us-te-**kin**-yoo-mab)
Stelara

Classification
Therapeutic: antipsoriatics
Pharmacologic: interleukin antagonists monoclonal antibodies

Indications

Treatment of adults with moderate-to-severe plaque psoriasis who are candidates for phototherapy or systemic therapy.

Action

Binds to the p40 protein subunit used by both the interleukin-12 (IL-12) and IL-23 cytokines. These cytokines that are involved in inflammatory and immune responses, including natural killer cell activation and CD4+ T-cell differentiation and activation. Binding to interleukins antagonizes their effects, disrupting IL-12– and IL-23–mediated signaling and cytokine cascades. **Therapeutic Effects:** ↓ in area and severity of psoriatic lesions.

Adverse Reactions/Side Effects

CNS: fatigue, headache. **Local:** erythema. **Misc:** INFECTION, REVERSIBLE POSTERIOR LEUKOENCEPHALOPATHY SYNDROME.

PHYSICAL THERAPY IMPLICATIONS

Examination and Evaluation

- Be alert for signs of reversible posterior leukoencephalopathy. Signs include headache, confusion, memory lapses, decreased cognition, vision loss, and seizures. Report these signs to the physician immediately.
- Watch for signs of infection, including fever, sore throat, chills, nausea, vomiting, diarrhea, and localized inflammation. Notify physician immediately.
- Periodically assess skin condition to document whether drug therapy is successful in decreasing the size and severity of psoriatic lesions.
- Monitor injection site for redness and warmth. Report prolonged or excessive injection-site reactions to the physician.

Interventions

- Implement ultraviolet light therapy when indicated to help treat psoriasis and augment the effects of drug therapy.

Patient/Client-Related Instruction

- Instruct patient to guard against infection (frequent hand washing, etc.), and to avoid crowds and contact with persons with contagious diseases.
- Instruct patient to report other troublesome side effects, including severe or prolonged headache or fatigue.

Pharmacokinetics

Absorption: Well absorbed following SC administration.
Distribution: Unknown.
Metabolism and Excretion: Broken down by catabolic processes into peptides and amino acids.
Half-life: 15–46 days.

TIME/ACTION PROFILE

ROUTE	ONSET	PEAK*	DURATION
45 mg SC	unknown	13.5 days	12 wk
90 mg SC	unknown	7 days	12 wk

*Blood levels.

Contraindications/Precautions

Contraindicated in: Active untreated infection.
Use Cautiously in: History of known malignancy or tuberculosis (possibility of reactivation); OB: Use during pregnancy only if potential benefit justifies potential risk to the fetus. Lactation: Use cautiously in nursing women; unknown risks to infant from gastrointestinal/systemic exposure should be weighed against known benefits of breast-feeding. Pedi: Safe and effective use in patients <18 yr not established.
Exercise Extreme Caution in: Chronic infection or history of recurrent infection.

Interactions

Drug-Drug: May ↓ antibody response to and ↑ risk of adverse reactions from **live vaccines;** May ↓ desired antibody response to **nonlive vaccines;** May affect the activity of CYP450 drug-metabolizing enzymes; when treatment is started during concurrent **CYP450 substrates,** especially those with a narrow therapeutic indices, including

warfarin and **cyclosporine;** appropriate monitoring and dose adjustment should be carried out.

Route/Dosage

SC (Adults ≤100 kg): 45 mg initially and 4 wk later, then 45 mg q 12 wk.

SC (Adults >100 kg): 90 mg initially and 4 wk later, then 90 mg q 12 wk.

Availability

Solution for SC injection: 45 mg/0.5-mL vial, 90 mg/1-mL vial.

valacyclovir (val-a-sye-kloe-veer)

Valtrex

Classification
Therapeutic: antivirals
Pharmacologic: purine analogues

Indications

Treatment of herpes zoster (shingles). Treatment/suppression of genital herpes. Reduction of transmission of genital herpes. Treatment of chickenpox. Treatment of herpes labialis (cold sores).

Action

Rapidly converted to acyclovir. Acyclovir interferes with viral DNA synthesis. **Therapeutic Effects:** Inhibited viral replication, ↓ viral shedding, reduced time to healing of lesions. Reduced transmission of genital herpes.

Adverse Reactions/Side Effects

CNS: <u>headache</u>, dizziness, weakness. **GI:** <u>nausea</u>, abdominal pain, anorexia, constipation, diarrhea. **Hemat:** THROMBOTIC THROMBOCYTOPENIC PURPURA/HEMOLYTIC UREMIC SYNDROME (VERY HIGH DOSES IN IMMUNOSUPPRESSED PATIENTS).

PHYSICAL THERAPY IMPLICATIONS

Examination and Evaluation

- Monitor signs of thrombotic thrombocytopenic purpura (purplish spots on the skin, decreased consciousness, fatigue, weakness, shortness of breath on exertion, tachycardia) and hemolytic uremic syndrome (bloody diarrhea and vomiting, decreased urine output). Report these signs to the physician immediately.
- Assess dizziness or weakness that might affect gait, balance, or other functional activities (See Appendix C). Report balance problems and functional limitations to the physician, and caution the patient and family/caregivers to guard against falls and trauma.
- Assess skin and mucosal lesions to help document whether drug therapy is successful in controlling infection.

Interventions

- Avoid contact with cutaneous or mucosal lesions when treating patient.
- Always wash hands thoroughly and disinfect equipment (whirlpools, electrotherapeutic devices, treatment tables, and so forth) to help prevent the spread of infection. Use universal precautions as indicated for specific patients.

Patient/Client-Related Instruction

- Advise patient to take medication as directed. Valacyclovir should not be used more frequently or longer than prescribed.
- Remind patient that valacyclovir does not cure herpes infections. The virus lies dormant in the ganglia, and valacyclovir will not prevent the spread of infection to others.
- Instruct patient and family/caregivers to report other troublesome side effects, including severe or prolonged headache or GI problems (nausea, diarrhea, constipation, loss of appetite, abdominal pain).

Pharmacokinetics

Absorption: 54% bioavailable as acyclovir after oral administration of valacyclovir.
Distribution: CSF concentrations of acyclovir are 50% of plasma concentrations. Acyclovir crosses placenta; enters breast milk.
Metabolism and Excretion: Rapidly converted to acyclovir via intestinal/hepatic metabolism.
Half-life: 2.5–3.3 hr; up to 14 hr in renal impairment (acyclovir).

TIME/ACTION PROFILE (blood levels*)

ROUTE	ONSET	PEAK	DURATION
PO	unknown	1.5–2.5 hr	8–24 hr

*Acyclovir.

Contraindications/Precautions

Contraindicated in: Hypersensitivity to valacyclovir or acyclovir.
Use Cautiously in: Renal impairment (dose reduction/↑ dosing interval recommended if CCr <50 mL/min); Geri: Dose ↓ may be necessary; OB/Lactation: Pregnancy, lactation; Pedi: Children <2 yr (safety not established).

Interactions

Drug-Drug: Probenecid and **cimetidine** ↑ blood levels; significant only in renal impairment.

Route/Dosage

Herpes Zoster

PO (Adults): 1 g tid for 7 days.

Genital Herpes

PO (Adults): *Initial treatment*—1 g bid for 10 days. *Recurrence*—500 mg bid for 3 days. *Suppression of recurrence*—1 g once daily or 500 mg once daily in patients experiencing <10 recurrences/yr. *Suppression of recurrence in HIV-infected patients*—500 mg q 12 hr. *Reduction of transmission*—500 mg once daily for source partner.

Herpes Labialis

PO (Adults and Children ≥12 yr): 2 g, then 2 g 12 hr later.

Chickenpox

PO (Children ≥2 yr): 20 mg/kg tid for 5 days (not to exceed 1 g tid).

Renal Impairment

PO (Adults): *CCr 30–49 mL/min*—1 g q 12 hr for herpes zoster treatment, no reduction required for treatment of genital herpes; 1 g, then 1 g 12 hr later for herpes labialis. *CCr 10–29 mL/min*—1 g q 24 hr for initial treatment of genital herpes, 500 mg q 24 hr for treatment of recurrent episodes of genital herpes, 500 mg q 48 hr for suppression of genital herpes in patients with 9 or fewer recurrences/yr, 500 mg q 24 hr for suppression of genital herpes in patients with ≥10 recurrences/yr or HIV-infected patients, 1 g q 24 hr for treatment of herpes zoster; 500 mg then 500 mg 12 hr later for herpes labialis. *CCr <10 mL/min*—500 mg q 24 hr for initial treatment of genital herpes, 500 mg q 24 hr for treatment of recurrent episodes of genital herpes, 500 mg q 48 hr for suppression of genital herpes in patients with 9 or fewer recurrences/yr, 500 mg q 24 hr for suppression of genital herpes in patients with ≥10 recurrences/yr or HIV-infected patients, 500 mg q 24 hr for treatment of herpes zoster; single 500-mg dose for herpes labialis.

Availability

Tablets: 500 mg, 1 g.

valganciclovir

(val-gan-**sye**-kloe-veer)

Valcyte

Classification

Therapeutic: antivirals

Pharmacologic: guanine nucleoside analogues

Indications

Treatment of cytomegalovirus (CMV) retinitis in patients with AIDS. Prevention of CMV disease in kidney, kidney/pancreas, and heart transplant patients at risk.

Action

Valganciclovir is a prodrug which is rapidly converted to ganciclovir by intestinal and hepatic enzymes. CMV virus converts ganciclovir to its active form (ganciclovir phosphate) inside host cell, where it inhibits viral DNA polymerase. **Therapeutic Effects:** Antiviral effect directed preferentially against CMV-infected cells.

Adverse Reactions/Side Effects

CNS: SEIZURES, headache, insomnia, agitation, confusion, dizziness, hallucinations, psychosis, sedation. **GI:** abdominal pain, diarrhea, nausea, vomiting. **GU:** renal impairment. **Hemat:** NEUTROPENIA, THROMBOCYTOPENIA, anemia, aplastic anemia, bone marrow depression, pancytopenia. **Neuro:** ataxia, paresthesia, peripheral neuropathy. **Misc:** fever, hypersensitivity reactions, infections.

PHYSICAL THERAPY IMPLICATIONS

Examination and Evaluation

- Be alert for new seizures or increased seizure activity, especially at the onset of drug treatment. Document the number, duration, and severity of seizures, and report these findings to the physician immediately.
- Monitor signs of neutropenia (fever, sore throat, signs of infection), thrombocytopenia (bruising, nose bleeds, and bleeding gums), or unusual weakness and fatigue that might be due to anemias or other blood dyscrasias. Report these signs to the physician immediately.
- Monitor signs of hypersensitivity reactions, including pulmonary symptoms (tightness in the throat and chest, wheezing, cough, dyspnea) or skin reactions (rash, pruritus, urticaria). Report these reactions to the physician.
- Monitor signs of paresthesia and peripheral neuropathy (numbness, tingling). Perform objective tests (nerve conduction, monofilaments) to document any neuropathic changes.
- Be alert for dizziness or ataxia that might affect gait, balance, or other functional activities. Report balance problems and functional limitations to the physician and nursing staff, and caution the patient and family/caregivers to guard against falls and trauma.
- Be alert for agitation, confusion, sedation, hallucinations, psychosis, or other alterations in mental status. Notify the physician promptly if these symptoms develop.

Interventions

- Always wash hands thoroughly and disinfect equipment (whirlpools, electrotherapeutic devices, treatment tables, and so forth) to help prevent the spread of infection. Use universal precautions as indicated for specific patients.

Patient/Client-Related Instruction

- Instruct patient to report signs of kidney impairment, including blood or pus in the urine, increased urinary frequency, cloudy urine, and decreased urine output.
- Instruct patient and family/caregivers to report other troublesome side effects, including severe or prolonged fever, infection, or GI problems (diarrhea, nausea, vomiting, abdominal pain).

Pharmacokinetics

Absorption: 59.4% absorbed following oral administration; rapidly converted to ganciclovir.

Distribution: Unknown.
Metabolism and Excretion: Rapidly converted to ganciclovir; ganciclovir is mostly excreted by the kidneys.
Half-life: 4.1 hr (intracellular half-life of ganciclovir phosphate is 18 hr).

TIME/ACTION PROFILE (ganciclovir blood levels)

ROUTE	ONSET	PEAK	DURATION
PO	rapid	2 hr	12–24 hr

Contraindications/Precautions

Contraindicated in: Hypersensitivity to valganciclovir or ganciclovir; OB: Pregnancy or planned pregnancy; OB: Lactation; Hemodialysis; Patients undergoing liver transplantation.
Use Cautiously in: Renal impairment (dosage reduction recommended if CCR <60 mL/min); Preexisting bone marrow depression; Previous or concurrent myelosuppressive drug therapy or radiation therapy; Geriatric patients (age-related ↓ in renal function requires dosage reduction); Pedi: Children (safety not established).

Interactions

Drug-Drug: ↑ risk of hematologic toxicity with **zidovudine.** Blood levels and effects may be ↑ by **probenecid.** Patients with renal impairment may experience accumulation of metabolites of **mycophenolate** and valganciclovir. ↑ blood levels and risk of toxicity from **didanosine.**
Drug-Food: Food ↑ absorption.

Route/Dosage

Treatment of CMV Disease

PO (Adults): *Induction*—900 mg bid for 21 days; *maintenance treatment or patients with inactive CMV retinitis*—900 mg once daily.

Renal Impairment

CCr 40–59 mL/min: (Adults): *Induction*—450 mg bid for 21 days; *maintenance treatment or patients with inactive CMV retinitis*—450 mg once daily.

Renal Impairment

CCr 25–39 mL/min: (Adults): *Induction*—450 mg once daily for 21 days; *maintenance treatment or patients with inactive CMV retinitis*—450 mg q 2 days.

Renal Impairment

CCr 10–24 mL/min: (Adults): *Induction*—450 mg q 2 days for 21 days; *maintenance treatment or patients with inactive CMV retinitis*—450 mg twice weekly.

Prevention of CMV Disease in Transplant Patients

PO (Adults): 900 mg once daily, starting 10 days prior to transplant and continued for 100 days after.

Renal Impairment

PO (Adults): *CCr 40–59 mL/min*—450 mg once daily; *CCr 25–39 mL/min*—450 mg q 2 days; *CCr 12–24 mL/min*—450 mg twice weekly.

Availability

Tablets: 450 mg.

VALPROATES

divalproex sodium
(dye-val-**proe**-ex **soe**-dee-um)
Apo-Divalproex, Depakote, Depakote ER, DOM-Divalproex, ✱Epival, Gen-Divalproex, Novo-Divalproex, Nu-Divalproex, PHL-Divalproex, PMS-Divalproex

valproate sodium
(val-**proe**-ate **soe**-dee-um)
Depacon

valproic acid (val-**proe**-ik **as**-id)
Apo-Valproic, Depakene, DOM-Valproic Acid, PHL-Valproic Acid, PMS-Valproic Acid, Ratio-Valprox, Stavzor

Classification
Therapeutic: anticonvulsants, vascular headache suppressants

V

Indications

Monotherapy and adjunctive therapy for simple and complex absence seizures. Monotherapy and adjunctive therapy for complex partial seizures. Adjunctive therapy for patients with multiple seizure types, including absence seizures. **Divalproex sodium only:** Manic episodes associated with bipolar disorder, Prevention of migraine headache.

Action

Increase levels of gamma-aminobutyric acid (GABA), an inhibitory neurotransmitter in the CNS. **Therapeutic Effects:** Suppression of seizure activity; ↓ manic episodes; ↓ frequency of migraine headaches.

Adverse Reactions/Side Effects

CNS: SUICIDAL THOUGHTS, agitation, dizziness, headache, insomnia, sedation, confusion, depression. **CV:** peripheral edema. **EENT:** visual disturbances. **GI:** HEPATOTOXICITY, PANCREATITIS, abdominal pain, anorexia, diarrhea, indigestion, nausea, vomiting, constipation, increased appetite. **Derm:** alopecia, rashes. **Endo:** weight gain.

Hemat: leukopenia, thrombocytopenia. **Metab:** HYPERAMMONEMIA. **Neuro:** HYPOTHERMIA, tremor, ataxia.

PHYSICAL THERAPY IMPLICATIONS

Examination and Evaluation

- Watch for signs of hepatotoxicity (anorexia, abdominal pain, severe nausea and vomiting, yellow skin or eyes, fever, sore throat, malaise, weakness, facial edema, lethargy, unusual bleeding or bruising), or pancreatitis (upper abdominal pain after eating, indigestion, weight loss, oily stools). Report these signs to the physician immediately.
- Be alert for suicidal thoughts and ideology; notify physician immediately if patient exhibits signs of depression or other changes in mood and behavior.
- Monitor signs of hypothermia, including shivering, confusion, drowsiness, slurred speech, incoordination, weak pulse, shallow slow breathing, and progressive loss of consciousness. Notify physician immediately, and request emergency assistance if these signs occur.
- Be alert for signs of increased ammonia levels (hyperammonemia), including anxiety, irritability disorientation, combativeness, loss of appetite, vomiting, lethargy, somnolence, and decreased consciousness that can progress to coma and death. Report these signs to the physician immediately.
- Document the number, duration, and severity of seizures to help document whether this drug is effective in reducing seizure activity.
- Be alert for signs of leukopenia (fever, sore throat, mucosal lesions, signs of infection) or thrombocytopenia (bruising, nose bleeds, bleeding gums). Report these signs to the physician immediately.
- Assess dizziness, ataxia, or tremor that might affect gait, balance, and other functional activities (See Appendix C). Report balance problems and functional limitations to the physician, and caution the patient and family/caregivers to guard against falls and trauma.
- Monitor daytime drowsiness, confusion, or anxiety. Repeated or excessive symptoms may require change in dose or medication.
- Assess peripheral edema using girth measurements, volume displacement, and measurement of pitting edema (See Appendix N). Report increased swelling in feet and ankles or a sudden increase in body weight due to fluid retention.
- If divalproex sodium is used to suppress migraines, assess the frequency and severity of headaches, and document whether drug therapy is successful in decreasing migraine attacks.
- If divalproex sodium is used to treat bipolar disorder, monitor the patient's mood and behavior, and report changes in manic symptoms (excitement, agitation) to help document drug effectiveness.
- Periodically assess body weight and other anthropometric measures (body mass index, body composition). Report a rapid or unexplained weight gain or increased body fat.

Interventions

- Guard against falls and trauma (hip fractures, head injury, and so forth), especially if dizziness affects gait and balance. Implement fall prevention strategies, especially if balance is impaired (See Appendix E).

Patient/Client-Related Instruction

- Advise patient to avoid alcohol and other CNS depressants because of the increased risk of sedation and adverse effects.
- Advise patients on prolonged antiseizure therapy not to discontinue medication without consulting their physician. Abrupt withdrawal may cause increased seizures.
- Advise patient about the risk of daytime drowsiness and decreased attention and mental focus. Use care if driving or in other activities that require strong concentration and fast responses.
- Instruct patient and family/caregivers to report other troublesome side effects such as severe or prolonged headache, sleep loss, vision problems, skin reactions (rash, hair loss), or GI problems (nausea, vomiting, diarrhea, constipation, indigestion, change in appetite, abdominal pain).

Pharmacokinetics

Absorption: Well absorbed following oral administration; divalproex is enteric coated, and absorption is delayed. ER form produces lower blood levels. IV administration results in complete bioavailability.
Distribution: Rapidly distributed into plasma and extracellular water. Crosses blood-brain barrier and placenta; enters breast milk.
Protein Binding: 80–90%; ↓ in neonates, elderly, renal impairment, or chronic hepatic disease.
Metabolism and Excretion: Mostly metabolized by the liver; minimal amounts excreted unchanged in urine.
Half-life: Adults: 9–16 hr.

TIME/ACTION PROFILE (onset = anticonvulsant effect; peak = blood levels)

ROUTE	ONSET	PEAK	DURATION
PO—liquid	2–4 days	15–120 min	6–24 hr
PO—capsules	2–4 days	1–4 hr	6–24 hr
PO—delayed-release products	2–4 days	3–5 hr	12–24 hr
PO—extended-release products	2–4 days	7–14 hr	24 hr
IV	2–4 days	end of infusion	6–24 hr

Contraindications/Precautions

Contraindicated in: Hypersensitivity; Hepatic impairment; Known/suspected urea cycle disorders (may result in fatal hyperammonemic encephalopathy).

Use Cautiously in: All patients (may ↑ risk of suicidal thoughts/behaviors); Bleeding disorders; History of liver disease; Organic brain disease; Bone marrow depression; Renal impairment; Geri: ↑ risk of adverse effects; OB: Use during pregnancy is linked to congenital anomalies, neural tube defects, clotting abnormalities, and hepatic dysfunction in the neonate. Use with extreme caution. Lactation: Pass into breast milk. Consider discontinuing nursing when valproates are administered to the nursing mother; Pedi: Children, especially <2 yr (at ↑ risk for potentially fatal hepatotoxicity).

Interactions

Drug-Drug: ↑ risk of bleeding with **warfarin.** Blood levels and toxicity may be ↑ by **aspirin, carbamazepine, chlorpromazine, cimetidine, erythromycin,** or **felbamate.** ↑ CNS depression with other **CNS depressants,** including **alcohol, antihistamines, antidepressants, opioid analgesics, MAO inhibitors,** and **sedative/hypnotics. MAO inhibitors** and other **antidepressants** may ↓ seizure threshold and ↓ effectiveness of valproate. **Carbamazepine, meropenem, phenobarbital, phenytoin,** or **rifampin** may ↓ valproate blood levels. Valproate may ↑ toxicity of **carbamazepine, diazepam, amitriptyline, nortriptyline, ethosuximide, lamotrigine, phenobarbital, phenytoin, topiramate,** or **zidovudine.** Concurrent use with **topiramate** may ↑ risk of hypothermia. **Ertapenem, imipenem,** or **meropenem** may ↓ valproate blood levels.

Route/Dosage

Regular-release and delayed-release formulations usually given in 2–4 divided doses daily; extended-release formulation (Depakote ER) usually given once daily.

Anticonvulsant

PO (Adults and Children >10 yr): *Single-agent therapy (complex partial seizures)*—Initial dose of 10–15 mg/kg/day in 1–4 divided doses; ↑ by 5–10 mg/kg/day weekly until therapeutic response achieved (not to exceed 60 mg/kg/day); when daily dose exceeds 250 mg, give in divided doses. *Polytherapy (complex partial seizures)*—Initial dose of 10–15 mg/kg/day; ↑ by 5–10 mg/kg/day weekly until therapeutic response achieved (not to exceed 60 mg/kg/day); when daily dosage exceeds 250 mg, give in divided doses.

PO (Adults and Children >2 yr [>10 yr for Depakote ER and Stavzor]): *Simple and complex absence seizures*—Initial dose of 15 mg/kg/day in 1–4 divided doses; ↑ by 5–10 mg/kg/day weekly until therapeutic response achieved (not to exceed 60 mg/kg/day); when daily dose exceeds 250 mg, give in divided doses.

IV (Adults and Children): Give same daily dose and at same frequency as was given orally; switch to oral formulation as soon as possible.

Rect (Adults and Children): Dilute syrup 1:1 with water for use as a retention enema. Give 17–20 mg/kg load; maintenance 10–15 mg/kg/dose q 8 hr.

Mood Stabilizer

PO (Adults): *Depakote and Stavzor*—Initial dose of 750 mg/day in divided doses initially; titrated rapidly to desired clinical effect or trough plasma levels of 50–125 mcg/mL (not to exceed 60 mg/kg/day). *Depakote ER*—Initial dose of 25 mg/kg once daily; titrated rapidly to desired clinical effect of trough plasma levels of 85–125 mcg/mL (not to exceed 60 mg/kg/day).

Migraine Prevention

PO (Adults and Children ≥16 yr): *Depakote and Stavzor*—250 mg bid (up to 1000 mg/day). *Depakote ER*—500 mg once daily for 1 wk, then ↑ to 1000 mg once daily.

Availability

Valproic Acid (generic available)

Capsules: 250 mg, 500 mg. **Delayed-release capsules:** 125 mg, 250 mg, 500 mg. **Syrup:** 250 mg/5 mL.

Valproate Sodium (generic available)

Injection: 100 mg/mL in 5-mL vials.

Divalproex Sodium (generic available)

Delayed-release tablets (Depakote): 125 mg, 250 mg, 500 mg. **Capsules-sprinkle:** 125 mg. **Extended-release tablets (Depakote ER):** 250 mg, 500 mg.

V

valsartan (val-sar-tan)

Diovan

Classification

Therapeutic: antihypertensives

Pharmacologic: angiotensin II receptor antagonists

Indications

Alone or with other agents in the management of hypertension. Treatment of heart failure (New York Heart Association classes II–IV). Reduction of risk of death from cardiovascular causes in patients with left ventricular systolic dysfunction following myocardial infarction.

Action

Blocks the vasoconstrictor and aldosterone-secreting effects of angiotensin II at various receptor sites, including vascular smooth muscle and the adrenal glands. **Therapeutic Effects:** Lowering of blood pressure in patients with hypertension. Decreased risk of heart-failure–related hospitalizations in patients with heart failure. ↓ risk of death from cardiovascular causes in patients with left ventricular systolic dysfunction following myocardial infarction.

Adverse Reactions/Side Effects

CNS: dizziness, fatigue, headache. **CV:** hypotension, edema. **EENT:** rhinitis, sinusitis, pharyngitis. **F and E:** hyperkalemia. **GI:** abdominal pain, diarrhea, nausea. **GU:** impaired renal function. **MS:** arthralgia, back pain. **Misc:** ANGIOEDEMA.

PHYSICAL THERAPY IMPLICATIONS

Examination and Evaluation

- Monitor signs of angioedema, including rashes, raised patches of red or white skin (welts), burning/itching skin, swelling in the face, and difficulty breathing. Notify physician of these signs immediately.
- Assess blood pressure periodically and compare to normal values (See Appendix F) to help determine antihypertensive effects. Report low blood pressure (hypotension), especially if patient experiences dizziness or syncope.
- Assess signs and symptoms of CHF (dyspnea, rales/crackles, peripheral edema, jugular venous distention, exercise intolerance) to help document whether drug therapy is effective in reducing these symptoms.
- Assess peripheral edema using girth measurements, volume displacement, and measurement of pitting edema (See Appendix N). Report increased swelling in feet and ankles or a sudden increase in body weight due to peripheral vasodilation.
- Watch for signs of impaired renal function, including decreased urine output, cloudy urine, or sudden weight gain due to fluid retention. Report these signs to the physician.
- Monitor signs of high plasma potassium levels (hyperkalemia), including bradycardia, fatigue, weakness, numbness, and tingling. Notify physician because severe cases can lead to life-threatening arrhythmias and paralysis.
- Assess dizziness that might affect gait, balance, and other functional activities (See Appendix C). Report balance problems and functional limitations to the physician, and caution the patient and family/caregivers to guard against falls and trauma.
- Assess any back pain or joint pain to rule out musculoskeletal pathology; that is, try to determine if pain is drug induced rather than caused by anatomic or biomechanical problems.

Interventions

- Implement aerobic exercise and cardiac conditioning programs to augment drug therapy and maintain or improve cardiovascular pump function in patients with heart failure and other cardiac conditions.
- Use caution during aerobic exercise and other forms of therapeutic exercise in patients recovering from myocardial infarction. Assess exercise tolerance frequently (blood pressure, heart rate, fatigue levels), and terminate exercise immediately if any untoward responses occur (See Appendix L).
- Avoid physical therapy interventions that cause systemic vasodilation (large whirlpool, Hubbard tank). Additive effects of this drug and the intervention may cause a dangerous fall in blood pressure.
- To minimize orthostatic hypotension, patient should move slowly when assuming a more upright position.

Patient/Client-Related Instruction

- Remind patients to take medication as directed to control hypertension and other cardiac conditions even if they are asymptomatic.
- Instruct patients with heart failure to weigh themselves every day and call their physician if they gain 3 lb or more in 1 day or more than 5 lb in 1 wk. Sudden weight gain may indicate fluid buildup due to worsening heart failure.
- Counsel patients about additional interventions to help control blood pressure and cardiac dysfunction, such as regular exercise, weight loss, sodium restriction, stress reduction, moderation of alcohol consumption, and smoking cessation.
- Instruct patient or family/caregivers to report other troublesome side effects such as severe or prolonged headache, fatigue, upper respiratory tract inflammation, or GI problems (nausea, diarrhea, abdominal pain).

Pharmacokinetics

Absorption: 10–35% absorbed following oral administration.
Distribution: Crosses the placenta.
Protein Binding: 95%.
Metabolism and Excretion: Minor metabolism by the liver; 13% excreted in urine; 83% in feces.
Half-life: 6 hr.

TIME/ACTION PROFILE (antihypertensive effect)

ROUTE	ONSET	PEAK	DURATION
PO	within 2 hr*	4 wks†	24 hr†

*After single dose.
†Chronic dosing.

Contraindications/Precautions

Contraindicated in: Hypersensitivity; Pregnancy or lactation.
Use Cautiously in: Volume- or salt-depleted patients or patients receiving large doses of diuretics (correct deficits before initiating therapy or initiate at lower

doses); Black patients (may not be as effective); Impaired renal function due to primary renal disease or congestive heart failure (may worsen renal function); Hepatic impairment; Women of childbearing potential; Children <18 yr (safety not established).

Interactions

Drug-Drug: Additive hypotension with other **antihypertensives.** Excessive hypotension may occur with concurrent use of **diuretics.** ↑ risk of hyperkalemia with concurrent use of **potassium supplements, potassium-containing salt substitutes, angiotensin-converting enzyme inhibitors,** or **potassium-sparing diuretics.** Antihypertensive effect may be blunted by **NSAIDs.**

Route/Dosage

Hypertension

PO (Adults): 80 mg or 160 mg once daily when used as monotherapy in patients who are not volume depleted; may be ↑ up to 320 mg once daily.

Heart Failure

PO (Adults): 40 mg twice daily; dose may be titrated up to target dose of 160 mg bid, as tolerated.

Post-Myocardial Infarction

PO (Adults): 20 mg bid (may be initiated ≥12 hr after myocardial infarction); dose may be titrated up to target dose of 160 mg bid, as tolerated.

Availability

Tablets: 40 mg, 80 mg, 160 mg, 320 mg. ***In combination with:*** hydrochlorothiazide (Diovan HCT), amlodipine (Exforge). See Appendix B.

vancomycin (van-koe-**mye**-sin)

Lyphocin, Vancocin, Vancoled

Classification

Therapeutic: anti-infectives

Indications

IV: Treatment of potentially life-threatening infections when less toxic anti-infectives are contraindicated. Particularly useful in staphylococcal infections, including: Endocarditis, Meningitis, Osteomyelitis, Pneumonia, Septicemia, Soft-tissue infections in patients who have allergies to penicillin or its derivatives or when sensitivity testing demonstrates resistance to methicillin. **PO:** Treatment of staphylococcal enterocolitis or pseudomembranous colitis due to *Clostridium difficile*. **IV:** Part of endocarditis prophylaxis in high-risk patients who are allergic to penicillin.

Action

Binds to bacterial cell wall, resulting in cell death. **Therapeutic Effects:** Bactericidal action against susceptible organisms. **Spectrum:** Active against gram-positive pathogens, including Staphylococci (including methicillin-resistant strains of *Staphylococcus aureus*), Group A beta-hemolytic streptococci, *Streptococcus pneumoniae*, *Corynebacterium*, *Clostridium difficile*, *Enterococcus faecalis*, *Enterococcus faecium*.

Adverse Reactions/Side Effects

EENT: ototoxicity. **CV:** hypotension. **GI:** nausea, vomiting. **GU:** nephrotoxicity. **Derm:** rashes. **Hemat:** eosinophilia, leukopenia. **Local:** phlebitis. **MS:** back and neck pain. **Misc:** HYPERSENSITIVITY REACTIONS, INCLUDING ANAPHYLAXIS, chills, fever, "red man" syndrome (with rapid infusion), superinfection.

PHYSICAL THERAPY IMPLICATIONS

Examination and Evaluation

- Monitor signs of hypersensitivity reactions and anaphylaxis, including pulmonary symptoms (tightness in the throat and chest, wheezing, cough dyspnea) or skin reactions (rash, pruritus, urticaria). Notify physician or nursing staff immediately if these reactions occur.
- Assess blood pressure periodically and compare to normal values (See Appendix F). Report low blood pressure (hypotension), especially if patient experiences dizziness, fatigue, or other symptoms.
- Assess any back or neck pain to rule out musculoskeletal pathology; that is, try to determine if pain is drug induced rather than caused by anatomic or biomechanical problems.
- Monitor for signs of eosinophilia (fatigue, weakness, myalgia) or leukopenia (fever, sore throat, signs of infection). Report these signs to the physician.
- Monitor signs of ototoxicity (hearing loss, tinnitus, disturbed balance, vertigo). Report these signs to the physician.
- Report signs of "red man" syndrome, including a red, maculopapular rash that typically appears on the face, neck and upper torso, and may be accompanied by pruritus, urticaria, erythema, angioedema, tachycardia, hypotension, and muscle aches. These signs usually occur during or immediately after rapid IV infusion, and often resolve spontaneously within several hours. Some cases may develop cardiac toxicity, and they should therefore be monitored carefully.
- Monitor injection site for pain, swelling, and irritation. Report prolonged or excessive injection-site reactions to the physician.

V

Interventions

- Always wash hands thoroughly and disinfect equipment (whirlpools, electrotherapeutic devices, treatment tables, and so forth) to help prevent the spread of infection. Employ universal precautions or isolation procedures as indicated for specific patients.

Patient/Client-Related Instruction

- Instruct patient to notify physician immediately of signs of superinfection, including black, furry overgrowth on tongue, vaginal itching or discharge, and loose or foul-smelling stools.
- Advise patient to report signs of nephrotoxicity (blood or pus in urine, decreased urine output, weight gain from fluid retention, fatigue).
- Instruct patient and family/caregivers to report other troublesome side effects such as severe or prolonged fever, chills, skin rashes, or GI problems (nausea, vomiting).

Pharmacokinetics

Absorption: Poorly absorbed from the GI tract.
Distribution: Widely distributed. Some penetration (20–30%) of CSF; crosses placenta.
Metabolism and Excretion: Oral doses excreted primarily in the feces; IV vancomycin eliminated almost entirely by the kidneys.
Half-life: Neonates: 6–10 hr; Children 3 mo–3 yr: 4 hr; Children >3 yr: 2–2.3 hr; Adults: 5–8 hr (increased in renal impairment).

TIME/ACTION PROFILE (blood levels)

ROUTE	ONSET	PEAK	DURATION
IV	rapid	end of infusion	12–24 hr

Contraindications/Precautions

Contraindicated in: Hypersensitivity.
Use Cautiously in: Renal impairment (dosage reduction required if CCr ≤80 mL/min); Hearing impairment; Intestinal obstruction or inflammation (↑ systemic absorption when given orally); Pregnancy and lactation (safety not established).

Interactions

Drug-Drug: May cause additive ototoxicity and nephrotoxicity with other **ototoxic** and **nephrotoxic drugs (aspirin, aminoglycosides, cyclosporine, cisplatin, loop diuretics)**. May enhance neuromuscular blockade from **nondepolarizing neuromuscular blocking agents.** ↑ risk of histamine flush when used with **general anesthetics** in children.

Route/Dosage

Serious Systemic Infections

IV (Adults): 500 mg q 6 hr *or* 1 g q 12 hr (up to 4 g/day).
IV (Children >1 mo): 40 mg/kg/day divided q 6–8 hr. *Staphylococcal CNS infection*—60 mg/kg/day divided q 6 hr, maximum dose: 1 g/dose.
IV (Neonates 1 wk–1 mo): <1200 g: 15 mg/kg/day q 24 hr. 1200–2000 g: 10–15 mg/kg/dose q 8–12 hr. >2000 g: 15–20 mg/kg/dose q 8 hr.
IV (Neonates <1 wk): <1200 g: 15 mg/kg/day q 24 hr. 1200–2000 g: 10–15 mg/kg/dose q 12–18 hr. > 2000 g: 10–15 mg/kg/dose q 8–12 hr.
Intrathecal (Adults): 20 mg/day.
Intrathecal (Children): 5–20 mg/day.
Intrathecal (Neonates): 5–10 mg/day.

Endocarditis Prophylaxis in Penicillin-Allergic Patients

IV (Adults and Adolescents): 1-g single dose 1-hr preprocedure.
IV (Children): 20-mg/kg single dose 1-hr preprocedure.

Pseudomembranous Colitis

PO (Adults): 125–500 mg q 6 hr.
PO (Children): 40 mg/kg/day divided q 6 hr for 7–10 days (not to exceed 2 g/day).

Renal Impairment

IV (Adults): An initial loading dose of 750 mg–1 g (not less than 15 mg/kg); serum level monitoring is optimal for choosing maintenance dosage in patients with renal impairment; these guidelines may be helpful. *CCr 50–80 mL/min*— 1 g q 1–3 days; *CCr 10–50 mL/min*—1 g q 3–7 days; *CCr <10 mL/min*—1 g q 7–14 days.

Availability (generic available)

Capsules: 125 mg, 250 mg. **Oral solution:** 250 mg/5 mL, 500 mg/6 mL. **Injection:** 500-mg, 1-, 5-, 10-g vials.

vardenafil (var-den-a-fil)

Levitra

Classification
Therapeutic: vasodilators
Pharmacologic: phosphodiesterase type 5 inhibitors

Indications

Erectile dysfunction.

Action

Increases cyclic guanosine monophosphate (cGMP) levels by inhibiting phosphodiesterase type 5 (PDE5), an enzyme responsible for the breakdown of cGMP. cGMP produces smooth muscle relaxation of the corpus cavernosum, which in turn promotes increased blood flow and subsequent erection.

Therapeutic Effects: Enhanced blood flow to the corpus cavernosum and erection sufficient to allow sexual intercourse. Requires sexual stimulation.

Adverse Reactions/Side Effects

CNS: headache, amnesia, dizziness. **EENT:** HEARING LOSS, VISION LOSS, rhinitis, sinusitis. **CV:** arrhythmias. **GI:** dyspepsia, nausea. **GU:** priapism. **Derm:** flushing. **Misc:** flu syndrome.

PHYSICAL THERAPY IMPLICATIONS

Examination and Evaluation

- Be alert for sudden loss of vision or hearing, and seek emergency care for any changes in vision or hearing.
- Assess heart rate, ECG, and heart sounds, especially during exercise (See Appendices G, H). Report any rhythm disturbances or symptoms of increased arrhythmias, including palpitations, chest discomfort, shortness of breath, fainting, and fatigue/weakness.
- Assess dizziness that might affect gait, balance, and other functional activities (See Appendix C). Report balance problems and functional limitations to the physician, and caution the patient and family/caregivers to guard against falls and trauma.

Interventions

- Because of the risk of arrhythmias, use caution during aerobic exercise and other forms of therapeutic exercise. Assess exercise tolerance frequently (blood pressure, heart rate, fatigue levels), and terminate exercise immediately if any untoward responses occur (See Appendix L).

Patient/Client-Related Instruction

- Instruct patient to notify health care professional promptly if erection lasts longer than 4 hr or if he experiences a sudden decrease or loss of vision or hearing.
- Instruct patient and family/caregivers to report other bothersome side effects such as severe or prolonged headache, memory loss, nasal congestion/inflammation, flu-like symptoms, skin problems (flushing), or GI reactions (nausea, indigestion).

Pharmacokinetics

Absorption: 15% absorbed following oral administration; absorption is rapid.
Distribution: Extensive tissue distribution; penetrates semen.
Protein Binding: 95%.
Metabolism and Excretion: Mostly metabolized by the liver (mainly CYP3A4 enzyme system, minor metabolism by CYP2C). M1 metabolite has antierectile dysfunction activity. Parent drug and metabolites are mostly excreted in feces. 2–6% renally eliminated.
Half-life: 4–5 hr.

TIME/ACTION PROFILE

ROUTE	ONSET	PEAK	DURATION
PO	rapid	0.5–2 hr	4 hr

Contraindications/Precautions

Contraindicated in: Hypersensitivity; Concurrent use of nitrates or nitric oxide donors; Unstable angina, recent history of stroke, life-threatening arrhythmias, CHF or MI within 6 mo; End-stage renal disease requiring dialysis; Known hereditary degenerative retinal disorders; Severe hepatic impairment (Child-Pugh C); Congenital or acquired QT prolongation or concurrent use of Class IA or III antiarrhythmics; Pedi: Women, children or newborns.
Use Cautiously in: Other serious underlying cardiovascular disease or left ventricular outflow obstruction; Penile deformity; Underlying conditions predisposing to priapism, including sickle cell anemia, multiple myeloma, or leukemia; Bleeding disorders or active peptic ulcer diseases; History of sudden severe vision loss or nonarteritic ischemic optic neuropathy (NAION); may ↑ risk of recurrence; Strong inhibitors of the CYP3A4 enzyme system; Alpha-adrenergic blockers (patients should be on stable dose of alpha blockers before starting vardenafil); Geri: Have ↑ blood levels; ↓ dose required.

Interactions

Drug-Drug: Concurrent use of **nitrates** may cause serious, life-threatening hypotension and is contraindicated. Concurrent use of Class IA antiarrhythmics (such as **quinidine** or **procainamide**) or **Class III antiarrhythmics** (such as **amiodarone** or **sotalol**) ↑ risk of serious arrhythmias and should be avoided. Concurrent use of alpha-adrenergic blockers may cause serious hypotension; lowest doses of each should be used initially. Strong inhibitors of CYP3A4, including **protease inhibitor antiretrovirals** (including **ritonavir, saquinavir** and **indinavir**), **ketoconazole,** and **itraconazole,** ↑ effects and the risk of adverse reactions (dosage adjustments recommended). Concurrent use of moderate inhibitors of CYP2C, including **erythromycin,** may also ↑ effects. ↑ risk of hypotension with **alpha-adrenergic blockers** and acute ingestion of **alcohol.**

Route/Dosage

PO (Adults): 10 mg taken 1 hr prior to sexual activity (range 5–20 mg; not to exceed 1 dose/24 hr); *concurrent use of ritonavir*—single dose should not exceed

2.5 mg in any 72-hr period; *concurrent use of indinavir, ketoconazole 400 mg daily, or itraconazole 400 mg daily*—single dose should not exceed 2.5 mg/24 hr; *concurrent use of ketoconazole or itraconazole 200 mg daily or erythromycin*—single dose should not exceed 5 mg/24 hr.

PO (Geriatric Patients >65 yr): 5-mg initial dose; titrate as tolerated.

Hepatic Impairment

PO (Adults): *Moderate hepatic impairment (Child-Pugh B)*—May start with 5-mg dose; subsequent dosing should not to exceed 10 mg.

Availability

Tablets: 2.5 mg, 5 mg, 10 mg, 20 mg.

varenicline (ver-en-i-kline)

Chantix

Classification

Therapeutic: smoking deterrents

Pharmacologic: nicotine agonists

Indications

Treatment of smoking cessation; in conjunction with nonpharmacologic support (educational materials/counseling).

Action

Selectively binds to alpha$_4$ beta$_2$ nicotinic acetylcholine receptors, acting as a nicotine agonist; prevents the binding of nicotine to receptors. **Therapeutic Effects:** ↓ desire to smoke.

Adverse Reactions/Side Effects

CNS: ↓ attention span, anxiety, depression, insomnia, irritability, dizziness, restlessness, abnormal dreams, agitation, aggression, amnesia, disorientation, dissociation, migraine, psychomotor hyperactivity, suicidal thoughts/behaviors. **CV:** syncope. **GI:** diarrhea, gingivitis, nausea, ↑ appetite, constipation, dyspepsia, dysphagia, enterocolitis, eructation, flatulence, gallbladder disorder, GI bleeding, ↑ liver function tests, vomiting. **Derm:** flushing, hyperhidrosis, acne, dermatitis, dry skin. **Hemat:** anemia. **MS:** arthralgia, back pain, musculoskeletal pain, muscle cramps, myalgia, restless legs. **Misc:** chills, fever, hypersensitivity, mild physical dependence.

PHYSICAL THERAPY IMPLICATIONS

Examination and Evaluation

- Be alert for signs of depression or suicidal behaviors and ideology. Notify physician immediately if patient exhibits these signs.
- Watch for signs of anemia, including unusual fatigue, shortness of breath with exertion, bruising, and pale skin. Notify physician immediately if these signs occur.
- Monitor signs of hypersensitivity reactions, including pulmonary symptoms (tightness in the throat and chest, wheezing, cough, dyspnea) or skin reactions (rash, pruritus, urticaria). Notify physician if these reactions occur.
- Monitor anxiety, irritability, restlessness, agitation, decreased attention, increased aggression, hyperactivity, and other alterations in mood or behavior. Notify physician promptly if these symptoms develop.
- Assess any joint pain, back pain, or muscle pain/cramps to rule out musculoskeletal pathology; that is, try to determine if pain is drug induced rather than caused by anatomic or biomechanical problems.
- Assess dizziness and syncope that might affect gait, balance, and other functional activities (See Appendix C). Report balance problems and functional limitations to the physician, and caution the patient and family/caregivers to guard against falls and trauma.

Interventions

- Help patient explore nonpharmacologic methods to quit smoking (counseling, support groups, and so forth).

Patient/Client-Related Instruction

- Instruct patient to report other side effects such as severe or prolonged headache, sleep loss, restless legs, chills, fever, skin reactions (dermatitis, acne, flushing, increased sweating, dry skin), or GI problems (nausea, vomiting, diarrhea, constipation, indigestion, difficulty swallowing, abdominal pain, belching, flatulence).

Pharmacokinetics

Absorption: 100% absorbed following oral administration.

Distribution: 24 hr.

Metabolism and Excretion: Minimally metabolized; 92% excreted in urine unchanged.

Half-life: 24 hr.

TIME/ACTION PROFILE

ROUTE	ONSET	PEAK	DURATION
PO	unknown	3–4 hr	24 hr

Contraindications/Precautions

Contraindicated in: Hypersensitivity; Lactation: Lactation; Pedi: Children <18 yr (safety not established).

Use Cautiously in: Severe renal impairment (lower dose recommended if CCr <30 mL/min); Psychiatric illness; Geri: Consider age-related decline in renal function; OB: Use only if maternal benefit outweighs fetal risk.

Interactions

Drug-Drug: Smoking cessation may ↓ metabolism of **theophylline, warfarin,** and **insulin,** resulting in ↑ effects; careful monitoring is recommended. Risk of adverse reactions (nausea, vomiting, dizziness, fatigue, headache) may be ↑ with **nicotine** replacement therapy (nicotine transdermal patches).

Route/Dosage

PO (Adults): Treatment is started 1 wk prior to planned smoking cessation: 0.5 mg once daily on the first 3 days, then 0.5 mg bid for the next 4 days, then 1 mg bid.

Renal Impairment

PO (Adults): *CCr <30 mL/min*—0.5 mg daily; may increase to 0.5 mg bid.

Availability

Tablets: 0.5 mg, 1 mg.

vasopressin (vaye-soe-**pres**-in)

Pitressin, ✱Pressyn

Classification

Therapeutic: hormones

Pharmacologic: antidiuretic hormones

Indications

Central diabetes insipidus due to deficient antidiuretic hormone. **Unlabeled Use:** Management of pulseless VT/VF unresponsive to initial shocks, asystole, or pulseless electrical activity (PEA) (Advanced Cardiac Life Support guidelines). Septic shock.

Action

Alters the permeability of the renal collecting ducts, allowing reabsorption of water. Directly stimulates musculature of GI tract. In high doses, acts as a nonadrenergic peripheral vasoconstrictor. **Therapeutic Effects:** ↓ urine output and ↑ urine osmolality in diabetes insipidus.

Adverse Reactions/Side Effects

CNS: dizziness, "pounding" sensation in head. **CV:** MI, angina, chest pain. **GI:** abdominal cramps, belching, diarrhea, flatulence, heartburn, nausea, vomiting. **Derm:** paleness, perioral blanching, sweating. **Neuro:** trembling. **Misc:** allergic reactions, fever, water intoxication (higher doses).

PHYSICAL THERAPY IMPLICATIONS

Examination and Evaluation

- Continually monitor for signs of MI, including sudden chest pain, pain radiating into the arm or jaw, shortness of breath, dizziness, sweating, anxiety, and nausea. Seek immediate medical assistance if patient develops these signs.
- Assess heart rate, ECG, and heart sounds, especially during exercise (See Appendices G, H). Although intended to resolve severe arrhythmias, this drug can unmask or precipitate new arrhythmias (proarrhythmic effect). Report any rhythm disturbances or symptoms of increased arrhythmias, including palpitations, chest pain, shortness of breath, fainting, and fatigue/weakness.
- Monitor signs of excess fluid levels (water intoxication), including "pounding" headache, confusion, lethargy, irritability, decreased consciousness, and neuromuscular abnormalities (muscle weakness and cramps). Report these signs to the physician.
- Assess dizziness that might affect gait, balance, and other functional activities (See Appendix C). Report balance problems and functional limitations to the physician and nursing staff, and caution the patient and family/caregivers to guard against falls and trauma.
- Monitor signs of allergic reactions, including pulmonary symptoms (tightness in the throat and chest, wheezing, cough, dyspnea) or skin reactions (rash, pruritus, urticaria). Notify physician or nursing staff immediately if these reactions occur.

Interventions

- Because of the risk arrhythmias and MI, use extreme caution during aerobic exercise and other forms of therapeutic exercise. Assess exercise tolerance frequently (blood pressure, heart rate, fatigue levels), and terminate exercise immediately if any untoward responses occur (See Appendix L).

Patient/Client-Related Instruction

- Advise patient and family or caregivers about the signs of MI (see above under Examination and Evaluation), and to seek immediate medical assistance if these signs develop.
- Instruct patient and family/caregivers to report other troublesome side effects such as severe or prolonged fever, trembling, skin reactions (paleness, blanching around the mouth), or GI problems (nausea, vomiting, diarrhea, heartburn, belching, flatulence, abdominal cramps).

Pharmacokinetics

Absorption: IM absorption may be unpredictable.
Distribution: Widely distributed throughout extracellular fluid.
Metabolism and Excretion: Rapidly degraded by the liver and kidneys; <5% excreted unchanged by the kidneys.
Half-life: 10–20 min.

TIME/ACTION PROFILE (antidiuretic effect)

ROUTE	ONSET	PEAK	DURATION
IM, SC	unknown	unknown	2–8 hr
IV	unknown	unknown	30–60 min

Contraindications/Precautions

Contraindicated in: Chronic renal failure with ↑ BUN; Hypersensitivity to beef or pork proteins.
Use Cautiously in: Perioperative polyuria (↑ sensitivity to vasopressin); Comatose patients; Seizures; Migraine headaches; Asthma; Heart failure; Cardiovascular disease; Geri/Pedi: Geriatric patients and children (↑ sensitivity to vasopressin); Renal impairment.

Interactions

Drug-Drug: Antidiuretic effect may be ↓ by concurrent administration of **alcohol, lithium, demeclocycline, heparin,** or **norepinephrine.** Antidiuretic effect may be ↑ by concurrent administration of **carbamazepine, chlorpropamide, clofibrate, tricyclic antidepressants,** or **fludrocortisone.** Vasopressor effect may be ↑ by concurrent administration of **ganglionic blocking agents.**

Route/Dosage

IM, SC (Adults): 5–10 units bid–qid.
IM, SC (Children): 2.5–10 units bid–qid.
IV (Adults): *Pulseless VT/VF, asystole, or PEA (ACLS guidelines)*—40 units as a single dose (unlabeled). *Septic shock*—0.04 units/min infusion.

Availability (generic available)

Injection: 20 units/mL in 0.5- and 1-mL ampules and vials.

venlafaxine (ven-la-**fax**-een)

Effexor, Effexor XR

Classification

Therapeutic: antidepressants, antianxiety agents
Pharmacologic: selective serotonin/norepinephrine reuptake inhibitors

Indications

Major depressive disorder. Generalized anxiety disorder (Effexor XR only). Social anxiety disorder (Effexor XR only). Panic disorder (Effexor XR only). **Unlabeled Use:** Premenstrual dysphoric disorder.

Action

Inhibits serotonin and norepinephrine reuptake in the CNS. **Therapeutic Effects:** ↓ in depressive symptomatology, with fewer relapses/recurrences. ↓ anxiety. ↓ in panic attacks.

Adverse Reactions/Side Effects

CNS: NEUROLEPTIC MALIGNANT SYNDROME, SEIZURES, abnormal dreams, anxiety, dizziness, headache, insomnia, nervousness, weakness, abnormal thinking, agitation, confusion, depersonalization, drowsiness, emotional lability, worsening depression. **EENT:** rhinitis, visual disturbances, epistaxis, tinnitus. **CV:** chest pain, hypertension, palpitations, tachycardia. **GI:** abdominal pain, altered taste, anorexia, constipation, diarrhea, dry mouth, dyspepsia, nausea, vomiting, weight loss. **GU:** sexual dysfunction, urinary frequency, urinary retention. **Derm:** ecchymoses, itching, photosensitivity, skin rash. **Neuro:** paresthesia, twitching. **Misc:** SEROTONIN SYNDROME, chills, bleeding, yawning.

PHYSICAL THERAPY IMPLICATIONS

Examination and Evaluation

- Watch for signs of neuroleptic malignant syndrome, including hyperthermia, diaphoresis, generalized muscle rigidity, altered mental status, tachycardia, changes in blood pressure (BP), and incontinence. Symptoms typically occur within 4–14 days after initiation of drug therapy, but can occur at any time during drug use. Report these signs to the physician immediately.
- Monitor and immediately report signs of serotonin syndrome, including hyperthermia, rigidity, myoclonus, and autonomic instability with fluctuating vital signs and extreme agitation that may proceed to delirium and coma. Patients should not take venlafaxine with other drugs that increase serotonin levels (e.g., MAO inhibitors).
- Be alert for new seizures or increased seizure activity, especially at the onset of drug treatment. Document the number, duration, and severity of seizures, and report these findings to the physician immediately.
- Be alert for increased depression and suicidal thoughts and ideology, especially when initiating drug treatment, and in children and teenagers. Notify physician or other mental health care professional immediately if patient exhibits worsening depression.
- Monitor anxiety, nervousness, agitation, confusion, emotional lability, expression of abnormal thoughts, or other alterations in mood and behavior. Notify physician if these symptoms become problematic.
- Assess heart rate, ECG, and heart sounds, especially during exercise (See Appendices G, H). Report a rapid heart rate (tachycardia) or signs of other arrhythmias, including palpitations, chest discomfort, shortness of breath, fainting, and fatigue/weakness.

- Assess BP and compare to normal values (See Appendix F). Report a sustained increase in BP (hypertension).
- Assess signs of paresthesia (numbness, tingling) or muscle twitching. Perform objective tests including electroneuromyography and sensory testing to document any drug-related neuropathic changes.
- Assess dizziness and drowsiness that might affect gait, balance, and other functional activities (See Appendix C). Report balance problems and functional limitations to the physician, and caution the patient and family/caregivers to guard against falls and trauma.

Interventions

- Guard against falls and trauma (hip fractures, head injury, and so forth), and implement fall prevention strategies (See Appendix E).
- Causes photosensitivity; use care if administering UV treatments. Advise patient to avoid direct sunlight and use sunscreens and protective clothing.
- Help patient explore nonpharmacologic methods (exercise, counseling, support groups, and so forth) to reduce depression and anxiety.

Patient/Client-Related Instruction

- Advise patient that antidepressant effects may not occur immediately; it may take 2 wk or more before an improvement in mood is observed.
- Advise patient to avoid alcohol and other CNS depressants because of the increased risk of sedation and adverse effects.
- Instruct patient to report severe or prolonged GI problems, including nausea, vomiting, diarrhea, constipation, abdominal pain, altered taste, dry mouth, indigestion, and loss of appetite.
- Instruct patient to report other problematic side effects such as severe or prolonged headache, sleep loss, abnormal dreams, vision disturbances, ringing/buzzing in the ears (tinnitus), nasal irritation/bleeding, urinary problems, sexual dysfunction, chills, and skin reactions (rash, itching, bruising).

Pharmacokinetics

Absorption: 92–100% absorbed after oral administration.
Distribution: Extensive distribution into body tissues.
Metabolism and Excretion: Extensively metabolized on 1st pass through the liver. One metabolite, *O*-desmethylvenlafaxine (ODV), has antidepressant activity; 5% of venlafaxine is excreted unchanged in urine; 30% of the active metabolite is excreted in urine.
Half-life: *Venlafaxine*—3–5 hr; *ODV*—9–11 hr (both are increased in hepatic/renal impairment).

TIME/ACTION PROFILE (antidepressant action)

ROUTE	ONSET	PEAK	DURATION
PO	within 2 wk	2–4 wk	unknown

Contraindications/Precautions

Contraindicated in: Hypersensitivity; Concurrent MAO inhibitor therapy.
Use Cautiously in: Cardiovascular disease, including hypertension; Hepatic impairment (↓ dose recommended); Impaired renal function (↓ dose recommended); History of seizures or neurologic impairment; History of mania; History of ↑ intraocular pressure or angle-closure glaucoma; History of drug abuse; OB: Use only if clearly required during pregnancy weighing benefit to mother versus potential harm to fetus (potential for discontinuation syndrome or toxicity in the neonate when venlafaxine is taken during the 3rd trimester); Lactation: Potential for serious adverse reactions in infant; discontinue drug or discontinue breastfeeding; Pedi: ↑ risk of suicidal thinking and behavior (suicidality) in children and adolescents with major depressive disorder and other psychiatric disorders. Observe closely for suicidality and behavior changes.

Interactions

Drug-Drug: Concurrent use with **MAO inhibitors** may result in serious, potentially fatal reactions (wait at least 2 wk after stopping MAO inhibitor before initiating venlafaxine; wait at least 1 wk after stopping venlafaxine before starting MAO inhibitors). Concurrent use with **alcohol** or other **CNS depressants**, including **sedative/hypnotics, antihistamines,** and **opioid analgesics,** in depressed patients is not recommended. Drugs that affect serotonergic neurotransmitter systems, including **linezolid, tramadol,** and **triptans,** ↑ risk of serotonin syndrome. **Lithium** may have ↑ serotonergic effects with venlafaxine; use cautiously in patients receiving venlafaxine. ↑ blood levels and may ↑ effects of **desipramine** and **haloperidol. Cimetidine** may ↑ the effects of venlafaxine (may be more pronounced in geriatric patients, those with hepatic or renal impairment, or those with preexisting hypertension). **Ketoconazole** may ↑ the effects of venlafaxine. ↑ risk of bleeding with **NSAIDS, aspirin, clopidogrel,** or **warfarin.**
Drug-Natural: Concomitant use of **kava-kava, valerian, chamomile,** or **hops** can ↑ CNS depression. ↑ risk of serotonergic side effects, including serotonin syndrome with **St. John's wort** and **SAMe.**

Route/Dosage

Major Depressive Disorder

PO (Adults): *Tablets*—75 mg/day in 2–3 divided doses; may ↑ by up to 75 mg/day every 4 days, up to

V

225 mg/day (not to exceed 375 mg/day in 3 divided doses); *Extended-release (XR) capsules*—75 mg once daily (some patients may be started at 37.5 mg once daily) for 4–7 days; may ↑ by up to 75 mg/day at intervals of not less than 4 days (not to exceed 225 mg/day).

General Anxiety Disorder
PO (Adults): *Extended-release (XR) capsules*—75 mg once daily (some patients may be started at 37.5 mg once daily) for 4–7 days; may ↑ by up to 75 mg/day at intervals of not less than 4 days (not to exceed 225 mg/day).

Social Anxiety Disorder
PO (Adults): *Extended-release (XR) capsules*—75 mg once daily.

Panic Disorder
PO (Adults): *Extended-release (XR) capsules*—37.5 mg once daily for 7 days; may then ↑ to 75 mg once daily; may then ↑ by 75 mg/day every 7 days (not to exceed 225 mg/day).

Hepatic Impairment
PO (Adults): ↓ daily dose by 50% in patients with mild-to-moderate hepatic impairment.

Renal Impairment
PO (Adults): *CCr 10–70 mL/min*—↓ daily dose by 25–50%; *Hemodialysis*—↓ daily dose by 50%.

Availability (generic available)
Tablets: 25 mg, 37.5 mg, 50 mg, 75 mg, 100 mg. **Extended-release capsules:** 37.5 mg, 75 mg, 150 mg.

verapamil (ver-ap-a-mil)
Apo-Verap, Calan, Calan SR, Covera-HS, Isoptin, Isoptin SR, Novo-Veramil, Nu-Verap, Verelan, Verelan PM

Classification
Therapeutic: antianginals, antiarrhythmics (class IV), antihypertensives, vascular headache suppressants
Pharmacologic: calcium channel blockers

Indications
Management of hypertension, angina pectoris, and/or vasospastic (Prinzmetal's) angina. Management of supraventricular arrhythmias and rapid ventricular rates in atrial flutter or fibrillation. **Unlabeled Use:** Prevention of migraine headache. Management of cardiomyopathy.

Action
Inhibits the transport of calcium into myocardial and vascular smooth muscle cells, resulting in inhibition of excitation-contraction coupling and subsequent contraction. ↓ SA and AV conduction and prolongs AV node refractory period in conduction tissue. **Therapeutic Effects:** Systemic vasodilation resulting in ↓ blood pressure. Coronary vasodilation resulting in ↓ frequency and severity of attacks of angina. Suppression of ventricular tachyarrhythmias.

Adverse Reactions/Side Effects
CNS: abnormal dreams, anxiety, confusion, dizziness/lightheadedness, drowsiness, headache, jitteriness, nervousness, psychiatric disturbances, weakness. **EENT:** blurred vision, disturbed equilibrium, epistaxis, tinnitus. **Resp:** cough, dyspnea, shortness of breath. **CV:** ARRHYTHMIAS, CHF, bradycardia, chest pain, hypotension, palpitations, peripheral edema, syncope, tachycardia. **GI:** abnormal liver function studies, anorexia, constipation, diarrhea, dry mouth, dysgeusia, dyspepsia, nausea, vomiting. **GU:** dysuria, nocturia, polyuria, sexual dysfunction, urinary frequency. **Derm:** dermatitis, erythema multiforme, flushing, increased sweating, photosensitivity, pruritus/urticaria, rash. **Endo:** gynecomastia, hyperglycemia. **Hemat:** anemia, leukopenia, thrombocytopenia. **Metab:** weight gain. **MS:** joint stiffness, muscle cramps. **Neuro:** paresthesia, tremor. **Misc:** STEVENS-JOHNSON SYNDROME, gingival hyperplasia.

PHYSICAL THERAPY IMPLICATIONS

Examination and Evaluation
- Assess heart rate, ECG, and heart sounds, especially during exercise (See Appendices G, H). Although intended to treat certain arrhythmias, this drug can unmask or precipitate new arrhythmias (proarrhythmic effect). Report any rhythm disturbances or symptoms of increased arrhythmias, including palpitations, chest pain, shortness of breath, fainting, and fatigue/weakness.
- Monitor rashes or other skin reactions (hives, abnormal sweating, itching/burning, exfoliation). Notify physician immediately because certain skin reactions may indicate serious hypersensitivity reactions (Stevens-Johnson syndrome).
- Assess routinely for signs of CHF and pulmonary edema (dyspnea, cough, shortness of breath, rales/crackles, jugular venous distention). Report these signs to the physician.
- Assess blood pressure periodically and compare to normal values (See Appendix F) to help document antihypertensive effects.
- Assess episodes of angina pectoris at rest and during exercise. Document whether drug therapy is helpful in reducing the frequency and severity of anginal attacks.
- If used to prevent migraine headaches, monitor the incidence and severity of attacks to document whether verapamil is successful in helping manage this condition.

- Assess peripheral edema using girth measurements, volume displacement, and measurement of pitting edema (See Appendix N). Report increased swelling in feet and ankles or a sudden increase in body weight due to peripheral vasodilation.
- Watch for signs of hyperglycemia, including confusion, drowsiness, flushed/dry skin, fruit-like breath odor, rapid/deep breathing, polyuria, loss of appetite, and unusual thirst. Insulin dosages may need to be adjusted to prevent repeated episodes of hyperglycemia.
- Monitor and report signs of leukopenia (fever, sore throat, signs of infection), thrombocytopenia (bruising, nose bleeds and bleeding gums), or unusual weakness and fatigue that might be due to anemia.
- Assess signs of paresthesia (numbness, tingling) or muscle twitching. Perform objective tests including electroneuromyography and sensory testing to document any drug-related neuropathic changes.
- Assess any joint pain or muscle cramping to rule out musculoskeletal pathology; that is, try to determine if pain is drug induced rather than caused by anatomic or biomechanical problems.
- Assess dizziness and weakness that might affect gait, balance, and other functional activities (See Appendix C). Report balance problems and functional limitations to the physician, and caution the patient and family/caregivers to guard against falls and trauma.
- Monitor mood and personality changes, including anxiety, nervousness, confusion, memory loss, or other changes in behavior. Notify physician if these changes become problematic.

Interventions

- Design and implement aerobic exercise and endurance training programs to normalize blood pressure, improve coronary perfusion, reduce angina, and improve myocardial pumping ability.
- Because of the risk of cardiac arrhythmias and CHF, use caution during aerobic exercise and other forms of therapeutic exercise. Assess exercise tolerance frequently (blood pressure, heart rate, fatigue levels), and terminate exercise immediately if any untoward responses occur (See Appendix L).
- Guard against falls and trauma (hip fractures, head injury). Implement fall prevention strategies, especially if patient exhibits dizziness or disturbed equilibrium (See Appendix E).
- To minimize orthostatic hypotension, patient should move slowly when assuming a more upright position.
- Causes photosensitivity; use care if administering UV treatments.

Patient/Client-Related Instruction

- Remind patients to take medication as directed to control hypertension and other cardiac conditions even if they are asymptomatic.
- Counsel patients about additional interventions to help control blood pressure and cardiac dysfunction, including regular exercise, weight loss, sodium restriction, stress reduction, moderation of alcohol consumption, and smoking cessation.
- Advise patient about photosensitivity, and to use sunscreens, protective clothing, and avoid prolonged sun exposure. Advise patient to also report any rashes or other skin reactions.
- Instruct patient or family/caregivers to report other troublesome side effects such as severe or prolonged headache, nightmares, tremor, problems with urination, sexual dysfunction, breast enlargement in men (gynecomastia), or GI problems (nausea, vomiting, constipation, diarrhea, loss of appetite).

Pharmacokinetics

Absorption: 90% absorbed after oral administration, but much is rapidly metabolized, resulting in bioavailability of 20–25%.
Distribution: Small amounts enter breast milk.
Protein Binding: 90%.
Metabolism and Excretion: Mostly metabolized by the liver.
Half-life: 4.5–12 hr.

TIME/ACTION PROFILE (cardiovascular effects)

ROUTE	ONSET	PEAK	DURATION
PO	1–2 hr	30–90 min*	3–7 hr
PO-ER	unknown	5–7 hr	24 hr
IV	1–5 min†	3–5 min	2 hr†

*Single dose; effects from multiple doses may not be evident for 24–48 hr.
†Antiarrhythmic effects; hemodynamic effects begin 3–5 min after injection and persist for 10–20 min.

Contraindications/Precautions

Contraindicated in: Hypersensitivity; Sick sinus syndrome; 2nd- or 3rd-degree AV block (unless an artificial pacemaker is in place); BP <90 mmHg; CHF, severe ventricular dysfunction, or cardiogenic shock, unless associated with supraventricular tachyarrhythmias; Concurrent IV beta blocker therapy.
Use Cautiously in: Severe hepatic impairment (dose reduction recommended for most agents); Geri: Geriatric patients (dose reduction/slower IV infusion rates recommended for most agents; ↑ risk of hypotension); History of serious ventricular arrhythmias or CHF; OB/Lactation: Pregnancy or lactation (safety not established; verapamil is approved for use in children).

V

Interactions

Drug-Drug: Additive hypotension may occur when used concurrently with **fentanyl,** other **antihypertensives, nitrates,** acute ingestion of **alcohol,** or **quinidine.** Antihypertensive effects may be ↓ by concurrent use of **NSAIDs.** Serum **digoxin** levels may be ↑. Concurrent use with **beta blockers, digoxin, disopyramide,** or **phenytoin** may result in bradycardia, conduction defects, or CHF. May ↓ metabolism of and ↑ risk of toxicity from **cyclosporine, prazosin, quinidine,** or **carbamazepine.** May ↓ effectiveness of **rifampin.** ↑ the muscle-paralyzing effects of **nondepolarizing neuromuscular-blocking agents.** Effectiveness may be ↓ by coadministration with **vitamin D compounds** and **calcium.** May alter serum **lithium** levels.

Drug-Natural: ↑ **caffeine** levels with caffeine-containing herbs (**cola nut, guarana, mate, tea, coffee**).

Drug-Food: Grapefruit juice ↑ serum levels and effect.

Route/Dosage

PO (Adults): 80–120 mg tid; ↑ as needed. *Patients with poor ventricular function, hepatic impairment, or geriatric patients*—40 mg tid initially. *Extended-release preparations*—120–240 mg/day as a single dose; may be increased as needed (range 240–480 mg/day).

PO (Children up to 15 yr): 4–8 mg/kg/day in divided doses.

IV (Adults): 5–10 mg (75–150 mcg/kg); may repeat with 10 mg (150 mcg/kg) after 15–30 min.

IV (Children 1–15 yr): 2–5 mg (100–300 mcg/kg); may repeat after 30 min (initial dose not to exceed 5 mg; repeat dose not to exceed 10 mg).

IV (Children <1 yr): 0.75–2 mg (100–200 mcg/kg); may repeat after 30 min.

Availability (generic available)

Tablets: 40 mg, 80 mg, 120 mg. **Extended-release tablets (Isoptin SR, Covera HS):** 120 mg, 180 mg, 240 mg. **Extended-release capsules (Verelan PM):** 100 mg, 200 mg, 300 mg. **Extended-release capsules (Verelan):** 120 mg, 180 mg, 240 mg, 360 mg. **Solution for injection:** 2.5 mg/mL in 2- and 4-mL vials, ampules, and syringes. ***In combination with:*** trandolapril (Tarka). See Appendix B.

verteporfin (ver-te-**por**-fin)

Visudyne

Classification

Therapeutic: none assigned

Pharmacologic: photodynamic agents

Indications

Treatment of age-related macular degeneration in patients with predominantly classic subfoveal choroidal neovascularization.

Action

Verteporfin is activated by nonthermal red light in the presence of oxygen to form reactive oxygen radicals. The resultant compound produces local damage to neovascular epithelium and subsequent vessel occlusion. **Therapeutic Effects:** Improved visual acuity.

Adverse Reactions/Side Effects

CNS: headache, weakness. **EENT:** visual disturbances, cataracts, conjunctivitis/conjunctival injection, dry eyes, ocular itching, severe vision loss, subconjunctival/subretinal/vitreous hemorrhage. **Derm:** photosensitivity. **Local:** injection-site reactions, including extravasation and rashes. **MS:** back pain (during infusion). **Misc:** fever, flu-like syndrome.

PHYSICAL THERAPY IMPLICATIONS

Examination and Evaluation

- Assess any back pain, especially during or immediately after drug infusion. Try to determine if pain is drug-induced rather than caused by musculoskeletal pathology.
- Monitor IV injection site for pain, swelling, rash, or other local symptoms. Report prolonged or excessive injection site reactions to the physician.

Interventions

- Causes photosensitivity; avoid use of UV treatments for at least 5 days after drug infusion. Advise patient to avoid direct sunlight and wear protective clothing when outdoors.

Patient/Client-Related Instruction

- Instruct patient to report any vision disturbances, eye irritation, or loss of vision.
- Instruct patient to report other troublesome side effects such as severe or prolonged headache, fever, flu-like syndrome, or weakness.

Pharmacokinetics

Absorption: IV administration results in complete bioavailability.

Distribution: Transported by lipoproteins.

Metabolism and Excretion: Small amount of metabolism by the liver and plasma esterases; elimination is primarily fecal. Verteporfin in skin is inactivated by photobleaching from ambient indoor lighting.

Half-life: 5–6 hr.

TIME/ACTION PROFILE (improved visual acuity)

ROUTE	ONSET	PEAK	DURATION
IV	1–7 days	unknown	unknown

Contraindications/Precautions

Contraindicated in: Hypersensitivity; Porphyria; Exposure to direct sunlight.
Use Cautiously in: Moderate/severe hepatic impairment; Pregnancy, lactation or children (safety not established).

Interactions

Drug-Drug: Calcium channel blockers, polymyxin B, or **radiation therapy** may ↑ the rate of uptake by the vascular epithelium. Concurrent use of **other photosensitizing agents,** including **thiazide diuretics, sulfonylureas, phenothiazines, sulfonamides** or **tetracyclines,** may ↑ the risk of skin photosensitivity reactions. **Dimethyl sulfoxide, beta-carotene, alcohol, formate,** and **mannitol** may ↓ the activity of verteporfin.

Route/Dosage

IV (Adults): 6 mg/m^2 infused over 10 min, followed by appropriate laser light delivery initiated 15 min after the start of the infusion.

Availability

Lyophilized powder for reconstitution: 15 mg.

vigabatrin (vye-gab-a-trin)

Sabril

Classification
Therapeutic: anticonvulsants

Indications

Management (adjunctive) of refractory complex partial seizures in adults in patients who have responded inadequately to several alternative treatments; not a 1st-line treatment. Management of infantile spasms (ISs) in patients 1 mo–2 yr.

Action

Acts an irreversible inhibitor of γ-aminobutyric acid transaminase (GABA-T), the enzyme responsible for the metabolism of the inhibitory neurotransmitter GABA. This action results in increased levels of GABA in the central nervous system. **Therapeutic Effects:** ↓ incidence and severity of refractory complex partial seizures.

Adverse Reactions/Side Effects

CNS: SUICIDAL THOUGHTS, confusional state, memory impairment, drowsiness, fatigue. **CV:** edema. **EENT:** blurred vision, nystagmus, vision loss. **Hemat:** anemia. **Metab:** weight gain. **MS:** arthralgia. **Neuro:** abnormal coordination, tremor, peripheral neuropathy.

PHYSICAL THERAPY IMPLICATIONS

Examination and Evaluation

- Be alert for suicidal thoughts and ideology; notify physician immediately if patient expresses suicidal thoughts or exhibits suicidal behaviors.
- Document the number, duration, and severity of seizures to help determine if this drug is effective in reducing seizure activity.
- Assess incoordination and tremor that might affect gait, balance, and other functional activities. Report balance problems and functional limitations to the physician, and caution the patient and family/caregivers to guard against falls and trauma.
- Monitor signs of anemia, including unusual fatigue, shortness of breath with exertion, and bruising, and pale skin. Notify physician immediately if these signs occur.
- Assess signs of peripheral neuropathy such as numbness, tingling, and decreased muscle strength. Establish baseline electroneuromyographic values using EMG and nerve conduction at the beginning of drug treatment whenever possible, and reexamine these values periodically to document drug-induced changes in peripheral nerve function.
- Assess any joint pain to rule out musculoskeletal pathology; that is, try to determine if pain is drug induced rather than caused by anatomic or biomechanical problems.
- Monitor daytime drowsiness, confusion, hallucinations, memory impairment, or other changes in personality. Repeated or excessive symptoms may require change in dose or medication.
- Assess peripheral edema using girth measurements, volume displacement, and measurement of pitting edema (See Appendix N). Report increased swelling in feet and ankles or a sudden increase in body weight due to fluid retention.
- Periodically assess body weight and other anthropometric measures (body mass index, body composition). Report a rapid or unexplained weight gain.

Interventions

- Guard against falls and trauma (hip fractures, head injury, and so forth), especially if dizziness or ataxia affect gait and balance. Implement fall-prevention strategies, especially if balance is impaired (See Appendix E).

Patient/Client-Related Instruction

- Advise patient to avoid alcohol and other CNS depressants because of the increased risk of sedation and adverse effects.
- Advise patients on prolonged antiseizure therapy not to discontinue medication without consulting

V

their physician. Abrupt withdrawal may cause increased seizures.

- Advise patient about the risk of daytime drowsiness and decreased attention and mental focus. Use care if driving or in other activities that require strong concentration and fast responses.
- Instruct patient and family/caregivers to report other troublesome side effects such as severe or prolonged vision disturbances.

Pharmacokinetics

Absorption: Completely absorbed following oral administration.
Distribution: Enters breast milk; remainder of distribution unknown.
Metabolism and Excretion: Minimal metabolism, mostly eliminated unchanged in urine.
Half-life: 7.5 hr.

TIME/ACTION PROFILE (anticonvulsant effect)

ROUTE	ONSET	PEAK	DURATION
PO	unknown	1 hr*	12 hr†

*Blood level.
†Clinical benefit should be seen in 2–4 wk for ISs or within 3 mo for complex partial seizures.

Contraindications/Precautions

Contraindicated in: History or high risk of other types of irreversible vision loss unless benefits of treatment clearly outweigh risks; OB: Use only if the potential benefit justifies the potential risk to the fetus (may cause fetal harm); Lactation: Enters breast milk; breast-feeding should be avoided.
Use Cautiously in: Renal impairment (dose modification recommended for CCr <50 mL/min); History of suicidal ideation; Geri: Consider age-related ↓ in renal function adjust dose accordingly (↑ risk of sedation/confusion); Pedi: Abnormal MRI signal changes have been seen in infants.

Interactions

Drug-Drug: Should not be used concurrently with other **drugs having adverse ocular effects;** ↑ risk of additive toxicity; May ↓ **phenytoin** levels and effectiveness.

Route/Dosage

PO (Adults): 500 mg bid initially; may be ↑ in 500 mg increments every 7 days depending on response up to 1.5 g bid.

Renal Impairment

PO (Adults): *CCr >50–80 mL/min*—↓ dose by 25%; *CCr >30–50 mL/min*—↓ dose by 50%; *CCr >10–<30 mL/min*—↓ dose by 75%.
PO (Children 1 mo–2 yr): 50 mg/kg/day given in 2 divided doses initially, ↑ by 25–50 mg/kg/day increments every 3 days up to a maximum of 150 mg/kg/day; dosage adjustments are necessary for renal impairment.

Availability

Tablets: 500 mg; **Powder packets for oral solution:** 500 mg/packet.

vilazodone (vil-az-oh-done)

Viibryd

Classification

Therapeutic: antidepressants
Pharmacologic: selective norepinephrine reuptake inhibitors, benzofurans

Indications

Treatment of major depressive disorder.

Action

↑ serotonin activity in the CNS by inhibiting serotonin reuptake. **Therapeutic Effects:** Improvement in symptoms of depression.

Adverse Reactions/Side Effects

CNS: NEUROLEPTIC MALIGNANT-LIKE SYNDROME, SEIZURES, SUICIDAL THOUGHTS, insomnia, abnormal dreams, dizziness. **GI:** diarrhea, nausea, dry mouth, restlessness, vomiting. **Endo:** ↓ libido, sexual dysfunction, syndrome of inappropriate antidiuretic hormone (SIADH). **F and E:** hyponatremia. **Hemat:** bleeding. **Misc:** SEROTONIN SYNDROME.

PHYSICAL THERAPY IMPLICATIONS

Examination and Evaluation

- Be alert for increased depression and suicidal thoughts and ideology, especially when initiating drug treatment and in children and teenagers. Notify physician or other mental health care professional immediately if patient exhibits worsening depression or expresses thoughts of suicide.
- Watch for signs of neuroleptic malignant syndrome, including hyperthermia, diaphoresis, generalized muscle rigidity, altered mental status, tachycardia, changes in blood pressure (BP), and incontinence. Symptoms typically occur within 4–14 days after initiation of drug therapy, but can occur at any time during drug use. Report these signs to the physician immediately.
- Monitor and immediately report signs of serotonin syndrome, including hyperthermia, rigidity, myoclonus, and autonomic instability with fluctuating vital signs and extreme agitation that may proceed to delirium and coma. Patients should not take vilazodone with other drugs that increase serotonin levels (e.g., MAO inhibitors).
- Be alert for new seizures or increased seizure activity, especially at the onset of drug treatment. Document the number, duration, and severity of seizures, and report these findings immediately to the physician.

- Watch for signs of bleeding, such as bleeding gums, nosebleeds, unusual bruising, black/tarry stools, hematuria, and a fall in hematocrit or blood pressure. Notify physician immediately if these signs occur.
- Monitor signs of fluid-electrolyte imbalance due to syndrome of inappropriate antidiuretic hormone (SIADH). SIADH causes increased water retention that leads to relatively low sodium concentration (hyponatremia). Symptoms include confusion, lethargy, weakness, myoclonus, and depressed reflexes. Severe or sudden onset may also cause seizures, ataxia, nystagmus, tremor, dysarthria, dysphagia, and coma. Notify physician if these signs occur.
- Assess dizziness that might affect gait, balance, and other functional activities (See Appendix C). Report balance problems and functional limitations to the physician, and caution the patient and family/caregivers to guard against falls and trauma.

Interventions

- Guard against falls and trauma (hip fractures, head injury, and so forth), and implement fall-prevention strategies (See Appendix E).
- Help patient explore nonpharmacological methods reduce depression and other psychologic disorders (exercise, counseling, support groups, and so forth).

Patient/Client-Related Instruction

- Advise patient that antidepressant effects may not occur immediately; it may take 2 wk or more before an improvement in mood is observed.
- Advise patient to avoid alcohol and other CNS depressants because of the increased risk of sedation and adverse effects.
- Instruct patient to report other problematic side effects such as severe or prolonged insomnia, restlessness, abnormal dreams, decreased libido, sexual dysfunction, or GI problems (nausea, vomiting, diarrhea, dry mouth).

Pharmacokinetics

Absorption: 72% absorbed following oral administration with food.
Distribution: Unknown.
Protein Binding: 96–99%.
Metabolism and Excretion: Mostly metabolized by the liver, primarily by the CYP3A4 enzyme system; 1% excreted unchanged in urine.
Half-life: 25 hr.

TIME/ACTION PROFILE (blood levels)

ROUTE	ONSET	PEAK	DURATION
PO	unknown	4–5 hr	unknown

Contraindications/Precautions

Contraindicated in: Concurrent use or within 14 days of starting or stopping MOAIs; Severe hepatic impairment.
Use Cautiously in: History of seizure disorder; History of suicide attempt/suicidal ideation; Bipolar disorder; may ↑ risk of mania/hypomania; OB: Use during pregnancy only if maternal benefit outweighs fetal risk; use during 3rd trimester may result in need for prolonged hospitalization, respiratory support, and tube feeding; Lactation: Breast-feed only if maternal benefit outweighs newborn risk; Pedi: Safe and effective use in children not established; ↑ risk of suicidal thinking/behavior in children, adolescents, and young adults.

Interactions

Drug-Drug: Concurrent use with or use within 14 days of starting or stopping **MAOIs** may ↑ risk of neuroleptic malignant syndrome or serotonin syndrome and should be avoided; Concurrent use with **NSAIDs, aspirin, antiplatelet drugs**, or other **drugs that affect coagulation** may ↑ risk of bleeding; Concurrent use of **strong inhibitors of CYP3A4**, including **ketoconazole**, ↑ blood levels and the risk of adverse reactions/toxicity; daily dose should not exceed 20 mg; Concurrent use of **moderate inhibitors of CYP3A4**, including **erythromycin**, may require dose reduction to 20 mg daily if adverse reactions/toxicity occurs; Concurrent use with other **drugs that alter CNS serotonergic neurotransmitters**, including **SSRIs, SNRIs, triptans, buspirone, tramadol**, and **tryptophan products**, may ↑ risk of serotonin syndrome and should be undertaken with caution; Use cautiously with other **CNS-active drugs**.

Route/Dosage

PO (Adults): 10 mg once daily for 1 wk, then 20 mg once daily for 1 wk, then 40 mg once daily. *Concurrent use of strong inhibitors of CYP3A4*—daily dose should not exceed 20 mg.

Availability

Tablets: 10 mg, 20 mg, 40 mg.

HIGH ALERT

vinblastine (vin-**blas**-teen)

Velban, ✱Velbe

Classification

Therapeutic: antineoplastics
Pharmacologic: vinca alkaloids

Indications

Combination chemotherapy of Lymphomas, Nonseminomatous testicular carcinoma, Advanced breast cancer, Other tumors.

V

Action

Binds to proteins of mitotic spindle, causing metaphase arrest. Cell replication is stopped as a result (cell-cycle–specific for M phase). **Therapeutic Effects:** Death of rapidly replicating cells, particularly malignant ones. Has immunosuppressive properties.

Adverse Reactions/Side Effects

CNS: SEIZURES, mental depression, neurotoxicity, weakness. **Resp:** BRONCHOSPASM. **GI:** nausea, vomiting, anorexia, constipation, diarrhea, stomatitis. **GU:** gonadal suppression. **Derm:** alopecia, dermatitis, vesiculation. **Endo:** syndrome of inappropriate antidiuretic hormone (SIADH). **Hemat:** anemia, leukopenia, thrombocytopenia. **Local:** phlebitis at IV site. **Metab:** hyperuricemia. **Neuro:** neuritis, paresthesia, peripheral neuropathy.

PHYSICAL THERAPY IMPLICATIONS

Examination and Evaluation

- Be alert for new seizures or increased seizure activity. Document the number, duration, and severity of seizures, and report these findings to the physician immediately.
- Assess symptoms of bronchospasm (wheezing, coughing, tightness in chest) or other prolonged or severe respiratory problems (difficult or labored breathing). Perform pulmonary function tests to document suspected changes in ventilation and respiration (See Appendix I).
- Monitor signs of fluid-electrolyte imbalance due to syndrome of inappropriate antidiuretic hormone (SIADH). SIADH causes increased water retention that leads to relatively low sodium concentration (hyponatremia). Symptoms include confusion, lethargy, weakness, myoclonus, and depressed reflexes. Severe or sudden onset may also cause seizures, ataxia, nystagmus, tremor, dysarthria, dysphagia, and coma. Notify physician if these signs occur.
- Watch for signs of leukopenia (fever, sore throat, signs of infection), thrombocytopenia (bruising, nose bleeds, bleeding gums), or unusual weakness and fatigue that might be due to anemia. Report these signs to the physician.
- Be alert for signs of peripheral neuropathy or neuritis, including numbness, tingling, and decreased muscle strength. Establish baseline electroneuromyographic values using EMG and nerve conduction at the beginning of drug treatment whenever possible, and reexamine these values periodically to document drug-induced changes in peripheral nerve function.
- Monitor signs of mental depression, including confusion, disorientation, and impaired memory. Notify physician if these symptoms become problematic.
- Monitor IV injection site for pain, swelling, and inflammation (phlebitis). Report phlebitis or other prolonged or excessive injection site reactions to the physician.

Interventions

- For patients who are medically able to begin exercise, implement appropriate resistive exercises and aerobic training to maintain muscle strength and aerobic capacity during cancer chemotherapy or to help restore function after chemotherapy.
- Because of the risk of bronchospasm, use caution during aerobic exercise and other forms of therapeutic exercise. Assess exercise tolerance frequently (respiratory symptoms, blood pressure, heart rate, fatigue levels), and terminate exercise immediately if any untoward responses occur (See Appendix L).

Patient/Client-Related Instruction

- Instruct patient to guard against infection (frequent hand washing, etc.), and to avoid crowds and contact with persons with contagious diseases.
- Advise patient about the likelihood of GI reactions such as nausea, vomiting, diarrhea, constipation, loss of appetite, and irritation in or around the mouth. Instruct patient or family and caregivers to report severe or unexpected GI reactions.
- Advise patient that hair loss and other skin reactions (inflammation, blistering) are likely. Report other severe or unexpected skin reactions to the physician.

Pharmacokinetics

Absorption: Administered IV only, resulting in complete bioavailability.
Distribution: Does not cross the blood-brain barrier well.
Metabolism and Excretion: Converted by the liver to an active antineoplastic compound; excreted in the feces via biliary excretion, some renal elimination.
Half-life: 24 hr.

TIME/ACTION PROFILE (effects on white blood cell counts)

ROUTE	ONSET	PEAK	DURATION
IV	5–7 days	10 days	7–14 days

Contraindications/Precautions

Contraindicated in: Hypersensitivity; Pregnancy or lactation.
Use Cautiously in: Patients with childbearing potential; Infections; ↓ bone marrow reserve; Other chronic debilitating illnesses; Patients with impaired hepatic function (↓ dose by 50% if serum bilirubin >3 mg/dL).

Interactions

Drug-Drug: Additive bone marrow depression with other **antineoplastics** or **radiation therapy.**

Bronchospasm may occur in patients who have been previously treated with **mitomycin.** May ↓ antibody response to **live-virus vaccines** and ↑ risk of adverse reactions. May ↓ serum **phenytoin** levels.

Route/Dosage

Doses may vary greatly, depending on tumor, schedule, condition of patient, and blood counts.

IV (Adults): *Initial*—3.7 mg/m^2 (100 mcg/kg), single dose; increase weekly as tolerated by 1.8 mg/m^2 (50 mcg/kg) to maximum of 18.5 mg/m^2 (usual dose is 5.5–7.4 mg/m^2). *Maintenance*—10 mg 1–2 times/mo or 1 increment less than last dose q 7–14 days.

IV (Children): *Initial*—2.5 mg/m^2, single dose; increase weekly as tolerated by 1.25 mg/m^2 to maximum of 7.5 mg/m^2. *Maintenance*—1 increment less than last dose q 7 days.

Availability (generic available)

Solution for injection: 1 mg/mL in 10-mL vials. **Powder for injection:** 10 mg/vial.

HIGH ALERT

vincristine (vin-kris-teen)

Oncovin, Vincasar PFS

Classification

Therapeutic: antineoplastics

Pharmacologic: vinca alkaloids

Indications

Used alone and in combination with other treatment modalities (antineoplastics, surgery, or radiation therapy) in treatment of: Hodgkin's disease, Leukemias, Neuroblastoma, Malignant lymphomas, Rhabdomyosarcoma, Wilms' tumor, Other tumors.

Action

Binds to proteins of mitotic spindle, causing metaphase arrest. Cell replication is stopped as a result (cell-cycle–specific for M phase). Has little or no effect on bone marrow. **Therapeutic Effects:** Death of rapidly replicating cells, particularly malignant ones. Has immunosuppressive properties.

Adverse Reactions/Side Effects

CNS: agitation, insomnia, mental depression, mental status changes. **EENT:** cortical blindness, diplopia. **Resp:** bronchospasm. **GI:** nausea, vomiting, abdominal cramps, anorexia, constipation, ileus, stomatitis. **GU:** gonadal suppression, nocturia, oliguria, urinary retention. **Derm:** alopecia. **Endo:** syndrome of inappropriate antidiuretic hormone (SIADH). **Hemat:** anemia, leukopenia, thrombocytopenia (mild and brief). **Local:** phlebitis at IV site, tissue necrosis (from extravasation). **Metab:** hyperuricemia. **Neuro:** ascending peripheral neuropathy.

PHYSICAL THERAPY IMPLICATIONS

Examination and Evaluation

- Assess symptoms of bronchospasm (wheezing, coughing, tightness in chest), difficult or labored breathing, or other prolonged or severe respiratory problems. Perform pulmonary function tests to document suspected changes in ventilation and respiration (See Appendix I).
- Monitor signs of fluid-electrolyte imbalance due to SIADH. SIADH causes increased water retention that leads to relatively low sodium concentration (hyponatremia). Symptoms include confusion, lethargy, weakness, myoclonus, and depressed reflexes. Severe or sudden onset may also cause seizures, ataxia, nystagmus, tremor, dysarthria, dysphagia, and coma. Notify physician if these signs occur.
- Watch for signs of leukopenia (fever, sore throat, signs of infection), thrombocytopenia (bruising, nose bleeds, bleeding gums), or unusual weakness and fatigue that might be due to anemia. Report these signs to the physician.
- Be alert for signs of peripheral neuropathy or neuritis, including numbness, tingling, and decreased muscle strength. Establish baseline electroneuromyographic values using EMG and nerve conduction at the beginning of drug treatment whenever possible, and reexamine these values periodically to document drug-induced changes in peripheral nerve function.
- Monitor signs of agitation, mental depression, and changes in mental status including confusion, disorientation, and impaired memory. Notify physician if these symptoms become problematic.
- Monitor IV injection site for pain, swelling, and inflammation (phlebitis). Report phlebitis or other prolonged or excessive injection site reactions to the physician.

Interventions

- For patients who are medically able to begin exercise, implement appropriate resistive exercises and aerobic training to maintain muscle strength and aerobic capacity during cancer chemotherapy or to help restore function after chemotherapy.
- Because of the risk of bronchospasm, use caution during aerobic exercise and other forms of therapeutic exercise. Assess exercise tolerance frequently (respiratory symptoms, blood pressure, heart rate, fatigue levels), and terminate exercise immediately if any untoward responses occur (See Appendix L).

V

Patient/Client-Related Instruction

- Instruct patient to guard against infection (frequent hand washing, etc.), and to avoid crowds and contact with persons with contagious diseases.
- Instruct patient to report any vision disturbances including double vision or loss of vision.
- Advise patient about the likelihood of GI reactions such as nausea, vomiting, constipation, abdominal cramps, loss of appetite, and irritation in or around the mouth. Instruct patient or family and caregivers to report severe or unexpected GI reactions.
- Advise patient that hair loss is likely. Report other severe or unexpected skin reactions to the physician.
- Instruct patient to report severe or prolonged problems with urination, including urine retention or painful and difficult urination.

Pharmacokinetics

Absorption: Administered IV only, resulting in complete bioavailability.

Distribution: Rapidly and widely distributed; extensively bound to tissues.

Metabolism and Excretion: Metabolized by the liver and eliminated in the feces via biliary excretion.

Half-life: 10.5–37.5 hr.

TIME/ACTION PROFILE (effects on blood counts*)

ROUTE	ONSET	PEAK	DURATION
IV	unknown	4 days	7 days

*Usually mild.

Contraindications/Precautions

Contraindicated in: Hypersensitivity; Pregnancy or lactation.

Use Cautiously in: Patients with childbearing potential; Infections; ↓ bone marrow reserve; Other chronic debilitating illnesses; Hepatic impairment (50% dose reduction recommended if serum bilirubin >3 mg/dL).

Interactions

Drug-Drug: Bronchospasm may occur in patients who have been previously treated with **mitomycin. L-asparaginase** may ↓ hepatic metabolism of vincristine (give vincristine 12–24 hr prior to asparaginase). May ↓ antibody response to **live-virus vaccines** and ↑ risk of adverse reactions.

Route/Dosage

Many other protocols are used.

IV (Adults): 10–30 mcg/kg (0.4–1.4 mg/m^2); may repeat weekly (not to exceed 2 mg/dose).

IV (Children >10 kg): 1.5–2 mg/m^2 single dose; may repeat weekly.

IV (Children <10 kg): 50 mcg/kg single dose; may repeat weekly.

Availability (generic available)

Solution for injection: 1 mg/mL in 1-, 2-, 5-mL vials. **Powder for injection:** 5 mg/vial.

HIGH ALERT

vinorelbine (vin-oh-**rel**-been)

Navelbine

Classification

Therapeutic: antineoplastics

Pharmacologic: vinca alkaloids

Indications

Inoperable non–small-cell cancer of the lung in ambulatory patients (alone or with cisplatin).

Action

Binds to a protein (tubulin) of cellular microtubules, where it interferes with microtubule assembly. Cell replication is stopped as a result (cell-cycle–specific for M phase). **Therapeutic Effects:** Death of rapidly replicating cells, particularly malignant ones.

Adverse Reactions/Side Effects

CNS: fatigue. **Resp:** shortness of breath. **CV:** chest pain. **GI:** constipation, nausea, abdominal pain, anorexia, diarrhea, transient increase in liver enzymes, vomiting. **Derm:** alopecia, rashes. **F and E:** hyponatremia. **Hemat:** anemia, neutropenia, thrombocytopenia. **Local:** irritation at IV site, skin reactions, phlebitis. **MS:** arthralgia, back pain, jaw pain, myalgia. **Neuro:** neurotoxicity. **Misc:** pain in tumor-containing tissue.

PHYSICAL THERAPY IMPLICATIONS

Examination and Evaluation

- Monitor cardiopulmonary symptoms such as chest pain or shortness of breath. Report severe or unexpected cardiac and respiratory problems to the physician.
- Watch for signs of neutropenia (fever, sore throat, signs of infection), thrombocytopenia (bruising, nose bleeds, bleeding gums), or unusual weakness and fatigue that might be due to anemia. Report these signs to the physician.
- Assess any joint pain, muscle pain, or pain in the jaw or back to rule out musculoskeletal pathology; that is, try to determine if pain is drug induced rather than caused by anatomic or biomechanical problems.
- Be alert for signs of neurotoxicity and peripheral neuropathy, including numbness, tingling, and decreased muscle strength. Establish baseline electroneuromyographic values using EMG and nerve conduction at the beginning of drug treatment whenever possible, and reexamine these values periodically to document drug-induced changes in peripheral nerve function.
- Monitor signs of low sodium levels (hyponatremia), including headache, confusion, lethargy, irritability, decreased consciousness, and neuromuscular

abnormalities (muscle weakness and cramps). Report severe or prolonged signs to the physician.
- Monitor IV injection site for pain, swelling, and inflammation (phlebitis). Report phlebitis or other prolonged or excessive injection site reactions to the physician.

Interventions
- For patients who are medically able to begin exercise, implement appropriate resistive exercises and aerobic training to maintain muscle strength and aerobic capacity during cancer chemotherapy or to help restore function after chemotherapy.
- Use caution during aerobic exercise and other forms of therapeutic exercise. Assess exercise tolerance frequently (respiratory symptoms, blood pressure, heart rate, fatigue levels), and terminate exercise immediately if any untoward responses occur (See Appendix L).

Patient/Client-Related Instruction
- Instruct patient to guard against infection (frequent hand washing, etc.), and to avoid crowds and contact with persons with contagious diseases.
- Advise patient and family/caregivers that fatigue and weakness are likely and may be severe. Functional abilities may be limited, and patient may need to use assistive devices during ambulation.
- Advise patient about the likelihood of GI reactions such as nausea, vomiting, diarrhea, constipation, abdominal pain, and loss of appetite. Instruct patient or family and caregivers to report severe or unexpected GI reactions.
- Advise patient that hair loss and skin rashes are likely. Report other severe or unexpected skin reactions to the physician.

Pharmacokinetics
Absorption: IV administration results in complete bioavailability.
Distribution: Highly bound to platelets and lymphocytes.
Metabolism and Excretion: Mostly metabolized by the liver. At least 1 metabolite is active. Large amounts eliminated in feces; 11% excreted unchanged by the kidneys.
Half-life: 28–44 hr.

TIME/ACTION PROFILE (effect on WBCs)

ROUTE	ONSET	PEAK	DURATION
IV	unknown	7–10 days	7–15 days

Contraindications/Precautions
Contraindicated in: Hypersensitivity; Pregnancy or lactation; Active infections; ↓ bone marrow reserve; Other chronic debilitating illnesses.
Use Cautiously in: Patients with childbearing potential; Impaired hepatic function (dose reduction recommended if total bilirubin >2 mg/dL); Debilitated patients (↑ risk of hyponatremia); Granulocytopenic patients (temporarily discontinue or reduce dose); Pedi: Children (safe use not established).

Interactions
Drug-Drug: ↑ bone marrow depression with other **antineoplastics** or **radiation therapy.** Concurrent use with **cisplatin** ↑ risk and severity of bone marrow depression. Concurrent use with **mitomycin** or **chest radiation** ↑ risk of pulmonary reactions.

Route/Dosage
IV (Adults): 30 mg/m^2 once weekly.

Hepatic Impairment
IV (Adults): *Total bilirubin 2.1–3 mg/dL*—15 mg/m^2 once weekly; *total bilirubin >3 mg/dL*—7.5 mg/m^2 once weekly.

Availability (generic available)
Injection: 10 mg/mL.

voriconazole
(vor-i-**kon**-a-zole)
VFEND

Classification
Therapeutic: antifungals
Pharmacologic: triazoles

Indications
Serious systemic fungal infections, including candidemia, esophageal candidiasis, candidal deep tissue and skin infections, abdominal, kidney, bladder wall and wound infections, and aspergillosis.

Action
Inhibits fungal ergosterol synthesis leading to production of abnormal fungal plasma membrane.
Therapeutic Effects: Antifungal activity.

Adverse Reactions/Side Effects
CNS: dizziness, hallucinations, headache. **EENT:** visual disturbances, eye hemorrhage. **CV:** changes in blood pressure, tachycardia, peripheral edema. **GI:** HEPATOXICITY, abdominal pain, diarrhea, nausea, pancreatitis, vomiting. **Derm:** photosensitivity, rash. **F and E:** hypokalemia, hypomagnesemia. **Misc:** ALLERGIC REACTIONS, INCLUDING STEVENS-JOHNSON SYNDROME, chills, fever, infusion reactions.

PHYSICAL THERAPY IMPLICATIONS

Examination and Evaluation

- Be alert for signs of hepatotoxicity, including anorexia, abdominal pain, severe nausea and vomiting, yellow skin or eyes, fever, sore throat, malaise, weakness, facial edema, lethargy, and unusual bleeding or bruising. Notify physician of these signs immediately.
- Monitor rashes or other skin reactions such as exfoliation, hives, itching, raised patches of red or white skin (welts), burning, acne, and abnormal sweating. Notify physician immediately because certain skin responses may indicate serious allergic reactions such as Stevens-Johnson syndrome.
- Assess blood pressure (BP) and compare to normal values (See Appendix F). Report changes in BP, either a problematic decrease in BP (hypotension) or a sustained increase in BP (hypertension).
- Assess heart rate, ECG, and heart sounds, especially during exercise (See Appendices G, H). Report tachycardia or other rhythm disturbances, or symptoms of increased arrhythmias, including palpitations, chest discomfort, shortness of breath, fainting, and fatigue/weakness.
- Assess peripheral edema using girth measurements, volume displacement, and measurement of pitting edema (See Appendix N). Report increased swelling in feet and ankles or a sudden increase in body weight due to fluid retention.
- Monitor signs of low potassium levels (hypokalemia) such as muscle weakness, aches, or cramps, and signs of low magnesium levels (hypomagnesemia), such as lethargy, irritability, insomnia, muscle tremors, and confusion. Notify physician of these signs.
- Assess dizziness that might affect gait, balance, and other functional activities (See Appendix C). Report balance problems and functional limitations to the physician and nursing staff, and caution the patient and family/caregivers to guard against falls and trauma.
- Report allergy-like responses (wheezing, laryngeal edema, urticaria, other skin reactions) that occur during and after administration (infusion related reactions).

Interventions

- Always wash hands thoroughly and disinfect equipment (whirlpools, electrotherapeutic devices, treatment tables, and so forth) to help prevent the spread of infection. Employ universal precautions or isolation procedures as indicated for specific patients.
- Because of the risk of arrhythmias and abnormal BP responses, use caution during aerobic exercise and other forms of therapeutic exercise. Assess exercise tolerance frequently (BP, heart rate, fatigue levels), and terminate exercise immediately if any untoward responses occur (See Appendix L).
- Causes photosensitivity; use care if administering UV treatments. Advise patient to avoid direct sunlight and use sunscreens and protective clothing.

Patient/Client-Related Instruction

- Advise patient to take this drug as directed for the full course of treatment even if feeling better.
- Advise patient about the likelihood of GI reactions (diarrhea, nausea, vomiting, abdominal pain). Instruct patient to report severe or prolonged GI problems, or signs of pancreatitis such as upper abdominal pain (especially after eating), indigestion, weight loss, and oily stools.
- Instruct patient to report other troublesome side effects such as prolonged or severe headache, hallucinations, chills, fever, skin rash, or vision disturbances.

Pharmacokinetics

Absorption: Well absorbed following oral administration (96%); IV administration results in complete bioavailability.
Distribution: Extensive tissue distribution.
Metabolism and Excretion: Highly metabolized by the hepatic P450 enzymes (CYP2C19, CYP2C9, CYP3A4); <2% excreted unchanged in urine. Much individual variation in metabolism; metabolites are inactive.
Half-life: Dose dependent; increased in hepatic impairment.

TIME/ACTION PROFILE (blood levels)

ROUTE	ONSET	PEAK	DURATION
PO	rapid	1–2 hr	12 hr
IV	rapid	end of infusion	12 hr

Contraindications/Precautions

Contraindicated in: Concurrent use of ritonavir, rifampin, rifabutin, St. John's wort, carbamazepine, and phenobarbital (↓ antifungal activity); Concurrent use of sirolimus, pimozide, quinidine, ergotamine, and dihydroergotamine (↑ risk of toxicity of these agents); Tablets contain lactose and should be avoided in patients with galactose intolerance, Lapp lactase deficiency, or glucose-galactose malabsorption.
Use Cautiously in: Mild-to-moderate liver disease (Child-Pugh Classes A and B); maintenance dose reduction recommended; Renal impairment (CCr <50 mL/min); use only if justified by risk/benefit assessment (IV form should be avoided, use oral form only); OB/Lactation: Use only if benefits justify risk; Pedi: Children <12 yr (safety not established).

Interactions

Drug-Drug: Carbamazepine, ritonavir, phenobarbital, St. John's wort, rifabutin, and **rifampin**

↑ metabolism and ↓ antifungal activity of voriconazole; concurrent use is contraindicated. **Efavirenz** ↑ metabolism and ↓ antifungal activity of voriconazole; voriconazole also ↓ metabolism and ↑ risk of toxicity of **efavirenz;** if used together, ↑ dose of voriconazole to 400 mg q 12 hr and ↓ dose of efavirenz to 300 mg daily. ↓ metabolism and ↑ risk of toxicity from **dihydroergotamine, ergotamine, pimozide, rifabutin, quinidine,** and **sirolimus;** concurrent use is contraindicated. ↓ metabolism and ↑ risk of toxicity from **cyclosporine, HMG CoA reductase inhibitors,** some **benzodiazepines (alprazolam, midazolam, triazolam),** some **calcium channel blockers, sulfonylureas (glipizide, glyburide, tolbutamide), alfentanil, tacrolimus, warfarin,** and **vinca alkaloids (vincristine, vinblastine);** careful monitoring required during concurrent use. **Phenytoin** ↑ metabolism and ↓ antifungal activity of voriconazole; voriconazole ↑ **phenytoin** levels and may cause toxicity; careful monitoring required during concurrent use. ↑ blood levels of **omeprazole;** ↓ omeprazole dose by 50% during concurrent use. Similar effects may occur with other **proton-pump inhibitors.** May ↓ metabolism and ↑ blood levels and effects of **protease-inhibitor antiretrovirals** and **nonnucleoside reverse transcriptase inhibitor antiretrovirals;** frequent monitoring recommended. **Nonnucleoside reverse transcriptase inhibitor antiretrovirals;** may induce or inhibit the metabolism of voriconazole; frequent monitoring recommended.

Route/Dosage

IV (Adults and children >12 yr): *Loading dose*—6 mg/kg q 12 hr for 2 doses, followed by *maintenance dosing*—3–4 mg/kg q 12 hr. IV then switched to oral dosing when possible. If intolerance occurs, dose may be decreased to 3 mg/kg q 12 hr. If phenytoin is coadministered, ↑ maintenance dose to 5 mg/kg q 12 hr.

PO (Adults and children >12 yr and >40 kg): *Most infections*—(following IV loading dose) 200 mg q 12 hr; may be ↑ to 300 mg q 12 hr if response if inadequate. If phenytoin is coadministered, ↑ maintenance dose to 400 mg q 12 hr; *Esophageal candidiasis*—200 mg q 12 hr for 14 days or 7 days following symptom resolution.

PO (Adults and children >12 yr and <40 kg): *Most infections*—(following IV loading dose) 100 mg q 12 hr; may be increased to 150 mg q 12 hr if response is inadequate. If phenytoin is coadministered, increase maintenance dose to 200 mg q 12 hr; *E. candidiasis*—100 mg q 12 hr for 14 days or 7 days following symptom resolution.

Hepatic Impairment

IV (Adults and Children >12 yr): Use standard loading dose; ↓ maintenance dose by 50%.

Availability

Tablets: 50 mg, 200 mg. **Oral suspension (orange):** 40 mg/mL in 100-mL bottles. **Powder for injection (requires reconstitution):** 200 mg/vial.

vorinostat (vor-in-oh-stat)

Zolinza

Classification

Therapeutic: antineoplastics

Pharmacologic: enzyme inhibitors

Indications

Treatment of skin manifestations cutaneous T-cell lymphoma (CTCL) that has not responded to 2 systemic therapies.

Action

Acts as a histone deacetylase inhibitor which decreases gene transcription resulting in cell-cycle arrest. **Therapeutic Effects:** ↓ progression of CTCL.

Adverse Reactions/Side Effects

CNS: dizziness, headache. **CV:** PULMONARY EMBOLISM, deep vein thrombosis. **Resp:** cough. **GI:** anorexia, constipation, diarrhea, dry mouth, dysgeusia, nausea, vomiting. **GU:** proteinuria. **Derm:** alopecia, itching. **Endo:** hyperglycemia. **Hemat:** anemia, thrombocytopenia. **Metab:** weight loss. **MS:** muscle spasms. **Misc:** chills, fever.

PHYSICAL THERAPY IMPLICATIONS

Examination and Evaluation

- Monitor signs of deep vein thrombosis (lower extremity swelling, warmth, erythema, tenderness) and pulmonary embolism (shortness of breath, chest pain, cough, bloody sputum). Notify physician immediately, and request objective tests (Doppler ultrasound, lung scan, others) if thrombosis is suspected.
- Monitor signs of thrombocytopenia (bruising, nose bleeds, bleeding gums) or unusual weakness and fatigue that might be due to anemia. Report these signs to the physician or nursing staff.
- Be alert for signs of hyperglycemia, including confusion, drowsiness, flushed/dry skin, fruit-like breath odor, rapid/deep breathing, polyuria, loss of appetite, and unusual thirst. Patients with diabetes mellitus should check blood glucose levels frequently.
- Assess dizziness that might affect gait, balance, and other functional activities (See Appendix C). Report balance problems and functional limitations to the physician and nursing staff, and caution the patient

and family/caregivers to guard against falls and trauma.

- Assess any muscle spasms to rule out musculoskeletal pathology; that is, try to determine if spasms are drug induced rather than caused by anatomic or biomechanical problems.
- Periodically assess body weight and other anthropometric measures (body mass index, body composition). Report a rapid or unexplained weight loss or decreased body fat.

Interventions

- For patients who are medically able to begin exercise, implement appropriate resistive exercises and aerobic training to maintain muscle strength and aerobic capacity during cancer chemotherapy or to help restore function after chemotherapy.

Patient/Client-Related Instruction

- Advise patient about the likelihood of GI reactions such as nausea, vomiting, constipation, diarrhea, loss of appetite, dry mouth, and altered taste. Instruct patient to report severe or prolonged GI problems.
- Instruct patient to report other bothersome side effects such as severe or prolonged headache, cough, chills, fever, and skin reactions (rash, hair loss).

Pharmacokinetics

Absorption: Well absorbed following oral administration.
Distribution: Crosses the placenta.
Metabolism and Excretion: Mostly metabolized, <1% excreted unchanged in urine.
Half-life: 2 hr.

TIME/ACTION PROFILE (blood levels)

ROUTE	ONSET	PEAK ↑	DURATION
PO	unknown	4 hr	24 hr

Contraindications/Precautions

Contraindicated in: OB: Pregnancy or lactation.
Use Cautiously in: Renal/hepatic impairment; Geri: May be more sensitive to drug effects; Preexisting nausea, vomiting, diarrhea (treat symptomatically before initiating therapy); Pedi: Safe use in children not established.

Interactions

Drug-Drug: ↑ risk of thrombocytopenia and GI bleeding with **valproic acid.** May ↑ risk of bleeding with **warfarin.**

Route/Dosage

PO (Adults): 400 mg daily; if intolerance occurs, dose may be reduced to 300 mg daily or 300 mg daily for 5 consecutive days/wk.

Availability

Capsules: 100 mg.

HIGH ALERT

warfarin (war-fa-rin)
Coumadin, Warfilone

Classification
Therapeutic: anticoagulants
Pharmacologic: coumarins

Indications

Prophylaxis and treatment of Venous thrombosis, Pulmonary embolism, Atrial fibrillation with embolization. Management of myocardial infarction: ↓ risk of death, ↓ risk of subsequent MI, ↓ risk of future thromboembolic events. Prevention of thrombus formation and embolization after prosthetic valve placement.

Action

Interferes with hepatic synthesis of vitamin K–dependent clotting factors (II, VII, IX, and X). **Therapeutic Effects:** Prevention of thromboembolic events.

Adverse Reactions/Side Effects

GI: cramps, nausea. **Derm:** dermal necrosis.
Hemat: BLEEDING. **Misc:** fever.

PHYSICAL THERAPY IMPLICATIONS

Examination and Evaluation

- Watch for signs of bleeding and hemorrhage, including bleeding gums, nosebleeds, unusual bruising, coughing up blood, black/tarry stools, hematuria, or a fall in hematocrit or blood pressure. Notify physician or nursing staff immediately if warfarin causes excessive anticoagulation.
- Monitor any appreciable symptoms of DVT such as pain, swelling, warmth, and redness to determine if drug therapy is effective in preventing or reducing venous thrombosis. Request or administer objective tests (Doppler ultrasound) if symptoms increase.
- In patients with deep vein thrombosis (DVT), watch for signs of pulmonary embolism such as shortness of breath, chest pain, cough, and bloody sputum. Notify physician or nursing staff immediately if these signs occur.
- Monitor skin reactions, and report any severe or untoward reactions such as dermal necrosis.

Interventions

- Use caution with any physical interventions that could increase bleeding, including wound débridement, chest percussion, joint mobilization, and application of local heat.
- Recommend or implement other physical methods to decrease DVT and prevent thromboembolism, including graduated compression stockings and intermittent pneumatic compression pumps.
- Implement early mobilization and ambulation to reduce the risk of new or increased DVT. Early ambulation appears to be safe in patients with DVT if the patient is receiving adequate anticoagulant therapy (INR values in acceptable range), does not have an active pulmonary embolism, or have other risk factors that contraindicate ambulation.

Patient/Client-Related Instruction

- Instruct patient to immediately report signs of GI bleeding, including abdominal pain, vomiting blood, blood in stools, or black, tarry stools.
- Remind patient that excessive vitamin K intake negates warfarin's therapeutic effects. Refer patient to the physician or a nutritionist regarding appropriate dietary intake of foods rich in vitamin K (leafy green vegetables, dairy products, and so forth).
- Instruct patient or family/caregivers to report other troublesome side effects such fever, nausea, or stomach cramps.

Pharmacokinetics

Absorption: Well absorbed from the GI tract after oral administration.
Distribution: Crosses the placenta but does not enter breast milk.
Protein Binding: 99%.
Metabolism and Excretion: Metabolized by the liver.
Half-life: 42 hr.

TIME/ACTION PROFILE (effects on coagulation tests)

ROUTE	ONSET	PEAK	DURATION
PO, IV	36–72 hr	5–7 days*	2–5 days†

*At a constant dose.
†After discontinuation.

Contraindications/Precautions

Contraindicated in: Uncontrolled bleeding; Open wounds; Active ulcer disease; Recent brain, eye, or spinal cord injury or surgery; Severe liver or kidney disease; Uncontrolled hypertension; OB: Crosses placenta and may cause fatal hemorrhage in the fetus. May also cause congenital malformation.
Use Cautiously in: Malignancy; Patients with history of ulcer or liver disease; History of poor compliance; Women with childbearing potential; Pedi: Has been used safely but may require more frequent PT/INR assessments; Geri: Due to greater than expected anticoagulant response, initiate and maintain at lower dosages.

Interactions

Drug-Drug: Abciximab, androgens, capecitabine, cefoperazone, cefotetan, chloral hydrate,

W

chloramphenicol, clopidogrel, disulfiram, fluconazole, fluoroquinolones, itraconazole, metronidazole (including vaginal use), **thrombolytics, eptifibatide, tirofiban, ticlopidine, sulfonamides, quinidine, quinine, NSAIDs, valproates,** and **aspirin** may ↑ the response to warfarin and ↑ the risk of bleeding. Chronic use of **acetaminophen** may ↑ the risk of bleeding. Chronic **alcohol** ingestion may ↓ action of warfarin; if chronic **alcohol** abuse results in significant liver damage, action of warfarin may be ↑ due to ↓ production of clotting factor. **Barbiturates** and **hormonal contraceptives containing estrogen** may ↓ the anticoagulant response to warfarin. Acute **alcohol** ingestion may ↑ action of warfarin. **Many other drugs** may affect the activity of warfarin.
Drug-Natural: St. John's wort ↓ effect. ↑ bleeding risk with **anise, arnica, chamomile, clove, dong quai, fenugreek, feverfew, garlic, ginger, ginkgo, *Panax ginseng*, licorice,** and others.
Drug-Food: Ingestion of large quantities of **foods high in vitamin K content** may antagonize the anticoagulant effect of warfarin.

Route/Dosage

PO, IV (Adults): 2.5–10 mg/day for 2–4 days; then adjust daily dose by results of prothrombin time or international normalized ratio (INR). Initiate therapy with lower doses in geriatric or debilitated patients.
PO, IV (Children >1 mo): *Initial loading dose*—0.2 mg/kg (maximum dose: 10 mg) for 2–4 days then adjust daily dose by results of prothrombin time or international normalized ratio (INR); use 0.1 mg/kg if liver dysfunction is present. *Maintenance dose range*—0.05–0.34 mg/kg/day.

Availability (generic available)

Tablets: 1 mg, 2 mg, 2.5 mg, 3 mg, 4 mg, 5 mg, 6 mg, 7.5 mg, 10 mg. **Injection:** 5 mg/vial.

zafirlukast (za-feer-loo-kast)

Accolate

Classification

Therapeutic: antiasthmatics, bronchodilators

Pharmacologic: leukotriene antagonists

Indications

Long-term control agent in the management of asthma.

Action

Antagonizes the effects of leukotrienes, which are components of slow-reacting substance of anaphylaxis (SRSA). These substances mediate the following: Airway edema, Smooth muscle constriction, Altered cellular activity. Result is decreased inflammatory process that is part of asthma. **Therapeutic Effects:** ↓ frequency and severity of asthma.

Adverse Reactions/Side Effects

CNS: headache, dizziness, weakness. **GI:** HEPATOTOXICITY, abdominal pain, diarrhea, dyspepsia, nausea, vomiting. **MS:** arthralgia, back pain, myalgia. **Misc:** CHURG-STRAUSS SYNDROME, fever, infection (geriatric patients).

PHYSICAL THERAPY IMPLICATIONS

Examination and Evaluation

- Be alert for signs of eosinophilic conditions and allergic blood vessel reactions, including Churg-Strauss syndrome. Early signs include allergic rhinitis, sinusitis, asthma, or hay fever–like reactions. Symptoms can increase to include fever, skin rash, joint pain, severe pain and numbness (peripheral neuropathy), shortness of breath, coughing up blood, bloody urine, chest pain, arrhythmias, and GI problems (diarrhea, nausea, vomiting, GI bleeding). Notify physician immediately for further evaluation of any signs listed above.
- Watch for signs of hepatotoxicity, including anorexia, abdominal pain, severe nausea and vomiting, yellow skin or eyes, fever, sore throat, malaise, weakness, facial edema, lethargy, and unusual bleeding or bruising. Report these signs to the physician immediately.
- Assess pulmonary function at rest and during exercise (See Appendices I, J, K) to document effectiveness of medication in controlling bronchoconstriction and asthma attacks.
- Assess any back, joint, or muscle pain to rule out musculoskeletal pathology; that is, try to determine if pain is drug induced rather than caused by anatomic or biomechanical problems.
- Assess dizziness and weakness that might affect gait, balance, and other functional activities (See Appendix C). Report balance problems and functional limitations to the physician, and caution the patient and family/caregivers to guard against falls and trauma.

Interventions

- When implementing airway clearance techniques or respiratory muscle training, attempt to intervene when the airway is maximally bronchodilated. Patients should experience optimal effects after one week of recommended daily administration.

Patient/Client-Related Instruction

- Advise patient not to exceed the recommended dose or frequency of administration. Contact physician if bronchospasm is not adequately controlled by the current medication regimen, or if respiratory symptoms continue to worsen.
- Instruct patient and family/caregivers to report other troublesome side effects, including severe or prolonged headache, fever, infections, or GI problems (nausea, vomiting, diarrhea, indigestion, abdominal pain).

Pharmacokinetics

Absorption: Rapidly absorbed after oral administration.
Distribution: Enters breast milk.
Protein Binding: 99%.
Metabolism and Excretion: Mostly metabolized by the liver; 10% excreted unchanged by the kidneys.
Half-life: 10 hr.

TIME/ACTION PROFILE (improved symptoms of asthma)

ROUTE	ONSET	PEAK	DURATION
PO	unknown	1 wk	unknown

Contraindications/Precautions

Contraindicated in: Hypersensitivity; Lactation: Lactation.
Use Cautiously in: Acute attacks of asthma; Patients >55 yr (↑ risk of infection); Geri: Geriatric patients ≥65 yr or patients with hepatic impairment (may need lower doses); OB/Pedi: Pregnancy or children <7 yr (safety not established).

Interactions

Drug-Drug: Blood levels are ↑ by **aspirin.** Blood levels are ↓ by **erythromycin** and **theophylline.** ↑ effects and risk of bleeding with **warfarin.**
Drug-Food: Food (especially high-fat or high-protein meal) ↓ absorption.

Z

Route/Dosage

PO (Adults and Children ≥12 yr): 20 mg bid.
PO (Children 7–11 yr): 10 mg bid.

Availability

Tablets: 10 mg, 20 mg.

zaleplon (za-lep-lon)

Sonata

Classification

Therapeutic: sedative/hypnotics
Pharmacologic: pyrazolopyrimidines

Schedule IV

Indications

Short-term management of insomnia in patients unable to get at least 4 hr of sleep; especially useful in sleep initiation disorders.

Action

Produces CNS depression by binding to gamma-aminobutyric acid (GABA) receptors in the CNS. Has no analgesic properties. **Therapeutic Effects:** Sedation and induction of sleep.

Adverse Reactions/Side Effects

CNS: abnormal thinking, amnesia, anxiety, behavior changes, depersonalization, dizziness, drowsiness, hallucinations, headache, impaired memory (briefly following dose), impaired psychomotor function (briefly following dose), malaise, sleep driving, vertigo, weakness. **EENT:** abnormal vision, ear pain, epistaxis, hearing sensitivity, ocular pain, altered sense of smell. **CV:** peripheral edema. **GI:** abdominal pain, anorexia, colitis, dyspepsia, nausea. **GU:** dysmenorrhea. **Derm:** photosensitivity. **Neuro:** hyperesthesia, paresthesia, tremor. **Misc:** fever.

PHYSICAL THERAPY IMPLICATIONS

Examination and Evaluation

- Monitor daytime drowsiness, anxiety, behavior changes, short-term memory deficits, hallucinations, and "drugged" feelings. Repeated or excessive symptoms may require change in dose or medication.
- Assess dizziness and vertigo that affects gait, balance, and other functional activities (See Appendix C). Report balance problems and functional limitations to the physician, and caution the patient and family/caregivers to guard against falls and trauma.
- Assess signs of paresthesia (numbness, tingling), tremor, or abnormal sensitivity to touch or temperature (hyperesthesia). Perform objective tests, including electroneuromyography and sensory testing, to document any drug-related neuropathic changes.
- Assess peripheral edema using girth measurements, volume displacement, and measurement of pitting edema (See Appendix N). Report increased swelling in feet and ankles or a sudden increase in body weight due to fluid retention.

Interventions

- Guard against falls and trauma (hip fractures, head injury, and so forth). Implement fall-prevention strategies, especially in older adults or if drowsiness and dizziness carry over into the daytime (See Appendix E).
- Help patient explore nonpharmacologic methods to improve sleep, such as relaxation techniques, regular exercise, avoid caffeine, and so forth.
- Causes photosensitivity; use care if administering UV treatments. Advise patient to avoid direct sunlight and use sunscreens and protective clothing.

Patient/Client-Related Instruction

- Instruct patients on prolonged treatment not to discontinue medication without consulting their physician. Long-term use can cause tolerance and physical/psychologic dependence, and abrupt withdrawal after 2 or more weeks of use may result in fatigue, nausea, flushing, light-headedness, uncontrolled crying, vomiting, GI upset, panic attack, or nervousness.
- Advise patient about the risk of daytime drowsiness and decreased attention and mental focus. Use care if driving or in other activities that require strong concentration.
- Caution patient and family/caregivers that "sleepwalking" and other complex activities, including driving a car (sleep driving), may occur while completely asleep. Care should be taken to monitor such activities and prevent access to motor vehicles while under the influence of this drug.
- Advise patient to avoid alcohol and other CNS depressants because of the increased risk of sedation and adverse effects.
- Instruct patient and family/caregivers to report other troublesome side effects such as severe or prolonged headache, fever, vision or hearing disturbances, nosebleeds, altered sense of smell, menstrual irregularities, abnormal thoughts, or GI problems (nausea, abdominal pain, indigestion, loss of appetite).

Pharmacokinetics

Absorption: Rapidly absorbed following oral administration.
Distribution: Enters breast milk.
Metabolism and Excretion: Extensively metabolized in the liver (mostly by aldehyde oxidase and some by CYP4503A4 enzymes).

Half-life: Unknown.

TIME/ACTION PROFILE

ROUTE	ONSET	PEAK	DURATION
PO	within minutes	unknown	3–4 hr

Contraindications/Precautions

Contraindicated in: Hypersensitivity; OB/Lactation: Not recommended for use during pregnancy, lactation, or in patients with severe hepatic impairment.

Use Cautiously in: Mild-to-moderate hepatic impairment, age ≥65 yr or weight ≤50 kg or concurrent cimetidine therapy (initiate therapy at lowest dose); Impaired respiratory function; History of suicide attempt; Pedi: Safety not established.

Interactions

Drug-Drug: Cimetidine ↓ metabolism and ↑ effects (initiate therapy at a lower dose). Additive CNS depression with other **CNS depressants**, including **alcohol, antihistamines, opioid analgesics**, other **sedative/hypnotics, phenothiazines,** and **tricyclic antidepressants.** Effects may be ↓ by drugs that induce the CYP4503A4 enzyme system, including **rifampin, phenytoin, carbamazepine,** and **phenobarbital.**

Drug-Natural: Concomitant use of **kava-kava, valerian, chamomile,** or **hops** can ↑ CNS depression.

Drug-Food: Concurrent ingestion of a **high-fat meal** slows the rate of absorption.

Route/Dosage

PO (Adults <65 yr): 10 mg (range 5–20 mg) hs.

PO (Geriatric Patients or Patients <50 kg): Initiate therapy at 5 mg hs (not to exceed 10 mg hs).

Hepatic Impairment

PO (Adults): Initiate therapy at 5 mg hs (not to exceed 10 mg hs).

Availability (generic available)

Capsules: 5 mg, 10 mg.

zanamivir (zan-am-i-veer)

Relenza

Classification

Therapeutic: antivirals

Pharmacologic: neuramidase inhibitors

Indications

Treatment of uncomplicated acute illness caused by influenza virus in patients ≥7 yr who have been symptomatic ≤2 days. Prevention of influenza in patients ≥5 yr.

Action

Inhibits the enzyme neuramidase, which may alter virus particle aggregation and release. **Therapeutic Effects:** Reduced duration or prevention of flu-related symptoms.

Adverse Reactions/Side Effects

CNS: SEIZURES, abnormal behavior, agitation, delirium, hallucinations, nightmares. **Resp:** bronchospasm. **Misc:** allergic reactions.

PHYSICAL THERAPY IMPLICATIONS

Examination and Evaluation

- Be alert for new seizures or increased seizure activity, especially at the onset of drug treatment. Document the number, duration, and severity of seizures, and report these findings to the physician immediately.
- Monitor signs of allergic reactions, including pulmonary symptoms (tightness in the throat and chest, wheezing, cough, dyspnea) or skin reactions (rash, pruritus, urticaria). Notify the physician immediately if these reactions occur.
- Be alert for agitation, delirium, hallucinations, or other abnormal behaviors. Notify the physician promptly if these symptoms develop.
- Assess any breathing problems, and report signs of bronchospasm (wheezing, coughing, dyspnea, tightness in chest). Perform pulmonary function tests to quantify suspected changes in ventilation and respiration (See Appendices I, J, K).

Interventions

- Always wash hands thoroughly and disinfect equipment (whirlpools, electrotherapeutic devices, treatment tables, and so forth) to help prevent the spread of infection. Employ universal precautions as indicated for specific patients.

Patient/Client-Related Instruction

- Instruct patient and family/caregivers to report other troublesome side effects such as nightmares.

Pharmacokinetics

Absorption: 4–17% of inhaled dose is systemically absorbed.

Distribution: Unknown.

Protein Binding: <10%.

Metabolism and Excretion: Mainly excreted by kidneys as unchanged drug; unabsorbed drug is excreted in feces.

Half-life: 2.5–5.1 hr.

TIME/ACTION PROFILE (blood levels)

ROUTE	ONSET	PEAK	DURATION
inhalation	Rapid	1–2 hr	12 hr

Z

Contraindications/Precautions

Contraindicated in: Hypersensitivity to zanamivir or lactose.

Use Cautiously in: Chronic obstructive pulmonary disease or asthma (↑ risk of decreased lung function and/or bronchospasm); OB/Lactation: Safety not established; Children <7 yr (for treatment) or <5 yr (for prophylaxis) (safety not established; children may be at ↑ risk for neuropsychiatric events).

Interactions

Drug-Drug: None noted.

Route/Dosage

Treatment

Inhalation (Adults and children ≥7 yr): 10 mg (given as 2 inhalations of 5 mg each) bid for 5 days.

Prophylaxis

Inhalation (Adults and children ≥5 yr): 10 mg (given as 2 inhalations of 5 mg each) daily for 10 days (for household setting) (28 days for community outbreaks).

Availability

Powder for inhalation: 5 mg/blister.

ziconotide (zi-koe-noe-tide)

Prialt

Classification

Therapeutic: analgesics

Pharmacologic: n-type calcium channel blockers

Indications

Management of severe chronic pain when conventional therapies (analgesics or other adjunctive measures) have failed.

Action

Blocks spinal N-channel calcium channels, decreasing transmission of pain signals to the brain. Has no effect on opioid receptors. **Therapeutic Effects:** ↓ in severe pain.

Adverse Reactions/Side Effects

CNS: MENINGITIS, confusion, dizziness, drowsiness, headache, impaired memory, weakness, aphasia, ↓ alertness/responsiveness, cognitive impairment, hallucinations, psychiatric symptoms, speech disorder. **CV:** changes in blood pressure. **EENT:** nystagmus, abnormal vision. **GI:** nausea, anorexia, vomiting. **Local:** catheter/injection site reactions. **MS:** hypertonia, urinary retention, ↑ creatine kinase. **Neuro:** abnormal gait, ataxia. **Misc:** fever.

PHYSICAL THERAPY IMPLICATIONS

Examination and Evaluation

- Be alert for signs of meningitis, including severe headache, neck stiffness, nausea, vomiting, confusion, drowsiness, sensitivity to light, loss of appetite, high fever, skin rash, and seizures. Notify physician or nurse immediately if patient exhibits these signs.
- Use appropriate pain scales (visual analogue scales, others) to document whether this drug is successful in helping manage the patient's pain.
- Assess blood pressure (BP) and compare to normal values (See Appendix F). Report changes in BP, either a problematic decrease in BP (hypotension) or a sustained increase in BP (hypertension).
- Be alert for changes in mood and behavior, including hallucinations, impaired memory, speech problems, decreased cognition, and other psychiatric symptoms. Report these signs to the physician or nurse.
- Assess patient's gait and motor function periodically, and report any gait abnormalities or increased muscle tone.
- Assess dizziness or ataxia that might affect gait, balance, and other functional activities (See Appendix C). Report balance problems and functional limitations to the physician and nursing staff, and caution the patient and family/caregivers to guard against falls and trauma.
- Monitor intrathecal injection site and catheter placement for pain, swelling, and irritation. Report prolonged or excessive administration site reactions to the physician.

Interventions

- Implement appropriate manual therapy techniques, physical agents, and therapeutic exercises to reduce pain and help wean patient off analgesics as soon as possible.
- Help patient explore other nonpharmacologic methods to reduce chronic pain, such as relaxation techniques, exercise, counseling, and so forth.
- Guard against falls and trauma (hip fractures, head injury). Implement fall-prevention strategies (See Appendix E), especially if patient exhibits sedation, dizziness, ataxia, or blurred vision.

Patient/Client-Related Instruction

- Advise patient that analgesics are usually more effective if given before pain becomes severe; emphasize that adequate pain control will allow better participation in physical therapy.
- Advise patient to avoid alcohol and other CNS depressants because of the increased risk of sedation and decreased CNS function.
- Instruct patient to report other troublesome side effects such as severe or prolonged headache,

urinary retention, vision disturbances, or GI problems (nausea, vomiting, loss of appetite).

Pharmacokinetics

Absorption: IT administration results in complete bioavailability in the CSF. Minimal plasma distribution.
Distribution: Distributes in entire CSF volume.
Metabolism and Excretion: Degraded by enzymes in tissues and fluids.
Half-life: 4.6 hr (in CSF).

TIME/ACTION PROFILE

ROUTE	ONSET	PEAK	DURATION
IT	rapid	2–3 days	unknown

Contraindications/Precautions

Contraindicated in: Hypersensitivity; History of psychosis; Infection at microinfusion injection site; Uncontrolled bleeding; Spinal cord obstruction; Lactation.
Use Cautiously in: History of suicidal ideation/ psychiatric disorder; Geriatric patients (↑ susceptibility to adverse CNS effects); Children (safety not established); Pregnancy (use only if maternal benefit outweighs fetal risk).

Interactions

Drug-Drug: ↑ risk of CNS depression with other **CNS depressants,** including **anticonvulsants, phenothiazines, antipsychotics, antihistamines, opioids, sedatives,** or **diuretics.**

Route/Dosage

IT (Adults): up to 2.4 mcg/day initially (0.1 mcg/hr), may be gradually increased 2–3 times/week in increments of 2.4 mcg/day up to a maximum of 19.2 mcg/day (0.8 mcg/hr) over 21 days.

Availability

Solution for IT use: 25 mcg/mL in 20-mL vials, 100 mcg/mL in 1-, 2- or 5-mL vial.

zidovudine (zye-doe-vue-deen)

✱ Apo-Zidovudine, azidothymidine, AZT, ✱ Novo-AZT, Retrovir

Classification
Therapeutic: antiretrovirals
Pharmacologic: nucleoside reverse transcriptase inhibitors

Indications

HIV infection (with other antiretrovirals). Reduction of maternal/fetal transmission of HIV.

Action

Following intracellular conversion to its active form, inhibits viral RNA synthesis by inhibiting the enzyme DNA polymerase (reverse transcriptase). Prevents viral replication. **Therapeutic Effects:** Virustatic action against selected retroviruses. Slowed progression and ↓ sequelae of HIV infection. ↓ viral load and improved CD4 cell counts. ↓ transmission of HIV to infants born to HIV-infected mothers.

Adverse Reactions/Side Effects

CNS: SEIZURES, headache, weakness, anxiety, confusion, ↓ mental acuity, dizziness, insomnia, mental depression, restlessness, syncope. **GI:** abdominal pain, diarrhea, nausea, anorexia, drug-induced hepatitis, dyspepsia, oral mucosa pigmentation, vomiting. **Derm:** nail pigmentation. **Endo:** gynecomastia. **Hemat:** anemia, granulocytopenia, pure red-cell aplasia, thrombocytosis. **MS:** back pain, myopathy. **Neuro:** tremor.

PHYSICAL THERAPY IMPLICATIONS

Examination and Evaluation

- Be alert for new seizures or increased seizure activity, especially at the onset of drug treatment. Document the number, duration, and severity of seizures, and report these findings immediately to the physician.
- Assess any back pain, muscle tenderness, or weakness, especially if accompanied by fever, malaise, and dark-colored urine. These symptoms may represent drug-induced myopathy, and that myopathy can progress to severe muscle damage (rhabdomyolysis). Report any unexplained musculoskeletal symptoms to the physician immediately.
- Monitor signs of granulocytopenia (fever, sore throat, mucosal lesions, signs of infection, bruising, bleeding), thrombocytosis (headache, chest pain, dizziness, fainting, vision problems, numbness/ tingling in the hands and feet), or unusual weakness and fatigue that might be due to anemia and other blood dyscrasias. Report these signs to the physician.
- Assess dizziness or syncope that might affect gait, balance, and other functional activities (See Appendix C). Report balance problems and functional limitations to the physician and nursing staff, and caution the patient and family/caregivers to guard against falls and trauma.
- Be alert for anxiety, restlessness, confusion, decreased alertness, mental depression, or other alterations in mental status. Notify the physician promptly if these symptoms develop.

Interventions

- Implement resistive exercises and other therapeutic exercises as tolerated to maintain muscle strength and function, and prevent muscle wasting associated with HIV infection and AIDS.

Patient/Client-Related Instruction

- Emphasize the importance of taking zidovudine as directed even if the patient is asymptomatic, and that this drug must always be used in combination with other antiretroviral drugs. Do not take more than prescribed amount, and do not stop taking without consulting health care professional.
- Inform patient that zidovudine does not cure HIV or AIDS or prevent associated or opportunistic infections. Zidovudine does not reduce the risk of transmission of HIV to others through sexual contact or blood contamination. Caution patient to use a condom and avoid sharing needles or donating blood to prevent spreading the AIDS virus to others.
- Advise patient about the likelihood of GI reactions, including nausea, vomiting, diarrhea, and heartburn. Instruct patient to report severe or prolonged GI problems, or signs of hepatitis such as yellow skin or eyes, abdominal pain, severe nausea and vomiting, fever, sore throat, malaise, weakness, and facial edema.
- Instruct patient to report other troublesome side effects such as prolonged or severe headache, sleep loss, tremor, nail discoloration, or breast enlargement in men (gynecomastia).

Pharmacokinetics

Absorption: Well absorbed following oral administration.

Distribution: Widely distributed; enters the CNS. Crosses the placenta.

Metabolism and Excretion: Mostly (75%) metabolized by the liver; 15–20% excreted unchanged by the kidneys.

Half-life: 1 hr.

TIME/ACTION PROFILE (blood levels)

ROUTE	ONSET	PEAK	DURATION
PO	unknown	0.5–1.5 hr	4 hr
IV	rapid	end of infusion	4 hr

Contraindications/Precautions

Contraindicated in: Hypersensitivity; Lactation.

Use Cautiously in: ↓ bone marrow reserve (dosage reduction required for anemia or granulocytopenia); Severe hepatic or renal disease (dose modification may be required).

Interactions

Drug-Drug: ↑ bone marrow depression with other **agents having bone marrow–depressing properties, antineoplastics, radiation therapy,** or **ganciclovir.** ↑ neurotoxicity may occur with **acyclovir.** Toxicity may be ↑ by concurrent administration of **probenecid** or **fluconazole.** Zidovudine levels are ↓ by **clarithromycin.**

Route/Dosage

Management of HIV Infection

PO (Adults and Children >13 yr): 100 mg q 4 hr while awake or 200 mg tid or 300 mg bid (depends on combination and clinical situation).

PO (Children 3 mo–12 yr): 90–180 mg/m² every 6 hr (not to exceed 200 mg q 6 hr).

IV (Adults and Children >12 yr): 1 mg/kg infused over 1 hr q 4 hr. Change to oral therapy as soon as possible.

IV (Children): 120 mg/m² q 6 hr (not to exceed 160 mg/dose).

Prevention of Maternal/Fetal Transmission of HIV Infection

PO (Adults >14 wk Pregnant): 100 mg 5 times daily until onset of labor.

IV (Adults During Labor and Delivery): 2 mg/kg over 1 hr, then continuous infusion of 1 mg/kg/hr until umbilical cord is clamped.

IV (Infants): 1.5 mg/kg q 6 hr until able to take PO.

PO (Infants): 2 mg/kg q 6 hr, started within 12 hr of birth and continued for 6 wk.

Availability

Capsules: 100 mg, 300 mg. **Oral syrup:** 50 mg/5 mL. **Injection:** 200 mg/20 mL. ***In combination with:*** lamivudine (Combivir). See Appendix B.

zileuton (zye-loo-ton)

Zyflo CR

Classification

Therapeutic: bronchodilators

Pharmacologic: leukotriene antagonists

Indications

Long-term control agent in the management of asthma.

Action

Inhibits the enzyme 5-lipoxygenase that catalyzes to formation of leukotrienes. Leukotrienes are components of slow-reacting substance of anaphylaxis (SRSA) and mediate the following: Airway edema, Smooth muscle constriction, Altered cellular activity. Result is decreased inflammatory process that is part of asthma. **Therapeutic Effects:** ↓ incidence and severity of asthma.

Adverse Reactions/Side Effects

CNS: headache, dizziness, insomnia, malaise, nervousness, somnolence, weakness. **EENT:** conjunctivitis.

CV: chest pain. **GI:** abdominal pain, constipation, dyspepsia, flatulence, increased liver enzymes, nausea, vomiting. **GU:** urinary tract infection, vaginitis. **Derm:** pruritus. **MS:** arthralgia, myalgia, neck pain. **Neuro:** hypertonia. **Misc:** fever, lymphadenopathy.

PHYSICAL THERAPY IMPLICATIONS

Examination and Evaluation

- Assess pulmonary function at rest and during exercise (See Appendices I, J, K) to document effectiveness of medication in controlling bronchoconstriction and asthma attacks.
- Monitor any chest pain and attempt to determine if pain is drug-induced or caused by cardiovascular dysfunction (e.g., angina that occurs during exercise).
- Monitor changes in mood and behavior, including nervousness, malaise, unusual drowsiness, and other similar symptoms. Notify the physician if these changes become problematic.
- Assess any neck, joint, or muscle pain to rule out musculoskeletal pathology; that is, try to determine if pain is drug induced rather than caused by anatomic or biomechanical problems.
- Assess patient's muscle strength and motor function periodically, and report any increased muscle tone.
- Assess dizziness and weakness that might affect gait, balance, and other functional activities (See Appendix C). Report balance problems and functional limitations to the physician, and caution the patient and family/caregivers to guard against falls and trauma.

Interventions

- When implementing airway clearance techniques or respiratory muscle training, attempt to intervene when the airway is maximally bronchodilated. Peak responses typically occur about 60–90 min after oral administration.

Patient/Client-Related Instruction

- Advise patient to not exceed the recommended dose or frequency of administration. Contact physician if bronchospasm is not adequately controlled by the current medication regimen or if respiratory symptoms continue to worsen.
- Instruct patient and family/caregivers to report other troublesome side effects, including severe or prolonged headache, eye inflammation, itching skin, urinary tract infections, vaginal irritation, fever, swollen lymph nodes, or GI problems (nausea, vomiting, diarrhea, constipation, indigestion, flatulence, abdominal pain).

Pharmacokinetics

Absorption: Rapidly absorbed following oral administration.
Distribution: Unknown.
Protein Binding: 93%.
Metabolism and Excretion: Mostly metabolized by the liver.
Half-life: 2.5 hr.

TIME/ACTION PROFILE (improvement in pulmonary function)

ROUTE	ONSET	PEAK	DURATION
PO	unknown	1.7 hr	unknown

Contraindications/Precautions

Contraindicated in: Hypersensitivity; Active liver disease or transaminases ≥3 times upper limit of normal.
Use Cautiously in: Acute attacks of asthma; History of liver disease or alcohol consumption; OB/Lactation/Pedi: Pregnancy, lactation, or children <12 yr (safety not established).

Interactions

Drug-Drug: ↑ blood levels and effects of **theophylline, beta blockers, propranolol,** and **warfarin.**
Drug-Food: Food slows but does not alter extent of absorption.

Route/Dosage

PO (Adults and Children ≥12 yr): 1200 mg bid.

Availability

Extended-release tablet: 600 mg.

ziprasidone (zi-pras-i-done)

Geodon

Classification
Therapeutic: antipsychotics, mood stabilizers
Pharmacologic: piperazine derivatives

Z

Indications

Schizophrenia; IM form is reserved for control of acutely agitated patients. Bipolar mania (manic and manic/mixed episodes).

Action

Effects probably mediated by antagonism of dopamine type 2 (D2) and serotonin type 2 ($5\text{-}HT_2$). Also antagonizes α_2-adrenergic receptors. **Therapeutic Effects:** Diminished schizophrenic behavior.

Adverse Reactions/Side Effects

CNS: NEUROLEPTIC MALIGNANT SYNDROME, seizures, dizziness, drowsiness, restlessness, extrapyramidal reactions, syncope, tardive dyskinesia. **Resp:** cough/runny nose. **CV:** PROLONGED QT INTERVAL, orthostatic hypotension. **GI:** constipation, diarrhea, nausea, dysphagia. **Derm:** rash, urticaria.

PHYSICAL THERAPY IMPLICATIONS

Examination and Evaluation

- Be alert for signs of neuroleptic malignant syndrome, including hyperthermia, diaphoresis, generalized muscle rigidity, altered mental status, tachycardia, changes in blood pressure (BP), and incontinence. Symptoms typically occur within 4–14 days after initiation of drug therapy, but can occur at any time during drug use. Report these signs to the physician or nursing staff immediately.
- Assess heart rate, ECG, and heart sounds, especially during exercise (See Appendices G, H). Report arrhythmias (prolonged QT interval, others), or symptoms of rhythm disturbances including palpitations, chest discomfort, shortness of breath, fainting, and fatigue/weakness.
- Be alert for new seizures or increased seizure activity, especially at the onset of drug treatment. Document the number, duration, and severity of seizures, and report these findings immediately to the physician.
- Assess motor function, and be alert for extrapyramidal symptoms. Report these symptoms immediately, especially tardive dyskinesia, because this problem may be irreversible. Common extrapyramidal symptoms include:
  - Tardive dyskinesia (uncontrolled rhythmic movement of mouth, face, and extremities, lip smacking or puckering, puffing of cheeks, uncontrolled chewing, rapid or worm-like movements of tongue).
  - Pseudoparkinsonism (shuffling gait, rigidity, tremor, pill-rolling motion, loss of balance control, difficulty speaking or swallowing, mask-like face).
  - Akathisia (restlessness or desire to keep moving).
  - Other dystonias and dyskinesias (dystonic muscle spasms, twisting motions, twitching, inability to move eyes, weakness of arms or legs).
- Assess dizziness and drowsiness that might affect gait, balance, and other functional activities (See Appendix C). Report balance problems and functional limitations to the physician and nursing staff, and caution the patient and family/caregivers to guard against falls and trauma.
- Assess BP, and report a fall in BP when patient assumes a more upright position (lying to standing, sitting to standing, lying to sitting). Document orthostatic hypotension and contact physician when systolic BP falls >20 mm Hg, or diastolic BP falls >10 mm Hg.

Interventions

- Guard against falls and trauma (hip fractures, head injury, and so forth) caused by drowsiness, dizziness, syncope, or extrapyramidal symptoms; implement fall prevention strategies (See Appendix E).
- Because of the risk of arrhythmias and abnormal BP responses, use caution during aerobic exercise and other forms of therapeutic exercise. Assess exercise tolerance frequently (BP, heart rate, fatigue levels), and terminate exercise immediately if any untoward responses occur (See Appendix L).
- To minimize orthostatic hypotension, patient should move slowly when assuming a more upright position.
- Help patient and family/caregivers explore nonpharmacologic methods (exercise, counseling, support groups) to reduce schizophrenic episodes and other mood disorders.

Patient/Client-Related Instruction

- Advise patient to avoid alcohol and other CNS depressants because of the increased risk of sedation and adverse effects.
- Instruct patient to report other problematic side effects such as severe or prolonged cough, runny nose, skin reactions (rash, hives), or GI problems (nausea, diarrhea, constipation, difficulty swallowing).

Pharmacokinetics

Absorption: 60% absorbed following oral administration; 100% absorbed from IM sites.
Distribution: Unknown.
Protein Binding: 99%; potential for drug interactions due to drug displacement is minimal.
Metabolism and Excretion: 99% metabolized by the liver; <1% excreted unchanged in urine.
Half-life: *PO*—7 hr; *IM*—2–5 hr.

TIME/ACTION PROFILE (blood levels)

ROUTE	ONSET	PEAK	DURATION
PO	within hours	1–3 days*	unknown
IM	rapid	60 min	unknown

*Steady state achieved following continuous use.

Contraindications/Precautions

Contraindicated in: Hypersensitivity; History of QT prolongation (persistent QTc measurements >500 msec), arrhythmias, recent MI or uncompensated heart failure; Concurrent use of other drugs known to prolong the QT interval, including quinidine, dofetilide, sotalol, other class Ia and III antiarrhythmics, pimozide, sotalol, thioridazine, chlorpromazine, pentamidine, arsenic trioxide, mefloquine, dolasetron, tacrolimus, droperidol, and moxifloxacin; Hypokalemia or hypomagnesemia; Lactation: Discontinue drug or bottle-feed.
Use Cautiously in: Concurrent diuretic therapy or diarrhea (may ↑ the risk of hypotension,

hypokalemia, or hypomagnesemia); Significant hepatic impairment; History of cardiovascular or cerebrovascular disease; Hypotension, concurrent antihypertensive therapy, dehydration, or hypovolemia (may ↑ risk of orthostatic hypotension); OB: Use only if potential benefit outweighs potential risk to the fetus; Pedi: Safety not established; Geri: Alzheimer's dementia or age >65 yr (may ↑ risk of seizures). Geriatric patients (may require ↓ doses; ↑ risk of mortality in elderly patients treated for dementia-related psychosis); Patients at risk for aspiration pneumonia; History of suicide attempt.

Interactions

Drug-Drug: Concurrent use of **quinidine, dofetilide, other class Ia and III antiarrhythmics, pimozide, sotalol, thioridazine, chlorpromazine, pentamidine, arsenic trioxide, mefloquine, dolasetron, tacrolimus, droperidol, moxifloxacin,** or other agents that prolong the QT interval may result in potentially life-threatening adverse drug reactions (concurrent use contraindicated). Additive CNS depression may occur with **alcohol, antidepressants, antihistamines, opioid analgesics,** or **sedative/hypnotics.** Blood levels and effectiveness may be ↓ by **carbamazepine.** Blood levels and effects may be ↑ by **ketoconazole.**

Route/Dosage

PO (Adults): *Schizophrenia*—20 mg bid initially; dose increments may be made at 2-day intervals up to 80 mg bid; *Mania*—40 mg twice on 1st day, then 60 or 80 mg bid on 2nd day, then 40–80 mg bid.
IM (Adults): 10–20 mg as needed up to 40 mg/day; may be given as 10 mg q 2 hr or 20 mg q 4 hr.

Availability

Capsules: 20 mg, 40 mg, 60 mg, 80 mg. **Lyophilized powder for injection (requires reconstitution):** 20 mg/vial.

zoledronic acid
(zoe-le-**dron**-ik **as**-id)
Reclast, Zometa

Classification
Therapeutic: bone resorption inhibitors, electrolyte modifiers, hypocalcemics
Pharmacologic: bisphosphonates

Indications

Hypercalcemia of malignancy (Zometa only). Multiple myeloma and metastatic bone lesions from solid tumors (Zometa only). Paget's disease (Reclast only). Treatment of osteoporosis in postmenopausal women (Reclast only). Prevention of new clinical fractures in patients with recent low-trauma hip fracture (Reclast only).

Action

Inhibits bone resorption. Inhibits increased osteoclast activity and skeletal calcium release induced by tumors. **Therapeutic Effects:** ↓ serum calcium. ↓ serum alkaline phosphatase. ↓ fractures; radiation/surgery to bone, or spinal cord compression in patients with multiple myeloma or metastatic bone lesions. ↓ hip, vertebral, or nonvertebral osteoporosis-related fractures. ↓ new fractures in patients with recent low-trauma hip fractures.

Adverse Reactions/Side Effects

CNS: agitation, anxiety, confusion, insomnia. **EENT:** conjunctivitis. **CV:** hypotension, chest pain, leg edema. **GI:** abdominal pain, constipation, diarrhea, nausea, vomiting, dysphagia. **GU:** renal failure. **Derm:** pruritus, rash. **F and E:** hypophosphatemia, hypocalcemia, hypokalemia, hypomagnesemia. **Hemat:** anemia. **MS:** musculoskeletal pain, osteonecrosis (primarily of jaw). **Misc:** fever, flu-like syndrome.

PHYSICAL THERAPY IMPLICATIONS

Examination and Evaluation

- Assess any joint pain, muscle pain, or muscle spasms. Report persistent or increased musculoskeletal pain to determine presence of bone or joint pathology, including fracture. Be especially aware of possible mouth and jaw pain due to osteonecrosis of the jaw.
- Assess blood pressure periodically and compare to normal values (See Appendix F). Report low blood pressure (hypotension), especially if patient experiences dizziness, fatigue, or other symptoms.
- Assess peripheral edema using girth measurements, volume displacement, and measurement of pitting edema (See Appendix N). Report increased swelling in feet and ankles or a sudden increase in body weight due to fluid retention.
- Monitor any chest pain and attempt to determine if pain is drug induced or caused by cardiovascular dysfunction (e.g., angina that occurs during exercise).
- Monitor signs of anemia, including unusual fatigue, shortness of breath with exertion, and bruising, and pale skin. Notify physician immediately if these signs occur.
- Monitor signs of electrolyte imbalances (hypocalcemia, hypokalemia, etc.), including headache, lethargy, confusion, weakness, irritability, and muscle hyperexcitability, tremors, cramping, and tetany. Notify physician immediately if these signs occur.

- Monitor signs of renal failure, including decreased urine output, increased blood pressure, muscle cramps/twitching, edema/weight gain from fluid retention, yellowish brown skin, and confusion that progresses to seizures and coma. Report these signs immediately to the physician.
- Monitor and report anxiety, agitation, confusion, or other changes in mood and behavior.

Interventions

- Institute weight-bearing and resistance exercises as tolerated to maintain or increase bone mineral density. Start with low-impact or aquatic programs in patients with extensive demineralization, and increase exercise intensity slowly to prevent fractures.
- Protect against falls and fractures (See Appendix E). Modify home environment (remove throw rugs, improve lighting, etc.), and provide assistive devices (cane, walker) or other protective devices as needed to improve balance and prevent falls.

Patient/Client-Related Instruction

- Encourage patient to modify behaviors that increase the risk of osteoporosis (stop smoking, reduce alcohol consumption).
- Advise patient about the benefits of proper diet in sustaining bone mineralization. If necessary, refer patient for nutritional counseling about supplemental calcium and vitamin D.
- Instruct patient to report other side effects such as severe or prolonged headache, eye inflammation, sleep loss, fever, flu-like symptoms, skin reactions (rash, itching), or other GI problems (nausea, vomiting, diarrhea, constipation, difficulty swallowing, abdominal pain).

Pharmacokinetics

Absorption: IV administration results in complete bioavailability.
Distribution: Unknown.
Metabolism and Excretion: Mostly excreted unchanged by the kidneys.
Half-life: 167 hr.

TIME/ACTION PROFILE (effect on serum calcium)

ROUTE	ONSET	PEAK	DURATION
IV	within 4 days	4–7 days	30 days

Contraindications/Precautions

Contraindicated in: Hypersensitivity to zoledronic acid or other bisphosphonates.
Use Cautiously in: Severe renal impairment (not recommended if CCr <35 mL/min); History of aspirin-induced asthma; Concurrent use of loop diuretics or dehydration (correct deficits prior to use); Concurrent use of nephrotoxic drugs; Dental surgery (may ↑ risk of jaw osteonecrosis); OB/Lactation/Pedi: Safety not established.

Interactions

Drug-Drug: Concurrent use of **loop diuretics** or **aminoglycosides** ↑ risk of hypocalcemia.

Route/Dosage

Reclast

IV (Adults): *Paget's disease*—5 mg as a single dose (information regarding retreatment unknown); *Postmenopausal osteoporosis or patients with recent low-trauma hip fracture*—5 mg once yearly.

Zometa

IV (Adults): *Hypercalcemia of malignancy*—4 mg; may be repeated after 7 days; *Multiple myeloma and bone metastases from solid tumors*—4 mg q 3–4 wk (has been used for up to 15 mo).

Availability

Solution for IV infusion: 4 mg/5-mL vial. **Solution for IV infusion (premixed):** 5 mg/100 mL.

zolmitriptan (zole-mi-**trip**-tan)

Zomig, Zomig-ZMT

Classification
Therapeutic: vascular headache suppressants
Pharmacologic: 5-HT_1 agonists

Indications

Acute treatment of migraine headache.

Action

Acts as an agonist at specific 5-HT_1 receptor sites in intracranial blood vessels and sensory trigeminal nerves. **Therapeutic Effects:** Cranial vessel vasoconstriction with resultant decrease in migraine headache.

Adverse Reactions/Side Effects

CNS: dizziness, drowsiness, vertigo, weakness.
EENT: throat pain/tightness/pressure. **CV:** chest pain/pressure/tightness/heaviness, hypertension, palpitations.
GI: dry mouth, dyspepsia, dysphagia, nausea.
Derm: sweating, warm/cold sensation. **MS:** myalgia, myasthenia. **Neuro:** hypesthesia, paresthesia.
Misc: feeling of heaviness.

PHYSICAL THERAPY IMPLICATIONS

Examination and Evaluation

- Assess the duration and severity of headaches, and document whether drug therapy is successful in decreasing migraine attacks.
- Assess blood pressure (BP) and compare to normal values (See Appendix F). Report a sustained increase in BP (hypertension).
- Monitor any chest pain or other chest symptoms (pressure, tightness, heaviness, palpitations).

Attempt to determine if symptoms are drug induced or caused by cardiovascular dysfunction (e.g., angina that occurs during exercise).

- Assess any muscle pain or weakness to rule out musculoskeletal pathology; that is, try to determine if pain is drug induced rather than caused by anatomic or biomechanical problems.
- Assess signs of paresthesia (numbness, tingling) or hypesthesia (decreased sensation). Perform objective tests, including electroneuromyography and sensory testing, to document any drug-related neuropathic changes.
- Watch for dizziness and vertigo that affects gait, balance, and other functional activities (See Appendix C). Report balance problems and functional limitations to the physician, and caution the patient and family/caregivers to guard against falls and trauma.

Interventions

- Implement appropriate interventions (manual techniques, physical agents, therapeutic exercise) to manage headache pain and reduce the need for drug therapy. Help patient also explore other nonpharmacologic methods to reduce chronic headache pain (relaxation techniques, imagery, and so forth).
- If a headache occurs and drug treatment is needed during a rehabilitation session, allow patient to recover in a quiet, darkened room to allow the drug to achieve maximal effects.

Patient/Client-Related Instruction

- Advise the patient to bring this drug to each therapy session; this drug is most effective when taken at the first signs of a migraine attack. Make sure patients understand the correct administration techniques for intranasal inhalation.
- Advise patient to adhere to the correct dosing schedule, and to not exceed the recommended frequency and number of doses per 24-hr period.
- Instruct patient to report other troublesome side effects such as severe or prolonged headache, drowsiness, throat pain/tightness, skin reactions (sweating, warmth, cold, other strange sensations), or GI problems (nausea, dry mouth, indigestion, difficulty swallowing).

Pharmacokinetics

Absorption: Well absorbed (40%) following oral and intranasal administration.
Distribution: Unknown.
Metabolism and Excretion: Mostly metabolized by the liver; some conversion to metabolites that are more active than zolmitriptan. 8% excreted unchanged in urine.
Half-life: 3 hr (for zolmitriptan and active metabolite).

TIME/ACTION PROFILE (relief of headache)

ROUTE	ONSET	PEAK	DURATION
PO	unknown	1.5 hr*	Unknown
intranasal	unknown	3 hr	Unknown

*3 hr for orally disintegrating tablets.

Contraindications/Precautions

Contraindicated in: Hypersensitivity; Significant underlying heart disease (including ischemic heart disease, history of MI, coronary artery vasospasm, uncontrolled hypertension); Concurrent (or within 24 hr) use of other 5-HT agonists, ergotamine, or ergot-type medications; Concurrent (or within 2 wk) use of MAO inhibitors; Hemiplegic or basilar migraine; Symptomatic Wolff-Parkinson-White syndrome or other arrhythmias.
Use Cautiously in: Cardiovascular risk factors (hypertension, hypercholesterolemia, cigarette smoking, obesity, diabetes, strong family history, menopausal females or males >40 yr [use only if cardiovascular status has been evaluated and determined to be safe and 1st dose is administered under supervision]); Hepatic impairment (use lower doses); Pregnancy, lactation, or children (safety not established).

Interactions

Drug-Drug: Because of increased risk of cerebral vasospasm, avoid concurrent use of other **5-HT agonists (naratriptan, sumatriptan, rizatriptan)** and/or **ergot-type preparations (dihydroergotamine)**. Concurrent use of **MAO inhibitors** ↑ blood levels and risk of toxicity (avoid use within 2 wk of MAO inhibitors). Blood levels may be ↑ by **hormonal contraceptives. Cimetidine** ↑ half-life of zolmitriptan and its active metabolite. Concurrent use with **SSRI antidepressants** may result in weakness, hyperreflexia and incoordination.
Drug-Natural: ↑ risk of serotonergic side effects, including serotonin syndrome with **St. John's wort** and **SAMe.**

Route/Dosage

PO (Adults): 2.5 mg or less initially; if headache returns, dose may be repeated after 2 hr (not to exceed 10 mg/24 hr).
Intranasal (Adults): single 5-mg dose; may be repeated after 2 hr (not to exceed 10 mg/24 hr).

Availability

Tablets: 2.5 mg, 5 mg. **Orally disintegrating tablets:** 2.5 mg, 5 mg. **Nasal spray:** 5 mg/100 mcL unit-dose spray device (package of 6).

Z

zolpidem (zole-pi-dem)

Ambien, Ambien CR

Classification

Therapeutic: sedative/hypnotics

Pharmacologic: imidazopyridines

Schedule IV

Indications

Insomnia.

Action

Produces CNS depression by binding to gamma-aminobutyric acid (GABA) receptors. Has no analgesic properties. **Therapeutic Effects:** Sedation and induction of sleep.

Adverse Reactions/Side Effects

CNS: abnormal thinking, amnesia, behavior changes, daytime drowsiness, dizziness, "drugged" feeling, hallucinations, sleep driving. **GI:** diarrhea, nausea, vomiting. **Misc:** ANAPHYLACTIC REACTIONS, hypersensitivity reactions, physical dependence, psychologic dependence, tolerance.

PHYSICAL THERAPY IMPLICATIONS

Examination and Evaluation

- Monitor signs of hypersensitivity reactions and anaphylaxis, including pulmonary symptoms (laryngeal edema, wheezing, dyspnea) or skin reactions (rash, pruritus, urticaria). Notify physician immediately if these reactions occur.
- Monitor daytime drowsiness, anxiety, behavior changes, short-term memory deficits, hallucinations, and "drugged" feelings. Repeated or excessive symptoms may require change in dose or medication.
- Assess dizziness that might affect gait, balance, and other functional activities (See Appendix C). Report balance problems and functional limitations to the physician, and caution the patient and family/caregivers to guard against falls and trauma.

Interventions

- Guard against falls and trauma (hip fractures, head injury, and so forth). Implement fall-prevention strategies, especially in older adults or if drowsiness and dizziness carry over into the daytime (See Appendix E).
- Help patient explore nonpharmacologic methods to improve sleep, such as relaxation techniques, regular exercise, avoid caffeine, and so forth.

Patient/Client-Related Instruction

- Instruct patients on prolonged treatment not to discontinue medication without consulting their physician. Long-term use can cause tolerance and physical/psychologic dependence, and abrupt withdrawal after 2 or more weeks of use may result in fatigue, nausea, flushing, light-headedness, uncontrolled crying, vomiting, GI upset, panic attack, or nervousness.
- Advise patient about the risk of daytime drowsiness and decreased attention and mental focus. Use care if driving or in other activities that require strong concentration.
- Caution patient and family/caregivers that "sleep-walking" and other complex activities including driving a car (sleep driving) may occur while completely asleep. Care should be taken to monitor such activities and prevent access to motor vehicles while under the influence of this drug.
- Advise patient to avoid alcohol and other CNS depressants because of the increased risk of sedation and adverse effects.
- Instruct patient and family/caregivers to report other troublesome side effects such as severe or prolonged GI problems (nausea, vomiting, diarrhea), abnormal thoughts, or other bizarre behaviors.

Pharmacokinetics

Absorption: Rapidly absorbed following oral administration. Controlled-release formulation releases 10 mg immediately, then another 2.5 mg later.
Distribution: Minimal amounts enter breast milk; remainder of distribution not known.
Metabolism and Excretion: Converted to inactive metabolites, which are excreted by the kidneys.
Half-life: 2.5–2.6 hr (increased in geriatric patients and patients with hepatic impairment).

TIME/ACTION PROFILE (sedation)

ROUTE	ONSET	PEAK*	DURATION
PO	rapid	30 min–2 hr	6–8 hr
PO-ER	rapid	2–4 hr	6–8 hr

*Food delays peak levels and effects.

Contraindications/Precautions

Contraindicated in: Hypersensitivity; Sleep apnea.
Use Cautiously in: History of previous psychiatric illness, suicide attempt, drug or alcohol abuse; Geri: Geriatric patients and patients with impaired hepatic function (initial dose reduction recommended); Patients with pulmonary disease; OB/Pedi: Pregnancy, lactation, or children (safety not established).

Interactions

Drug-Drug: ↑ CNS depression may with **sedative/hypnotics, alcohol, phenothiazines, tricyclic antidepressants, opioid analgesics,** or **antihistamines.**
Drug-Natural: Concomitant use of **kava, valerian,** or **chamomile** can ↑ CNS depression.
Drug-Food: Food ↓ and delays absorption.

Route/Dosage

PO (Adults): *Tablets*—10 mg hs; *Extended-release tablets*—12.5 mg hs.
PO (Geriatric Patients, Debilitated Patients, or Patients with Hepatic Impairment): *Tablets*—5 mg hs initially, may be ↑ to 10 mg; *Extended-release tablets*—6.25 mg hs.

Availability (generic available)

Tablets: 5 mg, 10 mg. **Extended-release tablets:** 6.25 mg, 12.5 mg.

zonisamide (zoe-**nis**-a-mide)

Zonegran

Classification
Therapeutic: anticonvulsants
Pharmacologic: sulfonamides

Indications

Partial seizures in adults.

Action

Raises the threshold for seizures and reduces duration of seizures, probably by action on sodium and calcium channels. **Therapeutic Effects:** ↓ frequency of partial seizures.

Adverse Reactions/Side Effects

CNS: drowsiness, fatigue, agitation/irritability, depression, dizziness, psychomotor slowing, psychosis, weakness. **EENT:** amblyopia, tinnitus. **Resp:** cough, pharyngitis. **GI:** anorexia, nausea, vomiting. **GU:** kidney stones. **Derm:** oligohidrosis (↑ in children), rash. **Metab:** hyperthermia (↑ in children). **Neuro:** abnormal gait, hyperesthesia, incoordination, tremor.
Misc: ALLERGIC REACTIONS, INCLUDING STEVENS-JOHNSON SYNDROME.

PHYSICAL THERAPY IMPLICATIONS

Examination and Evaluation

- Monitor allergic responses, including skin reactions such as rash, itching/burning skin, hives, exfoliation, and dermatitis. Notify physician immediately about because certain skin reactions may indicate serious hypersensitivity reactions (Stevens-Johnson syndrome).
- Document the number, duration, and severity of seizures to help determine if this drug is effective in reducing seizure activity.
- Assess dizziness that might affect gait, balance, and other functional activities (See Appendix C). Report balance problems and functional limitations to the physician, and caution the patient and family/caregivers to guard against falls and trauma.
- Monitor daytime drowsiness, agitation, irritability, depression, psychosis, or other psychiatric disturbances. Repeated or excessive symptoms may require change in dose or medication.
- Assess any gait disturbances, incoordination, tremor, or increased sensation to pain/touch to rule out neuromuscular pathology; that is, try to determine if neurologic signs are drug induced rather than caused by neurologic pathology.
- Monitor and report signs of kidney stones, including severe pain in the side and back, pain on urination, bloody urine, and a persistent urge to urinate.

Interventions

- Guard against falls and trauma (hip fractures, head injury, and so forth), especially if dizziness or ataxia affect gait and balance. Implement fall-prevention strategies, especially if balance is impaired (See Appendix E).

Patient/Client-Related Instruction

- Advise patient to avoid alcohol and other CNS depressants because of the increased risk of sedation and adverse effects.
- Advise patients on prolonged antiseizure therapy not to discontinue medication without consulting their physician. Abrupt withdrawal may cause increased seizures.
- Advise patient about the risk of daytime drowsiness and decreased attention and mental focus. Use care if driving or in other activities that require strong concentration and fast responses.
- Instruct patient and family/caregivers to report other troublesome side effects such as severe or prolonged cough, pharyngeal irritation, vision problems, ringing/buzzing in the ears (tinnitus), skin reactions (rash, inadequate sweating), or GI problems (nausea, vomiting, loss of appetite).

Pharmacokinetics

Absorption: Well absorbed following oral administration.
Distribution: Binds extensively to red blood cells.
Metabolism and Excretion: Mostly metabolized by the liver; 35% excreted unchanged in urine. Some metabolism occurs via CYP3A4 enzyme system.
Half-life: 63 hr (plasma).

TIME/ACTION PROFILE (blood levels*)

ROUTE	ONSET	PEAK	DURATION
PO	unknown	2–6 hr	24 hr

*Requires 2 wk of dosing to achieve steady-state blood levels.

Contraindications/Precautions

Contraindicated in: Hypersensitivity to zonisamide or sulfonamides.

Use Cautiously in: Hepatic or renal disease (may require slower titration/more frequent monitoring); Pregnancy or lactation (use only if potential benefit justifies risk to fetus/infant); Children ≤16 yr (safety not established; ↑ risk of oligohidrosis/hyperthermia).

Interactions

Drug-Drug: Drugs that induce or inhibit CYP3A4 may alter blood levels and effects of zonisamide. Blood levels and effects may be ↓ by **phenytoin, carbamazepine, phenobarbital,** or **valproate.**

Route/Dosage

PO (Adults and Children >16 yr): 100 mg once daily initially for 2 wk, then ↑ to 200 mg daily for 2 wk; with subsequent increments of 100 mg made at 2-wk intervals as required (range 100–600 mg/day). Can be given as a single daily dose or in 2 divided doses.

Availability

Capsules: 25 mg, 50 mg, 100 mg.

COMPREHENSIVE INDEX*

*Entries for **generic** names appear in **boldface type.** Trade names appear in regular type, with Canadian trade names preceded by a maple leaf icon🍁.

*Entries for **generic names** appear in **boldface type**. Trade names appear in regular type, with Canadian trade names preceded by a maple leaf icon 🍁.

*Entries for **generic** names appear in **boldface type.** Trade names appear in regular type, with Canadian trade names preceded by a maple leaf icon.

*Entries for **generic** names appear in **boldface type**. Trade names appear in regular type, with Canadian trade names preceded by a maple leaf icon 🍁.

*Entries for **generic** names appear in **boldface type.** Trade names appear in regular type, with Canadian trade names preceded by a maple leaf icon (Canada).

*Entries for **generic** names appear in **boldface type.** Trade names appear in regular type, with Canadian trade names preceded by a maple leaf icon.

*Entries for **generic** names appear in **boldface type.** Trade names appear in regular type, with Canadian trade names preceded by a maple leaf icon 🍁.

*Entries for **generic** names appear in **boldface type.** Trade names appear in regular type, with Canadian trade names preceded by a maple leaf icon 🍁.

*Entries for **generic names appear in boldface type.** Trade names appear in regular type, with Canadian trade names preceded by a maple leaf icon 🍁.

*Entries for **generic** names appear in **boldface type.** Trade names appear in regular type, with Canadian trade names preceded by a maple leaf icon 🍁.

*Entries for **generic** names appear in **boldface type**. Trade names appear in regular type, with Canadian trade names preceded by a maple leaf icon 🍁.

*Entries for **generic** names appear in **boldface type**. Trade names appear in regular type, with Canadian trade names preceded by a maple leaf icon.

COMPREHENSIVE INDEX